Adler's Physiology of the Eye

Adler's Physiology of the Eye

Twelfth Edition

Leonard A. Levin, MD, PhD, FARVO

Distinguished James McGill Professor of Ophthalmology &
  Visual Sciences, Neurology & Neurosurgery
McGill University
Montreal, Quebec
Canada

Paul L. Kaufman, MD, FARVO

Emeritus Professor of Ophthalmology & Visual Sciences
Emeritus Ernst H. Bárány Professor of Ocular Pharmacology
Department Chair Emeritus
Department of Ophthalmology & Visual Sciences
School of Medicine & Public Health
University of Wisconsin-Madison
Madison, Wisconsin
USA

Mary Elizabeth Hartnett, MD, FACS, FARVO

Michael F. Marmor, M.D., Professor of Retinal Science and
  Disease
Vitreoretinal Surgery and Diseases
Director of Pediatric Retina
Principal Investigator, Hartnett Laboratory of Angiogenesis
Byers Eye Institute at Stanford University
Palo Alto, California
USA

ELSEVIER

ELSEVIER
1600 John F. Kennedy Blvd.
Ste 1800
Philadelphia, PA 19103-2899

ADLER'S PHYSIOLOGY OF THE EYE, TWELFTH EDITION   ISBN: 978-0-323-83406-3

...t Strategist: Kayla Wolfe
...lopment Specialist: Priyadarshini Pandey
...ager: Deepthi Unni
*...vagi Anandan

To our families, for providing the time and support for us to work on this project; to our readers, who are why this text exists; to our students, who we hope will continue to move our field forward to an even better understanding of ocular physiology in all its manifestations; and to our patients, who provide inspiration for advancing ocular physiology.

SECTION EDITORS

Julia V. Busik, PhD, FARVO
Professor and Chair
Department of Biochemistry and Physiology
Ed Miller Endowed Chair in Molecular Biology
University of Oklahoma Health Sciences Center
Oklahoma City, Oklahoma
USA

Melinda K. Duncan, PhD, FARVO
Professor
Department of Biological Sciences
Associate Vice President for Research
University of Delaware
Newark, Delaware
USA

Dennis M. Levi, OD, PhD
Distinguished Professor
Herbert Wertheim School of Optometry and Vision Science
University of California, Berkeley
Berkeley, California
USA

Linda K. McLoon, PhD
Professor
Department of Ophthalmology and Visual Neurosciences
University of Minnesota
Minneapolis, Minnesota
USA

Stuart Trenholm, PhD
Associate Professor
Montreal Neurological Institute
McGill University
Montreal, Quebec
Canada

Samuel M. Wu, PhD
Professor
Department of Ophthalmology
Baylor College of Medicine
Houston, Texas
USA

M. Carmen Acosta, PhD
Professor of Physiology
Department of Physiology
Universidad Miguel Hernández de Elche
San Juan de Alicante, Alicante
Spain
Principal Investigator
Instituto de Neurociencias
Universidad Miguel Hernández-CSIC
San Juan de Alicante, Alicante
Spain

José Manuel Alonso, MD, PhD
Distinguished Professor
Biological and Visual Sciences
SUNY College of Optometry
New York, New York
USA

Andrew J. Anderson, PhD, Msc, Bsc (Optom)
Associate Professor
Department of Optometry and Vision Sciences
The University of Melbourne
Parkville, Victoria
Australia

Marcus Ang, MBBS, MCI, MMED, FRCS, PhD
Senior Consultant
Cornea and Refractive Service
Singapore National Eye Center
Singapore
Associate Professor
Ophthalmology and Visual Sciences
DUKE-NUS
Singapore

Alessandra Angelucci, MD, PhD
Professor
Moran Eye Institute
University of Utah
Salt Lake City, Utah
USA

Daniel H. Baker, PhD, CSTAT
Professor
Department of Psychology
University of York
York, United Kingdom

Steven Barnes, PhD
Doheny Eye Institute
Departments of Ophthalmology and Neurobiology
David Geffen School of Medicine
University of California at Los Angeles
Los Angeles, California
USA

David M. Berson, PhD
Professor and Chair
Department of Neuroscience
Brown University
Providence, Rhode Island
USA

Catherine Bowes Rickman, PhD
George and Geneva Boguslavsky Distinguished Professor of
    Eye Research
Professor of Ophthalmology
Professor in Cell Biology
Duke University
Durham, North Carolina
USA

Nicholas C. Brecha, PhD
Distinguished Professor
Departments of Neurobiology, Ophthalmology and Medicine
David Geffen School of Medicine
University of California at Los Angeles
Los Angeles, California
Senior Research Career Scientist
Veterans Administration Greater Los Angeles Healthcare System
Los Angeles, California
USA

Leila Chew, MD
Resident
Department of Ophthalmology
University of California at Los Angeles
Los Angeles, California
USA

Yuzo M. Chino, PhD
Professor Emeritus
College of Optometry
University of Houston
Houston, Texas
USA

John Douglas Crawford, PhD
Distinguished Research Professor in Neuroscience
Department of Psychology
York University
Toronto, Ontario
Canada

Mary Ann Croft, MS
Distinguished Scientist III
Ophthalmology and Visual Sciences
University of Wisconsin-Madison
Madison, Wisconsin
USA

Kathleen E. Cullen, PhD
Professor
Department of Biomedical Engineering
The Johns Hopkins University
Baltimore, Maryland
USA

Darlene A. Dartt, AB, PhD
Senior Scientist
Professor of Ophthalmology
Schepens Eye Research Institute/Massachusetts Eye and Ear
Boston, Massachusetts
Professor
Professor of Ophthalmology
Harvard Medical School
Boston, Massachusetts
USA

Nicholas A. Delamere, PhD
Professor
Department of Physiology
University of Arizona
Tucson, Arizona
USA

Daniel Diniz, MD
Volunteer Professor
Department of Ophthalmology and Visual Sciences
Federal University of São Paulo
São Paul, São Paulo
Brazil

Paul James Donaldson, Bsc (Hons), PhD
Professor
Department of Physiology
School of Medical Sciences
New Zealand National Eye Centre
University of Auckland
Auckland, New Zealand

Thomas Euler, DR. RER. NAT
Professor
Centre for Ophthalmology / Centre for Integrative Neuroscience
University of Tübingen
Tübingen, Germany

Ione Fine, PhD
Professor
Department of Psychology
University of Washington
Seattle, Washington
USA

Laura J. Frishman, PhD
Professor and Associate Dean
Department of Vision Sciences
College of Optometry
University of Houston
Houston, Texas
USA

Juana Gallar, MD, PhD
Professor of Physiology
Department of Physiology
Universidad Miguel Hernández de Elche
San Juan de Alicante, Alicante
Spain
Principal Investigator
Instituto de Neurociencias
Universidad Miguel Hernández-CSIC
San Juan de Alicante, Alicante
Spain
Principal Investigator
Group 1-Neurosciences
Instituto de Investigación Sanitaria y Biomédica de Alicante
San Juan de Alicante, Alicante
Spain
Principal Investigator
NEUROTECH-EU
The European University of Brain and Technology

Jeffrey L. Goldberg, MD, PhD
Professor and Chair
Department of Ophthalmology
Byers Eye Institute at Stanford University
Palo Alto, California
USA

Gregory J. Griepentrog, MD, FACS
Associate Professor
Department of Ophthalmology and Visual Sciences
Division of Orbital and Ophthalmic Plastic Surgery
Medical College of Wisconsin
Milwaukee, Wisconsin
USA

Laura Hellinen, PhD Pharm
School of Pharmacy
Faculty of Health Sciences
University of Eastern Finland
Kuopio, Finland

Arlene A. Hirano, PhD
Researcher
Department of Neurobiology
David Geffen School of Medicine
University of California at Los Angeles
Los Angeles, California
Research Biologist
VAGLAHS
Los Angeles, California
USA

Chris A. Johnson, PhD, Dsc
Emeritus Professor
Department of Ophthalmology
University of Iowa
Iowa City, Iowa
USA

Bryan W. Jones, PhD
Associate Professor
Department of Ophthalmology
Moran Eye Center
University of Utah
Salt Lake City, Utah
USA

Randy H. Kardon, MD, PhD
Professor, Neuro-ophthalmology
Department of Ophthalmology and Visual Sciences
University of Iowa College of Medicine
Iowa City, Iowa
Director
Iowa City VA Center for the Prevention and Treatment of Visual Loss
Iowa City VA Health Care System
Iowa City, Iowa
USA

Paul L. Kaufman, MD
Ernst H. Bárány Professor of Ocular Pharmacology
Department Chair Emeritus
Department of Ophthalmology & Visual Sciences
School of Medicine & Public Health
University of Wisconsin-Madison
Madison, Wisconsin
USA

Vladimir J. Kefalov, PhD
Professor
Department of Ophthalmology
University of California Irvine
Irvine, California
USA

Heidi Kidron, PhD
Title of Docent
Divisions of Faculty of Pharmacy
University of Helsinki
Helsinki, Finland

Miriam Kolko, MD, PhD
Professor
Department of Drug Design and Pharmacology
University of Copenhagen
Copenhagen, Denmark
Chief Physician
Department of Ophthalmology
Copenhagen University Hospital
Rigshospitalet
Glostrup, Denmark

Arjun Krishnaswamy, PhD
Associate Professor
Department of Physiology
McGill University
Montreal, Quebec
Canada

Ronald Robert Krueger, MD, MSE
Chairman
Department of Ophthalmology
University of Nebraska Medical Center
Omaha, Nebraska
USA

James A. Kuchenbecker, PhD
Acting Research Assistant Professor
Department of Ophthalmology
University of Washington
Seattle, Washington
USA

Trevor D. Lamb, BE, ScD, FRS, FAA
Emeritus Professor
Eccles Institute of Neuroscience
John Curtin School of Medical Research
Australian National University
Canberra, ACT
Australia

Melissa A. Lee, PhD
Postdoctoral Research Scientist
Department of Neuroscience
Columbia University
New York, New York
USA

Dennis M. Levi, OD, PhD
Distinguished Professor
Herbert Wertheim School of Optometry and Vision Science
University of California
Berkeley, California
USA

Edward Linton, MD
Assistant Professor
Department of Ophthalmology
University of Iowa
Iowa City, Iowa
USA

Mark J. Lucarelli, MD, FACS
Dortzbach Professor of Oculofacial Plastic Surgery
Department of Ophthalmology and Visual Sciences
University of Wisconsin—Madison
Madison, Wisconsin
USA

Elke Lütjen-Drecoll, MD, PhD
Professor Emeritus
Department of Anatomy
University Erlangen-Nürnberg
Erlangen, Bavaria
Germany

Peter R. MacLeish, PhD
Professor
Department of Neurobiology
Morehouse School of Medicine
Atlanta, Georgia
USA

Clint L. Makino, PhD
Associate Professor
Pharmacology, Physiology and Biophysics
Boston University Chobanian and Avedisian School of Medicine
Boston, Massachusetts
USA

Katherine Mancuso, PhD
Department of Ophthalmology
University of Washington
Seattle, Washington
USA

Fabrice Manns, PhD
Professor
Department of Biomedical Engineering and Department of
   Ophthalmology
Bascom Palmer Eye Institute
University of Miami
Coral Gables, Florida
USA

Robert E. Marc, PhD
Distinguished Professor Emeritus
Department of Ophthalmology
University of Utah
Salt Lake City, Utah
CEO
Signature Immunologics Inc.
Torrey, Utah
USA

Carol Ann Mason, PhD
Professor of Pathology and Cell Biology, Neuroscience, and
   Ophthalmology
Vagelos College of Physicians and Surgeons
Columbia University
New York, New York
USA

Allison M. McKendrick, Bsc Optom, Msc OPTOM, PhD
Professor
Division of Optometry
Lions Eye Institute
The University of Western Australia
Crawley, Australia
Professorial Fellow
Department of Optometry and Vision Sciences
The University of Melbourne
Parkville, Australia

Linda K. McLoon, PhD
Professor
Department of Ophthalmology and Visual Neurosciences
University of Minnesota
Minneapolis, Minnesota
USA

Jodhbir S. Mehta, MBBS, PhD, FRCS(ED)
Professor
Cornea
Singapore National Eye Centre
Singapore

Janine D. Mendola, PhD
Associate Professor
Department of Ophthalmology and Vision Sciences
McGill University
Montreal, Quebec
Canada

Jay Neitz, PhD
Professor
Department of Ophthalmology
University of Washington
Seattle, Washington
USA

Maureen Neitz, PhD
Professor
Department of Ophthalmology
University of Washington
Seattle, Washington
USA

Anthony M. Norcia, PhD
Professor (Research)
Department of Psychology
Stanford University
Stanford, California
USA

Christopher C. Pack, PhD
Professor
Department of Neurology and Neurosurgery
School of Medicine
McGill University
Montreal, Quebec
Canada

Woon Ju Park, PhD
Research Scientist
Department of Psychology
University of Washington
Seattle, Washington
USA

Carlos R. Ponce, MD, PhD
Assistant Professor
Department of Neurobiology
Harvard Medical School
Boston, Massachusetts
USA

Ignacio Provencio, PhD
Professor
Department of Biology
Department of Ophthalmology
University of Virginia
Charlottesville, Virginia
USA

Eva Ramsay, PhD
Postdoctoral Researcher
Division of Pharmaceutical Biosciences
Faculty of Pharmacy, Helsinki
Finland

Amirsaman Sajad, PhD
Research Assistant Professor
Department of Psychology
Vanderbilt University
Nashville, Tennessee
USA

Valenteen Savage
Doctoral Candidate
Department of Psychology
University of Washington
Seattle, Washington
USA

Leopold Schmetterer, PhD
Professor
Singapore Eye Research Institute
Singapore
SERI-NTU Advanced Ocular Engineering (STANCE)
Singapore
Academic Clinical Program
Duke-NUS Medical School
Singapore
School of Chemical and Biomedical Engineering
Nanyang Technological University
Singapore

Clifton M. Schor, PhD, OD
Emeritus Professor of the Graduate Division
Herbert Wertheim School of Optometry and Vision Science
University of California
Berkeley, California
USA

Paulo Schor, MD, PhD
Associate Professor of Ophthalmology
Department of Ophthalmology of Escola Paulista de Medicina
Federal University of São Paulo

São Paulo, São Paulo
Brazil
Senior Coordinator for Innovation
Research for Innovation
The State of São Paulo Research Foundation
São Paulo, São Paulo
Brazil

Gregory W. Schwartz, PhD
Derrick T. Vail Associate Professor
Department of Ophthalmology and Neuroscience
Feinberg School of Medicine
Northwestern University
Chicago, Illinois
USA

J. Sebag, MD, FACS, FRCOphth, FARVO
Founding Director
Vitreo-Retinal Ophthalmology
VMR Institute for Vitreous Macula Retina
Huntington Beach, California
Senior Research Scientist
Doheny Eye Institute
Pasadena, California
Professor of Clinical Ophthalmology
Geffen School of Medicine
University of California at Los Angeles
Los Angeles, California
USA

W. Daniel Stamer, PhD
Professor
Department of Ophthalmology
Duke University
Durham, North Carolina
USA

Olaf Strauss, PhD
Professor
Experimental Ophthalmology
Department of Ophthalmology
Charite University Medicine Berlin
Berlin, Germany

Felipe Taguchi, MD
Department of Ophthalmology and Visual Sciences
Federal University of São Paulo
São Paulo, São Paulo
Brazil

Tetsuya Terasaki, PhD
Research Director
School of Pharmacy
University of Eastern Finland
Kuopio, Finland

Stuart Trenholm, PhD
Associate Professor
Montreal Neurological Institute
McGill University
Montreal, Quebec
Canada

Arto Urtti, PhD
Professor
School of Pharmacy
University of Eastern Finland
Kuopio, Finland
Professor
Faculty of Pharmacy
University of Helsinki
Helsinki, Finland

Rupali Vohra, MD, PhD
Department of Drug Design and Pharmacology
University of Copenhagen
Copenhagen, Denmark
Department of Veterinary and Animal Sciences
University of Copenhagen
Frederiksberg, Denmark
Department of Ophthalmology
Copenhagen University Hospital
Rigshospitalet-Glostrup
Glostrup, Denmark

Michael Wall, MD
Professor
Department of Ophthalmology and Neurology
University of Iowa
Iowa City, Iowa
Staff Physician
Ophthalmology
Iowa City VA Health Care System
Iowa City, Iowa
USA

Theodore G. Wensel, PhD
Professor
Department of Biochemistry and Molecular Biology
Baylor College of Medicine
Houston, Texas
USA

Kwoon Y. Wong, PhD
Associate Professor
Department of Ophthalmology and Visual Sciences
Department of Molecular, Cellular and Developmental Biology
University of Michigan
Ann Arbor, Michigan
USA

Renfeng Xu, MD, PhD
Resident
Department of Ophthalmology
University of Nebraska Medical Center
Omaha, Nebraska
USA

PREFACE

The 12th edition of *Adler's Physiology of the Eye* continues the reorganization of the 11th edition, in which the chapters are organized not by anatomy (used by the previous edition) but by function and function/structure relationships, whether of ocular cells, tissue, or organs. In addition, this new edition reinvigorates the author list to include many new leading experts in their respective fields and is now based on an additional level of contributions and editing by section editors. Other new areas included are imaging modalities and development, to provide an expanded comprehensive view of the topic. Finally, we hope that the callouts will serve to make the book easier to use and provide a rapid method to access critical information.

ACKNOWLEDGMENTS

We are grateful especially to our authors, who brought this edition up to date 13 years after the previous edition. Our new section editors were essential in ensuring that every chapter is both correct and timely, and we thank them for taking on this important task. Finally, we thank our editorial executive at Elsevier, Kayla Wolfe, for guiding this major revision of the text from concept to product. This new edition is proof of how the contributions of a small number of dedicated individuals can result in a product that is valuable for all.

ADP	adenosine-5′-diphosphate
ALDP (protein)	adrenoleukodystrophy protein
APE	Schiff base conjugate of retinaldehyde with phosphatidylethanolamine
BII	Binocular Interaction Index
CERP	cholesterol efflux regulatory protein
FL	left fovea
FR	right fovea
GAF	GTPase accelerating factor
GATE	German Adaptive Thresholding Estimation
GC1	guanylate cyclase-1
GGL	G protein-gamma-like, a domain found in RGS proteins
GRK1	GPRCR kinase-1
H&E	hematoxylin and eosin stain
HEK-293	human embryonic kidney cells
L-NAME	N(G)-nitro L-arginine methyl ester
L-NMMA	N(G)-monomethyl L-arginine
MEGF10	multiple EGF like domains 10
MERTK	MER proto-oncogene, tyrosine kinase
MerTK	TAM receptor tyrosine kinase
NADC3	sodium-dependent dicarboxylate transporter 3
NADH	nicotinamide adenine dinucleotide + hydrogen
OAT	organic anion transporter
OMIM	Online Mendelian Inheritance in Man
PDZ domain	a structural domain found in certain proteins that anchor postsynaptic signaling complexes
POU domain	a DNA-binding domain found in a family of eukaryotic transcription factors
ROS-GC1	rod outer segment guanylate cyclase-1
SIRPα	signal regulatory protein α
TOP	tendency oriented perimetry
UNC/DCC	un-coordinated and deleted in colorectal carcinoma
VIPAC	vasoactive intestinal peptide pituitary adenylate cyclase activating peptide receptor
ZEST	zippy estimation by sequential testing

CONTENTS

SECTION 1 Focusing of an Image on the Retina

1 **Optics,** 1
Daniel Diniz, Felipe Taguchi, and Paulo Schor
2 **Optical Aberrations and Wavefront Sensing,** 27
Renfeng Xu and Ronald Robert Krueger
3 **Accommodation,** 37
Mary Ann Croft, Paul L. Kaufman, Fabrice Manns, and
Elke Lütjen-Drecoll

SECTION 2 Physiology of Optical Media

4 **Cornea and Sclera,** 69
Jodhbir S. Mehta and Marcus Ang
5 **The Lens,** 124
Paul James Donaldson
6 **Vitreous,** 164
Leila Chew and J. Sebag

SECTION 3 Direction of Gaze

7 **The Extraocular Muscles,** 189
Linda K. McLoon
8 **Neural Control of Eye Movements,** 212
Kathleen E. Cullen
9 **Three-Dimensional Eye Movements: Kinematics, Control,
and Perceptual Consequences,** 236
John Douglas Crawford and Amirsaman Sajad

SECTION 4 Nutrition of the Eye

10 **Production and Flow of Aqueous Humor,** 245
W. Daniel Stamer, Paul L. Kaufman, and Nicholas A. Delamere
11 **Ocular Circulation,** 284
Leopold Schmetterer
12 **Metabolic Interactions Between Neurons and
Glial Cells,** 324
Rupali Vohra and Miriam Kolko
13 **The Function of the Retinal Pigment Epithelium,** 339
Catherine Bowes Rickman and Olaf Strauss

SECTION 5 Protection of the Eye

14 **Functions of the Orbit and Eyelids,** 347
Gregory J. Griepentrog and Mark J. Lucarelli
15 **Formation and Function of the Tear Film,** 363
Darlene A. Dartt
16 **Sensory Innervation of the Eye,** 378
Juana Gallar and M. Carmen Acosta
17 **Outward-Directed Transport,** 405
Eva Ramsay, Laura Hellinen, Heidi Kidron, Tetsuya Terasaki, and
Arto Urtti

SECTION 6 Photoreception

18 **Biochemical Cascade of Phototransduction,** 414
Theodore G. Wensel
19 **Photoresponses of Rods and Cones,** 432
Peter R. MacLeish and Clint L. Makino
20 **Light Adaptation in Photoreceptors,** 451
Trevor D. Lamb and Vladimir J. Kefalov

SECTION 7 Visual Processing in the Retina

21 **The Synaptic Organization of the Retina,** 464
Robert E. Marc and Bryan W. Jones
22 **Signal Processing in the Outer Retina,** 480
Nicholas C. Brecha, Arlene A. Hirano, and Steven Barnes
23 **Visual Processing in the Inner Retina,** 495
Gregory W. Schwartz and Thomas Euler
24 **Electroretinogram,** 506
Laura J. Frishman

SECTION 8 Non-Perceptive Vision

25 **Regulation of Light Through the Pupil,** 527
Randy H. Kardon and Edward Linton
26 **Ganglion-Cell Photoreceptors,** 549
Kwoon Y. Wong, David M. Berson, and Ignacio Provencio

SECTION 9 Visual Processing in the Brain

27 **Overview of the Central Visual Pathways,** 571
Janine D. Mendola
28 **Optic Nerve,** 578
Jeffrey L. Goldberg
29 **Processing in the Lateral Geniculate Nucleus,** 598
José Manuel Alonso and Arjun Krishnaswamy
30 **Primary Visual Cortex,** 612
Alessandra Angelucci and Stuart Trenholm
31 **Extrastriate Visual Cortex,** 627
Carlos R. Ponce and Christopher C. Pack

SECTION 10 Visual Perception

32 **Visual Processing of Spatial Form,** 638
Daniel H. Baker
33 **Visual Acuity,** 649
Dennis M. Levi
34 **Color Vision,** 668
Jay Neitz, Katherine Mancuso, James A. Kuchenbecker, and
Maureen Neitz
35 **The Visual Field,** 675
Chris A. Johnson and Michael Wall

36 **Binocular Vision,** 701
Dennis M. Levi and Clifton M. Schor

37 **Temporal Properties of Vision,** 721
Allison M. McKendrick and Andrew J. Anderson

SECTION 11 Development and Deprivation of Vision

38 **Development of Vision in Infancy,** 735
Anthony M. Norcia

39 **Development of Retinogeniculate Projections,** 748
Melissa A. Lee and Carol Ann Mason

40 **Developmental Visual Deprivation,** 755
Yuzo M. Chino

41 **The Effects of Visual Deprivation After Infancy,** 775
Ione Fine, Valenteen Savage, and Woon Ju Park

Index, 788

VIDEO TABLE OF CONTENTS

Video 3.1 Forward and inward movement of the ciliary muscle is required for accommodation to occur. The muscle pulls the ora serrata and the elastic network of the choroid forward by approximately 1.0 mm in the region of the ora serrata in the young monkey (age 4 years). These movements decline with age. *Cm*, Ciliary muscle.

Reprinted with permission from Croft MA, Nork TM, McDonald JP, Katz A, Lütjen-Drecoll E, Kaufman PL. Accommodative movements of the vitreous membrane, choroid, and sclera in young and presbyopic human and nonhuman primate eyes. *Invest Ophthalmol Vis Sci.* 2013;54:5049-5058

Video 3.2 Ultrasound biomicroscopy (UBM) image in the nasal *(left panel)* and temporal *(right panel)* quadrant of an iridectomized rhesus monkey eye (age 10 years old). During accommodation the triamcinolone particles *(white dots)*, suspended in the ocular fluid, flow around the lens equator and into the vitreous compartment toward the anterior hyaloid *(left and right panels)* and then further into the cleft between the intermediate vitreous zonule (vz) and pars plana (pp) *(right panel)*. When the *red dot* appears in the video clip *(left panel)*, or when the channel (CH) indicator *(right panel—lower left)* changes from 00 to 11, the stimulus to induce accommodation is on.

Reprinted with permission from Kaufman PL, Lütjen-Drecoll E, Croft MA. Presbyopia and glaucoma: Two diseases, one pathophysiology? The Friedenwald Lecture. *Invest Ophthalmol Vis Sci.* 2019;60(5):1801-1812.

Video 3.3 Ultrasound biomicroscopy (UBM) in the nasal and temporal quadrants of an iridic rhesus monkey eye (age 7 years old) injected with triamcinolone, which clings to the vitreous membranes. In the presence of the iris, the anterior hyaloid still bows backward during accommodation and does so in parallel with the accommodative backward bowing of the iris. For both *left and right panels*, when the *red dot* appears, the stimulus to induce accommodation is on. Reprinted with permission from Kaufman PL, Lütjen-Drecoll E, Croft MA. Presbyopia and glaucoma: Two diseases, one pathophysiology? The Friedenwald Lecture. *Invest Ophthalmol Vis Sci.* 2019;60(5):1801-1812.

Video 3.4 Typical ultrasound biomicroscopy (UBM) images in aniridic *(left panel)* and iridic *(right panel)* phakic eyes of the rhesus monkey. A *red dot* indicates when the stimulus to induce accommodation is on. The iris bows backward during accommodation and the posterior lens pole moves posteriorly while the anterior lens moves anteriorly becoming more sharply curved.

Reprinted with permission from: Kaufman PL, Lütjen-Drecoll E, Croft MA. Presbyopia and glaucoma: Two diseases, one pathophysiology? The Friedenwald Lecture. *Invest Ophthalmol Vis Sci.* 2019;60(5):1801-1812.

Video 3.5 Endoscopy in a 19-year-old rhesus monkey eye showing backward movement of the anterior hyaloid membrane during accommodation. Note anterior hyaloid configuration bowing toward the lens and pars plicata in the resting state, whereas in the accommodated state the anterior hyaloid bows in a posterior direction. Reprinted with permission from Croft MA, Nork TM, McDonald JP, Katz A, Lütjen-Drecoll E, Kaufman PL. Accommodative movements of the vitreous membrane, choroid, and sclera in young and

presbyopic human and nonhuman primate eyes. *Invest Ophthalmol Vis Sci.* 2013;54:5049-5058

Video 3.6, **3.7**, and **3.8** Ultrasound biomicroscopy (UBM) images in normal *(right panel*, iris and lens present), and aphakic and iridectomized *(left and middle panels)* rhesus monkey eyes following intravitreal injection of triamcinolone. During accommodation, the capsule bows backward following Extracapsular Lens Extraction (ECLE) (Video 3.6). Further, the central vitreous moves posteriorly following ECLE (Video 3.6) and Intracapsular Lens Extraction (ICLE) (Video 3.7; *thick green arrows*), and when the iris and the lens are in place (Video 3.8). Cloquet's canal also moves posteriorly during accommodation (Video 3.8). The anterior zonula (AZ) is attached to Wieger's ligament, possibly with capsular remnant (Video 3.7). A *red dot* indicates when the stimulus to induce accommodation is on for each respective video clip.

Reprinted with permission from Kaufman PL, Lütjen-Drecoll E, Croft MA. Presbyopia and glaucoma: Two diseases, one pathophysiology? The Friedenwald Lecture. *Invest Ophthalmol Vis Sci.* 2019;60(5):1801-1812.

Video 3.9 Ultrasound biomicroscopy (UBM) image in a normal (iris and lens present) rhesus monkey eye following intravitreal injection of triamcinolone. The central vitreous moves posteriorly during accommodation all the way to the optic nerve. Also, note the anterior hyaloid bows backward near the lens equator *(white arrow)*. A *red dot* indicates when the stimulus to induce accommodation is on. The speed is 3× real time as it is easier to discern the accommodative movements.

Video 3.10 During accommodation in the young eye, there is robust vitreous zonule/muscle forward movement. However, with increased age there would be reduced forward muscle movement, but centripetal movement would be maintained. This may place compression force to the cistern branch tips, cistern trunk, and thereby the choroid in the optic nerve region. The compression may intensify as the eye ages and there is decreased forward muscle movement while centrifugal muscle movement is maintained—fitting the cistern branches into a shorter anterior-posterior intravitreal space/distance, compressing/thinning the choroid in the ON region.

The *dots* moving posteriorly in the central vitreous during accommodation represent fluid flow toward the posterior pole of the eye and may add an additional compressive force to the retina/choroid. The movement is in the opposite direction during disaccommodation.

Also, note there is an iris pinch movement the pupil gives to the anterior pole of the lens, a trend that was noted by Croft M, Nork T, Heatley G, McDonald J, Katz A, Kaufman P. Intraocular accommodative movements in monkeys; relationship to presbyopia. *Exp Eye Res.* 2022;222:109029. EER 2022 and reported in a previous publication by other researchers. Montes-Mico R, Hernandez P, Fernandez-Sanchez V, Bonaque S, Lara F, Lopez-Gil N. Changes of the eye optics after iris constriction. *J Optometry.* 2010;3:212–218.

Reprinted with permission from Croft AM, Nork TM Heatley G, McDonald JP, Katz A, Kaufman PL. Intraocular accommodative movements in monkeys; relationship to presbyopia. *Exp Eye Res.* 2022:109029.

Optics

Daniel Diniz, Felipe Taguchi, and Paulo Schor

THE YOUNG EYE

Primate and human infants must normally pass head first through their mother's pelvis to accommodate the limited opening determined by the bony configuration. Therefore, the size of the mother's pelvis limits the head and brain size of the infant. Specifically, the brain of an infant ape is 55% of its full size, and the brain of a present-day human infant is only 23% of the adult size.[1] The result is a human infant who is neurologically immature.[2] Notice that the baby monkey can immediately cling tightly to the fur on its mother's stomach, whereas the human infant has poor muscle strength, has little motor control, and is completely dependent on the mother for survival. While immature, the human infant lives in a restricted and artificial reality, interacting primarily with the mother. The human infant interacts little with the forces of life in the outside world.

It is possible that this early immaturity and restricted world contact are naturally beneficial. The infant's restricted curriculum concentrates on a few priorities necessary for survival.

Without words, the infant must be able to announce all his or her needs and encourage a high level of motherly devotion. To communicate with the mother, the infant must be able to read facial expressions and respond with a nonverbal vocabulary. If this speculation is correct, what vision equipment does the infant have to perform these functions?

Relevant anatomy
Axial length

Larsen[3] noted that the axial length of the neonate's eye was 17 mm and that it increases 25% by the time the child reaches adolescence. Up to 6 months of age, it reaches around 19.7 mm and up to 1 year of age, 20.5 mm. Around 7 years old, on average it reaches 22.4 mm.[4] The size of the normal infant's eye is about three-quarters that of the adult size. Geometric optics teaches us that the retinal image of the normal infant eye is, therefore, about three-quarters the size of the adult's image.* A smaller image also means that much less fine detail is recorded. The small retinal image may be but one reason why an infant's visual acuity is poorer than that of an adult. In fact, experiments have shown that the neonate's visual appreciation for fine detail at birth is one-thirtieth,

or approximately 3%, of the development of the adult,[†] yet the neonate appreciates large objects (e.g., nose, mouth, eyes of close faces), as does the adult.

Fig. 1.1 shows that visual acuity swiftly improves, and by the age of 12 months, the infant's level of visual acuity is 25% (20/80) of optimal adult visual acuity. This improvement in acuity seems to parallel eyeball growth. By the age of 5 years, the child usually has 20/20 vision.[1,6–9] What other factors beyond eye size account for the young child's lowered visual acuity? As the eye grows, the optical power of the eye lens and cornea must weaken in a tightly coordinated fashion so that the world stays in sharp focus on the retina. Patients with myopia highlight the developmental process of balancing the growth of the eye while maintaining a sharp retinal image. In most cases of myopia the eye is elongated. The stretching and weakening of the sclera seems to depend on two major factors. First, that the intraocular pressure maintains a constant force on the sclera. Second, there is digestion of sclera architecture (collagen I fibers and extracellular matrix) by metalloproteinase enzymes.[10] This idea of strengthening the sclera to prevent myopic expansion is supported experimentally. In one series of experiments, 7-methylxanthine (a caffeine metabolite) was used to enhance concentration and thickness of collagen fibers in the posterior sclera of animals.[11] In humans, scleral collagen fibers were crosslinked using riboflavin activated by ultraviolet light.[12]

However, we do not know what activates the process of scleral weakening and stretching in myopia. Some human studies have shown that use of atropine drops in children partially inhibits the development of myopia. The reason is unclear. Some feel that atropine reduces the pull of the ciliary muscle on the sclera, which otherwise allows the sclera to elongate. Another theory suggests that the atropine reduces vitreous pressure, thus reducing the stretching force. However, atropine has the same effect in chickens that have a ciliary muscle unresponsive to the effects of atropine. Another school of thought is that retinal receptors somehow activate the process of scleral weakening (e.g., M1 muscarinic receptors present in the neural retina but not in muscle).

Animal experiments using specific M1 blockers such as pirenzepine show the same effects as atropine, without blockade of accommodation. The presence of pirenzepine-inhibited receptors within the choroid and retina could also explain why elongation in eyes with transected optic nerves is inhibited by pirenzepine. Human use of topical

---

*Specifically, the size of the retinal image depends on an entity known as the *nodal distance*, which averages 11.7 mm in the newborn and 16.7 mm in the adult emmetropic schematic eye, giving a ratio of adult to infant retinal images of 1.43.[5]

[†] The infant's visual acuity is about 20/600, versus the normal visual acuity of an adult, which is 20/20.

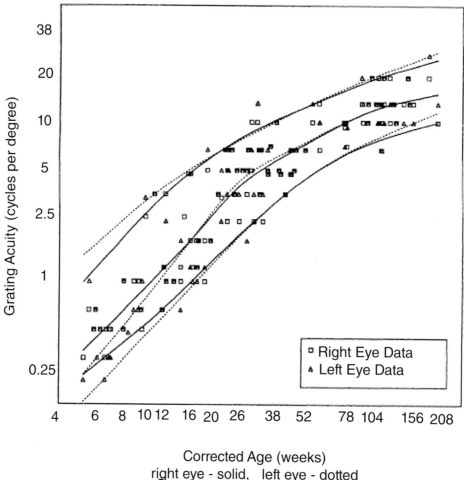

Fig. 1.1 A graph showing the improvement of visual acuity in the infant as it ages. The method of preferential viewing was used to achieve these results. The 30 cycles per degree is comparable to a 20/20 vision in adults. (From Chandna A. Natural history of the development of visual acuity in infants. *Eye*. 1991;5;20–26.)

pirenzepine was reported in two studies that showed a small but statistically significant reduction in myopia and axial length.[13] These data suggest that during childhood the retina can record information concerning the sharpness of the retinal image and then use this information to control the eye's axial length via scleral stretching.

If this tight coordination of growth fails, the infant may become nearsighted or farsighted. Because the coordination of eye length growth and the focusing power of the cornea and eye lens may be imperfect, is there some compensation provided, early in life, guaranteeing that almost every child can process a sharply focused retinal image of the world? Accommodation is the safety valve that can help provide a sharp image, even if all the ocular components are not perfectly matched. In the young child, the range of accommodation is greater than 20 diopters (D). This range, in addition to the farsightedness of almost all infants, means that most young eyes can focus almost any object by using part or all of this enormous focusing capacity.

Because of the infant's smaller pupil, a second factor that helps the infant achieve a sharper retinal image is an increased depth of focus.[6] Photographers use this principle when they use larger F-stops (F32, F64) to keep objects at different distances all in focus.

Fig. 1.2 shows the importance of the nodal point in determining the size of the retinal image in a typical human eye. To help us appreciate the basic optical principles operating within the human eye and

avoid being confused by their many details (e.g., the many different radii of curvature, the different indices of refraction), an all-purpose, simplified eye was developed. Such model eyes have many names (e.g., reduced, schematic, simplified eye) and were developed by some of the true giants of physiologic optics.*

Fig. 1.2 depicts such an eye with its cardinal points (the principal points, focal points, and nodal points). Knowing the location of the cardinal points of a lens system, the optical designer can calculate all of the relationships between an object and an image. For example, to determine the image size of the reduced eye, one simply traces the ray, starting from the top of the object, which goes undeviated through the nodal point and lands on the top of the inverted retinal image. As the distance between the nodal point and the retina increases, the image size increases. The addition of a plus spectacle lens to the eye's optic system moves the nodal point of the new system forward (increasing the nodal point to retina distance), thus magnifying the retinal image. The reverse is true with a negative spectacle lens. Therefore, a contact lens or a refractive cornea on which surgery has been performed enlarges the image size for a person with myopia who previously wore spectacles. The change in retinal image size should be taken into

---

* A partial list of giants of physiologic optics who have created schematic or reduced eyes includes Listing, Helmholtz, Wüllner, Tserning, Matthiessen, Gullstrand, Legrand, Ivanoff, and Emsley.

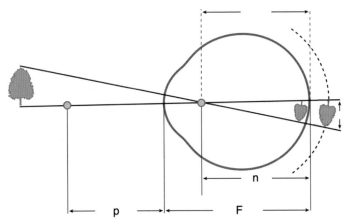

Fig. 1.2 A diagram of a reduced human eye. *F*, Focal points; *n*, nodal point; *p*, principal point. The *dotted line* represents the retina of an enlarged eye.

account when evaluating the visual acuity results after corneal refractive surgery. From an optical point of view, an 8-D hyperope exchanges a larger image produced by their +8 spectacle lens for a smaller image after corneal refractive surgery. Thus, they should theoretically lose a line of visual acuity after refractive surgery, but instead often gain a line. A possible reason is that the aberrations of the high plus spectacle lens cancel the effects of the larger retinal image, but this area requires further study.[14]

Emmetropization

The overall refractive state of the eye is determined by four components:
- Corneal power (mean, 43 D)
- Anterior chamber depth (mean, 3.4 mm)
- Crystalline lens power (mean, 21 D)
- Axial length (mean, 24 mm)

The coordination of the power of these components to process a sharp retinal image of a distant object is known as *emmetropization*.

Essentially, with age, cornea and lens must lose refractive power as the anterior chamber depth and axial length increase so that a sharp image remains focused on the retina.

The cornea, which averages 48 D of power at birth and has an increased elasticity, loses about 4 D by the time the child is 2 years of age.[15,16] One may assume that the spurt in growth of the sagittal diameter of the globe during this period pulls the cornea into a flatter curvature. The fact that the average corneal diameter is 8.5 mm at 34 weeks of gestation, 9 mm at 36 weeks, 9.5 mm at term, and about 11 mm in the adult eye supports this "pulling, flattening" hypothesis.[17]

However, other coordinated events also occur, such as the change of lens power and the coordinated increase in eye size (most important, an increase in axial length). The crystalline lens, which averages 45 D during infancy, loses about 20 D of power by age 6 years.[18,19] To compensate for this loss of lens power, the axial length increases by 5 to 6 mm in that same time frame.[3] (In general, 1 mm of change in axial length correlates with a 3-D change in refractive power of the eye.)

Now let us examine a possible mechanism that could account for most of the data.[18,20] As the cross-sectional area of the eye expands, there is an increased pull on the lens zonules and a subsequent flattening of the lens (the anterior lens surface is affected a bit more and the posterior lens surface a bit less), thus decreasing the overall lens power. There also may be a related decrease in the refractive index of the lens, which also contributes to the reduction in lens power. It seems, at final, that the various components cooperate to achieve a

higher-than-expected incidence of refractive state between 0 and +2 D.[21] It is now known that not only genetics but also the environment play an important role in regulating the final refractive state of human eye development. In other words, the genetic program can be tuned by environmental and intrinsic (i.e., intraocular) factors. Koretz et al.,[22] Laties and Stone,[23] and Stone et al.[9,22,24–28] have provided further insights into the biophysical and biochemical controls of emmetropization and their failure. The role of the environment is mainly demonstrated by three factors: deprivation myopia, deprivation myopia recovery, and lens-induced defocus compensation.

Experiments have shown that, after depriving an animal's eye of vision, for example, by suturing monkey eyelids, it was possible to induce axial myopia. After this experiment, it was found that the phenomenon occurred in several other animal species, including humans with unilateral eyelid ptosis, unilateral congenital cataract, or other pathologies that could deprive the vision of only one eye, generating axial anisometropia.[29,30] However, when removing the factor that generated the deprivation of sight, this eye tended to gradually reduce its myopia. This happened by the abrupt decrease in the growth rate of the vitreous chamber, while the cornea and lens followed their common flattening unaffected by the experiment. Another curious fact is that correcting deprivation-induced myopia with negative lenses prevented the expected hypermetropization after stopping vision deprivation.[29,30] It was also demonstrated in several species such as primates, pigs, and rats that the induction of hyperopia with negative lenses in emmetropic eyes caused an increase in the axial diameter and consequent induction of myopia equivalent to the power of the lens placed. Despite the limited evidence in humans, the fact that the human eye behaves similarly in other optical experiments suggests that the same occurs in our species. This is important knowledge that can be applied to address the increasing rates of myopia around the world.[29–34]

Retinal receptors

The cone photoreceptors of the retina are responsible for sharp vision under daylight conditions. For comparison and didactic purposes, an iPhone 13 Pro (Apple, California, EUA) has a resolution of 1170 × 2532 pixels, approximately 3 million pixels in total (460 pixels per inch), whereas the old iPhone 5 (Apple, California, EUA) had 1136 × 640 pixels, approximately 730,000 pixels (326 pixels per inch). Although it is not the only determining factor in image quality, it is known that the greater the number of pixels in a given space, the higher the quality of

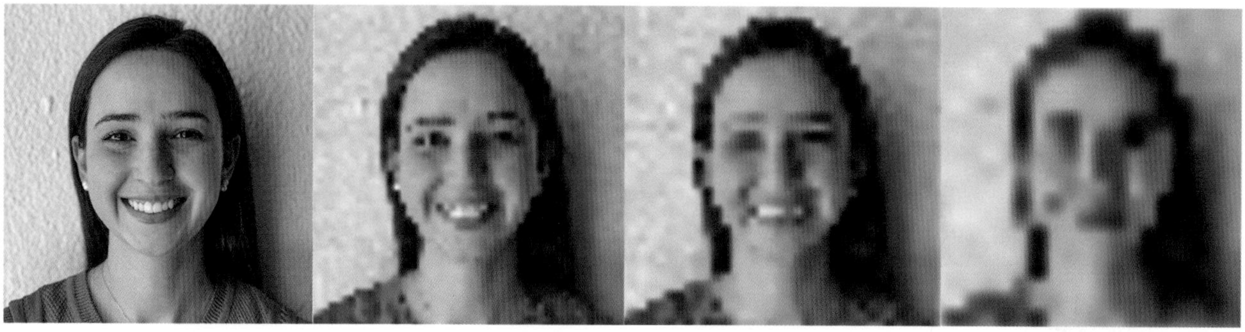

Fig. 1.3 A computer display of the face of a woman, with pixels of different sizes. (Courtesy of Gabriela Martines, MD.)

the screen image tends to be. Something similar happens in our retina. We have about 7 million cones, with a size of around 2.5 μm (micron), distributed irregularly. The areas where the denser number of cones are packed provide better image quality.

The most sensitive part of the retina is the fovea, the central region where the cones are even finer and are packed together even tighter. The fovea of the infant eye is packed less than one-quarter of the density of that of the adult. Furthermore, the synapse density in the neural portion of the retina, as well as the visual brain, is low at birth. The combination of these two anatomic configurations means that fewer fine details of the retinal image are recorded and sent to the brain.

Neural processing

Finally, the nerves that transmit visual information to the brain, as well as the nerve fibers at the various levels within the brain, are poorly myelinated in the infant. Myelin is the insulating wrap around each nerve fiber. A normally myelinated nerve can transmit nerve impulses swiftly and without static or "cross talk" from adjacent nerves. To use a computer analogy, one might think of the infant brain as being connected with poorly insulated wires. Therefore, sparks, short circuits, and static all slow or interfere with perfect transmission, and only the strongest messages get through. Fig. 1.3 represents an appropriate analogy. The face of a woman is shown with larger and larger pixels. The infant's early vision might be comparable to the picture with the biggest block pixels. With maturation of the brain-processing elements, the neurologic equivalent of pixel size gets smaller and more details can be registered. Thus, the equivalent of the photographic film grain size in the retina and the equivalent of pixel size in the brain processor both get smaller as the child grows. The immaturity of the infant's memory capacity may be one reason why its visual images have less detail. In other words, the coarseness of the infant visual system does not overtax the immature memory system.

Relevant early physiology

Experiments reveal that good color vision does not appear until about 3 months of age. After that, most infants are likely to be able to distinguish colors, while deuteranopes, tritanopes, and protanopes cannot. Some studies even suggest that development of color vision in humans may be faster in females, probably owing to faster maturation of the visual cortex.[35] However, little has been studied about the difference in sensory development between genders. The infant also takes longer to "make sense" of the retinal image. Specifically, the infant must stare for relatively long periods (1–3 minutes), blinking rarely during this period.[1,8]

Recognizing faces

The remarkable thing about the infant's eyesight is that the relatively poor level of resolution just described still allows the infant to recognize different faces and different facial expressions. We know this to be true in some newborn infants, who can accurately imitate the expressions of an adult (Fig. 1.4), almost as if the baby uses his or her own face as a canvas to reproduce the facial expression of the onlooker.

Experiments with infants demonstrate that infants prefer to look at faces or pictures of faces rather than look at other objects. Among the faces, the most important is that of the mother. Bushnell et al.[36] have reported that even newborns prefer to look at their mother's face than at strangers' faces. By the age of 6 weeks, infants can discern specific features of the face. For example, they can lock in on the mother's gaze. By age 6 months, they can also recognize the same face in different poses. In fact, they are experts at recognizing a face, be it upside down or right side up, till the age of 6 years. After age 6, infants actually lose their skill at quickly recognizing upside-down faces.[8]

A closer examination of the eye at 6 months of age is worthwhile because an unusual change has started to take place in the optics of the eye at this time. Gwiazda et al.[37] found that a significant amount of astigmatism develops in 56% of the infants studied. The degree of astigmatism is even greater in preterm babies and seems to be inversely related to birth weight.[38] This condition remains for only 1 to 2 years.[37,39–41]

The transient astigmatism just described tends to elongate tiny dots of the retinal image into lines. In essence, these create the equivalent of a line drawing of the retinal image. For example, think of a mime (i.e., a painted face with a few dark lines and spots for eyes and nose) as creating different line drawings of the face. What is astonishing is that, although made of only a few dark lines, the mime can recreate most human expressions. It seems reasonable to imagine that the mime presents faces similar to those seen by the young child or found in a child's drawing. The faces have no texture, no shadowing, and no creases—only a line for a mouth, circle for eyes, and occasionally a dot for a nose. Is it not then possible that infant astigmatism helps represent faces as line drawings to the infant visual system? Line drawings also save memory storage space, which would be an advantage for the small infant brain.* Fig. 1.5 illustrates this point in a different way. The face of the same woman is shown with a complete gray scale on the left and is shown as a line drawing (only black and white) on the right. Line drawing requires much less computing power than a face with texture and would be more compatible with the child's immature processing system.

Another theory is that transient astigmatism would diminish the "dead zone" of accommodation. The "dead zone" is a range of small defocus or loss of image contrast that is not enough to stimulate accommodation. In other words, an eye with astigmatism would always be in constant accommodative effort, in order to seek the best

---

* This idea was suggested by David Marr in "Early Processing of Visual Information," published in *Transactions of the Royal Society of London, Series B*, 1976; 275:483.

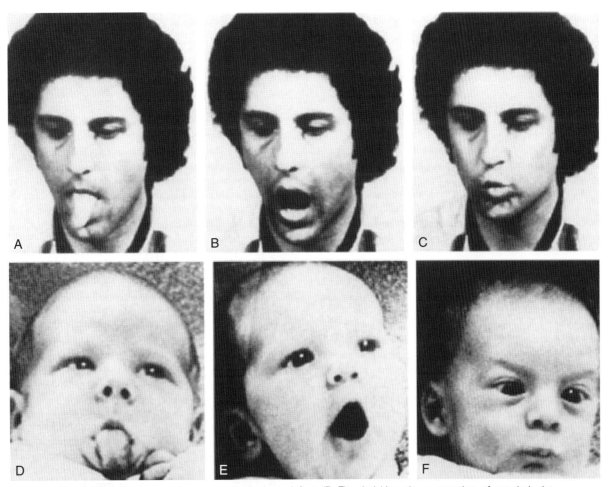

Fig. 1.4 These photos shows a recently born infant (**D–F**) mimicking the expression of psychologist Dr. A Meltzoff (**A–C**). The baby is obviously able to perceive the different expressions to mimic them. (From Klaus MH, Klaus PH. *The Amazing Newborn.* Reading, MA: Addison Wesley, 1985.)

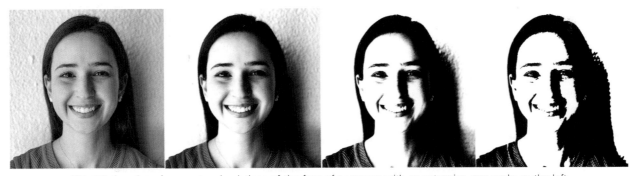

Fig. 1.5 A series of computer simulations of the face of a woman with an extensive gray scale on the left and only a two gray scale on the right, the latter being similar to a line drawing. (Courtesy of Gabriela Martines, MD.)

focus, inducing an activation and a "learning" of the accommodation mechanism in the first years of life.[42]

Line orientation receptors

As noted earlier, in many infants the amount of astigmatism can rise to a level of greater than 2 D in the first year of life. The orientation of the distortion is usually horizontal (180 degrees) initially. In the course of the next 2 years, the meridian of distortion rotates to the vertical and the amount of the astigmatism diminishes. This slow rotation of the axis of exaggeration can help activate different groups of brain cells, which become sensitive to features in the retinal image with different tilts. In

fact, the discovery of these brain cells with orientation selectively leads to a ground-breaking understanding of the functional architecture in the higher brain. In 1958 Torsten Wiesel and David Hubel, working in their laboratory at the Harvard Medical School, implanted electrodes in the visual cortex of an anesthetized cat to record cortical cell responses to patterns of light, which they projected onto a screen in front of the cat. After 4 hours of intense work, the two scientists put the dark spot slide into the projector, where it jammed. As the edge of the glass slide cast an angled shadow on the retina, the implanted cell in the visual cortex fired a burst of action potentials. Torsten Wiesel described that moment as the "door to all secrets." The pair went on to prove that cells in the cortex responded only to stimuli of a particular orientation. Similar responding cells were all located in the same part of the cortex. This work opened up the area of how and where the brain encodes specific features of the retinal image. Fittingly, Drs. Hubel and Wiesel were awarded the Nobel Prize for Medicine in 1981.[43]

Monitoring other's eye movements

Another function of great survival value to the infant is the ability to follow the eye movements of his or her caretakers. Consider this a near task involving the contrast discrimination of a 12-mm dark iris against a white sclera framed by the palpebral fissure; such a task can be accomplished with a visual acuity of 20/200.

The British psychologist Simon Baron-Cohen, in his book *Mindblindness*,* suggests that a major evolutionary advance has been the human's ability to understand and then interact with others in a social group (e.g., playing social chess). He further suggests that we accomplish this social intelligence primarily by following the eye movements of others, which begins at a young age. For example, an infant of 2 months begins to concentrate on the eyes of adults. Infants have been shown to spend as much time on the eyes as on all other features of an observer's face.

By 6 months of age, infants look at the face of an adult who is looking at them two to three times longer than an adult who is looking away. We also know that when infants achieve eye contact, a positive emotion is achieved (i.e., infants smile). By age 14 months, infants start to read the direction in which an adult is looking. Infants turn in that direction and then continue to look back at the adult to check that both are looking at the same thing. By age 2 years, infants typically can read fear and joy from eye and facial expression.

Recognizing movement

Infants are capable of putting up their arms to block a threatening movement. This act tells us that infants appreciate both movement and the implied threat of this particular movement.[6,44] Admittedly, infants cannot respond if the threat moves too quickly, probably because the immature myelinization of the nerves slows the neural circuits. Nevertheless, a definite appreciation of movement and threat exists.

For movement to be registered accurately, the infant retina probably records an object at point A. That image is then physiologically erased (in the brain and/or retina), and the object is now seen at point B. This physiologic erasure is important because without it movement would produce a smeared retinal image. Researchers think that the infant probably sees movement as a smoothed series of sharp images, not smears.[45] This hypothesis is supported by other experiments demonstrating that the infant can appreciate the on/off quality of a rapidly flickering light at an early age. It seems logical that the movement of an image across the retina (with the inherent erasures) is physiologically related to the rapid on/off registration of a flickering light.

A related reflex, the foveal reflex, is triggered by stimulation of the peripheral retina, activating the eye movement system so that the fovea is directed to the visual stimulus.

Summary—social seeing

Although the visual system of the infant is immature, some infants can recognize and respond to adult facial expressions on the first day of life and follow the mother's glances by 6 weeks of age. Clearly, the infant's top priority is to maintain a social relationship with his or her mother or other caring adults. This idea was described succinctly by the "language expert" Pinker[46]: "Most normally developing babies like to schmooze." As infants grow, they learn to see people and objects in the way that their culture demands and communicate in the expected manner, that is, "We don't see things as they are but as we are." Is it possible that the immature eye and visual system actually facilitate socially biased seeing? Perhaps the smaller, simpler retinal images, along with the less sophisticated brain processing, prevent the many other details of life from confusing the key message, that is, social interaction takes top priority.

Even in adulthood there is plasticity of the visual system, e.g., after the implantation of multifocal intraocular lenses (IOLs). These IOLs superimpose blurred near images on a sharply focused distant image. Thus, the patient's brain must filter and suppress the third, fourth, and so on blurred images from the scene. This is a time-dependent phenomenon that may take days to months to occur.[47]

THE IMAGE OF THE HUMAN ADULT EYE

The image quality of the human adult eye is far superior to that of the human infant, although probably inferior to certain predator birds. Its wide focusing range is smaller than that of certain diving birds, and its fine sensitivity to low light levels is weaker than spiders or animals with a tapetum lucidum. Its ability to repair itself is probably not as efficient as some animals (e.g., newts, which can form a new lens if the original is damaged). Finally, the human eye has the ability to transmit emotional information[48] (e.g., excitement by means of pupil dilation, sadness by means of weeping), but with less forcefulness than some fish, who uncover a pigmented bar next to the eye when they are about to attack,[49] or the horned lizard, which squirts a jet of blood from its eye when it is threatened.[50] Thus, in reading this chapter, one must appreciate the eye's level of performance in light of its large spectrum of functions.

Role of the cornea

The human cornea is a unique tissue. First, it is the most powerful focusing element of the eye, roughly twice as powerful as the lens within the eye. It is mechanically strong and transparent. Its strength comes from its collagen fiber layers. Some 200 fiber layers crisscross the cornea in different directions. These fibers are set in a thick, watery jelly called *glycosaminoglycan*. The jelly gives the cornea pliability. Normal corneas are aspherical, meaning flatter at the periphery than at the center. Scheimpflug-based technology has increasingly allowed for the accurate measurement of this corneal condition, important especially in the screening of pathologic situations. However, at normal levels, corneal asphericity is important as it counteracts the effects of paraxial light that are greater at peripheral areas of the cornea.[51] These light rays create a smeared focus because they behave differently to light rays from the central portion of the cornea. In other words, corneal asphericity decreases spherical aberration, a phenomenon that will be better explained later in this chapter.

For a long time, no one could convincingly explain the transparency of the cornea. No one could understand how nature combined tough, transparent collagen fibers (with their unique index of refraction) with the transparent glycosaminoglycan matrix, which had a different index of refraction, and still maintained clarity. Perhaps an everyday example of this phenomenon will help. When a glass is filled from the hot water tap, the solution looks cloudy. Looking closely, one can see many fine, clear expanded air bubbles (which have a unique index of refraction) within the water (which has different refractive properties). Conversely, cold water appears clear because its air bubbles are tiny. The normal corneal structure might be considered optically similar to the structure of the cold water (i.e., tiny components with different indices of refraction).

---

* In his book *Mindblindness: An Essay on Autism and Theory of Mind*, published by MIT Press in 1995, Baron-Cohen ferrets out the key features of "eye following" in the normal child by comparing them with those of the autistic child.

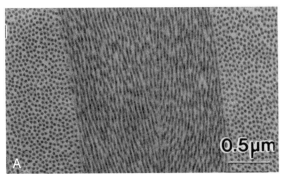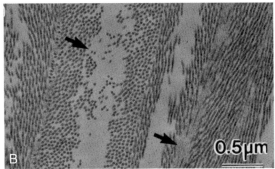

Fig. 1.6 Electron micrographs of the transparent (left) and opaque (right) calf cornea. In the normal cornea, there is an ordered, neat pattern of corneal collagen fibers. The black dots are the fibers cut on end and the spacing between them is less than a wavelength of light apart. In the opaque cornea, increased pressure resulted in defects that disrupted the normal short-range order of the fibrils. Large spaces between fibers are seen in this hazy cornea. (From Gisselberg M, Clark JI, Vaezy S, and Osgood TB. A quantitative evaluation of Fourier components in transparent and opaque calf cornea. *Am J Anat.* 1991;191:408–418. https://doi.org/10.1002/aja.1001910408.)

Miller and Benedek[52] were ultimately able to prove that if the spaces consisting of glycosaminoglycan and the size of the collagen fibers were smaller than one-half a wavelength of visible light, the cornea is clear, even if the fibers were arranged randomly. An orderly arrangement of the fibers also helps maintain corneal transparency.

Another way to explain it is to say that the cornea is basically transparent to visible light because its internal structures are tuned to the size of a fraction of the wavelengths of visible light. Fig. 1.6 is an electron micrograph showing the fibers of the human cornea. The black dots are cross-sections of collagen fibers embedded in the glycosaminoglycan matrix. In this specimen (Fig. 1.6A), the fibers are spaced closer than half a wavelength of visible light apart, and the fibers in each of the major layers are arranged in an orderly manner. In an edematous, hazy cornea, there are large spaces between collagen fibers (Fig. 1.6B).

This arrangement of corneal fibers serves a number of important functions. First, the arrangement offers maximal strength and resistance to injury from any direction. Second, the arrangement produces a transparent, stable optical element. Third, the spaces between the major layers act as potential highways for white blood cell migration if any injury or infection occurs. Horizontal arrangement of corneal lamellae, which can slide over each other during eye rubbing, facilitates the clinical development of pathologic conditions such as keratoconus. The lack of interlamellar adhesion and corneal thinning facilitates bulging under intraocular pressure and gravity. Enzymatic digestion seems to be the causative agent in the thinning, which eventually deforms the anterior surface of the cornea. This conical cornea is irregularly astigmatic and will produce multiple blurred images in the retina. Collagen crosslinking helps connect the adjacent lamellae, inducing greater corneal strength by resisting interlamellae sliding, and thus reduces the progression of keratoconus (Fig. 1.7).[53]

Role of the crystalline lens

Is it easier to see underwater with goggles?* Without goggles, the water practically cancels the focusing power of the cornea,† leaving objects blurred. The goggles ensure an envelope of air in front of the cornea, restoring its optical power. If water cancels optical power, how can we explain the focusing ability of the crystalline lens, which lies inside the eye and is surrounded by a fluid known as *aqueous humor*? The answer is that the focusing power resides in the unusually high protein content of the lens. The protein concentration may reach 50% or more in certain parts of the lens.‡ Such a high concentration increases the refractive index above that of water and allows the focusing of light. Now we are ready to appreciate the real secret of the lens.[52,54]

Normally, a 50% protein solution is cloudy, with precipitates floating about like curdled lumps of milk in a cup of coffee. However, the protein

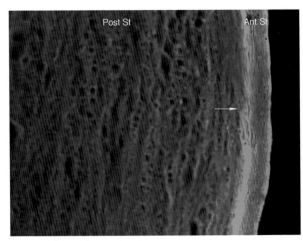

Fig. 1.7 Confocal microscopy (40x) of a bovine cornea that had been treated with a riboflavin (0.01%) solution, exposed to UV light (365 nm) to cross link stromal collagen, then subsequently immunostained for Collagen type I (Green). Note the connection between lamellae in the anterior stroma (ant st) compared to the laxity of the posterior stroma (post s). (Courtesy Bottos, Schor, Chamon, Regatieri, Dreyfuss, and Nader.)

complexes of the normal lens do not precipitate. In a manner not fully understood, the large protein complexes known as *crystallins* (ranging in size from 20 to 2000 kD) seem to repel each other, or at least prevent aggregation, to maintain tiny spaces between each other. The protein size and the spaces between them are equivalent to a small fraction of a light wavelength. Spaced as they are, one might say that they are tuned to visible light and allow the rays to pass through unimpeded. However, if some pathologic process occurs, the protein molecules aggregate and the lens

---

* Because the index of refraction of water is greater than air, objects underwater appear about one-third closer and thus one-third larger than they would in air (i.e., magnification = 1.33×).[55]

† The cornea is a focusing element for two reasons. First, it has a convex surface. Second, it has a refractive index greater than air. Actually, its refractive index is close to that of water. Thus, when one is underwater, the surrounding water on the outside and the aqueous humor inside the eye combine to neutralize the cornea's focusing power.

‡ The chemical composition of a focusing element such as the crystalline lens determines the refractive index. Water has a refractive index of 1.33. As the protein concentration of the lens rises, the index of refraction approaches 1.42.

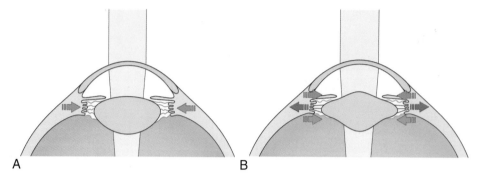

Fig. 1.8 Zonules and lens details as described by Helmholtz (**A**) and Schachar (**B**). (Courtesy of Francisco Irochima, MD.)

loses its clarity. When this happens, light is scattered as it passes through the lens. The result is a cataract. The amount of scatter more than doubles in the 60-year-old lens compared to a 20-year-old lens.[51]

Accommodation

If the emmetropic eye is in sharp focus for the distant world, it must refocus (accommodate) to see closer objects.[§] For example, the child's range of accommodation is large, as noted earlier. This allows the child to continue to keep objects in sharp focus from an infinite distance away to objects brought to the tip of the nose. The act of accommodation is fast, taking only about one-third of a second.

The contraction capacity of the ciliary muscle is called physiological accommodation, and the ability of the lens to change its shape is called physical accommodation.[51] The stimulus for accommodation is triggered by the human eye's attempt to focus on an object that is in a closer position than its far point, that is, the greatest distance at which a resting eye clearly sees an object. In emmetropes, this point is at infinity. According to Helmholtz (1856), under this stimulus, the ciliary muscle contracts, relaxing the zonule ligaments, which increases the antero-posterior diameter of the lens, increasing the dioptric power of the lens and the human eye, allowing focus at small distances (Fig. 1.8). Many theories have emerged since then, with new insights into the accommodation process. Schachar[57,58] proposed that, although the zonular tension decreases in the peripheral areas, it increases in the equatorial zone, causing the central region of the lens to curve, but the peripheral region to flatten (Fig. 1.8). Coleman[59,60] described the vitreous as applying force that produces changes on the posterior and anterior lens curvature, as well the role of the anterior displacement of the lens into the anterior chamber as an adjunct mechanism of accommodation.

With age, the lens enlarges and becomes denser and more rigid. In so doing, it progressively loses the ability to accommodate, generating presbyopia. Our range of accommodation decreases with each passing year, so by the age of 45, most of us are left with about 20% or less of the amplitude of accommodation we started with.

There are also theories that describe the contribution of changes in ciliary muscle strength or changes in the zonular attachments to the lens in presbyopia. However, it is accepted that the process of accommodation and the emergence of presbyopia is complex, and that probably no theory contemplates the exact explanation of all the events involving the dioptric changes in the power of the lens.

Parenthetically, the cornea of many birds, from pigeons to hawks, can change shape to accommodate.[61] The avian cornea does not change flexibility with age; therefore, these birds do not become presbyopic. However, there is no "free lunch" in nature. The human lens, sitting within the eye surrounded by protective fluid, is far less vulnerable to injury than the cornea.

Role of the retina

After light passes through the cornea, the aqueous humor, the lens, and the vitreous humor, it is focused onto the retinal photoreceptors. The light must pass through a number of retinal layers of nerve fibers, nerve cells, and blood vessels before striking the receptors. These retinal layers (aside from blood vessels) are transparent because of the small size of the elements and the tight packing arrangement.

The bird retina does not have blood vessels. The human retina has retinal blood vessels that cover some of the retinal receptors and produce fine angioscotomas (a blind spot or defect in the visual field produced by retinal vessels). A bird's retina obtains much of its oxygen and nutritive supply from a tangle of blood vessels (the pectin), which is covered with black pigment and sits in the vitreous in front of the retina and above the macula (so as to function as a visor). The negative aspect of such a vascular system is vulnerability to a direct blunt or penetrating injury that can lead to a vitreous hemorrhage and sudden blindness. Obviously, this is less probable in the bird because of its lifestyle.

Rhodopsin

The rods and cones are made up of a biologic molecule that absorbs visible light and then transluces that event into an electrical nerve signal. The rhodopsin molecule is an example of Einstein's photoelectric effect.[*] In fact, only one quanta (the smallest possible amount of light) of visible light[†] is needed to trigger the molecule, that is, snap the molecule into a new shape.[‡]

The internal structure of the molecule allows the wavelengths of visible light to resonate within its electron cloud and within 20 million millionths of a second, inducing the change in the molecule that starts the reaction.

Probably the earliest chemical relative of rhodopsin is to be found in a primitive purple-colored bacteria called *Holobacterium halobium*. Koji Nakanishi, a biochemist at Columbia University, in an article titled "Why 11-cis-Retinal?",[63] notes that this bacteria has been on the planet for the last 1.3 billion years.[64,65] Its preference for low oxygen and a salty environment places its origin at a time on earth when there was little

---

[§]The question "How does accommodation 'know' it has achieved the sharpest focus?" seems to be best answered by a sensing system in the brain. However, some have suggested that the system takes advantage of the naturally occurring chromatic aberration of the primate eye to fine-tune focusing.[56]

[*]Some wavelengths of light are powerful enough to knock electrons of certain molecules out of their orbits, thereby producing an electric current. Einstein was awarded the Nobel Prize for explaining the "photoelectric effect."
[†]In 1942, Selig Hecht and his coworkers in New York first proved that only one quanta of visible light could trigger rhodopsin to start a cascade of biochemical events eventuating in the sensing of light.
[‡]Photoactivation of one molecule of rhodopsin starts an impressive example of biologic amplification, in which hundreds of molecules of the protein transducer each activate a like number of phosphodiesterase molecules, which in turn hydrolyze a similar number of cyclic guanine monophosphate (cGMP) molecules, which then trigger a neural signal to the brain.[62]

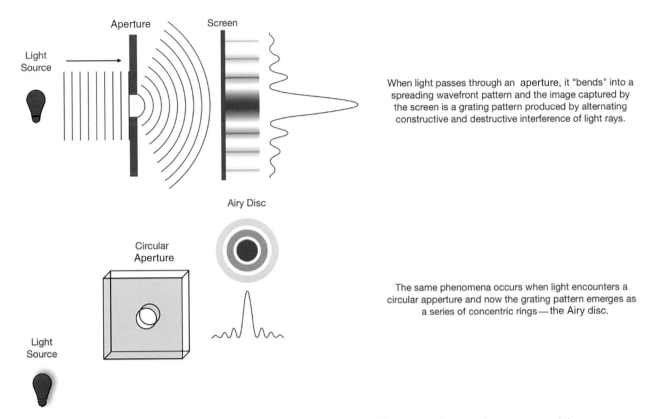

Fig. 1.9 Light passing through an aperture. Note that it "bends" into a spreading wavefront pattern, and the image captured by the screen is a grating pattern produced by alternating constructive and destructive interference of light rays. The same phenomena occurs when light encounters a circular aperture, and now the grating pattern emerges as a series of concentric rings—the Airy disc.

or no oxygen in the atmosphere and a high salt concentration in the sea. Although found in primeval bacteria, bacteriorhodopsin is a rather complicated molecule, containing 248 amino acids. It is thought that this bacteria probably used rhodopsin for photosynthesis, rather than light sensing. Time-resolved spectroscopic measurements have determined that this molecule changes shape within one trillionth of a second after light stimulation.[66] This early form of rhodopsin absorbs light most efficiently in the blue-green part of the spectrum, although it does respond to all colors.[67]

To function as the transducer for vision, the photopigment must capture light and then signal the organism's brain that the light has registered. As noted earlier, one molecule needs only one quanta to start the reaction. Even more amazing is the molecule's stability. Although only one quanta of visible light is necessary to trigger it, the molecule will not trigger accidentally. In fact, it has been estimated that spontaneous isomerization of retinal (the light-sensing chromophore portion of rhodopsin) occurs once in a thousand years.[66] If this were not so, we would see light flashes every time there is a rise in body temperature (a fever). To better understand the rhodopsin mechanism, one may picture a hair trigger on a pistol that takes only the slightest vibration (but only a special type of vibration) to be activated. As noted, the activating quanta must be of the proper energy level to "kick in" the reaction, that is, the quanta of light must be made of wavelengths of visible light.

Receptor size and spacing

Retinal receptor factors that influence the optical limits of visual acuity occur in the foveal component of the macula. The fovea itself subtends an arc of about 0.3 degrees. It is an elliptical area with a horizontal diameter of 100 μm. The area contains more than 2000 tightly packed cones. The distance between the centers of these tightly

packed cones is about 2 μm. The cone diameters themselves measure about 1.5 μm (a dimension comparable to three wavelengths of green light) and are separated by about 0.5 μm.[68–71] Therefore, the fine details of the retinal image occupy an elliptical area only about 0.1 mm in maximum width.

A discussion of the diffraction limits of resolution, in a theoretical emmetropic human eye, must involve the anatomic size of the photoreceptors and the pupil. A point or an object is focused on the retina as an Airy disc because of diffraction (Fig. 1.9). The angular size of the Airy disc is determined as follows:

$$\text{Angular size (in radians)} = 1.22 \times \text{wavelength (mm)} / \text{pupil diameter (mm)}$$

Let the wavelength be 0.00056 mm (560 nm; yellow/green light). Then

$$\text{Angular size} = 0.00068 \text{ radians/pupil diameter (mm)}$$

For a pupil of 2.4 mm (optimal balance between diffraction and spherical aberration in the human eye):

$$\text{Angular size} = 0.00028 \text{ radians, or about 1 minute of arc}$$

Given this angle of 1 minute, the actual size of the Airy disc can be calculated if the distance from the nodal point to the retina is known. The optimal distance depends on the diameter of the photoreceptors. Because these act as light guides, the theoretical limit is 1 to 2 μm. To obtain the maximum visual information available, Kirschfeld calculated that more than five receptors are required to scan the Airy disc.[52] Assume that each foveal cone is 1.5 μm in diameter and that there is an optimal space of 0.5 μm between receptors. The following equation describes the situation for three cones and two spaces (5.5 μm):

5.5 μm/Tan 1 minute = Nodal point to retina distance

Substituting 0.0003 from equation (2) into equation (3) gives equation (4):

5.5 μm/0.0003 = Nodal point to retina distance

From equation (4) the distance from the nodal point to the retina can be rounded off to 18.00 mm, which is close to the distance between the secondary nodal point and the retina in the schematic human eye.

How closely does optical theory agree with reality? The average visual acuity for healthy eyes in the age group younger than 50 was better than 20/16. In the distribution within the group younger than 40, the top 5% had an acuity of close to 20/10.[72]

Another related factor must be kept in mind. The fixating eye is in constant motion, as opposed to a camera on a tripod. Presumably, these movements prevent bleaching or fading within individual photoreceptors. These small movements, called either *tremors*, *drifts*, or *microsaccades*, range in amplitude from seconds to minutes of angular arc. Such movements tend to smear rather than enhance our traditional concept of visual resolution. It can only be presumed that to maintain high resolution within the context of this physiologic nystagmus, the visual system takes quick, short samples of the retinal image during these potentially smearing movements and then recreates an image of higher resolution.[73–75]

The unique essence of the vertebrate retina is that the structure of the transparent optical components, the rhodopsin molecule, and the size of the foveal cones are all tuned to interact optimally with wavelengths of visible light.[76,77] It is earth's unique atmosphere and its unique relationship to the sun that have allowed primarily visible light, a tiny band from the enormous electromagnetic spectrum of the sun, to rain down upon us at safe energy levels. Our eyes are a product of an evolutionary process that has tuned to these unique wavelengths at these levels of intensity.[78,79]

With this basic science background, we can discuss how functions such as visual acuity and contrast sensitivity are monitored in a clinical setting.

Visual acuity testing

The idea that the minimum separation between two point sources of light was a measure of vision dates back to Hooke in 1679, when he noted "tis hardly possible for any animal eye well to distinguish an angle much smaller than that of a minute: and where two objects are not farther distant than a minute, if they are bright objects, they coalesce and appear as one."[80] In the early nineteenth century, Purkinje and Young used letters of various sizes for judging the extent of the power of distinguishing objects. Finally, in 1863, Professor Hermann Snellen of Utrecht developed his classic test letters. He quantitated the lines by comparison of the visual acuity of a patient with that of his assistant, who had good vision. Thus, 20/200 (6/60) vision meant that the patient could see at 20 feet (6 m) what Snellen's assistant could see at 200 feet (60 m).[80]

The essence of correct identification of the letters on the Snellen chart is to see the clear spaces between the black elements of the letter. The spacing between the bars of the "E" should be 1 minute for the 20/20 (6/6) letter. The entire letter is 5 minutes high. To calculate the height of "x" (i.e., a 20/20 or 6/6 letter), use the following equation:

20 feet = 6,096 m

Tan 5 minutes = x/6,096

0,0015 = x/6,096

x = 0,0015 × 6,096 = 0,009144 meters
= 9,14 mm (0,36 inches)*

Chart luminance

Over a "normal" photopic range of 40 to 600 cd/m² (candela per square meter - a measure of luminance) the relation between the logarithm of the minimum angle of resolution (log MAR) and luminance (log L) can be approximated by a straight line.[81] In other words, visual acuity increases continuously as luminance increases, up to a limit of 600 cd/m². However, in clinical visual acuity testing, the chart luminance should represent typical real work photopic conditions (around 160 to 200 cd/m²).

Visual acuity as log MAR

If one looks at a standard Snellen acuity chart (Fig. 1.12), the lines of symbols progress as follows: 20/400, 20/200, 20/150, 20/120, 20/100, 20/80, 20/70, 20/60, 20/50, 20/40, 20/30, 20/25, 20/20, 20/15, and 20/10. Thus, the line-to-line decrease in symbol size varies from 25% (20/20 to 20/150) to 20% (20/120 to 20/100) to 16.7% (20/30 to 20/25).

Would it not be more logical to create a chart of uniform decrements, that is, a chart in which the line-to-line diminution in resolution angle were 0.1 steps? To create such a chart, one must first describe the spaces within a symbol (i.e., spaces between the bars of "E") in terms of "minutes of arc" (MAR) at 20 feet (6 m). Thus, the 20/20 line represents a resolution of 1 MAR. If we take the log to the base of 10 of 1 (minute), we get 0. A spacing of 1.25 MAR (the equivalent of 20/30) yields a log value of 0.2, whereas a spacing of 1.99 MAR (the equivalent of 20/40) yields a log MAR of 0.3. See Table 1.1 for a complete listing of equivalents (courtesy of Prof. Dr. Wallace Chamon).[82,83]

The Bailey-Lovie acuity chart (Fig. 1.13) uses the log MAR sizing system. Log MAR tests add precision to visual acuity testing. Thus, subtle individual variation may be identified under controlled conditions even in a high-contrast environment by counting the number of letters correctly identifiable by the subject.[84]

Visual acuity chart contrast

Clean printed charts using black characters on a white background usually have a character-to-background luminance contrast ratio between 1/20 and 1/33. For projected charts, the contrast ratio drops to a range of 1/5 to 1/10. Such a decrease in contrast is probably the result of the light scattering produced within the projector and the ambient light falling on the screen. Therefore, the test should be performed in a dark room or using retroilluminated charts or carefully calibrated screens.

Contrast sensitivity testing

Visual acuity testing is relatively inexpensive, takes little time to perform, and describes visual function with one notation, e.g., 20/40 (6/12 or 0.5). Best of all, for more than 150 years it has provided an end point for the correction of a patient's refractive error. However, contrast sensitivity testing, a time-consuming test born in the laboratory of the visual physiologist and described by a graph rather than a simple notation, has recently become a popular clinical test. It describes a number of subtle levels of vision, not accounted for by the visual acuity test; thus, it more accurately quantifies the loss of vision in cataracts, corneal edema, neuro-ophthalmic diseases, and certain retinal diseases. These assets have been known for a long time, but the recent enhanced popularity has arisen because

---

*The 20/200 (6/6) letter is 10 times larger than the 20/20 letter, or 3.6 inches (9.14 cm).

of cataract patients. As life span increases, more patients who have cataracts request medical help. Often, their complaints of objects that appear faded or objects that are more difficult to see in bright light are not described accurately by their Snellen acuity scores. Contrast sensitivity tests and glare sensitivity tests can quantitate these complaints. Several validated quality of life assessment questionnaires are also available.[85] They offer the possibility of evaluating vision-related symptoms in a comparable manner, either over a given time frame (pre vs. post operative period) or among different interventions and patients (presbyopic LASIK vs. multifocal IOL). A patient happy with his or her vision but with visual acuity worse than 20/20 has been

described as a "20/happy" patient. With physical evaluation alone it may not be possible to diagnose such "happiness," but subjective tests such as a quality-of-life questionnaire may help identify it. This is critically important when highly irregular astigmatism or highly aberrant human optical systems are to be evaluated, (e.g., intracorneal ring placement for treating keratoconic patients).

Definition and units

Resolution

As one point or object is focused as an Airy disc on the retina, the minimum distance between two points so that different perceivable images are formed is achieved when the center of one disc is aligned with the first minimum ring of the other (Fig. 1.10 & Fig. 1.11). This distance can be converted to an angle—the smallest angle of separation—that represents the limit of resolution or resolving power of an optical system.

Contrast

Whereas a black letter on a white paper is a scene of high contrast, a child crossing the white background road at dusk and a car looming up in a fog are also scenes of low contrast. Thus, contrast may be considered as the difference in the luminance of a target against the background:

$$\text{Contrast} = (\text{Target luminance} - \text{Background luminance})/$$
$$(\text{Target luminance} + \text{Background luminance})$$

To compute contrast, one uses a photometer to measure the luminance of a target against the background. For example, a background of 100 units of light and a target of 50 units of light yields the following:

$$\text{Contrast} = (50 - 100)/(50 + 100) = 50/150 = 33\%$$

Contrast sensitivity

Suppose the contrast of a scene is 33%, or one-third, which also represents the patient's threshold (i.e., the patient cannot identify targets of lower contrast). The patient's contrast sensitivity is the reciprocal of the fraction (i.e., 3). A young, healthy subject may have a contrast threshold

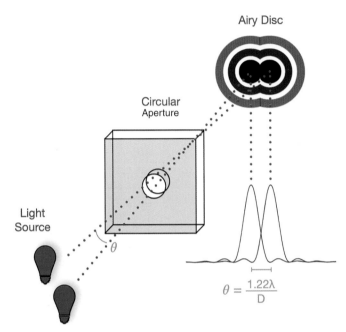

Fig. 1.10 The minimum distance between two points that can be detected by retina photoreceptors.

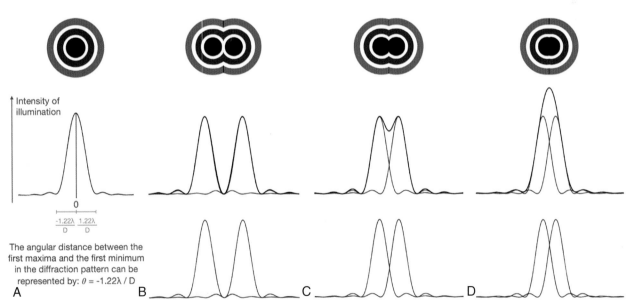

Fig. 1.11 (**A**) An Airy disc diffraction pattern can be represented by alternating peaks (maxima) and valleys (minima) that correspond to the light and dark rings of the disc. (**B**) Two points are seen as Airy discs. (**C**) At the minimum distance where they appear as distinct images. (**C**) When too close to each other, only one image is observed. (Courtesy of André Orlandi, PhD.)

TABLE 1.1   List of equivalent values for visual acuity measurements

	Decimal	Numerator base 20 (20/x)	Angle (Minutes of Arc)	Spacial Frequency	Log Numerator Base 20	LogMAR	Jaeger	American Point Type
HM 60c m	0.001	20,000	1000.00	0.03	4.30	3.00		
F 60c m	0.01	2000	100.00	0.30	3.30	2.00		
	0.03	800	40.00	0.75	2.90	1.60		
	0.05	400	20.00	1.50	2.60	1.30		
	0.06	320	16.00	1.88	2.51	1.20		
	0.08	250	12.50	2.40	2.40	1.10		
	0.10	200	10.00	3.00	2.30	1.00	14	23
	0.13	160	8.00	3.75	2.20	0.90	13	21
	0.16	125	6.25	4.80	2.10	0.80	12	14
	0.18	114	5.70	5.26	2.06	0.76	11	13
	0.20	100	5.00	6.00	2.00	0.70	10	12
	0.25	80	4.00	7.50	1.90	0.60	9	11
	0.30	67	3.33	9.00	1.82	0.52		
	0.32	63	3.15	9.51	1.80	0.50	8	10
	0.33	60	3.00	10.00	1.78	0.48	7	9
	0.40	50	2.50	12.00	1.70	0.40	6	8
	0.50	40	2.00	15.00	1.60	0.30	5	7
	0.60	33	1.67	18.00	1.52	0.22		
	0.63	32	1.59	18.90	1.50	0.20	4	6
	0.67	30	1.50	20.00	1.48	0.18	3	5
	0.70	29	1.43	21.00	1.46	0.15		
	0.80	25	1.25	24.00	1.40	0.10	2	4
	0.90	22	1.11	27.00	1.35	0.05		
	1.00	20	1.00	30.00	1.30	0.00	1	3
	1.10	18	0.91	33.00	1.26	−0.04		
	1.20	17	0.83	36.00	1.22	−0.08		
	1.25	16	0.80	37.50	1.20	−0.10		
	1.33	15	0.75	40.00	1.18	−0.12		
	1.50	13	0.67	45.00	1.12	−0.18		
	1.60	13	0.63	48.00	1.10	−0.20		
	2.00	10	0.50	60.00	1.00	−0.30		

Courtesy of Prof. Dr. Wallace Chamon.

of 1%, or 1/100 (i.e., a contrast sensitivity of 100). Occasionally, subjects have even better contrast thresholds. A subject could have a threshold of 0.003 (0.03%, or 1/1000), which converts into a contrast sensitivity of 3000. In the visual psychology literature, the contrast threshold is described in logarithmic terms. Therefore, a contrast sensitivity of 10 is 1, a contrast sensitivity of 100 is 2, and a contrast sensitivity of 1000 is 3.[86,87]

However, the video engineer describes contrast by using a gray scale that may contain more than 100 different levels of gray. A newspaper printer may use the term *halftones* in place of gray scale and may need more than 100 different half tones (densities of black dots) to describe the contrast of a scene.

Targets

Both the visual scientist and the optical engineer use a series of alternating black and white bars as targets (Fig. 1.14). The optical engineer describes the fineness of a target by the number of line pairs per millimeter (a line pair is a dark bar and the white space next to it): the higher the number of line pairs per millimeter, the finer the target. For example, about 100 line pairs per millimeter is equivalent to a space of 1 minute between two black lines, which is almost equivalent to the spacing of the 20/20 (6/6) letter. In experimental testing, 109 line pairs per millimeter is equivalent to 20/15 (6/4.5).

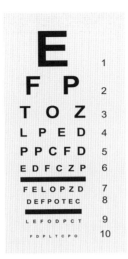

Fig. 1.12 The standard Snellen chart.

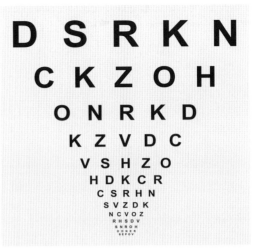

Fig. 1.13 Bailey-Lovie chart is another chart used to evaluate visual acuity.

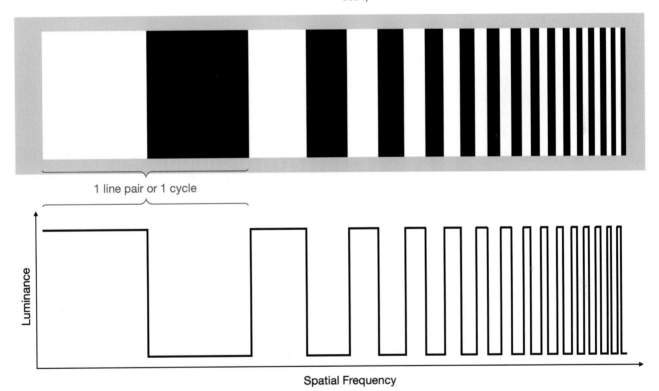

Fig. 1.14 A target example of alternating bar pattern. Spatial frequency can be represented in line pairs per millimeter or cycles per degree. A cycle is a dark bar and a white space.

The vision scientist describes the alternating bar pattern in terms of spatial frequency; the units are cycles per degree (cpd). A cycle is a black bar and a white space. To convert Snellen units into cpd, one must divide the Snellen denominator into 600, or 180 if meters are used, for example, 20/20 (6/6) converts to 30 cpd (600/20, or 180/6), and 20/200 (6/60) converts into 3 cpd (600/200, or 180/60).

Sine waves

So far, targets have been described as dark bars of different spatial frequency against a white background. These are also known as *square waves* or *Foucault gratings*. However, in optics, few images can be described as perfect square waves with perfectly sharp edges.

Diffraction tends to make most edges slightly fuzzy, as do spherical aberration and oblique astigmatism. If the light intensity is plotted across a black bar with fuzzy edges against a light background, a sine wave pattern results (Fig. 1.15). Sine wave patterns have great appeal because they can be considered the essential element from which any pattern can be constructed. The mathematician can break down any alternating pattern (be it an electrocardiogram or a trumpet's sound wave) into a unique sum of sine waves, known as a *Fourier transformation*. Joseph Fourier, a French mathematician, initially developed this waveform language to describe heat waves. Fourier's theorem states that a wave may be written as a sum of sine waves that has various spatial frequencies, amplitudes, and phases.

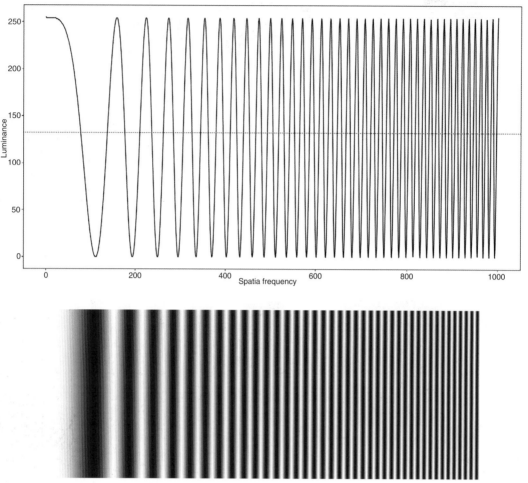

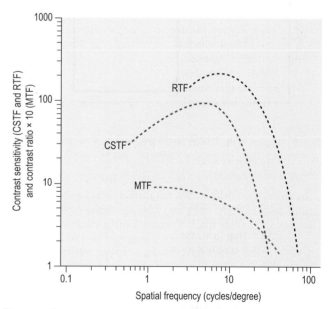

Fig. 1.15 A target example of sine wave pattern.

It also is thought that the visual system of the brain may operate by breaking down observed patterns and scenes into sine waves of different frequencies. The brain then adds them again to produce the mental impression of a complete picture.[88] Fourier transformations may be the method the visual system uses to encode and record retinal images. In fact, it has been shown that different cells or "channels" occur in the retina, lateral geniculate body, and cortex and selectively carry different spatial frequencies. It has also been shown that all channels respond to contrast. Interestingly, the cortex shows a linear relationship between the amplitude of the neuronal discharge and the logarithm of the grating contrast.[89] As a result of the preceding reasoning, most contrast sensitivity tests are based on sine wave patterns rather than square wave patterns of different frequency.

Recording contrast sensitivity

Fig. 1.16 shows a number of functions, including the contrast sensitivity testing function for a normal subject. The shape of the human contrast function is different from that of almost all good optical systems, which have a high contrast sensitivity for low spatial frequency. The contrast sensitivity gradually diminishes at the higher spatial frequencies, as diffraction and other aberrations make discrimination of finer details more difficult. The contrast sensitivity function for the purely optical portion of the visual system (cornea and lens) is the modulation transfer function. The human contrast sensitivity function is

Fig. 1.16 The normal human contrast sensitivity function (CSTF) is the sum of the contrast sensitivity of the purely optical contribution (MTF) and the neuroretinal enhancement system (RTF). (Mainster MA. Contemporary optics and ocular pathology. *Surv Ophthalmol.* 1978;23(2):135–142. https://doi.org/10.1016/0039-6257(78)90092-9.)

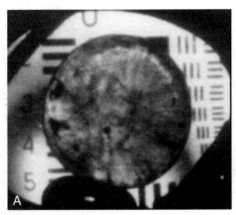
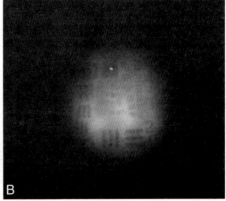

Fig. 1.17 **A.** Effect of a cataract (equivalent to a visual acuity of 20/200) on the image of a three-bar resolution target. **B.** Note how the addition of the inverse conjugate hologram allows you to see the resolution chart. The view is through the center of the cataract. (From David Miller, Joel L. Zuckerman, George O. Reynolds, Phase aberration balancing of cataracts using holography, *Experimental Eye Research*, 15 (2), 1973, 157–160. https://doi.org/10.1016/0014-4835(73)90114-0.)

different from the sum of its components because the retina-brain processing system is programmed to enhance the spatial frequencies in the range 2 to 6 Hz. Receptor fields, on/off systems, and lateral inhibition are the well-known physiologic mechanisms that influence the different spatial frequency channels and are responsible for such enhancement.

In Fig. 1.16, the wave labeled "retinal testing function" represents the retinal neural system performance.[89–91] Normal variations are found in the contrast sensitivity function. For example, contrast sensitivity decreases with age. Two factors appear to be responsible. First, the normal crystalline lens scatters more light with increasing age, which thus blurs the edges of targets and degrades the contrast. Second, the retina-brain processing system itself loses some ability to enhance contrast with increasing age. Illumination also plays an important role in contrast sensitivity. As retinal luminance drops, contrast sensitivity also decreases.

The contrast sensitivity function is also an accurate method by which to follow certain disease states. For example, the contrast sensitivity of a patient who has a cataract is diminished, as it is in another light-scattering lesion, corneal edema. Because the contrast sensitivity function depends on central nervous system processing, it is not surprising that conditions such as optic neuritis and pituitary tumors also characteristically have diminished contrast sensitivity functions.

Glare, tissue light scattering, and contrast sensitivity

When a transparent structure loses its clarity, the physicist describes it as a light *scatterer* rather than a light *transmitter*. This concept is foreign to the clinician, whose textbooks talk about opaque lenses and corneas. The word *opaqueness* conjures up the image of a cement wall that stops light. Of all the experiments demonstrating that most cataracts scatter light rather than stop light, the most graphic involves the science of holography. If it is true that a cataract splashes or scatters oncoming light, resulting in a poor image focused on the retina, it should theoretically be possible to collect all the scattered light with a special optical element and recreate a sharp image. The essence of such an optical element, one that would take the scattered light of the cataract and rescatter it so that a proper image could be formed, would be a special inverse hologram of the cataract itself. Fig. 1.17 shows how such a filter would work. Miller et al.[92] were able to demonstrate how an extracted

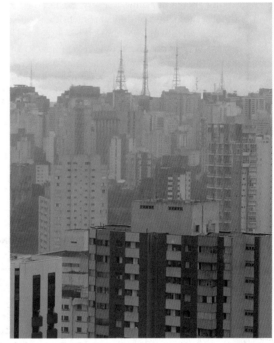

Fig. 1.18 A scene in a fog where the closer objects are sharp (good acuity through less cloudy media) and the more distant objects have poor contrast and resolution, as seen through a very cloudy media (i.e., cataract).)

cataract (the patient's visual acuity was worse than 20/200) would be made relatively transparent by registering a special inverse hologram of that specific cataract in front of the cataract.

To follow the progress of conditions such as cataracts or corneal edema, a measure of tissue transparency or tissue backscattering is useful. Although photoelectric devices can be used to quantitate the amount of light scattered by various ocular tissues, a subjective discrimination system is needed to evaluate patient complaints. The Snellen visual acuity test was the traditional index, but it is not sensitive enough. Fig. 1.18 shows a scene in a fog taken with a digital camera, where the closer objects are sharp (good acuity through less cloudy media)

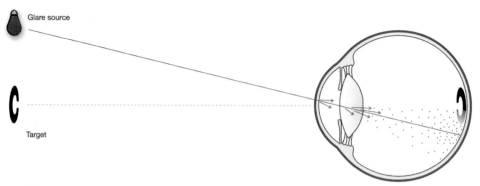

Fig. 1.19 Corneal edema scatters the light from the peripheral light source onto the fovea, decreasing the contrast of the foveal image.

and the more distant objects have poor contrast and resolution, as seen through a very cloudy media (i.e., cataract).

LeClaire et al.[93] observed that many patients with cataracts showed good visual acuity but had poor contrast sensitivity in the face of a glare source. In fact, this should not come as a surprise because the essence of vision is the discrimination of the light intensity of one object as opposed to another, often with a natural glare source present. Thus, a plane is seen against the sky because the retinal image of the plane does not stimulate the photoreceptors to the same degree that the sky does. Terms such as *contrast luminance* and *intensity discrimination* are used to describe differences in brightness between an object and its background.

How then can ocular light scattering, glare, and contrast sensitivity be linked together to give the clinician a useful index? An industrialist scientist named Holliday set the stage to solve this puzzle.[94] In 1926 Holliday developed the concept of glare and glare testing to measure the degrading effect of stray light. In the 1960s Wolfe, a visual physiologist working in Boston, realized that glare testing could be a useful way to describe the increase in light scattering seen in different clinical conditions.[95,96] How does increased light scattering produce a decrease in the contrast of the retinal image in the presence of a glare source? Fig. 1.19 shows how corneal edema splashes light from a naked light bulb onto the foveal image, reducing the contrast of the image of the target. In the mid-1970s Nadler observed that many of his cataract patients complained of annoying glare. His observations rekindled interest in glare testing and led to the first clinical glare tester—the Miller-Nadler glare tester.[92]

Clinical conditions affecting glare and contrast sensitivity
Optical conditions
This section describes how contact lenses, cataracts, opacified posterior capsules, displaced IOLs, and multifocal IOLs affect glare sensitivity and contrast. With the exception of IOLs, these conditions primarily diminish contrast sensitivity because of increased light scattering.

Corneal conditions
Corneal edema. Studies tracing the progression of corneal decompensation have shown that the stroma increases in thickness before the epithelium changes.[97] The stroma may increase in thickness by up to 30% before the epithelium becomes edematous. Studies have shown that an increase in stromal thickness above 30% need not influence Snellen visual acuity results if there is no epithelial edema.[98] Unlike Snellen visual acuity, both contrast sensitivity and glare sensitivity are compromised as soon as the stroma thickens. Mild edema affects only the middle and high frequencies of a contrast sensitivity test, sparing the low frequencies. With further edema, the sparing of the low frequencies disappears and contrast sensitivity is decreased throughout the spatial frequency spectrum.[92] Glare sensitivity measurements also detect early epithelial edema. A mildly edematous epithelium is roughly equivalent to an increase of 10% in stromal thickness, whereas moderate to significant epithelial edema has a profound effect on glare and contrast sensitivity.

Fuchs' endothelial corneal dystrophy. Is corneal guttae enough to impair the quality of vision? Studies have demonstrated increased light scattering and loss of contrast sensitivity in Fuchs' endothelial corneal dystrophy patients correlated with the severity of corneal guttae.[99–102] However, it may be difficult to distinguish whether this is a sole consequence of the presence of gutatta or other alterations such as mild corneal edema or corneal ultrastructural changes.

Contact lens wear. The wearing of contact lenses may reduce contrast sensitivity in a number of subtle ways. Patients with significant corneal astigmatism who wear thin, soft contact lenses experience blur that affects their contrast sensitivity. Aging of the plastic material itself or surface-deposit accumulations can affect soft lens hydration and ultimately influence acuity, glare, and contrast sensitivity. Most important, contact lens-induced epithelial edema produces increased glare disability and reduced contrast sensitivity.[92,103]

Keratoconus. Patients with keratoconus demonstrate attenuation of contrast sensitivity with relative sparing of low spatial frequencies despite normal Snellen visual acuity. However, once scarring develops in the keratoconic cornea, all frequencies become attenuated.[92] In addition, glare sensitivity may increase even without scarring.[104] Thus, contrast sensitivity testing at a number of spatial frequencies, with or without a glare source, may be an excellent way of following the progression of keratoconus.[105]

Penetrating keratoplasty. Contrast sensitivity or glare testing may also be useful in detecting the earliest signs of graft rejection. In such cases, the earliest corneal damage is corneal edema. Although visual acuity may remain normal, contrast and glare performance start to slip. As the edema progresses to involve the epithelium, the degradation of these visual functions is accentuated. Similarly, reversal of graft rejection may be followed by an improvement in the contrast sensitivity function.[92]

Refractive surgery. Some patients who have undergone radial keratotomy or photorefractive keratoplasty with postoperative corneal haze have been reported to experience increased glare sensitivity.[106,107] The extent of the problem and the number of patients complaining of heightened glare sensitivity varies from study to study and depends on the time elapsed since the surgery and the method by which the glare was assessed. Modern refractive surgery approaches the haze problem by attenuating the healing process either by the use of LASIK or mitomicyn-C and photorefractive keratectomy (PRK). Both techniques are effective and have their own indications. Glare owing to haze is nowadays less frequent than glare owing to postoperative spherical aberration.

Cataracts and opacified posterior capsules. Fig. 1.19 demonstrates the way that an edematous cornea or cataract scatters stray light onto the fovea and degrades contrast sensitivity, thereby heightening glare disability. Thus, measurements of contrast sensitivity are usually better correlated with patient complaints than with a visual acuity measurement. The addition of a glare source to a contrast sensitivity test causes a dramatic decrease in the contrast function. Of the various cataract types, posterior subcapsular cataract degrades the glare and contrast function the most. It should be noted that the presence of a glare light diminishes both visual acuity and contrast sensitivity in cataract patients. In the presence of a glare light, the contrast sensitivity function gradually diminishes as a simulated cataract increases in severity, whereas the visual acuity function holds steady until an 80% simulated cataract produces a dramatic drop in visual acuity.

Progressive opacification of the posterior capsule after cataract extraction produces a progressive increase in glare disability (Fig. 1.20).[108] A neodymium:yttrium-aluminum-garnet (Nd:YAG) laser capsulotomy in such cases improves visual function. The improvement of contrast and glare sensitivity after Nd:YAG laser treatment depends on the ratio of the area of the clear opening to the area of the remaining opaque capsule. Thus, a photopic pupil of 4 mm would require a 4-mm capsulotomy for best results in daylight. However, if the pupil dilates to 6 mm at night, an oncoming headlight would induce an annoying glare unless the capsulotomy were enlarged to 6 mm in diameter. Thus, the smallest capsulotomy is not necessarily the best from an optical point of view.

Modulation transfer function

Optical engineers generally evaluate optical systems by means of a system similar to contrast sensitivity called the *modulation transfer function* (MTF). The MTF is the ratio of image-to-object contrast as a function of spatial frequency, where the object is either a bar graph or a sinusoidal grating (Fig. 1.14 & 1.15). It gives more information than the parameter of resolving power. For example, two systems may have the same resolving power, but one might be unable to form useful images of low-contrast objects, which the other could readily form. A smaller pupillary aperture introduces diffraction interference, which makes it difficult to resolve fine detail (higher spatial frequencies). Thus, the spatial frequency cutoff occurs sooner with the small aperture system. In an MTF plot, the vertical axis is akin to contrast sensitivity (see Fig. 1.12). Because it represents the ratio of contrast of image against contrast of object, its values decrease from 1.0 to 0. The MTF is conceptually similar to the manner in which electronic engineers evaluate an amplifier. The performance of an amplifier is described by the output/input ratio, or the gain, for different sound frequencies. The MTF concept also may be useful in the comparison of the performance of the eye with that of optical and electronic instruments.

Campbell and Green[109] plotted the MTF of the human eye for various pupillary diameters and found that a smaller pupil system has a better contrast ratio than a larger pupil system. This probably reflects the opposing factors of a somewhat better performance with greater illumination and the degrading effect of spherical aberration with a larger pupil. As noted earlier, a pupil size in the range 2.0 to 2.8 mm gives the maximum MTF for high spatial frequencies.

Depth of focus

How can an insect or a small animal like a rat see objects clearly from 10 m to 10 cm without an accommodating mechanism? How does a pinhole allow a patient with presbyopia to read the newspaper without

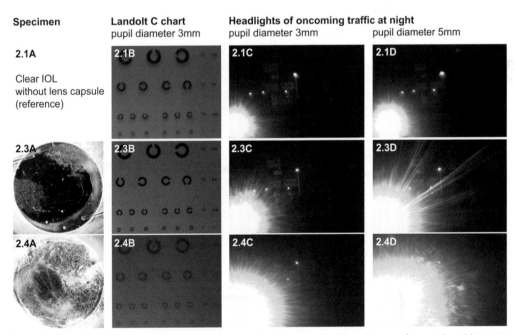

Fig. 1.20 Posterior capsule opacification specimens of varying severity (**A**) and images from real-world scenes captured through specimens: a Landolt C chart (3.0-mm aperture) (**B**) and a traffic scene at night with headlight simulation of oncoming traffic captured using 3.0-mm (**C**) and 5.0-mm (**D**) apertures. (Modified from van Bree MCJ, Kruijt B, van den Berg TJTP. Real-world scenes captured through posterior capsule opacification specimens: simulation of visual function deterioration experienced by PCO patients. *J Cataract Refract Surg.* 2013;39(1):144–147. https://doi.org/10.1016/j.jcrs.2012.10.024.)

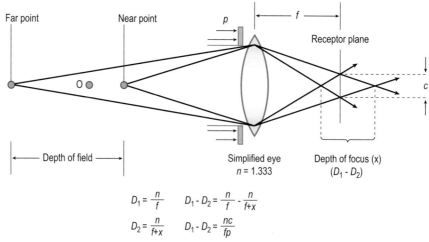

$$D_1 = \frac{n}{f} \qquad D_1 - D_2 = \frac{n}{f} - \frac{n}{f+x}$$

$$D_2 = \frac{n}{f+x} \qquad D_1 - D_2 = \frac{nc}{fp}$$

Fig. 1.21 A schematic representation of a single refracting surface model eye where ρ = pupillary diameter, f = focal length distance from the retina where image of near object falls, c = limiting photoreceptor cluster size (i.e., similar to grain or pixel size), n = refractive index, D1 = n/f dioptric power of eye when viewing infinite object, D2 = n/(f + x) (i.e., dioptric power of an eye when viewing near object). Thus, depth of focus = D1 − D2 = n/f − n/(f + x). Ultimately, we find D1 − D2 = nc/fρ.

a reading correction? The answer is that both situations rely on an optical system with an increased depth of focus.

Recall that an image can be thought of as being made up of an array of points. Thus, the finite size of the pixels or the photoreceptor clusters ultimately determine the fineness of details of the recorded image. This means that a blur of a focused point is tolerated if it is no bigger than the size of the receptor. Because a point of light is focused as an Airy disc, a cluster of two to five cones is considered the "limiting sensor size." Let us review two important definitions:

Depth of focus: *the amount of blur in diopters or millimeters from the retina that will be tolerated or go unnoticed.*

Depth of field: *the distance range, in object space, that an object can move toward or away from a fixed focus optical system and still be considered in focus.*

Fig. 1.21 is a schematic of the eye. For simplicity, we used a reduced eye with a biconvex lens representing the cornea and lens. Let:

- () = the object that can move from infinity to a near point N
- ρ = pupillary diameter
- *f* = focal length of the model eye
- *x* = distance from the retina that near point remains in focus
- c = limiting photoreceptor cluster size (i.e., limiting grain size or pixel size)
- N = refractive index of the model eye
- D_1 = n/f (i.e., dioptric power of eye when viewing a finite object)
- D_2 = n/f (i.e., dioptric power of eye when near object at N)

(In this case, the eye can be considered to have lengthened [theoretically] by a distance *x*.) Depth of focus is as follows:

$$D_1 - D_2 = n/f - n/f + x = nx(f + x) - nf/(f + x) = nx/f(f + x)$$

(but by similar triangles). Thus,

$$D_1 - D_2 = nc/fp$$

This equation tells us that the depth of focus in diopters ($D_1 - D_2$) is proportional to the index of refraction (*n*) and the limiting photoreceptor of grain size *c*. The depth of focus is also inversely proportional to the pupil size (ρ) or the focal length of the system (f).

For example, determine the depth of focus for a reduced human eye under the following conditions. Let:

- Pupil (ρ) = 3 mm, or 0.003 m
- Focal length (f) = 22.2 mm, or 0.0222 m
  Limiting cone cluster (c) = 5 cones. (Assume each cone is 1.5 μm in diameter, and spacing between cones is 0.5 μm. The total cluster of 5 cones + 4 spaces = 9.5 μm, or 0.0000095 m.)
- Index of refraction (n) = 1.333

$$\text{Depth of focus } (D_1 - D_2) = 1.33 \times 0.00000/0.0222 \times 0.003$$
$$= 0.189$$

Our calculation of 0.189 for the reduced (hypothetical) eye with a pupil of 3 mm is about half of the 0.40 D (Fig. 1.22A), which is the average value from four (real) human studies.[109–112] Thus, we may conclude that the normal eye has a modest depth of focus.

Interestingly, Fig. 1.22B represents a study in which artificial pupils (placed in front of the cornea) between 1 and 2 mm were used. Within this range of apertures, a depth of focus between 2 and 4 D was obtained.[52]

Do we ever see the equivalent of pupillary apertures of between 1 and 2 mm in human patients? Yes, we do in cases of trauma, disease, or use of strong miotics. Fig. 1.23 demonstrates two examples from pathologic conditions. Fig. 1.23A shows a 1- to 2-mm clear area within a corneal opacity. In Fig. 1.23B, we can see the equivalent of a reduced pupillary aperture produced by a ptosis or a conscious reduction of the palpebral fissure as a result of squinting. This could also be achieved by surgery, with the implant of corneal inlays (Box 1.1) or intraocular pinhole devices. It is comforting to know that in cases of trauma, disease, or significant refractive error, the human eye can call on a 2- to 3D depth of focus mechanism.

Optical aberrations

The famous nineteenth century German physiologist Herman von Helmholtz, in Volume 1 of his *Treatise on Physiologic Optics*,[113] wrote that the optical aberrations of the human eye are "of a kind that is not permissible in well-constructed instruments." The implication is that the optical design of the human eye would receive low marks if evaluated by someone from the optical industry. If we are to simply compare the optical quality of the living human eye with that of our best cameras and telescopes under ordinary static daylight conditions, then

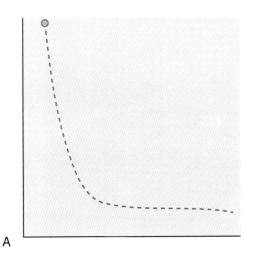

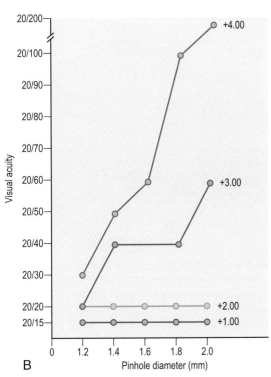

Fig. 1.22 (A) An averaged depth of focus versus pupil size function representing four different studies.[44,91,138,156] **(B)** Plot of visual acuity versus pinhole diameters (between 1 and 2 mm) using different blurring lenses (i.e., +1 diopter [D], +2 D, +3 D, and +4 D). Thus, for example, the subject could achieve a visual acuity of 20/40 through a 1.8-mm pinhole, but vision would be blurred by a 3-D lens. (Modified from Miller D. *Optics and Refraction: A User Friendly Guide*. St. Louis: Gower Medical; 1991.)

Helmholtz was correct. The optical imperfections noted by Helmholtz are discussed in the following sections.

Light scattering. Fingerprints on spectacle lenses scatter light, making small letters difficult to read. Raindrops or windshield wiper smears on the car windshield make the reading of street signs difficult. In a similar way, small bubbles from the warm water tap give a haze to a glass of water and make it difficult to see the details at the bottom of the glass. These are all examples of light scattering, which can obscure the details of any object.

As noted earlier, the cornea is clear, but technically speaking, it is not perfectly transparent. Its composition of fine collagen fibers, loaded into a watery matrix of glycosaminoglycans and populated by fine cells that

swim in the matrix, scatter a small percentage (10% of incident light) and create a slight haze. This is unquestionably a flaw, as opposed to the glass optical systems of cameras and telescopes. However, the "imperfect" corneal structure allows for healing. Thus, we can appreciate that a 10% level of light scatter is a fair price to pay for a self-healing system.

The lens of the eye is made up of tens of thousands of fine fibers (each a bag of clear protein solution) packed closely together. The living lens continually adds outside fibers and packs old cells in its nucleus throughout life, ultimately increasing its volume by a factor of three in the older eye. The refractive index of the fibers differs from that of the thin spaces between the fibers.

Thus, the young lens scatters about 20% of the incident light. Is there a practical advantage to the fiber structure of the lens? There are many ways that the lens may be injured, including inflammation from diseases inside the eye, blunt blows from fists or rocks, periods of malnutrition, poisoning, and osmotic upset from systemic disease. In all of these situations, the part of the lens being laid down at the time of the injury or disease loses transparency. This hazy section may also be lumpy in thickness. However, in a short time, new transparent layers cover and compress the hazy ones, smoothing and reducing the blurring effect of the injury. Again, we now understand that a small level of light scattering resulting from this fiber layering system is a fair price to pay for a self-repairing lens system.

Natural defenses against light scattering. The reader may have been led astray in thinking that the eye has no defense against normal light scattering. In fact, it does. For example, the birefringent capacity of the collagen fibers in the cornea, in combination with the birefringence of the fovea, may cancel out some annoying glare caused by light scattering through a process known as *destructive interference*, somewhat akin to the way polarizing sunglasses cancel annoying glare.

The retina has three defenses against the image-degrading effects of scattered light. To appreciate one of the defenses, one first must recognize that not all colors (wavelengths) are scattered equally. The fine components of eye tissue scatter blue light 16 times more than red light. This light produces lipofuscin-induced cell toxicity in in vitro experiments. It has also been proposed as a pathologic mechanism for cataract formation and retinal damage.[114] Yellow filter spectacles reduce chromatic aberration and sharpen the retinal image by reducing the number of wavelengths striking the retina.[115] However, a yellow filter makes the sky look gray rather than blue. This effect, although unnatural, enhances the contrast of objects seen against the sky.

Therefore, a defense that can reduce blue scattered light would be disproportionately helpful. Sprinkled throughout the ultrasensitive fovea and its immediate surround is yellow pigment. The yellow pigment is efficient at absorbing the scattered blue light, thus preventing much of it from degrading the retinal image.[52] Although light toxicity to the retina has been demonstrated in preclinical research, studies have not shown benefits of a blue light-filtering intraocular lens.[116] Long-term follow-up comparison of these lenses over "normal" IOLs have not demonstrated success in preventing retinal diseases such as macular degeneration.[117,118]

The second defense used by the retina involves the positioning of the rods and cones. Each rod or cone functions as a light guide. To enter the guide, light must enter at a specific angle.

Interestingly, normally focused light enters a photoreceptor at a different angle than does scattered light.[119] The photoreceptors of the retina are directed so that they primarily receive focused light, but not scattered light (Fig. 1.24). Stiles and Crawford established the fact that the human visual system has reduced sensitivity to light rays that enter near the edge of the pupil compared to those entering centrally. This effect, referred to as the psychophysical Stiles-Crawford effect, is the

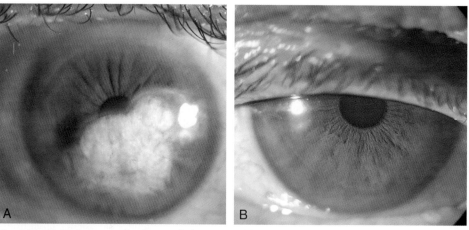

Fig. 1.23 (**A**) Clinical example of a small clear area within corneal opacity that operates as a pinhole. (**B**) The equivalent of a reduced aperture produced by a ptosis.

BOX 1.1   Corneal inlay and depth of focus

The picture represents the cornea of a 51-year-old female patient who had an Acufocus Presbyopic inlay implanted 45 days earlier. Unaided near visual acuity changed from J9 to J2 after surgery. Distance vision changed from 20/20 to 20/25.

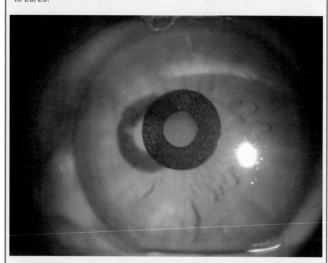

(Courtesy of the Refractive Surgery Section – Department of Ophthalmology – Paulista School of Medicine, Sao Paulo, Brazil.)

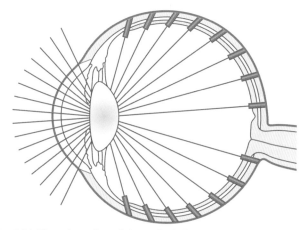

Fig. 1.24 The orientation of the retinal photoreceptors in the normal human eye. Note that they are directed to the second nodal point of the eye.

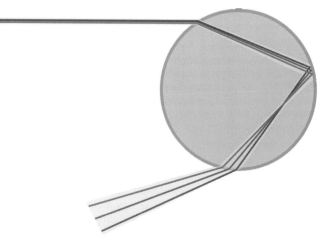

Fig. 1.25 The water droplet acts as a strong lens that refracts each wavelength differently. The resulting spread of different colors forms the rainbow.

---

result of the orientation of photoreceptors, which preferentially guide the central rays to the retina more efficiently than the peripheral rays.[120]

The dark brown pigment of the retinal pigment epithelium and the choroid absorbs any stray light that has passed through the retina and prevents such light from backscatter, which would reverberate among the neighboring photoreceptors. None of these defenses is perfect, but all work to reduce the annoyance of scattered light.

The brow and eyelid may also be thought of as blocking annoying glare sources such as the overhead sun. Interestingly, the Asian lid has a double fold and serves as a more effective thicker visor than the Caucasian lid, thereby more effectively blocking the glaring effect of the sun overhead.

Chromatic aberrations

A rainbow is produced by millions of tiny round droplets of water vapor that hover over the earth during or after rain. Each water droplet

functions as a tiny, powerful round lens. Such a powerful lens bends each wavelength of color differently. A rainbow is caused by the chromatic aberration of the water droplets (Fig. 1.25). Thus, like Newton's prism, the tiny droplets break up white light into the colors of the rainbow. The phenomenon of strong lenses producing colored fringes around a focused image is known as *chromatic aberration.*[121,122]

The optical components of the eye (cornea and lens), like the fine water droplets, also produce chromatic aberration. The total chromatic aberration of the photopic human eye is about 3 D. However, we do not see colored fringes around objects because significant colored fringes of red and blue are less likely to be seen as a result of the cones' relative insensitivity to the colors at the ends of the spectrum. Also, the visual processing in the retina and brain can sharpen the edges of the retinal image and "erase" the colored blur. Although we rarely consciously sense the chromatic aberration of the eye, some researchers believe that the retina may make use of the faint, colored fringes around images to help accommodation reach a precise end point.[56,123]

Spherical aberration

A major distortion produced by many high-powered optical systems such as the cornea or lens is called *spherical aberration*. Fig. 1.26 shows the results of this aberration. The rays at the edge of the lens are bent more than those going through the center of the lens, creating a smeared focus. The cornea (a strong optical element) is subject to spherical aberration. Fig. 1.26 shows that the cornea sits at the front of the eye like a small, strongly curved dome. The steeper the dome (the shorter its radius of curvature), the more spherical aberration created. We have known since the time of the French mathematician Descartes that spherical aberration can be controlled by flattening the curvature of the edge of a lens, thereby weakening the focusing power of the lens periphery. Descartes described such a surface as *aspheric*. Most cameras today use lenses with aspheric surfaces (Box 1.2).

The average cornea is also somewhat aspheric. It becomes slightly flatter at its periphery, allowing it to merge with the sclera more smoothly. However, there are some real-world considerations that make it advantageous to keep the cornea steeply curved. In the event of a direct blow to the eye by a blunt object, presumably the steep protruding cornea can absorb the blow, much like a spring. The steeper the cornea, the more it vaults over the rest of the eye and the greater the spring effect. Such a spring-dampening effect protects the deeper eye structures. How then does the eye satisfy both needs? In daylight, with the pupil being constricted, the iris tissue essentially blocks many of the light rays coming through the corneal periphery and effectively cancels most of the spherical aberration. Thus, spherical aberration from the cornea has an important degrading effect only when illumination is dim and the pupil is large. Night myopia can develop in these situations and is more of a problem when the corneal asphericity is greater. Such greater asphericity is often found after corneal refractive surgery.

Happily, in dim light, the human eye switches to the rod retinal system in which seeing fine details takes a lower priority than simply seeing large shapes.

The crystalline lens is also a powerful optical element and therefore is also vulnerable to spherical aberration. Although an aspheric surface corrects the aberration in cameras and telescopes, nature has chosen a different approach for the crystalline lens. Recall that refraction, or the bending of light, can be controlled by either the curvature of the lens surface or the index of refraction of the composition of the lens. The high index of refraction of the crystalline lens is the result of a high concentration of protein. The lens has a lower refractive index near its edge than at its center. Therefore, the lens periphery has a weaker focusing action and self-corrects spherical aberration, much as an aspheric surface.[49]

However, even with the aforementioned correction factors, the total spherical aberration of the human eye varies from 0.25 to 2.00 D. The corneal shape is the most important factor in the induction of spherical aberration.[124]

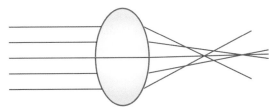

Fig. 1.26 An illustration of the smearing of sharp focus created by spherical aberration. Note that the peripheral rays are bent more than the paraxial rays of light.

BOX 1.2 Practical example of spherical aberration and its relationship with lens asphericity

A practical example is the comparison between the optical properties of the +20 diopter (D) trial frame lens and the aspheric indirect binocular ophthalmoscope (IBO) +20 D lens. Both lenses focus light coming from infinity to a focal point of 5 cm behind the lens.

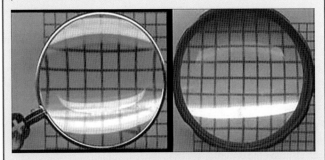

However, when analyzing the quality of the entire image, one can observe a deformity in the periphery of the image formed by the trial frame lens, which is not present with the aspheric lens. The higher the power of a lens, the more the distortion produced by spherical aberration. The figure on the right demonstrates the spherical aberration (i.e., peripheral distortion) produced by a typical + 20 D spectacle lens. The figure on the left demonstrates the reduced spherical aberration produced by an aspheric +20 D indirect ophthalmoscopy lens. [Right / left disparity!]

Abolition of spherical aberration not only sharpens focus but can be thought of as concentrating the light at the focus. Concentrating light energy at a focus makes it easier to see a dimly lit object. Therefore, cameras, or creatures with an optical system of minimal spherical aberration, function well in low illumination.

Some IOLs are aspheric. However, the degree of IOL asphericity must compensate for the patient's individual corneal asphericity to yield the sharpest retinal image of a distant object. On the other hand, the presence of some spherical aberration may blur a distant object but allow an object at an intermediate distance (1–2 meters) to be in focus. As yet, there is no IOL that produces completely sharp images for both distant and intermediate objects.

Light absorption

The lens of a typical 20-year-old absorbs about 30% of incident blue light. At age 60, the typical lens absorbs about 60% of incident blue light.[125] This increase in lens absorption of blue light results in both a decrease in subtle color discrimination and a decrease in chromatic aberration.

Summary—a compromise of eye function

The human eye (which is similar to the monkey eye) is a fairly good resolving optical instrument.[126-128] Admittedly, the eyes of certain birds are even better optical instruments, reaching the outer limits of the constraints of the laws of physics. One must appreciate that the evolution of better and better optics had to be balanced against other useful functions, such as glare prevention, injury prevention, injury repair, and use of the eyes for nonverbal communication.

THE AGING EYE

It is important to recognize that a high percentage of people live their entire lives with good vision—thanks to a number of positive compensations that help the aging eye. For example, the human macula is particularly vulnerable to damage from ultraviolet and blue light. Fortunately, a yellow pigment effectively absorbs or scatters away most of these harmful wavelengths, thus diminishing the potential damage to the macula.[129]

One of the more remarkable aspects of the aging eye is that the eye lens continually acquires new layers of fibers, becoming both progressively thicker and steeper. These changes would normally lead to an increase in lens focusing power and a tendency toward nearsightedness in older eyes. In fact, this does not happen universally because the index of refraction of the cortex of the lens decreases in a perfectly compensatory fashion,[130] so the lens power often stays constant.

Evolution of ocular components

Human eyes are fascinating examples of a potpourri of components seen all along the evolutionary trail. Indeed, human eyes contain components previously developed for other uses. For example, our retinal rhodopsin may have come from an ancient bacterium, which may have used the rhodopsin for photosynthesis. Also, many of the special crystallin proteins that have been identified in animal eye lenses are similar to metabolic enzymes found elsewhere in the body. Nonlenticular enzymes have been adapted to also function as special lens proteins, a process known as *gene sharing*. The term *gene sharing* simply names the phenomenon without giving us an idea of which function came first or what evolutionary pressures forced the new use of the molecules. For example, lactic dehydrogenase-β is similar to ε-crystallin found in the the lenses of birds and reptiles and arginosuccinate lyase is similar to δ-crystallin found in the bird lens.[131] α-Crystallin, a major lens protein (up to 40% of lens proteins), is found in all vertebrate lenses and is a member of the small heat shock protein family. αB-crystallin is overexpressed in various neurodegenerative diseases. It is also elevated in the ischemic heart and in other biologic systems where stress is introduced.[132] In summary, one might think of this entire process of nature as reaching into its dusty attic to find new uses for old creations as the ultimate in recycling efficiency.

Nonoptical brain mechanisms that enhance the retinal image

There is a group of visual phenomena in which the retinal image is enhanced or made complete by the brain.[133] They represent ways of improving the retinal image in nonoptical ways. One might think of these brain-processing effects as examples of methods of going beyond the limits of the laws of optics to bring out visual information (Box 1.3).[134]

Contrast enhancement

The visual brain has the ability to sharpen the contrast of elements in the retinal image. Fig. 1.27 presents two faces with the same degree of grayness. In the right figure, the face is seen against a black background, whereas in the left figure, it is seen against a white background. The gray face on the black background looks lighter (enhancing its contrast), whereas the gray face looks darker on the white background. This effect is reduced when the edges of the faces are fuzzy. One might speculate that a sharper edge on an object brings out a stronger contrast enhancement response.

Computer graphics professionals (the Joint Photographic Experts Group) have taken advantage of the knowledge of the physiology of human vision and released an image data compression format named after the group, i.e., JPEG. The JPEG compression process first separates the image into luminance and color signals. This step does not reduce the inherent quality of the image. The JPEG process then performs a variety of arithmetic procedures that separate out and remove small differences (in luminance and color) between adjacent pixels that would not be noticed by the human visual system. This process involves dividing the picture up into 8×8-pixel blocks and analyzing details contained in each block. The high-frequency (fine detail) information is then discarded. Such a process eliminates a great deal of data. The final process results in a very high compression ratio (i.e., often a 95% reduction in file size). As expected, such a trade-off results in a loss of high-frequency information (i.e., sharp transitions become blurred). Fortunately, our visual system accepts the slightly reduced image contrast.[135]

Edge sharpening

If an ametrope looks in the distance at a framed picture, the details within the picture will be fuzzy, yet the edges of the frame will be seen as a distinct boundary against the wall. The visual system places a priority on sharpening the edge of the retinal image, even though the details within remain hazy. One might suppose that in the case of the picture on the wall, recognizing the edges of the frame tells one that the fuzzy blob on the wall is a picture rather than a swarm of insects.

There is a second way that the brain processes the edge of a retinal image. If two objects of similar brightness are placed next to each other, they normally appear to merge into one object. However, if the connecting edge of one of these similar objects is slightly darker than the connecting edge of the other, the entire side with the darker edge appears darker than the lighter one. The greater contrast at the edge has spread across the whole panel.

This phenomenon, known as the Craik-Cornsweet O'Brien illusion, is seen in Fig. 1.28. If a pencil is placed between the two vertical rectangles (occluding the boundary), it becomes clear that they are actually the same brightness.

Vernier acuity

Earlier in this chapter, it was noted that a normal-sighted human being (with 20/20 visual acuity) can detect a separation between two objects as small as 1 minute of angular subtense. Interestingly, it was said that Ted Williams, the great outfielder of the Boston Red Sox, had a visual acuity of 20/10 (could detect a half minute of angular separation). However, there is a visual task (Vernier acuity), which has a threshold of about 5 seconds of arc (1/12th of a minute of arc). Indeed, as seen in Fig. 1.29, most normal-sighted people can line up dots or notice a discrepancy in the alignment of dots or lines as small as 5 seconds of arc or less. We know that the brain is involved in the processing because the experiment can be redesigned so that one eye is presented with the top and bottom dots (which are in alignment), while the other eye is allowed to see only the middle dot. Subjects show similar thresholds whether the experiment is done this way

BOX 1.3 Practical example of a nonoptical (brain) retinal image enhancement mechanism

Fig. A is an example of the "completing the picture" illusion. Because of our previous visual experience, we assume that the partially covered words represent "THE EYE." Wrong!

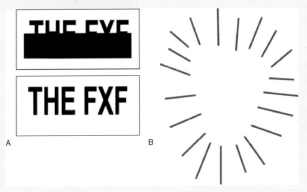

(A) Because of our previous visual experience, we assume the line covered words will spell "THE EYE."

On removal of the cover, we see we were wrong. If there is a discontinuity in an object, we almost always assume that the object is partially covered. We simply create a full impression of the covered object in our mind.

Suppose that the object of regard is not covered but that the observer has a brain lesion that has produced a small scotoma in the visual field. When such a patient is presented with a circle or square in which part of the figure resides inside the scotoma, after a brief period, the patient reports that the gap has filled in and the figure looks whole. The same phenomenon takes place if part of an image falls on the physiologic blind spot. It suggests that the visual system, faced with a gap in the information, hypothesizes (gambles) that the region surrounding the scotoma has the needed data and places that data within the scotoma to produce a complete scene.[162]

There is another series of illusions known as *gap figures*.[163] Fig. B shows an example of a gap illusion. The defect (gap) is strongly highlighted by the radiating lines as a footprint might appear highlighted to a skilled guide.

(B) A gap figure (modified from an Ehrenstein illusion). Note that the radiating lines seem to create the outline of a foot. A related phenomenon is presented in Conan Doyle's story *The Adventure of Silver Blaze*, in which Sherlock Holmes identifies the murderer when he concludes that the watchdog must have known the murderer because no barking was heard on the night of the murder. As in the gap figure, the gap in the expected pattern of the dog's behavior takes on a heightened importance. Hearst appropriately called this phenomenon "getting something for nothing."[164]

Vision suppression is present in pediatric patients with strabismus in order to avoid diplopia. Vitreous floaters (mostly seen in bright environments) are another example of the nervous system suppressing annoying visual effects. The floaters are structures which have a different index of refraction than the surrounding vitreous and so can cast a shadow onto the retina.

Floaters can be called a time domain phenomenon. They are often seen in postoperative refractive surgery patients, and usually disappear in 3 to 6 months.

Finally, mention should be made of a related temporal blocking of a visual scene, that is, our failure to notice the fleeting disappearance of an image during a blink, a twitch, a flicker, or a saccade.

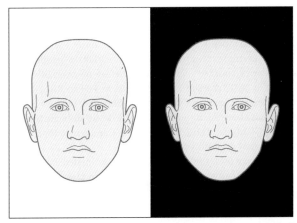

Fig. 1.27 *Right*: Gray face is seen against a black background. *Left*: Same gray face is seen against a white background. A contrast enhancement function makes the gray face look lighter on the black and darker on the white side. (Illusion created by R. Miller, F. Miller, and D. Miller.)

Fig. 1.28 The Craik–Cornsweet–O'Brien illusion. The perceived difference in the darkness of the vertical panels disappears if one places a pencil or finger along the border between panels. The effect persists even if the panel details are blurred.

or done monocularly. Clearly, the brain must be where the ultimate processing occurs in these experiments. Because a threshold of less than 5 seconds is well beyond the optical diffraction limit of the eye, Vernier acuity represents a special example of sophisticated brain processing. The challenge is to try to conceptualize some important task necessary for the survival of our *Homo sapiens* ancestors who required such precision. Incidentally, we also know that the macaque monkey demonstrates a high level of Vernier acuity. In fact, the adult monkey averages a threshold of about 13 seconds of arc.[136] Thus, it is possible that monkeys and early humans used Vernier acuity to detect the presence of an animal or an enemy hiding behind a stalk or a tree by noting a misalignment between the edge of the tree or stalk and the protruding body of the enemy. If that possible scenario were true, normal Vernier acuity might save a life. Once again, brain enhancement of the retinal image brings out details well beyond the limits of the best optical resolution.

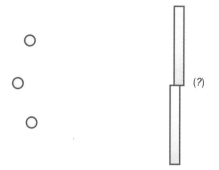

Fig. 1.29 Two typical targets for measuring Vernier acuity. The subject either notes misalignment of the vertical lines or of the three dots.

Refractive errors

Thus far, when pertinent, this chapter has covered the physiologic optics of the average emmetropic eye. However, the average refractive error in certain populations is not emmetropia. For example, in some Asian groups the incidence of myopia may be between 80% and 90%.[137]

Therefore, for a broader review of physiologic optics, this last section covers some of the essential epidemiologic aspects of the refractive errors.

Prevalence

Studies that tabulate the distribution of refractive errors are often taken from data on young army recruits.[138,139] Yang[140] reported a prevalence of 24% of myopes, 3% of hyperopes, and 72% of emmetropes. However, this group of healthy young men may not represent the general population. Because age, race, and education, among other factors, are related to refractive error distribution, comprehensive populational studies are ideal.

Pan,[141] studying a multiethnic adult population in the United States, found that overall 25% were myopes (4.6% high myopes), 38% were hyperopes, and 37% were emmetropes. Myopia was most prevalent in Chinese individuals (37.2%), and hyperopia was most common in Hispanic subjects. The European Eye Epidemiology Consortium (E3)[142] combined 15 studies in a meta-analysis and obtained age-standardized prevalences of 30.6% myopia (2.7% high myopia) and 25.2% hyperopia.

The spectacle-wearing population of a typical Western country provides a different focus on emmetropes. Bennett[143] surveyed the distribution of spectacles dispensed in England. His study of refractions carried out by the average eye clinician showed that about 20% are myopic refractions, and 75% of all refractions require prescriptions from −0.5 to +8.00 D.

Myopia

Higher prevalence of myopia is reported in younger ages and Asian people. According to Rim,[144] considering the population older than 5 years in Korea, myopia is found in almost 52% of subjects and high myopia in 5%. Wang[145] followed a cohort of junior high school students and identified a rise in myopia incidence and myopia prevalence reaching up to 79.4% of children at graduation.

This trend toward a higher prevalence of myopes has also been observed in Western countries. Analyses of over 1.5 million conscripts from Austria from 1983 to 2017 revealed that myopia prevalence rose from 13.8% to 24.4%.[140] Holden estimates that in 2050 approximately half of the global population will be myopic.[146] This increase is considered to result from multivariate factors, from gene susceptibility to lifestyle and environment changes. For instance, increasing time spent outdoors by children has been proposed as a simple strategy for reducing risk of myopia development.[147] Interestingly, inhabitants of the Amazon rainforest have an extremely low incidence of myopia. From an overall sample of 486 people, 259 indigenous people, and 78 Brazilians between 12 and 59 years of age, only 2.7% of eyes showed myopia of −1.00 D or more and 1.6% had bilateral myopia of −1.00 D or more.[148]

Pathologic myopia

Curtin[149] estimates that 2% to 3% of the population has pathologic myopia (a condition in which there is a significant enlargement of the eyeball with a lengthening of the posterior segment). This group falls into the group of patients with myopia of greater than 6 D. The term *pathologic* is used because these patients show significant choroidal and retinal degenerative changes, a high incidence of retinal detachment, glaucoma, and increased occurrence of staphyloma (a circumscribed outpouching of the wall of the globe). Severity of myopia and increasing age are risk factors for the development of pathologic changes.[150] As myopia prevalence rises worldwide, these degenerative changes may become the leading cause of irreversible vision loss in many communities.[151] High myopia (>6 D) is regarded as hereditary, and genetic factors are an important piece in its development. Some might be inherited in a complex fashion, and more than 22 loci for high myopia have been reported.[152]

Astigmatism

About 50% of term infants in their first years of life show astigmatism of more than 2 D.[153–155] This may arise from the influence of the recti muscles that pull on the delicate infant sclera, because the astigmatism seems to change in different gaze directions. Howland et al.[154] suggested that the high astigmatism helps the infant bracket the position of best focus while learning to accommodate. In previous studies,[141,142,144] 23% to 45% of the population was identified with 1 D or more of astigmatism.

Presbyopia

Although presbyopia is age related, its age of onset varies around the world. For example, presbyopia develops earlier in people who live closer to the equator.[156,157] Specifically, the age of onset of presbyopia was noted to be 37 years in India, 39 years in Puerto Rico, 41 years in Israel, 42 years in Japan, 45 years in England, and 46 years in Norway. Some studies show the important variable to be ambient temperature rather than latitude. Thus, the higher the ambient temperature, the earlier the onset of presbyopia.[158]

Around the world, 1.09 billion people are estimated to be affected by presbyopia. Difficulty in performing near vision tasks for daily activities introduces limitations to the routine and productivity losses.[159] To this day, uncorrected presbyopia is still a significant cause of vision impairment.[160] Seen in perspective, it constitutes about 65% of all who wear glasses in developed Western countries. Thus, it is of little surprise that the first spectacles produced sometime in the 14th century were created for persons with presbyopia.

Given the epidemiology, much has been discussed about new approaches in the treatment of presbyopia, being a major focus of the health industry. The coming years will be a period where much of the research and technology effort will be focused on developing eye drops or improving surgical approaches in addition to intraocular lens technology.

REFERENCES

1. Boothe RG, Dobson V, Teller DY. Post natal development of vision in human and non-human primates. *Ann Rev Neurosci.* 1985;8:495.
2. Collins D. *The Human Revolution: From Ape to Artist.* London: Phaidon; 1976.

3. Larsen JS. The sagittal growth of the eye: Ultrasonic measurements of axial length of the eye from birth to puberty. *Acta Ophthalmol.* 1971;49:872.
4. Bach A, Villegas VM, Gold AS, Shi W, Murray TG. Axial length development in children. *Int J Ophthalmol.* 2019;12(5):815–819.
5. Baldwin WR. *Some relationships between ocular, anthropometric and refractive variables in myopia. Doctoral thesis. Indianapolis.* University of Indiana; 1964.
6. Frantz RL. Visual perception from birth as shown by pattern selectivity. *Ann NY Acad Sci.* 1965;118:793.
7. Green DG, Powers MK, Banks MS. Depth of focus, eye size, visual acuity. *Vis Res.* 1980;20:827.
8. Reynolds CR, Fletcher F, Janzen E. *Handbook of clinical child neurophysiology.* New York: Plenum Press; 1989.
9. Teller DY. First glances: The vision of infants. *Invest Ophthalmol Vis Sci.* 1997;38:2183.
10. Rada JAS, Shelton S, Norton TT. The sclera and myopia. *Exp Eye Res.* 2006;82:185–200.
11. Cui D, Trier K, Zeng J, et al. Effects of 7-methylxanthine on the sclera in form deprivation myopia in guinea pigs. *Acta Ophthalmol.* 2011;89(4):328–334.
12. Guo P, Miao Y, Jing Y, et al. Changes in collagen structure and permeability of rat and human sclera after crosslinking. *Transl Vis Sci Technol.* 2020;9(9):45.
13. Siatkowski RM, Cotter SA, Crockett RS, et al. Study Group. Two-year multicenter, randomized, double-masked, placebo-controlled, parallel safety and efficacy study of 2% pirenzepine ophthalmic gel in children with myopia. *J Am Assoc Pediatr Ophthalmol Strabismus.* 2008;12:332–339.
14. Applegate RA, Howland HC. Magnification and visual acuity in refractive surgery. *Arch Ophthalmol.* 1993;111:1335–1342.
15. Inagaki Y. The rapid change of corneal curvature in the neonatal period and infancy. *Arch Ophthalmol.* 1986;104:1026.
16. Insler MS, et al. Analysis of corneal thickness and corneal curvature in infants. *CLAO J.* 1987;3:192.
17. Tucker SM, et al. Corneal diameter, axial length and intraocular pressure in premature infants. *Ophthalmology.* 1992;99:1296.
18. Mutti DO, et al. Optical and structural development of the crystalline lens in childhood. *Invest Ophthalmol Vis Sci.* 1997;39:120.
19. Wood ICJ, Mutti DO, Zadnik K. Crystalline lens parameters in infancy. *Ophthalmol Physiol Opt.* 1996;6:310.
20. Hofstetter HW. Emmetropization – biological process or mathematical artifact? *Am J Optom Arch Am Acad Optom.* 1969;46:447.
21. Sorsby A, et al. *Emmetropia and its aberrations. MRC Special Rep Serv Rep 293.* London: Medical Research Council; 1959.
22. Koretz JF, Rogot A, Kaufman PL. Physiological strategies for emmetropia. *Trans Am Ophthalmol Soc.* 1995;93:105.
23. Laties AM, Stone RA. Some visual and neurochemical correlates of refractive development. *Vis Neurosci.* 1991;7:125.
24. Stenstom S. Untersuchungen uber die variation fon kovariation des optishen elements des menschlichen auges. *Acta Ophthalmol.* 1946;26(suppl).
25. Iuvone PM, et al. Effects of apomorphine, a dopamine receptor agonist, on ocular refraction and axial elongation in a primate model of myopia. *Invest Ophthalmol Vis Sci.* 1991;32:1674.
26. Papastergiou GI, et al. Induction of axial eye elongation and myopic refractive shift in one-year old chickens. *Vis Res.* 1998;38:1883.
27. Stark L, Obrecht G. *Presbyopia: Recent Research and Reviews from the Third International Symposium.* New York: Professional Press; 1987.
28. Stone RA, et al. Postnatal control of ocular growth: Dopaminergic mechanisms. *Ciba Foundation Symposium.* 1990;155:45.
29. Troilo D, Smith EL III, Nickla DL, et al. IMI – report on experimental models of emmetropization and myopia. *Invest Ophthalmol Vis Sci.* 2019;60(3):M31–M88.
30. Huo L, Cui D, Yang X, et al. A retrospective study: Form-deprivation myopia in unilateral congenital ptosis. *Clin Exp Optom.* 2012;95:404–409.
31. Amedo AO, Norton TT. Visual guidance of recovery from lens-induced myopia in tree shrews (Tupaia glis belangeri). *Ophthalmic Physiol Opt.* 2012;32:89–99.
32. Wildsoet CF, Schmid KL. Optical correction of form deprivation myopia inhibits refractive recovery in chick eyes with intact or sectioned optic nerves. *Vision Res.* 2000;40(23):3273–3278.
33. Schaeffel F, Troilo D, Wallman J, Howland HC. Developing eyes that lack accommodation grow to compensate for imposed defocus. *Vis Neurosci.* 1990;4:177–183.
34. Diether S, Schaeffel F. Local changes in eye growth induced by imposed local refractive error despite active accommodation. *Vision Res.* 1997;37(6):659–668.
35. Mercer ME, Drodge SC, Courage ML, Adams RJ. A pseudoisochromatic test of color vision for human infants. *Vision Res.* 2014;100:72–77.
36. Bushnell I, Sai F, Mullin J. Neonatal recognition of mother's face. *British Journal of Developmental Psychology.* 2011;7:3–15.
37. Gwiazda J, et al. Astigmatism in children: Changes in axis and amount from birth to six years. *Invest Ophthalmol Vis Sci.* 1984;25:99.
38. Friling R, Weinberger D, Kremer I, Avisar R, Sirota L, Snir M. Keratometry measurements in preterm and full term newborn infants. *The British journal of ophthalmology.* 2004;88:8–10.
39. Zadnik K, Mutti DO. Development of ametropias. In: Benjamin WJ, ed. *Borish's Clinical Refraction.* Philadelphia: WB: Saunders; 1998.
40. Goss DA. Development of the ametropias. In: Benjamin WJ, ed. *Borish's Clinical Refraction.* Philadelphia: WB: Saunders; 1998.
41. Mohindra I, Held R, Gwiazda J. Astigmatism in infants. *Science.* 1978;202:329.
42. Howland HC. Infant eyes: Optics and accommodation. *Curr Eye Res.* 1982–1983;2(3):217–224.
43. Strickland C. *Torsten Wiesel, Winner of 1981 Nobel Prize for Vision Research.* San Francisco: American Academy of Ophthalmology; 1995.
44. Bower TG. *The Perceptual World of the Child.* Cambridge, MA: Harvard University Press; 1977.
45. Tronick E. Simultaneous control and growth of the infant's effective visual field. *Percep Psychophys.* 1972;11:373.
46. Pinker S. *The Language Instinct.* New York: Penguin Books; 1994.
47. Wilson SE. Wave-front analysis: Are we missing something? *Am J Ophthalmol.* 2003;136:340–342.
48. Kohda Y, Watanabe M. The aggression-releasing effect of the eye-like spot of the Oyanirami Coreopera kawamebari, a fresh water serranid fish. *Ethology.* 1990;84:162.
49. Fernald RD. Vision and behavior in an African cichlid fish. *Am Sci.* 1984;72:58.
50. Sherbrooke W. Personal communication, 1995.
51. Yanoff Myron, et al. Optics of the Human Eye. *Ophthalmology.* 5th ed. Edinburgh: Elsevier; 2019.
52. Miller D, Benedek G. *Intraocular Light Scattering.* Springfield. IL. Charles C Thomas; 1973.
53. Wollensak G, Wilsch M, Spoerl E, Seiler T. Collagen fiber diameter in the rabbit cornea after collagen crosslinking by riboflavin/UVA. *Cornea.* 2004;23:503–507.
54. Miles S. *Underwater Medicine.* Philadelphia: Heppesen Sandreson; 1966.
55. Mainster MD. Contemporary optics and ocular pathology. *Surv Ophthalmol.* 1978;23:135.
56. Aggurwala KR, Nowbotsing S, Kruger PB. Accommodation to monochromatic and white-light targets. *Invest Ophthalmol Vis Sci.* 1995;36:2695.
57. Schachar RA. Zonular function: A new hypothesis with clinical implications. *Ann Ophthalmol.* 1994;26:36–38.
58. Schachar RA. The mechanism of accommodation and presbyopia. *Int Ophthalmol Clin.* 2006;46:39–61.
59. Coleman DJ. Unified model for accommodative mechanism. *American Journal of Ophthalmology.* 1970;69:1063–1079.
60. Coleman DJ. On the hydraulic suspension theory of accommodation. *Trans Am Ophthalmol Soc.* 1986;84:846–868.
61. Pardue MT, Anderson ME, Sivak J. Accommodation in raptors. *Invest Ophthalmol Vis Sci.* 1996;37:725.
62. Stryer L. Mini review: Visual excitation and recovery. *J Biol Chem.* 1991;266:1071.
63. Nakanishi K. Why 11-cis-retinal? *Am Zool.* 1991;31:479.
64. Oesterhelt D, Stoeckenius W. Rhodopsin-like protein from the purple membrane of *Holobacterium halobium. Nature New Biol.* 1971;233:149.
65. Spudich JL, Bogomolni RD. Sensory rhodopsins of Halobacteria. Annu Rev. *Biophys Chem.* 1988;17:183.
66. Atkinson GH, et al. Picosecond time-resolved fluorescence spectroscopy of K-590 in the bacteriorhodopsin photocycle. *Biophys J.* 1989;55:263.
67. Yokoyama S, Yokoyama R. Molecular evolution of human visual pigment genes. *Mol Biol Evol.* 1989;6:186.
68. Campbell FW. The depth of field of the human eye. *Optica Acta.* 1957;4:157.
69. Fein A, Szutz EZ. *Photoreceptors: Their Role in Vision.* Cambridge: Cambridge University Press; 1982.
70. Snyder AW, Bossomaier TR, Hughes A. Optical image quality and the cone mosaic. *Science.* 1986;231:499.
71. Snyder AW, Menzal R. *Photoreceptor Optics.* Berlin: Springer-Verlag; 1975.
72. Elliott DB, Yang KGH, Whitaker D. Visual acuity changes throughout adulthood in normal healthy eyes seeing beyond 6/6. *Optom Vis Sci.* 1995;72:186.
73. Ratliff F. The role of physiologic nystagmus in monocular acuity. *J Exp Psychol.* 1952;43:163.
74. Riggs LA, et al. The disappearance of steadily fixated visual test objects. *J Opt Soc Am.* 1953;43:495.
75. Riggs LA. Visual acuity. In: Graham CH, ed. *Vision and Visual Perception.* New York: John Wiley & Sons; 1965.
76. Eakin RM. Evolution of photoreceptors. In: Robzhansky T, Hetch MK, Steere WC, eds. *Evolutionary Biology.* Vol 2. New York: Appleton-Century-Crofts; 1968.
77. Williams DR. Topography of the foveal cone mosaic in the living human eye. *Vis Res.* 1988;28:433.
78. Von Ditfurth H. *Children of the Universe.* New York: Athenaeum Press; 1976.
79. Zeilik M. *Astronomy: The Evolving Universe.* 3rd ed. New York: Harper & Row; 1982.
80. Levene JR. *Clinical Refraction and Visual Science.* London: Butterworths; 1977.
81. Sheedy JE, Bailey IL, Raasch TW. Visual acuity and chart luminance. *Am J Optom Physiol Opt.* 1984;61(9):595–600.
82. Bailey H, Lovie JE. New design principles for visual acuity letter charts. *Am J Optom Physiol Opt.* 1976;53:740.
83. Ferris FL, et al. New visual acuity charts for clinical research. *Am J Ophthalmol.* 1982;94:91.
84. Carkeet AD. Modeling logMAR visual acuity scores: Effects of termination rules and alternative forced-choice options. *Optom Vis Sci.* 2001;8:529–538.
85. Nunes LM, Schor P. Evaluation of the impact of refractive surgery on quality of life using the NEI-RQL (National Eye Institute Refractive Error Quality of Life) instrument. *Arq Bras Oftalmol.* 2005;68(6):789–794.
86. Pelli DG, Bex P. Measuring contrast sensitivity. *Vis Res.* 2013;90:10–14.
87. Richman J, et al. Contrast sensitivity basics and a critique of currently available tests. *J Cataract Refract Surg.* 2013;39(7):1100–1106.
88. Kauffmann L, et al. The neural bases of spatial frequency processing during scene perception. *Front Integr Neurosci.* 2014;8:37.
89. Maffei L, Fiorentini A. The visual cortex as a spatial frequency analyser. *Vis Res.* 1973;13:1255.
90. Campbell FW, Robson JG. Application of Fourier analysis to the visibility of gratings. *J Physiol.* 1968;197:551.
91. Campbell FW. The physics of visual perception. *Phil Trans R Soc Lond B Biol Sci.* 1980;290:5.
92. Miller D, Sanghvi S. Contrast sensitivity and glare testing in corneal disease. In: Nadler M, Miller D, Nadler DJ, eds. *Glare and Contrast Sensitivity for Clinicians.* New York: Springer-Verlag; 1990.
93. LeClaire J, et al. A new glare tester for clinical testing. *Arch Ophthalmol.* 1982;100:153.
94. Holliday LL. The fundamentals of glare and visibility. *J Opt Soc Am.* 1926;12A:492.

95. Wolfe E, Gardiner JS. Studies on the scatter of light in the dioptric median of the eye as a basis for visual glare. *Arch Ophthalmol.* 1963;37:450.
96. Wolfe E. Glare and age. *Arch Ophthalmol.* 1960;64:502.
97. Miller D, Dohlman CH. The effect of cataract surgery on the cornea. *Trans Am Acad Ophthalmol Otolaryngol.* 1970;74:369.
98. Lançon M, Miller D. Corneal hydration, visual acuity, and glare sensitivity. *Arch Ophthalmol.* 1973;90:227.
99. Watanabe S, et al. Relationship between corneal guttae and quality of vision in patients with mild Fuchs' endothelial corneal dystrophy. *Ophthalmology.* 2015;122(10):2103–2109.
100. Wacker K, et al. Corneal high-order aberrations and backscatter in Fuch's endothelial corneal dystrophy. *Ophthalmology.* 2015;122(8):1645–1652.
101. Augustin VA, et al. Influence of corneal guttae and nuclear cataract on contrast sensitivity. *Br J Ophthalmol.* 2021 Oct;105(10):1365–1370.
102. Gundlach E, et al. Recovery of contrast sensitivity after Descemet membrane endothelial keratoplasty. *Cornea.* 2021;40(9):1110–1116.
103. De Juan V, et al. Optical quality and intraocular scattering assessed with a double pass system in eyes with contact lens induced corneal swelling. *Cont Lens Anterior Eye.* 2014;37(4):278–284.
104. Jinabhai A, et al. Forward light scatter and contrast sensitivity in keratoconic patients. *Cont Lens Anterior Eye.* 2012 Feb;35(1):22–27.
105. Pesudovs K, Schoneveld P, Seto RJ, Coster DJ. Contrast and glare testing in keratoconus and after penetrating keratoplasty. *Br J Ophthalmol.* 2004;88(5):653–657.
106. Rowsey JJ, Balyeat HD. Preliminary results and complications of radial keratotomy. *Am J Ophthalmol.* 1982;93:437.
107. Waring GO, et al. Results of the progressive evaluation of radial keratotomy (PERK) study one year after surgery. *Ophthalmology.* 1985;92:177.
108. Koch D, et al. Glare following posterior chamber lens implantation. *J Cataract Refract Surg.* 1986;12:480.
109. Campbell FW, Green DG. Optical and retinal factors affecting visual resolution. *J Physiol.* 1965;181:576.
110. Charman WN, Whitefoot H. Pupil diameter and the depth-of-field of the human eye as measured by laser speckle. *Optica Acta.* 1977;24:1211.
111. Ogle KN, Schwartz JT. Depth of focus of the human eye. *J Opt Soc Am.* 1959;49:273.
112. Tucker J, Charman WN. The depth of focus of the human eye for Snellen letters. *Am J Optom Physiol Opt.* 1975;52:3.
113. Helmholtz H. *Handbuch der Physiologische Optik.* Leipzig: Hamburg University, 1909.
114. Fernandes BF, Marshall JCA, Burnier MN Jr. Blue light exposure and uveal melanoma. *Ophthalmology.* 2006;113:1062.
115. Pérez MJ, Puell MC, Sánchez C, Langa A. Effect of a yellow filter on mesopic contrast perception and differential light sensitivity in the visual field. *Ophthalmic Res.* 2003;35(1):54–59. https://doi.org/10.1159/000068202.
116. Vagge A, Ferro Desideri L, Del Noce C, Di Mola I, Sindaco D, Traverso CE. Blue light filtering ophthalmic lenses: A systematic review. *Semin Ophthalmol.* 2021;36(7):541–548.
117. Lee JS, Li PR, Hou CH, Lin KK, Kuo CF, See LC. Effect of blue light-filtering intraocular lenses on age-related macular degeneration: A nationwide cohort study with 10-year follow-up. *Am J Ophthalmol.* 2021;234:138–146.
118. Achiron A, Elbaz U, Hecht I, et al. The effect of blue-light filtering intraocular lenses on the development and progression of neovascular age-related macular degeneration. *Ophthalmology.* 2021;128(3):410–416.
119. Enoch JM. Retinal receptor orientation and the role of fiber optics in vision. *Am J Optometry.* 1972;49:455.
120. Snyder AW, Pask C. The Stiles-Crawford effect explanation and consequences. *Vision Res.* 1973;13:1115–1137.
121. Thisbos LN, Zhang X, Ye M, Bradley A. The chromatic eye: A new reduced-eye model of ocular chromatic aberration in humans. *Appl Opt.* 1992;31:3594.
122. Wald G, Griffin DR. The change in refractive power of the human eye in dim and bright light. *J Opt Soc Am.* 1947;37:321.
123. Troelstra A, et al. Accommodative tracking: A trial-and-error function. *Vis Res.* 1964;4:585.
124. Bennett AG, Rabbetts RB. *Clinical visual optics.* London: Butterworths; 1984.
125. Said FS, Weale RA. The variation with age of the human spectral transmissivity of the living human crystalline lens. *Gerontologia.* 1959;3:213.
126. Campbell FW, Gubisch RW. Optical quality of the human eye. *J Physiol.* 1966;186:558.
127. Barlow HB. Critical limiting factors in the design of the eye and visual cortex: The Ferrier lecture, 1980. *Proc R Soc Lond.* 1981;212B:1.
128. Katz M. The human eye as an optical system. In: Duane TD, ed. *Clinical Ophthalmology.* New York: Harper & Row; 1990.
129. Weiter JJ. Phototoxic changes in the retina. In: Miller D, ed. *Clinical Light Damage to the Eye.* New York: Springer-Verlag; 1987.
130. Hemenger RP, Garner LF, Ooi CS. Change with age of the refractive index gradient of the human ocular lens. *Invest Ophthalmol Vis Sci.* 1995;36:703.
131. Wistow GJ, Piatigorsky J. Recruitment of enzymes as lens structural proteins. *Science.* 1987;236:1554.
132. Horwitz J, Bova MP, Ding LL, Haley DA, Stewart PL. Lens alpha-crystallin: Function and structure. *Eye (Lond).* 1999;13(Pt 3b):403–408.
133. Frisby JP. *Seeing: Illusion, brain and mind.* Oxford: Oxford University Press; 1980.
134. Lee DN. The optic flow field: The foundation of vision. *Phil Trans R Soc London B Biol Sci.* 1980;290:169.
135. Zeng W, Daly S, Lei S. An overview of the visual optimization tools in JPEG 2000. *Signal Proc Image Commun.* 2002;17:85–104.
136. Tang C, Kiorpes L, Morshon JA. Stereoacuity and vernier acuity in macaque monkeys. *Invest Ophthal.* 1995;36:5365.
137. Lin LL, Shih YF, Hsiao CK, Chen CJ. Prevalence of myopia in Taiwanese schoolchildren: 1983 to 2000. *Ann Acad Med Singap.* 2004;33(1):27–33.
138. Sorsby A, Sheridan M, Leary GA, Benjamin B. Vision, visual acuity, and ocular refraction of young men. *Br Med J.* 1960;1:1394.
139. Stromberg E. Uber refraktion und Achsenlange des menchlicken Auges. *Acta Ophthalmol.* 1936;14:281.
140. Yang L, Vass C, Smith L, Juan A, Waldhör T. Thirty-five-year trend in the prevalence of refractive error in Austrian conscripts based on 1.5 million participants. *Br J Ophthalmol.* 2020;104(10):1338–1344.
141. Pan C-W, Klein BE, Cotch MF, et al. Racial variations in the prevalence of refractive errors in the United States: The multi-ethnic study of atherosclerosis. *Am J Ophthalmol.* 2013;155(6):1129–1138.
142. Williams KM, Verhoeven VJ, Cumberland P, et al. Prevalence of refractive error in Europe: The European Eye Epidemiology (E(3)) Consortium. *Eur J Epidemiol.* 2015;30(4):305–315.
143. Bennett AG, Rabbetts RB. *Clinical Visual Optics.* 2nd ed. London: Butterworth; 1989.
144. Rim TH, Kim SH, Lim KH, et al. Refractive Errors in Koreans: The Korea National Health and Nutrition Examination Survey 2008–2012. *Korean J Ophthalmol.* 2016;30(3):214–224.
145. Wang SK, Guo Y, Liao C, et al. Incidence of and factors associated with myopia and high myopia in Chinese children, based on refraction without cycloplegia. *JAMA Ophthalmol.* 2018;136(9):1017–1024.
146. Holden BA, Fricke TR, Wilson DA, et al. Global prevalence of myopia and high myopia and temporal trends from 2000 through 2050. *Ophthalmology.* 2016;123(5):1036–1042.
147. Sherwin JC, Reacher MH, Keogh RH, Khawaja AP, Mackey DA, Foster PJ. The association between time spent outdoors and myopia in children and adolescents: a systematic review and meta-analysis. *Ophthalmology.* 2012;119(10):2141–2151.
148. Thorn F, Cruz AA, Machado AJ, Carvalho RA. Refractive status of indigenous people in the northwestern Amazon region of Brazil. *Optom Vis Sci.* 2005;82:267–272.
149. Curtin BJ. *The Myopias: Basic Science and Clinical Management.* Philadelphia: Harper & Row; 1985.
150. Ohno-Matsui K, Lai TY, Lai CC, Cheung CM. Updates of pathologic myopia. *Prog Retin Eye Res.* 2016;52:156–187.
151. Fricke TR, Jong M, Naidoo KS, et al. Global prevalence of visual impairment associated with myopic macular degeneration and temporal trends from 2000 through 2050: Systematic review, meta-analysis and modelling. *Br J Ophthalmol.* 2018;102(7):855–862.
152. Li J, Jiang D, Xiao X, et al. Evaluation of 12 myopia-associated genes in Chinese patients with high myopia. *Invest Ophthalmol Vis Sci.* 2015;56(2):722–729.
153. Bennett AG. Lens usage in the supplementary ophthalmic service. *Optician.* 1965;149:131.
154. Howland HC, et al. Astigmatism measured by photorefraction. *Science.* 1978;202:331.
155. Mohundra I, et al. Astigmatism in infants. *Science.* 1978;202:329.
156. Miranda MH. The environmental factor in the onset of presbyopia. In: Stark L, Obrecht G, eds. *Presbyopia.* New York: Professional Press; 1987.
157. Klemstein RN. Epidemiology of presbyopia. In: Start L, Obrecht G, eds. *Presbyopia.* New York: Professional Press; 1987.
158. Nandi SK, Rankenberg J, Glomb MA, Nagaraj RH. Transient elevation of temperature promotes cross-linking of α-crystallin-client proteins through formation of advanced glycation endproducts: A potential role in presbyopia and cataracts. *Biochem Biophys Res Commun.* 2020;533(4):1352–1358.
159. Berdahl J, Bala C, Dhariwal M, Lemp-Hull J, Thakker D, Jawla S. Patient and economic burden of presbyopia: A systematic literature review. *Clin Ophthalmol.* 2020;14:3439–3450.
160. GBD 2019 Blindness and Vision Impairment Collaborators, Vision Loss Expert Group of the Global Burden of Disease Study. Trends in prevalence of blindness and distance and near vision impairment over 30 years: An analysis for the Global Burden of Disease Study. *Lancet Glob Health.* 2021;9(2):e130–e143.

2

Optical Aberrations and Wavefront Sensing

Renfeng Xu and Ronald Robert Krueger

Introduction

The purpose of the eye's optical system is to form an image on the retina. For a perfect eye, all rays of light from a single point in space will create a single image point on the photoreceptor layer to form a "sharp" image. This is called an "aberration-free eye." However, human eyes suffer from three types of optical imperfections, namely, diffraction, scatter, and aberrations, all of which degrade image quality, blurring the image and lowering retinal image contrast. This chapter will focus on optical aberrations and their impact on vision.

Optical aberrations are generally divided into lower- or higher-order aberrations. Lower-order aberrations include myopia, hyperopia, and astigmatism. We have been successfully providing excellent vision of 20/20 to the population by simply correcting the lower-order aberrations with spherocylindrical lenses for the past 200 years, so why should we even try to correct "higher-order aberrations" (HOAs)? Porter showed that over 90% of the total aberrations in eyes are due to lower-order aberrations.[1] There are the two main reasons to consider correcting HOAs. First, by correcting HOAs, vision quality of our patients could be further improved depending on the magnitude of the HOAs, which can be large in pathologic eyes, (i.e., keratoconic eyes). Secondarily, because the clinician's view of a patient's eye is created by the eye's optics, the image quality will improve if HOAs of the examined eye are corrected, even allowing a cell-level retinal fundus examination of retinal pathology[2,3] or a cell-level view of trabecular meshwork under gonioscopy.[4]

This chapter intends to provide the reader with a basic understanding of optical aberrations and the impact and clinical relevance of these aberrations on vision, with special attention paid to spherical aberration (SA).

OPTICAL ABERRATIONS

Optical aberrations include chromatic aberrations, monochromatic aberrations (lower-order aberrations and HOAs), and off-axis aberrations. All three play a significant role in ophthalmology.

Chromatic aberrations

Because the human eye is sensitive to a wide spectral range of light (approximately 400–750 nm) and because many optical instruments such as autorefractors and aberrometers employ infrared radiation, changes in optical properties of the eye across this large spectral range can affect retinal image quality, objective measures of refractive state, and measures of axial length by partial coherence interferometers, a technology employed in the clinical instrument called IOL Master. As is common to all transparent optical materials, the refractive indices of ocular tissues vary with wavelength, which creates a wavelength-dependent change with short wavelengths focusing in front of the long wavelengths along the horizontal optical axis (longitudinal chromatic

aberration [LCA], Fig. 2.1A), as well as wavelength-dependent variations in image size and location (transverse chromatic aberration [TCA], Fig. 2.1B). A generally well-centered pupil that lies close to the eye's nodal plane (which sits approximately just posterior to the lens[5]) minimizes the magnitude and impact of TCA.[6] Although LCA is large in dioptric terms (e.g., 2.5 diopters [D] across the visible spectrum[7]), its impact on quality of vision is small because visual sensitivity at both ends of the visible spectrum is very low.[8] Also, there are reports that the impact of LCA on polychromatic image quality[9] or contrast sensitivity[10] is further reduced by the presence of monochromatic aberrations. However, instruments that measure refractive state of the eye using infrared (IR) radiation[11] must include a correction factor to convert a near IR 850 nm measure to one that is visually relevant (e.g., 550 nm).

Although there are no simple ways to correct ocular chromatic aberrations, several clinical interventions have been implemented that either reduce or potentially increase chromatic aberrations. For example, different materials used for intraocular lenses (IOLs) have different refractive indices, and generally those with the higher refractive indices will have a larger change in index across the visible spectrum,[12] but these modest changes in chromatic dispersion have no measurable impact on polychromatic image quality. A more significant manipulation of LCA is generated by a type of lens called a "diffractive lens,"[13] which exhibits LCA opposite in sign to that of the human eye, and if the optical power of the diffractive lens is about +3 D, it can be used to correct the eye's LCA. Conveniently, +3 D is a typical add power used for a bifocal, and diffractive optics are routinely included in bifocal or trifocal IOLs[14] and contact lenses.[15] There is one optical correction that can amplify TCA by moving the entrance pupil anterior to the corneal plane (corneal inlays[16]), because TCA will scale with distance of the pupil from the eye's nodal point.

Aberrations that vary across the visual field

Although it is common to refer to the "image plane," such a plane only really exists for a small region of the visual field, and the true shape of the image surface is a three-dimensional curved surface (a "Petzval surface"[17]). Because the axial location of the image surface changes,[18] a focused image can only be present across the retina if it too has a curved shape, which, conveniently, it does.[19] Therefore, the curved retina generally matches the curved image surface over the central +/– 40 degrees of the visual field,[20] conveniently providing a focused image across a large area of the retina once the foveal image has been focused by standard refractive correction. Although eye shape can mostly correct for this "curvature of field," aberrations and off-axis astigmatism can be very large in the peripheral retina.[21-23] Although large optical aberrations are present in the peripheral image, the neural insensitivity to defocus[24] means that these off-axis aberrations likely play a minor role in peripheral vision. When we talk about defocus (either hyperopic or myopic), it simply means the image is out of focus. Hyperopic

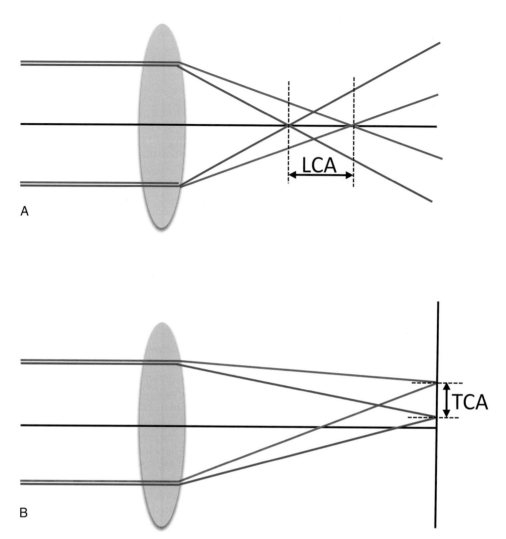

Fig. 2.1 Chromatic aberrations generated when white light passing through a positive lens. (**A**) Longitudinal chromatic aberration (*LCA*) manifested as separate focal points between different wavelengths along the horizontal plane. (**B**) Transverse chromatic aberration (*TCA*) manifested as separate focal points between different wavelengths along the vertical plane.

defocus means image focuses behind the retina as in uncorrected hyperopes, whereas myopic defocus means image focuses in front of the retina as in uncorrected myopes. Recent animal studies suggest that hyperopic defocus in the peripheral retina may play a significant role in the development of myopia.[25] Studies on interruption of hyperopic defocus or inducing myopic defocus peripherally have shown promising results on myopia prevention.[26–28]

Monochromatic aberrations

We usually describe myopic or hyperopic refractive errors of the eye with three numbers (sphere, cylinder, axis). Myopia, hyperopia, and astigmatism are refractive errors known as second-order aberrations. In myopia (Fig. 2.2B), light rays entering the eye focus anterior to the retina plane. This is most often seen in an elongated eye. In contrast, hyperopia (Fig. 2.2C) occurs in a less-powered eye where light rays tend to focus behind the retina plane. Astigmatism happens when the uneven curvatures of the cornea and lens cause light rays to focus at two different points. The location of two different points relative to the retina determines the type of astigmatism. When one focal line is located anterior to the retina and the other on the retina, it is termed

simple myopic astigmatism (Fig. 2.2D). When one focal line is located on the retina and the other behind it, it is termed simple hyperopic astigmatism. When both focal lines are before the retina but at two different locations, it is termed compound myopic astigmatism. When both focal lines are behind the retina but at two different locations, it is termed compound hyperopic astigmatism. When one focal line is in front of the retina and the other is behind the retina, it is termed mixed astigmatism. Both myopia and hyperopia can be corrected with spectacles, contact lenses, intraocular lenses, or refractive surgery. Astigmatism can be corrected with a cylindrical lens, a toric contact lens or IOL, or refractive surgery by counteracting the uneven curvature of the cornea or lens (Fig. 2.2).

For an aberration-free system, all rays at distance form at a single point (focal point) on the image plane (Fig. 2.3A). However, in the presence of optical aberrations, rays from a single object point intersect the image plane at different locations, causing the light to spread out over an area. As a result, there is no single focal point, as illustrated in Fig. 2.3B.

Clinicians often umbrella HOAs, including SA and coma, under "irregular astigmatism." When parallel light rays refract through a

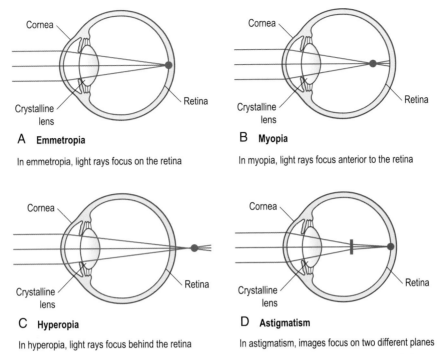

Fig. 2.2 Refractive states. (**A**) In emmetropia, light rays focus on the retina. (**B**) In myopia, light rays focus anterior to the retina. (**C**) In hyperopia, light rays focus behind the retina. (**D**) In astigmatism, variations in the surface of the cornea and lens cause light rays to focus at two different points. When one focal line is located anterior to the retina and the other on the retina, it is termed *myopic astigmatism*. When one focal line is located on the retina and the other behind it, it is termed *hyperopic astigmatism*.

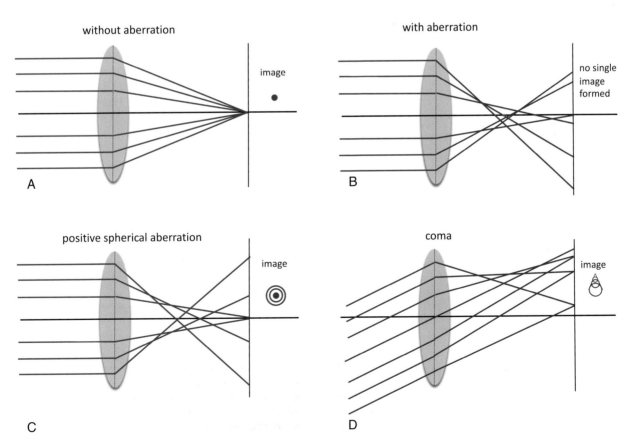

Fig. 2.3 The ray tracing and the corresponding image of the point light source for: (**A**) aberration-free system; (**B**) in the presence of aberration; (**C**) positive spherical aberration; (**D**) coma.

spherical lens with SA, the central rays will converge at the focal point of the lens, but the peripheral light rays fail to converge at the same focal point. Instead, in the presence of positive SA, the peripheral rays will refract more relative to the central rays (Fig. 2.3C), and the image of the point light source appears as concentric rings surrounding a central point. Coma is another example of an HOA, and causes light rays from an off-axis point of light to form an image with a comet-like tail (Fig. 2.3D).

The traditional sphere and cylinder lenses can no longer correct the optical error of the eye with these HOAs. A more complex numerical description is required to capture these HOAs.

Representation of aberrations

There are many ways to describe the shape of the wavefront, as schematically illustrated in Fig. 2.4: (1) we can draw rays perpendicular to every point on the wavefront to indicate the direction of propagation; (2) if we know the direction of each ray, we know the slope of the wavefront at every point, which means we can use the mathematical process of integration to determine the wavefront shape; (3) we can describe the extra distance light rays must travel when getting to each point on the wavefront, using the pupil plane as a reference—this extra distance is called the "optical path length difference"; (4) if light travels along paths of unequal length, then the phase will be different. This is very useful mathematically because a description of the phase of light at every point in the pupil plane is a major component of a pupil function (Pr). The pupil function is the product of amplitude and phase (Pr = $P_{amp} \times P_{phase}$). The amplitude factor of the pupil function is determined by the effective pupil area. The phase portion of pupil function is derived from the wavefront error (WFE) map, where WFE is relative to the perfect spherical wavefront required to focus an image on the retina.

Zernike polynomials

To reduce the dimensionality of an aberration map, we can mathematically fit the aberration map with a relatively small number of Zernike radial polynomials and describe aberrations in terms of the coefficients of each polynomial. Fig. 2.5 shows the first four radial orders of the Zernike pyramid used to describe the eye's wave aberrations. Zernike polynomials are the preferred method of representing wavefront aberrations for a couple of reasons. They are continuously orthogonal to or independent of one another, which will allow us to multiply one polynomial by another polynomial. They are reported as a single- or double-indexing scheme. The double-index notation is preferred because it minimizes the chance for confusion. The single-index notation is handy when making some types of plots, but it does not hold nearly as much information. For example, primary SA can be described

either as Z12 in the single index notation, or as Z subscript 4 superscript 0 (Z_4^0) in double index notation (Fig. 2.5).

In overview, each color map is a specific mode in the Zernike expansion through the fourth radial order. The second radial order defines the aberrations associated with defocus and astigmatism, in ophthalmic terms, sphere, cylinder, and axis. The third-order aberrations and above are collectively referred to as the HOAs. There are an infinite number of modes. The location of each mode in the tree is designated by the combination of a radial order and an angular frequency. When referring to a specific mode, a double index system is used. The Z is short for symbolizing all Zernike modes. The subscript and superscript designate each mode. The radial order is the subscript, and the angular frequency is the superscript. For example, Z subscript 4 superscript 0 (Z_4^0) refers to term number 12 in the single index notation, which is SA. The C is shorthand for the coefficient for each mode. The Zernike coefficients reveal how much of each mode is contributing to the total WFE, and these coefficients are typically specified in microns (short for micrometers; μm), or sometimes they are reported in the units of the wavelength of the light.

One drawback of the above standard Zernike polynomials is that higher-order modes involve lower-order modes (e.g., Z_4^0 contains an r^4 term and an embedded $-r^2$ term). To avoid this confusion, Gatinel et al.[29] proposed a new polynomial decomposition method by a low-order decomposition and higher-order decomposition that separates the orthogonality between low and high orders while maintaining orthogonality.

Standard metrics of optical quality

Although the Zernike coefficients are simpler than the wavefront map for describing the whole eye's optical imperfections, they remain a complex description and cannot directly correlate with vision. Therefore, we need standard metrics to summarize the overall optical quality and to simplify the complexity of the wavefront map. In the field of refractive ophthalmology, the most used metrics are root-mean-squared (RMS) WFE, point spread function (PSF), and modulation transfer function (MTF).

RMS. Computationally, RMS is simply the square root of the variance, that is, the standard deviation of the values of the WFE over the whole pupil. The unit of RMS is microns (micrometers; μm).

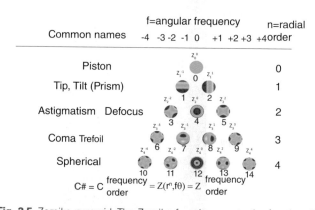

Fig. 2.5 Zernike pyramid. The Zernike functions up to the fourth radial order are represented. *n* represents the radial order and *f* the meridional frequency. Lower-order aberrations are those of the second radial order (astigmatism and defocus). Third radial order and higher are considered higher-order aberrations (HOAs). Clinically significant HOAs such as coma and trefoil are of the third radial order, and spherical aberrations are of the fourth radial order.

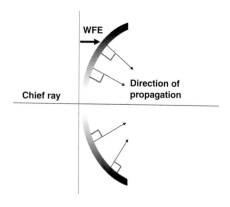

Fig. 2.4 Schematic representation of different ways to describe the shape of the wavefront. *WFE*, Wavefront error.

PSF. PSF is defined as the distribution of light intensity in the image plane for a point light source. To compute PSF, we first Fourier-transform the pupil function and then square it to get the PSF (PSF = FT $(P_r)^2$). Because the PSF is derived from the pupil function (phase × amplitude), both the pupil size and aberrations can influence the point source. The bigger the pupil and the larger the aberrations, the more irregular the shape of the point source imaged on the retina and therefore the worse the PSF (Fig. 2.6).

MTF. MTF is essentially the ratio of the image contrast to the object contrast. Fourier transformation of the PSF is known as the optical transfer function, which is composed of both MTF (the contrast attenuation) and phase transfer function (the amount of phase shift). Both modulation and phase transfer functions are spatial frequency dependent.

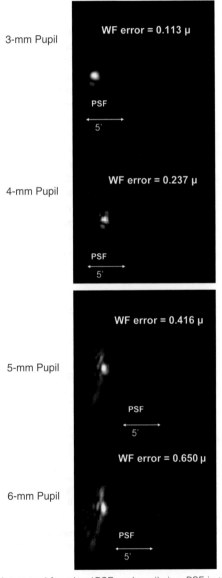

Fig. 2.6 Point spread function (*PSF*) and pupil size. PSF is the intensity with which an optical system focuses an image from a point source on the retina. Note how the blurring of the point source increases as the size of the pupil and aberration increases. *WF,* Wavefront. (Damien Gatinel, 9 – Wavefront analysis, in Azar DT. *Refractive Surgery,* 2nd ed. Mosby, 2007.)

Based on the above principal components, the team at Indiana University has developed 31 image quality metrics (i.e., area under MTF) to quantify the quality of the optical wavefront in either the pupil plane or retina plane.[30] These metrics have been widely used to compute the peak image quality and depth of focus on a variety of new intraocular lenses,[12,31–34] and in the field of myopia control and accommodation.[35,36]

THE IMPACT OF HOAs ON VISION

In the previous section we reviewed the basic concepts and fundamentals of aberrations. How much do HOAs affect human vision?

In normal eyes, wavefront aberrations are not a significant source of image quality degradation. Without correction of lower-order aberrations (sphere and astigmatism), only about 7% of RMS comes from HOAs in the normal population,[1] and 70% of these eyes have refractive error of 0.25 D or less after correction of lower-order aberrations. This is considered clinically nonsignificant because patients can tolerate 0.25 D with no noticeable perceptual difference.[37]

In contrast to normal eyes, visual quality can be significantly degraded by the elevated HOAs in some pathologic eyes; for examples, severe dry eye patients, keratoconus, and some postrefractive surgery eyes. Dry eye disease, one of the most common ocular diseases, affects over 16 million adults in the United States,[38] resulting in poor subjective[39,40] and objective[41] optical quality. Owing to the irregular tear film, SAs and coma increase about 2.5 times compared with normal controls,[42] which can be temporally improved with artificial tears.[43] In keratoconic patients, the HOAs can be 10 times higher than the normal population, predominantly due to coma and SA,[44] both of which can be significantly improved after successful treatment by crosslinking[45,46] or customized contact lens.[47] In postrefractive surgery eyes, the induction of pre-existing HOAs worsens as pupil size increases, (e.g., SA up to 1.7 microns for a 7-mm pupil).[48] The aberrated marginal optics around the edge of the ablation zone causes night vision disturbances or dysphotopsias such as "starbursts," "glare," and "halos."[49] SAs and coma are secondary effects of standard laser corneal ablations, which can be overcome with the optimized Femto-laser-assisted in situ keratomileusis (LASIK).[50]

Spherical aberration

Because primary SA is one of the most significant HOAs in humans and it has been most widely used clinically, in this section we will review the concept of SA.

As described by Snell's law, SA is generated as light refracts through any lens with a spherical surface resulting in a blur circle on the image plane. On-axis SA can be theoretically corrected with a perfect Cartesian oval[51] where all on-axis rays form an aberration-free single point on the image plane. The SA becomes positive when the surface is more spherical or oblate compared with the perfect Cartesian oval, and negative if the surface is more prolate.[51]

Unaccommodated human eyes typically have positive SA coming predominantly from the cornea, and become less positive (or more negative) during accommodation.[52] Ocular SA is general quite small for typical pupil sizes,[53] partly owing to the negative SA in the lens compensating for the positive SA in the cornea,[54] and partly because of the aspheric form of the cornea. However, SA becomes much larger with larger pupils (SA expands with fourth power of pupil), which can be up to 2.8 D more myopic peripherally compared with the paraxial for an unaccommodated eye with a fully dilated pupil.[55]

The impact of spherical aberration on vision

With the now routine control of SA levels by manipulating the wavefront profile on both IOLs and contact lenses, sometimes adding negative SA,[56–60] sometimes removing SA,[57,58,61,62] and sometimes introducing large amounts of SA to achieve multifocality,[63,64] it is important to understand the impact of SA manipulation on vision. In this section, we will review the impact of SA on refractive error, visual acuity, contrast sensitivity, depth of focus, and night vision.

Spherical aberration impact on refractive error

As mentioned, the aberration caused by distortion of light as it passes through an imperfect optical system can be expressed mathematically as polynomials. SA is typically defined in Seidel form $S_4^0 = C_4^0 \sqrt{5(6r^4)}$, which only contains the r^4 term, or Zernike form $Z_4^0 = C_4^0 \sqrt{5(6r^4 - 6r^2 + 1)}$, which contains an r^4 term and a negative r^2 term (–defocus), where C_4^0 is the Zernike coefficient of SA, and r is the radius of the pupil in mm. The key difference between the Seidel SA and Zernike SA is the embedded negative defocus term in Zernike form. Although the r^4 term is the distinguishing feature of the primary SA, without removing the $-r^2$ term, Zernike SA primary effect on refractive error is caused by the lower-order r^2 term embedded in this polynomial. For example, by adding positive Zernike SA $(+Z_4^0)$, refractive error becomes hyperopic due to the $-r^2$. On the other hand, after adding the C_2^0 (r^2 term) to achieve paraxial focus, Seidel SA effect on refractive error is caused by the higher-order r^4 term, that is, by adding positive Seidel SA $(+S_4^0)$, refractive error becomes myopic due to the $+r^4$ term. In the presence of positive Seidel SA, however, this myopic shift is mostly observed when viewing stimuli containing low spatial frequencies (e.g., contrast sensitivity charts with 2 cycles per degree grating stimuli). On the other hand, subjective refractions with high spatial frequency stimuli (e.g., high-contrast visual acuity charts) remain unchanged as the pupil expands.[65] Clinical refractions using the "darker" criterion ("Lens #1 vs. #2, which one makes the letter darker to you?") bias the patient to use lower spatial frequencies and thus prone to myopic bias, as most of unaccommodated human eyes have positive SA.[52] On the contrary, the "sharper" criterion ("Lens #1 vs. #2, which one is sharper to you?") favors the patient to use high spatial frequencies and generates reliable refractions that are minimally affected by the pupil size and the level of SAs.[66]

Spherical aberration impact on visual acuity

In general, correcting aberrations with adaptive optics (a technology that uses deformable mirrors to correct aberrations) improves visual acuity by 0.1 logMAR relative to subjective distance refraction, and human eyes can tolerate up to 0.1 microns of RMS without noticeable blurry vision.[67] However, by adding more Zernike SAs, visual acuity can be significantly affected even for high-contrast letters at photopic light level (retinal illuminance >50 Troland[68,69]). In general, detrimental impacts of Zernike SA on visual acuity varies from 0.3 logMAR/microns of SA to 0.8 logMAR/microns of SA.[67,70] After removing the r^2 term by adding C_2^0 (Seidel SA), the impact of Seidel SA on visual acuity is much smaller.[71,72] For low-contrast letters, visual acuity is on average 0.2 logMAR worse than high-contrast visual acuity for a given SA.[73]

Spherical aberration impact on contrast sensitivity

At photopic light levels, contrast sensitivity is maximal when aberrations are removed via adaptive optics, and contrast sensitivity decreases in the presence of SA.[74] Similar reduction in contrast sensitivity is seen for the *spherical* Sensar AR40e IOL compared with the *aspheric* Tecnis Z9000 IOL.[75] In post photorefractive keratectomy (PRK) eyes with significant amount of SAs, contrast sensitivity is much worse compared with the emmetropic control, especially at low light levels.[76] The reduced image contrast is presumably caused by the increased SA associated with larger pupils at low luminance levels.

Spherical aberration impact on night vision

Patients with high ocular aberrations routinely complain of vision disturbance (e.g., halos, starbursts) while driving at night. Studies from Xu et al.[77] showed that the starburst or halo size (in degrees) linearly correlates with the amount of SA (in microns) with a slope of 1.5 degrees/microns of SA for a fixed 7-mm pupil, a typical mesopic pupil size for the middle-aged population.[78] They also showed that focusing near the pupil margin minimizes starburst size, but a typical subjective refraction focuses a near paraxial region of the pupil;[65] therefore, starbursts exist in most eyes, especially those eyes with large amounts of SA. Also, significant positive SA generates myopic shift in refractive state when viewing high-contrast point sources at night[79]; this is commonly known as night myopia.[80]

Spherical aberration impact on depth of focus

Depth of focus (DOF) simply means the dioptric distance between the closest image and farthest image of an object that appears acceptably focused. There's no universal definition of DOF, and therefore the amount of DOF reported in the literature varies with the criteria used to define DOF. By convention, DOF can be defined by objective (e.g., the dioptric range over which a specific image quality exceeds certain criteria) or subjective criteria (e.g., the dioptric range over which visual acuity or contrast sensitivity meets a certain criterion level), both of which can be further grouped as relative (e.g., 50% of peak image quality) or absolute (e.g., 20/40 visual acuity). Although both primary (Z_4^0) and secondary SA (Z_6^0) can produce the double-peaked through-focus curves characteristic of true bifocals, this expansion of DOF is mostly absent if a strict image quality criterion is applied. The expansion of DOF observed with a low-image-quality criterion when opposite sign Z_4^0 and Z_6^0 are combined because of the elevated r^4 term. Although multifocality can be generated by adding primary SA alone or by adding opposite sign of Z_4^0 and Z_6^0, the former is more effective than the latter.[32]

TREATMENTS TO ALLEVIATE THE IMPACT OF HOAs

Fundamentally, there are two ways to alleviate the impact of HOAs on vision, either through manipulating the pupil amplitude function or via the phase function.

Reducing pupil size

Mathematically, Schwiegerling proved that Zernike polynomials scale to the power of their radial orders as pupil sizes change.[81] For example, 0.4 microns of SA (C_4^0) with a 6-mm diameter pupil will reduce to 0.4 × $(3/6)^4$ = 0.025 microns with a 3-mm diameter pupil. Clinically, reducing the impact of HOAs via reducing pupil size can be achieved with pinhole glasses,[82] contact lenses containing small artificial pupils,[49,83] miotic ophthalmic solutions,[84,85] or diaphragm IOLs.[86] All of these have proven successful at reducing night vision disturbance in highly aberrated eyes.

What is the optimal pupil size to minimize aberration effects associated with large pupils? This question becomes particularly interesting nowadays due to the ongoing development of multiple miotics as a treatment for presbyopia.[87,88] The traditional optical model taught us that a pupil size between 2 and 3 mm is optimal as a counterbalance between diffraction and aberration effects.[89] However, this is only true under photopic light levels (where Weber's law applies, meaning contrast sensitivity is unaffected by retinal illuminance[90]) and for a well-focused eye with average levels of ocular aberrations. The optimal pupil size is determined by the interactions between diffraction, amount of aberration, and photon noise effect.[91] As a result, a smaller pupil (e.g., <2 mm) is optimal in the presence of significant lower-order aberrations or HOAs at high light levels, while a larger pupil (e.g., >3 mm) is optimal at mesopic light levels, and the exact size depends on the amount of aberration and/or retinal illuminance.[92,93]

Reducing phase function from HOAs

Correcting HOAs with spectacles, contact lenses, and intraocular lenses

Spectacles. For wavefront-customized spectacles to work, they would have to be stable enough to not decenter with head movements, and they would have to be designed in such a way that the aberrations would be corrected in all fields of gaze and at different pupil sizes. Ophthonix, Inc. (Vista, CA) has designed a lens available for commercial use that consists of a three-layer structure with a refractive index of 1.6. The middle layer consists of a patented photopolymer in between two coated lenses. The lens corrects HOAs from the second to sixth order using wavefront-guided technology that corrects aberrations based on measurements from a built-in aberrometer.

Contact lenses. The use of customized contact lenses to correct HOAs is also possible.[94] There are rigid gas permeable (RGP) and soft contact lenses. In a clinical setting, RGP lenses are helpful in correcting refractive errors in highly irregular corneas. The smooth contour of their anterior and posterior curvatures, coupled with the tear film formed within the interface, provides a new refracting surface for the eye. These lenses are designed to move freely, reaching up to 1 mm of decentration from the visual axis of the eye with every blink,[95] which makes RGP lenses unable to correct HOAs, owing to decentration. Soft contact lenses, however, are much more stable and less likely to undergo misalignment relative to the visual axis. These lenses rotate less than 5 degrees with every blink, which is ideal for HOA correction because coma and astigmatism are tolerant to misrotations of up to 60 degrees.[96]

IOLs. Unlike young eyes in which the negative SA produced by the lens can compensate for the positive SA from the cornea, old eyes and pseudophakic eyes with spherical IOLs have significant positive SAs,[97] which has led to the dominance of aspheric IOLs. There are generally two types of aspheric IOLs: one with negative SAs and one with zero aberrations (aberration-free). The total aberration of a pseudophakic eye is the sum of the cornea aberration and the aberration from the inserted IOLs. Aspherical IOLs with *negative* SA are intended to neutralize the inherent positive SA of the cornea to achieve postoperatively aberration-free vision.[98] Because SA can expand DOF, sometimes aspherical *aberration-free* IOLs are used to preserve the inherent aberrations of the cornea to expand DOF.[99]

Some commercially available aspherical IOLs, such as the Tecnis-Z9000 (Pfizer, New York, NY) and SN60WF (Alcon, Fort Worth, TX), are designed with a prolate anterior surface, hence the term *aspheric*, and have the same radius of curvature at every point on the surface. The benefit of aspheric IOLs depends largely on their centration and stability within the capsular bag. The US Food and Drug Administration (FDA) approved the light adjustable IOL in 2017, which, once implanted in the eye, can be tuned to compensate for residual refractive errors, and even HOAs by irradiating the optic with blue light to polymerize monomers, setting up a diffusion gradient to alter lens shape.[100,101]

Corneal ablations

How can ablating cornea correct ocular aberrations? Let us start with lower-order aberration correction (e.g., myopia as an example). Myopia happens when an image focuses in front of the retina. LASIK can reshape the myopic cornea by flattening the central cornea so that the image can sharply focus on the retina. Similarly, to correct the HOAs, the preoperative and/or intraoperative aberrations can be measured using an aberrometer. Then this measured aberration profile can be loaded into a computerized laser system to generate a precise ablating profile that compensates for the pre-existing aberrations. For example, an eye with +0.2 microns of SA preoperatively requires induction of –0.2 microns of SA with corneal ablation to achieve postoperatively aberration-free vision.

The main focus of laser refractive surgery nowadays is to not only correct refractive errors such as defocus (myopia or hyperopia) and astigmatism, but to create customized ablations that compensate for induced HOAs (optimized ablation) and also correct pre-existing aberrations (customized ablation). There are several laser platforms utilized for corneal ablations. These range from the simple conventional treatments to the more sophisticated topographical guided and wavefront-customized ablations. Differences in these treatment modalities lie in the type of beam delivery, spot size, treatment zone, and amount of tissue ablated for each diopter of refractive error treated. For the purpose of this chapter, we will only discuss wavefront-customized corneal ablations.

There are two types of wavefront-customized ablations: wavefront-guided ablations[102] and wavefront-optimized ablations,[103] both of which aim to correct for HOAs in the eye. In wavefront-guided ablations, the treatment is aimed to correct HOAs that exist preoperatively. The wavefront-optimized ablations profile corrects expected HOAs for an average eye and those that are anticipated as a result of the surgery. Therefore, unlike wavefront-optimized ablations, which apply population-based mean aberration levels to individual eye, wavefront-guided ablations may be better at correcting eyes with extremely high preoperative HOAs. Consistently, studies[104] found that wavefront-guided ablations induced fewer HOAs and had better contrast sensitivity after surgery than wavefront-optimized ablations. However, a recent study showed that owing to the intraoperative induction of HOAs especially associated with LASIK, the beneficial effect of wavefront-guided ablations was mainly found in PRK-treated eyes, not LASIK-treated eyes.[102]

WAVEFRONT SENSING

In the previous sections, we explained the concepts of optical aberrations and their impact on human eyes. In this section, we will review how we measure these aberrations in both laboratory and clinic settings.

Evolution of aberrometers

Wavefront sensing is a technique originally developed by astronomers to improve their vision to see stars in space. In the 1600s a German astronomer, Christopher Scheiner, set the stage for modern aberrometry and wavefront-sensing devices with the invention of the Scheiner disc. He reasoned that an optically imperfect eye would form two separate images on the retina when looking at a distant light source through a disc containing two pinholes (Fig. 2.7). If the eye's imperfection is a simple case of defocus,

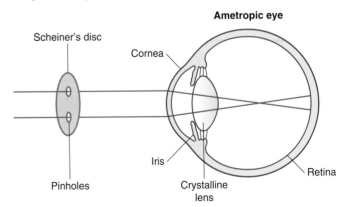

Fig. 2.7 Scheiner's disc. An ametropic eye forms two separate retinal images when viewing a distant light source through a disc with two pinholes.

then the double retinal images can be brought into register by viewing through a spectacle lens of the appropriate power. However, if a simple lens cannot bring the two retinal images into coincidence, a more complex device is needed for quantifying the imperfection.

In 1895 Tscherning[105] developed an instrument to measure aberrations of the eye consisting of a grid with lots of holes (vs. two holes in the Scheiner disc), which allowed him to measure multiple rays simultaneously. However, the resolution of these fundus images was poor due to the low light levels and aberrations of the eye. This eventually led to the invention of the Shack-Hartmann aberrometer, in which the pinholes were removed and replaced with small lenslets that allow more light into the eye, making the device more sensitive. The modern Shack-Hartmann technique was first introduced into the field of vision science by Liang and Williams[106] at Manchester University.

How does the Shack-Hartmann aberrometer work?

The shape of the aberrated wavefront is a fundamental description of the optical quality of the eye called the "wavefront aberration function." This function lies at the heart of a rich optical theory that allows us to calculate the retinal image of any object, to assess the quality of that retinal image quantitatively, and ultimately to predict visual performance on visual tasks.

However, to apply this wonderful optical theory we need to analyze the wavefront as soon as it passes through the eye's pupil. To do this, we use a pair of relay lenses which focus the lenslet array onto the pupil of the eye. Optically, then, the lenslet array appears to reside inside the eye, right in the pupil plane where it can subdivide the reflected wavefront immediately as it emerges from the eye's pupil. This final configuration is the basic form of the modern Hartmann-Shack aberrometer described by Liang in 1994 (Fig. 2.8).

For a perfect eye, the reflected plane wave will be focused into a perfect lattice of point images, each image falling on the optical axis of the corresponding lenslet (Fig. 2.9A). By contrast, the aberrated eye reflects a distorted wavefront. The local slope of the wavefront is now

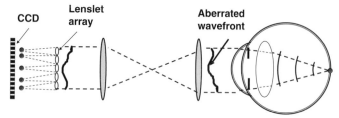

Fig. 2.8 The Shack-Hartmann sensor. Light is reflected on the retina from a point source, and the emerging wave from the eye is transmitted through an array of lenslets that focus the wavefront on a charge-coupled device (CCD) device and processed in a computer to produce a two-dimensional image. (Thibos LN, Applegate R. Assessment of optical quality. In: MacRae SM, Krueger RR, Applegate RA, eds. *Customized Corneal Ablation: The Quest for Super Vision.* Thorofare, NJ: Slack; 2001:67–78.)

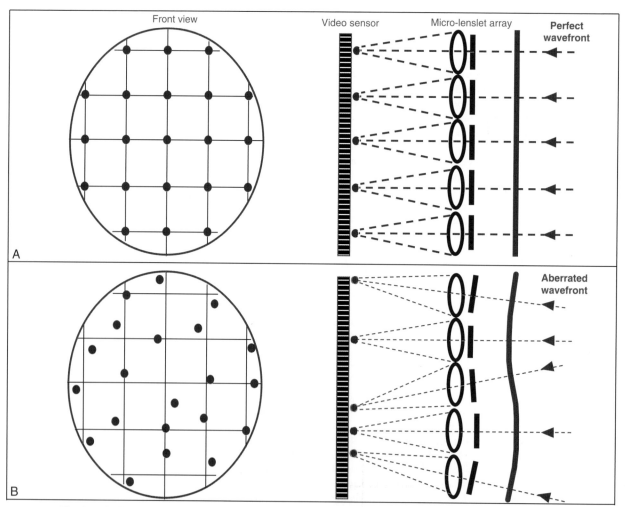

Fig. 2.9 (**A**) For a perfect eye the reflected plane wave focuses into a perfect lattice of point images, each image falling on the optical axis of the corresponding lenslet. (**B**) The aberrated eye reflects a distorted wavefront. (Thibos LN, Applegate R. Assessment of optical quality. In: MacRae SM, Krueger RR, Applegate RA, eds. *Customized Corneal Ablation: The Quest for Super Vision.* Thorofare, NJ: Slack; 2001:67–78.)

different for each lenslet, and therefore the wavefront will be focused into a disordered collection of spot images. By analyzing the displacement of each spot from its corresponding lenslet axis, we can deduce the slope of the aberrated wavefront when it entered the corresponding lenslet. Mathematical integration of this slope information yields the shape of the aberrated wavefront (Fig. 2.9B).

Wavefront-sensing devices

There are multiple wavefront-sensing devices commercially available thanks to the recent increase in demand for customized laser refractive surgery. Clinical aberrometers can be grouped into four categories:

1. Hartman-Shack systems: Alcon, Visx—Wavescan, Bausch & Lomb—Zywave, Meditec, Schwind, Topcon—Wavefront Analyzer, Wavefront Sciences—COAS, Johnson & Johnson Vision—COAS-HD (no longer being manufactured), and Zeiss-Meditec—Asclepion WASCA.

2. Tscherning / ray-tracing systems: Schwind—ORK Wavefront Aberrometer, Lumenis/WaveLight—Wavefront Aberrometer, Tracey—Refractometer, and Interwave—Interwave Scanner.

3. Dynamic skiascopy systems: Nidek (Nidek OPD) uses a mechanism to measure aberrations called slit skiascopy,[107] in which a slit of light scans the eye along different axes. Photodetectors then determine the timing and scan rate of the light reflected to construct the wavefront.

4. A newly developed pyramidal wavefront sensor-based aberrometer, Osiris by Costruzione Strumenti Oftalmici (Firenze, Italy), with high sampling density of 41 microns, and wide dynamic with a frame rate of up to 33 images per second.[108]

In conclusion, the "Quest for Super-Vision," as described by Drs. Applegate and Thibos[109] in the field of wavefront technology, holds a promising and exciting future. In the last decade, significant contributions to the field have been made and continue to flourish. The clinician must be aware of these rapid changes to provide patients with state-of-the-art technology to improve their quality of vision and life. Currently, there is no perfect way to treat HOAs. Both small pupils and customized corneal ablations offer a stable form of HOA correction, and the industry is working diligently at developing miotic drops and perfecting customized lenses.

REFERENCES

1. Porter J, Guirao A, Cox IG, Williams DR. Monochromatic aberrations of the human eye in a large population. *J Opt Soc Am A Opt Image Sci Vis.* 2001;18:1793–1803.
2. Liang J, Williams DR, Miller DT. Supernormal vision and high-resolution retinal imaging through adaptive optics. *J Opt Soc Am A Opt Image Sci Vis.* 1997;14:2884–2892.
3. Liu Z, Kurokawa K, Zhang F, Lee JJ, Miller DT. Imaging and quantifying ganglion cells and other transparent neurons in the living human retina. *Proc Natl Acad Sci U S A.* 2017;114:12803–12808.
4. King BJ, Burns SA, Sapoznik KA, Luo T, Gast TJ. High-resolution, adaptive optics imaging of the human trabecular meshwork in vivo. *Transl Vis Sci Technol.* 2019;8:5.
5. Atchison DA, Thibos LN. Optical models of the human eye. *Clin Exp Optom.* 2016;99:99–106.
6. Thibos LN, Bradley A, Still DL, Zhang X, Howarth PA. Theory and measurement of ocular chromatic aberration. *Vision research.* 1990;30:33–49.
7. Thibos LN, Ye M, Zhang X, Bradley A. The chromatic eye: A new reduced-eye model of ocular chromatic aberration in humans. *Appl Opt.* 1992;31:3594–3600.
8. Bradley A. Glenn A. Fry Award Lecture 1991: perceptual manifestations of imperfect optics in the human eye: attempts to correct for ocular chromatic aberration. *Optom Vis Sci.* 1992;69:515–521.
9. Yoon GY, Williams DR. Visual performance after correcting the monochromatic and chromatic aberrations of the eye. *J Opt Soc Am A Opt Image Sci Vis.* 2002;19:266–275.
10. Ravikumar S, Thibos LN, Bradley A. Calculation of retinal image quality for polychromatic light. *Journal of the Optical Society of America. A, Optics, image science, and vision.* 2008;25:2395–2407.
11. Mallen EA, Gilmartin B, Wolffsohn JS, Tsujimura S. Clinical evaluation of the Shin-Nippon SRW-5000 autorefractor in adults: an update. *Ophthalmic Physiol Opt.* 2015;35:622–627.
12. Bradley A, Xu R, Wang H, Jaskulski M, Hong X, Brink N, Van Noy S. The impact of IOL Abbe number on polychromatic image quality of pseudophakic eyes. *Clin Ophthalmol.* 2020;14:2271–2281.
13. Simpson MJ. Diffractive multifocal intraocular lens image quality. *Appl Opt.* 1992;31:3621–3626.
14. Mojzis P, Kukuckova L, Majerova K, Liehneova K, Piñero DP. Comparative analysis of the visual performance after cataract surgery with implantation of a bifocal or trifocal diffractive IOL. *J Refract Surg.* 2014;30:666–672.
15. Atchison DA, Thibos LN. Diffractive properties of the Diffrax bifocal contact lens. *Ophthalmic Physiol Opt.* 1993;13:186–188.
16. Langenbucher A, Goebels S, Szentmáry N, Seitz B, Eppig T. Vignetting and field of view with the KAMRA corneal inlay. *BioMed research international.* 2013;2013:154593.
17. Escudero-Sanz I, Navarro R. Off-axis aberrations of a wide-angle schematic eye model. *Journal of the Optical Society of America A-Optics Image Science and Vision.* 1999;16:1881–1891.
18. Atchison DA, Jones CE, Schmid KL, Pritchard N, Pope JM, Strugnell WE, Riley RA. Eye shape in emmetropia and myopia. *Invest Ophthalmol Vis Sci.* 2004;45:3380–3386.
19. Atchison DA, Pritchard N, Schmid KL, Scott DH, Jones CE, Pope JM. Shape of the retinal surface in emmetropia and myopia. *Invest Ophth Vis Sci.* 2005;46:2698–2707.
20. Atchison DA. The Glenn A. Fry Award Lecture 2011: Peripheral optics of the human eye. *Optom Vis Sci.* 2012;89:E954–E966.
21. Atchison DA, Scott DH. Monochromatic aberrations of human eyes in the horizontal visual field. *J Opt Soc Am A Opt Image Sci Vis.* 2002;19:2180–2184.
22. Liu T, Thibos LN. Customized models of ocular aberrations across the visual field during accommodation. *J Vis.* 2019;19:13.
23. Charman WN, Mathur A, Scott DH, Hartwig A, Atchison DA. Specifying peripheral aberrations in visual science. *J Biomed Opt.* 2012;17:025004.
24. Wang B, Ciuffreda KJ. Depth-of-focus of the human eye in the near retinal periphery. *Vision Research.* 2004;44:1115–1125.
25. Smith EL III, Kee C-S, Ramamirtham R, Qiao-Grider Y, Hung L-F. Peripheral vision can influence eye growth and refractive development in infant monkeys. *Invest Ophthalmol Vis Sci.* 2005;46:3965–3972.
26. Benavente-Perez A, Nour A, Troilo D. Short interruptions of imposed hyperopic defocus earlier in treatment are more effective at preventing myopia development. *Sci Rep.* 2019;9:11459.
27. Berntsen DA, Kramer CE. Peripheral defocus with spherical and multifocal soft contact lenses. *Optom Vis Sci.* 2013;90:1215–1224.
28. Jiang BC, Bussa S, Tea YC, Seger K. Optimal dioptric value of near addition lenses intended to slow myopic progression. *Optom Vis Sci.* 2008;85:1100–1105.
29. Gatinel D, Malet J, Dumas L. Polynomial decomposition method for ocular wavefront analysis. *J Opt Soc Am A Opt Image Sci Vis.* 2018;35:2035–2045.
30. Applegate RA, Marsack JD, Thibos LN. Metrics of retinal image quality predict visual performance in eyes with 20/17 or better visual acuity. *Optom Vis Sci.* 2006;83:635–640.
31. Bradley A, Nam J, Xu R, Harman L, Thibos L. Impact of contact lens zone geometry and ocular optics on bifocal retinal image quality. *Ophthalmic Physiol Opt.* 2014;34:331–345.
32. Xu R, Bradley A, López Gil N, Thibos LN. Modelling the effects of secondary spherical aberration on refractive error, image quality and depth of focus. *Ophthalmic Physiol Opt.* 2015;35:28–38.
33. Xu R, Wang H, Jaskulski M, Kollbaum P, Bradley A. Small-pupil versus multifocal strategies for expanding depth of focus of presbyopic eyes. *J Cataract Refract Surg.* 2019;45:647–655.
34. Artal P, Marcos S, Navarro R, Miranda I, Ferro M. Through focus image quality of eyes implanted with monofocal and multifocal intraocular lenses. *Opt Eng.* 1995;34:772–779.
35. Altoaimi BH, Almutairi MS, Kollbaum PS, Bradley A. Accommodative behavior of young eyes wearing multifocal contact lenses. *Optom Vis Sci.* 2018;95:416–427.
36. López-Gil N, Martin J, Liu T, Bradley A, Díaz-Muñoz D, Thibos LN. Retinal image quality during accommodation. *Ophthalmic Physiol Opt.* 2013;33:497–507.
37. Atchison DA, Fisher SW, Pedersen CA, Ridall PG. Noticeable, troublesome and objectionable limits of blur. *Vision Research.* 2005;45:1967–1974.
38. Farrand KF, Fridman M, Stillman IO, Schaumberg DA. Prevalence of diagnosed dry eye disease in the United States among adults aged 18 years and older. *Am J Ophthalmol.* 2017;182:90–98.
39. Herbaut A, Liang H, Rabut G, Trinh L, Kessal K, Baudouin C, Labbe A. Impact of dry eye disease on vision quality: An optical quality analysis system study. *Transl Vis Sci Technol.* 2018;7:5.
40. Uchino M, Schaumberg DA. Dry eye disease: Impact on quality of life and vision. *Curr Ophthalmol Rep.* 2013;1:51–57.
41. Koh S, Maeda N, Kuroda T, et al. Effect of tear film break-up on higher-order aberrations measured with wavefront sensor. *Am J Ophthalmol.* 2002;134:115–117.
42. Montes-Mico R, Caliz A, Alio JL. Wavefront analysis of higher order aberrations in dry eye patients. *J Refract Surg.* 2004;20:243–247.
43. Lu N, Lin F, Huang Z, He Q, Han W. Changes of corneal wavefront aberrations in dry eye patients after treatment with artificial lubricant drops. *J Ophthalmol.* 2016; 2016:1342056.
44. Colak HN, Kantarci FA, Yildirim A, Tatar MG, Goker H, Uslu H, Gurler B. Comparison of corneal topographic measurements and high order aberrations in keratoconus and normal eyes. *Cont Lens Anterior Eye.* 2016;39:380–384.
45. Iselin KC, Baenninger PB, Bachmann LM, Bochmann F, Thiel MA, Kaufmann C. Changes in higher order aberrations after central corneal regularization - a comparative two-year analysis of a semi-automated topography-guided photorefractive keratectomy combined with corneal cross-linking. *Eye Vis (Lond).* 2020;7:10.
46. Kosekahya P, Koc M, Tekin K, et al. Evaluation of the shifting of the line of sight and higher order aberrations of eyes with keratoconus after corneal cross-linking. *Cont Lens Anterior Eye.* 2017;40:311–317.
47. Katsoulos C, Karageorgiadis L, Vasileiou N, Mousafeiropoulos T, Asimellis G. Customized hydrogel contact lenses for keratoconus incorporating correction for vertical coma aberration. *Ophthalmic Physiol Opt.* 2009;29:321–329.
48. Fang L, Wang Y, He X. Effect of pupil size on residual wavefront aberration with transition zone after customized laser refractive surgery. *Optics express.* 2013;21:1404–1416.
49. Villa C, Gutiérrez R, Jiménez JR, González-Méijome JM. Night vision disturbances after successful LASIK surgery. *British Journal of Ophthalmology.* 2007;91:1031–1037.

50. Au JD, Krueger RR. Optimized femto-LASIK maintains preexisting spherical aberration independent of refractive error. *J Refract Surg.* 2012;28:S821–S825.
51. Calossi A. Corneal asphericity and spherical aberration. *J Refract Surg.* 2007;23:505–514.
52. López-Gil N, Fernández-Sánchez V. The change of spherical aberration during accommodation and its effect on the accommodation response. *Journal of Vision.* 2010;10:12.
53. Thibos LN, Bradley A, Hong X. A statistical model of the aberration structure of normal, well-corrected eyes. *Ophthalmic Physiol Opt.* 2002;22:427–433.
54. Artal P, Guirao A, Berrio E, Piers P, Norrby S. Optical aberrations and the aging eye. *International Ophthalmology Clinics.* 2003;43:63–77.
55. Thibos LN, Ye M, Zhang X, Bradley A. Spherical aberration of the reduced schematic eye with elliptical refracting surface. *Optom Vis Sci.* 1997;74:548–556.
56. Toto L, Falconio G, Vecchiarino L, et al. Visual performance and biocompatibility of 2 multifocal diffractive IOLs: Six-month comparative study. *J Cataract Refract Surg.* 2007;33:1419–1425.
57. Pepose JS, Wang D, Altmann GE. Comparison of through-focus image quality across five presbyopia-correcting intraocular lenses (an American Ophthalmological Society thesis). *Transactions of the American Ophthalmological Society.* 2011;109:221–231.
58. McKelvie J, McArdle B, McGhee C. The influence of tilt, decentration, and pupil size on the higher-order aberration profile of aspheric intraocular lenses. *Ophthalmology.* 2011;118:1724–1731.
59. Lindskoog Pettersson A, Mårtensson L, Salkic J, Unsbo P, Brautaset R. Spherical aberration in relation to visual performance in contact lens wear. *Cont Lens Anterior Eye.* 2011;34:12–16. quiz 50–11.
60. Gifford P, Cannon T, Lee C, Lee D, Lee HF, Swarbrick HA. Ocular aberrations and visual function with multifocal versus single vision soft contact lenses. *Cont Lens Anterior Eye.* 2013;36:66–73. quiz 103–104.
61. Denoyer A, Denoyer L, Halfon J, Majzoub S, Pisella PJ. Comparative study of aspheric intraocular lenses with negative spherical aberration or no aberration. *J Cataract Refract Surg.* 2009;35:496–503.
62. De Brabander J, Chateau N, Bouchard F, Guidollet S. Contrast sensitivity with soft contact lenses compensated for spherical aberration in high ametropia. *Optom Vis Sci.* 1998;75:37–43.
63. Plainis S, Ntzilepis G, Atchison DA, Charman WN. Through-focus performance with multifocal contact lenses: Effect of binocularity, pupil diameter and inherent ocular aberrations. *Ophthalmic Physiol Opt.* 2013;33:42–50.
64. Plakitsi A, Charman WN. Ocular spherical aberration and theoretical through-focus modulation transfer functions calculated for eyes fitted with two types of varifocal presbyopic contact lens. *Cont Lens Anterior Eye.* 1997;20:97–106.
65. Xu R, Bradley A, Thibos LN. Impact of primary spherical aberration, spatial frequency and Stiles Crawford apodization on wavefront determined refractive error: A computational study. *Ophthalmic Physiol Opt.* 2013;33:444–455.
66. Bradley A, Xu R, Thibos L, Marin G, Hernandez M. Influence of spherical aberration, stimulus spatial frequency, and pupil apodisation on subjective refractions. *Ophthalmic Physiol Opt.* 2014;34:309–320.
67. Rocha KM, Soriano ES, Chamon W, Chalita MR, Nose W. Spherical aberration and depth of focus in eyes implanted with aspheric and spherical intraocular lenses: A prospective randomized study. *Ophthalmology.* 2007;114:2050–2054.
68. Stockman A, Sharpe LT. Into the twilight zone: the complexities of mesopic vision and luminous efficiency. *Ophthalmic Physiol Opt.* 2006;26:225–239.
69. Xu R, Gil D, Dibas M, Hare W, Bradley A. The effect of light level and small pupils on presbyopic reading performance. *Invest Ophthalmol Vis Sci.* 2016;57:5656–5664.
70. Yi F, Iskander DR, Collins M. Depth of focus and visual acuity with primary and secondary spherical aberration. *Vision Research.* 2011;51:1648–1658.
71. Cheng X, Bradley A, Ravikumar S, Thibos LN. Visual impact of Zernike and Seidel forms of monochromatic aberrations. *Optom Vis Sci.* 2010;87:300–312.
72. Applegate RA, Marsack JD, Ramos R, Sarver EJ. Interaction between aberrations to improve or reduce visual performance. *J Cataract Refract Surg.* 2003;29:1487–1495.
73. Li J, Xiong Y, Wang N, et al. Effects of spherical aberration on visual acuity at different contrasts. *J Cataract Refract Surg.* 2009;35:1389–1395.
74. Piers PA, Fernandez EJ, Manzanera S, Norrby S, Artal P. Adaptive optics simulation of intraocular lenses with modified spherical aberration. *Invest Ophthalmol Vis Sci.* 2004;45:4601–4610.
75. Packer M, Fine IH, Hoffman RS, Piers PA. Improved functional vision with a modified prolate intraocular lens. *J Cataract Refract Surg.* 2004;30:986–992.
76. Montes-Mico R, Charman WN. Mesopic contrast sensitivity function after excimer laser photorefractive keratectomy. *J Refract Surg.* 2002;18:9–13.
77. Xu R, Kollbaum P, Thibos L, López-Gil N, Bradley A. Reducing starbursts in highly aberrated eyes with pupil miosis. *Ophthalmic Physiol Opt.* 2018;38:26–36.
78. Winn B, Whitaker D, Elliott DB, Phillips NJ. Factors affecting light-adapted pupil size in normal human subjects. *Invest Ophthalmol Vis Sci.* 1994;35:1132–1137.
79. Marin-Franch I, Xu R, Bradley A, Thibos LN, López-Gil N. The effect of spherical aberration on visual performance and refractive state for stimuli and tasks typical of night viewing. *Journal of Optometry.* 2018;11:144–152.
80. Levene JR. Nevil Maskelyne and the discovery of night myopia. *Notes and Records of the Royal Society of London.* 1965;20:100–108.
81. Schwiegerling J. Scaling pseudo-Zernike expansion coefficients to different pupil sizes. *Opt Lett.* 2011;36:3076–3078.
82. Kim WS, Park IK, Chun YS. Quantitative analysis of functional changes caused by pinhole glasses. *Invest Ophthalmol Vis Sci.* 2014;55:6679–6685.
83. Freeman E. Pinhole contact lenses. *American Journal of Optometry and Archives of American Academy of Optometry.* 1952;29:347–352.
84. O'Brart DP, Lohmann CP, Fitzke FW, Smith SE, Kerr-Muir MG, Marshall J. Night vision after excimer laser photorefractive keratectomy: haze and halos. *European journal of ophthalmology.* 1994;4:43–51.
85. Randazzo A, Nizzola F, Rossetti L, Orzalesi N, Vinciguerra P. Pharmacological management of night vision disturbances after refractive surgery: Results of a randomized clinical trial. *J Cataract Refract Surg.* 2005;31:1764–1772.
86. Muñoz G, Rohrweck S, Sakla HF, Altroudi W. Pinhole iris-fixated intraocular lens for dysphotopsia and photophobia. *J Cataract Refract Surg.* 2015;41:487–491.
87. Abdelkader A. Improved presbyopic vision with miotics. *Eye & Contact Lens.* 2015;41:323–327.
88. Xu R, Gil D, Dibas M, et al. Time-course of the visual Impact on presbyopes of a low dose miotic. *Ophthalmic Physiol Opt.* 2021;41:73–83.
89. Campbell FW, Gregory AH. Effect of size of pupil on visual acuity. *Nature.* 1960;187:1121–1123.
90. Van Nes FL, Bouman MA. Spatial modulation transfer in the human eye. *Journal of the Optical Society of America.* 1967;57:401–406.
91. Xu R, Wang H, Thibos LN, Bradley A. Interaction of aberrations, diffraction, and quantal fluctuations determine the impact of pupil size on visual quality. *J Opt Soc Am A Opt Image Sci Vis.* 2017;34:481–492.
92. Xu R, Thibos L, Bradley A. Effect of Target Luminance on Optimum Pupil Diameter for Presbyopic Eyes. *Optom Vis Sci.* 2016;93:1409–1419.
93. J. Pepose and R. Xu, What is the optimal pupil size?, *Cataract & Refractive Surgery Today* (2022).
94. Chen M, Sabesan R, Ahmad K, Yoon G. Correcting anterior corneal aberration and variability of lens movements in keratoconic eyes with back-surface customized soft contact lenses. *Opt Lett.* 2007;32:3203–3205.
95. Knoll HA, Conway HD. Analysis of blink-induced vertical motion of contact lenses. *Am J Optom Physiol Opt.* 1987;64:153–155.
96. Guirao A, Williams DR, Cox IG. Effect of rotation and translation on the expected benefit of an ideal method to correct the eye's higher-order aberrations. *J Opt Soc Am A Opt Image Sci Vis.* 2001;18:1003–1015.
97. Holladay JT, Van Dijk H, Lang A, et al. Optical performance of multifocal intraocular lenses. *J Cataract Refract Surg.* 1990;16:413–422.
98. Holladay JT, Piers PA, Koranyi G, van der Mooren M, Norrby NES. A new intraocular lens design to reduce spherical aberration of pseudophakic eyes. *Journal of Refractive Surgery.* 2002;18:683–691.
99. Madrid-Costa D, Ruiz-Alcocer J, Ferrer-Blasco T, García-Lázaro S, Montés Micó R. *In vitro* optical performance of a new aberration-free intraocular lens. *Eye (Lond).* 2014;28:614–620.
100. Moshirfar M, Duong AA, Shmunes KM, Castillo-Ronquillo YS, Hoopes PC. Light adjustable intraocular lens for cataract surgery after radial keratotomy. *J Refract Surg.* 2020;36:852–854.
101. Patnaik JL, Kahook MY. Long-term follow-up and clinical evaluation of the light-adjustable intraocular lens implanted after cataract removal: 7-year results. *J Cataract Refract Surg.* 2020;46:929.
102. Russo A, Filini O, Salvalai C, et al. Two-year changes in corneal spherical aberration after laser-assisted in situ keratomileusis and photorefractive keratectomy in regular and wavefront-guided ablations. *Ophthalmol Ther.* 2021;10:1003–1014.
103. Smadja D, Santhiago MR, Mello GR, Touboul D, Mrochen M, Krueger RR. Corneal higher order aberrations after myopic wavefront-optimized ablation. *J Refract Surg.* 2013;29:42–48.
104. Padmanabhan P, Mrochen M, Basuthkar S, Viswanathan D, Joseph R. Wavefront-guided versus wavefront-optimized laser in situ keratomileusis: Contralateral comparative study. *J Cataract Refract Surg.* 2008;34:389–397.
105. Tscherning M, Weiland C (translation). *Physiologic Optics.* Philadelphia, PA: Keystone; 1900.
106. Liang J, Grimm B, Goelz S, Bille JF. Objective measurement of wave aberrations of the human eye with the use of a Hartmann-Shack wave-front sensor. *J Opt Soc Am A Opt Image Sci Vis.* 1994;11:1949–1957.
107. MacRae S, Fujieda M. Slit skiascopic-guided ablation using the Nidek laser. *J Refract Surg.* 2000;16:S576–S580.
108. Singh NK, Jaskulski M, Ramasubramanian V, et al. Validation of a clinical aberrometer using pyramidal wavefront sensing. *Optom Vis Sci.* 2019;96:733–744.
109. Applegate RA, Thibos LN, Hilmantel G. Optics of aberroscopy and super vision. *J Cataract Refract Surg.* 2001;27:1093–1107.

3

Accommodation

Mary Ann Croft, Paul L. Kaufman, Fabrice Manns, and Elke Lütjen-Drecoll

Introduction

"There is no other portion of physiological optics where one finds so many differing and contradictory ideas as concerns the accommodation of the eye, where in the most recent time have we actually made observations, where previously everything was left to the play of hypotheses."

Hermann von Helmholtz (1909)

It is primarily due to Helmholtz[1] that we owe our current "basic" understanding of the accommodative mechanism of the human eye (Fig. 3.1). His insight came from his own work and from pioneers before him. Thomas Young[2] was instrumental in demonstrating that accommodation occurs, not through changes in corneal curvature or axial length as those before him believed,[3] but through changes in the curvature of the lens. Young's painstaking anatomical investigations were insufficient for him to rule out the possibility that the crystalline lens received direct innervation from a branch of the ciliary nerves to allow it to contract as a muscle. It was only after the work of Crampton,[4] who first described the ciliary muscle from his investigation of bird eyes, that a mechanistic description of how the ciliary muscle might alter lens curvatures was proposed by Müller.[5] Understanding of human accommodation was mired by confusion from numerous investigations of the eyes of birds and other vertebrates, studied for their comparatively large size to gain insight into the human accommodative mechanism (Box 3.1). However, these species are now known to accommodate through mechanisms quite different from humans.[6-8] Current understanding of human accommodation stems from the work of many early investigators including Brücke,[9] Cramer,[10] Hess,[11] Müller,[5] Helmholtz,[1] and Gullstrand.[12] This path was made tortuous by the diversity of accommodative mechanisms of the various vertebrates studied. The wide diversity of avian visual habitats (aerial, aquatic, terrestrial), eye shapes (tubular, globose, and flattened), and feeding behaviors in all likelihood dictates their accommodative needs. Corneal accommodation, of considerable value to terrestrial birds, is of no value to aquatic birds where the corneal optical power is neutralized under water. The evolutionarily divergent accommodative mechanisms, or the absence of accommodation in other vertebrates, is, by reasonable conjecture, determined by feeding behaviors. Herbivorous animals (sheep, horses, cows, etc.), those that forage and dig for food primarily using olfactory cues (pigs), or those with nocturnal eyes and relatively poor visual abilities (mice, rats, rabbits) have little need for accommodation. Carnivores have better-developed ciliary muscles than these other species, but still have relatively little accommodative ability; the raccoon is the only nonprimate terrestrial mammal with substantial accommodative amplitude.[13] Cats are suggested[14-16] and raccoons[13] and fish shown to translate the lens forward without lenticular thickening.[17-19] Other adaptations in the lens, iris, or retina allow other lower vertebrates functional near and distance vision, although these cannot be classified as true accommodation as they rely on static optical adaptations. Among the vertebrates that do accommodate, amplitudes vary considerably. Diving birds have among the largest amplitudes, with cormorants having ~50 diopters (D)[11] and diving ducks suggested to have 70 to 80 D.[20] Among the mammals, vervet and cynomolgus monkeys have approximately 20 D,[21-23] young rhesus as much as 40 D[24] and raccoons about 20 D.[13] Humans, for only a few short childhood years, may have a maximum of about 10 to 15 D measured subjectively[25] or about 7 to 8 D measured objectively,[26] but find much less accommodation adequate for most visual tasks. Although accommodative amplitude gradually declines until completely lost by about age 50 years, to most individuals the deficit appears to be of sudden onset when the accommodative amplitude is diminished to a few diopters as presbyopia develops. Although full presbyopes may read at intermediate distances, this is almost certainly due to depth of field (see section Depth of Field) resulting from pupil constriction rather than active accommodation. The word presbyopia (Greek, presbys meaning an aged person and opsis meaning vision) possibly derives from Aristotle's use of the term presbytas to describe "those who see well at distance, but poorly at near."[27] Historically the term was used to describe the condition in which the near point has receded too far from the eye due to a diminution in the range of accommodation.[28] Despite the wealth of studies of accommodation on vertebrates, only primates are shown to systematically lose the ability to accommodate with increasing age. It may be no coincidence that although absolute life spans differ considerably, the relative age course of the progression of presbyopia is similar in humans and monkeys (Fig. 3.2).

ACCOMMODATION

Accommodation is a dynamic optical change in the dioptric power of the eye allowing the point of focus of the eye to be changed from distant to near objects. Accommodation changes the focus of the eye from the far point to the near point. The far point is the position of the object that is imaged sharply on the retina when the eye is unaccommodated. The near point is the position of the object that is imaged sharply on the retina when the eye is under maximal accommodation. In primates this is mediated through a contraction of the ciliary muscle, release of resting zonular tension around the lens equator, a decrease in lens equatorial diameter, and a "rounding up" of the crystalline lens through the force exerted on the lens by the lens capsule. The increased optical power of the lens is achieved through increased anterior and posterior surface curvatures and overall increased thickness. In an emmetropic eye (an eye without refractive error), the far point is a distant object located at or beyond what is considered optical infinity for the eye (6 m or 20 ft). When an object is brought closer to the eye, the eye must accommodate to maintain a clearly focused image on the retina. Myopic eyes, typically too long for the optical power of

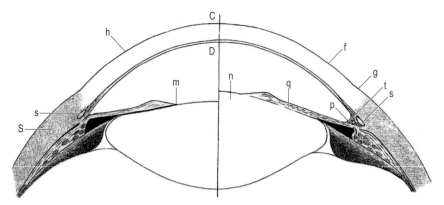

Fig. 3.1 Diagram showing the mechanism of accommodation of the human eye as described by Helmholtz. The *left half* depicts the eye in the unaccommodated state and the *right half* depicts the eye in the accommodative state. Helmholtz described an increase in lens thickness, an increase in the anterior surface curvature, an anterior movement of the anterior lens surface, but no posterior movement of the posterior lens surface. S, Sclera; *s*, Schlemm's canal; *h*, cornea; *F*, configuration for far vision; *m*, unaccommodated lens; *n*, accommodated lens; *q*, iris; *p*, trabecular meshwork; *f*, clear cornea; *g*, limbus; *N*, configuration for near vision; *C–D*, optical axis). (From Von Helmholtz HH. Helmholtz's Treatise on Physiological Optics. Translation edited by Southall JPC in 1924 (original German in 1909). New York: Dover; 1962: vol. 1, ch. 12.)

BOX 3.1   Accommodative Mechanism

- Accommodation is a dioptric change in optical power of the eye due to ciliary muscle contraction.
- The basic mechanism of accommodation occurs largely in accordance with the mechanism originally proposed by Helmholtz.
- Ciliary muscle contraction moves the apex of the ciliary body towards the axis of the eye and releases resting zonular tension around the lens equator.
- When zonular tension is released, the elastic lens capsule molds the young lens into a more spherical and accommodated form.
- During accommodation, lens diameter decreases, lens thickness increases, the anterior lens surface moves anteriorly, the posterior lens surface moves posteriorly, and the lens anterior and posterior surface curvatures increase; the thickness of the nucleus increases, but without a change in thickness of the cortex.
- The increase in curvature of the lens anterior and posterior surfaces results in an increase in optical power of the lens.
- The physical changes in the lens and eye result in an increase in optical power of the eye to focus on near objects.
- During accommodation the ciliary muscle pulls forward the vitreous zonule, the PVZ-INS-LE and the cistern branch tips while the anterior hyaloid bows backward and the central vitreous moves backward, including the central cistern.

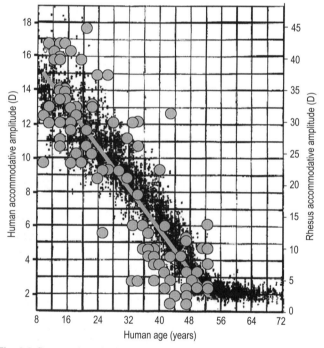

Fig. 3.2 Progression of presbyopia in humans (Duane, 1912, *small solid black symbols*) as measured subjectively using a push-up test, and in rhesus monkeys (Bito et al. 1982, *larger gray symbols* and *solid line*) as measured objectively with a Hartinger coincidence refractometer following topical application of the cholinergic agonist pilocarpine. The horizontal axis is in human years and the rhesus data are scaled to human years such that 20 rhesus years is equivalent to 50 human years, as the life span is ~75 years for humans and 30 years for rhesus monkeys. Analogously, the maximum magnitude of accommodation in rhesus monkeys is ~2.5 times higher than in humans, not surprising given the shorter arms and the closer in the monkeys hold their targets. In humans and rhesus monkeys, presbyopia progresses at the same rate relative to the absolute age span of each species. D, Diopter. (From Bito LZ, De Rousseau CJ, Kaufman PL, Bito JW. Age-dependent loss of accommodative amplitude in rhesus monkeys: an animal model for presbyopia. *Invest Ophthalmol Vis Sci.* 1982;23:23-31 and Duane A. Normal values of the accommodation at all ages. *J Am Med Assoc.* 1912;59:1010. Reproduced with permission from Association for Research in Vision and Ophthalmology.)

the lens and cornea combined, are unable to attain a sharply focused image for objects at optical infinity unless optical compensation is provided, such as through negative-powered spectacle lenses. The far point of young myopes is an object at a distance closer to the eye than optical infinity, i.e., myopes can see sharply at a near distance when the eye in unaccommodated. Young hyperopic eyes, however, are typically too short for the optical power of the lens and cornea and require correction with a positive spectacle lens to view objects at infinity sharply. Young hyperopes can focus on objects at optical infinity by increasing the optical power of the eye through accommodation.

Optics of the eye

Light from the environment enters the eye at the cornea and, in an emmetropic eye, is brought to a focus on the retina through the combined optical power of the cornea and the lens (see Chapter 1). Specific details for schematic eyes are given in Bennett and Rabbetts.[29] Accommodation is caused by a change in power of the lens. In the unaccommodated eye, the lens represents approximately 30% of the total power of the eye. The lens power is determined by the curvature of the anterior and posterior surfaces and by the presence of a refractive index gradient inside the lens. The lens refractive index progressively increases from ~1.379 at the surface of the cortex to ~1.410 at the center of the nucleus of the lens. The gradient refractive index (GRI) of the lens adds additional optical power because the gradient results in refraction of light throughout the lens. This results in light taking a curved path rather than a straight path through the lens. For simplified optical calculations, the more complex GRI of the lens is often substituted with a single equivalent refractive index value. An equivalent refractive index lens would need to have a value that is greater than the highest refractive index value at the center of the GRI lens, in order to have the same shape and optical power as the GRI lens.

The posterior lens surface is more steeply curved, and therefore has higher refractive power than the anterior surface. The lens anterior and posterior radii of curvature and the GRI change with age because of continuous lens growth, with a more pronounced change in the anterior surface. It is these surfaces that become more steeply curved to allow the accommodative increase in optical power of the lens to occur. Historically, it was suggested that the posterior lens surface does not move[1] and that the posterior lens surface curvature does not change appreciably with accommodation.[1,30,31] However, it is now known that the posterior lens surface does undergo an increase in curvature and moves posteriorly during accommodation as the lens thickness increases.[32–39] Gullstrand[12] suggested that the lens equivalent refractive index must change during accommodation. As the lens shape, axial thickness, and equatorial diameter change during accommodation, this dictates that the form of the GRI of the lens must also change during accommodation.[40,41] However, this does not require a change in the equivalent refractive index of the lens during accommodation, at least to the extent that resolution limits of currently available technology can detect.[42]

THE OPTICAL REQUIREMENTS FOR ACCOMMODATION

The optical power of the crystalline lens increases (i.e., the lens focal length decreases) during accommodation. As a consequence, the eye changes focus from distance to near so the image of a near object is brought to focus on the retina. The dioptric change in power of the eye defines accommodation, and accommodation is measured in units of diopters (D). A diopter is a reciprocal meter and is a measure of the vergence of light. Light rays from a point object diverge and are by convention designated to have negative vergence. Light rays converging toward a point image are designated to have positive vergence (see Chapter 1). An object at optical infinity subtends zero vergence at the cornea. The optical interfaces of the eye (the cornea and lens) add positive vergence to draw light rays toward a focus on the retina (Fig. 3.3). When an object is moved from infinity to a point closer to the eye, the near object subtends divergent rays on the cornea. To focus on the near object, the optical power of the eye must increase to add positive vergence to the now divergent rays to bring the refracted rays to a focus on the retina. When an emmetropic eye is focused on a distant object the eye is considered unaccommodated. If the eye accommodates from an object at optical infinity to an object 1.0 m in front of the eye, this represents 1.0 D of accommodation. If the eye accommodates from infinity to 0.5 m in front of the eye, this is 2 D of accommodation; from infinity to 0.1 m is 10 D, and so on. The accommodative amplitude (in

diopters) is close to, but not exactly equal, to the increase in optical power of the eye.

DEPTH OF FIELD

Clinically, the nearest point of clear vision is typically measured subjectively in an eye corrected for distance vision. This is done using the push-up test: a near reading chart is moved toward the eyes while the subject is asked to report when they can no longer sustain clear vision on the near target or when the near target first becomes blurred.

Although the reciprocal of this near reading distance expressed in meters is clinically referred to as the accommodative amplitude, this is technically inaccurate. The push-up test is a subjective measure of the near point expressed in units of diopters. However, this is not a measure of the true dioptric change in power of the eye because the eye's depth of field results in an overestimation of the dioptric change in the eye's optical power by about 1 to 2 D compared with the objectively measured accommodative response amplitude.[43–46] Subjective testing of this nature in complete presbyopes might lead one to believe that about 1 D of accommodation is present, but this is not a true change in optical power of the eye and is sometimes called pseudoaccommodation.[44,46,47]

VISUAL ACUITY

In addition to the depth of field of the eye, acuity and contrast sensitivity of the eye affect the subjective measurement of the near point of clear vision. Increased illumination provides higher contrast on the target, thus, smaller changes in focus or blur of the target are more easily detected. While increasing the level of illumination will help to improve the contrast sensitivity and acuity, this will also decrease the pupil size and will thereby increase the depth of field of the eye, resulting in a nearer point of perceived clear vision. Further, in cases of cataract or other opacities of the ocular optical media, the image of a near object is not seen clearly, thus small changes in the focus of the image are less readily detected. With increasing age, the optical clarity of the lens decreases and the prevalence of cataract increases. Retinal disease can also affect visual acuity. Elderly patients often have reduced visual acuity and/or reduced contrast sensitivity, not solely owing to decreased optical performance.[48]

THE ANATOMY OF THE ACCOMMODATIVE APPARATUS

Grossly, the accommodative apparatus of the eye consists of the ciliary body (including the ciliary muscle and the ciliary pigmented and nonpigmented epithelium), the choroid, the anterior and posterior zonular fibers, the lens capsule, and the crystalline lens (Fig. 3.4). The ciliary muscle forms the active component of the accommodative apparatus. This specialized smooth muscle, with cellular elements of fast striated muscle[49] (see section The ciliary muscle) is attached anteriorly to Schwalbe's line by collagenous tendons and posteriorly to the choroid by elastic tendons. These elastic tendons then insert into the elastic lamina of Bruch's membrane and the choroid, and thus includes their ultimate functional insertion into the elastic ring around the optic nerve head. The muscle is comprised of three muscle fiber groups, oriented respectively longitudinally, radially (obliquely), and circularly in the outer, middle, and inner portions of the ciliary muscle. Contraction of the muscle stretches the posterior elastic tendons, the muscle moves anteriorly and inwardly along the curved inner scleral surface, and the muscle's circular portion thickens so that the distance between lens and ciliary body shortens. The elastic zonula between the ciliary body and lens equator is thus relaxed, loosening the tension at the lens equator.

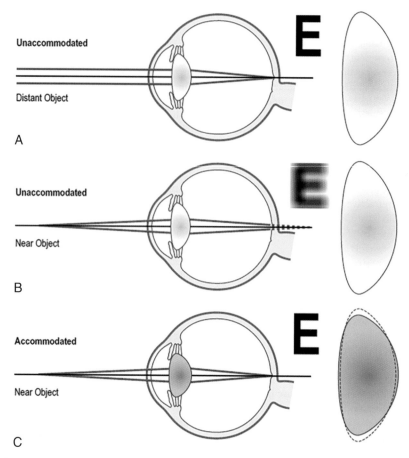

Fig. 3.3 The accommodative optical changes in the eye occur through an increase in optical power of the crystalline lens. (A) The unaccommodated emmetropic eye is focused on a distant object, with the lens in an unaccommodated state. (B) A near object subtends divergent rays and, in the unaccommodated eye, the image would be formed behind the retina and is therefore out of focus when the lens remains unaccommodated. (C) In the accommodated eye, the in-focus image of the near object is formed on the retina when the lens is in an accommodated state.

The crystalline lens, consisting of a central nucleus, a surrounding cortex, and an outer collagenous elastic lens capsule, "rounds up," thereby increasing optical power. In addition to lens rounding a recent study in human subjects demonstrated that the lens equator moves forward during accommodation and is correlated with accommodative amplitude.[50]

Improved optical methods have shown that the zonula consists of different portions, serving different functions. The anterior zonular fibers span the circumlental space extending from the valleys of the ciliary processes and inserting all around the lens equator and the anterior vitreous membrane. They constitute the suspensory elements of the crystalline lens. The posterior zonular fibers (or pars plana zonules that line the inner aspect of the pars plana[51–54]) intermingle with the anterior zonula at the transition between posterior pars plicata and anterior pars plana (zonular plexus), and extend from the plexus and the pars plana to the region of the ora serrata and the vitreous membrane facing the pars plana (Fig. 3.4). Presumably, the posterior zonula tenses as the anterior zonula relaxes, helping to prevent and smooth larger movements of the ora serrata during anterior movement of the ciliary muscle. The posterior zonula is distinct from zonular fibers inserting into the outer vitreous membrane (intermediate vitreous zonule) thus forming a fluid-filled cleft between the vitreous and the pars plana zonule, (Figs. 3.4 and 3.5). Attached posteriorly at the insertion zone (near the ora serrata), both the intermediate vitreous zonules and the

PVZ-INS LE (Fig. 3.6)[55] extend forward in a straight course to attach to the zonular plexus *or* the posterior lens equator, respectively (Fig. 3.4A). The cleft between the pars plana zonule of the ciliary body and the vitreous membrane is bridged by bands of intermediate vitreous zonule fibers. The cleft could provide a low-friction interface between the ciliary epithelium/pars plana zonule and vitreous membrane when the ciliary muscle moves anteriorly and posteriorly during accommodation and disaccommodation, increasing the efficiency of the system. Thus, the vitreous zonula allows a sliding of the ciliary body during accommodation/disaccommodation, with only a little friction.

Theoretical suggestions that the vitreous plays a role in accommodation exist,[56–59] although empirical evidence implies no need for the vitreous in accommodation.[60–62] A recent study found evidence, including quantifiable intravitreal accommodative movements, indicating a vitreous role in the mechanism of accommodation (also see section The vitreous).[63] In addition, accommodative choroidal movements that extend to the optic nerve region have been quantified.[64]

The ciliary body

The ciliary body occupies a triangular-shaped region that lies between the scleral spur and retina. It is bounded on its outer surface by the anterior sclera and on its inner surface by the nonpigmented ciliary epithelium. The anterior ciliary body begins at the scleral spur at the angle of the anterior chamber. The base of the iris inserts into the

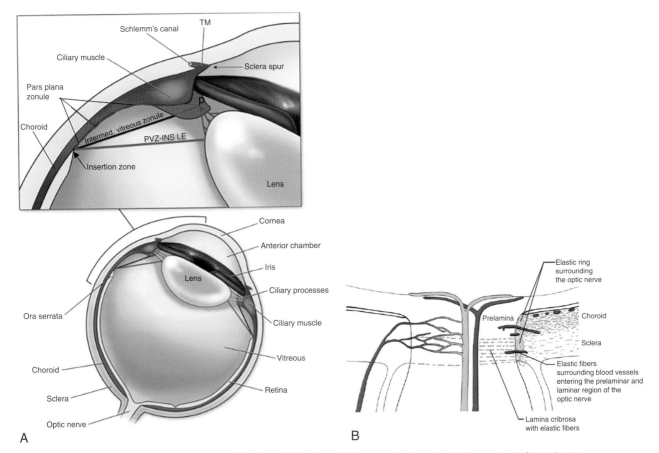

Fig. 3.4 The ciliary muscle and the choroid functionally form an elastic network that extends from the trabecular meshwork (*TM*) to the back of the eye (A) and ultimately attaches to the elastic fiber ring that surrounds the optic nerve and to the lamina cribrosa, through which the nerve passes (B). In (A) PVZ-INS LE is the vitreous strand that extends from the posterior insertion zone of the vitreous zonule to the lens equator. (A is reprinted with permission from Kaufman PL, Lütjen-Drecoll E, Croft MA. Presbyopia and glaucoma: Two diseases, one pathophysiology? The Friedenwald Lecture. *Invest Ophthalmol Vis Sci.* 2019;60(5):1801-1812.) (B is reprinted with permission from Croft MA, Kaufman PL, Lütjen-Drecoll E. Age-related posterior ciliary muscle restriction—A link between trabecular meshwork and optic nerve head pathophysiology. Exp Eye Res. 2016;158:187-189; and Tektas O, Lütjen-Drecoll E, Scholz M. Qualitative and quantitative morphologic changes in the vasculature and extracellular matrix of the prelaminar optic nerve head in eyes with POAG. *Invest Ophthalmol Vis Sci.* 2010;51:5083-5091.)

anterior ciliary body. Posterior to the iris, the ciliary processes are found at the anterior-innermost point of the ciliary body and form the corrugated pars plicata of the ciliary body. The smooth surface of the ciliary body, the pars plana, is posterior to the pars plicata. The most posterior aspect of the ciliary body is joined to the ora serrata of the retina. The outer surface of the ciliary body beneath the anterior sclera is the suprachoroidal lamina, or supraciliarus, and is formed by a thin layer of collagen fibers, fibroblasts, and melanocytes.[65] The ciliary epithelium has two layers of secretory cells. The inner layer, the nonpigmented epithelium (NPE), is made up of columnar cells and faces the posterior chamber and the vitreous body. The NPE is apposed apex-to-apex to the outer layer of ciliary epithelium made up of cuboidal cells, the highly pigmented epithelium (PE). The PE and the NPE express ultrastructural differences that seem to result from different functional demands.[65] Ultrastructural differences exist between the ciliary NPE cells at the tips of the processes and those in the valleys, the former being adapted for fluid secretion and the latter for mechanical anchoring of the zonule.[66] The length of the ciliary body, from the tips of the ciliary processes to the ora serrata, is longest temporally and shortest nasally.[67]

The ciliary muscle

The ciliary muscle occupies a triangular-shaped region within the ciliary body beneath the anterior sclera (Fig. 3.7).[68] It has an anterior origin at the scleral spur in close proximity to Schlemm's canal.[67,69] Anterior ciliary muscle tendons insert into the scleral spur, the elastic network of the trabecular meshwork, the inner wall endothelia of Schlemm's canal, and Schwalbe's line, which collectively serve as a fixed anterior anchor against which the ciliary muscle contracts.[65] Posterior to the scleral spur, the outer surface of the ciliary muscle is attached only loosely to the inner surface of the anterior sclera,[65] allowing the muscle to slide forward and backward as it contracts and relaxes during accommodation and disaccommodation. The posterior ciliary muscle attaches to the stroma of the choroid. Here the muscle forms true elastic tendons, which insert into the choroidal elastic network. The anterior and inner surfaces of the ciliary muscle are bounded anteriorly by the stroma of the pars plicata and posteriorly by the pars plana of the ciliary body. The ciliary muscle fiber bundles beneath the sclera are oriented such that a contraction of the ciliary muscle results in a forward and inward redistribution of the mass of the ciliary body and a narrowing of the ciliary ring diameter owing to sliding ciliary muscle movement along the

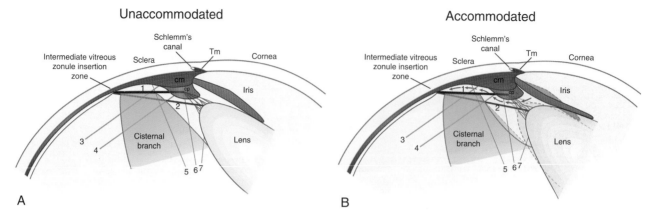

Unaccommodated   Accommodated

A   B

Fig. 3.5 Accommodation ciliary muscle, lens, iris, and cisternal branch tip close-up. (A) Unaccommodated state. *Thick black line* (1) represents the intermediate vitreous zonule that extends between the intermediate vitreous zonule posterior insertion zone and the zonular plexus (which resides between the walls of the ciliary processes). *Thick blue line* (2) represents the vitreous strand that extends from the intermediate vitreous zonule posterior insertion zone and attaches to the posterior lens equator (PVZ-INS LE).[55] *Thin green lines* represent other vitreous strands that extend from the posterior vitreous body to the pars plana region (3) or the pars plicata region (4). *Thin orange lines* (5, 6, 7) represent vitreous strands that extend from the anterior vitreous to the pars plana (5), the pars plicata (6), or the posterior lens surface (7). (B) Accommodated state. Legend as for (A) but structures are now in the accommodated state. Note backward bowing of the iris and anterior hyaloid. The lens is thickened, and the lens equator has moved away from the sclera. The muscle apex is in a more forward and inward position. Fluid flows around the lens equator toward the anterior hyaloid and then further into the cleft between the intermediate vitreous zonule and the pars plana region during accommodation, as represented by the red arrows. (Reprinted with permission from Kaufman PL, Lütjen-Drecoll E, Croft MA. Presbyopia and glaucoma: Two diseases, one pathophysiology? The Friedenwald Lecture. *Invest Ophthalmol and Vis Sci.* 2019;60(5):1801-1812.)

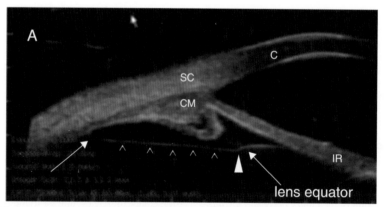

Fig. 3.6 (A) Ultrasound biomicroscopy (UBM) images (50 mHz, UBM-ER) in the nasal quadrant of a 19-year-old male human. Note the connection between the posterior insertion zone of the vitreous zonule *(arrow)* and the posterior aspect of the lens equator *(large arrowhead)*, seen in all 12 human subjects, termed PVZ-INS LE strand *(arrowheads)*. *CM,* Ciliary muscle; *IR,* iris; *C,* cornea; *SC,* sclera. (Reprinted with permission from Croft MA, Nork TM, McDonald JP, et al. Accommodative movements of the vitreous membrane, choroid, and sclera in young and presbyopic human and nonhuman primate eyes. *Invest Ophthalmol and Vis Sci.* 2013;54:5049-5058.)

inner surface of the sphere formed by the anterior sclera. This causes the choroid to be pulled forward not only in the region of the ora serrata, but also in the region of the optic nerve, perhaps putting tension on the optic nerve.[64,70,71]

The three muscle fiber groups that comprise the ciliary muscle, identified by their relative positions and orientations as detailed previously, form a morphologically and functionally integrated three-dimensional structure.[65] The major group of muscle fibers is the peripheral meridional or longitudinal fibers, or Brücke's muscle.[9] They extend longitudinally between the scleral spur and the choroid adjacent to the sclera.

Located inward to the longitudinal fibers are the reticular or radial fibers. These fibers are branching V- or Y-shaped fibers and constitute a relatively smaller proportion of the ciliary muscle. They are attached anteriorly to the scleral spur and the peripheral wall of the anterior ciliary body at the insertion of the iris. Beneath the radial fibers and positioned more anteriorly in the ciliary body and closest to the lens are the equatorial or circular fibers, or Müller's muscle. These constitute the smallest proportion of the ciliary muscle. The division of the ciliary muscle into three muscle fiber groups is somewhat artificial. In reality, there is a gradual transition from the outermost longitudinal muscle

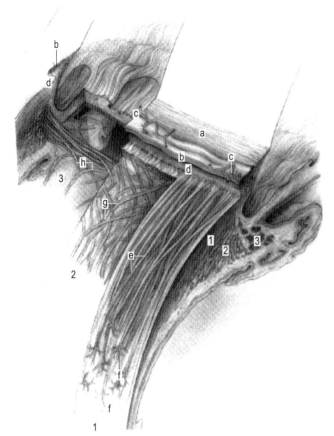

Fig. 3.7 Drawing of the ciliary body showing the ciliary muscle and its components. The cornea and sclera have been dissected away but the trabecular meshwork (a), Schlemm's canal (b) and two external collectors (c), as well as the scleral spur (d), have been left undisturbed. The three components of the ciliary muscle are shown separately, viewed from the outside and sectioned meridionally. Section 1 shows the *longitudinal* ciliary muscle; in section 2 the longitudinal ciliary muscle has been dissected away to show the *radial* ciliary muscle; in section 3 only the innermost *circular* ciliary muscle is shown. According to Calasans (1953)[68] the ciliary muscle originates in the ciliary tendon, which includes the scleral spur (d) and the adjacent connective tissue. The cells originate as paired V-shaped bundles. The *longitudinal* muscle forms long V-shaped trellises (e) which terminate in the epichoroidal stars (f). The arms of the V-shaped bundles formed by the *radial* muscle meet at wide angles (g) and terminate in the ciliary processes. The V-shaped bundles of the circular muscle originate at such distant points in the ciliary tendon that their arms meet at a very wide angle (h). The iridic portion is shown at (i) joining the circular muscle cells. (Reproduced with permission from Hogan MJ, Alvarado JA, Weddell JE. *Histology of the human eye. An atlas and textbook*. Philadelphia: WB Saunders, 1971.)

fibers to the radial fibers to the innermost circular muscle fibers, with some intermingling of the different fiber types. A contraction of the ciliary muscle results in a contraction of all three muscle fiber groups together. When the ciliary muscle contracts there is a gradual rearrangement of the muscle bundles, with an increase in thickness of the circular portion and a decrease in thickness of the radial and longitudinal portions of the muscle.[65] Contraction of the ciliary muscle as a whole pulls the anterior choroid forward (inducing centrifugal choroidal movements around the optic nerve[64,70]), resulting in a forward and inward redistribution of the mass of the ciliary body and a narrowing of the ciliary ring diameter. The valleys of the ciliary processes with the inserted zonules move toward the lens equator and serve the

primary function of releasing resting zonular tension at the lens equator to allow accommodation to occur. The ciliary muscle bundles, each containing around 6 to 12 individual muscle fibers, collectively are surrounded/bound by a sheath composed of thin flattened fibroblasts or connective tissue cells.[65,72]

The ciliary muscle is a smooth muscle, with a dominant parasympathetic innervation causing accommodative contraction mediated by M3 muscarinic receptors.[73] Upon disaccommodation, there is β2-adrenergic receptor–mediated relaxation of the ciliary muscle,[74–77] so that the posterior elastic tendons and the elastic choroid can pull the muscle backward. The stretched tendons and choroid retract, the muscle is pulled backward, and the inner circular edge of the muscle is diminished.

Only in the inner circular portion are there nitrergic ganglia that innervate the circular muscle cells.[78] Connections to mechanoreceptors in the inner ciliary body facing the attachment of anterior zonular fibers indicate that this innervation is important for fine regulation of accommodation.[78–80]

In general the ciliary muscle is atypical for smooth muscles in its speed of contraction, the large size of its motor neurons, the distance between the muscle and the motor neurons, and the unusual ultrastructure throughout the ciliary muscle cells, which in some ways resembles skeletal muscles[49] (indeed, in birds of prey it is a striated skeletal muscle). There are also regional differences in ultrastructure and histochemistry of the primate ciliary muscle, suggesting that the longitudinal portion may be acting like a fast skeletal muscle to "set" or "brace" the system rapidly, for the contraction of the inner portion to be most effective.[49] Thus, the ciliary muscle fibers have some intracellular elements analogous to fast striated muscle; indeed, in primates this is the fastest smooth muscle in the body.[49]

In the young eye both forward (anterior; Fig. 3.8A) and inward (centripetal; Fig. 3.8B) muscle movement is required for efficient and maximal accommodation to occur (Video 3.1; Fig. 3.8C).[81] The amount of centripetal lens equator movement parallels the centripetal ciliary muscle movement, but the amount of centripetal muscle movement required is greater than centripetal lens equator movement.[82] Thus, the system requires a greater amount of centripetal muscle movement than centripetal lens equator movement.[82] The amount of muscle movement in both vectors is similar in humans and monkeys.[50,81,82]

The zonular fibers

The zonular apparatus is a complex meshwork of fibrils 70 to 80 nm in diameter[83] and grouped into fiber bundles, which are estimated to be between 4 to 6 and 40 to 50 microns (μm) in diameter.[83,84] From these bundles fine fibrils separate to attach to the basement membrane (inner limiting membrane) of the nonpigmented ciliary epithelium. The principal constituent of the zonule is fibrillin-1, but there are also noncollagenous carbohydrate–protein mucopolysaccharide and glycoprotein complexes that are secreted by the ciliary epithelium. The fibrillin-rich elastic zonular microfibrils are thought to be much more elastic than the lens capsule. Their primary function is to stabilize the lens and allow accommodation. Because the zonule is not a continuous tissue but is composed of fibers, it allows fluid flow from the posterior chamber behind the iris to the vitreous chamber.

Anterior zonule. The attachment of the zonular fibers to the lens capsule is superficial, with few fibers penetrating into the capsule to form a mechanical (possibly similar to Velcro) or chemical union.[85] From scanning electron microscopy this anterior zonule crossing the circumlental space and extending to the lens is alternatively described as:

(1) consisting of three fiber strands running to the anterior, equatorial, and posterior lens surfaces,[86] or

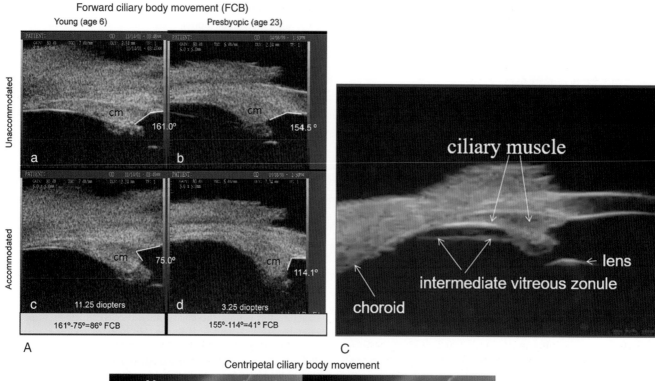

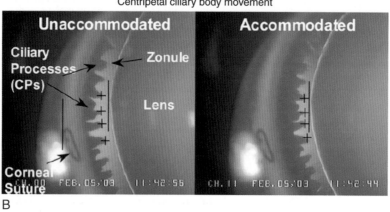

Fig. 3.8 (A) Ultrasound biomicroscopy (UBM): UBM images of two normal monkey eyes, aged 6 years (a, c) and 23 years (b, d), in the unaccommodated and accommodated states. The change in angle between the anterior aspect of the ciliary body and the inner aspect of the cornea during supramaximal central stimulation was used as a surrogate indicator of forward ciliary body movement (FCB). *cm*, ciliary muscle. (Panels a and c modified with permission from Croft MA, McDonald JP, Nadkarni NV, Lin T, Kaufman PL. Age-related changes in centripetal ciliary body movement relative to centripetal lens movement in monkeys. *Exp Eye Res.* 2009;89:824-832. Panels b and d adapted with permission from Croft MA, Glasser A, Heatley G, et al. Accommodative ciliary body and lens function in rhesus monkeys I. Normal lens, zonule, and ciliary process configuration in the iridectomized eye. *Invest Ophthalmol Vis Sci.* 2006;47:1076-1086; copyright Association for Research in Vision and Ophthalmology (ARVO).). **(B)** Goniovideography images of normal lens and ciliary process (CP) configuration in the accommodated and unaccommodated states. To obtain quantitative measurements, a 9-0 nylon suture placed at the corneoscleral limbus served as a reference point (*left solid vertical line*) from which to measure distances to the lens equator (*right solid vertical line*) and the CPs (*cross-hairs*) for each image during a 2.2-second stimulus period. (Reprinted with permission from Croft MA, Glasser A, Heatley G, et al. Accommodative ciliary body and lens function in rhesus monkeys I. Normal lens, zonule, and ciliary process configuration in the iridectomized eye. *Invest Ophthalmol Vis Sci.* 2006; 47:1076-1086; copyright Association for Research in Vision and Ophthalmology (ARVO).) **(C)** UBM overview image in a live rhesus monkey shows a prominent straight line *(arrow)* extending from the pars plicata region of the ciliary body to the ora serrata region and separated from the pars plana epithelium by a cleft. (Reprinted with permission from Lütjen-Drecoll E, Kaufman PL, Wasielewski R, Lin T, Croft MA. Morphology and accommodative function of the vitreous zonule in human and monkey eyes. *Invest Ophthalmol Vis Sci.* 2010;51:1554-1564. See also Video 3.1.)

(2) fibers that insert along a circular line on the anterior and posterior surface of the lens with some fibers inserting directly on the equator,[83,84,87] or

(3) a zonular fork with two main fiber groups extending to the lens anterior and posterior surfaces with finer bundles seemingly of relative unimportance running to the lens equator,[52] or

(4) successive sagittal lines of insertion from lens anterior to posterior surface and two coronal lines of insertion, one where the fibers insert onto the capsule around the anterior surface and another where the fibers insert onto the capsule around the posterior surface.[88]

Although no systematic crossing of anterior zonular fiber was observed by McCulloch,[88] crossing of anterior zonular fibers has been observed in other preparations[61,83,84] and was documented in early diagrams from histology (Fig. 3.9) and in live monkeys in which the iris was totally removed and a fluorescent dye injected into the anterior chamber.[89] From histologic preparations, when an appropriate plane of section is obtained, a continuous line of zonular insertion into the entire lens equator is seen.[88] Unfixed, dissected human eye specimens show a continuous meshwork of fibers uniformly covering the entire lens equator, and show crossing of zonular fibers.[61]

Zonular plexus and posterior zonule. In the attachment zone, the lateral walls of the ciliary processes and the transition zone between pars plicata and pars plana, the zonular fibers form broad, flattened strands crossing and joining each other and the attaching posterior zonular fibers to form the zonular plexus. This plexus functions as a fulcrum. During disaccommodation the fulcrum moves posterolaterally, exerting traction directly to the anterior zonular fibers. During

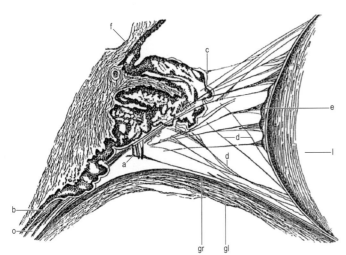

Fig. 3.9 Owing to the delicate nature of the zonule and the difficulties in observing it, descriptions of the insertion of the anterior zonule onto the lens equator differ. Early anatomists with relatively crude methods produced remarkably accurate diagrams of the structure of the anterior zonule showing crossing of zonular fibers, fiber bundles of varying thickness and insertion into a thickened region of the capsule at the lens equator. Some clumping of zonular bundles is evident in this depiction which is not seen in unfixed specimens. *l*, Lens; *gl*, vitreous humor; *gr*, anterior boundary layer; *o*, orbicular space; *i*, iris root; *a*, short strong fibrous attachments of the posterior ligament of the zonule; *b*, fibers of the zonule arising behind from the hyaloid membrane; *c*, fibers of the zonule arising anteriorly from the ciliary processes; *d*, fibers of the zonule arising from the ciliary processes which cross the ligaments of the zonule and partly attach to them; *e*, space between the capsule of the lens and the pericapsular membrane. (From Helmholtz von HH. Treatise on Physiological Optics. Translation edited by Southall JPC in 1924 (original German in 1909). New York: Dover, 1962: vol. 1, ch. 12 and pp 408.)

accommodation the pars plana zonule (tension fibers) is stretched, relaxing the anterior zonule.[52]

Anteriorly located zonule as a tool for fine regulation in accommodation. An additional system of fine zonular fibers derive from the valleys of the anterior pars plicata, opposite to structures resembling mechanosensors in the ciliary body, and join the main anterior zonule at their insertion to the lens. Changes in tension of these fibers can stimulate the mechanoreceptors that show nervous connections to the nitrergic nerve cells, relaxing innervation of the circular portion of the muscle. This zonular system could help to fine-regulate accommodation.[79,80]

Vitreous zonule. The vitreous zonule connects the vitreous membrane in the region of the ora serrata with the ciliary plexus (intermediate vitreous zonule), as well as the plexus with the anterior vitreous membrane posterior to the lens capsule (anterior vitreous zonule). Observations of the ciliary region during accommodation show that the posterior ciliary body slides forward against the curvature of the anterior sclera, moving the posterior insertion zone of the intermediate vitreous zonular fibers forward (Figs. 3.4 and 3.5; Video 3.1). In addition, contraction of the ciliary muscle pulls the muscle's posterior attachment forward owing to forward and inward movement of the ciliary muscle and ciliary process tips. This suggests that in addition to allowing nearly resistance-free gliding of the muscle during contraction, the intermediate vitreous zonular fibers may similarly assist in pulling the ciliary muscle back to the unaccommodated configuration after cessation of an accommodative effort.

The PVZ-INS LE strand. In addition to the insertion to the vitreous membrane there are strands of vitreous zonules attaching to the lens equator (PVZ-INS LE). The PVZ-INS LE strand is attached to the vitreous membrane at the insertion zone posteriorly (near the region of the ora serrata) and extends forward to attach directly to the posterior lens equator (Fig. 3.4A).[50,55] The PVZ-INS LE strand is pulled/pushed forward by the ciliary muscle during accommodation and remains straight during the accommodative response (i.e., it does not relax) (Figs. 3.4 and 3.6).[55] The lens equator also moves forward during the accommodative response.[50] The vitreous is partially composed of collagen type materials[90–93] and the PVZ-INS LE may be "stiff," thereby supplying forward push to the lens equator as the muscle, the PVZ-INS LE, and insertion zone move forward during accommodation.[55] In an older eye with decreased accommodative forward muscle movement, the PVZ-INS LE not only supplies less "forward push," but may also provide a direct drag against its forward movement and thereby against lens thickening during accommodation.[94]

The vitreous

Recent advances have allowed visualization of the vitreous by ultrasound biomicroscopy, contrast agents (in nonhuman primates) (Fig. 3.10; Video 3.2 and 3.3), and endoscopy (Fig. 3.11; Video 3.4) during dynamic imaging of the accommodative response, providing empirical evidence for a role of the vitreous in accommodation.[63,64,95] There are numerous connections between the vitreous and the accommodative apparatus, from the front to back of the eye.[63,64,71,95] Histologic and other research has examined the vitreous structure[58–60,90–93,96–103] and its possible role in accommodation and presbyopia.[63,64,95,104] Jongbloed and Worst[96] reported on the cistern structure within the vitreous compartment. The base of the cistern resides in the optic nerve region and the branches of the cistern extend forward to the anterior vitreous.[96] In the rhesus monkey the tips of the cistern branches in the anterior vitreous attach to the intermediate vitreous zonule[63,95] (Figs. 3.12 and 3.13; Video 3.2 and 3.3). As the ciliary muscle contracts and moves forward and inward, the lens thickens (the anterior lens pole moves anteriorly and becomes more sharply curved and the central posterior

Pre-Triamcinolone

Post-Triamcinolone

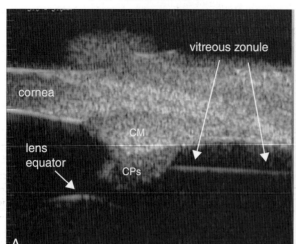 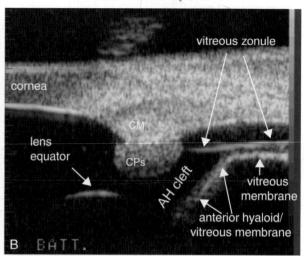

Fig. 3.10 (A) Typical ultrasound biomicroscopy (UBM) image in an 8-year-old rhesus monkey prior to injection of triamcinolone (Triesence). The vitreous zonule was clearly visible but the anterior hyaloid/vitreous membrane was not visualized. (B) UBM image 24 hours after injection of triamcinolone in the same monkey eye and quadrant as in Panel A. The location of the vitreous membrane and anterior hyaloid (AH) portion of the vitreous membrane are now clearly visible as the triamcinolone clings to the vitreous membranes. There is a cleft between the ciliary processes (pars plicata region) and the anterior hyaloid membrane, termed the AH cleft. *CPs*, Ciliary processes; *CM*, ciliary muscle. (Reprinted with permission from Croft MA, Nork TM, McDonald JP, et al. Accommodative movements of the vitreous membrane, choroid and sclera in young and presbyopic human and non human primate eyes. *Invest Ophthalmol and Vis Sci.* 2013;54:5049-5058.)

Unaccommodated

Accommodated

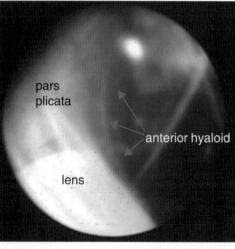 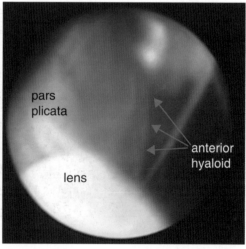

Fig. 3.11 See Video 3.5 for movement of the vitreous membrane during accommodation visualized using an endoscopic camera in a 19-year-old rhesus monkey eye. Note anterior hyaloid configuration bowing toward the lens and pars plicata in the resting state, whereas in the accommodated state the anterior hyaloid bows in a posterior direction. An aminofluorescein dye was used as a contrast agent to facilitate visualization of the vitreous membrane or zonula. (Reprinted with permission from Croft MA, Nork TM, McDonald JP, et al. Accommodative movements of the vitreous membrane, choroid, and sclera in young and presbyopic human and nonhuman primate eyes. *Invest Ophthalmol Vis Sci.* 2013; 54:5049-5058.)

lens pole/capsule moves backward [Fig. 3.14; Video 3.5]),[55,71,103] and the fibrillar structures within the central vitreous[70] (including the anterior hyaloid,[95] Cloquet's canal, and possibly the cistern trunk[96]) move posteriorly toward the optic nerve head (Figs. 3.12, 3.13, 3.15, and 3.16; Video 3.2, 3.3, 3.4–3.9).[63] The accommodative posterior movements of the central vitreous correlate with accommodative amplitude; the greater the accommodative posterior movement of the central vitreous the higher the accommodative amplitude (Fig. 3.17). These movements have been quantified (Table 3.1; Figs. 3.17 and 3.18)[63] and decline significantly with age (Fig.3.17). The accommodative posterior movement of the central vitreous includes the region of the vitreous very near the optic nerve head (Video 3.6–3.9). This strongly suggests that there is a

Rhesus monkey: accommodation and fluid flow in the iridectomized eye

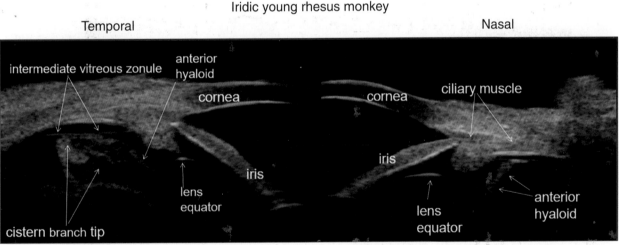

Fig. 3.12 See Video 3.2. Ultrasound biomicroscopy image in the nasal *(left panel)* and temporal *(right panel)* quadrant of a 10-year-old iridectomized rhesus monkey eye. During accommodation the triamcinolone particles *(white dots)*, suspended in the ocular fluid, flow around the lens equator and into the vitreous compartment toward the anterior hyaloid *(left and right panels)* and then further into the cleft between the intermediate vitreous zonule (vz) and pars plana (pp) *(right panel)*. When the *red dot* appears in the video clip *(left panel)*, or when the channel (CH) indicator *(right panel, lower left)* changes from 00 to 11, the stimulus to induce accommodation is on. (Reprinted with permission from: Kaufman PL, Lütjen-Drecoll E, Croft MA. Presbyopia and glaucoma: Two diseases, one pathophysiology? The Friedenwald Lecture. *Invest Ophthalmol and Vis Sci.* 2019;60(5):1801-1812.)

Iridic young rhesus monkey

Fig. 3.13 See Video 3.3. Ultrasound biomicroscopy in the nasal and temporal quadrants of a 7-year-old iridic rhesus monkey eye injected with triamcinolone, which clings to the vitreous membranes. In the presence of the iris, the anterior hyaloid still bows backward during accommodation and does so in parallel with the accommodative backward bowing of the iris. For both *left* and *right* panels, when the *red dot* appears, the stimulus to induce accommodation is on. (Reprinted with permission from Kaufman PL, Lütjen-Drecoll E, Croft MA. Presbyopia and glaucoma: Two diseases, one pathophysiology? The Friedenwald Lecture. *Invest Ophthalmol and Vis Sci.* 2019;60(5):1801-1812.)

fluid wave—and consequently a pressure change—impacting the nerve head. Simultaneously, the fibrillar peripheral vitreous, some of which is attached to the intermediate vitreous zonule (including the tips of the cistern branches near the anterior vitreous[96]; Video 3.2 and 3.3), moves anteriorly (Fig. 3.18) and inwardly.[63,95] The accommodative forward movement of the cistern branch tips correlate with accommodative amplitude; the greater the forward movement of the cistern

branch tips, the higher the accommodative amplitude (Fig. 3.18).[63] These movements are reversed in disaccommodation.[63] The accommodative forward movement of the cistern branch tips tends to decline with age (Fig. 3.18). In addition to pressure gradients, the fluid movements may generate shear stress at the nerve head. Whether these vitreal forces are bad, good, or irrelevant for the nerve is impossible to say, but they likely gradually *decrease* with age (see further in this section)

Accommodation: rhesus monkey

Aniridic

Iridic

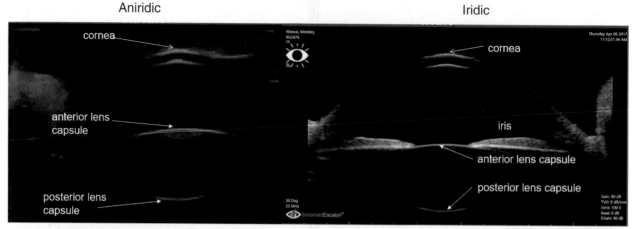

Fig. 3.14 See Video 3.4. Typical ultrasound biomicroscopy images taken from two separate phakic rhesus monkeys: one with an aniridic eye (*left panel*; age 6) and the other monkey with an iridic (*right panel*; age 7) eye. A *red dot* indicates when the stimulus to induce accommodation is on. The iris bows backward during accommodation and the posterior lens pole moves posteriorly. (Left panel reprinted with permission from Kaufman PL, Lütjen-Drecoll E, Croft MA. Presbyopia and glaucoma: Two diseases, one pathophysiology? The Friedenwald Lecture. *Invest Ophthalmol and Vis Sci.* 2019;60(5):1801-1812.)

Aniridic, ECLE

Aniridic, ICLE

One day post triamcinolone iris and lens present

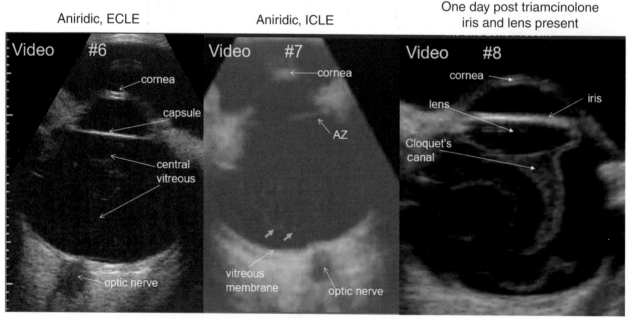

Fig. 3.15 See Video 3.6, 3.7, and 3.8. Ultrasound biomicroscopy images in normal (*right panel*, iris and lens present), and aphakic and iridectomized (*left and middle*) rhesus monkey eyes following intravitreal injection of triamcinolone. Ages of monkeys posted on the figure and videos. During accommodation following extracapsular lens extraction (ECLE) (Video 3.6), the capsule bows backward and the central vitreous moves posteriorly following ECLE (Video 3.6) and intracapsular lens extraction (ICLE) (Video 3.7; *thick green arrows*), and also when the iris and the lens are in place (Video 3.8). Cloquet's canal also moves posteriorly during accommodation (Video 3.8). *AZ*, Anterior zonula attached to Wieger's ligament possibly with capsular remnant (Video 3.7). A *red dot* indicates when the stimulus to induce accommodation is on for each respective video clip. (Reprinted with permission from: Kaufman PL, Lütjen-Drecoll E, Croft MA. Presbyopia and glaucoma: Two diseases, one pathophysiology? The Friedenwald Lecture. *Invest Ophthalmol and Vis Sci.* 2019;60(5):1801-1812.)

and become small once presbyopia becomes complete, again at about the age when primary open angle glaucoma begins to appear.[105,106] Of course, the above effects may not be on the nerve directly, but rather on the astrocytes and other glial elements associated with the nerve head and the lamina.[107] Several other phenomena occur with age in addition to the likely significant reduction in accommodative vitreal movements, including an age-related increase in lens thickness. In the older eye the anterior lens pole encroaches on the anterior chamber, and the posterior lens pole is in a more rearward position, encroaching on the anterior central vitreous. With age, there is a large decrease in the forward movement of the ciliary muscle (65% and 85% loss in monkeys and humans, respectively), but less reduction in movement in the centripetal direction (i.e., ~20%).[81,82] Furthermore, the central vitreous liquifies with age,[108] perhaps allowing more pressure on the optic nerve via the fluid current, lens position, and accommodative pressure spikes. In the older eye, to achieve zonular relaxation and maximum accommodation, the ciliary muscle moves more in a centripetal direction (rather than forward direction), forcing the tips of the cistern branches backward. Thus, the cistern trunk would be pressed backward toward the optic nerve head (i.e., the hypotenuse of the right triangle (cistern branch) fits into a smaller space).[63]

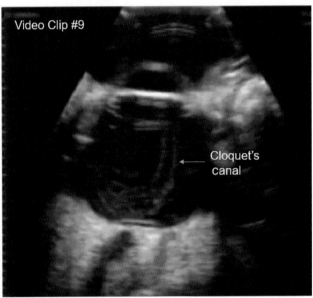

Fig. 3.16 See Video 3.9. Ultrasound biomicroscopy image in a normal (iris and lens present) rhesus monkey eye (age 19) following intravitreal injection of triamcinolone. The central vitreous moves posteriorly during accommodation all the way to the optic nerve. A *red dot* indicates when the stimulus to induce accommodation is on.

The sclera

During accommodation in both monkeys and humans, there is a slight change (a small notch) in the scleral contour in the region of the limbus when they are young (Fig. 3.19).[95] In the older resting eye, there is inward bowing of the sclera in the region of the limbus (increased concavity), and with it, significant changes in the geometry of the ciliary muscle/sclera/lens complex. The inward bowing of the sclera in the resting older eye is more pronounced during accommodation.[95]

The anterior hyaloid

Dynamic imaging of the anterior hyaloid membrane during accommodation in the rhesus monkey showed that the anterior hyaloid bows backward (Figs. 3.11–3.13; Video 3.2, 3.3, 3.5, and 3.9[63,95]). Burian and Allen[109] noted similar observations in two human subjects via gonioscopy (i.e., backward bowing/relaxation of the anterior hyaloid membrane during accommodation). The backward bowing of the anterior hyaloid during accommodation, as shown in in vivo images[63,95] (Video Clips 3.2, 3.3, and 3.5), was quantified and correlated with accommodative amplitude; the higher the accommodative amplitude, the greater the backward bowing of the anterior hyaloid (Fig. 3.20).

Fluid flows from the anterior chamber angle around the lens equator toward the anterior hyaloid and then into the cleft between the posterior vitreous zonule and the pars plana (Figs. 3.5 and 3.12 right panel; Video 3.2 right panel).[63,71] This indicates a change in anterior chamber pressure and volume induced by lens thickening and the redistribution of lens mass, as proposed by other researchers.[110] Although the function of the anterior hyaloid during accommodation may not be as previously proposed by Cramer's theory[111] or by the catenary theory of accommodation,[59,110] it is clearly reconfigured in a "dose-dependent" (i.e., accommodative amplitude-dependent) manner during the accommodative/disaccommodative response and may play a role in accommodation.[63]

The lens capsule

The crystalline lens is surrounded by the lens capsule (Fig. 3.21). This is a thin, transparent elastic membrane secreted by the lens epithelial cells and is largely composed of collagen type IV.[112] Fincham[113] was the first to attribute the accommodative change in shape of the lens to the forces exerted on the young lens by the lens capsule. Fincham studied the capsule in histologic sections and found it to be of relatively uniform thickness in nonaccommodating mammals. However, in nonhuman primates Fincham found it to be thickest at the midperipheral anterior

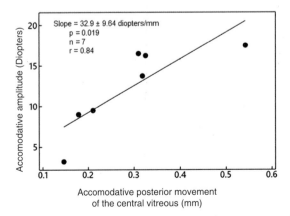

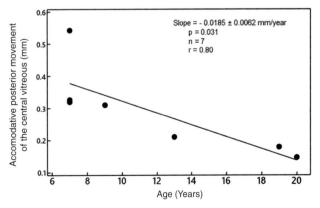

Fig. 3.17 Accommodative posterior movement of the central vitreous with respect to the retina plotted vs accommodative amplitude *(left panel)* or age *(right panel)* in seven rhesus monkeys. Triamcinolone particles were not visualized in the central vitreous in one additional monkey post injection, thus *n* = 7. (Reprinted with permission from Croft MA, Nork TM, Heatley G, et al. Intraocular accommodative movements in monkeys; relationship to presbyopia. *Exp Eye Res*. 2022;222:109029.)

TABLE 3.1   Intravitreal Accommodative Movements

		Accommodative Backward Bowing of the Anterior Hyaloid		Accommodative Posterior Movements of the Central Vitreous		Accommodative Movements of the Lacunae Peripheral () Tips			
						Forward Movement		Centripetal Movement	
		(mm)	paired t	(mm)	paired t	(mm)	paired t	(mm)	paired t
Young	Mean	0.29	p=0.001	0.34	p=0.003	0.540.54	p=0.008	0.15	p=0.014
Ages 7-13yr	s.e.m.n	0.025		0.055		0.115		0.045	
Older	Mean	0.21	p=0.029	0.15	p=0.030	0.22	p=0.052	0.13	p=0.30
Ages 19-25yr	s.e.m.n	0.043		0.012		0.053		0.023	
Young vs. Older two sample-t		N.S.		p=0.025		p=0.049		N.S.	
Young+Older	Mean	0.26	p=0.001	0.29	P=0.001	0.42	p=0.003	0.14	p=0.001
	s.e.m.n	0.028		0.057		0.098		0.028	

Data are mean standard error of the mean accommodative backward movements of the anterior hyaloid and central vitreous, and accommodative forward and centripetal movements of the peripheral lacunae (cistern branch) tips in the rhesus monkey eye. The young vs. older age groups were compared using an unpaired two-tailed two-sample t-test. *N.S*, Not significant. Reprinted with permission from Croft, MA, Nork TM, Heatley G, et al. Intraocular accommodative movements in monkeys; relationship to presbyopia. *Exp Eye Res.* 222;2022.

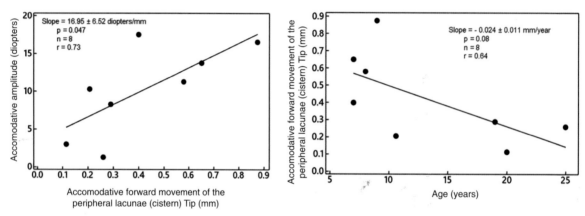

Fig. 3.18 Accommodative forward movement of the peripheral lacunae (cistern) tip with respect to the scleral spur plotted vs accommodative amplitude *(left panel)* or age *(right panel)* in eight rhesus monkeys. (Reprinted with permission from Croft MA, Nork TM, Heatley G, et al. Intraocular accommodative movements in monkeys; relationship to presbyopia. *Exp Eye Res.* 2022;222:109029.)

surface, thinner toward the lens equatorial region, with a posterior peripheral thickening, and thinnest at the region of the posterior pole of the lens[32] (Fig. 3.21). Several aspects of Fincham's idealized description of the capsule have been largely confirmed in a more recent study, although with some age-related changes in thickness.[112] The human lens capsule is about 11- to 15-μm thick at the anterior pole, and there is an anterior, midperipheral additional thickening of the capsule of about 13.5 to 16 μm that is located more central to the region of zonular insertion into the capsule around the lens equator. The equatorial region of the capsule, to which the anterior zonular fibers insert, is about 7-μm thick at the lens equator and does not appear to change systematically with age. The posterior capsule thickness decreases to a minimum of about 4 μm at the posterior pole, without posterior midperipheral thickening.[112]

In vivo experiments in the rhesus monkey model following extracapsular lens extraction showed that the posterior pole of the capsule bows backward during accommodation in a dose-dependent manner.[55] The higher the stimulus to accommodate, the greater the backward bowing of the capsule. The capsule bowed backward whether the eye was facing upward toward the ceiling or facing forward, indicating that these capsular movements were due to accommodative function and were independent of gravity.

The crystalline lens

The lens consists largely of lens fiber cells, which compose the nucleus and cortex. On the anterior lens surface, beneath the capsule, is a layer of lens epithelial cells, the deeper layers of which differentiate to become lens fiber cells. Lens epithelial cells just anterior to the equator undergo mitosis, and the cells migrate to the posterior equator where they differentiate and elongate (see Chapter 5). The proliferation of lens epithelial cells and their differentiation into lens fiber cells continues throughout life. The embryonic nucleus remains at the center of the lens throughout life as the cortex grows progressively around it by the addition of layers of lens fiber cells. Because the lens is contained within the capsule, lens epithelial cells do not slough off as do epithelial cells in other organ systems, such as those lining the skin and gut; thus, the lens continues to grow throughout life. After adolescence the human lens undergoes a linear increase in mass[114] and thickness[115,116] with increasing age, resulting in increases in anterior and posterior surface curvatures.[117,118] Also, there is a rapid growth of the lens in childhood, predominantly in the

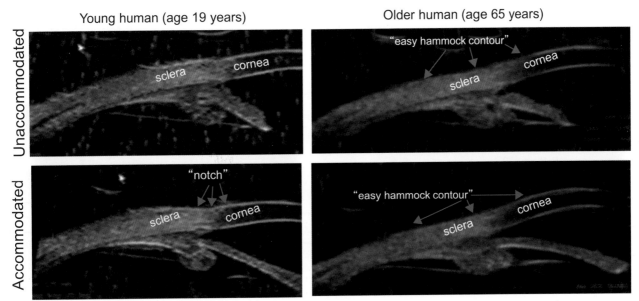

Fig. 3.19 Age-related change in the geometry of the sclera, ciliary body, and zonula: human. Note the deformation of the outer limbus ("notch"; *arrow*) in the accommodated young eye compared with the unaccommodated eye. In the older eye there is a discernable depression or "easy hammock" contour to the sclera. The notch appearance in the young sclera and the "easy hammock" appearance of the older sclera occur in the nasal but not the temporal quadrant. In the older eye there is not much difference between the unaccommodated and accommodated state with regard to the ciliary body/muscle shape. The young accommodated muscle is clearly in the anterior inward position and the lens equator is farther from Schwalbe's line compared with the unaccommodated eye.[95] The "easy hammock" appearance is also present in the monkey eye, but has not been observed as frequently due to iatrogenic conjunctival swelling in the monkey eye. (Reprinted with permission from Croft MA, Nork TM, McDonald JP, et al. Accommodative movements of the vitreous membrane, choroid, and sclera in young and presbyopic human and non human primate eyes. *Invest Ophthalmol and Vis Sci.* 2013;54:5049-5058.)

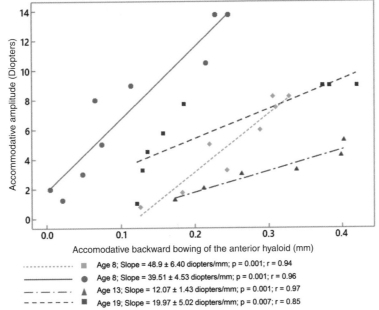

.... ■ Age 8; Slope = 48.9 ± 6.40 diopters/mm; p = 0.001; r = 0.94
——— ● Age 8; Slope = 39.51 ± 4.53 diopters/mm; p = 0.001; r = 0.96
—·—·— ▲ Age 13; Slope = 12.07 ± 1.43 diopters/mm; p = 0.001; r = 0.97
– – – – ■ Age 19; Slope = 19.97 ± 5.02 diopters/mm; p = 0.007; r = 0.85

Fig. 3.20 Accommodative backward bowing of the anterior hyaloid with respect to the scleral spur vs accommodative amplitude in one eye of each of four rhesus monkeys, aged 8, 8, 13, and 19 years old. Accommodative backward bowing of the anterior hyaloid was significantly related to accommodative amplitude; as the accommodative amplitude increased the backward bowing of the anterior hyaloid increased. (Reprinted with permission from Croft MA, Nork TM, Heatley G, et al. Intraocular accommodative movements in monkeys; relationship to presbyopia. *Exp Eye Res.* 2022;222:109029.)

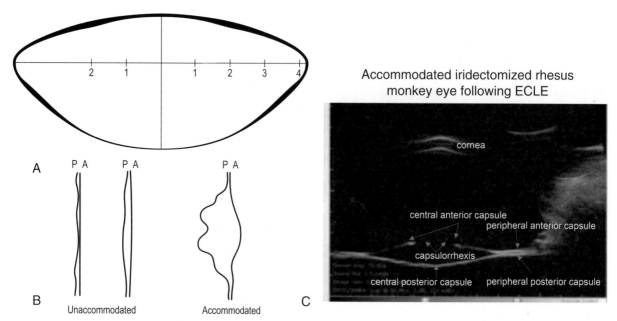

Fig. 3.21 (A) Fincham's idealized depiction of the regional variations in thickness of the human lens capsule, showing the anterior midperipheral thickening. The equatorial region of the capsule, to which the zonular fibers insert, show regional thinning. This idealized depiction is supported by more recent results, albeit with some age-related regional variations. (B) Appearance of the anterior (A) and posterior (P) capsule in the eye of a patient in whom the lens was displaced and lost from the eye after ocular injury. When the patient focused with the contralateral eye on a distant object *(left)* the capsule was relatively taut. When the patient focused on a near object *(middle)*, capsule became more flaccid; but still somewhat taut. After contraction of the ciliary muscle *(right)* with eserine, the capsule became completely flaccid. Observation by Graves of the behavior of the empty capsule in this aphakic patient eye served as the basis for Fincham's recognition of the role of the capsular tension holding the lens in a flattened and unaccommodated state when the ciliary muscle is relaxed, and the capsule rounding the lens into a more spherical and accommodated form when the ciliary muscle contracts. (From Fincham EF. The mechanism of accommodation. *Br J Ophthalmol*. 1937; Monograph VIII:7-80.) (**C**) Typical ultrasound biomicroscopy image of the accommodated capsule shape following extracapsular lens extraction (*ECLE*) in a rhesus monkey eye. When the muscle is contracted the capsule is progressively freer to mold the lens into a more spherical configuration. (Reprinted with permission from Croft MA, Nork TM, Heatley G, et al. Intraocular accommodative movements in monkeys; relationship to presbyopia. *Exp Eye Res*. 2022;222:109029.)

equatorial direction, with a significant increase in diameter and a progressive decrease in thickness. Then sometime during adolescence it transitions to a linear increase in lens thickness.[115,116,118] However, there is no systematic age-related change in unaccommodated adult lens diameter (see section Growth of the crystalline lens).[116,118,119]

The crystalline lens has a GRI of 1.379 near the poles and 1.410 at the center of the nucleus. The lens is not optically homogeneous, and when viewed through a slit lamp, several optical zones of discontinuity are observed that allow visual differentiation of the lens nucleus from the surrounding lens cortex. The unaccommodated young adult human lens is roughly 9.0 mm in diameter and 3.6-mm thick. The lens thickness increases by approximately 0.5 mm with 8 D of voluntary accommodation in young eyes (ages 19–31 years old), based on infrared photorefraction.[34] Pharmacologically induced accommodation in young human subjects (ages 19–23 years) produced 0.4-mm increase in lens thickness with an average of 12 D accommodation measured by Hartinger coincidence refractometry.[50]

THE MECHANISM OF ACCOMMODATION IN THE LENS AND EYE

The "basic" understanding of the accommodative mechanism is still largely in accord with the description provided by Helmholtz in

1855,[1,120] (Fig. 3.22), although Fincham[113] and more recent investigations have added further understanding. When the young eye is unaccommodated and focused for distance, the ciliary muscle is relaxed. Resting tension on the zonular fibers spanning the circumlental space and inserting around the lens equator (collectively called the anterior zonular fibers[52]) apply an outward directed tension around the lens equator through the lens capsule holding the lens in a relatively flattened and unaccommodated state. For the eye to focus at near, the ciliary muscle contracts and the inner apex of the ciliary muscle and body move forward and inward toward the axis of the eye[121] (Figs. 3.8 and 3.13; Video 3.1–3.4). This inward movement of the ciliary muscle apex stretches the choroid, which is attached to the ciliary muscle, pulling the intermediate vitreous zonule forward and releasing resting tension on all zonular fibers that are attached to the lens equator. The lens capsule then molds the lens into a more accommodated (thickened and rounded) form (Video 3.4).[61,71,113] The capsule provides the force that causes the lens to become accommodated.[61,113,114] A clear role for the lens capsule in accommodation stems from observations by Graves of the effect of accommodation on the empty lens capsule in an otherwise healthy aphakic eye.[122,123] When the patient looked at a distant object, the anterior and posterior capsule was taut and flat (Fig. 3.21B, left hand side). When the patient focused on a near object, the capsule became mildly flaccid, and the surfaces separated (Fig. 3.21B, middle).

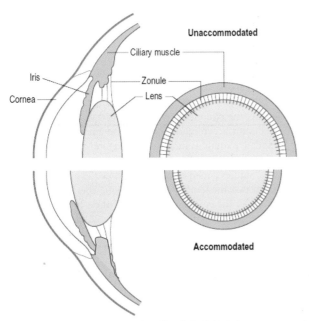

Fig. 3.22 Diagram showing the "basic" Helmholtz accommodative mechanism. In the *upper half* of the diagram the eye is in the unaccommodated state; in the *lower half* the eye is in the accommodated state. The *left side* shows a sagittal section and the *right side* a frontal section through the anterior segment of the eye. In the unaccommodated state resting tension on the zonule at the lens equator holds the lens in a relatively flattened and unaccommodated state. When the ciliary muscle contracts, this resting zonular tension is released and the lens is allowed to round up through the force exerted on the lens substance by the lens capsule. Lens axial thickness increases, lens equatorial diameter decreases, anterior chamber depth decreases and vitreous chamber depth decreases with accommodation The lens anterior and posterior surface curvatures increase to increase the optical power of the lens. (Redrawn from Koretz JF, Handelman GH. How the Human Eye Focuses. *Sci Am.* 1988; July:92–99.)

An eserine-stimulated contraction of the ciliary muscle resulted in a completely slack capsule (Fig. 3.21B, right hand side). Similar results were seen in the monkey eye in vivo (Fig. 3.21C), where the anterior and posterior capsule separated from each other. Fincham[113] concluded that resting zonular tension at the lens equator pulls outward on the capsule to hold the lens in the unaccommodated state, and that when the eye is accommodated, the resting tension on the zonular fibers is released to allow the capsule to mold the lens into the accommodated form. Further evidence of the role of the capsule comes from in vitro experiments. Upon dissecting a young human or monkey eye the isolated young lens with the intact capsule assumes a maximally accommodated form when the zonular fibers around the lens equator are cut. If the capsule is then cut and carefully removed from the isolated lens, the young decapsulated lens substance assumes a maximally unaccommodated form.[113,114,124] Furthermore, mechanical stretching studies of partially dissected young human and monkey eyes show that applying an outward directed stretching force to the lens via the capsule and anterior zonular fibers pulls the lens into a flattened and unaccommodated state, and releasing the zonular tension will allow the lens to become accommodated through the forces exerted by the capsule on the lens. Such in vitro mechanical stretching studies reliably and reproducibly produce accommodative optical changes in the lens that match the accommodative optical changes in the living eye.[61,62,125–127] During accommodation, the lens diameter decreases systematically in response to voluntary accommodation, brain-stimulated accommodation, or pharmacologically stimulated accommodation.[119,128–131]

Lens thickness,[34–36,39,132] the central anterior surface curvature, and to a lesser extent the central posterior surface curvature all increase during accommodation.[37–39] These physical changes are relatively linearly correlated with the accommodative optical changes in the eye. The increased lens surface curvatures result in an increase in the optical power of the lens. Anterior chamber depth decreases owing to the forward movement of the anterior lens surface, and the vitreous chamber depth decreases owing to the posterior movement of the posterior lens surface[34,35,39] (Video 3.4).[71] About 75% of the increase in lens thickness is accounted for by the forward movement of the anterior lens surface and about 25% is accounted for by a backward movement of the posterior lens surface.[34,35] When the accommodative effort ceases, the ciliary muscle relaxes and the elasticity of the posterior attachment of the choroid pulls the ciliary muscle back into its flattened and unaccommodated configuration. The outward movement of the apex of the ciliary body once again increases the tension on the anterior zonular fibers around the lens equator to pull the lens via the capsule into a flattened and unaccommodated form. Variants on the Helmholtz accommodative mechanism have been suggested to include a role for the vitreous and differential pressure changes in the eye.[58,59,103] However, accommodation still occurs after vitrectomy,[60] and mechanical stretching studies of dissected eyes in which the vitreous was absent and thus no pressure differential could exist between the vitreous and the anterior chamber resulted in normal accommodative optical changes to the lens,[61,125,127] thereby theoretically obviating a role for the vitreous or for differential pressure changes in the eye. A revisionist theory of accommodation, originally proposed by Tscherning[133] and espoused by others,[134–136] was contradicted by the Helmholtz accommodative mechanism in that Tscherning paradoxically required an increase in lens equatorial diameter during accommodation, a flattening of the peripheral lens surfaces and an increase in curvature of the lens central surfaces. However, there is no experimental evidence supporting the supposed accommodative increase in lens diameter, and numerous studies demonstrate that lens diameter decreases systematically during accommodation.[119,121128,129,131,137]

ACCOMMODATIVE OPTICAL CHANGES IN THE LENS AND EYE

For the unaccommodated emmetropic eye to focus on a near object, an increase in the eye's optical power, which occurs through an increase in the optical power of the lens is required. The latter comes from an increase in anterior and, to a lesser extent, posterior lens surface curvatures. Several other physical changes that have optical effects also occur in the eye and lens during accommodation. Lens thickness increases, the lens asphericity changes, and the pupil constricts (Video 3.4). In addition, because the lens has a GRI, the form of which is constrained by the lens shape and size, the lens changes shape, and so too must the form of the lens. However, there is evidence from magnetic resonance imaging (MRI) studies that the refractive index profile can be closely fit with a power function that remains constant with accommodation, except for scaling to account for the accommodative thickness change.[41] The outer cortex and nuclear index remain unchanged with accommodation.[41] In addition, the changes in shape of the lens also produce changes in ocular aberrations of the eye.

Simple paraxial vergence calculations show that, for parallel rays incident on a simple biconvex lens, if lens thickness alone is increased, lens power decreases. However, if the lens thickens in an eye, this must occur in conjunction with either a decrease in anterior chamber depth or an increase in anterior segment length consequent to the increase in lens thickness. For a distant object, the lens inside the eye does not have parallel light incident on it, but rather convergent light owing to refraction by the cornea. Simple paraxial schematic eye calculations show that if lens thickness alone is increased without a change in lens curvatures, but with a resultant decrease in anterior chamber depth, the result is an overall increase in the power of the eye. The accommodative increase in the optical power of the lens, however, is primarily due to an increase in the lens surface curvatures. Most of the change in curvature with accommodation is in the anterior lens surface. The posterior lens surface changes only slightly with accommodation. Thus, most of the power change is due to the change in the anterior lens surface shape.

The accommodative optical increase in the power of the eye is therefore ultimately due to a complex combination of optical and physical changes in the lens and the eye. This results not only in an increase in optical power of the eye, but also accommodative changes in ocular aberrations of the eye and lens.[125,126,138–140] In addition, the iris constricts during accommodation, which decreases the diameter of the entrance pupil of the eye. Simply decreasing the entrance pupil diameter results in an overall reduction in optical aberrations and increase in depth of focus.[126] Further, human eyes typically have negative spherical aberration (i.e., central rays are focused further away from the the lens than peripheral rays). Rays passing through the periphery of the pupil will therefore contribute to moving the the position of the sharpest focus away from the lens. By removing the most peripheral rays, pupil constriction therefore results in a shift of the sharpest focus toward the lens, effectively increasing the optical power.[126] When accommodation occurs in a young eye, these various optical changes occur in concert.

THE STIMULUS TO ACCOMMODATE

Eyes have some residual (or resting) level of accommodation amounting to approximately 0.5 to 1.5 D when at rest. This is called tonic accommodation, a lead of accommodation, or night myopia. In a young eye, the effort to focus on near objects causes three physiological responses: the eyes accommodate, the pupils constrict, and the eyes converge. Together these three physiologic functions are referred to as the accommodative triad or the near reflex. These three actions are neuronally coupled through the preganglionic parasympathetic innervation extending from the Edinger-Westphal (EW) nucleus in the brain. The intraocular muscles (iris and ciliary muscle) are innervated by the postganglionic ciliary nerves entering the sclera. The extraocular muscles of the eyes are innervated by the oculomotor (III), trochlear (IV), and abducens (VI) nerves. The axons of these nerves originate from motor nerve nuclei in the brainstem, which receive impulses from the EW nucleus. Accommodation and convergence, and the accompanying pupil constriction, are neuronally coupled in the brain and thus in the two eyes. An accommodative stimulus, such as minus lens–induced blur or a proximal stimulus presented monocularly to one eye, results in binocular accommodation, convergence, and pupil constriction. Similarly, a convergence stimulus presented monocularly to one eye results in pupil constriction, convergence, and accommodation in both eyes. Accommodation can be stimulated in a variety of ways. It can be driven by blur cues alone, such that if myopic blur is presented to one or both eyes by placing a negative-powered lens in front of the eye(s), both eyes will accommodate to attempt to overcome the imposed defocus. If convergence is stimulated in a young eye by having the subject fixate on a distant target and placing base-out prisms in front of the eyes, for example, pupil constriction and accommodation will occur. In an emmetropic eye, blur and vergence-driven accommodation can be induced simultaneously with a proximal stimulus. If a near object is presented, coupled accommodation and convergence occur. As the accommodative stimulus increases, the objectively measured accommodative response is typically less than the magnitude of the stimulus. This is called the lag of accommodation. Studies in which the accommodative response is measured with a wavefront

aberrometer show that calculated retinal image quality for the near object actually improves when the lag of accommodation is taken into account.[141] Therefore, although the overall refraction of the eye lags the accommodative stimulus, the lag may serve to maximize retinal image quality for near objects, owing to the eye's ocular aberrations. As the stimulus amplitude increases, there is a linear increase in the accommodative response, although the slope is less than 1 due to the accommodative lag. As the stimulus is increased further, the lag increases until the maximum accommodative response amplitude is reached. The accommodative stimulus function is therefore "S" shaped with the initial lead, the intermediate linear region with some lag, and the final plateau region. Studies aimed at addressing how the eye detects defocus have shown that the longitudinal chromatic aberration (LCA) of the eye plays a role. The eye's imperfect optics cause considerable LCA such that shorter wavelengths of light are focused closer to the lens than longer wavelengths. Removing the LCA by using monochromatic light or optically neutralizing or reversing the LCA disrupts the normal accommodative reflex response.[142–145] Accommodation can also be pharmacologically stimulated. Topical application of muscarinic cholinergic agonists, such as pilocarpine, results in direct pharmacologic stimulation of the ciliary muscle.[46,47,146] In rhesus monkeys, pharmacologically stimulated accommodation results in higher amplitudes than centrally stimulated accommodation.[147–149] This is attributed to a supramaximal pharmacologic contraction of the ciliary muscle and iris, which is greater than the contraction due to a parasympathetically driven stimulus from the brain.[150] In addition, drug-stimulated accommodation ultimately produces a net forward movement of the natural lens that does not occur with centrally stimulated accommodation in monkeys[151] or with voluntary accommodation in humans.[152] Rapid and strong pupil constriction also occurs with pharmacologic stimulation, but convergence does not. Anticholinesterases such as echothiophate iodide produce a resting tonus of accommodation when applied topically, owing to their breakdown of the neurotransmitter acetylcholine normally released at the neuromuscular junction.[23] Accommodative esotropia, which often occurs in uncorrected hyperopes because of the need to accommodate to focus on distant objects, can be treated with topical echothiophate. By producing increased accommodative tonus without increased neuronal input, the stimulus for convergence is reduced, and the accommodation convergence/accommodation ratio is reduced, helping to alleviate the accommodative esotropia.[153] Anticholinesterases produce a long response to a single administration and so are more therapeutically useful than shorter-acting cholinomimetics like pilocarpine.

THE PHARMACOLOGY OF ACCOMMODATION

Accommodation occurs when the postganglionic parasympathetic innervation to the ciliary muscle releases the neurotransmitter acetylcholine at the neuromuscular junctions.

Acetylcholine, the natural neuromuscular cholinergic neurotransmitter, is a muscarinic agonist that binds with the ciliary muscle muscarinic receptors to cause the ciliary muscle to contract. Topically applied muscarinic agonists, such as pilocarpine, also bind to the muscarinic receptors and cause ciliary muscle contraction, and thus accommodation.[46,47,146,152] This involuntary monocular accommodative response, which in some individuals can be of higher amplitude than voluntary accommodation, is greater in eyes with lighter-colored irides (e.g., blue) than in eyes with darker-colored irides (e.g., brown).[47] Dark-eyed individuals are less sensitive to topically applied cholinomimetic drugs because the pigmented cells in the iris and ciliary muscle bind the drugs and decrease their bioavailability. This also applies to the ocular hypotensive response to cholinomimetics.[154] Accommodation and miosis can be pharmacologically blocked temporarily by paralyzing the ciliary muscle (cycloplegia) and the pupillary sphincter (mydriasis) with topical application of muscarinic antagonists such as atropine, cyclopentolate, or tropicamide. These agents competitively bind to and block the muscarinic receptors in the ciliary muscle and the iris. There are at least five muscarinic receptor subtypes (M1–M5). Outflow facility (ciliary muscle contraction), accommodation (ciliary muscle contraction), and miosis (pupillary sphincter contraction) are all mediated by the M3 subtype.

MEASUREMENT OF ACCOMMODATION

Although objective methods are available for measurement of accommodation (Box 3.2), unfortunately, clinically the subjective measurement of the near point of clear vision is most often used. The subjective push-up method requires the patient to gradually move a near letter chart toward the eyes and report when a near letter chart can no longer be maintained in clear, sharp focus. The reciprocal of the distance from the eyes and the near reading chart is then used as a measure of accommodative amplitude in diopters. Subjective push-up measurements of accommodation are fraught with missteps and are discussed in sections Depth of Field and Visual Acuity in this chapter and Chapters 1 and 2 of this book. Subjective measurements overestimate the true accommodative optical change in power of the eye, and there are many reasons why they should be avoided. The end point of the subjective push-up test requires a subjective evaluation of the best image focus by the subject, and this end point varies between individuals. Subjective evaluation of the point of best focus can be influenced by depth of focus, visual acuity, contrast sensitivity of the eye, and contrast of the image, for example. A dimly illuminated reading chart may provide a poor stimulus to accommodate or may not allow an accurate recognition of defocus. Different levels of illumination alter pupil diameter and therefore depth of focus of the eye, thus influencing the near point of clear vision. Subjective push-up measurements are also confounded by the increasing angular subtense of the object. As a reading chart is brought closer to the eye, the retinal image size increases, and hence the legibility of the letters increases as they are brought closer. Although this can be avoided by carefully controlling the image angular magnification with scaled letter sizes, this is not done with the subjective push-up test.

Subjective measurement of accommodative amplitude can also be done by placing negative-powered trial lenses in front of one or both eyes to blur a distant letter chart. The optically induced blur stimulates accommodation in an attempt to maintain a sharp focused image on the retina. The negative lens power is progressively increased until the smallest legible letter line of a distance Snellen letter chart can no longer be maintained in clear focus.[155] Accommodative amplitude is determined by the strongest-powered negative lens through which the smallest legible Snellen letter line can still be read clearly. This is still a subjective test and prone to the same sources of errors as the subjective push-up test.

Subjective tests are also an inaccurate measure of accommodative amplitude because of the lag of accommodation. The accommodative optical response of the eye lags behind the stimulus and this lag increases as the stimulus amplitude increases; therefore, the dioptric vergence of the stimulus is expected to be less than the accommodative response. Subjective methods traditionally used for evaluating accommodative amplitude are inherently inaccurate and overestimate true accommodative amplitude. The ability to read at near does not unequivocally imply that accommodation occurs, and subjective methods to measure accommodation cannot differentiate between true accommodation, depth of field, or optical compensation such as with multifocal optics.

Accommodation can be measured objectively because it results in a change in the optical refractive power of the eye. Objective methods provide a true measure of accommodative amplitude, and accurate objective measurement of accommodation can be done statically[44,155,156] or dynamically.[157–161] Autorefractors, refractometers, and aberrometers are suitable instruments for objective measurement of accommodation. These instruments provide a measure of the refraction of the eye as the eye changes focus between a distant and a near target. The accommodative response amplitude is then considered as the difference between the refraction when looking at a distant target and the refraction when looking at a near target. Subjective measurements in presbyopes may suggest that some accommodation is present, but when objective methods are used, a complete loss of active accommodation is demonstrated at the endpoint of presbyopia.[45,46] The success of objective instruments to measure maximal accommodation relies on the accuracy of the instrument, as well as on the ability to elicit the maximum accommodative response from the subject and whether the near target can be viewed monocularly or binocularly by the subject. To stimulate accommodation, the subject must be presented with a compelling accommodative stimulus and the subject must elicit an accommodative response. If the subject does not produce an accommodative response, no accommodation can be measured.

The objective accommodative response can be recorded for instance by stimulating accommodation in one eye and measuring the consensual accommodative response in the contralateral eye. In this case, accommodation can be stimulated by placing a negative trial lens in front of the eye while the eye views a distant target.[46,47] This method suffers the disadvantage that the convergence response accompanying accommodation occurs entirely in the eye being measured because the eye being stimulated maintains a primary gaze position as it fixates on the distant letter chart. Unless the instrument being used to measure accommodation is realigned with the optical axis of the converged eye, an off-axis refraction measurement will result, which can introduce inaccuracies. Accommodation can also be stimulated by topically applied muscarinic agonists (e.g., pilocarpine) and the resulting accommodative response measured periodically over 30 to 45 minutes using a refractometer or an autorefractor until the maximal accommodative response is attained.[46,47] This is a slow time course for an accommodative response, but if the refraction is measured frequently enough the maximum accommodative response amplitude can be determined. The accommodative amplitude measured in this way is independent of a visual accommodative stimulus and of patient subjectivity because the application of the drug produces the accommodative response. However, the magnitude of the accommodative response depends on drug concentration, intraocular pharmacokinetics, iris pigmentation,

---

BOX 3.2 Measurement of Accommodation

- Subjective measurement of accommodation relies on a subject's perception of the clarity of focus of a visual target as the target is moved towards the eyes.
- Subjective estimation of near reading distance overestimates the accommodative response amplitude, largely owing to depth of field of the eye.
- Depth of field of the eye increases as the pupil constricts, and since the pupil constricts during accommodation, this will further increase the depth of field of the eye.
- Objective measurement of accommodation can be accomplished by measuring the refractive change in optical power of the eye with an objective instrument such as an autorefractor or an aberrometer as the eye changes focus from a distant target to a near target.

and other nonaccommodative factors that influence how much drug or how quickly the drug reaches the ciliary muscle.

PRESBYOPIA

Presbyopia (Box 3.3) is the loss of near visual function, typically noticeable at around age 40 to 50 years, that is due to the gradual age-related loss of accommodation amplitude that begins early in life and ultimately culminates in a complete loss of accommodation by about 50 years of age.[45,46,162] Subjective measurements of accommodation suggest that about 1 D of accommodation remains after approximately 50 years of age.[25,45,46] This small remaining apparent response is due to depth of field effects that are inherent in the subjective measurement of accommodation. Objective measurement of accommodation shows a linear decline of about 2.5 D per decade, reaching zero at about 50 to 55 years of age.[45,46,162] Presbyopia results in the complete loss of the normal physiologic function of accommodation roughly two-thirds of the way through the human life span. Few other normal physiologic functions undergo such a profound and systematic deterioration so soon and with such certainty. Presbyopia is likely a consequence of age-related changes in the accommodative apparatus that begin early in life and continue beyond the point at which accommodation is ultimately completely lost, possibly continuing until death. Two-thirds of human accommodative amplitude is lost by age 35 years, but at this age most people do not yet notice the loss. Studies of subjects between the ages of 15 and 45 years may be of the most interest for trying to understand the progression of presbyopia, but the age-related changes that continue beyond 50 years of age may also provide important insights.

FACTORS CONTRIBUTING TO PRESBYOPIA

Because the accommodative apparatus is composed of many different tissues and systems and accommodation is a complex interaction of these components, there are potentially many factors that contribute to the accommodative loss. Aging affects many of these tissues and

---

BOX 3.3   Presbyopia

- Presbyopia is the age-related loss of accommodative amplitude.
- The accommodative optical change in power of the eye with an effort to focus at near is completely lost by about 55 years of age.
- Many aspects of the accommodative apparatus of the eye change with increasing age
- Lens thickness increases, the lens anterior surface curvature increases, anterior segment length increases, the apex of the unaccommodated ciliary body progressively moves inward towards the axis of the eye, and the elastic modulus of the capsule increases.
- Lens stiffness increases exponentially with increasing age.
- The stiffness gradient of the human lens increases with increasing age. In the young lens, the nucleus is softer than the cortex, but with increasing age the nucleus undergoes a greater increase in stiffness than the cortex such that in the older lens the nucleus becomes stiffer than the cortex.
- Ultimately, the human lens completely loses the ability to undergo accommodative changes in optical power.
- Presbyopia is, at its end point, due to a complete loss in accommodative ability of the lens.
- Although the ciliary muscle retains the ability to contract, the mobility of the muscle decreases with age owing to posterior restriction, more so in the forward vector than in the centripetal vector, and may play a role in presbyopia.
- The vitreous may also play a role in accommodation and thereby presbyopia.

---

systems to differing extents, thus the reasons why accommodation is lost are potentially many and complex. Although several fundamental changes occur, such as stiffening of the lens, that have profound impacts on the ability of the eye to accommodate, other aspects of ocular aging may also impact accommodative amplitude. Furthermore, many studies show age-related changes in the accommodative structures that progress well beyond the age at which accommodation is lost. Ultimately, at its end point, presbyopia is due to a loss of the fine balance of forces that permit the accommodative structures to cause a change in optical power of the lens. In the following sections, age-related changes in the ciliary muscle, lens, lens capsule, zonule, and associated tissues are considered in terms of their possible roles in presbyopia.

Age-related changes in rhesus ciliary muscle

Because accommodation is lost with increasing age, and accommodation is mediated by the ciliary muscle, the question arises whether presbyopia is due to a loss in ability of the ciliary muscle to contract. Pupillary constriction and convergence are part of the near reflex but do not decrease with increasing age; therefore, this suggests that generalized loss of muscle contractility is not a normal part of presbyopia.[163] The iris continues to contract to light stimulus on the retina and with an accommodative effort even in presbyopes; thus it is likely that the ciliary muscle also continues to contract with an accommodative effort in presbyopes. Accommodative excursion of the ciliary muscle is reported to be reduced in presbyopic rhesus monkeys, as seen from both direct observation in surgically aniridic animals in which accommodation is stimulated by an electrode placed in the EW nucleus,[164] and from histologic study of ciliary muscle topography in eyes fixed in the presence of pilocarpine or atropine[165] (Fig. 3.23). The posterior attachment of the rhesus ciliary muscle, comprising elastic tendons continuous with elastic lamina of Bruch's membrane, shows structural changes with increasing age.[166] Whereas the elastic tendons of the young monkey eye stain strongly for actin and desmin, in the aging eye there is less elastin and this region exhibits increased collagen fibers that adhere to and fix the elastic fibers to Bruch's membrane, along with thickening of the elastic tendons and increased microfibrils.[166] These anatomical changes may lead to decreased compliance of the posterior attachment of the ciliary muscle and the choroid. This is supported by the observation that in aged rhesus monkey eyes, in which the posterior attachment of the ciliary muscle is severed prior to accommodative stimulation, a configurational change occurs that is otherwise absent.[54,167,168] However, the contractile force of isolated rhesus ciliary muscle strips to pilocarpine stimulation is not reduced with increasing age[169] (Fig. 3.24). Although there is some loss of ciliary muscle mass, there is no loss of muscarinic receptor number or binding affinity, and no change in cholineacetyltransferase or acetylcholinesterase activity, the enzymes that respectively synthesize and degrade the muscarinic cholinergic transmitter.[170] These histologic, histochemical, and ultrastructural studies collectively show that the reduced ciliary muscle accommodative movement in presbyopic monkey eyes is due to a loss of elasticity of the muscle's posterior elastic tendons, Bruch's membrane, and perhaps the entire choroid, and not to any degenerative changes in the ciliary muscle itself.

Studies comparing the accommodative movements of the ciliary muscle and lens equator in iridectomized monkeys show that both ciliary muscle and lens edge movements are reduced with increasing age and the loss of accommodation. However, some argue that accommodative movements of the ciliary muscle are always greater than accommodative movements of the lens edge, irrespective of age[82,171] (Fig. 3.25) and that ciliary muscle movements are also greater than lens edge movements, even in young monkeys.[171] They argue that lens

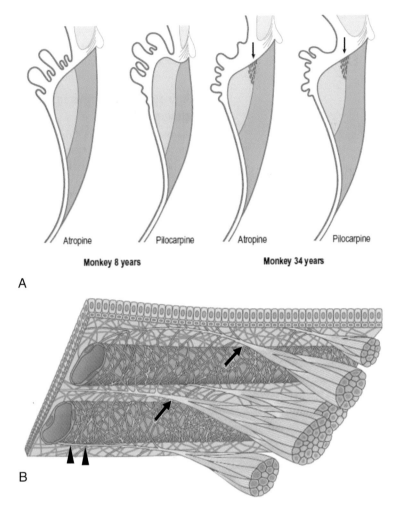

Atropine   Pilocarpine   Atropine   Pilocarpine

Monkey 8 years   **Monkey 34 years**

A

B

Fig. 3.23 (A) Diagrams of the configuration of the ciliary muscle from an 8-year-old (*left pair of images*) and a 34-year-old (*right pair of images*) enucleated rhesus monkey eye after each globe was bisected with one half (*left*) placed in an atropine solution and the other half (*right*) placed in a pilocarpine solution. Representative sections based on histologic specimens. In the young, but not the old eye, the pilocarpine treated ciliary muscle (CM) showed a configurational accommodative change. The CM from the older eye fails to undergo an accommodative configurational change, owing to the loss of elasticity of the posterior attachment of the CM to the choroid. The 8-year-old rhesus monkey exhibits essentially no intramuscular connective tissue, whereas the 34-year-old rhesus monkey exhibits connective tissue (*arrows*) only anteriorly between longitudinal and reticular zones of the ciliary muscle. (B) Diagram of the posterior attachment of the CM in rhesus monkeys. The meridional muscle fiber bundles (*arrows*) are attached to the elastic layer of Bruch's membrane via the elastic tendons. Smaller elastic fibers (*arrowheads*) connect the tendons of different bundles to the elastic network that surrounds the vessels of the pars plana. (Panel B from Tamm, Lutjen-Drecoll, Jungkunz & Rohen. Posterior attachment of ciliary muscle in young, accommodating old, presbyopic monkeys. *Invest Ophthalmol Vis Sci.* 1991;32:1680, with permission from the Association for Research in Vision and Ophthalmology and from the author.)

movement, not ciliary body movement, limits the accommodative amplitude at all ages and that at the end point of presbyopia, ciliary muscle movement still occurs even in the absence of accommodative movements of the lens.[82] Thus, the proponents of a lens-centered reason for presbyopia argue that although accommodative movement of the ciliary muscle may be systematically reduced with increasing age in rhesus monkey eyes, it is not the reduced ciliary body movements that limit accommodative amplitude in rhesus monkeys. However, one must recall that a greater amount of centrifugal muscle movement than centrifugal lens movements is required to induce accommodation (See section Age-related changes in ciliary muscle accommodative movements) and that age-related changes of the lens and muscle may *both*

play a role in presbyopia. In addition, one must consider the vector/direction of ciliary muscle accommodative movement (see section Age-related changes in ciliary muscle accommodative movements).

Age-related changes in human ciliary muscle

With increasing age, the human ciliary muscle shows a loss of muscle fibers and an increase in connective tissue.[167,172,173] Despite this, studies using impedance cyclography[174,175] or modeling[176] to indirectly infer force of contraction of the human ciliary muscle suggest that human ciliary muscle contractile force does not decrease, but indeed may increase and reach a maximum at the age at which presbyopia is manifest. These findings are consistent with observations of

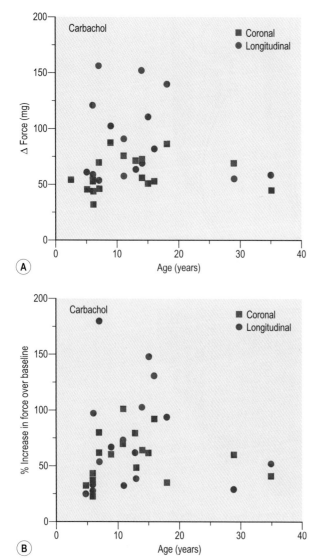

Fig. 3.24 (A) Force of contraction and (B) percent increase in force of contraction over baseline of longitudinal *(circles)* and coronal *(squares)* strips of isolated rhesus monkey ciliary muscle strips stimulated with muscarinic agonists aceclidine (50 μm) or carbachol (1 μm). No age dependence in force of contraction of the isolated ciliary muscle was observed. (Graphs modified with data from Poyer JF, Kaufman PL, Flügel C. Age does not affect contractile responses of the isolated rhesus monkey ciliary muscle to muscarinic agonists. *Curr Eye Res.* 1993;12:413-422, with permission from Swetz & Zeitlinger Publishers.)

continued accommodative movement of the ciliary body with accommodative effort in human presbyopes and pseudophakic eyes.[137,177,178] Histologic study of the atropinized human ciliary muscle shows that total area, area of longitudinal and reticular portion, and length of the muscle decrease with age. In addition, there is a decrease in ciliary ring diameter[137] and the inner apex of the unaccommodated ciliary muscle resides further forward and inward toward the anterior/posterior (A/P) axis in the aging eye so that the configuration of the older unaccommodated ciliary muscle appears more like that of the young accommodated ciliary muscle[167] (Fig. 3.26). This is due to the age-related loss of elasticity of the posterior ciliary muscle tendons, which are not tightly fixed to Bruch's membrane but connect to the elastic net of the choroid, which also loses elasticity with age. Thus, the relaxed muscle is not pulled backward as much as in young eyes but retains a somewhat contracted shape in presbyopic eyes. Whether

this is a cause or a consequence of the anterior zonule gradually pulling the ciliary muscle inward is not clear. Based on this result it has been suggested that, at rest, the aged human ciliary muscle may be less able to hold or pull the crystalline lens into its flattened and unaccommodated configuration.[163]

Age-related changes in ciliary muscle accommodative movements

Accommodation in the human and monkey eye occurs with the forward (anterior) and centripetal (inward) movement of the ciliary muscle during contraction, releasing tension on the zonula that are attached to the lens, allowing the lens to thicken and increase in curvature. By middle age in the monkey eye (ages 12–16.5 years) centripetal muscle movement declines by only 19%, whereas forward muscle movement declines by ~50%.[81] Similar results are seen in the human eye.[50] Forward muscle movement declines by 61% and 85% in the older presbyopic monkey (Fig. 3.27) and human eyes, respectively (monkey, ages 17–26 years; human, ages 50–65 years).[50,81,168] A study utilizing the monkey eye demonstrated that severing the posterior attachment restored forward movement of the muscle.[168,179] At around 3 D of accommodation in the monkey eye, the amount of centripetal lens movement required did not significantly change with age; however, the amount of centripetal ciliary body movement required significantly increased with age, while the amount of forward ciliary body movement significantly decreased with age.[81] In the middle-aged animals (12–16.5 years), a greater amount of centripetal ciliary body movement was required to induce a given level of lens movement, and thereby a given level of accommodation, compared with the young animals (6–10 years). Collectively, the data suggest that, with age, the accommodative system may be attempting to compensate for the loss of forward ciliary body movement by increasing the amount of centripetal ciliary body movement. This, in turn, would allow enough zonular relaxation to achieve the magnitude of centripetal lens movement necessary for a given amplitude of accommodation.[81] The system adapts.

Age-related changes in the zonule

The anterior zonular attachment all around the equatorial region of the lens serves a fundamental role in the accommodative process. It is the outward force directed through these zonular fibers and the resulting tension on the lens capsule that maintains the unaccommodated lens in its flattened state. The release of this resting tension during accommodation allows the capsule to mold the lens into its more spherical and accommodated form.[113] Thus, any age-related changes that may affect this zonular attachment are likely to impact the accommodative process and may contribute to presbyopia. The anterior zonula is a very fine, delicate network of fibers and is especially difficult to study; thus relatively few studies have been done on this tissue. Zonular spring constants determined indirectly by stretching human tissues show no correlation with age.[180] Scanning electron microscopic studies of human eyes over a range of ages show an anterior zonular/capsular shift on the lens with increasing age.[181] The distance from the zonular/capsule insertion to the lens equator increases, the distance from the zonular/capsule insertion to the ciliary processes does not change, and the circumlental space decreases with age (see further in this section). In addition, rate of increase in distance from zonular/capsular insertion to lens equator remains relatively constant until the fifth decade and then increases dramatically.[181] The constancy of the distance between the zonular/capsular insertion and the ciliary body suggests that there would be no change in zonular length or zonular tension with increasing age, provided zonular elasticity remains unchanged. It is therefore possible that the decreased circumlental space is due to

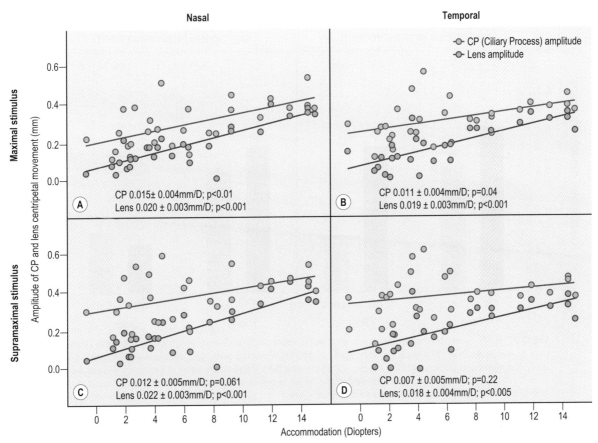

Fig. 3.25 Graphs showing the accommodative excursions of the ciliary processes *(pink symbols)* and lens edge *(blue symbols)* from the eyes of live iridectomized rhesus monkeys. Quantitative goniovideographic analysis of the accommodative movements from the nasal *(left)* and temporal *(right)* sides of the monkey eyes for Edinger-Westphal stimulated accommodative responses to either maximal *(top)* or supramaximal *(bottom)* stimulus amplitudes. Accommodative movements of the lens and ciliary processes are reduced with the age-related loss of accommodative amplitude, but in all eyes the magnitude of ciliary process movement exceeds the magnitude of the lens edge movements. (From Croft MA, Glasser A, Heatley G, et al. Accommodative Ciliary Body and Lens Function in Rhesus Monkeys, I: Normal Lens, Zonule and Ciliary Process Configuration in the Iridectomized Eye. *Invest Ophthalmol Vis Sci.* 2006;47:1076-1086. Reproduced with permission from The Association for Research in Vision and Ophthalmology.)

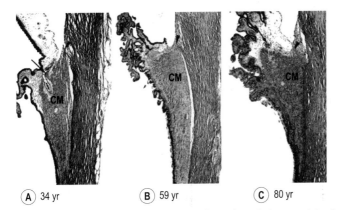

Fig. 3.26 Age-related changes in the configuration of the atropinized human ciliary muscle. Histologic sections from (A) a 34-year-old, (B) a 59-year-old, and (C) an 80-year-old human donor eye. The aging, atropinized human ciliary muscle looks more like a young accommodated ciliary muscle with the inner apex of the ciliary muscle moving forward and toward the axis of the eye. (Reprinted from Tamm S, Tamm E, Rohen JW. Age-related changes of the human ciliary muscle. A quantitative morphometric study. *Mechanisms Ageing Development* 1992;62:209-221, with permission from Elsevier Science Ltd.)

centripetal pulling of the ciliary body by the zonule as the zonule/capsular shift occurs with increasing lens thickness, or due to the inward expansion of the ciliary muscle.[167,182] The decreased circumlental space is not due to an age-related increase in equatorial diameter of the lens because lens diameter does not increase systematically with age (see section Growth of the Crystalline Lens). Farnsworth and Shyne[181] theorized that the anterior zonular shift occurs because the capsule is thinner on the posterior lens surface and is stretched more than the anterior capsule as the lens continues to grow within the capsule.[112,113] In older eyes, as a consequence of this zonular/capsular shift, the attachment of the anterior zonular fibers to the lens is anterior to the equator, the fine zonular fibers that reside at the lens equator in the young eye are found anterior to the equator, and there are fewer zonular fibers at the equator.[181] This would result in diminution of the outward directed force on the lens equator by the anterior zonular fibers as a whole and is suggested as a contributing factor in the age-related loss of accommodation.[181] Measurements on unfixed human eyes from which the lens substance was removed by phacoemulsification also show an age-dependent increase in the distance from the anterior zonular/capsular insertion to the equatorial edge of the capsular bag, a decrease in circumlental space, and an age-dependent increase in the distance from the anterior zonular/capsular insertion to the ciliary body.[183] However,

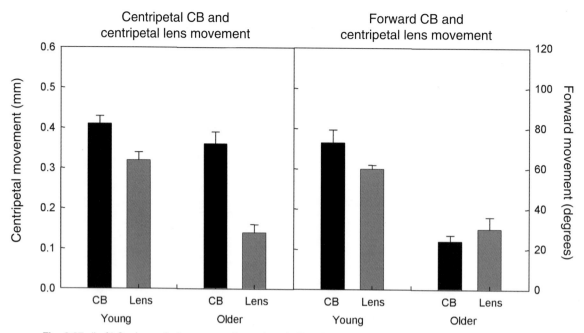

Fig. 3.27 *(Left)* Gonioscopically measured centripetal ciliary body (CB) and lens movement (mm) in young (*n* = 6) and older (*n* = 16) rhesus monkey eyes. *(Right)* Ultrasound biomicroscopy–measured forward ciliary body (degrees) and gonioscopically measured centripetal lens (mm) movement in young (*n* = 5) and older (*n* = 11) rhesus monkey eyes. The narrowing of the angle between the anterior aspect of the ciliary body and the inner aspect of the cornea was used as a surrogate indicator of forward ciliary body movement during accommodation. (Reprinted with permission from Croft MA, Kaufman PL. Accommodation and presbyopia: Neuromuscular and biophysical aspects. *Ophthalmol Clin North Am.* 2006;19:13-24.)

absence of the lens substance from the capsular bag complicates interpretation of these measurements.

Age-related changes in the capsule

The thickness of the anterior lens capsule has been reported to increase from around 11 microns (μm) at birth to approximately 20 μm at 60 years of age and decreases slightly thereafter.[184] Krag[185] found an increase in the thickness of the anterior lens capsule from 11 to 33 μm up to age 75 years and a slight decrease thereafter. More recent results show an increase in the thickness of the anterior midperipheral capsule and a thinning of the midperipheral posterior capsule with increasing age.[112] Fisher[184] measured the extensibility of the human lens capsule by applying a fluid pressure behind the central part of the anterior lens capsule clamped between two rings and found it to be 29% and age-independent. Despite the increased capsular thickness with increasing age, Fisher[184] showed a decrease in Young's modulus of elasticity of the capsule from 6×10^7 dyn/cm^2 in infancy to 2×10^7 dyn/cm^2 in old age. Fisher suggests that the force that can be transmitted per unit thickness of the capsule decreases by half by age 60 years, but that the increased thickness offers some compensation for the loss of elasticity. The age-related change in lens volume may account for the variations in thickness of the capsule at a specified region on the lens. Measurements by Krag et al.[185] of extensibility of a ring cut from the anterior capsule show that whereas the young capsule can be stretched to 108% of its unstretched length, there is a linear decline in strain to 40% by age 98 years. The force required to break the capsular ring remained constant until age 35 years and decreased linearly thereafter. In the 0% to 10% strain level, the level of strain relevant for accommodation, there is a linear increase in elastic modulus of the anterior lens capsule up to about 35 years of age and a slight decrease after this age. With increasing age the capsule gets thicker, less extensible, and more brittle.[185,186]

Growth of the crystalline lens

The crystalline lens continues to grow throughout life. In humans, this results in a linear increase in the mass of the isolated lens between 5 and 96 years of age.[114] The human lens also undergoes an increase in axial thickness as a consequence of the addition of lens fiber cells.[45,187–189] However, lens equatorial diameter in the unaccommodated state does not increase systematically with increasing age[116,119,137,189] Scheimpflug slit-lamp phakometry and MRI measurements have shown that anterior lens surface curvatures increase systematically with increasing age, whereas posterior lens surface curvature was found to increase in some studies, but not in others.[39,189,190] The increase in axial thickness of the lens results in a decrease in anterior chamber depth and an increase in anterior segment length.[189] The distance between the cornea and the center of the lens does not change with increasing age.[191] Qualitatively similar age-related changes have been described in the anterior segment of the rhesus monkey eye.[119,192] Because the thickness and anterior surface curvature of the lens increases with increasing age, and if the posterior lens surface also increases with increasing age but the lens equatorial diameter does not, the external shape of the aged lens begins to look more like that of an accommodated lens. However, the increased axial thickness with age is due to an increase in thickness of the anterior and posterior cortex, whereas accommodation in a young lens is due to an increase in thickness of the nucleus.[30,190,191] In addition, with increasing age, the cortical layers of the lens increase to a greater extent than the nucleus.[191] Although the surface curvatures in the aging lens appear to be more like an accommodated lens, the presbyopic eye is clearly not focused for near because presbyopia results in a loss of near vision.

The incongruity between the increasing lens surface curvatures and the gradual loss of near vision has been termed the *lens paradox*.[193] The reason that the presbyopic eye does not become nearsighted, despite the increasing lens surface curvatures, is due to a gradual age-related decrease in the equivalent refractive index of the lens.[117,189,194] The optical changes in the lens with accommodation and aging differ in several respects. Whereas accommodation results in an increase in the extent of the negative spherical aberration of young lenses, aging results in a systematic change in sign of spherical aberration from negative to positive.[61,114] The increased axial thickness of the lens also tends to reduce the lens refractive power if no other changes occur in the lens. Although the refractive index value at the center of the lens does not change systematically with increasing age, the shape of the lens GRI does change with increasing age, resulting in a larger plateau in the refractive index in the central regions of the lens and a steeper change in the GRI in the more peripheral lens cortical regions.[41]

It has been suggested that lens equatorial diameter increases systematically with increasing age[195-197] and that this may be the primary cause of presbyopia.[198] The only evidence cited in support of an age-related increase in lens diameter is data from an original study by Priestly Smith in 1883 in which lens equatorial diameter was measured in isolated human lenses.[199] Smith and others[61,113,114] recognized that when the zonular fibers were cut and the lens was isolated and removed from the eye and from external zonular traction forces, younger lenses tended to become accommodated and decreased in equatorial diameter, whereas older presbyopic lenses did not undergo any change in shape,[113,114] Thus the diameter of the isolated lenses was relatively smaller in young than in older isolated lenses. Although such studies showed an age-dependent increase in lens diameter, this trend was not due to age but rather to the different accommodative states of the isolated lenses because the equatorial diameter measurements of young accommodated lenses were being compared with those of older unaccommodated lenses.[199] Measurements from isolated adult lenses do not reflect the equatorial diameter of the lens in vivo. Recent studies have measured lens thickness and equatorial diameter in living human[116,137,189] and monkey[119] eyes. These studies showed that although lens growth occurs, as is evident from the increase in lens axial thickness, the progression of presbyopia occurs without a systematic increase in lens equatorial diameter.[119,137]

Loss of ability of the human lens to accommodate

In vitro studies have shown that the human lens progressively loses the ability to undergo accommodative changes. Fisher subjected isolated human lenses to high-speed rotational forces designed to simulate the forces that act on the lens, to hold it in an unaccommodated state in the living eye.[200] The results showed an age-dependent decline in deformability of the human lens. For a given rotational stress, the equatorial and polar strain (change in lens diameter and thickness) decreased by about one-third between the ages of 15 and 65 years. Fisher's[200] calculated Young's modulus of polar and equatorial elasticity showed a more than three-fold increase over this age range. From these studies Fisher suggested that a decrease in elastic modulus of the capsule, an increase in elastic modulus of the lens substance, and a flattening of the lens were sufficient to account for the loss of accommodation by the age of 61 years.[201] However, because Fisher's assumptions of no age-related change in lens shape or zonular insertion onto the lens were inaccurate[181,190] the theoretical assumptions on which the calculations were based are questionable.[202] Although Fisher's calculated Young's modulus values may be inaccurate, his experiments do demonstrate reduced deformability of the aging human lens owing to rotational forces.

Mechanical stretching experiments have shown that young human lenses undergo 12 to 16 D of change in optical power from stretching

forces applied through the intact zonular apparatus.[61] These mechanically induced changes in optical power of the lens correspond well with the accommodative dioptric change in power of the young eye in vivo. The change in optical power that the human lens undergoes with mechanical stretching gradually decreases with increasing age[61,176] (see Fig. 3.28). Presbyopic human lenses are unable to undergo any change in optical power from forces exerted on the lenses either through zonular traction or rotational forces.[61,200]

By about 55 years of age, human lenses are unable to undergo any change in optical power with the same degree of stretching that produces a 12 to 16 D of change in young lenses.[61] Phacoemulsification and aspiration of the presbyopic lens and injection of a soft silicone polymer to refill the capsule restores the ability of the refilled lens to undergo accommodative changes in optical power with mechanical stretching.[127] These experiments show that regardless of what other age-related changes occur in the human accommodative apparatus, the human lens ultimately completely loses the ability to undergo accommodative optical changes, and that this is due to the increased stiffness of the lens.

In the young eye, after the zonule is cut and the lens is removed from the eye, the isolated lens is in a maximally accommodated form due to the forces exerted by the lens capsule.[113,114,199] When the lens capsule is removed from the isolated young lens, the decapsulated lens substance takes on an unaccommodated form.[113,114] Removing the capsule from young lenses results in a decrease in optical power, but removing the capsule from lenses over about 50 years of age results in no change in optical power.[114] This, together with the results from mechanical stretching experiments,[61] shows that the lens substance of older human lenses is ultimately incapable of undergoing the capsule-induced optical alterations required for accommodation and disaccommodation.

High resolution MRI studies in living human eyes provide insights on aging of the accommodative apparatus.[137] When subjects are presented with an 8 D accommodative stimulus, there is an accommodative increase in lens thickness and decrease in lens equatorial diameter in young subjects, but these accommodative changes in the lens decline with age, reaching zero by about age 50 years (see Fig. 3.28). However, an accommodative decrease in ciliary ring diameter still occurs even in the oldest subjects, which demonstrates that the effort to focus at near results in ciliary muscle contraction and accommodative movements of the ciliary body in presbyopes, but without the required accommodative changes in the lens. Therefore, presbyopia results in a failure of the crystalline lens to undergo accommodative changes. However, that does not preclude changes in other parts of the accommodative apparatus (see previously).

Age-related increase in stiffness of the human lens

The human lens undergoes an exponential age-related increase in stiffness.[114,203,204] In the young lens, the nucleus is softer than the cortex, but with increasing age, there is a relatively greater increase in the stiffness of the nucleus[203,204] (Fig. 3.29). In the young eye, accommodation occurs through an increase in thickness of the lens nucleus, but not the cortex. It may be that the relatively stiffer cortical layers surrounding the nucleus mold the nucleus to change shape during accommodation. With increasing age, the rate of stiffening of the nucleus exceeds that of the cortex, and the nucleus stiffness begins to exceed that of the cortex by about 35 years of age.[203] There is a stiffness gradient to the lens (Fig. 3.30). In the young lens, stiffness progressively decreases from the surface of the cortex to the center of the nucleus, whereas in older lenses the stiffness gradient increases from the surface of the cortex to the center of the nucleus. It may be that this change in stiffness gradient that leads to an age-related change in the fine balance of forces that ultimately results in a loss of accommodation.[204,205] It is an

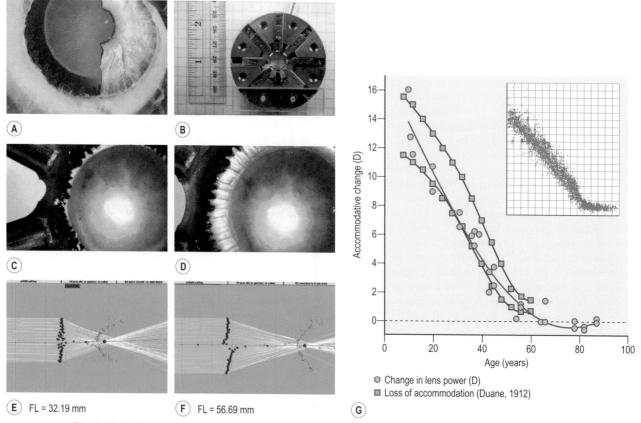

Fig. 3.28 (A) The anterior segment of a partially dissected 54-year-old human donor eye glued to (B), the arms of a mechanical stretching apparatus. The zonule can be completely relaxed (C) allowing the lens to become maximally accommodated, or (D) the zonule stretched to disaccommodate the lens. (E) Scanning laser measurements of the focal length of a 10-year-old human lens measured in the unstretched, accommodated state (focal length = 34.39 mm) and (F) in the maximally stretched and unaccommodated state (focal length = 57.69 mm). Parallel laser beams enter the lens, are refracted by the lens (at *red symbols, left*), and cross the optical axis *(dark horizontal line)* at the position identified *(yellow symbols, right)*. The distance from the lens *(red symbols, left)* to the average focus of all rays *(blue symbol)* represents the lens focal length. (G) The change in focal length converted to diopters *(red line and circles)* as a function of the applied stretch shows that young lenses undergo 12–16 D of change in power with stretching, but that by age 60, the same extent of applied stretch results in no change in lens power. The data from the human lenses are plotted in the inset in G, together with Duane's (1912) data *(blue lines, diamonds)* showing the range of accommodative amplitudes from some 1500 subjects as measured with a push-up technique. *D*, Diopters. (A-F: Reprinted from Glasser A, Campbell MCW. Presbyopia and the optical changes in the human crystalline lens with age. *Vis Res.* 1998;38(2):209-229. https://doi.org/10.1016/S0042-6989(97)00102-8.)

essential requirement that if accommodation is to occur, the lens substance must remain sufficiently pliable for capsular and zonular forces to flatten the lens to hold it in an unaccommodated form, and for capsular forces to increase the surface curvatures to mold the lens into an accommodated form. Because accommodation relies on forces exerted by the capsule on the lens, a small change in the fine balance of capsular and lens nuclear and cortical elastic forces would diminish the accommodative ability of the lens. Although presbyopia results in a complete loss of accommodation by the age of about 50 years, the stiffness of the human lens continues to increase beyond this age throughout the remaining years of the human life span. The age-related stiffening of the lens may simply represent a continuation of the age-related changes that ultimately lead to cataract.

The progressive loss of compliance of the lens from early in life parallels the decline in accommodative amplitude. If no other age-related changes were to occur in the accommodative apparatus of the eye, increased stiffness of the lens and a change in the stiffness gradient of the lens could completely account for the loss of accommodation with

advancing age. Presbyopia has classically been attributed to the hardening or "sclerosis" of the lens. Some confusion may exist regarding the meaning of the term "lenticular sclerosis." Evidence suggests that there is a gradual and progressive increase in stiffness of the lens, with a relatively greater increase in the stiffness of the nucleus than in the stiffness of cortex, that occurs throughout life, ultimately leading to an inability of the lens to undergo the optical changes required for accommodation. However, other parts of the accommodation apparatus also degrade with aging (i.e., ciliary muscle mobility restriction), so that even a flexible lens would not necessarily preclude presbyopia.

The mechanism of accommodation—update

Beyond the "basic" mechanism of accommodation, we can now propose, based on recent information from real time in vivo experiments in rhesus monkeys and corroborated by a small data set in live humans,[50,55,63,64,95] a new and more complete description of accommodation (Fig. 3.31; Video 3.10). The ciliary muscle contracts, releasing tension on the anterior zonula, allowing the capsule/lens to become

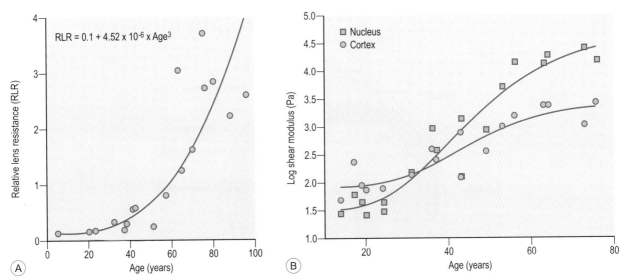

Fig. 3.29 Age-related increase in stiffness of human lenses. (A) Nineteen human lenses ranging in age from 5 to 96 years show an exponential increase in stiffness with an over four-fold increase in stiffness over the human life span that continues well after the age at which accommodation is completely lost. (B) The nuclear regions of young lenses have a lower sheer modulus than the cortex, but there is an exponential increase in stiffness of both the nucleus and the cortex of the lens with a relatively greater increase in sheer modulus of the nucleus. (Panel A from Glasser A, Campbell MCW. Biometric, optical and physical changes in the isolated human crystalline lens with age in relation to presbyopia. *Vis Res.* 1999;39:1991-2015. https://doi.org/10.1016/S0042-6989(98)00283-1. Panel B from Heys KR, Cram SL, Truscott RJ. Massive increase in the stiffness of the human lens nucleus with age: the basis for presbyopia? *Mol Vis.* 2004;10:956-963.)

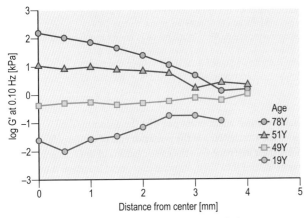

Fig. 3.30 In younger human lenses, lens stiffness is lowest nearer the center of the nucleus and increases toward the periphery of the cortex. With increasing age, there is a progressive change in stiffness gradient of the lens. In the oldest lenses, the stiffness gradient has altered such that the center of the nucleus is stiffer than the periphery of the cortex. Thus, lens stiffness of the 19-year-old is lowest at the center of the nucleus and increases with increasing distance from the center; however, in the old eye (age 78 years) the reverse is true. (From Weeber HA, Eckert G, Pechhold W, van der Heijde RGL. Stiffness gradient in the crystalline lens. *Graefe's Arch Clin Exp Ophthalmol.* 2007; 245:1357-1366 with kind permission of Springer Science + Business Media.)

branch tips are pulled forward and centripetally during accommodation and the central vitreous moves posteriorly facilitating posterior lens pole movement and lens shape change.[63,71] During accommodation in the young eye, the muscle moves forward and inward, placing tension on the elastic choroid all the way back to the optic nerve region and pulling the choroid centrifugally with the force centered around the optic nerve.[64,70] In the older eye, the choroid stiffens, dampening muscle forward mobility, but muscle contractility remains, and the stiffening of the choroid may increase accommodative tension spikes on the optic nerve as the muscle contracts. Forward muscle movement is diminished more than centripetal movement because the restriction is from the posterior direction in direct opposition to forward muscle movement. Thus, centripetal movement is still available and largely maintained in the older eye, and the need for centripetal movement is increased to achieve a given level of zonular relaxation and accommodative amplitude. Geometrically, the increased demand for centripetal muscle movement may also generate more pressure toward the optic nerve during accommodation owing to the attachments of the cisternal structure to the vitreous zonule/muscle complex, that is, as if fitting the "hypotenuse" formed by the cisternal branches into a shorter A/P distance to the optic nerve region, displacing vitreous fluid posteriorly toward the optic nerve head. The base of the cistern may also be subject to the accommodative tensional forces exerted by the choroid at the optic nerve region.

The *dots moving posteriorly* in the central vitreous during accommodation represent fluid flow toward the posterior pole of the eye and may add an additional compressive force to the retina/choroid. The movement is in the opposite direction during disaccommodation.

Also, note there is an iris pinch movement the pupil gives to the anterior pole of the lens, a trend that was noted by Croft et al. and reported in a previous publication by other researchers (Montes-Mico et al. 2010)[206]. (Reprinted with permission from Croft MA, Nork TM, Heatley G, et al. Intraocular accommodative movements in monkeys; relationship to presbyopia. *Exp Eye Res.* 2022;222:109029.)

more spherical and the iris and the anterior hyaloid to bow backward.[71] During accommodation, the ciliary muscle pulls all of these structures forward and centripetally: (1) the vitreous zonule; (2) the PVZ-INS LE[55]; (3) the cisternal branch tips[63]; and (4) the choroid at the ora serrata. The PVZ-INS LE acts like a strut to the posterior lens equator and facilitates forward lens equator movement and lens shape change.[55] The cistern

Young monkey

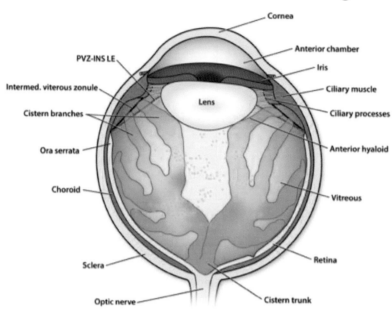

Fig. 3.31 See Video 3.10. During accommodation in the young eye, there is robust vitreous zonule/muscle forward movement. However, with increased age there would be reduced forward muscle movement, but centripetal movement would be maintained. This may place compression force to the cistern branch tips, cistern trunk, and thereby the choroid in the optic nerve region. The compression may intensify as the eye ages and there is decreased forward muscle movement while centripetal muscle movement is maintained—fitting the cistern branches into a shorter anterior/posterior intravitreal space/distance, compressing/thinning the choroid in the ON region. The dots moving posteriorly in the central vitreous during accommodation represent fluid flow toward the posterior pole of the eye and may add an additional compressive force to the retina/choroid. The movement is in the opposite direction during disaccommodation. Also, note there is an iris pinch movement the pupil gives to the anterior pole of the lens (See Video 3.4).; a trend that was noted in Croft et al. 2022 and reported in a previous publication by other researchers (Montes-Mico et al. 2010).[206] (Reprinted with permission from Croft MA, Nork TM, Heatley G, et al. Intraocular accommodative movements in monkeys; relationship to presbyopia. *Exp Eye Res.* 2022;222:109029.)

The accommodative movements of the lens/capsule complex cannot explain the accommodative movements within the vitreous, given the small amount of force that can be generated by the capsule and given that the vitreous movements occur in absence of the lens/capsule complex. Rather, we hypothesize that, in addition to the capsule molding the lens, the accommodative movements of the vitreous (driven by ciliary muscle contraction) also facilitate accommodative lens thickening. The anterior lens pole moves anteriorly, the anterior chamber shallows, and the posterior lens pole moves posteriorly during accommodation.[50,55,95] For this to happen, the accommodative central vitreous movement has to allow for, or perhaps even facilitate, the posterior movement of the lens posterior pole, while at the same time the PVZ-INS LE provides accommodative forward strut-like support to the peripheral posterior lens[55] to support the accommodative forward movement of the lens equator and lens shape change (thickening).[55]

Accommodation, presbyopia, and accommodative pressure and tension spikes

Although forward muscle movements are reduced in older eyes, a substantial amount of centripetal muscle movement remains. The posterior lens pole, being positioned more posteriorly with age, coupled with the inward bowing of the sclera and the presence of the cisternal trunk in the region of the optic nerve (with the branches of the cistern extending to and attaching to the vitreous zonule), may contribute to a greater pressure spike toward the optic nerve during accommodation in the aged eye.

Here we must again point out that the accommodative mechanism includes the attachments at the posterior end of the muscle—the elastic tendons, their insertion into the elastic lamina of Bruch's membrane and the choroid, and thus their ultimate functional insertion into the elastic ring around the optic nerve head (Fig. 3.4). Focusing requires a continuous "zeroing in" on the target, much as a gunner acquires a target's range. This constant, high-frequency micro contraction/relaxation generates its own force fluctuations on the surrounding structures and fluidics, which may also affect the optic nerve and may diminish with age.

The anterior longitudinal region of the ciliary muscle, with its tendinous attachment to the scleral spur, trabecular meshwork (TM), inner wall of Schlemm's canal (SC), and Schwalbe's line, is also affected by aging.[207–211] The TM stiffens[211–218] and forward ciliary muscle (CM) movement is severely restricted[81] (more than is the centripetal vector) by the posterior stiffening,[179] so that the TM deformation and recovery associated with accommodation and disaccommodation is progressively lost. The deformation/recovery cycle may contribute to the "self-cleaning" ascribed to the TM,[219–221] and thus its loss may contribute to TM stiffening[215,216] and accumulation of collagen and other extra cellular matrix materials seen with aging,[206,221] especially in glaucomatous eyes.[214,215] These changes may impede the outflow of aqueous humor, as evidenced by, and perhaps accounting for, the age-related increase in outflow resistance seen in both monkeys[211,222] and (at least in Western) human[146,224] populations. We do not know whether the intrinsic contraction/relaxation mechanisms possessed by the TM/SC[223] might change with age and affect CM movement and thereby the optic nerve.

Although all of the biomechanics at play are not clear, altered forces and decreased deformation of the TM during accommodative effort seem likely to contribute to increased outflow resistance.

CONCLUSIONS

The ocular anterior and posterior segments are linked both structurally and functionally, and their intellectual separation in both the clinical and research enterprises is counterproductive to advances. The accommodative mechanism and its aging are much more complex than generally realized, and extralenticular changes with age may play an important role in the pathophysiology of presbyopia, glaucomatous optic neuropathy, impaired aqueous outflow, and the frustrating inability of intraocular lenses to provide more than 1.75 to 2.00 D of dynamic accommodation[225,226]—not quite enough for fine near vision in subpar lighting conditions.

ACKNOWLEDGMENTS

The work on this chapter was supported in part by National Eye Institute (NEI) grants R01 EY025359-01A1, RO1 EY10213, R21 EY018370-01A2, and R21 EY018370-01A2S1; the Ocular Physiology Research & Education Foundation (OPREF); the Wisconsin National Primate Research Center National Institutes of Health (NIH) Grant # 5P51 RR 000167, University of Wisconsin-Madison NIH base grant # P51 RR OD011106; OPREF and NIH Core Grant for Vision Research grant #P30 EY016665; and Research to Prevent Blindness Unrestricted Departmental Challenge Grant.

REFERENCES

1. von Helmholtz H.. In: Southall JPC, ed. *Helmholtz's treatise on physiological optics, in Mechanism of accommodation*. New York: Dover Publications; 1909:143–172.
2. Young T. On the mechanism of the eye. *Phil Trans R.Soc Lond*. 1801;91:23.
3. Home E. The Croonian lecture on the muscular motion. *Phil Trans R.Soc Lond*. 1795;85:1.
4. Crampton P. Thr description of an organ by which the eyes of birds are accommodated to the different distances of objects. *Thompson's Annals of of Philosophy*. 1813;1:170.
5. Müller H. Ueber den accommodations-apparat im auge der vogel, besonders den falken. *Archiv für Ophthalmologie*. 1857;3:25.
6. Glasser A, Troilo D, Howland H. The mechanism of corneal accommodation in chicks. *Vision Res*. 1994;34:1549.
7. Glasser A, Howland HC. A history of studies of visual accmmodation in birds. *Q Rev Biol*. 1996;71:475.
8. Glasser A, C. Murphy D. Troilo and a. et, *The mechanism of lenticular accommodation in the chick eye*. Vision Res. 1995;35:1525.
9. Brücke E. Uber den musculus Cramptonianus und den spannmuskel der choroidea. *Archiv für Anatomie, Physiologie und Wissenschaftliche*. 1846;1:370.
10. Cramer A. Het accommodatievermogen der oogen,physiologisch toegelicht. *Hollandsche Maatschappij der Wetenschappen te Haarlem: De Erven Loosjes*. 1853;1:139.
11. Hess C. Vergleichende Untersuchungen über den Einfluss der Accommodation auf den Augendruck in der Wirbelthierreihe. *Archiv fur Augenheilkunde*. 1909;63:88.
12. Gullstrand A. *Helmholtz's Treatise on physiological optics*. New York: Dover; 1909.
13. Rohen JW, Kaufman PL, Eichhorn M, Goeckner PA, Bito LZ. Functional morphology of accommodation in the raccoon. *Experimental Eye Research*. 1989;48:523–537.
14. Armaly M. Studies on intraocular effects of the orbital parasympathetic pathway. I. Techniques and effects on morphology. *AMA Arch Ophthalmol*. 1959;61:14.
15. Vakkur G. The schematic eye in the cat. *Vision Res*. 1963;3:357.
16. O'Neill W, Brodkey J. A non-linear analysis of the mechanics of accommodation. *Vision Res*. 1970;10:375.
17. Sivak J, Howland H. Accommodation in the northern rock bass (Ambloplites rupestris rupestris) in response to natural stimuli. *Vision Res*. 1973;13:2059.
18. Andison M, Sivak J. The naturally occuring accommodative response of the oscar, Astronotus ocellatus, to visual stimuli. *Vision Res*. 1996;36:3021.
19. Beer T. Die accommodation des fischauges. *Pfluegers Arch fuer die Gesamte Physiologie des Menschen und der Tiere*. 1894;58:523.
20. Sivak J, Hildebrand T, Lebert C. Magnitude and rate of accommodation in diving and nondiving birds. *Vision Res*. 1985;25:925.
21. Törnqvist G. Effect on refraction of intramuscular pilocarpine in two species of monkey (Ceropithecus aethiops and Macaca irus). *Invest Ophthalmol*. 1965;4(2):211.
22. Törnqvist G. Effect of topical carbachol on the pupil and refraction in young and presbypic monkeys. *Invest Ophthalmol Vis Sci*. 1966;5(2):186.
23. Kaufman PL, Bárány EH. Subsensitivity to pilocarpine in primate ciliary muscle following topical anticholinesterase treatment. *Investigative Ophthalmology*. 1975;14:302–306.
24. Bito LZ, DeRousseau CJ, Kaufman PL, Bito JW. Age-dependent loss of accommodative amplitude in rhesus monkeys: an animal model for presbyopia. *Investigative Ophthalmology and Visual Science*. 1982;23:23–31.
25. Duanne A. Normal values of accommodation at all ages. *J Am Med Assoc*. 1912;59:1010.
26. Anderson H, Hentz G, Glasser A, Stuebing K, Manny R. Minus-lens-stimulated accommodative amplitudes from age 3. *Invest Ophthalmol Vis Sci*. 2008;49:2919.
27. Hirschberg J. *The history of ophthalmology*. Ostend Belgium: Wayenborgh Publishing,; 1982.
28. Donders F. *On the annomalies of accommodation and refraction of the eye with a preliminary essay on physiologcal dioptrics*. London: The New Sydenham Society; 1864.
29. Rabbetts R. *Bennett and Rabbetts' Clinical visual optics*. 3rd edn. Boston: Butterworth Heinemann; 1998.
30. Koretz JF, Handelman GH, Brown NP. Analysis of human crystalline lens curvature as a function of accommodative state and age. *Vision Research*. 1984;24:1141–1151.
31. Strenk S, Strenk LM, Koretz JF. The mechanism of presbyopia. *Progress in Retinal and Eye Research*. 2005;24:379–393.
32. Fincham E. The changes in the form of the crystalline lens in accommodation. *Trans Optical Soc*. 1825;26:240.

33. Garner L, Yap M. Changes in ocular dimensions and refraction with accommodation. *Ophthalmic and Physiol Optics*. 1997;17:12.
34. Bolz M, Prinz A, Drexler W, Findl O. Linear relationship of refractive and biometric lenticular changes during accommodation in emmetropic and myopic eyes. *Br. J. Ophthalmol*. 2007;91:360.
35. Vilupuru A, Glasser A. The relationship between refractive and biometric changes during Edinger-Westphal stimulated accommodation in rhesus monkey. s. *Exp Eye Res*. 2005;80(3):349–360.
36. Drexler W, Baumgartener A, Findl Oea, Hitzenberger C, Fercher A. Biometric investigation of changes in the anterior eye segment during accommodation. *Vision Res*. 1997;37:2789.
37. Rosales P, Wendt M, Marcos S, Glasser A. Changes in crystalline lens radii of curvature and lens tilt and decentration during dynamic accommodation in rhesus monkeys. *J Vis*. 2008;8:18.
38. Rosales P. Crystalline lens radii of curvature from Purkinje and Scheimpflug imaging. *J Vis*. 2006;6:1057.
39. Dubbleman M, van der Heijde G, Weeber H. Change in shape of the aging human crystalline lens with accommodation. *Vision Res*. 2005;45:117.
40. Garner L, Smith C. Changes in equivalent and gradient refractive index of the crystaline lens with accommodation. *Optom Vis Sci*. 1997;74:114.
41. Kasthurirangan S, Markwell E, Atchison D, Pope J. In vivo study of changes in refractive index distribution in the human crystalline lens with age and accommodation. *Invest Ophthalmol Vis Sci*. 2008;49:2531.
42. Hermans E, Dubbleman M, van der Heijde R, Heethaar R. Equivalent refractive index of the human lens upon accommodative response. *Optom Vis Sci*. 2008;85:1179.
43. Duane A. Studies in monocular and binocular accommodation with their clinical applications. *Am J Ophthalmol*. 1922;5:867–877.
44. Win-Hall D, Glasser A. Objective accommodation measurement in presbyopic eyes using an autorefractor and an aberrometer. *J Cataract Refract Surg*. 2008;34:774.
45. Koretz JF, Kaufman PL, Neider MW, Goeckner PA. Accommodation and presbyopia in the human eye - aging of the anterior segment. *Vis Res*. 1989;29:1685–1692.
46. Ostrin L, Glasser A. Accommodation measurements in a prepresbyopic and presbyopic population. *J Cataract Refract Surg*. 2004;30:1435.
47. Wold J, Hu A, Chen S, Glasser A. Subjective and objective measurement of human accommodative amplitude. *J Cataract Refract Surg*. 2003;29:1878.
48. Calver R, Cox M, Elliot D. Effect of aging on the monochromatic aberration of the human eye. *J Vis Opt Soc Am A Opt Image Sci Vis*. 1999;16:2069.
49. Flügel C, Bárány EH, Lütjen-Drecoll E. Histochemical differences within the ciliary muscle and its function in accommodation. *Experimental Eye Research*. 1990;50:219–226.
50. Croft MA, McDonald JP, Katz A, Lin TL, Lütjen-Drecoll E, Kaufman PL. Extralenticular and lenticular aspects of accommodation and presbyopia in human versus monkey eyes. *Invest Ophthalmol and Vis Sci*. 2013;54:5035–5048. PMC3726241.
51. Glasser A, Croft MA, Brumback L, Kaufman PL. Ultrasound biomicroscopy of the aging rhesus monkey ciliary region. *Opt Vis Sci*. 2001;78:417–424.
52. Rohen JW. Scanning electron microscopic studies of the zonular apparatus in human and monkey eyes. *Investigative Ophthalmology and Visual Science*. 1979;18:133–144.
53. Ludwig K, Wegscheider E, Hoops JP, Kampik A. In vivo imaging of the human zonular apparatus with high-resolution ultrasound biomicroscopy. *Graefes Archive for Clinical and Experimental Ophthalmology*. 1999;237:361–371.
54. Lütjen-Drecoll E, Kaufman P, Wasielewski R, Ting-Li L, Croft M. Morphology and accommodative function of the vitreous zonule in human and monkey eyes. *Invest Ophthalmol and Vis Sci*. 2010;51(3):1554–1564. PMC2829378.
55. Croft MA, Heatley G, McDonald JP, Alexander. K, Kaufman PL. Accommodative movements of the lens/capsule and the strand that extends between the posterior vitreous zonule insertion zone & the lens equator, in relation to the vitreous face and aging. *Ophthalmic and Physiologic Optics*. 2016;36:21–32. PMC4755275.
56. Koretz JF, Handelman GH. A model for accommodation in the young human eye: the effects of lens elastic anisotropy on the mechanism. *Vision Research*. 1983;23:1679–1686.
57. Coleman D, Rondeau M. *Current aspects of human accommodation II*. Heidelberg: Kaden Verlag; 2003.
58. Coleman DJ, Fish SK. Presbyopia, accommodation, and the mature catenary. *Ophthalmology*. 2001;108(9):1544–1551.
59. Coleman DJ. On the hydraulic suspension theory of accommodation. *Transactions of the American Ophthalmological Society*. 1986;84:846–868.

60. Fisher RF. *Is the vitreous necessary for accommodation in man?* Br. J Ophthalmology. 1983;67:206.

61. Glasser A, Campbell MCW. Presbyopia and the optical changes in the human crystalline lens with age. *Vis Res.* 1998;38(2):209–229.

62. Manns F, Parel J, Denham D, Billotte C, Ziebarth N, Borja D, Fernandez V, Aly M, Arrieta E, Ho A, Holden B. Optomechanical response of human and monkey lenses in a lens stretcher. *Invest Ophthalmol Vis Sci.* 2007;43:3260.

63. Croft M, Nork T, Heatley G, McDonald J, Katz A, Kaufman P. Intraocular accommodative movements in monkeys; relationship to presbyopia. *Exp Eye Res.* 2022;222:109029. https://doi.org/10.1016/j.exer.2022.109029.

64. Croft M, Peterson J, Smith C, Kiland J, Nork T, McDonald J, Katz A, Hetzel S, Lütjen-Drecoll E, Kaufman P. Accommodative movements of the choroid in the optic nerve head region of human eyes, and their relationship to the lens. *Exp Eye Res.* 2022;222:109124 https://doi.org/10.1016/j.exer.2022.109124.Online ahead of print. PMID: 35688214.

65. Tamm E, Lütjen-Drecoll E. Ciliary body. *Microscopy Research and Technique.* 1996;33: 390–439.

66. Hara K, Lütjen-Drecoll E, Prestele H, Rohen JW. Structural differences between regions of the ciliary body in primates. *Investigative Ophthalmology and Visual Science.* 1977;16:912–924.

67. Hogan M, Alvarado J, Weddell J. *Histology of the human eye; an atlas and a textbook.* Philadelphia: WB Saunders; 1971.

68. Calasans O. The architechture of the ciiary muscle of man. *Ann Fac Med Univ Sao Paolo.* 1953;27:3.

69. Lütjen-Drecoll E. Functional morphology of the trabecular meshwork in primate eyes. *Prog Retin Eye Res.* 1998;18:91.

70. Croft MA, Lütjen-Drecoll E, Kaufman PL. Age-related posterior ciliary muscle restriction - a link between trabecular meshwork and optic nerve head pathophysiology. *Exp Eye Res.* 2016;158:187–189. PMC5253323.

71. Kaufman PL, Lütjen-Drecoll E, Croft MA. Presbyopia and Glaucoma: Two diseases, one pathophysiology? The Friedenwald Lecture. *Invest Ophthalmol and Vis Sci.* 2019;60(5):1801–1812. PMC6540935.

72. Ishikawa T. Fine structure of the human ciliary muscle. *Invest Ophthalmol.* 1962;1:587–608.

73. Gabelt BT, Kaufman PL. Inhibition of outflow facility, accommodative, and miotic responses to pilocarpine in rhesus monkeys by muscarinic receptor subtype antagonists. *Journal of Pharmacology and Experimental Therapeutics.* 1992;263(3):1133–1139.

74. Bill A. Conventional and uveo-scleral drainage of aqueous humor in the cynomolgus monkey (Macaca irus) at normal and high intraocular pressures. *Experimental Eye Research.* 1966;5:45–54.

75. Bill A. Effects of norepinephrine, isoproterenol and sympathetic stimulation on aqueous humour dynamics in vervet monkeys. *Exp Eye Res.* 1970;10:31–46.

76. Bill A. Effects of atropine on aqueous humor dynamics in the vervet monkey (cercopithecus ethiops). *Experimental Eye Research.* 1969;8:284–291.

77. Alm A, Nilsson S. Uveoscleral outflow – A review. *Experimental Eye Research.* 2009;88:760–768.

78. Tamm ER, Lütjen-Drecoll E. Nitrergic nerve cells in the primate ciliary muscle are only present in species with a fovea centralis. *Ophthalmologica.* 1997;211:201–204.

79. Flügel-Koch C, Neuhuber WL, Kaufman PL, Lütjen-Drecoll E. Morphologic indication for proprioception in the human ciliary muscle. *Investigative Ophthalmology and Visual Science.* 2009;50(12):5529–5536.

80. Flügel-Koch C, Croft MA, Kaufman PL, Lütjen-Drecoll E. *Anteriorly located zonular fibers as a tool for fine regulation in accommodation. Ophthalmic and Physiological Optics.* Ophthalmic and Physiological Optics. 2016;36(1):13–20. PMC4715652.

81. Croft M, McDonald JP, Nadkarni NV, Lin TL, Kaufman PL. Age-related changes in centripetal ciliary body movement relative to centripetal lens movement in monkeys. *Exp Eye Res.* 2009;89:824–832. PMC278077.

82. Croft MG, Heatley A, McDonald G, Ebbert J, Kaufman, PL T. Accommodative ciliary body and lens function in rhesus monkeys. I. Normal lens, zonule and ciliary process configuration in the iridectomized eye. *Invest Ophthalmol and Vis Sci.* 2006;47:1076–1086.

83. Farnsworth PN, Burke P. Three dimensional architecture of suspensory apparatus of lens of rhesus monkey. *Experimental Eye Research.* 1977;25:563–576.

84. Davenger M. The suspensory apparatus of the lens. The surface of the ciliary body. A scanning electron microscopic study. *Acta Ophthalmol.* 1975;53:19.

85. Farnsworth P, Mauriello J, Burke-Gadomski P, Kulyk T, Cinotti A. Surface ultrastructure of the human lens capsule and zonular attachments. *Invest Ophthalmol Vis Sci.* 1976;15(1):36.

86. Marshall J, Beaconsfield M, Rothery S. The anatomy and development of the human lens and zonules. *Trans Ophthal Soc UK.* 1982;102(3):423.

87. Bernal A, Parel JM, Manns F. Evidence for Posterior Zonule Fiber Attachment on the Anterior Hyaloid Membrane. *Investigative Ophthalmology and Visual Science.* 2006;47(11):4708–4713.

88. McCulloch C. The zonule of Zinn: Its origin, course, and insertion, and its relation to neighboring structures. *Trans. Am. Ophth.Soc.* 1954;52:525–585.

89. Bito LZ, Kaufman PL, Neider M, Miranda OC, Antal P. *The dynamics of accommodation (ciliary muscle contraction, zonular relaxation and lenticular deformation) as a function of stimulus strength and age in iridectomized rhesus eyes,* in. *Investigative Ophthalmology and Visual Science.* 1987;318.

90. Sebag J.. In: hart WM, ed. *The vitreous, in Adler's Physiology of the Eye.* St. Louis, MO: G.F. Stamathis; 1992:268–347.

91. Sebag J. Vitreous: from biochemistry to clinical relevance. In: Tasman W, Jaeger EA, eds. *Duane's Foundations of Clinical Ophthalmology.* Philadelphia: Lippincott Williams &Wilkins; 1998:1–67.

92. Sebag J, Balazs EA. Human Vitreous Fibers and Vitreoretinal Disease. *Trans. Ophthalmol. Soc. U.K.* 1985;104:123–128.

93. Kaczerowski MI. The surface of the vitreous. *Am. J. Ophth..* 1967;3:419.

94. Croft MA, McDonald JP, Katz A, Lin TL, Lütjen-Drecoll E, Kaufman PL. Extralenticular and lenticular aspects of accommodation and presbyopia in human versus monkey eyes. *Invest Ophthalmol Vis Sci.* 2013;54:5035–5048. PMCID3726241.

95. Croft MA, Nork TM, McDonald JP, Katz A, Lütjen-Drecoll E, Kaufman PL. Accommodative movements of the vitreous membrane, choroid and sclera in young and presbyopic human and nonhuman primate eyes. *Invest Ophthalmol and Vis Sci.* 2013;Vol 54:5049–5058. PMC3726242.

96. Jongbloed WL, Worst JGF. The cisternal anatomy of the vitreous body. *Doc Ophthalmol.* 1987;67:183.

97. Sebag J. *Chptr VI Development and Aging of the Vitreous in: The Vitreous.* 73. New York: Springer- Verlag; 1989;95.

98. Eisner G. Clinical examination of the vitreous. *Trans. Ophthalmol. Soc. U.K.* 1975;95: 360–363.

99. Eisner G. Clinical anatomy of the vitreous. In: Tasman W, Jaeger EA, eds. *Duanne's foundations of clinical Ophthalmology.* Philadelphia: Lippincott Williams & Wilkins; 2005:1–34.

100. Fine BS, Ben S. *The vitreous body In Ocular Histology: A Text and Atlas.* Hagerstown, MD: Harper and Row; 1979:131–145 Medical Dept.

101. Lund-Anderson H, Sander B.. In: Kaufman PLAA, ed. *Vitreous. In Adler's Physiology of the Eye.* St. Louis, MO: Mosby; 2003:293–316.

102. Peyman GA, R.C. Cheema MD, Fang T. Triamcinolone acetonide as an aid to visualization of the vitreous and the posterior hyaloid during pars plana vitrectomy. *Retina.* 2000;20: 554–555.

103. Coleman DJ. Unified model for accommodative mechanism. *Am J Ophthalmol.* 1970;69:1063–1079.

104. Smith RC, Smith GT, Wong D. Refractive Changes in Silicone Filled Eyes. *Eye.* 1990;4: 230–234.

105. Tuck MW, Crick RP. The age distribution of primary open angle glaucoma. *Ophthalmic Epidemiology.* 1998;5:173–183.

106. Hitzl W, Hornykewycz K, Grabner G, Reitsamer HA. On the relationship between age and prevalence and/or incidence of primary open-angle glaucoma in the "Salzburg- Moorfields Collaborative Glaucoma Study". *Klin Monbl Augenheilkd.* 2007;224:115–119.

107. Miao H, Crabb AW, Hernandez MR, Lukas TJ. Modulation of factors affecting optic nerve head astrocyte migration. *Investigative Ophthalmology and Visual Science.* 2010;51: 4096–4103.

108. Balazs EA, Denlinger JL. Aging changes in the vitreous. In: Sekuler R, Kline D, Dismukes K, eds. *Aging and the human visual function.* New York: A.R. Liss; 1982:45–57.

109. Burian HM, Allen L. Mechanical changes during accommodation observed by gonioscopy. *Arch Ophthalmol.* 1955;54:66–72.

110. Coleman DJ, S.K F. Presbyopia, accommodation, and the mature catenary. *Ophthalmology.* 2001;108(9):1544–1551.

111. Cramer, A., *Tijdschrift der Maatshappij vor Geneeskunde Nederlandisch Lancet 1851. Cited in Fincham, The mechanism of accommodation. Brit. J Ophth. 8 (Suppl.): 9 1937.* 1851.

112. Barraquer R, Michael R, Abrue R, Lamarca J, Tresserra F. Human lens capsule thickness as a function of age and location along the saggital lens perimeter. *Invest Ophthalmol Vis Sci.* 2006;47:2053.

113. Fincham E. The mechanism of accommodation. *British Journal of Ophthalmology.* 1937;8:7–80.

114. Glasser A, Campbell MCW. Biometric, optical and physical changes in the isolated human crystalline lens with age in relation to presbyopia. *Vis Res.* 1999;39:1991–2015.

115. Dubbleman M, van der Heijde GL, Weeber HA. The thickness of the aging human lens obtained from corrected Scheimpflug images. *Optometry and Vision Science.* 2001;78: 411–416.

116. Jones C, Atchison D, Pope J. Changes in lens dimension and refractive index with age and accommodation. *Optom Vis Sci.* 2007;84:990.

117. Dubbleman M, van der Heijde GL. The shape of the aging human lens: curvature, equivalent refractive index and the lens paradox. *Vision Research.* 2001;41:1867–1877.

118. Augusteyn R. On the growth and internal structure of the human lens. Review. *Exp Eye Res.* 2010;90:643–654.

119. Wendt M, Croft M, McDonald J, Kaufman P, Glasser A. Lens diameter and thickness as a function of age and pharmacologically stimulated accommodation in rhesus monkeys. *Experimental Eye Research.* 2008;86:746–752.

120. von Helmholtz HH. Uber die Accommodation des Auges. *Arch für Ophthalmologie.* 1855;1:1.

121. Glasser A, Kaufman PL. The mechanism of accommodation in primates. *Ophthalmology.* 1999;106:863–872.

122. Graves B. Change of tension on the lens capsule during accommodation and under the influence of various drugs. *Br Med J.* 1926;1:46.

123. Graves B. The response of the lens capsule in the act of accommodation. *Trans Am Ophthalmol Soc.* 1925;23:184.

124. Glasser A, Croft MA, Kaufman PL. Aging of the human crystalline lens and presbyopia. *International Ophthalmology Clinics.* 2001;41(Presbyopia):1–15.

125. Roorda A, Glasser A. Wave aberrations of the isolated crystalline lens. *Journal of Vision.* 2004;4:250–261.

126. Vilupuru AS, Roorda A, Glasser A. Spatially variant changes in lens power during ocular accommodation in a rhesus monkey eye. *Journal of Vision.* 2004;4:299–309.

127. Koopmans SA, Terwee T, Barkhof J, Haitjema HJ, Kooijman AC. Polymer refilling of presbyopic human lenses in vitro restores the ability to undergo accommodative changes. *Investigative Ophthalmology and Visual Science.* 2003;44:250–257.

128. Glasser A, Wendt M, Ostrin L. Accommodative changes in lens diameter in rhesus monkeys. *Investigative Ophthalmology and Visual Science.* 2006;47(1):278–286.

129. Wilson RS. Does the lens diameter increase or decrease during accommodation? Human accommodation studies: a new technique using infared retro-illumination video photography and pixel unit measurements. *Transactions of the American Ophthalmological Society.* 1997;95:261–270.

130. Grossmann K. The mechansim of accommodation in man. *Br Med J.* 1903;2:726.

131. Grossmann K. The mechansim of accommodation in man. *Ophthal Rev.* 1904;23:1.

132. Beauchamp R, Mitchell B. Ultrasound measures of vitreous chamber depth during ocular accommodation. *Am J Optom and Physiol Optics*. 1985;62:523.
133. Tscherning ML. *Dioptrics of the eye, functions of the retina, ocular movements, and binocular vision, in Physiologic Optics*. Keystone: Philadelphia; 1904:160–189.
134. Tscherning ML. *Accommodation, in Physiologic Optics*. Keystone: Philadelphia; 1920: 192–228.
135. Schachar R. Cause and treatment of presbyopia with a method for increasing the amplitude of accommodation. *Ann Ophth*. 1992;24:445.
136. Schachar RA, Black TD, Kash RL, Cudmore MS, Schanzlin DJ. The mechanism of accommodation and presbyopia in the primate. *Annals of Ophthalmology*. 1995;27(2): 59–67.
137. Strenk SA, Semmlow JL, Strenk IM, Munoz P, Gronlund-Jacob J, DeMarco JK. Age-related changes in human ciliary muscle and lens: a magnetic resonance imaging study. *Investigative Ophthalmology and Visual Science*. 1999;40:1162–1169.
138. Cheng H, Barnett J, Vilupuru A, Marsack J, Kasthurirangan S, Applegate R, Roorda A. A population study on changes in wave abberations with accommodation. *J Vis*. 2004;4:272.
139. He J, Burns S, Marcos S. Monochromatic abberrations in the accommodated human eye. *Vision Res*. 2000;40:41.
140. Lopez-Gil N, Fernandez-Sanchez V. R.e.a. Legras, R. Montés-Micó, F. Lara and J. Nguyen-Khoa, *Accommodation-related changes in monochromaticabberations of the human eyeas a function of age. Invest Ophthalmol Vis Sci*. 2008;49:1736.
141. Buehren T, Collins M. Accommodation stimulus response function and retinal image quality. *Vision Res*. 2006;46:1633.
142. Kruger P, Nowbotsing S, Aggarwala K, Mathews S. Small amounts of chromatic abberation influence dynamic accommodation. *Optom Vis Sci*. 1995;72:656.
143. Aggarawala K, Nowbotsing S, Kruger P. Accommodation to monochromatic and white-light targets. *Invest Ophthalmol Vis Sci*. 1995;36:2695.
144. Aggarwala K, Kruger E, Mathews S, Kruger P. Spectral bandwidth and ocular accommodation. *J Opt Soc Am A*. 1995;12:450.
145. Kruger P, Mathews S, Aggarwala Kea, Yager, ES DK. Accommodation responds to changing contrast of long, middle, and short spectral-waveband components of the retinal image. *Vision Res*. 1995;35:2415.
146. Croft MA, Oyen MJ, Gange SJ, Fischer MR, Kaufman PL. Aging effects on accommodation and outflow facility responses to pilocarpine in humans. *Arch Ophthalmol*. 1996;114: 586–592.
147. Koretz JF, Bertasso AM, Neider MW, Gabelt BT, Kaufman PL. Slit-lamp studies of the rhesus monkey eye: II. Changes in crystalline lens shape, thickness and position during accommodation and aging. *Experimental Eye Research*. 1987;45:317–326.
148. Vilupuru AS, Glasser A. Dynamic accommodation in rhesus monkeys. *Vision Research*. 2002;42:125–141.
149. Crawford K, Terasawa E, Kaufman PL. Reproducible stimulation of ciliary muscle contraction in the cynomolgus monkey via a permanent indwelling midbrain electrode. *Brain Research*. 1989;503:265–272.
150. Crawford K, Kaufman P, Bito L. The role of the iris in accommodation of rhesus monkeys. *Investigative Ophthalmology and Visual Science*. 1990;31:2185–2190.
151. Ostrin L, Glassaer A. Comparison between pharmacologically and Edinger-Westphl stimulated accommodation in rhesus moneys. *Invest Ophthalmol Vis Sci*. 2005;46:609.
152. Koeppl C, Findl O, Kriechbaum K, Drexler W. Comparison of pilocarpine-induced and stimulus-driven accommodation in phakic eyes. *Exp Eye Res*. 2005;80:795.
153. Owens P, Amos D. *Clinical ocular pharmacology*. Boston: Butterworth-Heinemann; 1995.
154. Harris LS, Galin MA. Effect of ocular pigmentation on hypotensive response to pilocarpine. *American Journal of Ophthalmology*. 1971;72:923–925.
155. Win-Hall D, Glasser A. Objective accommodation measurement in pseudophakic subjects using an autorefractor and an abberometer. *J Cataract Refract Surg*. 2009;35:282.
156. Win-Hal D, Ostrin L, Kasthurirangan S, Glasser A. Objective accommodation measurement with the Grand Seiko and Hartinger coincidence refractometer. *Optom Vis Sci*. 2007;84:879.
157. Kasthurirangan S, Vilupuru A, Glasser A. Amplitude dependence accommodative dynamics in humans. *Vision Res*. 2003;43:2945.
158. Seidemann A, Schaeffel F. An evaluation of the lag of accommodation using photorefraction. *Vision Res*. 2003;43:419.
159. Schaeffel F, Wilhelm H, Zrenner E. Inter-individual variability in the dynamics of natural accommodation in humans: Relation to age and refractive errors. *Journal of Physiology (London)*. 1993;461:301–320.
160. Mathews S. Scleral expansion does not restore accommodation in human presbyopia. *Ophthalmology*. 1999;106(5):873–877.
161. Bharadwaj S, Schor C. Acceleration characteristics of human ocular accommodation. *Vision Res*. 2005;45
162. Hamasaki D, Ong J, Marg E. The amplitude of accommodayion in presbyopia. *Am J Optom Arch Am Acad Optom.*. 1956;33:3.
163. Bito LZ, Miranda OC.. In: Reinecke RD, ed. *Accommodation and presbyopia, in Ophthalmology Annual*. New York: Raven Press; 1989:103–128.
164. Neider MW, Crawford K, Kaufman PL, Bito LZ. In vivo videography of the rhesus monkey accommodative apparatus. Age-related loss of ciliary muscle response to central stimulation. *Arch Ophthalmol*. 1990;108:69–74.
165. Lütjen-Drecoll E, Tamm E, Kaufman PL. Age-related loss of morphologic responses to pilocarpine in rhesus monkey ciliary muscle. *Archives of Ophthalmology*. 1988;106:1591–1598.
166. Tamm E, Lütjen-Drecoll E, Jungkunz W, Rohen JW. Posterior attachment of ciliary muscle in young, accommodating old, presbyopic monkeys. *Invest Ophthalmol Vis Sci*. 1991;32(5):1678–1692.
167. Tamm S, Tamm E, Rohen JW. Age-related changes of the human ciliary muscle. A quantitative morphometric study. *Mechanisms of Ageing and Development*. 1992;62:209–221.
168. Wasielewski R, McDonald JP, Heatley G, Lütjen-Drecoll E, Kaufman PL, Croft MA. Surgical intervention and accommodative responses, II. Forward ciliary body accommodative movement is facilitated by zonular attachments to the lens capsule. *Invest Ophthalmol and Vis Sci*. 2008;49:5495–5502. PMC2798153.
169. Poyer JF, Kaufman PL, Flügel C. Age does not affect contractile response of the isolated monkey ciliary muscle to muscarinic agonists. *Current Eye Research*. 1993;12:413–422.
170. Gabelt BT, Kaufman PL, Polansky JR. Ciliary muscle muscarinic binding sites, choline acetyltransferase and acetylcholinesterase in aging rhesus monkeys. *Investigative Ophthalmology and Visual Science*. 1990;31:2431–2436.
171. Ostrin L, Glasser A. Edinger-Westphal and pharmacologically stimulated accommodative refractive changes and lens and ciliary process movements in rhesus monkeys. *Exp Eye Res*. 2007;84:302.
172. Nishida S, Mizutani S. Quantitative and morphometric studies of age-related changes in human ciliary muscle. *Jpn J Ophthalmol*. 1992;36:380.
173. Pardue MS, JG Age-related changes in human ciliary muscle. *Optometry and Vision Science*. 2000;77:204–210.
174. Swegmark G. Studies with impedance cyclography on human ocular accommodation at different ages. *Acta Ophthalmologica*. 1969;47:1186–1206.
175. Saladin JJ, Stark L. Presbyopia: new evidence from impedence cyclography supporting the Hess-Gulstrand theory. *Vision Research*. 1975;15:537–541.
176. Fisher RF. The force of contraction of the human ciliary muscle during accommodation. *Journal of Physiology (London)*. 1977;270:51–74.
177. Strenk SA, Strenk LM, Guo S. Magnetic resonance imaging of aging, accommodating, phakic, and pseudophakic ciliary muscle diameters. *Journal of Cataract and Refractive Surgery*. 2006;32:1792–1798.
178. Stachs O, Martin H, Kirchhoff A, Stave J, Terwee T, Guthoff R. Monitoring accommodative ciliary muscle function using three-dimensional ultrasound. *Graefe's Arch Clin and Exp Ophthalmol*. 2002;240:906.
179. Tamm E, Croft MA, Jungkunz W, Lütjen-Drecoll E, Kaufman PL. Age-related loss of ciliary muscle mobility in the rhesus monkey: role of the choroid. *Arch Ophthalmol*. 1992;110:871–876.
180. van Alphen GWHM, Graebel WP. Elasticity of tissues involved in accommodation. *Vision Research*. 1991;31:1417–1438.
181. Farnsworth PN, Shyne SE. Anterior zonular shifts with age. *Experimental Eye Research*. 1979;28:291–297.
182. Croft MA, Glasser A, Heatley G, McDonald J, Ebbert T, Nadkarni NV, Kaufman PL. The zonula, lens, and circumlental space in the normal iridectomized rhesus monkey eye. *Invest Ophthalmol and Vis Sci*. 2006;47:1087–1095.
183. Sakabe I, Oshika T, Lim S, Apple D. Anterior shift of zonular insertion onto the anterior surface of human crystalline lens with age. *Ophthalmology*. 1998;105:295.
184. Fisher RF. Elastic constants of the human lens capsule. *Journal of Physiology (London)*. 1969;201:1–19.
185. Krag S, Olsen T, Andreassen TT. Biomechanical characteristics of the human anterior lens capsule in relation to age. *Investigative Ophthalmology and Visual Science*. 1997;38:357–363.
186. Krag S, Andreassen TT. Mechanical properties of the human lens capsule. *Progress in Retinal and Eye Research*. 2003;22(6):749–767.
187. Sorsby A, Leary G, Richards M. Ultrasonographic measurements of the components of ocular refraction in life-2. *Clinical procedures. Vision Research*. 1963;3:499.
188. Weekers, R., Y. Delmarcelle, J. Luyckx-Bacus and et.al. *The human lens in relation to cataract. Morphological changes of the lens with age and cataract*. in Ciba Foundation Symposium. 1973.
189. Atchison D, Markwell E, Kasthurangan S, Pope J, Smith G, Swann P. Age-related changes in optical and biometric charateristics of emmetropic eyes. *J Vis*. 2008:29.
190. Brown NP. The change in lens curvature with age. *Experimental Eye Research*. 1974;19:175–183.
191. Dubbleman M, van der Heijde G, Weeber H. Change in internal structure of the human crystalline lens with age and accommodation. *Vision Res*. 2003;43:2363.
192. Koretz JF, Neider MW, Kaufman PL, Bertasso AM, DeRousseau CJ, Bito LZ. Slit- lamp studies of the rhesus monkey eye: I. Survey of the anterior segment. *Experimental Eye Research*. 1987;44:307–318.
193. Koretz JF, Handelman GH. *The "lens paradox" and image formation in accommodating human eyes*, in *The lens: Transparency and cataract*. In: Duncan G, ed. *Topics in aging research in Europe*. Rijswijk; 1986:57–64.
194. Moffat B, Atchison D, Pope J. Eplanation of the lens parafox. *Optom Vis Sci*. 2002;79:148.
195. Schachar RA. Cause and treatment of presbyopia with a method for increasing the amplitude of accommodation *Annals of Ophthalmology*. 241992445–452.
196. Weale RA. *A biography of the eye - development, growth, age*. London: HK Lewis; 1982.
197. Rafferty NS.. In: Maisel H, ed. *Structure, function, and pathology, in The ocular lens*. New York: Marcel Dekker; 1985:1–60.
198. Schachar RA. *Presbyopia: a surgical textbook*. Thorofare, NJ: SLACK Inc; 2002.
199. Smith P. Diseases of the crystalline lens and capsule: on the growth of the crystalline lens. *Transactions of the Ophthalmological Societies of the United Kingdom*. 1883;3:79.
200. Fisher RF. The elastic constants of the human lens. *Journal of Physiology (London)*. 1971;212:147–180.
201. Fisher RF. Presbyopia and the changes with age in the human crystalline lens. *Journal of Physiology (London)*. 1973;228:765–779.
202. Burd H, Wilde G, Judge S. Can reliable values of Young's modulus be deduced from Fisher's (1971) spinning lens measurements? *Vision Res*. 2006;46:1346.
203. Heys KR, Cram SL, Truscott RJ. Massive increase in the stiffness of the human lens nucleus with age: the basis for presbyopia? *Molecular Vision*. 2004;10:956–963.
204. Weeber H, Eckert G, Pechhold W, van der Heijde R. Stiffness gradient in the crystalline lens. *Graefe's Arch Clin and Exp Ophthalmol*. 2007;245:1357.
205. Weeber H, van der Heijde R. On the relationship between lens stiffness and accommodative amplitude. *Exp Eye Res*. 2007;85:602.
206. Montes-Mico R, Hernandez P, Fernandez-Sanchez V, Bonaque S, Lara F, Lopez-Gil N. Changes of the eye optics after iris constriction. *J Optometry*. 2010;3:212–218.

207. Lütjen-Drecoll E, Shimizu T, Rohrbach M, Rohen JW. Quantitative analysis of 'plaque material' in the inner- and outer wall of Schlemm's canal in normal- and glaucomatous eyes. *Exp Eye Res*. 1986;42:443–455.
208. Lütjen-Drecoll E, Deitl T, Futa R, Rohen JW. Age changes of the trabecular meshwork, a preliminary morphometric study. In: Hollyfield JG, ed. *The structure of the eye*. New York, Amsterdam, Oxford: Elsevier Biomedical; 1982:341–348.
209. Stamer WD, Braakman ST, Zhou EH, Ethier CR, Fredberg JJ, Overby DRJ, M Biomechanics of Schlemm's canal endothelium and intraocular pressure reduction *Progress in Retinal Eye Research*. 44201586–98.
210. Saccà SC, Gandolfi S, Bagnis A, Manni G, Damonte G, Traverso CE, Izzotti A. From DNA damage to functional changes of the trabecular meshwork in aging and glaucoma. *Ageing Res Rev*. 2016;29:26–41.
211. Liu B, McNally S, Kilpatrick JI, Jarvis SP, O'Brien CJ. Aging and ocular tissue stiffness in glaucoma. *Surv Ophthalmol*. 2018;63:57–74.
212. Gabelt BT, Gottanka J, Lütjen-Drecoll E, Kaufman PL. Aqueous humor dynamics and trabecular meshwork and anterior ciliary muscle morphologic changes with age in rhesus monkeys. *Investigative Ophthalmology and Visual Science*. 2003;44:2118–2125.
213. Morgan JT, Raghunathan VK, chang YR, Murphy CH, Russell P. The intrinsic stiffness of human trabecular meshwork cells increases with senescence. *Oncotarget*. 2015;6(17):15362–15374.
214. Wang K, Read AT, Sulchek T, Ethier CR. Trabecular meshwork stiffness in glaucoma. *Exp Eye Res*. 2017;158:3–12.
215. Last JA, Pan T, Ding Y, Reilly CM, Keller K, Acott TS, Fautsch MP, Murphy CJ, Russell P. Elastic modulus determination of normal and glaucomatous human trabecular meshwork. *Invest Ophthalmol Vis Sci*. 2011;52:2147–2152.
216. Russell P, Johnson M. Elastic modulus determination of normal and glaucomatous human trabecular meshwork. *Invest Ophthalmol Vis Sci*. 2012;53(1):117.
217. Dismuke WM, Liang J, Overby DR, Stamer WD. Concentration-related effects of nitric oxide and endothelin-1 on human trabecular meshwork cell contractility. *Exp Eye Res*. 2014;120:28–35.
218. Overby DR, Bertrand J, Schicht M, Paulsen F, Stamer WD, Lütjen-Drecoll E. The structure of the trabecular meshwork, its connections to the ciliary muscle, and the effect of pilocarpine on outflow facility in mice. *Invest Ophthalmol Vis Sci*. 2014;55:3727–3736.
219. Bill A. Basic physiology of the drainage of aqueous humor. *Experimental Eye Research*. 1977;25(Suppl):291–304.
220. Bill A, Phillips I. Uveoscleral drainage of aqueous humor in human eyes. *Experimental Eye Research*. 1971;21:275–281.
221. Bill A. Aqueous humor dynamics in monkeys (Macaca irus and Cercopithecus ethiops). *Experimental Eye Research*. 1971;11:195–206.
222. Rohen JW, Futa R, Lütjen-Drecoll E. The fine structure of the cribriform meshwork in normal and glaucomatous eyes as seen in tangential sections. *Investigative Ophthalmology and Visual Science*. 1981;21:574–585.
223. Tian B, Gabelt BT, Geiger B, Kaufman PL. The role of the actomyosin system in regulating trabecular fluid outflow. *Exp Eye Res*. 2009;88:713–717.
224. Becker B. Decline in aqueous secretion and outflow facility with age. *American Journal of Ophthalmology*. 1958;46:731–736.
225. Koeppl C, Findl O, Menapace R. Pilocarpine-induced shift of an accommodating intraocular lens: AT-45 Crystalens. *J Cataract Refract Surg*. 2005;31:1290–1297.
226. Pepose JS, Burke JS, Qazi MA. Accommodating Intraocular Lenses. *Asia-Pac J Ophthalmol*. 2017;6:350–357.

Cornea and Sclera

Jodhbir S. Mehta and Marcus Ang

Introduction

The outermost, fibrous tunic of the human eye consists of the cornea and the sclera (Fig. 4.1A,B).[1–5] Both are soft connective tissues that provide structural integrity to the globe and protect the inner components of the eye from physical injury. The clear, transparent cornea (Fig. 4.1A,C) covers the anterior one-sixth of the total surface area of the globe, and the white, opaque sclera (Fig. 4.1A) covers the remaining five-sixths. The cornea and the lens are the eye's primary refractive structures and both have two key optical properties to this end—refractive power (light refraction) and transparency (light transmission). The presence of a healthy cornea is essential for good vision as it is basically the window of the eye. The cornea is most analogous to the external lens of a compound lens camera. By comparison, the sclera predominantly serves more of a biomechanical function and is analogous to the housing of the camera and lens.

The normal human cornea is between 500 and 650 microns (μm) thick and is arranged in five basic layers—epithelium, Bowman's layer, stroma, Descemet's membrane, and endothelium (Fig. 4.1D), each having distinctly different structural and functional characteristics.[6] It also is composed of three major cell types—epithelial, stromal keratocyte, and endothelial cells. However, there are several other cell types found in the stroma, (e.g., Langerhans cells, nonmyelinated Schwann cells, and dendritic cells).[6] Two of these, epithelium and endothelium, form cellular barrier layers to the stroma. Thus, their resistance to diffusion of solutes and bulk fluid flow are of considerable importance to maintaining normal corneal function (resistance to diffusion of solutes and fluid flow: epithelium [2000] >> endothelium [10] > stroma [1]).[6] All three can replicate through mitosis, but vary considerably in their in vivo proliferative capacity, with epithelial cells having the highest rates of cell division and endothelial cells being the least renewable. This fact is seen clinically because epithelial cells can completely regenerate after injury (e.g., corneal abrasions), whereas endothelial cells, as a result of limited in vivo proliferation, are most commonly involved in age-related disease (e.g., Fuchs' dystrophy) or injury-related disease (e.g., pseudophakic bullous keratopathy [PBK]), ultimately resulting in corneal edema and bullous keratopathy. However, more recently, an early proliferative progenitor endothelial cell has been described in the transition zone.[7] Corneal stromal keratocytes are a middle ground compromise between these two extremes. One major disadvantage of the epithelium's high proliferative potential is that it can occasionally go unchecked, resulting in cancer (e.g., squamous cell cancers of the cornea), whereas keratocytes and endothelial cells do not have this risk.[7]

The sclera is 0.3- to 1.35-mm thick and is arranged into three layers—episclera, scleral stroma proper, and lamina fusca; each having distinctly different structural and functional characteristics. The sclera is composed of only one major cell type, the sclera fibrocyte, which has moderate proliferative potential, like that of the corneal stromal keratocyte. Because the sclera has no cellular barrier layers, its permeability properties are quite similar to those of the corneal stroma. The sclera is an excellent example of a tissue made for biomechanical stability, as it is stiff, strong, and tough. As such, disease of the sclera commonly results in loss of structural strength, abnormal size owing to dysregulated growth, and inflammatory conditions that commonly also affect the joints in the body. Many animals have a very rigid sclera that is often supported by bone or cartilage. Humans deviate from this extreme in that their sclera is a less rigid fibrous connective tissue, perhaps reflecting its need to maintain an even blood flow to the choroid and retina during large excursions in eye motility.

This chapter reviews and explains the structure and function of the cornea and sclera, providing a framework for understanding normal health and disease of each tissue with an emphasis on function.

CORNEA

Embryology, growth, development, and aging in human eyes

Between 4 and 5 weeks' gestation (27–36 days), surface ectodermal cells left behind after vesicle separation become the primitive, undifferentiated corneal epithelium, which is composed initially of two cell layers.[7] The primitive corneal epithelium immediately produces a primary acellular corneal stroma, or postepithelial layer.[8,9] This is seen as the gradual subepithelial addition of diagonal and then randomly oriented fibrillar elements, which later thicken into collagen fibrils that are slightly smaller in diameter than stromal collagen fibrils.[8] The Bowman's layer is thought to be a distinct, dense anterior-most remnant of this embryologic layer, which is first detectable by light microscopy around 20 weeks' gestation.[9] Around 12 weeks' gestation, a time period between eyelid fusion at 8 weeks' gestation and eyelid opening at 26 weeks' gestation, the epithelium differentiates to become a stratified, squamous epithelium, four cell layers thick, which then produces an epithelial basement membrane. It remains four cell layers thick until approximately 6 months after birth when it reaches adult levels of four to six cell layers thick. Early in gestation, the epithelial basement membrane and anchoring complexes on the basal surface of the epithelium are absent. Rudimentary epithelial basement membrane and anchoring complexes only become detectable by 17 weeks' gestation. With further

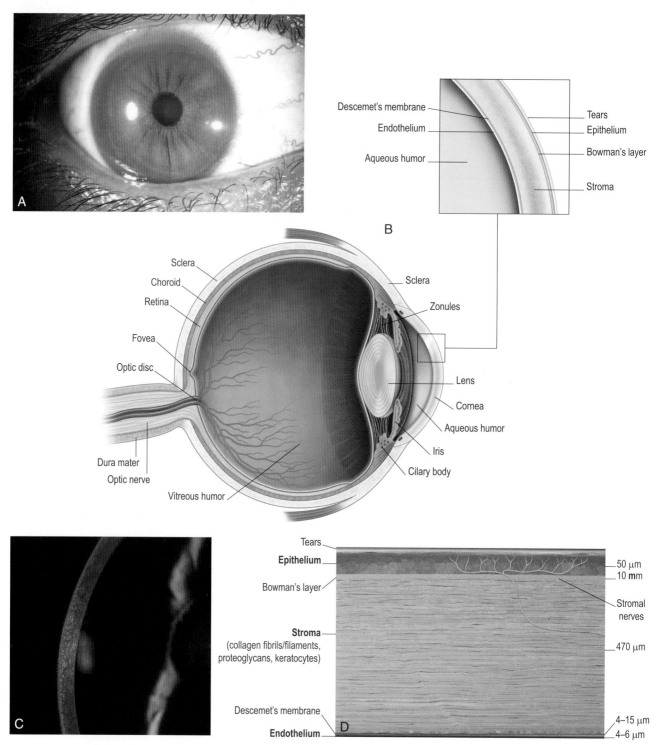

Fig. 4.1 (**A**) Diffuse illumination slit-lamp image of the human cornea and sclera. (**B**) Main anatomical components of the globe with detailed emphasis on the corneal and scleral components. (**C**) Slit-beam illumination of the human cornea shows an optical section of the tissue. Notice the slight light scattering that occurs in the tissue, mainly from cellular components in cornea. (**D**) Histologic section of the human cornea labeling the five main cellular and extracellular matrix layers (toluidine blue ×25).

development in utero, the thickness and number of these structures gradually increase.

A first wave of neural crest-derived mesenchymal cells begins to migrate beneath the corneal epithelial cells from the limbus around 5 weeks' gestation (33 days); these cells form the primitive endothelium. The primitive endothelium is initially composed of two cell layers. By 8 weeks' gestation, it becomes a monolayer that starts to

produce Descemet's membrane, which becomes recognizable on light microscopy at 3 to 4 months' gestation. The epithelium and endothelium remain closely opposed until 7 weeks' gestation (49 days), when a second wave of mesenchymal cells begins to migrate centrally from the limbus between the epithelium and endothelium invading below and into most of the primary acellular stroma. The cells do not enter the anterior-most 10 μm of stroma, which lacks keratocan, a proteoglycan core protein signal thought to be required for cellular invasion.[9] This second wave of cells forms the stroma proper, or secondary cellular corneal stroma, as production of lamellar collagen begins within a few days in a posterior-to-anterior fashion. It is believed that the invading mesenchymal cells, destined to become keratocytes, use the primary acellular stroma as a scaffold, primarily in the anterior third of stroma proper. This concurs with the significant lamellar interweaving and oblique lamellar orientation in the anterior third of postnatal human corneal stroma, as well as each successive lamellar layer being rotated 1 to 2 degrees clockwise. This directional rotation is the same in both right and left eyes. In the posterior two-thirds of the stroma, the corneal stroma is composed of essentially orthogonal lamellae. By 3 months' gestation, corneal nerves invade the stroma and eventually penetrate through the Bowman's layer so that nerve endings develop in the epithelium. Studies also suggest that by 5 months' gestation, tight junctions form around all the corneal endothelial cells and by 5 to 7 months' gestation the in-utero cornea becomes transparent as the density of functioning endothelial Na^+/K^+-ATPase metabolic pump sites increases to adult levels.[10] By 7 months' gestation, the cornea resembles that of the adult in most structural characteristics other than size. At birth in the full-term infant, the horizontal corneal diameter is about 9.8 mm and the corneal surface area is around 102 mm². The cornea of the newborn infant is approximately 75% to 80% of the size of the adult human cornea (Fig. 4.2A–C), whereas the posterior segment is less than 50% of adult size (Fig. 4.2D).[11] At birth, the cross-sectional thickness of the four cell layer epithelium averages 50 µm, the Bowman's layer averages 10 µm, the central stroma proper averages 500 µm, Descemet's membrane averages 4 µm, and the endothelium averages 6-µm thick (total mean central corneal thickness ~570 µm).[12–15]

During infancy, the cornea continues to grow, reaching adult size around 2 years of age with a horizontal diameter of 11.7 mm, surface area of 138 mm², anterior surface curvature of 44.1 diopters (D) (Fig. 4.2A), and mean central corneal thickness of 544 µm (Fig. 4.2C).[12] Thereafter, it changes very little in size, shape, transparency, or curvature, although a shift from with-the-rule to against-the-rule astigmatism has been associated with aging (Fig. 4.2B). This means that if we consider the cornea as a sphere, "with-the-rule" astigmatism is where the curvature is steepest is near the 90-degree meridian, whereas "against-the-rule" is astigmatism in which the steepest curve lies near the 180-degree meridian (Fig. 4.2B).[16–18] Postnatal aging is associated with several structural changes to the corneal tissue including: (1) epithelial basement membrane growth or thickening of an additional 100 to 300 nm or a rate of approximately 30 nm per decade of life; (2) decreased keratocyte, sub-basal nerve fiber, and endothelial cell density, presumably from stress-induced premature senescence; (3) increased stiffness, strength, and toughness of the stroma, from enzymatic maturation and nonenzymatic age-related glycation-induced crosslinking of collagen fibrils; (4) Descemet's membrane thickening of an additional 6 to 11 µm or a rate of approximately 1 µm per decade of life; and (5) possible degeneration of extracellular matrix structures.[19] These structural and cellular changes, however, minimally affect the optical and barrier functions of the cornea and perhaps improve its mechanical function. For example, corneal ectasia from natural causes such as keratoconus is rarely seen after 40 years of age. Only three documented functional consequences are associated with aging—impaired corneal wound healing, decreased corneal sensation, and decreased extensibility of its tissue.[20–22] In elderly individuals or younger individuals with lipid abnormalities, the cornea often becomes yellowish in the periphery of the cornea due to a fine deposition of lipid. This condition is called arcus senilis.[23]

Major corneal reference points and measurements

When viewed anteriorly in the living eye, the adult human cornea appears elliptical (Fig. 4.3A), as the largest diameter is typically in the horizontal meridian (mean 11.7 mm) and the smallest is in the vertical meridian (mean 10.6 mm).[1] This elliptical configuration is brought about by anterior extension of the opaque sclera superiorly and inferiorly. When viewed from the posterior surface, the cornea is actually circular (Fig. 4.3A), with an average horizontal and vertical diameter of 11.7 mm. The average radius of curvature of the anterior and posterior corneal surface is 7.8 mm and 6.5 mm, respectively, which is significantly less than the 11.5-mm average radius of curvature of the sclera. This results in a small 1.5- to 2-mm transition zone that forms an external and internal surface groove, or scleral sulcus, where the steeper cornea meets the flatter sclera (Fig. 4.3A). This sulcus typically is not obvious clinically because it is filled in by overlying episclera and conjunctiva externally. The tissue in this transition zone is known as the limbus (Fig. 4.3B), which averages 1.5-mm wide in the horizontal meridian and 2-mm wide in the vertical meridian. It is important because it contains adult corneal stem cell populations, contains the trabecular meshwork, which is the conventional outflow pathway for the aqueous humor, and is the inciting site of pathology in a few immunologic diseases. The limbus is also a major anatomic reference point for planning surgical entry into the anterior segment because it appears clinically as a blue transition zone. Therefore, an incision placed anterior to the blue zone is anatomically in the peripheral cornea, safely inside the trabecular meshwork and stem cells. The cornea is thinner in the center, measuring on average 544 ± 34 µm (range: 440–650 µm) with ultrasound-based corneal thickness measurements (ultrasound pachymetry), and increasing in thickness in the periphery to approximately 700 µm as it reaches the limbus.[1–4,6] A meta-analysis of all cross-sectional and longitudinal corneal thickness studies over a 30-year time period showed that no significant age-related change in central corneal thickness occurred beyond the infant years.[12]

The central cornea is overlying the entrance pupil, which is a virtual image of the real pupil and is typically located 0.5-mm anterior to, and is 14% larger than, the real pupil. It contains the central or effective optical zone of the cornea (Fig. 4.3C). The central optical zone is the portion of the cornea that can successfully refract a cone-like bundle of light from a distant or near fixation target through the pupil of the eye, and it then directly refracts it onto the fovea. The central location and size of this central optical zone dynamically changes according to the location of the fixation target in relation to the cornea (e.g., more distant fixation target = larger-diameter central optical zone, off-center fixation target = off-center central optical zone) and the aperture of the real pupil in various lighting conditions. This is because the bundle of light has the same cross-sectional shape as the pupil (e.g., an oval pupil results in an oval central optical zone) and its diameter is defined by the pupil's diameter, as well as the location of fixation target. The central optical zone's diameter typically averages 3.6 ± 0.8 mm in photopic lighting and 5.8 ± 0.9 mm in scotopic light, with a range between 1.5 and 9.0 mm depending on the lighting condition.[24,25] The remaining cornea peripheral to this central optical zone is the peripheral optical zone, which can refract light through the entrance pupil; however, it does so at such an acute angle that it only affects the more peripheral aspects of the retina (Fig. 4.3C)—it rarely directly impacts foveal vision.

Within the central optical zone are three major corneal reference points (Fig. 4.3D) that are extremely useful in determining the shape, refractive power, and biomechanical properties of the cornea, as they are statically fixed reference points.[26] The first is called the corneal apex; it is defined as the steepest point or area of the cornea. Its exact location on the cornea is referenced in relation to the corneal intercept of an imaging device's optical axis (Fig. 4.3E).[27] The corneal intercept of the imaging device's optical axis is termed the device's axis point (DAP). On average, the corneal apex is usually located 0.8-mm temporal and 0.2-mm superior to the DAP or 0.5-mm temporal and 0.5-mm superior to the corneal intercept of the line of sight of the eye (Fig. 4.3D), but considerable

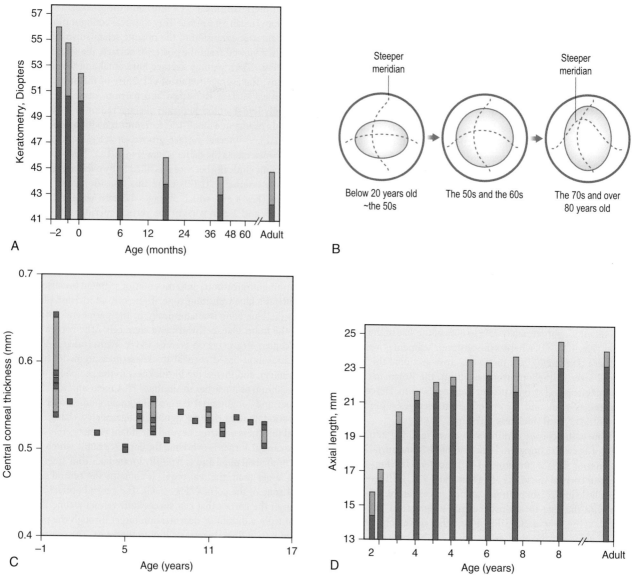

Fig. 4.2 (**A**) Keratometry values plotted with respect to age on a logarithmic scale. Negative numbers represent months of prematurity; dot = mean value for each age group and bar = standard deviation. (Data from Gordon RA, Donzis PB. Refractive development of the human eye. *Arch Ophthalmol.* 1985;103(6): 785–789.) (**B**) Changes in corneal shape associated with aging showing the shift from with-the-rule astigmatism to against-the-rule astigmatism. (Hayashi K, Hayashi H, Hayashi F. Topographic analysis of the changes in corneal shape due to aging. *Cornea.* 1995;14:527–532.) (**C**) Scatterplot showing the relationship between age and central corneal thickness from various studies in the published literature. (Doughty MJ, Laiquzzaman M, Müller A, Oblak E, Button NF. Central corneal thickness in European (white) individuals, especially children and the elderly, and assessment of its possible importance in clinical measures of intra-ocular pressure. *Ophthalm Physiol Optics.* 2002;22:491–504. https://doi.org/10.1046/j.1475-1313.2002.00053.x.) (**D**) Axial length plotted with respect to age. *Dots* = mean values for age group; *bars* = standard deviation. (Data from Gordon RA, Donzis PB. Refractive development of the human eye. *Arch Ophthalmol.* 1985;103(6):785–789.)

Fig. 4.3 (**A**) Coronal views show the elliptical shape of the right cornea when viewed anteriorly (*upper left*) and the circular shape when viewed posteriorly (*lower left*). Superior axial view (*right*) illustrates how the right globe deviates from a perfect sphere. *Dashed lines* = theoretical spherical globe; *solid lines* = actual contour of the globe. (Modified from Bron AJ, Tripathi R, Tripathi B. In: *Wolff's Anatomy of the Eye and Orbit*, 8th ed. London, UK: Chapman & Hall; 1997.) (**B**) Locations of the peripheral cornea, limbus, sclera, episclera, and conjunctiva (peripheral anterior synechiae (PAS) × 20). (**C**) The cornea overlying the entrance pupil, known as the central or effective optical zone, directly impacts foveal vision, whereas the cornea peripheral to the entrance pupil, known as the peripheral optical zone, primarily impacts peripheral vision. (Modified from Uozato H, Guyton D. Centering corneal surgical procedures. *Am J Ophthalmol.* 1987;103:264–275.) (**D**) The clinically definable principal axes of the eye (*left*), line of sight and pupillary axis, and major corneal reference points of the cornea (*right [right cornea shown]*), corneal sighting center (*CSC*), corneal apex, and thinnest corneal point (*TCP*) are illustrated in reference to the theoretical, but not practically useful, visual axis. The line of sight is the line from the fixation target to the CSC that typically continues through the cornea into the eye, at or near the center of the entrance pupil, where it is refracted by the cornea and lens to finally reach the fovea. The light rays from the fixation target (*shown by shaded areas*) are usually centered on or near the entrance pupil, E,

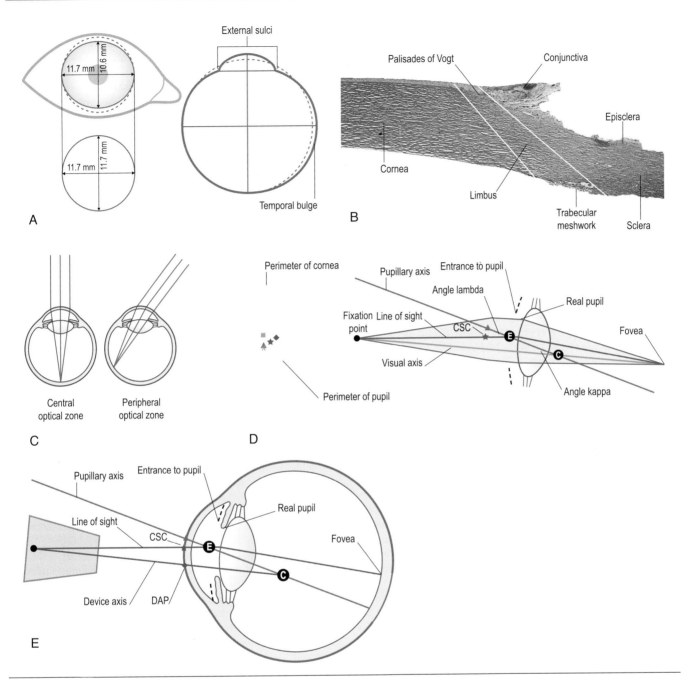

and are nearly symmetric around the line of sight. The line of sight is often confused with a theoretical principal axis of the schematic eye called the visual axis. Technically, there is no visual axis of the real human eye because the noncentered optics of the real eye do not allow a single straight line to describe this theoretical pathway of chief light rays, defined as a line from the fixation target that directly passes through the nodal points of the eye and ultimately onto the fovea. The visual axis is used for calculating the relation between object and image sizes using Gaussian optics and Gullstrand's schematic eye. The pupillary axis is an easily definable line from the center of the real pupil to the perpendicular or normal surface of the cornea, which is aligned with the center of curvature of the cornea, C_1. Angle kappa is the angle between real pupillary axis and theoretical visual axis; angle lambda is the angle between the real pupillary axis and real line of sight. In the clinical setting, it is the angle lambda that is measured by observing the displacement of the coaxially viewed corneal reflex from the pupil center of a fixating eye, even though it is erroneously called angle kappa. Usually angle lambda measures between 3 and 6 degrees. The visual axis and line of sight are often assumed to be parallel, but this is only true for very distant objects near infinity. *Pink dot* = pupillary axis intercept with cornea; *blue dot* = line of sight intercept with cornea or CSC; *yellow dot* = corneal apex; *violet dot* = imaging device's axis point (DAP); *gray dot* = TCP. (**E**) The standard alignment position for all imaging devices occurs when a patient directly looks at a luminous fixation point centered in the circular rings of the imaging device and its reflected image is then aligned by the examiner so that it is centered in the operator's screen of the device. When in standard alignment position, the imaging device's optical axis is aimed perpendicular or vertex normal to the surface of cornea and directed toward the center of curvature of the cornea, C; it also is approximately twice the distance from the pupillary axis as the line of sight. The anterior corneal surface intercept with the device axis is the device axis point (*DAP*). The center of the circular rings of the imaging device's operator screen and the reflected first Purkinje image of the luminous fixation target are perfectly aligned in the standard alignment position. Only if angle lambda is zero will standard alignment position coincide with the line of sight and the corneal sighting center. E = center of entrance pupil. (Modified from Mandell R, Horner D. In: Gills J, Sanders D, Thornton S, et al., eds. *Corneal Topography: The State of the Art.* Thorofare, New Jersey: Slack; 1995.)

interindividual variability is found in the location of the corneal apex in comparison to the average.[27] The clinical utility of the corneal apex is that it is of paramount importance in the selection and fitting of contact lenses and in determining the geometric aspheric shape of the cornea.[26] Significant decentration of the corneal apex from the DAP may give a false interpretation of corneal shape (e.g., asymmetric shape). The easiest way to clarify whether this is real or due to artifact is to aim the imaging device's optical axis directly at the corneal apex, which is more cumbersome and difficult to do than using a standard alignment position.

The second major corneal reference point is the corneal intercept of the line of sight, also known as the corneal sighting center (CSC).[28] The line of sight is an actual principal axis of the real eye as opposed to a theoretical construct of a schematic eye (e.g., visual axis), and it is defined as the principal axis joining a distant fixation point to the fovea. Theoretically, it is always thought to cross the center of the entrance pupil, which may not be true in the real eye because it is known that the center of the entrance pupil dynamically and unpredictably shifts up to 0.7 mm in direction with changes in pupil diameter, whereas the line of sight is a statically fixed axis line. Thus, the line of sight is perhaps best thought of as a line that connects the fixation target to the CSC on the anterior surface of the cornea and then, via an unknown nonlinear pathway, is refracted in the cornea and by the lens to focus on the fovea. It is of utmost importance to know the location of the line of sight and CSC in certain clinical situations, to obtain the best visual results with keratorefractive surgery. This is particularly so with retreatments and customized ablations, and for calculating the proper posterior chamber intraocular lens (PCIOL) power to put in during cataract extraction (CE), especially after previous refractive surgery or with anterior surface irregularities. As subclinical decentrations 0.5 mm (or more) or torsional misalignments 15 degrees (or more) can yield unwanted visual symptoms (e.g., coma or other higher-order aberrations [HOAs]).[28-31] On average, the CSC is 0.4-mm nasal and 0.3-mm superior to the dynamically, unfixed pupillary axis or 0.5-mm inferior and 0.5-mm nasal to the static, fixed corneal apex reference point (Fig. 4.3D), but its location overall is highly variable between different individuals.[28] Using a keratographer, topographer, or tomographer in nonstandard alignment position, the CSC can be directly determined by having the patient directly look at a luminous fixation point centered in the circular rings of the imaging device. It is then marked in reference to the center of the operator's screen. Because of practical difficulties in nonstandard alignment, some clinicians approximate the CSC's position using the coaxially sighted corneal reflex. With this method, the patient looks directly at a luminous fixation point centered in the circular rings of the imaging device. The anterior corneal surface's first Purkinje image, i.e., the reflection of the light on the exterior corneal surface, is used to approximate the location of the CSC.[28] This approximation method reportedly locates a point on average 0.02 ± 0.17 mm (range: −0.43 mm to +0.68 mm) from the actual CSC in normal eyes; this, however, may not be the case in diseased or surgically altered corneas.[28]

The third major and newest corneal reference point is called the thinnest corneal point (TCP), defined as the thinnest point or zone of the entire cornea. It is measured using various tomography instruments, which enable a mathematical three-dimensional reconstruction of the in vivo pachymetric distribution map, allowing one to evaluate the spatial variation of the thickness profile over the entire cornea. In the normal cornea, the average location and value of the TCP is 0.4-mm inferior and 0.4-mm temporal to CSC and 5-μm less thick than the central corneal thickness at the CSC.

Optical properties

Light refraction

The main optical measurements that determine the total refractive power of the eye are the anterior and posterior curvatures of both the central cornea and lens, the depth of the anterior chamber, and the axial length of the eye (Fig. 4.4A). Because this chapter is strictly about the cornea and sclera, we will focus only on the optical properties of the cornea. Refractive power and aberrations induced by the optics of the cornea are primarily due to corneal curvature and contour, respectively. Both are descriptors of corneal shape. The contour of the anterior corneal surface is basically of an aspheric geometry. The corneal apex defines the point of greatest refractive power or steepest curvature, and it then gradually and variably flattens from the apex to the periphery.[32] Corneal asphericity has been known for over 100 years and has been modeled by various mathematical formulas in order to derive a quantitative approximation of contour.[33] The central optical zone of the anterior corneal surface best corresponds to that of a conic section using the following formula, which requires knowing only two conic fit parameters—Q and R.[34]

$$Q = p - 1 = \left(\frac{b}{a}\right)^2 - 1 = \frac{R}{a} - 1 = \left(1 - e^2\right) - 1$$

Q is a unitless asphericity factor or expression of the rate of curvature change from the apex of the cornea to the periphery (Fig. 4.4B); p is a geometric form factor; a and b are horizontal and vertical semimeridian hemi-axes; R is the apical radius of curvature; and e is the eccentricity. Q averages −0.4 in early childhood, but then gets gradually slightly less negative with age such that the central optical zone has a mean Q of −0.2 in adulthood (range: −0.81 to +0.47).[35,36] $Q < 0$ describes a prolate contour where the rate of curvature change from the apex is less than that of a sphere (Fig. 4.4C); most normal corneas are prolate, which is advantageous in that it compensates for spherical aberrations induced by larger pupil sizes, which project misaligned peripheral rays of light on the fovea. $Q = 0$ describes a spherical contour where the rate of curvature change from the apex to the periphery is zero, and $Q > 0$ describes an oblate contour where the rate of curvature change from the apex is more than that of a sphere (Fig. 4.4C). Oblate contours are typically present in 20% or less of the normal population. Interestingly, asphericity can significantly change after surgery, especially excimer laser keratorefractive surgery, usually resulting in various oblate contours. Although the contour of the central optical zone of the anterior corneal surface is the most important for directly impacting foveal vision and on-axis aberrations (spherical aberrations, coma, and other HOAs), recent study has also shown that the peripheral optical zone is important for off-axis aberrations (e.g., glare, halos, starbursts). This peripheral optical zone does not fit a conic section well, but rather fits a ninth-order polynomial formula best and has a measured Q of −0.4 in adulthood when the central 10 mm of cornea is best fit to this formula.[37] A few reports on the posterior corneal surface suggest it also has a prolate contour with a Q of −0.4, but its contribution to the total optical aberrations of the eye is less well known.[35]

The actual total corneal dioptric power of the central 4.0 mm of cornea reportedly averages 42.4 ± 1.5 D (range: 38.4–46.3 D) of the eye's total dioptric power of 60 D.[38] The location of the corneal apex compared with the CSC (generally <1 mm from the CSC and on average 0.7 D steeper than that at the CSC), the degree of asphericity of the anterior corneal surface, and the degree of anterior corneal surface-to-posterior corneal surface ratios can vary widely from one individual to another or even change with age in an individual.[39-41] For these reasons, it is difficult to take these general population-averaged results as empirically useful values. An individual's total corneal power along the line of sight of the eye should probably best be measured using the Gaussian optics formula:

$$P_{totalcornea} = \frac{n_c - n_{air}}{r_{ant}} + \frac{n_a - n_c}{r_{post}}\left(\frac{d}{n_c} \times \left(\frac{n_c - n_{air}}{r_{ant}}\right) \times \left(\frac{n_a - n_c}{r_{post}}\right)\right)$$

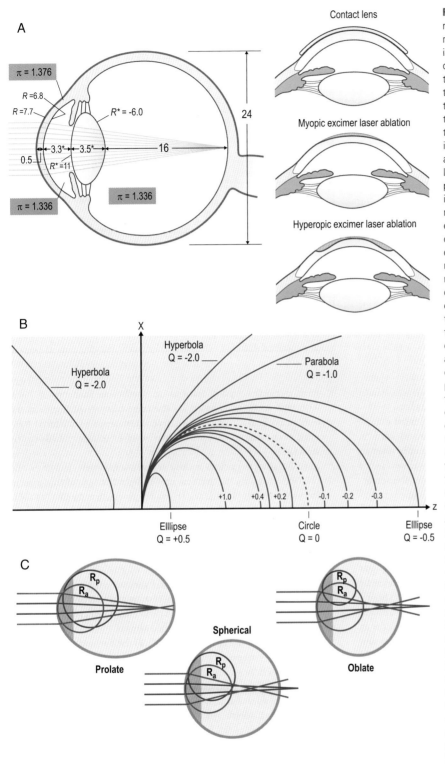

Fig. 4.4 (A) Diagram of the schematic eye with representative average dimensions in millimeters and refractive indices of the relaxed, nonaccommodating eye. The starred values change with accommodation. These dimensions are average values used to construct a schematic eye—all dimensions of the eye vary greatly between individuals and from these average values. *Upper-right* diagram shows that the principle of corneal contact lens wear is to make the anterior corneal surface ineffective as it is now bathed with aqueous tears, and the new anterior refractive surface is the air-anterior contact lens interface. *Middle-right* diagram shows that the principle of myopic correction using the excimer laser is based on a graded removal of central anterior corneal tissue to decrease the central anterior corneal curvature, analogous to the removal of a biologic contact lens that is thicker in the center. *Lower-right* diagram shows that the principle of hyperopic correction using the excimer laser is based on a graded removal of a peripheral and paracentral concave lenticule of tissue to increase the central anterior corneal curvature (i.e., a donut-shaped trough) analogous to the removal of a biologic contact that is thicker in the periphery and of no or minimal thickness in the center. **(B)** Variations in conicoid shape for different asphericities, or Q-factors, with the same radius of curvature. **(C)** Schematic diagrams showing the three possible anterior corneal surface contours with ray tracings from a distant fixation point being refracted onto the retina. Upper left diagram is of a prolate cornea (Q factor < 0), which has a larger peripheral radius of curvature than at the apex ($R_p > R_a$). Lower middle diagram is of a spherical cornea (Q factor = 0), which has equal peripheral and apical radii of curvature ($R_a = R_p$). Upper-right diagram is of an oblate cornea (Q factor > 0), which has a smaller peripheral radius of curvature than at the apex ($R_a > R_p$). As a prolate cornea reduces spherical aberrations, its image is more tightly or precisely focused than spherical or, lastly, oblate corneas. The mean value of the Q factor for normal healthy adult corneas is −0.2, which reduces natural spherical aberration by about half; a Q factor of −0.50 eliminates all spherical aberration. Thus, the human cornea typically is not designed to induce zero spherical aberrations. In fact, the human lens is optically coupled to the cornea in such a way that spherical aberrations are reduced close to zero in youth because during childhood and young adulthood the lens has negative asphericity. Lens asphericity dynamically changes with aging, usually resulting in a Q of zero around age 40 and then has positive asphericity after age 40 years. The overall effect on the optical properties of the human eye is that it gains progressively more spherical and other optical aberrations with increasing age, which perhaps best explains the direct association of deterioration of visual performance and quality with aging. Most degradation of image quality is due to age-related changes in the lens. (Modified from Gatinel D, Haouat M, Hoang-Xuan T. [A review of mathematical descriptors of corneal asphericity]. *J Fr Ophthalmol.* 2002;25:81–90.)

Where $P_{totalcornea}$ equals diopters of optical power; n_{air}, n_c, and n_a are the indices of refraction in air (1.000), cornea (1.376), and aqueous humor (1.336), respectively; r_{ant} and r_{post} are the radii of curvature of the anterior (0.0078) and posterior (0.0065) corneal surface in meters, respectively; and d is the central corneal thickness (0.00054) in meters.

$$42.18D = \frac{1.376-1}{0.0078} + \frac{1.336-1.376}{0.0065} - \left(\frac{0.00054}{1.376} \times \left(\frac{1.376-1}{0.0078}\right) \times \left(\frac{1.336-1.376}{0.0065}\right)\right)$$

Therefore, the calculated total optical power of the cornea using known average major reference values is $48.21 - 6.15 + 0.12 = 42.18$ D, which agrees closely with the actual mean of 42.4 D found in the study cited previously.

Because the cornea is thinner in the center than in the periphery, it should act as a minus lens, but functions as a plus lens because the aqueous humor neutralizes most of the minus optical power on the posterior corneal surface. If we compute the power of the posterior corneal surface in air, we find the following:

$$P_{postcornea} = \frac{n_a - n_c}{r_{post}} = \frac{1-1.376}{0.0065} = -57.85$$

The resulting calculated total optical power of the cornea would then be $48.21 - 57.85 + 1.12 = -8.52$ D, which is a minus lens.

From the foregoing calculations, it is obvious that the most important refractive surface for humans is the anterior corneal surface. However, if a large air bubble is placed in the anterior chamber so that it contacts the corneal endothelium or if the anterior surface of the cornea is submerged in water, tremendous changes in the refractive power of the eye occur. For example, when the eye is open underwater during swimming, the optical imagery is extremely blurred; the index of refraction of water (1.333) is quite similar to that of the tear film and cornea (1.376). Thus, most of the optical power of the anterior corneal surface is lost. If the air-tear film interface is maintained by the use of a mask or goggles, then underwater vision is as sharp and clear as normal terrestrial vision. If the central optical zone of the anterior corneal surface is regular, yet not uniformly spherical in each meridian, the condition of astigmatism usually results. With astigmatism, a distant fixation point is refracted by the cornea and lens to become two focal lines rather than a sharp image point. However, if the central optical zone is irregular, then irregular astigmatism usually results. In adult humans, the conjunctival surface area has been measured at approximately 17.65 cm² and the corneal surface area measures 1.38 cm², giving a conjunctival-to-corneal surface area ratio of 12.8, which is important for drug delivery calculations.[1]

Light transmission

The cornea is an excellent example of the structural characteristics that a tissue needs to fulfill its dual role of transparency and mechanical support. Tissue transparency is rarely seen in the animal kingdom outside the eye.[2] In fact, the only structures in humans where this property is seen are in the eye (e.g., cornea, lens). Corneal transparency has occupied scientists for over half a century and initial transparency theories focused on the extracellular stromal matrix while ignoring the cells of the stroma.[42] Corneal transparency is now thought to be attributable to both the lattice-like arrangement of collagen fibrils in the corneal stroma and the transparency of cells that reside in the cornea.[42-44] In summary, all currently viable transparency theories agree with these major points:

TABLE 4.1 Composition of cornea and sclera

Component	Wet weight (%)	Dry weight (%)
Cornea		
Water	78	–
Matrix	*66*	
Cellular	*12*	
Collagen	15	71
Proteoglycans	1	9
Keratocytes	1	10
Other	5	10
Sclera		
Water	68	–
Collagen	27	77
Elastin	1	2
Proteoglycans	1	3
Fibrocytes	1	3
Other	2	6

1. Each corneal collagen fibril is an ineffective scatterer of light. Although inefficient, based on the large number of fibrils in the human corneal stroma, destructive interference of scattered light must occur due to the short-range order of collagen fibrils in the stroma.
2. Each keratocyte nucleus mildly scatters some light. However, the cell body is an ineffective scatterer of light because of transparent intracellular cytoplasmic water-soluble corneal crystallins, its thinness, and because keratocytes are evenly distributed in the corneal stroma through a clockwise circular arrangement, so light transmission is hardly affected.
3. Scattering of light is minimal in the cornea because it is thin.
4. If an increased refractive index imbalance occurs between fibrils, keratocytes, or extrafibrillar matrix, light scattering can increase tremendously in the corneal stroma, resulting in loss of transparency.

To understand these theories and generalized principles, one needs to start with the structure of the corneal stroma.

The corneal stroma accounts for 90% of the corneal thickness. It is predominantly composed of water (3.5-gram H_2O/gram dry weight) that is stabilized by an organized structural network of insoluble and soluble extracellular and cellular substances (Table 4.1).[32] The dry weight of the adult human corneal stroma is made up of collagen, keratocyte constituents, proteoglycans, corneal nerve constituents, glycoproteins, and salts (Table 4.1).[32] Overall, these corneal components work together to maintain and establish a transparent cornea. Although the cornea primarily absorbs most ultraviolet (UV) light, it transmits almost all visible (400–700 nm) and infrared (IR) light up to a wavelength of 2500 nm, with its peak transmission rate of 85% to 99% in the visible spectrum (Fig. 4.5A).[45] The remaining portion (1%–15%) is scattered in all directions by the cornea in a wavelength-dependent fashion, with violet light being most affected.[46] Clinical slit-lamp examination and in vivo confocal microscopy suggest that most of the light scatter is due to cellular components in the cornea rather than extracellular matrix. Relative amounts of light scattering owing to each stromal constituent are the following: endothelial cells > epithelial cells > nerve cells > keratocytes >> collagen fibrils or extracellular matrix (Fig. 4.5B).[47,48] In fact, the in vivo confocal

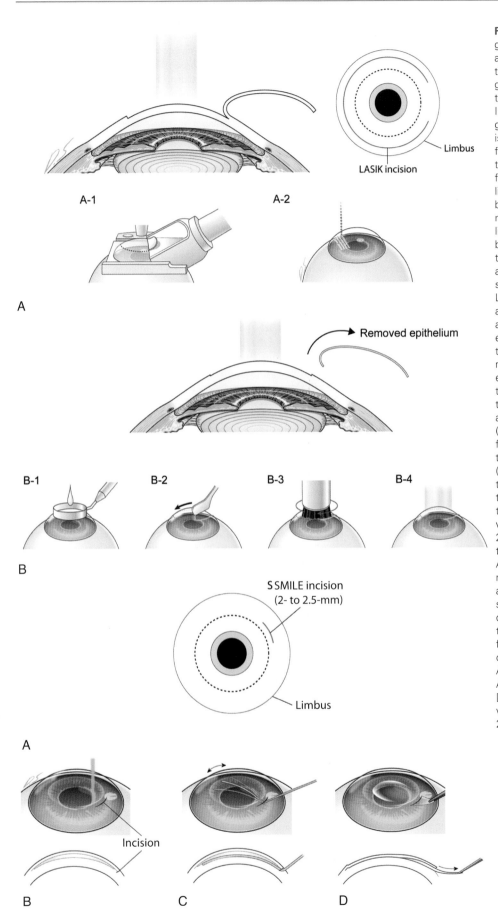

Fig. 4.5 Part 1: In lamellar refractive surgery, a corneal flap is created and lifted after which an excimer laser is applied to the inner stromal tissue. With LASIK surgery, the corneal flap is created by cutting the corneal tissue, leaving a hinge area (**A**). In traditional mechanical LASIK, a hand-guided, oscillating blade (microkeratome) is used to create the corneal flap (**A-1**). In femtosecond laser-assisted LASIK surgery, the femtosecond laser moves back and forth, emitting short, rapid bursts of laser light that create a series of minute bubbles at a predetermined depth (**A-2**). The mechanical- or laser-created flap is then lifted, exposing the region of the cornea to be ablated. With surface ablation, the epithelium is removed and the excimer laser is applied to the corneal surface (**B**). There are several methods of epithelium removal. For LASEK surgery, the trephine is centered and pressed onto the corneal epithelium, and diluted alcohol is applied to loosen the epithelium. The thin flap of loosened epithelium is detached before an excimer laser reshapes the cornea to correct refractive errors (**B-1**). With photorefractive keratectomy (PRK), a blunt blade is used to scrape the epithelium (**B-2**). An Amoils brush can also be used to assist epithelium removal (**B-3**). With transepithelial PRK, a laser profile of a PTK and laser treatment for refractive correction are performed in one step (**B-4**). Part 2: Small-incision lenticule extraction (SMILE) eliminates the same tissue that is eliminated by excimer laser ablation through a smaller corneal incision and without creating a flap. With SMILE, a 2- to 2.5-mm incision is generated using a femtosecond laser for lenticule extraction (**C**). A femtosecond laser creates the intrastromal lenticule within the cornea, as well as a small incision at the side (**C1**). A round-tip spatula is inserted through the incision to dissect the disc-shaped lenticule beneath the cap without touching the corneal surface (**C2**). The dissected lenticule is pulled out through the incision (**C3**). (From Kim TI, Alió Del Barrio JL, Wilkins M, Cochener B, Ang M. Refractive surgery. *Lancet*. 2019;393 [10185]:2085–2098.) (A and B, Reprinted with permission from Elsevier. The Lancet, 2019 May 18;393[10185]:2085–2098.).

microscope shows that the highest area of the light scatter occurs where differences in the indices of refraction are high, such as at the air-tear film interface of the epithelium.[47] Within the corneal stroma, light scatter predominantly comes from the stroma-plasma membrane interface of nerve cells and the cytoplasm-nuclear interface of keratocytes. With corneal edema or corneal scarring, loss of corneal transparency has been found to be primarily due to changes in the light-scattering characteristics of keratocytes rather than alterations in the extracellular matrix.[47] In these conditions, keratocytes scatter considerably more light than normal corneas, particularly their cell bodies and dendritic processes (Box 4.1).

Collagen. Collagen is a structural protein organized into a relatively inextensible scaffold of water-insoluble fibrils that form the basic structural framework of a connective tissue. The corneal collagens are functionally important in establishing tissue transparency and in resisting tensile loads, ultimately defining the size and shape of the tissue. Collagen molecules measure 1.5 nm in width by 300 nm in length and are composed of a triple helix of three alpha chains.[49] Of the 28 different types of collagen, currently 13 are known to occur in the human cornea.[50,51] Upon secretion from the cell, the propeptide form of the collagen molecule is cleaved and the monomer of the collagen molecule is assembled into fibril-forming, nonfibril-forming, or fibril-associated collagens with interrupted terminals (FACIT) in a surface recess on the keratocyte or, sometimes, begins assembly inside the cell.

The most common collagen molecule in the cornea is type I (58%), which usually aggregates into structural, banded fibrils (Fig. 4.6B), as seen on transmission electron microscopy, by ordering into a quarter-staggered parallel arrangement that is further stabilized in position by covalent intramolecular and head-to-tail intermolecular immature divalent crosslinks in a posttranslational enzymatic step using lysyl oxidase (Fig. 4.6A and 4.6C1–3).[51] With increasing maturity, a spontaneous conversion to mature crosslinks occurs in which intramolecular, intermolecular, and interfibrillar mature trivalent crosslinks replace the immature divalent ones resulting in corneal collagen fibrils with improved mechanical properties (Fig. 4.6C, middle diagram). Both immature and mature crosslinks occur between lysine and hydroxylysine side-chains.[51] After maturation, the turnover or half-life of collagen molecules and fibrils becomes very slow; the concentration of mature crosslinks, however, remains stable, whereas high levels of random intramolecular, intermolecular, and interfibrillar nonenzymatic

glycation crosslinks accumulate, predominantly between lysine and arginine residues (Fig. 4.6C, bottom diagram).[51] These nonenzymatic age- or diabetes-related glycation crosslinks initially enhance the mechanical properties of fibrils, resulting in stiffer, stronger, and tougher fibrils than normal, but occasionally they can go too far, making the tissue too brittle or inextensible to function normally. Type I fibrils are generally heterotypic (type I and type V [15%] collagen molecules) as they are composed of two or more types of collagen molecules (Fig. 4.6B). This may serve as a fine-tuning mechanism for controlling a fibril's structural characteristics, such as fibril size and interfibrillar connectivity.

Type I fibrils usually reach certain specific diameters based on their composition and ratio of heterotypic collagen molecular types. They are restricted from further lateral accretion or growth and are permitted to fuse and grow axially due to interactions with small leucine-rich proteoglycans covalently bound to their external surface. Through surface interactions, they connect to various other fibril-forming, nonfibril-forming, or FACIT collagens, which overall link different levels of structural organization (Fig. 4.6). Thus, the surface properties of type I fibrils are a major determinant of intrafibrillar and interfibrillar biomechanical properties of the tissue. The other major determinants are the direction of the fibrils and the suprafibrillar architectures of the tissue, which overall define the hierarchical structure of the tissue. They typically form uniform 25-nm diameter fibrils in the stroma proper with only slight variability. (Note: the diameters used in this chapter are based on transmission electron microscopic [TEM] data; x-ray scattering of ex vivo unprocessed human tissue suggests that a 24% to 36% shrinkage artifact occurs by fixing and processing tissue for TEM studies.)[52,53] Bowman's layer is the main exception as it has uniform 22-nm diameter type I fibrils, which are epithelial in origin as opposed to keratocyte in origin. The diameter of type I fibrils remains constant across most of the central cornea (mean: 25 ± 2 nm; range: 18–32 nm), but then gradually thickens another 4 nm at about 5.5 mm from the center of the cornea, eventually increasing to up to 50 nm at the limbus.[54] Similarly, interfibrillar spacing between nearest neighbor type I fibrils remains constant in the central cornea (mean: 20 ± 5 nm; range: 5–35 nm), then gradually increases another 5 nm at about 4.5 to 5 mm from the center of the cornea before increasing even more rapidly up to the limbus.[54] Type I fibril diameters and interfibrillar spaces do not seem to vary significantly with depth in the cornea.[54] Although the refractive index of type I fibrils (1.47) is different from that of the extrafibrillar matrix (1.35), the highly uniform small size and highly uniform small interfibrillar spaces, along with the predominantly parallel directionality of these fibrils, results in a highly ordered lattice-like arrangement. This arrangement is not a true crystalline lattice, but more of a short-range order that allows transparency of the cornea owing to destructive interference (Fig. 4.7).

Type VI collagen (24%) is the second most common type of collagen in the corneal stroma. It is present in an unusually high amount compared with most other connective tissues in the body, but it is also unique in that it is only able to aggregate into repeating tetramers of type VI molecules that are stabilized by disulfide crosslinks (Fig. 4.8A).[55,56] Thus, it forms 10- to 15-nm diameter nonbanded filaments with 20- to 30-nm diameter beaded ovals having a periodicity of 100 nm. Functionally, type VI filaments act as a bridging structure in the interlamellar space, as they bind corneal lamellae together diffusely throughout the stroma where they directly cross one another (Fig. 4.8B,C). Along with type XII and XIV FACIT collagens, type VI collagen may bridge fibrils together in the interfibrillar space (Fig. 4.8D).[56] Overall, this suprafibrillar architecture results in a one-dimensionally ordered Bowman's layer and a three-dimensionally ordered stroma proper.[57–59]

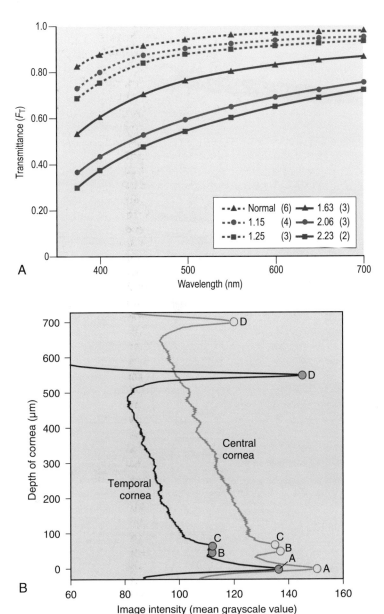

Fig. 4.6 (**A**) Experimental values for the percentage of light transmitted through normal and edematous rabbit corneas as a function of wavelength. The ratio of the thickness of the edematous corneas to normal thickness values and the number of corneas used for each curve are given in the key. (From Farrell RA, McCally RL, Tatham PER. Wave-length dependencies of light scattering in normal and cold swollen rabbit corneas and their structural implications*. *J Physiol.* 1973;233:589–612. https://doi.org/10.1113/jphysiol.1973.sp010325.) (**B**) In vivo confocal microscopy back-scattered light intensity profile from the central and temporal portions of a 25-year-old normal, healthy human cornea. Intensity peaks correspond to the (**A**) epithelium, (**B**) sub-basal nerve plexus, (**C**) most anterior keratocyte layer, and (**D**) endothelium. (Data from Patel SV, McLaren JW, Hodge DO, Bourne WM. Normal human keratocyte density and corneal thickness measurement by using confocal microscopy in vivo. *Invest Ophthalmol Vis Sci.* 2001;42(2):333–339.)

Although difficult to count precisely, the central corneal stroma reportedly consists of approximately 300 corneal lamellae, while the peripheral cornea consists of approximately 500.[57] Although most corneal stromal lamellae extend from limbus to limbus and cross adjacent lamellae at various angles, randomly in the anterior stroma and nearly orthogonal to one another in the posterior two-thirds, various regional differences in lamellar size, directionality, and amount of interweaving are also found (Figs. 4.9 and 4.10). The anterior third of the stroma proper has thinner (0.2- to 1.2-μm thick), narrower (0.5- to 30-μm wide), and mostly obliquely oriented lamellae (mean 18 ± 11 degrees [range 0–36 degrees]) with extensive vertical and horizontal interweaving (Fig. 4.9A). The posterior two-thirds has thicker (1- to 2.5-μm thick), wider (100- to 200-μm wide), and mostly parallel-oriented lamellae (mean 1 ± 2 degrees [range 0–5 degrees]) with only slight horizontal interweaving (Figs. 4.9B and 4.10B,C).[60] In the most superficial layers of the stroma, the interwoven lamellae actually attach or possibly seem to originate from the posterior surface of Bowman's layer in a polygonal fashion, creating an anterior corneal mosaic pattern

(Fig. 4.9A, inset) that can be seen on the anterior corneal surface under certain circumstances. The attached fibrils to Bowman's layer seem to be homologous to sutural fibers in the shark cornea and embryologically may be remnants of the primary acellular stroma. Those attaching or originating fibril bundles are usually oriented obliquely to Bowman's layer, but are sometimes noted to be almost perpendicular to it.[61] Finally, excepting those fibrils and lamellae in the anterior-most region of the stroma that attach to Bowman's layer, the remaining type I fibrils and corneal lamellae stretch across the cornea from limbus to limbus in a belt-like fashion, where they turn and form a circumferential annulus approximately 1.0- to 2.5-mm wide around the cornea. This annulus is thought to maintain the curvature of the cornea, while blending with limbal collagen fibrils.[62,63]

Keratocytes. Keratocytes make up the second major component of the corneal stroma's dry weight. They are sandwiched between collagenous lamellae, forming a closed, highly organized syncytium. They function as modified fibroblasts during neonatal life, forming most of the extracellular matrix of the stroma. Subsequently, they

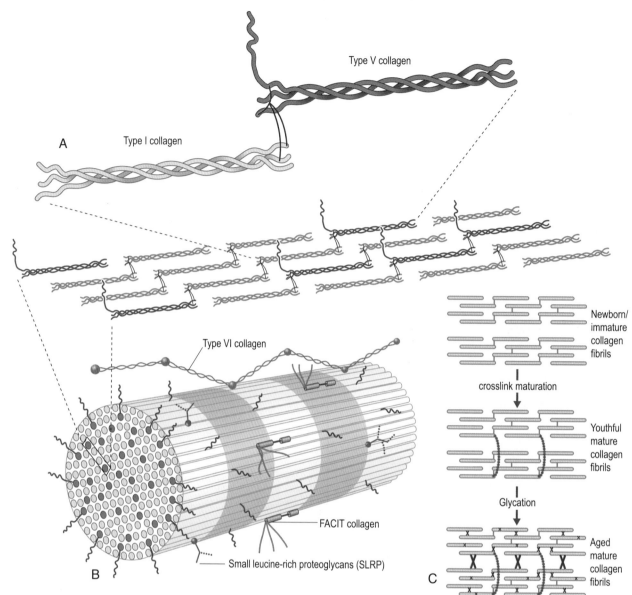

Fig. 4.7 (A,B) Cross-sectional oblique view of a 25-nm diameter, heterotypic, banded (periodicity = 65nm) corneal stromal collagen fibril composed of type I (*white*) and V (*blue*) collagen molecules (*bottom*). The amino-terminal domains on the type V collagen molecules appear to be important in regulating collagen fibril diameter as they project externally to the fibril surface and presumably block further accretion of collagen molecules through steric and/or electrostatic hindrance effects. The collagen molecules on longitudinal view are aligned in a parallel, quarter-staggered (68-nm) arrangement with 40-nm gaps between molecules (*middle*). The longitudinal view also clearly shows that the ends of the alpha chains in each collagen molecule form intermolecular crosslinks with adjacent collagen molecules, as well as intramolecular crosslinks (*top*). (**C**) With maturity, these immature divalent crosslinks become mature trivalent crosslinks with the addition of interfibrillar crosslink branches. Finally, with aging, intramolecular, intermolecular, and interfibrillar nonenzymatic glycation crosslinks form.

remain in the cellular stroma throughout life as modified fibrocytes, where they maintain the extracellular matrix of the corneal stroma. Keratocytes can become metabolically activated or fibroblastic again if the corneal stroma is wounded. The adult human corneal stroma has approximately 2.4 million keratocytes communicating with each other through gap junctions present on their long dendritic processes (Figs. 4.11A).[64,65] In adulthood, keratocytes occupy 10% of the stromal volume, decreasing from 20% in infancy, and on two-dimensional cross-sectional views appear to be sparse, flattened, and quiescent (scant intracytoplasmic organelles) cells lying between corneal lamella (Fig. 4.11B).[66] In actuality, keratocytes are three-dimensional stellate-shaped cells composed of a 15- to 20-μm diameter cell body with numerous dendritic processes that extend up to 50μm from the cell body. Tangential sections of the normal cornea suggest that these cells more densely populate the stroma than originally thought and are more metabolically active in the resting state than initially presumed, as in tangential section, an abundance of cytoplasmic organelles are commonly seen (Fig. 4.11C,D).[67]

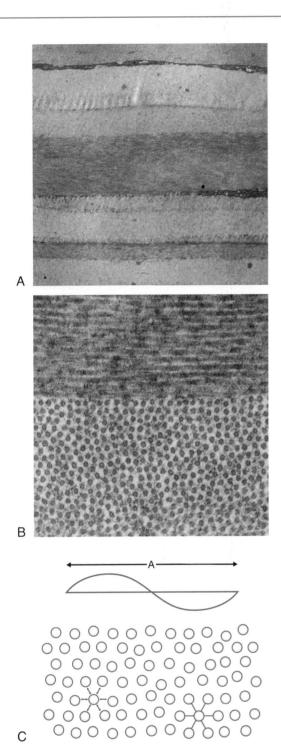

Fig. 4.8 (A) Low-magnification (×4750) transmission electron micrograph (TEM) of predominantly orthogonally stacked lamellae in the middle third of stroma proper. **(B)** Higher magnification (×72,500) TEM of two lamellae in the middle third of stroma proper. One lamella is in longitudinal view (*top portion*) and the other is in cross-sectional view (*bottom portion*). Notice the uniform 25-nm diameter type I collagen fibrils and uniform 20-nm diameter interfibrillar spaces, which demonstrate only a short-range order, but not a true crystalline lattice arrangement. **(C)** Cross-sectional diagram of collagen fibrils arranged in a true crystalline lattice arrangement. Size of a wavelength of light is shown above for comparison. (Maurice DM. The structure and transparency of the cornea. *J Physiol.* 1957;136. https://doi.org/10.1113/jphysiol.1957.sp005758.).

Tangential sections show that the anterior stromal keratocytes contain twice the number of mitochondria as the posterior two-thirds of the stroma, which correlates with the higher oxygen tension of the anterior stroma.[68] It has also been demonstrated that a higher stromal cell density occurs in the anterior stroma than in the mid- or posterior stroma, whereas a higher cell volume-to-extracellular matrix ratio occurs in the posterior stroma compared with the anterior- or midstroma.[67] These views also show that in all levels the keratocytes are highly spatially ordered as they turn in a clockwise direction like a cork-screw. In vivo confocal microscopy of normal human corneas has shown stromal cell densities averaging around 20,000 keratocytes/mm³, with a focal zone of increased cell density directly under Bowman's layer, averaging 35,000 keratocytes/mm³ in the anterior-most layer that gradually tapers to 20,000 keratocytes/mm³ over the initial 60 to 100 μm in depth. Confocal microscopy has also shown that stromal cell density decreases with age at a rate of approximately 0.5% per year of life with the anterior stroma declining 0.9% per year, midstroma 0.3% per year, and posterior stroma 0.3% per year.

Studies using immunohistochemistry or electron microscopy suggest that not all the cells in the corneal stroma are actually keratocytes, but some are one of three types of bone marrow-derived immune cells: "professional" dendritic cells, "nonprofessional" dendritic cells, and histiocytes.[67,69,70] Recent studies also found evidence of a small resident subpopulation of adult stromal stem cells, also known as keratocyte progenitor cells/corneal stromal stem cells, primarily in the periphery of the corneal stroma near the limbus.[71,72] The immune cells appear to play a pivotal role in the induction of immune tolerance versus immune initiation in cell-mediated immunity, and the stromal histiocytes have a role in innate immunity as phagocytic effector cells. The presence of adult stromal stem cells helps explain how the slow replacement and renewal of keratocytes occurs after injury, surgery (e.g., epikeratophakia or penetrating keratoplasty [PK]), or toxicity to the central corneal stroma (e.g., mitomycin C or refractive surgery)[73] (Box 4.2).

Proteoglycans. Proteoglycans make up the third major component of the corneal stroma's dry weight. They are water-soluble glycoproteins made up of a core protein with a covalently attached anionic polysaccharide side-chain called a glycosaminoglycan (GAG). The core proteins are noncovalently attached to collagen fibrils uniformly throughout the tissue, whereas the GAG side-chains extend into the interfibrillar space where they act as a pressure-exerting polyelectrolyte gel.[74–76] The cornea collapses to approximately 20% of its original volume if the proteoglycans of the corneal stroma are precipitated out with cetylpyridinium.[76] It has become apparent that the primary functions of proteoglycans are to provide tissue volume, maintain spatial order of collagen fibrils, resist compressive forces, and give viscoelastic properties to the tissue, as well as having a secondary role in regulating collagen fibril assembly.[74] Corneal proteoglycans were previously referred to as extrafibrillar amorphous ground substance, as their water-soluble state made it difficult to fully delineate them with light and electron microscopy (Fig. 4.12A). It was not until an electron-dense cationic dye called cupromeronic blue and a critical electrolyte concentration of 0.1 M $MgCl_2$ were used in combination to specifically stain for the sulfate-ester groups on corneal proteoglycans that the shape, size, arrangement, and location of this material were observed with light and electron microscopy (Fig. 4.12B).[77]

Since that discovery, it has become apparent that corneal proteoglycans are not amorphous, but rather tadpole-shaped molecules

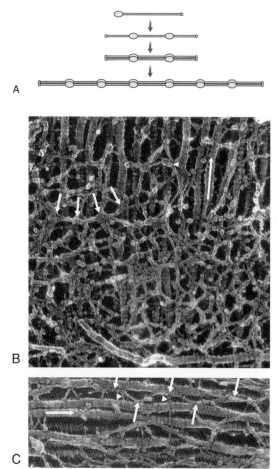

Fig. 4.9 (**A**) Diagram of a type VI collagen molecule showing how it assembles into filaments by aggregating into repeating tetramers of type VI molecules with a periodicity of 100 nm. (**B**) High-magnification (×115,000) quick-freeze, deep-etched electron micrograph showing a loose meshwork of interlamellar beaded (type VI) filaments with a periodicity of 100 nm (*thick arrows*) that appear to bind to collagen fibrils (*long arrow*) by their beads (*arrowhead*) and bridge fibrils from separate lamellae together. (**C**) Very-high-magnification (×185,000) quick-freeze, deep-etched electron micrograph of intralamellar collagen fibrils (*long arrows*) with beaded (type VI) filaments (*thick arrows*) crisscrossing between fibrils in the interfibrillar space and projecting three finger-like structures (FACIT collagens) (*arrowheads*), which both appear to function in joining neighboring fibrils together. (B and C are from Hirsch M, Prenant G, Renard G. Three-dimensional supramolecular organization of the extracellular matrix in human and rabbit corneal stroma, as revealed by ultrarapid-freezing and deep-etching methods. *Exp Eye Res.* 2001;72(2):123–135. https://doi.org/10.1006/exer.2000.0935.)

composed of a 10- to 15-nm diameter globular core protein with a covalent attached that is 7-nm wide × 45 to 70 nm in length. The GAG side-chain attaches to the covalent. They are arranged in the corneal stroma perpendicular to collagen fibrils with a constant spacing of around 65 nm between each other along the collagen fibrils. Their core proteins noncovalently bind to collagen fibrils in specific gap zones along the peripheral portions of the collagen fibril. The core proteins with dermatan sulfate side-chains bind to "d" and "e" gap zones and those with keratan sulfate side-chains bind to "a" and "c" gap zones.[78] GAGs are highly negatively charged stiff polymers that extend into the interfibrillar space and form antiparallel

duplexes with adjacent GAG side-chains (Fig. 4.12C), thereby linking different next-nearest-neighbor collagen fibrils together by forming dumbbell-like structures. The genes that produce the core proteins have been cloned, and four types of corneal stromal proteoglycan core proteins have been identified: decorin, lumican, keratocan, and mimecan. Decorin contains a single dermatan sulfate GAG side-chain (Fig. 4.12D), whereas lumican and mimecan have a single keratan sulfate GAG side-chain and keratocan has three keratan sulfate GAG side-chains (Fig. 4.12D). Thus, there are four known types of proteoglycan core proteins and only two types of GAGs, keratan sulfate (60%) and dermatan sulfate (40%), found in the human corneal stroma. GAGs are polymers of repeating disaccharide units of galactose and N-acetylglucosamine or iduronic acid and N-acetylgalactosamine, respectively.[78]

Because the core protein tail and their associated GAG side-chains are post-translationally added to core proteins in the Golgi apparatus, there seems to be some flexibility in how long or how sulfated they can become depending on the function of the connective tissue producing them. The human cornea is unique in that the core protein tail and its associated GAG side-chains are fibril-associated and small in length (keratan sulfate ~45 nm and dermatan sulfate ~70 nm), with a higher amount over-sulfated compared with other connective tissues. A comparative study of corneas from 12 mammalian species suggests that dermatan sulfate is the preferred proteoglycan in oxygen-rich environments, such as in the thin cornea of mice, or is seen predominantly in the anterior portion of the thicker cornea of mammals, such as humans or rabbits. Keratan sulfate is a functional substitute produced through an alternate metabolic pathway in thicker corneas, especially in the posterior portion where oxygen levels may drop precipitously.[79] Functionally, this duality is quite useful because dermatan sulfate appears to be more efficient at holding water; it absorbs less water than keratan sulfate, but holds most of it in a tightly bound, non-freezable state.[80] This is consistent with the fact that dermatan sulfate is more abundant in the anterior corneal stroma in humans, which is the region of highest oxygen tension and most affected by evaporation. In contrast, keratan sulfate is more abundant in the posterior corneal stroma (Fig. 4.13). This is the region of lowest oxygen tension, least affected by evaporation, and the area where the need for loosely bound water is required for transport across the endothelium via the metabolic pumps.

Corneal nerves. The epithelium of the cornea is the most richly innervated tissue of the body with about 16,000 nerve terminals/mm² (~2.2 million nerve endings), about 300 to 400 times more dense than skin.[81–83] Most of the nerve fibers in the cornea are sensory in origin, responding to mechanical, chemical, and temperature stimuli, and are derived from the ophthalmic branch of the trigeminal nerve (CN III₁) (Fig. 4.14A).[84] Refer to Chapter 16 (Sensory Innervation of the Eye) for full details of the innervation pathway of the cornea. Although all mammalian species receive variable proportions of nerve fibers in the cornea from the sympathetic and parasympathetic autonomic nervous system, human corneas appear to be on the extreme end of this spectrum as their corneas have a very small proportion of their nerve fibers derived from the autonomic nervous system.[84]

Electrophysiological studies have shown that the cornea's receptive nerve field is composed primarily of polymodal nociceptors (70%) followed by mechanonociceptors (20%) and then cold-sensitive nociceptors (10%).[85] Using in vivo laser confocal microscopes, one can only evaluate morphologically the corneal nerves from the main nerve trunks up to sub-basal plexus (SBP) as the resolution and contrast of these images is not capable of visualizing the final nerve branches and free nerve terminals in the corneal epithelium.[86]

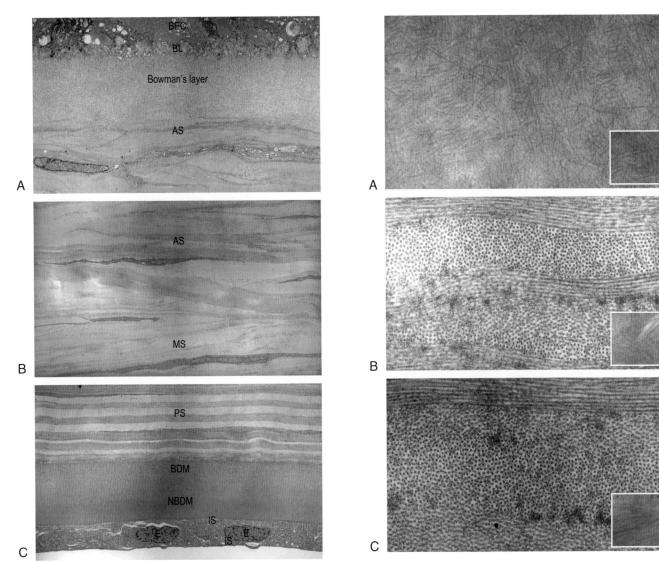

Fig. 4.10 (**A**) The acellular Bowman's layer and anterior-most portion of the stroma proper are shown. The type I fibrils and interweaving lamellae in this region branch extensively and some insert into the posterior surface of the Bowman's layer. This arrangement causes an anterior corneal mosaic pattern to occur on the anterior corneal surface after applying digital pressure through the eyelid and instilling fluorescein. (**B**) The anterior third of the stroma proper has predominantly oblique lamellar orientation and extensive vertical lamellar branching and interweaving. (**C**) The posterior third of the stroma proper along with Descemet's membrane and endothelium is shown. The parallel-oriented, orthogonal arrangement of lamellae in this region of corneal stroma is clearly apparent. Although some collagen fibrils randomly insert into Descemet's membrane, no interweaving or significant attachment occurs in this region of the cornea. (TEM ×4750.) *AS*, Anterior stroma; *BDM*, banded portion of Descemet's membrane; *BEC*, basal epithelial cells; *BL*, basal lamina; *E*, endothelial cells; *IS*, intercellular space of the endothelium; *MS*, midstroma; *PS*, posterior stroma; *NBDM*, nonbanded portion of Descemet's membrane; *TEM*, transmission electron micrograph.

Fig. 4.11 (**A**) The acellular Bowman's layer in cross-section (*main photo*) and tangential section (*inset*). Notice the random directionality of the 22-nm diameter collagen fibrils in Bowman's layer. (**B**) The transition zone between the anterior third and mid-third of the stroma proper in cross-section (*main photomicrograph*) and tangential section (*inset*). The thin and more obliquely oriented lamellae in this region of the corneal stroma and its lattice-like arrangement of 25-nm diameter type I collagen fibrils are shown. (**C**) The posterior third of the stroma proper in cross-section (*main photomicrograph*) and tangential section (*inset*). The thick and parallel-oriented lamellae in this region of the cornea stroma and its lattice-like arrangement of 25-nm diameter collagen fibrils are shown. Compare the orthogonal nature of crossing lamellae (*inset*) to that in the inset B. (TEM ×72,500.). *TEM*, transmission electron micrograph.

Because corneal nerve fibers ultimately terminate in the brainstem, it appears that interneuron intermediate pathways must relay the information to the sensation areas of cerebrum. Additionally, there must be intermediate relays to efferent systems that trigger the reflex pathways of involuntary blinking via orbicularis motor innervation from CN VII and reflex tearing via parasympathetic innervation of lacrimal gland.

The intricate central nervous system (CNS) details of these specific pathways are currently unknown.

Corneal sensitivity is a valuable clinical measure of corneal health, as corneal nerves directly maintain the health of corneal epithelium through direct trophic factors. Corneal sensitivity also serves a protective role in warning the host of possible dangers to the normal healthy state

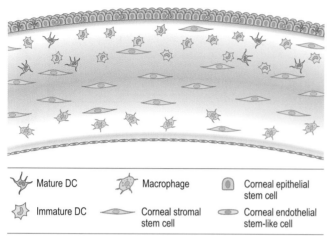

Mature DC

Immature DC

Macrophage

Corneal stromal
stem cell

Corneal epithelial
stem cell

Corneal endothelial
stem-like cell

Fig. 4.12 The mouse cornea suggests that 5% to 10% of the cells in the cellular corneal stroma are actually one of three types of bone marrow-derived immune cells. The anterior-third of the cellular corneal stroma contains professional (major histocompatibility complex [MHC]-positive) dendritic antigen-presenting cells in periphery of the cornea, while nonprofessional (MHC-negative) dendritic cells are present in both the periphery and center of the anterior cornea. The posterior-most regions of the cellular corneal stroma appear to contain macrophages in the periphery and center of the cornea. (Modified from Hamrah P, Liu Y, Zhang Q, Dana MR. The corneal stroma is endowed with a significant number of resident dendritic cells. *Invest Ophthalmol Vis Sci.* 2003;44(2):581–589. https://doi.org/10.1167/iovs.02-0838.).

and in maintaining an adequate basal tear secretion rate.[87] It is usually tested clinically in a semiquantitative fashion with a Cochet and Bonnet esthesiometer, which is a thin (0.12-mm diameter) flexible nylon filament of variable length (0–6 cm).[87–89] When the filament is long, it applies very little pressure to the corneal surface because it bends easily, whereas when short it applies a proportionally higher pressure before bending. The length is converted into pressure using a conversion table with a range of touch pressures between 11 and 200 mg/mm². Corneal sensitivity is defined as the reciprocal of corneal touch threshold. It can be evaluated subjectively by asking patients when they feel touch upon the cornea, or objectively when a reflexive blink response is triggered. Refer to Chapter 16 for full details on the subjective and objective threshold in normal healthy corneas and those with disease or after surgery.

Corneal sensation also variably decreases with corneal disease (e.g., herpes simplex keratitis, diabetes, corneal dystrophies, keratoconus); following surgical procedures on the anterior segment of the eye and sometimes the posterior segment (e.g., panretinal photocoagulation); after application of certain topical medications (e.g., anesthetics, nonsteroidal anti-inflammatory drugs); and even after contact lens wear.[90,91] As nerve regeneration occurs at the rate of approximately 1 mm per month, it may take up to 3 to 12 months or longer for corneal reinnervation and sensation to maximally recover, depending on the type and degree of surgical injury.[87] After maximal recovery, the sensitivity in the portion of the cornea involved by the procedure often is less than that present prior to surgery, which means there is a potential for neurotrophic keratitis.[73]

It has been discovered recently that after corneal nerve injury, microneuromas can develop during the regeneration process.[92] These microneuromas, as well as injured corneal nerves themselves, exhibit

altered functional properties where responsiveness to normal stimuli is impaired, yet paradoxically display abnormal intrinsic electrical excitability (i.e., spontaneous impulses or even abnormal responsiveness to normally minimal stimuli).[92] Overall, this may produce hyperalgesia and/or dysesthesia, which may continue long term after surgery despite some attenuation. These neuropathic pain impulses are often perceived by the patient as dryness, foreign body sensation, and irritation after surgery, yet are not due to actual dryness or irritation of the cornea. These undesired, unpleasant sensations may best respond to ion channel antagonists rather than dry eye lubricating medications.[92]

The mechanisms by which corneal nerves maintain the ocular surface and promote healing after eye injuries are currently under active research in several laboratories. Corneal nerves secrete neuropeptides, such as substance P and calcitonin gene-related protein, and neurotransmitters, such as acetylcholine, vasoactive intestinal polypeptide, and neurotensin, which are believed to be important in corneal epithelial function and proliferation.[84,93]

Corneal stromal wound healing. The first published report specifically addressing the cellular reactions in the corneal stroma after injury appeared in 1958.[94] It described the morphologic changes of stromal cells after different types of trauma and found that stromal cells lose their interconnecting dendritic processes immediately after injury, with many cells subsequently developing signs of degeneration. That report also described the appearance of morphologically unique, spindle-shaped corneal fibroblastic cells invading into the wound region during later stages of stromal healing. Since that time, many excellent animal-model studies of corneal wound healing have further addressed the changes in the extracellular matrix and the stromal cells after stromal injury.[95–101] They suggest that corneal stromal injury is immediately followed by keratocyte apoptosis in the zone around the site of stromal injury, with a subsequent influx of transient mixed acute and chronic inflammatory cells; proliferation and migration of surviving keratocytes; and, finally, differentiation of the keratocytes into transiently metabolically activated cell types called activated keratocytes. This latter cell type is functionally important because it synthesizes and deposits the extracellular matrix of the stromal scar, while also degrading and remodeling the damaged cellular and extracellular tissues around the wound. Epithelial injury alone can also cause transient cellular injury to the underlying stroma, presumably from exposure of stroma to tear-related factors, resulting in apoptosis, proliferation, and differentiation into migratory keratocytes, as well as resulting in some anterior stromal edema.[102–104] However, it does not appear to cause differentiation into activated keratocytes, hypercellularity, differentiation into myofibroblasts, or the stimulation of extracellular matrix production—all of which are seen with corneal stromal injury, whether by incision or excision.[102–104] Myofibroblasts are characterized by the intracellular cytoplasmic appearance of α-smooth muscle actin, which helps impart contractile properties to the cell.[104]

A number of studies have looked into the expression of cytokines and growth factors in normal and injured corneas.[105,106] These studies tried to assess the relative importance of each specific factor in cornea wound healing, as it was known clinically and experimentally that epithelial-stromal interactions increase the number of proliferative and migratory keratocytes within the stromal wound compared with deeper corneal stromal injury, some of which differentiated beyond the activated keratocyte stage into myofibroblasts.[107–110] Some studies focused even more specifically on strictly epithelial or tear-related cytokines or growth factors, as the epithelium and aqueous tears were found to be a major source of cytokines and growth factors.[111–115] The major cytokines and growth factors studied to date include epithelial growth factor (EGF), fibroblast growth factor (FGF), interleukin-1, nerve growth factor (NGF), transforming growth factor beta (TGF-β),

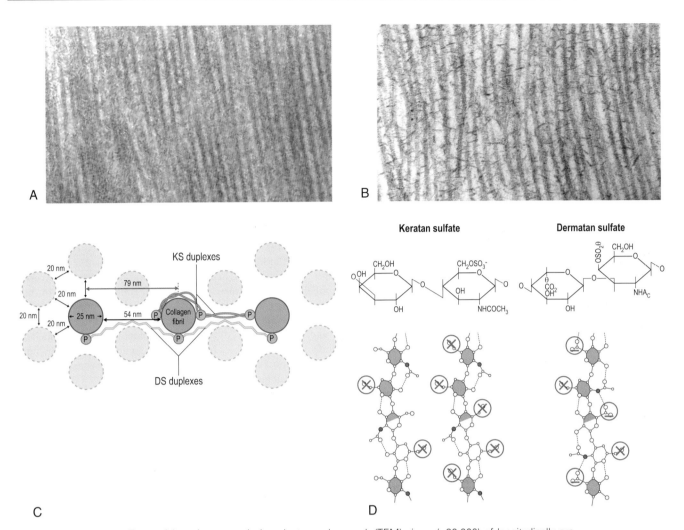

Fig. 4.13 Tangential-section transmission electron micrograph (TEM) views (×90,000) of longitudinally running type I corneal stromal collagen fibrils in a lamellae without (**A**) and with (**B**) cupromeronic blue staining. Notice the scattered "amorphous ground substance" in the interfibrillar spaces in (**A**), while in (**B**) duplexes of proteoglycans are clearly seen bridging next-nearest neighbor collagen fibrils. (**C**) Diagram of how proteoglycans attach along the periphery of type I fibrils via their core proteins (P) and how the core protein tail/glycosaminoglycans (GAGs) duplex in an antiparallel fashion in the interfibrillar space between next-nearest neighbor collagen fibrils. (**D**) Diagram of the polymer backbones of keratan sulfate and dermatan sulfate. The top portion shows the primary structure of the repeating disaccharide units of keratan sulfate (KS; *top left*) and dermatan sulfate (DS; *top right*). The bottom portion of the diagram shows the secondary structures of each proteoglycan. In the human cornea, around 50% of KS is in the normal-sulfated state (*left*), while the other roughly 50% is in the over-sulfated state (*center*). All three displayed proteoglycan polymers have similar backbones and, therefore, form similar secondary structures of a twofold helix (*right*). Anionic charges = sulfate esters (X) and carboxylic acid (−). (**C** and **D**, modified from Scott JE. Proteoglycan: collagen interactions and corneal ultrastructure. *Biochem Soc Trans.* 1991;19(4):877–881. https://doi.org/10.1042/bst0190877.)

insulin, retinol, and Lysophosphatidic acid (LPA). TGF-β is currently thought to be the most important growth factor of this group with regard to stimulating a fibrotic reparative stromal scar phenotype.[115,116] A recent study, however, has shown that local cytokine and growth factor-related influence on normal corneal stromal wound repair is predominantly an early wound-healing phenomenon, as cell-matrix interactions seem to take over in the later stages of wound healing.[116] For example, integrity or return of a complete epithelial cell basement membrane after stromal injury seems to regulate epithelial-stromal interactions long term, as it decreases the production and, more importantly, the release of TGF-β from epithelial cells into the stroma.[115] One gap in this area of research is how mechanotransduction pathways (mechanical load-induced intracellular signals) fit into this scheme,

particularly in maintaining myofibroblast differentiation long term and thus corneal haze. Other cytokines and growth factors of this group were also found to have some minor complementary or even competing roles with TGF-β, and in other cases they had no role at all in corneal wound healing. For example, NGF is complementary to TGF-β, as it too is known to stimulate myofibroblastic cellular transformation independent of TGF-β, but it does so without enhancing keratocyte proliferation or extracellular matrix deposition.[114] In another example, all-*trans* retinol (vitamin A), which is reflexively secreted in the aqueous tears from its storage location in the lacrimal gland, has a completely different role than wound healing, as it maintains the moist, mucosal ocular surface phenotype via gene transcription regulation; thus, it ultimately controls the rate of ocular surface cell proliferation

The principle of using contact lenses to correct refractive errors is that one essentially replaces the powerful anterior corneal refractive surface to that of the anterior contact lens surface (Fig. 4.4A, *right top diagram*). Upon application of a contact lens, the cornea's anterior surface is rendered ineffective as it is bathed with aqueous tears and the air-contact lens interface now becomes the predominate refractive surface of the eye.[314] Soft contact lenses are typically used to treat spherical and regular astigmatism and rarely cause any permanent pathologic changes or alterations to the cornea unless there is a complication, such as corneal infection, infiltrate, or toxic conjunctivitis.

The prevalence of complications in contact lens wearers is currently about 5% per year of wear.[314] Soft contact lenses, however, have been noted to cause some acute physiologic changes to the cornea, including epithelial thinning, hypoesthesia, superficial punctate keratitis, epithelial abrasions, stromal edema, and endothelial blebs. They also cause chronic changes including corneal vascularization, stromal thinning, corneal shape alterations, and endothelial cell polymegathism and pleomorphism (signs of endothelial cell stress).[314] These are all thought to result from the contact lens-induced hypoxia and/or hypercapnia of the tissue.

Most of these physiologic alterations, particularly the chronic ones, are markedly less common now with the introduction of daily-wear high oxygen transmissibility lenses, such as silicone hydrogel contact lenses. In contrast, hard contact lenses treat spherical, regular astigmatism, and even some cases of irregular astigmatism. Hard contact lenses cause the same acute and chronic physiologic changes to cornea as soft contact lenses, although they do more commonly cause corneal shape alterations to occur because they induce more mechanical pressure on the anterior corneal surface. In fact, this is the basis for the practice of deliberately fitting tight, overly flat rigid gas-permeable contact lenses with the aim of flattening the central cornea to reduce myopia in a technique known as orthokeratology.[315] The fitting of contact lenses is highly empirical. Considerable trial and error can be involved in adjusting variables such as contact lens material, size, curvature, and other patient-related factors that are used to arrive at an appropriate correction and comfort level for each individual contact lens wearer.

and differentiation (i.e., prevents keratinization and squamous metaplasia).[117,118] Once activated, keratocytes exhibit a wide range of cellular responses, including increased tritiated thymidine uptake (indicating increased proliferation); initiation of protease and collagenase activity; phagocytosis; interferon, prostaglandin, and complement factor 1 production; and fibronectin, collagen, and proteoglycan secretion.[90,119–121]

Human studies of stromal wound healing concur with animal studies on most issues, with the following notable differences: adult human corneas heal less aggressively, more slowly, and not as completely as animal corneas.[91,122,123] However, both animal and human studies show that corneal stromal wounds heal in two distinct phases: (1) an active phase, which results in the production of a stromal scar over the first 6 months after injury in humans, and (2) a remodeling phase, which improves corneal transparency and increases wound strength. This second phase occurs up to 3 to 4 years after injury in humans. Overall, the long-term result in human corneas is the production of a hypercellular fibrotic stromal scar in wound regions where epithelial-stromal interactions occur and a hypocellular primitive stromal scar in wound regions where keratocyte injury pathways occur. These two histologic wound types have functional differences, as the hypercellular fibrotic stromal scar is strong, but can look clinically hazy because of myofibroblastic cells populating this scar type.[99] In contrast, the hypocellular primitive stromal scar is transparent, but it is very weak in tensile and cohesive strength sand serves as a potential space for fluid, inflammatory cells, and microbes.[124] An additional variable to consider in this

scheme is that more precisely realigned wounds, such as sutured and unsutured wounds with minimal gaping and no epithelial cell plugging, heal better than poorly aligned wounds, such as wounds with wide wound gaping, epithelial plugging, or incarceration of Bowman's layer, Descemet's membrane, or uvea.[124–127]

Barrier properties
Low-permeability barrier: the corneal epithelium

The external surface of the human cornea is covered by a stratified squamous epithelium (see Fig. 4.1D).[1] Unlike other epithelial surfaces, the corneal epithelium is specialized to exist over a moist, transparent, refractive avascular surface, and thus it is smooth and nonkeratinized. The corneal epithelium is composed of 4 to 6 cell layers about 50 μm in total thickness across the entire anterior corneal surface (Fig. 4.16). It is continuous with the epithelium of the limbus (see Fig. 4.3B). The basal epithelial cells actively secrete a basement membrane, around 90-nm thick at birth, composed of type IV collagen fibrils, laminin, heparan sulfate, and fibronectin. The corneal epithelial basement membrane, or basal lamina, increases in thickness with age, measuring around 300-nm thick in late adulthood.[19] By electron microscopy, the basal lamina appears to be composed of two distinct layers: a 20- to 30-nm thick more anterior lamina lucida and a 30- to 60-nm thick more posterior lamina densa. Its function is similar to most basement membranes in that it serves as a scaffold for epithelial cell movement and attachment.

The cytoplasm of all epithelial cells contains mainly cytoskeletal intermediate filaments and has sparse cytoplasmic organelles. This aids in maintaining transparency. The predominant cytoplasmic protein is keratin, and actin filaments and microtubules are the other major ones. The basal cell layer stores large glycogen granules as a source of metabolic energy for times of stress during hypoxia or wound healing. The epithelial cells are held together by desmosomes, while the basal surface of the epithelium adheres to the basal lamina and underlying Bowman's layer through an anchoring complex composed of hemidesmosomes, type VII collagen anchoring fibrils, and anchoring plaques (Fig. 4.17). The epithelial cells differentiate from the basal layer to form one to three midepithelial layers of wing cells and finally to form one to two superficial squamous cell layers (Fig. 4.16). The most superficial squamous cells at the external surface form a high-resistance (8–16 kΩ·cm^2) barrier to the external environment because they are all surrounded by a continuous band of apical zonula occludens tight junctions at their peripheral intercellular margins (Fig. 4.18).[128,129]

Zonula occludens tight junctions are characterized by fusion of the adjacent cell membranes resulting in obliteration of the intercellular space over variable distances, and they are made up of the tight junction proteins ZO-1, JAM-A, occludin, and claudin-1, as well as some other claudin subtypes.[130] This barrier prevents the movement of ions and thus fluid from the tears into the stroma, reduces some evaporation, and protects the cornea from infectious pathogens. A clinical test to determine if this barrier is disrupted uses the vital dye fluorescein, which is topically instilled on the external surface of the cornea and stains the corneal surface if there is a breakdown in the epithelial tight junctions. The apical surface of the corneal epithelium has microplicae and microvilli (Fig. 4.16) that are covered with a wettable, smooth glycocalyx layer, consisting of membrane-associated mucins (Fig. 4.18), MUC1, MUC4, and MUC16.[131–133] These mucins are produced by surface epithelial cells and conjunctival goblet cells forming a 1.0-μm thick mucinous layer of the tear film.[2] The healthy total tear film typically measures 7 μm in thickness and contains three layers: mucinous, aqueous, and lipid (Fig. 4.18B). Recently, the aqueous layer of the tear film has also been found to contain other membrane-spanning, gel-forming mucins, MUC5AC and MUC2, along with lysozyme, immunoglobulin

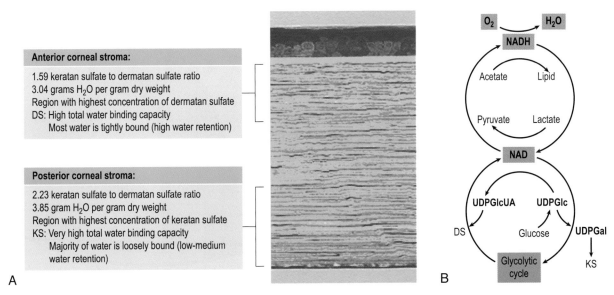

Anterior corneal stroma:

1.59 keratan sulfate to dermatan sulfate ratio
3.04 grams H_2O per gram dry weight
Region with highest concentration of dermatan sulfate
DS: High total water binding capacity
　Most water is tightly bound (high water retention)

Posterior corneal stroma:

2.23 keratan sulfate to dermatan sulfate ratio
3.85 gram H_2O per gram dry weight
Region with highest concentration of keratan sulfate
KS: Very high total water binding capacity
　Majority of water is loosely bound (low-medium
　water retention)

A

B

Fig. 4.14 (**A**) The regional differences in the corneal stroma for the proportion of the two types of corneal gly-cosaminoglycans (GAGs) and the water-absorbing properties in these regions are shown. (**B**) Diagram of the metabolic pathways for dermatan sulfate and keratan sulfate production. The supply of oxygen is the primary factor determining whether dermatan sulfate is made through an aerobic pathway or whether keratan sulfate is made through an anaerobic alternative pathway. (Modified from Scott JE. Oxygen and the connective tissues. *Trends Biochem Sci,* 1992;17(9):340–343. https://doi.org/10.1016/0968-0004(92)90307-U.)

A, transferrin, defensin, and trefoil factor.[98] Overall, the tear film functions in maintaining a healthy ocular surface by preventing evaporation, friction during eye blinking, and ocular infections. It is also of paramount importance in forming a moist, smooth optical surface on the cornea required for clear vision. Deficiencies in the components of tear film potentially can cause ocular surface disease. For example, loss of the lipid layer, which is produced by the meibomian glands, results in the condition of evaporative dry eye disease owing to increased evaporative loss from the anterior corneal surface (from the normal baseline rate of $3\,\mu L/h\ cm^2$ up to a maximum of $40\,\mu L/h\ cm^2$).[134] In another example, loss of the aqueous layer, which is produced by the lacrimal glands, results in the condition of aqueous tear-deficiency dry eye disease. For more information about dry eye disease, including the pathophysiology, classification, diagnosis, and management, see references or refer to Chapter 15.[135–137]

The corneal epithelium is in a state of constant renewal, as the most superficial squamous cells are continuously shed into the tear film. It is estimated that the cell layers of the corneal epithelium turn over every 7 to 10 days. The epithelial surface is maintained by basal epithelial cells, which can usually undergo mitosis once, resulting in two daughter cells that are found anterior to the basal cell layer, which transform into two wing cells and eventually into two squamous cells (Fig. 4.19).[138–140] A delicate balance of shedding followed by proliferation is critical in maintaining a smooth and uniform epithelial surface. The shedding step is induced primarily by friction that occurs from involuntary or voluntary eyelid blinking, which happens on average every 7 seconds, or 6 to 15 times/minute. The signal for basal epithelial cell proliferation probably comes via the gap junctions, especially in the basal cell layer because the basal cells express the gap junction protein connexin 43.[141] In addition to basal epithelial cell mitosis (vertical proliferation), the corneal epithelium is maintained by migration of new basal epithelial cells into the cornea from the limbus (horizontal proliferation). The

cells migrate centripetally at a rate of approximately $120\,\mu m$/week and originate from a subpopulation of proliferative limbal progenitor epithelial cells (Fig. 4.19).[142–144] It appears that the corneal epithelium is maintained by a balance among the processes of limbal cell horizontal proliferation and migration; basal corneal epithelial cell horizontal migration and vertical terminal proliferation; and shedding of superficial squamous corneal epithelial cells.[144,145] This concept has been coined the X, Y, Z hypothesis by Thoft,[146] where X (basal corneal epithelial cell proliferation) + Y (limbal cell proliferation) = Z (epithelial cell loss on the anterior surface from eyelid blinking). When this equilibrium is disrupted, corneal epithelial cell wound healing typically begins. After injury, these processes typically return to equilibrium with a degree of flexibility. For instance, after epithelial and stromal injury, if a stromal deficit occurs (e.g., a healed corneal ulcer) then the epithelium can still maintain a smooth anterior corneal surface by developing elongated hypertrophic basal epithelial cells in mild defects and/or by developing epithelial hyperplasia (> six cell layers) in moderate to severe defects.[147]

The subpopulation of limbal basal progenitor epithelial cells are called adult corneal epithelial stem cells.[148] Epithelial stem cells have the characteristics of being undifferentiated, slow cycling, and extremely long lived with a high proliferative potential. They are an excellent source for corneal epithelial cell reconstruction. In humans, stem cells are located in a well-defined, protective niche microenvironment called the palisades of Vogt (see Fig. 4.3B) and are controlled via delicate regulatory mechanisms.[149–151] The progeny of these epithelial stem cells are referred to as transient amplifying (TA) cells, which are the basal epithelial cells of the limbus or peripheral cornea that migrate centripetally (Fig. 4.19). These TA cells divide more frequently than stem cells and undergo mixed (horizontal or vertical) proliferation. They do, however, have a finite proliferative potential, usually replicating at least twice, which is in marked distinction to the stem cells from which they are derived. Once TA cells reach the end of their proliferative capacity,

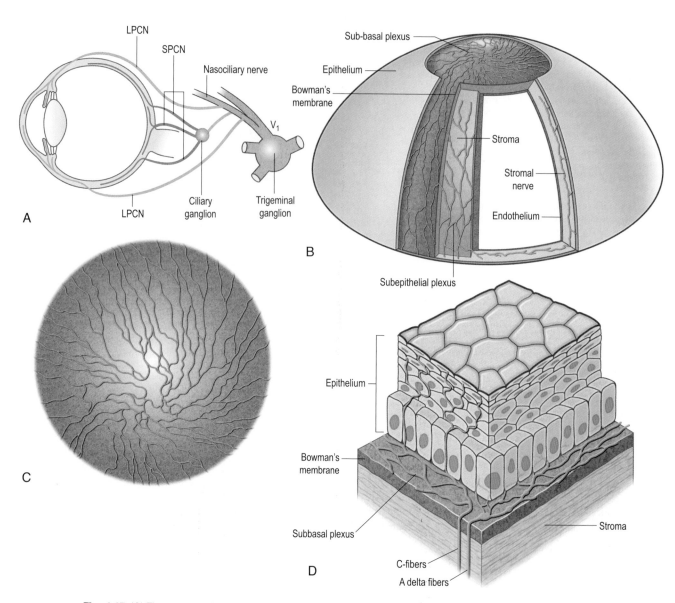

Fig. 4.15 (**A**) The nerves of the cornea and sclera are mixed (motor, sensory, and autonomic) and come from the nasociliary branch of the first division of cranial nerve V, which branch to form two long (LPCN) and several short posterior ciliary nerves (SPCN). The SPCN supply the posterior sclera, whereas the LPCN supply the cornea and equatorial and anterior sclera. The nerve supply of the cornea is the richest in the body and the sclera also has numerous nerves, commonly with many free nerve terminal endings found in the most vascular portions of the episclera, presumably to regulate blood flow in the anterior segment and to influence aqueous humor outflow. (Modified from Watson PG, Hazelman B, Pavesio C, Green WR. *The Sclera and Systemic Disorders*, 2nd ed. Edinburgh, UK: Butterworth Heinemann; 2004.) (**B**) and (**C**) Distribution of corneal nerves in the stroma including the subepithelial plexus (SEP) and the sub-basal plexus (SBP). (**B**, Müller LJ, Marfurt CF, Kruse F, Tervo TMT. Corneal nerves: structure, contents and function. *Exp Eye Res.* 2003;76(5):521–542. https://doi.org/10.1016/S0014-4835(03)00050-2.; **C**, Modified from Patel DV, McGhee CNJ. Mapping of the normal human corneal sub-basal nerve plexus by in vivo laser scanning confocal microscopy. *Invest Ophthalmol Vis Sci.* 2005;46[12]:4485–4488). (**D**) The architecture of the nerve bundles in the SBP (*arrow*) contain both straight and beaded fibers. The straight C fibers branch and turn upwards to extend into the epithelium. (Modified from Guthoff RF, Wienss H, Hahnel C, Wree A. Epithelial innervation of human cornea: A three-dimensional study using confocal laser scanning fluorescence microscopy. *Cornea.* 2005;24(5):608–613. https://doi.org/10.1097/01.ico.0000154384.05614.8f).

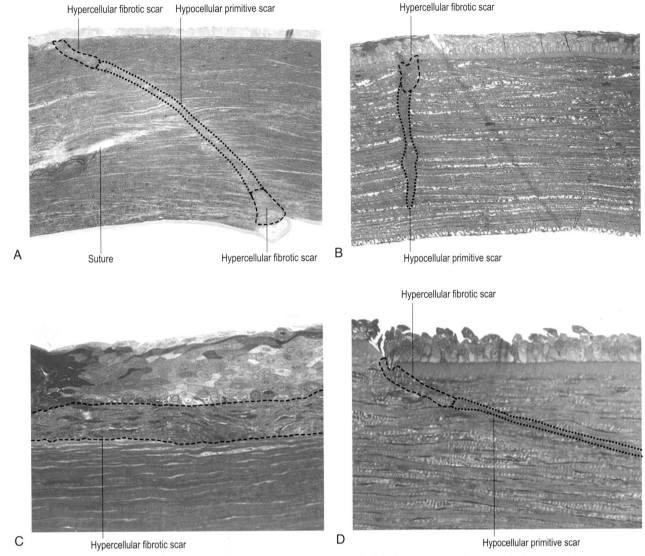

Fig. 4.16 Long-term wound-healing findings of corneas that had undergone sutured, temporal, clear corneal cataract extraction surgery (**A**), astigmatic keratotomy (**B**), photorefractive keratectomy (**C**), and laser in situ keratomileusis (**D**). All corneas shown are greater than 4 years after surgery (toluidine blue ×15 for [**A**], ×25 for [**B**], and ×100 for [**C**] and [**D**]). (Modified Newton RH, Meek KM. Circumcorneal annulus of collagen fibrils in the human limbus. *Invest Ophthalmol Vis Sci.* 1998;39:1125–34.)

usually when near the center of the cornea, they become basal epithelial cells, which terminally differentiate just once into two daughter wing cells (vertical proliferation). Limbal stem cell theory forms the basis for several surgical procedures using transplanted or cultured limbal stem cells to restore vision in patients with limbal stem cell deficiency.[152,153]

Finally, it has been shown in both animal and human specimens that the corneal epithelium is devoid of melanocytes but does contain immune cells. The basal epithelial cell layer of the peripheral cornea along with the limbus and conjunctiva appear to have a subpopulation of cells that are bone marrow-derived immune surveillance cells with high constitutive expression of major histocompatibility complex (MHC) type II antigen and costimulatory molecules.[154] This type of immune cell has previously been termed a Langerhans cell, which functions as a "professional" antigen-presenting cell with an extraordinary capacity to initiate T-cell lymphocyte-dependent responses.[155] The functional steps of this cell type include the uptake and processing of antigens and migration out of the cornea to lymph nodes where they stimulate naïve T-lymphocyte-mediated immune responses by presenting antigens and overexpressing costimulatory molecules. Recently, the central corneal epithelium has also been found to have a similar subpopulation of immune cells that are apparently all "immature" Langerhans cells because their constitutive expression of MHC type II antigen and costimulatory molecules is low.[156] These "immature" Langerhans cells or "nonprofessional" antigen-presenting cells under certain circumstances, such as inflammation or trauma, may develop the requisite signals for T-cell priming.[156]

High-permeability barrier: the corneal endothelium

The primary function of the corneal endothelium is to maintain corneal transparency by regulating corneal hydration and nutrition through a "leaky" barrier and metabolic pump function. The "pump-leak" hypothesis basically suggests that an equilibrium is needed in the amount of passive fluid flow into the cornea and energy expended pumping out excess fluid for maintenance of corneal transparency and

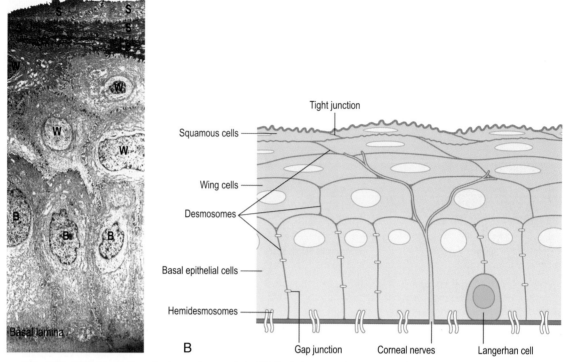

Fig. 4.17 (**A**) Transmission electron micrograph (×3500) of the central corneal epithelium with a summary diagram (**B**). Microvilli project from the anterior corneal surface into the tear film. *B*, Basal epithelial cells; *S*, squamous cells; *W*, wing cells. (**B** modified from Hogan MJ, Alvarado JA, Esperson Weddell J. *Histology of the Human Eye*. Philadelphia: WB Saunders; 1971.)

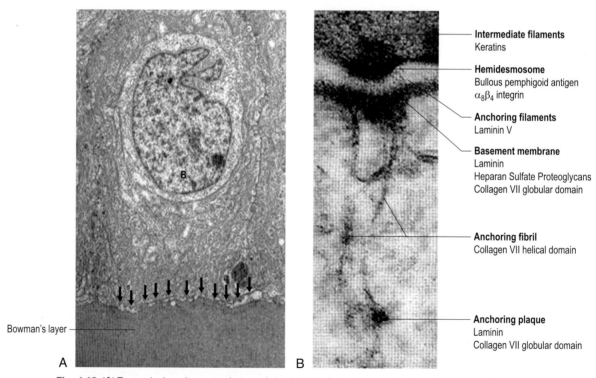

Fig. 4.18 (**A**) Transmission electron micrograph (×10,000) of the basal epithelial cells showing the adhesion complexes (*arrows*) that anchor it in place into the Bowman's layer and a summary diagram (**B**). *B*, Basal epithelial cell. Bar = 1 μm. (B from Gipson I, Joyce N. In: Albert D, Miller J, eds. *Principles and Practice of Ophthalmology*, 3rd ed. Philadelphia: WB Saunders; 2008).

Mucinous layer of the tear film

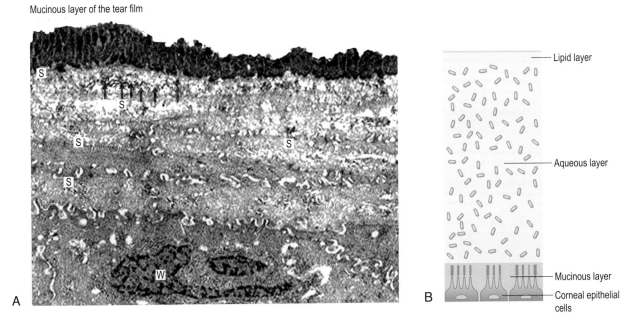

Fig. 4.19 (**A**) Transmission electron micrograph (×10,000) of surface epithelium from a specimen specially preserved in glutaraldehyde and cetylpyridium chloride and specially stained with tannic acid to show the mucinous layer of the tear film (glycocalyx + membrane-bound mucins). (**B**) Summary diagram showing how the tear film layers interact with the microvilli of the surface squamous epithelial cells and mucinous layer. *Arrows* = zonula occludens tight junctions. *S*, Squamous cells; *W*, wing cells.

relative dehydration of the corneal stroma. Secondarily, the endothelium is also known to secrete an anteriorly located basement membrane called Descemet's membrane and a posterior-located glycocalyx layer.

The endothelium of the infant cornea is composed of a monolayer of approximately 500,000 neural crest-derived cells, each measuring around 6 μm in thickness by 20 μm in diameter or covering a surface area of 250 μm^2 (Figs. 4.20A and 4.21A).[157] The cells lie on the posterior surface of the cornea and form an irregular polygonal mosaic. The tangential apical or inner surface of each corneal endothelial cell is uniquely irregular but are hexagons of uniform size when viewed en face. The hexagon is the most energy-efficient geometric shape in order to cover a surface completely without leaving gaps, thus minimizing intercellular boundary exposure to the aqueous humor.[157] They abut one another in an undulating, interdigitating fashion with a 20-nm wide intercellular space between each other, which serves to increase the internal surface area of the lateral cell membranes, making the length of the intercellular space sometimes at least 10 times the width of the cell itself (Fig. 4.20A,B).[158] This is clearly seen on the endothelium's tangential basal or outer surface, as corneal endothelial cells form an extremely complex jigsaw shape here as opposed to the six-sided hexagon on the inner surface.[159] The intercellular space is known to contain apical macula occludens tight junctions and lateral gap junctions (Fig. 4.20C,D), thereby forming an incomplete barrier with a preference for the diffusion of small molecules (Fig. 4.21B,C). The corneal endothelial cells have numerous cytoplasmic organelles, particularly mitochondria, and thus have been inferred to have the second highest aerobic metabolic rate of all the cells in the eye next to the retinal photoreceptors (Fig. 4.20B).

At birth, the central endothelial cell density (ECD) of the cornea is around 5000 cells/mm^2.[157] Postnatally, the corneal endothelium of primates and humans mature and lose most of their proliferative capacity. The human corneal endothelium has very limited innate in

vivo proliferative capacity. This is due to contact inhibition, high aqueous humor concentrations of TGF-β, and gradual age-related cellular senescence. Particularly in the central regions of the cornea and in part through the activity of the cyclin-dependent kinase inhibitor p21, there is a well-documented decline in central ECD with age that typically involves two phases: a rapid and a slow component.[160–162] In fact, recent studies suggest that an adult stem cell population of corneal endothelial cells exists beyond Schwalbe's line of the limbus, which is a transition zone between the trabecular meshwork and the corneal endothelial periphery, and these proliferate in a limited fashion, particularly after injury.[163,164] Owing to corneal growth and developmentally selective cell death, during the fast component, the central ECD decreases rapidly to about 3500 cells/mm^2 by age 5 and 3000 cells/mm^2 by age 14 to 20 years (Fig. 4.22A).[162] Thereafter, a slow component occurs where central ECD decreases to a linear steady rate of 0.3% to 0.6% per year, resulting in central ECDs around 2500 cells/mm^2 in late adulthood (Fig. 4.22A).[162] Because the corneal endothelium maintains its continuity by migration and expansion or thinning of surviving cells to cover a larger surface area, it is not surprising that the percentage of hexagonal cells decreases (pleomorphism) and the coefficient of variation of cell area increases (polymegathism) with age.[162]

When reviewing normal physiologic variability of the corneal endothelium, realize that these average central ECDs are primarily from White US populations. Several studies reveal that important ethnic differences exist, as the corneas of Japanese, Filipino, and Chinese people have been found to have higher central ECDs than White people at all ages, whereas corneas of people from India have lower central ECDs (Table 4.2).[165–168] It is hypothesized that this ethnic variance of central ECDs may be predominantly due to population differences in mean corneal diameter and thus mean endothelial surface area between these groups (the horizontal cornea diameters of the corneas of Japanese and White people and people from India averaged 11.2,

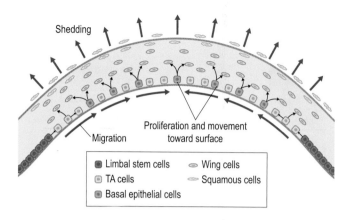

Fig. 4.20 The basal epithelial cells of the cornea, which undergo vertical proliferation (both daughter cells move into the middle layers of the epithelium), are continually replenished by a stem cell population that resides in basal layer of the limbus. The transient amplifying (*TA*) basal epithelial cells, which are two horizontal progeny from the stem cells, migrate forward from the limbus to the periphery of the cornea and commonly to reach the center of the cornea. The TA cells undergo mixed (one daughter cell retained in the basal cell layer and the other moves into the middle layers of the epithelium) proliferation. The final or terminal cell cycle of mitosis is the vertical proliferation step, in which the two daughters continually move toward the surface, eventually being shed in the tear film. (Modified from Thoft RA, Friend J. The X, Y, Z hypothesis of corneal epithelial maintenance. *Invest. Ophthalmol. Vis. Sci.* 1983;24(10):1442–1443.)

11.7, and 12.0 mm, respectively), but genetic and environmental factors cannot be excluded and thus need further study.[169–171] Additionally, these data apply only to central ECD, as a recent study has shown that higher ECDs can typically be found in the periphery of the cornea (Figs. 4.21A and 4.22B).[172] This finding has been reported previously, but the recent study was the only one that was thorough enough in detail to document how the variance applies to the entire posterior corneal surface. In addition, radial furrows from the peripheral endothelium, guiding cells toward the central cornea, have also been recently described.[173–176] Therefore, it appears that total corneal endothelial cell numbers and ECDs decrease on average about 50% from birth to death in normal subjects without causing corneal disease or pathology.[177] Because corneal decompensation typically does not occur until central ECDs reach 500 cells/mm² (Fig. 4.23A,B), which is a 90% decrease in central ECD from birth or an 80% decrease from healthy adulthood levels, there appears to be plenty of cellular reserve remaining after an average human life span of 75 to 80 years.[162] Estimates suggest that healthy, normal human corneal endothelium should maintain corneal clarity up to a minimum of 224 to 277 years of life—if humans could live that long (Box 4.3).

Leaky barrier function. The barrier function of the corneal endothelium is dependent upon a sufficient number of endothelial cells to cover the posterior surface of the cornea (Fig. 4.21A) and intact macula occludens tight junctions (Fig. 4.21B,C) between the endothelial cells, resulting in a low electrical resistance (25 Ω·cm²) barrier to aqueous humor flow. Macula occludens tight junctions are characterized by partial obliteration of the intercellular space and partial retention of a 10-nm wide intercellular space.[158] Clinically, the barrier function of the cornea can be assessed by using the specular microscope or the confocal microscope to measure ECD, and fluorophotometry to measure permeability.[178] In healthy human corneas, this barrier prevents the bulk flow of fluid from the aqueous humor to the corneal stroma, but it does still allow moderate diffusion of small nutrients, water, and other

metabolites to cross into the stroma through the 10-nm wide intercellular spaces.[178]

The leakiness of the endothelial barrier may initially seem inefficient and counterproductive; however, most nutrients for all layers of the cornea come from the aqueous humor. Thus, leakiness of the endothelial cell monolayer is essential for corneal health due to the fact that the cornea is avascular and contains no lymph vessels or other channels for bulk fluid flow. Despite the loss of endothelial cells that occurs with aging, there appears to be no significant increase in the permeability of normal, healthy aged corneas.[179,180] Only when the endothelial cell junctions are disrupted does permeability increase, usually up to a maximum of sixfold higher than baseline (Fig. 4.21B).[179] Corneal endothelial permeability does, however, gradually increase as central ECD decreases below 2000 cells/mm², but compensatory metabolic pump mechanisms keep the cornea at its normal dehydrated state until a central ECD of 500 cells/mm² is reached.

A number of factors acutely affect the barrier function of the endothelium, including reversible disruption of cell junctions during irrigation with calcium-free solutions or glutathione-restricted solutions, mechanical damage during intraocular surgery, or chemical injury due to introduction of nonphysiologic or toxic solutions into the anterior chamber. Fortunately, the remaining viable cells are often able to migrate and recover the posterior corneal surface by spreading out over a larger surface area, reestablishing the intercellular cell junctions. Thus, the barrier function of the corneal endothelium is efficiently restored.

Metabolic pump function. In the early days of corneal transplantation, it was observed that when donor corneas were refrigerated, corneal thickness increased and transparency decreased.[181] When the cornea was brought back to its normal temperature of 35°C, a temperature reversal occurred during which the cornea returned to its normal thickness and regained clarity. In vitro perfusion studies of the cornea showed that temperature reversal can take place in the absence of the epithelium, leading to the conclusion that active metabolic processes in the endothelium are responsible for maintaining corneal dehydration.[181] Subsequent studies demonstrated that transporters, located primarily in the endothelial cell's basolateral cell membrane, transport ions, principally sodium (Na^+) and bicarbonate (HCO_3^-), out of the stroma and into the aqueous humor (Fig. 4.21C).[181] An osmotic gradient is created, and water is thus osmotically drawn from the stroma into the aqueous humor. This osmotic gradient can be maintained only if the endothelial barrier is intact. A major transport protein found to be essential for endothelial metabolic pump function is Na^+/K^+-ATPase.[182] The number and density of Na^+/K^+-ATPase sites have been quantified using [3H]-ouabain, which binds specifically in a one-to-one ratio to Na^+/K^+-ATPase pump sites.[183] These studies have shown that approximately 3 million Na^+/K^+-ATPase pump sites are present in the basolateral membrane of a single corneal endothelial cell. This corresponds to an average pump site density of 4.4 trillion sites/mm² along the lateral plasma membrane of an intact endothelial cell.[183] Clinically, the metabolic pump function of the corneal endothelium can be assessed in vivo using pachymetry to measure how quickly the corneal thickness recovers after being purposefully swollen by the wearing of an oxygen-impermeable contact lens or, secondarily, by measuring the degree of diurnal fluctuation in corneal thickness.[184]

A number of factors alter endothelial pump function, including pharmacologic inhibition of Na^+/K^+-ATPase, decreased temperature, lack of bicarbonate, carbonic anhydrase inhibitors, and a chronic reduction in ECD from mechanical injury, chemical injury, or disease states. Fortunately, with regard to the latter, compensatory metabolic pump mechanisms prevent corneal edema from occurring to a certain degree when central ECDs are between 2000 and 750 cells/mm²

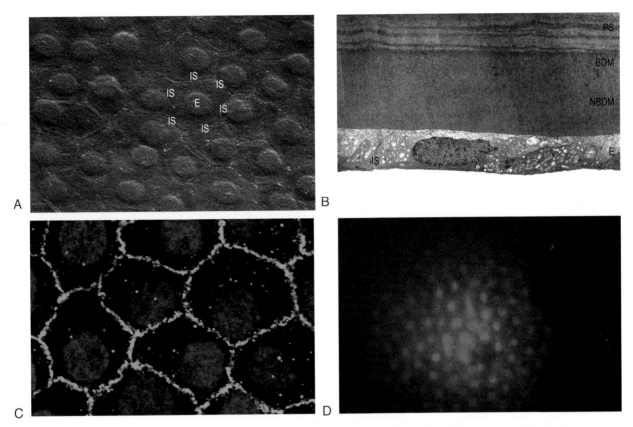

Fig. 4.21 (**A**) Scanning electron micrograph (TEM, ×1000) of the posterior surface of the corneal endothelium from a 65-year-old patient with healthy corneas. Note how the hexagonal endothelial cells form a uniform monolayer with small 20-nm intercellular spaces between adjacent endothelial cells. (**B**) TEM (×4750) of the posterior corneal stroma, Descemet's membrane, and corneal endothelium from a 65-year-old patient with healthy corneas. (**C**) Immunofluorescent laser confocal microscopic photomicrograph (×2000) of human corneal endothelial macula occludens tight junctional complexes stained with immunolabeled monoclonal antibodies to junctional adhesion molecule-A (*green*). Nuclei are counterstained with TO-PRO (*blue*). (Courtesy of Kenneth J. Mandell.) (**D**) Photomicrograph (×400) of fluorescein dye spreading between many adjacent endothelial cells in a human cornea, which demonstrates the intimate importance of gap junctions in how endothelial cells communicate with one another. (Courtesy of Mitchell A. Watsky, PhD.) *BDM*, Banded portion of Descemet's membrane; *E*, endothelial cells. *IS*, intercellular space; *NBDM*, nonbanded portion of Descemet's membrane; *PS*, posterior stroma.

(Fig. 4.23A,B). This occurs by either increasing the metabolic activity of pump sites already present, which requires more ATP production by the cell, and/or by increasing the total number and density of pump sites on the lateral membranes of endothelial cells.[183] A similar phenomenon occurs in the proximal tubule of the human kidney to adjust for an increased salt load. For example, in Fuchs' endothelial dystrophy, the cornea remains clear and of normal thickness despite having focal areas of very low ECD and increased endothelial monolayer permeability to fluorescein.[185] Apparently, this occurs because the metabolic activity and density of the Na^+/K^+ pump sites increase in adjacent healthier areas to compensate for the focal areas of increased permeability.[185] The point at which compensatory mechanisms ultimately fail is when the central ECD reaches approximately 500 cells/mm^2 or less.[186] At this low ECD, the permeability has increased to a point where the endothelial cells are spread so thin that they do not have enough room on their lateral cell membranes for more metabolic pump sites, and all the existing pump sites are maximally active (Fig. 4.23A,B). At this point, the metabolic pump fails to balance the leak and corneal edema results.

A summary of the entire corneal endothelial cell transport system was reviewed by Bonanno.[187] When the corneal endothelial barrier and metabolic pump are functioning normally, the corneal stroma has a total Na^+ concentration of 179 mM (134.4 mM free and 44.6 mM bound to stromal Prostaglandins (PGs)), while the aqueous humor has a total Na^+ concentration of 142.9 mM (all free).[188] Therefore, after accounting for chloride activity and stromal imbibition pressure, an osmotic gradient of +30.4 mmHg exists, causing water to diffuse from the stroma into the aqueous humor.

Corneal edema. Corneal edema is a term often used loosely and nonspecifically by clinicians, but it literally refers to a cornea that is more hydrated than its normal physiologic state of 78% water. The Donnan effect states that the swelling pressure in a charged gel, like the corneal stroma, results from ionic imbalances. The fixed negative or anionic charges on the corneal stromal proteoglycan GAG side-chains have a central role in this effect. The antiparallel GAG duplexes (tertiary structure) produce long-range electrostatic repulsive forces that induce an expansive force termed swelling pressure (SP). Because the corneal stroma has cohesive and tensile stiffness (elasticity) that resists expansion, the normal SP is around +55 mmHg.[189,190] If the stroma is compressed as occurs with increasing intraocular pressure (IOP) or mechanical applanation, or is expanded as occurs with corneal edema, the SP will correspondingly increase or decrease. Conversely, the

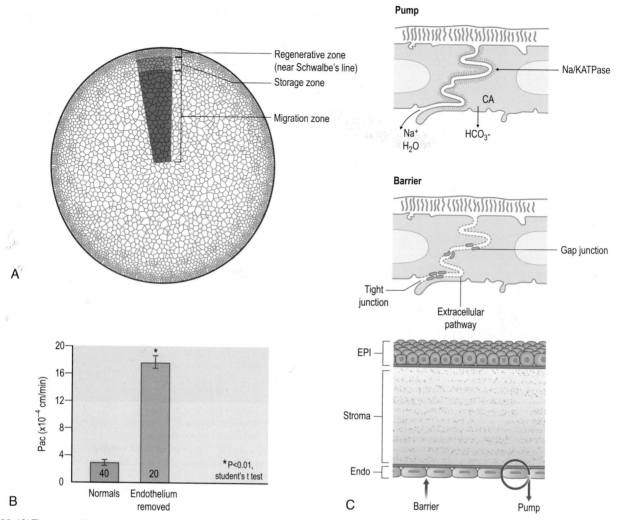

Fig. 4.22 (**A**) The normal barrier function of corneal endothelium is due to endothelial cells covering the entire posterior corneal surface without gaps and the focal, discontinuous tight junctions in its apical intercellular space. (**B**) shows the normal permeability of the human endothelial cell monolayer to carboxyfluorescein (2.26×10^{-4} cm/min) compared with that without endothelium (12.85×10^{-4} cm/min), which resulted in a sixfold increase in permeability. (Modified from Watsky MA, McDermott ML, Edelhauser HF. In vitro corneal endothelial permeability in rabbit and human: The effects of age, cataract surgery, and diabetes. *Exp Eye Res.* 1989;49(5):751–767. https://doi.org/10.1016/S0014-4835(89)80036-3.) (**C**) The opposing forces of the leaky corneal endothelial barrier and the metabolic pump sites are shown. When the leak rate equals the metabolic pump rate, the corneal stroma is 78% hydrated and the corneal thickness and transparency is maintained. (Waring GO, Bourne WM, Edelhauser HF, Kenyon KR. The corneal endothelium: Normal and pathologic structure and function. *Ophthalmology.* 1982;89(6):531–590. https://doi.org/10.1016/S0161-6420(82)34746-6.).

TABLE 4.2   Comparison of endothelial cell density in Indian, American, Chinese, Filipino, and Japanese populations

Age groups (years)	Indian[a]		American[b]		Chinese[c]		Filipino[d]		Japanese[b]	
	# of eyes	Cell density (cells/mm²)	# of eyes	Cell density (cells/mm²)	# of eyes	Cell density (cells/mm²)	# of eyes	Cell density (cells/mm²)	# of eyes	Cell density (cells/mm²)
20–30	104	2782 ± 250	11	2977 ± 324	100	2988 ± 243	114	2949 ± 270	18	3893 ± 259
31–40	96	2634 ± 288	6	2739 ± 208	100	2920 ± 325	112	2946 ± 296	10	3688 ± 245
41–50	97	2408 ± 274	11	2619 ± 321	97	2935 ± 285	112	2761 ± 333	10	3749 ± 407
51–60	98	2438 ± 309	13	2625 ± 172	97	2810 ± 321	102	2555 ± 178	10	3386 ± 455
61–70	88	2431 ± 357	8	2684 ± 384	90	2739 ± 316	114	2731 ± 299	6	3307 ± 330
>70	54	2360 ± 357	15	2431 ± 339	83	2778 ± 365	86	2846 ± 467	15	3289 ± 313

[a]Rao SK, Ranjan Sen P, Fogla R, et al. Corneal endothelial cell density and morphology in normal Indian eyes. *Cornea.* 2000; 19:820–823.
[b]Matsuda M, Yee RW, Edelhauser HF. Comparison of the corneal endothelium in an American and a Japanese population. *Arch Ophthalmol.* 1985;103:68–70.
[c]Yunliang S, Yuqiang H, Ying-Peng L, et al. Corneal endothelial cell density and morphology in healthy Chinese eyes. *Cornea.* 2007;26:130–132.
[d]Padilla MD, Sibayan SA, Gonzales CS. Corneal endothelial cell density and morphology in normal Filipino eyes. *Cornea.* 2004; 23:129–135.

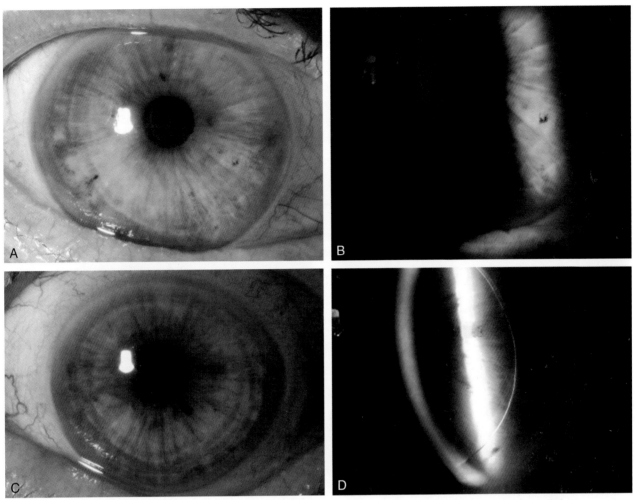

Fig. 4.23 Part 1: Postoperative slit-lamp photographs comparing endothelial keratoplasty techniques **(A)**. Descemet membrane endothelial keratoplasty **(B)**. Descemet membrane endothelial keratoplasty with graft edge barely visible **(C)**. Descemet stripping automated endothelial keratoplasty with visible graft edge **(D)**.

negatively charged GAG side-chains also form a double-folded helix in aqueous solution (secondary structure) that attracts and binds Na^+ cations, resulting in an osmotic effect, leading to the diffusion and subsequent absorption of water. Thus, the central corneal thickness is maintained at an average value of 544 μm because the fixed negatively charged proteoglycans induce a constant SP through anionic repulsive forces, yet it still tends to imbibe more water via its cationic attractive forces.[191]

Under normal circumstances, the negative pressure drawing fluid into the cornea, called the imbibition pressure (IP) of the corneal stroma, is approximately −40 mmHg.[191] This implies that the negative charges on corneal proteoglycan GAG side-chains are just over one-quarter saturated or bound with Na^+, and that the remaining unbound proportion is still available to bind more Na^+ and absorb more water if given the opportunity. Normally, the highly impermeable epithelium and the mildly impermeable endothelium keep the diffusion of electrolytes and fluid flow in the stroma to such a low level that the endothelium's metabolic pumps can maintain stromal hydration in the normal range of 78% without significant effort. Although IP = SP when corneas are in the ex

vivo state, IP is lower than SP in the in vivo state because the hydrostatic pressure induced by IOP must now be accounted. This is best represented by the equation IP = IOP − SP and explains why the hydration level of a patient's cornea is not only dependent on having normal barrier function, but also on having a normal IOP.[191] Therefore, a loss of corneal barrier function, an IOP ≥55 mmHg, or a combination of the two typically results in the clinical appearance of corneal edema (Fig. 4.24).[192]

The topic of corneal edema is important for clinicians to understand because it affects the function of the corneal stroma and the epithelium. With minor (<5%) hydration changes, the corneal thickness changes have minimal effect on the refractive, transparency, and mechanical functions of the cornea. For example, during sleep, a diurnal increase in hydration occurs causing on average a 6% ± 3% increase in corneal thickness of the cornea (range: 2%–13%; stromal = 6% and epithelial = 8%), mainly because of reduced oxygen levels (from 155 to 55 mmHg) caused by eyelid closure and secondarily from decreased evaporative loss (from 3 μL/h cm² to 0 μL/h cm²) caused by eyelid closure.[193,194] Upon awakening and eyelid opening, the corneal hydration and thickness reverts back to normal within 1 to 2 hours.

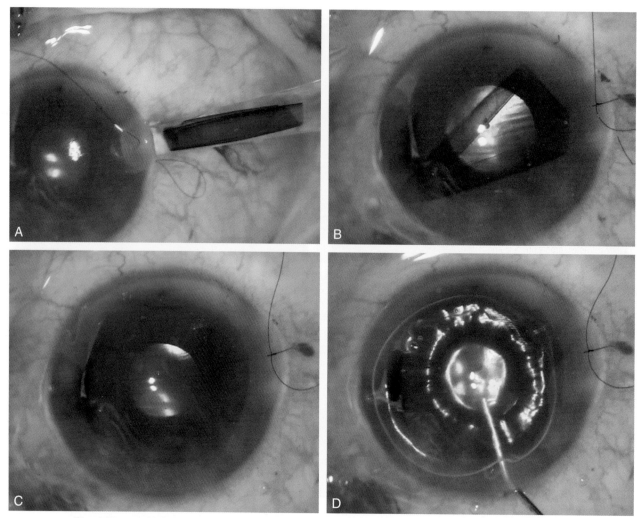

Fig. 4.23, cont'd Part 2: Descemet membrane endothelial keratoplasty donor insertion technique. (**A**) Insertion of donor via glass injector through temporal 3.2-mm clear corneal tunnel. (**B**) Double scroll formation with endothelium rolled upwards. (**C**) Donor unscrolled in shallow anterior chamber. (**D**) 20% SF6 gas combination with air injected under donor for full air fill with inferior peripheral iridectomy. (From Ang M, Wilkins MR, Mehta JS, Tan D. Descemet membrane endothelial keratoplasty. *Br J Ophthalmol.* 2016;100[1]:15–21.)

If the cornea becomes hydrated by 5% or more above its normal physiologic level of 78%, it begins to scatter significant amounts of light and loses its transparency. Some loss of refractive function may also occur, particularly if the epithelial surface becomes too irregular. Clinically, mild to moderate cases of epithelial edema cause the epithelium to appear hazy and microcystic, significantly decreasing vision and increasing glare. It also can cause the development of large, painful subepithelial bullae in severe cases. These changes correlate histopathologically with hydropic basal epithelial cell degenerative changes owing to intraepithelial fluid accumulation and the development of interepithelial cellular fluid-filled spaces, known as cysts and bullae. If bullae are chronically present, a fibrocollagenous degenerative pannus will often form in the subepithelial space, decreasing vision further, but, paradoxically, this reduces the pain. In comparison, corneal stromal edema appears clinically as a painless, hazy thickening of the corneal stroma, resulting in a mild to moderate reduction in visual acuity and an increase in glare. At the same time, Descemet's membrane folds commonly appear on the posterior corneal surface. Histopathologically, these changes correlate with the light microscopic

findings of thickening of the corneal stroma in the posterior cross-sectional direction, with loss of the normally present artifacteous interlamellar stromal clefting.[195] Ultrastructural and biochemical studies have further shown that stromal edema results in an increase in the interfibrillar distance and disruption of the spatial order between collagen fibrils, a decrease in the refractive index of the extracellular matrix, loss of proteoglycans, and, perhaps most importantly, hydropic degenerative changes or cell lysis in the resident keratocyte population.[196–198]

Although depth-related differences in the concentration of the two types of negatively charged proteoglycans may account for the higher hydration levels in the posterior stroma compared with the anterior stroma, it appears that the directional orientation of the collagen fibrils and the degree of lamellar interweaving have the greatest influence on the amount of regional stromal thickening from edema-related swelling.[199] Because the collagen fibrils in the cornea run from limbus to limbus, the corneal stroma highly resists circumferential expansion; however, it can expand anterior-posteriorly, mostly in the posterior direction. The depth-related differences in lamellar interweaving explain why the anterior third of the cornea mildly swells and actually

BOX 4.3 Refractive surgery

Several keratorefractive surgical procedures have been developed to permanently alter the curvature of the anterior corneal surface, thereby reducing refractive errors.[316] The procedures most commonly performed today use the 193-nm argon fluoride (ArF) excimer laser and include laser in situ keratomileusis (LASIK), a thin-flap variant of LASIK known as sub-Bowman's keratomileusis (SBK), and surface ablation techniques of photorefractive keratectomy (PRK), laser-assisted subepithelial keratectomy (LASEK), and EpiLASIK.[317] The excimer laser reshapes the curvature and contour of the anterior corneal surface by removing anterior corneal stroma in a microscopically precise process known as ablative photodecomposition. This results in nonthermal, photochemical breakage of carbon-carbon covalent molecular bonds in the corneal tissue with submicron accuracy. Thus, excimer laser-based keratorefractive surgery is a very accurate, precise, and safe means to permanently change the curvature and contour of the anterior cornea surface. In fact, it has become the most commonly performed refractive procedure performed in the US since it was approved by the US Food and Drug Administration (FDA) in 1995.

The main reason that photoablation of stroma is effective is that the corneal stroma does not regenerate after it is ablated. It only undergoes reparative stromal scarring that at most replaces 5% to 20% of the ablated stromal tissue.[318] Excimer laser-based keratorefractive surgery has been used to successfully treat myopic and hyperopic refractive errors with mild to moderate degrees of astigmatism resulting in stable long-term (>10 years) uncorrected visual outcomes. However, it still is known to potentially deteriorate visual quality due to induction of on- or off-axis aberrations.[319] This occurs mainly because:

1. the actual laser ablation profile is sometimes different from the intended profile
2. the laser ablation profile is based on spherical geometry, whereas the preoperative anterior corneal surface is an aspheric ellipse
3. the myopic ablation profile makes the cornea more oblate in shape with a flatter curvature in the center and a steeper one in the periphery

4. visually significant subclinical lateral decentrations or torsional misalignments occasionally occur
5. the ablation zone is sometimes less than the diameter of the entrance pupil, particularly under low lighting conditions[320]

The basic principle of myopic correction is based on the graded removal of central tissue to flatten or increase the radius of curvature of the anterior corneal surface (Fig. 4.4A, right middle).[320] In contrast, the correction of spherical hyperopia involves the graded removal of peripheral and paracentral tissue to steepen or decrease the radius of curvature of the anterior corneal surface (Fig. 4.4A, right bottom).[320] Finally, the goal behind various astigmatic ablations is to reshape the anterior corneal surface to bring the two focal points of the eye to the same plane and then ultimately onto the retina with a subsequent second spherical treatment step, if needed.[320] The first step requires selective flattening of the steep meridian and/or steepening of the flat meridian, usually using plus or minus cylinder formats depending on which one removes the least amount of tissue.

Recent advances in femtosecond laser technology have led to the development of refractive lenticule extraction.[321] Small-incision lenticule extraction (SMILE) uses only the femtosecond laser to delineate a refractive lenticule within the stroma, which is removed via a keyhole wound without a flap. Thus, SMILE brings two main advantages over LASIK: faster dry eye symptom recovery and better spherical aberration control, owing to the minimally invasive incision with maximal retention of anterior corneal innervation, as well as structural integrity.[322–324] SMILE has reduced dry eye, owing to corneal nerve regeneration[325] and recovery of corneal sensitivity.[326] SMILE offers a theoretical advantage over LASIK by preservation of the stronger anterior stromal lamellae using finite element modeling.[327,328] This leads to reduction in spherical aberration induction compared with LASIK,[329] allowing for increase in the optical zone diameter without compromising the corneal biomechanics in SMILE.[330] Clinical trials support that SMILE is safe, effective, and predictable for treating moderate myopia and modest levels of astigmatism,[331] with postoperative visual outcomes comparable to that of femtosecond LASIK.[332,333]

---

maintains the anterior corneal curvature even when the remaining posterior two-thirds swells up to three times its normal thickness. Because fibrotic corneal scars have random directionally oriented collagen fibrils, they too have been found to resist swelling under edematous conditions.[200] Therefore, although it is commonly stated that corneal thickness and interfibrillar spacing increase linearly with increasing hydration of the corneal stroma, this relationship mainly applies to the posterior two-thirds of the corneal stroma.[192]

Finally, although epithelial and stromal edema commonly coexist together, there are two notable exceptions. Because the epithelium has much weaker cohesive and tensile strengths than the corneal stroma, its state of hydration is mainly dictated by IOP levels.[201] Conversely, because collagen fibrils in the corneal stroma are anchored at the limbus for 360 degrees, they exert increasing or decreasing cohesive strength on the corneal stroma (i.e., compression or decompression of stromal tissue) as the IOP elevates above or decreases below normal, respectively. This results in the transmission of stromal edema to the epithelial surface in cases of high IOP or into the stroma in cases of low IOP. Therefore, if IOP is 55 mmHg or more with normal endothelial barrier and metabolic pump function, epithelial edema usually occurs by itself. In comparison, if endothelial cell dysfunction and hypotony (IOP ~0 mmHg) occur together, then stromal edema occurs alone (Fig. 4.24).

Basement membrane and glycocalyx. A secondary function of the corneal endothelium is its ability to secrete a basement membrane, called Descemet's membrane, along its basal surface, which is continuously deposited throughout life (Fig. 4.20B). Although some collagen fibrils from the posterior stroma are embedded in the Descemet's

membrane, it really has no major junctional or adhesional complexes to the posterior stroma other than a 0.5-μm-thick layer of fibronectin. Descemet's membrane is highly extensible and tough, but less strong and stiff than the posterior stroma because it is primarily composed of type IV and VIII collagen fibrils, as well as the glycoproteins fibronectin, laminin, and thrombospondin. At birth, it averages 4-μm thick. On electron microscopy, the fetal Descemet's membrane is composed of many wide-spaced, 110-nm banded collagen fibrils (see Fig. 4.20B).[202] Postnatally, collagen is gradually added posteriorly to this initial fetal layer throughout life, being notably different in morphology from the fetal layer, as it is nonbanded and contains small-diameter collagen fibrils that are arranged into a hexagonal lattice (see Fig. 4.20B).[202] Typically, at the end of a normal life span, Descemet's membrane measures around 10- to 15-μm thick (a 4-μm-thick banded layer and a 6- to 11-μm-thick nonbanded layer). With disease (e.g., Fuchs' dystrophy) or injury (e.g., trauma or surgery), Descemet's membrane may become focally (corneal guttae) or diffusely thicker than normal, from abnormal collagen deposition. This newly deposited abnormal basement membrane is called the posterior collagenous layer of the Descemet's membrane and is classified into one of three types: banded, fibrillar, or fibrocelluar.[203] Excess basement membrane deposition is a common strategy used by cells attempting to recover from injury, allowing them to remain attached to a tissue's scaffolding. Finally, the endothelium is also known to secrete a 0.7-μm-thick glycocalyx layer on its apical or posterior surface.[157] Functionally, it is thought that the glycocalyx layer may protect the internal (or posterior) surface membrane of the endothelium.

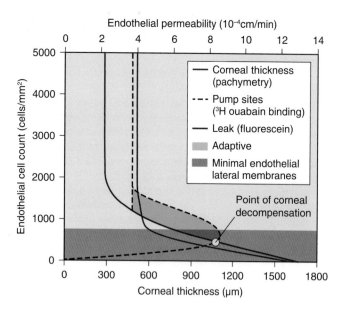

Fig. 4.24 Graph illustrating the central, paracentral, and peripheral corneal ECDs for healthy, normal subjects of different ages. (Data from Edelhauser HF. The Balance between Corneal Transparency and Edema: The proctor lecture. *Invest. Ophthalmol. Vis. Sci.* 2006;47(5): 1755–1767.)

Mechanical properties

Because the cornea is a pressurized, thick-walled, partially woven, unidirectionally fibril-reinforced laminate biocomposite, it represents an excellent compromise between stiffness, strength, extensibility, and therefore toughness to withstand internal and external forces that may stress it, distort its shape, or threaten its integrity.[204] The biologic behavior of a soft fibrous connective tissue such as the human cornea is usually much stronger in the direction of its collagen fibrils than perpendicular to it. These fibrils are assembled into various hierarchical structures, which give the tissue anisotropic mechanical properties, (i.e., these mechanical properties are direction dependent).[205] Maturity and age-acquired covalent collagen crosslinks serve to bolster the stiffness, strength, and toughness of these hierarchical structures, usually without significantly compromising extensibility (Fig. 4.6C).[206] Because the biomechanical properties of the cornea are dominated by the stroma, the macro-, micro-, and nanomechanical behaviors of the cornea are due primarily to the hierarchical structure of, essentially, four composite-like regions: Bowman's layer, the anterior third of the stroma proper, the posterior two-thirds of the stroma proper, and Descemet's membrane (Fig. 4.26).[207–212] Like most composites, the cornea is biomechanically strong, light in weight (when dehydrated), and has an extraordinary capacity to absorb energy owing to its fluid-like matrix gel. However, it also has a composite's shortcomings in that its dynamic three-dimensional state of stress is difficult to definitively quantify, and its biomechanical failure process is complex, as it appears to break down at the nano- and micromechanical level.

When a biologic tissue is subjected to force (or load), it will typically deform (elongate, compress, or shear) in the direction of the applied force. The *stress* acting on a material is the force divided by the cross-sectional area of the applied stress (N/m²), whereas the degree of deformation in the direction of the applied stress is called *strain*. The ratio of the stress and strain (i.e., the slope of the stress-strain curve)

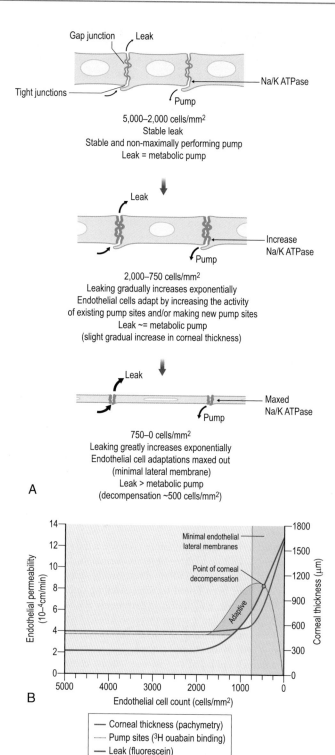

Fig. 4.25 (**A**) and (**B**) The relationship between central endothelial cell density, barrier function, metabolic pump sites, and pachymetry is shown. Note that the pump sites are not all maximally used in the normal state (5000–2000 cells/mm²). With increased permeability (2000–750 cells/mm²), there is an adaptive phase in which the endothelial cells can maximally use all their pump sites or can make more pump sites to offset the leak up to a certain point. When the surface area of the corneal endothelial cell's lateral membranes becomes too small (750–0 cells/mm²), these adaptations max out and eventually decline. The point at which endothelial cell pump site adaptations intersect with permeability (500 cells/mm²) is typically when corneal decompensation occurs. (A and B, Dawson DG, Watsky MA, Geroski DH, Edelhauser HF. *Duane's Foundation of Clinical Ophthalmology on CD-ROM*, Vol. 2c. Philadelphia: Lippincott Williams & Wilkins; 2006;41–76)

TABLE 4.3 Composition of aqueous humor compared with various intraocular irrigating solutions

Ingredient	Human aqueous humor	BSS Plus	BSS
Sodium	162.9	160.0	155.7
Potassium	2.2–3.9	5.0	10.1
Calcium	1.8	1.0	3.3
Magnesium	1.1	1.0	1.5
Chloride	131.6	130.0	128.9
Bicarbonate	20.15	25.0	–
Phosphate	0.62	3.0	–
Lactate	2.5–4.5	–	–
Glucose	2.7–3.7	5.0	–
Ascorbate	1.06	–	–
Glutathione	0.002–0.010	0.3	–
Citrate	–	–	5.8
Acetate	–	–	28.6
pH	7.38	7.6	7.4
Osmolarity (mOsm)	304	305	298
Protein	0.135–0.237	–	–

All concentrations are expressed in millimoles per liter or millequivalents per liter of solution.

TABLE 4.4 Causes of toxic anterior segment syndrome

1. *Irrigating solutions or viscoelastic devices*
   - Incomplete chemical composition
   - Incorrect pH (<6.7 or >8.1)
   - Incorrect osmolality (<270 mOsm or >350 mOsm)
   - Preservatives or additives (e.g., antibiotics, dilating medications)
2. *Ophthalmic instrument contaminants*
   - Detergent residues (ultrasonic, soaps, enzymatic cleaners)
   - Bacterial Lipopolysaccharides (LPS) or other endotoxin residues
   - Metal ion residues (copper and iron)
   - Denatured viscoelastics?
3. *Ocular medications*
   - Incorrect drug concentration
   - Incorrect pH (<6.7 or >8.1)
   - Incorrect osmolality (<270 mOsm or >350 mOsm)
   - Vehicle with wrong pH or osmolality
   - Preservatives in medication solution
4. *Contaminated water sources*
   - Water baths
   - Autoclave reservoirs
   - Nonsterile or nonpyrogen-free water
5. *Intraocular lenses*
   - Polishing compounds
   - Cleaning and sterilizing compounds

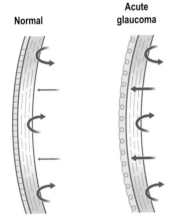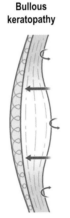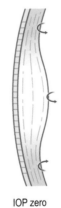

Normal — IOP normal, Normal epithelium, Normal stroma, Normal endothelium

Acute glaucoma — IOP high, Epithelial edema, Normal stroma, Normal endothelium

Bullous keratopathy — IOP normal, Epithelial edema, Stromal edema, Abnormal endothelium

Phthisis — IOP zero, Normal epithelium, Stromal edema, Abnormal endothelium

Fig. 4.26 The delicate balance between stromal swelling pressure, endothelial barrier, metabolic pump function, and intraocular pressure (*IOP*) is illustrated. Usually if endothelial cell pump function fails and IOP remains at normal physiologic levels, both stromal and epithelial edema occur (*center right*). Only when IOP increases above the swelling pressure of the stroma and the endothelium functions normally, does epithelial cell edema occur by itself (*center left*); and only when IOP is around zero and the endothelium functions abnormally does stromal edema occur by itself (*farther right*). (Hatton MP, Perez VL, Dohlman CH. Corneal oedema in ocular hypotony. *Exp Eye Res.* 2004;78(3):549–552. https://doi.org/10.1016/j.exer.2003.06.003.).

is called the elastic modulus or Young's modulus of the tissue, that is, a representation of tissue elasticity that relates the force (stress) required to generate a certain fractional deformation (strain). Stiff materials are needed to transmit forces and are especially crucial in resisting bending or buckling from compression. The strength of a material is defined as the maximum stress it can sustain before breaking. Strong materials are needed to carry a load. The extensibility of a tissue is defined as the maximum strain it can sustain before rupturing. Extensible materials need to reversibly change elastic shape instantaneously and then return to their original shape without damage. Toughness is defined as the ability of the material's micro- and nanostructure to dissipate deformation energy without initiation or propagation of a critical crack. Toughness is a common characteristic of a tissue that deforms to dissipate energy on impact (i.e., not brittle) and/or has natural crack-stopping mechanisms so that it avoids initiation and/or propagation of a critical crack (i.e., work of extension [work per volume or work per unit mass] or work of fracture [work per surface area created]). The area under the stress-strain curve or the energy needed to elongate a pre-existing crack both correspond to the toughness of the material, with the former describing crack initiation and the latter crack propagation. Strength and toughness are both highly influenced by internal defects in a tissue's structure or material components, whereas stiffness and extensibility are not.

Corneal stress. The dome-like cornea encounters three types of loads or stresses: (1) transmural pressure, i.e., pressure through the full thickness of the cornea, (2) piercing, and (3) crushing. The static net internal pressure constantly stressing the cornea in an outward direction is the IOP (16 ± 3 standard deviation [SD] mmHg above external atmospheric pressure [760 mmHg] and the external resting tension from the eyelids).[213,214] Additional dynamic stressors that can occur as a result of normal variability or external environmental stress include various causes of increased IOP such as accommodation (4 mmHg); turning the eyes (10 mmHg); arterial pulsation (1–2 mmHg); diurnal changes (5 mmHg); respiration (5 mmHg); Valsalva maneuver (8 mmHg) and recumbent or inverted positions; external eyelid blinking (normal blinks = 5–10 mmHg; hard squeeze blinks = 50–110 mmHg; eye rubbing (increases IOP [light digital rubbing = 5–20 mmHg, hard knuckle grinding/rubbing = 25–135 mmHg], induces shear and transverse compression on the corneal stroma, and may actually indent the cornea); or accidental eye impact.[215] An increase in internal pressure causes the cornea's stress behavior to be dominated by transmural longitudinal tension, which is usually very well tolerated because the net vector direction of stress is essentially parallel to the direction of most of the collagen fibrils in the structure. In contrast, external pressure, such as from eye rubbing (back and forth or circular pressure and friction), nocturnal external eye pressure, or direct blunt impact trauma, causes radial compressive stress, circumferential tensile stress, and/or deformation. As the net vector direction of stress is oblique to the direction of most collagen fibrils in the cornea, external stress is more likely to initiate or propagate internal defects due to fatigue-related damage in the corneal stroma than internal stress. Moreover, eye rubbing's often repetitive or oscillatory ECM shearing and subsequent cellular damage result in both transmural pressure and crush-related injury.

Based on mechanical physics, the cornea should theoretically obey Pascal's principle, which states that the pressure is the same everywhere inside an enclosed system or vessel at equilibrium, in addition to contributions from static fluid pressure. Despite this constant IOP, differences in wall tension exist according to the law of Laplace, that is, the tension in the walls of an enclosed vessel is directly dependent on the pressure in the system and its radius of curvature and is inversely dependent on the thickness of the vessel wall. For example, in an isotropic, thin-walled (wall thickness to cavity diameter ratio ≤0.1) elastic vessel, the law of Laplace would be simplified to the following equation:

$$T = PR/2t$$

where T equals the radial wall tension or stress of a spherical vessel wall, P equals the internal pressure in the vessel (IOP), R equals the radius of curvature of the wall (the curvature of the posterior corneal surface), and t equals the thickness of the wall in meters (corneal thickness). Unfortunately, the law of Laplace is not a perfect approximation of stress in the corneal eye wall, as the cornea is actually anisotropic, inhomogeneous, asymmetric, and thick-walled (Fig. 4.26). Thus, although static stress can be approximated (Fig. 4.27A), the dynamic temporal stresses acting upon the corneal eye wall are quite complex and difficult to definitively characterize, particularly because they overlap with one another in real time.[216]

Corneal stiffness, strength extensibility, and toughness. The two principal structural characteristics of the human cornea that help maintain its stiffness (rigidity or elasticity), strength (ultimate fracture stress), extensibility (ultimate fracture strain), and toughness (durability or unbreakability) are its thickness and innate biomechanical properties (hierarchical structure and degree of collagen fibril crosslinking).[217] Although corneal thickness can be directly measured accurately in vivo, a major challenge in the field of ophthalmology has been an adequate measurement or even an accurate approximation of its innate biomechanical properties.[218] The current understanding of the cornea's biomechanical properties still mainly relies on ex vivo experiments, primarily from strip extensiometry and inflation testing.[219]

The cornea is an important biologic *mechanotransducer* of stress due to its viscoelastic properties (i.e., solids with some characteristics of a fluid), which helps prevent premature biomechanical failure via energy dissipation. The property of viscoelasticity complicates our understanding of corneal biomechanical behavior as it contains both elastic and viscous component properties that overlap one another over time when forming the stress-strain curve. Thus, the cornea exhibits a time-dependent response to perturbation and a deformation in response to an applied force (loading), differing from its response to unloading. Elasticity is related to time-independent energy storage due to stretching or strain of the flexible domains of collagen molecules (potential

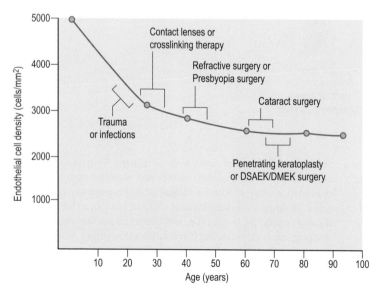

Fig. 4.27 The normal decrease in central endothelial cell density (ECD) that occurs with aging is shown. Located along the line graph are major endothelial cell stressors that commonly may occur in a person's lifetime, which potentially could decrease the central ECD more than normal.

energy), and deformation or transfer of energy to the sclera and other portions of the eye due to the rigid domains of collagen molecules (kinetic energy). In essence, elasticity is a time-independent physical property of a solid that allows the cornea to return to its original shape after stress or, if significantly damaged, to be permanently altered in shape. Viscosity is related to time-dependent energy dissipation due to the sliding of interfibrillar collagen fibrils, filaments, and lamellae past one another in a hydrated proteoglycan matrix (mechanicothermal energy transduction). In essence, viscosity is a time-dependent physical property of a fluid that allows the cornea to deflect some input energy away from its elastic components, and it allows the cornea the possibility to reversibly or permanently change its elastic shape with time.

Ex vivo experiments show that the human cornea has J-shaped, nonlinear stress-strain loading and unloading curves.[220] The cornea's stress-strain curves have an immediate elastic response dominated initially by the low strain behavior of the cornea's noncollagenous matrix and the act of removing slack from its collagen fibrils (fibril uncrimping), as well as the reorientation of its collagen fibrils to the direction of the stress (fibril recruitment) at the lower part of the "J." This is followed by the high strain behavior of collagen fibrils that are maximally taut and oriented in the direction of stress in the upper part of the J. Finally, a slower, time-dependent viscous response occurs in addition to the immediate J-shaped response, owing to interlamellar and interfibrillar slippage resulting in time-dependent strain (creep) or stress (stress relaxation) curves.

Creep is defined as a time-dependent elongation that occurs in three stages: (1) primary creep with its associated decelerating strain rate, (2) secondary creep with its associated constant strain rate, and (3) tertiary creep with its accelerating strain rate until rupture.

Primary and secondary creep are reversible viscoelastic responses without accompanying damage, whereas tertiary creep is associated with an irreversible reduction in the strength and toughness of the structure due to damage by irreversible slippage or cracking. The cornea's unloading stress-strain curve does not overlap with the loading curve, being variably less dependent on the load or strain rate. The difference in area between the two curves represents the energy dissipated via viscous friction (i.e., hysteresis) during a single mechanical cycle.[220] As the cornea has very small collagen fibril diameters and lengths compared with other connective tissues (e.g., skin and bone), and has biomechanical properties similar to that between skin and ligament, it is reported that the cornea converts approximately 35% of its total input energy into energy dissipation and the other 65% into energy storage, energy transmission, or deformation. However, it should be pointed out that a single stress-strain curve has limited meaning when evaluating a structure's total dynamic, temporal biomechanical properties because each curve is either load or strain rate dependent over a specific time interval and represents only one of several different material components or orientations of the structure itself.

Based on the hierarchical structure of the corneal stroma (Fig. 4.26), it has been inferred that the anterior woven portion of the cornea is much stiffer and stronger than the posterior nonwoven portion. This has been qualitatively supported by both clinical and experimental studies, which show that the posterior two-thirds of the corneal stroma is easier to bluntly dissect in a lamellar fashion than the anterior third, whereas the anterior corneal curvature remains relatively constant at various physiologic IOPs and stromal hydration levels compared with the posterior corneal curvature.[221-224] After induction of corneal edema in an ex vivo setting, ultrastructural studies by Müller and associates[197] showed that the 10 μm-thick Bowman's layer and the underlying anterior 100 to 120 μm of the stroma proper are the most stiff regions of the cornea as they did not swell significantly, even when stromal edema resulted in total central stromal thicknesses of up to 1200 μm.

Quantitative ex vivo direct measurements of human corneal stiffness are very consistent with these initial observations and inferences. Seiler and associates[208] showed, using uniaxial strip extensiometry, that removing the Bowman's layer with an excimer laser reduced the longitudinal (x- and y-axis length-wise dimension) Young's modulus on average by 4.75%. This was similar to findings discussed in a 1989 National Eye Institute-sponsored corneal biophysics workshop that described the longitudinal Young's modulus of Bowman's layer as about 50 MPa/mm² and that of the stroma proper as ranging between 2 to 10 MPa/mm².

Uniaxial strip extensiometry further demonstrated that the anterior third of the corneal stroma is two- to threefold stiffer and stronger than the posterior two-thirds.[225] Using inflation tests, Descemet's membrane was measured to have a longitudinal Young's modulus of 0.5 to 2.6 MPa/mm² depending on the physiologic stress levels used during testing, which overall is less than that of the corneal stroma.[226] Uniaxial strip extensiometry measurements show considerable regional and directional anisotropy in the longitudinal cornea, as vertical and horizontal strips were stiffer (53% and 40%, respectively) and stronger (25% and 13%, respectively) than diagonal strips.[227] Cohesive or transverse (z-axis thickness-wise dimension) strength measurements, using modified strip extensiometry techniques, showed that Bowman's layer averages 50 g/mm, the anterior third of stroma proper averages 34 g/mm, the posterior two-thirds of stroma proper averages 20 g/mm, and Descemet's membrane averages 7 g/mm. This same study importantly documented a depth-dependent decrease in the cohesive strength in the corneal stroma, with a maximum at Bowman's layer and then a rapid decrease until reaching a plateau at approximately 40% to 80% in depth into the stroma before decreasing again in the posterior-most 20%. An approximately twofold increase in cohesive strength was also found comparing the peripheral cornea to central cornea. Interestingly, these z-directional cohesive strength measurements were quantitatively five- to fiftyfold less than the longitudinal x- and y-direction tensile strengths.

Inflation studies have further shown that cutting or ablating Bowman's layer and anterior corneal stroma down to approximately 150-μm depth results in anterior corneal flattening and peripheral corneal thickening, whereas deeper cuts or ablations into the stroma result in progressively more anterior corneal steepening rather than flattening.[228,229] According to Hjortdal,[230] after taking into account load-induced volume change, shallow ablations resulted in anterior corneal flattening because of similar inward inner and outer corneal wall strains. In contrast, deeper ablations result in anterior corneal steepening because outward outer corneal wall strains can be twofold higher than inward inner corneal wall strains.[230] Their conclusion was that this difference between outer and inner corneal wall strains was due to less shear resistance in the posterior two-thirds of the corneal stroma. Finally, using inflation testing, increasing age and increasing IOP have both been shown associated with increased stiffness of the human cornea, presumably owing to age-related crosslinking of the collagen fibrils and the changes in the viscoelastic properties of the interfibrillar matrix with increasing IOP.[229] In summary, measuring the viscoelastic biomechanical properties of the cornea is complicated, given its heterogeneous and anisotropic structure.[220] Further information about the innate biomechanical material properties of the human cornea are still needed, as the current information is far from complete.

Chronic biomechanical failure of the cornea—ectasia. In classical mechanics, acute damage and rupture occur when the stress reaches a critical value, which is called the ultimate tensile stress (UTS). In addition to overload-induced acute rupture, if you dissect a tendon and hang a lesser load (below the UTS) from it while keeping it moist, the tendon will become damaged or fatigued in a chronic, time-dependent fashion and eventually will rupture. This occurs because of tertiary creep and its associated micro- and nanostructural pathogenesis of interfibrillar crack initiation and propagation (known as "slippage" for biologic tissues). In fact, susceptibility to fatigue is a universal phenomenon in biologic tissues, which typically fail through constant static load (time-dependent damage owing to magnitude of the constant load and time of application of this load). In comparison, man-made structural materials typically fail through dynamic oscillatory loads (cycle-dependent damage owing to magnitude of the load and frequency of the cycling time). Cycling of the load may also accelerate the time-to-rupture of biologic tissues.

The human cornea's innate biomechanical properties depend on the composition and organization of collagen fibrils, as well as the matrix structures involved in force transmission between successive lamellar and fibrillar layers of collagenous tissue. This framework is essentially composed of 25-nm diameter, heterotypic type I collagen fibrils. The exact mechanical properties of these individual corneal collagen fibrils have not been evaluated or measured specifically. However, rat tendon studies found that individual 50-nm diameter, heterotypic type I collagen fibrils are moderately stiff, strong, and tough with only slight (~10%) extensibility, which is usually only evident when loaded under extreme physiologic stress. This suggests that corneal type I collagen fibrils do not stretch much under normal physiologic conditions or stressors. This seems to imply, at least from a theoretical perspective, that the matrix structures involved in force transmission between lamellar and fibrillar layers are the primary structures of the corneal stroma that are vulnerable to fatigue (tertiary creep or irreversible slippage) under physiologic circumstances.[231] Ultrastructural and x-ray scattering studies in corneal ectasia such as keratoconus or post-LASIK ectasia suggest that a chronic two-phase biomechanical matrix failure process of the stroma proper is the initiating and evolving pathophysiology, resulting in irreversible interlamellar slippage as opposed to collagen fibril failure (Fig. 4.28).[232–237]

In the scientific field of composite sciences, man-made laminate polymer matrix composites that are most similar to that of the human cornea (e.g., woven and nonwoven unidirectional fiber-reinforced laminate composites made of ductile matrix material) are known to undergo two similar chronic types of biomechanical matrix (or resin) failure processes, known as delamination and interfiber fracture (IFF).[238] These lead to breakdown of the matrix between lamina or fibers, respectively, causing redistribution of stresses within the laminate structure.[238] The quantitative amount of stress that causes this damage is the sum of the cycling rate of the stresses acting on the structure, the duration of time exposed to this stress, the temperature of the structure, the curvature and thickness of the structure, the laminate stacking sequence of the individual plies, and the innate biomechanical properties of the fibers and binding matrix. Nano- and micromechanical damage usually result from transverse compression or transverse shear stresses as opposed to transverse tension or longitudinal shear. Further damage can occur, eventually resulting in macroscopic interlaminar delamination between two layers and full-thickness intralaminar fractures of a layer. In essence, delamination and IFF cause concentrations of internal stress throughout the laminate composite, and accumulation of these damage sites can reduce the strength and toughness of the material without detectable thinning or bulging.[235]

Eventually, once the biomechanical failure process progresses to at least a moderate stage, the structure begins to become thinner. It typically only begins to bulge or undergo pathologic shape changes once a significant reduction in stiffness or significant increase in extensibility at late or severe stages occurs, before ultimately undergoing total structural failure during the end stage. Moreover, during the redistribution

of stress phase, further damage to other adjacent layers may occur even without significant external or internal increases in wall stress. Thus, from a composite science perspective, corneal ectasia essentially is the biologic equivalent of both delamination and IFF in the stroma proper. It is essentially a stereotypic, nonspecific chronic biomechanical failure response to multiple different specific stimuli, such as eye rubbing, LASIK surgery, family history (genetic conditions associated with environmental or behavioral eye rubbing), or possibly external nocturnal eye pressure.[239] The irreversible slippage caused by delamination and IFF can either be benign or harmful to the overall cornea, with the latter causing a gradual, progressive biomechanical failure process eventually leading to the ultimate failure of the structure through loss of shape and loss of refractive function. Although both delamination and IFF are universally seen in the nonwoven posterior two-thirds of the stroma proper, they can progress into the woven anterior third of the stroma proper. However, the woven anterior third of the stroma has a natural crack-stopping mechanism owing to the highly interwoven nature of its lamellae. This perhaps also explains why keratoconus rarely results in spontaneous rupture of the eye. Although the exact biomechanical changes in keratoconus are not completely understood, finite element modeling has suggested that incremental focal weaknesses can lead to the cone shape seen in keratoconus, further suggesting that focal weakening might be the common pathway in the multifactorial pathogenesis of keratoconus.[240]

Other functions
Drug delivery
Although there are several drug delivery routes into the anterior segment of the eye (Fig. 4.29A), topical instillation of ophthalmic drugs is the most common method used to administer treatments for ocular disease—evidenced by the fact that 90% of ophthalmic drug formulations are geared for topical drop use. The barriers to productive topical absorption of drugs into the anterior chamber are well documented, with the two major pathways to permeate these barriers being the transcorneal and transconjunctival pathways. The primary absorption pathway for small, lipophilic drugs is the transcorneal route and the primary absorption pathway for large, hydrophilic drugs is the transconjunctival (conjunctiva-sclera-ciliary body) route.[241] In order to understand these pathways, and therefore predict the drug's biologic effects on targeted anterior segment tissues, knowledge of the physicochemical properties of the drug and the pharmacokinetics of the tissues the drug must traverse is essential. Physicochemical properties describe the relationship between the chemical structure of the drug and its biologic effects. Various physicochemical properties of a drug—such as its molecular size (radii, weight, and shape), lipophilicity or hydrophilicity, degree of ionization—may optimize its biologic effects in the targeted tissue and/or may improve its pharmacokinetic profile. For example, positively charged molecules may exhibit permeability presumably owing to their binding to the negatively charged proteoglycan matrix within the conjunctiva.[242] Pharmacokinetics describes the process of absorption, distribution, metabolism, and elimination of a drug in a tissue, organ, or entire body, depending on the drug delivery route and its absorption pathways. It is a function of the intrinsic physicochemical properties of the drug being applied, the applied concentration and dosing frequency of the drug, the static permeability properties of the tissue, the dynamic metabolic and elimination mechanisms of the tissues it permeates, and the bioavailability of the administered drug at its target tissue site. Bioavailability describes how much of an instilled concentration of a drug actually reaches the target tissue (Box 4.4).

The advantages of topical drug delivery are its convenience and noninvasiveness, its avoidance of first-pass metabolism in the liver,

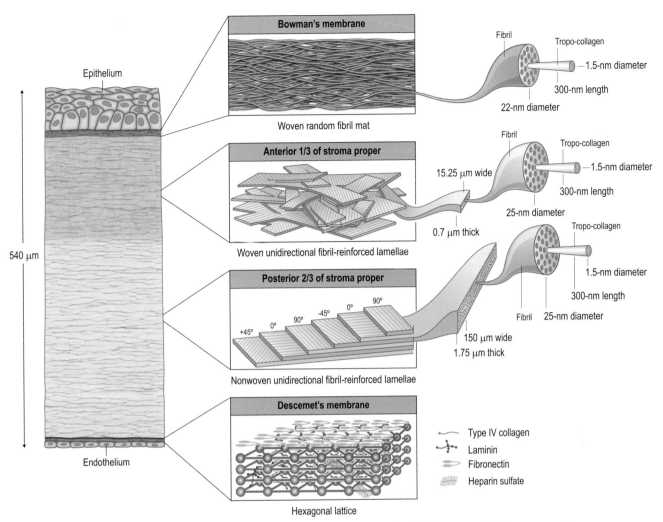

Fig. 4.28 The hierarchical structure of the cornea showing that it is basically composed of three composite-like regions. A fourth composite-like region, the Descemet's membrane, is included for completion's sake. The macroscopic to microscopic to nanoscopic features are emphasized (*from left to right*) to help illustrate the various interactions between the tissue components. The Bowman's layer is essentially a random fibril, woven mat composite, which maximizes multiaxial stiffness and strength. The underlying anterior third of the stroma proper is a lamellar interwoven fabric composed of unidirectional (UD) fibril-reinforced lamellae. This architectural hierarchy is much more reinforced against z-axis deformations compared to nonwoven UD laminates. In the human body, it is most similar to that of pericardium, which serves in mechanically preventing aneurysm formation of the heart. The posterior two-thirds of the stroma is essentially a nonwoven, UD fibril-reinforced lamellar composite, which maximizes longitudinal x- and y-axis stiffness and strength but has weak transverse z-axis stiffness and strength. In the human body, it is most similar to that of the annulus fibrosis of intervertebral disc, which functions efficiently as a cushioning mechanism for the spine but is prone to chronic biomechanical failure. The UD orientation of collagen fibrils in each lamella is important because this arrangement prevents fibril undulation and thus maximizes the initial axial tensile strength of each individual fibril. Descemet's membrane forms a hexagonal lattice. In toto, these composite-like regions characterize the overall stiffness, strength, extensibility, and toughness of the cornea. They also help explain how the cornea biomechanically behaves normally after surgery, disease, or injury.

and its ability to locally target cornea and anterior segment tissues with high drug concentrations. The main disadvantages of this route are its high dynamic drug clearance rates, and the static anatomic and physiologic permeability barriers to drug absorption, both of which contribute to low bioavailability.[241] On average, usually less than 5% to 10% of instilled topical drugs (average topical drop ~50 μL) reach the aqueous humor or even the corneal stroma (Fig. 4.29B), whereas the major portion (50%–99%) goes to the systemic circulation, primarily via absorption in the conjunctiva vasculature and lymphatics and/

or via absorption in the nasal mucosal vasculature owing to drainage in the nasolacrimal duct. Moreover, a drug resides in the conjunctival cul-de-sac for only about 5 to 6 minutes before being removed by the precorneal tear clearance mechanism (tear film volume 7–10 μL; tear turnover rate of 0.5–2.2 μL/min).[241] Even if the topical drug does get into the anterior or posterior chamber via the transcorneal or transconjunctival route, respectively, it usually only stays there briefly unless it is retained in depot form on the external surface or binds to proteins in the tissues it traverses because the aqueous humor removes it through

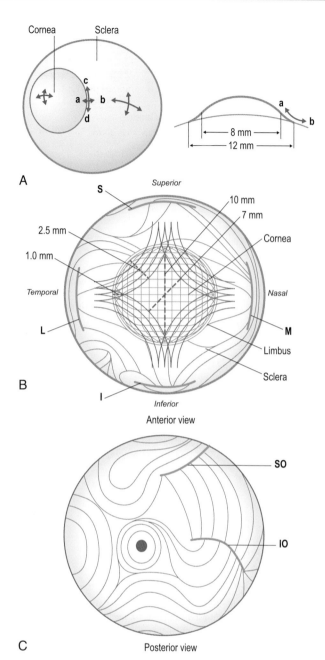

A

B

C

Anterior view

Posterior view

Fig. 4.29 The stress on the coats of the eye wall (*red lines with double-headed arrows* are shown in **A**) and the preferential orientation of the collagen fibrils (*solid gray and blue lines*) are shown in (**B**) and (**C**). (**A**) The lowest radial stress is in the cornea due to its smaller radius of curvature; the largest radial stress is under the rectus muscle insertion sites or at the equator of the globe due to its large radius of curvature and the fact that these are the thinnest regions of the sclera. The largest circumferential stress is at the limbus due to the sudden change in curvature going from the cornea to the sclera, which doubles the stress in the circumferential direction compared with the radial direction. (**B**) The central 4 to 5 mm of the cornea has collagen fibrils that are relatively uniformly directed in either the superior-inferior or the nasal-temporal direction. These fibrils appear to bend in the periphery of the cornea to coalesce and form the circumferential annulus. The diamond-shaped appearance of the central orthogonal collagen fibrils suggests that additional anchoring collagen fibrils come in from the sclera and limbus at one of the principal meridians (inferior, nasal, etc.), then curve within the peripheral cornea to exit an adjacent principal meridian 90 degrees away. Overall, this arrangement would aid in maintaining the peripheral flattening of the cornea and resisting the higher stress in that region of the cornea. It secondarily would not interfere with the central optical zone of the cornea. (**C**) The preferential direction of the sclera's collagen fibrils is radial in the anterior sclera, particularly in relation to the muscle insertion sites, whereas those at the equator are circumferential and those at the posterior sclera form circular whirls. The deep layers of sclera, which are not shown, form a net- or rhomboid-like layer diffusely throughout all regions of the sclera. *IO,* Inferior Oblique; *SO,* Superior Oblique. (Modified from Meek KM. In: Frazl P, ed. *Collagen: Structure and Mechanics.* New York: Springer; 2008:359–396; Aghamohammadzadeh H, Newton RH, Meek KM. X-ray scattering used to map the preferred collagen orientation in the human cornea and limbus. *Structure,* 2004;12[2]:249–256; and Watson PG, Hazelman B, Pavesio C, Green WR. *The Sclera and Systemic Disorders,* 2nd ed. Edinburgh, UK: Butterworth Heinemann; 2004.)

the trabecular meshwork (aqueous humor turnover rate 2–3 μL/min) or venous blood flow removes it through the porous anterior uvea.

After topical drug instillation, the peak concentration in the aqueous humor, or even the corneal stroma, is usually reached 30 minutes to 3 hours after application, but the bioavailability or concentration of drug in the corneal stroma or aqueous humor is reduced to approximately 1/1500th for lipophilic drugs and 1/150,000th for hydrophilic drugs compared with the original concentration of the eye drop.[243] From the aqueous humor, the drug has easy access to the uvea (iris and ciliary body). Here, the drug may bind to melanin, which may form a reservoir source that gradually releases the drug to the surrounding cells, thereby prolonging the drug activity (e.g., beta-blockers).[244,245] Drug distribution to the lens is much slower than to the uvea since it is composed of tightly packed lens proteins without melanin; however, sequestration of lipophilic drugs in cell membranes of the lens may serve as another potential depot reservoir source.[246] Topical drugs also reportedly can sometimes reach the vitreous cavity, most likely

via the conjunctival-scleral-choroid-retinal pigment epithelium (RPE)-retina or possibly the conjunctival-orbital-optic nerve head routes, where bioavailability is approximately one-millionth of the original concentration of the eye drop (Fig. 4.29B).[246] Various modifications can be made to topical drugs in order to increase their corneal absorption and bioavailability: (1) drug formulations are made to increase residence time in the conjunctival cul-de-sac (e.g., gels, suspensions, ointments, and inserts), or (2) compounds are added to topical drug solutions to increase corneal penetration (e.g., benzalkonium chloride [BAK], other preservatives, epithelial scraping [when treating fungal ulcers with antifungal drops]).[247]

In addition to dynamic clearance mechanisms, topical drug delivery is also hampered by various anatomic and physiologic barriers that affect the permeability properties of the tissue.[248] Topical drug delivery via the transcorneal route (Fig. 4.29A) is challenging because the drug needs to be small (<5 kDa) and lipophilic (e.g., prednisolone acetate) to bypass the intercellular zonula occludens tight junctions of the

Wound healing variability after common ophthalmic surgeries

The location of scar types along with the variable degree of wound healing responses in the human cornea is best exemplified when one reviews published human histopathology studies that describe findings in corneas that have had common ophthalmic procedures such as cataract extraction (CE), penetrating keratoplasty (PK), radial keratotomy (RK), astigmatic keratomy (AK), photorefractive keratectomy (PRK), or Laser-assisted in situ keratomileusis (LASIK) (Fig. 4.15). It is also apparent from these cases that acellular barrier layers, such as Bowman's layer, are not reformed if damaged or excised, whereas acellular basement membranes, such as the epithelial basement membrane and Descemet's membrane, can be regenerated.[334] Sutured and unsutured clear corneal CE wounds are corneal stromal incisions constructed at oblique angles to the corneal surface so that they self-seal. They usually heal with well-aligned external wound margins and wound edges, resulting in a small (50–75 μm in depth) subepithelial zone of hypercellular fibrotic stromal scarring and a remaining deeper zone of hypocellular primitive scarring (Fig. 4.15A).[318]

Occasional small epithelial plugs are found in the external wound of unsutured clear corneal cataract wounds, and sometimes Descemet's membrane is found partially detached or poorly realigned along the internal wound margin so that stromal ingrowth occurs. In marked contrast, limbal and scleral tunnel CE incisions heal because fibrovascular granulation tissue from the episclera completely grows into the wound by 15 days after surgery, with remodeling up to 2.5 years after surgery (early wound repair mechanisms in vascularized tissue are controlled by bioactive substances released by platelets at the wound site, such as platelet-derived growth factor and as opposed to epithelial-derived factors, such as TGF-β, seen in the avascular cornea).[335,336] PK wounds heal similarly to sutured clear corneal cataract wounds, with the notable differences of having significant wound compression because of the oversized nature of the donor button (usually 0.25–0.5mm) and wound edge mismatch caused by the irregular, asymmetric nature of the trephine wound found between donor and host wound edges. Additionally, a high percentage of PK cases have overriding external or internal wound edges with Bowman's layer or Descemet's membrane incarceration, which serves to cause weak areas in the hypercellular fibrotic scar or regenerated Descemet's membrane.[337]

Although of partial thickness (70%–95% depth) and being constructed perpendicular to the corneal surface, RK and AK incisions heal similarly to unsutured clear corneal cataract wounds.[338–340] The most notable difference from unsutured CE wounds is the more commonly present and more widely variable degree of external wound gaping found in these corneas, which commonly leads to epithelial ingrowth or plugging that rarely goes away long term (Fig. 4.15B).[340] PRK heals entirely under the influence of epithelial-stromal interactions. Therefore, a disc-shaped hypercellular fibrotic stroma scar is produced (Fig. 4.15C), which is usually 12% to 20% in thickness of the amount initially ablated.[341,342] In contrast, LASIK heals similar to that of unsutured clear corneal cataract incisions (Fig. 4.15D). A subepithelial zone of hypercellular fibrotic scarring occurs at the flap wound margin and the remainder heals by producing a hypocellular primitive stromal scar, usually with a thickness around 5% to 10% of the amount initially ablated.[343–345] However, a notable difference from unsutured CE wounds was that approximately 50% of the LASIK corneas were found to have at least some microscopic epithelial plugging present.

most superficial squamous corneal epithelial cells. In fact, on average, 90% of the corneal barrier to hydrophilic drug penetration is due to the resistance of the paracellular (intercellular) pathway. In contrast, on average, the corneal epithelium accounts for only 10% of the resistance to lipophilic drug permeation, as these drugs can penetrate the

epithelium via the transcellular (intracellular) pathway. In comparison to the epithelium, the corneal stroma is highly permeable to most lipophilic and hydrophilic drugs, although the main rate-limiting criterion is the molecular radius (size), owing to the 20-nm wide interfibrillar spaces.[249] Of note, although no significant changes in permeability have been reported with aging, the interfibrillar space of the corneal stroma does decrease 15% with aging. Also, interfibrillar spacing in the corneal stroma dynamically changes depending on tissue hydration and IOP levels of the eye. The corneal endothelium has static permeability properties for hydrophilic drugs that are only slightly less than that of the lipophilic drugs, reflecting the 10-nm wide intercellular spaces or discontinuities in the macula occludens tight junctions. As the static permeability properties of the corneal endothelium and stroma are actually quite similar, the corneal epithelium is the main barrier for drug absorption using the transcorneal route—which can be overcome quite easily if the drug molecules are small and lipophilic.

On the other hand, the transconjunctival route (Fig. 4.29A) allows passive diffusion of larger (<20 to 40kDa) or more hydrophilic molecules (e.g., beta-adrenergic antagonists, carbonic anhydrase inhibitors) than the transcorneal route because of its diffusely scattered goblet cell population, which contains leakier tight junctions, and a surface area nearly 18 times greater than that of the cornea.[249] Thus, the static permeability properties of the conjunctival epithelium are 50- to 100-times greater than the corneal epithelium.[246]

Other possible anterior segment drug delivery options include intrastromal, intracameral, and subconjunctival injections (Fig. 4.29A). Although all three of these routes produce the highest peak concentrations of drugs in the cornea or anterior segment, the major disadvantage is that the peak is often followed by low and persistent trough concentrations, unless given repeatedly and frequently.[249] Thus, the overall biologic efficacy of the drug may be less than optimal using these routes compared with topical drug delivery's moderate, but sustained drug concentrations in the targeted tissues, which are needed for therapeutic effects against corneal or anterior segment infection.[249]

Ultraviolet light filtration

The external surface of the human body is exposed to terrestrial sunlight that contains UV (∼295–400-nm wavelengths), visible (400–800nm), and infrared (IR; 800–1200nm) light.[250] Solar UV light undergoes significant scattering and absorption in the Earth's atmosphere such that most of the harmful, shortest wavelengths (<290nm), or all of the UVC rays (100–280nm) and 70% to 90% of the UVB rays (280–315nm) do not reach the Earth's surface. UV light contains more energy than visible or IR light and consequently has more potential to cause a photochemical injury or damage. When this radiation reaches the eye, the proportion absorbed by different structures depends on its wavelength and angle of incidence, with maximal absorption occurring when UV light rays are parallel to the pupillary axis. Although the cornea is more sensitive to UV light injury than the skin because it has no melanin, individuals seldom experience acute UV sunburns unless direct high exposure occurs. Such injuries occur in "snow blindness" (this is common when skiing at midday without goggles, as snow reflects 85% of incident UV light as opposed to only 1%–2% from grass) or when welding without UV eye protection since welding arcs emit harmful UV-C and UV-B radiation.

There also is considerable variability in UV light exposure to the eye as the terrestrial UV-B exposure spectrum varies enormously with solar elevation in the sky and other exposure-related factors, such as the albedo ratio (percentage reflectance of UV light) from the ground surface.[251] As human photoreceptors and corneal nerves cannot detect UV light, suprathreshold and, more importantly, repeated subthreshold UV light injury can take place without the individual knowing it.

This can cause acute photokeratitis of the epithelial surface or chronic irreversible keratopathies to the epithelium and anterior parts of the corneal stroma. The cornea absorbs 100% of incident UV-C, 90% of incident UV-B, and 60% of incident UV-A radiation (Fig. 4.30).[250] It, therefore, is the major filter of UV light for wavelengths of 200 to 300 nm, protecting the lens and retina from damage.[252] All UV-C radiation is absorbed in the corneal epithelium due to its high ascorbic acid content. UV-B is absorbed primarily in the anterior 100 μm of the human cornea, especially the epithelium and Bowman's layer, owing to high amounts of tryptophan residues in the proteins of the Bowman's layer and anterior stroma and the previously mentioned high ascorbic acid content in the epithelium.[253–256] UV-A (315–400 nm) is only partially attenuated by the cornea (Fig. 4.30), but the transmitted portion is nearly all absorbed by the lens so that only a minor percentage (<3%) reaches the retina. Short visible wavelengths, such as violet (~400 nm) and blue (~475 nm) light, pass through the cornea and lens predominantly unattenuated (85%–90% transmittance) before being absorbed by the retina and RPE. These wavelengths are less harmful to biologic tissues than UV light, but are still capable of photochemical injury and damage, particularly if the duration of exposure is long or cumulative. Evidence to support the detrimental health effects of UV light on the eye with the acute and chronic ocular conditions for which UV light has been suggested to be a causative agent is listed in Table 4.5 and includes several conjunctival, corneal, iris, lens, and possible retinal disorders.[250]

Acute overexposure to UV-B and UV-C damages the corneal epithelium by causing apoptosis, or programmed cell death.[257] UV-B and UV-C exposure directly activates signaling molecules and enzymes in corneal epithelia, including JNK, SEK, p53, caspase 9, and caspase 3, all of which lie in the pathway that leads to classic apoptotic events such as DNA fragmentation and formation of apoptotic bodies.[258–260] This culminates in massive shedding of corneal epithelial cells within hours of exposure. Studies of corneal epithelial cells in culture show that a very early event leading to apoptosis is activation of K^+ channels by UV. This activation of channels occurs within minutes of exposure and apoptosis can be prevented by K^+ channel blockers. In contrast, chronic overexposure to UV-B and UV-A best explains the high frequency and variable degree of acquired cytogenic DNA damage found in the keratocytes of normal adult corneas.[252]

A second injury mechanism by which UV, violet, and blue light works is through the generation of reactive oxygen species (ROS), such as hydrogen peroxide, singlet oxygen, and oxygen free radicals (superoxide anions and hydroxyl radicals), which cause cellular and extracellular damage by reacting with lipids, proteins, and DNA. Under normal physiologic conditions, the cornea and anterior segment protect themselves from ROS by producing and maintaining sufficient antioxidant levels, including several low-molecular-weight (ascorbic acid, glutathione and alpha-tocopherol) and high-molecular-weight (catalase, superoxide dismutase, glutathione peroxidase, and reductase) antioxidants.[252] Ascorbic acid is thought to be the primary antioxidant in the cornea and anterior segment of the human eye as it is produced in such high concentrations in the aqueous humor.[261] The danger to the cornea from ROS appears to stem from excessive UV-B exposure (as opposed to UV-A or UV-C exposure), as experiments have shown that only UV-B excess leads to profound decreases in corneal antioxidants. Thus, an imbalance in the pro-oxidant to antioxidant ratio can take place in the anterior 100 μm of the cornea, which may lead to oxidative eye injury and inflammation as the tissue components of the cornea then become the predominant absorbers of UV light.[262]

SCLERA

The human sclera is a relatively avascular, white, rigid, dense connective tissue that covers the globe posterior to the cornea (see Fig. 4.1A,B; 4.3A; and 4.31A).[263] Evidence demonstrates that although the sclera has low baseline metabolic requirements, it constantly remodels throughout life to maintain its functions and thus is far from inert.[264,265] In comparison to the cornea, major differences in the sclera are that it (1) has variably larger collagen fibril diameters and interfibrillar spaces (compare Fig. 4.32B to Fig. 4.10A–C); (2) is more opaque, interwoven (Fig. 4.33D), and rigid; (3) has a regional zone of vascularity in the episclera (Fig. 4.33D); and (4) does not have adjacent external or internal cellular barrier layers. The color of the sclera is opaquely white because it scatters all frequencies of visible light owing to spatial fluctuations in the refractive index of the tissue, which have dimensions that are greater than a half-wavelength of visible light (Fig. 4.32B and C).[265,266] The opaqueness reduces internal light scattering, but some light actually does transmit through the sclera, evidenced when transilluminating the globe. The interwoven rigidity helps maintain a stable shape because deformation of the sclera could lead to poor vision or internal injury (Fig. 4.32D). It is also notable for containing a moderately rich nerve supply (Fig. 4.14A), predominantly around episcleral blood vessels, and it has no lymphatic channels, albeit the overlying conjunctiva has two well-formed lymphatic layers (Fig. 4.33C,D). The cornea limbus represents the junction between the avascular cornea that should be devoid of lymphatics, and the transition to the corneosclera, sclera, and episcleral, which have blood and lymphatic vessels.[267] The episclera is a thin, dense layer of connective tissue consisting mainly of collagen bundles that run circumferentially and merge with the stroma, sparsely populated with elastic fibers, melanocytes, and macrophages.[263] The principal functions of the sclera are to provide a strong, tough external framework to protect the delicate intraocular structures and to maintain the shape of the globe so that the retinal image is undisturbed. Secondarily, it serves as a stable expansive-resistant semispherical structure to the forces generated by IOP, facilitates appropriate aqueous outflow, and provides stable attachment sites for the extraocular muscles to rotate the globe and for the ciliary muscle to accommodate the lens. It also provides a conduit for vascular and neural pathways, and plays a critical role in determining the axial length of the eye, thereby the refractive error of the eye.

Embryology, growth, development, and aging

The sclera is predominantly neural crest-derived, except for a small temporal portion that comes from the mesoderm. The development of the sclera begins by 6.5 weeks of gestation in humans and proceeds in an anterior-to-posterior and inside-to-outside fashion as the anterior periocular mesenchyme, derived from the second wave of neural crest cell invasion, condenses anteriorly on the optic cup. This anterior mesenchyme subsequently differentiates into an inner vascular layer that develops into the uvea (iris, ciliary body, and choroid) and an outer fibrous layer that develops into the sclera. The RPE and/or the choroid is directly responsible for embryonic scleral development—if the RPE or choroid is absent or not in contact with the sclera, the sclera does not develop (e.g., chorioretinal colobomas) or will not grow, respectively. The anterior sclera fully differentiates by 7 weeks' gestation followed by the equatorial sclera at 8 weeks' gestation and the posterior sclera by 11 weeks' gestation. It gradually increases in thickness and extracellular matrix denseness during the remaining months of gestation. Initially it is primarily composed of scleral fibroblasts, collagen fibrils, and proteoglycans; elastin fibers are acquired mainly after birth. At birth,

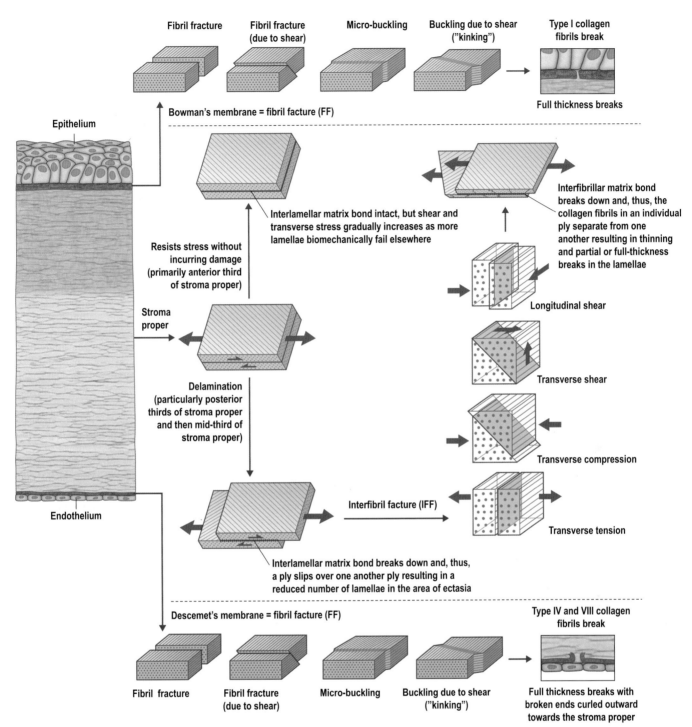

Fig. 4.30 Diagram illustrating how the four composite-like regions of the cornea biomechanically fail when undergoing ectasia. In essence, ectasia appears to be a stereotypic chronic biomechanical failure response to multiple different stimuli. According to Alfred Puck's theory, laminated fiber polymer matrix composites, such as the corneal stroma, biomechanically fail through three pathways: fibril fracture (FF), interfibril fracture (IFF), and/or delamination. Although FFs are seen in Bowman's layer and Descemet's membrane in late stages of ectatic disease, they are not the cause of the ectasia, but are rather secondary events to the biomechanical failure process going on in the stroma proper. The initiating and evolving pathology causing the ectasia is due to delamination and subsequent IFF, which is seen in the stroma proper, particularly in the posterior-most regions of the cornea. This two-step biomechanical failure process leads to ectasia through gradual cumulative damage rather than an acute event. Interestingly, delamination and subsequent IFF can also occur in a benign fashion, depending on type and degree of stress. Although delamination and IFF both take place and are clearly seen using ultrastructure studies in the posterior two-thirds of the corneal stroma, it does progress to the anterior third of the stroma proper. However, in the anterior third of the stroma proper, ultrastructurally IFF appears to dominate as the interlamellar slippage resulting from the delamination step is minimized by crack-stopping mechanisms due to the interwoven nature of lamellae in this region of the stroma proper. FF usually is associated with acute ultimate failure of its individual composite-like layer, which results in acute loss of biomechanical and barrier function in that specific layer. For example, FF of Bowman's layer results in the clinical appearance of subepithelial fibrotic scarring, which is seen histopathologically as full-thickness breaks in Bowman's layer with outgrowth of hypercellular fibrotic stromal scar tissue. In another example, FF of Descemet's membrane results in the acute clinical appearance of corneal hydrops owing to loss of endothelial barrier function, which is seen histopathologically as full-thickness Descemet's membrane breaks with curled outward fracture edges and endothelial cell discontinuity. Delamination may be seen clinically at the slit lamp as Vogt's striae, which are often found during early to moderate stages of ectasia in the posterior-most regions of the corneal stroma. (Modified from Knops M. *Analysis of Failure in Fiber Polymer Laminates: The Theory of Alfred Puck*. Heidelberg, Germany: Springer; 2008; and Reifsnider K. In: McNicol L, Strahlman E, eds. *Corneal Biophysics Workshop. Corneal Biomechanics and Wound Healing*. Bethesda, MD: NEI; 1989.)

TABLE 4.5   Ocular diseases potentially due to ultraviolet radiation exposure

	Strength of evidence
EXTERNAL:	
Photokeratitis	High
Climatic droplet keratopathy	Medium
Pterygium	Medium
Pinguecula	Low
Carcinoma in situ/conjunctival squamous cell carcinoma	Low
IRIS:	
Melanoma	Low
LENS:	
Cataract	Medium
Exfoliation (more likely related to infrared light)	None
Anterior lens capsule changes	Medium
CHOROID/RETINA:	
Solar retinopathy	High
Photomaculopathy (more likely related to blue or visible violet light)	None
Uveal melanoma	Low
Age-related macular degeneration (AMD)	Low

matrix of the sclera to undergo constant remodeling during childhood eye growth, continuing to some extent into adult life—albeit to a lesser degree.[264] This visual feedback mechanism serves to guide childhood eye growth toward emmetropia and the attainment of adult eye size. Interestingly, this visual feedback mechanism is not dependent on the CNS. In animal studies, transection of the optic nerve or blocking ganglion cell action potentials does not prevent the development or the recovery of experimentally induced myopia.[264] Rather, it is directly dependent on paracrine cytokine or growth factor pathways (e.g., dopamine, acetylcholine) originating from the retina and/or RPE.[264] Animal experiments that pharmacologically damage the retinal photoreceptors or RPE prevent visual deprivation myopia. Epidemiologic studies suggest that environmental visual stimuli (e.g., lack of outdoor time with excessive near work),[270] or genetic factors may alter this visual feedback mechanism resulting in physiologic or pathologic myopia.[271]

A breakdown of this emmetropization process may result in refractive error progression outside the normal period of eye growth, such as adolescent-onset (16–20 years of age) or adult-onset (second to fourth decades of life) myopia, owing to further axial length and posterior scleral elongation.[272-274] The exact pathogenesis of myopia is still not completely understood, but myopia induction in mammalian animal models using various visual deprivation stimuli suggests that the earliest biochemical and structural remodeling changes begin with reduced scleral fibrocyte proliferation and altered metabolism resulting in reduced type I collagen fibril synthesis, increased collagen degradation (increased matrix metalloproteinase-2 expression), reduced proteoglycan synthesis, scleral tissue volume loss (loss of both scleral wet and dry weight), and posterior scleral thinning.[275] Chronic biochemical and structural remodeling includes reduction of mean type I collagen fibril diameters, particularly in the outer layers of the sclera. In advanced or late stages, localized areas of circumscribed outpouching of the posterior sclera known as staphyloma may form, especially at the optic nerve or the macula.[275] Although some studies have suggested that annular arrangement of the scleral collagen bundles around the optic nerve head and the fovea would increase the local susceptibility of the sclera to deformation, the exact mechanism of staphyloma formation in pathologic myopia may not rely entirely on scleral mechanisms.[276]

All of these biochemical and structural changes appear to be guided by a retino-RPE-scleral visual signaling pathway, which dynamically controls scleral extensibility under the stress of normal IOP and thus controls the innate biomechanical properties of the sclera.[271] Biomechanical testing of myopic human eyes by Avetisov and associates[269] supports this theory, as the thinned posterior sclera was 30% to 40% biomechanically weaker in tensile strength than normal eyes. Animal studies by McBrien and associates[264] have also shown that posterior scleral creep rates during acute periods of myopia induction are significantly higher in myopic eyes compared with normal control eyes. Interestingly, using animal models, after removal of the myopia-inducing visual deprivation stimulus, recovery to normal eye size is quite rapid and is thought to be due to scleral keratocyte differentiation into contractile myofibroblasts and possibly due to resumption of normal proteoglycan synthesis.[264] In contrast to animals allowed to recover naturally, some myopic animals had their myopia corrected with optical devices (analogous to spectacles in humans). The myopic biomechanical scleral phenotype persisted and thus recovery from the induced myopic state was aborted—although the eyes did return to a more normal stable growth rate.[264] Such a finding may have important implications for the correction of myopia in humans as prevention of the aberrant remodeling process seems to be the key to any potentially successful medical or optical therapy for myopia.[277] Another promising medical treatment option is that of crosslinking the sclera in a manner that might serve to stabilize or halt myopic progression.[278] Currently,

the sclera is relatively thin, highly distensible (in infancy, the sclera is on average one-quarter as stiff as it is in adulthood), and translucent (explaining why the blue color from the underlying uvea often shows through the infant sclera).

Postnatal growth and maturation continue in a similar anterior-to-posterior fashion. During the first 3 years of life, the sclera grows rapidly in diameter and thickness, gradually losing some of its high distensibility (owing to increased thickness, decreased cellularity, increased extracellular matrix denseness, and proportionally increased type I collagen fibril deposition), but it still remains relatively translucent. This early loss of distensibility explains why the sclera can expand from increased IOP (e.g., infantile glaucoma) only from birth to around an age of 3 years old, resulting in a buphthalmic "ox" eye. Thereafter, the sclera distends only slightly from increased IOP, mainly in the lamina cribosa. After age 3 years, the sclera thickens further, becomes more opaque, and grows in diameter at a much slower rate than during the first 3 years of life, reaching adult size by 13 to 16 years of age.[268] During this growth period, the anterior sclera develops and matures much more quickly (adult size by 2 years of age) than the equatorial (adult size by 13 years of age) and the posterior sclera (adult size by 13–16 years of age). The sclera continues to become less distensible and more rigid with advancing age, primarily because of maturation and age-related glycation-induced crosslinking of collagen fibrils (scleral stiffness reportedly increases two- to threefold from age 3 to 20 years, and then another twofold from age 20 to 78 years), typically resulting in no further eye or scleral growth after age 16 years.[269]

Normal eye growth is thought to be controlled in part by a visual feedback mechanism that depends on the quality of the retinal image. This feedback influences the scleral fibrocytes and thus the extracellular

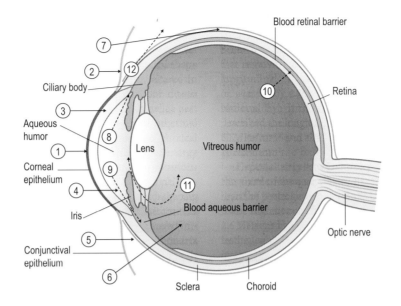

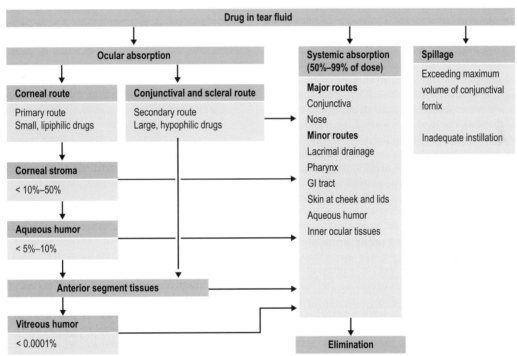

Fig. 4.31 (**A**) Diagram of the eye with common drug delivery routes (*solid arrows*) and clearance pathways (*dotted arrows*) illustrated. The numbers refer to the following processes: (1) transcorneal route from the tear film across the cornea into the anterior chamber; (2) transconjunctival route across the conjunctiva, sclera, and anterior uvea into the posterior chamber; (3) intrastromal route directly into corneal stroma; (4) intracameral route directly into anterior chamber; (5) subconjunctival route from the anterior subconjunctival space across the sclera and anterior uvea into the posterior chamber or across the sclera, choroid, retinal pigment epithelium (RPE), and retina into the anterior vitreous; (6) intravitreal drug injection directly into the vitreous; (7) sub-Tenon route from the posterior sub-Tenon space across the sclera, choroid, RPE, and retina into the posterior vitreous; (8) elimination of drug in the aqueous humor across the trabecular meshwork and Schlemm's canal into the systemic vascular circulation; (9) elimination of drug in the aqueous humor across the uvea into the systemic vascular circulation; (10) elimination of drug in the vitreous humor across the blood-retinal barrier to the systemic vascular circulation; (11) drug elimination from the vitreous across anterior hyaloid face to the posterior chamber or vice versa; (12) drug elimination from subconjunctival and/or episcleral space to systemic lymphatic or vascular circulation. (From Urtti A. Challenges and obstacles of ocular pharmacokinetics and drug delivery. *Adv Drug Deliv Rev.* 2006;58(11):1131–1135). (**B**) Pharmacokinetics of topical eye drop drug delivery. (Modified from Cruysberg L. Novel methods of ocular drug delivery. Ph.D thesis. University of Maastricht; 2008.)

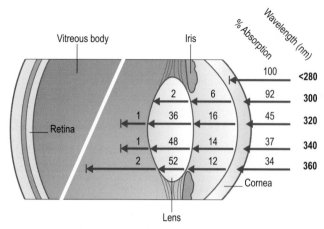

Fig. 4.32 The UV light absorption spectra for different structures in the eye. (From Johnson G. The environment and the eye. *Eye.* 2004;18:1235–1250. https://doi.org/10.1038/sj.eye.6701369.)

the proposed mechanism of axial elongation in myopia involves scleral remodeling, that is, the rearrangement of existing material owing to microdeformations that retain scleral volume, rather than scleral growth.[264]

Age-related changes to the sclera involve changes to its structure and composition, leading to increased stiffness.[279] In elderly individuals, the sclera often becomes somewhat yellowish due to a fine deposition of lipid. Another common finding is a small rectangular area of grayish-blue translucency just anterior to the insertion of the medial and lateral rectus muscles. These changes are known as senile scleral plaques and are associated with deposition of calcium in scleral regions that are under strain and exposed to the environment.[263] They are never found adjacent to unexposed superior or inferior rectus muscles (Box 4.5).

Major scleral reference points and measurements

The sclera is an incomplete sphere (Fig. 4.31A,B), resulting in an average outer surface area of 16.3 cm², an average outer diameter of 24 mm, and an average inner diameter of 23 mm (mean radius of curvature = 11.5 mm).[263] Knowing the topographic curvature of the anterior sclera is important for fitting scleral contact lenses, which can have certain advantages over corneal contact lenses, including the ability to optically neutralize almost any corneal topographical shape as the lens is borne solely by the sclera and not the cornea. They can be more comfortable than some corneal contact lenses, as the edge of the lenses do not touch the eyelids and can be better for some forms of aqueous dry eye deficiency because a large precorneal tear film reservoir is trapped between the lens and the entire corneal surface. On average, the sclera is thickest posteriorly near the optic nerve (1.0–1.35 mm), decreasing gradually as it approaches the equator of the globe (0.4–0.6 mm), before typically becoming thinnest under the rectus muscles just before it reaches its insertion sites (0.3 mm) (Fig. 4.31C).[280] It then gradually increases in thickness at the actual muscle insertion sites (0.6 mm) and continues getting thicker up to the limbus (0.8 mm), where it blends with the cornea (Fig. 4.31C).[280] However, these average scleral thickness measurements are subject to great variation amongst individuals, especially in eyes with myopia[276] (Box 4.6).

There are two major openings in the sclera: the anterior scleral foramen (13.7-mm diameter; circumscribes the area of the cornea

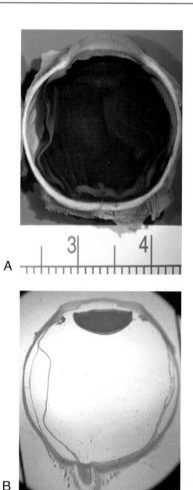

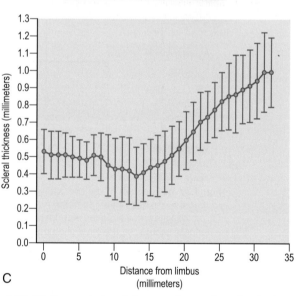

Fig. 4.33 (A) Gross photo of the superior section of a horizontally bisected normal globe demonstrating the cross-sectional appearance of the sclera, limbus, and cornea. **(B)** Photomicrograph of a normal globe showing the cross-sectional appearance of the sclera, limbus, and cornea (PAS, ×2). **(C)** Line graph summarizing the average scleral thickness (± standard deviation) vs. distance from the limbus in normal eyes (n = 55). (From Olsen TW, Aaberg SY, Geroski DH, Edelhauser HF. Human sclera: Thickness and surface area. *Am J Ophthalmol.* 1998;125(2):237–241. https://doi.org/10.1016/S0002-9394(99)80096-8.)

BOX 4.5 Endothelial cell injury

There are many exogenous stresses that could potentially damage the corneal endothelium (Fig. 4.25). Although accidental trauma and infection are perhaps the most common, they usually are preventable or are difficult to prognosticate because so many variables need to be considered. Several common interventions that might stress a person's corneal endothelium are contact lens wear, excimer laser-based keratorefractive surgery, and intraocular surgery.

Contact lenses

Contact lens wear does not cause loss of endothelial cell density (ECD), but it can cause acute reversible corneal edema and, in the long term, increased polymegathism and decreased pleomorphism.[157] The corneal endothelium utilizes the same carbohydrate metabolic pathways as the corneal epithelium. However, the transport function of the endothelial cell is higher than that of the epithelial cell due to its high baseline metabolic rate, which requires oxidative activity that is five to six times that of the epithelial cell.[157] Atmospheric oxygen is the primary source of oxygen to the endothelium. Interruption of this oxygen supply by low oxygen transmissibility contact lenses or a low oxygen environment (e.g., eyelid closing) will result in a shift to anaerobic metabolism, a concurrent increase in stromal lactic acid and CO_2 production, and a drop in stromal pH.[346] Hypoxia can also stimulate epithelial production of 12(R)HETE, a potent inhibitor of the endothelial Na^+/K^+-ATPase pump sites.[346] Acute reversible endothelial changes observed with hypoxia include stromal swelling, endothelial dysfunction, and endothelial blebbing. Chronic hypoxia can eventually lead to irreversible endothelial polymegathism and pleomorphism. In fact, Polse and associates[347] have shown that chronic corneal hypoxia in humans alters the endothelium's ability to reverse induced swelling.

Surgical injury

Excimer laser-based keratorefractive surgery has been found to induce acute loss of barrier function and reversible endothelial cell stress (increased polymegathism and decreased pleomorphism) only if performed on a cornea with a residual stromal bed thickness $\leq 200\,\mu m$, owing to the shockwave effect from photoablation. As refractive surgeons rarely or never ablate to this depth because of concerns for the risk of ectasia, there appear to be no short- or long-term endothelial effects from this type of surgery in the current clinical setting.[346]

By comparison, all intraocular surgeries have been found to cause varying degrees of both acute and, perhaps more importantly, chronic damage to the corneal endothelium. Modern small-incision cataract surgery ($\leq$1.5-mm incisions for microincision cataract surgery [MICS]; ~3.5-mm incisions for phacoemulsification) may have advantages over larger incision techniques (~7- to 12-mm incisions for extracapsular cataract extraction [ECCE]).[348,349] However, phacoemulsification can cause significant endothelial cell injury owing to a number of factors, such as corneal distortion, ricocheting of nuclear fragments, intraocular lens or intraocular instrument contact, and release of free radicals.[350] A randomized controlled trial showed that phacoemulsification caused an exponential reduction in central ECD up to 1 year after surgery, with ECD loss averaging 10.5%.[350] However, no significant changes in polymegathism or pleomorphism were found.[350] This fast-component period of cell loss is statistically similar to that observed following ECCE, another common surgical alternative technique used for performing cataract surgery, particularly in developing countries, which results in an average 9.1% reduction in ECD at 1 year after surgery.[350] Long-term endothelial cell loss data suggest that an annual cumulative cell loss rate of 2.5% exists from 1 to 10 years after ECCE surgery (fourfold higher than normal physiologic annual cell loss rates).[350,351] However, there is currently no significant evidence to support ECCE over phacoemulsification or to support one cataract technique over another (e.g., divide-and-conquer vs. phaco-chop) from an ECD loss standpoint as they all seem to be statistically similar.[352,353]

Data on two phakic refractive intraocular lens (IOL) procedures commercially available in the US, Verisyse (Ophthec, Gronigen, The Netherlands/AMO, Santa Ana, California) and the foldable Visian Implantable Collamer Lens (ICL, Visian ICL 4; STAAR Surgical Co., Monrovia, California), show less acute component damage than standard cataract surgery (Verisyse: ~7% ECD loss and Visian ICL: ~3% ECD at 1 year after surgery).[354,355] However, just as with ECCE, a chronic, slow-component annual cumulative cell loss rate is found from 1 to 5 years postoperatively, which is approximately four- to fivefold higher than normal physiologic cell loss rates (Verisyse: ~2.7% ECD loss/year and Visian ICL: 2.5% ECD loss/year between 1 and 5 years after surgery).

Corneal transplantation surgery (e.g., PK) has been found associated with significant long-term ECD loss, perhaps because of the peripheral loss of stem-like cells or the peripheral storage zone (Fig. 4.21A).[172] Long-term longitudinal studies up to 20 years after PK surgery show that ECD loss occurs in two phases, i.e., early and late postoperative.[356] During the early postoperative phase, the central ECD decreases exponentially with 36.7% ECD loss at 1 year and 8.4% ECD loss/year up to 5 years after surgery. Thereafter, a slow late postoperative phase occurs in which central ECD loss decreases to a linear rate of 4.2% ECD loss/year.[356] Concurrently, polymegathism gradually increases and pleomorphism gradually decreases throughout the longitudinal follow-up period.

Over the last decade, surgical techniques for corneal transplantation have changed markedly as techniques such as posterior lamellar keratoplasty (PLK), deep lamellar endothelial keratoplasty (DLEK), Descemet's stripping endothelial keratoplasty (DSEK), Descemet's stripping automated endothelial keratoplasty (DSAEK), and Descemet's membrane endothelial keratoplasty (DMEK) have evolved to take the place of PK for endothelial cell disorders.[297,357] Currently, DSAEK has become the surgical technique of choice for corneal endothelial diseases, compared with the more traditional full-thickness PK surgery.[358,359] The preferred approach of DSAEK, however, may soon be supplanted by DMEK.[360] However, long-term endothelial cell loss leading to late endothelial failure remains a concern in both DSAEK and DMEK,[361,362] although studies show similar short-term rates of ECD loss (35%–39% central ECD cell loss at 1 year postoperatively) to those observed after PK.[361,362]

Finally, there are other surgical adjuvants or new procedures on the horizon that could affect the corneal endothelium. The surgical adjuvant that is currently of most interest is topical mitomycin C (MMC) application, which is applied after excimer laser-based keratorefractive surface surgery to prevent or treat corneal haze caused by subepithelial scarring. Currently, there appears to be no evidence of short- or long-term ECD loss or keratocyte toxicity, if a single local application of MMC is used at a concentration of 0.02% to 0.002% for an exposure duration of 12 seconds to 2 minutes.[363,364] The medical procedure that is currently of most interest is corneal collagen crosslinking with riboflavin and UVA light (CXL), which is a promising treatment option for the disease of corneal ectasia.[365,366] Currently, no evidence of endothelial cell damage has been found, but most of the studies are short-term and small in number, and are under strict research protocols.[366,367]

Pharmacologic toxicity

In addition to surgical injury, the corneal endothelium can also be influenced by pharmacologic toxicity.[368] Past studies that helped guide the development of intraocular irrigating solutions found that the best were those most similar to aqueous humor in composition. BSS Plus (Alcon Laboratories, Ft. Worth, TX, USA) is currently the most physiologically compatible intraocular solution (Table 4.3); BSS is probably the next best alternative (Table 4.3). The main ingredients required for intraocular solutions to be biologically compatible with the corneal endothelium are electrolyte levels matching those in the aqueous humor, glucose as an energy source, bicarbonate as a buffer, and glutathione as an antioxidant/free radical scavenger. Intraocular tissues, particularly the corneal endothelium,

(Continued)

BOX 4.5 Endothelial cell injury—cont'd

require a pH between 6.7 and 8.1 and an osmolality between 270 and 350 mOsm. Furthermore, any medication used intraocularly needs to be at a nontoxic concentration and contain no preservatives. Pharmacologic toxicity to the anterior segment tissues of the eye, including the corneal endothelium, has become better understood through the discovery of a condition known as toxic anterior segment syndrome (TASS).[368] TASS is a sterile postoperative inflammatory reaction caused by a noninfectious substance that enters the anterior segment, resulting in toxic damage to intraocular tissues. Most cases are severe, resulting in >50% loss of central ECD. The injury typically starts 12 to 48 hours after cataract or anterior segment surgery and is limited to the anterior segment of the eye. It is always Gram stain and culture negative and usually improves with steroid treatment. The primary differential diagnosis is infectious endophthalmitis.

The possible causes of TASS include intraocular solutions with an inappropriate chemical composition, drug concentration, pH, or osmolality. It can also be caused by preservatives, enzymatic detergents, bacterial endotoxin, oxidized metal deposits and residues, and factors related to intraocular lens processing, such as retained residues from polishing or sterilizing the lenses (Table 4.4).[368] Because TASS is an environmental and toxic control issue, it has made anterior segment surgeons and surgical staff more aware that maintaining the health of the corneal endothelium requires a thorough understanding of all medications and fluids used during surgery. Additionally, it has helped all involved in surgical eye care understand the importance of proper cleaning and sterilization of intraocular instruments since most cases of TASS appear to be directly caused by retained detergents or contaminated water sources.

and limbus) and the posteronasally located fenestrated posterior scleral foramen or scleral canal (1.5- to 2.0-mm internal diameter and 3.5-mm external diameter). The inner third of the sclera forms a fenestrated scaffold in the scleral canal called the lamina cribosa that supports the optic nerve axons, whereas the outer posterior two-thirds of the sclera merge with the dura mater of the optic nerve, leaving the outer posterior two-thirds of the scleral canal essentially free of any scleral support. Traditionally, it has been postulated that elevated IOP deforms the lamina cribosa, leading to ganglion cell injury and resultant optic neuropathy. However, peripapillary scleral thickness also plays a big role in optic nerve head biomechanics, with decreased thickness resulting in increased maximum strain in the lamina cribosa—whereas chronic raised IOP has been shown to cause scleral remodeling and stiffening of the peripapillary sclera.[279] There are also other numerous minor openings in the sclera, including 30 to 40 emissary channels for ciliary arteries, veins, and nerves, and 4 to 7 vortex vein channels. The outer surface of the sclera is smooth, except where the tendons of the extraocular muscles insert (spiral of Tillaux and oblique muscle insertion sites) and where Tenon's capsule adheres (within 1 mm of limbus, over rectus muscle insertion sites, and around the optic nerve)—depicted in Fig. 4.33. The superficial layer of the sclera, called the episclera, is a thin, highly vascularized, dense connective tissue. It is around 15- to 20-μm thick near the limbus, progressively thinning as it extends into the posterior aspect of the eye.[279] The scleral stroma proper is a white, avascular, dense connective tissue accounting for more than 95% of the total scleral thickness. Finally, the inner surface of the sclera is a brown, avascular, 5-μm-thick layer called the lamina fusca, which contains a large number of elastin fibers and melanocytes.

Mechanical properties

The mechanical behavior of the sclera is most dependent on its thickness and innate biomechanical properties (hierarchical structure of collagen and its associated crosslinks). Because of its toughness, cohesiveness, and tightly interwoven architecture, the sclera is not easily dissected in a blunt fashion. The sclera is predominantly composed of water (68%) that is stabilized in a disorganized structural network of insoluble and soluble extracellular proteins with fewer fibrocytes than the cornea (see Table 4.1).[263] The posterior sclera is more hydrated than the equatorial and anterior sclera (71% vs. 62%).[281] The dry weight of the adult human sclera (see Table 4.1) is comprised of collagen, proteoglycans, fibrocyte constituents, elastin, blood vessel constituents,

BOX 4.6 Clinical biomechanical testing

Recently, the study of in vivo corneal biomechanics has rapidly evolved. Traditionally, corneal topography and tomography (two- and three-dimensional reconstruction of thickness profiles) indirectly infer information about the innate biomechanical properties of the cornea based on shape and thickness changes, respectively.[238] However, recent improvements in imaging have improved the ability to predict the probability of ectasia after corneal refractive surgery, progression in keratoconus patients and improve accuracy of tonometry measurements. The Ocular Response Analyzer (ORA; Reichert Corporation; Depew, USA) was the first commercial device that measures the corneal response to indentation with an air pulse (principally similar to air pulse noncontact tonometry).[369,370] This is the first instrument that purportedly directly measures the innate biomechanical properties of the cornea in vivo. The two biomechanical properties that it currently measures are corneal hysteresis (CH) and corneal resistance factor (CRF). CH is reported to be intraocular pressure (IOP)-dependent and predominantly reflects the viscous properties of the cornea, whereas the CRF correlates with the elasticity of the cornea. However, discrepancies compared with expected results with these measures (e.g., a decrease in these properties with aging and no change in these properties after CXL treatment) suggest that further work is needed to determine precisely what these two properties measure or represent so that they are clinically meaningful to the clinician.[371–373] The Corneal Visualisation Scheimpflug Technology (Corvis ST, CVS, Oculus Optikgeräte GmbH, Germany) is a dynamic Scheimpflug analyzer that uses a concentric air puff to deform the central cornea, while monitoring its deformation using an ultra-high-speed camera.[93] The system captures 140 images of the central horizontal meridian of the cornea over 32 milliseconds, and the images are analyzed in real time to produce dynamic corneal response (DCR) parameters. These DCR parameters correlated with corneal stiffness in keratoconic, glaucoma, and postrefractive surgery eyes, leading to the development of the Corvis Biomechanical Index (CBI), which has been shown to be highly sensitive and specific to separate keratoconic from healthy eyes.[374] A combination of Scheimpflug-based corneal tomography and biomechanics assessment led to the development of the Tomographic and Biomechanical Index (TBI) to enhance ectasia detection.[375] Finally, despite its limitations, Brillouin microscopy has provided some insights into corneal biomechanical responses, and a commercial system Brillouin Optical Scattering System (BOSS; Intelon Optics Inc., Lexington, MA, USA) may soon become available.[376]

and other substances (lipids, salts, glycoproteins, etc.). The biomechanical properties of the sclera are dominated by the scleral stroma proper, which has a similar composite-like structure to that of the anterior third of the corneal stroma, albeit it is more disorganized and highly irregular (Fig. 4.32D).

Collagen is the major water-insoluble extracellular protein of the scleral stroma proper (80% type I, 5% type III, and minor amounts of types V, VI collagen); elastin is a minor component.[263] In contrast to the cornea, the sclera's heterotypic type I collagen fibrils are composed of types I, III, and V collagen molecules, are larger and more variable in diameter (mean diameter: 100 ± 30 nm; range: 25–300 nm), are more irregularly spaced (mean center-to-center interfibrillar distances: 150 ± 40 nm; range: 30–375), and are arranged in variably sized (0.5- to 6-μm thick; 1- to 50-μm wide), highly interwoven, irregularly directed lamellar collagen bundles.[263] The arrangement of collagen fibrils in the individual bundles is more random and they intermingle in a more wavy fashion than that of the cornea. Also, the bundles do not form a plywood-like stacking sequence, like that seen in the posterior two-thirds of the corneal stroma. Topographically, the sclera varies not only in thickness, but also in size, compactness, and angle of weave of its collagen bundles.[282] The anterior sclera consists of medium- to small-sized, moderately compact collagen bundles with wide-angle weave, whereas the equatorial sclera consists of small-sized, very compact collagen bundles with narrow-angle weave.[282] The posterior sclera consists of medium- to large-sized, loose collagen bundles with a wide-angle weave.[282]

No significant differences in the number of collagen bundles or elastin fibers have been reported when comparing these three topographic regions. There also are depth-related changes in the scleral stroma proper as the more superficial collagen fibrils are on average further apart from one another and are larger in diameter than the deeper layers where they are more compact and smaller in diameter. Additionally, the collagen bundles are thinner, narrower, and form whorl-like patterns superficially, whereas they are thicker, wider, and form a net- or rhomboid-like pattern in the deeper layers. The scleral proteoglycans and their covalently linked GAG side-chains differ markedly from the corneal stroma as they are about one-quarter the concentration and consist of the following: core proteins—decorin, biglycan, aggrecan, and GAGs—dermatan sulfate (36%), chondroitin sulfate (35%), hyaluronic acid (23%), and heparan sulfate (6%).[263] The scleral stroma proper also contains a syncytium of fibrocytes, like the corneal stroma, albeit at a much lower level of cellularity. Although the scleral stroma proper is traversed by ciliary blood vessels and nerves, it has no direct blood, lymph, or nerve supply.[263] It derives its nutrition solely by diffusion from the overlying episcleral and underlying choroidal vascular networks.

The most superficial layer of the sclera, called the episclera, differs from the scleral stroma proper in that its collagen bundles are more loosely arranged; it contains melanocytes and a few resident histiocytes. It also has a rich nerve supply with many unmyelinated and myelinated free nerve terminals (see Fig. 4.14A), which are most densely populated near the rich direct blood supply in the episclera (Fig. 4.34A) and lymph vasculature in the overlying conjunctiva (Fig. 4.34D), presumably to help regulate blood supply and to influence aqueous outflow. The episcleral venous system drains aqueous humor from the conventional outflow route via anastomosis with the aqueous collector channels.[283] Thus, outflow and IOP are dependent on the pressure gradient between IOP and episcleral venous pressure (EVP). The lamina fusca serves as a transition zone from the sclera to the choroid.

Although the sclera is constantly under stress from the IOP, which dynamically varies considerably, it acts in a similar manner to systemic muscular arteries in the body. It also typically displays a limited ability to distend in adulthood (range: 0.58%–6.68% strain), termed scleral distensibility. Considering the different possible topographical thicknesses and internal curvatures of the sclera, marked regional differences in wall stress can occur depending on each individual globe (see law of Laplace, described in section "Corneal stress"). Thus, accurately calculating regional wall stress of the sclera is very complex and perhaps even more difficult to do than for the cornea. In general, the anterior sclera under the rectus muscle insertion sites and the equatorial sclera should have the highest internal wall radial stress as they are the thinnest areas with comparable internal curvatures to the rest of the sclera, whereas the limbus should have the highest circumferential wall stress because a twofold higher amount of stress is required to sustain the curvature change from the cornea to the sclera (see Fig. 4.27A). Thus, when under acute extreme stress, such as direct blunt impact to the globe, there is a tendency for the globe to rupture in these areas. However, these regions also have the highest innate biomechanical properties, which were measured using ex vivo strip extensiometry or inflation tests—which may explain why the thinning of the posterior sclera in myopia or changes of the lamina cribosa seen in glaucoma are not observed in these regions. In fact, structural alterations in the sclera caused by myopia or the glaucoma may considerably change the expected normal stress distribution in the scleral wall (e.g., posterior scleral stress may increase up to fourfold with severe myopic globe elongation). Ex vivo studies have shown that the biomechanical properties of the sclera differ with age, race, glaucoma, and myopia.[279]

Using inflation testing and finite element modeling, the longitudinal Young's modulus of the adult human sclera averages 1.7×10^7 dyne/cm^2 (Fig. 4.35E).[284] This is approximately 3.7-fold stiffer than the cornea and 5.3-fold stiffer than the lamina cribosa (Fig. 4.35E).[284] Using uniaxial strip extensiometry, cohesive strength measurements of the anterior sclera averaged 55 g/mm, which was approximately twofold stronger than the cornea. Human uniaxial strip extensiometry testing has also shown topographical differences in the sclera's longitudinal Young's modulus as the equatorial sclera was the stiffest at 23 ± 8 g/mm^2 and the posterior sclera was the least stiff at 3 ± 1 g/mm^2; the anterior sclera was between these at 4 ± 1 g/mm^2.[282] The greater extensibility of the posterior sclera had previously led to a "dual function" theory of the sclera in which the anterior and equatorial sclera were thought to be essential for the rigid support and stability of the globe, whereas that of the posterior sclera served to act as a mechanical buffer or cushion against acute increases in IOP, which could be injurious to the delicate globe.[282] More recently, in vivo biomechanical measurements of the sclera have been studied using scleral deformations with inverse computational approaches, which require further development.[279]

The sclera's elastic stress-strain curve exponentially or nonlinearly increases with higher elevations in IOP or stress and then, because of viscosity, shows a time-dependent decrease with time. The J-shaped stress-strain curve of the sclera involves an immediate elastic response dominated initially by elastin, noncollagenous matrix, and collagen fibrils at the lower part of the J and then later by collagen fibrils in the upper part of the J. Overall, the nonlinearity arises from the gradual loading of highly extensible elastin fibers and the wavy collagen fibrils that take up slack initially, followed by gradually increasing in resistance to stress as maximal recruitment is attained. Finally, a slower, time-dependent viscous response results over time, where the resistance to stress gradually decreases with time owing to creep. The viscoelastic properties of the sclera also mean the loading or unloading stress-strain curves do not overlap, with the unloading curve being less than the loading curve—depending on the loading rate. This allows energy dissipation via viscous friction during the mechanical cycle and, ultimately, the return of the original shape of the material in a

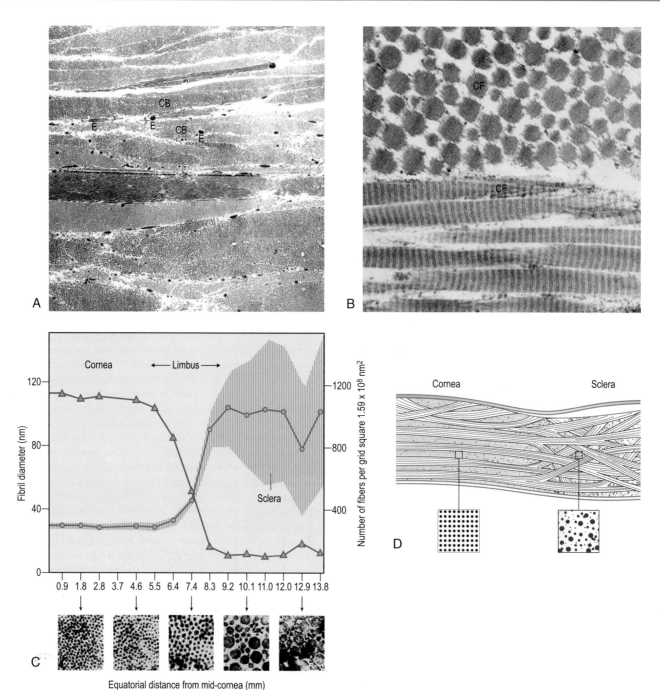

Fig. 4.34 (**A**) Low- (×4750) and (**B**) high-magnification (×72,500) transmission electron micrographs of the human sclera in the region of the stroma proper. Compare these to Figs. 4.9 and 4.10A–C to see how much more variably larger or irregular the collagen fibril diameters, interfibrillar spaces, and collagen bundles of the scleral stroma proper are to the corneal stroma. *CB,* Collagen bundle; *CF,* collagen fibril; *E,* elastin fibers. (**C**) Diagram comparing the collagen fibril diameters (red circles) and densities (blue triangles) in the cornea, limbus, and sclera. (From Borcherding MS, Blacik LJ, Sittig RA, et al. Proteoglycans and collagen fibre organization in human corneoscleral tissue. *Exp Eye Res.* 1975;21(1):59–70. https://doi.org/10.1016/0014-4835(75)90057-3.) (**D**) Diagram illustrating the greater degree of interweave of collagen bundles in the sclera than collagen lamellae in the corneal stroma. Additionally, the sclera has larger and more varied in collagen fibril diameters and interfibrillar spacing. (From Bron AJ, Tripathi R, Tripathi B. In: *Wolff's anatomy of the eye and orbit,* 8th edn. London, UK: Chapman & Hall, © 1997. Reproduced by permission of Taylor & Francis Group.)

Fig. 4.35 (**A**) The arterial supply of the anterior segment comes from the anterior ciliary arteries (ACA) and from the terminal branches of the long posterior ciliary arteries (LPCA). These vessels form two sagittal arterial circles (between superior or inferior ACA and LPCA arteries) and also anastomose together superficially and deeply to form two coronal arterial circles, called the episcleral arterial circle (EAC) superficially and the greater circle of the iris (GCI) deeply. In the anterior episclera (*inset*), the deep perforating branches of the LPCA anastomose with the ACA, together forming the EAC. The blood flow in the EAC typically comes from LPCA (inside outwards) rather than from ACA. The EAC supplies both a superficial and a deep episcleral plexus (deep plexus not shown). The conjunctival artery derives from the EAC, passing posteriorly, while also giving off an anteriorly directed branch called the limbal artery, which subsequently forms the limbal arcade. Blood flow in the EAC (*inset*) is continuous near the rectus muscle insertion sites but oscillates rather than flows between the rectus muscle insertion sites. (Modified from Watson PG, Hazelman B, Pavesio C, Green WR. *The Sclera and Systemic Disorders,* 2nd ed. Edinburgh, UK: Butterworth Heinemann; 2004.) (**B**) Diagram shows a schematic of the arterial circulation of

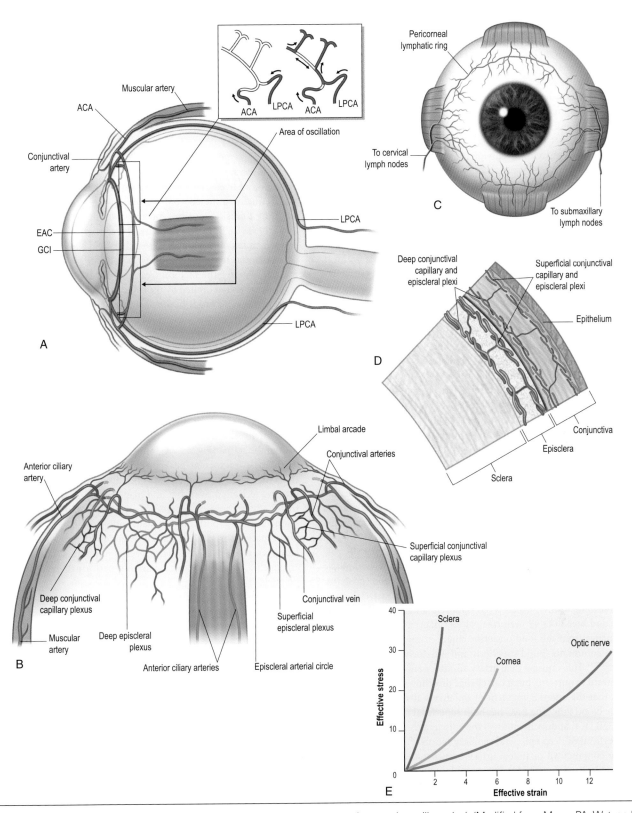

the episcleral and conjunctival, which both have superficial and deep components that supply capillary plexi. (Modified from Meyer PA, Watson PG. Low dose fluorescein angiography of the conjunctiva and episclera. *Br J Ophthalmol.* 1987;71:2–10.) (**C**) Schematic diagram showing the distribution of lymphatics (*green*) in relation to the blood vessels in the conjunctiva. Centripetal branches collect into a larger circular lymphatic ring, called the pericorneal lymphatic ring, which then drains medially or laterally into regional lymph nodes. (**D**) A cross-sectional representation of the conjunctiva and episclera, and sclera shows the episcleral and sclera are devoid of lymphatic networks, while the conjunctiva has two lymphatic plexi—a superficial plexus (below the epithelium) and a deep plexus (within Tenon's fascia, but just above the episcleral). Blood vessel plexi are found in the superficial and deep conjunctiva and episclera. (C and D from Robinson MR, Lee SS, Kim H, et al. A rabbit model for assessing the ocular barriers to the transscleral delivery of triamcinolone acetonide. *Exp Eye Res.* 2006;82(3):479–487. https://doi.org/10.1016/j.exer.2005.08.007.) (**E**) Exponential approximations of trilinear stress-strain curves for sclera, cornea (stroma), and lamina cribosa (optic nerve). (From Woo SL-Y, Kobayashi AS, Schlegel WA, Lawrence C. Nonlinear material properties of intact cornea and sclera. *Exp Eye Res.* 1972;14(1):29–39. https://doi.org/10.1016/0014-4835(72)90139-X.)

slow, time-dependent fashion. Therefore, the amount of distension of the sclera is not fixed, but determined by the level of the pressure changes and how long they have acted on the sclera—but also on the thickness and innate biomechanical properties of the sclera.[285]

A good example of this is when measuring IOP by indentation methods. The pressure measurement recorded by indentation initially increases the IOP of the eye by indenting the cornea inward (immediate elastic response), but by the time the measurement is made several seconds later it is typically back to normal levels (slow viscous response). However, in some individuals (e.g., high myopes or severely thinned sclera from scleral malacia perforans), the sclera will distend much more than normal because of the lower innate biomechanical properties or thinner sclera—which may result in false low readings. In contrast, false high readings may occur in the cases of more rigid scleras (e.g., scleral buckles). Therefore, applanation tonometry techniques have become the standard for IOP measurements, which are based on the Imbert-Fick principle (i.e., the pressure inside an ideal, dry, thin-walled sphere equals the force necessary to flatten its surface divided by the area of flattening). The IOP is determined by varying the applanating force or the area of cornea flattened by the device, for example, the Goldmann applanation tonometer measures the force necessary to flatten a corneal area of 3.06-mm diameter, currently considered the "gold standard" of IOP measurement.

Scleral dehydration and edema. Hydration of the sclera is most closely associated with the extracellular proteoglycan concentrations in the sclera. Because the normal healthy sclera has one-quarter the concentration of proteoglycans (scleral SP of 20–30 g/cm) between collagen fibrils than the cornea, it is not surprising that it contains less water (68%) than the cornea (78%). However, if the normal water content of sclera is reduced to less than 40%, it becomes somewhat translucent. This is a common observation made during long surgical procedures on the sclera when scleral flaps are dissected and sometimes inadvertently exposed to air for prolonged time periods, which reduces the hydration level through evaporation. Similarly, if the water content is increased to more than 80%, the sclera again becomes somewhat translucent due to the hydration of scleral proteoglycans.

Episcleral vasculature. The blood supply of the episclera is particularly prominent along a 4-mm zone anterior to the rectus muscle insertion sites, while being markedly less vascular in more posterior aspects.[286–288] The former area is called the episcleral arterial circle (EAC) (see Fig. 4.35A), which is fed by seven anterior ciliary arteries (ACAs) and several (≤12 per principal meridian) anastomotic terminal branches from the long posterior ciliary arteries (LPCA), which are more commonly found superiorly and inferiorly than medially or laterally.[263,289] This unusual dual artery-to-artery anastomosis typically flows inward to outward, but it can change direction if needed and thus ensures that the anterior segment of the eye is always supplied with adequate blood flow. The EAC has both superficial and deep branches (Fig. 4.35B,D) that directly nourish the episclera through corresponding superficial or deep episcleral capillary plexus.[290] The EAC also has separate conjunctival or limbal artery branches that have their own capillary plexus (Fig. 4.33B,D). For example, with severe corneal infection or inflammation, the limbal plexus is notable for dilating and causing a limbal ciliary flush pattern to appear around the periphery of the cornea on slit-lamp examination.[291]

Wound healing. Although injury converts scleral fibrocytes to metabolically active fibroblasts, similar to the cornea, superficial lacerations of the sclera heal more aggressively and completely than the cornea because episcleral fibrovascular granulation tissue migrates into and fills the wound.[292] Similarly, lacerations involving the inner portion of the sclera also heal predominantly through fibrovascular granulation tissue, which grows outward from the choroid. Penetrating scleral lacerations typically heal because fibrovascular granulation tissue grows from both of these sites. Such healing is usually very strong because it causes fibrovascular scarring. As time passes, a gradual remodeling or reorganization occurs to this scar; however, it can always be identified histologically by the abrupt change in scleral collagen fibril orientation, the persistent vascularity, or the disorganization of the surrounding tissue architecture.

Drug delivery

Although most of the bulk transport of fluid out of the eye takes place through the anterior segment's trabecular meshwork/Schlemm's canal system or via uveoscleral outflow, an appreciable amount is also drained transretinally to the choroid where it can get into the systemic circulation by diffusion into the choroidal vasculature or can travel extraocularly via the transscleral pathway (see Fig. 4.29A). The transscleral pathway is very intriguing to researchers and clinicians as it may serve as a potential route for noninvasive delivery of medications into the eye.[293] Currently, the medical treatment for posterior segment disease is to a large extent limited by the difficulty in delivering therapeutically effective doses of drugs to the posterior segment tissues (vitreous and retina). Unfortunately, the topical drug delivery route does not consistently or even efficiently yield therapeutic drug levels in posterior segment tissues.[294] Although systemic administration (oral or intravenous routes) can deliver drugs to the choroidal vasculature at therapeutic levels, the duration of choroidal drug delivery is too brief (usually less than 30 minutes) to result in meaningful intraocular drug levels and the large systemic doses necessary are often associated with significant systemic side effects or toxicities.

Intravitreal injection delivers agents directly into the vitreous and next to the retina (Fig. 4.29A). Thus, it has the advantages of achieving the highest intraocular peak drug levels, while minimizing systemic exposure.[295] However, it also has the disadvantage of being the most invasive technique available, and may need to be given repeatedly and frequently because drugs are usually rapidly eliminated via anterior segment and/or posterior segment bulk flow. The intravitreal route places patients at risk for high IOP, endophthalmitis, and cataract.[296] However, given its minimal risks, serial intravitreal injections of antiangiogenic drugs are now commonly performed in routine clinical practice.[295]

Periocular drug delivery is an alternative, minimally invasive approach to drug delivery to the posterior segment as it commonly delivers moderately sustained concentrations of drugs.[297] The various periocular techniques include subconjunctival, retrobulbar, peribulbar, and sub-Tenon's injections (see Fig. 4.29A). They are far less invasive than the direct intravitreal route, but they do have notable shortcomings, mainly from having to permeate more static anatomical barriers and from encountering enhanced dynamic clearance mechanisms. In general, periocular drug delivery involves placing the drug, usually by needle injection, into the tissue surrounding or adjacent to the posterior segment of the eye. Corticosteroids are the most common drugs given by these techniques (e.g., sub-Tenon's triamcinolone injection). The feasibility of using these techniques depends, to a large extent, on the permeability of the sclera to the drugs and the accuracy of the clinician in injecting the drug to the desired location. In fact, although three possible absorption pathways exist (transscleral, systemic hematogenous circulation, and anterior routes) for the various periocular drug delivery techniques, the transscleral pathway has been proven to be the main route for delivering sufficient drug concentrations into the choroid, RPE, retina, and vitreous.[293] Ghate and associates,[293] performing in vivo dynamic periocular drug delivery studies in rabbits, reported that sub-Tenon's injection resulted in the highest and most persistent vitreous concentrations with the least systemic exposure of the various periocular techniques. Subconjunctival injection resulted in the highest and most persistent anterior segment concentrations, with slightly lower vitreous concentrations than sub-Tenon's injection, and some higher risk for systemic exposure.[293]

Although preliminary studies several decades ago suggested that it might be possible to exploit the transscleral route for drug delivery to intraocular tissues in the posterior segment, renewed interest has arisen after the introduction of anti-vascular endothelial growth factor (VEGF) drug therapy for wet age-related macular degeneration.[298] Of these initial studies, Barza[299] was the first to clearly establish that drugs could permeate through various ocular tissues including the sclera when they were administered by either subconjunctival or retrobulbar injection. Anders Bill[300] further demonstrated that albumin or dextran injected into the suprachoroidal space of the rabbit eye could diffuse across the sclera and accumulate in extraocular tissues. In vitro permeability studies on human sclera by Olsen and associates[301] further demonstrated that the tissue was permeable to drugs up to a molecular weight of 70 kDa. Scleral permeability is expressed as a pharmacokinetic volume transfer coefficient known as its K^{trans} (cm/sec), which reflects the tissue's surface area permeability to a specific perfusion flow of the drug.[301] A number of permeability studies have been published, using essentially comparable methods, and have shown that the sclera is quite permeable to a wide range of drugs (Table 4.6).[302] Collectively, the results indicate that scleral permeability is 5 to 15 times higher than that of the corneal stroma, depending on the molecular radius of the drug studied. The sclera shares a similar ultrastructure and composition to corneal stroma, albeit the sclera has variably larger interfibrillar spaces (50 nm [range: 5–120 nm] vs. 20 nm [range: 5–35 nm]) one-quarter the ground substance, one-fifth the cellularity, a 10% less hydration level, and a much more variable thickness profile.[243]

Like the corneal stroma, the primary transportation route through the sclera is by passive diffusion through the interfibrillar spaces. Also, as in corneal stroma, scleral permeability was found to be primarily dependent on the molecular radius of the drug (scleral permeability declines roughly exponentially with increasing molecular radius, and drugs of molecular radius of 8 nm or less have been successfully shown to permeate the sclera) and secondarily dependent on the shape and molecular weight of the drug.[303] As the scleral stroma is hypocellular and is essentially devoid of melanin, it has no intercellular barriers, few proteolytic enzymes, and few protein-binding sites to interfere with drug permeation. Thus, it shows no preference for hydrophilic or lipophilic drugs. Several studies have found no significant changes in scleral permeability to small molecules as a function of aging, tissue hydration, or various IOP levels. However, the hydration level and interfibrillar space of the scleral stroma decrease 35% and 20% with age, respectively, owing to the effects of age-related collagen fibril crosslinking rather than an age-related change in the concentration of proteoglycans. The interfibrillar spaces also dynamically change based on the IOP of the eye (i.e., high IOP compresses the

TABLE 4.6 Known scleral permeability values for certain drugs or agents

Drug	Molecular weight (g/mol)	K_{trans} (cm/sec)	Source
Polymyxin B	1800	$3.90 \pm 0.59 \times 10^{-7}$	2
Doxil	580	$4.74 \pm 0.73 \times 10^{-7}$	8
Vancomycin boron-dipyrromethene (BODIPY)	1723	$6.66 \pm 1.46 \times 10^{-7}$	2
SS fluorescein-labeled oligonucleotide	7998.3	$7.67 \pm 1.8 \times 10^{-7}$	3
Dexamethasone-fluorescein	841	$1.64 \pm 0.17 \times 10^{-6}$	4
Rhodamine	479	$1.86 \pm 0.39 \times 10^{-6}$	4
Penicillin G	661.46	$1.89 \pm 0.21 \times 10^{-6}$	2
Methotrexate-fluorescein	979	$3.36 \pm 0.62 \times 10^{-6}$	4
Doxorubicin hydrochloride	580	$3.50 \pm 0.31 \times 10^{-6}$	8
Nanoparticle doxorubicin	580	$4.97 \pm 0.19 \times 10^{-6}$	8
Fluorescein	332	$5.21 \pm 0.71 \times 10^{-6}$	4
Vinblastine boron-dipyrromethene-Fluorscein (BODIPY FL)	1043	$5.88 \pm 1.2 \times 10^{-6}$	-
Cisplatin in collagen matrix	300.05	$8.3 \pm 1.2 \times 10^{-6}$	5
Carboxyfluorescein	317	$9.93 \pm 3.5 \times 10^{-6}$	6
Carboplatin in fibrin sealant	371.25	$13.7 \pm 2.3 \times 10^{-6}$	7
Cisplatin in balanced Salt Saline (BSS)	300.05	$20.1 \pm 1.8 \times 10^{-6}$	5
Carboplatin in BSS	371.25	$27.0 \pm 1.7 \times 10^{-6}$	7
Water (H$_2$O)	18	$51.8 \pm 18 \times 10^{-6}$	6

From Zhang L, Gu FX, Chan JM, et al. Nanoparticles in medicine: Therapeutic applications and developments. *Clin Pharmacol Ther.* 83(5):761–769; Kao JC, Geroski DH, Edelhauser HF. Trans-scleral permeability of fluorescent-labeled antibiotics. *J Ocul Pharmacol Ther.* 2005;21:1–10; Shuler RK Jr, Dioguardi PK, Henjy C, et al. Scleral permeability of a small single-stranded oligonucleotide. *J Ocul Pharmacol Ther.* 2004;20:159–168; Cruysberg LPJ, Nuijts RMMA, Geroski DH, et al. In vitro human scleral permeability of fluorescein, dexamethasone-fluorescein, methotrexate-fluorescein, and rhodamine 6G and the use of a coated coil as a new drug delivery system. *J Ocul Pharmacol Ther.* 2002; 18:559–569; Gilbert JA, Simpson AE, Rudnick DE, et al. Transscleral permeability and intraocular concentrations of cisplatin from a collagen matrix. *J Control Release.* 2003;89:409–417; Rudnick DE, Noonan JS, Geroski DH, et al. The effect of intraocular pressure on human and rabbit scleral permeability. *Invest Ophthalmol Vis Sci.* 1999; 40:3054–3058; Simpson AE, Gilbert BS, Rudnick DE, et al. Transscleral diffusion of carboplatin: An in vitro and in vivo study. *Arch Ophthalmol.* 2002;120:1069–1074; Kim ES, Lee SJ, Zaffos JA, et al. Transscleral delivery of doxorubicin: A comparison of hydrophilic and lipophilic nanoparticles. ARVO E-Abstract A590.

sclera and narrows the interfibrillar spaces, and vice versa).[304,305] Thus, the effect of aging, tissue hydration, or IOP may affect scleral permeability to large macromolecules (e.g., monoclonal antibodies, vectors for gene-based therapy).

Periocular drug delivery using the transscleral diffusion route is able to deliver drugs to the choroid efficiently as this pathway is highly permeable to most ophthalmic drugs. However, this comes with the important caveat that the clearance mechanisms in the subconjunctival space near the limbus appear to be superb (Fig. 4.29A), which can affect the retention time of the drug depot that is available for absorption transsclerally—especially when given via subconjunctival injection. In fact, knowing a specific drug's scleral permeability properties is now known to be insufficient information to accurately predict the drug delivery rate to the retina or vitreous humor, particularly for large hydrophilic drugs.[306] The choroid and Bruch's membrane are rather porous as their permeation properties are better than that of the sclera,[307] although the permeability properties of Bruch's membrane gradually decline with age owing to lipid accumulation. The major rate-limiting step for retinal or vitreous targeted drug delivery via the periocular route has recently been determined to be the RPE, which forms the outer part of the blood-retinal barrier owing to the apical zonula occludens tight junctions found in its intercellular space (most similar to that of the corneal epithelium).[307] This is ten- to a hundred-fold less permeable than the human sclera and fourteen- to sixteenfold less permeable than the choroid or Bruch's membrane for large, hydrophilic drugs, whereas comparably similar to sclera, choroid, or Bruch's membrane for lipophilic drugs.[307]

Although drug metabolism does not appear to be a major source of drug removal in the posterior segment, dynamic drug clearance via orbital blood vessels and lymphatics, conjunctival blood vessels and lymphatics, episcleral blood vessels, and the choroidal vasculature are confirmed inhibitory factors for successful periocular drug delivery.[308] Currently, animal studies show that the orbital (~25% drug removal rate from retrobulbar injections as drugs disperse throughout the orbit) and conjunctival (~5% to 80% drug removal rate using sub-Tenon's injection as drugs disperse circumferentially around the eye) clearance mechanisms are of more importance than that of the choroid (~2% to 20% drug removal rate from sub-Tenon's injections).[308,309] Therefore, for large, hydrophilic drugs, the major barrier to drug entry into the retina or vitreous is the RPE, whereas small, lipophilic drugs are relatively unaffected because they transverse RPE quite easily using the intracellular (transcellular) route. Overall then, the rate-limiting factors for posterior segment drug delivery using this drug delivery route come down to avoiding or abrogating the dynamic physiologic clearance mechanisms and the individual physiochemical properties of the drug itself—predominantly the molecular radius (≤8-nm molecular radii drugs) and the lipophilicity of the drug, and, secondarily, its shape, molecular weight (MW), protein-binding properties, and ionic charge (Box 4.7).

In summary, there is now definitive in vitro and in vivo evidence to suggest that periocular drug delivery is the most efficient means to treat choroidal and RPE disease without significant systemic or intraocular risk because it diffuses through the static permeability barriers of the sclera and choroid quite easily. However, the drug depot site must have a drug release rate that exceeds the dynamic tissue clearance rates stated previously. The feasibility of treating retinal or vitreous diseases is less certain, but is promising, likely depending more on the molecular size and lipophilicity of the drug being administered. Studies on static permeability properties of the sclera, choroid, Bruch's membrane, and RPE suggest how the posterior segment is amenable to pharmacologic interventions other than direct intravitreal injection. One promising drug delivery technology is that of minimally invasive drug-eluting microneedles (<1-mm diameter) that deliver drugs into

The precapillary arterioles and postcapillary venules of the superficial and deep episcleral, limbus, and conjunctiva capillary plexus are notable for having continuous nonfenestrated endothelium without intercellular tight junctions (20-nm intercellular spaces).[287] Therefore, these vessels are leaky and are highly permeable to small molecules but do at least resist bulk fluid flow. Since the precapillary arterioles of the anterior segment do not have a smooth muscle wall, they tend to be thrown into tortuous folds resulting in areas of turbulent blood flow.[288] This, combined with the fact that a notable disadvantage to having artery-to-artery anastomosis is that regions between the rectus muscles may not have continuous high arterial perfusion pressures, but rather oscillatory blood flow, then it should not be surprising that extravasation of fluid or stagnation of cells commonly occurs in these regions. If the individuals have systemic infections or autoimmune diseases (such as hepatitis viral infections, systemic lupus erythematosus, rheumatoid arthritis, or Wegener's granulomatosis), deposition of antigens or immune complexes occurs in this region of stagnation, resulting in inflammatory microangiopathy (e.g., peripheral ulcerative keratitis, episcleritis, scleritis, Mooren's ulcers).[263,286] Moreover, as some of these regions (sclera and peripheral cornea) are far from lymphatic drainage sites, which are efficient mechanisms for removal of unwanted antigens or immune complexes, chronic problems often follow.[263]

the cornea, sclera, or suprachoroidal space.[310,311] Preliminary animal studies suggest that by circumventing the subconjunctival/episcleral clearance mechanism, microneedle-based drug delivery markedly improves (eightyfold) the intraocular bioavailability and moderately improves (threefold) the duration of action over periocular drug delivery techniques. Because of our improved understanding of the pharmacokinetics involved in periocular drug delivery, optimizing the physiochemical properties of existing drugs to prolong residence time or enhance penetration into the retina and vitreous may be the future of ocular drug delivery.[312]

REFERENCES

1. Dawson D, Watsky M, Geroski D, Edelhauser H. *Duane's Foundation of Clinical Ophthalmology on CD-ROM Vol. 2c.* Philadelphia: Lippincott Williams & Wilkins; 2006.
2. Gipson I, Joyce N, Zieske J. The anatomy and cell biology of the human cornea, limbus, conjunctiva, and adnexa. In: Foster CS, AD Dohlman CH, eds. *Smolin and Thoft's The Cornea: Scientific Foundations and Clinical Practice.* 4th ed. Philadelphia: Lippincott Williams & Wilkins; 2005.
3. Klyce S. Corneal Physiology. In: Foster CSAD, Dohlman CH, eds. *Smolin and Thoft's The Cornea: Scientific Foundations and Clinical Practice.* 4th ed. Philadelphia: Lippincott Williams & Wilkins; 2005.
4. Nishida T. Cornea. In: Krachmer JH, Holland EJ, eds. *Cornea. Fundamental, Diagnosis, and Management.* 2nd ed. Philadelphia: Elsevier Mosby; 2005.
5. Rada J, Johnson JSclera. In: Krachmer JH, Holland EJ, eds. *Cornea. Fundamental, diagnosis, and management.* 2nd ed. Philadelphia: Elsevier Mosby; 2005.
6. Ligocki AJ, Fury W, Gutierrez C, et al. Molecular characteristics and spatial distribution of adult human corneal cell subtypes. *Sci Rep.* 2021;11:16323.
7. Sie NM, Yam GH, Soh YQ, et al. Regenerative capacity of the corneal transition zone for endothelial cell therapy. *Stem Cell Res Ther.* 2020;11:523.
8. Hay ED. Development of the vertebrate cornea. *Int Rev Cytol.* 1980;63:263–322.
9. Quantock AJ, Young RD. Development of the corneal stroma, and the collagen-proteoglycan associations that help define its structure and function. *Dev Dyn.* 2008; 237:2607–2621.
10. Stiemke MM, McCartney MD, Cantu-Crouch D, Edelhauser HF. Maturation of the corneal endothelial tight junction. *Invest Ophthalmol Vis Sci.* 1991;32:2757–2765.
11. Gordon RA, Donzis PB. Refractive development of the human eye. *Arch Ophthalmol.* 1985;103:785–789.
12. Doughty MJ, Zaman ML. Human corneal thickness and its impact on intraocular pressure measures: A review and meta-analysis approach. *Surv Ophthalmol.* 2000;44:367–408.
13. Pan C-W, Cheng C-Y, Sabanayagam C, et al. Ethnic variation in central corneal refractive power and steep cornea in Asians. *Ophthalmic Epidemiol.* 2014;21:99–105.
14. Sng CC, Ang M, Barton K. Central corneal thickness in glaucoma. *Curr Opin Ophthalmol.* 2017;28:120–126.
15. Ehlers N, Sorensen T, Bramsen T, Poulsen EH. Central corneal thickness in newborns and children. *Acta Ophthalmol (Copenh).* 1976;54:285–290.

16. Niederer RL, Perumal D, Sherwin T, McGhee CN. Age-related differences in the normal human cornea: A laser scanning in vivo confocal microscopy study. *Br J Ophthalmol.* 2007;91:1165–1169.

17. Faragher RG, Mulholland B, Tuft SJ, et al. Aging and the cornea. *Br J Ophthalmol.* 1997; 81:814–817.

18. Hayashi K, Hayashi H, Hayashi F. Topographic analysis of the changes in corneal shape due to aging. *Cornea.* 1995;14:527–532.

19. Alvarado J, Murphy C, Juster R. Age-related changes in the basement membrane of the human corneal epithelium. *Invest Ophthalmol Vis Sci.* 1983;24:1015–1028.

20. Malik NS, Moss SJ, Ahmed N, et al. Ageing of the human corneal stroma: Structural and biochemical changes. *Biochim Biophys Acta.* 1992;1138:222–228.

21. Kanai A, Kaufman HE. Electron microscopic studies of corneal stroma: Aging changes of collagen fibers. *Ann Ophthalmol.* 1973;5:285–287.

22. Moller-Pedersen T. A comparative study of human corneal keratocyte and endothelial cell density during aging. *Cornea.* 1997;16:333–338.

23. Ang M, Wong W, Park J, et al. Corneal arcus is a sign of cardiovascular disease, even in low-risk persons. *Am J Ophthalmol.* 2011;152:864–871.e1.

24. Cheng AC, Rao SK, Cheng LL, Lam DS. Assessment of pupil size under different light intensities using the Procyon pupillometer. *J Cataract Refract Surg.* 2006;32:1015–1017.

25. Winn B, Whitaker D, Elliott DB, Phillips NJ. Factors affecting light-adapted pupil size in normal human subjects. *Invest Ophthalmol Vis Sci.* 1994;35:1132–1137.

26. Mandell RB, Chiang CS, Klein SA. Location of the major corneal reference points. *Optom Vis Sci.* 1995;72:776–784.

27. Edmund C. Location of the corneal apex and its influence on the stability of the central corneal curvature. A photokeratoscopy study. *Am J Optom Physiol Opt.* 1987;64:846–852.

28. Pande M, Hillman JS. Optical zone centration in keratorefractive surgery. Entrance pupil center, visual axis, coaxially sighted corneal reflex, or geometric corneal center? *Ophthalmology.* 1993;100:1230–1237.

29. Uozato H, Guyton DL. Centering corneal surgical procedures. *Am J Ophthalmol.* 1987; 103:264–275.

30. Bueeler M, Mrochen M, Seiler T. Maximum permissible lateral decentration in aberration-sensing and wavefront-guided corneal ablation. *J Cataract Refract Surg.* 2003;29:257–263.

31. Bueeler M, Mrochen M, Seiler T. Maximum permissible torsional misalignment in aberration-sensing and wavefront-guided corneal ablation. *J Cataract Refract Surg.* 2004; 30:17–25.

32. Kaye GI. Stereologic measurement of cell volume fraction of rabbit corneal stroma. *Arch Ophthalmol.* 1969;82:792–794.

33. Gatinel D, Haouat M, Hoang-Xuan T. [A review of mathematical descriptors of corneal asphericity]. *J Fr Ophtalmol.* 2002;25:81–90.

34. Consejo A, Llorens-Quintana C, Radhakrishnan H, Iskander DR. Mean shape of the human limbus. *J Cataract Refract Surg.* 2017;43:667–672.

35. Dubbelman M, Sicam VA, Van der Heijde GL. The shape of the anterior and posterior surface of the aging human cornea. *Vision Res.* 2006;46:993–1001.

36. Davis WR, Raasch TW, Mitchell GL, et al. Corneal asphericity and apical curvature in children: A cross-sectional and longitudinal evaluation. *Invest Ophthalmol Vis Sci.* 2005; 46:1899–1906.

37. Read SA, Collins MJ, Carney LG, Franklin RJ. The topography of the central and peripheral cornea. *Invest Ophthalmol Vis Sci.* 2006;47:1404–1415.

38. Ho JD, Tsai CY, Tsai RJ, et al. Validity of the keratometric index: Evaluation by the Pentacam rotating Scheimpflug camera. *J Cataract Refract Surg.* 2008;34:137–145.

39. Khoramnia R, Rabsilber TM, Auffarth GU. Central and peripheral pachymetry measurements according to age using the Pentacam rotating Scheimpflug camera. *J Cataract Refract Surg.* 2007;33:830–836.

40. Navarro R, Gonzalez L, Hernandez JL. Optics of the average normal cornea from general and canonical representations of its surface topography. *J Opt Soc Am A Opt Image Sci Vis.* 2006;23:219–232.

41. Dingeldein SA, Klyce SD. The topography of normal corneas. *Arch Ophthalmol.* 1989; 107:512–518.

42. Meek KM, Leonard DW, Connon CJ, et al. Transparency, swelling and scarring in the corneal stroma. *Eye (Lond).* 2003;17:927–936.

43. Jester JV, Moller-Pedersen T, Huang J, et al. The cellular basis of corneal transparency: Evidence for 'corneal crystallins'. *J Cell Sci.* 1999;112(Pt 5):613–622.

44. Piatigorsky J. Enigma of the abundant water-soluble cytoplasmic proteins of the cornea: The "refracton" hypothesis. *Cornea.* 2001;20:853–858.

45. Lerman S. Biophysical aspects of corneal and lenticular transparency. *Curr Eye Res.* 1984;3:3–14.

46. Farrell RA, McCally RL, Tatham PE. Wave-length dependencies of light scattering in normal and cold swollen rabbit corneas and their structural implications. *J Physiol.* 1973;233:589–612.

47. Moller-Pedersen T. Keratocyte reflectivity and corneal haze. *Exp Eye Res.* 2004;78:553–560.

48. van den Berg TJ, Tan KE. Light transmittance of the human cornea from 320 to 700 nm for different ages. *Vision Res.* 1994;34:1453–1456.

49. Ihanamaki T, Pelliniemi LJ, Vuorio E. Collagens and collagen-related matrix components in the human and mouse eye. *Prog Retin Eye Res.* 2004;23:403–434.

50. Robert L, Legeais JM, Robert AM, Renard G. Corneal collagens. *Pathol Biol (Paris).* 2001; 49:353–363.

51. Meek KM, Fullwood NJ. Corneal and scleral collagens—a microscopist's perspective. *Micron.* 2001;32:261–272.

52. Birk DE. Type V collagen: Heterotypic type I/V collagen interactions in the regulation of fibril assembly. *Micron.* 2001;32:223–237.

53. White J, Werkmeister JA, Ramshaw JA, Birk DE. Organization of fibrillar collagen in the human and bovine cornea: Collagen types V and III. *Connect Tissue Res.* 1997;36:165–174.

54. Borcherding MS, Blacik LJ, Sittig RA, et al. Proteoglycans and collagen fibre organization in human corneoscleral tissue. *Exp Eye Res.* 1975;21:59–70.

55. Cho HI, Covington HI, Cintron C. Immunolocalization of type VI collagen in developing and healing rabbit cornea. *Invest Ophthalmol Vis Sci.* 1990;31:1096–1102.

56. Hirsch M, Prenant G, Renard G. Three-dimensional supramolecular organization of the extracellular matrix in human and rabbit corneal stroma, as revealed by ultrarapid-freezing and deep-etching methods. *Exp Eye Res.* 2001;72:123–135.

57. Komai Y, Ushiki T. The three-dimensional organization of collagen fibrils in the human cornea and sclera. *Invest Ophthalmol Vis Sci.* 1991;32:2244–2258.

58. Meek KM, Boote C. The organization of collagen in the corneal stroma. *Exp Eye Res.* 2004;78:503–512.

59. Ojeda JL, Ventosa JA, Piedra S. The three-dimensional microanatomy of the rabbit and human cornea. A chemical and mechanical microdissection-SEM approach. *J Anat.* 2001;199:567–576.

60. Dawson DG, Grossniklaus HE, McCarey BE, Edelhauser HF. Biomechanical and wound healing characteristics of corneas after excimer laser keratorefractive surgery: is there a difference between advanced surface ablation and sub-Bowman's keratomileusis? *J Refract Surg.* 2008;24:S90–S96.

61. Mathew JH, Bergmanson JP, Doughty MJ. Fine structure of the interface between the anterior limiting lamina and the anterior stromal fibrils of the human cornea. *Invest Ophthalmol Vis Sci.* 2008;49:3914–3918.

62. Newton RH, Meek KM. Circumcorneal annulus of collagen fibrils in the human limbus. *Invest Ophthalmol Vis Sci.* 1998;39:1125–1134.

63. Newton RH, Meek KM. The integration of the corneal and limbal fibrils in the human eye. *Biophys J.* 1998;75:2508–2512.

64. Moller-Pedersen T, Ledet T, Ehlers N. The keratocyte density of human donor corneas. *Curr Eye Res.* 1994;13:163–169.

65. Watsky MA. Keratocyte gap junctional communication in normal and wounded rabbit corneas and human corneas. *Invest Ophthalmol Vis Sci.* 1995;36:2568–2576.

66. Hahnel C, Somodi S, Weiss DG, Guthoff RF. The keratocyte network of human cornea: a three-dimensional study using confocal laser scanning fluorescence microscopy. *Cornea.* 2000;19:185–193.

67. Müller LJ, Pels L, Vrensen GF. Novel aspects of the ultrastructural organization of human corneal keratocytes. *Invest Ophthalmol Vis Sci.* 1995;36:2557–2567.

68. Yam GHF, Riau AK, Funderburgh ML, et al. Keratocyte biology. *Exp Eye Res.* 2020; 196:108062.

69. Hamrah P, Liu Y, Zhang Q, Dana MR. The corneal stroma is endowed with a significant number of resident dendritic cells. *Invest Ophthalmol Vis Sci.* 2003;44:581–589.

70. Poole CA, Brookes NH, Clover GM. Keratocyte networks visualised in the living cornea using vital dyes. *J Cell Sci.* 1993;106(Pt 2):685–691.

71. Du Y, Funderburgh ML, Mann MM, et al. Multipotent stem cells in human corneal stroma. *Stem Cells.* 2005;23:1266–1275.

72. Du Y, Sundarraj N, Funderburgh ML, et al. Secretion and organization of a cornea-like tissue in vitro by stem cells from human corneal stroma. *Invest Ophthalmol Vis Sci.* 2007; 48:5038–5045.

73. Stewart S, Liu YC, Lin MT, Mehta JS. Clinical applications of in vivo confocal microscopy in keratorefractive surgery. *J Refract Surg.* 2021;37:493–503.

74. Hedblom EE. The role of polysaccharides in corneal swelling. *Exp Eye Res.* 1961;1:81–91.

75. Bettelheim FA, Plessy B. The hydration of proteoglycans of bovine cornea. *Biochim Biophys Acta.* 1975;381:203–214.

76. Scott JE. Proteoglycan: Collagen interactions and corneal ultrastructure. *Biochem Soc Trans.* 1991;19:877–881.

77. Scott JE. Proteoglycan histochemistry—a valuable tool for connective tissue biochemists. *Coll Relat Res.* 1985;5:541–575.

78. Scott JE. Extracellular matrix, supramolecular organisation and shape. *J Anat.* 1995; 187(Pt 2):259–269.

79. Scott JE, Bosworth TR. The comparative chemical morphology of the mammalian cornea. *Basic Appl Histochem.* 1990;34:35–42.

80. Castoro JA, Bettelheim AA, Bettelheim FA. Water gradients across bovine cornea. *Invest Ophthalmol Vis Sci.* 1988;29:963–968.

81. Guthoff RF, Wienss H, Hahnel C, Wree A. Epithelial innervation of human cornea: a three-dimensional study using confocal laser scanning fluorescence microscopy. *Cornea.* 2005;24:608–613.

82. Rozsa AJ, Beuerman RW. Density and organization of free nerve endings in the corneal epithelium of the rabbit. *Pain.* 1982;14:105–120.

83. Schimmelpfennig B. Nerve structures in human central corneal epithelium. *Graefes Arch Clin Exp Ophthalmol.* 1982;218:14–20.

84. MüllerLJ, Marfurt CF, Kruse F, Tervo TM. Corneal nerves: Structure, contents and function. *Exp Eye Res.* 2003;76:521–542.

85. Belmonte C, Acosta MC, Gallar J. Neural basis of sensation in intact and injured corneas. *Exp Eye Res.* 2004;78:513–525.

86. Stachs O, Zhivov A, Kraak R, et al. In vivo three-dimensional confocal laser scanning microscopy of the epithelial nerve structure in the human cornea. *Graefes Arch Clin Exp Ophthalmol.* 2007;245:569–575.

87. Lawrenson JG. Corneal sensitivity in health and disease. *Ophthalmic Physiol Opt.* 1997; 17(Suppl 1):S17–22.

88. Cochet P, Bonnet R. [Corneal esthesiometry. Performance and practical importance]. *Bull Soc Ophtalmol Fr.* 1961;6:541–550.

89. Brennan NA, Bruce AS. Esthesiometry as an indicator of corneal health. *Optom Vis Sci.* 1991;68:699–702.

90. Johnson MK, Gebhardt BM, Berman MB. Appearance of collagenase in pneumolysin-treated corneal fibroblast cultures. *Curr Eye Res.* 1988;7:951–953.

91. Maurice DM. The biology of wound healing in the corneal stroma. Castroviejo lecture. *Cornea.* 1987;6:162–168.

92. Belmonte C. Eye dryness sensations after refractive surgery: Impaired tear secretion or "phantom" cornea? *J Refract Surg.* 2007;23:598–602.

93. Yang K, Xu L, Fan Q, et al. Repeatability and comparison of new Corvis ST parameters in normal and keratoconus eyes. *Sci Rep.* 2019;9:15379.
94. Wolter JR. Reactions of the cellular elements of the corneal stroma; a report of experimental studies in the rabbit eye. *AMA Arch Ophthalmol.* 1958;59:873–881.
95. Cintron C, Hassinger LC, Kublin CL, Cannon DJ. Biochemical and ultrastructural changes in collagen during corneal wound healing. *J Ultrastruct Res.* 1978;65:13–22.
96. Hassell JR, Cintron C, Kublin C, Newsome DA. Proteoglycan changes during restoration of transparency in corneal scars. *Arch Biochem Biophys.* 1983;222:362–369.
97. Cintron C, Covington HI, Kublin CL. Morphologic analyses of proteoglycans in rabbit corneal scars. *Invest Ophthalmol Vis Sci.* 1990;31:1789–1798.
98. Mohan RR, Hutcheon AE, Choi R, et al. Apoptosis, necrosis, proliferation, and myofibroblast generation in the stroma following LASIK and PRK. *Exp Eye Res.* 2003;76:71–87.
99. Jester JV, Petroll WM, Cavanagh HD. Corneal stromal wound healing in refractive surgery: the role of myofibroblasts. *Prog Retin Eye Res.* 1999;18:311–356.
100. Wilson SE, Mohan RR, Mohan RR, et al. The corneal wound healing response: cytokine-mediated interaction of the epithelium, stroma, and inflammatory cells. *Prog Retin Eye Res.* 2001;20:625–637.
101. Netto MV, Mohan RR, Ambrosio R Jr, et al. Wound healing in the cornea: a review of refractive surgery complications and new prospects for therapy. *Cornea.* 2005;24:509–522.
102. Zhao J, Nagasaki T, Maurice DM. Role of tears in keratocyte loss after epithelial removal in mouse cornea. *Invest Ophthalmol Vis Sci.* 2001;42:1743–1749.
103. Wilson SE, Mohan RR, Hong J, et al. Apoptosis in the cornea in response to epithelial injury: Significance to wound healing and dry eye. *Adv Exp Med Biol.* 2002;506:821–826.
104. Zieske JD, Guimarães SR, Hutcheon AE. Kinetics of keratocyte proliferation in response to epithelial debridement. *Exp Eye Res.* 2001;72:33–39.
105. Fini ME. Keratocyte and fibroblast phenotypes in the repairing cornea. *Prog Retin Eye Res.* 1999;18:529–551.
106. Fini ME, Stramer BM. How the Cornea heals: Cornea-specific repair mechanisms affecting surgical outcomes. *Cornea.* 2005;24:S2–S11.
107. Jester JV, Barry-Lane PA, Cavanagh HD, Petroll WM. Induction of alpha-smooth muscle actin expression and myofibroblast transformation in cultured corneal keratocytes. *Cornea.* 1996;15:505–516.
108. Wilson SE, Liu JJ, Mohan RR. Stromal-epithelial interactions in the cornea. *Prog Retin Eye Res.* 1999;18:293–309.
109. Meltendorf C, Burbach GJ, Bühren J, et al. Corneal femtosecond laser keratotomy results in isolated stromal injury and favorable wound-healing response. *Invest Ophthalmol Vis Sci.* 2007;48:2068–2075.
110. Meltendorf C, Burbach GJ, Ohrloff C, et al. Intrastromal keratotomy with femtosecond laser avoids profibrotic TGF-beta1 induction. *Invest Ophthalmol Vis Sci.* 2009;50:3688–3695.
111. Lim M, Goldstein MH, Tuli S, Schultz GS. Growth factor, cytokine and protease interactions during corneal wound healing. *Ocul Surf.* 2003;1:53–65.
112. Klenkler B, Sheardown H. Growth factors in the anterior segment: Role in tissue maintenance, wound healing and ocular pathology. *Exp Eye Res.* 2004;79:677–688.
113. Klenkler B, Sheardown H, Jones L. Growth factors in the tear film: role in tissue maintenance, wound healing, and ocular pathology. *Ocul Surf.* 2007;5:228–239.
114. Micera A, Lambiase A, Puxeddu I, et al. Nerve growth factor effect on human primary fibroblastic-keratocytes: Possible mechanism during corneal healing. *Exp Eye Res.* 2006;83:747–757.
115. Stramer BM, Zieske JD, Jung JC, et al. Molecular mechanisms controlling the fibrotic repair phenotype in cornea: Implications for surgical outcomes. *Invest Ophthalmol Vis Sci.* 2003;44:4237–4246.
116. Girard MT, Matsubara M, Fini ME. Transforming growth factor-beta and interleukin-1 modulate metalloproteinase expression by corneal stromal cells. *Invest Ophthalmol Vis Sci.* 1991;32:2441–2454.
117. Ubels JL, Foley KM, Rismondo V. Retinol secretion by the lacrimal gland. *Invest Ophthalmol Vis Sci.* 1986;27:1261–1268.
118. Tsubota K. Tear dynamics and dry eye. *Prog Retin Eye Res.* 1998;17:565–596.
119. Woost PG, Brightwell J, Eiferman RA, Schultz GS. Effect of growth factors with dexamethasone on healing of rabbit corneal stromal incisions. *Exp Eye Res.* 1985;40:47–60.
120. Kirschner SE, Ciaccia A, Ubels JL. The effect of retinoic acid on thymidine incorporation and morphology of corneal stromal fibroblasts. *Curr Eye Res.* 1990;9:1121–1125.
121. Kenney MC, Chwa M, Escobar M, Brown D. Altered gelatinolytic activity by keratoconus corneal cells. *Biochem Biophys Res Commun.* 1989;161:353–357.
122. Lemp MA. Cornea and sclera. *Arch Ophthalmol.* 1976;94:473–490.
123. Binder PS. Barraquer lecture. What we have learned about corneal wound healing from refractive surgery. *Refract Corneal Surg.* 1989;5:98–120.
124. Schmack I, Dawson DG, McCarey BE, et al. Cohesive tensile strength of human LASIK wounds with histologic, ultrastructural, and clinical correlations. *J Refract Surg.* 2005;21:433–445.
125. Fournié PR, Gordon GM, Dawson DG, et al. Correlations of long-term matrix metalloproteinase localization in human corneas after successful laser-assisted in situ keratomileusis with minor complications at the flap margin. *Arch Ophthalmol.* 2008;126:162–170.
126. Morrison JC, Swan KC. Bowman's layer in penetrating keratoplasties of the human eye. *Arch Ophthalmol.* 1982;100:1835–1838.
127. Morrison JC, Swan KC. Full-thickness lamellar keratoplasty. A histologic study in human eyes. *Ophthalmology.* 1982;89:715–719.
128. Klyce SD, Crosson CE. Transport processes across the rabbit corneal epithelium: A review. *Curr Eye Res.* 1985;4:323–331.
129. McLaughlin BJ, Caldwell RB, Sasaki Y, Wood TO. Freeze-fracture quantitative comparison of rabbit corneal epithelial and endothelial membranes. *Curr Eye Res.* 1985;4:951–961.
130. Ban Y, Dota A, Cooper LJ, et al. Tight junction-related protein expression and distribution in human corneal epithelium. *Exp Eye Res.* 2003;76:663–669.
131. Gipson IK, Yankauckas M, Spurr-Michaud SJ, et al. Characteristics of a glycoprotein in the ocular surface glycocalyx. *Invest Ophthalmol Vis Sci.* 1992;33:218–227.
132. Nichols BA, Chiappino ML, Dawson CR. Demonstration of the mucous layer of the tear film by electron microscopy. *Invest Ophthalmol Vis Sci.* 1985;26:464–473.
133. Argüeso P, Gipson IK. Epithelial mucins of the ocular surface: Structure, biosynthesis and function. *Exp Eye Res.* 2001;73:281–289.
134. Mishima S. Some physiological aspects of the precorneal tear film. *Arch Ophthalmol.* 1965;73:233–241.
135. The definition and classification of dry eye disease: Report of the Definition and Classification Subcommittee of the International Dry Eye WorkShop (2007). *Ocul Surf.* 2007;5:75–92.
136. Behrens A, Doyle JJ, Stern L, et al. Dysfunctional tear syndrome: A Delphi approach to treatment recommendations. *Cornea.* 2006;25:900–907.
137. Perry HD. Dry eye disease: Pathophysiology, classification, and diagnosis. *Am J Manag Care.* 2008;14:S79–S87.
138. Friedenwald JS, Buschke W. Some factors concerned in the mitotic and wound-healing activities of the corneal epithelium. *Trans Am Ophthalmol Soc.* 1944;42:371–383.
139. Hanna C, Bicknell DS, O'Brien JE. Cell turnover in the adult human eye. *Arch Ophthalmol.* 1961;65:695–698.
140. Hanna C, O'Brien JE. Cell production and migration in the epithelial layer of the cornea. *Arch Ophthalmol.* 1960;64:536–539.
141. Williams K, Watsky M. Gap junctional communication in the human corneal endothelium and epithelium. *Curr Eye Res.* 2002;25:29–36.
142. Buck RC. Measurement of centripetal migration of normal corneal epithelial cells in the mouse. *Invest Ophthalmol Vis Sci.* 1985;26:1296–1299.
143. Kinoshita S, Friend J, Thoft RA. Sex chromatin of donor corneal epithelium in rabbits. *Invest Ophthalmol Vis Sci.* 1981;21:434–441.
144. Schermer A, Galvin S, Sun TT. Differentiation-related expression of a major 64K corneal keratin in vivo and in culture suggests limbal location of corneal epithelial stem cells. *J Cell Biol.* 1986;103:49–62.
145. Sharma A, Coles WH. Kinetics of corneal epithelial maintenance and graft loss. A population balance model. *Invest Ophthalmol Vis Sci.* 1989;30:1962–1971.
146. Thoft RA, Friend J. The X, Y, Z hypothesis of corneal epithelial maintenance. *Invest Ophthalmol Vis Sci.* 1983;24:1442–1443.
147. Dillon EC, Eagle RC Jr, Laibson PR. Compensatory epithelial hyperplasia in human corneal disease. *Ophthalmic Surg.* 1992;23:729–732.
148. Cotsarelis G, Cheng SZ, Dong G, et al. Existence of slow-cycling limbal epithelial basal cells that can be preferentially stimulated to proliferate: Implications on epithelial stem cells. *Cell.* 1989;57:201–209.
149. Tseng SC. Concept and application of limbal stem cells. *Eye (Lond).* 1989;3(Pt 2):141–157.
150. Lavker RM, Tseng SC, Sun TT. Corneal epithelial stem cells at the limbus: Looking at some old problems from a new angle. *Exp Eye Res.* 2004;78:433–446.
151. Boulton M, Albon J. Stem cells in the eye. *Int J Biochem Cell Biol.* 2004;36:643–657.
152. Nakamura T, Kinoshita S. [Current regenerative therapy for the cornea]. *Nihon Rinsho.* 2008;66:955–960.
153. Koizumi N, Nishida K, Amano S, Kinoshita S. [Progress in the development of tissue engineering of the cornea in Japan]. *Nippon Ganka Gakkai Zasshi.* 2007;111:493–503.
154. Gillette TE, Chandler JW, Greiner JV. Langerhans cells of the ocular surface. *Ophthalmology.* 1982;89:700–711.
155. Steinman RM. The dendritic cell system and its role in immunogenicity. *Annu Rev Immunol.* 1991;9:271–296.
156. Hamrah P, Zhang Q, Liu Y, Dana MR. Novel characterization of MHC class II-negative population of resident corneal Langerhans cell-type dendritic cells. *Invest Ophthalmol Vis Sci.* 2002;43:639–646.
157. Edelhauser HF. The resiliency of the corneal endothelium to refractive and intraocular surgery. *Cornea.* 2000;19:263–273.
158. Iwamoto T, Smelser GK. Electron microscopy of the human corneal endothelium with reference to transport mechanisms. *Invest Ophthalmol.* 1965;4:270–284.
159. Hirsch M, Renard G, Faure JP, Pouliquen Y. Study of the ultrastructure of the rabbit corneal endothelium by the freeze-fracture technique: Apical and lateral junctions. *Exp Eye Res.* 1977;25:277–288.
160. Joyce NC. Cell cycle status in human corneal endothelium. *Exp Eye Res.* 2005;81:629–638.
161. Mimura T, Joyce NC. Replication competence and senescence in central and peripheral human corneal endothelium. *Invest Ophthalmol Vis Sci.* 2006;47:1387–1396.
162. Yee RW, Matsuda M, Schultz RO, Edelhauser HF. Changes in the normal corneal endothelial cellular pattern as a function of age. *Curr Eye Res.* 1985;4:671–678.
163. McGowan SL, Edelhauser HF, Pfister RR, Whikehart DR. Stem cell markers in the human posterior limbus and corneal endothelium of unwounded and wounded corneas. *Mol Vis.* 2007;13:1984–2000.
164. Whikehart DR, Parikh CH, Vaughn AV, et al. Evidence suggesting the existence of stem cells for the human corneal endothelium. *Mol Vis.* 2005;11:816–824.
165. Matsuda M, Yee RW, Edelhauser HF. Comparison of the corneal endothelium in an American and a Japanese population. *Arch Ophthalmol.* 1985;103:68–70.
166. Rao SK, Ranjan Sen P, Fogla R, et al. Corneal endothelial cell density and morphology in normal Indian eyes. *Cornea.* 2000;19:820–823.
167. Padilla MD, Sibayan SA, Gonzales CS. Corneal endothelial cell density and morphology in normal Filipino eyes. *Cornea.* 2004;23:129–135.
168. Yunliang S, Yuqiang H, Ying-Peng L, et al. Corneal endothelial cell density and morphology in healthy Chinese eyes. *Cornea.* 2007;26:130–132.
169. Yuen LH, He M, Aung T, et al. Biometry of the cornea and anterior chamber in Chinese eyes: An anterior segment optical coherence tomography study. *Invest Ophthalmol Vis Sci.* 2010;51:3433–3440.
170. Ang M, Chong W, Tay WT, et al. Anterior segment optical coherence tomography study of the cornea and anterior segment in adult ethnic South Asian Indian eyes. *Invest Ophthalmol Vis Sci.* 2012;53:120–125.

171. Tan DK, Chong W, Tay WT, et al. Anterior chamber dimensions and posterior corneal arc length in Malay eyes: An anterior segment optical coherence tomography study. *Invest Ophthalmol Vis Sci.* 2012;53:4860–4867.
172. Amann J, Holley GP, Lee S-B, Edelhauser HF. Increased endothelial cell density in the paracentral and peripheral regions of the human cornea. *Am J Ophthalmol.* 2003;135:584–590.
173. Irvine AR, Irvine AR Jr. Variations in normal human corneal Endothelium: A preliminary report of pathologic human corneal endothelium. *Am J Ophthalmol.* 1953;36:1279–1285.
174. Schimmelpfennig BH. Direct and indirect determination of nonuniform cell density distribution in human corneal endothelium. *Invest Ophthalmol Vis Sci.* 1984;25:223–229.
175. Daus W, Völcker HE, Meysen H, Bundschuh W. [Vital staining of the corneal endothelium—increased possibilities of diagnosis]. *Fortschr Ophthalmol.* 1989;86:259–264.
176. Daus W, Völcker HE, Meysen H. [Clinical significance of age-related regional differences in distribution of human corneal endothelium]. *Klin Monbl Augenheilkd.* 1990;196:449–455.
177. He Z, Campolmi N, Gain P, et al. Revisited microanatomy of the corneal endothelial periphery: New evidence for continuous centripetal migration of endothelial cells in humans. *Stem Cells.* 2012;30:2523–2534.
178. Bourne WM, McLaren JW. Clinical responses of the corneal endothelium. *Exp Eye Res.* 2004;78:561–572.
179. Watsky MA, McDermott ML, Edelhauser HF. In vitro corneal endothelial permeability in rabbit and human: The effects of age, cataract surgery and diabetes. *Exp Eye Res.* 1989;49:751–767.
180. Carlson KH, Bourne WM, McLaren JW, Brubaker RF. Variations in human corneal endothelial cell morphology and permeability to fluorescein with age. *Exp Eye Res.* 1988;47:27–41.
181. Harris JE. Symposium on the cornea. Introduction: Factors influencing corneal hydration. *Invest Ophthalmol.* 1962;1:151–157.
182. Lim JJ. Na+ transport across the rabbit corneal endothelium. *Curr Eye Res.* 1981;1:255–258.
183. Geroski DH, Matsuda M, Yee RW, Edelhauser HF. Pump function of the human corneal endothelium. Effects of age and cornea guttata. *Ophthalmology.* 1985;92:759–763.
184. Bourne WM. Clinical estimation of corneal endothelial pump function. *Trans Am Ophthalmol Soc.* 1998;96:229–239; discussion 239–242.
185. Burns RR, Bourne WM, Brubaker RF. Endothelial function in patients with cornea guttata. *Invest Ophthalmol Vis Sci.* 1981;20:77–85.
186. Mishima S. Clinical investigations on the corneal endothelium—XXXVIII Edward Jackson Memorial Lecture. *Am J Ophthalmol.* 1982;93:1–29.
187. Bonanno JA. Identity and regulation of ion transport mechanisms in the corneal endothelium. *Prog Retin Eye Res.* 2003;22:69–94.
188. Stiemke MM, Roman RJ, Palmer ML, Edelhauser HF. Sodium activity in the aqueous humor and corneal stroma of the rabbit. *Exp Eye Res.* 1992;55:425–433.
189. Hedbys BO, Dohlman CH. A new method for the determination of the swelling pressure of the corneal stroma in vitro. *Exp Eye Res.* 1963;2:122–129.
190. Klyce SD, Dohlman CH, Tolpin DW. In vivo determination of corneal swelling pressure. *Exp Eye Res.* 1971;11:220–229.
191. Hedbys BO, Mishima S, Maurice DM. The imbibition pressure of the corneal stroma. *Exp Eye Res.* 1963;2:99–111.
192. Ytteborg J, Dohlman CH. Corneal edema and intraocular pressure. II. Clinical results. *Arch Ophthalmol.* 1965;74:477–484.
193. Harper CL, Boulton ME, Bennett D, et al. Diurnal variations in human corneal thickness. *Br J Ophthalmol.* 1996;80:1068–1072.
194. Feng Y, Varikooty J, Simpson TL. Diurnal variation of corneal and corneal epithelial thickness measured using optical coherence tomography. *Cornea.* 2001;20:480–483.
195. Van Horn DL, Doughman DJ, Harris JE, et al. Ultrastructure of human organ-cultured cornea. II. Stroma and epithelium. *Arch Ophthalmol.* 1975;93:275–277.
196. Meek KM, Dennis S, Khan S. Changes in the refractive index of the stroma and its extrafibrillar matrix when the cornea swells. *Biophys J.* 2003;85:2205–2212.
197. Müller LJ, Pels E, Vrensen GF. The specific architecture of the anterior stroma accounts for maintenance of corneal curvature. *Br J Ophthalmol.* 2001;85:437–443.
198. Kangas TA, Edelhauser HF, Twining SS, O'Brien WJ. Loss of stromal glycosaminoglycans during corneal edema. *Invest Ophthalmol Vis Sci.* 1990;31:1994–2002.
199. Cristol SM, Edelhauser HF, Lynn MJ. A comparison of corneal stromal edema induced from the anterior or the posterior surface. *Refract Corneal Surg.* 1992;8:224–229.
200. Connon CJ, Meek KM. The structure and swelling of corneal scar tissue in penetrating full-thickness wounds. *Cornea.* 2004;23:165–171.
201. Hatton MP, Perez VL, Dohlman CH. Corneal oedema in ocular hypotony. *Exp Eye Res.* 2004;78:549–552.
202. Johnson DH, Bourne WM, Campbell RJ. The ultrastructure of Descemet's membrane. I. Changes with age in normal corneas. *Arch Ophthalmol.* 1982;100:1942–1947.
203. Waring GO III. Posterior collagenous layer of the cornea. Ultrastructural classification of abnormal collagenous tissue posterior to Descemet's membrane in 30 cases. *Arch Ophthalmol.* 1982;100:122–134.
204. Hayes S, Boote C, Lewis J, et al. Comparative study of fibrillar collagen arrangement in the corneas of primates and other mammals. *Anat Rec (Hoboken).* 2007;290:1542–1550.
205. Silver FH, Kato YP, Ohno M, Wasserman AJ. Analysis of mammalian connective tissue: Relationship between hierarchical structures and mechanical properties. *J Long Term Eff Med Implants.* 1992;2:165–198.
206. Dupps WJ Jr, Wilson SE. Biomechanics and wound healing in the cornea. *Exp Eye Res.* 2006;83:709–720.
207. Elsheikh A, Alhasso D, Rama P. Assessment of the epithelium's contribution to corneal biomechanics. *Exp Eye Res.* 2008;86:445–451.
208. Seiler T, Matallana M, Sendler S, Bende T. Does Bowman's layer determine the biomechanical properties of the cornea? *Refract Corneal Surg.* 1992;8:139–142.
209. Avetisov SE, Mamikonian VR, Zavalishin NN, Neniukov AK. [Experimental study of mechanical characteristics of the cornea and the adjacent parts of the sclera]. *Oftalmol Zh.* 1988:233–237.
210. Jue B, Maurice DM. The mechanical properties of the rabbit and human cornea. *J Biomech.* 1986;19:847–853.
211. Meek KM, Newton RH. Organization of collagen fibrils in the corneal stroma in relation to mechanical properties and surgical practice. *J Refract Surg.* 1999;15:695–699.
212. Bron AJ. The architecture of the corneal stroma. *Br J Ophthalmol.* 2001;85:379–381.
213. Chihara E. Assessment of true intraocular pressure: The gap between theory and practical data. *Surv Ophthalmol.* 2008;53:203–218.
214. Miller D. Pressure of the lid on the eye. *Arch Ophthalmol.* 1967;78:328–330.
215. Coleman DJ, Trokel S. Direct-recorded intraocular pressure variations in a human subject. *Arch Ophthalmol.* 1969;82:637–640.
216. McPhee TJ, Bourne WM, Brubaker RF. Location of the stress-bearing layers of the cornea. *Invest Ophthalmol Vis Sci.* 1985;26:869–872.
217. Roberts C. Biomechanics of the cornea and wavefront-guided laser refractive surgery. *J Refract Surg.* 2002;18:S589–S592.
218. Ethier CR, Johnson M, Ruberti J. Ocular biomechanics and biotransport. *Annu Rev Biomed Eng.* 2004;6:249–273.
219. Elsheikh A, Anderson K. Comparative study of corneal strip extensometry and inflation tests. *J R Soc Interface.* 2005;2:177–185.
220. Blackburn BJ, Jenkins MW, Rollins AM, Dupps WJ. A review of structural and biomechanical changes in the cornea in aging, disease, and photochemical crosslinking. *Front Bioeng Biotechnol.* 2019;7:66.
221. Maloney RK. Effect of corneal hydration and intraocular pressure on keratometric power after experimental radial keratotomy. *Ophthalmology.* 1990;97:927–933.
222. Simon G, Small RH, Ren Q, Parel JM. Effect of corneal hydration on Goldmann applanation tonometry and corneal topography. *Refract Corneal Surg.* 1993;9:110–117.
223. Simon G, Ren Q. Biomechanical behavior of the cornea and its response to radial keratotomy. *J Refract Corneal Surg.* 1994;10:343–351; discussion 351–356.
224. Ousley PJ, Terry MA. Hydration effects on corneal topography. *Arch Ophthalmol.* 1996;114:181–185.
225. Kohlhaas M, Spoerl E, Schilde T, et al. Biomechanical evidence of the distribution of cross-links in corneas treated with riboflavin and ultraviolet A light. *J Cataract Refract Surg.* 2006;32:279–283.
226. Danielsen CC. Tensile mechanical and creep properties of Descemet's membrane and lens capsule. *Exp Eye Res.* 2004;79:343–350.
227. Elsheikh A, Brown M, Alhasso D, et al. Experimental assessment of corneal anisotropy. *J Refract Surg.* 2008;24:178–187.
228. Gilbert ML, Roth AS, Friedlander MH. Corneal flattening by shallow circular trephination in human eye bank eyes. *Refract Corneal Surg.* 1990;6:113–116.
229. Elsheikh A, Wang D, Brown M, et al. Assessment of corneal biomechanical properties and their variation with age. *Curr Eye Res.* 2007;32:11–19.
230. Hjortdal JO, Ehlers N. Effect of excimer laser keratectomy on the mechanical performance of the human cornea. *Acta Ophthalmol Scand.* 1995;73:18–24.
231. Provenzano PP, Vanderby R Jr. Collagen fibril morphology and organization: Implications for force transmission in ligament and tendon. *Matrix Biol.* 2006;25:71–84.
232. Patey A, Savoldelli M, Pouliquen Y. Keratoconus and normal cornea: A comparative study of the collagenous fibers of the corneal stroma by image analysis. *Cornea.* 1984;3:119–124.
233. Pouliquen YJ. 1984 Castroviejo lecture. Fine structure of the corneal stroma. *Cornea.* 1984;3:168–177.
234. Meek KM, Tuft SJ, Huang Y, et al. Changes in collagen orientation and distribution in keratoconus corneas. *Invest Ophthalmol Vis Sci.* 2005;46:1948–1956.
235. Dawson DG, Randleman JB, Grossniklaus HE, et al. Corneal ectasia after excimer laser keratorefractive surgery: Histopathology, ultrastructure, and pathophysiology. *Ophthalmology.* 2008;115:2181–2191.e1.
236. Andreassen TT, Simonsen AH, Oxlund H. Biomechanical properties of keratoconus and normal corneas. *Exp Eye Res.* 1980;31:435–441.
237. Edmund C. Corneal topography and elasticity in normal and keratoconic eyes. A methodological study concerning the pathogenesis of keratoconus. *Acta Ophthalmol Suppl.* 1989;193:1–36.
238. Swartz T, Marten L, Wang M. Measuring the cornea: The latest developments in corneal topography. *Curr Opin Ophthalmol.* 2007;18:325–333.
239. Bron AJ. Keratoconus. *Cornea.* 1988;7:163–169.
240. Sinha Roy A, Dupps WJ Jr. Patient-specific computational modeling of keratoconus progression and differential responses to collagen cross-linking. *Invest Ophthalmol Vis Sci.* 2011;52:9174–9187.
241. Gause S, Hsu K-H, Shafor C, et al. Mechanistic modeling of ophthalmic drug delivery to the anterior chamber by eye drops and contact lenses. *Adv Colloid Interface Sci.* 2016;233:139–154.
242. Gaudana R, Ananthula HK, Parenky A, Mitra AK. Ocular drug delivery. *AAPS J.* 2010;12:348–360.
243. Prausnitz MR, Noonan JS. Permeability of cornea, sclera, and conjunctiva: A literature analysis for drug delivery to the eye. *J Pharm Sci.* 1998;87:1479–1488.
244. Urtti A. Challenges and obstacles of ocular pharmacokinetics and drug delivery. *Adv Drug Deliv Rev.* 2006;58:1131–1135.
245. Salazar-Bookaman MM, Wainer I, Patil PN. Relevance of drug-melanin interactions to ocular pharmacology and toxicology. *J Ocul Pharmacol.* 1994;10:217–239.
246. Maurice DM. Drug delivery to the posterior segment from drops. *Surv Ophthalmol.* 2002;47(Suppl 1):S41–52.
247. Kang-Mieler JJ, Rudeen KM, Liu W, Mieler WF. Advances in ocular drug delivery systems. *Eye (Lond).* 2020;34:1371–1379.
248. Ustundag Okur N, Caglar ES, Siafaka PI. Novel ocular drug delivery systems: An update on microemulsions. *J Ocul Pharmacol Ther.* 2020;36:342–354.
249. Ghate D, Edelhauser HF. Ocular drug delivery. *Expert Opin Drug Deliv.* 2006;3:275–287.
250. Johnson GJ. The environment and the eye. *Eye (Lond).* 2004;18:1235–1250.
251. Sliney DH. Exposure geometry and spectral environment determine photobiological effects on the human eye. *Photochem Photobiol.* 2005;81:483–489.

252. Cejková J, Stípek S, Crkovská J, et al. UV rays, the prooxidant/antioxidant imbalance in the cornea and oxidative eye damage. *Physiol Res.* 2004;53:1–10.

253. Ringvold A. Corneal epithelium and UV-protection of the eye. *Acta Ophthalmol Scand.* 1998;76:149–153.

254. Brubaker RF, Bourne WM, Bachman LA, McLaren JW. Ascorbic acid content of human corneal epithelium. *Invest Ophthalmol Vis Sci.* 2000;41:1681–1683.

255. Mitchell J, Cenedella RJ. Quantitation of ultraviolet light-absorbing fractions of the cornea. *Cornea.* 1995;14:266–272.

256. Kolozsvári L, Nógrádi A, Hopp B, Bor Z. UV absorbance of the human cornea in the 240- to 400-nm range. *Invest Ophthalmol Vis Sci.* 2002;43:2165–2168.

257. Ren H, Wilson G. The effect of ultraviolet-B irradiation on the cell shedding rate of the corneal epithelium. *Acta Ophthalmol (Copenh).* 1994;72:447–452.

258. Shimmura S, Tadano K, Tsubota K. UV dose-dependent caspase activation in a corneal epithelial cell line. *Curr Eye Res.* 2004;28:85–92.

259. Wang L, Li T, Lu L. UV-induced corneal epithelial cell death by activation of potassium channels. *Invest Ophthalmol Vis Sci.* 2003;44:5095–5101.

260. Lu L, Wang L, Shell B. UV-induced signaling pathways associated with corneal epithelial cell apoptosis. *Invest Ophthalmol Vis Sci.* 2003;44:5102–5109.

261. Rose RC, Richer SP, Bode AM. Ocular oxidants and antioxidant protection. *Proc Soc Exp Biol Med.* 1998;217:397–407.

262. Kennedy M, Kim KH, Harten B, et al. Ultraviolet irradiation induces the production of multiple cytokines by human corneal cells. *Invest Ophthalmol Vis Sci.* 1997;38:2483–2491.

263. Watson PG, Young RD. Scleral structure, organisation and disease. A review. *Exp Eye Res.* 2004;78:609–623.

264. McBrien NA, Gentle A. Role of the sclera in the development and pathological complications of myopia. *Prog Retin Eye Res.* 2003;22:307–338.

265. Vaezy S, Clark JI. A quantitative analysis of transparency in the human sclera and cornea using Fourier methods. *J Microsc.* 1991;163:85–94.

266. Vaezy S, Clark JI. Quantitative analysis of the microstructure of the human cornea and sclera using 2-D Fourier methods. *J Microsc.* 1994;175:93–99.

267. Palme C, Ahmad S, Romano V, et al. En-face analysis of the human limbal lymphatic vasculature. *Exp Eye Res.* 2020;201:108278.

268. Jones LA, Mitchell GL, Mutti DO, et al. Comparison of ocular component growth curves among refractive error groups in children. *Invest Ophthalmol Vis Sci.* 2005;46:2317–2327.

269. Avetisov ES, Savitskaya NF, Vinetskaya MI, Iomdina EN. A study of biochemical and biomechanical qualities of normal and myopic eye sclera in humans of different age groups. *Metab Pediatr Syst Ophthalmol.* 1983;7:183–188.

270. Ang M, Flanagan JL, Wong CW, et al. Review: Myopia control strategies recommendations from the 2018 WHO/IAPB/BHVI Meeting on Myopia. *Br J Ophthalmol.* 2020;104:1482–1487.

271. Ohno-Matsui K, Wu PC, Yamashiro K, et al. IMI pathologic myopia. *Invest Ophthalmol Vis Sci.* 2021;62:5.

272. McBrien NA, Millodot M. A biometric investigation of late onset myopic eyes. *Acta Ophthalmol (Copenh).* 1987;65:461–468.

273. McBrien NA, Adams DW. A longitudinal investigation of adult-onset and adult-progression of myopia in an occupational group. Refractive and biometric findings. *Invest Ophthalmol Vis Sci.* 1997;38:321–333.

274. Lanca C, Foo LL, Ang M, et al. Rapid myopic progression in childhood is associated with teenage high myopia. *Invest Ophthalmol Vis Sci.* 2021;62:17.

275. Rada JA, Shelton S, Norton TT. The sclera and myopia. *Exp Eye Res.* 2006;82:185–200.

276. Ohno-Matsui K, Jonas JB. Posterior staphyloma in pathologic myopia. *Prog Retin Eye Res.* 2019;70:99–109.

277. Jonas JB, Ang M, Cho P, et al. IMI prevention of myopia and its progression. *Invest Ophthalmol Vis Sci.* 2021;62:6.

278. Wollensak G, Spoerl E. Collagen crosslinking of human and porcine sclera. *J Cataract Refract Surg.* 2004;30:689–695.

279. Boote C, Sigal IA, Grytz R, et al. Scleral structure and biomechanics. *Prog Retin Eye Res.* 2020;74:100773.

280. Olsen TW, Aaberg SY, Geroski DH, Edelhauser HF. Human sclera: Thickness and surface area. *Am J Ophthalmol.* 1998;125:237–241.

281. Boubriak OA, Urban JP, Bron AJ. Differential effects of aging on transport properties of anterior and posterior human sclera. *Exp Eye Res.* 2003;76:701–713.

282. Curtin BJ. Physiopathologic aspects of scleral stress-strain. *Trans Am Ophthalmol Soc.* 1969;67:417–461.

283. Lee WD, Devarajan K, Chua J, et al. Optical coherence tomography angiography for the anterior segment. *Eye Vis (Lond).* 2019;6:4.

284. Woo SL, Kobayashi AS, Schlegel WA, Lawrence C. Nonlinear material properties of intact cornea and sclera. *Exp Eye Res.* 1972;14:29–39.

285. St Helen R, McEwen, WK. Rheology of the human sclera. 1. Anelastic behavior. *Am J Ophthalmol.* 1961;52:539–548.

286. Hau SC, Devarajan K, Ang M. Anterior segment optical coherence tomography angiography and optical coherence tomography in the evaluation of episcleritis and scleritis. *Ocul Immunol Inflamm.* 2021;29:362–369.

287. Meyer PA, Watson PG. Low dose fluorescein angiography of the conjunctiva and episclera. *Br J Ophthalmol.* 1987;71:2–10.

288. Ang M, Sim DA, Keane PA, et al. Optical coherence tomography angiography for anterior segment vasculature imaging. *Ophthalmology.* 2015;122:1740–1747.

289. Ang M, Foo V, Ke M, et al. Role of anterior segment optical coherence tomography angiography in assessing limbal vasculature in acute chemical injury of the eye. *Br J Ophthalmol.* 2022;106:1212–1216.

290. Tan ACS, Tan GS, Denniston AK, et al. An overview of the clinical applications of optical coherence tomography angiography. *Eye (Lond).* 2018;32:262–286.

291. Ang M, Cai Y, Tan AC. Swept source optical coherence tomography angiography for contact lens-related corneal vascularization. *J Ophthalmol.* 2016;2016:9685297.

292. Atta G, Tempfer H, Kaser-Eichberger A, et al. The lymphangiogenic and hemangiogenic privilege of the human sclera. *Ann Anat.* 2020;230:151485.

293. Ghate D, Brooks W, McCarey BE, Edelhauser HF. Pharmacokinetics of intraocular drug delivery by periocular injections using ocular fluorophotometry. *Invest Ophthalmol Vis Sci.* 2007;48:2230–2237.

294. Sripetch S, Loftsson T. Topical drug delivery to the posterior segment of the eye: Thermodynamic considerations. *Int J Pharm.* 2021;597:120332.

295. Reibaldi M, Fallico M, Avitabile T, et al. Frequency of intravitreal anti-vascular endothelial growth factor injections and risk of death: A systematic review with meta-analysis. *Ophthalmol Retina.* 2021

296. Li T, Sun J, Min J, et al. Safety of receiving anti-vascular endothelial growth factor intravitreal injection in office-based vs operating room settings: A meta-analysis. *JAMA Ophthalmol.* 2021;139:1080–1088.

297. Woo J-H, Ang M, Htoon HM, Tan D. Descemet membrane endothelial keratoplasty versus Descemet stripping automated endothelial keratoplasty and penetrating keratoplasty. *Am J Ophthalmol.* 2019;207:288–303.

298. Ahmed I, Patton TF. Importance of the noncorneal absorption route in topical ophthalmic drug delivery. *Invest Ophthalmol Vis Sci.* 1985;26:584–587.

299. Barza M, Kane A, Baum J. Intraocular penetration of gentamicin after subconjunctival and retrobulbar injection. *Am J Ophthalmol.* 1978;85:541–547.

300. Bill A. Movement of albumin and dextran through the sclera. *Arch Ophthalmol.* 1965;74:248–252.

301. Olsen TW, Edelhauser HF, Lim JI, Geroski DH. Human scleral permeability. Effects of age, cryotherapy, transscleral diode laser, and surgical thinning. *Invest Ophthalmol Vis Sci.* 1995;36:1893–1903.

302. Ambati J, Canakis CS, Miller JW, et al. Diffusion of high molecular weight compounds through sclera. *Invest Ophthalmol Vis Sci.* 2000;41:1181–1185.

303. Lawrence MS, Miller JW. Ocular tissue permeabilities. *Int Ophthalmol Clin.* 2004;44:53–61.

304. Rudnick DE, Noonan JS, Geroski DH, et al. The effect of intraocular pressure on human and rabbit scleral permeability. *Invest Ophthalmol Vis Sci.* 1999;40:3054–3058.

305. Anderson OA, Jackson TL, Singh JK, et al. Human transscleral albumin permeability and the effect of topographical location and donor age. *Invest Ophthalmol Vis Sci.* 2008;49:4041–4045.

306. Pitkänen L, Ranta V-P, Moilanen H, Urtti A. Permeability of retinal pigment epithelium: Effects of permeant molecular weight and lipophilicity. *Invest Ophthalmol Vis Sci.* 2005;46:641–646.

307. Moore DJ, Clover GM. The effect of age on the macromolecular permeability of human Bruch's membrane. *Invest Ophthalmol Vis Sci.* 2001;42:2970–2975.

308. Robinson MR, Lee SS, Kim H, et al. A rabbit model for assessing the ocular barriers to the transscleral delivery of triamcinolone acetonide. *Exp Eye Res.* 2006;82:479–487.

309. Kim SH, Lutz RJ, Wang NS, Robinson MR. Transport barriers in transscleral drug delivery for retinal diseases. *Ophthalmic Res.* 2007;39:244–254.

310. McAllister DV, Allen MG, Prausnitz MR. Microfabricated microneedles for gene and drug delivery. *Annu Rev Biomed Eng.* 2000;2:289–313.

311. Jiang J, Gill HS, Ghate D, et al. Coated microneedles for drug delivery to the eye. *Invest Ophthalmol Vis Sci.* 2007;48:4038–4043.

312. Simpson AE, Gilbert JA, Rudnick DE, et al. Transscleral diffusion of carboplatin: An in vitro and in vivo study. *Arch Ophthalmol.* 2002;120:1069–1074.

313. Konstantopoulos A, Hossain P, Anderson DF. Recent advances in ophthalmic anterior segment imaging: A new era for ophthalmic diagnosis? *Br J Ophthalmol.* 2007;91:551–557.

314. Liesegang TJ. Physiologic changes of the cornea with contact lens wear. *CLAO J.* 2002;28:12–27.

315. Swarbrick HA. Orthokeratology (corneal refractive therapy): What is it and how does it work? *Eye Contact Lens.* 2004;30:181–185; discussion 205–26.

316. Kim TI, Alio Del Barrio JL, Wilkins M, et al. Refractive surgery. *Lancet.* 2019;393:2085–2098.

317. Ang M, Gatinel D, Reinstein DZ, et al. Refractive surgery beyond 2020. *Eye (Lond).* 2021;35:362–382.

318. Dawson DG, Edelhauser HF, Grossniklaus HE. Long-term histopathologic findings in human corneal wounds after refractive surgical procedures. *Am J Ophthalmol.* 2005;139:168–178.

319. Kohnen T, Bühren J, Cichocki M, et al. [Optical quality after refractive corneal surgery]. *Ophthalmologe.* 2006;103:184–191.

320. Mrochen M, Hafezi F, Jankov M, Seiler T. [Ablation profiles in corneal laser surgery. Current and future concepts]. *Ophthalmologe.* 2006;103:175–183.

321. Ang M, Mehta JS, Chan C, et al. Refractive lenticule extraction: Transition and comparison of 3 surgical techniques. *J Cataract Refract Surg.* 2014;40:1415–1424.

322. Vestergaard AH, Grauslund J, Ivarsen AR, Hjortdal JØ. Efficacy, safety, predictability, contrast sensitivity, and aberrations after femtosecond laser lenticule extraction. *J Cataract Refract Surg.* 2014;40:403–411.

323. Sekundo W, Gertnere J, Bertelmann T, Solomatin I. One-year refractive results, contrast sensitivity, high-order aberrations and complications after myopic small-incision lenticule extraction (ReLEx SMILE). *Graefes Arch Clin Exp Ophthalmol.* 2014;252:837–843.

324. Moshirfar M, McCaughey MV, Reinstein DZ, et al. Small-incision lenticule extraction. *J Cataract Refract Surg.* 2015;41:652–665.

325. Denoyer A, Landman E, Trinh L, et al. Dry eye disease after refractive surgery: Comparative outcomes of small incision lenticule extraction versus LASIK. *Ophthalmology.* 2015;122:669–676.

326. Reinstein DZ, Archer TJ, Gobbe M, Bartoli E. Corneal sensitivity after small-incision lenticule extraction and laser in situ keratomileusis. *J Cataract Refract Surg.* 2015;41:1580–1587.

327. Seven I, Vahdati A, Pedersen IB, et al. Contralateral eye comparison of SMILE and flap-based corneal refractive surgery: Computational analysis of biomechanical impact. *J Refract Surg.* 2017;33:444–453.

328. Sinha Roy A, Dupps WJ Jr, Roberts CJ. Comparison of biomechanical effects of small-incision lenticule extraction and laser in situ keratomileusis: Finite-element analysis. *J Cataract Refract Surg.* 2014;40:971–980.
329. Pedersen IB, Ivarsen A, Hjortdal J. Changes in astigmatism, densitometry, and aberrations after SMILE for low to high myopic astigmatism: A 12-month prospective study. *J Refract Surg.* 2017;33:11–17.
330. Damgaard IB, Ang M, Mahmoud AM, et al. Functional optical zone and centration following SMILE and LASIK: A prospective, randomized, contralateral eye study. *J Refract Surg.* 2019;35:230–237.
331. Shen Z, Shi K, Yu Y, et al. Small incision lenticule extraction (SMILE) versus femtosecond laser-assisted in situ keratomileusis (FS-LASIK) for myopia: A systematic review and meta-analysis. *PLoS One.* 2016;11:e0158176.
332. Ang M, Farook M, Htoon HM, Mehta JS. Randomized clinical trial comparing femtosecond LASIK and small-incision lenticule extraction. *Ophthalmology.* 2020;127:724–730.
333. Ang M, Ho H, Fenwick E, et al. Vision-related quality of life and visual outcomes after small-incision lenticule extraction and laser in situ keratomileusis. *J Cataract Refract Surg.* 2015;41:2136–2144.
334. Obata H, Tsuru T. Corneal wound healing from the perspective of keratoplasty specimens with special reference to the function of the Bowman layer and Descemet membrane. *Cornea.* 2007;26:S82–S89.
335. Flaxel JT, Swan KC. Limbal wound healing after cataract extraction. A histologic study. *Arch Ophthalmol.* 1969;81:653–659.
336. Flaxel JT. Histology of cataract extractions. *Arch Ophthalmol.* 1970;83:436–444.
337. Lang GK, Green WR, Maumenee AE. Clinicopathologic studies of keratoplasty eyes obtained post mortem. *Am J Ophthalmol.* 1986;101:28–40.
338. Deg JK, Binder PS. Wound healing after astigmatic keratotomy in human eyes. *Ophthalmology.* 1987;94:1290–1298.
339. Melles GR, Binder PS. A comparison of wound healing in sutured and unsutured corneal wounds. *Arch Ophthalmol.* 1990;108:1460–1469.
340. Jester JV, Villaseñor RA, Schanzlin DJ, Cavanagh HD. Variations in corneal wound healing after radial keratotomy: Possible insights into mechanisms of clinical complications and refractive effects. *Cornea.* 1992;11:191–199.
341. Wu WC, Stark WJ, Green WR. Corneal wound healing after 193-nm excimer laser keratectomy. *Arch Ophthalmol.* 1991;109:1426–1432.
342. Taylor DM, L'Esperance FA Jr, Del Pero RA, et al. Human excimer laser lamellar keratectomy: A clinical study. *Ophthalmology.* 1989;96:654–664.
343. Anderson NJ, Edelhauser HF, Sharara N, et al. Histologic and ultrastructural findings in human corneas after successful laser in situ keratomileusis. *Arch Ophthalmol.* 2002;120:288–293.
344. Kramer TR, Chuckpaiwong V, Dawson DG, et al. Pathologic findings in postmortem corneas after successful laser in situ keratomileusis. *Cornea.* 2005;24:92–102.
345. Dawson DG, Kramer TR, Grossniklaus HE, et al. Histologic, ultrastructural, and immunofluorescent evaluation of human laser-assisted in situ keratomileusis corneal wounds. *Arch Ophthalmol.* 2005;123:741–756.
346. Edelhauser HF, Geroski DH, Woods WD, et al. Swelling in the isolated perfused cornea induced by 12(R)hydroxyeicosatetraenoic acid. *Invest Ophthalmol Vis Sci.* 1993;34:2953–2961.
347. Polse KA, Brand RJ, Cohen SR, Guillon M. Hypoxic effects on corneal morphology and function. *Invest Ophthalmol Vis Sci.* 1990;31:1542–1554.
348. Minassian DC, Rosen P, Dart JK, et al. Extracapsular cataract extraction compared with small incision surgery by phacoemulsification: A randomised trial. *Br J Ophthalmol.* 2001;85:822–829.
349. Ang M, Evans JR, Mehta JS. Manual small incision cataract surgery (MSICS) with posterior chamber intraocular lens versus extracapsular cataract extraction (ECCE) with posterior chamber intraocular lens for age-related cataract. *Cochrane Database Syst Rev.* 2014;2014:CD008811.
350. Bourne RR, Minassian DC, Dart JK, et al. Effect of cataract surgery on the corneal endothelium: Modern phacoemulsification compared with extracapsular cataract surgery. *Ophthalmology.* 2004;111:679–685.
351. Bourne WM, Nelson LR, Hodge DO. Continued endothelial cell loss ten years after lens implantation. *Ophthalmology.* 1994;101:1014–1022; discussion 1022–1023.
352. Crema AS, Walsh A, Yamane Y, Nosé W. Comparative study of coaxial phacoemulsification and microincision cataract surgery. One-year follow-up. *J Cataract Refract Surg.* 2007;33:1014–1018.
353. Storr-Paulsen A, Norregaard JC, Ahmed S, et al. Endothelial cell damage after cataract surgery: Divide-and-conquer versus phaco-chop technique. *J Cataract Refract Surg.* 2008;34:996–1000.
354. Srinivasan S. Phakic intraocular lenses: Lessons learned. *J Cataract Refract Surg.* 2019;45:1529–1530.
355. Vargas V, Alio JL. Refractive outcomes and complications following angle supported, iris fixated, and posterior chamber phakic intraocular lenses bilensectomy. *Curr Opin Ophthalmol.* 2021;32:25–30.
356. Bourne WM. Cellular changes in transplanted human corneas. *Cornea.* 2001;20:560–569.
357. Straiko MD, Shamie N, Terry MA. Endothelial keratoplasty: Past, present, and future directions. *Int Ophthalmol Clin.* 2010;50:123–135.
358. Price MO, Price FW. Descemet's stripping endothelial keratoplasty. *Curr Opin Ophthalmol.* 2007;18:290–294.
359. Bose S, Ang M, Mehta JS, et al. Cost-effectiveness of Descemet's stripping endothelial keratoplasty versus penetrating keratoplasty. *Ophthalmology.* 2013;120:464–470.
360. Ang M, Wilkins MR, Mehta JS, Tan D. Descemet membrane endothelial keratoplasty. *Br J Ophthalmol.* 2016;100:15–21.
361. Ang M, Soh Y, Htoon HM, et al. Five-year graft survival comparing Descemet stripping automated endothelial keratoplasty and penetrating keratoplasty. *Ophthalmology.* 2016;123:1646–1652.
362. Ang M, Mehta JS, Lim F, et al. Endothelial cell loss and graft survival after Descemet's stripping automated endothelial keratoplasty and penetrating keratoplasty. *Ophthalmology.* 2012;119:2239–2244.
363. Lacayo GO III, Majmudar PA. How and when to use mitomycin-C in refractive surgery. *Curr Opin Ophthalmol.* 2005;16:256–259.
364. Arranz-Marquez E, Katsanos A, Kozobolis VP, et al. A critical overview of the biological effects of mitomycin C application on the cornea following refractive surgery. *Adv Ther.* 2019;36:786–797.
365. Kohlhaas M. [Collagen crosslinking with riboflavin and UVA-light in keratoconus]. *Ophthalmologe.* 2008;105:785–793; quiz 794.
366. Raiskup F, Theuring A, Pillunat LE, Spoerl E. Corneal collagen crosslinking with riboflavin and ultraviolet-A light in progressive keratoconus: Ten-year results. *J Cataract Refract Surg.* 2015;41:41–46.
367. Raiskup-Wolf F, Hoyer A, Spoerl E, Pillunat LE. Collagen crosslinking with riboflavin and ultraviolet-A light in keratoconus: Long-term results. *J Cataract Refract Surg.* 2008;34:796–801.
368. Mamalis N. Toxic anterior segment syndrome update. *J Cataract Refract Surg.* 2010;36:1067–1068.
369. Luce DA. Determining in vivo biomechanical properties of the cornea with an ocular response analyzer. *J Cataract Refract Surg.* 2005;31:156–162.
370. Kotecha A. What biomechanical properties of the cornea are relevant for the clinician? *Surv Ophthalmol.* 2007;52(Suppl 2):S109–S114.
371. Kotecha A, Elsheikh A, Roberts CR, et al. Corneal thickness- and age-related biomechanical properties of the cornea measured with the ocular response analyzer. *Invest Ophthalmol Vis Sci.* 2006;47:5337–5347.
372. Ortiz D, Piñero D, Shabayek MH, et al. Corneal biomechanical properties in normal, post-laser in situ keratomileusis, and keratoconic eyes. *J Cataract Refract Surg.* 2007;33:1371–1375.
373. Moreno-Montañés J, Maldonado MJ, García N, et al. Reproducibility and clinical relevance of the ocular response analyzer in nonoperated eyes: corneal biomechanical and tonometric implications. *Invest Ophthalmol Vis Sci.* 2008;49:968–974.
374. Vinciguerra R, Ambrósio R Jr, Elsheikh A, et al. Detection of keratoconus with a new biomechanical index. *J Refract Surg.* 2016;32:803–810.
375. Ambrósio R Jr, Lopes BT, Faria-Correia F, et al. Integration of Scheimpflug-based corneal tomography and biomechanical assessments for enhancing ectasia detection. *J Refract Surg.* 2017;33:434–443.
376. Antonacci G, Beck T, Bilenca A, et al. Recent progress and current opinions in Brillouin microscopy for life science applications. *Biophys Rev.* 2020;12:615–624.

5

The Lens

Paul James Donaldson

INTRODUCTION

The optical properties of the ocular lens are a critical determinant of overall vision quality.[1,2] As a transparent specialized epithelial tissue, the lens contributes to the overall and dynamic focusing power of the eye and corrects for optical errors introduced by the cornea. To perform these functions, the lens needs not only to be transparent to avoid light scattering but also to have a higher refractive index than the medium in which it is suspended. It also needs to have refractive surfaces with the appropriate curvature to ensure that light is correctly focused on the retina. Furthermore, to compensate for its own spherical aberration (see Box 5.1) and that of the cornea, the lens generates a gradient of refractive index (GRI) that improves overall vision quality. Thus, the critical tissue level parameters that determine the focusing power of the lens are its surface curvature (geometry) and GRI. However, as might be expected of a living tissue, these parameters change as we grow. Therefore the transparent (light scattering) and the refractive (optical power and dynamic focusing) properties of the lens are not constant and change throughout life. Some of these changes are compensated for by alterations to lens power to ensure that the focal point and vision quality of the eye remains remarkably constant despite the continual growth of the lens. However, other age-dependent changes to the lens reduce the dynamic focusing or accommodative ability of the lens that manifests as presbyopia in middle age, while increased light scattering produces a loss of transparency that leads to cataract formation in the elderly. Together these two lens pathologies are by far the leading causes of uncorrected refractive error and blindness, respectively, in the world today.

At the molecular and cellular levels, the transparency and refractive properties of the lens are established by a specialized tissue architecture that is first established in utero, and which is maintained throughout life by a unique physiology. This chapter provides an overview of how lens development, growth, metabolism, and physiology establish and maintain the optical properties of the normal lens. It also explores how age-related changes in these processes contribute to the observed change in lens power that occurs with age, the onset of presbyopia in middle age, and the formation of different forms of cataract in the elderly. Information about the human lens is emphasized, although studies using animals are included when human data are unavailable. The unsolved issues in the biology and pathology of the lens are highlighted throughout. References to comprehensive reviews and original source material are included to assist the reader. The citations provided are not meant to be inclusive, but to highlight articles of special relevance.

THE ORGANIZATION, DEVELOPMENT, AND GROWTH OF THE LENS

Because the lens grows throughout life and consequently changes its geometry and therefore its optical power, we will initiate our discussion of the organization of the lens by considering the lens from a typical adult subject that can accommodate. At this stage of life, the unaccommodated lens of a young adult typically exhibits a flattened oblate spheroid shape with a diameter of approximately 9 mm, a thickness of approximately 4.5 mm, and anterior and posterior surface radii of curvature of some 10 mm and 5.5 mm, respectively.[3] This lens contributes around 20 diopters (D) of optical power to the emmetropic eye, corrects for corneal spherical aberration, and can accommodate. It is located in the eye behind the iris, and its position in the optical pathway is maintained by the zonules of Zinn that attach the lens to the ciliary body (Fig. 5.1). During the process of accommodation, contraction of the ciliary muscle causes the ciliary attachments of these zonular fibers to move forward and inward, thereby allowing the elastic, collagen-rich capsule that surrounds the lens to mold its shape.[4-7] Thus, in our typical young adult, the accommodated lens assumes a rounder shape and increases its optical power by approximately 10 to 12 D to enable focusing on near objects.[8-10] The cellular organization of this typical young adult lens will be first considered before discussing the processes during embryonic development and growth that establish the structural features of the adult lens.

Cellular organization of the adult human lens

The zonules that suspend the lens within the eye originate in the nonpigmented layer of the ciliary epithelium and insert into the lens capsule that surrounds the lens near the equator (Fig. 5.2).[11] Examination of the insertion of zonular fibers into the lens capsule that surrounds the lens shows that these fibers are intimately interwoven with the components of the collagenous lens capsule.[12-14] The extracellular matrix that forms the lens capsule is continuously secreted by epithelial and superficial fiber cells.[15,16] It is composed predominantly of type IV collagen, laminin, entactin (nidogen), and the heparan sulfate proteoglycan perlecan.[17-21] The capsule is composed of multiple laminae, as if the basal lamina had been replicated many times,[19] and the different laminae appear to have distinctive compositions in different regions. At the lens equator, collagen IV and nidogen span the capsule depth, while laminin and perlecan are located in two separate lamellae located at the innermost and outermost capsule domains.[21] The lamina structure of the capsule suggest that it is synthesized from the inside out. This

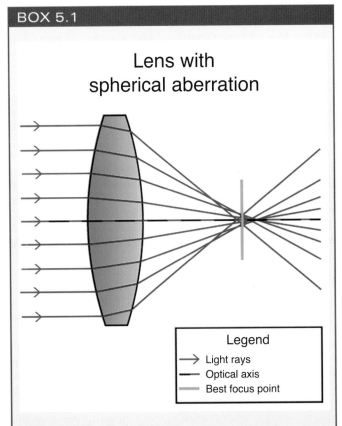

BOX 5.1

Lens with spherical aberration

Legend
→ Light rays
— Optical axis
— Best focus point

Spherical aberration is an example of a subtle optical imperfection or higher-order aberration that results in a loss of clarity of images formed by the eye and is more complex than simple refractive errors such as astigmatism, near-sightedness, and far-sightedness. Spherical aberration is a specific type of optical aberration. It occurs when light rays passing through the periphery of the cornea and lens come to a focus at a slightly different location than light rays passing through the center of the cornea and lens. This results in decreased image quality. Spherical aberration tends to increase with pupil size and is therefore more noticeable in low light conditions than in bright sunlight. Visually, spherical aberration causes blur, loss of contrast, and halos around lights.

contention has been supported by studies of the synthesis of the lens capsule in experimental animals. These have shown that newly synthesized capsular materials are originally deposited close to the basal ends of epithelial and fiber cells, but over time move farther away from the surface of the cells as they are displaced by successive layers of newly synthesized capsular material.[22] These observations suggest that the rate of synthesis of components of the capsule at its inner surface and the rate of degradation at its outer surface regulate capsule thickness. The enzymes that are responsible for the degradation or remodeling of the capsule have not been identified.

The rest of the lens is formed from two populations of cells. A sheet of cuboidal cells, the lens epithelium, covers the surface of the lens closest to the cornea, while the bulk of the lens consists of concentric layers of elongated fiber cells that are at different stages of differentiation (Fig. 5.3). The outer shells of fiber cells extend from just beneath the anterior epithelium to the posterior lens surface, a distance of over 1 cm in adults. In the adult lens, most epithelial cells and all fiber cells are nondividing. Only cells near the equatorial margin of the lens epithelium, in a region called the germinative zone, undergo a slow proliferation (Fig. 5.3A,B). Most of the cells produced by mitosis in this region migrate toward the posterior of the lens and differentiate into fiber cells at the lens equator.[23] These new differentiating fiber cells undergo extensive elongation and express a number of fiber-specific proteins. It needs to be remembered, however, that fiber cells are essentially elongated epithelial cells that retain their distinct apical and basal membrane domains but have dramatically elongated lateral membranes (Fig. 5.3C). To adopt the hexagonal cross-sectional shape used by fiber cells to achieve an orderly packing that minimizes their extracellular space, lateral membranes of fiber cells are further subdivided into distinct broad- and narrow-side membrane domains (Fig. 5.3D).

During elongation, the posterior (basal) ends of the fiber cells migrate along the inner surface of the capsule, and their anterior (apical) ends migrate beneath the epithelium until they meet elongating cells from the other side of the lens near the posterior and anterior midlines to form the lens sutures.[24,25] In some species, all fiber cells meet near the midline of the lens, forming an "umbilical" suture. In most species, the sutures form along planes. In human embryos, elongated lens fiber cells meet at three planes, forming an upright "Y" at their anterior ends (with respect to the superior-inferior axis of the eye)

Fig. 5.1 Diagram showing the relationship of the lens and zonules to the other structures in the adult eye.

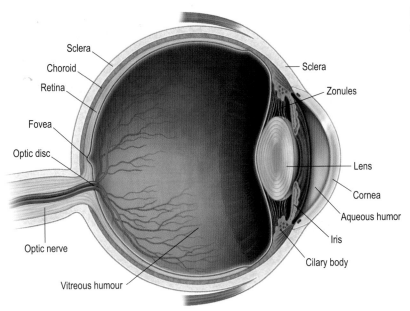

Sclera
Choroid
Retina
Fovea
Optic disc
Optic nerve
Vitreous humour
Sclera
Zonules
Lens
Cornea
Aqueous humor
Iris
Cilary body

and an inverted "Y" posteriorly (Fig. 5.4A). As the human lens grows, the suture planes formed by more superficial shells of fibers become increasingly complex. The first evidence of this typically occurs soon after birth, when two new suture planes form at the ends of each of the three branches of the Y sutures (Fig. 5.4B). As new fibers are added during lens growth, the branch points of the newly formed sutures gradually "migrate" toward the center, eventually forming a six-pointed "star" suture (Fig. 5.4C).[24] Branching again occurs at the tips of each of these six planes, eventually forming a total of 12 suture planes at the anterior and posterior surfaces of the lens (Fig. 5.4D,E).[24] The increasing geometric complexity of the suture patterns in older human lenses

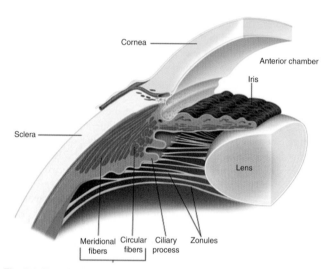

Fig. 5.2 Zonular fibers attach to the outer layer of the lens capsule (the zonular lamella) and hold the lens in place. Zonular fibers originate in the basal lamina of the pars plana and pars plicata of the ciliary body and insert on the equatorial region of the lens. (Images from the National Eye Institute.)

results in lenses with better optical properties than in species that maintain a simple Y suture pattern throughout life.[26]

Once fiber cells reach the sutures, they stop elongating and their basal ends detach from the capsule. Soon after reaching the sutures, fiber cells degrade all intracellular membrane-bound organelles, including their nuclei, mitochondria, and endoplasmic reticulum.[27–30] Organelle-free mature fiber cells are gradually buried deeper in the lens as successive generations of fibers elongate and differentiate. In this way, the lens continues to increase in size and cell number throughout life.[23] Because protein synthesis ceases just before organelle degradation,[31] the components of mature fiber cells must be much more stable than those in cells found in other parts of the body. In fact, since the fiber cells in the center of the lens are present at birth and persist until death (or cataract surgery), their constituent proteins and membranes may last for more than 100 years. Because this process occurs throughout life, a gradient of fiber cell age is established, with the oldest mature fiber cells in the lens nucleus having been laid down during embryogenesis.

Development of the embryonic lens

The adult lens is formed by cells that were originally part of the surface ectoderm covering the head of the embryo. Interactions between the future lens cells and nearby tissues during early development give these cells a "lens forming bias."[32] As a result of these interactions, patches of cells that lie on either side of the head are marked by expression of the transcription factor, Pax6, which is a master regulator of lens and eye development.[33] At the same time, neural epithelial cells on either side of the diencephalon in the embryonic forebrain bulge laterally to form the optic vesicles, which eventually contact the surface ectoderm cells (Fig. 5.5A). The cells of the optic vesicle also express Pax6, and Pax6 function in these cells is essential for eye formation.[34,35] Many of the genes that regulate and are regulated by Pax6 during the early stages of eye formation are now known and have been extensively reviewed.[36,37] Hence, in this section we will concentrate only on the morphologic changes that occur during embryonic development to first establish the structure of the lens that is maintained throughout life.

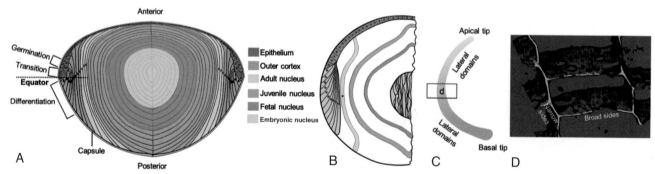

Fig. 5.3 (**A**, **B**) Schematic diagrams showing the morphologically distinct regions of the human lens established during lens development and growth. The epithelial cells that cover the anterior surface of the lens divide and proliferate in the germinative zone before migrating in the transition zone, where they begin their transformation into fiber cells. Differentiating fiber cells undergo extensive elongation until they reach the anterior and posterior poles where fibers from the opposing lens hemispheres meet to form the lens sutures. During the differentiation process, fiber cells undergo extensive remodeling, progressively losing their nuclei and other organelles as they become internalized to create an inherent age gradient that encapsulates all stages of fiber cell differentiation. (**C**) An isolated elongated fiber cell depicting the apical and basal tips that form the anterior and posterior sutures, respectively, and the greatly elongated lateral membranes. (**D**) Three-dimensional volume rendered image taken from an equatorial section through the lens, labeled with the membrane marker wheat germ agglutin showing the hexagonal cross-sectional profile adopted by differentiating fiber cells, which consists of distinct narrow- and broad-side membrane domains.

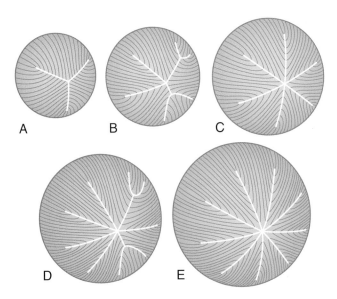

Fig. 5.4 Diagram illustrating the increasing complexity of the sutures as the lens grows. The sizes of the lenses depicted are to scale. (**A–C**) The tripartite "Y" suture that forms during embryogenesis as a result of secondary fiber cell formation is converted into a six-pointed star suture by the continued deposition of new fiber cells. If one were to peel away the fibers from the lens depicted in (**C**), the initial tripartite suture pattern would be revealed. (**D, E**) Further growth results in the formation of additional suture planes.

After they make contact, the optic vesicles and the prospective lens ectoderm cells secrete an extracellular matrix that causes these cell layers to adhere tightly to each other (Fig. 5.5B).[38] The surface epithelial cells then elongate, forming the thickened lens placode (Fig. 5.5B).[39] Soon afterward, the lens placode and the adjacent cells of the optic vesicle buckle inward to form the lens pit (Fig. 5.5C).[40] This morphologic transformation is accompanied by the formation of the bilayered optic cup. The invaginated lens placode soon separates from the surface ectoderm by a process involving the death of the cells in the connecting stalk between the cells of the surface ectoderm and the lens (Fig. 5.5D).[41] The Pax6-expressing ectodermal cells adjacent to the lens placode that remain on the surface of the eye become the corneal and conjunctival epithelium.[42] During lens invagination, the extracellular matrix between the optic vesicle and the lens begins to diminish and the two tissues separate (Fig. 5.5E).[18,38] The space that is formed between them is rapidly filled with a loose extracellular matrix, the primary vitreous body, that is secreted by the cells of the inner layer of the optic cup (Fig. 5.5E).[43]

The epithelial cells that give rise to the lens vesicle originally lie on a thin basal lamina. During the process of invagination, this basal lamina surrounds the lens vesicle. It gradually thickens by the deposition of successive layers of basal lamina material to form the lens capsule.[15–17] Soon after the lens vesicle separates from the surface ectoderm, the cells in the portion of the vesicle that are closest to the retina begin to elongate. The elongation of these primary fiber cells soon obliterates the lumen of the vesicle as their apical ends contact the apical ends of the anterior epithelial cells (Fig. 5.5E,F). Primary fiber cell formation establishes the fundamental structure of the lens, with epithelial cells covering the anterior surface and elongated fiber cells filling the bulk of the lens.

At early stages of lens formation, most of the lens epithelial cells are actively proliferating. Cells at the margin of the epithelium are displaced posteriorly and migrate toward the equator, where they are stimulated to differentiate into secondary fiber cells by growth factors present in the vitreous body.[44–47] As the secondary fibers elongate and their basal and apical ends migrate toward the poles of the lens, they displace the central primary fibers from their attachments with the capsule and the lens epithelium. This process buries the primary fiber cells in the center of the lens to form the embryonic nucleus (Fig. 5.3A).

Because this process of secondary fiber cell differentiation and internalization of existing cells occurs throughout life, the lens increases in size over time with either a monophasic or biphasic growth rate that is species specific.[48–51] For most species, lens growth is monophasic, being characterized by a period of rapid growth during early development that slows postnatally to approach an asymptotic maximum by the end of the life span.[50] In contrast, the human lens exhibits a biphasic growth rate in which lens growth in utero and in the immediate postnatal period is asymptotic, but thereafter the lens grows linearly (but slowly) at a rate of about 1.38 mg/year.[23] This generates two distinct compartments, the prenatal and the postnatal. The prenatal growth mode leads to the formation of an adult nuclear core of fixed dimensions and the postnatal to an ever-expanding cortex.[52] The nuclear core and the cortex have different properties and can readily be physically separated. In addition, the composition (dry matter to wet matter) of the lens tends to change over time as the lens grows. By simply weighing lenses of different ages before and after drying, the rate of increase in dry weight compared with the increase in wet weight can be calculated. This analysis showed that the proportion of dry weight increases significantly with age in many species.[50] This phenomenon is believed to reflect the time-dependent compaction of fiber cells in the lens interior, suggesting that this process is driven by the removal of water from the cytosol of the inner fibers, leading to elevated protein concentrations. This in turn contributes to the development of the GRI.[53]

In most species, lens shape appears to scale with growth, in that its aspect ratio (sagittal thickness/equatorial diameter) remains relatively constant across the life span.[23] However, consistent with its biphasic growth pattern, the shape of human lens does not simply scale with growth (Fig. 5.6). Early in embryonic development, the human lens is almost spherical (Fig. 5.6A) and remains that way until shortly after birth when, as part of the emmetropization process, it becomes increasingly elliptical, eventually losing approximately 20 D of refractive power by adulthood (Fig. 5.6B). This shape change is the result of an increase in the equatorial diameter and, remarkably, a decrease in sagittal thickness (Fig. 5.6C), which suggests the changes in the shape of the human lens during childhood and puberty reflect both compaction and remodeling of fiber cells in the lens interior.[54] Then, during adulthood (>20 years of age), the continued growth of the lens produces similar increases in both the sagittal thickness and equatorial diameter (Fig. 5.6D) such that the aspect ratio remains fairly constant throughout adulthood.[3]

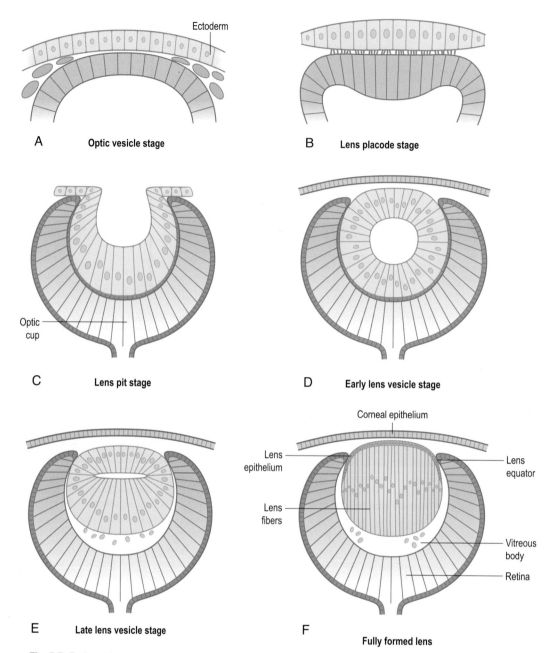

Fig. 5.5 Embryonic development of the lens. (**A**) The lens vesicle contacts the surface ectoderm. (**B**) The optic vesicle adheres to the surface ectoderm and the prospective lens cells elongate to form the lens placode. (**C**) The lens placode and the outer surface of the optic vesicle invaginate to form the lens pit and the optic cup, respectively. (**D**) The lens vesicle separates from the surface ectoderm. (**E**) The primary lens fibers elongate and begin to occlude the lumen of the vesicle. The posterior of the lens vesicle separates from the inner surface of the optic cup. Capillaries from the hyaloid artery invade the primary vitreous body. (**F**) The configuration of the lens as it begins to grow. Secondary fiber cells have not yet developed, and organelles are still present in all fiber cells. (Modified from McAvoy J. Developmental biology of the lens. In: Duncan G, ed. *Mechanism of Cataract Formation.* Academic Press; 1981:7–46. Copyright Elsevier 1981.[493])

Differentiation of secondary fiber cells

At the edge of the epithelium, near the lens equator, epithelial cells differentiate continuously into fiber cells (Fig. 5.3 A,B). In the germinative zone (GZ) of the epithelium, daughter cells produced by mitosis are eventually displaced (or migrate) into the transition zone (TZ).[55] Cells in this TZ are postmitotic and have not yet begun to elongate, but as they move posteriorly, they are exposed to growth factors contained in the vitreous, which appear to be secreted from the retina, that stimulate their elongation. Several growth factors are capable of initiating lens fiber cell differentiation when added to cultured lens epithelia or, in some cases, when overexpressed in the lens in vivo. Among these are members of the fibroblast growth factor (FGF) and insulin-like growth factor (IGF) families.[47,56–66] Studies using mouse lenses deficient in three of the four FGF receptors have conclusively demonstrated that FGF signaling is required for the formation of lens fiber cells.[67] In contrast, other soluble factors, especially members of the bone morphogenic

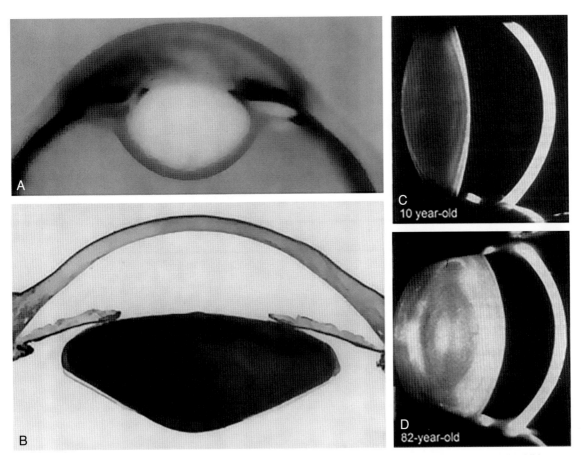

Fig. 5.6 Age-dependent changes in lens shape and size. Midsagittal ocular section from a 3-month-old child (**A**) and an adult (**B**). Note the marked increase in aspect ratio in the older lens. Scheimpflug images of the lens of a child (**C**) and an elderly man (**D**). Note the increase in lens thickness in the older eye. (From Bassnett S, Šikić H. The lens growth process. *Prog Retin Eye Res.* 2017;60:181–200.)

protein (BMP) family, appear to modulate or potentiate the effects of FGFs on lens fiber cell differentiation.[68–71] This work has led to the development of the lens gradient hypothesis (Fig. 5.7A), in which the vitreous contains higher levels of FGF and associated enhancers of FGF signaling than the aqueous.[72] However, there are other considerations, including the presence of recently identified growth factor signaling inhibitors, Sef, Sprouty, and Spreds, in the epithelium.[73] Thus, while the FGF gradient hypothesis provides a good explanation for the initiation of the process of fiber differentiation, questions remain around the interaction of FGF with other growth factors and signaling pathways that sustain fiber cell differentiation so that the correct three-dimensional cell architecture of the lens is obtained.

In this regard, several additional signal transduction pathways are activated at different times during fiber cell differentiation and maturation to ensure that fiber cells elongate with the correct curvature, lose their organelles, and change their junctional morphology and hence cellular shape—all changes required to establish the optical properties of the lens.[37,74–76] One such pathway that appears to coordinate the extension of the fiber cells is the planar cell polarity (PCP) mechanism that involves Wnt/Frz signaling.[75] Differentiating fiber cells contain a cilium/centrosome that is polarized toward the side that faces the anterior pole (Fig. 5.7B), and depletion of multiple protein components of the PCP pathway disrupt cilium orientation and fiber cell morphology, which alters the surface curvature and hence optical properties of the lens.[75,77] Cadherins, integrins, Rho-GTP proteins, and tropomodulin are all involved in the regulation of the lens cell cytoskeleton, the reorganization of which is associated with the change in cell morphology

that occurs as fiber cells differentiate and elongate.[76] However, the degradation of fiber cell nuclei, mitochondria, and other subcellular organelles[28] appears to be driven by autophagy and mitophagy,[78–80] with the inhibition of full apoptosis in fiber cells regulated by the IGF-1R/NF-κB pathway[81] and β1-integrin signaling.[82] More recently, Eph-ephrin signaling has been associated with cataract formation.[83] The binding of Eph receptor tyrosine kinases to ephrin ligands leads to a bidirectional signaling pathway that controls many cellular processes. In the lens, EphA2 and ephrin-A5 have been shown to be involved in determining fiber cell shape, organization and patterning, as well as the overall optical and biomechanical properties of the whole lens. In summary, it appears that a variety of signaling pathways interact to coordinate the differentiation and maturation of fiber cells to order, to establish a level of cellular organization that results in the correct optical properties at the whole tissue level.

STRUCTURAL DETERMINANTS OF THE TRANSPARENT AND REFRACTIVE PROPERTIES OF THE LENS

The transparent properties of the lens are the result of several structural adaptations that occur at the molecular and cellular levels in the different regions of the lens, all of which are designed to minimize light scatter. These adaptations include the loss of the lens-associated vasculature, the elimination of light-scattering intracellular organelles, an ordered cellular architecture in the peripheral lens, changes to fiber cell

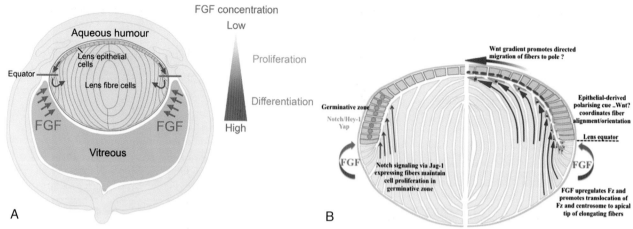

Fig. 5.7 (**A**) The fibroblast growth factor (*FGF*) gradient model showing how anterior to posterior differences in FGF concentration in the ocular media drive fiber cell differentiation. (**B**) When epithelial cells (*pink*) shift below the lens equator, fiber (*light blue*) differentiation is initiated in response to FGF in the posterior segment. *Left-hand side* shows that where Jag-1-expressing cortical fibers (*red arrows*) abut the epithelium determines the germinative zone (*orange star*), which expresses the Notch-Jagged effector, Hey-1, and Yap. *Right-hand side* shows the upregulation of Wnt-Frizzle (Fz) signaling components along with pathway activation that plays a key role in fiber elongation and differentiation. This response also involves translocation of Fz (*green*) and the centrosome (*red spot*) to the apical tips of elongating fiber cells, which acts as the organizing center for cytoskeletal assembly and dynamics. Early in the elongation process the fibers have concave curvature (*concave blue arrows*) as they orient toward overlying epithelia in response to an epithelial-derived polarizing cue (*pink-purple dashed line* in epithelium). As elongation progresses, the fibers take on convex curvature (*convex blue arrows*) as they undergo directed migration toward the pole, possibly in response to a Wnt concentration gradient. (From McAvoy JW, Dawes LJ, Sugiyama Y, Lovicu FJ. Intrinsic and extrinsic regulatory mechanisms are required to form and maintain a lens of the correct size and shape. *Exp Eye Res* 2017;156:34–40.)

morphology to form a barrier to extracellular diffusion, and the matching of the refractive index of the membranes and cytoplasm of fiber cells in the lens nucleus. These cellular level adaptations also manifest as changes to the refractive properties of the lens at the whole tissue level that alter the geometry and the GRI, the two key parameters that determine the focusing power of the lens.

Loss of the lens vasculature

Soon after its formation, the embryonic lens becomes covered with a meshwork of capillaries. The portion of this network encasing the posterior lens, the tunica vasculosa lentis, arises from the hyaloid artery. The capillaries found at the anterior side of the lens, the anterior pupillary membrane, arise from blood vessels of the developing iris stroma. These capillary networks join with each other near the lens equator. It has been assumed the fetal vasculature is important for normal lens development, although similar vessels are never present around the lenses of nonmammalian species. Deletion of vascular endothelial growth factor (VEGF-A) from the lens prevented the formation of the fetal vasculature, resulting in smaller lenses with transient nuclear cataracts.[84] Since mouse lens cells express functional VEGF receptors,[85] further studies are required to determine whether these cataracts were due to loss of VEGF signaling in lens cells, the absence of the fetal vasculature, or both.

During the second trimester of human development, the capillaries of the tunica vasculosa lentis and the anterior pupillary membrane regress.[86] Hence, by the fetal period, the lens is devoid of a blood supply, and therefore the avascular lens relies on the aqueous and vitreous humor for nutrients.[87] Decreasing levels of plasma-derived VEGF may be one of the factors involved in the normal regression of these vessels.[88] Macrophages in the vitreous body also appear to play an essential role in capillary regression.[86,89] In mice, these macrophages cause the programmed death of the endothelial cells by secreting the morphogen, Wnt7b.[90] A number of hereditary and acquired ocular diseases are accompanied by persistence of the fetal vasculature (see review[91]). At present, it is not clear why the fetal vasculature fails to regress in so many different syndromes and hereditary diseases. Better understanding of the factors that regulate vascular regression in normal ocular development is needed to address this question. However, regardless of the exact molecular mechanisms, loss of lens-associated vasculature is essential to establish normal vision by ensuring that light is not absorbed by heme pigments within the visual axis.[2]

Loss of nuclei and cellular organelles

The degree to which lens organelles scatter light depends largely on the difference in refractive index between the organelle and the surrounding cytoplasm.[2] However, as the refractive index of the cytoplasm is not matched to that of the organelles, the lens possesses a coordinated strategy for degrading organelles throughout the course of lens fiber cell differentiation, such that the majority of the fiber cells situated in the light path completely lack organelles. Soon after elongating, fiber cells detach from the posterior capsule and suddenly degrade all of their membrane-bound organelles, including their mitochondria, endoplasmic reticulum, and nuclei.[28–30,92] This process of organelle degradation occurs very rapidly, being completed within a few hours.[29] The loss of cell organelles from differentiating fiber cells produces a central organelle-free zone (OFZ) that consists of mature fiber cells that are incapable of protein synthesis or turnover of existing proteins, so that they are maintained throughout life.[29] Disruptions to the formation of the OFZ are accompanied by the persistence of organelles in lens fiber cells,[93] which in animal models have been shown to increase light scattering and contribute to cataract formation.[94] In adult primates, the outer shell of fiber cells that contain organelles is only about 100 microns wide. These organelle-containing cells are located, for the most part, outside of the optical axis of the lens.[27] Thus, the programmed removal of organelles in mature fibers enhances lens transparency by eliminating potential light-scattering elements.[95] However, organelle removal also renders mature fiber cells in the center of the lens incapable of de novo protein synthesis.

The mechanisms underlying the process in which organelle systems are rapidly degraded initially appeared similar to apoptosis (programmed cell death), since chromatin condensation and marginalization occur, as well as DNA fragmentation between nucleosomes.[92,96] However, unlike apoptosis, the cytoskeleton is maintained in lens fiber cells, even though organelles have fully disappeared.[29] This indicates that the underlying mechanisms that control organelle loss in differentiating lens fiber cells, relative to cells undergoing apoptosis, are different. Indeed, in recent years it has emerged that the process of organelle degradation has more in common with the processes of autophagy and mitophagy, which are designed to ensure cell survival, rather than the cellular mechanisms that drive apoptotic cell death.[97]

Autophagy is a cellular process whereby damaged or excess organelles and macromolecules are degraded in a stepwise program.[98–100] Originally considered a specific response to cellular starvation or stress, it is now recognized that autophagy plays a major part in the regulation of cellular development and differentiation, as well as the ongoing maintenance of cellular homeostasis.[101–104] Classic autophagy begins with the formation of a phagophore, a membrane that surrounds cellular materials or organelles targeted for degradation. Phagophores expand to become autophagosomes, which then fuse with lysosomes to form autophagolysosomes or autolysosomes where final degradation of the contents takes place. A plethora of signaling and regulatory molecules are required not just to initiate phagophore formation and complete autophagy but also to target specific cellular organelles/macromolecules for degradation.[99,100,105,106] Indeed, it appears that each organelle has a specific autophagy pathway for its degradation, with mitophagy the selective autophagy process in which mitochondria are degraded.[107] Hence, the elucidation of the complex repertoire of pathways and events leading to lens organelle elimination is an ongoing area of research. Current results suggest, however, that distinct but coordinated mechanisms function to regulate the elimination of the nucleus, mitochondria, endoplasmic reticulum, and Golgi apparatus that occurs during fiber cell differentiation so that these light-scattering elements are removed from the optical pathway in the deeper lens.[97]

Ordered cellular architecture of lens fiber cells

It has long been thought that, in addition to the removal of light-scattering elements, the ordered cellular architecture of the "crystalline" lens is a major contributor to lens transparency. However, this ordered cellular structure is only really evident in differentiating fiber cells in the outer cortex, and as fiber cells undergo further differentiation and become internalized deeper into the lens, they exhibit changes to their morphology that disrupt this initial cellular order (Fig. 5.8). Hence, the relative contribution of fiber cell morphology to lens transparency changes between the cortex and the nucleus. These regional differences in fiber cell morphology are thought to be driven by age-dependent changes to the cytoskeletal and junctional proteins that modulate fiber morphology.[2,74] The distinctive hexagonal fiber cell morphology found in the outer cortex is the net result of the interaction of a variety of junctional and cytoskeletal proteins, and this complement of proteins changes as fiber cells differentiate and become internalized within the lens. In differentiating fiber cells, these changes in protein expression can be initially achieved via de novo protein synthesis of a specific complement of proteins required at that specific stage of the differentiation process. However, once a fiber cell enters the OFZ and loses its

ability to synthesize new proteins, any further changes in cellular components required to elicit the observed changes in fiber cell morphology and function in the OFZ needs to be driven by post-translational modifications to the existing pool of lens proteins.

Differentiation-dependent changes to membrane junctions

Lens cells express many of the proteins that form the junctions (i.e., adherens junctions and gap junctions) typically found in other cell types. The lens also contains a number of unique membrane specializations that are comprised of distinct junctional complexes that contribute to the distinctive morphology of lens fiber cells. Because fiber cell morphology changes from the outer cortex to deeper nucleus, so does the complement of cell junctions and membrane specializations (Table 5.1). In the lens cortex, adherens junctions, immunoglobulin superfamily (IgSF) proteins, and gap junctions are the predominant junction-forming proteins. However, as fiber cells differentiate and become internalized, adherens junctions disappear, the morphology of gap junction plaques changes, ball-and-sockets are less prevalent, and tongue-and-groove membrane interdigitations and membrane fusions become the dominant features in mature fiber cells in the lens nucleus.

Differentiation-dependent changes to the composition and ultrastructure of fiber cells junctions

The adherens junctions found between cortical fiber cells are composed of the calcium-dependent cadherin proteins that complex with catenin proteins to link the actin cytoskeleton of neighboring cells together.[108] N-cadherin is the most prominent cadherin present in lens fiber cells.[109] Previously, it has been proposed that the large lateral fiber cell domains represent a tissue-specific adherens junctional structure, termed the cortex adhaerens. In this structure, cytoskeletal interacting proteins are localized to narrow- or broad-side membranes to maintain cortical fiber cell structure.[110] Also present in cortical fibers are gap junctions, which contain connexin (Cx) protein isoforms and form not only cell-to-cell adhesions but communicating channels between adjacent cells.[111] Cx46 and Cx50 are abundant in lens fiber cells, and are found in large plaques on the broad sides of differentiating fiber cells in the outer cortex.[112] IgSF proteins that facilitate calcium-independent adhesion are also present in the membranes of elongating fiber cells.[113,114]

Cortical fiber cell membrane interdigitations appear as cellular projections along the vertices of the large lateral membrane domain (Fig. 5.9A,B). These edge protrusions are regularly arrayed along the length of fibers and fit into complementary-shaped pockets formed between neighboring lens fiber cells. It is speculated that these structures, which are present in lens fiber cells of all ages, physically interlock cells and may be important to resist the shear forces that are generated during lens accommodation.[2] Smaller membrane interdigitations are also found emanating from broad face surfaces in a random pattern. These are characterized by cellular outpocketings, or balls, that consist of a globular portion attached by a short cylindrical cytoplasmic stalk and fit into complementary sockets in fiber cells of neighboring growth rings (Fig. 5.9C,D). Ball-and-socket joints are thought to play a role in the interlocking of fiber cells to minimize extracellular space and therefore light scattering.

Mature secondary lens fiber cells exhibit a markedly different morphology and complement of cell junctions and membrane specializations in comparison to cortical fibers. Adherens junctions are generally absent, probably owing to the degradation of the N-cadherin protein in lens development and aging.[109] In addition, the large broad-side gap junction plaques have fragmented and instead are distributed throughout the cell membrane.[115–120] In addition to the breakup and

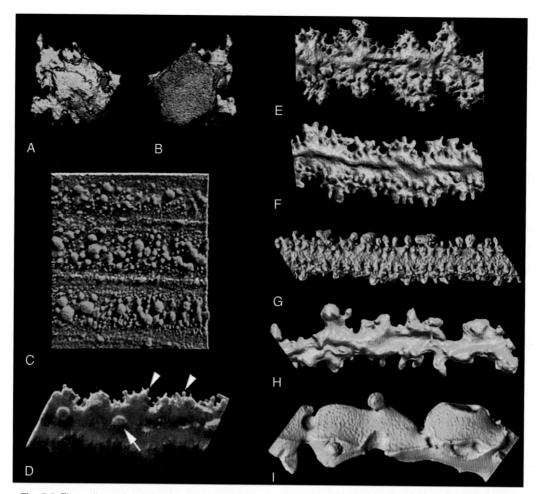

Fig. 5.8 Three-dimensional structure of mouse lens cells at various stages of differentiation as revealed by confocal microscopy. (**A, B**). Lens epithelial cells showing basal (**A**) or apical (**B**) surfaces. (**C**) Young elongating fiber cells located near the surface of a 2-month-old mouse lens. The fibers are initially smooth and ribbon-like. Their membrane surface features a large number of gap junction plaques (*green*) visualized here by immuno-fluorescence with anti-Cx50. (**D**) At this stage, the fiber cell is in the process of losing its organelles. At the membrane surface, ball-and-socket processes (enriched with Cx50) are formed on the broad face of the lateral membrane (*arrow*). Smaller, finger-like structures protrude from the narrow membrane faces (*arrowheads*). (**E**) With the disappearance of organelles the fibers take on an undulating appearance. (**F–I**) Fiber cells dissected from progressively deeper cell layers. The primary fiber cells from the center of the lens (**I**) are characterized by a very irregular structure. (From Bassnett S, Shi Y, Vrensen GF. Biological glass: structural determinants of eye lens transparency. *Philos Trans R Soc Lond B Biol Sci* 2011;366(1568):1250–1264.)

dispersal of gap junction plaques, ball-and-sockets are less prevalent in the highly compacted lens nucleus, while other morphologically distinct membrane structures are present. The tongue-and-groove membrane interdigitations (Fig. 5.9E,F), also known as microplicae,[121,122] are frequent membrane ridges that form close membrane appositions, and are prominent in the lens nucleus.[123] Tongue-and-groove interdigitations cover the surface of the nuclear fibers and stain asymmetrically for AQP0, the most abundant lens integral membrane protein. Square arrays that are a feature of the tongue-and-groove interdigitations are thought to contain AQP0 and/or its cleavage products.[120,124,125] The morphology of these arrays suggests a role for AQP0 in cell-to-cell adhesion.[115] These observations suggest that post-translational changes to junctional proteins in different regions of the lens alter not only the morphology of individual fiber cells but also the intracellular and extracellular interactions between cells.

EFFECT OF CHANGES IN FIBER CELL JUNCTIONS ON REGIONAL DIFFERENCES IN LENS STRUCTURE

The changes in the composition and ultrastructure of membrane junctions described in the previous section serve to adapt fiber cell structure to establish the key structural features in the different regions of the lens required to maintain the transparent, optical, and biomechanical properties of the whole lens. As fiber cells differentiate, they change their classical hexagonal shape and exhibit several distinct features that alter the morphology and therefore the function of deeper fiber cells. Again, it should be remembered that many of these changes occur in mature fiber cells that are incapable of de novo protein synthesis and therefore involve the post-translational modification of existing proteins to modify their membrane localization, interaction with other proteins, and regulation.

TABLE 5.1 Summary of regional differences in fiber cell junction morphology and function[a]

Lens region	Fiber cell junctional feature	Main associated protein(s)	Cell membrane localization	Proposed function
Cortex	Cortex adhaerens	N-cadherin, α-/β-catenin, plakoglobin, p120ctn, vinculin[109,110,494]	Narrow side	Cell adhesion, actin cytoskeleton linking, intermediate and beaded filament linking
		Ezrin, periplakin, periaxin, desmoyokin[110]	Broad side	Cell adhesion, actin cytoskeleton linking, intermediate and beaded filament linking
	Gap junction[495,496]	Cx46, Cx50	Broad side	Cell adhesion, cell communication
	Immunoglobulin Superfamily adhesion proteins[113,114]	Nr-Cam, Cadm1, N-Cam	All	Cell adhesion
	Edge protrusions[2]		Cell vertices	Cell interlocking
	Ball-and-sockets[497-499]	Cx46, Cx50	Broad side	Cell interlocking
Nucleus	Gap junction[115,116,119,120]	Cx46 (C-terminally truncated), Cx50 (C-terminally truncated)	All	Cell adhesion, cell communication
	Tongue-and-grooves (microplicae)[121,122]	AQP0 (C-terminally truncated)	All	Cell interlocking
	Square arrays[115,120,124,125]	AQP0 (C-terminally truncated)	All	Cell adhesion
	Compaction folds[53,132,500]		All, orthogonal to fiber cell long axis	Cell shortening
	Cell fusions[141–144]	MP20	All	Cell communication

Table modified from Donaldson PJ, Grey AC, Heilman BM, Lim JC, Vaghefi E. The physiological optics of the lens. *Prog Retin Eye Res.* 2017;56: e1–e24. https://doi.org/10.1016/j.preteyeres.2016.09.002.

Large gap junction plaques on the broad sides of cortical fiber cells undergo a process of fragmentation and dispersion as fiber cells differentiate,[115-120] which has been shown to correlate with a change in the direction of the flow of solutes between cells.[112] In peripheral fiber cells, the large broad-side plaques serve to preferentially direct solute flows within fiber cell columns toward the lens surface, while the subsequent fragmentation and dispersal of the plaques promotes a more isotropic flow of solutes between deeper mature fiber cells. In addition, the cleavage of the cytoplasmic tails of Cx46 and Cx50[126,127] alters the function and pH regulation of gap junction channels in the lens nucleus.[128,129] These observations suggest that changes to the ultrastructural organization of the gap junctional plaques and the subsequent cleavage of the pH-sensitive C-terminal tails of Cx46 and Cx50 are post-translational modifications designed to modify the direction of solute flows within the lens, as well as to ensure that the normally pH-sensitive gap junctions can operate in the low pH environment established by anaerobic metabolism in the lens nucleus.[130]

Fiber cell compaction is a morphologic feature that occurs in nuclear fiber cells that correlates with the observed loss of cell volume.[53] Scheimpflug imaging suggests that fiber cell compaction is initiated in the lens nucleus but also occurs in the lens inner cortex, and is most rapid in young lenses.[131] Accordion-like "compaction folds" oriented orthogonal to the long axis of primary fiber cells are evident in the embryonic nucleus,[132] while inner cortical fiber cells display numerous tongue-and-groove or microplicae junctions that become increasingly numerous with depth and completely cover the surface of nuclear fibers.[122] The close apposition of the plasma membranes of neighboring cells ensures that the topology of the microplicae on one cell is matched by a complementary series of folds on the neighboring cell. In the absence of cellular organelles, it appears the remodeling of the fiber cell membrane is driven by a reduction in cell volume that causes fiber cell membranes to become folded and compacted. This compaction of fiber cells means that despite the constant growth of the lens throughout life, the lens can still be fit within the eye that stops growing.[53]

A barrier to extracellular diffusion has been observed in the inner cortex of lenses in a number of species.[133-136] This extracellular diffusion barrier has been proposed to restrict the movement of solutes into the lens and acts to direct nutrients and antioxidants into the lens core via the suture at both poles.[135] The formation of this barrier appears to be associated with significant membrane and cytoskeletal protein remodeling.[134,136,137] At the ultrastructural level, a number of structures could be involved in this observed closure of the extracellular space. Previous electron microscopy data suggested that the reduction of lenticular intercellular space was correlated with the formation of square array and membrane undulations.[115,138] Thus, square arrays might potentially drive the formation of complicated membrane interdigitations and serve to maintain an extremely narrow extracellular space. In addition, it has been reported that gap junction plaques on the broad side of the outer fiber cells restrict penetration of larger solutes through the extracellular space.[139] More recently, spatial resolved proteomic analysis of the region of the lens where the extracellular barrier forms have shown that AQP0 and its interacting partners, ezrin and radixin,[140] are upregulated in this barrier region.[136] Because ezrin and radixin link AQP0 to the cytoskeleton, these data suggest that changes in the membrane distribution of AQP0 may play an important role in controlling the narrowing of the extracellular spaces between fiber cells.[136]

Membrane fusions between adjacent fiber cells have been observed in the deeper regions of a variety of lenses.[141] These membrane fusions have subsequently been shown to form a functional pathway for the diffusion of large proteins between mature fiber cells within discrete growth rings.[142,143] Interestingly, in the mouse lens, the formation of this lens syncytium was dependent on the presence of the abundant integral membrane protein MP20.[144] These fusions have implications for the establishment of the GRI (see further discussion in this chapter).

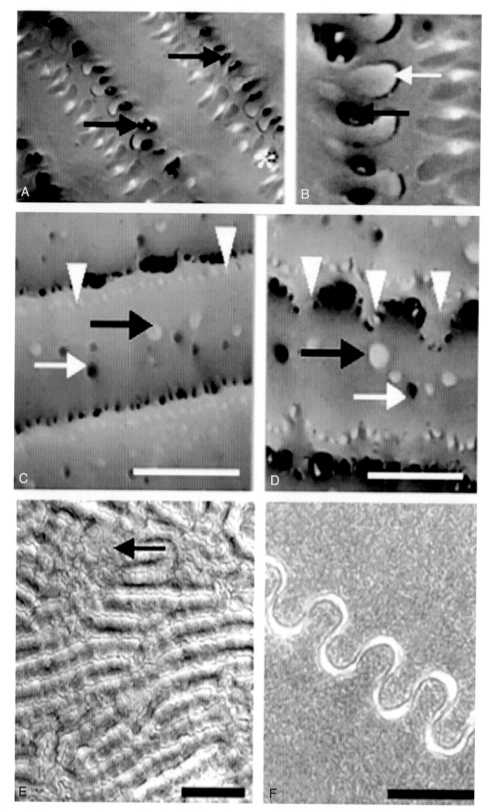

Fig. 5.9 Membrane junctions found between fiber cells. (**A, B**) Scanning electron microscopy images of interlocking edge protrusions (*asterisk, white* and *black arrows*) between superficial lens fibers. (**C, D**) In deeper cortical regions the edge protrusions (*arrowheads*) become tortuous, and ball-and-socket junctions (*black* and *white arrows*) appear. (**E, F**) In freeze fracture images of deep cortical regions (**E**), lens fiber membranes show grooves and ridges (microplicae) on their surface that correspond to undulating membranes of neighboring fibers as shown in transmission electron microscopy images (**F**). (Modified and reproduced with permission from Bassnett S, Shi Y, Vrensen GF. Biological glass: structural determinants of eye lens transparency. *Philos Trans R Soc Lond B Biol Sci* 2011;366(1568):1250–1264.)

Differentiation-dependent changes to cytoskeletal proteins

The lens is a specialized tissue that is specifically reliant on the establishment of a precise cytoarchitecture to determine and maintain structure that, in turn, is critical for its function, transparency, and biomechanical properties.[145] This structure is determined by cytoskeletal networks, including microtubules, intermediate filaments, and actin microfilaments, and their interactions with cell adhesion junctions and fiber cell–specific membrane specializations.[74] These cytoskeletal networks also act synergistically to regulate lens structure and, consequently, function.[145,146]

Microtubules: Microtubules are abundant beneath the plasma membranes of lens fiber cells where they probably play an important role in stabilizing the fiber cell membrane.[147] Microtubules may also be important for transporting vesicles to the apical and basal ends of elongating fiber cells, although neither function has been demonstrated in vivo. Microtubules are poorly expressed in the lens epithelium and nuclear fiber cells but are localized in lengthwise arrays in the peripheral cytoplasm of cortical fiber cells,[148] which suggests they may contribute to the processes associated with fiber cell elongation. As in other cells, microtubules in the lens also mediate vesicle trafficking, through kinesin and dynein motors, to both lens poles, which is likely important to establishing polarity during lens development. For example, they are known to transport vesicles harboring membrane proteins, such as aquaporin 0 (AQP), during fiber cell differentiation and elongation.[149] They may also facilitate the formation of the OFZ, which is crucial for continued transparency. A mutation in a mediator of microtubule plus end-directed vesicle transport, FYVE And Coiled-Coil Domain Autophagy Adaptor 1 (FYCO1), causes a form of autosomal-recessive congenital cataract.[150] As FYCO1 is known to associate with autophagosomes in other cells, microtubules may participate in autophagosome trafficking.[151]

Recently it was noted that the stabilized (acetylated) population of microtubules, localized close to the epithelial–fiber cell interface, was specifically involved in fiber cell elongation, as loss of the dynamic microtubule population alone did not affect lens fiber cell elongation or the directionality of their migration.[145] Interestingly, this function was mediated through the regulation of myosin 2 activation.[145] Moreover, through their association with N-cadherin junctions, specifically in elongating fiber cells, stable microtubules regulate N-cadherin junction organization along the lateral borders.[145] As these junctions are epicenters of actin organization, this interaction suggests that stable microtubules may impact actin organization during lens morphogenesis.[145]

Actin: The actin cytoskeleton in the lens interacts closely with fiber cell membranes to maintain epithelial cell morphology and polarity, and to influence fiber cell differentiation.[76] Complexes of F-actin and adherens junctions can be found at epithelial–epithelial, epithelial–fiber, and cortical fiber–fiber cell membrane contacts.[76] Of the different actin networks, the spectrin-actin skeleton is the best characterized in the lens.[76,146] It consists of actin filaments crosslinked by $\alpha_2\beta_2$-spectrin, stabilized along their sides by γ-tropomyosin (γTM), and capped at their barbed and pointed ends by adducin and tropomodulin 1 (Tmod1), respectively. The meshwork is thought to be anchored at the fiber cell membrane via the interaction of spectrin with ankyrin-B, which, in turn, is linked to cadherin-based adherens junctions and the ezrin, periplakin, periaxin, and desmoyokin (EPPD) anchorage complex.[76] The relationship between the N-cadherin junctions and actin cytoskeleton appears to be reciprocal in that the cytoskeleton determines cadherin junction maturation, while independent maturation of cadherin junctions also appears to drive organization of the cortical actin cytoskeleton and elongation of fiber cells.[152]

Rearrangement of the basal network of actin (actin-rich lamellipodia and stress fibers) in the anterior epithelial cells, which tethers them to the lens capsule, is necessary to drive fiber cell elongation and differentiation, and ends in the formation of a terminal web that stabilizes the ends of fiber cells at the sutures.[76,148] Upon differentiation, this previously discontinuous and irregular spectrin-actin network becomes smooth and continuous along fiber cell membranes, likely due to stabilization via Tmod1.[76] Unlike other organelles or proteins that are degraded or, indeed, cytoskeletal elements that are proteolyzed/modified, both F-actin and Tmods remain undegraded and associated with mature fiber cell membranes. This suggests that the actin network has a fundamental role in stabilizing and maintaining overall membrane integrity.[76]

Tmod1 and γTM-mediated stabilization of the spectrin-actin network is critical for its long-range connectivity in fiber cells.[153] In this way, the network is essential for maintaining regular hexagonal fiber cell morphology and packing geometry.[76,153] Loss of Tmod1 leads to F-actin disassembly, reduced levels of γTM, and widespread disruption of the spectrin-actin lattice in differentiating fiber cells, including abnormal membrane protrusions and cell shapes and disordered packing geometry. This demonstrates the importance of the actin cytoskeleton in establishing fiber cell architecture during differentiation.[153] However, transparency remains unaffected in Tmod1-null lenses.[153] Maintenance of the actin cytoskeleton in mature fiber cells may rely on appropriate interactions with lens crystallins, particularly β- and γ-crystallins.[76] γ-crystallins may stabilize F-actin in mature lens fiber cells by protecting against depolymerization.[76] Additionally, optimal levels of HSPB1, a heat shock protein and molecular chaperone that interacts with and stabilizes the actin cytoskeleton, appears to be essential in preventing cataractous changes.[154] The RNA granule component, TDRD7, is necessary to maintain optimal HSPB1 levels, as reduced levels of HSPB1 in $Tdrd7-/-$ lenses results in abnormal membrane morphology in mature fiber cells and precedes cataract.[154] Moreover, mutations in TDRD7 cause pediatric cataract.[155]

Intermediate filaments: In the lens, intermediate filaments are key regulators of fiber cell architecture and mechanical properties (Fig. 5.10), with vimentin and "beaded filament" proteins, CP49 (Beaded Filament Structural Protein 1 (BFSP1)/phakinin) and filensin (BFSP2), being the most highly expressed.[156] Vimentin filaments are tightly associated with the plasma membrane of lens epithelial and differentiating fiber cells, but are not present in nuclear fiber cells.[157] In contrast, beaded filaments are predominantly associated with fiber cell membranes. This association is, however, dependent on the stage of fiber cell differentiation and can be influenced by proteolytic fragmentation and phosphorylation of the filaments. Accordingly, in the deeper cortex, these proteins become more cytoplasmic.[146] CP49 or filensin gene deletion leads to subtle, age-dependent opacification and loss of optical quality in mice, as detected by slit-lamp examination and laser ray tracing.[158] However, mutations in CP49/BFSP2 protein lead to hereditary cataracts in humans and mice.[159] In contrast, whereas loss of vimentin does not elicit phenotypic changes, vimentin overexpression does induce cataract formation.[160] It is likely that tight regulation of intermediate filaments via post-translational modifications and membrane-cytoplasmic shifts is critical in maintaining the optical properties of the lens.

Intermediate filaments can serve as mechanical support and scaffolding for membrane-associated proteins. Through their plasma membrane associations they are able to maintain the correct spatial organization and plasma membrane profile of fiber cells in the lens (Fig. 5.10).[156] Indeed, the plasma membranes of lens fiber cells are enriched in potential intermediate filament–binding proteins.[156] Changes to the complement of intermediate filament proteins in the lens, seen as a sharp transition from vimentin to beaded filament expression in the lens cortex, appears to be associated with the remodeling of the plasma membrane. Indeed, post-translational modifications and truncations of filensin are observed following its

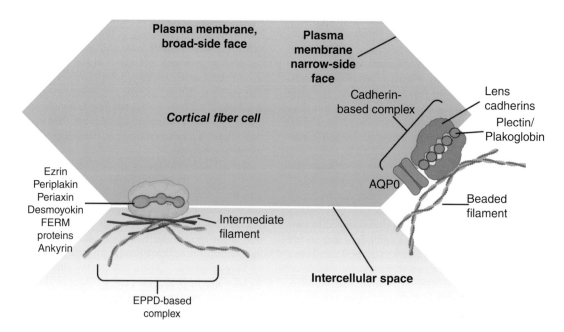

Fig. 5.10 Schematic showing the links between beaded and other intermediate (vimentin) filaments at different plasma membrane sites in lens fiber cells. Beaded filaments interact with the plasma membranes of lens fiber cells via cadherins and EPPD-based (ezrin, periplakin, periaxin, desmoyokin) complex, located on the narrow- and broad-side faces, respectively, of fiber cells. Plakoglobin and plectin are potential linkers for intermediate and beaded filaments to the cadherin complex. On the broad-sides of the fiber cells, such as ankyrin and a number of proteins that contain the four-point-one ezrin-radixin-moesin homology (FERM) domain link the intermediate and beaded filaments to the plasma membrane have been identified, but the identity of the transmembrane proteins has yet to be determined although band 3 has been implicated. (Redrawn from Song S, Landsbury A, Dahm R, Liu Y, Zhang Q, Quinlan RA. Functions of the intermediate filament cytoskeleton in the eye lens. *J Clin Inves.* 2009;119(7):1837–1848.)

expression in the inner cortex of the bovine lens.[161] In the human lens, this transition occurs rapidly in the remodeling zone (RZ),[160] a narrow area of regulated differentiation in the lens cortex in which fiber cells undergo extreme morphologic changes.[134] The expression of beaded filaments in the RZ[160] may indicate their involvement in membrane deformation/remodeling and/or the establishment of ball-and-socket joints (see further), which first arise in the RZ.[134,137] Alternatively, alterations in membrane-filament attachments, for example, through AQP0,[162] may also allow undulating membranes to develop.[137] Moreover, deletion of CP49 or filensin does not alter outer cortical radial fiber cell alignment or formation of membrane protrusions, but fiber cells in the inner cortex display striking morphologic abnormalities, such as failing to maintain their paddle-like membrane protrusions, leading to their gross misalignment.[158,163] This suggests that intermediate filaments are necessary for the maintenance, but not establishment, of interdigitations and long-range stacking of fiber cells.[163] Therefore, beaded filaments appear to become more associated with the membrane to establish interlocking domains, and the switch between intermediate filaments may be an important tool for the remodeling of membranes observed as a function of fiber cell differentiation.[160]

Intermediate filaments help to maintain lens transparency through their association with protein chaperones.[156] Indeed, α-crystallins appear to be critical for the assembly, maintenance, and remodeling of beaded filaments.[148] The dramatic cellular rearrangements that occur in the human RZ are also most likely due to alterations in crystallin associations with beaded filaments.[137] In turn, this association stabilizes the high protein concentrations, which are essential in creating the GRI,

thereby maintaining protein homeostasis and transparency.[156] Indeed, recent work has shown that CP49 and filensin proteins are essential components of the super molecular structure in the lens core.[164] Mutations in the CP49 gene or filensin KO prevented the formation of reversible cold cataracts in the lens core at 25°C and reduced the severity of the cataracts at 4°C, suggesting that aggregation or accumulation of these proteins was necessary to precipitate cataractous changes. Interestingly, beaded filaments were not necessary for cold cataracts that extended to the inner fiber cells.[164]

Interactions between cytoskeletal networks: Given their overlap in expression and function, it is perhaps not surprising that the spectrin-actin network and beaded filaments work in functional synergy to regulate three-dimensional hexagonal fiber cell packing, lens transparency, and mechanical stiffness.[146] First, the spectrin-actin network and beaded filament cytoskeleton are biochemically coupled as Tmod1, actin, CP49, and filensin, and they coexist in a protein complex. Second, both networks are also functionally coupled, as deletion of both Tmod1 and CP49 causes defects in fiber cell organization, light scattering, and compressive mechanical properties that are distinct from those defects arising from loss of either Tmod1 or CP49 alone.[146] Both proteins are also needed for the normal formation or stabilization of the small protrusions at the vertices of mature fiber cells.[153] The cytoskeleton also seems to influence the biomechanical properties of the lens in response to application of an external load. The spectrin-actin membrane skeleton appears to mechanically stiffen the lens at low loads and strains, while beaded filaments provide fortification at high loads and strains.[146] Based on these experiments, it has been speculated that the distinct cytoskeletal architectures of the lens epithelium, superficial cortex, deep cortex, and nucleus give rise to radially variable and depth-dependent recruitment of cytoskeletal scaffolding during tissue compression, resulting in radial heterogeneity in the compressive modulus.[146] These networks also appear to synergize in promoting the formation of large gap junction plaques that are crucial for normal lens ion and fluid homeostasis in differentiating fiber cells.[165] Gap junction plaques rest in gaps within the spectrin-actin network along fiber cell membranes, suggesting that the actin skeleton plays a role in the accretion or stability of large gap junction plaques.[165]

Taken together, the observed age-dependent changes in cytoskeletal architecture and the complement of membrane junctions, which alter fiber cell morphology at the ultrastructural and cellular level in different regions of the lens, have the potential to significantly influence the overall optical properties of the lens at the tissue level.

EFFECTS OF REGIONAL DIFFERENCES IN FIBER CELL MORPHOLOGY ON LENS TRANSPARENCY, OPTICS, AND BIOMECHANICS

Light scattering in biological tissue occurs at boundaries between compartments of differing refractive index, such as at the cell border or within the cell, where cellular organelles tend to have different (usually higher) refractive indices.[2] It might be expected therefore that light passing through the lens would be scattered at every interface between cellular and extracellular compartments, and consequently that the lens would be opaque. This is not the case in the outer cortex because differentiating secondary lens fiber cells are initially packed in a geometrically ordered array that helps to minimize light scattering and promote tissue transparency. This level of cellular organization is facilitated by the characteristic flattened hexagonal cross-section profile of fiber cells (Fig. 5.11A,B), which serves to not only minimize the extracellular space but also to form a lattice-like structure that acts like a diffraction grating.[166] The regular spacing of fiber cells results in individual light scattering-centers that produce constructive interference in the forward direction and destructive interference at other angles (Fig. 5.11C). In this way, extracellular space is minimized and tissue transparency is facilitated, despite the presence of a refractive index mismatch between the cortical fiber cell plasma membrane and the cytosol of cortical fiber cells.[166-169]

However, the ordered architecture of cells in the outer cortex is not as apparent in the deeper regions of all lenses, with this change in cellular order being most noticeable in humans. In the human lens, the regular cellular order seen in the outer cortex is abruptly disrupted as differentiating fiber cells enter the RZ where fiber cells lose their characteristic hexagonal profile and cell interfaces become unusually interdigitated and irregular.[134,170] However, cell integrity and gap junctional interactions are not compromised, indicating that this abrupt transition is a highly regulated process.[137] After exiting this lens region, secondary lens fiber cells continue to differentiate, becoming more deeply buried in the lens. Cross-sectional profiles of these mature fiber cells

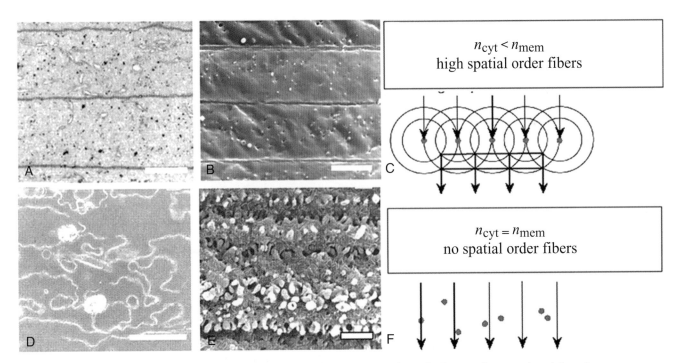

Fig. 5.11 Refractive index matching of lens membranes and cytoplasm. Explanatory figure on the relation of spatial lens fiber order and light scattering, considering differences in refractive index between lens fiber membranes in the lens cortex and nucleus. Images from transmission electron microscopy (**A, D**) and scanning electron microscopy (**B, E**) of human lens fibers of the superficial cortex (**A, B**) and in the lens nucleus (**B, E**). Schematic diagram of resultant light scattering from regularly spaced scattering centers (**C**) and irregularly spaced fiber cells (**F**). Scale bar is 5 μm. (Reproduced with permission from Bassnett S, Shi Y, Vrensen GF. Biological glass: structural determinants of eye lens transparency. *Philos Trans R Soc Lond B Biol Sci* 2011; 366(1568):1250–1264.)

become increasingly circular, the columnar arrangement becomes less apparent,[134,171] and central fiber cells undergo compaction and exhibit a reduction in the number of fiber cell interdigitations.[53] Hence, in the lens nucleus, fiber cells have little spatial order and exhibit irregular membrane surfaces (Fig. 5.11D,E), and the minimization of light scattering is no longer a result of an ordered cellular architecture (Fig. 5.12F). Instead, the reduction in light scattering is thought to be the consequence of proteomic and lipidomic changes that occur during lens fiber cell maturation,[172] which produces more closely matched refractive indices between the cytoplasm and plasma membrane of mature fiber cells, thus removing the physical basis for light scattering in the lens nucleus.[166] Overall, it appears that the spatial order of fiber cells is important to establish lens transparency in the outer cortex, whereas it is less important in the deeper regions of the lens.

Establishment of a gradient of refractive index

The GRI contributes to the optical power of the lens and is essential for sharp vision,[173,174] since it generates a negative spherical aberration to compensate for the positive spherical aberration (see Box 5.1) introduced by the cornea and its own geometry.[175] The shape and magnitude of the GRI changes throughout life. In early childhood, the GRI adopts a parabolic shape, but with advancing age a gradual flattening of GRI profile gradient occurs that results in the formation of a central plateau that contributes to an age-related reduction in overall lens power. The GRI is established by varying the ratio of water to protein in the different regions of the lens (Fig. 5.12A). This is achieved by a combination of the age-dependent expression of a variety of crystallin proteins that exhibit different refractive increments (dn/dc),[176] the formation of membrane fusions that normalize protein concentrations between growth rings,[2] and the active removal of water from the lens nucleus.[177]

Contribution of the crystallin proteins to the gradient of refractive index

The synthesis and accumulation of very large amounts of crystallin proteins is a major characteristic of lens fiber cell differentiation. As much as 40% of the wet weight of the lens fiber cell can be accounted for by crystallins,[167] a protein concentration that is about three times higher than in the cytoplasm of typical cells. Crystallin proteins can be classified as either "classical" or "taxon-specific." Taxon-specific crystallins,[178,179] as the name implies, are found in the lenses of different taxonomic groups. Taxon-specific crystallins can be functional enzymes or proteins that are structurally very similar to enzymes but with little or no enzymatic activity. The classical crystallins that are found in all vertebrate lenses are comprised of two α-crystallins and several members of the beta/gamma (β/γ)-crystallin superfamily. These classical crystallins can be distinguished by their refractive index increment, dn/dc, a variable that defines the contribution of a given concentration of protein to the refractive index of the whole solution,[180] and their intramolecular packing properties, which promotes their solubility in the highly compacted lens nucleus.

α-Crystallin: The human lens expresses two α-crystallin genes, αA and αB. Examination of the protein structure of the α-crystallins revealed that they are members of the widely distributed family of small heat shock proteins.[181-183] Small heat shock proteins can act as chaperones that stabilize proteins that are partially unfolded and prevent them from aggregating. The ability of α-crystallins to act as a chaperone and prevent protein aggregation and precipitation has been demonstrated in experiments performed in vitro.[184] A similar in vivo role for αA-crystallin has been inferred in mice in which the αA-crystallin gene was disrupted.[185] The function of the α-crystallins in preventing protein aggregation has obvious importance for the lens, because the proteins in lens fiber cells must persist for the life of the individual, and excessive protein aggregation could lead to light scattering and cataract formation.

α-Crystallins are also enzymes because they possess serine-threonine auto-kinase activity.[186] It is not yet clear whether the α-crystallins phosphorylate other proteins in lens fiber cells. The α-crystallins are themselves normally phosphorylated in vivo and can be phosphorylated in vitro; however, the factors that regulate the phosphorylation of α-crystallins and the importance of this phosphorylation for the function of the α-crystallins in the living lens has yet to be determined (see ref 187).

α-Crystallin proteins normally associate in the lens cell cytoplasm to make high-molecular-weight complexes containing approximately

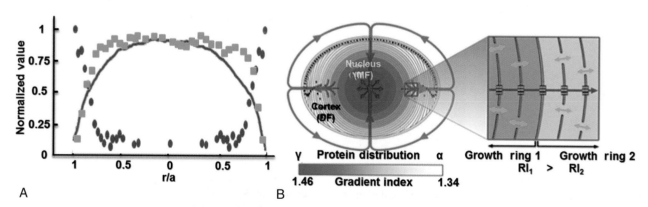

Fig. 5.12 Establishment of the gradient of refractive index in the lens. (**A**) Equatorial profiles of the refractive index *(blue)*, water content of a young human lens *(red)*, and dry mass distribution of a 24-year-old lens *(green)* are normalized in magnitude, superimposed, and plotted against normalized distance from the surface of the lens (r/a). (**B**) A model two-dimensional gradient of refractive index (GRI) profile of the lens superimposed on its geometry, where it is established by the removal of water from its nucleus by the microcirculation system. The refractive gradient shells are established and homogenized over multiple fiber layers, via macromolecular fusion channels. (Reproduced with permission from Donaldson PJ, Grey AC, Heilman BM, Lim JC, Vaghefi E. The physiological optics of the lens. *Prog Retin Eye Res* 2017;56:e1–e24.)

30 subunits. The structure of these complexes has been revealed by cryoelectron microscopy.[188] These observations show that native α-crystallin complexes can be assembled in a number of configurations, indicating that there is substantial flexibility in the way the subunits associate. α-Crystallin monomers also readily exchange between high-molecular-weight complexes, further supporting the view that α-crystallin complexes are quite plastic.[189]

The phenotype of αA-crystallin knockout mice provides insight into the function of α-crystallins in vivo.[185] The lenses of these animals are slightly smaller than normal but structurally quite similar to the normal lens. Mature fiber cells contain aggregates of proteins that lead to the formation of cataracts, beginning a few weeks after birth. Analysis of these aggregates shows that they contain large amounts of αB-crystallin and smaller amounts of other proteins. These results suggest that, in the fiber cell cytoplasm, αA-crystallin is partly responsible for preventing αB from aggregating. In addition, when lens epithelial cells from these animals were cultured in vitro, they grew more slowly than normal cells, were more sensitive to stress, and had a higher rate of apoptosis, accounting for the smaller size of the knockout lenses.[190] Therefore, αA-crystallin appears to be important for the normal function of lens epithelial and fiber cells. A naturally occurring mutation in the αB-crystallin gene (CRYAB) leads to the formation of cataracts and "desmin-related" myopathy.[191] In vitro tests showed that the mutant form of the protein had no chaperone activity and even enhanced the aggregation of test proteins.[192] These studies suggest that αB-crystallin has important chaperone functions in the lens and in other cells of the body. However, the fact that the mutant protein accelerated the denaturation of test proteins leaves open the possibility that the mutant is a gain-of-function. In this case, the cataracts and myopathy seen in individuals carrying this mutation could be due to the destabilizing function of the protein, rather than loss of its function as a chaperone. However, additional mutations in CRYAB, which do not have myopathy as part of their phenotype, support the view that loss of its chaperone function contributes to cataract.[193]

β- and -γ crystallins: The β/γ crystallin superfamily is more diverse than the α-crystallins. Originally thought to be two distinct protein families, subsequent protein sequencing of the β- and γ-crystallins shows them to be closely related.[194] The major difference in these proteins is the tendency for most of the β-crystallins to form multimers, whereas the γ-crystallins exist as monomers. Solving the three-dimensional structure of these molecules confirmed their close structural relationship. It also confirmed that the N- and C-terminal extensions of the β-crystallins provided a structural rationale for why these family members form higher-order complexes.[195,196] There are six β-crystallin polypeptides (βA1, βA3, βA4, βB1, βB2, βB3) and three gamma (γ) crystallins (γS, γC, γD) expressed in the human lens,[197] although the β A1 and βA3 polypeptides are derived from the same gene (CRYBA1).[198] β- and γ-crystallins bind calcium in vitro and may buffer this important cation in the lens fiber cell cytoplasm.[199-201]

γ-crystallins are thought to function in the lens as structural proteins,[201] and γ-crystallin has the highest dn/dc increment (~0.199 versus ~0.193 for α-crystallin) of the classical crystallin proteins.[202] Because γ-crystallins are differentially expressed in the lens nucleus during prenatal growth, they are the predominant crystallin protein expressed in the nucleus of the human lens.[203] It is likely that this expression pattern combined with their inherently higher dn/dc values ensures that the refractive index is highest in the lens nucleus.[204]

In addition, structural features of γ-crystallins allow intramolecular packing that results in a highly compact form[205] facilitating the short-range spatial order that supports lens transparency.[206] Interestingly, using a model of noninteracting hard spheres, Zhao and

colleagues[207] showed that the higher macromolecular dn/dc afforded by the γ-crystallins can significantly reduce the concentration of protein required to achieve the GRI, which then has the effect of reducing osmotic pressure generated by the proteins and their propensity to aggregate. As such, this property of γ-crystallins allows these extremely long-lived proteins to remain soluble in the highly compacted lens nucleus while delivering the required refractive power. γ-crystallins are also known to have unusually low frictional ratios, suggesting that they may have lower tendencies for "sticky" interactions with other proteins, which is relevant in a polydisperse and crowded lenticular environment.[208] This property is likely due to highly conserved tertiary features and the close packing of surface side chains. Therefore, a key role for γ-crystallins may involve acting as a "molecular lubricant" to maintain short-range order by separating distinct components of the lens.[208] This avoids the formation of light-scattering groups through protein unfolding, aggregation, or phase separation. Moreover, the high level of intracellular crowding in the lens leaves little space for protein unfolding and can provide additional stabilizing forces.[208]

In addition, it has recently been suggested that the short-range order of γ-crystallins can be modulated by the presence of other molecules.[209] For instance, ATP can act as a hydrotropic molecule that helps prevent protein aggregation, in addition to its established role as a cellular energy source.[210] Hydrotropes are amphiphilic molecules that at millimolar concentrations solubilize hydrophobic molecules, preventing protein aggregation in aqueous solution. By shielding the hydrophobic regions of protein molecules, ATP provides a hydrophilic interfacial surface comprised of the negatively charged triphosphate side chains of ATP molecule. This hydrophilic surface in turn forms an interfacial dynamic water layer that has been proposed to separate adjacent lens fiber cell proteins, keeping them from aggregating.[209] The hydrotropic function of ATP in preventing protein aggregation would perhaps provide an explanation for the extremely high concentrations of ATP found in the lens, and an age-related decline in ATP concentrations in the center of the lens could contribute to the protein aggregation observed in nuclear cataract in the elderly.[209]

The higher-order structure and dn/dc properties of proteins are the result of their primary amino acid structure.[204] In this regard, lens crystallins have highly unusual amino acid compositions compared with other proteins. β/γ-crystallins contain Greek key motif domains that are enriched with the amino acids lysine and glutamic acid, which exhibit higher dn/dc values than classical Greek motifs containing arginine and aspartic acid residues with lower dn/dc values.[180,202,204,208] These substitutions may allow for more hydrogen bonding and possibly more compact structures.[204] Additionally, mammalian β/γ-crystallins have a higher proportion of interstrand salt bridges compared with other proteins, suggestive of long-range structural stabilization and interactive potential, highly relevant properties for such long-lived proteins.[204]

In addition to the amino acid composition, it is important to consider the effect that other factors such as protein hydration can have on the high refractivity of lens proteins.[211] The layer of water around a protein, known as its hydration shell, is dynamic and heterogenous.[211] Protein surface solvation provides a large energetic deterrent for protein-protein contacts that may lead to protein aggregation, thereby contributing to protein solubility.[205] Indeed, some cataract-forming mutants of human γ-crystallin are due to changes in local solvation properties rather than protein structure.[205,212] The behavior of the hydration shell, as it forms hydrogen bonds with multiple exposed amino acid residues, is distinct from that of a solution of its component amino acids and can also be reasonably expected to contribute to the refractive index.[211,213] Current hypotheses propose that the arrangement of exposed hydroxyl groups on the protein surface may affect protein hydration and, thus, the dipole moment and polarizability.[211] In addition, or alternatively, short-range interactions between highly polarizable amino acids with pi-bonding systems, a feature common in lens crystallins, may cause local regions of anisotropic polarizability.[211,213] Indeed, accounting for cation-pi and pi-pi interactions improves the agreement between predicted and measured refractive indices.[211]

Role of membrane fusion in the establishment of the gradient of refractive index

The lens consists of a series of discrete growth rings that contain fiber cells, which at specific stages of cell differentiation become metabolically linked by membrane fusions.[144] It has been proposed that these intracellular linkages allow for the exchange of large proteins such as the crystallins within, but not between, adjacent growth rings.[2] This intercellular diffusion of crystallins via membrane fusions serves to equalize the protein concentration, and therefore the refractive index, between cells within a growth ring. However, the lack of fusions between adjacent growth rings ensures that differences in refractive index are maintained between adjacent rings (Fig. 5.12B). The presence of discrete concentric growth rings, plus the differential expression of α-, β- and γ-crystallin subtypes with different refractive indices, forms the structural basis for the establishment of the GRI. Although not connected by membrane fusions, adjacent growth rings are coupled by gap junctions channels.[214] Gap junction channels, although not permeable to crystallin proteins, allow the flow of ions and water between adjacent growth rings. It follows, therefore, that the removal of water from the lens nucleus[177,215] would not only steepen the GRI by increasing the concentration of crystallin proteins but also smoothen the GRI profile established by stepwise regional differences in crystallin subtype expression between the individual concentric growth rings (Fig. 12B). This active maintenance of the GRI and its effect on the refractive properties of the lens are discussed in the next section.

Biomechanical properties of the lens

The mammalian lens appears to exhibit a radial stiffness gradient, with cortical fiber cells gradually stiffening as they age and becoming displaced toward the lens nucleus.[146] The spectrin-actin network is integral for developing and maintaining this mechanical stiffness. Although mechanical loading appears to be distributed throughout the lens capsule, epithelium, and fiber cells, specific microstructures have different propensities to bear and recover from load.[216] For example, despite bearing high levels of axial strain, mouse lens epithelial cell area, capsule thickness, and fiber cell widths recover when the load is removed.[216] The load-bearing properties of epithelial cells may be conferred by the hexagonal actomyosin array, which generates tensional forces. General actomyosin disruption can affect the whole (chick) lens biomechanical response to bear load.[217] In contrast, the separation of fiber cell tips is irreversible at high loads, leading to incomplete recovery of the suture gap area and incomplete whole-lens resilience.[216] Tropomyosins (Tpms) such as Tpm3.5, directly by associating with F-actin and indirectly by promoting Tmod1 and α-actinin association, stabilize the actin network associated with fiber cell membranes.[218] Decreased levels of Tpm3.5 and the accompanying dissociation of Tmod1 led to rearrangement of F-actin networks that decreased lens resilience, i.e., the ability of the lens to resume its original shape after removal of a compressive mechanical load.[218] Curiously, fiber cell organization and morphology remained unaffected.[218] Alternatively, loss of Tmod1 resulted in loss of large fiber cell undulations, or paddles, in mature fiber cells, which was correlated with a decrease in lens stiffness, even at low mechanical loads.[219] In contrast, very old mouse lenses, despite misalignment/loss of characteristic hexagonal profile of outer cortical fiber cells, continue to exhibit an age-dependent increase

in stiffness, suggesting that fiber cells packing in this region may not contribute to the biomechanical properties of the lens.[220]

Intermediate filaments are also thought to influence the biomechanical properties of the lens.[146] When subjected to ramp compression and decompression cycles, young CP49-null lenses showed decreased stiffness and slightly increased resilience compared with wild-type lenses.[221] Loss of one or both alleles of aquaporin-0, a beaded filament–binding partner in the lens, led to a significant reduction in the load-bearing ability of the lens, suggesting that aquaporin-0 is required to provide sufficient anchorage for beaded filaments to establish normal lens biomechanics. Interestingly, loss of aquaporin-5 did not affect the compressive load-bearing capacity of the mouse lens.[222] In contrast, loss of Cx46, which forms gap junctions in both the lens cortex and nucleus, resulted in increased stiffness of the mouse lens at young and old ages.[223] This increase in stiffness was alleviated in young, but not old, lenses that lacked CP49. Overall, the appropriate and combined interaction of beaded filaments with plasma membrane–associated proteins and junctional complexes appears to be important in maintaining the biomechanical properties of the lens as it ages, although the exact mechanisms linking these molecular changes to gross morphology remains unknown.

METABOLIC DETERMINANTS OF THE TRANSPARENT AND REFRACTIVE PROPERTIES OF THE LENS

While the structural organization of the lens establishes its transparent and refractive properties, the lens is not a passive optical element,[1] but a biologic tissue that requires the input of energy to drive the structural and function processes that actively maintain its optical properties. Because of its position in the eye beyond the eye-blood barrier (Fig. 5.1) and its internal structural organization into morphologically distinct regions (Fig. 5.3), the different regions of the lens do not have equal access to the nutrients supplied to it via the aqueous and vitreous humors and thus exhibit different metabolic requirements. Fiber cells in the outer cortex are closer to the nutrient supply and contain functional mitochondria, which allows them to use aerobic metabolism to meet the higher energy demands required to perform the multitude of cellular processes associated with the massive elongation of these differentiating cells. In contrast, deeper mature fiber cells that are internalized within the lens are further from the nutrients in the humors that bathe the surface of the lens and, having lost their mitochondria, rely on anaerobic glycolytic metabolism to produce the concentrations of ATP and other reducing equivalents for the antioxidant enzyme systems that operate to preserve the solubility of the crystallin proteins.[224-226] How nutrients are delivered to different regions of the lens from the surrounding humors is considered later in the chapter, but first the major metabolic functions of the different lens regions are outlined.

Glucose metabolism

The primary source of energy for the lens is glucose, which in the absence of a blood supply is supplied to the lens directly from the surrounding aqueous and vitreous humors, which in humans have glucose concentrations of approximately 3.2 mM[227] and 3.0 mM,[228] respectively. Although the normal concentration of glucose within the lens varies between species, it is in the order of 10 mg/100 g tissue.[229] Like in other tissues, glucose in the lens is primarily metabolized by three pathways: glycolysis,[230] the pentose phosphate pathway (hexose monophosphate shunt),[224] and the polyol pathway.[231,232] However, it appears that the relative activity of these pathways may vary in the different lens regions. As the initial step in a number of metabolic pathways, glycolysis is essential for the maintenance of lens physiologic function and tissue transparency over many decades of life, since perturbations to major enzyme-mediated steps in glycolysis result in lens swelling and cataract.[230,233] Owing to the differentiation-dependent degradation of cellular organelles, aerobic glycolysis and metabolism via the citric acid cycle is possible only in the lens epithelium and peripheral fiber cells that still contain mitochondria.

Hence, aerobic metabolism only accounts for approximately 20% to 30% of the total lens ATP production while consuming only around 3% of the glucose supplied to the lens.[234,235] The remaining 70% of lens glucose metabolism is carried out under anaerobic conditions,[236] which produces lactate that is thought to contribute to a measurable pH gradient from the periphery to the center of the lens.[130] In addition, owing to the lack of a blood supply, the oxygen concentration within and around the lens is much lower than in most other parts of the body.[237-241] This, in combination with the consumption of oxygen by mitochondria in epithelial and differentiating fiber cells, means that an oxygen gradient is established across the lens with the negligible oxygen levels being measured in the lens nucleus.[241]

In the lens, the pentose phosphate pathway uses glucose to produce a number of reducing equivalents (NADPH) that help protect against oxidative stress by reducing oxidized glutathione (GSSG) to regenerate glutathione (GSH).[224] NAPDH is also used in the human lens by the polyol (sorbitol) pathway.[231,232] In this pathway, sorbitol is formed from glucose by aldose reductase (AR) using NADPH as a cofactor, which is then converted to fructose by a second enzyme, polyol (sorbitol) dehydrogenase, using nicotinamide adenine dinucleotide (NAD^+) as a coenzyme. Under normal physiologic conditions, almost one-third of the glucose entering the human lens is metabolized through this sorbitol pathway.[242] In the human lens, the majority of AR, and its activity, is present predominantly in the epithelium.[242] In diabetes, the elevated levels of glucose in the blood, and hence the aqueous humor,[227] have been linked to hyperglycemia-related changes to the lens and cortical cataract formation.[236] Sorbitol is osmotically active, and therefore an overabundance of sorbitol can draw additional water inside fiber cells, which, by causing cellular swelling and damage, disrupts the ordered tissue architecture of the lens and results in light scattering. Whereas this mechanism has been demonstrated in species such as dogs[243] and rats,[244] AR activity in the human lens is lower.[242] Hence, the exact mechanism of diabetic cataract in humans is less clear and is thought to involve an oxidative component in addition to osmotic stress.[245,246]

Antioxidant defense systems

Molecular oxygen is, directly or indirectly, the source of most oxidative damage. If cells could survive in an atmosphere free of oxygen, most oxidative damage would be avoided. For most cells this is not possible, but the oxygen tension around the lens in the living eye is quite low, less than 15 mmHg (~2% O_2) just anterior to the lens and less than 9 mmHg (~1.3% O_2) near its posterior surface.[237-240,247,248] Oxygen levels within the human lens are even lower (<2 mmHg).[241] The low oxygen tension around and within the lens helps to protect lens proteins and lipids from oxidative damage. However, even with this low level of oxygen, the lens normally derives a proportion of its ATP from oxidative phosphorylation,[225] a process that inherently generates free oxygen radicals.[249]

Hydrogen peroxide is another molecule that has been suggested to cause oxidative stress to the lens. Hydrogen peroxide is produced in mitochondria by the enzyme superoxide dismutase acting on superoxide anions, a by-product of oxidative phosphorylation. Hydrogen peroxide can also be produced during the oxidation of ascorbic acid, which is present at high levels in the aqueous and vitreous humors (~1.5–2.5 mM) that bathe the lens. Both processes may contribute to the resting hydrogen peroxide levels that have been reported within both intraocular fluids and the lens itself.[250,251] The level of hydrogen peroxide in the aqueous humor has been reported to average over 30 mM and to exceed 200 mM in about one-third of cataract patients.[250,252] The lens has two enzyme systems to detoxify hydrogen peroxide. Lens epithelial cells have abundant levels of catalase, which converts hydrogen peroxide to water,[253] and GSH peroxidase, an enzyme that couples the reduction of hydrogen peroxide to the oxidation of GSH. Studies on cultured lenses and lens epithelial cells suggest that GSH peroxidase provides most of the protection against the potential damaging effects of physiologic levels of hydrogen peroxide, as catalase is only effective against relatively high concentrations of peroxide.[254]

The lens has a number of antioxidants, but the principal antioxidant in the lens is GSH.[255] It has been shown that the maintenance of GSH in the lens nucleus is critical to the prevention of protein crosslinking, crystallin aggregation, and light scattering.[256] GSH is a tripeptide of the amino acids glutamine, cysteine, and glycine, and provides most of the protection against oxidative damage in the lens. It can prevent the oxidation of components of the lens cytoplasm because its concentration in the lens is very high, approximately 4 to 6 mM, and its sulfhydryl group is readily oxidized. These high intracellular GSH levels are maintained by a combination of pathways (Fig. 5.13), which includes (1) synthesis of GSH from its precursor amino acids, cysteine, glutamate, and glycine, by the sequential actions of the enzymes glutamate cysteine ligase (GCL) and GSH synthetase; (2) transport of GSH from outside the cell via specific carriers; (3) regeneration of GSH from oxidized GSH (GSSG) by the enzyme GSH reductase (GR) and nicotinamide adenine dinucleotide phosphate (NADPH) generated via the pentose phosphate pathway; and (4) the export of GSH, followed by its degradation into constituent amino acids by γ-glutamyl transpeptidase (GGT) to ensure GSH turnover.[257] In the absence of GSH synthesis in the lens nucleus, GSH needs to be regenerated from GSSG. GSH can form disulfide bonds with the oxidized sulfhydryl groups of proteins. These GSH-protein mixed disulfides can then be reduced by a second molecule of GSH, a process that is facilitated by the enzyme thioltransferase.[258] This regenerates the protein sulfhydryl and forms GSSG, which can then be subsequently reduced to regenerate GSH. When GSH levels have been lowered in lens epithelial cells or whole lenses, cell damage and cataract formation follow rapidly.[259-261] Furthermore, it has been shown in human and rat lenses that GSH-dependent enzymes protect and restore protein-thiol groups in their reduced state to prevent protein crosslinking.[262]

In addition to GSH, ascorbic acid is used to protect the lens against oxidative damage. Ascorbate is actively transported from the blood to the aqueous humor by a sodium-dependent transporter located in the ciliary epithelium[263] and reaches concentrations in the aqueous humor that are 40 to 50 times higher than levels in the blood.[264] The ascorbate levels in the lens and other intraocular tissues are also substantial.[265,266] Dehydroascorbate (DHA), the oxidized form of ascorbic acid, enters lens cells by way of the glucose transporter (GLUT), where it is reduced by GSH-dependent processes.[264,267] Like GSH, ascorbate is readily oxidized, forming DHA in the process. Therefore ascorbate can react with free radicals and other oxidants in the aqueous humor and the lens, preventing these molecules from damaging lens lipids, proteins, and nucleic acids. However, if DHA accumulates in the lens, its metabolites can react with lens proteins, increasing lens color and decreasing protein stability.[266] The high GSH levels in the lens likely maintain the majority of ascorbate in its reduced state, thereby avoiding much of this potential damage.

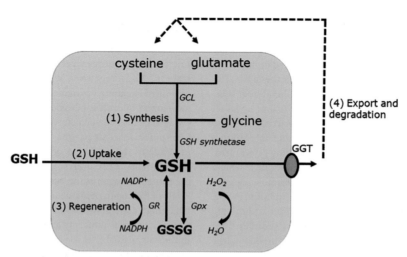

Fig. 5.13 Maintenance of intracellular glutathione (*GSH*) levels. High cellular levels of GSH are maintained by a dynamic balance between four distinct pathways. **(1)** Intracellular synthesis from precursor amino acids cysteine, glutamate, and glycine. The enzyme glutamate cysteine ligase (GCL) catalyzes the reaction between cysteine and glutamate to form gamma-glutamylcysteine (γ-GC), which in turn reacts with glycine to form GSH, a reaction catalyzed by the enzyme glutathione synthetase. **(2)** Direct uptake of GSH via GSH uptake transporters. **(3)** Regeneration of GSH from GSSG. GSH is used as a cofactor for GSH peroxidase (Gpx) in the process of detoxifying H_2O_2 into H_2O and is in turn oxidized to GSSG. GSH reductase (GR) is used in combination with NADPH to help recycle GSSG back to GSH. **(4)** Export of GSH followed by degradation into its precursor amino acid by GGT and subsequent reuptake of amino acids for GSH synthesis. (Reproduced with permission from Lim JC, Grey AC, Zahraei A, Donaldson PJ. Age-dependent changes in glutathione metabolism pathways in the lens: New insights into therapeutic strategies to prevent cataract formation: a review. *Clin Experimen Ophthalmol* 2020;48(8):1031–1042.)

Ultraviolet protection

Lens antioxidant defense systems are also important to support the human lens' role as an ultraviolet (UV) filter that works in conjunction with the cornea to protect the retina against light-induced damage from wavelengths of light in the UV range (250–400 nm). While the cornea restricts the transmission of wavelengths less than 290 nm,[268,269] the remaining harmful solar radiation is absorbed by UV filters in the lens that absorb light in the 295 to 400 nm range.[270,271] These filters are small molecules formed through tryptophan metabolism and, although present in many mammals, are predominantly found in primates and humans.[272,273]

The major UV filter compounds found in the human lens are kynurenine (Kyn), 3-hydroxykynurenine (3-OHK), and 3-hydroxykynurenine O-β-D-glucoside (3-OHKG). They are found at higher concentrations in the nucleus than the cortex, and their concentrations decline with advancing lens age.[274] These compounds can undergo spontaneous deamination to produce the structurally related UV filters, which follow the same age-related concentration changes observed for the kynurenine UV filters.[275] Some of these UV filters are unstable at physiologic pH and undergo spontaneous degradation or react with a range of other small molecules found in the lens. For example, 3-OHKG can undergo deamination to produce deamidated 3-hydroxykynurenine O-β-D-glucoside (3OHKG-D) and 3-hydroxykynurenine O-β-D-glucoside yellow (3OHKG-Y). For example, GSH reacts with 3-OHKG to form glutathionyl-3-hydroxykynurenine glucoside (GSH-3-OHKG), a UV filter and lens fluorophore[276] that increases concentration in the lens nucleus with increasing lens age. In addition, UV filters are present in cataractous tissue at concentrations higher than age-matched controls,[274] and in modified forms.[277] For this reason, they have been implicated in cataract formation, possibly through their modification of crystallin proteins,[278,279] and subsequent action as photosensitizers that increase oxidative stress in the aging lens.[280]

PHYSIOLOGICAL DETERMINANTS OF THE TRANSPARENT AND REFRACTIVE PROPERTIES OF THE LENS

The structural and metabolic adaptations described previously that establish the transparent and refractive properties of the lens in turn impose a number physiologic constraints on the lens.[281] As a consequence of these constraints, the lens requires a specialized transport system that can: (1) rapidly deliver nutrients/antioxidants to, and remove metabolic wastes from, deeper-lying fiber cells, so that the solubility of lens crystallins is maintained and protein aggregation prevented; (2) impose the negative membrane potential that is required to maintain the steady-state volume of the fiber cells, which is necessary to prevent changes in their cellular morphology and light scatter; and (3) prevent alterations to the GRI by countering water influx into the lens generated by the high concentrations of the lens crystallins needed for the lens to refract light while immersed in aqueous media. Our understanding of how the cellular physiology of the lens regulates these key features has evolved over recent decades as advances in histologic and electrophysiological techniques, utilized to study fluid transport in other epithelial tissues, have been applied to the lens.[282,283] A major early milestone came from the work of Robinson and Patterson[284] who used vibrating probe measurements to show that a standing flow of ionic current, which was directed inward at the poles and outward at the equator, was a common feature of different species of vertebrate lenses.[285,286] Utilizing a combination of electrical impedance measurements and theoretical modeling, Mathias[281] subsequently proposed that these currents measured at the lens surface represent the external portion of a circulating ionic current that drives a unique internal microcirculatory system, which operates to maintain fiber cell homeostasis and therefore lens transparency. Although the microcirculation model of lens transport was not initially accepted by all,[287,288] in recent years the application of other experimental techniques to the lens has allowed researchers to actually measure and visualize the solute and fluid fluxes original predicted by the microcirculation system model.[1] These findings have significantly strengthened and expanded our current understanding of how the underlying cellular physiology of the lens actively maintains its transparency and refractive properties.

An overview of the lens microcirculation system

Mathias et al.[281] originally proposed a working model in which circulating Na^+ currents, initially identified by vibrating probe measurements,[284] enter the lens at both the anterior and posterior poles via an extracellular pathway located between fiber cells (Fig. 5.14A). Na^+ eventually crosses the fiber cell membranes, and then flows from cell to cell toward the surface via an intracellular pathway mediated by gap junction channels. Because the gap junction coupling conductance in the outer shell of differentiating fibers is concentrated at the equatorial plane of the lens,[112,289] this intracellular current is directed toward the equatorial surface of the lens where epithelial and peripheral fiber cells that contain the highest densities of Na^+/K^+ pumps are located, to actively transport Na^+ out of the lens.[289-292] The driving force for these fluxes is hypothesized to be the difference in the electromotive potential of surface cells and inner fiber cells (Fig. 5.14B, top panel). Data from ion substitution experiments performed on both intact lenses[281] and isolated fiber cells[293] have shown that the surface cells, including epithelial cells and newly differentiating fiber cells, contain Na^+/K^+ pumps, and K^+-channels, which together generate a negative electromotive potential. Fiber cells deeper in the lens lack functional Na^+/K^+ pumps, and K^+-channels and their permeability is dominated by nonselective cation[294] and Cl^- conductances.[295,296] In these inner cells, the negative membrane potential that helps maintain the steady-state volume of the fiber cells is imposed on deeper fiber cells by virtue of their connection to surface cells via gap junctions.[281] This electrical connection, together with the different membrane properties of the surface and inner cells, causes the standing current to flow.

In this model, the circulating Na^+ current creates a net flux of solute that in turn generates fluid flow (Fig. 5.14B, middle panel). This fluid flow has two main consequences. First, the extracellular flow of water convects nutrients and antioxidants toward the deeper-lying fiber cells (Fig. 5.14B, bottom panel), which have been shown to express multiple membrane transporters, enabling them to take up nutrients convected by the microcirculation system.[297] Many of these transport proteins are Na^+-dependent secondary active transporters and utilize the energy stored in the Na^+ electrochemical gradient established by the active removal of Na^+ at the lens equatorial surface.[298] Second, the intracellular flow of water from the nucleus to the lens surface through gap junction channels generates a substantial hydrostatic pressure (0–330 mmHg) gradient that drives the intracellular flow of fluid from the central cells to the surface cells.[299] This pressure gradient drives the removal of water from the lens nucleus, and has important implications for the maintenance of the transparent and refractive properties of the lens.[1] Hence, the ability of the microcirculation system to deliver nutrients and actively regulate lens water content is the key contributor to the homeostatic mechanisms that maintain the transparency and refractive properties of the lens.

Delivery of nutrients and antioxidants to the lens core

In the absence of a vasculature, the lens needs a mechanism to deliver nutrients and antioxidants to the fiber cells in the different regions of the lens that have distinctly different energy requirements. Differentiating fiber cells in the periphery of the lens, which have the

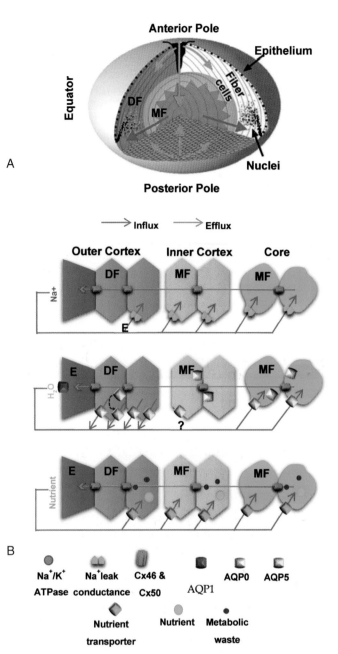

Fig. 5.14 Lens structure and function **(A)** 3-D representation of the microcirculation model, showing ions and fluid fluxes that enter the lens at both poles via the extracellular space (blue arrows) before crossing fiber cell membranes and exiting the lens at the equator via an intracellular pathway (red arrows) mediated by gap junctions. **(B)** Equatorial cross-sections showing how the spatial differences in the distribution of ion channels and transporters between the epithelium (E), differentiating (DF) and mature (MF) fiber cells that generate the circulating flux of Na+ ions (top) that drives isotonic fluid fluxes (middle) which in turn deliver nutrients to and remove metabolic waste from the MF cells (bottom). (From Braakhuis AJ, Donaldson CI, Lim JC, Donaldson PJ. Nutritional strategies to prevent pens cataract: Current status and future strategies. *Nutrients.* 2019;11:1186. https://doi.org/10.3390/nu11051186.)

highest energy demand, can source their nutrients directly from the surrounding humors. However, fiber cells located deeper in the lens are too far from the surface to rely on the passive diffusion to provide an adequate supply of nutrients and antioxidants to establish the reductive environment necessary to maintain lens transparency in the deeper regions of the lens.[298] Two different views have emerged of how nutrients and antioxidants are delivered to the deeper regions of the lens and subsequently taken up and utilized in mature fiber cells.[257]

Based on the observation that levels of GSH fall in the lens nucleus in age-related nuclear cataract but are maintained relatively constant in the outer cortical regions of the lens (Fig. 5.15A), Truscott[300] hypothesized that nuclear cataract is a transport problem. To explain this phenomenon, Truscott proposed that the delivery of glucose and GSH to the nucleus of the lens occurs by an intracellular route mediated via diffusion through gap junctions.[300-302] In this model, the relatively higher concentrations of GSH and other metabolites in the outer cortex relative to the nucleus creates a concentration gradient that is thought to drive the diffusion of reduced GSH to the lens nucleus via the extensive network of gap junction found in the lens (Fig. 5.15B). Once delivered to the nucleus, GSH is proposed to be oxidized to GSSG, before the GSSG diffused from the nucleus back to the cortex via the same gap junction–mediated pathway, where it is then reduced back to GSH. Under this model, the low concentration of GSH observed in the aged lens nucleus was proposed to be caused by the age-dependent development of an intracellular diffusion barrier that becomes apparent in middle age, which acts to impede the intracellular diffusion of small molecules into the nucleus.[300,302] In support of this model, Slavi et al.[303]

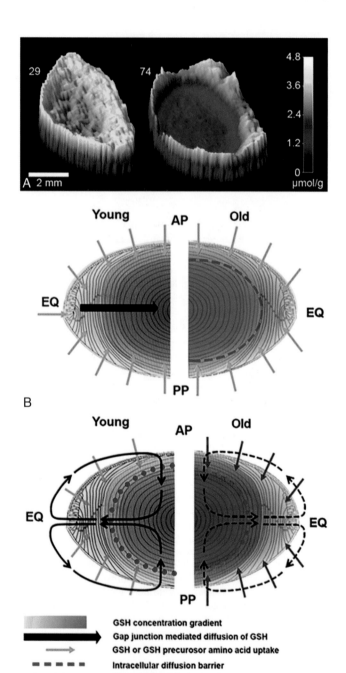

Fig. 5.15 Alternative views to the delivery of GSH to the lens nucleus. (**A**) Quantitative matrix-assisted laser desorption ionization (MALDI) imaging mass spectrometry of 29- and 74-year-old human lenses that show that while cortical GSH levels remain relatively constant, the nuclear GSH concentration drops significantly with age. (Modified from Grey AC, Demarais NJ, West BJ, Donaldson PJ. A quantitative map of glutathione in the aging human lens. *Int J Mass Spect.* 2019;437:58–68.) (**B, C**) Alternative functional models to explain the age-dependent drop in glutathione (GSH) levels shown in (**A**). In these models, the GSH gradient is depicted as a color gradient and the changes in GSH levels are shown for a young (*left panels*) and old (*right panels*) lens. Direct GSH uptake and/or the uptake of precursor amino acids is indicated by the *green arrows*. (**B**) In this model, GSH passively diffuses to the nucleus via an intracellular route mediated by gap junctions (*black arrow in young lens*). However, in older lenses, it is proposed that a barrier to intercellular diffusion develops (*blue dotted line in old lens*), impeding the movement of GSH from its site of synthesis and regeneration in the cortex to produce the observed localized depletion of GSH in the lens nucleus. (**C**). In this second model, the extracellular movement of GSH into the lens nucleus is prevented by an extracellular diffusion barrier (*red dots*). However, this barrier can be bypassed via the lens microcirculation system (*continuous black arrows in the young lens*), which acts to direct ion and water fluxes into *the lens* nucleus mediated *via the sutures*. The inflow of *water* along the extracellular spaces *within the lens* carries *nutrients* and antioxidants such as GSH deep into the lens and removes waste products toward the equator via an intracellular outflow pathway mediated by gap junctions. With increasing age, the microcirculation systems declines (*dotted black arrows in older lens*) resulting in reduced delivery of GSH to the lens nucleus. *AP*, anterior pole; *EQ*, equator; *PP*, posterior pole (Reproduced with permission from Lim JC, Lam L, Li B, Donaldson PJ. Molecular identification and cellular localization of a potential transport system involved in cystine/cysteine uptake in human lenses. *Exp Eye Res* 2013;116:219–226.)

have shown that the lens gap junctional proteins Cx46 and Cx50 exogenously expressed in cell lines form gap junction channels that were permeable to GSH, albeit at low levels.[303] In experiments using Cx46 and Cx50 knockout mice, GSH levels in the nucleus were markedly reduced in Cx46 knockout lens, but were unaffected in the Cx50 knockout, suggesting that GSH diffuses from cortical fiber cells to the nucleus via gap junction channels formed from Cx46. However, in these same studies, GSSG was shown not to permeate lens gap junctions,[303] suggesting that the regeneration of GSH from GSSG has to occur locally in the nucleus of the mouse lens. Furthermore, although GSH can diffuse between isolated pairs of cells, whether this passive cell-to-cell diffusion of GSH is sufficient to deliver sufficient GSH across the many cell layers that comprise the whole lens is unclear. Model calculations have suggested that owing to the distances involved, passive diffusion would not be fast enough to deliver sufficient antioxidants to maintain the reductive environment in the lens.[298]

The alternative view is that nutrients and antioxidants such as glucose and GSH are supplied to the nucleus via an extracellular pathway that uses the circulating ion and water fluxes generated by the microcirculation system to deliver nutrients faster than would occur by passive diffusion alone (Fig. 5.15C). Transporters specific for GSH and glucose present in the membranes of mature fiber cells can then accumulate the nutrients supplied to them, which in the case of glucose can then be metabolized locally to supply the reducing equivalent NADPH required to regenerate GSH.[224] In support of this model, Vaghefi et al.[135,304] utilized magnetic resonance imaging (MRI) contrast agents as extracellular space tracers, and monitored their penetration into organ-cultured bovine lenses using confocal reflectance microscopy and T1-weighted imaging. This real-time MRI showed that contrast agents below a specific molecular size cutoff were able to be delivered to the lens nucleus at a rate that was significantly faster than could be achieved by passive diffusion alone, and furthermore that this enhanced rate of delivery was abolished by inhibiting the lens microcirculation system.[304] The pattern of contrast agent penetration into the lens also revealed an area in the inner cortex of the bovine lens from which the contrast agent was excluded,[135,304] which appeared to be equivalent to the formation of a barrier to extracellular space diffusion first identified in the rat lens using fluorescent dyes.[133] Reflection imaging of lens sections loaded with MRI contrast agents showed that the agents crossed this barrier at the anterior and posterior poles and were delivered to the lens nucleus via an extracellular pathway associated with the sutures.[135] Although these experiments provide support for this model of extracellular delivery of solutes to the lens nucleus, it needs to be stressed that the MRI contrast agents used in these experiments are exogenous tracers, and these results need to be repeated using more metabolically relevant endogenous molecules.

Despite this caveat, there is considerable evidence showing that the membranes of mature fiber cells contain an array of transporters that are capable of taking up nutrients delivered via the extracellular space by the microcirculation system.[305] Molecular studies have shown that differentiating and mature fiber cells both express a variety of transporters capable of mediating the uptake of glucose[306-308] and amino acids involved in the synthesis of GSH,[309-313] but in some cases the complement of transporters found in plasma membranes of fiber cells was found to change between the outer cortex and the nucleus.[297] In differentiating fiber cells, which are capable of de novo protein synthesis, nutrient transport proteins exist as two distinct pools: a pool associated with the plasma membrane and a second storage pool of cytoplasmic vesicles.[297] Trafficking between these two pools determines the abundance of transporters in the membrane and hence the rate of uptake of nutrients from the extracellular space. It appears that this trafficking to the membrane is under differential control.[297] In the outer

cortex, changes in nutrient levels such as observed in hyperglycemia can induce dynamic changes in the membrane insertion of GLUT3 to increase glucose uptake in the rat lens.[307] In contrast to this dynamic substrate-induced insertion, a more programmed differentiation-dependent irreversible insertion of a variety of nutrient transporters into the membrane has also been observed.[306,307,310,312] This process has been proposed to change the complement of transporter proteins in the membranes of mature fiber cells, which have lost their ability to synthesize new membrane proteins but need to adapt to the different metabolic environment they now experience in the lens nucleus.[297]

This differentiation-dependent change in the complement of nutrient transporters can be illustrated by considering how the amino acids cysteine, glycine, and glutamate that are required for GSH synthesis accumulate in the different regions of the lens. Cysteine is the rate-limiting substrate for GSH synthesis[314-317] and is first taken up from the aqueous humor as cystine, the dimeric oxidized form of cysteine that is more stable and abundant than cysteine in the aqueous.[318,319] In rat[310] and human[313] lenses, the uptake of cystine from the aqueous humor is mediated by the amino acid transporter, Xc-, which exchanges extracellular cystine for intracellular glutamate (Fig. 5.16). This exchange system relies on the maintenance of a high intracellular glutamate concentration, and in other tissues this is mediated by members of the X_{AG} amino acid transport family.[320,321] The X_{AG} transporters are a multigene family of Na^+-dependent amino acid transporters, which include the excitatory amino acid transporters (EAAT1–5) and the alanine serine cysteine transporters (ASCT1–2).[322] In the rat lens Xc- is expressed in combination with different members of the X_{AG} family (Fig. 5.16C,D). In the outer cortex, Xc- expression was shown to overlap with EAAT4/5 expression (Fig. 5.16A,C), while in the core (Fig. 5.16B,D), Xc- expression colocalized with ASCT2 expression.[310,312] The observed switch in glutamate uptake mechanisms from EAAT4/5 to ASCT2 may reflect the ability of ASCT2 to preferentially accumulate glutamate at the low intracellular pH,[323] which, because of anaerobic metabolism and the production of lactate, prevails in the lens nucleus.[324]

The lack of capacity of the lens nucleus to synthesize GSH from its precursor amino acids raised questions around why this region of the lens engages in cystine/cysteine uptake. Since the sulfhydryl moiety of cysteine gives GSH its antioxidant properties, it has been proposed that cysteine itself may act directly as a small-molecular-weight antioxidant by maintaining the free sulfhydryl groups of proteins in their reduced state.[262] Another possible role of cystine is to act as a source for the formation of protein mixed disulfides (PSSC), which act to protect sulfhydryl groups of proteins/enzymes from irreversible damage by oxidation until thioltransferases can dethiolate the PSSC and restore protein/enzyme function. Thus, cystine delivery to and uptake by the nucleus may constitute a low-molecular-mass antioxidant defense system.[313]

To facilitate the uptake of glycine, the rat lens expresses two high-affinity Na^+-dependent glycine uptake transporters, GLYT1 and GLYT2.[312] GLYT1 has a stoichiometry of $2Na^+/Cl^-$/glycine, whereas GLYT2 has a stoichiometry of $3Na^+/Cl^-$/glycine.[325,326] A difference of one more Na^+ in ionic coupling implies that the available driving force for glycine uptake for GLYT2 is two orders of magnitude larger than for GLYT1 under physiologic conditions.[327] This difference affords GLYT2 with a greater ability relative to GLYT1 to accumulate glycine to concentrations that exceed those found in the extracellular spaces. Furthermore, GLYT2 has a consistently higher affinity for glycine than GLYT1.[326] As a result, the differential expression of the GLYTs in the lens establishes a gradient of transporter affinities, which increases with distance into the lens and allows deeper fiber cells to take up glycine from the extracellular space, where the glycine concentration diminishes with distance into the lens. Although both isoforms are

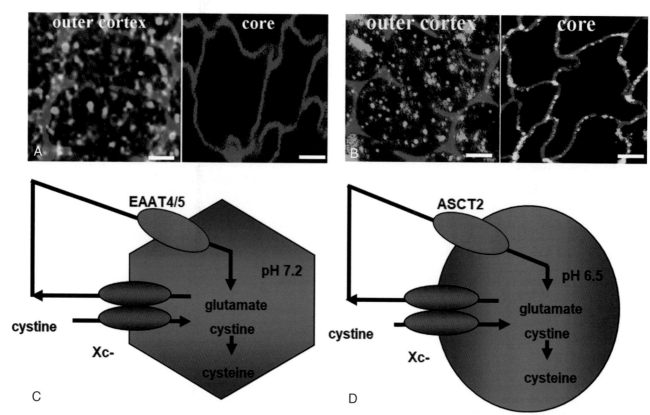

Fig. 5.16 Differential expression of glutamate transporters in the cortex and core of the rat lens. (**A**) EAAT4 labeling *(green)* in the outer cortex is associated with the cytoplasm and the membranes *(red)* but is absent from the core of the lens. (**B**) ASCT2 labeling *(green)* in the outer cortex is predominately associated with cytoplasm, while in the lens core ASCT2 labeling is not only detected but localizes with the membrane *(red)*. (**C, D**) Models showing how the uptake of cystine by Xc- in exchange for glutamate utilizes EAAT4/5 in the outer cortex (**C**), but ASCT2 (**D**) in the core to recycle the glutamate removed by Xc- in order to restore the intracellular glutamine concentration gradient. This switch from EAAT4/5 to ASCT2 is proposed to be due to the ability of ASCT2 to preferentially accumulate glutamate at the low intracellular pH environment found in the lens core. (From Lim J, Lorentzen KA, Kistler J, Donaldson PJ. Molecular identification and characterisation of the glycine transporter (GLYT1) and the glutamine/glutamate transporter (ASCT2) in the rat lens. *Exp Eye Res* 2006;83(2):447–455.)

expressed in differentiating fiber cells and are likely to mediate glycine uptake in the outer cortex, only the higher-affinity transporter GLYT2 is present in the lens nucleus and is therefore thought to be responsible for the accumulation of glycine observed in the center of the lens.[311] Like the observed change in the glutamate recycling partner for Xc- from EAAT4/5 to ASCT2, it has been proposed that the dominance of GLYT2 function in the lens nucleus is an adaptation that allows the uptake of glycine to occur in the low pH environment found in the inner regions of the lens,[311] as the histidine residue at position 421 in GLYT1 that reduces its ability to uptake glycine at low pH (pH <7.0) is not conserved in GLYT2.[328] The resulting accumulation of glycine in the lens nucleus has been proposed to afford protection against protein glycation, as glycine can protect human lens proteins from glycation by efficiently scavenging glucose.[311,329] Because advanced-stage glycation products often accumulate during aging,[330] enhancing the uptake of glycine by the lens could help prevent cataract.

Taken together, these results indicate that the lens has evolved a very sophisticated system that employs the differential use of nutrient transporters to match their functional properties to the environmental conditions and the nutrient supply that prevails in different regions of the lens. Because lens fiber cells mature further after they lose their organelles, this differential expression is achieved in the absence of

de novo protein synthesis via the insertion of previously synthesized transporters located in cytoplasmic vesicles into the plasma membrane. This ensures that deeper-lying fiber cells are capable of nutrient uptake under low pH conditions and when nutrient concentrations become marginal. This increased understanding of regional differences in nutrient delivery and uptake pathways opens new avenues to understanding how the age-dependent decline in these pathways could lead to observed decreases in the reductive environment in the lens that precedes the onset of nuclear cataract.

Dynamic regulation of lens water content

A prediction of the original microcirculation model was that the outflow of water through gap junction channels would generate a corresponding change in hydrostatic pressure.[331] Using a microelectrode-based manometer method, this prediction was subsequently confirmed and a substantial hydrostatic pressure (0–330 mmHg) gradient was measured, the magnitude of which could be altered using different strains of transgenic mice with different degrees of gap junction coupling.[299,332,333] Subsequent experiments also showed that a decline in gap junction coupling observed in older mouse lenses resulted in an increase in the hydrostatic pressure gradient that appeared to be mediated by a degradation of the lens gap junction proteins, Cx46

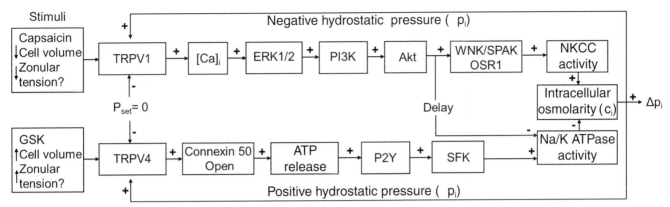

Fig. 5.17 The dual feedback control system that maintains hydrostatic pressure in the lens. Lens surface pressure (pset) is maintained by the competing activities of the two arms of a dual feedback system that regulate ion transporters that control the intracellular osmolarity of cells at the lens surface. Increases in pressure (Δp_i), hypo-osmotic stress, increased zonular tension, and the TRPV4 agonist GSK all work via TRPV4 to activate one arm of feedback system. This arm uses a signaling pathway that involves the release of ATP via Cx50 hemichannels and the subsequent activation of P2Y receptors and the Src family of protein tyrosine kinases (SFK), to increase the activity of the Na/K- ATPase and decrease lens pressure. Decreases in pressure (Δp_i), hyperosmotic stress, decreased zonular tension, and the TRPV1 agonist capsaicin all work via TRPV1 to activate the other arm of the feedback system. This arm utilizes a signalling pathway consisting of extracellular signal–regulated kinase 1/2 (ERK1/2), phosphatidylinositol 3-kinase (PI3/Akt), and WNK-SPAK/OSR1 to directly activate. NKCC1 and eventually reduce the activity of the Na⁺/K-ATPase to effect an increase in surface pressure. (Reproduced with permission from Nakazawa Y, Petrova RS, Sugiyama Y, Nagai N, Tamura H, Donaldson PJ. Regulation of the membrane trafficking of the mechanosensitive ion channels TRPV1 and TRPV4 by zonular tension, osmotic stress and activators in the mouse lens. *Int J Mol Sci* 2021;22(23).)

and Cx50.[334] Furthermore, this observed age-dependent decrease in gap junction coupling appears to be mediated by oxidative stress, as a similar degradation of Cx46 and Cx50 was observed in mouse lenses in which oxidative stress was increased by the knockout of the antioxidant enzyme GSH peroxidase 1 (GPX-1).[335] Interestingly, this pressure gradient is remarkably conserved between species of lenses of dramatically different sizes,[332] and its magnitude is maintained relatively constant due to a dual feedback system (Fig. 5.17), which utilizes mechanosensitive TRP channels to sense changes in pressure at the surface of the lens.[336,337] Pressure decreases or increases sensed by TRPV1 or TRPV4, respectively, utilize distinct signaling pathways to modulate Na⁺ pump and sodium-potassium-chloride cotransporter (NKCC1) activity, which in turn regulates the microcirculation system to ensure a constant hydrostatic pressure is maintained. Because this highly regulated hydrostatic pressure gradient is generated by the outflow of water from the lens, it implies that water transport and therefore water content in the different regions of the lens are similarly regulated.

Regulation of water content and fiber cell volume in the outer cortex

Any change to the water content in the periphery of the lens will alter the high spatial order of differentiating fiber cells that contributes to the establishment of lens transparency in the outer cortex (see Fig. 5.11). Hence, any failure of these fiber cells to maintain their water content will swell or shrink them, disrupting local spatial order to induce an increase in light scattering.[338,339] To minimize such changes in water content, differentiating fiber cells utilize a variety of ion channels and transporters to actively maintain their cell volume and therefore overall lens volume.[338,339] This ability of the lens to regulate its volume was first studied by incubating lenses in anisomotic solutions.[340-342] Lenses exposed to hypo-osmotic challenge media exhibited an initial swelling before undergoing a regulatory volume decrease (RVD) mediated via the efflux of K⁺ and Cl⁻ ions to generate an associated loss of internal water and subsequent reduction in lens volume. In contrast,

lenses placed in a hyperosmotic media underwent an initial shrinkage, which was subsequently restored by a regulatory volume increase (RVI) driven by the intracellular accumulation of K⁺, Na⁺, and Cl⁻ ions and, consequently, water influx.

In other tissue cell types, the sodium-potassium-chloride cotransporter (NKCC1) and potassium chloride cotransporters (KCC1–4), which all belong to the cation chloride cotransporter (CCC) family,[343] dynamically interact to regulate the intracellular concentration of Cl⁻ that in turn plays a vital role in the maintenance of cell volume. NKCC1 uses the energy of the Na⁺ electrochemical gradient to drive the uptake of Cl⁻,[344] while the direction of Cl⁻ transport mediated by the KCC is determined by the sum of the chemical potential differences for K⁺ and Cl⁻. Normally, owing to the K⁺ gradient produced by Na⁺-K⁺ pump, KCCs mediate the efflux of Cl⁻ out of cells. However, under circumstances in which the membrane potential is depolarized, this gradient is reversed and KCC can mediate the uptake of Cl⁻.[343,345]

Subsequent studies on rat lenses cultured under isosmotic conditions in the presence of reagents that modulate the activity of Cl⁻ channels and CCC transporters have shown that a constitutively active flux of Cl⁻ ions exists in the lens cortex that regulates steady-state fiber cell volume.[338] The histologic analysis of these lenses revealed that blocking Cl⁻ transport induced spatially distinct damage phenotypes that are due to the inhibition of Cl⁻ influx and efflux in deeper and peripheral fiber cells in the lens cortex, respectively.[296,346-348] Since these influx and efflux zones are coupled together by gap junctions, it is thought that they generate a circulating flux of Cl⁻ ions, which contributes to the maintenance of steady-state lens volume.[338]

In other cell types, the activity of NKCC1 and KCCs is reciprocally regulated by a signaling pathway that modulates their phosphorylation status to ensure that at steady state, cell volume is held constant.[349] This pathway involves members of the With No Lysine Kinases (WNK1–4) family.[350] WNKs respond to osmotic stress by phosphorylating and activating two closely related kinases: the Ste-20-like Proline Alanine Rich Kinase (SPAK) and Oxidative Stress Response Kinase 1 (OXSR1).[351]

These kinases directly phosphorylate and thus activate NKCC1 while inactivating KCC. The phosphorylation of these cotransporters is reversible through the actions of phosphatases PP1 and PP2A. Thus, the current view of the mechanism underlying cell volume regulation is that WNK kinases act as sensors while SPAK/OSR1 act as transducers that reciprocally regulate phosphorylation levels of the CCCs that affect changes in cell volume.[351]

CCC transporters have been identified in the lenses of a variety of species.[346,352,353] A spatially distinct expression pattern for NKCC1 was observed in both rat[346,352] and bovine lenses,[354] with NKCC1 being localized only to the outer cortical regions, suggesting that NKCC1-mediated ion uptake in the lens is localized to peripheral fiber cells. As in other tissues, hypertonic challenge results in phosphorylation and activation of NKCC1 activity via the WNK-SPAK/OSR1 kinase signaling pathway.[354,355] More recently, TRPV1 has been shown to respond to hyperosmotic-induced cell shrinkage by phosphorylating and activating NKCC1 to induce an RVI response that restores lens volume.[355] This response was prevented by the addition of the TRPV1 antagonist A-88,[355] and has been recently confirmed in mice using both WT and TRPV1[-/-] mouse models.[337]

Conversely, TRPV4 channels can sense and respond to hypoosmotic stress by triggering ATP release and increasing Na$^+$/K$^+$ ATPase activity in the lens.[356,357] In other cell types, a transient increase in Na$^+$/K$^+$ ATPase activity plays an important role in RVD, which mediates recovery from swelling.[358] Because mechanosensitive TRPV4 is considered to be a volume-regulated cation channel,[359] it is not surprising that the TRPV4 channel mediates the lens RVD process to restore lens volume. Whether TRPV4 also activates KCC activity to facilitate RVD in the lens is currently unknown but is highly likely. Thus, this activation of TRPV1 in response to cell shrinking contrasts with the response of TRPV4 to cell swelling. This suggests the existence of potential synergistic involvement of these two Transient Receptor Potential Vanilloid (TRPV) channels in reciprocal activation of ion transporters involved in the maintenance of cellular and tissue volume homeostasis in response to localized osmotic perturbations.[355,360]

In addition to their roles in the regulation of lens volume, NKCC and Na$^+$/K$^+$ ATPase are also actively involved in lens pressure regulation.[336,337,361] This indicates that the cotransporters are involved in both lens volume and pressure regulation and suggests that a dynamic volume regulation response could be triggered by changes to the lens surface pressure as shown in Fig. 5.18. Under this scenario, any change in lens pressure will initiate a transport of ions (Na$^+$, K$^+$, Cl$^-$) either into or out of the surface cells through NKCC1 or Na$^+$/K$^+$ ATPase (and potentially KCC activity), increasing or minimizing the transmembrane water flux and thus returning cell volume/pressure to steady state. Furthermore, because both NKCC1[346,352,354] and Na$^+$/K$^+$ ATPase[290-292] expression is more concentrated in the lens equator, one might speculate that this dynamic volume regulation is more significant in the

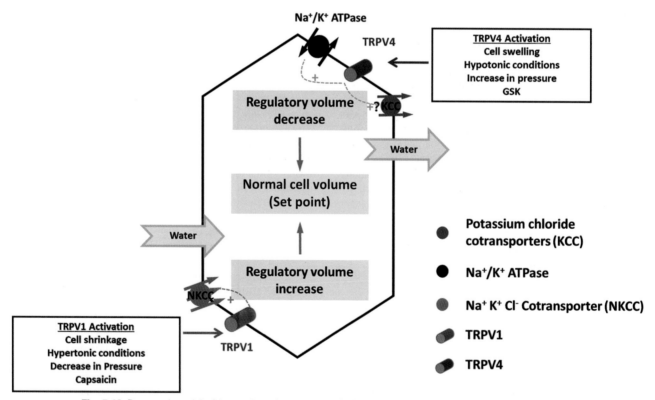

Fig. 5.18 Proposed model of lens volume/pressure regulation that actively maintains the fiber cell order in the lens outer cortex. In this model TRPV1 and TRPV4 channels act as transducers that sense cell shrinkage and swelling, respectively, and activate signaling pathways that return cell volume back to normal (set point) volume. Activation of TRPV1 channels leads to an increase in NKCC and reduction in Na$^+$/K$^+$ ATPase activity to produce a regulatory volume increase that increases ion and water influx that increases intracellular osmolality and surface pressure. TRPV4 activation increases Na$^+$/K$^+$ ATPase, and potentially KCC, activity to produce a regulatory volume decrease that increases ion and water efflux in peripheral fiber cells and thereby decreases intracellular osmolality and surface pressure. These changes in volume can be detected as changes in surface pressure.

outer regions of the lens where the transparency of the lens is more dependent on the maintenance of the ordered structure of the fiber cells to reduce light scattering (see Fig. 5.11).

Regulation of water content and refractive index in the lens nucleus

Because the matching of refractive index between the membrane and cytoplasm, rather than the spatial order of the cells, establishes the transparent properties of the central lens (see Fig. 5.11F), having a mechanism to regulate the water content of the lens nucleus to protect against changes in refractive index would be necessary to maintain the overall optical properties of the lens. Consistent with this view, impeding the removal of water from the lens by blocking the lens microcirculation system has been shown to increase the water content[215] and alter the gradient of refractive index[177] in the lens nucleus. In addition, the realization that the removal of water from the lens nucleus generates a hydrostatic pressure gradient that is subjected to feedback regulation[336] shows that water content in the lens nucleus is tightly controlled. However, unlike the lens cortex that uses a collection of volume-sensitive ion channels and transporters to buffer changes in water content, it appears that the lens nucleus relies on so-called syneretic processes to buffer changes in water content.[362,363] In cells, most of the water is largely unstructured and exists as the "free" water pool. In contrast, "bound" water in cells consists of multiple layers of water molecules that are tightly bound to cellular macromolecules (proteins, phospholipids, polysaccharides, and fat) and thus have restricted motion.[364,365] Syneresis is defined as the physical process that occurs when bound water is released from the hydration layers of these cellular macromolecules to become free water, whereas "inverse syneresis" is the process in which free water becomes bound water (Box 5.2).

Because most of the mass of the lens, particularly in the nucleus, consists of crystallin proteins, the supposition that syneretic processes play a role in the modulation of lens water content is highly likely. Indeed, in 1999, Bettelheim first proposed on theoretical grounds the idea that a reversible syneretic response may be present in the lens as a defensive response to osmotic challenge.[362] To his hypothesis, Bettelheim applied a variety of experimental approaches to show that whereas the application of high external pressure (1–3 atm) to organ-cultured lens had no effect on total (free + bound) water content, the ratio of free water to bound water decreased in a linear fashion with increasing pressure, and furthermore this syneretic response was more significant in the lens nucleus relative to the cortex.[363,366-368] The relevance of this so-called protein syneresis was not fully recognized at the time, as the pressure values tested were larger than those experienced by the lens in vivo.[369] The subsequent discovery of a substantial internal lens hydrostatic pressure gradient subject to feedback regulation[336] suggests that changes in the lens pressure gradient could indeed affect protein syneresis, especially in the lens nucleus where the pressure and protein concentrations are the highest. Furthermore, recent findings in the mouse lens that show changes to zonular tension altering the lens pressure gradient[370] suggest that the tension applied at the lens surface can modulate protein syneresis to change the amount of free water in the lens nucleus. Syneretic regulation of lens water content would therefore be expected to modulate the refractive index via a simple change in protein concentration. However, as outlined previously, changes to protein hydration induced by syneresis can have other effects on the refractivity of γ-crystallin that is highly expressed in the lens nucleus.[211,213] How changes to the cell physiology of the lens interact at molecular level with lens crystallins to control their local refractive properties, and therefore the overall power of the lens, will be an interesting area for future study.

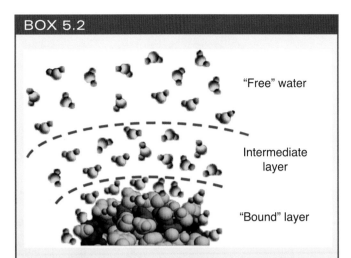

BOX 5.2

Syneresis is defined as the physical process that occurs when bound water is released from the hydration layer of biopolymers to become free water. Conversely, "inverse syneresis" is the process in which free water becomes water that is bound to a biopolymer. In gels, syneresis affects the activity of water and can change the colligative properties of the gel. In cells, most of the water is largely unstructured and exists as the "free" water pool. In contrast, "bound" water in cells consists of multiple layers of water molecules that are tightly bound to cellular macromolecules (proteins, phospholipids, polysaccharides, and fat) and thus have restricted motion. There is also an intermediate layer of water molecules with characteristics between the free and bound forms. Although not directly visualized, these bound water molecules can undergo dipolar interactions and chemical exchange with those in the free water pool.[364,365] This idea that a reversible syneretic response may be present in the lens as a defensive response to osmotic challenge was first proposed on theoretical grounds by Bettelheim.[362]

Taken together, these findings suggest that the water content of the lens is determined by a combination of water flow through the lens, plus the localized control of free water content via pressure-sensitive syneretic processes in the lens nucleus, and in the outer cortex via volume-sensitive ion transporters that modulate fiber cell volume (Fig. 5.19). Under this revised model, modulating the water transport generated by the lens microcirculation will affect free water content in the lens nucleus. This occurs, directly, by modulating the rate of water outflow from the nucleus and, indirectly, by volume regulation of fiber cells in the outer cortex and by changing the magnitude of the pressure gradient that will in turn alter the amount of water bound to the high concentration of proteins in the nucleus.

Regulation of lens power

Although the lens microcirculation system actively maintains the water content in different regions of the lens,[215] inhibiting the lens microcirculation did not immediately compromise lens transparency.[177] Instead, the alteration in lens water content induced by inhibiting the microcirculation system affects lens geometry and GRI, the two key parameters that set the optical power of the lens. MRI studies have been used to extract measurements of overall lens geometry and T2 value maps (T2 is inversely proportional to refractive index and can be obtained from T2 using a calibration factor[371]) from bovine lenses incubated in the absence and presence of conditions that inhibit the microcirculation system.[177] The extracted geometric parameters (front and back radii of curvature, conic constants, axial length, and equatorial radius) and the GRI were then used by an optical modeling

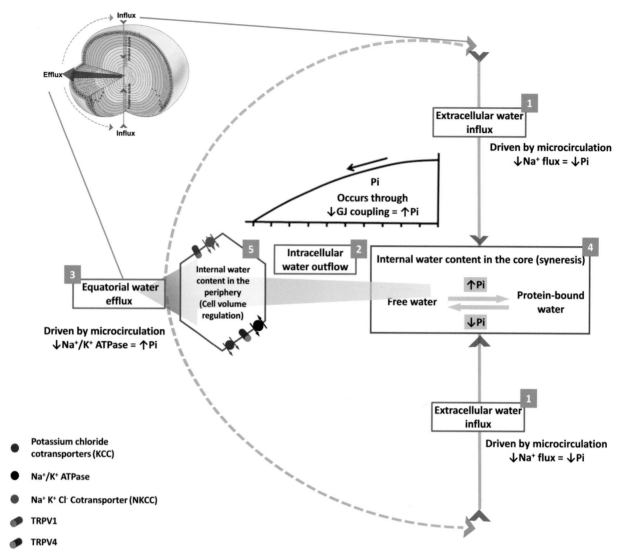

Potassium chloride
cotransporters (KCC)

Na⁺/K⁺ ATPase

Na⁺ K⁺ Cl⁻ Cotransporter (NKCC)

TRPV1

TRPV4

Fig. 5.19 A working model to explain how water content is regulated in the different regions of the lens. (**1**) The circulation of Na⁺ ions established by the Na⁺/K⁺ ATPase activity at the lens surface creates a local osmotic gradient that directs an extracellular flow of water via both poles into the core of the lens where the water enters the deeper mature fiber cells. (**2**) The movement of water through an intracellular outflow pathway mediated by gap junctions channels generates a hydrostatic pressure (Pi) gradient that drives water outflow from the lens and lowers the free water content of the lens core. (**3**) Intracellular water flow is directed to the lens equator where Na⁺/K⁺ ATPase activity is concentrated and water exits the lens. (**4**) In the lens core, the combination of high protein concentrations and pressure mean that syneretic processes (see Box 5.2) can buffer changes in water transport/pressure by altering the amount of water bound to lens proteins. (**5**) In the outer cortex, volume-sensitive ion transporters (NKCC and KCC) and the Na⁺/K⁺ ATPase, whose activity is reciprocally modulated by TRPV1/4 channels, modulate fiber cell volume.

software to calculate the lens power and spherical aberration, plus the contribution of the lens to overall vision quality in a model bovine eye. Using this approach, Vaghefi et al.[177] showed that inhibiting the lens microcirculation system by depolarizing the lens potential by incubating lenses in high extracellular K⁺, or blocking the Na⁺ pump by exposure of lenses to ouabain, caused an increase in lens power. This caused a myopic shift in overall vision quality, with the biggest changes being associated with the addition of ouabain. Furthermore, exposing bovine lenses to hyperbaric oxygen (HBO), which serves as a model of lens aging, had opposite effects on lens geometry and GRI to those observed in response to the ouabain-induced inhibition of the microcirculation system.[177,372] In contrast to the ouabain-induced change in lens geometry, increase in GRI, and myopic shift, HBO exposure did not significantly alter lens geometry but did significantly decrease

GRI, a change that resulted in a decrease in lens power and produced a hyperopic shift in the overall optics of the bovine lens.[372] The differential effects of these two manipulations on the refractive properties of the bovine lens tend to support the timeline of age-related nuclear (ARN) cataract development in humans (see Fig. 5.21B).

In summary, it appears that the transparency and refractive properties of the adult lens are the net result of structural adaptations that are first initiated during embryonic development and continue throughout the postnatal growth of the lens. However, the lens is not a passive optical element and utilizes an internal microcirculation system to maintain both its transparency and refractive properties. Having determined how the optical properties of a young adult human lens are established and maintained, how these properties change with advancing age will now be considered.

EFFECTS OF AGE ON THE TRANSPARENT AND REFRACTIVE PROPERTIES OF THE LENS

When humans reach adulthood, the eye stops growing but the lens continues to grow, and this age-dependent increase in lens size is associated with changes to the baseline optical power of the lens, the ability of the lens to accommodate, and ultimately a loss in lens transparency. Since the optical properties of the lens are the net result of its cellular structure and function, age-dependent changes to lens water content, stiffness, shape, and GRI are thought to be major contributors to observed decreases in lens power, the onset of presbyopia, and the development of cataract in the elderly.

Age-dependent changes to lens refractive power

Unlike other ocular refractive structures, the lens grows throughout adulthood, becoming thicker and rounder with age.[373-375] This change in lens geometry should *theoretically* make the lens more powerful and increase its relative contribution to the refractive power of the eye. However, aging of the eye in adulthood has, in general, been associated with a hyperopic rather than myopic shift.[91,376-381] This discrepancy in the relationship between lens shape and refractive power such that the steepening of lens curvatures with age is not accompanied by an increase in lens power has been termed the "lens paradox."[382,383] Theoretical modeling has predicted that the lens paradox can be explained by an age-dependent reduction in refractive index variation across the GRI and/or a flattening of the GRI profile.[384-387] Subsequent experimental studies have confirmed these predictions and shown both a gradual flattening of GRI profile through the formation a central plateau of constant index[176] and a decline in lens nuclear refractive index[388,389] with advancing age.

Several hypotheses have been advanced to explain how this observed age-dependent flattening of the GRI profile occurs at the cellular level. The first possibility is that because of the continual addition, internalization, and compaction of fiber cells that occurs throughout life, the number of cells per unit area in the adult nucleus increases.[53] This increased compaction has been proposed to increase the crystallin concentration and therefore the refractive index of the more central regions of the lens.[390,391] This addition of compacted fiber cells with increased refractive index in the inner lens regions adds a shoulder to the GRI profile. Over time the addition of this shoulder both flattens the GRI across the central nuclear region and steepens the interface between the outer and inner lens regions. However, this change in profile may not be the only explanation for the change in GRI, as the absolute value for refractive index in the nucleus also falls as the GRI flattens with age.[388,389] Although the mechanism that causes this drop in refractive index remains unclear, it should be noted that it is the interaction between water and proteins that determines the conformational state a protein will adopt,[392] and this interaction is considered integral to the ability of a protein to maintain its dn/dc. Therefore, any change in the ratio of free and bound water within the lens would be expected to produce downstream effects on the refractive properties of the lens. Indeed, a progressive increase in the ratio of free to bound water has been observed to occur with age,[393-395] and this has been correlated to a concurrent decrease in the refractive index of the lens, especially in the nucleus.[176,388,389]

Because it appears that the water content of the lens nucleus is determined by a balance between the active removal of water that generates the hydrostatic pressure gradient and the pressure-sensitive binding of water to the high concentration of crystallin proteins found in the nucleus (Fig. 5.19), it is highly likely that the observed increase in free water content and decrease in refractive index changes is due to an age-dependent failure in this integrated system. The lifelong exposure to oxidative stress and the subsequent accumulation of post-translational modifications to lens proteins[396-398] can be reasonably expected to impair the ability of lens proteins to bind water. This would in turn cause the observed increase in free water content in the deeper areas of the lens where long-lived crystallin proteins are concentrated.

Development of presbyopia

Presbyopia is the loss of near visual function that results from the gradual loss of accommodative amplitude with age.[399-402] Symptoms of presbyopia commence in human emmetropes at around 40 to 50 years of age, and in 2020 it was estimated that presbyopia affected 2.1 billion people.[403] This age-related loss of visual performance[404] requires the need for both distant and near vision correction.[405,406] Although the ultimate cause of presbyopia is still unknown, three major theories—the extra-lenticular,[407,408] the geometric,[409,410] and the lens and capsule[4,411,412]—have been proposed to explain how accommodative capacity is lost with advancing age. The lens and capsule theory, which attributes the cause of presbyopia to a stiffening of the crystalline lens with age, is currently the most widely accepted.

In this theory of presbyopia, the observed age-dependent stiffening of the lens was variously attributed to changes to the biomechanical properties of lens owing to an increased sclerosis of the lens fibers,[413,414] changes in the mechanical properties of the capsule,[5] and/or an increased incidence of protein crosslinking,[415,416] events that were all associated with advancing age. However, in a study conducted by Fisher[6,417] on ex vivo human lenses subjected to rotational forces, the elasticity of the human lens capsule was found to decrease with age, which, counterintuitively, may be a result of the increased capsule thickness of aged lenses.[6,418] Interestingly, these experiments revealed that the stiffness of the lens nucleus and that of the cortex increase at different rates with age,[417,419-421] becoming similar between the ages of 35 and 45 years.[420] Thus, it appears that the cortex is initially stiffer than the nucleus in young lenses, whereas the nucleus is stiffer than the cortex in older lenses.[422] Hence there is an emerging consensus that it is the age-dependent increase in the stiffness of the lens nucleus that is the initiating cause of presbyopia in humans.[423,424] This was further confirmed by stretching ex vivo human lenses through the ciliary body/zonular complex and observing that the lens becomes increasingly resistant to the effects of applied stretching forces with age.[425] Therefore a decreased elasticity of the lens capsule, which fails to reshape an increasingly stiffer lens nucleus during accommodation, appears to render the lens presbyopic.[426]

These changes to the biomechanical properties (stiffness) of the lens have been traditionally attributed to the observed age-related changes to the structural proteins and/or lipids in the different regions of the lens, or to the fiber cell compaction that occurs in older lenses as they grow.[412,415] In addition to these structural changes, parallel increases in the free water content of the human lens with age have been observed,[168,393,395,426,427] but the relevance of these changes to the onset of presbyopia has not been fully appreciated. However, the emerging evidence that the water content in the lens nucleus is controlled by a pressure-sensitive syneretic process (Fig. 5.19) suggests that the age-dependent failure of this system should be considered as a possible contributor to the underlying causes for the onset of presbyopia in middle age. In this system, the ability of the nonaccommodating mouse lens to alter its hydrostatic pressure gradient via the pharmacologic modulation of zonular tension[370] raises the possibility that similar changes in zonular tension in young accommodating human lenses would also dynamically alter lens pressure. This change in pressure wave via syneresis would result in a change in the free water distribution and/or content of the lens to drive the shape changes associated with accommodation.[375,428,429] Hence, it is possible that presbyopia occurs as a consequence of the diminished ability of the aging human lens to compensate for changes in zonular tension, and therefore hydrostatic pressure, during accommodation. The age-dependent accumulation of oxidative damage to proteins involved in mediating water transport and water binding would not only explain the observed age-dependent increase in free water proportion within the lens but also be expected to have implications on the stiffness and accommodative ability of the lens.[430] Validating this new hypothesis has the potential to deliver new approaches to avert the onset of presbyopia.

Development of cataract

As we age, there is an increase in the degree of light scattering in the lens that eventually manifests as cataract, a loss of lens transparency that becomes clinically significant when the opacification interferes with visual function. Globally, lens cataract is the leading cause of visual impairment and blindness,[431,432] with estimates suggesting that approximately 68% of people over 79 years of age have some form of reduced lens transparency or cataract.[433] Clinically, four main forms of lens cataract are recognized: subcapsular (anterior or posterior), cortical, nuclear, and mixed (nuclear and cortical). Of these classes, cortical cataract and ARN cataract are the most common. Thankfully, cataract can be treated by a surgical procedure that replaces the cataractous lens with a plastic intraocular lens implant (Box 5.3). However, despite the existence of a safe and effective surgical treatment, it is estimated that unoperated cataracts are responsible for the loss of sight of more than 20 million people worldwide.[432,434] Furthermore, a percentage of cataract patients experience posterior cataract opacification (see Box 5.4) that requires a second (albeit noninvasive laser) procedure to restore vision. Given our globally aging population, the increased incidence of diabetes, and the social and economic costs of lens cataract, the demand for cataract surgery is expected to only increase. Hence, to reduce the demand for cataract surgery, alternative medical therapies to delay cataracts are urgently required, particularly as it has been predicted that delaying the onset of cataract by 10 years will halve its incidence and associated costs.[435] To facilitate this search for such anticataract therapies, a more in-depth understanding of the epidemiology and pathophysiology of different types of lens cataract is required.

Cataract epidemiology

Not surprisingly, age is the primary risk factor for the most common kinds of cataract, but other risk factors also influence its onset and progression. Lower socioeconomic status can predispose individuals to nutritional deficiencies, increased exposure to diseases, poor general health status, and increased occupational exposure to cataractogenic agents. However, it is difficult to determine the specific aspects of lower socioeconomic status that are important for cataract formation. Gender is also an important influence on the incidence of cataract. Women are at increased risk for most kinds of cataract.[436-442] Conversely, studies have suggested that estrogen protects against cataract formation in humans and animals and that cataracts may be delayed by late menopause.[443-448] Lowering estrogen function with the antiestrogen tamoxifen increased the risk of cataracts when used for long duration.[449,450] The protective effect of estrogen suggested by these studies makes the increased overall levels of cataract in women harder to understand, although a recent report found that sex-specific differences in the lens transcriptome of mice become more pronounced with age.[451] If estrogen is protective, other factors, as yet unknown, must strongly predispose women to cataract formation. Alternatively, higher levels of male sex steroids may be protective against cataract.

When the influences of age, sex, and socioeconomic status are removed, specific risks for different types of cataracts are revealed. Smoking and high alcohol consumption have been identified in several studies as dose-dependent risk factors for nuclear and, in some cases, cortical cataracts.[442,452-454] Dark iris color is often associated with a higher incidence of all types of lens opacities,[442,455,456] a finding that may also be related to higher levels of cortical cataract in different ethnic groups.[438] Exposure to anti-inflammatory steroids and ionizing radiation is a well-recognized risk for posterior subcapsular cataracts, while ocular injury and even intense eye rubbing are risks for anterior subcapsular cataract. Finally, several studies have found an association between lens thickness and the most common types of age-related cataract, with cortical cataracts being correlated with thinner and nuclear

---

BOX 5.3

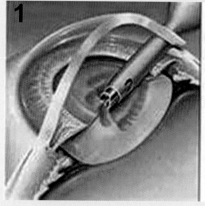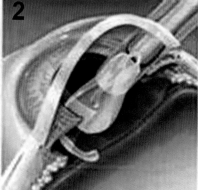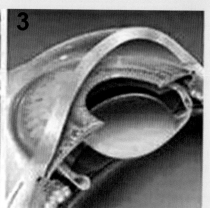

Cataract surgery via a process called phacoemulsification is the most frequently performed surgical procedure in people over 60 years of age. Briefly, after the pupil is dilated, a corneal paracentesis is made and viscoelastic is inserted to stabilize the anterior chamber and protect ocular structures. A second corneal microincision is made at the margin through which a capsulorrhexis (continuous circular opening in the anterior lens capsule) is created. The ultrasound phacoemulsification probe (1) is then inserted to break the cataractous lens into smaller pieces that can be easily aspirated. The capsular bag is thoroughly cleaned to ensure all lens pieces (2), including adherent epithelial cells, are removed and an intraocular lens inserted in place of the crystalline lens (3).

BOX 5.4

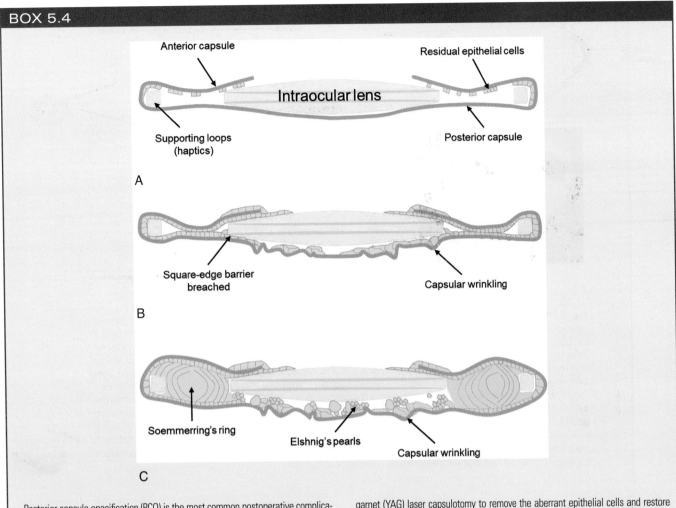

Posterior capsule opacification (PCO) is the most common postoperative complication of cataract surgery and can occur in up to 20% of eyes in the first 3 years post-surgery. PCO occurs owing to the abnormal proliferation and migration of residual lens epithelial cells from the anterior capsule to the posterior capsule, because of a wound-healing response induced by the surgical trauma of cataract surgery. This response induces wrinkling of the capsule that obscures the central visual axis, which presents as blurred vision or glare and requires a erbium-doped yttrium aluminium garnet (YAG) laser capsulotomy to remove the aberrant epithelial cells and restore vision. The process of PCO has been shown to involve an increase in the level of growth factors and cytokines, which result in epithelial cell proliferation, migration, and fiber cell differentiation that indicate the lens is attempting to regenerate itself.[492] Continuing technical advances in cataract surgery and improvements in intraocular lens design and pharmacologic approaches have emerged over the past few decades that have reduced the incidence of PCO.

cataracts with thicker lenses.[457-460] These differences tend to indicate that the pathophysiology of cortical and nuclear cataracts is distinctly different.

The pathophysiology of diabetic cortical cataract

Population growth, sedentary lifestyles, unhealthy diets, and an increasing prevalence of obesity are increasing the number of people with diabetes mellitus.[461] A frequent complication of both type 1 and type 2 diabetes is diabetic cortical cataract, which is the best-understood form of cortical cataract. Cortical lens opacification occurs two to five times more frequently in patients with diabetes, with the onset of the cataract also occurring at an earlier age compared with nondiabetics.[462] Clinically, cortical cataract presents as wedge-shaped or radial spoke opacifications in the lens cortex (Fig. 5.20A), and is particularly prevalent in the elderly or diabetic patients.[463] These distinctive opacifications are caused by a discrete localized zone of tissue liquefaction that is surrounded by fiber cells that have a normal morphologic structure.[464] Cortical cataracts induce significant astigmatic shifts in vision[465] that are caused by asymmetrical refractive index changes within the lens cortex.[466]

Early insights into the pathophysiology of diabetic cataract came from animal models that utilized streptozotocin (STZ) treatment and galactose feeding to induce type 1 and type 2 diabetes, respectively, in the rat. Both models were effective in inducing the formation of "fast" sugar cataracts, and the consensus view from these studies was that high levels of the impermeable osmolyte, sorbitol, produced from excess glucose by the enzyme AR, initiated an osmotic stress that caused fluid accumulation, fiber cell swelling, and subsequent tissue liquefaction.[467-469] Based on this view, considerable attention was focused on the development and testing of AR inhibitors, which were proven to be very successful in ameliorating diabetic cataract in rats and dogs[470] but have been shown to be ineffective in humans. The failure of AR inhibitors to slow the progression of cataract in humans lies with the differences in AR activity and polyol accumulation between rats and humans, with humans exhibiting low levels of AR activity relative to rat. In addition, the acute animal models replicate the fast development

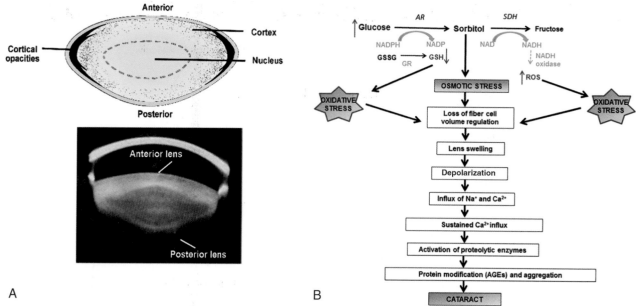

Fig. 5.20 Cortical cataracts. (**A**) Location of the cortical cataract subtype. *Top panel:* diagram showing the opacities that form in the lens cortex. *Lower panel:* Scheimpflug slit-lamp photographic image revealing a cortical cataract. (**B**) Molecular mechanisms involved in the pathogenesis of diabetic cortical cataract. An increase in glucose leads to a decrease in GSH and an increase in reactive oxygen species as indicated by the *red arrows.* The induced osmotic and oxidative stress work synergistically to inhibit the ability of fiber cells to regulate their volume. This leads to cell swelling, depolarization, and an influx of sodium and calcium ions. The accumulation of calcium ions results in the activation of calcium-dependent proteases, which target cytoskeletal and crystallin proteins. Furthermore, proteins are modified by the formation of advanced glycation end (*AGE*) products, which are known to alter the structure and function of crystallins, resulting in an increase in insoluble proteins, the formation of high-molecular-weight aggregates, and cataract. (Reproduced with permission from Braakhuis AJ, Donaldson CI, Lim JC, Donaldson PJ. Nutritional strategies to prevent lens cataract: Current status and future strategies. *Nutrients* 2019;11(5).)

of cataract that occurs in diabetic patients with uncontrolled hyperglycemia. However, with access to modern medical care, most diabetic patients can control their blood glucose reasonably well, so such acute cataract development is rarely seen today. Instead, the majority of adult diabetic patients typically develop cataract after having suffered from diabetes for several years. Therefore, while the initiating mechanism in the development of diabetic cataract is osmotic stress, it is now believed that oxidative stress generated by polyol pathway activity[471] impairs the ability of the lens over time to regulate its volume, resulting in the slower development of tissue damage observed in this type of cortical cataract.[245,246]

Although it now appears that osmotic and oxidative stress work synergistically to cause a loss of cell volume regulation that eventually manifests as tissue liquefaction in the outer cortex of the diabetic lens (Fig. 5.20B), it is unknown why the observed damage is only restricted to a localized zone of damaged fiber cells in the outer cortex of the lens. The reciprocal roles played by cation chloride cotransporters KCC1–4 and NKCC1 in regulating fiber cell volume in the lens cortex have been offered as a potential explanation.[338] Under normal glucose levels, the coordinated action of these transporters produces a net efflux of ions and water in peripheral cortical fiber cells and a net influx of ions and water into fiber cells located in a deeper zone of the lens outer cortex.[338] Since the influx and efflux zones are connected by gap junctions, ion influx and efflux in the two zones are balanced by the coordinated regulation of KCC and NKCC activity, through reciprocal modulation of their phosphorylation status.[349] However, in the diabetic lens, osmotic and/or oxidative stress imposes an imbalance in the relative activities of kinases and phosphatases that modulate transporter activity, resulting

in a dephosphorylation of the two transporters that increases KCC and decreases NKCC activity. Because the K+ and Cl− gradients that determine the direction of KCC-mediated ion transport reverse with radial distance into the lens, any increase of KCC activity would be expected to increase ion efflux from peripheral fiber cells, but increase ion influx into fiber cells in the influx zone.[348] This alteration in KCC transport activity would in turn result in peripheral cell shrinkage and localized cell swelling in the ion influx zone. In support of this prediction, it was shown that incubating rat lenses in the presence of N-ethylmaleimide (NEM),[347] a reagent known to stimulate KCC transporter activity via thiol inactivation of the two kinases that control KCC activity,[472] mimicked the diabetic cataract damage phenotype. This localized swelling of fiber cells in the influx zone, initiated by the dephosphorylation of KCC to increase its activity, is thought to be exacerbated by the activation of stretch-activated nonselective cation channels in the influx zone.[473] In isolated fiber cells, this influx of Na+ and Ca2+ has been shown to activate Ca2+-dependent proteases (Fig. 5.20B), which cause fiber cells to undergo a process of vesiculation that resembles the tissue liquefaction observed in diabetic cataract.[474-476] Thus, the oxidative and osmotic stress sensed by the phosphoregulatory pathway is transduced into the overactivation of KCC, which in the influx zone causes cell swelling that activates a cascade of events (Fig. 5.20B) that ultimately produce the localized damage phenotype observed in diabetic cataract.

The pathophysiology of nuclear cataract

ARN cataract is initiated in the central core of the lens (Fig. 5.21A), which contains primary fiber cells that were initially laid down during embryonic development (Fig. 5.5). Clinically, ARN cataract can appear

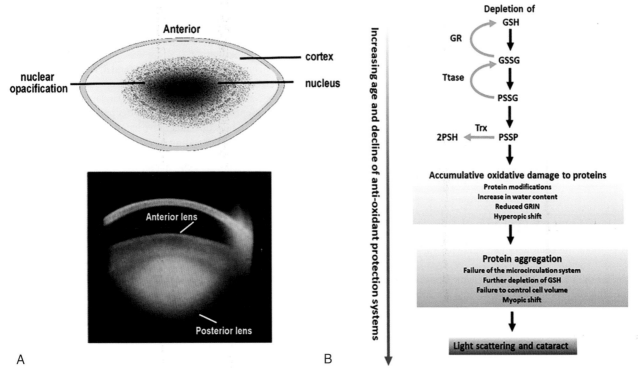

Fig. 5.21 Nuclear cataracts. (**A**) Location of the nuclear cataract subtype. *Top panel:* diagram showing the opacities that form in the lens nucleus. *Bottom panel:* Scheimpflug slit-lamp photographic image revealing a nuclear cataract. (Modified from Braakhuis AJ, Donaldson CI, Lim JC, Donaldson PJ. Nutritional strategies to prevent lens cataract: Current status and future strategies. *Nutrients* 2019;11(5).) (**B**) Molecular mechanisms involved in the pathogenesis of age-related nuclear cataract. The lens utilizes glutathione (*GSH*) as a primary defense mechanism against oxidative stress. However, with chronic oxidative stress, a decrease of GSH occurs resulting in an imbalance of the GSH/GSSG ratio. The accumulation of GSSG, thiolates protein thiols to form protein-GSH conjugates (*PSSG*), which can be dethiolated by thioltransferase (Ttase). If dethiolation is impaired due to oxidation overload, PSSGs can form protein-protein disulfides (*PSSP*), which can be reduced by thioredoxin (*Trx*) to break these disulfide linkages. Over time however, accumulated damage to proteins results in changes to protein structure and function, an increase in free water content, and a concomitant decrease in the GRI leading to a hyperopic shift. An age-dependent failure of the microcirculation systems compromises the ability of the system to maintain lens volume (geometry) that manifests as the observed myopic shift in lens power. It results in further depletion of nuclear GSH levels below a critical threshold that leads to the protein aggregation that causes the light scattering associated with the development of full-blown nuclear cataract formation. (Modified from Lim JC, Grey AC, Zahraei A, Donaldson PJ. Age-dependent changes in glutathione metabolism pathways in the lens: New insights into therapeutic strategies to prevent cataract formation-A review. *Clin Exper Ophthalmol* 2020;48(8):1031–1042.)

as a browning or brunescence of the lens nucleus.[477] In contrast to cortical cataract, the morphology of the cells in the lens nucleus from nuclear cataract patients reveals no major structural distortions.[170,478,479] Instead, nuclear cataract is associated with the extensive loss of protein sulfhydryl groups, with over 90% of cysteine residues and ~50% of methionine residues being found oxidized in nuclear proteins in lenses obtained from patients with ARN.[480-483] Accompanying the loss of protein sulfhydryl groups is an increase in protein-thiol mixed disulfides,[484,485] and protein deamidation and cleavage, which likely lead to an increase in the water insoluble fraction,[483,486] culminating in the formation of protein-protein disulfides (PSSP), and other crosslinkages that lead to protein aggregation and light scattering (Fig. 5.21B). This series of biochemical changes has been extensively reviewed,[262,487,488] and there is general agreement that oxidative stress is the major contributing factor to ARN cataract formation.

Furthermore, based on the observation that cortical fiber cells are able to maintain their GSH levels in ARN cataract whereas fiber cells in the nucleus do not,[302,489] there is now an emerging consensus that

ARN cataract is caused by an inability to maintain GSH levels in the lens nucleus due to a failure to deliver GSH to the central regions of the lens.[300] As outlined in Fig. 5.15, two different mechanisms for the delivery and regeneration of GSH in the lens nucleus have been proposed. However, only the model that utilizes the microcirculation system to deliver GSH allows for the occurrence of GSH regeneration from GSSG in the lens nucleus, through the local production of NADPH from glucose via the pentose phosphate pathway (Fig. 5.15C). If this pathway is indeed the one used to maintain the reductive environment (GSH:GSSG) of the lens nucleus, which is so critical for maintaining the crystallin solubility and therefore lens transparency, then an age-dependent failure of the microcirculation to deliver nutrients to the lens nucleus is a potential cause of ARN cataract.

In support of this contention, it has been shown in human lenses that the observed age-dependent decline in GSH levels in the lens nucleus is accompanied by an increase in intracellular Na+ concentration and a depolarization of the lens membrane potential.[490] These are signs of a failure of the microcirculation system to maintain lens ionic homeostasis. Because the specific conductivity of the fiber cell membrane is initially very low,[289] this observed age-dependent increase in Na^+ and Ca^{2+} permeability has been attributed to the activation of a nonselective cation channel (or channels).[490,491] More recently, in animal studies, Gao et al.[334] have shown that with advancing age there was a similar depolarization of the intracellular voltage, and an increase in the intracellular concentration of Na^+ that was attributed to a down-regulation of gap junction coupling. In both instances, the resultant age-dependent decline in the electrochemical gradient for Na^+ would result in a reduction to the transmembrane driving force for the uptake of key nutrients and antioxidants by Na^+-dependent membrane transporters.[298] Thus, with advancing age, the underlying physiology of the lens, and therefore its ability to maintain an environment that protects nuclear proteins against oxidative stress, deteriorates, resulting in increased oxidative damage, crystallin aggregation, and, ultimately, increased light scattering.

In conclusion, the lens is a complex and dynamic tissue that requires an understanding of how regional differences in lens cell biology, biochemistry, and physiology at the cellular level interact to maintain the transparent and refractive properties of the lens at the tissue level. Understanding how this integrative lens biology controls lens function will be key to understanding how the optics of the lens change with age and to developing new therapies to combat the age-related lens pathologies presbyopia and cataract.

ACKNOWLEDGMENTS

Many thanks to the colleagues and students whose stimulating discussions and exciting results have laid the foundation for the ideas expressed in this chapter. I especially thank Drs. Julie Lim and Angus Grey for critically reading this chapter and Dr. Ankita Umapathy for editorial support and her research of literature. Support for preparing this manuscript was derived from the Health Research Council of New Zealand, the Marsden Fund, Auckland Medical Research Foundation, and NIH Grants EY02691106, and EY013462.

REFERENCES

1. Donaldson PJ, Grey AC, Heilman BM, Lim JC, Vaghefi E. The physiological optics of the lens. *Prog Retin Eye Res*. 2017;56:e1–e24.
2. Bassnett S, Shi Y, Vrensen GF. Biological glass: structural determinants of eye lens transparency. *Philos Trans R Soc Lond B Biol Sci*. 2011;366(1568):1250–1264.
3. Rosen AM, Denham DB, Fernandez V, Borja D, Ho A, Manns F, et al. In vitro dimensions and curvatures of human lenses. *Vision Research*. 2006;46(6–7):1002–1009.
4. Charman WN. The eye in focus: accommodation and presbyopia. *Clinical and Experimental Optometry*. 2008;91(3):207–225.
5. Fincham E. The mechanism of accommodation. *British Journal of Ophthalmology, Monograph Supplement VIII, Pulman & Sons Ltd London*. 1937:7–76.
6. Fisher RF. The significance of the shape of the lens and capsular energy changes in accommodation. *The Journal of physiology*. 1969;201:21.
7. Glasser A, Kaufman PL. The mechanism of accommodation in primates. *Ophthalmology*. 1999;106:863–872.
8. Duane A. Are the current theories of accommodation correct? *American Journal of Ophthalmology*. 1925;8:196–202.
9. Glasser A, Campbell MC. Biometric, optical and physical changes in the isolated human crystalline lens with age in relation to presbyopia. *Vision research*. 1999;39:1991–2015.
10. Kasthurirangan S, Markwell EL, Atchison DA, Pope JM. In vivo study of changes in refractive index distribution in the human crystalline lens with age and accommodation. *Investigative ophthalmology & visual science*. 2008;49:2531–2540.
11. Bassnett S. Zinn's zonule. *Prog Retin Eye Res*. 2021;82:100902.
12. Wheatley HM, Traboulsi EI, Flowers BE, Maumenee IH, Azar D, Pyeritz RE, et al. Immunohistochemical localization of fibrillin in human ocular tissues: relevance to the Marfan syndrome. *Archives of Ophthalmology*. 1995;113(1):103–109.
13. Streeten BW. The zonular insertion: a scanning electron microscope study. *Investigative Ophthalmology and Visual Science*. 1977;16(4):364–375.
14. Farnsworth PN, Mauriello JA, Burke-Gadomski P, Kulyk T, Cinotti AA. Surface ultrastructure of the human lens capsule and zonular attachments. *Investigative Ophthalmology and Visual Science*. 1976;15(1):36–40.
15. Parmigiani C, McAvoy J. The roles of laminin and fibronectin in the development of the lens capsule. *Current Eye Research*. 1991;10(6):501–511.
16. Silver P, Wakely J. The initial stage in the development of the lens capsule in chick and mouse embryos. *Experimental Eye Research*. 1974;19(1):73–77.
17. Danysh BP, Duncan MK. The lens capsule. *Experimental Eye Research*. 2009;88(2):151–164.
18. Parmigiani C, McAvoy J. Localisation of laminin and fibronectin during rat lens morphogenesis. *Differentiation*. 1984;28(1):53–61.
19. Cammarata PR, Cantu-Crouch D, Oakford L, Morrill A. Macromolecular organization of bovine lens capsule. *Tissue & Cell*. 1986;18(1):83–97.
20. Onodera S. Presence of the basement membrane component-heparan sulfate proteoglycan-in bovine lens capsules. *Chemical Pharmaceutical Bulletin*. 1991;39(4):1059–1061.
21. DeDreu J, Walker JL, Menko AS. Dynamics of the lens basement membrane capsule and its interaction with connective tissue-like extracapsular matrix proteins. *Matrix Biology*. 2021;96:18–46.
22. Young RW, Ocumpaugh DE. Autoradiographic studies on the growth and development of the lens capsule in the rat. *Investigative Ophthalmology and Visual Science*. 1966;5(6):583–593.
23. Bassnett S, Šikić H. The lens growth process. *Prog Retin Eye Res*. 2017;60:181–200.
24. Kuszak J. The development of lens sutures. *Progress in Retinal and Eye Research*. 1995;14(2):567–591.
25. Kuszak JR, Zoltoski RK, Tiedemann CE. Development of lens sutures. *International Journal of Developmental Biology*. 2004;48(8–9):889–902.
26. Kuszak J, Peterson K, Sivak J, Herbert K. The interrelationship of lens anatomy and optical quality II. Primate lenses. *Experimental Eye Research*. 1994;59(5):521–535.
27. Bassnett S. Mitochondrial dynamics in differentiating fiber cells of the mammalian lens. *Current Eye Research*. 1992;11(12):1227–1232.
28. Bassnett S. Lens organelle degradation. *Experimental Eye Research*. 2002;74(1):1–6.
29. Bassnett S, Beebe DC. Coincident loss of mitochondria and nuclei during lens fiber cell differentiation. *Developmental Dynamics*. 1992;194(2):85–93.
30. Kuwabara T. The maturation of the lens cell: a morphologic study. *Experimental Eye Research*. 1975;20(5):427–443.
31. Shestopalov VI, Bassnett S. Exogenous gene expression and protein targeting in lens fiber cells. *Investigative Ophthalmology and Visual Science*. 1999;40(7):1435–1443.
32. Henry JJ, Grainger RM. Early tissue interactions leading to embryonic lens formation in Xenopus laevis. *Developmental Biology*. 1990;141(1):149–163.
33. Shaham O, Menuchin Y, Farhy C, Ashery-Padan R. Pax6: a multi-level regulator of ocular development. *Prog Retin Eye Res*. 2012;31(5):351–376.
34. Walther C, Gruss P. Pax-6, a murine paired box gene, is expressed in the developing CNS. *Development*. 1991;113(4):1435–1449.
35. Hill RE, Favor J, Hogan BL, Ton CC, Saunders GF, Hanson IM, et al. Mouse small eye results from mutations in a paired-like homeobox-containing gene. *Nature*. 1991;354(6354):522–525.
36. Cvekl A, Duncan MK. Genetic and epigenetic mechanisms of gene regulation during lens development. *Prog Retin Eye Res*. 2007;26(6):555–597.
37. Cvekl A, McGreal R, Liu W. Chapter 10: Lens development and crystallin gene expression. In: Hejtmancik JF, Nickerson JM, eds. *Progress in Molecular Biology and Translational Science*. 134: Academic Press; 2015:129–167.
38. Hendrix RW, Zwaan J. The matrix of the optic vesicle-presumptive lens interface during induction of the lens in the chicken embryo. *Journal of Embryology and Experimental Morphology*. 1975
39. Hendrix R, Zwaan J. Cell shape regulation and cell cycle in embryonic lens cells. *Nature*. 1974;247(5437):145–147.
40. Schook P. A review of data on cell actions and cell interaction during the morphogenesis of the embryonic eye. *Acta Morphologica Neerlando-Scandinavica*. 1978;16(4):267–286.
41. Garcí-Porrero JA, Colvée E, Ojeda JL. The mechanisms of cell death and phagocytosis in the early chick lens morphogenesis: a scanning electron microscopy and cytochemical approach. *The Anatomical Record*. 1984;208(1):123–136.
42. Koroma BM, Yang J-M, Sundin OH. The Pax-6 homeobox gene is expressed throughout the corneal and conjunctival epithelia. *Investigative Ophthalmology and Visual Science*. 1997;38(1):108–120.
43. Smith GN, Linsenmayer TF, Newsome DA. Synthesis of type II collagen in vitro by embryonic chick neural retina tissue. *Proceedings of the National Academy of Sciences*. 1976;73(12):4420–4423.
44. Coulombre JL, Coulombre AJ. Lens development: fiber elongation and lens orientation. *Science*. 1963;142(3598):1489–1490.
45. Coulombre JL, Coulombre AJ. Lens development. IV. Size, shape, and orientation. *Investigative Ophthalmology and Visual Science*. 1969;8(3):251–257.
46. Beebe DC, Feagans DE, Jebens H. Lentropin: a factor in vitreous humor which promotes lens fiber cell differentiation. *Proceedings of the National Academy of Sciences*. 1980;77(1):490–493.
47. Schulz MW, Chamberlain CG, de Iongh RU, McAvoy JW. Acidic and basic FGF in ocular media and lens: implications for lens polarity and growth patterns. *Development*. 1993;118(1):117–126.

48. Augusteyn RC. Growth of the human eye lens. *Molecular Vision*. 2007;13:252–257.
49. Augusteyn RC. Growth of the lens: in vitro observations. *Clinical and Experimental Optometry*. 2008;91:226–239.
50. Augusteyn RC. Growth of the eye lens: I. Weight accumulation in multiple species. *Molecular Vision*. 2014;20:410–426.
51. Augusteyn RC. Growth of the eye lens: II. Allometric studies. *Molecular Vision*. 2014;20:427–440.
52. Augusteyn RC. On the growth and internal structure of the human lens. *Experimental Eye Research*. 2010;90(6):643–654.
53. Bassnett S, Costello MJ. The cause and consequence of fiber cell compaction in the vertebrate lens. *Exp Eye Res*. 2017;156:50–57.
54. Augusteyn RC. On the contribution of the nucleus and cortex to human lens shape and size. *Clinical and Experimental Optometry*. 2018;101(1):64–68.
55. Shi Y, De Maria A, Lubura S, Šikić H, Bassnett S. The penny pusher: a cellular model of lens growth. *Invest Ophthalmol Vis Sci*. 2014;56(2):799–809.
56. Chamberlain CG, McAvoy JW. Evidence that fibroblast growth factor promotes lens fibre differentiation. *Current Eye Research*. 1987;6(9):1165–1168.
57. McAvoy J, Chamberlain C. Fibroblast growth factor (FGF) induces different responses in lens epithelial cells depending on its concentration. *Development*. 1989;107(2):221–228.
58. Liu J, Chamberlin CG, Mcavoy JW. IGF enhancement of FGF-induced fibre differentiation and DNA synthesis in lens explants. *Experimental Eye Research*. 1996;63(6):621–629.
59. Chamberlain C, McAvoy J, Richardson N. The effects of insulin and basic fibroblast growth factor on fibre differentiation in rat lens epithelial explants. *Growth Factors*. 1991;4(3):183–188.
60. Leenders W, Van Genesen S, Schoenmakers J, Van Zoelen E, Lubsen N. Synergism between temporally distinct growth factors: bFGF, insulin and lens cell differentiation. *Mechanisms of Development*. 1997;67(2):193–201.
61. Robinson ML, Overbeek PA, Verran DJ, et al. Extracellular FGF-1 acts as a lens differentiation factor in transgenic mice. *Development*. 1995;121(2):505–514.
62. Robinson ML, Ohtaka-Maruyama C, Chan C-C, et al. Disregulation of ocular morphogenesis by lens-specific expression of FGF-3/int-2 in transgenic mice. *Developmental Biology*. 1998;198(1):13–31.
63. Chow RL, Roux GD, Roghani M, et al. FGF suppresses apoptosis and induces differentiation of fibre cells in the mouse lens. *Development*. 1995;121(12):4383–4393.
64. Stolen CM, Griep AE. Disruption of lens fiber cell differentiation and survival at multiple stages by region-specific expression of truncated FGF receptors. *Developmental Biology*. 2000;217(2):205–220.
65. Lang RA. Which factors stimulate lens fiber cell differentiation in vivo? *Investigative Ophthalmology and Visual Science*. 1999;40(13):3075–3078.
66. Le A-CN, Musil LS. FGF signaling in chick lens development. *Developmental Biology*. 2001;233(2):394–411.
67. Zhao H, Yang T, Madakashira BP, et al. Fibroblast growth factor receptor signaling is essential for lens fiber cell differentiation. *Developmental Biology*. 2008;318(2):276–288.
68. Beebe D, Garcia C, Wang X, et al. Contributions by members of the TGFbeta superfamily to lens development. *International Journal of Developmental Biology*. 2004;48(8–9):845–856.
69. Rajagopal R, Dattilo LK, Kaartinen V, et al. Functions of the type 1 BMP receptor Acvr1 (Alk2) in lens development: cell proliferation, terminal differentiation, and survival. *Investigative Ophthalmology and Visual Science*. 2008;49(11):4953–4960.
70. Boswell BA, Lein PJ, Musil LS. Cross-talk between fibroblast growth factor and bone morphogenetic proteins regulates gap junction-mediated intercellular communication in lens cells. *Molecular Biology of the Cell*. 2008;19(6):2631–2641.
71. Shu DY, Lovicu FJ. Insights into bone morphogenetic protein-(BMP-) signaling in Ocular Lens Biology and Pathology. *Cells*. 2021;10:10.
72. Lovicu FJ, McAvoy JW, de Iongh RU. Understanding the role of growth factors in embryonic development: Insights from the lens. *Philosophical Transactions of the Royal Society B: Biological Sciences*. 2011;366(1568):1204–1218.
73. Lovicu FJ, Shin EH, McAvoy JW. Fibrosis in the lens. Sprouty regulation of TGFβ-signaling prevents lens EMT leading to cataract. *Experimental Eye Research*. 2016;142:92–101.
74. Audette DS, Scheiblin DA, Duncan MK. The molecular mechanisms underlying lens fiber elongation. *Exp Eye Res*. 2017;156:41–49.
75. McAvoy JW, Dawes LJ, Sugiyama Y, Lovicu FJ. Intrinsic and extrinsic regulatory mechanisms are required to form and maintain a lens of the correct size and shape. *Exp Eye Res*. 2017;156: 34-40.
76. Cheng C, Nowak RB, Fowler VM. The lens actin filament cytoskeleton: Diverse structures for complex functions. *Experimental Eye Research*. 2017;156:58–71.
77. Sugiyama Y, Stump RJW, Nguyen A, et al. Secreted frizzled-related protein disrupts PCP in eye lens fiber cells that have polarised primary cilia. *Developmental Biology*. 2010;338(2):193–201.
78. Basu S, Rajakaruna S, Reyes B, Van Bockstaele E, Menko AS. Suppression of MAPK/JNK-MTORC1 signaling leads to premature loss of organelles and nuclei by autophagy during terminal differentiation of lens fiber cells. *Autophagy*. 2014;10(7):1193–1211.
79. Chauss D, Basu S, Rajakaruna S, et al. Differentiation state-specific mitochondrial dynamic regulatory networks are revealed by global transcriptional analysis of the developing chicken lens. *G3 Bethesda*. 2014;4(8):1515–1527.
80. Costello MJ, Brennan LA, Basu S, et al. Autophagy and mitophagy participate in ocular lens organelle degradation. *Experimental eye research*. 2013;116:141–150.
81. Basu S, Rajakaruna S, Menko AS. Insulin-like growth factor receptor-1 and nuclear factor κB are crucial survival signals that regulate caspase-3-mediated lens epithelial cell differentiation initiation. *Journal of Biological Chemistry*. 2012;287(11):8384–8397.
82. Samuelsson AR, Belvindrah R, Wu C, Müller U, Halfter W. β1-integrin signaling is essential for lens fiber survival. *Gene Regulation*. 2007;1117762500700100016.
83. Murugan S, Cheng C. Roles of eph-ephrin signaling in the eye lens cataractogenesis, biomechanics, and homeostasis. *Front Cell Dev Biol*. 2022:10.
84. Garcia CM, Shui Y-B, Kamath M, et al. The function of VEGF-A in lens development: formation of the hyaloid capillary network and protection against transient nuclear cataracts. *Experimental Eye Research*. 2009;88(2):270–276.
85. Shui Y-B, Wang X, Hu JS, et al. Vascular endothelial growth factor expression and signaling in the lens. *Investigative Ophthalmology and Visual Science*. 2003;44(9):3911–3919.
86. Zhu M, Madigan MC, van Driel D, et al. The human hyaloid system: cell death and vascular regression. *Experimental Eye Research*. 2000;70(6):767–776.
87. Moore, K.L., Persaud, T.V.N., Torchia, M.G., 2018. The Developing Human - Clinically Oriented Embryology, 11 ed. Elsevier.
88. Meeson AP, Argilla M, Ko K, Witte L, Lang RA. VEGF deprivation-induced apoptosis is a component of programmed capillary regression. *Development*. 1999;126(7):1407–1415.
89. Diez-Roux G, Argilla M, Makarenkova H, Ko K, Lang RA. Macrophages kill capillary cells in G1 phase of the cell cycle during programmed vascular regression. *Development*. 1999;126(10):2141–2147.
90. Lobov IB, Rao S, Carroll TJ, et al. WNT7b mediates macrophage-induced programmed cell death in patterning of the vasculature. *Nature*. 2005;437(7057):417–421.
91. Goldberg MF. Persistent fetal vasculature (PFV): an integrated interpretation of signs and symptoms associated with persistent hyperplastic primary vitreous (PHPV) LIV Edward Jackson Memorial Lecture. *American Journal of Ophthalmology*. 1997;124(5):587–626.
92. Bassnett S, Mataic D. Chromatin degradation in differentiating fiber cells of the eye lens. *The Journal of Cell Biology*. 1997;137(1):37–49.
93. Zandy AJ, Bassnett S. Proteolytic mechanisms underlying mitochondrial degradation in the ocular lens. *Invest Ophthalmol Vis Sci*. 2007;48(1):293–302.
94. Wride MA. Lens fibre cell differentiation and organelle loss: many paths lead to clarity. *Philosophical transactions of the Royal Society of London Series B, Biological sciences*. 2011;366(1568):1219–1233.
95. Nishimoto S, Kawane K, Watanabe-Fukunaga R, et al. Nuclear cataract caused by a lack of DNA degradation in the mouse eye lens. *Nature*. 2003;424(6952):1071–1074.
96. Nagata S. DNA degradation in development and programmed cell death. *Annual review of immunology*. 2005;23:853–875.
97. Brennan L, Disatham J, Kantorow M. Mechanisms of organelle elimination for lens development and differentiation. *Experimental Eye Research*. 2021;209:108682.
98. Cuervo AM. Autophagy's top chef. *Science*. 2011;332(6036):1392–1393.
99. Yang Z, Klionsky DJ. Eaten alive: A history of macroautophagy. *Nature Cell Biology*. 2010; 12(9):814–822.
100. Yang Z, Klionsky DJ. Mammalian autophagy: Core molecular machinery and signaling regulation. *Current Opinion in Cell Biology*. 2010;22(2):124–131.
101. Boya P, Esteban-Martínez L, Serrano-Puebla A, Gómez-Sintes R, Villarejo-Zori B. Autophagy in the eye: Development, degeneration, and aging. *Progress in Retinal and Eye Research*. 2016;55:206–245.
102. Lampert MA, Orogo AM, Najor RH, et al. BNIP3L/NIX and FUNDC1-mediated mitophagy is required for mitochondrial network remodeling during cardiac progenitor cell differentiation. *Autophagy*. 2019;15(7):1182–1198.
103. Mizushima N, Levine B. Autophagy in mammalian development and differentiation. *Nature Cell Biology*. 2010;12(9):823–830.
104. Nezis IP, Vaccaro MI, Devenish RJ, Juhász G. Autophagy in development, cell differentiation, and homeodynamics: From molecular mechanisms to diseases and pathophysiology. *BioMed Research International*. 2014;2014
105. Nakatogawa H. Mechanisms governing autophagosome biogenesis. *Nature Reviews Molecular Cell Biology*. 2020;21(8):439–458.
106. Yang Z, Klionsky DJ. An overview of the molecular mechanism of autophagy. In: Levine B, Yoshimori T, Deretic V, eds. *Autophagy in Infection and Immunity*. Berlin, Heidelberg: Springer Berlin Heidelberg; 2009:1–32.
107. Ashrafi G, Schwarz TL. The pathways of mitophagy for quality control and clearance of mitochondria. *Cell Death and Differentiation*. 2013;20(1):31–42.
108. Padmanabhan A, Rao MV, Wu Y, Zaidel-Bar R. Jack of all trades: functional modularity in the adherens junction. *Current Opinion in Cell Biology*. 2015;36:32–40.
109. Atreya PL, Barnes J, Katar M, Alcala J, Maisel H. N-cadherin of the human lens. *Curr Eye Res*. 1989;8(9):947–956.
110. Straub BK, Boda J, Kuhn C, et al. A novel cell-cell junction system: the cortex adhaerens mosaic of lens fiber cells. *J Cell Sci*. 2003;166(Pt 24):4985–4995.
111. Mathias R.T., Gao J., Sun X., Moore L., White T.W., Brink P.R. The circulation of sodium and fluid through lens gap junctions ARVO abstract. 2010.
112. Jacobs MD, Soeller C, Sisley AM, Cannell MB, Donaldson PJ. Gap junction processing and redistribution revealed by quantitative optical measurements of connexin46 epitopes in the lens. *Invest Ophthalmol Vis Sci*. 2004;45(1):191–199.
113. Moré MI, Kirsch FP, Rathjen FG. Targeted ablation of NrCAM or ankyrin-B results in disorganized lens fibers leading to cataract formation. *J Cell Biol*. 2001;154(1):187–196.
114. Watanabe M, Kobayashi H, Rutishauser U, Katar M, Alcala J, Maisel H. NCAM in the differentiation of embryonic lens tissue. *Dev Biol*. 1989;135(2):414–423.
115. Costello MJ, McIntosh TJ, Robertson JD. Distribution of gap junctions and square array junctions in the mammalian lens. *Invest Ophthalmol Vis Sci*. 1989;30(5):975–989.
116. Gruijters WTM, Kistler J, Bullivant S. Formation, distribution and dissociation of intercellular junctions in the lens. *Journal of Cell Science*. 1987;88(Pt 3):351–359.
117. Gruijters WTM, Kistler J, Bullivant S, Goodenough DA. Immunolocalization of MP70 in lens fiber 16-17-nm intercellular junctions. *Journal of Cell Biology*. 1987;104(3):565–572.
118. Jacobs MD, Donaldson PJ, Cannell MB, Soeller C. Resolving morphology and antibody labeling over large distances in tissue sections. *Microsc Res Tech*. 2003;62(1):83–91.
119. Tenbroek E, Arneson M, Jarvis L, Louis C. The distribution of the fiber cell intrinsic membrane proteins MP20 and connexin46 in the bovine lens. *Journal of Cell Science*. 1992;103(Pt 1):245–257.
120. Zampighi GA, Hall JE, Ehring GR, Simon SA. The structural organization and protein composition of lens fiber junctions. *Journal of Cell Biology*. 1989;108(6):2255–2275.
121. Dickson DH, Crock GW. Interlocking patterns on primate lens fibers. *Investigative Ophthalmology*. 1972;11:809–815.
122. Kuszak JR, Ennesser CA, Umlas J, Macsai-Kaplan MS, Weinstein RS. The ultrastructure of fiber cells in primate lenses: a model for studying membrane senescence. *J Ultrastruct Mol Struct Res*. 1988;100:60–74.

123. Zampighi G, Simon S, Hall J, et al. The specialized junctions of the lens. *Int Rev Cytol.* 1992;136:185–225.
124. Kistler J, Bullivant S. Lens gap junctions and orthogonal arrays are unrelated. *FEBS Letters.* 1980;111(1):73–78.
125. Zampighi G, Simon SA, Robertson JD, McIntosh TJ, Costello MJ. On the structural organization of isolated bovine lens fiber junctions. *Journal of Cell Biology.* 1982;93(1): 175–189.
126. Kistler J, Evans C, Donaldson P, et al. Ocular lens gap junctions: Protein expression, assembly, and structure-function analysis. *Microscopy Research Technique.* 1995;31(5): 347–356.
127. Lin JS, Fitzgerald S, Dong Y, Knight C, Donaldson P, Kistler J. Processing of the gap junction protein connexin50 in the ocular lens is accomplished by calpain. *Eur J Cell Biol.* 1997;73(2):141–149.
128. Baldo GJ, Gong X, Martinez-Wittinghan FJ, Kumar NM, Gilula NB, Mathias RT. Gap junctional coupling in lenses from alpha(8) connexin knockout mice. *J Gen Physiol.* 2001;118(5):447–456.
129. Lin JS, Eckert R, Kistler J, Donaldson P. Spatial differences in gap junction gating in the lens are a consequence of connexin cleavage. *European Journal of Cell Biology.* 1998;76(4):246–250.
130. Bassnett S, Croghan P, Duncan G. Diffusion of lactate and its role in determining intracellular pH in the lens of the eye. *Experimental Eye Research.* 1987;44(1):143–147.
131. Brown NAP, Sparrow JM, Bron AJ. Central compaction in the process of lens growth as indicated by lamellar cataract. *British Journal of Ophthalmology.* 1988;72(7):538–544.
132. Al-Ghoul KJ, Nordgren RK, Kuszak AJ, Freel CD, Costello MJ, Kuszak JR. Structural evidence of human nuclear fiber compaction as a function of ageing and cataractogenesis. *Experimental Eye Research.* 2001;72(3):199–214.
133. Grey AC, Jacobs MD, Gonen T, Kistler J, Donaldson PJ. Insertion of MP20 into lens fibre cell plasma membranes correlates with the formation of an extracellular diffusion barrier. *Exp Eye Res.* 2003;77(5):567–574.
134. Lim JC, Walker KL, Sherwin T, Schey KL, Donaldson PJ. Confocal microscopy reveals zones of membrane remodeling in the outer cortex of the human lens. *Investigative Ophthalmology and Visual Science.* 2009;50(9):4304–4310.
135. Vaghefi E, Walker K, Pontre BP, Jacobs MD, Donaldson PJ. Magnetic resonance and confocal imaging of solute penetration into the lens reveals a zone of restricted extracellular space diffusion. *American journal of physiology.* 2012;302(11):R1250–R1259.
136. Wang Z, Cantrell LS, Schey KL. Spatially resolved proteomic analysis of the lens extracellular diffusion barrier. *Investigative Ophthalmology & Visual Science.* 2021;62(12):25.
137. Costello MJ, Mohamed A, Gilliland KO, Fowler WC, Johnsen S. Ultrastructural analysis of the human lens fiber cell remodeling zone and the initiation of cellular compaction. *Experimental Eye Research.* 2013;116:411–418.
138. Lo WK, Harding CV. Square arrays and their role in ridge formation in human lens fibers. *J Ultrastruct Res.* 1984;86(3):228–245.
139. Hu Z, Shi W, Riquelme MA, et al. Connexin 50 functions as an adhesive molecule and promotes lens cell differentiation. *Sci Rep.* 2017;7(1):5298.
140. Wang Z, Schey KL. Aquaporin-0 interacts with the FERM domain of ezrin/radixin/moesin proteins in the ocular lens. *Invest Ophthalmol Vis Sci.* 2011;52(8):5079–5087.
141. Kuszak J, Macsai M, Bloom K, Rae J, Weinstein RS. Cell-to-cell fusion of lens fiber cellsin situ: Correlative light, scanning electron microscopic, and freeze-fracture studies. *Journal of Ultrastructure Research.* 1985;93(3):144–160.
142. Shestopalov VI, Bassnett S. Expression of autofluorescent proteins reveals a novel protein permeable pathway between cells in the lens core. *Journal of Cell Science.* 2000;113(11):1913–1921.
143. Shestopalov VI, Bassnett S. Development of a macromolecular diffusion pathway in the lens. *Journal of Cell Science.* 2003;116(20):4191–4199.
144. Shi Y, Barton K, De Maria A, Petrash JM, Shiels A, Bassnett S. The stratified syncytium of the vertebrate lens. *J Cell Sci.* 2009;122(10):1607–1615.
145. Logan CM, Bowen CJ, Menko AS. Functional role for stable microtubules in lens fiber cell elongation. *Experimental Cell Research.* 2018;362(2):477–488.
146. Gokhin DS, Nowak RB, Kim NE, et al. Tmod1 and CP49 synergize to control the fiber cell geometry, transparency, and mechanical stiffness of the mouse lens. *PLoS One.* 2012;7(11):e48734.
147. Kuwabara T. Microtubules in the lens. *Archives of Ophthalmology.* 1968;79(2):189–195.
148. Hejtmancik JF, Riazuddin SA, McGreal R, Liu W, Cvekl A, Shiels A. Lens biology and biochemistry. *Progress in Molecular Biology and Translational Science.* 2015;134:169–201.
149. Lo W-K, Wen X-J, Zhou C-J. Microtubule configuration and membranous vesicle transport in elongating fiber cells of the rat lens. *Experimental Eye Research.* 2003;77(5):615–626.
150. Chen J, Ma Z, Jiao X, et al. Mutations in FYCO1 cause autosomal-recessive congenital cataracts. *The American Journal of Human Genetics.* 2011;88(6):827–838.
151. Logan CM, Menko AS. Microtubules: Evolving roles and critical cellular interactions. *Experimental Biology and Medicine.* 2019;244(15):1240–1254.
152. Leonard M, Zhang L, Zhai N, et al. Modulation of N-cadherin junctions and their role as epicenters of differentiation-specific actin regulation in the developing lens. *Dev Biol.* 2011;349(2):363–377.
153. Nowak RB, Fischer RS, Zoltoski RK, Kuszak JR, Fowler VM. Tropomodulin1 is required for membrane skeleton organization and hexagonal geometry of fiber cells in the mouse lens. *Journal of Cell Biology.* 2009;186(6):915–928.
154. Barnum CE, Al Saai S, Patel SD, et al. The Tudor-domain protein TDRD7, mutated in congenital cataract, controls the heat shock protein HSPB1 (HSP27) and lens fiber cell morphology. *Human Molecular Genetics.* 2020;29(12):2076–2097.
155. Lachke SA, Alkuraya FS, Kneeland SC, et al. Mutations in the RNA granule component TDRD7 cause cataract and glaucoma. *Science.* 2011;331(6024):1571–1576.
156. Song S, Landsbury A, Dahm R, Liu Y, Zhang Q, Quinlan RA. Functions of the intermediate filament cytoskeleton in the eye lens. *J Clin Inves.* 2009;119(7):1837–1848.
157. Blankenship TN, Hess JF, FitzGerald PG. Development-and differentiation-dependent reorganization of intermediate filaments in fiber cells. *Investigative Ophthalmology and Visual Science.* 2001;42(3):735–742.
158. Sandilands A, Prescott AR, Wegener A, et al. Knockout of the intermediate filament protein CP49 destabilises the lens fibre cell cytoskeleton and decreases lens optical quality, but does not induce cataract. *Experimental Eye Research.* 2003;76(3):385–391.
159. Jakobs PM, Hess JF, FitzGerald PG, Kramer P, Weleber RG, Litt M. Autosomal-dominant congenital cataract associated with a deletion mutation in the human beaded filament protein gene BFSP2. *The American Journal of Human Genetics.* 2000;66(4):1432–1436.
160. Wenke JL, McDonald WH, Schey KL. Spatially directed proteomics of the human lens outer cortex reveals an intermediate filament switch associated with the remodeling zone. *Investigative Ophthalmology and Visual Science.* 2016;57(10):4108–4114.
161. Wang Z, Ryan DJ, Schey KL. Localization of the lens intermediate filament switch by imaging mass spectrometry. *Experimental Eye Research.* 2020;198:108134.
162. Rose KML, Gourdie RG, Prescott AR, Quinlan RA, Crouch RK, Schey KL. The C terminus of lens aquaporin 0 interacts with the cytoskeletal proteins filensin and CP49. *Investigative Ophthalmology and Visual Science.* 2006;47(4):1562–1570.
163. Yoon K-h, Blankenship T, Shibata B, FitzGerald PG. Resisting the effects of aging: a function for the fiber cell beaded filament. *Investigative Ophthalmology and Visual Science.* 2008;49(3): 1030–1036.
164. Li Y, Liu X, Xia C-h, et al. CP49 and filensin intermediate filaments are essential for formation of cold cataract. *Molecular Vision.* 2020;26:603.
165. Cheng C, Nowak RB, Gao J, et al. Lens ion homeostasis relies on the assembly and/or stability of large connexin 46 gap junction plaques on the broad sides of differentiating fiber cells. *American Journal of Physiology-Cell Physiology.* 2015;308(10):C835–C847.
166. Michael R, van Marle J, Vrensen GFJM, van den Berg TJTP. Changes in the refractive index of lens fibre membranes during maturation—impact on lens transparency. *Experimental Eye Research.* 2003;77(1):93–99.
167. Fagerholm PP, Philipson BT, Lindström B. Normal human lens—the distribution of protein. *Experimental Eye Research.* 1981;33(6):615–620.
168. Siebinga I, Vrensen GF, De Mul FF, Greve J. Age-related changes in local water and protein content of human eye lenses measured by Raman microspectroscopy. *Experimental eye research.* 1991;53:233–239.
169. Smith G, Pierscionek BK. The optical structure of the lens and its contribution to the refractive status of the eye. *Ophthalmic and Physiological Optics.* 1998;18:21–29.
170. Costello MJ, Oliver TN, Cobo LM. Cellular architecture in age-related human nuclear cataracts. *Invest Ophthalmol Vis Sci.* 1992;33(11):3209–3227.
171. Al-Ghoul KJ, Costello MJ. Light microscopic variation of fiber cell size, shape and ordering in the equatorial plane of bovine and human lenses. *Mol Vis.* 1997;3:2.
172. Greiner JV, Auerbach DB, Leahy CD, Glonek T. Distribution of membrane phospholipids in the crystalline lens. *Invest Ophthalmol Vis Sci.* 1994;35:3739–3746.
173. Kasthurirangan S, Markwell EL, Atchison DA, Pope JM. In vivo study of changes in refractive index distribution in the human crystalline lens with age and accommodation. *Investigative Ophthalmology and Visual Science.* 2008;49(6):2531–2540.
174. Moffat BA, Pope JM. The interpretation of multi-exponential water proton transverse relaxation in the human and porcine eye lens. *Magnetic Resonance Imaging.* 2002;20: 83–93.
175. Birkenfeld J, De Castro A, Ortiz S, Pascual D, Marcos S. Contribution of the gradient refractive index and shape to the crystalline lens spherical aberration and astigmatism. *Vision research.* 2013;86:27–34.
176. Pierscionek B, Bahrami M, Hoshino M, Uesugi K, Regini J, Yagi N. The eye lens: age-related trends and individual variations in refractive index and shape parameters. *Oncotarget.* 2015;6(31):30532–30544.
177. Vaghefi E, Kim A, Donaldson PJ. Active maintenance of the gradient of refractive index is required to sustain the optical properties of the lens. *Invest Ophthalmol Vis Sci.* 2015;56(12):7195–7208.
178. Wistow G, Piatigorsky J. Recruitment of enzymes as lens structural proteins. *Science.* 1987; 236(4808):1554–1556.
179. Piatigorsky J, Wistow GJ. Enzyme/crystallins: gene sharing as an evolutionary strategy. *Cell.* 1989;57(2):197–199.
180. Zhao H, Brown PH, Magone MT, Schuck P. The molecular refractive function of lens γ-crystallins. *Journal of Molecular Biology.* 2011;411(3):680–699.
181. Klemenz R, Fröhli E, Steiger RH, Schäfer R, Aoyama A. Alpha B-crystallin is a small heat shock protein. *Proceedings of the National Academy of Sciences.* 1991;88(9):3652–3656.
182. Ingolia TD, Craig EA. Four small Drosophila heat shock proteins are related to each other and to mammalian alpha-crystallin. *Proceedings of the National Academy of Sciences.* 1982; 79(7):2360–2364.
183. Piatigorsky J, Sasaki H. Molecular biology: Recent studies on enzyme/crystallins and α-crystallin gene expression. *Experimental Eye Research.* 1990;50(6):725–727.
184. Horwitz J. Alpha-crystallin can function as a molecular chaperone. *Proceedings of the National Academy of Sciences.* 1992;89(21):10449–10453.
185. Brady JP, Garland D, Duglas-Tabor Y, Robison WG, Groome A, Wawrousek EF. Targeted disruption of the mouse αA-crystallin gene induces cataract and cytoplasmic inclusion bodies containing the small heat shock protein αB-crystallin. *Proceedings of the National Academy of Sciences.* 1997;94(3):884–889.
186. Kantorow M, Piatigorsky J. Alpha-crystallin/small heat shock protein has autokinase activity. *Proceedings of the National Academy of Sciences.* 1994;91(8):3112–3116.
187. Muranova LK, Sudnitsyna MV, Gusev NB. αB-Crystallin phosphorylation: Advances and problems. *Biochemistry (Moscow).* 2018;83(10):1196–1206.
188. Horwitz J, ed. *The function of alpha-crystallin in vision. Seminars in Cell & Developmental Biology.* Elsevier; 2000.
189. Bova MP, Ding L-L, Horwitz J, Fung BK-K. Subunit exchange of αA-crystallin. *Journal of Biological Chemistry.* 1997;272(47):29511–29517.
190. Andley UP, Song Z, Wawrousek EF, Bassnett S. The molecular chaperone αA-crystallin enhances lens epithelial cell growth and resistance to UVA stress. *Journal of Biological Chemistry.* 1998;273(47):31252–31261.
191. Vicart P, Caron A, Guicheney P, et al. A missense mutation in the αB-crystallin chaperone gene causes a desmin-related myopathy. *Nature Genetics.* 1998;20(1):92–95.

192. Bova MP, Yaron O, Huang Q, et al. Mutation R120G in αB-crystallin, which is linked to a desmin-related myopathy, results in an irregular structure and defective chaperone-like function. *Proceedings of the National Academy of Sciences.* 1999;96(11):6137–6142.

193. Berry V, Francis P, Reddy MA, et al. Alpha-B crystallin gene (CRYAB) mutation causes dominant congenital posterior polar cataract in humans. *The American Journal of Human Genetics.* 2001;69(5):1141–1145.

194. Driessen HP, Herbrink P, BloemendaL H, de Jong WW. Primary structure of the bovine β-crystallin bp chain: internal duplication and homology with γ-crystallin. *European Journal of Biochemistry.* 1981;121(1):83–91.

195. Bax B, Lapatto R, Nalini V, et al. X-ray analysis of βB2-crystallin and evolution of oligomeric lens proteins. *Nature.* 1990;347(6295):776–780.

196. Kroone R, Elliott G, Ferszt A, Slingsby C, Lubsen N, Schoenmakers J. The role of the sequence extensions in β-crystallin assembly. *Protein Engineering, Design Selection.* 1994;7(11):1395–1399.

197. Lampi KJ, Ma Z, Shih M, et al. Sequence analysis of βA3, βB3, and βA4 crystallins completes the identification of the major proteins in young human lens. *Journal of Biological Chemistry.* 1997;272(4):2268–2275.

198. McDermott JB, Peterson CA, Piatigorsky J. Structure and lens expression of the gene encoding chicken βA3/A1-crystallin. *Gene.* 1992;117(2):193–200.

199. Jobby MK, Sharma Y. Calcium-binding to lens βB2 and βA3-crystallins suggests that all β-crystallins are calcium-binding proteins. *The FEBS journal.* 2007;274(16):4135–4147.

200. Rajini B, Shridas P, Sundari CS, et al. Calcium binding properties of γ-crystallin: calcium ion binds at the Greek key βγ-crystallin fold. *Journal of Biological Chemistry.* 2001;276(42):38464–38471.

201. Bloemendal H, de Jong W, Jaenicke R, Lubsen NH, Slingsby C, Tardieu A. Ageing and vision: structure, stability and function of lens crystallins. *Progress in Biophysics Molecular Biology.* 2004;86(3):407–485.

202. Zhao H, Brown PH, Schuck P. On the distribution of protein refractive index increments. *Biophysical Journal.* 2011;100(9):2309–2317.

203. Thomson JA, Augusteyn RC. Ontogeny of human lens crystallins. *Experimental eye research.* 1985;40:393–410.

204. Mahendiran K, Elie C, Nebel J-C, Ryan A, Pierscionek BK. Primary sequence contribution to the optical function of the eye lens. *Scientific Reports.* 2014;4(1):1–8.

205. Zhao H, Chen Y, Rezabkova L, Wu Z, Wistow G, Schuck P. Solution properties of γ-crystallins: Hydration of fish and mammal γ-crystallins. *Protein Science.* 2014;23(1):88–99.

206. Delaye M, Tardieu A. Short-range order of crystallin proteins accounts for eye lens transparency. *Nature.* 1983;302(5907):415–417.

207. Zhao H, Magone MT, Schuck P. The role of macromolecular crowding in the evolution of lens crystallins with high molecular refractive index. *Physical Biology.* 2011;8(4):046004.

208. Chen Y, Zhao H, Schuck P, Wistow G. Solution properties of γ-crystallins: Compact structure and low frictional ratio are conserved properties of diverse γ-crystallins. *Protein Science.* 2014;23(1):76–87.

209. Greiner JV, Glonek T. Hydrotropic function of ATP in the crystalline lens. *Experimental Eye Research.* 2020;190:107862.

210. Patel A., Malinovska L., Saha S., et al. ATP as a biological hydrotrope. 2017;356(6339):753–6.

211. Khago D, Bierma JC, Roskamp KW, Kozlyuk N, Martin RW. Protein refractive index increment is determined by conformation as well as composition. *Journal of Physics: Condensed Matter.* 2018;30(43):435101.

212. Pande A, Annunziata O, Asherie N, Ogun O, Benedek GB, Pande J. Decrease in protein solubility and cataract formation caused by the Pro23 to Thr mutation in human γD-crystallin. *Biochemistry.* 2005;44(7):2491–2500.

213. Roskamp KW, Paulson CN, Brubaker WD, Martin RW. Function and aggregation in structural eye lens crystallins. *Accounts of Chemical Research.* 2020;53(4):863–874.

214. Cheng C, Xia C, Li L, White TW, Niimi J, Gong X. Gap junction communication influences intercellular protein distribution in the lens. *Experimental eye research.* 2008;86:966–974.

215. Vaghefi E, Pontre BP, Jacobs MD, Donaldson PJ. Visualizing ocular lens fluid dynamics using MRI: manipulation of steady state water content and water fluxes. *Am J Physiol Regul Integr Comp Physiol.* 2011;301(2):R335–R342.

216. Parreno J, Cheng C, Nowak RB, Fowler VM. The effects of mechanical strain on mouse eye lens capsule and cellular microstructure. *Molecular Biology of the Cell.* 2018;29(16):1963–1974.

217. Won G.-J., Fudge D.S., Choh V.J.Mv The effects of actomyosin disruptors on the mechanical integrity of the avian crystalline lens. 2015;21:98.

218. Cheng C, Nowak RB, Amadeo MB, Biswas SK, Lo W-K, Fowler VM. Tropomyosin 3.5 protects the F-actin networks required for tissue biomechanical properties. *Journal of Cell Science.* 2018;131(23):jcs222042.

219. Cheng C, Nowak RB, Biswas SK, Lo W-K, FitzGerald PG, Fowler VM. Tropomodulin 1 regulation of actin is required for the formation of large paddle protrusions between mature lens fiber cells. *Investigative Ophthalmology and Visual Science.* 2016;57(10):4084–4099.

220. Cheng C, Parreno J, Nowak RB, et al. Age-related changes in eye lens biomechanics, morphology, refractive index and transparency. *Aging.* 2019;11(24):12497.

221. Fudge DS, McCuaig JV, Van Stralen S, et al. Intermediate filaments regulate tissue size and stiffness in the murine lens. *Investigative Ophthalmology and Visual Science.* 2011;52(6):3860–3867.

222. Kumari SS, Gupta N, Shiels A, et al. Role of Aquaporin 0 in lens biomechanics. *Biochemical and Biophysical Research Communications.* 2015;462(4):339–345.

223. Stopka W, Libby T, Lin S, Wang E, Xia C-h, Gong X. Age-related changes of lens stiffness in wild-type and Cx46 knockout mice. *Experimental Eye Research.* 2021;108777.

224. Giblin FJ, Nies DE, Reddy VN. Stimulation of the hexose monophosphate shunt in rabbit lens in response to the oxidation of glutathione. *Experimental eye research.* 1981;33(3):289–298.

225. Winkler BS, Riley MV. Relative contributions of epithelial cells and fibers to rabbit lens ATP content and glycolysis. *Investigative Ophthalmology and Visual Science.* 1991;32(9):2593–2598.

226. Yan H, Harding JJ, Xing K, Lou MF. Revival of glutathione reductase in human cataractous and clear lens extracts by thioredoxin and thioredoxin reductase, in conjunction with α-crystallin or thioltransferase. *Current Eye Research.* 2007;32(5):455–463.

227. Davies PD, Duncan G, Pynsent PB, Arber DL, Lucas VA. Aqueous humour glucose concentration in cataract patients and its effect on the lens. *Experimental Eye Research.* 1984;39(5):605–609.

228. Kokavec J, Min SH, Tan MH, et al. Biochemical analysis of the living human vitreous. *Clinical and Experimental Ophthalmology.* 2016;44(7):597–609.

229. Kuck Jr. JF. Carbohydrates of the lens in normal and precataractous states. *Invest Ophthalmol.* 1965;4:638–642.

230. Kinoshita JH. Carbohydrate metabolism of Lens. AMA. *Archives of Ophthalmology.* 1955;54(3):360–368.

231. Dvornik D, Simard-Duquesne N, Krami M, et al. Polyol accumulation in galactosemic and diabetic rats: control by an aldose reductase inhibitor. *Science.* 1973;182(4117):1146–1148.

232. Kinoshita JH. A thirty year journey in the polyol pathway. *Experimental Eye Research.* 1990;50(6):567–573.

233. Hejtmancik JF, Riazuddin SA, McGreal R, Liu W, Cvekl A, Shiels A. Chapter 11: Lens biology and biochemistry. In: Hejtmancik JF, Nickerson JM, eds. *Progress in Molecular Biology and Translational Science.* 134: Academic Press; 2015:169–201.

234. Hockwin O, Blum G, Korte I, Murata T, Radetzki W, Rast F. Studies on the citric acid cycle and its portion of glucose breakdown by calf and bovine lenses in vitro. *Ophthalmic Research.* 1971;2(3–4):143–148.

235. Trayhurn P, Van Heyningen R. The role of respiration in the energy metabolism of the bovine lens. *The Biochemical journal.* 1972;129(2):507–509.

236. Bron AJ, Sparrow J, Brown NAP, Harding JJ, Blakytny R. The lens in diabetes. *Eye.* 1993;7(2):260–275.

237. Helbig H, Hinz J, Kellner U, Foerster M. Oxygen in the anterior chamber of the human eye. *German Journal of Ophthalmology.* 1993;2(3):161–164.

238. Holekamp NM, Shui Y-B, Beebe D. Lower intraocular oxygen tension in diabetic patients: possible contribution to decreased incidence of nuclear sclerotic cataract. *American Journal of Ophthalmology.* 2006;141(6):1027–1032.

239. Holekamp NM, Shui Y-B, Beebe DC. Vitrectomy surgery increases oxygen exposure to the lens: a possible mechanism for nuclear cataract formation. *American Journal of Ophthalmology.* 2005;139(2):302–310.

240. McLaren JW, Dinslage S, Dillon JP, Roberts JE, Brubaker RF. Measuring oxygen tension in the anterior chamber of rabbits. *Investigative Ophthalmology and Visual Science.* 1998;39(10):1899–1909.

241. McNulty R, Wang H, Mathias RT, Ortwerth BJ, Truscott RJW, Bassnett S. Regulation of tissue oxygen levels in the mammalian lens. *The Journal of Physiology.* 2004;559(3):883–898.

242. Jedziniak JA, Chylack Jr. LT, Cheng HM, Gillis MK, Kalustian AA, Tung WH. The sorbitol pathway in the human lens: aldose reductase and polyol dehydrogenase. *Invest Ophthalmol Vis Sci.* 1981;20(3):314–326.

243. Murata M, Ohta N, Sakurai S, et al. The role of aldose reductase in sugar cataract formation: aldose reductase plays a key role in lens epithelial cell death (apoptosis). *Chemico-Biological Interactions.* 2001;130–132:617–625.

244. Kador P, Randazzo J, Babb T, et al. Topical aldose reductase inhibitor formulations for effective lens drug delivery in a rat model for sugar cataracts. *Journal of ocular pharmacology and therapeutics: the official journal of the Association for Ocular Pharmacology and Therapeutics.* 2007;23:116–123.

245. Chan AW, Ho YS, Chung SK, Chung SS. Synergistic effect of osmotic and oxidative stress in slow-developing cataract formation. *Exp Eye Res.* 2008;87(5):454–461.

246. Lee A.Y.W., Chung S.S.M. Contributions of polyol pathway to oxidative stress in diabetic cataract. 1999;13(1):23–30.

247. Kwan M, Niinikoski J, Hunt TK. In vivo measurements of oxygen tension in the cornea, aqueous humor, and anterior lens of the open eye. *Investigative Ophthalmology and Visual Science.* 1972;11(2):108–114.

248. Shui Y-B, Fu J-J, Garcia C, et al. Oxygen distribution in the rabbit eye and oxygen consumption by the lens. *Investigative Ophthalmology and Visual Science.* 2006;47(4):1571–1580.

249. Turrens JF, Alexandre A, Lehninger AL. Ubisemiquinone is the electron donor for superoxide formation by complex III of heart mitochondria. *Archives of Biochemistry and Biophysics.* 1985;237(2):408–414.

250. Spector A, Garner WH. Hydrogen peroxide and human cataract. *Experimental Eye Research.* 1981;33(6):673–681.

251. Devamanoharan PS, Ramachandran S, Varma SD. Hydrogen peroxide in the eye lens: radioisotopic determination. *Current Eye Research.* 1991;10(9):831–838.

252. Spector A. Oxidative stress-induced cataract: mechanism of action. *The FASEB Journal.* 1995;9(12):1173–1182.

253. Reddan JR, Steiger CA, Dziedzic DC, Gordon SR. Regional differences in the distribution of catalase in the epithelium of the ocular lens. *Cellular and Molecular Biology.* 1996;42(2):209–219.

254. Giblin FJ, Reddan JR, Schrimscher L, Dziedzic DC, Reddy VN. The relative roles of the glutathione redox cycle and catalase in the detoxification of H2O2 by cultured rabbit lens epithelial cells. *Experimental Eye Research.* 1990;50(6):795–804.

255. Braakhuis AJ, Donaldson CI, Lim JC, Donaldson PJ. Nutritional strategies to prevent lens cataract: Current status and future strategies. *Nutrients.* 2019;11(5):1186.

256. Giblin FJ. Glutathione: A vital lens antioxidant. *Journal of Ocular Pharmacology & Therapeutics.* 2000;16(2):121.

257. Lim JC, Grey AC, Zahraei A, Donaldson PJ. Age-dependent changes in glutathione metabolism pathways in the lens: New insights into therapeutic strategies to prevent cataract formation—A review. *Clin Exper Ophthalmol.* 2020;48(8):1031–1042.

258. Lou MF. Thiol regulation in the lens. *Journal of Ocular Pharmacology Therapeutics.* 2000;16(2):137–148.

259. Reddan JR, Giblin FJ, Kadry R, Leverenz VR, Pena JT, Dziedzic DC. Protection from oxidative insult in glutathione depleted lens epithelial cells. *Experimental Eye Research.* 1999;68(1):117–127.

260. Calvin HI, Medvedovsky C, David J, et al. Rapid deterioration of lens fibers in GSH-depleted mouse pups. *Investigative Ophthalmology and Visual Science.* 1991;32(6):1916–1924.

261. Reddy VN. Glutathione and its function in the lens—an overview. *Experimental Eye Research.* 1990;50(6):771–778.

262. Lou MF. Redox regulation in the lens. *Progress in Retinal and Eye Research.* 2003;22(5): 657–682.

263. Tsukaguchi H, Tokui T, Mackenzie B, et al. A family of mammalian Na⁺-dependent L-ascorbic acid transporters. *Nature.* 1999;399(6731):70–75.

264. Rose R.C., Bode A.M. Ocular ascorbate transport and metabolism. Comparative Biochemistry Physiology Part A: Physiology. 1991;100(2):273–85.

265. Kern H, Zolot S. Transport of vitamin C in the lens. *Current Eye Research.* 1987;6(7): 885–896.

266. Fan X, Reneker LW, Obrenovich ME, et al. Vitamin C mediates chemical aging of lens crystallins by the Maillard reaction in a humanized mouse model. *Proceedings of the National Academy of Sciences.* 2006;103(45):16912–16917.

267. Winkler BS, Orselli SM, Rex TS. The redox couple between glutathione and ascorbic acid: a chemical and physiological perspective. Free Radical Biology Medi. cine. 1994;17(4): 333–349.

268. Beems EM, Van Best JA. Light transmission of the cornea in whole human eyes. *Experimental Eye Research.* 1990;50(4):393–395.

269. Lerman, S.J. 1984. *Biophysical aspects of corneal and lenticular transparency.* Current eye research 3, 3–14.

270. Collier, R., Zigman, S. 1987. *The gray squirrel lens protects the retina from near-UV radiation damage.* Progress in clinical biological research 247, 571–585.

271. Zigman, S., Paxhia, T. 1988. *The nature and properties of squirrel lens yellow pigment.* Experimental eye research 47, 819–824.

272. Van Heyningen R. Fluorescent glucoside in the human lens. *Nature.* 1971;230(5293): 393–394.

273. Van Heyningen R. The glucoside of 3-hydroxykynurenine and other fluorescent compounds in the human lens. Ciba Foundation Symposium 19. *The Human Lens—in Relation to Cataract.* 1973:151–171.

274. Streete, I.M., Jamie, J.F., Truscott, R.J.W. 2004. *Lenticular levels of amino acids and free UV filters differ significantly between normals and cataract patients.* Investigative ophthalmology visual science 45, 4091–4098.

275. Truscott, R.J.W., Wood, A.M., Carver, J.A., et al. 1994. A new UV-filter compound in human lenses. FEBS letters 348, 173–176.

276. Garner, B., Vazquez, S., Griffith, R., Lindner, R.A., Carver, J.A., Truscott, R.J.W. 1999. *Identification of glutathionyl-3-hydroxykynurenine glucoside as a novel fluorophore associated with aging of the human lens.* Journal of Biological Chemistry 274, 20847–20854.

277. Snytnikova, O.A., Fursova, A.Z., Chernyak, E.I., Vasiliev, V.G., Morozov, S.V., Kolosova, N.G., Tsentalovich, Y.P., 2008. Deaminated UV filter 3-hydroxykynurenine O-β-d-glucoside is found in cataractous human lenses. Experimental eye research 86, 951–956.

278. Aquilina, J.A., Truscott, R.J.W., 2001. Kynurenine binds to the peptide binding region of the chaperone αB-crystallin. J Biochemical Biophysical Research Communications 285, 1107–1113.

279. Vazquez, S., Aquilina, J.A., Sheil, M.M., Truscott, R.J.W., Jamie, J.F., 2002. Novel protein modification by kynurenine in human lenses. Journal of Biological Chemistry 277, 4867–4873.

280. Mizdrak J., Hains P.G., Truscott R.J., Jamie J.F., Davies M.J. Tryptophan-derived ultraviolet filter compounds covalently bound to lens proteins are photosensitizers of oxidative damage. 2008;44(6):1108–19.

281. Mathias R, Rae J, Baldo G. Physiological properties of the normal lens. *Physiological Reviews.* 1997;77(1):21–50.

282. Donaldson PJ, Webb KF. Ionic permeability and currents in the lens. In: Dartt DA, ed. *Encyclopedia of the Eye.* Oxford: Academic Press; 2010:477–486.

283. Mathias RT, Rae JL. The lens: local transport and global transparency. *Experimental eye research.* 2004;78(3):689–698.

284. Robinson KR, Patterson JW. Localization of steady currents in the lens. *Current Eye Research.* 1982;2(12):843–847.

285. Parmelee JT. Measurement of steady currents around the frog lens. *Experimental Eye Research.* 1986;42(5):433–441.

286. Wind BE, Walsh S, Patterson JW. Equatorial potassium currents in lenses. *Experimental Eye Research.* 1988;46(2):117–130.

287. Beebe DC, Truscott RJ. Counterpoint: The lens fluid circulation model—a critical appraisal. *Invest Ophthalmol Vis Sci.* 2010;51(5):2306–2310. discussion 10-2.

288. Donaldson PJ, Musil LS, Mathias RT. Point: A critical appraisal of the lens circulation model—an experimental paradigm for understanding the maintenance of lens transparency? *Invest Ophthalmol Vis Sci.* 2010;51(5):2303–2306.

289. Baldo GJ, Mathias RT. Spatial variations in membrane properties in the intact rat lens. *Biophys J.* 1992;63(2):518–529.

290. Candia OA, Zamudio AC. Regional distribution of the Na(+) and K(+) currents around the crystalline lens of rabbit. *American journal of physiology Cell physiology.*2002;282(2): C252–C262.

291. Gao J, Sun X, Yatsula V, Wymore RS, Mathias RT. Isoform-specific function and distribution of Na/K pumps in the frog lens epithelium. *J Membr Biol.* 2000;178(2): 89–101.

292. Tamiya S, Dean WL, Paterson CA, Delamere NA. Regional distribution of Na,K-ATPase activity in porcine lens epithelium. *Invest Ophthalmol Vis Sci.* 2003;44(10):4395–4399.

293. Webb KF, Donaldson PJ. Differentiation-dependent changes in the membrane properties of fiber cells isolated from the rat lens. *American journal of physiology Cell physiology.* 2008;294(5):C1133–C1145.

294. Gunning SJ, Chung KK, Donaldson PJ, Webb KF. Identification of a nonselective cation channel in isolated lens fiber cells that is activated by cell shrinkage. *American journal of physiology Cell physiology.* 2012;303(12):C1252–C1259.

295. Tong JJ, Acharya P, Ebihara L. Calcium-activated chloride channels in newly differentiating mouse lens fiber cells and their role in volume regulation. *Invest Ophthalmol Vis Sci.* 2019; 60(5):1621–1629.

296. Webb KF, Merriman-Smith BR, Stobie JK, Kistler J, Donaldson PJ. Cl- influx into rat cortical lens fiber cells is mediated by a Cl- conductance that is not ClC-2 or -3. *Invest Ophthalmol Vis Sci.* 2004;45(12):4400–4408.

297. Donaldson PJ, Lim J. Membrane transporters: new roles in lens cataract. In: Rizzo JF, Tombran-Tink J, Barnstable CJ, eds. *Ocular Transporters in Ophthalmic Diseases and Drug Delivery.* Totowa, NJ: Humana Press Inc; 2008:83–104.

298. Mathias RT, Kistler J, Donaldson P. The lens circulation. *The Journal of Membrane Biology.* 2007;216(1):1–16.

299. Gao J, Sun X, Moore LC, White TW, Brink PR, Mathias RT. Lens intracellular hydrostatic pressure is generated by the circulation of sodium and modulated by gap junction coupling. *The Journal of General Physiology.* 2011;137:507–520.

300. Truscott RJ. Age-related nuclear cataract: a lens transport problem. *Ophthalmic Research.* 2000;32(5):185–194.

301. Truscott RJ. Age-related nuclear cataract—oxidation is the key. *Experimental Eye Research.* 2005;80(5):709–725.

302. Sweeney MH, JWTR. An impediment to glutathione diffusion in older normal human lenses: a possible precondition for nuclear cataract. *Experimental Eye Research.* 1998;67(5):587–595.

303. Slavi N, Rubinos C, Li L, et al. Connexin 46 (cx46) gap junctions provide a pathway for the delivery of glutathione to the lens nucleus. *J Biol Chem.* 2014;289(47):32694–32702.

304. Vaghefi E, Donaldson PJ. The lens internal microcirculation system delivers solutes to the lens core faster than would be predicted by passive diffusion. *American journal of physiology Regulatory, integrative and comparative physiology.* 2018;315(5):R994–R1002.

305. Donaldson PJ, Lim JC. Membrane transporters. In: Tombran-Tink J, Barnstable CJ, eds. *Ocular Transporters In Ophthalmic Diseases And Drug Delivery: Ophthalmology Research.* Humana Press; 2008.

306. Lim JC, Perwick RD, Li B, Donaldson PJ. Comparison of the expression and spatial localization of glucose transporters in the rat, bovine and human lens. *Exp Eye Res.* 2017; 161:193–204.

307. Merriman-Smith BR, Krushinsky A, Kistler J, Donaldson PJ. Expression patterns for glucose transporters GLUT1 and GLUT3 in the normal rat lens and in models of diabetic cataract. *Invest Ophthalmol Vis Sci.* 2003;44(8):3458–3466.

308. Merriman–Smith R, Donaldson P, Kistler J. Differential expression of facilitative glucose transporters GLUT1 and GLUT3 in the lens. *Investigative Ophthalmology and Visual Science.* 1999;40(13):3224–3230.

309. Li L, Lim J, Jacobs MD, Kistler J, Donaldson PJ. Regional differences in cystine accumulation point to a sutural delivery pathway to the lens core. *Invest Ophthalmol Vis Sci.* 2007;48(3):1253–1260.

310. Lim J, Lam YC, Kistler J, Donaldson PJ. Molecular characterization of the cystine/glutamate exchanger and the excitatory amino acid transporters in the rat lens. *Invest Ophthalmol Vis Sci.* 2005;46(8):2869–2877.

311. Lim J, Li L, Jacobs MD, Kistler J, Donaldson PJ. Mapping of glutathione and its precursor amino acids reveals a role for GLYT2 in glycine uptake in the lens core. *Invest Ophthalmol Vis Sci.* 2007;48(11):5142–5151.

312. Lim J, Lorentzen KA, Kistler J, Donaldson PJ. Molecular identification and characterisation of the glycine transporter (GLYT1) and the glutamine/glutamate transporter (ASCT2) in the rat lens. *Exp Eye Res.* 2006;83(2):447–455.

313. Lim JC, Lam L, Li B, Donaldson PJ. Molecular identification and cellular localization of a potential transport system involved in cystine/cysteine uptake in human lenses. *Exp Eye Res.* 2013;116:219–226.

314. Beutler E. Nutritional and metabolic aspects of glutathione. *Annu Rev Nutr.* 1989;9: 287–302.

315. Burdo J, Dargusch R, Schubert D. Distribution of the cystine/glutamate antiporter system Xc- in the brain, kidney and duodenum. *J Histochem Cytochem.* 2006;54(5):549–557.

316. Davis MA, Wallig MA, Eaton D, Borroz KI, Jeffery EH. Differential effect of cyanohydroxybutene on glutathione synthesis in liver and pancreas of male rats. *Toxicol Appl Pharmacol.* 1993;123:257–264.

317. Deneke SM, Fanburg BL. Regulation of cellular glutathione. *Am J Physiol.* 1989;257: L163–L173.

318. Mackic JB, Kannan R, Kaplowitz N, Zlokovic BV. Low de novo glutathione synthesis from circulating sulfur amino acids in the lens epithelium. *Exp Eye Res.* 1997;64:615–626.

319. Wang XF, Cynader MS. Astrocytes provide cysteine to neurons by releasing glutathione. *J Neurochem.* 2000;74:1434–1442.

320. McBean GJ. Cerebral cystine uptake: a tale of two transporters. *Trends Pharmacol Sci.* 2002; 23(7):299–302.

321. McBean GJ, Flynn J. Molecular mechanisms of cystine transport. *Biochem Soc Trans.* 2001; 29(Pt 6):717–722.

322. Gegelashvili G, Schousboe A. High affinity glutamate transporters: regulation of expression and activity. *Mol Pharmacol.* 1997;52(1):6–15.

323. Utsunomiya-Tate N, Endou H, Kanai Y. Cloning and functional characterization of a system ASC-like Na⁺ dependent neutral amino acid transporter. *J Biol Chem.* 1996;271: 14883–14890.

324. Bassnett S, Duncan G. Direct measurement of pH in the rat lens by ion-sensitive micro-electrodes. *Experimental Eye Research.* 1985;40(4):585–590.

325. Aragon MC, Gimenez C, Mayor F. Stoichiometry of sodium- and chloride-coupled glycine transport in synaptic plasma membrane vesicles derived from rat brain. *FEBS Lett.* 1987;212(1).

326. Lopez-Corcuera B, Martinez-Maza R, Nunez E, Roux M, Supplisson S, Aragon C. Differential properties of two stably expressed brain-specific glycine transporters. *J Neurochem.* 1998;71(5):2211–2219.

327. Supplisson S, Roux MJ. Why glycine transporters have different stoichiometries. *FEBS Lett.* 2002;259(1):93–101.

328. Aubrey KR, Mitrovic AD, Vandenberg RJ. Molecular basis for proton regulation of glycine transport by glycine transporter subtype 1b. *Mol Pharmacol.* 2000;58(1):129–135.

329. Ramakrishnan S, Sulochana KN. Decrease in glycation of lens proteins by lysine and glycine by scavenging of glucose and possible mitigation of cataractogenesis. *Exp Eye Res.* 1993;57(5):623–628.

330. Oimomi M, Maeda Y, Hata F, et al. Glycation of cataractous lens in non-diabetic senile subjects and in diabetic patients. *Exp Eye Res.* 1988;46(3):415–420.

331. Mathias, R.T., White, T.W., Brink, P.R., 2008. The role of gap junction channels in the ciliary body secretory epithelium. Current topics in membranes 62, 71–96.

332. Gao J, Sun X, Moore LC, Brink PR, White TW, Mathias RT. The effect of size and species on lens intracellular hydrostatic pressure. *Invest Ophthalmol Vis Sci.* 2013;54(1):183–192.

333. Sellitto C, Li L, Gao J, et al. AKT activation promotes PTEN hamartoma tumor syndrome-associated cataract development. *J Clin Invest.* 2013;123(12):5401–5409.

334. Gao J, Wang H, Sun X, et al. The effects of age on lens transport. *Invest Ophthalmol Vis Sci.* 2013;54(12):7174–7187.

335. Wang H, Gao J, Sun X, et al. The effects of GPX-1 knockout on membrane transport and intracellular homeostasis in the lens. *J Membr Biol.* 2009;227(1):25–37.

336. Gao J, Sun X, White TW, Delamere NA, Mathias RT. Feedback regulation of intracellular hydrostatic pressure in surface cells of the lens. *Biophys J.* 2015;109(9):1830–1839.

337. Shahidullah M, Mandal A, Mathias RT, et al. TRPV1 activation stimulates NKCC1 and increases hydrostatic pressure in the mouse lens. *American journal of physiology Cell physiology.* 2020;318(5):C969–C980.

338. Donaldson PJ, Chee KS, Lim JC, Webb KF. Regulation of lens volume: implications for lens transparency. *Exp Eye Res.* 2009;88(2):144–150.

339. Jacob TJ. The relationship between cataract, cell swelling and volume regulation. *Prog Retin Eye Res.* 1999;18(2):223–233.

340. Duncan G, Croghan PC. Mechanisms for the regulation of cell volume with particular reference to the lens. *Experimental Eye Research.* 1969;8(4):421–428.

341. Patterson JW. Lens volume regulation in hypertonic medium. *Experimental Eye Research.* 1981;32(2):151–162.

342. Patterson JW, Fournier DJ. The effect of tonicity on lens volume. *Investigative Ophthalmology & Visual Science.* 1976;15(10):866–869.

343. Gamba G. Molecular physiology and pathophysiology of electroneutral cation-chloride cotransporters. *Physiol Rev.* 2005;85(2):423–493.

344. Lang, F., Busch, G.L., Ritter, M., et al. 1998. Functional significance of cell volume regulatory mechanisms. Physiological reviews 78, 247–306.

345. Adragna, N., Fulvio, M.D., Lauf, P., 2004. Regulation of K-Cl cotransport: from function to genes. Journal of membrane biology 201, 109–137.

346. Chee KN, Vorontsova I, Lim JC, Kistler J, Donaldson PJ. Expression of the sodium potassium chloride cotransporter (NKCC1) and sodium chloride cotransporter (NCC) and their effects on rat lens transparency. *Mol Vis.* 2010;16:800–812.

347. Chee KS, Kistler J, Donaldson PJ. Roles for KCC transporters in the maintenance of lens transparency. *Invest Ophthalmol Vis Sci.* 2006;47(2):673–682.

348. Young MA, Tunstall MJ, Kistler J, Donaldson PJ. Blocking chloride channels in the rat lens: localized changes in tissue hydration support the existence of a circulating chloride flux. *Investigative ophthalmology visual science.* 2000;41(10):3049–3055.

349. Kahle KT, Rinehart J, Lifton RP. Phosphoregulation of the Na–K–2Cl and K–Cl cotransporters by the WNK kinases. *Biochimica et Biophysica Acta.* 2010;1802(12):1150–1158.

350. Huang CL, Cha SK, Wang HR, Xie J, Cobb MH. WNKs: protein kinases with a unique kinase domain. *Experimental & molecular medicine.* 2007;39(5):565–573.

351. Alessi DR, Zhang J, Khanna A, Hochdörfer T, Shang Y, Kahle KT. The WNK-SPAK/OSR1 pathway: master regulator of cation-chloride cotransporters. *Science signaling.* 2014;7(334):re3.

352. Alvarez LJ, Candia OA, Turner HC, Polikoff LA. Localization of a Na+-K+-2Cl− cotransporter in the rabbit lens. *Experimental Eye Research.* 2001;73(5):669–680.

353. Lauf PK, Warwar R, Brown TL, Adragna NC. Regulation of potassium transport in human lens epithelial cells. *Experimental Eye Research.* 2006;82(1):55–64.

354. Vorontsova I, Donaldson PJ, Kong Z, Wickremesinghe C, Lam L, Lim JC. The modulation of the phosphorylation status of NKCC1 in organ cultured bovine lenses: Implications for the regulation of fiber cell and overall lens volume. *Exp Eye Res.* 2017;165:164–174.

355. Shahidullah M, Mandal A, Delamere NA. Activation of TRPV1 channels leads to stimulation of NKCC1 cotransport in the lens. *American journal of physiology Cell physiology.* 2018;315(6):C793–C802.

356. Shahidullah M, Mandal A, Beimgraben C, Delamere NA. Hyposmotic stress causes ATP release and stimulates Na,K-ATPase activity in porcine lens. *J Cell Physiol.* 2012;227(4):1428–1437.

357. Shahidullah M, Mandal A, Delamere NA. TRPV4 in porcine lens epithelium regulates hemichannel-mediated ATP release and Na-K-ATPase activity. *American journal of physiology Cell physiology.* 2012;302(12):C1751–C1761.

358. Andersson R.M., Aizman O., Aperia A., Brismar H. Modulation of Na+,K+-ATPase activity is of importance for RVD. 2004;180(4):329–34.

359. Clapham DE. TRP channels as cellular sensors. *Nature.* 2003;426(6966):517–524.

360. Mandal A, Shahidullah M, Delamere NA. TRPV1-dependent ERK1/2 activation in porcine lens epithelium. *Exp Eye Res.* 2018;172:128–136.

361. Delamere NA, Shahidullah M, Mathias RT, et al. Signaling between TRPV1/TRPV4 and intracellular hydrostatic pressure in the mouse lens. *Invest Ophthalmol Vis Sci.* 2020;61(6):58.

362. Bettelheim FA. Syneretic response to pressure in ocular lens. *Journal of Theoretical Biology.* 1999;197(2):277–280.

363. Bettelheim FA, Lizak MJ, Zigler Jr. JS. Syneretic response of aging normal human lens to pressure. *Invest Ophthalmol Vis Sci.* 2003;44(1):258–263.

364. Levy Y, Onuchic JN. Water and proteins: a love-hate relationship. Proc Natl Acad Sci U S A. 2004 Mar 9;101(10):3325-6. doi: 10.1073/pnas.0400157101. Epub 2004 Mar 1. PMID: 14993602; PMCID: PMC373459.

365. Zhang L, Wang L, Kao YT, et al. Mapping hydration dynamics around a protein surface. Proc Natl Acad Sci U S A. 2007 Nov 20;104(47):18461-6. doi: 10.1073/pnas.0707647104. Epub 2007 Nov 14. PMID: 18003912; PMCID: PMC2141799.

366. Bettelheim FA, Lizak MJ, Zigler JS. NMR relaxation studies of syneretic response to pressure change in bovine lenses. *Current Eye Research.* 2001;22(6):438–445.

367. Bettelheim FA, Zigler Jr. JS. Pressure-induced syneretic response in rhesus monkey lenses. *Invest Ophthalmol Vis Sci.* 1999;40(6):1285–1288.

368. Lizak MJ, Zigler Jr. JS, Bettelheim FA. Syneretic response to incremental pressures in calf lenses. *Curr Eye Res.* 2005;30(1):21–25.

369. Schachar RA. Letter to the Editor: Accommodation, presbyopia, and the lenticular syneretic response. *Current Eye Research.* 2005;30(11):927–.

370. Chen Y, Gao J, Li L, et al. The ciliary muscle and zonules of zinn modulate lens intracellular hydrostatic pressure through transient receptor potential vanilloid channels. *Invest Ophthalmol Vis Sci.* 2019;60(13):4416–4424.

371. Jones CE, Pope JM. Measuring optical properties of an eye lens using magnetic resonance imaging. *Magnetic Resonance Imaging.* 2004;22(2):211–220.

372. Lim JC, Vaghefi E, Li B, Nye-Wood MG, Donaldson PJ. Characterization of the effects of hyperbaric oxygen on the biochemical and optical properties of the bovine lens. *Investigative Ophthalmology & Visual Science.* 2016;57(4):1961–1973.

373. Atchison DA, Markwell EL, Kasthurirangan S, Pope JM, Smith G, Swann PG. Age-related changes in optical and biometric characteristics of emmetropic eyes. *J Vis.* 2008;8(4):29 1-0.

374. Bron AJ, Vrensen GF, Koretz J, Maraini G, Harding JJ. The ageing lens. *Ophthalmologica.* 2000;214(1):86–104.

375. Dubbelman M, Van der Heijde GL, Weeber HA, Vrensen GF. Changes in the internal structure of the human crystalline lens with age and accommodation. *Vision Res.* 2003;43(22):2363–2375.

376. Bomotti, S., Lau, B., Klein, B.E.K., et al. 2018. Refraction and change in refraction over a 20-year period in the Beaver Dam Eye Study. Investigative ophthalmology visual science 59, 4518–4524.

377. Fotedar, R., Mitchell, P., Burlutsky, G., Wang, J.J., 2008. Relationship of 10-year change in refraction to nuclear cataract and axial length: findings from an older population. Ophthalmology 115, 1273-1278. e1271.

378. Gudmundsdottir, E., Arnarsson, A., Jonasson, F., 2005. Five-year refractive changes in an adult population: Reykjavik Eye Study. Ophthalmology 112, 672–677.

379. Guzowski, M., Wang, J.J., Rochtchina, E., Rose, K.A., Mitchell, P., 2003. Five-year refractive changes in an older population: the Blue Mountains Eye Study. Ophthalmology 110, 1364–1370.

380. Lee KE, Klein BE, Klein R. Changes in refractive error over a 5-year interval in the Beaver Dam Eye Study. *Invest Ophthalmol Vis Sci.* 1999;40(8):1645–1649.

381. Lee, K.E., Klein, B.E.K., Klein, R., Wong, T.Y., 2002. Changes in refraction over 10 years in an adult population: the Beaver Dam Eye study. *Invest Ophthalmol Vis Sci.* 43, 2566–2571.

382. Brown N. The change in lens curvature with age. *Experimental Eye Research.* 1974;19(2):175–183.

383. Brown, N.P., Koretz, J.F., Bron, A.J., 1999. The development and maintenance of emmetropia. Eye 13, 83–92.

384. Díaz, J.A., Pizarro, C., Arasa, J.J., 2008. Single dispersive gradient-index profile for the aging human lens. JOSA A 25, 250–261.

385. KORETZ, JANE F. COOK, CHRISTOPHER A. Aging of the Optics of the Human Eye: Lens Refraction Models and Principal Plane Locations. Optometry and Vision Science 78(6):p 396-404, June 2001.

386. Smith, G., Atchison, D.A., Pierscionek, B.K., 1992. Modeling the power of the aging human eye. JOSA A 9, 2111–2117.

387. Smith, G., Pierscionek, B.K., Atchison, D.A., 1991. The optical modelling of the human lens. Ophthalmic Physiological Optics 11, 359–369.

388. Moffat B, Atchison D, Pope J. Age-related changes in refractive index distribution and power of the human lens as measured by magnetic resonance micro-imaging in vitro. *Vision Research.* 2002;42(13):1683–1693.

389. Moffat, B.A., Atchison, D.A., Pope, J.M., 2002. Explanation of the lens paradox. Optometry vision science 79, 148–150.

390. Philipson B. Distribution of protein within the normal rat lens. *Invest Ophthalmol Vis Sci.* 1969;8:258–270.

391. Pierscionek B, Smith G, Augusteyn RC. The refractive increments of bovine α-, β-and γ-crystallins. *Vision research.* 1987;27:1539–1541.

392. Bellissent-Funel, M.-C., Hassanali, A., Havenith, M., et al. 2016. Water determines the structure and dynamics of proteins. Chemical reviews 116, 7673–7697.

393. Bettelheim FA, Lizak MJ, Zigler JS. Relaxographic studies of aging normal human lenses. *Experimental eye research.* 2002;75:695–702.

394. Heys KR, Friedrich MG, Truscott RJW. Free and bound water in normal and cataractous human lenses. *Investigative Ophthalmology & Visual Science.* 2008;49(5):1991–1997.

395. Lahm D, Lee LK, Bettelheim FA. Age dependence of freezable and nonfreezable water content of normal human lenses. *Investigative ophthalmology & visual science.* 1985;26:1162–1165.

396. Bloemendal H, de Jong W, Jaenicke R, Lubsen NH, Slingsby C, Tardieu A. Ageing and vision: structure, stability and function of lens crystallins. *Progress in biophysics and molecular biology.* 2004;86(3):407–485.

397. Hains PG, Truscott RJW. Post-translational modifications in the nuclear region of young, aged, and cataract human lenses. *Journal of Proteome Research.* 2007;6(10):3935–3943.

398. Wilmarth PA, Tanner S, Dasari S, Nagalla SR, Riviere MA, Bafna V, et al. Age-related changes in human crystallins determined from comparative analysis of post-translational

modifications in young and aged lens: does deamidation contribute to crystallin insolubility? *J Proteome Res.* 2006;5(10):2554–2566.

399. Kaufman L, Kramer D, Crooks L, Ortendahl D. Measuring signal-to-noise ratios in MR imaging. *Radiology.* 1989;173:265–267.
400. Weale RA. Presbyopia. *The British journal of ophthalmology.* 1962;46:660.
401. Weale RA. *The aging eye: Hoeber Medical Division.* Harper & Row; 1963.
402. Weale RA. On potential causes of presbyopia. *Vision research.* 1999;39:1263–1265.
403. Holden BA, Fricke TR, Ho SM, Wong R, Schlenther G, Cronjé S, et al. Global vision impairment due to uncorrected presbyopia. *Archives of Ophthalmology.* 2008;126(12):1731–1739.
404. Westheimer G, Liang J. Influence of ocular light scatter on the eye's optical performance. *Journal of the Optical Society of America. A, Optics, Image Science, and Vision.* 1995;12:1417–1424.
405. Hofstetter HW. A survey if practices in prescibing presbyopic adds. *Optometry & Vision Science.* 1949;26:144–160.
406. Pointer JS. The presbyopic add. II. Age-related trend and a gender difference. *Ophthalmic and Physiological Optics.* 1995;15:241–248.
407. Neider MW, Crawford K, Kaufman PL, Bito LZ. In vivo videography of the rhesus monkey accommodative apparatus: age-related loss of ciliary muscle response to central stimulation. *Archives of Ophthalmology.* 1990;108:69–74.
408. Tamm S, Tamm E, Rohen JW. Age-related changes of the human ciliary muscle. A quantitative morphometric study. *Mechanisms of ageing and development.* 1992;62:209–221.
409. PEDDIE, W. Helmholtz's Treatise on Physiological Optics . Nature 116, 88–89 (1925).
410. Herranz RM, Herran RMC. *Ocular Surface: Anatomy and Physiology, Disorders and Therapeutic Care.* CRC Press; 2012:374.
411. Glasser A. Restoration of accommodation: surgical options for correction of presbyopia. *Clinical & experimental optometry.* 2008;91(3):279–295.
412. Truscott RJ. Presbyopia. Emerging from a blur towards an understanding of the molecular basis for this most common eye condition. *Experimental Eye Research.* 2009;88(2):241–247.
413. Gullstrand A. Mechanism of accommodation. In: Helmholtz von HH, ed. *Handbuch der physiologischen optik (appendix IV.* New York: J. P. C. Southall, Trans.: Helmholtz's treatise in physiological optics); 1909:383–415.
414. Helmholtz Hv Ueber die Accommodation des Auges. *Archiv für Ophthalmologie.* 1855;1(2):1–74.
415. Michael R, Bron A. The ageing lens and cataract: a model of normal and pathological ageing. *Philosophical Transactions of the Royal Society B: Biological Sciences.* 2011;366:1278.
416. Roy D, Spector A. Absence of low-molecular-weight alpha crystallin in nuclear region of old human lenses. *Proceedings of the National Academy of Sciences.* 1976;73(10):3484–3487.
417. Fisher R. The elastic constants of the human lens. *The Journal of Physiology.* 1971;212(1):147–180.
418. Krag S, Andreassen TT. Mechanical properties of the human lens capsule. *Progress in retinal and eye research.* 2003;22:749–767.
419. Pau H, Kranz J. The increasing sclerosis of the human lens with age and its relevance to accommodation and presbyopia. *Graefe's Archive for Clinical Experimental Ophthalmology.* 1991;229(3):294–296.
420. Weeber HA, Eckert G, Pechhold W, van der Heijde RG. Stiffness gradient in the crystalline lens. *Graefe's Archive for Clinical Experimental Ophthalmology.* 2007;245(9):1357–1366.
421. Wilde GS, Burd HJ, Judge SJ. Shear modulus data for the human lens determined from a spinning lens test. *Experimental Eye Research.* 2012;97(1):36–48.
422. Heys KR, Truscott RJ. The stiffness of human cataract lenses is a function of both age and the type of cataract. *Experimental Eye Research.* 2008;86(4):701–703.
423. Burd H, Wilde G, Judge S. An improved spinning lens test to determine the stiffness of the human lens. *Experimental eye research.* 2011;92(1):28–39.
424. Sheppard AL, Davies LN. The effect of ageing on in vivo human ciliary muscle morphology and contractility. *Investigative Ophthalmology & Visual Science.* 2011;52(3):1809–1816.
425. Fisher R. The force of contraction of the human ciliary muscle during accommodation. *The Journal of Physiology.* 1977;270(1):51–74.
426. Fisher RF, Pettet BE. Presbyopia and the water content of the human crystalline lens. *The Journal of physiology.* 1973;234:443.
427. Bettelheim FA, Ali S, White O, Chylack JLT. Freezable and non-freezable water content of cataractous human lenses. *Investigative Ophthalmology & Visual Science.* 1986;27(1):122–125.
428. Hermans E, Dubbelman M, van der Heijde R, Heethaar R. The shape of the human lens nucleus with accommodation. *J Vis.* 2007;7(10).
429. Koretz JF, Cook CA, Kaufman PL. Accommodation and presbyopia in the human eye. Changes in the anterior segment and crystalline lens with focus. *Invest Ophthalmol Vis Sci.* 1997;38(3):569–578.
430. Lie AL, Pan X, White TW, Vaghefi E, Donaldson PJ. Age-dependent changes in total and free water content of in vivo human lenses measured by magnetic resonance imaging. *Invest Ophthalmol Vis Sci.* 2021;62(9):33.
431. Hobbs RP, Bernstein PS. Nutrient supplementation for age-related macular degeneration, cataract, and dry Eye. *Journal of ophthalmic & vision research.* 2014;9(4):487–493.
432. Pascolini D, Mariotti SP. Global estimates of visual impairment: 2010. *British Journal of Ophthalmology.* 2012;96(5):614–618.
433. Weikel KA, Garber C, Baburins A, Taylor A. Nutritional modulation of cataract. *Nutrition Reviews.* 2014;72(1):30–47.
434. Bourne RPA, GAS, White RA, et al. Causes of vision loss worldwide, 1990–2010: A systematic analysis. *Lancet Global Health.* 2013;1(6):e339–e349.
435. Brian G, Taylor H. Cataract blindness—challenges for the 21st century. *Bulletin of the World Health Organization.* 2001;79(3):249–256.
436. Leske MC, Connell AM, Wu S-Y, Hyman L, Schachat A. Prevalence of lens opacities in the Barbados Eye Study. *Archives of Ophthalmology.* 1997;115(1):105–111.
437. Hiller R, Sperduto RD, Ederer F. Epidemiologic associations with nuclear, cortical, and posterior subcapsular cataracts. *American Journal of Epidemiology.* 1986;124(6):916–925.

438. Leske MC, Wu S-Y, Nemesure B, et al. Incidence and progression of lens opacities in the Barbados Eye Studies. *Ophthalmology.* 2000;107(7):1267–1273.
439. Klein BE, Klein R, Lee KE. Incidence of age-related cataract: the Beaver Dam Eye Study. *Archives of Ophthalmology.* 1998;116(2):219–225.
440. Klein BE, Klein R, Moss SE. Incident cataract surgery: the Beaver Dam eye study. *Ophthalmology.* 1997;104(4):573–580.
441. Carlsson B, Sjöstrand J. Increased incidence of cataract extractions in women above 70 years of age: a population based study. *Acta Ophthalmologica Scandinavica.* 1996;74(1):64–68.
442. Delcourt C, Cristol J-P, Tessier F, Leger CL, Michel F. Papoz LaPSg. Risk factors for cortical, nuclear, and posterior subcapsular cataracts: the POLA study. *American Journal of Epidemiology.* 2000;151(5):497–504.
443. Klein B. Lens opacities in women in Beaver Dam, Wisconsin: Is there evidence of an effect of sex hormones? *Transactions of the American Ophthalmological Society.* 1993;91:517.
444. Klein BE, Klein R, Ritter LL. Is there evidence of an estrogen effect on age-related lens opacities?: The Beaver Dam Eye Study. *Archives of Ophthalmology.* 1994;112(1):85–91.
445. Bigsby RM, Cardenas H, Caperell-Grant A, Grubbs CJ. Protective effects of estrogen in a rat model of age-related cataracts. *Proceedings of the National Academy of Sciences.* 1999;96(16):9328–9332.
446. Hales AM, Chamberlain CG, Murphy CR, McAvoy JW. Estrogen protects lenses against cataract induced by transforming growth factor-β (TGFβ). *The Journal of Experimental Medicine.* 1997;185(2):273–280.
447. Cumming RG, Mitchell P. Hormone replacement therapy, reproductive factors, and cataract The Blue Mountains Eye Study. *American Journal of Epidemiology.* 1997;145(3):242–249.
448. Benitez del Castillo JM, del Rio T, Garcia-Sanchez J. Effects of estrogen use on lens transmittance in postmenopausal women. *Ophthalmology.* 1997;104(6):970–973.
449. Paganini-Hill A, Clark LJ. Eye problems in breast cancer patients treated with tamoxifen. *Breast Cancer Research Treatment.* 2000;60(2):167–172.
450. Gorin MB, Day R, Costantino JP, et al. Long-term tamoxifen citrate use and potential ocular toxicity. *American Journal of Ophthalmology.* 1998;125(4):493–501.
451. Faranda AP, Shihan MH, Wang Y, Duncan MK. The effect of sex on the mouse lens transcriptome. *Exp Eye Res.* 2021;209:108676.
452. Phillips C, Clayton R, Cuthbert J, Qian W, Donnelly C, Prescott R. Human cataract risk factors: significance of abstention from, and high consumption of, ethanol (U-curve) and non-significance of smoking. *Ophthalmic Research.* 1996;28(4):237–247.
453. Hodge WG, Whitcher JP, Satariano W. Risk factors for age-related cataracts. *Epidemiologic Reviews.* 1995;17(2):336–346.
454. West SK, Valmadrid CT. Epidemiology of risk factors for age-related cataract. *Survey of Ophthalmology.* 1995;39(4):323–334.
455. Cumming RG, Mitchell P, Lim R. Iris color and cataract: The blue mountains eye study. *American Journal of Ophthalmology.* 2000;130(2):237–238.
456. Hammond Jr BR, Nanez JE, Fair C, Snodderly DM. Iris color and age-related changes in lens optical density. *Ophthalmic Physiological Optics.* 2000;20(5):381–386.
457. Klein B, Klein R, Moss SE. Correlates of lens thickness: the Beaver Dam Eye Study. *Investigative Ophthalmology and Visual Science.* 1998;39(8):1507–1510.
458. Klein BE, Klein R, Moss SE. Lens thickness and five-year cumulative incidence of cataracts: the Beaver Dam Eye Study. *Ophthalmic Epidemiology.* 2000;7(4):243–248.
459. Wong TY, Foster PJ, Johnson GJ, Seah SK. Refractive errors, axial ocular dimensions, and age-related cataracts: the Tanjong Pagar survey. *Investigative Ophthalmology and Visual Science.* 2003;44(4):1479–1485.
460. Praveen M, Vasavada A, Shah S, et al. Lens thickness of Indian eyes: impact of isolated lens opacity, age, axial length, and influence on anterior chamber depth. *Eye.* 2009;23(7):1542–1548.
461. Wild S., Roglic G., Green A., Sicree R., King H. Global prevalence of diabetes. Estimates for the year 2000 and projections for 2030. 2004;27(5):1047–53.
462. Klein BE, Klein R, Wang Q, Moss SE. Older-onset diabetes and lens opacities. The Beaver Dam Eye Study. *Ophthalm Epid.* 1995;2:49–55.
463. Michael R. Cortical cataract. Encyclopedia of the eye [Internet]. Oxford, UK: Academic Press; 2010:532–536.
464. al-Ghoul KJ, Costello MJ. Morphological changes in human nuclear cataracts of late-onset diabetics. *Exp Eye Res.* 1993;57(4):469–486.
465. Pesudovs K, Elliott DB. Refractive error changes in cortical, nuclear, and posterior subcapsular cataracts. *The British journal of ophthalmology.* 2003;87(8):964–967.
466. Planten JT. Changes of refraction in the adult eye due to changing refractive indices of the layers of the lens. *Ophthalmologica.* 1981;183(2):86–90.
467. Kinoshita JH. Pathways of glucose metabolism in the lens. *Investigative Ophthalmology.* 1965;4:619–628.
468. Kinoshita JH. Cataracts in galactosemia. The Jonas S. Friedenwald Memorial Lecture. Investigative. *Ophthalmology.* 1965;4:786–799.
469. Kinoshita JH. Mechanisms initiating cataract formation. Proctor Lecture. *Invest Ophthalmol.* 1974;13(10):713–724.
470. Kador PF, Wyman M, Oates PJ. Aldose reductase, ocular diabetic complications and the development of topical Kinostat*. *Progress in Retinal and Eye Research.* 2016
471. Chung SS, Ho EC, Lam KS, Chung SK. Contribution of polyol pathway to diabetes-induced oxidative stress. *Journal of the American Society of Nephrology.* 2003;14(8 Suppl 3):S233–S236.
472. Lauf PKK. Cl cotransport: sulfhydryls, divalent cations, and the mechanism of volume activation in a red cell. *J Memb Biol.* 1985;88:1–13.
473. Wang LF, Dhir P, Bhatnagar A, Srivastava SK. Contribution of osmotic changes to disintegrative globulization of single cortical fibers isolated from rat lens. *Exp Eye Res.* 1997;65(2):267–275.
474. Bhatnagar A, Ansari NH, Wang L, Khanna P, Wang C, Srivastava SK. Calcium-mediated disintegrative globulization of isolated ocular lens fibers mimics cataractogenesis. *Exp Eye Res.* 1995;61(3):303–310.

475. Bond J, Green C, Donaldson P, Kistler J. Liquefaction of cortical tissue in diabetic and galactosemic rat lenses defined by confocal laser scanning microscopy. *Invest Ophthalmol Vis Sci.* 1996;37(8):1557–1565.

476. Wang L, Christensen BN, Bhatnagar A, Srivastava SK. Role of calcium-dependent protease(s) in globulization of isolated rat lens cortical fiber cells. *Invest Ophthalmol Vis Sci.* 2001;42(1):194–199.

477. Pirie A. Color and solubility of the proteins of human cataracts. *Investigative Ophthalmology and Visual Science.* 1968;7(6):634–650.

478. Al-Ghoul K, Costello M. Fiber cell morphology and cytoplasmic texture in cataractous and normal human lens nuclei. *Current Eye Research.* 1996;15(5):533–542.

479. Al-Ghoul K, Lane C, Taylor V, Fowle W, Costello M. Distribution and type of morphological damage in human nuclear age-related cataracts. *Experimental Eye Research.* 1996;62(3):237–252.

480. Garner MH, Spector A. Sulfur oxidation in selected human cortical cataracts and nuclear cataracts. *Exp Eye Res.* 1980;31(3):361–369.

481. Garner MH, Spector A. Selective oxidation of cysteine and methionine in normal and senile cataractous lenses. *Proc Natl Acad Sci U S A.* 1980;77(3):1274–1277.

482. Spector A, Roy D. Disulfide-linked high molecular weight protein associated with human cataract. *Proc Natl Acad Sci U S A.* 1978;75(7):3244–3248.

483. Truscott RJ, Augusteyn RC. The state of sulphydryl groups in normal and cataractous human lenses. *Exp Eye Res.* 1977;25(2):139–148.

484. Lou MF, Dickerson Jr. JE, Garadi R. The role of protein-thiol mixed disulfides in cataractogenesis. *Exp Eye Res.* 1990;50(6):819–826.

485. Lou MF, Dickerson Jr. JE, Tung WH, Wolfe JK, Chylack Jr. LT. Correlation of nuclear color and opalescence with protein S-thiolation in human lenses. *Exp Eye Res.* 1999;68(5):547–552.

486. Pirie A. Color and solubility of the proteins of human cataracts. *Invest Ophthalmol.* 1968;7(6):634–650.

487. Lim JC, Umapathy A, Donaldson PJ. Tools to fight the cataract epidemic: A review of experimental animal models that mimic age related nuclear cataract. *Experimental Eye Research.* 2016;145:432–443.

488. Truscott RJ, Augusteyn RC. Oxidative changes in human lens proteins during senile nuclear cataract formation. *Biochimica et Biophysica Acta.* 1977;492(1):43–52.

489. Rathbun WB, Murray DL. Age-related cysteine uptake as rate-limiting in glutathione synthesis and glutathione half-life in the cultured human lens. *Exp Eye Res.* 1991;53:205–212.

490. Duncan G, Hightower K, Gandolfi S, Tomlinson J, Maraini G. Human lens membrane cation permeability increases with age. *Investigative Ophthalmology and Visual Science.* 1989;30(8):1855–1859.

491. Gandolfi SA, Maraini G. Increased ion traffic through non-specific cation pathways in the ageing human lens. Evidence from radiotracer fluxes studies. *Exp Eye Res.* 1991;52(1):1–4.

492. Wormstone IM, Wormstone YM, Smith AJO, Eldred JA. Posterior capsule opacification: What's in the bag? *Prog Retin Eye Res.* 2021;82:100905.

493. McAvoy J. Developmental biology of the lens. In: Duncan J, ed. *Mechanism of Cataract Formation.* London: Academic Press; 1981:7–46.

494. Xu L, Overbeek PA, Reneker LW. Systematic analysis of E-, N- and P-cadherin expression in mouse eye development. *Exp Eye Res.* 2002;74(6):753–760.

495. Jiang JX, Goodenough DA. Heteromeric connexons in lens gap junction channels. *Proc Natl Acad Sci U S A.* 1996;93(3):1287–1291.

496. Konig N, Zampighi GA. Purification of bovine lens cell-to-cell channels composed of connexin44 and connexin50. *J Cell Sci.* 1995;108(Pt 9):3091–3098.

497. Biswas SK, Lee JE, Brako L, Jiang JX, Lo WK. Gap junctions are selectively associated with interlocking ball-and-sockets but not protrusions in the lens. *Mol Vis.* 2010;16:2328–2341.

498. Kuszak J, Alcala J, Maisel H. The surface morphology of embryonic and adult chick lens-fiber cells. *American Journal of Anatomy.* 1980;159(4):395–410.

499. Paul DL, Goodenough DA. Preparation, characterization, and localization of antisera against bovine MP26, an integral protein from lens fiber plasma membrane. *J Cell Biol.* 1983;96(3):625–632.

500. Taylor VL, al-Ghoul KJ, Lane CW, Davis VA, Costello MJ. JRK. Morphology of the normal human lens. *Invest Ophthalmol Vis Sci.* 1996;37(7):1396–1410.

6

Vitreous

Leila Chew and J. Sebag

INTRODUCTION

The vitreous body is the largest single structure of the human eye, comprising approximately 80% of the eye's volume (Fig. 6.1). Anteriorly, it is delineated by and adjoins the ciliary body, the zonules, and the lens. Posteriorly, the vitreous body is adjacent to the retina and optic disc. Vitreous has important physiologic functions that including providing structural support, serving as a diffusion barrier between the anterior and the posterior segments of the eye, providing metabolic buffering against oxidative stress, and maintaining optical transparency. This chapter focuses on those aspects of vitreous physiology and pathophysiology that have clinical importance, by reviewing relevant biochemistry, anatomy, and biophysics.

BIOCHEMISTRY

Vitreous is an extracellular matrix in the form of a clear viscous gel that is composed of 98% water; 15% to 20% of the water is bound to glycosaminoglycans, primarily hyaluronan (HA). The gel structure of vitreous results from the arrangement of long, nonbranching collagen fibrils integrated in a network of HA, which stabilizes the gel structure and the conformation of the collagen fibrils (Fig. 6.2). Changes in vitreous HA and collagen alter the viscosity of the gel and destabilize the vitreous body. In myopia and aging, this contributes to posterior vitreous detachment which can result in retinal detachment, when anomalous. Persistent attachment to the retina can exacerbate diabetic retinopathy and age-related macular degeneration (see further in chapter).

Glycosaminoglycans

Glycosaminoglycans are polysaccharides with repeating disaccharide units that are characteristic for each glycosaminoglycan. The relative amounts and molecular sizes of various glycosaminoglycans are tissue specific.[1] Three major glycosaminoglycans of the vitreous body are hyaluronan, chondroitin sulfate, and heparan sulfate.

Hyaluronan

HA was initially termed hyaluronic acid due to its colorless nature ("hyalos" meaning glass in Greek) and its composition that includes uronic acid.[2] In 1986 this term was replaced with "hyaluronan" to be more consistent with nomenclature conventions for polysaccharides and to reflect that HA can be found in either its protonated acid form (hyaluronic acid) or base salt form (sodium hyaluronate) based on the surrounding pH.[3] HA plays an essential role in many physiologic processes. Importantly for vision, HA promotes transparency via its anti-inflammatory and anticicatrical (scarring) properties.[4]

HA is a long, unbranched polymer of repeating D-glucuronic acid and N-acetyl-D-glucosamine that forms a linear threefold helix.[5,6] It is unique as a glycosaminoglycan in that it is nonsulfated.[7] It can assume vastly different configurations and volumes depending on its environment, particularly if it is surrounded by water or ionic charges. The volume of nonhydrated HA is 0.66 cm³/g, in contrast with the volume of its hydrated form of 2000 to 3000 cm³/g.[8] When surrounded by high ionic charges, the charged HA molecule can contract, thus resulting in contraction of the vitreous body and tractional forces on adjacent ocular structures, such as the retina. The HA molecule forms large, open coils with its anionic sites spread apart. This arrangement of small-diameter fibers separated by highly hydrated glycosaminoglycan chains permits the transmission of light to the retina with minimal scattering.[9] Furthermore, these open coils can become highly entangled in the vitreous body with many electrostatic interactions. These interactions can influence osmotic pressure, ion transport and distribution, electric potentials within the vitreous, and vitreous collagen fibril assembly.[10,11]

Hyaluronan-collagen binding. Type II collagen binds to HA with a binding affinity of 755 nM.[12] It has been proposed that HA stabilizes vitreous gel via long-range spacing, but studies using HA lyase found that the gel structure was not destroyed.[13] Vitreous collagen fibrils are believed to form a crosslinked polymer system with HA, with collagen providing structural support, and osmotically active HA adding bulk to the gel.

Hyaluronan lipid binding. In addition to collagen, HA might bind to vitreous phospholipids, thereby disrupting their physiologic interaction with collagen and promoting undesirable vitreous liquefaction. Based on the binding affinity of HA and phospholipids, however, only about 4% of the hydrophobic hydrogens of the HA molecules in human vitreous would be expected to bind to phospholipids; thus, it is unclear whether this amount of binding has significant effects on vitreous liquefaction (Fig. 6.3).[14] Interestingly, diabetic patients who have earlier than expected vitreous liquefaction were found to have higher vitreous levels of lipids.[15,16] This could contribute to exacerbation of diabetic retinopathy (see further in chapter). As a corollary, it might be interesting to determine phospholipid levels in myopic eyes that have precocious vitreous liquefaction to determine if HA binding to phospholipids might play a role in disrupting normal vitreous physiology.

Chondroitin sulfate

Vitreous contains two chondroitin sulfate proteoglycans. The minor type is type IX collagen. The major type is versican, which forms complexes with HA and microfibrillar proteins such as fibulin-1 and fibulin-2.[17] Chondroitin sulfate protects against vitreous liquefaction by preventing collagen degradation, thus preserving gel vitreous structure.[18]

Heparan sulfate

Heparan sulfate is a sulfated galactosamine-containing glycosaminoglycan present in vitreous in small amounts. It is thought to be important in maintaining transparency by ensuring an adequate distance between vitreous collagen fibrils.[19]

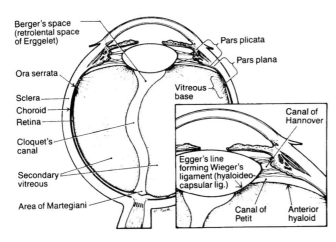

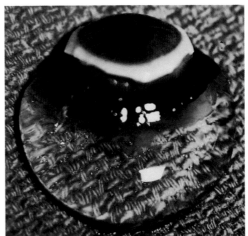

Fig. 6.1 Human vitreous body. *Right:* The sclera, choroid, and retina were dissected (postmortem) off the vitreous body in a 9-month-old child. Still attached to the anterior segment and situated on a surgical towel exposed to room air, the vitreous body maintains its solid gel state owing to the young age of the donor. *Left:* Schematic diagram of the human vitreous demonstrates important relations to surrounding tissues. Wieger's ligament is the attachment of vitreous to the lens. Berger's space and Cloquet's canal are the former sites of the embryonic hyaloid artery. The vitreous base straddles the ora serrata and is important in retinal detachments and proliferative vitreo-retinopathy. The area of Martegiani can be identified on swept source optical coherence tomography imaging. The posterior vitreous cortex is important in various vitreo-maculopathies (as discussed in the chapter text).

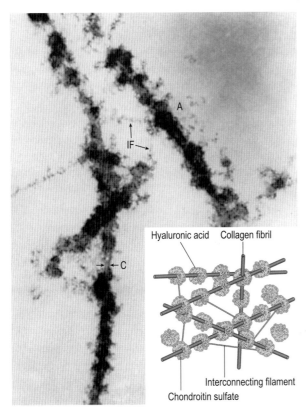

Fig. 6.2 Ultrastructure of hyaluronan/collagen interaction. Postmortem specimen was fixed in glutaraldehyde/paraformaldehyde and stained with ruthenium red. Collagen fibrils (C) are coated with amorphous material (A) believed to be hyaluronan (HA). The amorphous material may connect to the collagen fibril via another glycosaminoglycan, possibly chondroitin sulfate (see inset). Interconnecting filaments (IF) appear to bridge between collagen fibrils, inserting or attaching at sites of HA adhesion to collagen fibrils (bar = 0.1 μm). (From Asakura A. Histochemistry of hyaluronic acid of the bovine vitreous body as studied by electron microscopy. *Acta Soc Ophthalmol J.* 1985;89:179.)

Vitreous collagens

Vitreous collagen fibrils are thin, with diameters of approximately 10 to 20 nm. They are composed primarily of type II collagen (75%) surrounding a central core of a hybrid of types V/XI (10%), with chondroitin sulfate side-chains of type IX collagen (15%) located on the surface of the fibril (Fig. 6.4). At physiologic pH, vitreous collagen undergoes fibrillization with crosslinkages between lysyl and hydroxylysyl residues, catalyzed by copper-dependent lysyl oxidase. This fibrillization and crosslinkage adds tensile strength and mechanical stability.[20] At higher ionic strengths, collagen fibrils increase in size and decrease in concentration, which may be relevant to the pathophysiology of vitreous collagen aggregation during age-related fibrous liquefaction.[11]

Type II collagen

Type II collagen is the most prevalent type of collagen found in human vitreous. It is composed of three identical alpha chains that form a triple helix. This helix is stabilized by hydrogen bonds between opposing residues in different chains.[21,22] Although the cell type responsible for vitreous collagen synthesis is not known (retinal Müller cells, hyalocytes, and ciliary body epithelial cells are candidates), type II collagen is first synthesized as a soluble procollagen and excreted into the extracellular space, where it is then cleaved by *N*-proteinase and *C*-proteinase enzymes. The resulting collagen molecule is reduced in solubility and able to form fibrils through covalent crosslinkages. On the surface of the fibril are *N*-propeptides, which bind growth factors such as transforming growth factor (TGF)-β_1 and bone morphogenic protein-2.[23] This affinity for growth factors may contribute to proliferative vitreo-retinal disorders.[24] Additionally, alternative splicing of type II collagen propeptides is important in the pathogenesis of hereditary vitreo-retinopathies, most commonly Stickler syndrome, which is the most frequent inherited cause of retinal detachment.[21]

Type IX collagen

Type IX collagen is a disulfide bonded heterotrimer that is secreted as a mature collagen and does not undergo processing prior to incorporation onto the surfaces of the major collagen fibrils. It contains both

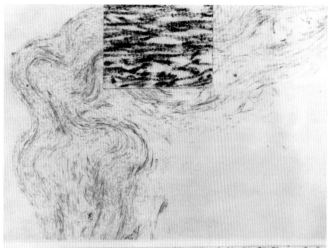

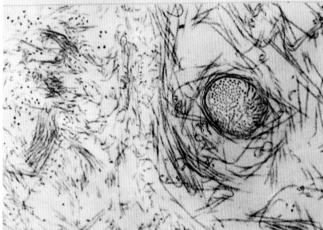

Fig. 6.3 Ultrastructure of human vitreous. *Upper:* Transmission electron microscopy of human vitreous showing the organization of collagen fibrils into larger fibers. Inset demonstrates the striated pattern of collagen. (From Sebag J, Niemeyer M, Koss M. Anomalous PVD & vitreoschisis. In: Sebag J, ed. *Vitreous: in Health and Disease.* New York: Springer; 2014:241–265.) *Lower:* Postmortem specimens centrifuged to concentrate structural elements but containing no membranes or membranous structures. Only collagen fibrils detected, at times organized in bundles of parallel collagen fibrils such as the one shown here in cross-section (*to right*). (From Sebag J, Balazs EA. Morphology and ultrastructure of human vitreous fibers. *Invest Ophthalmol Vis Sci.* 1989; 30:1867–1871.)

collagenous and noncollagenous regions, as well as a covalently linked chondroitin sulfate glycosaminoglycan chain, allowing the molecule to assume a proteoglycan form.[25] Type IX collagen modulates the spatial arrangement of collagen fibrils by both bridging together and spacing apart individual fibers.[20] Age-related changes in type IX collagen may play an important role in the age-related aggregation of vitreous collagen fibrils. There are also reports of mutations in type IX collagen causing ocular manifestations in some forms of Stickler syndrome.[26,27]

Type V/XI collagen

Collagen types V and XI are found complexed into a "hybrid" configuration located in the core of the major vitreous collagen fibrils (Fig. 6.4).[28] These collagens are secreted as procollagens with subsequent processing removing the C-propeptide and partially removing the N-propeptide.[29] The hybrid type V/XI collagen forms heterotypic fibrils, with type V collagen playing an essential role in the initiation

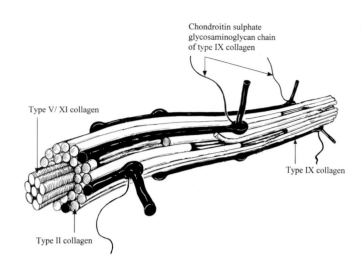

Fig. 6.4 **Human vitreous collagen fibril.** Type II collagen surrounds a core of type V/XI collagen. Chondroitin sulfate chains of type IX collagen are found on the surface, likely mediating interactions with other components of vitreous. (Reprinted from Bishop PN. The biochemical structure of the mammalian vitreous. *Eye.* 1996;10:664–670.)

of collagen fibril formation.[30] This suggests that hybrid V/XI collagen could also play an important role in vitreous fibril assembly.

Type VI collagen

Type VI collagen is found in small amounts within the vitreous body. It can bind both type II collagen and HA, suggesting a potential role for organizing the supramolecular structure of vitreous. It may also play a role in promoting vitreo-retinal adhesion because type VI collagen has been identified at the vitreo-retinal interface and is known to bind vitreous type II collagen, as well as type IV collagen found in the inner limiting membrane of the retina.[31]

Type VII collagen

Type VII collagen has been found at the vitreo-retinal interface, suggesting a role in mediating vitreo-retinal adhesion.[32]

Non-collagenous structural proteins
Fibrillins

Fibrillin-1 and fibrillin-2 are found in vitreous, but it is unknown whether these microfibrils contribute significantly to vitreous structure.[20] Mutations in fibrillin-1 cause Marfan syndrome, which features ocular manifestations of lens dislocation, myopia, and rhegmatogenous retinal detachment.

Fibulins

Fibulins are a family of extracellular matrix glycoproteins that are thought to have bridging roles in extracellular matrix assembly, including interactions with versican and fibronectin.[20] However, it is not known whether fibulins contribute significantly to the structural stability of vitreous.

Versican

Versican is a large chondroitin sulfate proteoglycan with an N-terminal domain that binds to HA. Mutations in the gene encoding versican can cause "*versican vitreo-retinopathy*" with retinal detachment and dystrophy.[33] Wagner syndrome of erosive vitreo-retinopathy is a hereditary condition with vitreous abnormalities caused by splice site mutations in the versican gene.[34,35]

Opticin

Opticin is a small leucine-rich repeat proteoglycan that is bound to the surface of heterotypic collagen fibrils and is expressed by nonpigmented ciliary epithelium.[36,37] Opticin has antiangiogenic properties by coating collagen fibrils and weakening integrin-mediated endothelial cell adhesion to collagen, thereby inhibiting integrin-mediated signaling required for angiogenesis.[20] Opticin also plays a role in preventing the aggregation of collagen fibrils in vitreous, thus promoting transparency.

Supramolecular organization

Vitreous collagen fibrils are widely spread apart with significant amounts of proteoglycans between fibrils. The average mesh size through which endogenous or exogenous materials can diffuse through the vitreous body is 550 ± 50 nm.[38] The surface of the fibril has N-propeptide extensions of the hybrid V/XI collagen and type IX collagen with extensions of its chondroitin sulfate chains, which mediate interactions with other extracellular matrix molecules.[21] Throughout the vitreous body, collagen fibrils interpenetrate complexes of HA molecules, forming a crosslinked polymer system.[39] Studies have shown that if collagen is removed, the remaining HA forms a viscous solution, whereas if HA is removed, the gel shrinks.[10] This suggests that collagen fibrils provide structure to the vitreous, which is then "inflated" by the osmotic contribution of hydrophilic HA. Both collagen and HA contribute to vitreous viscoelasticity.[40] Collagen, HA, and other proteoglycans all work synergistically to maintain vitreous stiffness, with HA as the key mediator of vitreous adhesivity.[41]

Dissolved substances

Dissolved substances in the vitreous body are inorganic and organic compounds as shown in Table 6.1, where serum values are given for comparison.[42,43]

Vitreous plasma gradients

Gradients of salts and organic substances exist in both directions between vitreous and plasma (Table 6.1).[44] These gradients result from several mechanisms: blood-aqueous and blood-retinal barriers, metabolism in the retina and ciliary body, and diffusion through the vitreous body,[45-49] especially for small molecules.

Regional differences

Oxygen tension is lower in the center of the vitreous body, due to oxygen flux from the retina toward vitreous corresponding to arterioles; the flux goes in the opposite direction corresponding to venules.[50,51] Glucose concentration is highest in the center, followed by the posterior vitreous body, with the lowest concentrations anteriorly.[52] Lactate is found at highest concentrations in the posterior vitreous, with decreasing concentrations more anteriorly.[52]

ANATOMY

The vitreous body

The mature vitreous body is a transparent gel (Fig. 6.1, right) occupying the center of the eye. It is almost spherical, except for the anterior part, which is concave, corresponding to the presence of the crystalline lens. The mean vitreous chamber volume is 4.65 ± 0.43 mm³ for women and 4.97 ± 0.47 mm³ for men, with a significant positive correlation with axial length, and a negative correlation between age and vitreous (gel) volume.[53] Histologic studies of vitreous structure introduce artifacts owing to specimen dehydration; thus, dark-field slit microscopy has been instrumental in the study of vitreous anatomy (Fig. 6.5).

TABLE 6.1 Concentration of chemical substances in the vitreous body

	Vitreous	Serum
Sodium (mmol/L)	146.7	139.7
Potassium (mmol/L)	5.73	4.25
Chloride (mmol/L)	121.6	104.4
Calcium (mmol/L)	1.128	2.368
Magnesium (mmol/L)	0.900	0.871
Glucose (mmol/L)	2.97	6.16
Lactate (mmol/L)	3.97	0.84
Copper (µmol/L)	0.519	16.35[a]
Zinc (µmol/L)	1.95	9.73[a]
Selenium (µmol/L)	0.1035	1.00[a]
Iron (µmol/L)	3.11	19.95[a]
Ferritin (µg/L)	19.5	101[b]
Transferrin (g/L)	0.0878	0.2394[b]

[a]Data from Baudry J, Kopp JF, Boeing H, Kipp AP, Schwerdtle T, Schulze MB. Changes of trace element status during aging: Results of the EPIC-Potsdam cohort study. *Eur J Nutr.* 2020;59(7):3045–3058.
[b]Data from *National Report on Biochemical Indicators of Diet and Nutrition in the U.S. Population 1999–2002*. Department of Health and Human Services, Centers for Disease Control and Prevention; 2008:1–155. Accessed January 5, 2022. https://www.cdc.gov/nutrition report/99-02/pdf/nutrition_report.pdf.
All other data from Kokavec J, Min SH, Tan MH, et al. Biochemical analysis of the living human vitreous. *Clin Experiment Ophthalmol.* 2016;44(7):597–609.

Anterior and posterior vitreous cortex

The outermost part of the vitreous, called the *cortex* (not *"hyaloid"*, which is a term that should only be used to refer to the embryonic artery), is divided into an anterior cortex ("hyaloid face") and a posterior cortex, the latter being approximately 100-µm thick. The cortex consists of densely packed collagen fibrils. Vitreous base collagen fibers insert anterior to the ora serrata (linear junction between the retina and the pars plana ciliaris) forming the anterior loop. In youth, the peripheral and posterior vitreous cortex can be seen as a thin, membranous structure that is continuous from the ora serrata to the posterior pole with greater light scattering than in the central vitreous (Fig. 6.6; Fig. 6.7, top panel). By middle age, there are visible fibers that arise from the vitreous base and course continuously to the posterior pole of the fundus (Fig. 6.7, middle panel). In addition to vitreous fibrils, there are larger fibers oriented perpendicular to the retina that insert into the extracellular matrix between the retina and vitreous body.[54] By old age, these fibers become aggregated and tortuous, associated with liquid vitreous (Fig. 6.7, bottom panel).

Hyalocytes. Hyalocytes are mononuclear cells embedded in the posterior vitreous cortex (Fig. 6.8A) anterior to the inner limiting membrane (ILM) of the retina (Fig. 6.8C). Although there are similarities with microglia due to a common embryologic origin, microglia are cells of the retina, while hyalocytes are cells of the vitreous body.[55,56] Sized about 10 to 15 µm in diameter, hyalocytes are oval-, spindle-, or star-shaped, depending upon their state of activity, (i.e., dormant, activated, phagocytosing, migrating, etc).[55,56] The highest density of hyalocytes is near the vitreous base, followed by the posterior pole, with the lowest density at the equator of the ocular fundus.[55,56] Utilizing staining and confocal imaging modalities, hyalocytes have historically been studied *ex vivo* (Fig. 6.8A,B). But recent technologic advances[56] have enabled hyalocyte imaging in vivo via B-scan optical coherence

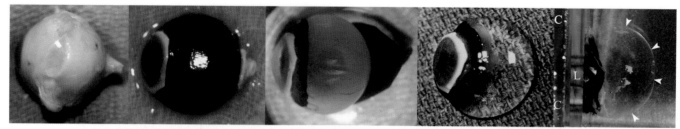

Fig. 6.5 Human vitreous dissection. The sclera, choroid, and retina were dissected off the vitreous body, which remains attached to the anterior segment. A band of gray tissue can be seen posterior to the ora serrata. This is peripheral retina that is firmly adherent to the vitreous base and could not be dissected. The specimen is mounted on a lucite frame (L) using sutures through the limbus and is then immersed in a lucite chamber (C) containing an isotonic, physiologic solution that maintains the turgescence of the vitreous and avoids collapse and artifactual distortion of vitreous structure (*white arrowheads*). (From Sebag J, Silverman RH, Coleman DJ. To see the invisible—the quest of imaging vitreous. In: Sebag J, ed. *Vitreous: in Health and Disease.* New York: Springer; 2014:193–222.)

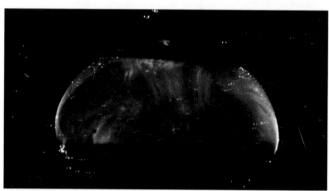

Fig. 6.6 Human vitreous structure during childhood. Dark-field slit microscopy of the dissected vitreous body from a 6-year-old child demonstrates light scattering from the dense collagen matrix of the mid-peripheral/equatorial vitreous cortex with embedded hyalocytes (highly refractile pin-point spots). No visible fibers are present in the central vitreous body. (From Sebag J. *The Vitreous: Structure, Function, and Pathobiology.* New York: Springer-Verlag; 1989:79.)

tomography (OCT) (Fig. 6.8C) and adaptive optics scanning light ophthalmoscopy (AO-SLO) in the coronal plane (*en face*) (Fig. 6.8D, top). Such studies in humans revealed hyalocytes in the temporal retina and near the optic disc with regular spatial separation in healthy subjects, which contrasted with nonuniform distribution and altered morphology in patients with retinopathies.[57,58] Coronal plane imaging in vivo has also led to the observation that these cells migrate over time (Fig. 6.8D, bottom).

Physiologic functions of hyalocytes include phagocytosis and antigen processing, as well as recruitment of circulating monocytes in response to antigens.[59,60] Transcriptional analysis has shown strong gene expression for processes related to antigen processing, presentation, and immune modulation, including the *SPP1*, *FTL*, *CD74*, and *HLA-DRA* genes.[61] Compared with other myeloid cell lines, the main differences in hyalocytes were the significantly increased expression of genes related to immune privilege of the eye, including *POMC*, *CD46*, and *CD86*.[61] Other potential hyalocyte physiologic functions relate to metabolism, including ongoing synthesis and metabolism of glycoproteins, as well as possible synthesis of collagen and enzymes.[52,62–64] Hyalocytes have been found to be located in the regions with the highest concentration of HA, suggesting they may be responsible for

vitreous HA synthesis.[65] Enzymes for HA synthesis have been found within hyalocytes, and hyalocytes have been shown to take up and internalize labeled intermediates for HA synthesis.[63,65] In turn, HA may have a regulatory effect on hyalocyte phagocytic activity.[55]

Pathologically, hyalocytes can induce collagen gel contraction in response to platelet-derived growth factor and other cytokines, causing tangential vitreo-retinal traction.[66,67] Hyalocytes might also play a role in retinal neovascularization. Boneva et al.[68] analyzed samples of retinal neovascularization from patients with proliferative diabetic retinopathy and found increased M2 macrophages within fibrovascular membranes, postulated to be derived from vitreous hyalocytes. This hypothesis was supported by the staining of cultivated vitreous hyalocytes, which revealed a strong expression of α-smooth muscle actin (α-SMA). As α-SMA is a marker for myofibroblasts, these results suggest that hyalocytes can differentiate into myofibroblasts and might therefore comprise part of the fibrovascular membrane in neovascularization.[68]

Vitreous base

The vitreous base is a three-dimensional zone, best conceived as a "doughnut" or "bagel" straddling the ora serrata. It extends from approximately 2-mm anterior to the ora serrata to about 3-mm posterior to the ora serrata, and it is several millimeters thick. Collagen fibrils are densely packed in this region, inserting anterior and posterior to the ora serrata (Fig. 6.9, left). Fibers can be seen within the vitreous base that course over the ora serrata, forming the "anterior loop" (Fig. 6.9. right), an important structure in anterior proliferative vitreo-retinopathy.

The vitreo-retinal interface

The vitreo-retinal interface is defined as the fascial (sheet-like) apposition of the outer surface of the posterior vitreous cortex and the inner surface of the ILM of the retina (Fig. 6.10).[69–73]

Inner limiting membrane of the retina

The ILM is 1- to 3-μm thick, consisting of type IV collagen (more abundant on the vitreous side) and laminin (more abundant on the retinal side)[74] (Fig 6.10B). There are also glycoproteins, type VI collagen, which may contribute to vitreo-retinal adhesion, and type XVIII collagen, which binds opticin and prevents cell migration from the retina into the vitreous body.[23,75–79] The ILM is multilayered and can be considered the basal lamina of Müller cells, the foot processes of which insert into the interface (Fig. 6.11). Adjacent to Müller cell footplates is

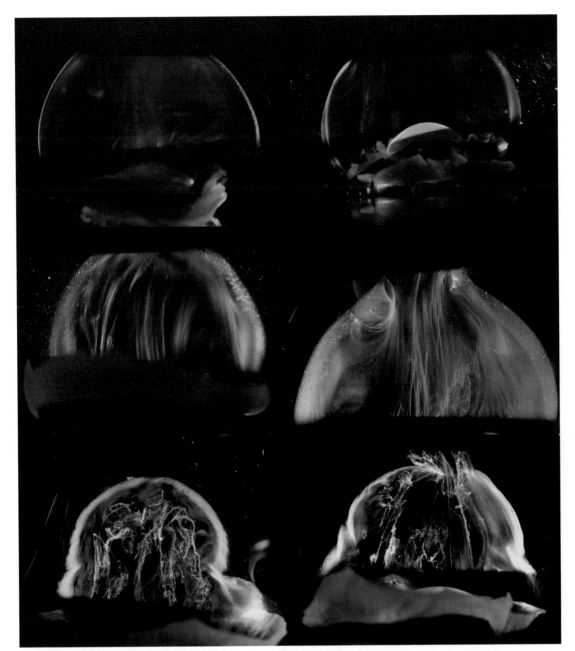

Fig. 6.7 Dark-field slit microscopy of human vitreous body. *Top:* Dark-field slit microscopy of the vitreous body in children is devoid of light-scattering structures except for dense collagen matrix of the peripheral vitreous cortex. *Middle:* In middle age, there are macroscopic fibers oriented anteroposteriorly. *Bottom:* By old age, vitreous fibers become thickened and tortuous, associated with areas of liquefied vitreous. (From Sebag J, ed. *Vitreous: in Health and Disease*. New York: Springer; 2014:245.)

the lamina rara externa that is 0.03- to 0.06-μm thick with no changes related to topography or age. The lamina densa (central lamella) is thinnest at the fovea (0.01–0.02 μm).

Posterior vitreous cortex/inner limiting membrane adhesion

The vitreous cortex is firmly attached to the ILM in the vitreous base region, around the optic disc (Weiss ring), along retinal blood vessels, and in the area surrounding the fovea to a diameter of 500 μm.[80,81] There is no vitreous cortex over the optic disc, and the cortex is thin over the macula. Vitreo-retinal adhesion is strong in young individuals, and dissection of the retina from vitreous often leaves inner retinal tissue adherent to the vitreous cortex.[76,80,82,83] (Fig. 6.11) Under pathologic conditions, the strong adhesion between the posterior vitreous cortex and the retinal ILM plays an important role, as is discussed next.

Intervening extracellular matrix. The interface between vitreous and adjacent structures consists of a complex formed by the outer vitreous complexed with basal laminae, which are firmly attached to their cells.[84] It is currently believed that an extracellular matrix "glue" of fibronectin, laminin, and other extracellular matrix components exists between vitreous and retina, causing adhesion to be fascial (sheet-like), as opposed to focal or linear.[66,85,86] Chondroitin sulfate is present at the

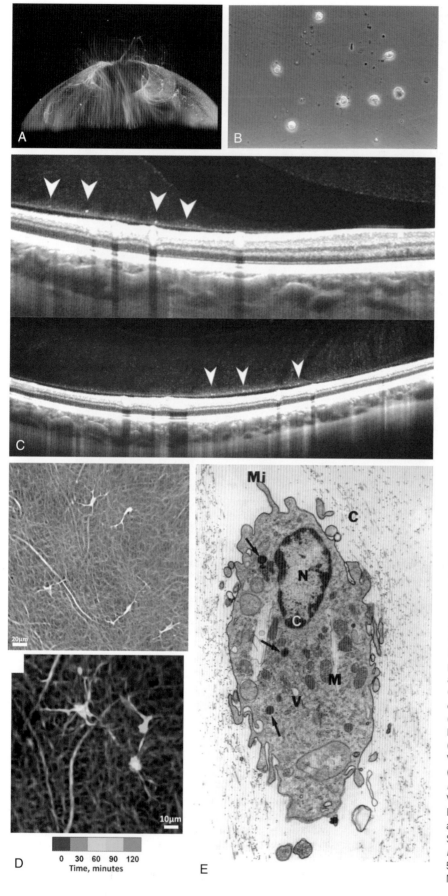

Fig. 6.8 Human hyalocytes. Hyalocytes can be seen in the posterior vitreous cortex by dark-field slit microscopy (**A**), phase contrast microscopy (**B**), B-scan optical coherence tomography (OCT) (**C**), coronal plane adaptive optics OCT imaging (**D**), and transmission electron microscopy (**E**). (**D**) *Top:* in vivo coronal plane (*en face*) AO-SLO imaging of human hyalocytes. Note the different morphologic appearances—star-shaped, spindle-like, and ameboid. *Bottom:* superimposed coronal plane OCT images with point-to-point registration demonstrate the migration of hyalocytes over 2 hours. (**E**) *Black* C: collagen fibrils of the vitreous cortex; N: lobulated nucleus with dense marginal chromatin (*white* C); M: mitochondria; *arrows:* dense granules; V: vacuoles; Mi: microvilli. Magnification = 11,670×. (A,B: From Sebag J. *The Vitreous: Structure, Function, and Pathobiology.* New York: Springer-Verlag; 1989:49; C: Courtesy of M. Engelbert, MD, PhD, New York; D: Courtesy of Toco Y. P. Chui, PhD and Richard B. Rosen, MD, New York; E: From Sebag J. *The Vitreous: Structure, Function, and Pathobiology.* New York: Springer-Verlag; 1989: 50; courtesy of JL Craft and DM Albert, Harvard Medical School, Boston, Mass.)

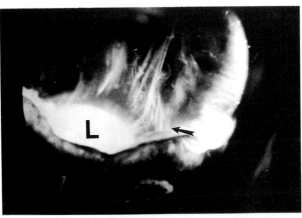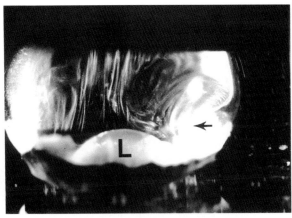

Fig. 6.9 Dark-field slit microscopy of anterior human vitreous. *Left*: Fibers course from the peripheral vitreous across the ora serrata forming the "anterior loop" (*arrow*), which is important in the pathophysiology of anterior proliferative vitreo-retinopathy. L, Crystalline lens. (From Sebag J. *The Vitreous: Structure, Function, and Pathobiology*. New York: Springer-Verlag; 1989:42.) *Right*: Fibers splay out to insert into the vitreous base both anterior and posterior to the ora serrata, forming the anterior loop (*arrow*). L, Crystalline lens. (From Sebag J. *The Vitreous: Structure, Function, and Pathobiology*. New York: Springer-Verlag; 1989:41.)

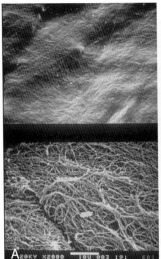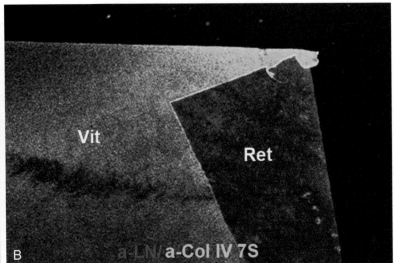

Fig. 6.10 Vitreo-retinal interface. (A) The vitreo-retinal interface consists of two major components: the outer surface of the posterior vitreous cortex, composed of a dense matrix of collagen (primarily type II) fibrils (*lower image*) and the inner surface of the inner limiting membrane (ILM) of the retina (*upper image*). The ILM is composed of three parts: the lamina rara interna, lamina densa, and lamina lucida. Between the ILM and the posterior vitreous cortex is a "glue" composed of typical extracellular matrix components. (Upper image from Sebag J, Hageman G. *Interfaces*. Rome: Fondazione G. B. Bietti and Farina Publishing; 2000:48; Lower image from Sebag J. *The Vitreous: Structure, Function, and Pathobiology*. New York: Springer-Verlag; 1989:47.) **(B)** Immunofluorescence of human vitreo-retinal interface demonstrates the predominance of laminin (*green*) on the vitreal side and type IV collagen (*red*; 7 S domain of coll IVα3) on the retinal side of the interface. (From Halfter W, Cunningham ET, Sebag J. Vitreo-retinal interface and ILM. In: Sebag J. *Vitreous: in Health and Disease*, New York: Springer; 2014:179.)

sites of strong vitreo-retinal adhesion such as the vitreous base and optic disc, forming the rationale for pharmacologic vitreolysis using avidin-biotin complex chondroitinase.[87,88]

Topographic variations
Strength of vitreo-retinal adhesion
Vitreous is attached to all contiguous structures but is most firmly adherent at the vitreous base.[70] There are also topographic differences posteriorly, with greater adhesion at the posterior pole than the equator.[76]

Peripheral fundus and vitreous base
There is a high density of collagen fibrils oriented at right angles to the inner surface of the ciliary epithelium and peripheral retina. Vitreous fibrils attach to the basement membrane of the nonpigmented epithelium of the pars plana portion of the ciliary body and the ILM of the peripheral retina, interwoven with the intervening extracellular matrix.[89] Within the vitreous base, there are several anatomic variations where vitreo-retinal adhesion is firm, predisposing to peripheral retinal breaks.[90–92]

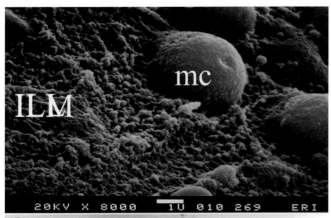

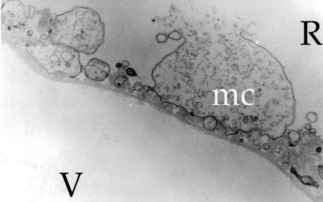

Fig. 6.11 Human Müller cell footplates. Transmission electron microscopy of human vitreo-retinal interface demonstrates the insertion of the footplates of Müller cells (mc) into the vitreo-retinal interface. *V*, Vitreous; *R*, retina. (From Sebag J. *Vitreous – in Health & Disease.* New York: Springer; 2014:248.)

Interface along major retinal blood vessels

The ILM thins and is sometimes absent over major retinal vessels.[93,94] At such points, vitreous may be embedded within the retina, directly continuous with perivascular tissue. These form attachments called "vitreo-retinovascular bands" or "spider-like bodies," that are vitreous fibrils traversing the ILM to coil about retinal vessels.[95,96]

Vitreo-macular interface

Attachment of vitreous to the macula occurs in an irregular, annular zone of 3- to 4-mm diameter, generally not visible by clinical examination in normal adults but possibly evident in fetal and young adult eyes and in pathologic conditions.[55] The posterior vitreous cortex is thinner over the macula in a disc-shaped area about 4 to 5 mm in diameter. Discontinuity of the ILM in the fovea may be a site where glial cells extend into the vitreo-retinal interface.[97]

Vitreo-papillary interface

The ILM ceases at the rim of the optic disc, although the membrane continues as the inner limiting membrane of Elschnig.[71] This 50-nm thick membrane is believed to be the basal lamina of the astroglia in the optic nerve head. At the central-most portion of the optic disc the membrane thins to 20 nm, follows the irregularities of the underlying cells of the optic disc, and is composed only of glycosaminoglycans and no collagen (central meniscus of Kuhnt). Given that the ILM prevents the passage of cells, the thinness and chemical composition of the central meniscus of Kuhnt and the membrane of Elschnig may account for frequent cell proliferation from or near the optic disc.[98]

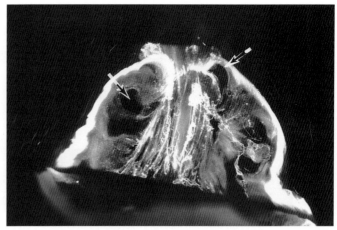

Fig. 6.12 Human vitreous structure in old age. Dark-field slit microscopy of dissected vitreous body in an 88-year-old woman demonstrates advanced fibrous liquefaction with pockets of liquid vitreous, called lacunae (*arrows*). (From Sebag J. *The Vitreous: Structure, Function, and Pathobiology.* New York: Springer-Verlag; 1989:88.)

Vitreous attachment to the optic disc may persist even though vitreous is detached elsewhere. Vitreo-papillary adhesion may be fortified by epipapillary membranes.[99,100] The entire complex may subsequently detach, resulting in a Weiss ring which can cause floaters, and when extensive, results in *vision degrading myodesopsia.*

VITREOUS BIOPHYSICS

Transvitreous transport

As mentioned previously, the average mesh size through which endogenous or exogenous materials can diffuse is 550 ± 50 nm.[38] Intravitreal drug injection is one of the most common ophthalmic procedures performed to introduce exogenous substances for medicinal purposes. Pharmacotherapy via intravitreal injection would theoretically be greatly improved if more were known about how substances traverse vitreous to access the fundus. Unfortunately, there is a paucity of such information. Furthermore, there is no consideration given to controlling the location of drug injection during clinical treatments. It stands to reason that drug distribution will be very different if introduced into an area of gel vitreous as opposed to a pocket of liquid vitreous, called a *lacuna* (Fig. 6.12). Assuming a homogeneous structure in the vitreous body, (which is probably not true because common conditions like myopia, diabetes, and aging substantially alter vitreous structure), injected substances may move through the vitreous body by two different processes: diffusion or convective flow. Both diffusion and convective flow are inversely related to vitreous viscosity.[101]

Diffusion

Transvitreous diffusion has been examined in humans using fluorescein as a tracer to measure the biophysical behavior of the gel during vitreous fluorophotometry (Fig. 6.13). Although this testing modality generated considerable interest in the past, there have never been clinical applications that resulted in enhanced care. One possible reason is that the models do not take into consideration the profound heterogeneity in vitreous structure with age, myopic vitreopathy, and diabetic vitreopathy (see further in chapter), which are likely to impact the physiology of transvitreous diffusion and the pharmacokinetics and pharmacodynamics of drugs injected into the vitreous body. It is generally believed that diffusion is the primary mechanism of drug delivery during intravitreal pharmacotherapy.[94] However, this is likely

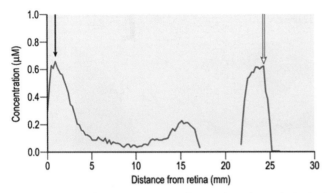

Fig. 6.13 Vitreous fluorophotometry. A scan along the optical axis of the eye was obtained 60 min after intravenous injection of fluorescein. The *black arrow* indicates the retina, the *open arrow* the fluorescein concentration in the anterior chamber. The autofluorescence signal from the lens has been removed. Note a small peak behind the lens (~15 mm from the retina) due to fluorescein leaking from the anterior chamber into the vitreous body. (From Lund-Andersen H, Sander B. The Vitreous. In: *Adler's Physiology of the Eye*. Saunders; 2011:169.)

to be an oversimplification because the distribution of a particular molecule in the vitreous gel versus time occurs according to the diffusion properties of that molecule. The mesh size of bovine vitreous has been estimated to be about 500 nm, which is much larger than the biologics typically used in intravitreal injections (typically <10 nm).[38,102] Thus, vitreous is believed to allow relatively unrestricted diffusion for smaller particles.[103] However, the diffusion of positively charged molecules is restricted in vitreous, due to the overall negative charge of the vitreous body.[103] Liquefaction (myopia, diabetes, aging, or vitrectomy) causes the viscosity of vitreous to approach that of water promoting modest increase in particle diffusion. This is likely significant for larger molecules, although the effects of vitreous liquefaction may be less significant for smaller drug molecules given that the mesh size prior to liquefaction already does not restrict diffusion.[103] The presence of ocular barriers to the systemic circulatory system is the probable explanation for why transient changes in systemic circulating drug levels are reflected slowly in the vitreous body.

The rate of change of the vitreous body concentration of various substances, most notably potassium, can be used in forensic medicine to rapidly and reliably assist with postmortem time of death determination.[45,104–108] Postmortem analyses can also reveal electrolyte abnormalities and hyperglycemia, which can help elucidate contributing causes of death.[106] Zilg et al.[106] found that samples from the left vs. right eye, and center vs. whole vitreous samples, all gave similar results. The time constants for many substances are of the same magnitude as those describing glucose transport between blood and brain; that is, half of the maximum is achieved in approximately 10 minutes.[109]

Convective flow

In addition to diffusion, molecules can move through the vitreous via convective flow, also referred to as bulk flow. Convective flow occurs as aqueous permeates posteriorly through the vitreous body.[110] Low-molecular-weight substances move faster, diffusing in all directions, and are virtually unaffected by convective flow. However, high-molecular-weight substances move through the vitreous body more via convective flow.[110,111] The velocity of posteriorly directed convective fluid flow in rabbit eyes has been estimated at 2×10^{-5} cm/min.[112]

Half-lives of intravitreal drugs range from less than 10 hours for small molecule drugs, to around 1 week for biologics.[113] Drug

elimination from the vitreous body can occur via anterior elimination through aqueous humor outflow and posterior elimination via the blood-ocular barriers,[103] which consist of tight junctions with a pore size of about 2 nm.[103] The permeability of the blood-ocular barriers appears to be the rate-limiting step for smaller molecules, with small lipophilic drugs exhibiting higher rates of clearance.[103,114] There are conflicting reports in the literature about whether biologics are primarily eliminated via the anterior or posterior pathway, but more recent modeling studies and findings of rabbit and human studies of bevacizumab concentrations in aqueous humor indicate that proteins such as anti-vascular endothelial growth factor (anti-VEGF) molecules are likely mainly eliminated via the anterior pathway.[103,115–117] Strategies to reverse this might increase drug levels at the macula and possibly improve efficacy, as well as decrease the need for frequent reinjection. Drugs can also be taken up by the retina via receptor-mediated endocytosis by Müller cells, which may play an important role in retinal pharmacokinetics.[103] Lastly, endogenous proteases might also play a role in drug degradation.

Traditional compartmental pharmacokinetic models assume a homogenous drug concentration, but this is likely not realistic given the heterogeneous nature of the vitreous body at different ages and in different diseases. Finite element modeling (FEM)-based models build upon the traditional compartmental model by using three-dimensional models with thousands of microscopic compartments that are associated with specific tissues and incorporate tissue-specific physiologic data.[118,119] These newer models have afforded helpful insights into vitreous pharmacokinetics. Studies by Zhang et al.[120] have shown that significant mixing occurs immediately after injection, with intravitreal drugs occupying 2 to 10 times their initial injected volume. The exact degree of mixing likely varies depending on viscosity of the drug and vitreous viscosity, which may vary based on factors such as age, myopia, diabetes, and prior ocular procedures.[120] Peak intravitreal drug concentrations vary depending on injection factors such as needle position, needle gauge, and speed of injection.[110,120] However, the long-term drug concentration profiles are apparently less impacted by initial distribution and depend primarily on the injected dose.[118,120] In these studies, clearance of intravitreal drugs depended on molecular size, and retinal delivery of drugs depended on RPE and ILM permeability, consistent with the aforementioned.

EMBRYOLOGY AND DEVELOPMENT

The vitreous body develops through two embryologic stages called the primary and secondary vitreous. Older literature speaks of a tertiary vitreous, but this is actually the zonular system of the lens composed of elastin and not vitreous collagen. A significant limitation in our understanding of vitreous embryology is the lack of a clear understanding about which cells synthesize various components of the vitreous body and at what time points in development.

Primary vitreous

In early stages, the optic cup is mainly occupied by the lens vesicle. As the cup grows, it is filled by fibrillar material, presumably secreted by the cells of the embryonic retina, but possibly the ciliary epithelium. Later, with penetration of the hyaloid artery, more fibrillar material apparently originating from the cells of the walls of the embryonic vasculature and adjacent cells (hyalocytes?) fills the space between the developing lens and retina.[5,121–124]

Inner limiting membrane and Bruch's membrane continuity

During invagination of the optic vesicle the primary vitreous forms between the lens and the ILM of the retina. It is noteworthy that the

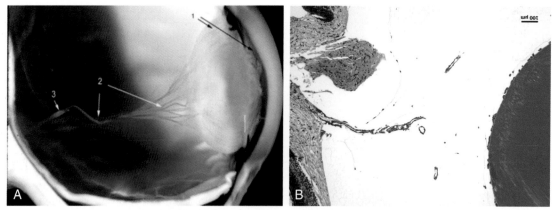

Fig. 6.14 Fetal vitreous vasculature. The hyaloid artery arises from the optic disc, branches throughout the vitreous body as the vasa hyaloidea propria, and anastomoses with the tunica vasculosa lentis. **(A)** Photomicrograph: 1 = tunica vasculosa lentis, 2 = vasa hyaloidea propria, 3 = hyaloid artery. (From Yee K, et al. Vitreous cytokines and regression of the fetal vasculature. In: *Vitreous: in Health and Disease*. New York: Springer; 2014:42.) **(B)** Histologic section with H&E staining (bar = 100 μm). (Courtesy of Greg Hageman, PhD.)

ILM is continuous with Bruch's membrane (Fig. 6.14), demonstrating a common embryologic origin with analogous molecular composition and structure, suggesting important similarities later in life.[75,125]

Secondary vitreous

The *secondary vitreous* appears at the end of the 6th week, associated with increasing size of the vitreous body and regression of the hyaloid vasculature. Primordial cells of the primary vitreous differentiate into hyalocytes and fibroblasts in the secondary vitreous.

Regression of hyaloid vascular system

A unique aspect of vitreous development is growth (Fig. 6.15) and regression (Fig. 6.16) of the fetal hyaloid vasculature during the first two trimesters of human embryogenesis. Vitreous vascularization begins with the hyaloid artery entering the nascent eye through the optic cup. By 10 weeks' gestation (WG), the hyaloid system is well established, branching to form the vessels of the vasa hyaloidea propria, which anastomose to a dense capillary network surrounding the lens, the tunica vasculosa lentis.[126] Maximal development of the hyaloid vasculature is reached by 12 to 13 WG.[125] Regression of the fetal hyaloid vasculature results from downregulation of cell metabolism driven by reactive oxygen species-induced apoptosis, and concurrent upregulation of connective tissue synthesis in the extracellular space (Fig. 6.16).[127]

In a proteomics study[128] of vitreous bodies from 17 human embryos aged 14 to 20 WG, 1217 proteins were detected, of which 768 proteins were not previously identified in the literature. After quantile normalization and variance filtering, 206 unique proteins were analyzed, finding that the peptide counts of 37 proteins changed significantly from 14 to 20 WG: 9 decreased while 28 increased. Among those with decreased expression were cofilin-1, which has been shown to promote/mediate angiogenesis; peroxiredoxin, which may play an antioxidant protective role; and the glycolytic enzyme enolase. Notable in the group that increased were pigment epithelium-derived factor, which has been shown to be important in antiangiogenesis, and cytochrome C, a known mediator of developmental apoptosis. Immunohistochemistry localized proteins to the hyaloid artery, vasa hyaloidea propria, and tunica vasculosa lentis (Fig. 6.17), and changes were noted during this period of vitreous embryogenesis. For example, clusterin and cadherin were not detected in 14 WG vitreous but did appear in the hyaloid

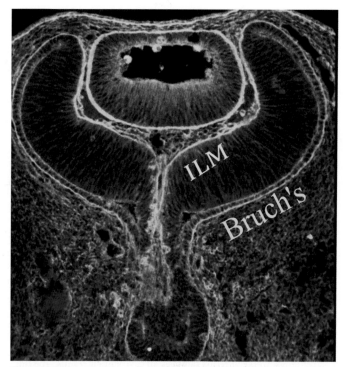

Fig. 6.15 Human embryonic eye. After invagination of the optic cup, vitreous begins to form between the lens and retina. At this time there is continuity between the inner limiting membrane of the retina and Bruch's membrane. (From Sebag J, Hageman G. *Interfaces*. Rome: Fondazione G. B. Bietti & Farina Publishing; 2000, cover photo.)

vasculature by 18 WG. This is consistent with the increase in peptide counts detected in the proteomic analyses.

Fetal hyaloid vessels show clear signs of regression by 13 to 15 WG, beginning in the vasa hyaloidea propria followed by the tunica vasculosa lentis, and then the pupillary membrane.[24,126] This regression may be induced by decreased levels of VEGF along with autophagy and apoptosis.[129–131] Blood flow in the hyaloid artery ceases at the 240-mm stage (7 months' gestation).[125] Regression of the vessel begins with glycogen and lipid deposition in the endothelial cells and

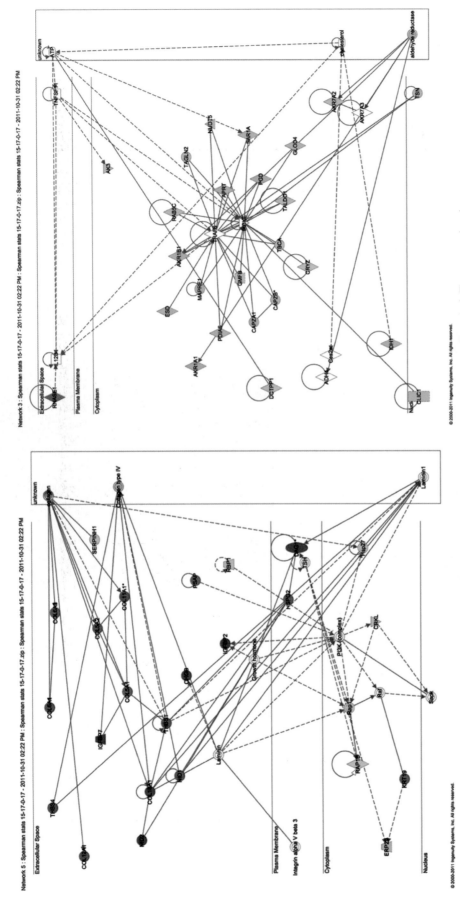

Fig. 6.16 Bioinformatics of human embryonic vitreous proteomic profiles. *Left:* The connective tissue pathway is upregulated, consistent with the formation of a collagenous secondary vitreous ($P < 10^{-56}$). The overwhelming majority of this activity occurs in the extracellular space (*red* = upregulated). *Right:* The small molecule biochemistry pathway shows reduced activity, suggesting a role for reactive oxygen species–driven apoptosis and a reduction in cellular processes as the acellular secondary vitreous is formed and the hyaloid vasculature regresses ($P < 10^{-42}$) (*green* = downregulated). (From Yee KMP, Feener E, Gao B, Aiello LP, Madigan MC, Provis J, Ross-Cisneros F, Sadun AA, Sebag J. Vitreous cytokines and regression of the fetal hyaloid vasculature. In: Sebag J, ed. *Vitreous: in Health and Disease.* New York: Springer; 2014: 41–56.)

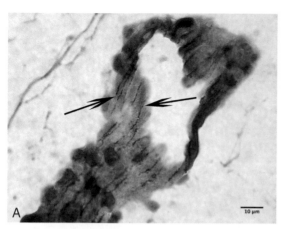
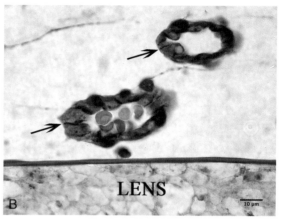

Fig. 6.17 Immunohistochemistry of human fetal vasculature. Dystroglycan is a transmembrane scaffold protein (laminin receptor dystrophin-associated glycoprotein) involved in adhesion-mediated signaling. This is important in the formation of glio-vascular connections, cerebral vascularization, and formation of the blood-brain barrier. Immunostaining confirmed the presence of dystroglycan on cell membranes and cell junctions of the endothelial cells in the hyaloid vessels of a 14 weeks' gestation human. (A) Hyaloid artery. (B) Tunica vaculosa lentis. (From Yee KMP, Feener E, Gao B, Aiello LP, Madigan MC, Provis J, Ross-Cisneros F, Sadun AA, Sebag J. Vitreous cytokines and regression of the fetal hyaloid vasculature. In: Sebag J, ed. *Vitreous: in Health and Disease.* New York: Springer; 2014:41–56.)

pericytes of the hyaloid vessels.[132] Endothelial cell processes fill the lumen, and macrophages form a plug that occludes the vessel. The cells in the vessel wall then undergo necrosis and are phagocytosed by hyalocytes.[133] Dying endothelial cells project into the capillary lumen and interfere with blood flow, stimulating synchronous apoptosis of downstream endothelial cells ("secondary apoptosis") and ultimately obliteration of the vessel.[134] Vessel atrophy begins posteriorly, leading to the prevailing concept that posterior development of the avascular secondary vitreous induces regression of the vascular primary vitreous in a posterior to anterior direction through displacement and compression. However, this prevailing concept has recently been challenged by Bu et al.,[135] who suggested that interactive remodeling of the developing vitreous may be the case, rather than displacement by the secondary vitreous.

After fetal hyaloid vessel regression, the main hyaloid artery leaves in its wake a tubular structure surrounded by the secondary vitreous. This courses from the retrolental space of Berger to the optic nerve (area of Martegiani) and is called *Cloquet's canal* (Fig. 6.1, right; Fig. 6.18). The studies of Jan Worst, who defined this as one of the cisterns within the vitreous body, suggest that this is a liquid-filled canal, which is likely to be true. Thus, the (intentional or incidental) injection of drugs into this structure might result in preferential transport to the optic disc, which might be beneficial or deleterious, depending upon the circumstances.

Growth

During childhood the vitreous body undergoes significant growth. The length in the newborn eye is approximately 10.5 mm, and by the age of 13 years, axial length increases to 16.1 mm in the male.[136] The average adult vitreous is 16.5 mm long.[53,137,138] Recent studies[53] using computed tomography (CT) imaging to measure the volume of the human vitreous "chamber" (not the vitreous body) found a volume of 4.65 ± 0.4 mm³ for women and 4.97 ± 0.5 mm³ for men. There was a significant correlation between vitreous chamber volume and age, as well as axial length. Although this study did improve upon previous ones by excluding contributions of the retina and choroid, the state of the actual vitreous body was not assessed; specifically, there was no

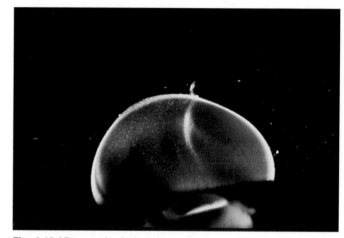

Fig. 6.18 Vitreous body in a human embryo. Dark-field slit microscopy of dissected vitreous body in a 33 weeks' gestational age human demonstrates intense light scattering from the vitreous cortex. Other than the remnant of the hyaloid artery, there is no light scattering within the central vitreous. (From Sebag J. *The Vitreous: Structure, Function, and Pathobiology.* New York: Springer-Verlag; 1989:77.)

consideration given to the presence or absence of posterior vitreous detachment and how that influences volumetric measurements of the vitreous body itself.

Developmental anomalies

Developmental anomalies can arise from inherited genetic abnormalities, irregular vitreous development, or abnormal regression of fetal hyaloid vessels,[139] resulting in persistent fetal vasculature (PFV) syndrome, which accounts for 4.8% of blindness in infants.[140] Abnormal fetal vasculature regression occurs in 95% of premature infants and 3% of full-term infants, owing to multiple causes.[141,142] The majority of cases are sporadic, but some are inherited. Studies have found that the germline deletion of Bim, a proapoptotic factor, results in persistent hyaloid vasculature, increased retinal vascular density, and stunted retinal vessel regression in response to hyperoxia.[143] Astrocytes have been shown to ensheath persistent hyaloid arteries in cases of PFV, suggesting a role in the persistence of these fetal vitreous vessels.[144] Many other genes, growth factors, and molecular pathways have been implicated, including the Wnt signaling pathway, VEGF, and apoptotic factors such as p53 and angiopoietin 2.[145] Incomplete regression of the hyaloid vasculature might underlie the presence of branching linear structures within the vitreous body that sometimes cause floaters and vision degrading myodesopsia (see section: Symptomatic posterior vitreous detachment). Indeed, given that both incomplete embryonic vessel regression and myopia are developmental abnormalities, there may be shared pathogenetic aspects that underlie myopic vitreopathy, a leading cause of vision degrading myodesopsia.[125,146]

VITREOUS AGING

The vitreous body undergoes considerable physiologic changes during life that have great impacts on its structure and function. The fundamental aging change is fibrous liquefaction of the gel structure. This process begins early in life and progresses until about 70% of patients develop advanced, symptomatic, fibrous liquefaction by their eighth decade of life.[147] (Fig. 6.19)

Molecular mechanisms of vitreous aging

Fibrous vitreous liquefaction likely begins as a result of changes in both HA and collagen that alter the interaction of these two macromolecules. The apparent molecular weight of vitreous collagen increases with age because of the formation of new covalent crosslinks between the peptide chains, equivalent to the aging process of collagen elsewhere in the body.[148] Bundles of collagen fibrils become biomicroscopically visible as coarse linear opacities.[149] The etiologic importance of HA is suggested by the finding that eyes with posterior vitreous detachment (PVD) have a lower concentration of HA than eyes with an attached vitreous.[150] Vitreous dehydration from a decrease in HA concentration with age has been proposed as causative, since HA concentrations increase from anterior to posterior and are inversely correlated with viscosity.[151] However, some investigators have challenged this assertion, demonstrating that even if more than 90% of vitreous

HA is depolymerized, the vitreous body does not liquefy, although the volume of the gel decreases.[13]

Aging processes that are common in skin and other connective tissue of the body are likely also important in vitreous. In particular, the cumulative effect(s) of light exposure and nonenzymatic glycation seem relevant. Both HA and collagen may be affected by free radicals in the presence of a photosensitizer such as riboflavin (present in the eye), which has been shown to induce vitreous liquefaction after irradiation with white light.[152] Enzymatic and nonenzymatic crosslinking of vitreous proteins have also been demonstrated with aging and diabetes.[153–155] Other studies have identified breakdown products of type II collagen, as well as proteolytic enzymes such as trypsin-1 and trypsin-2 in human vitreous.[156–158] Nonenzymatic glycation induces a Maillard reaction forming covalent bonds between amino groups and glucose leading to insolubilized proteins, known as advanced glycation end-products (AGEs), and protein crosslinking. Slow-turnover proteins of the lens and vitreous accumulate AGEs over years resulting in significant structural abnormalities.[83,159,160] There are also physiologic consequences, as evidenced by a decrease in vitreous permeability to fluorescein (Fig. 6.13).[161] It is not known how the concurrence of age-related or myopia-associated vitreous gel liquefaction influences this phenomenon. This aging process is promoted by ultraviolet light[162] and accelerated in patients with diabetes[153–155] whose vitreous glucose concentration is doubled compared with controls.[48]

Other mechanisms are probably involved. Although type IX collagen only accounts for 15% of total human vitreous collagen, its location on the surface of vitreous collagen fibrils could make it very important for the maintenance of the gel structure by mediating interactions with other extracellular matrix components, most notably HA.[163] In the adult there is no evidence of physiologic (only pathologic) synthesis of vitreous collagen. With aging, there is a loss of type IX collagen from the surface of these fibrils,[164] which has been shown to cause type II collagen aggregation.[164] Type II collagen has alternative splicing within the second exon where mutations result in significant vitreous liquefaction in Stickler syndrome.[20,165] Such mechanisms may also be important in age-related liquefaction. Additionally, the network density of collagen decreases in childhood owing to the growth of the eye, which could destabilize the gel. On the other hand, HA concentration is increased, promoting gel stabilization.[22] The concentration of electrolytes, soluble protein, and other substances such as metalloproteinases may change.[166,167] The soluble protein concentration increases with age owing to an increase in the leakage through the blood-retinal barrier, which may play a role both in the normal aging process and in pathologic conditions such as diabetic vitreo-retinopathy.[5]

Structural changes
Fibrous liquefaction

Vitreous gel liquefies throughout life (Fig. 6.19). The structural correlates of vitreous liquefaction are fibers, which can be observed *in vivo* with slit-lamp biomicroscopy and *in vitro* using dark-field microscopy (Figs. 6.7, 6.9, 6.12). Ultrasonography has great utility in characterizing vitreous structure *in vivo* (Figs. 6.20, 6.21),[168] and OCT imaging is being developed to provide more detailed assessments.[169] In youth, the vitreous body is optically empty apart from the posterior and peripheral vitreous cortex (Fig. 6.6; Fig. 6.7, top panel; Fig. 6.18). Following HA dissociation from collagen, vitreous collagen fibrils crosslink, fusing laterally into increasingly larger aggregates (Figs. 6.7, 6.9), and with increasing age these fibers become thickened[149] and associated with pockets of liquid vitreous called *lacunae*,[55] which coalesce over time (Fig. 6.12). These parallel fibers have an anterior-posterior orientation (Fig. 6.7, middle panel) circumferential with the vitreous cortex, inserting into the vitreous base peripherally (Fig. 6.9). Ponsioen et al.[170] have postulated that the formation of fibrous aggregates in the vitreous

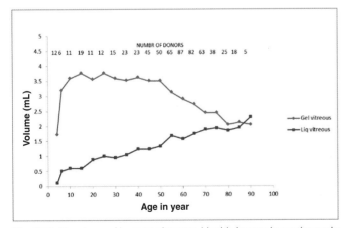

Fig. 6.19 Rheology of human vitreous. Liquid vitreous is continuously formed throughout life, attaining more than 50% of total vitreous volume by old age. (Modified from Balazs EA, Denlinger JL. Aging changes in the vitreous. In: *Aging and Human Visual Function*. New York: Alan R. Liss; 1982:45–57.)

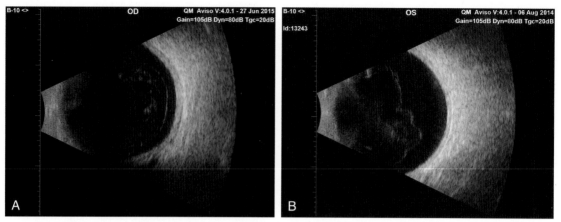

Fig. 6.20 Ultrasonography of posterior vitreous detachment. (A) Vertical B-scan of posterior vitreous detachment (PVD) demonstrating the posterior vitreous cortex positioned anterior to the retina (*left of fundus in this image*). **(B)** Vertical B-scan of PVD showing the posterior vitreous cortex positioned anterior to the retina, but considerably farther from the fundus than in (**A**).

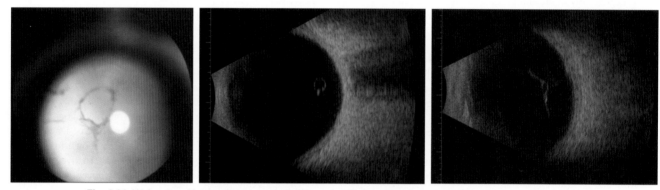

Fig. 6.21 Weiss ring. Fundus photography (*left image*) and ultrasonography (*middle image*) demonstrate the appearance of a Weiss ring in vivo. This develops following posterior vitreous detachment when peripapillary tissue is torn away by the detaching posterior vitreous cortex (*right image*).

body is the result of active, enzyme-mediated remodeling and not necessarily a degenerative process. The formation of large collagenous vitreous fibers could also result from fibrosis, a major cause of aging throughout the body.[171,172] In the vitreous body, this could be mediated by fibroblasts that constitute 10% of the vitreous cell population.[173] Gärtner[174] suggested that fibroblasts are responsible for aging changes in the collagen network of the vitreous base; thus, they may also play a role in the vitreous body itself.

Fibrous vitreous liquefaction occurs earlier and more extensively in myopic eyes,[175] but can be accelerated by inflammation, trauma, and in arthro-ophthalmopathies.[176–178] In a series of investigations using India ink injection in the vitreous body, Worst[179–181] showed that the adult vitreous body is composed of cisterns, the most prominent being the bursa premacularis. Using fluorescein staining, Kishi and Shimizu[182] confirmed the presence of this liquefied premacular structure. Associations between the bursa premacularis of Worst and myopia have been described.[183] The presence and magnitude of this premacular bursa could influence intravitreal pharmacotherapy of the macula and optic nerve if the drug is injected into a lacuna or cistern, as this will likely affect pharmacokinetics and result in altered pharmacodynamics.[97,184] This approach could potentially be improved with a more individualized assessment of vitreous anatomy and enhanced localization of intravitreal drug administration.

Weakening of vitreo-retinal adhesion

In youth, there is firm adhesion between the posterior vitreous cortex and ILM of the retina.[76,185–187] Vitreo-retinal adhesion is often reported to be greater at the equator than the posterior pole, but greatest at the vitreous base. Using a rotational peel device in human autopsy eyes, Creveling et al.[186] determined that the maximum peel force at the equator was greater than in the posterior pole, especially in younger eyes (donors 30–39 years of age). After 60 years of age, there was a significant decrease in equatorial and posterior pole adhesion. The factors underlying these observations are not known, because little is known about the actual mechanisms of vitreo-retinal adhesion. With aging, there is a significant increase in ILM thickness, which may play a role in the weakening of vitreo-retinal adhesion with age.[187] Russell[188] proposed that vitreous maintains adhesion to the retina via interactions between the ILM, a vitreous proteoglycan protein core, chondroitin sulfate glycosaminoglycans, opticin, and type II collagen of the posterior vitreous cortex. Ponsioen et al.[170] suggested dynamic remodeling with collagen synthesis and deposition at the interface, beginning very early and continuing throughout life. Oxidative stress and neurodegeneration have also been implicated.[189,190]

Peripheral fundus

Teng and Chi[191] found that the radial width of the vitreous base posterior to the ora serrata increases with age to over 3.0 mm. There is also posterior migration of the posterior border of the vitreous base with age, mostly temporally.[192] Additionally, there is the aforementioned lateral aggregation of collagen fibrils in the vitreous base of older individuals.[193] These changes all play important roles in the pathogenesis of peripheral retinal breaks and rhegmatogenous retinal detachment.

Posterior pole degenerative remodeling

Foos[194] defined a spectrum of changes in the ILM as "degenerative remodeling." Features include detachment and discontinuity of the ILM with vitreous collagen beneath the ILM, cellular debris with macrophages, and absence of Müller cell attachment plaques. In larger lesions, vitreous can insinuate into degenerative crypts and adhere to the cell membrane of the lining Müller cells that have no basal lamina. In the peripapillary area, retinal glial cells extend from the optic disc and are continuous with a glial epipapillary membrane that has vitreous fiber incarceration. Roth and Foos[100] observed nasal epipapillary membranes associated with Bergmeister papillae in 27.6% of autopsy cases.

Posterior vitreous detachment

PVD is defined as separation of the posterior vitreous cortex from the optic disc and ILM of the retina (Fig. 6.20).[195] PVD is believed to begin at the posterior pole in the perifoveal region,[196] although recent studies proposed that the onset location of PVD is more peripheral.[197] Innocuous PVD is a clean separation between the ILM and the cortical vitreous.[198] Whereas it is widely held that PVD is an "abnormal" event, it is possible that PVD may be a "preprogrammed" event that mitigates the risks of an attached vitreous, as in patients with pathologies such as diabetic retinopathy or age-related macular degeneration where an attached vitreous is more deleterious than a PVD.[195,199] Fortunately, PVD is innocuous in most cases and only anomalous in some instances (see further in this chapter).

Epidemiology

PVD is the most common event to occur in the human vitreous body, but its exact epidemiology is not known because the clinical diagnosis is unreliable, even when a Weiss ring (the circular defect in the posterior vitreous cortex that was the former site of vitreo-papillary adhesion) is seen on clinical evaluation by physical examination and imaging.[195,200] Estimates for PVD prevalence vary between studies depending upon the diagnostic modality used, but there is a gradual increase in prevalence with increasing age in all studies. The prevalence estimates are 1% to 2% in the fourth decade of life, increasing to 51% to 65% in the seventh decade of life, and further increasing to 72% to 100% in the ninth decade of life.[147,200–202] A study comparing PVD prevalence between White and Japanese patients found no differences between the two groups.[203]

Perifoveal PVD is a slow process occurring over many years, with only 10% of stages 1 and 2 PVD progressing to complete PVD over the course of 30 months.[196] One study found that after PVD in one eye, the fellow eye developed PVD within 3 years in 90% of cases.[204,205] Yonemoto and associates[206] determined that, in the general population, the average age of PVD onset was 61 years for emmetropia, with a younger age of onset at increasing levels of myopia. From these data, they determined that for each diopter of myopic refractive error, 0.91 years could be subtracted from the average age of PVD onset in emmetropic eyes. This was confirmed by Itakura and associates,[207] who used swept source OCT and found that highly myopic subjects with partial and complete PVD were younger than controls ($P < .0001$). It should be pointed out, however, that OCT is not an accurate way to diagnose PVD, as comparison with intraoperative findings determined a

predictive value of only 53%, leading the authors to recommend ultrasonography be used to diagnose PVD.[208]

Risk factors for PVD are age, myopia, female gender (attributed to postmenopausal loss of estrogen influencing HA metabolism and the accumulation of advanced glycation end-products), surgical aphakia, hereditary disorders of collagen metabolism, trauma, inflammation, retino-vascular disorders, and vitreous hemorrhage.[209–213] Decreased vitreous HA levels with aging have indeed been detected.[214]

Symptomatic posterior vitreous detachment

The most common effect of PVD is the onset of the visual phenomenon of *floaters*, or *myodesopsia* (derived from Greek: myiodes = fly-like, opsis = vision). According to a smartphone survey (possibly biased by a young demographic), floaters were reported in 76% of individuals, with 33% reporting visual impairment.[215] Studies have found that floaters have a significant negative impact on quality of life,[168] likely owing to a significant reduction in contrast sensitivity.[125,216] Floaters occur in late-stage PVD and typically result from shadows cast by aggregates of central vitreous fibers, the posterior vitreous cortex, and/or the Weiss ring (Fig. 6.21). Type IV collagen has been identified in the posterior vitreous of eyes with PVD, most likely derived from the ILM.[217] This suggests that in some cases of PVD there is unusually firm adhesion between the posterior vitreous cortex and the ILM, resulting in splitting between the lamellae of the ILM.[218] Greater amounts of ILM on the detached posterior vitreous might induce more light scattering and result in more bothersome floaters. An additional factor potentially causing light scattering in PVD is that once the posterior vitreous is detached, it occupies a smaller surface area with resultant folding of the posterior vitreous cortical surface (Fig. 6.22). This concept is supported by the fact that increased gel liquefaction is associated with PVD, likely because increased liquefaction leads to further anterior displacement and more surface folding.[125]

Floaters might also be influenced by differences in vitreous viscosity. During head turning and ocular saccades there is movement of the vitreous opacities that induce floaters, characterized by a lag and overshoot before coming to rest. Ultrasound studies of vitreous motion and

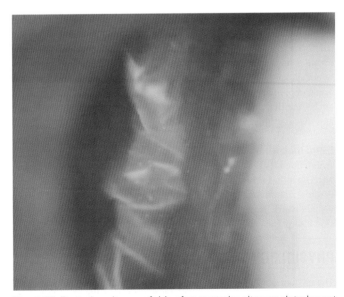

Fig. 6.22 Posterior vitreous folds after posterior vitreous detachment (PVD). Still photo from a slit-lamp video showing folds in the posterior vitreous of an eye with PVD. (Courtesy of Martin Snead MD. Director of Vitreoretinal Research. University of Cambridge, England.)

viscosity have demonstrated that the vitreous body of subjects younger than 46 years of age had significantly less speckle density and less overshoot time compared with older subjects.[219] These findings are consistent with the experience of older patients with acute symptomatic PVD whose symptoms likely arise from both opacities in the central vitreous body as well as movement of the detached and folded posterior vitreous cortex.

Anomalous posterior vitreous detachment

Anomalous PVD is the result of vitreous gel liquefaction without separation at the vitreo-retinal interface, resulting in persistent vitreo-retinal adhesion, or damage to the interface structures.[74,97] The resulting deleterious effects depend on where vitreous is most adherent to retina and which areas of the vitreous body are most liquefied (Fig. 6.23).

Full-thickness vitreo-retinal adhesion

Persistent vitreo-retinal adhesion that includes the entire thickness of the vitreous cortex can result in retinal tears in the peripheral fundus or traction at the posterior pole. Peripherally, vitreous remains attached to the retinal flap, which pulls away with movement of fluid, influenced by intraocular currents.[220] These retinal breaks can progress to retinal detachments, at rates that vary in the literature from 2% to 18%.[221,222] Full-thickness vitreous adhesion posteriorly can induce axial vitreo-macular traction with structural alteration of the underlying neural retina,[223–225] or tangential traction (see next section). Vitreo-macular adhesion is a risk factor for exudative age-related macular degeneration[226,227] and macular edema.[228]

Partial-thickness vitreo-retinal adhesion

Vitreoschisis occurs when the posterior vitreous cortex splits and the outer cortex remains attached to the peripheral retina or the posterior pole.[229] In the periphery, vitreoschisis leaves hyalocytes attached to the retina where they promote proliferative vitreo-retinopathy, as described by van Overdam.[58] Posteriorly, the pathologic manifestations depend on the level of the split in the posterior vitreous cortex. If the split is anterior to hyalocytes, these cells remain attached to the macula and recruit monocytes (from the circulation) and glial cells (from the retina), resulting in a hypercellular membrane.[97] This typically is accompanied by separation of the vitreous from the optic disc (present in ~90% of cases), with tangential traction directed inward toward the fovea (centripetal tangential traction), inducing retinal folds and macular pucker. If vitreoschisis occurs posterior to hyalocytes, a thin hypocellular membrane remains attached to the macula.[230] This often is accompanied by persistent adhesion of the vitreous to the optic disc, anchoring that produces outward (centrifugal) vitreo-macular traction and macular holes.[230,231]

Optic disc effects

Anomalous PVD with persistent adhesion to the optic disc can cause vitreo-papillary traction with resulting hemorrhage,[232] worsening neovascularization in proliferative diabetic retinopathy,[233] and gaze-evoked visual disturbances.[234] As mentioned previously, vitreo-papillary adhesion also plays a role in the formation of macular holes and cysts.[230]

PHYSIOLOGY

The normal physiologic functions of the vitreous body can be divided into four categories:

- Structural support
- Diffusion barrier between the anterior and the posterior segments of the eye

- Metabolic buffer against oxidative stress
- Optical transparency

Structural support

Vitreous may be important in modulating growth of the eye by generating internal swelling pressure. If so, then irregularities in this process might play a role in the development of myopia. In blunt trauma, an intact vitreous body can absorb external forces and reduce mechanical deformation of the globe. The viscoelasticity of vitreous has always seemed important as a shock absorber, a phenomenon that has recently been studied experimentally.[235–237]

Diffusion barrier between anterior and posterior segments
Normal conditions

Because the healthy, young vitreous body is a solid gel, it has considerable barrier properties for bulk flow of substances between the anterior and posterior segments of the eye. Substances in the anterior segment of the eye will have difficulty reaching high concentrations in the posterior segment of the eye when the vitreous body is intact, because diffusion is slow and movement by bulk flow is very limited in a gel. An intact vitreous gel will also prevent topically administered substances from reaching the retina and the optic nerve in significant concentrations. Entrance of antibiotics from the bloodstream to the center of the vitreous will also be impeded by normal vitreous gel structure. The distribution of injected substances throughout the vitreous body varies according to the viscosity of the drug, the vitreous viscosity, and injection factors (see previously).[120] Vitreous viscosity is altered by factors such as age, myopia, and prior ocular procedures. Injection factors include needle position, needle gauge, and speed of injection.[110,120]

Pathologic conditions

If the vitreous body is partly removed, degenerated, or collapsed, the exchange between the anterior and posterior segments of the eye may be much faster. Such is the case when the lens is removed and anterior vitrectomy has been performed. Substances that are produced in the anterior segment of the eye or given topically enter the vitreous body through the violated barrier systems of the anterior segment (blood-aqueous barrier) and can be expected to reach the retina in higher concentrations than in eyes with an intact vitreous and an intact iridolenticular barrier.

Increased transit following liquefaction of the gel vitreous, whether from aging or from vitrectomy, has important consequences in many pathologies. For example, molecules such as VEGF can clear from the vitreous body/chamber faster and reduce the VEGF concentration to which the retina is exposed.[101] Accordingly, vitrectomy can improve conditions in ischemic retinopathies such as proliferative diabetic vitreo-retinopathy and retinal vein occlusions, reducing macular edema and retinal neovascularization, presumably by increasing intravitreal oxygen levels.[101,238–243]

Multiple studies have found higher rates of posterior vitreous attachment in patients with age-related macular degeneration (AMD),[214,226,227,244,245] with one study finding surgical evidence of vitreo-retinal attachment in 80% of patients undergoing vitrectomy for subretinal neovascularization.[246] Adherent vitreous over the macula may not allow VEGF and other cytokines to be cleared from the posterior segment, worsening disease.[101,247] Vitreo-macular adhesion can also lead to chronic low-grade inflammation, further contributing to macular pathologies.[248] While vitrectomy can promote egress of vasoproliferative factors from the posterior segment via the anterior segment, this can lead to neovascularization in the anterior segment

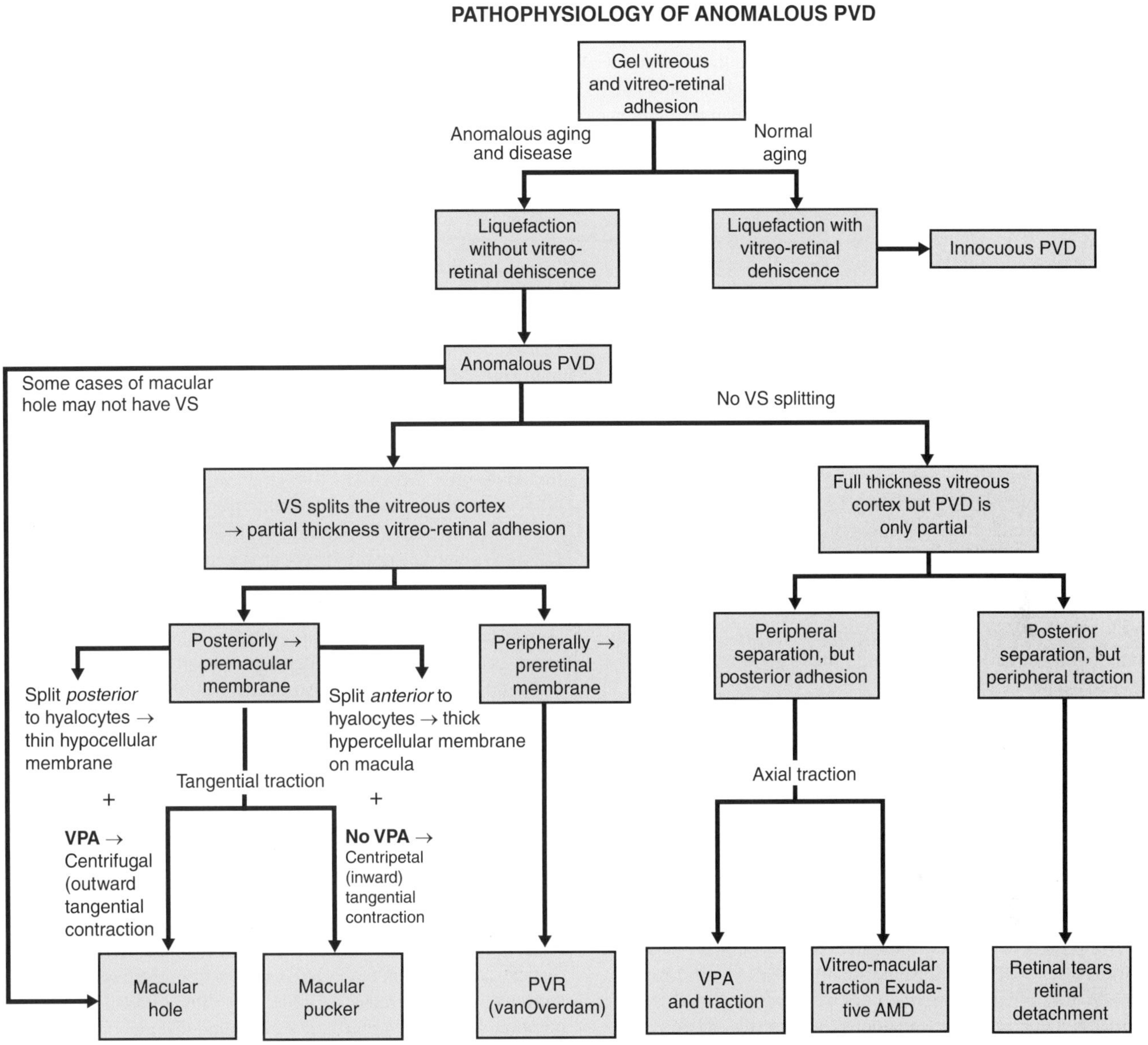

PATHOPHYSIOLOGY OF ANOMALOUS PVD

Fig. 6.23 Anomalous posterior vitreous detachment (APVD). The various possible manifestations of APVD are demonstrated in this flow diagram. When gel liquefaction and weakening of vitreo-retinal adhesion occur concurrently, the vitreous body separates away from the retina without sequelae (*top section of diagram*). If the gel liquefies without concurrent vitreo-retinal dehiscence, there can be various untoward consequences. If separation of vitreous from retina is full thickness but topographically incomplete, there can be different forms of partial PVD (*right side of diagram*). Posterior separation with persistent peripheral vitreo-retinal attachment can induce retinal breaks and detachments. Peripheral vitreo-retinal separation with persistent full-thickness attachment of vitreous to the retina posteriorly can induce traction upon the macula, where it promotes neovascular age-related macular degeneration (AMD), and optic disc, where it contributes to neovascularization and vitreous hemorrhage in ischemic retinopathies. If during PVD the posterior vitreous cortex splits (vitreoschisis), there can be different effects depending on the level of the split (*left side of diagram*). VPA, Vitreo-papillary adhesion; VS, vitreoschisis; PVD, proliferative vitreo-retinopathy.

and neovascular glaucoma. Indeed, patients with vitrectomized eyes, and especially vitrectomized/lensectomized eyes, were found to have increased rates of iris neovascularization.[249]

Vitreous can also influence the efficacy of pharmacologic substances. Whether this has major clinical significance is not known, but the condition of the vitreous body should be taken into consideration relative to ocular pharmacokinetics, both for topically and systemically applied agents. There is increasing evidence that the state of

vitreous has an effect on the therapeutic efficacy of pharmaceuticals, particularly for anti-VEGF therapy in AMD. Multiple studies have shown anti-VEGF therapy to be significantly less effective in the presence of vitreo-macular adhesion, necessitating more intensive therapy to prevent vision loss in these patients.[184,247,250–252] The attached vitreo-macular interface may inhibit the diffusion of anti-VEGF molecules across the dense collagen matrix of the vitreous into the retina, contributing to decreased efficacy. One postulated reason for decreased efficacy is the development of leaky blood vessels, which may affect the permeability of the blood-ocular barrier and thus affect the clearance of therapeutic drugs. Animal studies have shown that vitrectomy increased the clearance of $VEGF_{165}$ (tenfold in the rabbit)[253] and anti-VEGF drugs (fourfold greater clearance of bevacizumab in the monkey).[254] However, a review of pharmacokinetics in various pathologic conditions including choroidal neovascularization, diabetic retinopathy, cytomegalovirus retinitis, and postoperative endophthalmitis with and without core vitrectomy found only a modest effect on drug clearance (less than 1.5-fold).[103] While the animal studies strongly suggest that vitreous has an influence, further studies are needed to elucidate the exact mechanisms by which vitreous might influence posterior segment pharmacotherapy.

Oxygen transport

Vitreous contains oxygen gradients, with higher oxygen tension near the vascularized retina and pars plana, and lower oxygen tension in the central vitreous body.[255,256] Following liquefaction, oxygen transport is enhanced in areas with faster fluid currents.[101] Coupled with decreased vitreous oxygen consumption in liquefied vitreous, as described below the result is overall higher oxygen tension in liquefied vitreous and lack of significant oxygen gradients following vitrectomy.[255,256] This is supported by findings that preretinal oxygen tension is higher in diabetic patients, and oxygen content increases near the posterior lens after vitrectomy.[256-258] Finite element modeling of oxygen transport and consumption in vitreous by Filas et al.[255] found good reproduction of experimental data in humans.

Metabolic buffer against oxidative stress
Normal conditions

Because of the close anatomic relationship to the ciliary body and retina, the vitreous body can act as a metabolic buffer and, to a certain extent, a reservoir for metabolism in the ciliary body and retina. The ILM and the posterior vitreous cortex do not act as a diffusion barrier for smaller molecules, but because of the tight blood-retinal barrier, water-soluble substances in the retina have easier access to the vitreous body than to the bloodstream. Substances present in or produced by the retina are thus diluted by diffusing into the vitreous body. Likewise, glucose and glycogen in the vitreous body can support retinal metabolism, especially during anoxic conditions. Additionally, the footplates of Müller cells have close contact with the posterior vitreous (Fig. 6.11), so vitreous can act as a buffer in the physiologic functions of Müller cells. For example, vitreous plays a role in the buffering of potassium, which flows from the retina through the Müller cells and into the vitreous body.[259,260] This modulates potassium concentrations within the retina, important in neurotransmission.

Vitreous oxygen levels play an important role in lens physiology and cataract formation, vitreous surgery, AMD, and macular edema.[101,261-263] An important aspect of how vitreous modulates oxygen free radical damage is the presence of ascorbate. Studies of vitreous oxygen consumption have found that the vitreous consumes oxygen via an ascorbate-dependent chemical reaction.[264] Although synthesized by the ciliary body, ascorbate levels are higher in the posterior vitreous than centrally, presumably to protect the retina and optic disc from oxygen free radicals.[264,265] Many additional substances with antioxidant properties are found in vitreous, including riboflavin, glutathione, crystallin, cysteine, tyrosine, albumin, transferrin, pigment epithelium-derived factor (PEDF), selenium, zinc, and uric acid.[44,266-277] The vitreous body also contains enzymatic vitreous antioxidants, including superoxide dismutase, glutathione peroxidase, and catalase.[266,271,278,279] Moreover, proteomic studies have shown a high degree of spatial organization comparing four different areas of the human vitreous, suggesting that these proteins likely localize to different vitreous substructures to variably protect intraocular tissues from infection, oxidative stress, and energy disequilibrium.[280]

Pathologic conditions

Because normal retinal function is preserved following vitrectomy, the metabolic buffer functions of vitreous do not seem to play a major role in this aspect of ocular physiology. However, the condition of vitreous plays an important role in the concentration gradients of substances in the eye, as previously described in this chapter (section: Diffusion barrier between anterior and posterior segments). This appears to be quite important with respect to oxygen, owing to its significant downstream effects. Vitreous degeneration is associated with increased oxidative stress biomarkers, as well as proteolytic enzymes in vitreous.[155,280] Increased oxidative stress can exacerbate diabetic retinopathy and AMD.[266] Another effect of higher intravitreal oxygen tension is increased exposure of the lens to oxidative damage and the accelerated formation of nuclear cataracts.[256,258] Thus, although vitrectomy can increase oxygenation of hypoxic tissues and improve conditions such as diabetic retinopathy,[101] the removal of vitreous can have other untoward effects. It is known that gel vitreous has a higher concentration of ascorbate compared to liquefied vitreous, so that loss of gel vitreous via aging, pharmacologic vitreolysis, or vitrectomy results in an overall higher oxygen tension in the vitreous body, which can lead to oxidative damage to nearby structures.[255,256,262,264] Mitigating this to prevent postoperative cataract formation was the rationale underlying the strategy to preserve 3 to 4mm of intact gel vitreous behind the lens during vitrectomy for vision degrading myodesopsia.[125,281]

Another concern has been the question of an increased risk of open-angle glaucoma in patients following vitrectomy, with studies ranging from 15% to 20% and higher rates among pseudophakic compared with phakic eyes.[282-285] This may be due to increased oxidative damage to the trabecular meshwork, which can lead to increased intraocular pressure and glaucoma.[286] However, Stefansson[101] pointed out that the oxygen tension in the anterior chamber decreases after vitrectomy, as the transit of oxygen increases from the more oxygen-rich aqueous into the vitreous chamber, thus calling this mechanism into question. Indeed, a Mayo Clinic study found that among the cohort of patients who developed glaucoma, 27% had normal-tension glaucoma, suggesting that reduced aqueous outflow via the trabecular meshwork with increased intraocular pressure did not play a role.[282] Others have also disagreed with the postulate that vitrectomy induces chronic open-angle glaucoma.[287,288]

Vitreous oxygen and cataracts. As previously mentioned, vitreous oxygen promotes cataracts via the action of reactive oxygen species inducing crosslinking and aggregation of lens crystallins.[256,261] PVD and vitrectomy are known to increase intravitreal levels of oxygen. Thus, it was hypothesized that a limited approach to vitrectomy would not increase levels of intravitreal oxygen as much as extensive vitrectomy (Fig. 6.24). Thus, in performing limited vitrectomy for vision degrading myodesopsia (clinically significant vitreous floaters) in phakic patients, surgical PVD is avoided and 3 to 4 mm of retrolental gel vitreous is left intact.[289] Employing this limited approach, the incidence of cataract surgery in the total group of one study was 18%; average follow-up = 20 months. At 24 months after limited vitrectomy the incidence was 35%, compared with 87% after extensive vitrectomy.[281] The time to cataract surgery was also significantly longer following limited vitrectomy than after extensive vitrectomy. Another study with an average follow-up of 32.6 months found that

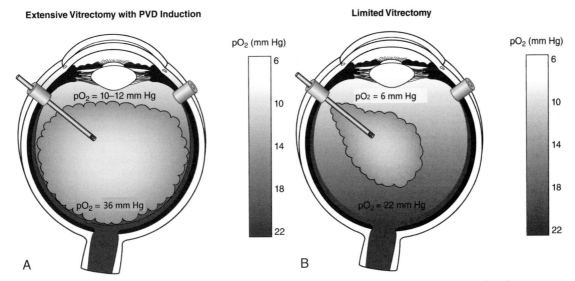

Extensive Vitrectomy with PVD Induction

pO₂ (mm Hg)

$pO_2 = 10\text{--}12$ mm Hg

$pO_2 = 36$ mm Hg

A

Limited Vitrectomy

pO₂ (mm Hg)

$pO_2 = 6$ mm Hg

$pO_2 = 22$ mm Hg

B

Fig. 6.24 Postvitrectomy oxygen levels. Following extensive vitrectomy with surgical posterior vitreous detachment (PVD) induction (**A**), intravitreal oxygen levels are considerably higher than following limited vitrectomy without PVD induction (**B**). Additionally, leaving intact gel vitreous behind the lens retains endogenous vitreous antioxidants that mitigate against the untoward effects of reactive oxygen species, further protecting against cataract formation. (From Huang LC, Yee KMP, Wa CA, Nguyen JN, Sadun AA, Sebag J. Vitreous floaters and vision – current concepts and management paradigms. In: Sebag J, ed. *Vitreous: in Health and Disease*. New York: Springer; 2014:771–788.)

the incidence of cataract surgery was only 16.9%.[290] The mean age of those requiring cataract surgery was 63 years, and no patient under the age of 53 years has required cataract surgery following limited vitrectomy.

Optical transparency
Normal conditions
Among the various physiologic functions of the vitreous body, transparency is key. Vitreous optical transparency is primarily due to the low concentration of structural macromolecules (<0.2% w/v) and soluble proteins (see previously). The scattering properties of the vitreous are anisotropic, and scatter decreases when the vitreous swells.[9] Transparency is maintained by the specific collagen/HA configuration, as well as various physiologic properties that inhibit intravitreal cell migration and proliferation. Indeed, HA specifically inhibits vascular endothelial cell proliferation[291] mitigating intravitreal angiogenesis, as well as the migration and proliferation of other cells.[292–296]

Pathologic conditions
Proangiogenic stimuli resulting from ischemia and inflammation can override the aforementioned physiologic properties that maintain vitreous transparency. Age-related fibrous liquefaction/degeneration of the vitreous body with the formation of vitreous opacities is a common process that interferes with the path of light. This is accentuated by PVD, as mentioned previously. However, not all patients with vitreous opacities experience overly bothersome floaters. When there is a negative impact on quality of life, as well as measurable alteration of the vitreous structure and degradation in vision, the term *vision degrading myodesopsia* applies.[125] Other examples of pathologic conditions that interfere with the normal path of light through the vitreous body include vitreous hemorrhage,[297] posterior uveitis,[298] myopic vitreopathy,[146] and diabetic vitreopathy.[299]

A major undesired effect of vitreous opacification is reduction in quality of life and vision[168] due to the degradation of contrast sensitivity,[125,300] which is exacerbated by PVD in both emmetropes[301] and

myopes.[146] Opacities in ocular media increase measurable ocular straylight, which is the spreading of light around a bright light source.[302] Patients perceive straylight effects as haziness, decreased color and contrast, difficulty recognizing faces, and glare hindrance.[303] However, some clinical conditions that fill vitreous with opacities, such as asteroid hyalosis, often do not impact vision.[302] It has been postulated that this is because the smooth surfaces of asteroid bodies do not scatter light in as disturbing a manner as the tortuous aggregates of vitreous fibers with nodularities and the folded detached posterior vitreous cortex with its dense matrix of collagen fibrils.[125,303,304]

CONCLUSIONS
Vitreous plays an important role in the physiology and pathophysiology of the eye. The former is emphasized in this chapter while the latter is only briefly reviewed here because it is explored in greater detail in other comprehensive writings.[125,305,306] The major physiologic functions are to provide structural support, to serve as a diffusion barrier between the anterior and the posterior segments of the eye, to provide metabolic buffering against oxidative stress, and to maintain optical transparency. Alterations in these important physiologic functions occur perinatally, with aging, in myopia, and as a result of diabetes, inflammation, and other conditions, all resulting in significant pathologic effects.[305,306] Future advances will require a better understanding of vitreous physiology to develop preventive strategies intended to mitigate the role of vitreous in ocular pathologies, for example, by inhibiting fibrous vitreous degeneration/liquefaction and anomalous PVD. Alternatively, strategies such as pharmacologic vitreolysis could be developed to induce an innocuous PVD in patients at high risk of anomalous PVD.[307–310] Another future consideration will be improving/expanding posterior segment pharmacotherapy via intravitreal drug application and release, including the optimization of vitreous influences on the use of viral vectors for gene therapy.[311] This will require a deeper understanding of vitreous biochemistry and structure to better understand effects on pharmacodynamics and pharmacokinetics.

ACKNOWLEDGMENTS

Support provided by the VMR Research Foundation, Newport Beach, CA (JS).

REFERENCES

1. Toledo OMS, Dietrich CP. Tissue specific distribution of sulfated mucopolysaccharides in mammals. *Biochim Biophys Acta BBA - Gen Subj.* 1977;498(1):114–122.
2. Meyer K, Palmer JW. The polysaccharide of the vitreous humor. *J Biol Chem.* 1934;107(3):629–634.
3. Balazs EA, Laurent TC, Jeanloz RW. Nomenclature of hyaluronic acid. *Biochem J.* 1986;235(3):903.
4. Nečas J, Bartošíková L, Brauner P, Kolar J. Hyaluronic acid (hyaluronan): A review. *Vet Med (Praha).* 2008(8):53.
5. Swann DA. Chemistry and biology of the vitreous body. *Int Rev Exp Pathol.* 1980;22:1–64.
6. Sheehan JK, Atkins EDT, Nieduszynski IA. X-ray diffraction studies on the connective tissue polysaccharides: Two-dimensional packing schemes for threefold hyaluronate chains. *J Mol Biol.* 1975;91(2):153–163.
7. Fraser JR, Laurent TC, Laurent UB. Hyaluronan: Its nature, distribution, functions and turnover. *J Intern Med.* 1997;242(1):27–33.
8. Balazs EA, Denlinger JL. The vitreous. In: Davson H, ed. *The Eye. Third Edition.* Cambridge, MA: Academic Press; 1984:533–589.
9. Bettelheim FA, Balazs EA. Light-scattering patterns of the vitreous humor. *Biochim Biophys Acta.* 1968;158(2):309–312.
10. Comper WD, Laurent TC. Physiological function of connective tissue polysaccharides. *Physiol Rev.* 1978;58(1):255–315.
11. Morozova S, Muthukumar M. Electrostatic effects in collagen fibril formation. *J Chem Phys.* 2018;149(16):163333.
12. Peng Y, Yu Y, Lin L, et al. Glycosaminoglycans from bovine eye vitreous humour and interaction with collagen type II. *Glycoconj J.* 2018;35(1):119–128.
13. Bishop PN, McLeod D, Reardon A. Effects of hyaluronan lyase, hyaluronidase, and chondroitin ABC lyase on mammalian vitreous gel. *Invest Ophthalmol Vis Sci.* 1999;40(10):2173–2178.
14. Ewurum A, Alur AA, Glenn M, Schnepf A, Borchman D. Hyaluronic acid-lipid binding. *BMC Chem.* 2021;15(1):36.
15. Schnepf A, Yappert MC, Borchman D. In-vitro and ex-situ regional mass spectral analysis of phospholipids and glucose in the vitreous humor from diabetic and non-diabetic human donors. *Exp Eye Res.* 2020;200:108221.
16. Schnepf A, Yappert MC, Borchman D. Regional distribution of phospholipids in porcine vitreous humor. *Exp Eye Res.* 2017;160:116–125.
17. Bishop PN. Structural macromolecules and supramolecular organisation of the vitreous gel. *Prog Retin Eye Res.* 2000;19(3):323–344.
18. Zhang Q, Filas BA, Roth R, et al. Preservation of the structure of enzymatically degraded bovine vitreous using synthetic proteoglycan mimics. *Invest Ophthalmol Vis Sci.* 2014;55(12):8153–8162.
19. Balazs EA, Sundblad L, Toth LZJ. In vitro formation of hyaluronic acid by cells in the vitreous body and by comb tissue. *Abstr Fed Proc.* 1958;17:184.
20. Bishop PN. Vitreous proteins. In: Sebag J, ed. *Vitreous: in Health and Disease.* New York: Springer; 2014:3–12.
21. Le Goff MM, Bishop PN. Adult vitreous structure and postnatal changes. *Eye.* 2008;22(10):1214–1222.
22. Sebag J. Macromolecular structure of the corpus vitreum. *Prog Polym Sci.* 1998;23:415.
23. Reardon A, Sandell L, Jones CJP, McLeod D, Bishop PN. Localization of pN-type IIA procollagen on adult bovine vitreous collagen fibrils. *Matrix Biol.* 2000;19(2):169–173.
24. Zhu M, Madigan MC, van Driel D, et al. The human hyaloid system: Cell death and vascular regression. *Exp Eye Res.* 2000;70(6):767–776.
25. Bishop PN, Crossman MV, McLeod D, Ayad S. Extraction and characterization of the tissue forms of collagen types II and IX from bovine vitreous. *Biochem J.* 1994;299(2):497–505.
26. Nikopoulos K, Schrauwen I, Simon M, et al. Autosomal recessive Stickler syndrome in two families is caused by mutations in the COL9A1 gene. *Invest Ophthalmol Vis Sci.* 2011;52(7):4774–4779.
27. Nixon TRW, Alexander P, Richards A, et al. Homozygous Type IX collagen variants (COL9A1, COL9A2, and COL9A3) causing recessive Stickler syndrome—Expanding the phenotype. *Am J Med Genet A.* 2019;179(8):1498–1506.
28. Zhidkova NI, Justice SK, Mayne R. Alternative mRNA processing occurs in the variable region of the pro-α1(XI) and pro-α2(XI) collagen chains. *J Biol Chem.* 1995;270(16):9486–9493.
29. Smith SM, Birk DE. Focus on molecules: Collagens V and XI. *Exp Eye Res.* 2012;98:105–106.
30. Wenstrup RJ, Florer JB, Brunskill EW, Bell SM, Chervoneva I, Birk DE. Type V collagen controls the initiation of collagen fibril assembly. *J Biol Chem.* 2004;279(51):53331–53337.
31. Ponsioen TL, van Luyn MJA, van der Worp RJ, van Meurs JC, Hooymans JMM, Los LI. Collagen distribution in the human vitreoretinal interface. *Invest Ophthalmol Vis Sci.* 2008;49(9):4089–4095.
32. Wullink B, Pas HH, Van der Worp RJ, Kuijer R, Los LI. Type VII collagen expression in the human vitreoretinal interface, corpora amylacea and inner retinal layers. *Plos One.* 2015;10(12):e0145502.
33. Tang PH, Velez G, Tsang SH, Bassuk AG, Mahajan VB. VCAN canonical splice site mutation is associated with vitreoretinal degeneration and disrupts an MMP proteolytic site. *Invest Ophthalmol Vis Sci.* 2019;60(1):282–293.
34. Rothschild P-R, Burin-des-Roziers C, Audo I, Nedelec B, Valleix S, Brézin AP. Spectral-domain optical coherence tomography in Wagner syndrome: Characterization of vitreo-retinal interface and foveal changes. *Am J Ophthalmol.* 2015;160(5):1065–1072.e1.
35. Araújo JR, Tavares-Ferreira J, Estrela-Silva S, et al. Wagner syndrome: Anatomic, functional and genetic characterization of a Portuguese family. *Graefe's Arch Clin Exp Ophthalmol.* 2018;256(1):163–171.
36. Reardon AJ, Le Goff M, Briggs MD, et al. Identification in vitreous and molecular cloning of opticin, a novel member of the family of leucine-rich repeat proteins of the extracellular matrix. *J Biol Chem.* 2000;275(3):2123–2129.
37. Bishop PN, Takanosu M, Le Goff M, Mayne R. The role of the posterior ciliary body in the biosynthesis of vitreous humour. *Eye Lond Engl.* 2002;16(4):454–460.
38. Xu Q, Boylan NJ, Suk JS, et al. Nanoparticle diffusion in, and microrheology of, the bovine vitreous ex vivo. *J Controlled Release.* 2013;167(1):76–84.
39. Tokita M, Fujiya Y, Hikichi K. Dynamic viscoelasticity of bovine vitreous body. *Biorheology.* 1984;21(6):751–756.
40. Sharif-Kashani P, Hubschman J-P, Sassoon D, Pirouz Kavehpour H. Rheology of the vitreous gel: Effects of macromolecule organization on the viscoelastic properties. *J Biomech.* 2011;44(3):419–423.
41. Filas BA, Zhang Q, Okamoto RJ, Shui YB, Beebe DC. Enzymatic degradation identifies components responsible for the structural properties of the vitreous body. *Invest Ophthalmol Vis Sci.* 2014;55(1):55–63.
42. Baudry J, Kopp JF, Boeing H, Kipp AP, Schwerdtle T, Schulze MB. Changes of trace element status during aging: Results of the EPIC-Potsdam cohort study. *Eur J Nutr.* 2020;59(7):3045–3058.
43. National Report on Biochemical Indicators of Diet and Nutrition in the U.S. *Population 1999–2002.* Department of Health and Human Services, Centers for Disease Control and Prevention; 2008:1–155. Accessed January 5, 2022. https://www.cdc.gov/nutritionreport/99-02/pdf/nutrition_report.pdf.
44. Kokavec J, Min SH, Tan MH, et al. Biochemical analysis of the living human vitreous. *Clin Experiment Ophthalmol.* 2016;44(7):597–609.
45. McNeil AR, Gardner A, Stables S. Simple method for improving the precision of electrolyte measurements in vitreous humor. *Clin Chem.* 1999;45(1):135–136.
46. Andersen MV. Changes in the vitreous body pH of pigs after retinal xenon photocoagulation. *Acta Ophthalmol.* 1991;69(2):193–199.
47. Reddy DVN, Kinsey VE. Composition of the vitreous humor in relation to that of plasma and aqueous humors. *AMA Arch Ophthalmol.* 1960;63(4):715–720.
48. Lundquist O, Osterlin S. Glucose concentration in the vitreous of nondiabetic and diabetic human eyes. *Graefe's Arch Clin Exp Ophthalmol.* 1994;232(2):71–74.
49. Riley MV. Intraocular dynamics of lactic acid in the rabbit. *Invest Ophthalmol Vis Sci.* 1972;11(7):600–607.
50. Stefansson E, Peterson JI, Wang YH. Intraocular oxygen tension measured with a fiber-optic sensor in normal and diabetic dogs. *Am J Physiol.* 1989;256(4 Pt 2):H1127–H1133.
51. Sakaue H, Negi A, Honda Y. Comparative study of vitreous oxygen tension in human and rabbit eyes. *Invest Ophthalmol Vis Sci.* 1989;30(9):1933–1937.
52. Hoffmann K, Bourwieg H, Riese K. On a content and distribution of low- and high-molecular substances in the vitreous body. II. High-molecular substances (LDH, MDH, GOT) (author's transl). *Graefe's Arch Clin Exp Ophthalmol.* 1974;191(3):231–238.
53. Azhdam AM, Goldberg RA, Ugradar S. In vivo measurement of the human vitreous chamber volume using computed tomography imaging of 100 eyes. *Transl Vis Sci Technol.* 2020;9(1):2.
54. Gal-Or O, Ghadiali Q, Dolz-Marco R, Engelbert M. In vivo imaging of the fibrillar architecture of the posterior vitreous and its relationship to the premacular bursa, Cloquet's canal, prevascular vitreous fissures, and cisterns. *Graefes Arch Clin Exp Ophthalmol.* 2019;257(4):709–714.
55. Sebag J. *The Vitreous: Structure, Function, and Pathobiology.* New York: Springer-Verlag; 1989:43–46 (hyalocytes); 47–54 (vitreo-retinal interface); 80-90 (aging & lacunae).
56. Wieghofer P, Engelbert M, Chui TYP, Rosen RB, Sakamoto T, Sebag J. Hyalocyte origin, structure, and imaging. *Exp Rev Ophthalmol.* 2022;17(4):233–248.
57. Castanos MV, Zhou DB, Linderman RE, et al. Imaging of macrophage-like cells in living human retina using clinical OCT. *Invest Opthalmol Vis Sci.* 2020;61(6):48.
58. Jones CH, Gui W, Schumann RG, et al. Hyalocytes in proliferative vitreo-retinal diseases. *Exp Rev Ophthalmol.* 2022;17(4):263–280.
59. Kita T, Sakamoto T, Ishibashi T. Hyalocytes: Essential vitreous cells in vitreo-retinal health and disease. In: Sebag J, ed. *Vitreous: in Health and Disease.* New York: Springer; 2014:151–164.
60. Boneva S, Wolf J, Wieghofer P, Sebag J, Lange C. Hyalocyte function and immunology. *Exp Rev Ophthalmol.* 2022;17:249–262.
61. Boneva SK, Wolf J, Rosmus DD, et al. Transcriptional profiling uncovers human hyalocytes as a unique innate immune cell population. *Front Immunol.* 2020;11:567274.
62. Rhodes RH, Mandelbaum SH, Minckler DS, Cleary PE. Tritiated fucose incorporation in the vitreous body, lens and zonules of the pigmented rabbit. *Exp Eye Res.* 1982;34(6):921–931.
63. Jacobson B. Identification of sialyl and galactosyl transferase activities in calf vitreous hyalocytes. *Curr Eye Res.* 1984;3(8):1033–1041.
64. Newsome DA, Linsenmayer TF, Trelstad RL. Vitreous body collagen. Evidence for a dual origin from the neural retina and hyalocytes. *J Cell Biol.* 1976;71(1):59–67.
65. Osterlin SE. The synthesis of hyaluronic acid in the vitreous. IV. Regeneration in the owl monkey. *Exp Eye Res.* 1969;8(1):27–34.
66. Kita T, Hata Y, Kano K, et al. Transforming growth factor-beta2 and connective tissue growth factor in proliferative vitreoretinal diseases: Possible involvement of hyalocytes and therapeutic potential of Rho kinase inhibitor. *Diabetes.* 2007;56(1):231–238.

67. Hirayama K, Hata Y, Noda Y, et al. The involvement of the rho-kinase pathway and its regulation in cytokine-induced collagen gel contraction by hyalocytes. *Invest Ophthalmol Vis Sci.* 2004;45(11):3896–3903.

68. Boneva SK, Wolf J, Hajdú RI, et al. In-depth molecular characterization of neovascular membranes suggests a role for hyalocyte-to-myofibroblast transdifferentiation in proliferative diabetic retinopathy. *Front Immunol.* 2021;12:757607.

69. Heegaard S. Morphology of the vitreoretinal border region. *Acta Ophthalmol Scand Suppl.* 1997;222:1–31.

70. Fine BS, Tousimis AJ. The structure of the vitreous body and the suspensory ligaments of the lens. *Arch Ophthalmol.* 1961;65:95–110.

71. Heegaard S. Structure of the human vitreoretinal border region. *Ophthalmologica.* 1994; 208(2):82–91.

72. Heegaard S, Jensen OA, Prause JU. Structure and composition of the inner limiting membrane of the retina. SEM on frozen resin-cracked and enzyme-digested retinas of Macaca mulatta. *Graefe's Arch Clin Exp Ophthalmol.* 1986;224(4):355–360.

73. Pedler C. The inner limiting membrane of the retina. *Br J Ophthalmol.* 1961;45(6):423–438.

74. Sebag J. Anomalous posterior vitreous detachment: A unifying concept in vitreo-retinal disease. *Graefe's Arch Clin Exp Ophthalmol.* 2004;242(8):690–698.

75. Sebag J, Hageman GS. Interfaces. *Eur J Ophthalmol.* 2000;10(1):1–3.

76. Sebag J. Age-related differences in the human vitreoretinal interface. *Arch Ophthalmol.* 1991;109(7):966–971.

77. Kefalides NA. The chemistry and structure of basement membranes. *Arthritis Rheum.* 1969;12(4):427–443.

78. Fukai N, Eklund L, Marneros AG, et al. Lack of collagen XVIII/endostatin results in eye abnormalities. *EMBO J.* 2002;21(7):1535–1544.

79. Hindson VJ, Gallagher JT, Halfter W, Bishop PN. Opticin binds to heparan and chondroitin sulfate proteoglycans. *Invest Ophthalmol Vis Sci.* 2005;46(12):4417–4423.

80. Hogan MJ, Alvarado JA, Weddell JE. *Histology of the Human Eye: An Atlas and Textbook.* Philadelphia: Saunders; 1971.

81. Schubert HD. Cystoid macular edema: The apparent role of mechanical factors. *Prog Clin Biol Res.* 1989;312:277–291.

82. Kishi S, Demaria C, Shimizu K. Vitreous cortex remnants at the fovea after spontaneous vitreous detachment. *Int Ophthalmol.* 1986;9(4):253–260.

83. Sebag J. Abnormalities of human vitreous structure in diabetes. *Graefe's Arch Clin Exp Ophthalmol.* 1993;231(5):257–260.

84. Cohen AI. Electron microscopic observations of the internal limiting membrane and optic fiber layer of the retina of the Rhesus monkey (M. mulatta). *Am J Anat.* 1961;108:179–197.

85. Russell SR, Shepherd JD, Hageman GS. Distribution of glycoconjugates in the human retinal internal limiting membrane. *Invest Ophthalmol Vis Sci.* 1991;32(7):1986–1995.

86. Nishitsuka K, Kashiwagi Y, Tojo N, et al. Hyaluronan production regulation from porcine hyalocyte cell line by cytokines. *Exp Eye Res.* 2007;85(4):539–545.

87. Russel S, Hageman G. Chondroitinase as a vitreous interfactant. *Vitreous: in Health and Disease.* New York: Springer; 2014:881–894.

88. Sebag J. Pharmacologic vitreolysis. *Vitreous: in Health and Disease.* New York: Springer; 2014:799–816.

89. Hogan MJ. The vitreous, its structure, and relation to the ciliary body and retina: Proctor Award Lecture. *Invest Ophthalmol Vis Sci.* 1963;2(5):418–445.

90. Spencer LM, Foos RY, Straatsma BR. Meridional folds, meridional complexes, and associated abnormalities of the peripheral retina. *Am J Ophthalmol.* 1970;70(5):697–714.

91. Byer NE. Cystic retinal tufts and their relationship to retinal detachment. *Arch Ophthalmol.* 1981;99(10):1788–1790.

92. Spencer L, Straatsma B, Foos R. Tractional degenerations of the peripheral retina. *Transactions of the New Orleans Academy of Ophthalmology, Symposium on Retina and Retinal Surgery.* Maryland Heights: Mosby; 1969.

93. Foos RY. Vitreoretinal juncture over retinal vessels. *Graefe's Arch Clin Exp Ophthalmol.* 1977;204(4):223–234.

94. Wolter JR. Pores in the internal limiting membrane of the human retina. *Acta Ophthalmol.* 1964;42:971–974.

95. Kuwabara T, Cogan DG. Studies of retinal vascular patterns. I. Normal architecture. *Arch Ophthalmol.* 1960;64:904–911.

96. Mutlu F, Leopold IH. The structure of human retinal vascular system. *JAMA Ophthalmol.* 1964;71(1):93–101.

97. Sebag J. Vitreous and vitreoretinal interface. In: Wilkinson CP, Hinton DR, Sadda SR, Wiedemann P, Schachat AP, eds. *Ryan's Retina.* 6th ed. Elsevier Health Sciences; 2017: 544–581.

98. Grabner G, Boltz G, Förster O. Macrophage-like properties of human hyalocytes. *Invest Ophthalmol Vis Sci.* 1980;19(4):333–340.

99. Foos RY, Roth AM. Surface structure of the optic nerve head. 2. Vitreopapillary attachments and posterior vitreous detachment. *Am J Ophthalmol.* 1973;76(5):662–671.

100. Roth AM, Foos RY. Surface structure of the optic nerve head. 1. Epipapillary membranes. *Am J Ophthalmol.* 1972;74(5):977–985.

101. Stefánsson E. Physiology of vitreous surgery. *Graefe's Arch Clin Exp Ophthalmol.* 2009; 247(2):147–163.

102. Peeters L, Sanders NN, Braeckmans K, et al. Vitreous: A barrier to nonviral ocular gene therapy. *Invest Ophthalmol Vis Sci.* 2005;46(10):3553–3561.

103. del Amo EM, Rimpelä A-K, Heikkinen E, et al. Pharmacokinetic aspects of retinal drug delivery. *Prog Retin Eye Res.* 2017;57:134–185.

104. Madea B, Henssge C. Determination of the time since death. III. Potassium in vitreous humour. Rise of precision by use of an "inner standard." *Acta Med Leg Soc (Liege).* 1988; 38(1):109–114.

105. Ortmann J, Markwerth P, Madea B. Precision of estimating the time since death by vitreous potassium—Comparison of 5 different equations. *Forensic Sci Int.* 2016;269:1–7.

106. Zilg B, Alkass K, Kronstrand R, Berg S, Druid H. A rapid method for postmortem vitreous chemistry—deadside analysis. *Biomolecules.* 2021;12(1):32.

107. Zilg B, Bernard S, Alkass K, Berg S, Druid H. A new model for the estimation of time of death from vitreous potassium levels corrected for age and temperature. *Forensic Sci Int.* 2015;254:158–166.

108. Cordeiro C, Ordóñez-Mayán L, Lendoiro E, Febrero-Bande M, Vieira DN, Muñoz-Barús JI. A reliable method for estimating the postmortem interval from the biochemistry of the vitreous humor, temperature and body weight. *Forensic Sci Int.* 2019;295:157–168.

109. Lund-Andersen H. Transport of glucose from blood to brain. *Physiol Rev.* 1979;59(2): 305–352.

110. Jooybar E, Abdekhodaie MJ, Farhadi F, Cheng Y-L. Computational modeling of drug distribution in the posterior segment of the eye: Effects of device variables and positions. *Math Biosci.* 2014;255:11–20.

111. Fatt I. Flow and diffusion in the vitreous body of the eye. *Bull Math Biol.* 1975;37(1):85–90.

112. Araie M, Maurice DM. The loss of fluorescein, fluorescein glucuronide and fluorescein isothiocyanate dextran from the vitreous by the anterior and retinal pathways. *Exp Eye Res.* 1991;52(1):27–39.

113. Hutton-Smith LA, Gaffney EA, Byrne HM, Maini PK, Schwab D, Mazer NA. A mechanistic model of the intravitreal pharmacokinetics of large molecules and the pharmacodynamic suppression of ocular vascular endothelial growth factor levels by ranibizumab in patients with neovascular age-related macular degeneration. *Mol Pharm.* 2016;13(9):2941–2950.

114. Del Amo EM, Vellonen KS, Kidron H, Urtti A. Intravitreal clearance and volume of distribution of compounds in rabbits: In silico prediction and pharmacokinetic simulations for drug development. *Eur J Pharm Biopharm.* 2015;95:215–226.

115. Bakri SJ, Snyder MR, Reid JM, Pulido JS, Singh RJ. Pharmacokinetics of intravitreal bevacizumab (Avastin). *Ophthalmology.* 2007;114(5):855–859.

116. Krohne TU, Eter N, Holz FG, Meyer CH. Intraocular pharmacokinetics of bevacizumab after a single intravitreal injection in humans. *Am J Ophthalmol.* 2008;146(4):508–512.

117. Meyer CH, Krohne TU, Holz FG. Intraocular pharmacokinetics after a single intravitreal injection of 1.5 mg versus 3.0 mg of bevacizumab in humans. *Retina.* 2011;31(9):1877–1884.

118. Lamminsalo M, Karvinen T, Subrizi A, Urtti A, Ranta V-P. Extended pharmacokinetic model of the intravitreal injections of macromolecules in rabbits. Part 2: Parameter estimation based on concentration dynamics in the vitreous, retina, and aqueous humor. *Pharm Res.* 2020;37(11):226.

119. Missel PJ. Simulating intravitreal injections in anatomically accurate models for rabbit, monkey, and human eyes. *Pharm Res.* 2012;29(12):3251–3272.

120. Zhang Y, Bazzazi H, Lima E Silva R, et al. Three-dimensional transport model for intravitreal and suprachoroidal drug injection. *Invest Ophthalmol Vis Sci.* 2018;59(12):5266–5276.

121. Davson D. *Physiology of the Eye.* 3rd ed. Edinburgh: Churchill Livingstone; 1972.

122. Duke-Elder F. *Textbook of Ophthalmology.* London: Henry Kimpton; 1938.

123. Gloor B, Moses RA, Hart WM. In: The vitreous. *Adler's Physiology of the Eye,* 8th ed. Maryland Heights: Mosby; 1981.

124. Sebag J. Surgical anatomy of the vitreous and the vitreoretinal interface. *Duane's Clinical Ophthalmology.* Philadelphia: Tasman W. Lippincott; 1994. http://www.oculist.net/downaton502/prof/ebook/duanes/pages/v6/v6c051.html.

125. Sebag J. Vitreous and vision degrading myodesopsia. *Prog Retin Eye Res.* 2020;79:100847.

126. Kingston ZS, Provis JM, Madigan MC II.A. Development and developmental disorders of vitreous. In: Sebag J, ed. *Vitreous: in Health and Disease.* New York: Springer; 2014:95–111.

127. Yee KMP, Feener EP, Gao B, et al. Vitreous cytokines and regression of the fetal hyaloid vasculature. In: *Vitreous: in Health and Disease.* New York: Springer; 2014:41–55.

128. Yee KMP, Feener EP, Madigan M, et al. Proteomic analysis of embryonic and young human vitreous. *Invest Ophthalmol Vis Sci.* 2015;56(12):7036–7042.

129. Gogat K, Le Gat L, Van Den Berghe L, et al. VEGF and KDR gene expression during human embryonic and fetal eye development. *Invest Ophthalmol Vis Sci.* 2004;45(1):7–14.

130. Shui YB, Wang X, Hu JS, et al. Vascular endothelial growth factor expression and signaling in the lens. *Invest Ophthalmol Vis Sci.* 2003;44(9):3911–3919.

131. Kim JH, Kim JH, Yu YS, Mun JY, Kim K-W. Autophagy-induced regression of hyaloid vessels in early ocular development. *Autophagy.* 2010;6(7):922–928.

132. Jack RL. Regression of the hyaloid vascular system: An ultrastructural analysis. *Am J Ophthalmol.* 1972;74(2):261–272.

133. McMenamin PG, Djano J, Wealthall R, Griffin BJ. Characterization of the macrophages associated with the tunica vasculosa lentis of the rat eye. *Invest Ophthalmol Vis Sci.* 2002; 43(7):2076–2082.

134. Meeson A, Palmer M, Calfon M, Lang R. A relationship between apoptosis and flow during programmed capillary regression is revealed by vital analysis. *Development.* 1996;122(12): 3929–3938.

135. Bu SC, Kuijer R, van der Worp RJ, Li XR, Hooymans JMM, Los LI. The ultrastructural localization of type II, IV, and VI collagens at the vitreoretinal interface. *PLOS ONE.* 2015;10(7):e0134325.

136. Sebag J: The vitreous. In: *Adler's Physiology of the Eye.* 9th ed. (WM Hart, Jr, ed). Mosby, St. Louis, 1992.

137. Fledelius HC. Ophthalmic changes from age of 10 to 18 years. A longitudinal study of sequels to low birth weight. IV. Ultrasound oculometry of vitreous and axial length. *Acta Ophthalmol (Copenh).* 1982;60(3):403–411.

138. Oksala A. Ultrasonic findings in the vitreous body at various ages. *Graefe's Arch Klin Exp Ophthalmol.* 1978;207(4):275–280.

139. Asanad S, Sebag J: Vitreous and developmental vitreo-retinopathies. In: *Pediatric Retina* 3rd ed (Hartnett, ed.) Lippincott Williams & Wilkins, Phila, 2020.

140. Mets MB. Childhood blindness and visual loss: An assessment at two institutions including a "new" cause. *Trans Am Ophthalmol Soc.* 1999;97:653–696.

141. Hartnett ME. *Pediatric Retina: Medical and Surgical Approaches.* Philadelphia: Lippincott Williams & Wilkins; 2004.

142. Fineman MS, Ho AC. *Retina: Color Atlas and Synopsis of Clinical Ophthalmology.* 2nd ed. Philadelphia: Lippincott Williams & Wilkins; 2012.

143. Grutzmacher C, Park S, Elmergreen TL, et al. Opposing effects of bim and bcl-2 on lung endothelial cell migration. *Am J Physiol Lung Cell Mol Physiol.* 2010;299(5):L607–L620.

144. Zhang C, Gehlbach P, Gongora C, et al. A potential role for beta- and gamma-crystallins in the vascular remodeling of the eye. *Dev Dyn Off Publ Am Assoc Anat*. 2005;234(1):36–47.
145. Thomas DM, Kannabiran C, Balasubramanian D. Identification of key genes and pathways in persistent hyperplastic primary vitreous of the eye using bioinformatic analysis. *Front Med*. 2021;8:690594.
146. Nguyen JH, Nguyen-Cuu J, Mamou J, Routledge B, Yee KMP, Sebag J. Vitreous structure and visual function in myopic vitreopathy causing vision-degrading myodesopsia. *Am J Ophthalmol*. 2021;224:246–253.
147. Foos RY, Wheeler NC. Vitreoretinal juncture. Synchysis senilis and posterior vitreous detachment. *Ophthalmology*. 1982;89(12):1502–1512.
148. Akiba J, Ueno N, Chakrabarti B. Age-related changes in the molecular properties of vitreous collagen. *Curr Eye Res*. 1993;12(10):951–954.
149. Sebag J, Balazs EA. Morphology and ultrastructure of human vitreous fibers. *Invest Ophthalmol Vis Sci*. 1989;30(8):1867–1871.
150. Larsson L, Osterlin S. Posterior vitreous detachment. A combined clinical and physiochemical study. *Graefe's Arch Clin Exp Ophthalmol*. 1985;223(2):92–95.
151. Bettelheim FA, Zigler JS. Regional mapping of molecular components of human liquid vitreous by dynamic light scattering. *Exp Eye Res*. 2004;79(5):713–718.
152. Ueno N, Sebag J, Hirokawa H, Chakrabarti B. Effects of visible-light irradiation on vitreous structure in the presence of a photosensitizer. *Exp Eye Res*. 1987;44:863–870.
153. Sebag J, Buckingham B, Charles MA, Reiser K. Biochemical abnormalities in vitreous of humans with proliferative diabetic retinopathy. *Arch Ophthalmol*. 1992;110(10):1472–1476.
154. Sebag J, Nie S, Reiser K, Charles MA, Yu NT. Raman spectroscopy of human vitreous in proliferative diabetic retinopathy. *Invest Ophthalmol Vis Sci*. 1994;35(7):2976–2980.
155. Stitt AW. Advanced glycation: An important pathological event in diabetic and age-related ocular disease. *Br J Ophthalmol*. 2001;85(6):746–753.
156. Vaughan-Thomas A, Gilbert SJ, Duance VC. Elevated levels of proteolytic enzymes in the aging human vitreous. *Invest Ophthalmol Vis Sci*. 2000;41(11):3299–3304.
157. Van Deemter M, Kuijer R, Harm Pas H, van der Worp RJ, Hooymans JMM, Los LI. Trypsin-mediated enzymatic degradation of type II collagen in the human vitreous. *Mol Vis*. 2013;19:1591–1599.
158. Los LI, van der Worp RJ, van Luyn MJA, Hooymans JMM. Age-related liquefaction of the human vitreous body: LM and TEM evaluation of the role of proteoglycans and collagen. *Invest Ophthalmol Vis Sci*. 2003;44(7):2828–2833.
159. Kasai K, Nakamura T, Kase N, et al. Increased glycosylation of proteins from cataractous lenses in diabetes. *Diabetologia*. 1983;25(1):36–38.
160. Sebag J, Ansari RR, Dunker S, Suh SI. Dynamic light scattering of diabetic vitreopathy. *Diabetes Technology & Therapeutics*. 1999;1:169–176.
161. Lee O-T, Good SD, Lamy R, Kudisch M, Stewart JM. Advanced glycation end-product accumulation reduces vitreous permeability. *Invest Ophthalmol Vis Sci*. 2015;56(5):2892–2897.
162. Sander B, Larsen M. Photochemical bleaching of fluorescent glycosylation products. *Int Ophthalmol*. 1994;18(4):195–198.
163. Bos KJ, Holmes DF, Meadows RS, Kadler KE, McLeod D, Bishop PN. Collagen fibril organisation in mammalian vitreous by freeze etch/rotary shadowing electron microscopy. *Micron*. 2001;32(3):301–306.
164. Bishop PN, Holmes DF, Kadler KE, McLeod D, Bos KJ. Age-related changes on the surface of vitreous collagen fibrils. *Invest Ophthalmol Vis Sci*. 2004;45(4):1041–1046.
165. Richards AJ, Martin S, Yates JRW, et al. COL2A1 exon 2 mutations: Relevance to the Stickler and Wagner syndromes. *Br J Ophthalmol*. 2000;84(4):364–371.
166. Brown DJ, Bishop P, Hamdi H, Kenney MC. Cleavage of structural components of mammalian vitreous by endogenous matrix metalloproteinase-2. *Curr Eye Res*. 1996;15(4):439–445.
167. Jin M, Kashiwagi K, Iizuka Y, Tanaka Y, Imai M, Tsukahara S. Matrix metalloproteinases in human diabetic and nondiabetic vitreous. *Retina, Phila Pa*. 2001;21(1):28–33.
168. Mamou J, Wa CA, Yee KMP, et al. Ultrasound-based quantification of vitreous floaters correlates with contrast sensitivity and quality of life. *Invest Ophthalmol Vis Sci*. 2015;56(3):1611–1617.
169. Ruminski D, Sebag J, Toledo RD, et al. Volumetric optical imaging and quantitative analysis of age-related changes in anterior human vitreous. *Invest Ophthalmol Vis Sci*. 2021;62(4):31.
170. Ponsioen TL, Hooymans JMM, Los LI. Remodelling of the human vitreous and vitreoretinal interface – a dynamic process. *Prog Retin Eye Res*. 2010;29(6):580–595.
171. Wynn TA, Ramalingam TR. Mechanisms of fibrosis: therapeutic translation for fibrotic disease. *Nat Med*. 2012;18(7):1028–1040.
172. Zeisberg M, Kalluri R. Cellular mechanisms of tissue fibrosis. 1. Common and organ-specific mechanisms associated with tissue fibrosis. *Am J Physiol-Cell Physiol*. 2013;304(3):C216–C225.
173. Balazs EA, Toth LZ, Ozanics V. Cytological studies on the developing vitreous as related to the hyaloid vessel system. *Graefe's Arch Clin Exp Ophthalmol*. 1980;213(2):71–85.
174. Gärtner J. The fine structure of the vitreous base of the human eye and pathogenesis of pars planitis. *Am J Ophthalmol*. 1971;71(6):1317–1327.
175. Gale J, Ikuno Y. Myopic vitreopathy. In: Sebag J, ed. *Vitreous: in Health and Disease*. New York: Springer; 2014:113–130.
176. Goldmann H. Senile changes of the lens and the vitreous. *Am J Ophthalmol*. 1964;57:1–13.
177. Takahashi M, Jalkh A, Hoskins J, Trempe CL, Schepens CL. Biomicroscopic evaluation and photography of liquefied vitreous in some vitreoretinal disorders. *Arch Ophthalmol*. 1981;99(9):1555–1559.
178. Maumenee IH. Vitreoretinal degeneration as a sign of generalized connective tissue diseases. *Am J Ophthalmol*. 1979;88(3 Pt 1):432–449.
179. Worst JG. Cisternal systems of the fully developed vitreous body in the young adult. *Trans Ophthalmol Soc U K*. 1977;97(4):550–554.
180. Jongebloed WL, Humalda D, Worst JFG. A SEM-correlation of the anatomy of the vitreous body: Making visible the invisible. *Doc Ophthalmol*. 1986;64(1):117–127.
181. Jongebloed WL, Worst JF. The cisternal anatomy of the vitreous body. *Doc Ophthalmol Adv Ophthalmol*. 1987;67(1–2):183–196.
182. Kishi S, Shimizu K. Posterior precortical vitreous pocket. *Arch Ophthalmol*. 1990;108(7):979–982.
183. She X, Ye X, Chen R, Pan D, Shen L. Characteristics of posterior precortical vitreous pockets and Cloquet's canal in patients with myopia by optical coherence tomography. *Invest Ophthalmol Vis Sci*. 2019;60(14):4882–4888.
184. Sebag J. Vitreous in age-related macular degeneration therapy – the medium is the message. *Retina*. 2015;35(9):1715–1718.
185. Gandorfer A, Putz E, Welge-Lüssen U, Grüterich M, Ulbig M, Kampik A. Ultrastructure of the vitreoretinal interface following plasmin assisted vitrectomy. *Br J Ophthalmol*. 2001;85(1):6–10.
186. Creveling CJ, Colter J, Coats B. Changes in vitreo-retinal adhesion with age and region in human and sheep eyes. *Front Bioeng Biotechnol*. 2018;6:153.
187. Halfter W, Cunningham E, Sebag J. Vitreo-retinal interface and inner limiting membrane. In: Sebag J, ed. *Vitreous: in Health and Disease*. New York: Springer; 2014:165–191.
188. Russell SR. What we know (and do not know) about vitreo-retinal adhesion. *Retina*. 2012;32:S181.
189. Wert KJ, Velez G, Cross MR, et al. Extracellular superoxide dismutase (SOD3) regulates oxidative stress at the vitreo-retinal interface. *Free Radic Biol Med*. 2018;124:408–419.
190. Öhman T, Tamene F, Göös H, Loukovaara S, Varjosalo M. Systems pathology analysis identifies neurodegenerative nature of age-related vitreoretinal interface diseases. *Aging Cell*. 2018;17(5):e12809.
191. Teng CC, Chi HH. Vitreous changes and the mechanism of retinal detachment. *Am J Ophthalmol*. 1957;44(3):335–356.
192. Wang J, McLeod D, Henson DB, Bishop PN. Age-dependent changes in the basal retino-vitreous adhesion. *Invest Ophthalmol Vis Sci*. 2003;44(5):1793–1800.
193. Gärtner J. Electron microscopic observations on the cilio-zonular border area of the human eye with particular reference to the aging changes. *Z Anat Entwicklungsgesch*. 1970;131(3):263–273.
194. Foos RY. Vitreoretinal juncture; topographical variations. *Invest Ophthalmol*. 1972;11(10):801–808.
195. Sebag J. Posterior vitreous detachment. *Ophthalmology*. 2018;125(9):1384–1385.
196. Johnson MW. Posterior vitreous detachment: Evolution and complications of its early stages. *Am J Ophthalmol*. 2010;149(3):371–382.e1.
197. Tsukahara M, Mori K, Gehlbach PL, Mori K. Posterior vitreous detachment as observed by wide-angle OCT imaging. *Ophthalmology*. 2018;125(9):1372–1383.
198. Foos RY. Ultrastructural features of posterior vitreous detachment. *Graefe's Arch Clin Exp Ophthalmol*. 1975;196(2):103–111.
199. Sebag J. Vitreous: The resplendent enigma. *Br J Ophthalmol*. 2009;93(8):989–991.
200. Tozer K, Johnson M, Sebag J. Vitreous aging and posterior vitreous detachment. In: Sebag J, ed. *Vitreous: in Health and Disease*. New York: Springer; 2014:131–150.
201. Favre M, Goldmann H. Zur Genese der hinteren Glaskörperabhebung. *Ophthalmologica*. 1956;132(2):87–97.
202. Palacio AC, Gupta A, Nesmith BL, Jadav PR, Schaal Y, Schaal S. Vitreomacular adhesion evolution with age in healthy human eyes. *Retina*. 2017;37(1):118–123.
203. Hikichi T, Hirokawa H, Kado M, et al. Comparison of the prevalence of posterior vitreous detachment in Whites and Japanese. *Ophthalmic Surg Lasers Imaging Retina*. 1995;26(1):39–43.
204. Hikichi T, Yoshida A. Time course of development of posterior vitreous detachment in the fellow eye after development in the first eye. *Ophthalmology*. 2004;111(9):1705–1707.
205. Hikichi T. Time course of posterior vitreous detachment in the second eye. *Curr Opin Ophthalmol*. 2007;18(3):224–227.
206. Yonemoto J, Ideta H, Sasaki K, Tanaka S, Hirose A, Oka C. The age of onset of posterior vitreous detachment. *Graefe's Arch Clin Exp Ophthalmol*. 1994;232(2):67–70.
207. Itakura H, Kishi S, Li D, Nitta K, Akiyama H. Vitreous changes in high myopia observed by swept-source optical coherence tomography. *Invest Ophthalmol Vis Sci*. 2014;55(3):1447–1452.
208. Hwang ES, Kraker JA, Griffin KJ, Sebag J, Weinberg DV, Kim JE. Accuracy of spectral-domain OCT of the macula for detection of complete posterior vitreous detachment. *Ophthalmol Retina*. 2020;4(2):148–153.
209. Novak MA, Welch RB. Complications of acute symptomatic posterior vitreous detachment. *Am J Ophthalmol*. 1984;97(3):308–314.
210. Chuo JY, Lee TYY, Hollands H, et al. Risk factors for posterior vitreous detachment: A case-control study. *Am J Ophthalmol*. 2006;142(6):931–937.
211. Van Deemter M, Ponsioen TL, Bank RA, et al. Pentosidine accumulates in the aging vitreous body: A gender effect. *Exp Eye Res*. 2009;88(6):1043–1050.
212. Hayreh SS, Jonas JB. Posterior vitreous detachment: Clinical correlations. *Ophthalmologica*. 2004;218(5):333–343.
213. Snead M, Richards A. Hereditary vitreo-retinopathies. In: Sebag J, ed. *Vitreous: in Health and Disease*. New York: Springer; 2014:21–40.
214. Itakura H, Kishi S, Kotajima N, Murakami M. Decreased vitreal hyaluronan levels with aging. *Ophthalmologica*. 2009;223(1):32–35.
215. Webb BF, Webb JR, Schroeder MC, North CS. Prevalence of vitreous floaters in a community sample of smartphone users. *Int J Ophthalmol*. 2013;6(3):402–405.
216. Sebag J, Yee KMP, Wa CA, Huang LC, Sadun AA. Vitrectomy for floaters: Prospective efficacy analyses and retrospective safety profile. *Retina*. 2014;34(6):1062–1068.
217. Fincham GS, James S, Spickett C, et al. Posterior vitreous detachment and the posterior hyaloid membrane. *Ophthalmology*. 2018;125(2):227–236.
218. Henrich PB, Monnier CA, Halfter W, et al. Nanoscale topographic and biomechanical studies of the human internal limiting membrane. *Invest Ophthalmol Vis Sci*. 2012;53(6):2561–2570.
219. Walton KA, Meyer CH, Harkrider CJ, Cox TA, Toth CA. Age-related changes in vitreous mobility as measured by video B scan ultrasound. *Exp Eye Res*. 2002;74(2):173–180.
220. Machemer R. The importance of fluid absorption, traction, intraocular currents, and chorioretinal scars in the therapy of rhegmatogenous retinal detachments. XLI Edward Jackson memorial lecture. *Am J Ophthalmol*. 1984;98(6):681–693.
221. Davis MD. Natural history of retinal breaks without detachment. *Arch Ophthalmol*. 1974;92(3):183–194.

222. Neumann E, Hyams S. Conservative management of retinal breaks. A follow-up study of subsequent retinal detachment. *Br J Ophthalmol.* 1972;56(6):482–486.
223. Duker JS, Kaiser PK, Binder S, et al. The International Vitreomacular Traction Study Group classification of vitreomacular adhesion, traction, and macular hole. *Ophthalmology.* 2013;120(12):2611–2619.
224. Sebag J. Pathophysiologie der partiellen PVD und vitreomakulären traktion. In: Maier M, ed. *Die Vitreomakuläre Traktion (VMT).* Uni-Med Berlin; 2014:19–32.
225. Bottós JM, Elizalde J, Rodrigues EB, Maia M. Current concepts in vitreomacular traction syndrome. *Curr Opin Ophthalmol.* 2012;23(3):195–201.
226. Krebs I, Brannath W, Glittenberg C, Zeiler F, Sebag J, Binder S. Posterior vitreomacular adhesion: A potential risk factor for exudative age-related macular degeneration? *Am J Ophthalmol.* 2007;144(5):741–746.
227. Robison CD, Krebs I, Binder S, et al. Vitreomacular adhesion in active and end-stage age-related macular degeneration. *Am J Ophthalmol.* 2009;148(1):79–82.e2.
228. Khoshnevis M, Sebag J. Management of macular edema in vitreo-maculopathies. In: Schaal S, Kaplan H, eds. *Cystoid Macular Edema.* New York: Springer; 2016:91–120.
229. Sebag J. Vitreoschisis. *Graefe's Arch Clin Exp Ophthalmol.* 2008;246(3):329–332.
230. Wang MY, Nguyen D, Hindoyan N, Sadun AA, Sebag J. Vitreo-papillary adhesion in macular hole and macular pucker. *Retina.* 2009;29(5):644–650.
231. Nguyen JH, Yee KMP, Nguyen-Cuu J, Sebag J. Structural and functional characteristics of lamellar macular holes. *Retina.* 2019;39(11):2084–2089.
232. Cibis GW, Watzke RC, Chua J. Retinal hemorrhages in posterior vitreous detachment. *Am J Ophthalmol.* 1975;80(6):1043–1046.
233. Kroll P, Wiegand W, Schmidt J. Vitreopapillary traction in proliferative diabetic vitreoretinopathy. *Br J Ophthalmol.* 1999;83(3):261–264.
234. Katz B, Hoyt WF. Gaze-evoked amaurosis from vitreopapillary traction. *Am J Ophthalmol.* 2005;139(4):631–637.
235. Shah NS, Beebe DC, Lake SP, Filas BA. On the spatiotemporal material anisotropy of the vitreous body in tension and compression. *Ann Biomed Eng.* 2016;44(10):3084–3095.
236. Maeda N, Tano Y. Intraocular oxygen tension in eyes with proliferative diabetic retinopathy with and without vitreous. *Graefe's Arch Clin Exp Ophthalmol.* 1996; 234(Suppl 1):S66–S69.
237. Blankenship GW, Machemer R. Long-term diabetic vitrectomy results: Report of 10 year follow-up. *Ophthalmology.* 1985;92(4):503–506.
238. Nasrallah FP, Jalkh AE, Van Coppenolle F, et al. The role of the vitreous in diabetic macular edema. *Ophthalmology.* 1988;95(10):1335–1339.
239. Lewis H. The role of vitrectomy in the treatment of diabetic macular edema. *Am J Ophthalmol.* 2001;131(1):123–125.
240. Hoerle S, Poestgens H, Schmidt J, Kroll P. Effect of pars plana vitrectomy for proliferative diabetic vitreoretinopathy on preexisting diabetic maculopathy. *Graefes Arch Clin Exp Ophthalmol.* 240(3):197–201.
241. Takahashi MK, Hikichi T, Akiba J, Yoshida A, Trempe CL. Role of the vitreous and macular edema in branch retinal vein occlusion. *Ophthalmic Surg Lasers.* 1997;28(4):294–299.
242. Kumagai K, Furukawa M, Ogino N, Uemura A, Larson E. Long-term outcomes of vitrectomy with or without arteriovenous sheathotomy in branch retinal vein occlusion. *Retina.* 2007;27(1):49–54.
243. Lindberg C, Larsson J. Vitrectomy for non-ischaemic macular oedema in retinal vein occlusion. *Acta Ophthalmol Scand.* 2006;84(6):812–814.
244. Weber-Krause B, Eckardt U. [Incidence of posterior vitreous detachment in eyes with and without age-related macular degeneration. An ultrasonic study]. *Ophthalmol Z Deutsch Ophthalmol Ges.* 1996;93(6):660–665.
245. Ondeş F, Yilmaz G, Acar MA, Unlü N, Kocaoğlan H, Arsan AK. Role of the vitreous in age-related macular degeneration. *Jpn J Ophthalmol.* 2000;44(1):91–93.
246. Lambert HM, Capone A, Aaberg TM, Sternberg P, Mandell BA, Lopez PF. Surgical excision of subfoveal neovascular membranes in age-related macular degeneration. *Am J Ophthalmol.* 1992;113(3):257–262.
247. Lee SJ, Koh HJ. Effects of vitreomacular adhesion on anti-vascular endothelial growth factor treatment for exudative age-related macular degeneration. *Ophthalmology.* 2011;118(1):101–110.
248. Anderson DH, Mullins RF, Hageman GS, Johnson LV. A role for local inflammation in the formation of drusen in the aging eye. *Am J Ophthalmol.* 2002;134(3):411–431.
249. Rice TA, Michels RG, Maguire MG, Rice EF. The effect of lensectomy on the incidence of iris neovascularization and neovascular glaucoma after vitrectomy for diabetic retinopathy. *Am J Ophthalmol.* 1983;95(1):1–11.
250. Waldstein SM, Ritter M, Simader C, Mayr-Sponer U, Kundi M, Schmidt-Erfurth U. Impact of vitreomacular adhesion on ranibizumab mono- and combination therapy for neovascular age-related macular degeneration. *Am J Ophthalmol.* 2014;158(2):328–336.e1.
251. Houston SK III, Rayess N, Cohen MN, Ho AC, Regillo CD. Influence of vitreomacular interface on anti-vascular endothelial growth factor therapy using treat and extend treatment protocol for age-related macular degeneration (Vintrex). *Retina.* 2015;35(9):1757–1764.
252. Krishnan R, Arora R, De Salvo G, et al. Vitreomacular traction affects anti-vascular endothelial growth factor treatment outcomes for exudative age-related macular degeneration. *Retina.* 2015;35(9):1750–1756.
253. Lee SS, Ghosn C, Yu Z, et al. Vitreous VEGF clearance is increased after vitrectomy. *Invest Ophthalmol Vis Sci.* 2009;51:2135–2138.
254. Kakinoki M, Sawada O, Sawada T, et al. Effect of vitrectomy on aqueous VEGF concentration and pharmacokinetics of bevacizumab in macaque monkeys. *Invest Ophthalmol Vis Sci.* 2012;53(9):5877–5880.
255. Filas BA, Shui YB, Beebe DC. Computational model for oxygen transport and consumption in human vitreous. *Invest Ophthalmol Vis Sci.* 2013;54(10):6549–6559.
256. Holekamp NM, Shui Y-B, Beebe DC. Vitrectomy surgery increases oxygen exposure to the lens: A possible mechanism for nuclear cataract formation. *Am J Ophthalmol.* 2005;139(2): 302–310.
257. Stefánsson E. The therapeutic effects of retinal laser treatment and vitrectomy. A theory based on oxygen and vascular physiology. *Acta Ophthalmol Scand.* 2001;79(5):435–440.
258. Harocopos GJ, Shui YB, McKinnon M, Holekamp NM, Gordon MO, Beebe DC. Importance of vitreous liquefaction in age-related cataract. *Invest Ophthalmol Vis Sci.* 2004; 45(1):77–85.
259. Brew H, Attwell D. Is the potassium channel distribution in glial cells optimal for spatial buffering of potassium? *Biophys J.* 1985;48(5):843–847.
260. Newman EA. Regulation of potassium levels by Müller cells in the vertebrate retina. *Can J Physiol Pharmacol.* 1987;65(5):1028–1032.
261. Beebe DC, Holekamp NM, Siegfried C, Shui YB. Vitreoretinal influences on lens function and cataract. *Philos Trans R Soc B Biol Sci.* 2011;366(1568):1293–1300.
262. Stefánsson E, Geirsdóttir Á, Sigurdsson H. Metabolic physiology in age related macular degeneration. *Prog Retin Eye Res.* 2011;30(1):72–80.
263. Jonsdottir KD, Einarsdottir AB, Stefánsson E. Why does vitreoretinal traction create macular oedema? *Acta Ophthalmol.* 2018;96(4):e533–e534.
264. Shui YB, Holekamp NM, Kramer BC, et al. The gel state of the vitreous and ascorbate-dependent oxygen consumption: Relationship to the etiology of nuclear cataracts. *Arch Ophthalmol.* 2009;127(4):475–482.
265. Murali K, Kang D, Nazari H, et al. Spatial variations in vitreous oxygen consumption. *PLoS ONE.* 2016;11(3):e0149961.
266. Ankamah E, Sebag J, Ng E, Nolan JM. Vitreous antioxidants, degeneration, and vitreo-retinopathy: Exploring the links. *Antioxidants.* 2019;9(1):7.
267. Duarte TL, Lunec J. Review: When is an antioxidant not an antioxidant? A review of novel actions and reactions of vitamin C. *Free Radic Res.* 2005;39(7):671–686.
268. McGahan MC. Ascorbic acid levels in aqueous and vitreous humors of the rabbit: Effects of inflammation and ceruloplasmin. *Exp Eye Res.* 1985;41(3):291–298.
269. Park SW, Ghim W, Oh S, et al. Association of vitreous vitamin C depletion with diabetic macular ischemia in proliferative diabetic retinopathy. *PloS One.* 2019;14(6):e0218433.
270. Philpot FJ, Pirie A. Riboflavin and riboflavin adenine dinucleotide in ox ocular tissues. *Biochem J.* 1943;37(2):250–254.
271. Sulochana KN, Biswas J, Ramakrishnan S. Eales' disease: Increased oxidation and peroxidation products of membrane constituents chiefly lipids and decreased antioxidant enzymes and reduced glutathione in vitreous. *Curr Eye Res.* 1999;19(3):254–259.
272. Cicik E, Tekin H, Akar S, et al. Interleukin-8, nitric oxide and glutathione status in proliferative vitreoretinopathy and proliferative diabetic retinopathy. *Ophthalmic Res.* 2003; 35(5):251–255.
273. Géhl Z, Bakondi E, Resch MD, et al. Diabetes-induced oxidative stress in the vitreous humor. *Redox Biol.* 2016;9:100–103.
274. Diederen RMH, La Heij EC, Deutz NEP, et al. Increased glutamate levels in the vitreous of patients with retinal detachment. *Exp Eye Res.* 2006;83(1):45–50.
275. Heinämäki AA, Muhonen AS, Piha RS. Taurine and other free amino acids in the retina, vitreous, lens, iris-ciliary body, and cornea of the rat eye. *Neurochem Res.* 1986;11(4):535–542.
276. Krizova L, Kalousova M, Kubena A, et al. Increased uric acid and glucose concentrations in vitreous and serum of patients with diabetic macular oedema. *Ophthalmic Res.* 2011;46(2): 73–79.
277. Ouchi M, West K, Crabb JW, Kinoshita S, Kamei M. Proteomic analysis of vitreous from diabetic macular edema. *Exp Eye Res.* 2005;81(2):176–182.
278. González de Vega R, Fernández-Sánchez ML, González Iglesias H, et al. Quantitative selenium speciation by HPLC-ICP-MS(IDA) and simultaneous activity measurements in human vitreous humor. *Anal Bioanal Chem.* 2015;407(9):2405–2413.
279. Mayer U. Comparative investigations of catalase activity in different ocular tissues of cattle and man. *Graefe's Arch Clin Exp Ophthalmol.* 1980;213(4):261–265.
280. Skeie JM, Roybal CN, Mahajan VB. Proteomic insight into the molecular function of the vitreous. *PloS One.* 2015;10(5):e0127567.
281. Yee KM, Tan S, Lesnick-Oberstein SY, et al. Incidence of cataract surgery after vitrectomy for vitreous opacities. *Ophthalmology Retina.* 2017;1: 154–157.
282. Mansukhani SA, Barkmeier AJ, Bakri SJ, et al. The risk of primary open-angle glaucoma following vitreoretinal surgery—a population-based study. *Am J Ophthalmol.* 2018;193: 143–155.
283. Koreen L, Yoshida N, Escariao P, et al. Incidence of, risk factors for, and combined mechanism of late-onset open-angle glaucoma after vitrectomy. *Retina.* 2012;32(1):160–167.
284. Luk FOJ, Kwok AKH, Lai TYY, Lam DSC. Presence of crystalline lens as a protective factor for the late development of open angle glaucoma after vitrectomy. *Retina.* 2009;29(2):218–224.
285. Wu L, Berrocal MH, Rodriguez FJ, et al. Intraocular pressure elevation after uncomplicated pars plana vitrectomy: Results of the Pan American Collaborative Retina Study Group. *Retina.* 2014;34(10):1985–1989.
286. Siegfried CJ, Shui YB, Holekamp NM, Bai F, Beebe DC. Oxygen distribution in the human eye: Relevance to the etiology of open-angle glaucoma after vitrectomy. *Invest Ophthalmol Vis Sci.* 2010;51(11):5731–5738.
287. Lalezary M, Kim SJ, Jiramongkolchai K, Recchia FM, Agarwal A, Sternberg P Jr. Long-term trends in intraocular pressure after pars plana vitrectomy. *Retina.* 2011;31(4):679–685.
288. Yu AL, Brummeisl W, Schaumberger M, Kampik A, Welge-Lussen U. Vitrectomy does not increase the risk of open-angle glaucoma or ocular hypertension—a 5-year follow-up. *Graefe's Arch Clin Exp Ophthalmol A.* 2010;248(10):1407–1414.
289. Sebag J. Vitrectomy for vision degrading myodesopsia. *Ophthalmol Retina.* 2021;5(1):1–3.
290. Sebag J, Yee KMP, Nguyen JH, Nguyen-Cuu J. Long-term safety and efficacy of vitrectomy for vision degrading myodesopsia from vitreous floaters. *Ophthalmol Retina.* 2018;2:881–887.
291. West DC, Kumar S. Hyaluronan and angiogenesis. *Ciba Found Symp.* 1989;143:187–201.
292. Forrester JV, Wilkinson PC. Inhibition of leukocyte locomotion by hyaluronic acid. *J Cell Sci.* 1981;48:315–331.
293. Sebag J, Balazs EA, Eakins KE, Kulkarni PS. The effect of Na-hyaluronate on prostaglandin synthesis and phagocytosis by mononuclear phagocytes in vitro. *Invest Ophthalmol Vis Sci.* 1981;20(ARVO):33.

294. Dübe B, Lüke HJ, Aumailley M, Prehm P. Hyaluronan reduces migration and proliferation in CHO cells. *Biochim Biophys Acta*. 2001;1538:283–289.

295. Alaniz L, Rizzo M, Malvicini M, et al. Low molecular weight HA inhibits colorectal carcinoma by decreasing tumor cell proliferation and stimulating immune response. *Cancer Lett*. 2009;278:9–16.

296. Wang R, Zhou W, Wang J, et al. Role of hyaluronan and glucose on 4-methylumbelliferone-inhibited cell proliferation in breast carcinoma cells. *Anticancer Res*. 2015;35:4799–4805.

297. Spraul CW, Grossniklaus HE. Vitreous hemorrhage. *Surv Ophthalmol*. 1997;42(1):3–39.

298. Mahendradas P, Madhu S, Kawali A, et al. Enhanced vitreous imaging in uveitis. *Ocul Immunol Inflamm*. 2019;27(1):148–154.

299. Sebag J. Diabetic vitreopathy. *Ophthalmology*. 1996;103(2):205–206.

300. Garcia G, Khoshnevis M, Nguyen-Cuu J, et al. The effects of aging vitreous on contrast sensitivity function. *Graefe's Arch Clin Exp Ophthalmol*. 2018;256:919–925.

301. Garcia G, Khoshnevis M, Yee KM, Nguyen-Cuu J, Nguyen JH, Sebag J. Degradation of contrast sensitivity following posterior vitreous detachment. *Am J Ophthalmol*. 2016;172:7–12.

302. van den Berg TJTP, Franssen L, Kruijt B, Coppens JE. History of ocular straylight measurement: A review. *Z Für Med Phys*. 2013;23:6–20.

303. Huang LC, Yee KMP, Wa CA, Nguyen JN, Sadun AA, Sebag J. Vitreous floaters and vision: Current concepts and management paradigms. In: Sebag J, ed. *Vitreous: In Health and Disease*. New York: Springer; 2014:771–788.

304. Khoshnevis M, Rosen S, Sebag J. Asteroid hyalosis—a comprehensive review. *Surv Ophthalmol*. 2019;64(4):452–462.

305. Sebag J. Vitreous and vitreo-retinal interface. In: Schachat A, ed. *Ryan's Retina*. 7th ed. Oxford: Elsevier; 2022.

306. Sebag J. *Vitreous: in Health and Disease*. New York: Springer; 2014.

307. Sebag J. Pharmacologic vitreolysis. [guest editorial]. *Retina*. 1998;18:1–3.

308. Sebag J. Is pharmacologic vitreolysis brewing? [guest editorial]. *Retina*. 2002;22:1–3.

309. Sebag J. Molecular biology of pharmacologic vitreolysis. *Trans Am Ophthalmol Soc*. 2005;103:473–494.

310. Sebag J. Pharmacologic vitreolysis—premise and promise of the first decade. [guest editorial]. *Retina*. 2009;29:871–874.

311. Dosmar E, Walsh J, Doyel M, et al. Targeting ocular drug delivery: An examination of local anatomy and current approaches. *Bioengineering*. 2022;9(1):41.

The Extraocular Muscles

Linda K. McLoon

INTRODUCTION

The extraocular muscles (EOM) are a complex group of skeletal muscles located within the bony orbit. They function in a highly coordinated manner to perform conjugate eye movements, maintain primary gaze position, and provide visuomotor fusion—maintaining corresponding visual elements within the binocular field to fall on corresponding retinal loci. In addition, the eyes are able to follow moving objects, called smooth pursuit, and accomplish rapid changes in fixation, called saccades. This is accomplished by a very highly organized oculomotor control system in the brain, with the EOM forming the final effector tissues. Understanding how the EOM adapt to changing visual demands is critical to the development of improved treatment strategies to realign the eyes when the system fails, as in strabismus or nystagmus.

The EOM have many distinct and complex properties that distinguish them from noncranial skeletal muscles, many of which are normally associated with developing or regenerating muscle. This includes a population of multiply and polyneuronally innervated myofibers, retained expression of the immature subunit of the acetylcholine receptor, neural cell adhesion molecule, and "immature" myosin heavy chain isoforms. The EOM also have the capacity to remodel continuously throughout life. From a clinical perspective, the EOM have a distinct propensity for or sparing from a number of skeletal muscle diseases. EOM share some of their unusual characteristics with other craniofacial muscles, such as the laryngeal muscles, and the potential developmental basis for their unusual properties and disease profiles is presented.

THE BONY ORBIT

The eyes and other orbital contents are protected in deep bony orbits that are roughly pyramidal in shape (Fig. 7.1). The orbit is largest just inside the orbital margin at its anterior extent and smallest at its posterior extent, the apex. The orbital margins are composed of the frontal bone superiorly, the zygomatic process of the frontal bone and the frontal process of the zygomatic bone laterally, the zygoma and the maxillary bone inferiorly, and the frontal process of the maxillary bone, the lacrimal bone and the maxillary process of the frontal bone medially (Fig. 7.1). However, direct impact to the bony margin can result in fracture of the bones within the orbit (see Box 7.1). The bony orbit has a thick bony roof composed of frontal bone and a portion of the lesser wing of the sphenoid bone. The lateral wall is composed of the zygomatic bone and the greater wing of the sphenoid. The relatively thin floor is composed of the maxillary bone, a small and variable part of the palatine bone, and the zygomatic bone. The thin medial wall is composed of the maxillary, the lacrimal, ethmoid, and sphenoid bones, from anterior to posterior respectively.[1] As a result of this bony configuration, the globe is relatively protected from injury caused by direct impacts to the face and orbital margins, particularly if there are no bony fractures.

An understanding of the geometry of the bony anatomy relative to maintenance of eye position is critically important. The medial walls are parallel to each other, while the plane of the lateral wall in each orbit is 45 degrees from the sagittal plane formed by the medial wall (Figs. 7.1 and 7.2). Additionally, the geometry of the orbital bones requires that both globes need to be partially adducted in the primary position of gaze, which is looking directly straight ahead. Maintenance of eye position in primary gaze thus requires a constant steady-state level of tension in all the EOM, referred to as tonus.[2]

The apex of the bony orbit has three major foramina: the optic foramen, and the superior and inferior orbital fissures. The nerves and blood vessels to the majority of structures within the orbit enter or exit through these foramina. A number of small foramina also open into the orbit, allowing entry and exit of nerves and vasculature to a wide array of structures in the orbit and head.[3]

EXTRAOCULAR MUSCLE ANATOMY

There are six EOM in each orbit whose function is to move the eyes: four rectus muscles, superior, medial, inferior, and lateral; and two oblique muscles, inferior and superior (Fig. 7.3). In addition there is a seventh skeletal muscle in each orbit, the levator palpebrae superioris, which inserts into the upper eyelid and functions in elevating the palpebral fissure. Although its cranial nerve innervation is similar to the EOM, functionally and metabolically it is distinct, and will not be discussed further in this chapter.

The four rectus muscles take their origin in part from the bones at the apex of the orbit, but also from a connective tissue ring called the tendinous annulus. They course anteriorly to insert into the sclera anterior to the equator of the globe, a key factor when considering their functional effects on eye movements. Classically, this insertion is described as directly external to the ora serrata; however, recent studies demonstrate that insertions of the rectus muscles range from 2.25-mm posterior to 2.25-mm anterior to the ora serrata, with 90% of the insertions within 1 mm.[4] Generally considered to be tendinous at the insertion site into the globe, the medial and lateral rectus muscles in humans may contain myofibers that extend directly to the sclera,[5] an important consideration for incisional strabismus surgery. The insertions of the four rectus muscles increase in distance from the corneal limbus circumferentially, with the medial rectus closest and the superior rectus

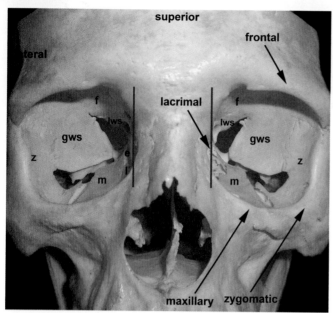

Fig. 7.1 Bony orbit (*anterior view*). The medial walls of the two orbits are parallel to each other and in the sagittal plane (*blue vertical lines*). The walls form a pyramidal shape with the apex pointing posteriorly. *e*, Ethmoid bone; *f*, frontal bone; *gws*, greater wing of the sphenoid; *l*, lacrimal bone; *lws*, lesser wing of the sphenoid; *m*, maxillary bone; *z*, zygomatic bone.

BOX 7.1   Blowout fractures

Bony fractures of the thin orbital walls can occur with blunt impact to the orbital margins. The increased force causes the bone to "blowout" into the sinuses, with the inferior and medial walls most susceptible to fracture. Sometimes the EOM become entrapped at the fracture site, as evidenced by restricted movements in the range of function of the entrapped muscle. These must be surgically repaired.[1]

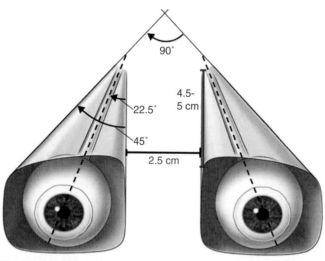

Fig. 7.2 Geometry of the orbit. The orbit is a pyramid-shaped structure with the base anterior and the apex posterior. The medial walls of the two orbits are parallel to each other and in the sagittal plane. The lateral walls are angled 45 degrees relative to the medial wall. The lateral walls of both orbits form a 90-degree angle. The optic nerve emerges at an angle of 22.5 degrees from the medial wall. The eyes in the primary gaze position results in adduction of the globe 22.5 degrees. The orbital volume is, on average, 30 mL, with 6.5 mL filled by the globe.

furthest. The distances were originally determined on cadaveric material[6]; however, recent analyses on living adult patients during strabismus surgery show that the average distances from the corneal limbus to the rectus muscle insertions have large interindividual variations.[7–10] In part, this explains the disparate measurements seen in the literature. One typical study measured the distances from the limbus to muscle insertion as 6.2 ± 0.6 mm for the medial rectus, 7.0 ± 0.6 mm for the inferior rectus, 7.7 ± 0.7 mm for the lateral rectus, and 8.5 ± 0.7 mm for the superior rectus.[10] Distances can vary up to 4 mm, even between the same muscles in both eyes of one individual; these differences do not correlate with the primary position of the eye or surgical success for strabismus patients.[11] Thus, there is a significant amount of variation in rectus muscle insertions, and this variability has important consequences for incisional surgery of the EOM.

The superior and inferior oblique muscles have distinct paths compared with the rectus muscles. The superior oblique takes its origin from the dense connective tissue periosteum lining the orbit just superior and medial to the attachment of the tendinous annulus, and courses anteriorly along the border between the orbital roof and the medial orbital wall. Approximately 10 to 15 mm posterior to the orbital margin it becomes tendinous and enters the trochlea, a cartilaginous and dense connective tissue structure attached to the orbital periosteum. Emerging from the trochlea, the superior oblique muscle passes posteriorly at a 51-degree angle to the axis of the eye in primary position and inserts into the sclera. The trochlea thus serves as the "de facto" origin, creating the vector of force that moves the globe. The insertion of the superior oblique is on the superior pole deep to the superior rectus muscle, but in contrast to the rectus muscles, inserts posterior to the equator of the globe (Fig. 7.3). The inferior oblique muscle is the only EOM that does not take its origin from the apex of the orbit; instead, it originates from the anteromedial orbital floor (Fig. 7.3). The inferior oblique muscle courses posteriorly and inferior to the inferior rectus and inserts into the sclera posterior to the equator of the globe, running in a parallel direction to the superior oblique muscle.

The shape, size, and orientation of the EOM from origin to insertion form the basis for the eye movements that result from their contraction (Table 7.1). Although the effect of contraction of each EOM will be described separately, it is important to remember that they work in a coordinated fashion, maintaining significant tension or "tonus" even when the eye is in primary position and thus presumably "at rest."[2,12]

Eye movements in the horizontal plane are controlled by the medial and lateral rectus muscles, agonist-antagonist pairs with opposing primary functions; the medial rectus adducts the eye, and the lateral rectus abducts the eye. Vertical movements are more complex. The superior and inferior rectus muscles have a more complex action on the direction of eye movements because the bony orbits are not parallel to each other (Fig. 7.2). In primary gaze, both the superior and inferior recti are angled laterally at approximately 22.5 degrees from the sagittal plane. The primary action of the superior rectus muscle is elevation, but it also adducts and intorts the eye (Table 7.1; Fig. 7.4). Intorsion is where the superior pole of the eye rotates medially. Thus, if the superior rectus muscle was acting alone, the direction of gaze would be superior and medial, that is, up and in toward the nose. The inferior rectus is parallel to the superior rectus but inserts on the inferior surface of the globe. It primarily depresses the eye, but also adducts and extorts (Fig. 7.4); extorsion is rotation of the superior pole of the eye laterally.

Owing to its insertion posterior to the equator of the globe, as well as the vector of force directed by the position of the trochlea in the superior and medial orbit, the superior oblique mainly intorts the eye (Table 7.1; Fig. 7.4). It also depresses and abducts. Thus, working unilaterally, gaze would be directed down and out. As the inferior oblique muscle parallels the superior oblique, but inserts on the inferior surface

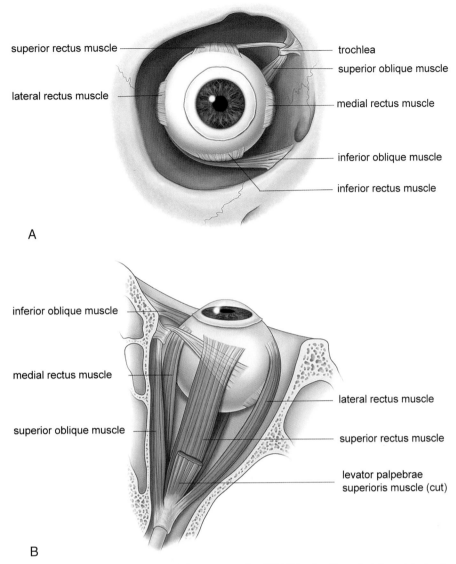

Fig. 7.3 (**A**) Anterior view of the extraocular eye muscles (EOM) in situ. Note that the origin for the inferior oblique is in the inferomedial aspect of the orbit and not the apex. (**B**) Superior view of the EOM in situ. Note the parallel arrangements of the horizontal muscles (medial and lateral rectus); the vertical muscles (superior and inferior rectus); and the insertional tendons of the superior and inferior oblique muscles. (Modified from Doxanas MT, Anderson RL, eds. *Clinical Orbital Anatomy*. Baltimore: William and Wilkins; 1984.)

TABLE 7.1	**Extraocular muscle function: Primary and secondary actions**				
Muscle	**Primary Action**	**Secondary Action**	**Motor Innervation**	**Antagonists**	**Synergists**
Lateral rectus	Abduction	None	Abducens nerve (CN VI)	Medial rectus	Superior and inferior oblique muscle
Medial rectus	Adduction	None	Oculomotor nerve (CN III, inferior division)	Lateral rectus	Superior and inferior rectus muscle
Superior rectus	Elevation	Adduction Intorsion	Oculomotor nerve (CN III, superior division)	Inferior rectus	Medial and inferior rectus muscle Superior oblique muscle
Inferior rectus	Depression	Adduction Extorsion	Oculomotor nerve (CN III, inferior division)	Superior rectus	Medial and superior rectus muscle Inferior oblique and superior rectus muscle
Superior oblique	Intorsion	Depression Abduction	Trochlear nerve (CN IV)	Inferior oblique	Inferior rectus muscle Lateral rectus and inferior oblique muscle
Inferior oblique	Extorsion	Elevation Abduction	Oculomotor nerve (CN III, inferior division)	Superior oblique	Superior rectus muscle Medial rectus and superior oblique muscle

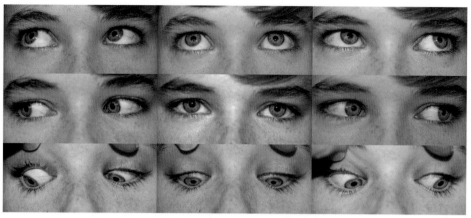

Fig. 7.4 Composite photograph showing a subject looking in the nine cardinal positions of gaze. *Center panel*: Primary gaze straight ahead. *Top panels*: up gaze. *Bottom panels*: down gaze. *Left panels*: gaze to the right. *Right panels*: gaze to the left. (From Christiansen SP and McLoon LK. Extraocular muscles: Functional assessment in the clinic. In: *Elsevier's Encyclopedia of the Eye*. Dartt D [ed.]. Elsevier; 2010).

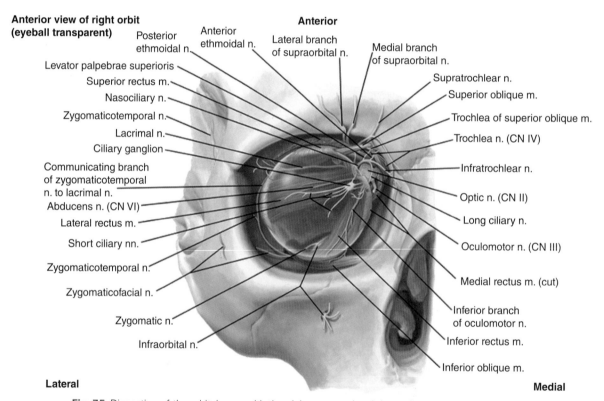

Fig. 7.5 Dissection of the orbital apex with the globe removed and the optic nerve sectioned to allow visualization of the orbital nerves. All motor nerves except the trochlear nerve enter the muscles they innervate on their deep surfaces in the posterior third of their length. (Frank H. Netter MD. *Head and Neck*. Netter Atlas of Human Anatomy: Classic Regional Anatomy Approach. 2, 25–196.e19. © 2022 by Elsevier Inc.).

of the globe, its primary function is extorsion of the eye (Table 7.1; Fig. 7.4); it also elevates and abducts. For accurate positioning of the visual world on the fovea, activity of all the EOM must be highly coordinated by the ocular motor control systems in the brain.

Cranial nerve innervation

The optic foramen is located within the lesser wing of the sphenoid bone at the orbital apex, through which runs the optic nerve (cranial nerve II, CN II) and the ophthalmic artery. Between the greater and lesser wings of the sphenoid bone is the superior orbital fissure. The structures entering the orbit through this fissure are divided by the tendinous annulus (formerly the annulus of Zinn). Structures that enter the orbit superior to the annulus are the lacrimal and frontal nerves, both sensory branches of the ophthalmic division of the trigeminal nerve (CN V); the trochlear nerve (CN IV), motor nerve to the superior oblique muscle; and the superior ophthalmic veins (Fig. 7.5). A large number of structures course through the annulus, entering into an area within what is referred to as the muscle cone. These vessels and nerves are surrounded by the EOM and their connective tissue ensheathments. Within the annulus, the superior orbital fissure admits the superior and inferior divisions of the oculomotor nerve (CN III), which is the motor nerve to the inferior rectus, inferior oblique, medial rectus, superior rectus and levator palpebrae superioris muscles, and the abducens nerve (CN VI), the motor nerve to the lateral rectus muscle.[3] The nasociliary nerve is also located in this region, and it is a sensory branch of the ophthalmic division of the trigeminal nerve (CN V). Entering the orbit through the superior orbital fissure inferior to the annulus is the inferior ophthalmic vein that communicates with the pterygoid plexus of veins inferiorly. On the floor of the orbit is the inferior orbital fissure, which admits small branches of the zygomatic nerve, a sensory nerve innervating the lateral midface as well as lacrimal rami, carrying parasympathetic innervation from the facial nerve (CN VII) to the lacrimal gland.[13]

Once inside the bony orbit, the motor nerve branches of CN III, CN IV, and CN VI course anteriorly toward the muscles they innervate. The superior division of CN III innervates the superior rectus muscle and continues superiorly to innervate the levator palpebrae superioris. The inferior division of CN III innervates the medial and inferior rectus muscles, and the latter branch continues inferiorly to innervate the inferior oblique. All nerve branches of CN III enter the muscles on their deep surfaces within the muscle cone. CN VI also enters the lateral rectus muscle on its deep surface. Of the motor nerves, only the trochlear nerve, CN IV, enters the orbit outside the tendinous annulus innervating the superior oblique muscle on its superior or lateral surface (Fig. 7.5). All motor nerves that innervate the EOM enter the body of the muscles at their posterior third (Fig. 7.5).

Neuromuscular junctions (NMJs) are the specialized sites of communication between a nerve and the myofibers it innervates. In noncranial skeletal muscle, NMJs usually form in the middle one-third of each myofiber. The NMJs formed by the cranial motor nerves with individual EOM myofibers display some distinct differences compared with those in noncranial skeletal muscle. Similar to body muscles, the EOM have singly innervated myofibers with NMJs referred to as "*en plaque*" endings (Fig. 7.6). However, the *en plaque* NMJs in EOM are smaller and less complicated structurally than those in noncranial skeletal muscles.[14] In addition, the EOM have multiply innervated myofibers with neuromuscular junctions referred to as "*en grappe*" endings (Fig. 7.6).[15] These are a linear array of small synaptic contacts often found toward the ends of individual myofibers, but can be continuous along the length of individual myofibers.[16] The *en grappe* NMJ contacts are structurally simple.[17] Thus, in EOM a single myofiber can have an *en plaque* NMJ somewhere along the middle one-third and also have multiple *en grappe* endings along the tapered ends (Fig. 7.6). Some myofibers in EOM that express the slow tonic myosin heavy chain isoform (MYH14) have *en grappe* endings along their entire myofiber length and do not have an *en plaque* ending.

Acetylcholine receptors found within NMJs in skeletal muscle are composed of five subunits. In developing noncranial muscle there are two alpha, one beta, one gamma, and one delta subunits ($\alpha2\beta\gamma\delta$), and in the adult the gamma subunit is replaced with the epsilon subunit.[18] This subunit pattern is found in most *en plaque* endings within the extraocular muscles. In contrast, in adult EOM the majority of the *en grappe* endings express the "immature" gamma subunit, rather than the epsilon subunit of mature endings.[19,20] Both the *en plaque* and *en grappe* endings in the EOM can coexpress both the epsilon and gamma subunits[21]; this appears to be unique to EOM based on studies performed thus far. Owing to the nature of EOM myofiber length, as discussed in a following section, NMJs can be seen throughout the origin-to-insertional length of EOM in most species where this has

been examined.[22,23] This is in contrast to most limb skeletal muscles, which have a motor endplate zone, an NMJ band that is fairly contained within a defined area in the midbelly region of the muscle.

It has generally been assumed that the multiply innervated myofibers are innervated by a single motor neuron, but polyneuronally innervated myofibers are also present.[24,25] This means that more than one motor neuron can innervate a single myofiber. This has important implications for EOM physiology and will be discussed in that section.

Orbital connective tissue

A complex framework of connective tissue exists throughout the orbit, and this network has a clear structural organization and consistent pattern (Fig. 7.7).[26] These connective tissue septa contain nerves, vessels, and smooth muscle, and are postulated to play a role in supporting eye movements. Recent studies have confirmed and extended these initial detailed analyses of orbital connective tissue septa to include thickenings around individual EOM called orbital pulleys (Fig. 7.7).[27] These connective and smooth muscle septa and bands constrain the paths of the EOM, changing the vector of force as the EOM contract and stabilize muscle position during movement.[28]

Recent studies demonstrated extensive interconnections between muscle fibers, muscle fascicles, and the muscle epimysium (Fig. 7.8).[29] This meshwork of interconnected peri- and epimysial elements results in demonstrable lateral force transmission during muscle fiber contraction, as evidenced by direct *in vitro* measurements (Fig. 7.8).[29] These are likely involved in the nonadditive properties of force development, described in more detail in the following section.

Histologic anatomy and physiologic implications

The EOM have a complex anatomy at the microscopic level. The overall cross-sectional areas of their myofibers are extremely small compared to noncranial skeletal muscle. Each EOM is composed of two layers: an outer orbital layer composed of myofibers of extremely small cross-sectional area and an inner global layer with myofibers larger than in the orbital layer but still extremely small compared to noncranial skeletal muscle (Fig. 7.9). Further descriptions will concentrate on human muscle, but the EOM of other mammals have the same general features despite some variations in detail.

In noncranial skeletal muscles, two general fiber types are described, fast and slow, referring mainly to the myosin heavy chain isoforms (MyHC) they express, which in turn determines their shortening velocity.[30] Whether a fiber is "fast" or "slow" is due, in part, to their complement of contractile proteins. Noncranial skeletal muscles that are largely fast MyHC-positive, such as the extensor digitorum longus, have an oxidative metabolism, rapid shortening velocities, and rapid fatigue with activation. Slow MyHC-positive myofibers in noncranial skeletal muscle have a glycolytic metabolism, slower shortening velocities, larger force generation, and are fatigue resistant. The EOM also have these two basic myofiber types. About 85% of the myofibers in both layers in adult EOM are fast MyHC-positive (Fig. 7.9).[31,32] The other 15% of the EOM myofibers are positive for the slow MyHC. In contrast to noncranial skeletal muscle, however, the EOM have extremely fast contractile characteristics, yet are also extremely fatigue resistant.[33] Several factors support these apparently contradictory characteristics. Although the vast majority of noncranial skeletal muscles express one of four MyHCs, fast fiber types IIa (*myh2*), IIx (*myh1*) and IIb (*myh4*), and slow type I (*myh7*) EOM myofibers can contain up to eleven MyHCs with multiple myosins, even within single fibers.[34-37]

The MyHC expressed in EOM include fast types IIa (*myh2*), IIx (*myh1*), and IIb (*myh4*); MyHCs associated with immaturity in limb

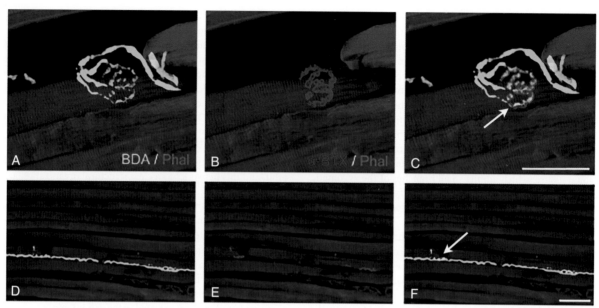

Fig. 7.6 Three-dimensional projections from stacks of confocal laser scanning microscope images showing two types of neuromuscular junctions in extraocular muscles. Neuromuscular junctions were visualized with the tracer biotinylated dextran amine (*green*) injected into the oculomotor nucleus in the brain and α-bungarotoxin labeling (*red*). **A–F**, Triple fluorescence staining with streptavidin (*green*), α-bungarotoxin (*red*), and phalloidin (*blue*) of a medial rectus muscle. Tracer-positive axons establishing neuromuscular contacts resembling en plaque motor terminals (**A–C**) and *en grappe* motor terminals (**D–F**). **B, E**, En plaque and *en grappe* motor terminals, respectively, after α-bungarotoxin labeling. **C, F**, Overlays in yellow mixed color confirming that tracer-positive *en plaque-like* and *en grape-like* endings bind α-bungarotoxin. Scale bars, 50 μm. (From Zimmerman L, Morado-Díaz CJ, Davis-López de Carrizosa MA, et al. Axons giving rise to the palisade endings of feline extraocular muscles display motor features. *J Neurosci.* 2013;33(7):2784–2793. By Elsevier Inc.).

and body skeletal muscles—embryonic (developmental) (*myh3*) and neonatal (fetal) (*myh8*); slow or type I (which is the same as beta-cardiac myosin in the heart) (*myh7*); alpha-cardiac (*myh6*); EOM-specific (*myh13*); and the slow tonic myosin (*myh7b* or *myh14*). Two additional novel myosins also are found in EOM. The first MyHC isoform was found to be expressed in extraocular muscles MYH15 (*myh15*), but only in orbital layer fibers and muscle spindles.[38] In addition, approximately 20% of the global layer slow MyHC-positive fibers were shown to express the nonmuscle myosin IIB (*myh10*).[39] This large array of expressed MyHC within the EOM helps explain why its dynamic physiologic properties are significantly different than those in limb muscles.[40] It should be noted that patterns of MyHC composition vary between each EOM, with lateral rectus being the most different.[41] Support for the idea that the MyHC composition may be critical for understanding control of force generation is the physiologic demonstration that there are significant contractile differences between individual muscles. For example, when comparing the medial and lateral rectus muscles, motor units in the medial rectus generate faster twitch contractions and those in lateral rectus generate greater tonic tensions.[42] This concept is critical in understanding the central nervous system (CNS) control of eye movements, as well as eye movement disorders like strabismus.

The expression patterns of EOM myofibers for these MyHC differ significantly between the global and orbital layers (Fig. 7.9). For example, the vast majority of the orbital layer myofibers are positive for developmental myosin (MYH3), yet the global layer only has scattered fibers that immunostain for this isoform (Fig. 7.9). Distinct patterns of differential staining are seen for all other MyHC present in EOM. From a physiologic perspective, this issue becomes even more complex. Approximately 25% of the analyzed cat single lateral rectus motor units, defined as all the fibers innervated by a single motor neuron, had

myofibers in both the orbital and global layers.[42,43] These bilayer motor units were stronger and faster than motor units contained within single EOM layers, and they tended to be fatigable. Approximately 54% of the global motor units examined were stronger and faster than orbital layer units, in part a reflection of the properties imbued upon the individual myofibers by their contractile proteins.

The expression of individual MyHC also varies along the origin-to-insertional length of each muscle.[41,44,45] In part this is because many of the EOM myofibers do not run from origin to insertion in both the orbital and global layers[23,24,41,45–47]; they can be arranged in parallel or in series, and many branched and/or split myofibers exist (Fig. 7.10).[23] These short myofiber lengths have functional consequences. For example, in a series of studies examining summation of motor forces, individual cat and monkey motor units were stimulated, and the forces each unit produced in the lateral rectus muscle were determined. Then, using simultaneous stimulation, the evoked unit force of other motor units was added to the single motor unit force. In about 25% of the cases in cat and about 85% of the cases in monkey, the measured forces did not add linearly.[48,49] Thus, force is "lost" as multiple myofibers are activated, partly due to force dissipation laterally through myomyous junctions and myoconnective tissue connections formed by short myofibers (Fig. 7.8).[29]

In addition, the serial or parallel arrangement of myofibers with different myofibrillar isoforms would significantly affect contractile behavior. This was elegantly demonstrated using sets of single myofibers in vitro, one fast and one slow, that were tied together in series or in parallel.[50] In any given combination of one fast and one slow myofiber, the paired fibers showed a range of forces with greater or lesser fast or slow characteristics. In a fast/slow combination, the fast fiber began to contract prior to the slow fiber, which was then

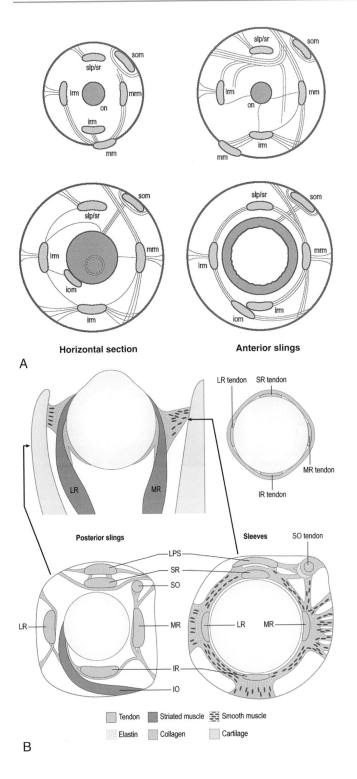

Fig. 7.7 (A) Connective tissue septa at different levels in the orbit. *Top left*, near the orbital apex. *Top right*, hallway between apex and rear surface of the globe. *Bottom left*, near the rear surface of the globe. *Bottom right*, area near the equator of the globe. *iom*, Inferior oblique muscle; *irm*, inferior rectus muscle; *slp/sr*, superior *levator* palpebrae/superior rectus complex; *lrm*, lateral rectus muscle; *mm*, Muller's muscle; *mrm*, medial rectus muscle; *som*, superior oblique muscle; *on*, optic nerve. (Redrawn from Koornneef L. *Spatial Aspects of Orbital Musculo-fibrous Tissue in Man: A New Anatomical and Histological Approach*. Amsterdam: Swets and Zeitlinger; 1976.) **(B)** Diagrammatic representation of orbital connective tissues. The three coronal views are represented at the levels indicated by *arrows* in the horizontal section. *IR*, Inferior rectus; *SO*, superior oblique; *SR*, superior rectus ; *LR*, lateral rectus; *MR*, medial rectus; *SR*, superior rectus; *LPS*, levator palpebrae superioris; *IO*, inferior oblique. (Modified from Demer JL, Miller JM, Poukens V, Vinters HV, Glasgow BJ. Evidence for fibromuscular pulleys of the recti extraocular muscles. *Invest Ophthalmol Vis Sci.* 1995;36:1125–1136, with permission from the Association of Research in Vision and Ophthalmology.)

slack and therefore not at its optimal length to generate its full force. Based on these studies, serial or parallel arrangements of myofibers with disparate MyHC isoform composition would result in a range, or continuum, of forces produced by their coactivation. These data suggest that a distributed model of motor recruitment at the CNS level is needed to address the nonlinearity of the effector arm of the system, the EOM themselves.[51]

Individual EOM myofibers are polymorphic and can express more than one MyHC in different regions of each fiber.[34,44,45,52–54] This is true for a wide variety of species, including human EOM.[34] For example,

in both singly and multiply innervated myofibers in the orbital layer in rats, the fiber ends expressed the neonatal MyHC (*myh8*), but this isoform was completely eliminated at the position of the NMJ, where the fibers immunostained for fast MyHC.[44] In the orbital layer, individual myofibers expressed the embryonic MyHC (*myh3*) at their fiber ends and the EOM-specific MyHC (*myh13*) in the NMJ region. Orbital multiply innervated myofibers were found that expressed slow MyHC (*myh7*) along their entire length, but also expressed embryonic MyHC (*myh3*) at the fiber ends.[45] Single myofibers in the global layer were found that expressed EOM-specific MyHC (*myh13*) at the

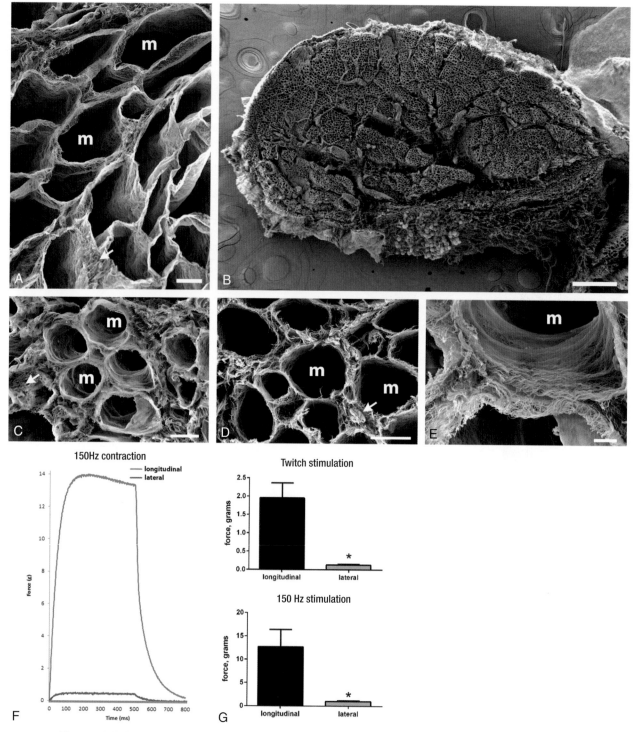

Fig. 7.8 (**A–E**) Scanning electron micrographs of rabbit gastrocnemius muscle (**A**) and human medial rectus (**B–E**). Notice that myofibers (m; here seen as the tubular cavities corresponding to the digested myofibers) in the limb muscle share the connective tissue sleeve forming the endomysium with the adjacent myofibers. The whole extraocular muscle cross-section shows the impressive connective tissue network interconnecting both layers and extending all the way from the fibers to the perimysium and the epimysium (**B**). At higher magnifications (**C–E**), a very generous network of curvilinear fibrils surrounds each myofiber (m) separately (**C**) or as a common boundary between adjacent myofibers (**D**). The network widely anchors the myofibers across the interstitial space between them and extends to the perimysium (*arrows*). *Scale bars*: 20 μm (**A**), 500 μm (**B**), 10 μm (**C,D**), 2 μm (**E**). (**F**) Example of the force in grams of one muscle stimulated at 150 Hz. The *blue trace* is in the longitudinal orientation, and the *red trace* depicts force in the medial to lateral (lateral) dimension. (**G**) Mean force in grams after a single twitch stimulation ($n = 4$). *Significant difference from the force generated in the longitudinal direction. (**H**) Mean force in grams after a 150-Hz stimulation ($n = 4$). *Significant difference from the force generated in the longitudinal direction. (From McLoon LK, Vincente A, Fitzpatrick KR, Lindstrom M, Pedrosa Domellöf F. Composition, architecture, and functional implications of the connective tissue network of the extraocular muscles. *Invest Ophthalmol Vis Sci.* 2018;59:322–329, with permission from the Association of Research in Vision and Ophthalmology.)

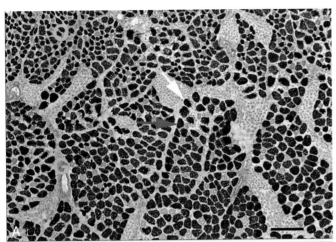

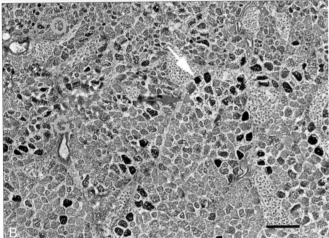

Fig. 7.9 Photomicrographs of two serial sections from a normal monkey lateral rectus muscle immunostained for (**A**) fast MyHC and (**B**) neonatal MyHC. The orbital layer is on the *top* (O) and global layer on the *bottom* (G). *Arrows* point to two myofibers: one positive for both fast and neonatal MyCH and one positive for fast but negative for neonatal MyHC. Bar is 100 µm.

NMJ region, as well as fast MyHC IIb and/or IIx (*myh1* and *myh4*).[53] In human EOM, orbital layer myofibers were found that expressed type I MyHC (*myh7*), and of these (Fig. 7.11), some also expressed slow tonic MyHC (*myh14*), alpha-cardiac (*myh6*), and/or embryonic (*myh3*) or EOM-specific (*myh13*).[32,36,54] Physiologic examination of individual multiply innervated myofibers from the orbital layer of rats showed that contractile velocity varied along the length of the fiber, with tonic characteristics at the fiber end and twitch characteristics in the central region near the endplate, the only location where fast MyHC was expressed.[24]

Thus, physiologic properties of the EOM motor units, when activated singly or collectively, reflect these MyHC isoform complexities, as well as differences in individual myofiber length and branching patterns.[49] It should be noted that the EOM show significant activity at all times, even when the eye is directed in what would be considered the off-direction for muscle action.[2] In addition, all motor units participate in all types of eye movements, and there appear to be no motor units that specialize in rapid saccades or slow vergence movements, for example.[55] Presumably, the MyHC composition is a reflection of demands placed on the EOM by the oculomotor control system, and this view is supported by the observation that altering the stimulation

frequency to a muscle causes significant changes in MyHC expression.[56] Functional denervation also affects MyHC composition.[57] It is reasonable to suggest that a complex "conversation" is constantly occurring between EOM myofibers and the neurons innervating them, helping them to adapt to ever-changing physiologic demands. Because of these complex MyHC expression patterns and physiologic characteristics, past attempts to classify EOM myofibers into simple groups ultimately fail. Classically, myofibers in noncranial skeletal muscles have been described by their MyHC expression profile (e.g., type IIa or type I). Even in noncranial skeletal muscles, it is becoming increasingly clear that single myofiber MyHC polymorphism is more common than was previously believed.[58,59] Another fiber type, called "mismatched," has been described in both noncranial and cranial skeletal muscle.[58,60] Mismatched myofibers include those with "mixed" fast and slow characteristics, and can include fibers with mixtures of fast and slow MyHC or fast or slow MyHC with various regulatory protein such as troponin[61] or myosin-binding protein C[62] that are not of the same "type." This complexity of protein expression and the heterogeneity of individual myofibers in EOM cannot be overstated. What these studies suggest is that rather than specific "types" of myofibers (Fig. 7.12) in EOM, there is, in fact, a continuum of myofiber types. Each myosin heavy and light chain isoform results in a distinct shortening velocity,[63] which allows for an incredible plasticity in the control of muscle force generation. The modulation of the MyHC patterns with alterations in hormones or innervational changes also compounds the heterogeneity of the EOM myofibers. These adaptive protein changes are extremely rapid, and the control may be at the level of histone modifications[64] or at the translational level controlled by microRNA—known to be upregulated in the EOM.[65] The EOM myofiber continuum hypothesis was suggested previously for other skeletal muscles, including plantaris[66] and masseter.[67] This continuum of myofiber types in EOM combined with the nonlinearity of eye muscle contractile properties[49] would allow CNS control of eye movement position and velocity to be finely tuned as the eyes are moved into an infinite number of positions.

Metabolism

The physiologic properties of the EOM derive their dynamic and unusual characteristics from (1) their expression of specific contractile proteins including, but not limited to, isoforms of MyHC, myosin light chains, tropomyosin, and troponin; (2) the presence of myofibers shorter than the total origin-to-insertional length of each EOM, resulting in fibers connected in parallel or in series; (3) the presence of singly, multiply, and polyneuronally innervated individual myofibers; and (4) adaptations of their metabolic pathways.

The most studied metabolic property in EOM is their calcium handling. Calcium plays a critical role in controlling the duration of muscle contractions. In part, this is controlled by the sarcoplasmic reticulum Ca^{2+}-ATPases (SERCA1 and SERCA2) in fast and slow myofibers, respectively, in noncranial skeletal muscle. In contrast to limb skeletal muscle, in the EOM SERCA1 and SERCA2 are coexpressed in the majority of individual myofibers.[68] The EOM contain an abundance of mitochondria, and EOM myofibers appear to use their mitochondria as fast calcium sinks to aid in regulation of calcium.[69] This effectively widens the dynamic range of EOM force production. Owing to their efficient calcium handling, EOM myofibers are resistant to pathologic elevations of intracellular calcium levels.[70]

EOM are resistant to injury and oxidative stress and contain higher levels of superoxide dismutases and glutathione peroxidase activity than limb skeletal muscle.[71] These properties are concordant with the highly aerobic nature of the EOM. Only cardiac muscle has a higher blood

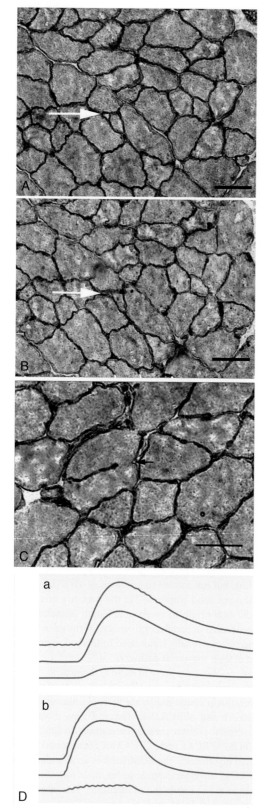

Fig. 7.10 (A) and **(B)** Cross-sections through rabbit superior rectus muscle immunostained for dystrophin. Arrows indicate a myofiber present in one section that ended before the next section 24-μm distant. Bar is 20 μm. **(C)** Interconnected myofibers (*arrow*) in normal extra-ocular muscles (EOM) immunostained for dystrophin. Bar is 20 μm. **(D)** Physiologic demonstration of nonadditive muscle forces in extraocular eye muscles using (a) twitch and (b) tetanic responses after stimulation. (a) Muscle responses to stimulation of one motor neuron (*bottom trace*, 45.9 mg), muscle responses to stimulation of several motor units (*middle trace*, 209.5 mg), and activation of a single motor unit plus nerve responses (*upper trace*, 257.5 mg). The twitch responses are additive; no force is "lost." (b) Muscle responses of the same motor unit to tetanic stimulation. Muscle responses from tetanic stimulation of a single motor unit (*bottom trace*, 398.7 mg), several motor units (*middle trace*, 4066 mg) and the single motor unit plus nerve responses (*upper trace*, 4226 mg). This unit loses 40% of its force upon tetanic stimulation. Horizontal bar, 50 msec. Vertical bar, 917 mg. (From Goldberg SJ, Wilson KE, Shall ME. Summation of extraocular motor unit tensions in the lateral rectus muscle of the cat. *Muscle Nerve* 1997; 20:1229–1235, with permission from Wiley)

flow rate.[72] Despite their highly oxidative metabolism, the EOM are also extremely fatigue-resistant.[73] Unlike noncranial muscles, EOM do not depend on creatine kinase activity for their fatigue resistance[74]; instead, EOM can utilize lactate as a metabolic substrate during times of increased contractile activity.[75] This further illustrates how the EOM can maintain a highly oxidative metabolism and fatigue resistance simultaneously. Additionally, these two opposite metabolic demands are met by the expression in individual EOM myofibers of both succinate dehydrogenase and alpha-glycerophosphate dehydrogenase, enzymes in the oxidative and glycolytic pathways, respectively.

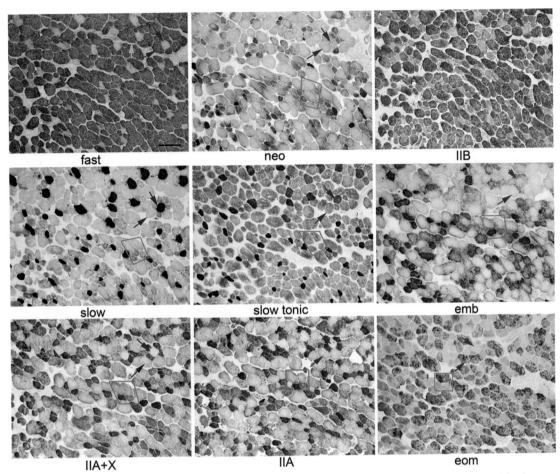

Fig. 7.11 Photomicrograph of serial sections of the orbital layer of a superior rectus muscle from normal adult rabbit immunostained for each of the following MyHC isoforms: fast, neonatal, MyHCI (slow) (from Vector) and type IIB (BF-F3), slow-tonic (S46), embryonic (F1.652), type IIA (SC-71), and type IIX(6H1) (from Hybridoma Bank). Six individ-ual myofibers are followed in the 8 serial sections, each identified with a single colored arrow (*green, blue, red, yellow, purple, and orange*). Black and maroon arrows indicate fibers that are differentially positive for slow and slow-tonic antibody staining. Bar represents 20 μm. (From McLoon LK, Park H, Kim JH, Pedrosa-Domellof F, Thompson LV. A continuum of myofibers in adult rabbit extraocular muscle: force, shortening velocity, and patterns of myosin heavy chain co-localization. *J Appl Physiol.* 2011;111(4):1178–1189. By Elsevier Inc.).

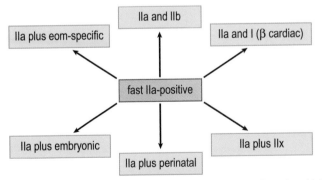

Fig. 7.12 Schematic of human single myofiber coexpression of multiple MyHC isoforms. Myofibers can express MyHCIIA only or coexpress any one of the six MyHC isoforms shown, creating seven myofiber "types." However, single myofibers can coexpress three, four, or more MyHC isoforms, increasing the possible number of "fiber types." This diagram only considers MyHC expression patterns. (Based on coexpression data found in Kjellgren D, Thornell LE, Andersen J, Pedrosa-Domellöf F. Myosin heavy chain isoforms in human extraocular muscles. *Invest Ophthalmol Vis Sci.* 2003;44:1419-1425 and Kranjc BS, Smerdu V, Erzen I. Histochemical and immunohistochemical profile of human and rat ocular medial rectus muscles. *Graefes Arch Clin Exp Ophthalmol.* 2009;247:1505–1515.)

In contrast, these two enzymes are fiber-type specific in limb skeletal muscle.[76] This supports the view that skeletal muscles consist of distinct allotypes relative to body and limb skeletal muscles,[77] and the EOM represent the extreme end relative to its anatomy, innervation, metabolism, and physiologic function.

Another distinctive aspect of EOM function is their ability to undergo a significant level of myonuclear addition and subtraction throughout life,[78,79] while simultaneously maintaining their overall size, morphology, and function. Using labeling with the thymidine analog bromodeoxyuridine, activated satellite cells, the myogenic precursor cells of adult muscle, are seen; with sufficient postlabeling intervals, labeled myonuclei are present within existing myofibers in normal adult EOM of rabbits and mice (Fig. 7.13). These new myonuclei are located peripherally, not centrally, indicating that this process of myonuclear addition is different from what occurs during muscle regeneration. This was validated using a PAX7 reporter mouse line, where tdTomato was expressed in PAX7 cells. Myonuclear addition is seen by red fluorescence in fibers where this process has occurred (Fig. 7.13B).[80] Although a low level of myonuclear addition occurs in the noncranial muscles examined thus far, it is not at the level of the EOM (Fig. 7.13B). The process of myofiber remodeling continues throughout life even in human EOM, as the presence of activated satellite cells, identified by the myogenic lineage marker MYOD,[81] is seen in the EOM specimens from elderly humans.[82] Ongoing and significant levels of myofiber remodeling occurs in other craniofacial muscles as well,[83] suggesting that the differences in genes involved in the development of cranial muscles may play a role in retention of this dynamic process in adult EOM.[84] The control of this process in the adult EOM is unknown.

In contrast to noncranial skeletal muscles, EOM continue to express a number of myogenic growth factors and functional receptors for these growth-promoting molecules.[85,86] PITX2, a mitogen and repressor of differentiation,[87,88] is a signaling factor expressed in adult EOM[87] and may play a role in maintaining a proliferative state in adult EOM. A conditional knockout of PITX2 in adult EOM results in alteration of the adult EOM phenotype to resemble that of limb skeletal muscle, with a loss of EOM-specific MyHC.[89] This is another aspect of the unusual biology of the EOM.

EOM are also set apart from noncranial skeletal muscles in their resiliency to injury and/or denervation. Botulinum toxin A, a muscle paralytic agent used to treat strabismus and focal dystonias such as blepharospasm,[90] causes myofiber atrophy in limb skeletal muscle. However, botulinum toxin A treatment in EOM actually causes some myofiber hypertrophy,[91] short-term activation of satellite cell proliferation,[57] and shifts in MyHC composition,[57] but few long-term effects except for decreases of the EOM-specific MyHC isoform.[92] Recalcitrance to injury is also seen after injection of the local anesthetic bupivacaine. Bupivacaine is a potent myotoxin and causes massive myofiber degeneration when injected into limb skeletal muscles; however, in the EOM of primates minimal lesions were seen after retrobulbar injection.[93,94] Surprisingly, denervation of adult EOM causes relatively little histologic change;[95–97] the multiply innervated myofibers actually hypertrophy in the denervated EOM.[95]

Using a denervation/reinnervation animal model, previously denervated EOM actually have more myofibers than the nonoperated control side.[98] These data illustrate two very important features of the adult EOM: they are remarkably resistant to various forms of injury, and they are incredibly adaptive under a variety of perturbations.

Proprioception and proprioceptors

Proprioception in limb skeletal muscle is largely the job of muscle spindles, sensory receptors that detect changes in muscle length; this information is conveyed to the CNS, which responds by regulating muscle tension to resist stretch. In the EOM, the role of proprioception is a matter of some controversy. Primate EOM does not appear to have a stretch reflex.[99] Deafferentation of the EOM bilaterally does not result in eye position or eye movement changes.[100] However, when the EOM of a cat is stretched, neurons within the brain respond, despite the fact that cat EOM lack muscle spindles.[101] The brain has access to eye position, because even in total darkness humans perceive passive changes in eye position.[101] Visual cortex responses are modulated by changes in eye position also,[102] and primary somatosensory cortex possesses proprioceptive representation of eye position.[103] What are the sensory organs, then, that receive and transmit this proprioceptive input?

The presence of muscle spindles has been histologically demonstrated only in the EOM of man, monkey, and even-toed ungulates. Muscle spindles are composed of two types of specialized intrafusal myofibers within a connective tissue sheath (Fig. 7.14): nuclear chain and nuclear bag fibers. Only nuclear chain fibers are common in human EOM. Intrafusal fibers receive sensory innervation at their equatorial region and motor innervation at their spindle poles, and they are surrounded by an acidic mucopolysaccharide-containing fluid (Fig. 7.14).[104] In human EOM, the number and placement of muscle spindles vary quite significantly in the different muscles.[105] In general,

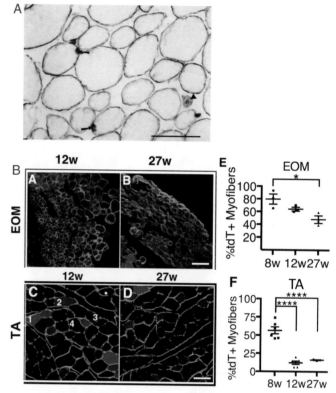

Fig. 7.13 (A). Normal extraocular muscles (*EOM*) incorporated the thymidine analog bromodeoxyuridine (brdU) into dividing satellite cells, and these were incorporated into normal myofibers in adults. In this case, the rabbit was injected once per day with brdU for 7 days, followed by 14 days brdU-free. Arrows indicate brdU-positive myonuclei. Myofibers were counterstained with an antibody to dystrophin for visualization of the inner side of the sarcolemma. Bar is 100 μm. (From McLoon LK, Wirtschafter JD. Continuous myonuclear addition to single extraocular myofibers in uninjured adult rabbits. *Muscle Nerve.* 2002;25:348–358 with permission from Wiley.) **(B)** Satellite cell contribution to EOM (a,b,e) did not plateau with age, as many tdTomato expressing myofibers were present at both 12 and 27 weeks of age. Quantification showed high percentages of red myofibers overtime. In contrast, in the leg muscle tibialis anterior (*TA*) (c,d,f), a significant contribution of tdTomato expressing PAX7 satellite cells was seen at 8 weeks of age but dropped to extremely low percentages (f) by 27 weeks of age. Scale bar is 50 μm. (Modified from Pawlikowski B, Pulliam C, Betta ND, Kardon G, Olwin BB. Pervasive satellite cell contribution to uninjured adult muscle fibers. *Skelet Mus.* 2015;5:42, with permission from Springer Nature.)

they are higher in density in the more proximal and distal portions of the EOM and relatively devoid of spindles in the midbelly region. The density varies between the individual EOM. The inferior rectus contains the most, with approximately 34 in the entire muscle. Superior oblique has twofold more spindles than the other three rectus muscles. Inferior oblique has the fewest, averaging only four spindles which are located in the midbelly region, rather than toward the origin and insertion.[105] Despite their well-described nature, the role muscle spindles play in the control of eye movements is unclear; one hypothesis suggests that they monitor static length and play no role in velocity monitoring, as no stretch reflex is present in the EOM of monkey, for example.[99]

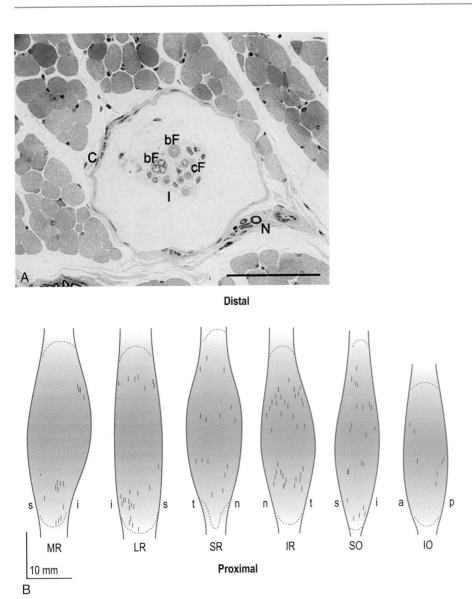

Distal

Proximal

MR   LR   SR   IR   SO   IO

10 mm

B

Fig. 7.14 (**A**) Cross-section through the equatorial region of a cow muscle spindle. The muscle spindle contains two nuclear bag fibers (bF) and five nuclear chain fibers (cF). In one nuclear bag fiber the bag region containing several nuclei is visible. In some nuclear chain fibers, their central nuclei are seen. Bag fibers have a larger diameter than chain fibers. An inner capsule (I) surrounds the intrafusal myofibers. Capsule (C), nerve (N). Scale bar, 100 μm. (From Blumer R, Konakci KZ, Brugger PC et al. Muscle spindles and Golgi tendon organs in bovine calf extraocular muscle studied by means of double-fluorescent labeling, electron microscopy, and three-dimensional reconstruction. *Exp Eye Res.* 2003;77(4):447–462. Copyright Elsevier 2003). (**B**) Reconstructions from camera lucida drawings illustrating the exact positions and relative lengths of muscle spindles projected into one plane for all six extraocular muscles of the same orbit (72-year-old woman). *IO,* Inferior oblique; *IR,* inferior rectus; *MR,* medial rectus; *LR,* lateral rectus; *SO,* superior oblique; *SR,* superior rectus. *a,* anterior; *i,* inferior; *n,* nasal; *p,* posterior; *s,* superior; *t,* temporal. Scale, 12.5. (Modified from Lukas JR, Aigner M, Blumer R, Heinzl H, Mayr R. Number and distribution of neuromuscular spindles in human extraocular muscles. *Invest Ophthalmol Vis Sci.* 1994; 35:4317–4327, with permission from the Association for Research in Vision and Ophthalmology.)

A second structure that has been associated with proprioception is palisade endings (formerly called myotendinous cylinders), present in all mammalian EOM examined thus far, including man (Fig. 7.15).[106] These endings appear to be unique to the EOM.[107] They are found in the distal myotendinous region, where nerve fibers exit the muscle and then turn back to form synaptic contacts on the distal muscle tips of multiply innervated myofibers (Fig. 7.15).[108] The synapses of palisade endings are now considered to have a motor function rather than sensory (Fig. 7.15).[15,109] This view is amply supported by experiments lesioning the oculomotor nucleus, which results in loss of both myofiber NMJs and those in the palisade endings[110] and tracing studies showing they take their origin from motor neurons of the ocular motor system.[111] These endings have exocytotic machinery within them, but only those associated with *en grappe* endings expressed acetylcholinase activity.[112] Thus, palisade endings have an effector function and lack the central connections that would provide sensory feedback on eye position.[15,109]

Development

The distinct embryologic origin of EOM may explain retention of its many unusual characteristics. Although much more is understood about the early development of noncranial skeletal muscles, recent studies have shed light on the genetic control of myogenesis in extraocular and other craniofacial muscles.[113–115] The early control of craniofacial myogenesis involves a distinct set of genes and proteins compared with noncranial muscles (Fig. 7.16A),[114–116] and elucidating these differences helps lay the foundation for understanding clinical problems involving the EOM.

The EOM are derived from two sources of cranial mesoderm.[116,117] These early mesodermal precursor cells are not segmented, in contrast to the somites that give rise to noncranial skeletal muscles. Additionally, cranial mesoderm does not separate into distinct dermamyotomes and sclerotomes. Instead, EOM precursors arise from prechordal or paraxial mesoderm adjacent to the mes- and metencephalon, the

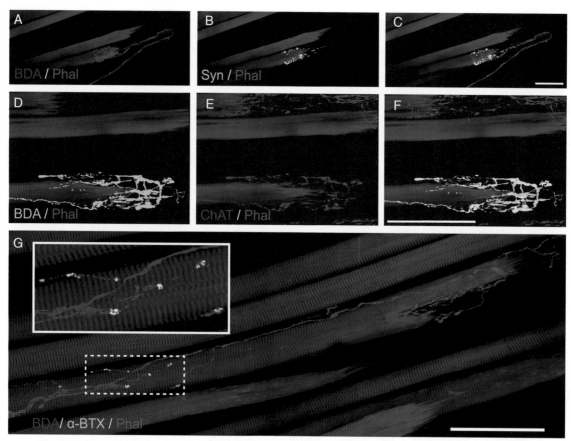

Fig. 7.15 Three-dimensional projections of stacks of CLSM images showing tracer-labeled palisade endings in muscle-tendon, whole-mount preparations. Tracer visualization was combined with fluorescence staining of other cellular molecules. **A–C**, Palisade ending in a lateral rectus muscle. The visualization of the anterograde tracer BDA with streptavidin (*red*) was combined anti-synaptophysin (*green*) and phalloidin (*blue*). **A**, A tracer-positive palisade ending. **B**, Palisade nerve terminals exhibit synaptophysin immunoreactivity. **C**, Overlay of **A** and **B**. Palisade nerve terminals appear in yellow mixed color. **D–F**, Palisade endings in a superior rectus muscle. Tracer visualization with avidin (*green*) was combined with anti-ChAT (*red*) and phalloidin (*blue*). **D**, A single tracer-positive palisade ending. **E**, Demonstrating two ChAT-positive palisade endings. **F**, Overlay in yellow mixed color exhibiting that tracer-positive palisade ending is ChAT-positive as well. The ChAT-positive palisade ending in the upper part of the image lacks tracer. **G**, Palisade ending in an inferior rectus muscle. Tracer visualization with streptavidin (*red*) was combined with α-bungarotoxin (*green*) and phalloidin (*blue*). The tracer-positive palisade ending is supplied by a nerve fiber that forms α-bungarotoxin-positive motor contacts along the muscle fiber. A detail of the motor contacts is shown in the inset. Scale bars, 100μm. (From Zimmerman L, Morado-Díaz CJ, Davis-López de Carrizosa MA, et al. Axons giving rise to the palisade endings of feline extraocular muscles display motor features. *J Neurosci.* 2013;33(7):2784–2793. By Elsevier Inc.).

future midbrain and hindbrain, respectively, and migrate to their final locations.[118] When the transcription factor PAX3 is knocked out in mice, despite a complete absence of body and limb skeletal muscle, EOM develop normally.[114] Other myogenic regulatory factors such as Sonic Hedgehog (SHH), WNT3a, and bone morphogenetic protein 4 (BMP4), which turn on myogenesis in somitic mesoderm, have an inhibitory effect on myogenesis in cranial mesodermal cells both in vitro and in vivo.[113] These proteins are generated by the developing brain and surface ectoderm, delaying myogenesis onset. Soon after identifiable EOM anlagen form, neural crest-derived cells migrate into them,[118] and this migration depends on BMP signaling.[119]

Recent studies show that the homeodomain transcription factor PITX2 is required for EOM development (Fig. 7.16A,B),[120,121] and the absence of this gene in development causes ocular defects such as

Rieger syndrome.[122] EOM morphogenesis is tightly regulated by *Pitx2* gene dose, so if there is a small reduction in *Pitx2*, no superior and inferior oblique muscles form but the rectus muscles develop normally.[123] If *Pitx2* levels are reduced further, the rectus muscles become smaller and more disorganized, and a total deletion of *Pitx2* results in the complete absence of all the EOM (Fig. 7.16B). *Pitx2* is a retinoic acid (RA)-responsive gene, and RA controls neural crest movement.[124] Neural crest infiltration into the EOM is required for their normal migration. In the absence of RA, the EOM form but do not successfully migrate.[124] Other signaling factors such as BARX2 and LBX1 are differentially expressed in early developing EOM, but not universally[115] (Fig. 7.16C), and their role in EOM formation is unclear.

After precursor migration, on a molecular level myogenesis proceeds similarly to that seen in noncranial skeletal muscle, but it differs quite significantly on a temporal level.[115] Muscles derived from somites express MYF5 and MYOD transcripts, early markers of muscle-specific differentiation, earlier in development than in craniofacial muscle precursors.[125] There is a prolonged period prior to expression of MyHC isoforms in craniofacial muscles compared with the timing between MYOD and MyHC expression in developing limb muscle. Neural crest cells express a number of signaling factors, including BMP, WNTs, and SHH, thought to be responsible for this early repression of myogenesis in developing craniofacial muscles,[113] whereas these same molecules promote muscle differentiation in somitic muscle precursors. The sequence and timing of MyHC expression also differs in cranial and noncranial skeletal muscle.[126,127]

In the EOM from human fetuses, only primary myotubes are present at early gestational ages, and coexpress two developmental isoforms of slow myosin (type I). In addition, they express the two "immature" isoforms, embryonic (*myh3*) and fetal (*myh8*). These developmental stages consistently lag behind limb skeletal muscle by 2 to 4 weeks.[128] When secondary myotube formation begins, the first type IIa (*myh2*) is expressed.[128,129] Even by 22 weeks of gestation in human fetuses, the alpha-cardiac (*myh6*) and EOM-specific (*myh13*) MyHC isoforms are not detected. This fiber type development and diversification in EOM occurs in the absence of morphologically mature endplates.[130] Studies in mouse embryos show that EOM position is dependent on cues from the local environment, but early EOM myogenesis is independent of

neural crest cells, target tissues, and nerves.[131] Modern molecular biologic tools are helping to answer the question of how EOM becomes EOM and what controls its collective unusual properties at the molecular level, yet there is much still unknown. This becomes rapidly apparent when congenital conditions involving the EOM are examined.

Disease propensity

From a clinical perspective, the preferential involvement or sparing of the EOM in disease represents critical unsolved questions. Diseases that involve the EOM can be divided into three basic categories: (1) clinical disorders related to the specific motor functions of EOM, (2) diseases with preferential sparing of the EOM compared to limb skeletal muscle, and (3) diseases where the EOM are either primarily or preferentially involved compared with limb skeletal muscle. An exhaustive review of all these clinical entities is beyond the scope of this chapter; however, each of these general categories will be discussed.

DISORDERS OF EYE MOVEMENTS

Three examples of conditions that manifest with abnormal eye position and/or movements are included: strabismus, nystagmus, and congenital cranial dysinnervation disorders (CCDD).

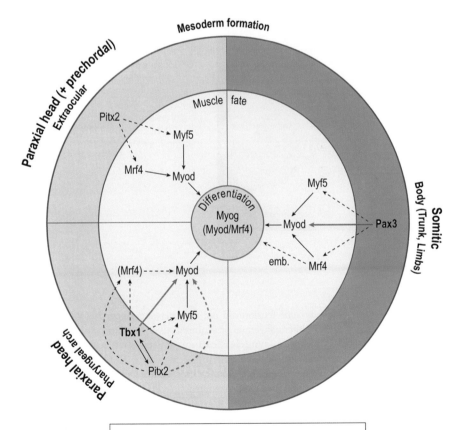

Fig. 7.16 (A) Extraocular muscles (EOMs) do not have complementary regulatory pathways. MYOD expression is not rescued in the absence of MYF5 and MRF4, and EOMs do not form. In pharyngeal (PA) muscles, TBX1 cooperates with MYRF5. In their combined absence, MYOD is not activated, and PA muscles are missing. In the body and EOMs, MRF4 determines embryonic but not fetal myogenic precursor cell fate. PITX2 may cooperate with TBX1 at this regulatory step in the PA. PAX3 acts as the complementary pathway for body myogenesis to rescue MYOD expression. (Amanda L. Zacharias, Mark Lewandoski, Michael A. Rudnicki, Philip J. Gage, Pitx2 is an upstream activator of extraocular myogenesis and survival, *Developmental Biology*. 349(2), 2011, 395–405, https://doi.org/10.1016/j.ydbio.2010.10.028.)

Extraocular: No major pathway complementary to core
Pharyngeal: Complementary to core → Tbx1
Trunk, limbs: Complementary to core → Pax3
Myf5, Mrf4, Myod: core determination genes
Myogenin: core MRF differentiation gene

A

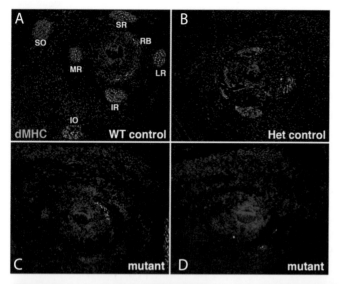

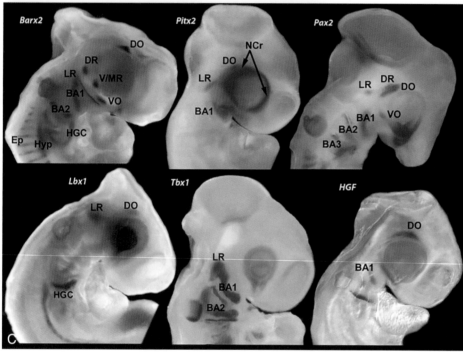

Fig. 7.16, cont'd Mesoderm-specific knockout of Pitx2 results in the absence of extraocular muscles. Sagittal sections behind the globe of the eye allow for visualization of all seven extraocular muscles at later developmental time points, such as e14.5 **(A)**. Immunohistochemistry for developmental myosin heavy chain (dMHC) shows T-Cre+; Pitx2flox/null mutant embryos have little **(C)** to no **(D)** differentiated extraocular muscle at e14.5, as compared to either T-Cre+; Pitx2+/+ (A) or T-Cre+; Pitx2+/null **(B)** controls. *SO*, superior oblique; *SR*, superior rectus; *MR*, medial rectus; *RB*, retractor bulbus; *LR*, lateral rectus; *IR*, inferior rectus; *IO*, inferior oblique. (From Zacharias AL, Lewandoski M, Rudnicki MA, Gage PJ. Pitx2 is an upstream activator of extraocular myogenesis and survival. *Dev Biol.* 2011;349 (2): 395–405. By Elsevier Inc.) **(C)** Genes expressed in all (*barx2, pax2*) or subsets of chick head muscles. *Lbx1* is, like *paraxis*, expressed in glossal and laryngeal myoblasts derived from occipital somites, and in the lateral rectus (and *lbx2* in the dorsal oblique). *Tbx2* is in all branchial myoblasts and also the lateral rectus and is expressed in other epithelial and mesenchymal cells of the head. *Pitx2* is present in the 1rst branchial arch muscle plate and also in several EOMs, plus periocular neural crest cells. Hepatocyte growth factor (HGF) is produced in the mandibular and dorsal oblique muscles, and serves as a neurotrophic factor for the mandibular and trochlear nerves. (From Noden DM, Francis-West P. The differentiation and morphogenesis of craniofacial muscles. *Dev Dyn.* 2006;235:1194–1218. Used with permission from Wiley.)

Strabismus

One of the most common motor disorders involving the EOM is strabismus, defined as misalignment of the eyes such that disparate images reach corresponding parts of each retina, disrupting binocular vision (see Chapter 36).[132]

Many studies have examined the oculomotor control of eye position in strabismus, but much less is understood about the EOM themselves in these conditions. Studies measuring EOM forces during eye movements in strabismic patients yielded quite disparate results.[2,133–136] In one study of adults with concomitant strabismus, whether convergent (esotropia) or divergent (exotropia), no differences in mechanical or contractile properties were seen.[2] All patients with superior oblique palsy showed reduced values for mean peak velocity in most directions of gaze compared with normal levels, whereas mean peak and steady-state tension did not vary between normal EOM and patients with either congenital or acquired superior oblique palsy.[137]

Studies of muscle structure in strabismic patients and animal models also yielded quite different results. Horizontal rectus muscle anatomy in naturally and artificially strabismic monkeys showed no differences in EOM size, structure, or innervation.[138] Interestingly, there was much less uniformity in cross-sectional area in the natural esotropes compared with those artificially induced. EOM obtained during strabismus surgery showed minimal changes at the light level, but an array of myofiber structural changes at the electron microscopic level, including fiber vacuolization and mitochondrial changes.[139,140] Others described minimal changes in the myofibers and their motor innervation, but significant pathology in the proprioceptive innervation at the myotendinous junctions.[141] However, after examination of

BOX 7.2 **Treatment of strabismus**

Eye deviations are first treated by patching the "good" eye, the one aligned in primary gaze. If this is ineffective, incisional surgery is performed on the muscles. Recession surgery is thought to weaken an "overacting" muscle, performed by moving the muscle's scleral insertion posteriorly. Resection surgery is thought to strengthen an "underacting" muscle, performed by removing a portion of the muscle and reattaching the muscle to its original site of insertion on the sclera.[134,135] If this misalignment is not corrected in early childhood, amblyopia may develop. Amblyopia is a condition of functional blindness in an otherwise normal eye.[132–135]

BOX 7.3 **Surgery for congenital nystagmus**

It has been suggested that tenotomy in congenital nystagmus patients, removal of the muscle from its scleral insertion and reattachment, results in reduced amplitude and intensity.[154] Other investigators found tenotomy increased the velocity and intensity of the nystagmus in a monkey model.[155] Recent work shows that surgery for nystagmus results in modest improvement of visual acuity.[212] Further studies are needed to clarify this issue; however, it is important to note that the myotendinous junctions thought to be disrupted by this procedure are motor, not sensory, as originally proposed.[111,112]

EOM from a number of different ocular motility disorders, some of the unusual features in the strabismic muscles appeared in the control muscles also.[142] Increased satellite cell numbers were present in the inferior oblique muscles from patients with inferior oblique overaction,[143] suggesting upregulated myofiber remodeling. Similarly, underacting medial rectus muscles from exotropes had twofold higher levels of activated satellite cells, whereas overacting medial rectus muscles from esotropes had fewer activated satellite cells compared with control.[144] These studies suggest that adaptive changes occur in strabismic muscles. Current treatments for strabismus can include patching, and surgery involving tightening (resection) or producing slack (recession) is routinely performed (see Box 7.2). Future approaches to strabismus treatment may be able to tap into the underlying mechanisms that are the underlying cause of the strabismus.

Nystagmus

Nystagmus is defined as a bilateral, involuntary, and conjugate oscillation of the eyes, and has primarily been considered to be a problem of oculomotor control within the brain. Patterns of eye movements in nystagmus patients are complex, and many different forms exist, including both congenital and acquired.[145,146] Nystagmus can be inherited genetically, such as in the case of a mutation in the gene *frmd7* (FERM domain containing 7),[147] or the albinism gene *TYR*,[148] and may have a sensory or motor origin.[145,146] However, many children with nystagmus have no known contributing factor. The complex waveforms of the oscillatory eye movements have been extensively studied,[149] but little is known about adaptive changes at the EOM level. Ultrastructural studies on human EOM from patients with congenital nystagmus show that myofibrillar orientation, as well as mitochondrial structure, are altered.[150,151] Recent studies demonstrated that muscle specimens from children with idiopathic infantile nystagmus (INS) have small neuromuscular junctions, with increased expression of the immature subunit of the acetylcholine receptor, as well as altered neurotrophic factor levels.[152] Although a variety of pharmacologic treatments have been suggested, controlled clinical trials are needed, as there is currently no cure for these uncontrolled oscillatory movements that often result in significant loss in visual acuity.[153] Surgery also is a common treatment option for these patients, particularly to correct head posture (Box 7.3),[149] but a four-muscle tenotomy approach is not uniformly accepted.[154,155]

Congenital cranial dysinnervation disorders

Several rare, nonprogressive inherited strabismic disorders have been described, and they are characterized by congenital fibrosis of one or more of the EOM resulting in an abnormal static eye position or directional impairment. The genetic basis for several of the CCDD, as they are now called, have been instructive in understanding EOM and cranial motor neuron development (Box 7.4, Fig. 7.17).[156–162] Each identified genetic mutation thus far causes distinct developmental defects of

the oculomotor (CN III), trochlear (CN IV), and/or abducens (CN VI) nerves.[157–162] Although patients with these CCDDs are rare, they demonstrate the incredible complexity in the genetic control of the EOM and their innervation.

MUSCLE DISEASES IN WHICH EXTRAOCULAR MUSCLES ARE PREFERENTIALLY SPARED

There are many skeletal muscle diseases in which the EOM are preferentially spared (Table 7.2). Duchenne muscular dystrophy (DMD) is a devastating X-linked genetic disorder characterized by the absence of dystrophin, repeated cycles of degeneration and regeneration, progressive muscle weakness, and ultimately an early death. The EOM are spared, both morphologically[163] and functionally.[164] The mechanism that allows for this sparing is not understood. None of the potential structural or metabolic characteristics examined thus far has proven to be mechanistic for this sparing, including, but not limited to, calcium handling, antioxidative enzymes, nitric oxide location, cation handling, and utrophin upregulation.[70,87,165–169]

The *constitutive* nature of EOM sparing is supported by the EOM being spared in other dystrophic diseases,[169] including Becker muscular dystrophy,[164] laminin alpha2-deficiency,[170] merosin-deficient muscular dystrophy,[171] sarcoglycan deficiency,[172] and congenital muscular dystrophy, where, despite some ultrastructural changes,[171] the EOM display full ocular motility.[173] EOM sparing has even been documented for inflammatory autoimmune diseases of skeletal muscle such as dermatomyositis.[174] This wide array of skeletal muscular dystrophies and degenerative disorders that spare the EOM suggests that the sparing mechanism must be intrinsic to the EOM. Two interesting hypotheses currently being tested as potential mechanisms for EOM sparing in various forms of muscular dystrophy suggest that either the EOM are inherently able to resist the necrosis caused by the "hostile" tissue milieu within dystrophic muscle, or they have the capacity for increased regenerative potential, an idea supported by their ability to remodel and repair throughout life.[175] Their inherent ability to survive denervation supports the first hypothesis.[91,92,97] The ability of the EOM to remodel even in aging muscle[82] and the relative absence in the EOM of the sarcopenia and other defects seen in aging noncranial skeletal muscle[176] suggest that the intrinsic regenerative capacity in adult EOM is sufficient to provide functional EOM throughout the lifetime of these patients. An understanding of the mechanism of sparing may lead to the development of new treatments for these fatal dystrophic diseases.

The EOM, and the motor neurons that innervate them, have long been considered spared in amyotrophic lateral sclerosis (ALS), with histopathologic examination of nerve roots as supporting evidence.[177] However, many studies cast doubt on this hypothesis, suggesting instead that the overall time course of the disease plays a role in whether eye movement disorders are apparent. Analysis of ocular

BOX 7.4   Congenital fibrosis of the extraocular muscles

Patients with congenital fibrosis of the extraocular muscles (EOM) type 1 (CFEOM1) have a defect in the development of the superior division of the CN III resulting in atrophic superior rectus and levator palpebrae superioris muscles.[156] The mutation is in the KIF21A gene, a developmentally expressed kinesin that presumably delivers a molecule critical for early neurite survival.[158] CFEOM2 has a recessive inheritance, and all EOM are missing except the lateral rectus, which is innervated by CN VI (Fig. 7.17). This disorder is due to mutations in the PHOX2A gene,[159] a transcription factor restricted to several classes of differentiating neurons. Its role in development is unclear;

however, in PHOX2A null mice, no oculomotor or trochlear neurons develop along with other brain abnormalities.[160] Duane's retraction syndrome is a congenital EOM disorder characterized by the lack of CN VI, and aberrant innervation of the lateral rectus from CN III is often seen (Fig. 7.17).[161] The genetic mutation in this disorder is the CHN1 gene, which encodes α1-chimaerin, a Rac guanosine triphosphatase-activating protein signaling protein. This mutation results in a gain-of-function causing increased α2-chimaerin on cell membranes,[162] and its overexpression in transgenic mice leads to pathfinding errors.

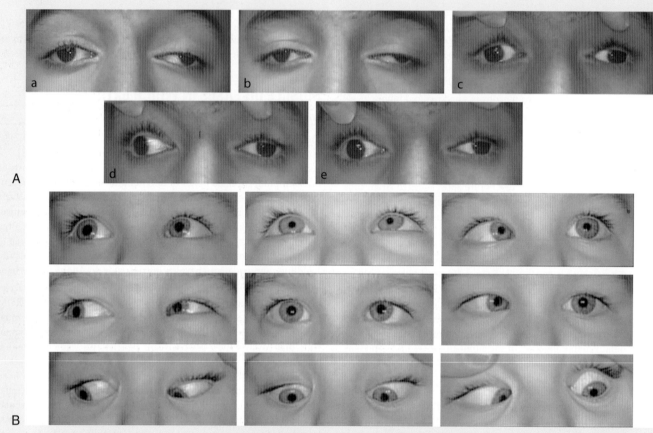

Fig. 7.17 (**A**) Patient with congenital fibrosis of the extraocular muscles type 2 (CFEOM2). In primary position, note eyelid ptosis and lack of fixation in either eye (b). Up gaze (a) and down gaze (c) show complete absence of vertical movement. Right gaze (d) and left gaze (e) show complete lack of adduction of the left eye with almost full abduction of the right eye but moderately reduced abduction of the left eye. (Reproduced with permission from Bosley TM, Oystreck DT, Robertson RL, al Awad A, Abu-Amero K, Engle EC. Neurological features of congenital fibrosis of the extraocular muscles type 2 with mutations in PHOX2A. *Brain*. 2006;129(9):2363–2374. https://doi.org/10.1093/brain/awl161.) (**B**) Child with Duane's retraction syndrome, the congenital absence of cranial nerve VI (CNVI) resulting in a paralytic lateral rectus muscle. In primary position (*center panel*), the child is esotropic. Note limited abduction (*middle row, far right*). (From Morad Y, Kraft SP, Mims JL 3rd. Unilateral recession and resection in Duane syndrome. *J AAPOS*. 2001;5(3):158–163. Copyright Elsevier 2001).

movements and muscle pathology is made difficult by the heterogeneity of the patient populations relative to onset and speed of decline. In a longitudinal study of eight patients, all but one showed changes in electro-oculography of the EOM; some were subclinical but most were progressive over time.[178] Differential vulnerability of cranial motor neurons innervating the EOM occurs in several mouse models of ALS, with differential loss or sparing of motor neurons in transgenic mice expressing the human mutation in the superoxide dismutase gene-1

compared with two spontaneous mouse models of ALS.[179] Direct examination of the EOM postmortem from two subsets of ALS patients, those with either a short- or long-time course of neuron loss, showed there were degenerative changes in the cranial motor nerves within the EOM from these patients, and differential sparing of myofibers in the two groups.[180] Recent studies have demonstrated that the EOM retain expression of a number of known neurotrophic factors at the neuromuscular junctions, which are downregulated in the neuromuscular

TABLE 7.2 Extraocular muscles have different disease profiles compared to limb skeletal muscle

Diseases where EOM are spared	Etiology	Limb muscle pathology
Duchenne muscular dystrophy	X-linked genetic mutation of dystrophin gene	Progressive; muscle wasting and weakness
Becker muscular dystrophy	X-linked genetic mutation of dystrophin gene, less severe phenotype than Duchenne	Progressive; muscle wasting and weakness
α, γ, and δ-sarcoglycan deficiency (limb girdle muscular dystrophy)	Mutation of the sarcoglycan gene	Progressive; muscle wasting and weakness
Laminin α2-congenital muscular dystrophy	Mutation of the laminin α2 gene	Progressive; muscle wasting and weakness
Amyotrophic lateral sclerosis	Mutations of the superoxide dismutase gene; mitochondriopathy	Progressive; muscle wasting and paralysis

Diseases where EOM are primarily or preferentially involved	Etiology	EOM pathology and/or symptoms
Graves' ophthalmopathy	Autoimmune disease of the EOM, resulting in enlargement; presumably due to one or more shared antigens with the thyroid gland	Inflammatory orbitopathy; myopathy
CPEO (chronic progressive external ophthalmoplegia}	Mitochondrial DNA deletion, mutation of DNA polymerase-gamma gene	Accumulation of mutant mitochondria leads to muscle paralysis
Kearns-Sayre syndrome	Longer mitochondrial DNA deletions than CPEO	Accumulation of mutant mitochondria leads to muscle paralysis
Ocular myasthenia gravis	Autoimmune disease to either the acetylcholine receptor or MuSK	EOM and levator palpebrae superioris muscle weakness
Myotonic dystrophy type I	Expansion of a CTG repeat within the DMPK gene	Saccadic slowing, optokinetic nystagmus
Myotonic dystrophy type 2	Expansion of a CCTG repeat expansion of the CNBP gene	Rebound nystagmus
Childhood strabismus	Unknown. Complex genetic cause?	Under- or overactive EOM with loss of binocularity and eye alignment in primary gaze
Congenital nystagmus	Missense mutation in FRMD7 gene; function unknown. Clinically heterogeneous; multiple genes involved.	Conjugate, horizontal eye oscillations, in primary or eccentric gaze
Miller-Fisher syndrome	Autoimmune disease against ganglioside GQIb/GTIa	EOM paralysis
Congenital cranial dysinnervation disorders	Specific gene mutation for each type	EOM weakness or absence

junctions in affected limb muscles.[181] These studies suggest possible new approaches for treatment of this fatal degenerative disease. The preferential sparing of the ocular motor neurons and the EOM in ALS patients may be in part temporal; if an individual lives sufficiently long, the ocular motor neurons and associated EOM do show some degenerative changes. Alternatively, eye movements may not be abnormal in these patients because even in the absence of 25% of the pool of cranial motor neurons, eye movements are completely unchanged.[182] In addition, polyneuronal innervation, where more than one neuron can control the same myofiber, may protect the eye movement system against disease; if one motor neuron is lost, there are others that can take over functionally.[25]

MUSCLE DISEASES WHERE EXTRAOCULAR MUSCLES ARE PREFERENTIALLY INVOLVED

There are many diseases where the EOM are exclusively or preferentially involved. One disorder with primary EOM involvement is thyroid eye disease (TED) or Graves' ophthalmopathy, an autoimmune disease with significant inflammatory cell invasion of the EOM (Fig. 7.18).[183–193] Despite many studies, the autoantigen responsible for this disease is still a matter of debate.[184–191] Eye findings include exophthalmos, lid retraction, periorbital edema, pain, and diplopia.[191,193] Significant

enlargement of the EOM can occur, and in severe cases causes compression of the optic nerve posteriorly, resulting in permanent vision loss (see Box 7.5). This is caused by the inability of the bony orbit to accommodate enlargement of soft tissues, resulting in compression injury and permanent vision loss if untreated.

Primary EOM involvement occurs with some mitochondrial myopathies, such as chronic progressive external ophthalmoplegia (CPEO). CPEO is not one specific disorder but a clinical set of symptoms associated with mitochondrial DNA deletions or mutations and primarily defined by paralysis or weakness of one or more of the EOM,[194,195] with no current treatments (see Box 7.6). CPEO is one of many diseases associated with clonal expansions of mitochondrial DNA mutations within myofiber segments.[195] Some mitochondrial myopathies affect both the EOM and other organs, including Kearns-Sayre syndrome (KSS) and myoclonic epilepsy associated with ragged red fibers (MERRF).[196,197] In KSS, patients have a more severe phenotype than seen with CPEO; in addition to ophthalmoplegia, patients have retinopathy, proximal muscle weakness, cardiac arrhythmia, and ataxia. In MERRF, chronic neurodegenerative changes also occur. Although it is still unclear why mitochondria with deletions would preferentially increase in the EOM and/or EOM and brain, both tissues are highly oxidative, with rates of mitochondrial function three to four times greater than limb skeletal muscles.[198] Mitochondrial mutations reduce

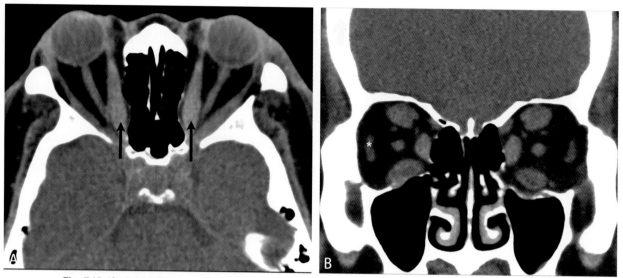

Fig. 7.18 (**A**) Axial MRI of a patient with thyroid eye disease (TED). Increased thicknesses of medial rectus muscles bilaterally (*arrow*) is prominent. (**B**) Coronal MRI of a patient with TED. Note that all rectus muscles are enlarged except the lateral rectus (*asterisk*). (Courtesy of Dr. Michael Lee, Department of Ophthalmology and Visual Neurosciences, University of Minnesota.)

BOX 7.5 Optic neuropathy of thyroid orbitopathy

Optic nerve compression in thyroid eye disease is a vision-threatening condition, and if the severity of the inflammation does not abate on its own and cannot be reduced medically with oral or intravenous pulse corticosteroids,[184] surgical decompression of the orbit by surgically produced transpalpebral orbital floor removal or endoscopic decompression is required to prevent permanent vision loss.[185]

BOX 7.6 Chronic progressive external ophthalmoplegia

Unfortunately, there are no proven effective therapies for chronic progressive external ophthalmoplegia (CPEO), Kearns-Sayre syndrome, and related mitochondrial cytopathies. In CPEO, for example, symptoms of strabismus, dry eye, and ptosis can only be managed, as is true for those patients with concomitant cardiac defects.[197]

BOX 7.7 Treating ocular myasthenia

There are a number of drug treatments available for ocular myasthenia gravis. For example, prednisone can reduce symptoms in ocular myasthenic patients, as well as significantly reduce the frequency of developing generalized myasthenia gravis both acutely and over the course of 4 or more years.[211]

---

energy production, a problem for the function of the highly oxidative EOM.[199] Aging has been associated with the clonal expansion of defective mitochondria in this disorder,[200] as mutated mitochondria can completely replace normal ones over time.[201,202] Interestingly, magnetic resonance imaging (MRI) of the EOM in CPEO patients demonstrates that the EOM are significantly smaller than in controls.[203] This can aid in the differential diagnosis of this condition.

Myasthenia gravis is an example of a condition that preferentially involves the EOM but can also involve multiple noncranial skeletal muscles. Myasthenia gravis is an autoimmune disease of the NMJ resulting in skeletal muscle weakness and fatigability caused by functional NMJ dropout.[204] Although EOM weakness occurs in 90% of patients with myasthenia gravis, approximately 15% have only ocular myasthenia without other muscle involvement.[204] Interestingly, in generalized myasthenia patients, 90% have serum antibodies to the nicotinic acetylcholine receptor, whereas only 65% of the ocular myasthenics are positive for this autoantigen.[205] Other possible autoantigens that have been implicated in this disease include muscle-specific kinase (MuSK),[206] the ryanodine receptor,[207] and a number of eye muscle-specific proteins.[208] The frequent involvement of the levator palpebrae superioris and the EOM in myasthenia gravis may be due to the distinct NMJ characteristics of EOM compared with noncranial skeletal muscles.[21,204] Early in the disease, slight weakness of the EOM results in lack of alignment of the visual world on the retina causing diplopia, blur, vertigo, and other ocular symptoms (see Box 7.7). The brain

oculomotor control system cannot quickly adapt to the asymmetric or variable EOM weakness.[209] Therefore, EOM weakness is discerned quickly by patients. However, when patients with ocular myasthenia are examined, many have measurable, albeit subclinical, weakness in other muscle groups as well. Differences in both classical and alternative complement-mediated immune response pathways in EOM may also increase their susceptibility to ocular myasthenic symptoms.[210,211]

CONCLUSION

The EOM are a specialized collection of craniofacial muscles with many distinctive characteristics compared to noncranial skeletal muscle. These muscles have a complex anatomy and physiology, which should be carefully considered when determining treatment of the motor disorders that affect them. The EOM are also highly adaptable, altering their protein expression and physiologic characteristics in response to hormones, denervation, and toxins. This adaptability should lend itself to pharmacologic manipulation of these muscles for the treatment of

EOM motor disorders. Furthermore, understanding the mechanisms that result in EOM sparing or preferential involvement in diseases of skeletal muscle will hopefully suggest new treatments for EOM diseases and for skeletal muscle diseases in general.

REFERENCES

1. Zaldivar RA, Lee MS, Harrison AR. Orbital anatomy and orbital fractures. In: Dartt D, editor. *Elsevier's Encyclopedia of the Eye*. Vol 3. London: Elsevier; 2010:210–218.
2. Lennerstrand G, Schiavi C, Tian S, Benassi M, Campos EC. Isometric force measured in human horizontal eye muscles attached to or detached from the globe. *Graefes Arch Clin Exp Ophthalmol.* 2006;244:539–544.
3. Anderson BC, McLoon LK. Cranial nerve and autonomic innervation. In: Dartt D, editor. *Elsevier's Encyclopedia of the Eye*. Vol 1. London: Elsevier; 2010:537–548.
4. White MH, Lambert HM, Kincaid MC, Dieckert JP, Lowd DK. The ora serrata and the spiral of Tillaux. Anatomic relationship and clinical correlation. *Ophthalmology.* 1989;96:508–511.
5. Jaggi GP, Laeng HR, Müntener M, Killer HE. The anatomy of the muscle insertion (scleromuscular junction) of the lateral and medial rectus muscle in humans. *Invest Ophthalmol Vis Sci.* 2005;46:2258–2263.
6. Fuchs E. Beiträge zur normulen Anatomie des Augapfels. *Graefes Arch Clin Exp Ophthalmol.* 1884;30:1–65.
7. Apt L, Call NB. An anatomical reevaluation of rectus muscle innervations. *Ophthalmic Surg.* 1982;13:108–112.
8. Souza-Dias C, Prieto-Díaz J, Uesugui CF. Topographical aspects of the insertions of the extraocular muscles. *J Pediatr Ophthalmol Strabismus.* 1986;23:183–189.
9. Stark N, Kuck H. Distance of muscle insertions in the corneal limbus. *Klin Monatsbl Augenheilkd.* 1986;189:148–153.
10. de Gottrau P, Gajisin S, Roth A. Ocular rectus muscle insertions revisited: An unusual anatomic approach. *Acta Anat.* 1994;151:268–272.
11. Otto J, Zimmermann E. Variations in the muscular insertion, the course and elasticity of the muscles in people suffering from squint. *Klin Monatsbl Augenheilkd.* 1979;175:418–427.
12. Robinson DA, O'Meara DM, Scott AB, Collins CC. Mechanical components of human eye movements. *J Appl Physiol.* 1969;26:548–553.
13. Ruskell GL. The fine structure of innervated myotendinous cylinders in extraocular muscles of rhesus monkeys. *J Neurocytol.* 1978;7:693–708.
14. Salpeter MM, McHenry FA, Feng HH. Myoneural junctions in the extraocular muscles of the mouse. *Anat Rec.* 1974;179:201–224.
15. Blumer R, Konakci KZ, Pomikal C, Wieczorek G, Lukas J-R, Streicher J. Palisade endings: Cholinergic sensory organs or effector organs? *Invest Ophthalmol Vis Sci.* 2009;50:1176–1186.
16. Kupfer C. Motor innervation of extraocular muscle. *J Physiol.* 1960;153:522–526.
17. Pilar G, Hess A. Differences in internal structure and nerve terminals of the slow and twitch muscle fibers in the cat superior oblique. *Anat Rec.* 1966;154:243–252.
18. Mishina M, Takai T, Imoto K, et al. Molecular distinction between fetal and adult forms of muscle acetylcholine receptor. *Nature.* 1986;321:406–411.
19. Oda K, Shibasaki H. Antigenic difference of acetylcholine receptor between single and multiple form endplates of human extraocular muscle. *Brain Res.* 1988;449:337–340.
20. Horton RM, Manfredi AA, Conti-Tronconi BM. The 'embryonic' gamma subunit of the nicotinic acetylcholine receptor is expressed in adult extraocular muscle. *Neurology.* 1993;43:983–986.
21. Kaminski HJ, Kusner LL, Block CH. Expression of acetylcholine receptor isoforms at extraocular muscle endplates. *Invest Ophthalmol Vis Sci.* 1996;37:345–351.
22. Mayr R, Gottschall J, Gruber H, Neuhuber W. Internal structure of cat extraocular muscle. *Anat Embryol.* 1975;148:25–34.
23. Harrison AR, Anderson BC, Thompson LV, McLoon LK. Myofiber length and three-dimensional localization of NMJs in normal and botulinum toxin treated adult extraocular muscles. *Invest Ophthalmol Vis Sci.* 2007;48:3594–3601.
24. Jacoby J, Chiarandini DJ, Stefani E. Electrical properties and innervation of fibers in the orbital layer of rat extraocular muscles. *J Neurophysiol.* 1989;61:116–125.
25. Dimitrova DM, Allman BL, Shall MS, Goldberg SJ. Polyneuronal innervation of single muscle fibers in cat eye muscles: Inferior oblique. *J Neurophysiol.* 2009;101:2815–2821.
26. Koornneef L. New insights in the human orbital connective tissue. *Arch Ophthalmol.* 1977;95:1269–1273.
27. Miller JM, Demer JL, Rosenbaum AL. Effect of transposition surgery on rectus muscle paths by magnetic resonance imagining. *Ophthalmology.* 1993;100:475–487.
28. Demer JL, Miller JM, Poukens V, Vinters HV, Glasgow BJ. Evidence for fibromuscular pulleys of the recti extraocular muscles. *Invest Ophthalmol Vis Sci.* 1995;36:1125–1136.
29. McLoon LK, Vicente A, Fitzpatrick KR, Lindström M, Pedrosa Domellöf F. Composition, architecture, and functional implications of the connective tissue network of the extraocular muscles. *Invest Ophthalmol Vis Sci.* 2018;59:322–329.
30. Lowey S, Waller GS, Trybus KM. Function of skeletal muscle myosin heavy and light chain isoforms by an in vitro motility assay. *J Biol Chem.* 1993;268:20414–20418.
31. Barmack NH. Laminar organization of the extraocular muscles of the rabbit. *Exp Neurol.* 1978;59:304–321.
32. Kjellgren D, Thornell L-E, Andersen J, Pedrosa-Domellöf F. Myosin heavy chain isoforms in human extraocular muscles. *Invest Ophthalmol Vis Sci.* 2003;44:1419–1425.
33. Robinson DA. Oculomotor unit behavior in the monkey. *J Neurophysiol.* 1970;33:393–403.
34. Wieczorek DF, Periasamy M, Butler-Browne GS, Whalen RG, Nadal-Ginard B. Co-expression of multiple myosin heavy chain genes, in addition to a tissue-specific one, in extraocular musculature. *J Cell Biol.* 1985;101:618–629.
35. Toniolo L, Maccatrozzo L, Patruno M, Caliaro F, Mascarello F, Reggiani C. Expression of eight distinct MHC isoforms in bovine striated muscles: Evidence for MHC–2B presence only in extraocular muscles. *J Exp Biol.* 2005;208:4243–4253.
36. Kranjc BS, Smerdu V, Erzen I. Histochemical and immunohistochemical profile of human and rat ocular medial rectus muscles. *Graefes Arch Clin Exp Ophthalmol.* 2009;247:1505–1515.
37. Bicer S, Reiser PJ. Myosin isoform expression in dog rectus muscles: Patterns in global and orbital layers and among single fibers. *Invest Ophthalmol Vis Sci.* 2009;50:157–167.
38. Rossi AC, Mammucari C, Argentini C, Reggiani C, Schiaffino S. Two novel/ancient myosins in mammalian skeletal muscles: MYH14/7b and MYH15 are expressed in extraocular muscles and muscle spindles. *J Physiol.* 2010;588:353–364.
39. Moncman CL, Andrade FH. Nonmuscle myosin IIB, a sarcomeric component in the extraocular muscles. *Exp Cell Res.* 2010;316:1958–1965.
40. Close RI, Luff AR. Dynamic properties of inferior rectus muscle of the rat. *J Physiol.* 1974;236:259–270.
41. McLoon LK, Rios L, Wirtschafter JD. Complex three-dimensional patterns of myosin isoform expression: Differences between and within specific extraocular muscles. *J Muscle Res Cell Motil.* 1999;30:771–783.
42. Meredith MA, Goldberg SJ. Contractile differences between muscle units in the medial rectus and lateral rectus muscles in the cat. *J Neurophysiol.* 1986;56:50–62.
43. Shall MS, Goldberg SJ. Lateral rectus EMG and contractile responses elicited by cat abducens motoneurons. *Muscle Nerve.* 1995;18:948–955.
44. Jacoby J, Ko K, Weiss C, Rushbrook JI. Systematic variation in myosin expression along extraocular muscle fibers of the adult rat. *J Muscle Res Cell Motil.* 1989;11:25–40.
45. Rubinstein NA, Hoh JFY. The distribution of myosin heavy chain isoforms among rat extraocular muscle fiber types. *Invest Ophthalmol Vis Sci.* 2000;41:3391–3398.
46. Alvarado-Mallart RM, Pincon-Raymond M. Nerve endings on the intramuscular tendons of cat extraocular muscles. *Neurosci Lett.* 1976;2:121–125.
47. Davidowitz J, Philips G, Breinin GM. Organization of the orbital surface layer in rabbit superior rectus. *Invest Ophthalmol Vis Sci.* 1977;16:711–729.
48. Goldberg SJ, Wilson KE, Shall ME. Summation of extraocular motor unit tensions in the lateral rectus muscle of the cat. *Muscle Nerve.* 1997;20:1229–1235.
49. Shall MS, Dimitrova DM, Goldberg SJ. Extraocular motor unit and whole-muscle contractile properties in the squirrel monkey. Summation of forces and fiber morphology. *Exp Brain Res.* 2003;151:338–345.
50. Lynch GS, Stephenson DG, Williams DA. Analysis of Ca^{2+} and Sr^{2+} activation characteristics in skinned muscle fibre preparations with different proportions of myofibrillar isoforms. *J Muscle Res Cell Motil.* 1995;16:65–78.
51. Dean P. Motor unit recruitment in a distributed model of extraocular muscle. *J Neurophysiol.* 1996;76:727–742.
52. Kranjc BS, Sketelj J, Albis AD, Ambroz M, Erzen I. Fibre types and myosin heavy chain expression in the ocular medial rectus muscle of the adult rat. *J Muscle Res Cell Motil.* 2000;21:753–761.
53. Briggs MM, Schachat F. The superfast extraocular myosin (MYH13) is localized to the innervation zone in both the global and orbital layers of rabbit extraocular muscle. *J Exp Biol.* 2002;205:3133–3142.
54. McLoon LK, Christiansen SP. Orbital anatomy: The extraocular muscles. In: Dartt D, editor. *Elsevier's Encyclopedia of the Eye*. Vol 2. London: Elsevier; 2010:89–98.
55. Keller EL, Robinson DA. Abducens unit behavior in the monkey during vergence movements. *Vision Res.* 1972;12:369–382.
56. Bacou F, Rouanet P, Barjot C, Janmot C, Vigneron P, d'Albis A. Expression of myosin isoforms in denervated, cross-reinnervated, and electrically stimulated rabbit muscles. *Eur J Biochem.* 1996;236:539–547.
57. Ugalde I, Christiansen SP, McLoon LK. Botulinum toxin treatment of extraocular muscles in rabbits results in increased myofiber remodeling. *Invest Ophthalmol Vis Sci.* 2005;46:4114–4120.
58. Stephenson GMM. Hybrid skeletal muscle fibres: A rare or common phenomenon? *Clin Exp Pharmacol Physiol.* 2001;28:692–702.
59. Caiozzo VJ, Baker MJ, Huang K, Chou H, Wu YZ, Baldwin KM. Single-fiber myosin heavy chain polymorphism: How many patterns and what proportions? *Am J Physiol Regul Integr Comp Physiol.* 2003;285:R570–R580.
60. Jacoby J, Ko K. Sarcoplasmic reticulum fast Ca^{2+} pump and myosin heavy chain expression in extraocular muscles. *Invest Ophthalmol Vis Sci.* 1993;34:2848–2858.
61. Briggs MM, Jacoby J, Davidowitz J, Schachat FH. Expression of a novel combination of fast and slow troponin T isoforms in rabbit extraocular muscles. *J Muscle Res Cell Motil.* 1988;9:241–247.
62. Kjellgren D, Stål P, Larsson L, Fürst D, Pedrosa-Domellöf F. Uncoordinated expression of myosin heavy chains and myosin-binding protein C isoforms in human extraocular muscles. *Invest Ophthalmol Vis Sci.* 2006;47:4188–4193.
63. McLoon LK, Park HN, Kim JH, Pedrosa-Domellöf F, Thompson LV. A continuum of myofibers in adult rabbit extraocular muscle: Force, shortening velocity, and patterns of myosin heavy chain localization. *J Appl Physiol.* 2011;111:1178–1189.
64. Pandorf CE, Haddad F, Wright C, Bodell PW, Baldwin KM. Differential epigenetic modifications of histones at the myosin heavy chain genes in fast and slow skeletal muscle fibers in response to muscle unloading. *Am J Physiol Cell Physiol.* 2009;297:C6–C16.
65. Zeiger U, Khurana TS. Distinctive patterns of microRNA expression in extraocular muscles. *Physiol Genomics.* 2010;41(3):289–296.
66. Bottinelli R, Schiaffino S, Reggiani C. Force-velocity relations and myosin heavy chain isoform compositions of skinned fibres from rat skeletal muscle. *J Physiol.* 1991;437:655–672.
67. Morris TJ, Brandon CA, Horton MJ, Carlson DS, Sciote JJ. Maximum shortening velocity and myosin heavy-chain isoform expression in human masseter muscle fibers. *J Dent Res.* 2001;80:1845–1848.
68. Kjellgren D, Ryan M, Ohlendieck K, Thornell LE, Pedrosa-Domellöf F. Sarco(endo)plasmic reticulum Ca^{2+} ATPases (SERCA1 and -2) in human extraocular muscles. *Invest Ophthalmol Vis Sci.* 2003;44:5057–5062.

69. Andrade FH, McMullen CA, Rumbaut RE. Mitochondria are fast Ca^{2+} sinks in rat extraocular muscles: A novel regulatory influence on contractile function and metabolism. *Invest Ophthalmol Vis Sci.* 2005;46:4541–4547.
70. Khurana TS, Prendergast RA, Alameddine HS, et al. Absence of extraocular muscle pathology in Duchenne's muscular dystrophy: Role for calcium homeostasis in extraocular muscle sparing. *J Exp Med.* 1995;182:467–475.
71. Ragusa RJ, Chow CK, St Clair DK, Porter JD. Extraocular, limb and diaphragm muscle group-specific antioxidant enzyme activity patterns in control and mdx mice. *J Neurol Sci.* 1996;139:180–186.
72. Wooten GF, Reis DJ. Blood flow in extraocular muscle of cat. *Arch Neurol.* 1972;26:350–352.
73. Fuchs AF, Binder MD. Fatigue resistance of human extraocular muscles. *J Neurophysiol.* 1983;49:28–34.
74. McMullen CA, Hayess K, Andrade FH. Fatigue resistance of rat extraocular muscles does not depend on creatine kinase activity. *BMC Physiol.* 2005;5:12.
75. Andrade FH, McMullen CA. Lactate is a metabolic substrate that sustains extraocular muscle function. *Pflugers Arch – Eur J Physiol.* 2006;452:102–108.
76. Asmussen G, Punkt K, Bartsch B, Soukup T. Specific metabolic properties of rat oculorotatory extraocular muscles can be linked to their low force requirements. *Invest Ophthalmol Vis Sci.* 2008;49:4865–4871.
77. Hoh JF, Hughes S. Myogenic and neurogenic regulation of myosin gene expression in cat jaw-closing muscles regenerating in fast and slow limb muscle beds. *J Muscle Res Cell Motil.* 1988;9:59–72.
78. McLoon LK, Wirtschafter JD. Continuous myonuclear addition to single extraocular myofibers in uninjured adult rabbits. *Muscle Nerve.* 2002;25:348–358.
79. McLoon LK, Rowe J, Wirtschafter JD, McCormick KM. Continuous myofiber remodeling in uninjured extraocular myofibers: Myonuclear turnover and evidence for apoptosis. *Muscle Nerve.* 2004;29:707–715.
80. Pawlikowski B, Pulliam C, Dalla Betta N, Kardon G, Olwin BB. Pervasive satellite cell contribution to uninjured adult muscle fibers. *Skelet Mus.* 2015;5:42.
81. Weintraub H, Tapscott SJ, Davis RL, et al. Activation of muscle-specific genes in pigment, nerve, fat, liver and fibroblast cell lines by forced expression of MyoD. *Proc Natl Acad Sci USA.* 1989;86:5434–5438.
82. McLoon LK, Wirtschafter JD. Activated satellite cells in extraocular muscles of normal adult monkeys and humans. *Invest Ophthalmol Vis Sci.* 2003;44:1927–1932.
83. Goding GS, Al-Sharif KI, McLoon LK. Myonuclear addition to uninjured laryngeal myofibers in adult rabbits. *Ann Otol Rhinol Laryngol.* 2005;114:552–557.
84. Shih HP, Gross MK, Kioussi C. Muscle development: Forming the head and trunk muscles. *Acta Histochem.* 2008;110:97–108.
85. Fischer MD, Gorospe JR, Felder E, et al. Expression profiling reveals metabolic and structural components of extraocular muscles. *Physiol Genomics.* 2002;9:71–84.
86. Anderson BC, Christiansen SP, Grandt S, Grange RW, McLoon LK. Increased extraocular muscle strength with direct injection of insulin-like growth factor-1. *Invest Ophthalmol Vis Sci.* 2006;47:2461–2467.
87. Zhou L, Porter JD, Cheng G, et al. Temporal and spatial mRNA expression patterns of TGF-β1, 2, 3 and TβRI, II, III in skeletal muscles of mdx mice. *Neuromusc Disord.* 2006;16:32–38.
88. Martínez-Fernandez S, Hernández-Torres F, Franco D, Lyons GE, Navarro F, Aránega AE. Pitx2C overexpression promotes cell proliferation and arrests differentiation in myoblasts. *Dev Dyn.* 2006;235:2930–2939.
89. Zhou Y, Cheng G, Dieter L, et al. An altered phenotype in a conditional knockout of Pitx2 in extraocular muscle. *Invest Ophthalmol Vis Sci.* 2009;50:4531–4541.
90. Scott AB. Botulinum toxin injection into extraocular muscles as an alternative to strabismus surgery. *J Pediatr Ophthalmol Strabismus.* 1980;17:21–25.
91. Spencer RF, McNeer KW. Botulinum toxin paralysis of adult monkey extraocular muscle. Structural alterations in orbital, singly innervated muscle fibers. *Arch Ophthalmol.* 1987;105:1703–1711.
92. Kranjc BS, Sketelj J, D'Albis A, Erzen I. Long-term changes in myosin heavy chain composition after botulinum toxin A injection into rat medial rectus muscle. *Invest Ophthalmol Vis Sci.* 2001;42:3158–3164.
93. Porter JD, Edney DP, McMahon EJ, Burns LA. Extraocular myotoxicity of the retrobulbar anesthetic bupivacaine hydrochloride. *Invest Ophthalmol Vis Sci.* 1988;29:163–174.
94. Carlson BM, Emerick S, Komorowski T, Rainin E, Shepard B. Extraocular muscle regeneration in primates. Local anesthetic-induced lesions. *Ophthalmology.* 1992;99: 582–589.
95. Asmussen G, Kiessling A. Hypertrophy and atrophy of mammalian extraocular muscle fibres following denervation. *Experientia.* 1975;31:1186–1188.
96. Ringel SP, Engel WK, Bender AN, Peters ND, Yee RD. Histochemistry and acetylcholine receptor distribution in normal and denervated monkey extraocular muscles. *Neurology.* 1978;28:55–63.
97. Porter JD, Burns LA, McMahon EJ. Denervation of primate extraocular muscle. A unique pattern of primate extraocular muscle. *Invest Ophthalmol Vis Sci.* 1989;30:1894–1908.
98. Baker RS, Christiansen SP, Madhat M. A quantitative assessment of extraocular muscle growth in peripheral nerve autografts. *Invest Ophthalmol Vis Sci.* 1990;31:766–770.
99. Keller EL, Robinson DA. Absence of a stretch reflex in extraocular muscles of the monkey. *J Neurophysiol.* 1971;34:908–919.
100. Lewis RF, Zee DS, Hayman MR, Tamargo RJ. Oculomotor function in the rhesus monkey after deafferentation of the extraocular muscles. *Exp Brain Res.* 2001;141: 349–358.
101. Donaldson IM, Dixon RA. Excitation of units in the lateral geniculate and contiguous nuclei of the cat by stretch of extrinsic ocular muscles. *Exp Brain Res.* 1980;38:245–255.
102. Wang X, Zhang M, Cohen IS, Goldberg ME. The proprioceptive representation of eye position in monkey primary somatosensory cortex. *Nature Neurosci.* 2007;10:640–646.
103. Zhang M, Wang X, Goldberg ME. Monkey primary somatosensory cortex has a proprioceptive representation of eye position. *Prog Brain Res.* 2008;171:37–45.
104. Blumer R, Konakci KZ, Streicher J, Hoetzenecker W, Blumer MJF, Lukas JR. Proprioception in the extraocular muscles of mammals and man. *Strabismus.* 2006;14:101–106.
105. Lukas JR, Aigner M, Blumer R, Heinzl H, Mayr R. Number and distribution of neuromuscular spindles in human extraocular muscles. *Invest Ophthalmol Vis Sci.* 1994;35: 4317–4327.
106. Richmond FJR, Johnston WSW, Baker RS, Steinbach MJ. Palisade endings in human extraocular muscle. *Invest Ophthalmol Vis Sci.* 1984;25:471–476.
107. Ruskell GL. The fine structure of innervated myotendinous cylinders in extraocular muscles of rhesus monkeys. *J Neurocytol.* 1978;7:693–708.
108. Lukas JR, Blumer R, Denk M, Baumgartner I, Neuhuber W, Mayr R. Innervated myotendinous cylinders in human extraocular muscles. *Invest Ophthalmol Vis Sci.* 2000;41:2422–2431.
109. Konakci KZ, Streicher J, Hoetzenecker W, et al. Palisade endings in extraocular muscles of the monkey are immunoreactive for choline acetyltransferase and vesicular acetylcholine transporter. *Invest Ophthalmol Vis Sci.* 2005;46:4548–4554.
110. Sas J, Schab R. Die sogennanten "Palisaden-Endigungen" der Augenmusklen. *Acta Morph Acad Sci Hung.* 1952;2:259–266.
111. Zimmerman L, Morado-Díaz CJ, Davis-López de Carrizosa MA, et al. Axons giving rise to the palisade endings of feline extraocular muscles display motor features. *J Neurosci.* 2013;33(7):2784–2793.
112. Blumer R, Streicher J, Carrero-Rojas G, Calvo PM, de la Cruz RR, Pastor AM. Palisade endings have an exocytotic machinery but lack acetylcholine receptors and distinct acetylcholinesterase activity. *Invest Ophthalmol Vis Sci.* 2020;61(14):31.
113. Tzahor E, Kempf H, Mootoosamy RC, et al. Antagonists of Wnt and BMP signaling promote the formation of vertebrate head muscle. *Genes Dev.* 2003;17:3087–3099.
114. Gage PJ, Rhoades W, Prucka SK, Hjalt T. Fate maps of neural crest and mesoderm in the mammalian eye. *Invest Ophthalmol Vis Sci.* 2005;46:4200–4208.
115. Sambasivan R, Gayraud-Morel B, Dumas G, et al. Distinct regulatory cascades govern extraocular and pharyngeal arch muscle progenitor cell fates. *Dev Cell.* 2009;16:810–821.
116. Tajbakhsh S, Rocancourt D, Cossu G, Buckingham M. Redefining the genetic hierarchies controlling skeletal myogenesis: Pax3 and Myf-5 act upstream of MyoD. *Cell.* 1997;89: 127–138.
117. Hacker A, Guthrie S. A distinct developmental programme for the cranial paraxial mesoderm in the chick embryo. *Development.* 1998;125:3461–3472.
118. Noden DM, Francis-West P. The differentiation and morphogenesis of craniofacial muscles. *Dev Dyn.* 2006;235:1194–1218.
119. Noden DM. Interactions and fates of avian craniofacial mesenchyme. *Development.* 1988;103(suppl):121–140.
120. Noden DM. Patterning of avian craniofacial muscles. *Dev Biol.* 1986;116:347–356.
121. Kanzler B, Foreman RK, Labosky PA, Mallo M. BMP signaling is essential for development of skeletogenic and neurogenic cranial neural crest. *Development.* 2000;127:1095–1104.
122. Kitamura K, Miura H, Miyagawa-Tomita S, et al. Mouse Pitx2 deficiency leads to anomalies of the ventral body wall, heart, extra- and periocular mesoderm and right pulmonary isomerism. *Development.* 1999;126:5749–5758.
123. Gage PJ, Suh H, Camper SA. Dosage requirement of Pitx2 for development of multiple organs. *Development.* 1999;126:4643–4651.
124. Gage PJ, Camper SA. Pituitary homeobox 2, a novel member of the bicoid-related family of homeobox genes, is a potential regulator of anterior structure formation. *Hum Mol Genet.* 1997;6:457–464.
125. Diehl AG, Zareparsi S, Qian M, Khanna R, Angeles R, Gage PJ. Extraocular muscle morphogenesis and gene expression are regulated by Pitx2 gene dose. *Invest Ophthalmol Vis Sci.* 2006;47:1785–1793.
126. Matt N, Ghyselinck NB, Pellerin I, Dupé V. Impairing retinoic acid signalling in the neural crest cells is sufficient to alter entire eye morphogenesis. *Dev Biol.* 2008;320:140–148.
127. Noden DM, Marcucio R, Borycki AG, Emerson CP Jr. Differentiation of avian craniofacial muscles: I. Patterns of early regulatory gene expression and myosin heavy chain synthesis. *Dev Dyn.* 1999;216:96–112.
128. Pedrosa-Domellöf F, Holmgren Y, Lucas CA, Hoh JF, Thornell LE. Human extraocular muscles: Unique pattern of myosin heavy chain expression during myotube formation. *Invest Ophthalmol Vis Sci.* 2000;41:1608–1616.
129. Marcucio RS, Noden DM. Myotube heterogeneity in developing chick craniofacial skeletal muscles. *Dev Dyn.* 1999;214:178–194.
130. Martinez AJ, McNeer KW, Hay SH, Watson A. Extraocular muscles: Morphogenetic study in humans. Light microscopy and ultrastructural features. *Acta Neuropath.* 1977;38:87–93.
131. Von Scheven G, Alvares LE, Mootoosamy RC, Dietrich S. Neural tube derived signals and FGF8 act antagonistically to specify eye versus mandibular arch muscles. *Development.* 2006;133:2731–2745.
132. Sengpiel F, Blakemore C, Harrad R. Interocular suppression in the primary visual cortex: A possible neural basis of binocular rivalry. *Vision Res.* 1995;35:179–195.
133. Birch EE, Stager DR. Long-term motor and sensory outcomes after early surgery for infantile esotropia. *J AAPOS.* 2006;10:409–413.
134. Wong AM. Timing of surgery for infantile esotropia: Sensory and motor outcomes. *Can J Ophthalmol.* 2008;43:643–651.
135. Kushner BJ. Perspective on strabismus, 2006. *Arch Ophthalmol.* 2006;124:1321–1326.
136. Collins CC, O'Meara D, Scott AB. Muscle tension during unrestrained human eye movements. *J Physiol Lond.* 1975;245:351–369.
137. Tian S, Lennerstrand G. Vertical saccadic velocity and force development in superior oblique palsy. *Vision Res.* 1994;34:1785–1798.
138. Narasimhan A, Tychsen L, Poukens V, Demer JL. Horizontal rectus muscle anatomy in naturally and artificially strabismic monkeys. *Invest Ophthalmol Vis Sci.* 2007;48:2576–2588.
139. Martinez AJ, Biglan AW, Hiles DA. Structural features of extraocular muscles of children with strabismus. *Arch Ophthalmol.* 1980;98:533–539.
140. Spencer RF, McNeer KW. Structural alterations in overacting inferior oblique muscles. *Arch Ophthalmol.* 1980;98:128–133.

141. Domenici-Lombardo L, Corsi M, Mencucci R, Scrivanti M, Faussone-Pelligrini MS, Salvi G. Extraocular muscles in congenital strabismus: Muscle fiber and nerve ending ultrastructure according to different regions. *Ophthalmologica*. 1992;205:29–39.
142. Berard-Badier M, Pellissier JF, Toga M, Mouillac N, Berard PV. Ultrastructural studies of extraocular muscles in ocular motility disorders. II. Morphological analysis of 38 biopsies. *Albracht v Graefes Arch Klin Exp Ophthal*. 1978;208:193–205.
143. Antunes-Foschini RM, Ramalho FS, Ramalho LN, Bicas HE. Increased frequency of activated satellite cells in overacting inferior oblique muscles from humans. *Invest Ophthalmol Vis Sci*. 2006;47:3360–3365.
144. Antunes-Foschini R, Miyashita D, Bicas HE, McLoon LK. Activated satellite cells in medial rectus muscles of patients with strabismus. *Invest Ophthalmol Vis*. 2008;49:215–220.
145. Stahl JS, Averbuch-Heller L, Leigh RJ. Acquired nystagmus. *Arch Ophthalmol*. 2000;118: 544–549.
146. Abadi RV, Bjerre A. Motor and sensory characteristics of infantile nystagmus. *Br J Ophthalmol*. 2002;86:1152–1160.
147. Tarpey P, Thomas S, Sarvananthan N, et al. Mutations in a novel member of the FERM family, *FRMD7* cause X-linked idiopathic congenital nystagmus (NYS1). *Nat Genet*. 2006;38:1242–1244.
148. Oetting WS. The tyrosinase gene and oculocutaneous albinism type I (OCA1): A model for understanding the molecular biology of melanin formation. *Pigment Cell Res*. 2000;13: 320–325.
149. Khanna S, Dell'Osso LF. The diagnosis and treatment of infantile nystagmus syndrome (INS). *Sci World J*. 2006;6:1385–1397.
150. Mencucci R, Domenici-Lombardo L, Cortesini L, Faussone-Pellegrini MS, Salvi G. Congenital nystagmus: Fine structure of human extraocular muscles. *Ophthalmologica*. 1995;209:1–6.
151. Peng GH, Zhang C, Yang JC. Ultrastructural study of extraocular muscle in congenital nystagmus. *Ophthalmologica*. 1998;212:1–4.
152. McLoon LK, Willoughby CL, Anderson JS, et al. Abnormally small neuromuscular junctions in the extraocular muscles from subjects with idiopathic nystagmus and nystagmus associated with albinism. *Invest Ophthalmol Vis Sci*. 2016;57:1912–1920.
153. McLean RJ, Gottlob I. The pharmacological treatment of nystagmus: A review. *Expert Opin Pharmacother*. 2009;10:1805–1816.
154. Hertle RW, Dell'Osso LF, FitzGibbon EJ, Thompson D, Yang D, Mellow SD. Horizontal rectus tenotomy in patients with congenital nystagmus: Results in 10 adults. *Ophthalmology*. 2003;110:2097–2105.
155. Wong AM, Tychsen L. Effects of extraocular muscle tenotomy on congenital nystagmus in macaque monkeys. *J AAPOS*. 2002;6:100–107.
156. Engle EC, Goumnerov BC, McKeown CA, et al. Oculomotor nerve and muscle abnormalities in congenital fibrosis of the extraocular muscles. *Ann Neurol*. 1997;41:314–325.
157. Engle EC. Genetic basis of congenital strabismus. *Arch Ophthalmol*. 2007;125:189–195.
158. Yamada K, Andrews C, Chan W-M, et al. Heterozygous mutations of the kinesin KIF21A in congenital fibrosis of the extraocular muscles type 1 (CFEOM1). *Nat Genet*. 2003;35:318–321.
159. Nakano M, Yamada K, Fain J, et al. Homozygous mutations in ARIX(PHOX2A) result in congenital fibrosis of the extraocular muscles type 2. *Nat Genet*. 2001;29:315–320.
160. Pattyn A, Morin X, Cremer H, Goridis C, Brunet JF. Expression and interactions of the two closely related homeobox genes Phox2a and Phox2b during neurogenesis. *Development*. 1997;124:4065–4075.
161. Demer JL, Clark RA, Lim KH, Engle EC. Magnetic resonance imaging evidence for widespread orbital dysinnervation in dominant Duane's retraction syndrome linked to the DURS2 locus. *Invest Ophthalmol Vis Sci*. 2007;48:194–202.
162. Miyake N, Chilton J, Psatha M, et al. Human CHN1 mutations hyperactivate alpha2-chimaerin and cause Duane's retraction syndrome. *Science*. 2008;321:839–843.
163. Karpati G, Carpenter S, Prescott S. Small-caliber skeletal muscle fibers do not suffer necrosis in mdx mouse dystrophy. *Muscle Nerve*. 1988;11:795–803.
164. Kaminski HJ, Al-Hakim M, Leigh RJ, Katirji MB, Ruff RL. Extraocular muscles are spared in advanced Duchenne dystrophy. *Ann Neurol*. 1992;32:586–588.
165. Ragusa RJ, Chow CK, Porter JD. Oxidative stress as a potential pathogenic mechanism in an animal model of Duchenne muscular dystrophy. *Neuromuscul Disord*. 1997;7:379–386.
166. Wehling M, Stull JT, McCabe TJ, Tidball JG. Sparing of mdx extraocular muscles from dystrophic pathology is not attributable to normalized concentration or distribution of neuronal nitric oxide synthase. *Neuromuscul Disord*. 1998;8:22–29.
167. Porter JD, Karathanasis P. Extraocular muscle in merosin-deficient muscular dystrophy: Cation homeostasis is maintained but is not mechanistic in muscle sparing. *Cell Tissue Res*. 1998;292:495–501.
168. Porter JD, Merriam AP, Khanna S, et al. Constitutive properties, not molecular adaptations, mediate extraocular muscle sparing in dystrophic mdx mice. *FASEB J*. 2003;17:893–895.
169. Andrade FH, Porter JD, Kaminski HJ. Eye muscle sparing by the muscular dystrophies: Lessons to be learned? *Microsc Res Tech*. 2000;48:192–203.
170. Nyström A, Holmblad J, Pedrosa-Domellöf F, Sasaki T, Durbeej M. Extraocular muscle is spared upon complete laminin α2 chain deficiency: Comparative expression of laminin and integrin isoforms. *Matrix Biol*. 2006;25:382–385.
171. Pachter BR, Davidowitz J, Breinin GM. A light and electron microscope study in serial sections of dystrophic extraocular muscle fibers. *Invest Ophthalmol*. 1973;12:917–923.
172. Porter JD, Merriam AP, Hack AA, Andrade FH, McNally EM. Extraocular muscle is spared despite the absence of an intact sarcoglycan complex in gamma- or delta-sarcoglycan-deficient mice. *Neuromuscul Disord*. 2001;11:197–207.
173. Mendell JR, Sahenk Z, Prior TW. The childhood muscular dystrophies: Diseases sharing a common pathogenesis of membrane instability. *J Child Neurol*. 1995;10:150–159.
174. Scoppetta C, Morante M, Casali C, Vaccario ML, Mennuni G. Dermatomyositis spares extraocular muscles. *Neurology*. 1985;35:141.
175. Kallestad KM, McDonald AA, Hebert SL, Daniel ML, Cu SR, McLoon LK. Sparing of extraocular muscle in aging and dystrophic skeletal muscle: A myogenic precursor cell hypothesis. *Exp Cell Res*. 2011;317(6):873–885.
176. McMullen CA, Ferry AL, Gamboa JL, Andrade FH, Dupont-Versteegden EE. Age-related changes of cell death pathways in rat extraocular muscle. *Exp Gerontol*. 2009;44:420–425.
177. Sobue G, Matsuoka Y, Mukai E, Takayanagi T, Sobue I, Hashizume Y. Spinal and cranial motor nerve roots in amyotrophic lateral sclerosis and X-linked recessive bulbospinal muscular atrophy: Morphometric and teased-fiber study. *Acta Neuropathol*. 1981;55:227–235.
178. Palmowski A, Jost WH, Prudlo J, et al. Eye movement in amyotrophic lateral sclerosis: A longitudinal study. *Ger J Ophthalmol*. 1995;4:355–362.
179. Haenggeli C, Kato AC. Differential vulnerability of cranial motoneurons in mouse models with motor neuron degeneration. *Neurosci Lett*. 2002;335:39–43.
180. Ahmadi M, Liu J-X, Brännström T, Andersen PM, Stål P, Pedrosa-Domellöf F. Human extraocular muscles in ALS. *Invest Ophthalmol Vis Sci*. 2010;51:3494–3501.
181. Liu J-X, Brännström T, Andersen PM, Pedrosa-Domellöf F. Distinct changes in synaptic protein composition at neuromuscular junctions of extraocular muscles versus limb muscles of ALS donors. *PLoS One*. 2013;8(2):e57473.
182. McClung JR, Cullen KE, Shall MS, Dimitrova DM, Goldberg SJ. Effects of electrode penetrations into the abducens nucleus of the monkey: Eye movement recordings and histopathological evaluation of the nuclei and lateral rectus muscles. *Exp Brain Res*. 2004;158:180–188.
183. Mizen TR. Thyroid eye disease. *Semin Ophthalmol*. 2003;18:243–247.
184. Stiebel-Kalish H, Robenshtok E, Hasanreisoglu M, Ezrachi D, Shimon I, Leibovici L. Treatment modalities for Graves' ophthalmopathy: Systemic review and metaanalysis. *J Clin Endocrinol Metab*. 2009;94:2708–2716.
185. Leong SC, Karkos PD, MacEwen CJ, White PS. A systemic review of outcomes following surgical decompression for dysthyroid orbitopathy. *Laryngoscope*. 2009;119:1106–1115.
186. Molnár I, Szombathy Z, Kovács I, Szentmiklósi AJ. Immunohistochemical studies using immunized Guinea pig sera with features of anti-human thyroid, eye and skeletal antibody and Graves' sera. *J Clin Immunol*. 2007;27:172–180.
187. Kloprogge SJ, Busuttil BE, Frauman AG. TSH receptor protein is selectively expressed in normal human extraocular muscle. *Muscle Nerve*. 2005;32:95–98.
188. Ohkura T, Taniguchi S, Yamada K, et al. Detection of the novel autoantibody (anti-UACA antibody) in patients with Graves' disease. *Biochem Biophys Res Commun*. 2004;321: 432–440.
189. Conley CA, Fowler VM. Localization of the human 64kD autoantigen D1 to myofibrils in a subset of extraocular muscle fibers. *Curr Eye Res*. 1999;19:313–322.
190. Feldon SE, Park DJ, O'Louglin CW, et al. Autologous T-lymphocytes stimulate proliferation of orbital fibroblasts derived from patients with Graves' ophthalmopathy. *Invest Ophthalmol Vis Sci*. 2005;46:3913–3921.
191. Khoo TK, Bahn RS. Pathogenesis of Graves' ophthalmopathy: The role of autoantibodies. *Thyroid*. 2007;17:1013–1018.
192. Nakase Y, Osanai T, Yoshikawa K, Inoue Y. Color Doppler imaging of orbital venous flow in dysthyroid optic neuropathy. *Jpn J Ophthalmol*. 1994;38:80–86.
193. Weber AL, Dallow RL, Sabates NR. Graves' disease of the orbit. *Neuroimaging Clin N Am*. 1996;6:61–72.
194. Hirano M, DiMauro S. ANT1, Twinkle, POLG, and TP. New genes open our eyes to ophthalmoplegia. *Neurology*. 2001;57:2163–2165.
195. Moslemi AR, Melberg A, Holme E, Oldfors A. Clonal expansion of mitochondrial DNA with multiple deletions in autosomal dominant progressive external ophthalmoplegia. *Ann Neurol*. 1996;40:707–713.
196. Schmiedel J, Jackson S, Schäfer J, Reichmann H. Mitochondrial cytopathies. *J Neurol*. 2003; 250:267–277.
197. Lee AG, Brazis PW. Chronic progressive external ophthalmoplegia. *Curr Neurol Neurosci Rep*. 2007;2:413–417.
198. Carry MR, Ringel SP, Starcevich JM. Mitochondrial morphometrics of histochemically identified human extraocular muscle fibers. *Anat Rec*. 1986;214:8–16.
199. Wallace DC. Mitochondrial DNA mutations and neuromuscular disease. *Trends Genet*. 1989;5:9–13.
200. Terman A, Brunk UT. Myocyte aging and mitochondrial turnover. *Exp Gerontol*. 2004;39: 701–705.
201. Richter C. Oxidative damage to mitochondrial DNA and its relationship to ageing. *Int J Biochem Cell Biol*. 1995;27:647–653.
202. Cao Z, Wanagat J, McKiernan SH, Aiken JM. Mitochondrial DNA deletion mutations are concomitant with ragged red regions of individual, aged muscle fibers: Analysis by laser-capture microdissection. *Nucleic Acids Res*. 2001;29:4502–4508.
203. Carlow TJ, Depper MH, Orrison WW Jr. MR of extraocular muscles in chronic progressive external ophthalmoplegia. *AJNR Am J Neuroradiol*. 1998;19:95–99.
204. Kaminski HJ, Maas E, Spiegel P, Ruff RL. Why are eye muscles frequently involved in myasthenia gravis? *Neurology*. 1990;40:1663–1669.
205. Zimmermann CW, Eblen F. Repertoires of autoantibodies against homologous eye muscle in ocular and generalized myasthenia gravis differ. *Clin Investig*. 1993;71:445–451.
206. Sanders DB, El-Salem K, Massey JM, McConville J, Vincent A. Clinical aspects of MuSK antibody positive seronegative MG. *Neurology*. 2003;60:1978–1980.
207. Takamori M, Motomura M, Kawaguchi N, et al. Anti-ryanodine receptor antibodies and FK506 in myasthenia gravis. *Neurology*. 2004;62:1894–1896.
208. Gunji K, Skolnick C, Bednarczuk T, et al. Eye muscle antibodies in patients with ocular myasthenia gravis: Possible mechanisms for eye muscle inflammation in acetylcholine-receptor antibody-negative patients. *Clin Immunol Immunopathol*. 1998;87:276–281.
209. Schmidt D, Dell'Osso LF, Abel LA, Daroff RB. Myasthenia gravis: dynamic changes in saccadic waveform, gain, and velocity. *Exp Neurol*. 1980;68:365–377.
210. Soltys J, Gong B, Kaminski HJ, Zhou Y, Kusner LL. Extraocular muscle susceptibility to myasthenia gravis: Unique immunological environment? *Ann NY Acad Sci*. 2008;1132: 220–224.
211. Kupersmith MJ. Ocular myasthenia gravis: Treatment successes and failures in patients with long-term follow-up. *J Neurol*. 2009;256:1314–1320.
212. Chang MY, Binenbaum G, Heidary G, Cavuoto KM, Morrison DG, TGrivedi RH, Kim SJ, Pineles SL. Surgical treatments to improve visual acuity in infantile nystagmus syndrome: A report by the American Academy of Ophthalmology. *Ophthalmology*. 2023;130: 331–344.

Neural Control of Eye Movements

Kathleen E. Cullen

INTRODUCTION

The brain controls the eyes to ensure optimal visual acuity as we navigate our environment throughout our daily lives. First, we make voluntary eye movements to explore our visual world and shift our focus attention from one object to another. Second, we can also voluntarily track an object as it moves through our environment. And third, as we move through space, our brains generate reflexive eye movements that reduce the motion of the visual surround relative to both retinas to ensure gaze stability. How the brain controls eye movements during all of these conditions is well understood, both in terms of the underlying neurophysiological mechanisms and anatomical organization.

Eye movements can be categorized into five classes (Table 8.1). Of these, three classes are voluntary eye movements made to redirect our gaze relative to the world. These voluntary eye movements include saccades, smooth pursuit, and smooth vergence. Specifically, *saccades*, which derive their name from the French word for "jerk," are rapid transient eye movements. Saccades are made to voluntary redirect gaze between stationary objects in the visual environment. By precisely positioning each eye, saccades effectively target the fovea so that an object can be viewed with the greatest acuity. *Smooth pursuit* eye movements are also foveating voluntary eye movements. However, in contrast to saccades, smooth pursuit eye movements are relatively slow and are made to track moving objects rather than shift gaze from one stationary object to another. Finally, animals with binocular vision such as humans make *smooth vergence* eye movements to track a target moving in depth and/or maintain fused binocular vision on a target.

The two remaining classes, namely the *vestibulo-ocular reflex* (VOR) and *optokinetic reflex* (OKR), are reflexive rather than voluntary eye movements. VOR and OKR eye movements are made to stabilize (rather than voluntarily redirect) gaze direction relative to the world. Specifically, the VOR functions to keep the visual world stationary on the retina during everyday activities such as walking and running by moving the eye in the opposite direction to the on-going head motion. Head motion is detected by the vestibular sensory organs of the inner ear, which in turn transmit commands to the brain that produce compensatory eye motion so that the visual world remains stationary on the retina. Correspondingly, the OKR also functions to stabilize gaze during everyday activities such as walking and running. However, in contrast to the VOR, OKR eye movements are driven by activation of the visual rather than vestibular system. The visual input from a large moving scene subtending much or all the visual field produces compensatory OKR eye movements that function to keep the visual scene stationary on the retina. The VOR is most effective for head motion at frequencies above 0.1 Hz, whereas the OKR reflex is most effective at lower frequencies, particularly below 0.1 Hz. Thus, in everyday life the VOR and OKR are complementary and work synergistically to stabilize gaze in response to head movements.

Traditionally, neurophysiological and behavioral experiments have studied and characterized each of the five classes of eye movements in isolation. As a result, as detailed in sections "Final common pathway" and "Premotor control of gaze redirection," we have an excellent understanding of the oculomotor pathways that generate each class of eye movement (Table 8.1). However, this experimental approach has also led to the prevailing (and incorrect) view that each of eye movement class is generated by separate and distinct neural pathways. Indeed, as discussed in section "Interactions between eye movement subsystems" the brain typically simultaneously employs two or more oculomotor "subsystems" to control gaze, and, most notably, vergence is generated by the same oculomotor pathways that generate saccades and smooth pursuit.

FINAL COMMON PATHWAY

To voluntarily move the eyes, a hierarchy of neural control exists within each of the functional categories of eye movements that plans, coordinates, and executes motor activity (Box 8.1). First, high-level structures, including regions of the cortex, basal ganglia, and cerebellum, underlie cognitive aspects of eye movements including visual attention and decision-making to plan where to next focus gaze (Box 8.1). Integration of such higher-level input by structures such as the superior colliculus is then required to trigger the planned eye movement. The superior colliculus activates premotor pathways that activate the motoneurons that control the extraocular muscles, which in turn move each eye about its center of rotation. These motor neurons are located in the three cranial nuclei that comprise the "final common pathway" for all classes of eye movements. Premotor pathways in the brainstem that mediate saccades, smooth pursuit, vergence, VOR and OKR eye movements all send the required motor commands to these motoneurons to generate eye movement. The next section, "The extraocular eye muscles and their motoneuron innervations," describes the final common pathway for all eye movements.

The extraocular eye muscles and their motoneuron innervations

To ensure a clear unified view of the world during our everyday activities, the brain must precisely coordinate the movement of our eyes so that both foveae are aligned on the same point in space. To do this the brain activates the six extraocular muscles that control the eye's movement and position. The six extraocular muscles are arranged in three antagonistic pairs (Fig. 8.1A) that together generate the net force required to rotate the eye to a new position. First, the relative activation of the paired lateral and medial recti muscles controls horizontal eye movement (i.e., the temporal-nasal rotation of each eye, respectively). Second, the relative activation of the paired superior and inferior recti muscles principally controls vertical movement (i.e., the up-down rotation [elevation] of each eye, respectively). Third, the relative activation of the paired superior and inferior oblique muscles controls the torsional rotation of each eye, as well as its elevation. Together, these three pairs of extraocular muscles allow the eye to rotate with three degrees of freedom (Fig. 8.1B). The VOR and OKR operate fully in three dimensions, while orbital mechanics and central mechanisms fundamentally restrict saccadic and smooth pursuit eye movements to two dimensions. This constraint on three-dimensional voluntary eye movements is referred to as Listing's law[1-3] (see Chapter 9).

To activate each of these six extraocular muscles, the brain sends commands to the motoneurons located within the three oculomotor cranial nerve nuclei (Fig. 8.2A, shaded red structures). These cranial nerve nuclei include the oculomotor (III), trochlear (IV), and abducens (VI) nuclei of the mesencephalon and pons. Notably, the oculomotor (III) nucleus is located in the midbrain and comprises four distinct anatomical regions in which motoneurons specifically control either the medial, superior or inferior recti, or inferior oblique. The trochlear (IV) nucleus is also located in the midbrain and its motoneurons

specifically control the superior oblique muscle. And finally, the abducens (VI) nucleus, which is located in the pons, controls the lateral rectus muscle. A shared feature across all three cranial nerve nuclei is that, in all cases, any given motoneuron only projects to a single extraocular muscle.

Additionally, some neurons within the cranial nerve nuclei controlling horizontal eye movements are actually not motoneurons, but instead project to the motoneurons controlling the antagonistic muscle of the other eye. These neurons, which are called internuclear neurons, encode similar eye movement-related information, as do the motoneurons. Thus, internuclear neurons are thought to facilitate the neural control of conjugate component of binocular eye movements, namely the component of the eye movement that is common to both eyes. For example, internuclear neurons within the abducens and oculomotor nucleus project via the medial longitudinal fasciculus (MLF) to the contralateral oculomotor and abducens nucleus, respectively.[4,5] Thus, the motoneurons of the left abducens nucleus project directly to the left lateral rectus, while the internuclear neurons of the left abducens project contralaterally to motoneurons in the right oculomotor (III) nucleus (Fig. 8.2B). The synchronous activations of both cell types thus serve to generate complementary temporally directed movement of the left eye and nasally directed movement of the right eye, such that both eyes effectively move in the same (i.e., leftward) direction. Correspondingly, the synchronous activations of motoneurons and internuclear neurons from oculomotor nucleus would function to generate complementary nasally directed movement of the left eye and temporally directed movement of the right eye, such that both eyes effectively move in the same (i.e., rightward) direction.

TABLE 8.1   Classification of eye movements

Eye movement classification	Function
Voluntary	
Saccades (conjugate/ disjunctive)	Fast gaze redirection between stationary far targets/stationary targets in depth
Smooth Pursuit	Slow eye movements used to track moving targets
Smooth Vergence	Slow eye movements used to track an object moving in depth/maintain fused binocular vision
Involuntary	
Vestibulo-ocular reflex	Uses vestibular information to hold images stationary on the retina as head moves
Optokinetic reflex	Uses visual information to stabilize gaze for low frequency head movements

BOX 8.1   Hierarchy of motor control

Subcortical oculomotor disorders are classified by lesion sites in the hierarchy of motor control:
- Supranuclear (motor planning stage)
- Internuclear (connections between nuclear and premotor sites)
- Premotor (coordinates combined actions of several muscles)
- Nuclear (cranial motor nuclei making up the final common pathway)
- Peripheral (cranial nerves and muscles)

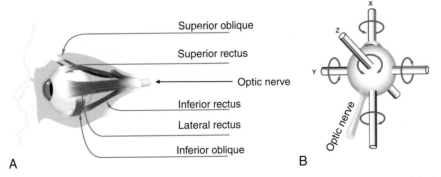

Fig. 8.1 The six extraocular muscles are arranged in three antagonistic pairs. (**A**) A lateral view of the left eye showing the global insertions of the extraocular motoneurons. (**B**) A posterosuperior view of the right eye shows the three axes of eye rotation. Rotation about the vertical "z" axis, controlled by the lateral and medial recti muscles, results in eye movements to left or right. Rotation about the transverse "y" axis, controlled by the superior and inferior recti muscles, elevates and depresses the eye. Finally, rotations about the anteroposterior "x" axis result in counterclockwise, as well as upwards and downwards, eye motion. (Modified from Kandel ER, Schwartz JH, Jessell TM, Siegelbaum SA and Hudspeth AJ. *Principles of Neural Science*. 2013; 5th Edition, McGraw-Hill Education, New York.)

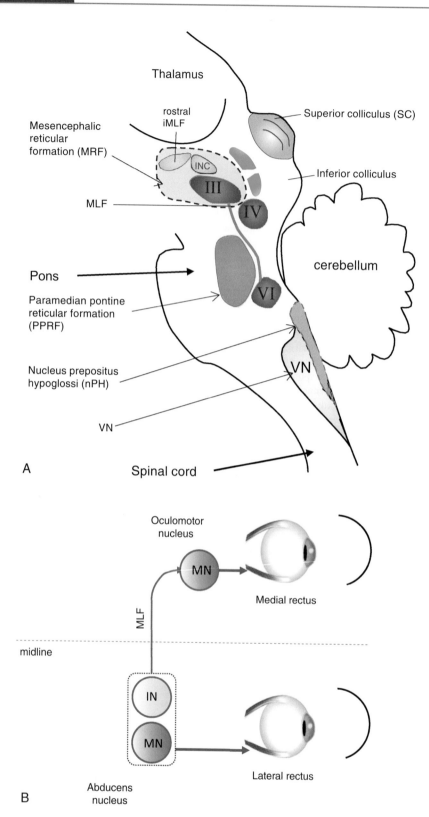

Fig. 8.2 The motor and premotor oculomotor nuclei. (**A**) A parasagittal slice through a rhesus monkey brain with motor (*red*) and premotor oculomotor nuclei indicated. *INC*, Interstitial nucleus of Cajal; *iMLF*, interstitial nucleus of the medial longitudinal fasciculus; *IN*, internuclear neurons; *MLF*, medial longitudinal fasciculus; *MN*, extraocular motoneurons; *VN*, vestibular nuclei. (**B**) Motoneurons in the abducens project to ipsilateral lateral rectus, while internuclear neurons in the abducens project contralaterally to the motoneurons in the oculomotor (III) nucleus.

Finally, it is noteworthy that there are two unique features of extraocular muscle. First, each of the six extraocular muscles is comprised of two distinct layers, a global layer and an orbital layer. These two layers contain fibers with different response properties (e.g., fatigability, fusion frequency, and contraction times; see Chapter 7) and in comparison to the muscles of the skeletal system, extraocular muscles in both the global and orbital layers have relatively fast contraction times.[6,7] Twitch fibers appear to receive stronger innervation from premotor pathways involved in the generation of fast eye movements (e.g., the saccadic burst generator), whereas nontwitch fiber innervation from premotor sources is involved in executing slow eye movements (e.g., pursuit, the VOR, OKN).[6,8] Second, in contrast to skeletal muscle, human extraocular muscles have muscle spindles but not Golgi tendon organs. In addition, extraocular muscles have a unique class of receptors—palisade endings—which are believed to serve as proprioceptors. Importantly, although human extraocular muscles process proprioceptor receptors, there is no evidence for a stretch reflex as is observed in skeletal muscle. The role of these receptors in extraocular muscles remains to be fully understood; however, there is reason to believe that they signal proprioceptive information from the extraocular muscles to the brain to ensure accurate visuomotor behavior.[9,10]

The biomechanics of eye movements and motor neuron activity

Mechanics of the oculomotor plant

To move the eye to a new position, the extraocular muscles must generate the active force necessary to overcome the passive restraining forces of the eyeball, extraocular muscles, and supporting tissues of the orbit. In his pioneering work, David Robinson[11] established that these passive forces are predominately governed by viscoelastic properties. Specifically, the eye's natural tendency to "spring" back to its center position when moved right/left or up/down defines its passive elasticity, whereas the finding that more force is required to move the eye at faster and faster velocities defines the eye's passive viscosity. In this same study, Robinson further made the surprising discovery that the eyeball has negligible inertia. Combined, the viscoelastic properties of the eye's passive restraining forces are central to our understanding of how motoneurons control eye movements. Notably, because the eyeball and its orbital tissues are dominated by viscoelastic properties and have negligible inertia, the active force required to move the eye can be well approximated by the simple first-order differential equation of the form:

$$F = kL + r(dL/dt) \qquad \textbf{(Eq. 8.1)}$$

where F is the force, k is the coefficient of elasticity, L is the length of the muscle, r is the coefficient of viscosity, and dL/dt is the rate of muscle length change (i.e., velocity). Given the anatomical complexity of the eyeball, extraocular muscles, and supporting tissues of the orbit, it is remarkable how well its mechanics are represented by such a simple equation. For example, Eq. 8.1 predicts that, when a constant external force is applied to the eye and then removed, the eye will passively drift back to the center position following a simple exponential characterized by the time constant r/k. Indeed, experiments confirming this prediction have established that the time constant of the return to center is around 250 ms (Fig. 8.3).

The relationship between motoneuron activity and eye movement

The simple relationship between force and eye movement represented by Eq. 8.1 has proven to be advantageous for understanding the neural control of eye movements. This is because motoneuron discharge is well related to active muscle force. Neural recordings made from individual extraocular motoneurons in alert-behaving monkeys demonstrated that the response of a given motoneuron, like force, is well approximated by Eq. 8.1.[12-14] This point is demonstrated in Fig. 8.4, which illustrates the activity of a typical inferior rectus motoneuron in different conditions. First, when the monkey held its eye stationary, approximately centered in the orbit (i.e., position = 0 degrees), the motoneuron discharged at a constant firing rate—namely its resting discharge (Fig. 8.4A: top, red arrow). Second, when the monkey made downward and upward eye movements to fixate target (Fig. 8.4A, top), the example motoneuron's firing rate increased and decreased, respectively, consistent with the pulling direction of the inferior rectus. The

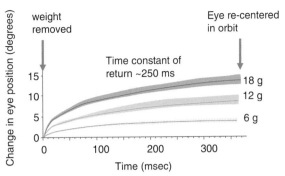

Fig. 8.3 The visco-elastic properties of the muscles and surrounding orbital tissues can be appreciated by the application of force to the eye, which initially causes it to move to an eccentric position. Once the force is removed at time = 0, the eye returns to the center position with a time constant of 250 ms. (Modified from Robinson DA. The mechanics of human saccadic eye movement. *J Physiol.* 1964;174:245–264.)

example motoneuron is typical in that its sustained change in firing rate was proportional to eye position—in this case, vertical eye position (Fig. 8.4A: bottom, red line). This same relationship is plotted for other example neurons in blue in Fig. 8.4A. Finally, the example extraocular motoneuron firing rate response was also related to eye velocity. This can be appreciated in Fig. 8.4B, in which the example neuron's activity is shown during vertical smooth pursuit eye movements. Comparison of the neurons' responses when the eye moves past the same orbital position reveals that firing rate is linearly related to the current velocity (Fig. 8.4B, red arrows).

Combining the findings of the experiments in Fig. 8.4 results in a first-order differential equation that well describes the relationship between motoneuron responses and eye movement across each of these three conditions:

$$FR(t) = b + k\ E(t - t_d) + r\dot{E}(t - t_d) \qquad \textbf{(Eq. 8.2)}$$

where FR(t) is the neuron's instantaneous firing rate, b, k, and r are constants that represent the neuron's resting rate when the eyes are pointing straight ahead (mean firing rate), and the neuron's eye position (slope of Fig. 8.4A, bottom) and eye velocity sensitivities (slope of Fig. 8.4B, bottom), respectively. Note b can take on negative values for motoneurons that are only recruited at eccentric eye positions in their preferred direction. t_d refers to the dynamic lead time, and $E(t)$ and $\dot{E}(t)$ refer to the instantaneous eye position and velocity, respectively.

Importantly, Eq. 8.2 is of the same form as Eq. 8.1, which described the biomechanics of the eye. Furthermore, the ratio characterizing average motoneuron discharges (r/k, Eq. 8.2) well approximates the 250-ms time constant of the extraocular plant (r/k, Eq. 8.1). In short, motoneuron discharge dynamics are proportional to the active force generated to move the eye, and thus effectively matched to the eye's biomechanics. Moreover, Eq. 8.2 can be used to describe eye movements not only during steady fixation, ocular fixation, and smooth pursuit, but also during all other eye movements, including the VOR and smooth vergence.[12-20] However, the parameters in Eq. 8.2 that correspond to motoneuron eye velocity and position sensitivities (i.e., r and k) decrease as a function of the eye's velocity.[12,21] Specifically, a given motoneuron's eye velocity and position sensitivities are greater for slower movements (e.g., pursuit) compared with faster movements (e.g., saccades).[12,22] This is likely due to nonlinearities in biomechanics of the extraocular plant that are generated by the velocity-dependent

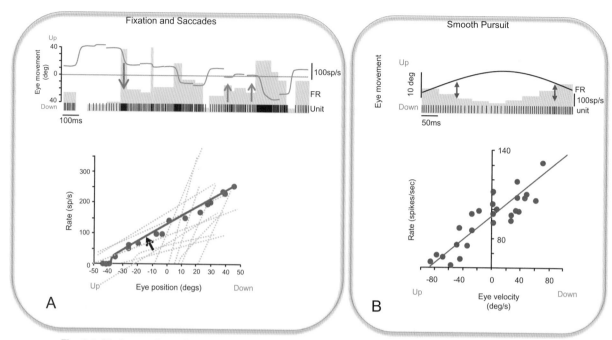

Fig. 8.4 Discharge of a typical motoneuron in the inferior rectus subdivision of the oculomotor (III) nucleus. (**A**) During target fixation, the motoneuron fires at a steady tonic rate that linearly increases with downward eye position. Times at which the eye is approximately centered in orbit are indicated by the two *blue arrows*. The *green arrow* indicates burst of activity during a downward saccade. **B.** During smooth pursuit, this same motoneuron also encodes eye velocity. Times at which the eye passed through the same orbital position at different velocities (in this case in opposite directions) are indicated by the two *red arrows*.

viscosity of the extraocular muscles.[23–25] As a result, faster eye movements such as saccades are ultimately met with less viscous resistance such that a smaller change in force (i.e., corresponding to smaller coefficients) is required to move the eye.

A pulse-step command is required to control saccadic eye movements

As explained previously, a simple first-order differential equation (Eq. 8.1) well describes the biomechanics of the eye. These dynamics have important implications regarding the motor commands that must be generated by the motoneurons to generate eye movements. For example, one might intuitively guess that a step change in motoneuron firing rate would be sufficient to generate a saccadic eye movement. However, this is not the case. Even large redirecting eye movement (i.e., amplitude >40 degrees) can be completed in less than 100 ms. In contrast, the dominant time constant of the biomechanics of the eye (Eq. 8.1) is around 250 ms. What this means is that a step change in motoneuron firing rate would produce an eye movement that would still be around 37% short of its final position after around 250 ms.[26]

Consequently, a step change in motoneuron firing rate is not sufficient to generate a saccadic eye movement. Instead, to generate saccades that move the eye to its final desired position in this shorter time frame, motoneurons must generate a burst (or "pulse") of action potentials. This burst of activity is required to offset for the eye's passive viscosity, represented by the eye velocity-dependent term (rE') in Eq. 8.2. Fig. 8.5A illustrates a schematic of the saccadic pulse-step command signal sent by motoneurons to extraocular muscles. Single unit recording studies in primates have demonstrated that the saccade-related bursts of motoneurons reach rates as high as 500 spikes/s. Once the saccade has been completed and the eye is oriented to focus on a new target of interest, motoneurons indeed continue to generate a sustained constant firing rate (or "step") to keep

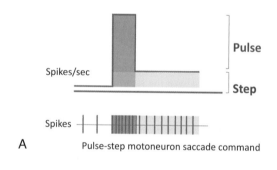

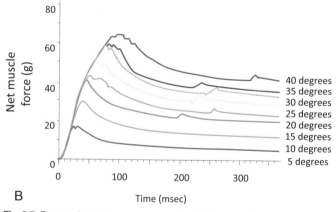

Fig. 8.5 Extraocular motoneurons generate a "pulse-step" command to drive saccades. (**A**) Schematic of the "pulse-step" command. (**B**) Measurement of muscle force generated in response to the extraocular motoneuron "pulse-step" command. The sustained force generated following the saccade by the "step" is required to hold the eye steady at its new position. (From Robinson DA. The mechanics of human saccadic eye movement. *J Physiol.* 1964;174:245–264. https://doi.org/10.1113/jphysiol.1964.sp007485.)

fixed in any eccentric location. This step of activity is required to offset for the eye's passive elasticity, represented by the eye position dependent term (kE) in Equation 2. Notably, this "pulse-step" pattern of motoneuron activity is evident in Fig. 8.4A. In this typical example, an inferior rectus motoneuron first produces a burst of spikes (the "pulse") to generate downward saccades. After this saccade-related burst, the same motoneuron then produces a sustained constant firing rate (or "step") which holds the eye stationary at this new location, to prevent it from drifting back to its centered location in the orbit. Correspondingly, as a result of this motoneuron pulse-step command signal, extraocular muscle tension first rises to a peak and then rapidly decays to a steady state level (Fig. 8.5B).

PREMOTOR CONTROL OF GAZE REDIRECTION

Having examined the properties of the motor neurons that control eye movements, the premotor circuits that command each class of eye movement when performed in isolation are now considered. This section will focus on the premotor pathways in the brainstem that mediate voluntary eye movements that are used to redirect the direction of gaze, namely saccades and smooth and vergence eye movements.

Neural control of saccadic eye movements

Saccades are rapid eye movements that are made to redirect the fovea to fixate a target of interest (Fig. 8.6). When exploring the visual world, humans routinely make two to three saccadic eye movements each second. Larger amplitude saccades are characterized by higher velocities, with the largest saccades reaching velocities up to 700 degrees/s for 40-degree saccades in humans. The consistent relationship between the saccadic duration, peak velocity, and amplitude is referred to as the "main sequence" (Box 8.2). For example, the relationship between amplitude and peak velocity is well described by a power law function.[27,28] Approximately 200 milliseconds are required to initiate a saccade in response to the appearance of an unexpected visual target.

Pathway overview

Higher-level structures, including regions of the cortex and cerebellum, play an essential role in visual attention and the decision-making process regarding where to next direct gaze. Integration of such higher-level input by structures such as the superior colliculus is then required to trigger the next saccadic eye movement. The superior colliculus, a bilateral structure located on the roof of the midbrain, plays an especially important role in visuo-oculomotor integration required for controlling saccades. This midbrain region effectively serves as an information "hub" that receives inputs from multiple cortical areas, including the frontal eye fields, posterior parietal cortex, and basal ganglia (Fig. 8.7). Cells in the deeper superior colliculus layers are arranged in a functional "motor map," with a series of iso-amplitude lines which run medial-laterally and a series of iso-direction lines that run rostral-caudally (Fig. 8.8).

Output neurons in these deeper layers of the superior colliculus send direct contralateral projections to three structures within the brainstem, which correspond to key nodes in the brainstem saccadic circuit, namely the paramedian pontine reticular formation (PPRF), rostral interstitial nucleus of medial longitudinal fasciculus (riMLF), and raphe interpositus nucleus (RIP).[29-31] The caudal superior colliculus preferentially targets the PPRF and riMLF, regions containing premotor saccadic burst neurons that project to the extraocular motoneurons to generate the horizontal and vertical/torsional components of saccadic eye movements, respectively. In contrast, the output neurons in the deeper layers of the rostral superior colliculus send direct projections to the RIP. As discussed further in the chapter, the nucleus raphe

---

BOX 8.2   Main sequence for saccades

Deviations from the main sequence (i.e., the relationships between duration, peak velocity, and amplitude of human saccades) can be used in patients to identify abnormalities in oculomotor pathways.

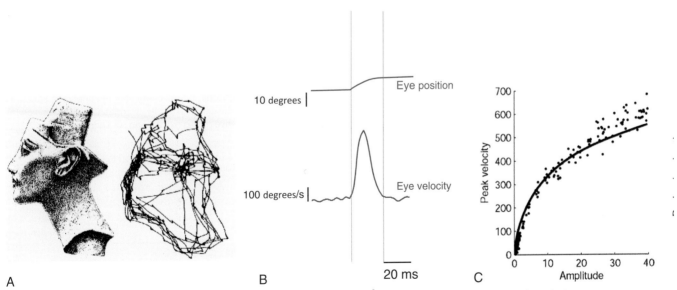

Fig. 8.6 Saccadic eye movements. (**A**) Saccadic eye movements made while a subject freely viewed a bust of Nefertiti. Saccades are largely directed to fixate the most salient features, including the nose, mouth, and eyes, and makes saccades between these features. (**B**) Saccades are rapid ballistic eye movements that can reach speeds >700 degrees/s in humans. (**C**) Saccades display well-defined kinematics, for example, there is a robust relationship between saccade amplitude and peak velocity—termed the saccadic "main sequence." (**A** from Yarbus AL. *Eye Movements and Vision*. New York: Springer; 1967; **C** from Harris CM, Wolpert DM. The main sequence of saccades optimizes speed-accuracy trade-off. *Biol Cybern*. 2006;95(1):21–9. https://doi.org/10.1007/s00422-006-0064-x. Epub 2006 Mar 23.)

pontis contains omnipause neurons that pause for saccades made in all directions. Accordingly, as shown in Fig. 8.9, the superior colliculus plays a role in both the generation of saccades and fixation via its caudal versus rostral connectivity to brainstem premotor circuits; neurons in the caudal superior colliculus trigger saccades, whereas those in the rostral superior colliculus have an active role in maintaining fixation.[31]

The superior colliculus' functional "motor map" was initially defined by microsimulation: Stimulating increasingly caudal sites produces larger and larger contralateral saccades, whereas stimulating sites that are increasing medial versus lateral to the midline produce saccades that are increasing downward versus upward (reviewed in[32]). Individual superior colliculus neurons display saccade-related burst activity with direction/amplitude tuning that correspond to their location on the motor map. Further, this saccadic burst activity predominately encodes motor, not sensory, information—neurons respond to saccadic eye movement of a particular amplitude rather the appearance of a target at a particular location on the retinal map.[33] A large population of coarsely tuned superior colliculus neurons comprise a "hill" of activity that drives a given saccade. If one only had access to the information encoded by a single superior colliculus neuron, there would be ambiguity in coding of both saccade amplitude and direction. Instead,

the direction and amplitude of a saccadic movement is read out from this population of neurons.[34] Finally, in addition to their descending projections to brainstem regions controlling eye movements, the output neurons of the superior colliculus have ascending projections that target forebrain structures including the basal ganglia and amygdala. Through these pathways, the superior colliculus also contributes to visual perception and cognition, for instance, playing an essential role in attention and decision-making, as well as motor control (reviewed in Zenon and Krauzlis, 2014; Basso et al., 2021[35,36]).

The superior colliculus sends descending projections to brainstem structures that produce the "pulse-step" motoneuron command

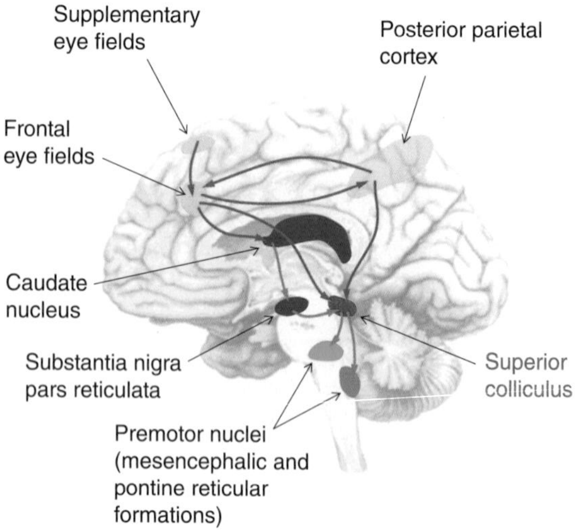

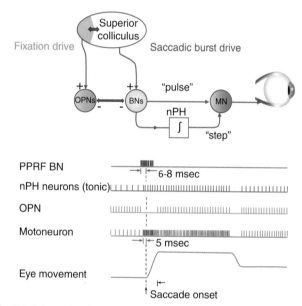

Fig. 8.9 Schematic of the premotor circuit for horizontal saccade generation. (Top panel) The superior colliculus plays a role in both the generation of saccades and fixation via its projections to brainstem premotor circuits. Neurons in the superior colliculus target areas that trigger saccades, whereas those in the rostral superior colliculus target areas involved in maintaining fixation. (Bottom panel) Saccadic burst neurons (BNs) in the paramedian pontine reticular formation (PPRF) send a "pulse" of activity to the extraocular motoneurons (MN) to drive the saccade. BNs also project to the nucleus prepositus (nPH), which in turn integrates this pulse input to compute the "step" command. nPH neurons send this "step" command to the extraocular MN. In contrast to BNs, omnipause neurons (OPN) are active during fixation and pause for saccades.

Fig. 8.7 Inputs from cortex (*yellow shading*) and basal ganglia (*purple shading*) to the superior colliculus (*red shading*) command the premotor circuitry in the mesencephalon and pons (*green and blue shading*) to produce saccades.

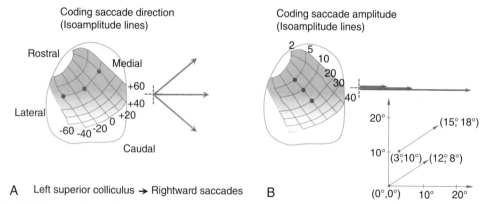

Fig. 8.8 The superior colliculus arranged topographically as a motor map on which the vector (direction location is indicated in *red*).

CHAPTER 8 Neural Control of Eye Movements 219

required to generate saccadic eye movements (see section "A pulse-step command is required to control saccadic eye movements"). Specifically, the "pulse-step" command is the consequence of the integration of two distinct premotor inputs at the level of the extraocular motoneurons (Fig. 8.9). For the horizontal component of saccades, premotor burst neurons in the PPRF provide the "pulse" command, while premotor neurons in the nucleus prepositus (nPH) provide the "step" command. A complementary and separate parallel circuit controls the vertical/torsional component of saccades; the pulse is provided by vertical burst neurons in the riMLF and the step is provided by premotor neurons in the interstitial nucleus of Cajal. This premotor saccadic circuitry is considered in more detail further for both the horizontal and vertical/torsional components of saccades.

The pulse of the "pulse-step" command for horizontal saccades

The premotor circuit generating the "pulse" command for the horizontal component of saccades is very well understood. To drive horizontal saccades, two classes of saccadic burst neurons work together: excitatory and inhibitory burst neurons. Excitatory burst neurons are located in the rostral PPRF and excite the agonist motoneurons (i.e., ipsilateral abducens), while inhibitory burst neurons are located in the caudal PPRF and inhibit the antagonist motoneurons (i.e., contralateral abducens)[37–42] (reviewed in[43,44]). Both excitatory and inhibitory saccadic burst neurons fire a burst of action potentials that precedes saccade onset by approximately 10–20 ms,[45–47] but are otherwise silent. For example, these neurons are silent during steady gaze, smooth pursuit, and smooth vergence, and during the slow phases of vestibular nystagmus.

The burst activity of both classes of saccadic burst neurons well correlates with measures of the saccadic movement (Fig. 8.10 A,B). Specifically, the duration of the burst and saccade are well correlated, as are the number of spikes within a burst and saccade amplitude.[38,39,46–51] Furthermore, the pattern of action potentials in the burst dynamically encodes saccadic eye velocity as a function of time.[46,47,52,53] Overall, the same first-order model for extraocular motoneurons discussed previously in the chapter (Eq. 8.2) can also be used to describe the time-varying saccadic burst neuron activity, by setting the position sensitivity to zero (i.e., k = 0). These response dynamics are consistent with the role of saccadic burst neurons in producing the "pulse" of the pulse-step command. Owing to its role in commanding horizontal saccades, chemical inactivation of the PPRF results in a substantial reduction in peak velocity and proportional increase in duration for ipsilateral saccades.[54]

The step of the "pulse-step" command for horizontal saccades

To hold the eye steady at its new horizontal location following a saccade, the nucleus prepositus sends a "step" command directly to the extraocular motoneurons[55] (reviewed in[56–59]). The mechanism by which this premotor control of "step" command is generated for horizontal saccades is also well understood. The nucleus prepositus receives direct input from the saccadic burst neurons in the PPRF. The nucleus prepositus in turn generates the "step" command by integrating (in the mathematical sense) its burst neuron input. Neural integration is performed within the nucleus prepositus itself via recurrent connectivity between individual neurons[60–63] that results in correlated firing activity between single neurons that varies as a function of distance.[58,64]

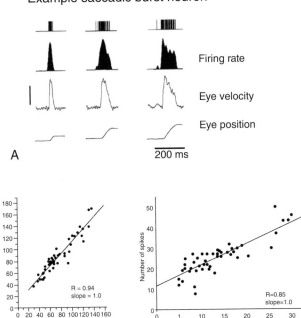

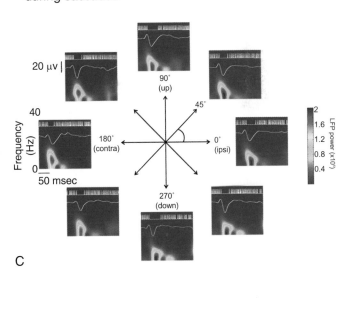

Fig. 8.10 Response dynamics of brainstem neurons that control horizontal saccade generation. (**A**) paramedian pontine reticular formation (PPRF) neurons fire a burst of activity during saccades. (**B**) This burst of activity dynamically encodes eye velocity and, as a result, the number of spikes in the saccade-related burst is correlated with saccade amplitude. (**C**) In contrast, omnipause neurons are inhibited during saccades, as demonstrated by their cessation of firing and negative local field potential (LFP) profiles. *Vertical line* in (**A**) 400 spikes/s, 400 degrees/s, and 40 degrees. (**A, C** Van Horn MR, Mitchell DE, Massot C, Cullen KE. Local neural processing and the generation of dynamic motor commands within the saccadic premotor network. *J Neurosci.* 2010;30(32):10905–10917. Copyright 2010 Society for Neuroscience; **B** Adapted from Cullen K, McCrea R. Firing behavior ofapte brain stem neurons during voluntary cancellation of the horizontal vestibuloocular reflex. I. Secondary vestibular neurons. *J Neurophysiol.* 1993;70(2):828–843.)

As a result of this integration, neurons in the nucleus prepositus predominately send a horizontal eye position signal to the extraocular motoneurons.[57] Thus, the same first-order model for motoneurons discussed previously in the chapter (Eq. 8.2) can also be used to describe nucleus prepositus neuron activity, where the position sensitivity (i.e., k) dominates, consistent with the role of these neurons in producing the "step" of the pulse-step command. In short, because the burst neuron "pulse" command encodes eye velocity, integration of this input within the nucleus prepositus effectively produces an eye position—or equivalently the required "step"—command. Owing to its role in controlling horizontal saccades, lesions of the nucleus prepositus result in the inability to hold the eyes at a new horizontal position after a saccade.[55]

The vertical/torsional "pulse-step" command for saccades

As noted previously, a parallel circuit, complementary to that described for the horizontal component of saccades, controls the vertical/torsional component of saccades. First the "pulse" command is provided by premotor neurons in the mesencephalic reticular formation (MRF). Specifically, individual neurons in the riMLF burst for upward or downward saccades, but are otherwise silent.[65,66] These burst neurons send this pulse of the "pulse-step" saccade command directly to the motoneurons in the oculomotor and trochlear nuclei that control vertical/torsional eye movements. Additionally, these burst neurons also project to the interstitial nucleus of Cajal, which integrates the pulse signal to produce the required "step" command.[67,68] In turn, interstitial nucleus of Cajal neurons send the step command directly to the motoneurons controlling the vertical/torsional eye motion. Accordingly, lesions of the riMLF and interstitial nucleus of Cajal lead to the impaired generation of vertical and torsional saccades.[67,69,70] These results show that burst neurons in the riMLF play a decisive role in generating rapid eye movements with a vertical and torsional component.

Together the riMLF and interstitial nucleus of Cajal generate the pulse and step commands required to control the vertical/torsional component of saccades. As a result, this premotor circuit and the parallel horizontal circuit described previously provide the required "pulse-step" input for saccades in all directions. It is noteworthy that the neural integration of the PPRF and riMLF pulse command by the nucleus prepositus and interstitial nucleus of Cajal is imperfect, such that the eyes will very gradually drift back to center position with a time constant of approximately 25 s following a saccade. However, this is typically not a major issue for visual stability, given that several saccades are made within each second during normal viewing.

The role of omnipause neurons

Omnipause neurons function to actively inhibit the generation of saccadic eye movements during fixation. They are located near the midline in the RIP, close to the rostral pole of the abducens nucleus.[71–73] While the output neurons within the caudal superior colliculus activate saccadic burst neurons in the PPRF and central mesencephalic nucleus to control saccades, the output neurons of the rostral zone of the superior colliculus are tonically active during fixation[74–78] and preferentially activate omnipause neurons.[31] Omnipause neurons, in turn, send direct inhibitory projections to saccadic burst neurons in the PPRF and in the MRF.[79–81] Consequently, omnipause neurons actively suppress the horizontal and vertical/torsional premotor saccade pathways during fixation. Correspondingly, omnipause neurons receive reciprocal inhibition from saccade burst neurons in the PPRF during saccades.[30,31,44]

The duration of an omnipause neuron's pause is well correlated to saccade duration.[50,49] Further, the hyperpolarizations that occur in association with saccade-related pauses similarly encode eye movement velocity for saccades in all directions (Fig. 8.10C[82,83]). The role

of omnipause neurons in active fixation and the inhibition of saccadic eye movements has been causally demonstrated in experiments showing that microsimulation of the omnipause region of the RIP causes complete cessation of eye movements.[50,84] How omnipause neurons function to gate the transition between fixation and saccadic eye movements by monosynaptically suppressing activity in premotor burst neurons during fixation and releasing them during saccades is shown schematically in Fig. 8.9.

The control of microsaccades by premotor saccadic neurons

To explore the visual world, we make voluntary saccadic eye movements that are interspersed with periods of fixation. However, even when our gaze is fixed, our eyes are not completely still. Instead, we generate small fixational eye movements called microsaccades (for reviews, see[85,86]). The direction and propensity of microsaccades can be biased by attention,[87–90] but, on average, microsaccades are corrective such that the eyes remain focused on the target.[85,86,91] Neural recordings in the saccadic pathway have established that the same premotor saccadic burst neurons that encode the size, duration, and velocity of saccades (i.e., Fig. 8.9), also encode these same measures during microsaccades.[92] Furthermore, the same simple first-order model provides an adequate description of the relationship between neural responses and eye motion. Finally, omnipause neurons cease firing (pause) during microsaccades as they do during saccades[92,93] and show a comparable robust relationship between the pause duration and microsaccade duration. Thus, the saccadic burst generator controls both saccades and microsaccades.

Neural control of pursuit

Smooth pursuit eye movements are made to track a moving visual target of interest, so that its image is stabilized on the fovea to provide high visual acuity. Such eye movements are typically considerably slower than saccades, rarely reaching velocities beyond 100 degrees/s as compared with 500 to 700 degrees/s. The neural basis of smooth pursuit eye movements involves the transformation of visual target motion information—a sensory signal produced by target motion relative to retina—into the eye movement motor command required to stabilize the moving target on the fovea. This visuomotor transformation is largely accomplished via a corticopontocerebellar pathway (reviewed in[94,95]) arising in areas of the extrastriate cortex and ending in the extraocular motoneurons (Fig. 8.11).

The smooth pursuit system is generally modeled as a negative feedback controller in which a retinal velocity error signal (i.e., the difference between target velocity and eye velocity) drives eye movements with a 100 ms delay (reviewed in[96]). This is because the fixed delays inherent to the corticopontocerebellar pathway, which controls smooth pursuit eye movements, result in a around 100-ms latency between visual target motion input and the resultant pursuit eye movement. Importantly, this delay places a limit on tracking performance. In conditions where target velocity changes dynamically as a function of time, the current tracking eye velocity will always be around 100 ms behind the actual target velocity. For this reason, smooth pursuit performance becomes increasingly inaccurate for more dynamic targets, notably those moving at frequencies greater than about 1 Hz. In addition to retinal velocity error, retinal position and acceleration error signals can also drive pursuit eye movements. However, their relative influence is far less than that of retinal velocity error. Finally, nonvisual mechanisms such as anticipation and target predictability can improve pursuit performance. As detailed further, this integration of higher-order extraretinal signals already begins early in the corticopontocerebellar pathway generating smooth pursuit, at the level of cortex.

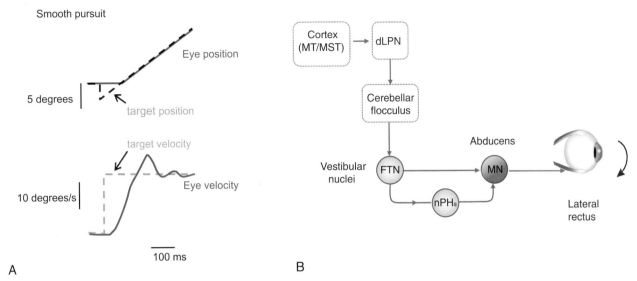

Fig. 8.11 Smooth pursuit eye movements. (**A**) To track moving targets in the visual world, animals with foveae generate smooth pursuit eye movements, the initiation of which lags target motion by ~90 ms. (**B**) Schematic of the neural pathway responsible for the generation of smooth pursuit movements. *dLPN*, Dorsolateral pontine nuclei; *FTN*, floccular target neuron; *MN*, extraocular motoneurons; *MT/MST*, medial temporal neocortical areas; *nPH*, nucleus prepositus.

The visuomotor transformation that controls smooth pursuit eye movements can be understood through analysis of the differences in neuronal responses seen at each stage of this corticopontocerebellar pathway. First, neurons in middle temporal cortex (area MT) of extrastriate cortex encode sensory information, namely the direction and velocity of visual target motion relative to the retina. Area MT sends this information on to both the medial superior temporal cortex (area MST) and smooth eye movement region of the frontal eye fields (FEF$_{SEM}$), where visual sensory signals begin the transformation to eye motor commands. Notably, area MST and FEF$_{SEM}$ neurons integrate extraretinal signals such as eye movement and predictive/anticipatory information with retinal sensory information to compute an estimate of the pursuit command required by downstream structures. These cortical areas then primarily transmit such information to the pursuit-related regions of the cerebellum via the dorsolateral pontine nucleus (dLPN).

The floccular lobe (flocculus and ventral paraflocculus) and oculomotor vermis comprise the pursuit-related regions of the cerebellum. These areas drive eye movements via their direct projections to premotor neurons in the brainstem. Specifically, cerebellar Purkinje cells in these regions of the cerebellum send inhibitory projections to target neurons located within the vestibular nuclei.[97–100] These vestibular nuclei neurons, which are known as eye-head (EH) neurons, in turn directly project to the extraocular motoneurons located in the III, IV, and VI cranial nuclei to drive pursuit eye movements. Whereas EH neurons provide the most significant input to drive the motoneurons during smooth pursuit eye movements,[101–103] neurons in other premotor brainstem nuclei, including the nucleus prepositus, also show clear modulation[57,101,104,105] and thus also contribute to generation of smooth pursuit eye movements.

Neurons at the final stages of the smooth pursuit pathway—both cerebellar Purkinje cells and EH premotor neurons—predominately encode motor signals. This finding indicates that visual sensory information (i.e., target motion relative to the retina) is successfully transformed into the required eye motor command by the smooth pursuit corticopontocerebellar pathway.[106–108] Moreover, the pursuit regions of the cerebellum not only serve as an essential node of the visuomotor

transformation required for pursuit eye movements, but also as a key site for guiding motor learning. Such cerebellar-dependent learning continuously calibrates that the eye movement motor commands relative to target motion to ensure that smooth pursuit remains accurate across our life span.

The neural control of voluntary binocular eye movements

Vergence eye movements are voluntarily made by foveated animals to redirect the gaze of both eyes between targets located at different distance (i.e., near versus far targets, or vice-versa). Notably, to precisely align the binocular gaze on a target located at a new distance, the two eyes must rotate by different amounts. The difference in the angles through which each of the two eyes rotate is termed the vergence eye movement. Specifically, any binocular eye movement can be described in terms of its vergence (vergence = left eye − right eye) versus conjugate (conjugate = [left eye + right eye]/2) components, where the left eye and right eye inputs in these computations can be either position or velocity signals. There are two types of *voluntary* vergence eye movements, which are each generated by distinct neural circuits. First, smooth vergence eye movements are relatively slow movements that are made to track and then fixate a target moving in depth. Second, disjunctive saccades are made to redirect our eye between targets in depth and comprise a vergence component that is much faster than that generated during smooth vergence. Additionally, there is also a type of reflexive vergence eye movement, termed accommodation vergence, which automatically generates convergence eye movements in response to changes in the refractive strength of the eye's lens to ensure proper binocular alignment (see Chapter 3). The two distinct premotor pathways that control voluntary smooth vergence versus disjunctive saccadic eye movements are described in detail next.

The neural control of voluntary smooth vergence

When gaze redirection between near and far targets is accomplished without a saccade, it is referred to as smooth vergence. In the laboratory, smooth vergence eye movements can be studied in conditions in which the gaze is redirected to track an object moving along the midsagittal plane. In this condition, each eye rotates by the same angle but in opposite directions, resulting in a symmetric vergence eye movement (Fig. 8.12A). As each eye rotates equally but in opposite directions, the eye movement has only a vergence but no conjugate component. The maximum smooth vergence velocities achieved in such conditions are typically less than 50 degrees/s (reviewed in[109]). Thus, smooth vergence eye movements are more sluggish than saccades. These voluntary smooth vergence movements can be further divided into two subclasses: fast fusional vergence, for example, the eye movements made to track a target moving in depth (consider a tennis player tracking a tennis ball),[110] and slow fusional vergence, for example, the eye movements made to maintain fused binocular vision on a near or far near target, which can be impaired in subjects with convergence insufficiency.[111]

The neural control of smooth vergence (Fig. 8.12B) involves a group of midbrain cells in the supraoculomotor area (SOA) of the midbrain reticular formation, termed "near-response neurons."[112-117] These neurons encode the eye velocity and position motor commands required to generate smooth vergence and project directly to the oculomotor motoneurons. Individual SOA near-response neurons will either increase or decrease their firing rate activity, proportional to vergence angle, when tracking visual targets located along the midline (i.e., symmetric vergence[115,118,119]). Accordingly, these neurons are further classified as either convergence or divergence neurons. Neurons in

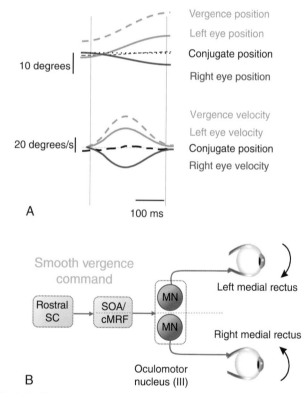

Smooth vergence

Vergence position

Left eye position

Conjugate position

10 degrees |

Right eye position

Vergence velocity

Left eye velocity

20 degrees/s |

Conjugate position

Right eye velocity

A   100 ms

Smooth vergence command

Rostral SC → SOA/cMRF → MN

Left medial rectus

MN

Right medial rectus

B   Oculomotor nucleus (III)

Fig. 8.12 Smooth vergence eye movements. (**A**) To track targets moving in depth along the midline, the two eyes must move in opposite directions. These smooth vergence eye movements are substantially slower than saccades. (**B**) Schematic of the neural pathway responsible for the generation of smooth vergence eye movements. *cMRF*, central mesencephalic reticular formation; *MN*, motoneurons; *SOA*, supraoculomotor area; *SC*, superior colliculus. (Modified from Van Horn MR, Cullen KE. Coding of microsaccades in three-dimensional space by premotor saccadic neurons. *J Neurosci*. 2012; 32[6]:1974–1980. https://doi.org/10.1523/JNEUROSCI.5054-11.2012.)

higher-order structures—including rostral superior colliculus—can also demonstrate preferential tuning to either near or far viewing. For example, a population of neurons in the rostral superior colliculus dynamically encode changes in vergence angle during symmetrical vergence tracking, similar to SOA neurons.[120] These neurons are distinct from the rostral superior colliculus neurons (described in section "Neural control of saccadic eye movements") that are active during target fixation. Projections from these higher-order structures to the SOA near-response neurons control smooth vergence eye movements, while parallel projections to the Edinger-Westphal (EW) nucleus control the accommodation reflex. Notably, SOA "near-response neurons" do not respond during either conjugate or disconjugate (also termed disjunctive) saccades.

The neural control of disjunctive saccades

In everyday life, we commonly generate saccades to redirect gaze between near and far targets in three-dimensional space. To binocularly fixate between such targets, the brain generates rapid disjunctive saccades. During such saccades, the two eyes generally rotate in the same direction but by different amounts, in a way that will depend on the relative eccentricity and distance of each target (Fig. 8.13A). Consequently, disjunctive saccades comprise both a vergence and conjugate component. The speed of the vergence component of disjunctive saccades is significantly faster than that which can be generated during smooth vergence eye movements, reaching velocities of above 150 degrees/s versus 50 degrees/s.[53,112,120-128]

Over the past two decades neurophysiological studies have firmly established that disjunctive saccadic eye movements are predominately generated by the saccadic pathway (Fig. 8.13B). Importantly, this discovery has overturned the widely accepted interpretation of Hering's law of equal innervation, which states that disjunctive saccades are produced by the linear addition of conjugate and vergence innervation commands produced by independent oculomotor subsystems: the saccadic subsystem (e.g., Fig. 8.9) and a separate subsystem (e.g., Fig. 8.12).[129,130] Instead, the same neurons that control conjugate saccades between far targets control disjunctive saccades between near and far targets. Specifically, the number of spikes generated during disjunctive saccades by burst neurons in the PPRF and nucleus prepositus neurons are best correlated with the movement of the ipsilateral eye, rather than conjugate eye movement.[13,52,53,131-134] Furthermore, the discharge dynamics of these premotor saccadic neurons preferentially encode the velocity of the ipsilateral eye.[13,52,53,132] Indeed, the vergence information encoded by the saccadic system provides the major premotor drive required to generate the vergence component of disjunctive saccades. Additionally, a small population of premotor midbrain reticular formation neurons that selectively respond during disjunctive but not conjugate saccades or pursuit appear to contribute to the neural control of disjunctive saccades.[135]

Binocular eye movements and the coding of disparity

In everyday life, the two distinct premotor pathways controlling smooth vergence versus disjunctive saccadic eye movements work together to redirect the direction of binocular gaze between targets at different distances. For example, the saccadic premotor circuitry drives the fast vergence eye movement to the new target, while the slow pathway comprising the premotor SOA serves to precisely align the fovea of each eye on a target after the saccade, thereby ensuring optimal binocular perception. Current research is now aimed at understanding how the coordinated inputs to these distinct saccadic and smooth vergence premotor pathways work together to ensure accurate binocular gaze positioning.

As reviewed previously in the chapter, the MRF and superior colliculus are two likely sources of vergence information for the binocular control of such eye movements (Figs. 8.12 and 8.13). In primates,

Disjunctive saccades

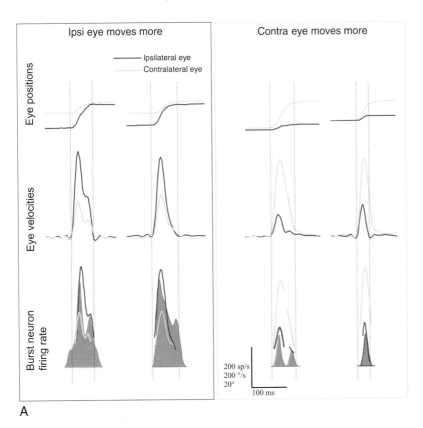

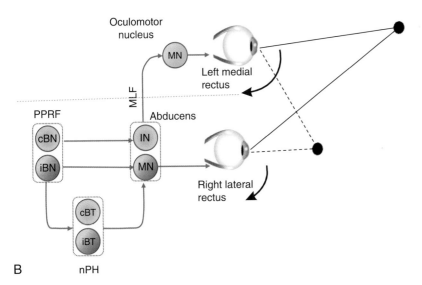

Fig. 8.13 Disjunctive saccadic eye movements. (**A**) To rapidly look between far and near targets, the two eyes must move different amounts. These eye movements are called disjunctive saccades and are characterized by a period of fast vergence that quickly redirects the eyes (i.e., *dashed box* labeled "fast"). The typical unit activity of motoneurons (motor; *gray* units) and saccadic burst neuron (premotor; *blue* units) associated with this movement are shown *below*. Both neurons encode the motion of the ipsilateral eye. (**B**) Schematic of the neural pathway responsible for the generation of disjunctive saccadic eye movements. The premotor saccadic pathway drives the fast component of the movement, while the smooth vergence pathway controls the subsequent smooth vergence that binocularly aligns the eyes. *cBN*, contralateral burst neurons; *cBT*, contralateral burst tonic neurons; *iBN*, ipsilateral burst neurons; *iBT*, ipsilateral burst tonic neurons; *MLF*, medial longitudinal fasciculus; *MN*, extraocular motoneurons; *nPH*, nucleus prepositus hypoglossi. (Modified from Cullen KE, Van Horn MR. The neural control of fast vs. slow vergence eye movements. *Eur J Neurosci.* 2011;33[11]:2147–2154.)

these structures receive inputs from disparity-sensitive cortical and subcortical regions (e.g.,[136–140]). Stimulation of either the MRF[141] or superior colliculus[142,143] can evoke vergence in primates. Furthermore, the responses of neurons in both structures encode vergence information (superior colliculus[120,144,145] and MRF[113,118,141,146]). Additionally, the cerebellum plays a vital role in the calibr'ation and fine-tuning of binocular eye movements required to maintain perception of a clear, single image over time (see, for example,[147]).

Once a target has been successfully foveated by both eyes, the brain can compute an estimate of target distance by calculating the difference in the image location when viewed by the left versus right eyes. The difference in location is referred to as binocular disparity and occurs owing to the eyes' horizontal separation (see Chapter 36). Evidence for the neural coding of disparity is found early in visual processing at the level of primary visual cortex (i.e., area V1), where single neurons show disparity-based tuning (reviewed in[148]). Area V1 in turn projects to regions of the ventral visual pathway, such as V2, V4, and IT, using disparity information to achieve perception of three-dimensional object shape (reviewed in[149]). Additionally, area V1 projects to regions of the dorsal visual pathway, most notably area MT, which, as noted previously, combines disparity signals with motion signals to estimate structure from motion or self-motion (reviewed in[150]). Neurons in cortical regions at the latter stages of the dorsal stream, including area MST, the lateral intraparietal area (LIP), and frontal eye fields (FEFs), combine retinal and extraretinal signals to transform visual disparity information into the neural commands required for accurate visuomotor control of binocular eye movements.

PREMOTOR CONTROL OF GAZE STABILIZATION: THE VESTIBULO-OCULAR AND OPTOKINETIC REFLEXES

In addition to the voluntary eye movements we make to purposefully redirect gaze to a target of interest, our brains also generate involuntary reflexive eye movements that function to keep the visual world stationary on the retina. Specifically, the brain generates reflexive stabilizing eye movements via the VOR and OKR. The VOR functions to provide stable gaze during everyday activities such as walking and running by moving the eye in the opposite direction to the on-going head motion. It is driven by head motion, sensed by the vestibular system, and is effective for the physiologically relevant frequencies that comprise our natural self-motion. The OKR also functions to provide stabile gaze by moving the eye in the opposite direction to on-going head motion. However, the OKR is driven by visual motion rather than vestibular input. In contrast to the VOR, OKR responses are not robust over most of the frequency range of natural self-motion. Instead, the OKR is most effective for lower frequency self-motion for which the VOR cannot effectively stabilize gaze (<0.1 Hz). Thus, the VOR and OKR work synergistically to ensure stable gaze over an extended range of head movements (see[151]).

The neural control of the vestibulo-ocular reflex

The function of the VOR is to generate eye motion of an equal amplitude but opposite direction to that of concurrent head motion. As a result of this compensatory eye movement, the visual axis of gaze remains directed at the same point in space. In conditions where head motion is sustained in one direction, the compensatory eye movements generated by the VOR can move the eye eccentrically toward its limit of excursion before the head movement is completed. In such conditions, the brain reflexively commands the eye to move back to a new, more centered starting position. The resulting pattern of alternating slow compensatory and rapid resetting eye movements (termed slow phases and quick phases, respectively) is referred to as vestibular nystagmus (see Fig. 8.15A). The quick phase uses some of the same neural machinery involved in the generation of voluntary saccades (see Fig. 8.9).

The VOR uses information from the vestibular sensory organs—the semicircular canals and otoliths—to generate compensatory eye movements during both head rotations and translations relative to space (Fig. 8.14). The three orthogonally oriented semicircular canals located on each side of the head (i.e., horizontal, superior, and posterior) together detect rotational motion in three dimensions. Correspondingly, the two otolith organs on each side of the head (i.e., the utricle and saccule) together detect linear translational motion in three dimensions. The most direct pathway mediating the VOR is a three-neuron arc.[152] Rotational and translational head movements are initially detected by the sensory hair cells in the semicircular canals and otoliths. This vestibular information is then transmitted from the sensory organs by vestibular nerve afferents (i.e., eighth cranial nerve) to vestibular nuclei neurons and then directly to the extraocular motoneurons that innervate the extraocular muscles of the eyes.

The angular vestibulo-ocular reflex

The VOR evoked in response to rotational head movements is more specifically referred to as the angular VOR (aVOR). During everyday activities, the rotational head motion experienced by humans and monkeys, as well as mice, has significant power up to 20 Hz.[153,154] Eye movements produced by the aVOR are robust and compensatory across the range of head movements generated during natural behaviors.[155,156] Importantly, because the most direct pathway mediating the VOR is a three-neuron arc, the aVOR has a remarkably fast response time (~5 ms) (Fig. 8.15B).[156,157] This 5-ms latency can be explained by known synaptic, neural, and muscle activation times within the aVOR pathway.[156,158]

Neurophysiological studies in nonhuman primates have established that a specific subclass of neurons within the vestibular nuclei comprise most of the intermediate leg of the aVOR pathway evoked by horizontal rotations (reviewed in[151]). These neurons are called position-vestibular pause (PVP) neurons based on the information that they encode during passive head rotations and eye movements. PVP neurons encode contralaterally directed eye position during steady fixation, respond to ipsilaterally directed head velocity stimulation during passive head movement, and stop firing action potentials (pause) for saccades and the quick phases of vestibular nystagmus.[101,105] These PVP neurons predominately send an excitatory projection to the motoneurons of the contralateral abducens nucleus but can also send excitatory projections to the ipsilateral medial rectus subdivision of the oculomotor nucleus (Fig. 8.15C). A minority of PVP neurons are inhibitory and send projections to the ipsilateral abducens nucleus.

Specifically, rightward head rotations will excite PVP neurons in the right vestibular nuclei. In turn, the axons of these PVP neurons predominantly cross the midline to activate neurons in the left abducens nucleus. In turn, left abducens nucleus motoneurons generate a compensatory (i.e., leftward) movement of the left eye via activation of the left lateral rectus. Additionally, internuclear neurons in the left abducens are activated. The axons of these internuclear neurons cross the midline to target motoneurons in the oculomotor nucleus and simultaneously generate leftward movement of the right eye via activation of the right medial rectus. Finally, it is noteworthy that the second class of PVP neurons do not mediate the direct VOR pathway, but instead support the inhibitory commissural pathways between the vestibular nuclei on each side of the brain (reviewed in[161]) that are essential for compensation following peripheral vestibular loss.[162–164] These PVP neurons are termed "type II" neurons as they are characterized by head and eye movement sensitivities that are opposite to those of the PVP neurons that mediate the direct VOR pathway (termed type I). Inhibitory inputs from saccadic burst neurons likely contribute to the pause-behavior of both type I and II PVP neurons during saccades and vestibular quick phases.[163]

The translational vestibulo-ocular reflex

The VOR evoked in response to translational head movements is more specifically referred to as the translational VOR (tVOR). The compensatory tVOR eye movements made during translation depend on both the eye's current position in the orbit and the viewing distance in a manner consistent with the geometrical requirements for holding a visual target stable on the two foveae (reviewed in[151]). For instance, effective compensation for the motion parallax typically experienced during translation requires scaling of the gain of the tVOR as a function of viewing distance. During everyday activities, translational head motion (like rotational head motion) has significant power up to 20 Hz.[153,154] However, the tVOR is not as effective as the aVOR in stabilizing gaze over this frequency range.[164,165] The tVOR's gain is not fully compensatory, and it has a longer response time latency compared

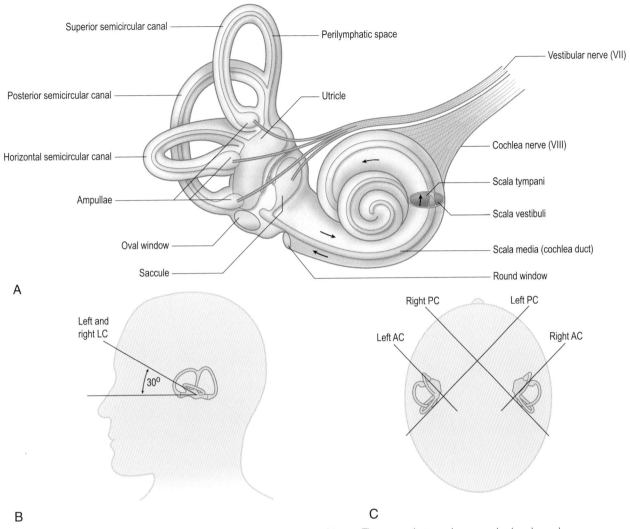

Fig. 8.14 Vestibular end-organs in the human temporal bone. Three canals transduce angular head acceleration and two otoliths, the sacculus and utricle, transduce linear acceleration and head orientation. Right labyrinth and cochlea are viewed from a horizontal aspect. (Drawings by Ernest W. Beck: courtesy Beltone Electronics Corp., Chicago, Ill.) The canals are in three orthogonal planes that are approximately parallel to a mirror image set of planes on the contralateral side of the head that lie roughly in the pulling direction of the three muscle planes. **(A)** Lateral canals. **(B,C)** Anterior and posterior vertical canals. *AC*, Anterior vertical canal; *LC*, lateral canal; *PC*, posterior vertical canal. (Modified from Levin L, ed. *Adler's Physiology of the Eye*, 11th ed. Elsevier; 2011.)

with the aVOR (>10 ms rather than 5 ms). The tVOR's latency is longer than that of the aVOR because it is largely mediated by polysynaptic pathways rather than a direct three-neuron arc. Notably, the PVPs that mediate the direct aVOR do not receive direct inputs from the otoliths and thus do not demonstrate otolith-related modulation during translational head motion. Thus, the three-neuron arc that mediates the aVOR pathway does not also function as the intermediate leg of the tVOR; instead, the tVOR is generated by more complex pathways.

The neural control of the optokinetic reflex

The optokinetic system uses visual rather than vestibular inputs to generate compensatory eye movements that function to help stabilize gaze relative to space. As noted previously, the response dynamics of the OKR are complementary to those of the VOR. Specifically, the OKR is generated in response to motion of the visual world across the retina (retinal slip) during low-frequency and constant-velocity head movements. In response to sustained visual motion, the OKR comprises

alternating slow compensatory and quick resetting eye movements in the opposite direction (Fig. 8.16A). The resultant pattern of slow and quick phases is referred to as optokinetic nystagmus. Following the start of visual motion, slow phase eye movements are initially generated within 100 to 200 ms, followed by a slower buildup of eye velocity. Following the offset of visual stimulation, the OKR pathway generates a slowly decaying optokinetic after-nystagmus (OKAN; Fig. 8.16B, top).

The same cortico-pontine-floccular circuit that generates smooth pursuit eye movement (Fig. 8.16C, blue) controls the initial OKR eye velocity generated following the onset of visual motion (reviewed in[151]). Briefly, cortical areas MT and MST and the FEFs project to the pontine nuclei, which in turn project to the cerebellar flocculus. In turn, floccular Purkinje cells target premotor neurons in the vestibular nuclei, which project directly to extraocular motoneurons. Accordingly, lesions of the cerebellar flocculus reduce the initial rise in OKR eye velocity,[166,167] as well as smooth pursuit. In contrast, the slower buildup in eye velocity that follows is mediated by subcortical pathways (Fig. 8.16C, green). Specifically,

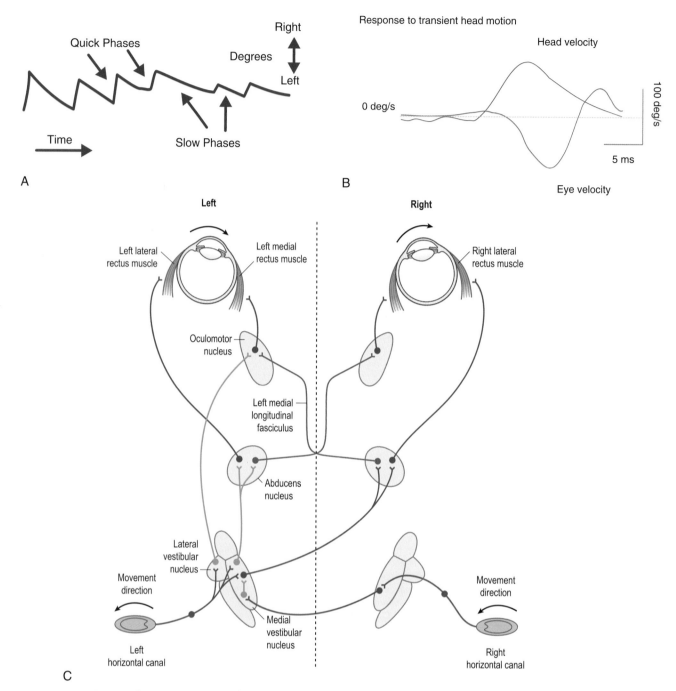

Fig. 8.15 (A) The resulting saw-tooth pattern of slow compensatory/rapid resetting eye movements (slow phases and quick phases, respectively) are referred to as vestibular nystagmus. **(B)** In response to head motion, the vestibulo-ocular reflex (VOR) produces an eye movement with a latency of 5 ms. This fast response is consistent with the minimal delays of the three-neuron pathway that control the reflex. **(C)** Pathways of the horizontal VOR in the brain stem for leftward head rotation. Inhibitory connections are shown as filled neurons, excitatory connections as unfilled neurons. Leftward head rotation stimulates the left horizontal canal and inhibits the right horizontal canal. This results in an increased discharge rate in the right lateral and left medial rectus and decreased discharge rate in the left lateral and right medial rectus. (B, adapted from Huterer M and Cullen K. Vestibuloocular reflex dynamics during high-frequency and high-acceleration rotations of the head on body in rhesus monkey. *J Neurophysiol.* 2002;88(1):13–28. C, from Goldberg ME, Eggers HM, Gouras D. The ocular motor system. In: Kandel ER, Schwartz JH, Jessell TM (eds). Principles of Neural Science, 3rd ed, Appleton and Lange 1991.

visually sensitive neurons in the nucleus of the optic tract and the accessory optic nuclei target premotor neurons in the vestibular nuclei and nPH, which again project directly to the extraocular motoneurons. Overall, the relative importance of different visual inputs (subcortical versus cortical)

to the OKR pathways varies across species. For example, whereas primates normally generate symmetric OKR responses, lesions to the visual cortex produce a marked asymmetry in their temporal and nasally directed OKR responses.[168] In contrast, lateral-eyed species such as rabbits

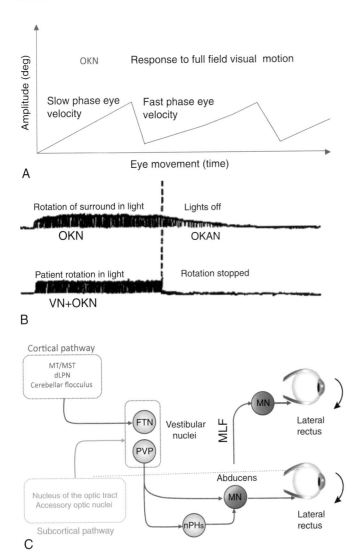

A

B

C

Fig. 8.16 (A) The optokinetic eye movement response (OKR) produced in response to full field visual motion stabilizes the visual world. In response to constant-velocity motion, these movements comprise two components: a slow compensatory movement and a fast resetting quick phase, termed optokinetic nystagmus (OKN). (B) optokinetic after-nystagmus (OKAN) following cessation of sustained rotation of the visual world. The after-nystagmus is in the direction opposite to that of visual stimulation and is suppressed by vestibular input evoked by head motion during actual self-motion. (C) The cortical and brainstem circuit for the generation of opto-kinetic eye movements. The pretectum targets the same premotor cells groups in the vestibular nuclei that control the vestibulo-ocular reflex. dLPN, Dorsolateral pontine nuclei; FTN, floccular target neuron; MLF, medial longitudinal fasciculus; MT/MST, medial temporal neocortical areas; nPH, nucleus prepositushypoglossi; PVP, position-vestibular pause; VN, vestibular nuclei. (B, modified from Waespe W, Henn V. Vestibular nuclei activity during optokinetic after-nystagmus (OKAN) in the alert monkey. Exp Brain Res. 1977;30[2–3]:323–330. https://doi.org/10.1007/BF00237259.)

normally show significant temporal-nasal asymmetries in their OKR responses,[169] suggesting that in these species the OKR is primarily driven by subcortical pathways.

The same neurons within the vestibular nuclei that generate the VOR (i.e., PVP neurons) also contribute to the optokinetic reflex.[170] Consistent with their role in OKR, the eye movement-sensitive neurons within the vestibular nuclei demonstrate a response that mirrors the decays of this OKAN response. In real-world situations, in which vestibular and optokinetic stimulation occur simultaneously—for

instance, walking down the street during the day—vestibular and visual information concurrently drives the VOR and OKR reflex pathways. The outputs of these two pathways are then integrated at the level of individual neurons in the vestibular nuclei to stabilize gaze relative to space. Because OKR and VOR response dynamics are complementary, during actual self-motion OKAN is suppressed by the corresponding VOR response to the abrupt cessation of head movement, resulting in stable gaze (Fig. 8.16B, bottom). To ensure stable gaze throughout life, the floccular lobe of the cerebellum functions to continuously calibrate the amplitude and dynamics of both the OKR and VOR (reviewed in[151]).

INTERACTIONS BETWEEN EYE MOVEMENT SUBSYSTEMS

The traditional approach of categorizing eye movements into five distinct classes (reference Table 8.1) has greatly advanced our understanding of the oculomotor "subsystems." The strategy of focusing research on the neural control of a given class of eye movement performed in isolation has been vital to establishing the pathways responsible for the sensory-motor transformations underlying both voluntary and reflexive eye movements. However, in everyday life the brain often simultaneously employs two or more oculomotor subsystems to control gaze. For instance, to rapidly look between two targets located at different eccentricities we typically make orienting head, as well as eye, movements to realign our gaze relative to visual space (gaze = eye-in-head + head-in-space). This common voluntary reorienting behavior is called a "gaze shift." During gaze shifts, the saccadic and VOR pathways do not function independently. Instead, the brain coordinates synergistic interactions between these two eye movement subsystems to efficiently ensure accurate gaze control. As detailed further in this section, recent work has established how the brain coordinates interactions between the VOR versus voluntary saccade and/or pursuit eye movements to accurately control gaze in everyday life.

Voluntary gaze shifts: interactions between saccadic and vestibulo-ocular reflex pathways

As noted previously, we commonly generate coordinated rapid eye and head movements—termed gaze shifts—to voluntarily redirect gaze to new targets. Because the head and eye movements are both directed toward the new target of interest, the compensatory eye movement generated by the VOR would actually be counterproductive to the behavioral goal. Specifically, if the brain generated a VOR in response to the orienting head movement, it would effectively command an eye movement in the direction opposite to that of the intended change in gaze. Instead, the brain suppresses the efficacy of the VOR pathway during gaze shifts (reviewed in[159]). Behavioral studies in humans and monkeys have shown that this efficacy reduction increases with increasing gaze shift amplitude, such that the VOR is nearly completely suppressed during large gaze shifts (>50 degrees). Moreover, this efficacy reduction is the strongest early in the gaze shift, with the VOR gain, then progressively recovering to reach normal values by gaze shift end.[171]

The neural mechanism underlying the powerful suppression of the VOR's efficacy during gaze shifts is well understood.[163,172] Saccadic burst neurons (Fig. 8.17A) in the PPRF are active during gaze shifts. The saccadic burst neurons located in the caudal PPRF send inhibitory projections to the vestibular nuclei,[37,41,42,173] which target the VOR pathway neurons (i.e., PVP neurons, Fig. 8.15C). This inhibition, in turn, effectively reduces the head velocity-related modulation of VOR pathway neurons.[163,172] Notably, the reduction occurs in an amplitude-dependent manner consistent with results from behavioral studies in humans and monkeys discussed previously. Thus, the VOR is not a hard-wired reflex, but rather is suppressed by the premotor saccadic pathway when the current gaze strategy is to redirect rather than stabilize gaze.

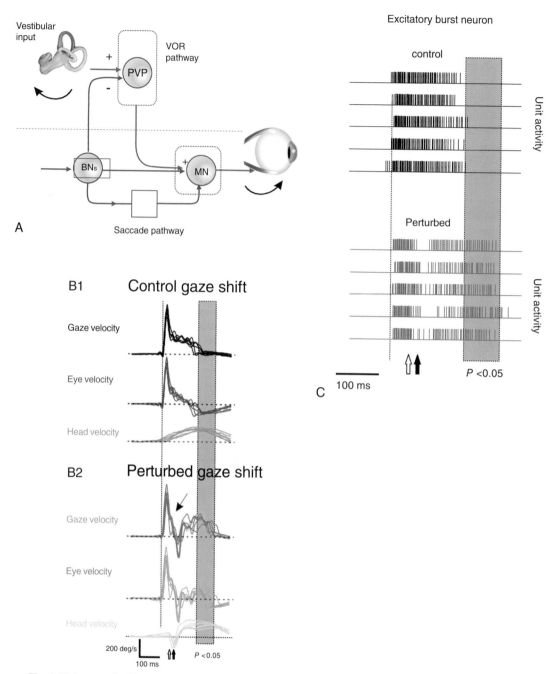

Fig. 8.17 In everyday life, we use coordinated eye and head movements to redirect our axis of gaze (gaze = eye-in-head + head-in-space). (**A**) A schematic of the interactions that occur between the vestibulo-ocular reflex (VOR; *blue*) and saccadic (*red*) premotor pathways during gaze shifts. The efficacy of the VOR pathway is suppressed via behaviorally dependent inputs that allow the head movement to contribute to the shifting the axis of visual gaze relative to space. (**B**) Matched control (**B1**) and perturbed (**B2**) gaze shifts. Vertical dashed line, gaze onset; shaded box, average increase in perturbed trials duration; open and filled arrows, average perturbation onset and time at which the resulting head perturbation reached maximum velocity, respectively. (**C**) Example burst neuron activity recorded during the control and perturbed trials shown in **B**. In the pertubed condition, firing rate and gaze shift duration increased in a complementary manner. *BNs*, burst neurons; *MN*, motoneurons; *PVP*, position-vestibular pause. (B, C; Modified from Sylvestre PA, Cullen KE. Premotor correlates of integrated feedback control for eye-head gaze shifts. *J Neurosci.* 2006:26(18):4922–4929.)

Integrated feedback control of eye-head gaze shifts and implications for upstream control

As reviewed in the previous section, the VOR is suppressed during gaze shifts such that the motion of both the eye-in-head and head-in-space contribute to shifting the axis of gaze relative to space. Thus, a fundamental question is: How are the motor commands to the eye and head musculature coordinated to ensure gaze accuracy? Behavioral and neurophysiological studies have shown that the brain uses a single integrated gaze controller to minimize gaze error, rather than two distinct controllers that separately control eye and head motion.[174–177] First, the output neurons of the caudal superior colliculus encode and control the direction and amplitude of gaze, rather than only its saccadic eye movement component.[175] Second, these neurons in turn directly target both the saccadic and neck brainstem premotor circuitry, thereby providing a physiologic substrate by which eye and head movements can be driven in a coordinated fashion during gaze shifts. Third, premotor burst neurons in the PPRF likewise encode the entire gaze shift, rather than only its saccadic component.[47,102,103,178,179] Finally, these PPRF responses show rapid "online" updating to applied head perturbations[178] (Fig. 8.17B). This updating occurs within 3 ms, indicating that the saccadic pathway is controlled online by head movement feedback (i.e., consistent with an integrated gaze controller). Thus, in everyday life, the saccadic system is more than just an eye-movement system. It is a gaze-control system that plays an integral role in coordinating head and eye movements to make rapid yet accurate gaze shifts.

Voluntary gaze pursuit: interactions between vestibulo-ocular reflex and pursuit pathways

In everyday life we also commonly make coordinated head and eye movements to voluntarily track a moving target of interest. During these coordinated eye-head movements—called gaze pursuit—the brain coordinates interactions between the smooth pursuit and VOR pathways. An intact VOR would be counterproductive during voluntary gaze pursuit for the same reason it is counterproductive during voluntary gaze shifts, namely that it would command an eye movement in the direction opposite to that of the intended tracking. Accordingly, the brain similarly suppresses the efficacy of the VOR pathway during voluntary smooth tracking (reviewed in[159]) via both rapid (<30-ms) nonvisual and slower visual pursuit-mediated mechanisms.[180,181]

The neural correlate underlying the suppression of the VOR during gaze pursuit, like that underlying gaze shifts, is well understood (reviewed in[159]). The head velocity-related modulation of the VOR pathway (i.e., PVP) neurons is reduced in a manner consistent with the observed parametric adjustment of VOR pathway efficacy.[102,102,172] In parallel, the cerebellar flocculus plays an essential role in driving the smooth pursuit pathway. Floccular Purkinje cells send inhibitory projections to the premotor neurons in the vestibular nuclei (EH neurons), which project to the extraocular motoneurons to control smooth pursuit eye movements (Fig. 8.11). Because these EH neurons also receive vestibular afferent input, their responses are well described by the summation of their gaze-related activity (measured during smooth pursuit) and their vestibular-related activity (measured during passive whole-body rotation in the dark). Overall, the smooth pursuit inputs mediated via premotor EH neurons function in parallel with the attenuation in the gain of the direct VOR pathways to further reduce VOR gain and generate coordinated head and eye movements to voluntarily redirect the axis of gaze to track a moving target of interest.

NEUROLOGIC DISORDERS OF THE OCULOMOTOR SYSTEM

The neural basis of numerous disorders of the oculomotor system is well established. The anatomical and neurophysiological studies, described earlier in this chapter, have provided a strong foundation for understanding many conditions responsible for the generation of abnormal eye movements in patients. Patients can display abnormal eye movements for many reasons, including abnormal weakness of the extraocular muscles, developmental disorders of normal central sensory-eye motor processing, as well as disorders that are acquired due to trauma or disease. Additionally, as eye movements provide a window into higher-level processes such as cognition, memory, volition, and reward, the analysis of eye movements has also proven useful for the evaluation of patients with neurologic disorders including schizophrenia, Alzheimer disease, and attention deficit/hyperactivity disorder.

BOX 8.3 Etiological classification of motor disorders

Motor anomalies are classified as congenital, developmental, and acquired.

BOX 8.4 Infantile strabismus syndrome

The infantile strabismus syndrome consists of asymmetric horizontal OKN and pursuit, dissociated vertical deviation (DVD), and latent nystagmus (LN).

Some eye movement disorders are present at birth and are congenital. Others develop or are acquired over time (Box 8.3) and may be associated with other problems, such as tumors, stroke, or injuries.[182] In this section the underlying causes of several common oculomotor disorders are reviewed. These disorders are organized in terms of those characterized by (1) misalignment of the two eyes (strabismus), (2) restricted motility of eye movement (gaze restrictions), (3) saccades with abnormal metrics—speed and/or amplitude (saccade disorders), and (4) difficulty maintaining fixation and abnormal nystagmus (pathologic nystagmus).

Strabismus

The misalignment of the two eyes is called strabismus. The underlying cause can vary and range from the impairment of the normal functionality of the eye muscles and/or oculomotor cranial nerves, to disorders in the central pathways that generate eye movements, to disorders of sensory processing resulting in a large refractive error. Strabismus is a common eye movement disorder in children and with a prevalence of 2% to 4% in children younger than 6 years of age. When misalignment of the two eyes is found at birth or during the first 6 months of life, the strabismus is characterized as congenital. Additionally, strabismus may not be present at birth but can develop in the first years of life. Strabismus that occurs after this age is referred to as developmental or acquired strabismus. If left uncorrected in children, both congenital and acquired strabismus can have serious long-term effects, including abnormal three-dimensional vision (impaired stereoacuity) that can ultimately result in permanent vision loss.

Strabismus can be categorized by the direction of the turned or misaligned eye, specifically: inward turning or "crossed-eyed" (esotropia), outward turning or "walleyed" (exotropia), upward turning (hypertropia), and downward turning (hypotropia). In childhood, esotropia is most common and can result in accommodative esotropia.[183] Another common early strabismus is infantile esotropia, which typically starts during the first 6 months of life and is characterized by marked inward turning of both eyes. Infantile esotropia is frequently associated with other eye movement abnormalities including asymmetric horizontal OKR and pursuit; vertical misalignment of the eyes when one eye is occluded—termed dissociated vertical deviation (DVD); a nystagmus when either eye is occluded that generates a slow phase in the direction of the occluded eye—termed a latent nystagmus; as well as a nasal/temporal asymmetry in the optokinetic eye movement response (Box 8.4).[184,185]

In adults, strabismus can be acquired due to the effect of disease on the efficacy of the eye muscles or oculomotor cranial nerves and motor nuclei, or by tumors, stroke, diseases, or injuries that impact the central pathways that generate eye movements. For example, a cranial nerve lesion that decreases the strength of the command to the extraocular muscle in one eye will produce a misalignment of the two eyes, which will increase as gaze is directed more and more into the affected muscle's field of action. This type of strabismus is referred to as a paralytic strabismus,[186] in which lesions of the third, fourth, and sixth cranial nerves are referred to as oculomotor palsy, trochlear palsy, and

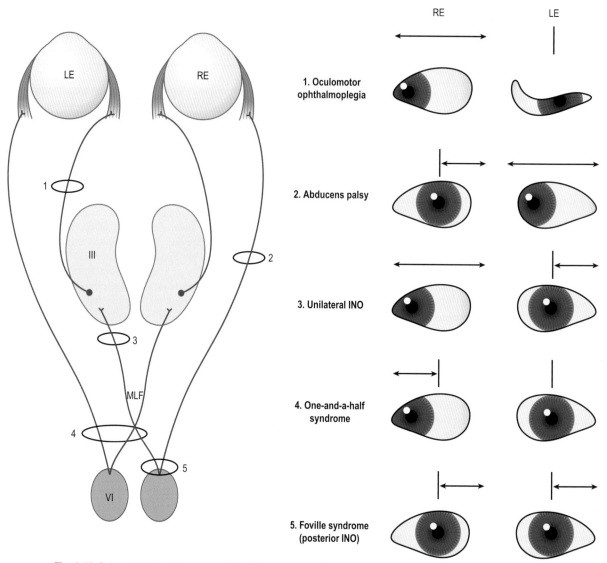

Fig. 8.18 Subcortical disorder: gaze palsies. Eye positions shown reflect attempted right gaze in each case, but the *arrows* show the full range of horizontal gaze for each eye. *INO*, Internuclear ophthalmoplegia; *LE*, Left eye; *MLF*, medial longitudinal fasciculus; *RE*, right eye. (Modified from original drawing by Scott B Stevenson, courtesy University of Houston, and sourced from Levin L, ed. *Adler's Physiology of the Eye*, 11th ed. Elsevier; 2011.)

abducens palsy, respectively. For example, an oculomotor palsy produces muscular weakness (paresis) of the extraocular muscles innervated by the third cranial nerve nucleus, namely the medial rectus, superior and inferior recti, and inferior oblique, resulting in a downward and abducted eye position for the affected versus normal eye. Additionally, an oculomotor palsy will produce weakness of the levator of the lid and the pupilloconstrictor muscle, and thus patients will also display fixed-dilated pupil and ptosis in the affected eye. Similarly, trochlear and abducens palsies are characterized by hyperdeviation in gaze during adduction and depression versus an increasing esotropia during abduction of the affected eye, respectively.

Early detection and treatment of strabismus is essential, as strabismus will result in reduced vision in one eye (amblyopia) that can, in turn, cause impaired binocular vision and stereoblindness, which are described in Chapter 36. Approximately 30% to 50% of children with strabismus develop amblyopia in which visual inputs from the affected eye are increasingly ignored. To prevent the development of serious amblyopia, clinical interventions for strabismus focus on surgery, botulinum toxin A muscle injections, and/or strategies to provide proper alignment of the visual axis.

BOX 8.5   Functional classification of motor disorders

- Peripheral and nuclear lesions are categorized as paresis and paralysis
- Premotor, internuclear, and supranuclear lesions are categorized as gaze restrictions or palsies

Disorders that restrict gaze

Lesions of the extraocular motor nuclei and/or the MLF, a fiber bundle that interconnects premotor regions with the III, IV, and VI cranial nuclei (Fig. 8.18), can restrict gaze (Box 8.5). Disorders in which lesions of the MLF sever projections from premotor pathways to the extraocular motor nuclei are referred to as ophthalmoplegias.[187] Disruption of the normal projections made by abducens internuclear neurons to the contralateral oculomotor abducens nucleus, via the MLF, is referred to as an internuclear ophthalmoplegia (INO). In this condition, the contralateral eye is unable to adduct normally. A lesion at or near the abducens nucleus results in Foville's syndrome. This condition produces a horizontal gaze palsy, in which abducting eye movements are blocked on the side of the lesion. In addition, because abducens interneurons project to the contralateral oculomotor nucleus, adducting eye movements of the contralateral eye are also affected. Correspondingly, lesions near the oculomotor nucleus can result in another gaze palsy termed Parinaud's syndrome.[188] In this condition, disruption of the projections from the riMLF and the interstitial nucleus of Cajal (INC) to the oculomotor nucleus limits vertical and torsional eye movement. Parinaud's syndrome is commonly produced by tumors of the pineal gland that compress the superior colliculus and pretectal structures. Because the extraocular motor nuclei are the final common pathway for all classes of eye movements, these conditions will alter all classes of eye movements: saccades, pursuit VOR, and OKR.

Additionally, lesions in higher-level structures can restrict gaze. Lesions of primary visual cortical areas such as MT and MST can produce a scotoma (i.e., a blind spot in the contralateral sensory visual field). Because this area is critical for processing visual motion information for smooth pursuit, patients will show impaired ability to track moving objects yet may still be able to make accurate saccades to stationary targets. Lesions of the FEF also restrict gaze function. Because this area contributes to the control of both saccades and smooth pursuit, patients show deficits for saccades to the contralateral side, as well as impaired pursuit. Finally, lesions to other cortical areas can influence cognitive aspects of eye movement control. For example, lesions of the supplementary eye fields impair the ability to perform memory-guided saccades, and lesions of the posterior parietal cortex causes attentional deficits that can impair patient pursuit and saccade performance.

Saccade disorders

Saccades are made to rapidly orient the visual axis of gaze on a target of interest. As reviewed previously in the chapter, saccades have well-defined kinematics for which there are robust relationships between saccade amplitude, peak velocity, and duration—termed the saccadic "main sequence" (see Fig. 8.6). Accordingly, quantification of saccade kinematics can be used to identify deviations from the main sequence in patients as a marker of specific impairments (Fig. 8.19). For example, saccades that are slower than those predicted by the main sequence could indicate either an extraocular muscle palsy (decreased strength) or a deficit in the pulse generated by the premotor pathways controlling the saccade eye movement.[182,189] In both cases, establishing the direction of the saccades that deviate from the main sequence can provide insight into the responsible eye muscle or central structure(s). For example, in patients with oculomotor, trochlear, or abducens palsies, saccades can be significantly slower than those of normal individuals along the direction corresponding to the affected muscle.

Moreover, quantification of saccade accuracy can be used to identify impairments in patients. As reviewed in sections: "The neural control of the vestibulo-ocular reflex," saccadic eye movements are driven by a pulse-step command that first rotates the eye to point its fovea at an object of interest, and then ensures that the eye is held stationary at this new position. In normal subjects, a small amount of saccadic hypometria (i.e., undershooting the target) is generally observed, particularly for larger saccades. In patients with damage to cerebellar and brainstem oculomotor pathways, saccades can demonstrate more inaccuracy (dysmetria), displaying either significantly greater undershoots (hypometria) or conversely being too large (hypermetria) (Box 8.6). For example, injury to the most medial of the deep cerebellar nuclei (i.e., the fastigial nucleus) produces hypermetric saccades.[182,190] Saccade dysmetria can in turn result in saccadic oscillations where the brain attempts to correct its fixation errors via the repeated back-to-back generation of inaccurate saccades. Dysmetria will occur if the pulse of the pulse-step command to the extraocular muscles is too small.

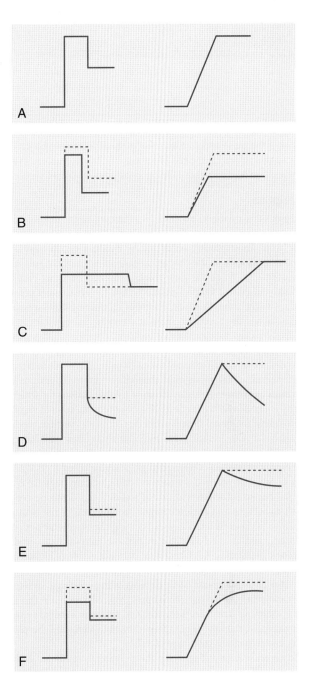

Fig. 8.19 Disorders of the saccadic pulse and step. Innervation patterns are shown on the *left*, and eye movements on the *right*. *Dashed lines* indicate the normal response. (**A**) Normal saccade. (**B**) Hypometric saccade: pulse amplitude (width X height) is too small but pulse and step are matched appropriately. (**C**) Slow saccade: decreased pulse height with normal pulse amplitude and normal pulse-step match. (**D**) Gaze-evoked nystagmus: normal pulse, poorly sustained step. (**E**) Pulse-step mismatch (glissade); step is relatively smaller than pulse. (**F**) Pulse-step mismatch owing to internuclear ophthalmoplegia: The step is larger than the pulse, and so the eye drifts onward after the initial rapid movements. (From Levin L, ed. *Adler's Physiology of the Eye*, 11th ed. Elsevier; 2011, and which was modified from Leigh JR, Zee DS. *The Neurology of Eye Movements*, 3rd ed. Oxford: Oxford University Press; 1999.)

BOX 8.6 Saccade disorders

Saccade disorders are of accuracy (dysmetria), velocity (glissades), and inappropriate timing (intrusions).

BOX 8.7   Waveform classification of nystagmus

Nystagmus can have pendular or jerk (saw-tooth) waveforms. Jerk nystagmus disorders are of the slow phase of unsteady fixation. Null point is the gaze distance and direction where nystagmus amplitude is minimal.

Further, if the pulse and step are mismatched, postabnormal saccadic drift can be observed at the end of the saccade. Inaccuracies in the step command can lead to a gaze-holding nystagmus, discussed next.

Nystagmus

Nystagmus is a rhythmic pattern of involuntary, rapid back and forth, oscillatory eye movements. The origin of the term nystagmus is from Greek word "nustagmos," which means nodding or drowsiness. As reviewed previously in the chapter, nystagmus is a normal subclass of eye movements. When the slow phases generated by either vestibular or optokinetic (visual field) stimulation rotate the eye to more eccentric positions in the orbit, the brain generates recentering quick-phase eye movements via the brainstem saccadic pathway. The resultant nystagmus displays a saw-tooth patterning because it comprises both slow- and quick-phase eye movements. By convention the direction of such nystagmus is defined by the direction of the quick phase. These eye movements are referred to as "jerk nystagmus" due to their patterning. Alternatively, nystagmus eye movements can comprise eye oscillations for which the velocity is equal in both directions. Notably, the application of vestibular or optokinetic rotational stimuli in one direction (e.g., vertical, torsional, or horizontal) can induce a bidirectional nystagmus with no quick phase, only oscillating directions of slow phase. The patterning of this latter type of nystagmus is referred to as "pendular" (Box 8.7).

In contrast to normal nystagmus, pathologic nystagmus is detrimental because it will impair visual stability and depth perception, as well as balance and accurate motor coordination of the oculomotor pathways. Lesions and diseases affecting the vestibular periphery, brainstem, and/or cerebellar eye movement pathways can underlie pathologic nystagmus. Additionally, impaired function of higher-order structures—such as cortical pathways that affect oculomotor function—can also contribute. Most patients with pathologic nystagmus report symptoms of vertigo, oscillopsia, blurred vision, or abnormal head positioning. Treatments for acquired nystagmus include surgery, pharmacologic therapy (e.g., gabapentin, baclofen, and botulinum toxin), and nystagmus treatment exercises.

However, precisely identifying the peripheral vestibular or brain abnormality that underlies pathologic nystagmus can be difficult.[182] For example, congenital nystagmus, a jerk waveform of nystagmus, is seen in children and appears early in life. Congenital nystagmus can be seen in patients with different disorders including albinism, aniridia, and congenital acromatopsia. Interestingly, congenital nystagmus generally has a "null point" eye position within the orbit for which the amplitude of the nystagmus is minimized. Affected individuals typically implement a viewing strategy in which they coordinate eye movements with head turns to keep their ocular position near this null point. The amplitude of congenital nystagmus can also be reduced during ocular convergence, and thus, individuals may also adopt esotropia to minimize their nystagmus. Latent nystagmus described previously in relation to strabismus is a developmental form of nystagmus that is also observed in children. Latent nystagmus is evidence of disrupted development of normal binocular vision in early onset esotropia. This binocular impairment can be demonstrated by the occlusion of one eye producing a slow phase in the direction of that eye, which is termed a latent nystagmus.

Nystagmus can also be acquired later in life, in adolescence, or even adulthood. Acquired forms of nystagmus generally indicate impairment of the vestibular periphery or central pathways that generate eye movements owing to trauma (e.g., head injury), disease (e.g., multiple sclerosis, brain tumor, metabolic disorder), or even alcohol or drug toxicity.[191] The ability to precisely measure and quantify eye movements in patients with peripheral and central damage has led to a clear understanding of the pathophysiology underlying several types of acquired nystagmus. For example, nystagmus owing to defective gaze holding is observed in patients with damage to the neural integrator.[192] As described in section "Neural control of saccadic eye movements," the nucleus prepositus hypoglossi and interstitial nucleus of Cajal ensure stable gaze following the horizontal and vertical/torsional components of saccadic eye movements. Additionally, the cerebellar flocculus contributes to calibrating the efficacy of the "neural integration." Thus, damage to any of these structures results in the inability to sustain eccentric gaze, resulting as a defective gaze-holding nystagmus. A variant of gaze-evoked nystagmus usually associated with cerebellar impairment is rebound nystagmus in which, after a subject recenters the eye to primary position, it drifts back toward the prior eccentric direction of gaze.

Finally, damage to the vestibular periphery or central pathways will also lead to nystagmus. Nystagmus is typically observed in the first week after unilateral peripheral vestibular damage due to the resulting imbalance of vestibular input to central pathways. Such nystagmus is then generally significantly reduced or resolved due to central compensatory mechanisms. In contrast, damage to central cerebellar and brainstem vestibular pathways can generate a more sustained nystagmus. For example, periodic alternating nystagmus is a jerk nystagmus in which the direction reverses every 2 minutes. This reversal is believed to reflect attempts by the cerebellum to correct an imbalance in central vestibular brainstem pathways. Downbeat nystagmus is another jerk nystagmus in which the eyes drift upward following a downward saccade that depends on the head's orientation relative to space. Finally, torsional nystagmus is characterized by fast phases of intorsion or extorsion that can be accompanied by horizontal or vertical components depending on the location of central damage. Whereas torsional nystagmus is generally conjugate, there is a subtype of torsional nystagmus termed seesaw nystagmus in which one eye elevates/intorts while the other depresses/extorts.

REFERENCES

1. Demer JL. Current concepts of mechanical and neural factors in ocular motility. *Curr Opin Neurol.* 2006;19(1):4–13.
2. Hess BJ. Control of ocular torsion in the rotational vestibulo-ocular reflexes. *Prog Brain Res.* 2008;171:199–206.
3. Klier EM, Meng H, Angelaki DE. Three-dimensional kinematics at the level of the oculomotor plant. *J Neurosci.* 2006;26(10):2732–2737.
4. Büttner-Ennever JA, Akert K. Medial rectus subgroups of the oculomotor nucleus and their abducens internuclear input in the monkey. *J Comp Neurol.* 1981;197(1):17–27.
5. Maciewicz R, Kaneko C, Highstein SM, Baker R. Morphophysiological identification of interneurons in the oculomotor nucleus that project to the abducens nucleus in the cat. *Brain Res.* 1975;96:60–65.
6. Büttner-Ennever J, Horn A, Scherberger H, D'Ascanio P. Motoneurons of twitch and nontwitch extraocular muscle fibers in the abducens, trochlear, and oculomotor nuclei of monkeys. *J Comp Neurol.* 2001;438:318–335.
7. Spencer RF, Porter JD. Structural organization of the extraocular muscles. *Rev Oculomot Res.* 1988;2:33–79.
8. Ugolini G, Klam F, Doldan Dans M, et al. Horizontal eye movement networks in primates as revealed by retrograde transneuronal transfer of rabies virus: Differences in monosynaptic input to "slow" and "fast" abducens motoneurons. *J Comp Neurol.* 2006;498(6):762–785.
9. Xu Y, Wang X, Peck C, Goldberg ME. The time course of the tonic oculomotor proprioceptive signal in area 3a of somatosensory cortex. *J Neurophysiol.* 2011;106(1):71–77.
10. Balslev D, Albert NB, Miall C. Eye muscle proprioception is represented bilaterally in the sensorimotor cortex. *Hum Brain Mapp.* 2011;32(4):624–631.

11. Robinson DA. The mechanics of human saccadic eye movement. *J Physiol.* 1964;174:245–264.
12. Sylvestre PA, Cullen KE. Quantitative analysis of abducens neuron discharge dynamics during saccadic and slow eye movements. *J Neurophysiol.* 1999;82(5):2612–2632.
13. Sylvestre PA, Cullen KE. Dynamics of abducens nucleus neuron discharges during disjunctive saccades. *J Neurophysiol.* 2002;88(6):3452–3468.
14. Van Horn MR, Cullen KE. Dynamic characterization of agonist and antagonist oculomotoneurons during conjugate and disconjugate eye movements. *J Neurophysiol.* 2009;102(1):28–40.
15. Mays LE, Porter JD. Neural control of vergence eye movements: Activity of abducens and oculomotor neurons. *J Neurophysiol.* 1984;52(4):743–761.
16. Robinson DA. Oculomotor unit behavior in the monkey. *J Neurophysiol.* 1970;33(3):393–403.
17. Robinson DA, Keller EL. The behavior of eye movement motoneurons in the alert monkey. *Bibl Ophthalmol.* 1972;82:7–16.
18. Skavenski AA, Robinson DA. Role of abducens neurons in vestibuloocular reflex. *J Neurophysiol.* 1973;36(4):724–738.
19. Keller EL. Accomodative vergence in the alert monkey. Motor unit analysis. *Vision Res.* 1973;13:1565–1575.
20. Keller EL, Robinson DA. Abducens unit behaviour in the monkey during vergence movements. *Vision Res.* 1972;12:369–382.
21. Fuchs AF, Scudder CA, Kaneko C. Discharge patterns and recruitment order of identified motoneurons and internuclear neurons in the monkey abducens nucleus. *J Neurophysiol.* 1988;60:1874–1895.
22. Stahl JS, Thumser ZC. Dynamics of abducens nucleus neurons in the awake mouse. *J Neurophysiol.* 2012;108(9):2509–2523.
23. Miller JM, Robins D. Extraocular muscle forces in alert monkey. *Vision Res.* 1992;32(6):1099–1113.
24. Collins C. *The Control of Eye Movements.* New York: American Press; 1971.
25. Collins CC, O'Meara D, Scott AB. Muscle tension during unrestrained human eye movements. *J Physiol.* 1975;245(2):351–369.
26. Cullen KE. In: Pfaff DW, ed. *Neuroscience in the 21st century: From Basic to Clinical.* Pfaff DW, Volkow ND & Rubenstein JL (eds.). 3rd ed. Springer Verlag GmbH.
27. Yarbus AL. *Eye Movements and Vision.* New York: Springer; 1967;103–113.
28. Lebedev S, Van Gelder P, Tsui WH. Square-root relations between main saccadic parameters. *Invest Ophthalmol Vis Sci.* 1996;37(13):2750–2758.
29. Sugiuchi Y, Izawa Y, Takahashi M, Na J, Shinoda Y. Physiological characterization of synaptic inputs to inhibitory burst neurons from the rostral and caudal superior colliculus. *J Neurophysiol.* 2005;93(2):697–712.
30. Takahashi M, Sugiuchi Y, Izawa Y, Shinoda Y. Commissural excitation and inhibition by the superior colliculus in tectoreticular neurons projecting to omnipause neuron and inhibitory burst neuron regions. *J Neurophysiol.* 2005;94(3):1707–1726.
31. Takahashi M, Sugiuchi Y, Na J, Shinoda Y. Brainstem circuits triggering saccades and fixation. *J Neurosci.* 2022;42(5):789–803.
32. Sparks DL, Mays LE. Signal transformations required for the generation of saccadic eye movements. *Annu Rev Neurosci.* 1988;13:309–336.
33. Mays LE, Sparks DL. Saccades are spatially, not retinocentrically, coded. *Science.* 1980;208(4448):1163–1165.
34. Lee C, Rohrer WH, Sparks DL. Population coding of saccadic eye movements by neurons in the superior colliculus. *Nature.* 1988;332(6162):357–360.
35. Zénon A, Krauzlis R. Superior colliculus as a subcortical center for visual selection. *Med Sci (Paris).* 2014;30(6–7):637-43.
36. Basso MA, Bickford ME, Cang J. Unraveling circuits of visual perception and cognition through the superior colliculus. *Neuron.* 2021, 109(6):918–937.
37. Sasaki S, Shimazu H. Reticulovestibular organization participating in generation of horizontal fast eye movement. *Ann N Y Acad Sci.* 1981;374:130–143.
38. Strassman A, Highstein SM, McCrea RA. Anatomy and physiology of saccadic burst neurons in the alert squirrel monkey. I. Excitatory burst neurons. *J Comp Neurol.* 1986;249(3):337–357.
39. Strassman A, Highstein SM, McCrea RA. Anatomy and physiology of saccadic burst neurons in the alert squirrel monkey. II. Inhibitory burst neurons. *J Comp Neurol.* 1986;249(3):358–380.
40. Yoshida K, McCrea R, Berthoz A, Vidal PP. Morphological and physiological characteristics of inhibitory burst neurons controlling horizontal rapid eye movements in the alert cat. *J Neurophysiol.* 1982;48(3):761–784.
41. Hikosaka O, Igusa Y, Nakao S, Shimazu H. Direct inhibitory synaptic linkage of pontomedullary reticular burst neurons with abducens motoneurons in the cat. *Exp Brain Res.* 1978;33:337–352.
42. Hikosaka O, Kawakami T. Inhibitory reticular neurons related to the quick phase of vestibular nystagmus—their location and projection. *Exp Brain Res.* 1977;27(3–4):377–386.
43. Scudder CA, Kaneko CS, Fuchs AF. The brainstem burst generator for saccadic eye movements: A modern synthesis. *Exp Brain Res.* 2002;142(4):439–462.
44. Shinoda Y, Sugiuchi Y, Izawa Y, Takahashi M. Neural circuits for triggering saccades in the brainstem. *Prog Brain Res.* 2008;171:79–85.
45. Scudder CA, Fuchs AF, Langer TP. Characteristics and functional identification of saccadic inhibitory burst neurons in the alert monkey. *J Neurophysiol.* 1988;59(5):1430–1454.
46. Cullen KE, Guitton D. Analysis of primate IBN spike trains using system identification techniques. I. Relationship to eye movement dynamics during head-fixed saccades. *J Neurophysiol.* 1997;78(6):3259–3282.
47. Cullen KE, Guitton D. Analysis of primate IBN spike trains using system identification techniques. II. Relationship to gaze, eye, and head movement dynamics during head-free gaze shifts. *J Neurophysiol.* 1997;78(6):3283–3306.
48. Van Gisbergen JA, Robinson DA, Gielen S. A quantitative analysis of generation of saccadic eye movements by burst neurons. *J Neurophysiol.* 1981;45(3):417–442.
49. Hepp K, Henn V. Spatio-temporal recoding of rapid eye movement signals in the monkey paramedian pontine reticular formation (PPRF). *Exp Brain Res.* 1983;52:105–120.
50. Keller EL. Participation of medial pontine reticular formation in eye movement generation in monkey. *J Neurophysiol.* 1974;37:316–332.
51. Luschei E, Fuchs AF. Activity of brain stem neurons during eye movements of alert monkeys. *J Neurophysiol.* 1972;35:445–461.
52. Van Horn M, Sylvestre PA, Cullen KE. The brain stem saccadic burst generator encodes gaze in three-dimensional space. *J Neurophysiol.* 2008;99(5):2602–2616.
53. Van Horn MR, Cullen KE. Dynamic coding of vertical facilitated vergence by premotor saccadic burst neurons. *J Neurophysiol.* 2008;100(4):1967–1982.
54. Barton EJ, Nelson JS, Gandhi NJ, Sparks DL. Effects of partial lidocaine inactivation of the paramedian pontine reticular formation on saccades of macaques. *J Neurophysiol.* 2003;90(1):372–386.
55. Cannon S, Robinson D. Loss of the neural integrator of the oculomotor system from brain stem lesions in monkey. *J Neurophysiol.* 1987;57(5):1383–1409.
56. McCrea RA. Neuroanatomy of the oculomotor system. The nucleus prepositus. *Rev Oculomot Res.* 1988;2:203–223.
57. Dale A, Cullen KE. The nucleus prepositus predominantly outputs eye movement-related information during passive and active self-motion. *J Neurophysiol.* 2013;109(7):1900–1911.
58. Dale A, Cullen KE. Local population synchrony and the encoding of eye position in the primate neural integrator. *J Neurosci.* 2015;35(10):4287–4295.
59. Fukushima K, Kaneko C, Fuchs AF. The neuronal substrate of integration in the oculomotor system. *Prog Neurobiol.* 1992;39:609–639.
60. McCrea RA, Baker R. Cytology and intrinsic organization of the perihypoglossal nuclei in the cat. *J Comp Neurol.* 1985;237(3):360–376.
61. McCrea RA, Baker R. Anatomical connections of the nucleus prepositus of the cat. *J Comp Neurol.* 1985;237(3):377–407.
62. Delgado-García JM, Vidal PP, Gómez C, Berthoz A. A neurophysiological study of prepositus hypoglossi neurons projecting to oculomotor and preoculomotor nuclei in the alert cat. *Neuroscience.* 1989;29(2):291–307.
63. Escudero M, de la Cruz RR, Delgado-García JM. A physiological study of vestibular and prepositus hypoglossi neurones projecting to the abducens nucleus in the alert cat. *J Physiol.* 1992;458:539–560.
64. Miri A, Daie K, Arrenberg AB, Baier H, Aksay E, Tank DW. Spatial gradients and multi-dimensional dynamics in a neural integrator circuit. *Nat Neurosci.* 2011;14(9):1150–1159.
65. Moschovakis AK, Scudder CA, Highstein SM. Structure of the primate oculomotor burst generator. I. Medium-lead burst neurons with upward on-directions. *J Neurophysiol.* 1991;65(2):203–217.
66. Moschovakis AK, Scudder CA, Highstein SM, Warren JD. Structure of the primate oculomotor burst generator. II. Medium-lead burst neurons with downward on-directions. *J Neurophysiol.* 1991;65(2):218–229.
67. Crawford JD, Cadera W, Vilis T. Generation of torsional and vertical eye position signals by the interstitial nucleus of Cajal. *Science.* 1991;252(5012):1551–1553.
68. Klier EM, Wang H, Crawford JD. Interstitial nucleus of cajal encodes three-dimensional head orientations in Fick-like coordinates. *J Neurophysiol.* 2007;97(1):604–617.
69. Waitzman DM, Silakov VL, DePalma-Bowles S, Ayers AS. Effects of reversible inactivation of the primate mesencephalic reticular formation. II. Hypometric vertical saccades. *J Neurophysiol.* 2000;83(4):2285–2299.
70. Helmchen C, Rambold H, Fuhry L, Büttner U. Deficits in vertical and torsional eye movements after uni- and bilateral muscimol inactivation of the interstitial nucleus of Cajal of the alert monkey. *Exp Brain Res.* 1998;119(4):436–452.
71. Büttner-Ennever JA, Cohen B, Pause M, Fries W. Raphe nucleus of the pons containing omnipause neurons of the oculomotor system in the monkey, and its homologue in man. *J Comp Neurol.* 1988;267(3):307–321.
72. Horn A, Büttner-Ennever J, Wahle P, Reichenberger I. Neurotransmitter profile of saccadic omnipause neurons in nucleus raphe interpositus. *J Neurosci.* 1994;14:2032–2046.
73. Langer TP, Kaneko CR. Brainstem afferents to the oculomotor omnipause neurons in monkey. *J Comp Neurol.* 1990;295(3):413–427.
74. Munoz DP, Wurtz RH. Fixation cells in monkey superior colliculus. I. Characteristics of cell discharge. *J Neurophysiol.* 1993;70(2):559–575.
75. Reyes-Puerta V, Philipp R, Lindner W, Hoffmann K-P. Role of the rostral superior colliculus in gaze anchoring during reach movements. *J Neurophysiol.* 2010;103(6):3153–3166.
76. Hafed ZM, Goffart L, Krauzlis RJ. A neural mechanism for microsaccade generation in the primate superior colliculus. *Science.* 2009;323(5916):940–943.
77. Hafed ZM, Krauzlis RJ. Goal representations dominate superior colliculus activity during extrafoveal tracking. *J Neurosci.* 2008;28(38):9426–9439.
78. Krauzlis RJ, Basso MA, Wurtz RH. Discharge properties of neurons in the rostral superior colliculus of the monkey during smooth-pursuit eye movements. *J Neurophysiol.* 2000;84(2):876–891.
79. Nakao S, Curthoys IS, Markham CH. Direct inhibitory projection of pause neurons to nystagmus-related pontomedullary reticular burst neurons in the cat. *Exp Brain Res.* 1980;40(3):283–293.
80. Strassman A, Evinger C, McCrea RA, Baker RG, Highstein SM. Anatomy and physiology of intracellularly labelled omnipause neurons in the cat and squirrel monkey. *Exp Brain Res.* 1987;67(2):436–440.
81. Furuya N, Markham CH. Direct inhibitory synaptic linkage of pause neurons with burst inhibitory neurons. *Brain Res.* 1982;245(1):139–143.
82. Yoshida K, Iwamoto Y, Chimoto S, Shimazu H. Saccade-related inhibitory input to pontine omnipause neurons: An intracellular study in alert cats. *J Neurophysiol.* 1999;82(3):1198–1208.
83. Van Horn MR, Mitchell DE, Massot C, Cullen KE. Local neural processing and the generation of dynamic motor commands within the saccadic premotor network. *J Neurosci.* 2010;30(32):10,905–10,917.

84. Gandhi NJ, Sparks DL. Dissociation of eye and head components of gaze shifts by stimulation of the omnipause neuron region. *J Neurophysiol.* 2007;98(1):360–373.

85. Hafed ZM. Mechanisms for generating and compensating for the smallest possible saccades. *Eur J Neurosci.* 2011;33(11):2101–2113.

86. Otero-Millan J, Macknik SL, Serra A, Leigh RJ, Martinez-Conde S. Triggering mechanisms in microsaccade and saccade generation: A novel proposal. *Ann N Y Acad Sci.* 2011;1233: 107–116.

87. Pastukhov A, Braun J. Rare but precious: Microsaccades are highly informative about attentional allocation. *Vision Res.* 2010;50(12):1173–1184.

88. Engbert R, Kliegl R. Microsaccades uncover the orientation of covert attention. *Vision Res.* 2003;43(9):1035–1045.

89. Hafed ZM, Clark JJ. Microsaccades as an overt measure of covert attention shifts. *Vision Res.* 2002;42(22):2533–2545.

90. Betta E, Turatto M. Are you ready? I can tell by looking at your microsaccades. *Neuroreport.* 2006;17(10):1001–1004.

91. Cornsweet TN. Determination of the stimuli for involuntary drifts and saccadic eye movements. *J Opt Soc Am.* 1956;46(11):987–993.

92. Van Horn MR, Cullen KE. Coding of microsaccades in three-dimensional space by premotor saccadic neurons. *J Neurosci.* 2012;32(6):1974–1980.

93. Brien DC, Corneil BD, Fecteau JH, Bell AH, Munoz DP. The behavioural and neurophysiological modulation of microsaccades in monkeys. *J Eye Mov Res.* 2009; 3:1–12.

94. Krauzlis RJ. Recasting the smooth pursuit eye movement system. *J Neurophysiol.* 2004; 91(2):591–603.

95. Lisberger SG. Visual guidance of smooth-pursuit eye movements: sensation, action, and what happens in between. *Neuron.* 2010;66(4):477–491.

96. Lisberger SG, Morris EJ, Tychsen L. Visual motion processing and sensory-motor integration for smooth pursuit eye movements. *Annu Rev Neurosci.* 1987;10:97–129.

97. Broussard D, Lisberger S. Vestibular inputs to brain stem neurons that participate in motor learning in the primate vestibuloocular reflex. *J Neurophysiol.* 1992;68(5):1906–1909.

98. Lisberger SG, Pavelko T. Brain stem neurons in modified pathways for motor learning in the primate vestibulo-ocular reflex. *Science.* 1988;242(4879):771–773.

99. Lisberger SG, Pavelko TA, Broussard DM. Neural basis for motor learning in the vestibuloocular reflex of primates. I. Changes in the responses of brain stem neurons. *J Neurophysiol.* 1994;72(2):928–953.

100. Lisberger SG, Pavelko TA, Broussard DM. Responses during eye movements of brain stem neurons that receive monosynaptic inhibition from the flocculus and ventral paraflocculus in monkeys. *J Neurophysiol.* 1994;72(2):909–927.

101. Scudder CA, Fuchs AF. Physiological and behavioral identification of vestibular nucleus neurons mediating the horizontal vestibuloocular reflex in trained rhesus monkeys. *J. Neurophysiol.* 1992;68:244–264.

102. Cullen KE, Chen-Huang C, McCrea RA. Firing behavior of brain stem neurons during voluntary cancellation of the horizontal vestibuloocular reflex. II. Eye movement related neurons. *J Neurophysiol.* 1993;70(2):844–856.

103. Cullen KE, Guitton D, Rey CG, Jiang W. Gaze-related activity of putative inhibitory burst neurons in the head-free cat. *J Neurophysiol.* 1993;70:2678–2683.

104. McCrea RA, Strassman EM, Highstein SM. Anatomical and physiological characteristics of vestibular neurons mediating the horizontal vestibulo-ocular reflex of the squirrel monkey. *Journal of Comparative Neurology.* 1987;264:547–570.

105. Cullen K, McCrea R. Firing behavior of brain stem neurons during voluntary cancellation of the horizontal vestibuloocular reflex. I. Secondary vestibular neurons. *J Neurophysiol.* 1993;70(2):828–843.

106. Roy JE, Cullen KE. Brain stem pursuit pathways: Dissociating visual, vestibular, and proprioceptive inputs during combined eye-head gaze tracking. *J Neurophysiol.* 2003;90(1):271–290.

107. Suh M, Leung HC, Kettner RE. Cerebellar flocculus and ventral paraflocculus Purkinje cell activity during predictive and visually driven pursuit in monkey. *J Neurophysiol.* 2000;84(4):1835–1850.

108. Leung HC, Suh M, Kettner RE. Cerebellar flocculus and paraflocculus Purkinje cell activity during circular pursuit in monkey. *J Neurophysiol.* 2000;83(1):13–30.

109. Cullen KE, Van Horn MR. The neural control of fast vs. slow vergence eye movements. *Eur J Neurosci.* 2011;33(11):2147–2154.

110. Troost BT. The neurology of eye movements. *Neurology.* 1984;34(6):845–845-c.

111. Alvarez TL, Scheiman M, Morales C, et al. Underlying neurological mechanisms associated with symptomatic convergence insufficiency. *Sci Rep.* 2021;11(1):6545.

112. Busettini C, Mays LE. Saccade-vergence interactions in macaques. II. Vergence enhancement as the product of a local feedback vergence motor error and a weighted saccadic burst. *J Neurophysiol.* 2005;94(4):2312–2330.

113. Mays LE, Porter JD, Gamlin PD, Tello CA. Neural control of vergence eye movements: Neurons encoding vergence velocity. *J Neurophysiol.* 1986;56(4):1007–1021.

114. Mays LE, Gamlin PD. A neural mechanism subserving saccade-vergence interactions. In: Findlay WRJ, Kentridge RW, eds. *Eye Movement Research: Mechanisms, Processes and Applications.* Amsterdam: Elsevier; 1995:215–223.

115. Zhang Y, Mays LE, Gamlin PD. Characteristics of near response cells projecting to the oculomotor nucleus. *J Neurophysiol.* 1992;67(4):944–960.

116. Gamlin PD. Neural mechanisms for the control of vergence eye movements. *Ann N Y Acad Sci.* 2002;956:264–272.

117. Gamlin PD, Gnadt JW, Mays LE. Abducens internuclear neurons carry an inappropriate signal for ocular convergence. *J Neurophysiol.* 1989;62(1):70–81.

118. Judge SJ, Cumming B. Neurons in monkey midbrain with activity related to vergence eye movement and accommodation. *J Neurophysiol.* 1986;55:915–930.

119. Mays LE. Neural control of vergence eye movements: Convergence and divergence neurons in midbrain. *J Neurophysiol.* 1984;51(5):1091–1108.

120. Van Horn MR, Waitzman DM, Cullen KE. Vergence neurons identified in the rostral superior colliculus code smooth eye movements in 3D space. *J Neurosci.* 2013;33(17): 7274–7284.

121. Maxwell JS, King WM. Dynamics and efficacy of saccade-facilitated vergence eye movements in monkeys. *J Neurophysiol.* 1992;68(4):1248–1260.

122. Ono H, Nakamizo S, Steinbach MJ. Nonadditivity of vergence and saccadic eye movement. *Vision Res.* 1978;18(6):735–739.

123. Oohira A. Vergence eye movements facilitated by saccades. *Jpn J Ophthalmol.* 1993;37(4): 400–413.

124. van Leeuwen AF, Collewijn H, Erkelens CJ. Dynamics of horizontal vergence movements: interaction with horizontal and vertical saccades and relation with monocular preferences. *Vision Res.* 1998;38(24):3943–3954.

125. Zee DS, Fitzgibbon EJ, Optican LM. Saccade-vergence interactions in humans. *J Neurophysiol.* 1992;68(5):1624–1641.

126. Collewijn H, Erkelens CJ, Steinman RM. Trajectories of the human binocular fixation point during conjugate and non-conjugate gaze-shifts. *Vision Res.* 1997;37(8):1049–1069.

127. Enright J. Changes in vergence mediated by saccades. *J Physiol.* 1984;350:9–31.

128. Enright JT. The remarkable saccades of asymmetrical vergence. *Vision Res.* 1992;32(12): 2261–2276.

129. Mays LE. Has Hering been hooked? *Nature Med.* 1998;4:889–890.

130. Hering E. *Lehre vom Binokularen Sehen. (The Theory of Binocular Vision) (1868).* New York: Plenum Press; 1977.

131. McConville KM, Tomlinson RD, King WM, Paige G, Na EQ. Eye position signals in the vestibular nuclei: Consequences for models of integrator function. *J. Vest. Res.* 1994;4: 391–400.

132. Sylvestre PA, Choi JT, Cullen KE. Discharge dynamics of oculomotor neural integrator neurons during conjugate and disjunctive saccades and fixation. *J Neurophysiol.* 2003;90(2): 739–754.

133. Zhou W, King WM. Ocular selectivity of units in oculomotor pathways. *Ann N Y Acad Sci.* 1996;781:724–728.

134. Zhou W, King WM. Premotor commands encode monocular eye movements. *Nature.* 1998; 393(6686):692–695.

135. Quinet J, Schultz K, May PJ, Gamlin PD. Neural control of rapid binocular eye movements: Saccade-vergence burst neurons. *Proc Natl Acad Sci U S A.* 2020;117(46):29,123–29,132.

136. Ferraina S, Pare M, Wurtz R. Disparity sensitivity of frontal eye field neurons. *J Neurophysiol.* 2000;83:625–629.

137. Genovesio A, Ferraina S. Integration of retinal disparity and fixation-distance related signals toward an egocentric coding of distance in the posterior parietal cortex of primates. *J Neurophysiol.* 2004;91(6):2670–2684.

138. Gnadt JW, Beyer J. Eye movements in depth: What does the monkey's parietal cortex tell the superior colliculus? *Neuroreport.* 1998;9:233–238.

139. Gnadt JW, Mays LE. Neurons in monkey parietal area LIP are tuned for eye-movement parameters in three-dimensional space. *J Neurophysiol.* 1995;73(1):280–297.

140. Mimeault D, Paquet V, Molotchnikoff S, Lepore F, Guillemot J-P. Disparity sensitivity in the superior colliculus of the cat. *Brain Res.* 2004;1010(1–2):87–94.

141. Waitzman DM, Van Horn MR, Cullen KE. Neuronal evidence for individual eye control in the primate cMRF. *Prog Brain Res.* 2008;171:143–150.

142. Chaturvedi V, Van Gisbergen J. Perturbation of combined saccade-vergence movements by microstimulation in monkey superior colliculus. *J Neurophysiol.* 1999;81:2279–2296.

143. Chaturvedi V, Van Gisbergen J. Stimulation in the rostral pole of monkey superior colliculus: Effects on vergence eye movements. *Exp Brain Res.* 2000;132:72–78.

144. Walton MM, Mays LE. Discharge of saccade-related superior colliculus neurons during saccades accompanied by vergence. *J Neurophysiol.* 2003;90(2):1124–1139.

145. Upadhyaya S, Das VE. Response properties of cells within the rostral superior colliculus of strabismic monkeys. *Invest Ophthalmol Vis Sci.* 2019;60(13):4292–4302.

146. Gamlin PD, Zhang Y, Clendaniel RA, Mays LE. Behavior of identified Edinger-Westphal neurons during ocular accommodation. *J Neurophysiol.* 1994;72(5):2368–2382.

147. Erkelens IM, Bobier WR, Macmillan AC, et al. A differential role for the posterior cerebellum in the adaptive control of convergence eye movements. *Brain Stimul.* 2020;13(1):215–228.

148. Henriksen S, Tanabe S, Cumming B. Disparity processing in primary visual cortex. *Philos Trans R Soc Lond B Biol Sci.* 2016;371(1697):20150255.

149. Verhoef B-E, Vogels R, Janssen P. Binocular depth processing in the ventral visual pathway. *Philos Trans R Soc Lond B Biol Sci.* 2016;371(1697):20150259.

150. Theys T, Romero MC, van Loon J, Janssen P. Shape representations in the primate dorsal visual stream. *Front Comput Neurosci.* 2015;22(9):43.

151. Goldberg JM, Wilson VJ, Cullen KE, et al. *The Vestibular System: a Sixth Sense.* Oxford: Oxford University Press; 2012.

152. Lorente de Nó R. Vestibulo-ocular reflex arc. *Arch Neur Psych.* 1933;30:245–291.

153. Carriot J, Jamali M, Chacron MJ, Cullen KE. Statistics of the vestibular input experienced during natural self-motion: Implications for neural processing. *J. Neurosci.* 2014;34:8347–8357.

154. Carriot J, Jamali M, Chacron MJ, Cullen KE. The statistics of the vestibular input experienced during natural self-motion differ between rodents and primates. *J. Physiol.* 2017;595:2751–2766.

155. Ramachandran R, Lisberger SG. Normal performance and expression of learning in the vestibulo-ocular reflex (VOR) at high frequencies. *J Neurophysiol.* 2005;93(4):2028–2038.

156. Huterer M, Cullen K. Vestibuloocular reflex dynamics during high-frequency and high-acceleration rotations of the head on body in rhesus monkey. *J Neurophysiol.* 2002;88(1): 13–28.

157. Minor LB, Lasker DM, Backous DD, Hullar TE. Horizontal vestibuloocular reflex evoked by high-acceleration rotations in the squirrel monkey. I. Normal responses. *J Neurophysiol.* 1999;82(3):1254–1270.

158. Hullar TE, Minor LB. High-frequency dynamics of regularly discharging canal afferents provide a linear signal for angular vestibuloocular reflexes. *J Neurophysiol.* 1999;82(4): 2000–2005.

159. Cullen KE, Roy JE. Signal processing in the vestibular system during active versus passive head movements. *J Neurophysiol.* 2004;91(5):1919–1933.

160. Mitchell DE, Della Santina CC, Cullen KE. Plasticity within non-cerebellar pathways rapidly shapes motor performance in vivo. *Nat Commun.* 2016;9(7):11,238.

161. Sadeghi SG, Minor LB, Cullen KE. Neural correlates of motor learning in the vestibulo-ocular reflex: Dynamic regulation of multimodal integration in the macaque vestibular system. *J. Neurosci.* 2010;30:10,158–10,168.

162. Sadeghi SG, Minor LB, Cullen KE. Neural correlates of sensory substitution in vestibular pathways following complete vestibular loss. *J. Neurosci.* 2012;32:14685–14695.

163. Roy JE, Cullen KE. A neural correlate for vestibulo-ocular reflex suppression during voluntary eye-head gaze shifts. *Nature Neuroscience.* 1998;1:404–410.

164. Paige GD, Seidman SH. Characteristics of the VOR in response to linear acceleration. *Ann N Y Acad Sci.* 1999;871:123–135.

165. Angelaki DE, McHenry MQ. Short-latency primate vestibuloocular responses during translation. *J. Neurophysiol.* 1999;871:136–147.

166. Waespe W, Cohen B. Flocculectomy and unit activity in the vestibular nuclei during visual-vestibular interactions. *Exp Brain Res.* 1983;51:23–35.

167. Waespe W, Cohen B, Raphan T. Role of the flocculus and paraflocculus in optokinetic nystagmus and visual-vestibular interactions: Effects of lesions. *Exp Brain Res.* 1983; 50:9–33.

168. Zee DS, Yamazaki A, Butler PH, Gücer G. Effects of ablation of flocculus and paraflocculus of eye movements in primate. *J Neurophysiol.* 1981;46(4):878–899.

169. Collewijn H, Holstege G. Effects of neonatal and late unilateral enucleation on optokinetic responses and optic nerve projections in the rabbit. *Exp Brain Res.* 1984;57(1):138–150.

170. Beraneck M, Cullen KE. Activity of vestibular nuclei neurons during vestibular and optokinetic stimulation in the alert mouse. *J Neurophysiol.* 2007;98(3):1549–1565.

171. Cullen KE, Huterer M, Braidwood DA, Sylvestre PA. Time course of vestibuloocular reflex suppression during gaze shifts. *J Neurophysiol.* 2004;92(6):3408–3422.

172. Roy JE, Cullen KE. Vestibuloocular reflex signal modulation during voluntary and passive head movements. *J. Neurophysiol.* 2002;87:2337–2357.

173. Igusa Y, Sasaki S, Shimazu H. Excitatory premotor burst neurons in the cat pontine reticular formation related to the quick phase of vestibular nystagmus. *Brain Res.* 1980;182(2):451–456.

174. Daye PM, Roberts DC, Zee DS, Optican LM. Vestibulo-ocular reflex suppression during head-fixed saccades reveals gaze feedback control. *J Neurosci.* 2015;35(3):1192–1198.

175. Galiana HL, Guitton D. Central organization and modeling of eye-head coordination during orienting gaze shifts. *Ann. NY Acad. Sci.* 1992;656:452–471.

176. Haji-Abolhassani I, Guitton D, Galiana HL. Modelling eye-head coordination without pre-planning—a reflex-based approach. *Annu Int Conf IEEE Eng Med Biol Soc.* 2012: 4583–4586.

177. Haji-Abolhassani I, Guitton D, Galiana HL. Modeling eye-head gaze shifts in multiple contexts without motor planning. *J Neurophysiol.* 2016;116(4):1956–1985.

178. Sylvestre PA, Cullen KE. Premotor correlates of integrated feedback control for eye-head gaze shifts. *J Neurosci.* 2006;26(18):4922–4929.

179. Cullen KE, Guitton D. Analysis of primate IBN spike trains using system identification techniques. III. Relationship to motor error during head-fixed saccades and head-free gaze shifts. *J Neurophysiol.* 1997;78(6):3307–3322.

180. Cullen KE, Belton T, McCrea RA. A non-visual mechanism for voluntary cancellation of the vestibulo-ocular reflex. *Exp Brain Res.* 1991;83:237–252.

181. Lisberger SG. Visual tracking in monkeys: Evidence for short-latency suppression of the vestibuloocular reflex. *J. Neurophysiol.* 1990;63:676–688.

182. Leigh RJ, Zee DS. *The Neurology of Eye Movements.* 5th ed. Oxford; New York: Oxford University Press; 2015.

183. Lembo A, Serafino M, Strologo MD, et al. Accommodative esotropia: The state of the art. *Int Ophthalmol.* 2019;39(2):497–505.

184. Hug D. Management of infantile esotropia. *Curr Opin Ophthalmol.* 2015;26(5):371–374.

185. Brodsky MC. Essential infantile esotropia: Potential pathogenetic role of extended subcortical neuroplasticity. *Invest Ophthalmol Vis Sci.* 2018;59(5):1964–1968.

186. Whitman MC. Axonal growth abnormalities underlying ocular cranial nerve disorders. *Annu Rev Vis Sci.* 2021;15(7):827–850.

187. Pierrot-Deseilligny C. Nuclear, internuclear, and supranuclear ocular motor disorders. *Handb Clin Neurol.* 2011;102:319–331.

188. Ortiz JF, Eissa-Garces A, Ruxmohan S, et al. Understanding Parinaud's syndrome. *Brain Sci.* 2021;11(11):1469.

189. Ramat S, Leigh RJ, Zee DS, Optican LM. What clinical disorders tell us about the neural control of saccadic eye movements. *Brain.* 2017;130(Pt 1):10–35.

190. Robinson FR, Straube A, Fuchs AF. Role of the caudal fastigial nucleus in saccade generation. II. Effects of muscimol inactivation. *J Neurophysiol.* 1993;70(5):1741–1758.

191. Tarnutzer AA, Straumann D. Nystagmus. *Curr Opin Neurol.* 2018;31(1):74–80.

192. Otero-Millan J, Colpak AI, Kheradmand A, Zee DS. Rebound nystagmus, a window into the oculomotor integrator. *Prog Brain Res.* 2019;249:197–209.

Three-Dimensional Eye Movements: Kinematics, Control, and Perceptual Consequences

John Douglas Crawford and Amirsaman Sajad

INTRODUCTION

For centuries it has been known that the eyes are capable of rotating in three dimensions (3D): horizontally (left-right), vertically (up-down), and *torsionally* (clockwise-counterclockwise, which for now we can define as rotation of the eye about the visual axis when looking straight ahead). For obvious reasons, visual and oculomotor scientists have tended to focus on the horizontal and vertical rotations because these have the most effect on visual gaze direction and ocular torsion is hard to see, let alone measure. Indeed, the 19th century scientists cited in the next section of this chapter discovered oculomotor rules that seem to purposefully minimize torsion (and thus tilting of retina relative to the world), presumably to simplify oculomotor control and minimize distortions in perception. This may have contributed to the notion that torsion is the "poor cousin" that could be ignored or added on as something of an afterthought. This perspective fit well with 20th century technologies for recording eye position and the highly influential control system theories of oculomotor control, espoused by David A. Robinson and others in the 20th century, because it fits well with linear systems math and analysis.

In parallel to those "two-dimensional (2D)" developments, there was a lesser but increasing awareness of 3D aspects of eye motion, such as the ocular torsion observed during head tilt or brainstem damage.[1] This advanced in the 1980s with the development of technologies for recording 3D eye orientation and axes of eye rotation.[2,3] This led to an increased awareness that the eye moves either with or without torsion, depending on the behavioral circumstances. Perhaps more importantly, theoretician Douglas Tweed pointed out that the mathematics of rotations are noncommutative, and thus (even during 2D motion) require modifications to standard models of oculomotor control.[4] This led to surprisingly fierce debates in the 1990s that largely focused on the role of the "oculomotor plant"—the tissues and muscles surrounding the eye—and whether this can rescue the brain from the problems of 3D rotational math. Although seemingly esoteric, this has important implications for neural control and the clinic because disorders affecting the vertical-pulling eye muscles have equal influence on torsion of the eye.

Although these debates have settled down and we have learned much in the 21st century, misunderstandings and knowledge gaps remain. The purpose of this chapter is to explain, in the simplest way possible (i.e., without math), how the eyes rotate in three dimensions, how the brain controls this, and the normal/pathologic consequences on vision. One take-home message is that, just as in 2D eye control, both muscles and neurons make important and necessary contributions to the special aspects of 3D eye control.

THREE-DIMENSIONAL OCULAR KINEMATICS

To measure eye motion and use these data to understand oculomotor control, and diagnose oculomotor deficits and their perceptual consequences, it is important to know something about *rotational kinematics*. Kinematics is the study of motion, typically measured in terms of position and velocity. In the case of 3D eye kinematics, we are mostly concerned with eye *orientation*, and angular motion about some axis of rotation. The eyes also translate very slightly within the head (and quite a bit in space when the head moves), but we will confine this chapter to rotations. To discuss 3D kinematics it is also necessary to define coordinates and reference frames. Coordinates can here be thought of as a set of mutually orthogonal axes (vertical axis for horizontal rotation, horizontal axis for vertical rotation, and a torsional axis) that can be used to express the components of position or motion. Sometimes in 3D eye recordings, orientations are expressed as rotation vectors relative to some central reference position (the origin in the coordinate system), where the rotation vector is parallel to the axis of rotation, scaled by the amount of rotation, and directed according to the *right-hand rule* (Fig. 9.1A; where the fingers curl in the direction of rotation and the thumb then points in the vector direction). These are then fixed within some rigid body called the reference frame. For example, for the retina, the natural reference frame is the eye. The eye muscles contract between fixed points on the eyes and skull, but being much lower in inertia, the eyes rotate and the head stays fixed, making the head the natural reference frame for eye motion. Using these concepts, we will first consider eye-in-head motion (with the head stable), and then briefly touch on what happens when the head moves freely.

EYE-IN-HEAD MOTION

Mechanically, the eyes are capable of rotating approximately ±50-degrees horizontally, ±45-degrees vertically, and ±30-degrees torsionally with the head. However, Donders, a 19th century Dutch physiologist, observed that only one torsional eye component is used for any given 2D gaze position when participants looked around with the head motionless.[5] Listing, a German mathematician, then somehow intuited the specific rule for this, now called *Listing's law* (LL).[6] A simple definition is that the eyes only assume orientations that could be reached from a central *primary position* through a rotation about a fixed axis that lies in *Listing's plane*, orthogonal to the primary gaze direction.[7] Thus, if we use rotation vectors (defined using the right-hand rule) to express eye orientations as rotations relative to primary position (the reference position), these vectors will line up in Listing's plane (Fig. 9.1B). This also provides a convenient coordinate system for

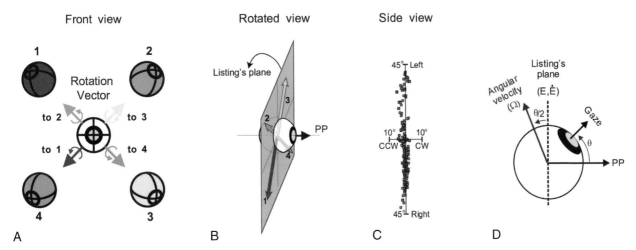

Fig. 9.1 (**A**) Front view of the eye when it is looking straight ahead (reference position) and four other orientations (*color-coded*) as shown. Each of these orientations (1–4) can be described by a single rotation vector (1–4) that would move the eye from the reference position to this orientation. These rotation vectors follow the right-hand rule convention. (**B**) A rotated view (close to a side view) of the eye showing these rotation vectors (in **A**) falling on a plane of zero torsion (*light brown*), known as the Listing's plane. (**C**) Scatterplot showing the side view of the rotation vector tips (*brown dots*) for several saccades, with the tail of the vector at the center (0,0). Here, the Listing's plane is the plane of the paper. (**D**) The half angle rule. In order to maintain the final eye position within Listing's plane, the angular velocity vector (Ω) that describes the rotation of the eye must tilt out of the Listing's plane by half of the angle (θ) by which the gaze deviates from the reference position. The derivative of eye position ($\dot{E} = dE/dt$) remains in Listing's plane (*dashed vertical line*), but $\dot{E}$ does not correctly describe the velocity of rotating objects owing to noncommutativity of rotations. *CCW*, Counterclockwise; *CW*, clockwise; *PP*, primary position.

describing eye orientations, where the horizontal and vertical axes lay in Listing's plane and the orthogonal torsional axis aligns with the primary gaze direction. Note that for now, these axes are fixed in the head, with the assumption that the head itself is motionless in some central position. An alternative is to define torsion as aligning with the visual axis, but this coordinate system results in so-called *false torsion*: clockwise rotation about the visual axis for up-left/down-right eye positions, counterclockwise rotation for up-right/down-left eye positions.[8]

Helmholtz confirmed that visual afterimages followed patterns predicted by LL, (i.e., tilting with false torsion),[6] and 20th century behavioral recordings allowed us to confirm and directly visualize Listing's plane (as 3D rotation vectors) during head-restrained saccades (Fig. 9.1C).[9–11] Human eye torsion varies within approximately 2 degrees of Listing's plane, whereas monkeys are even more precise (~1 degrees) and have been the most-used experimental model for studying the physiology of 3D eye rotation. It is noteworthy that the primary position, although near the center of the eye's mechanical range, varies considerably in humans and tends to be above center in monkeys (such that Listing's plane tilts back).

An important observation is that the actual axes of rotation (measured in angular velocity vectors, also following the right-hand rule convention) only align with Listing's plane for movements toward or away from primary position. For saccades passing orthogonal to primary position, the *half angle rule* applies, for example, the axis of a horizontal saccade must tilt by half the angle of gaze above or below primary position (Fig. 9.1D).

The latter, somewhat counterintuitive observation has caused a great deal of confusion, i.e., why would saccade axes tilt out of Listing's plane to keep eye position in Listing's plane? This tilt compensates for the noncommutative nature of eye rotations. For example, a horizontal rotation followed by a vertical rotation results in different final eye position than rotations in the opposite order.[4] All of this can be proven mathematically (or intuitively by careful manipulation of objects) but

for our purposes it must suffice to say that these observations have been confirmed experimentally many times.

LL thus provides an important organizing principle for understanding 3D eye movements and the perceptual consequences considered later in this chapter. As already noted, LL holds during head-restrained saccades and also smooth pursuit.[12,13] LL also holds during the translational vestibulo-ocular reflex (VOR),[14] where the binocular gaze point must remain fixed on some external point when the head shifts position. The common element is that these movements use a 3D system to aim 2D gaze, a classic "degrees of freedom problem" in motor control. LL is a control strategy that solves this problem in an orderly fashion.

In other oculomotor systems where there is no degrees of freedom problem, there is no LL. The ideal rotational VOR and optokinetic reflex should stabilize the retinal image by rotating the eye about the same 3D axis as the head but in the opposite direction, and they essentially do, with a somewhat lower torsional "gain" (amount of eye rotation/head rotation) and minor tilts/wiggles of the axis.[9,15,16] In other eye movements LL is modified. This obviously violates LL when the head rotates torsionally, but even pure horizontal/vertical rotation results in eye position-dependent violations, owing to the lack of a half angle rule. *Ocular counterroll* shifts Listing's plane torsionally by about 10% of the amount of static head tilt, whereas convergence causes the Listing's planes of the two eyes to rotate outward (counterintuitively) like "saloon doors."[9,17–19]

THREE-DIMENSIONAL KINEMATICS DURING HEAD-UNRESTRAINED GAZE SHIFTS

Finally, we must consider what happens to these rules in the real-world situation where both eye and head rotation contribute to final gaze position (Fig. 9.2). Here, Donders' law remains in place, with two exceptions.[20,21]

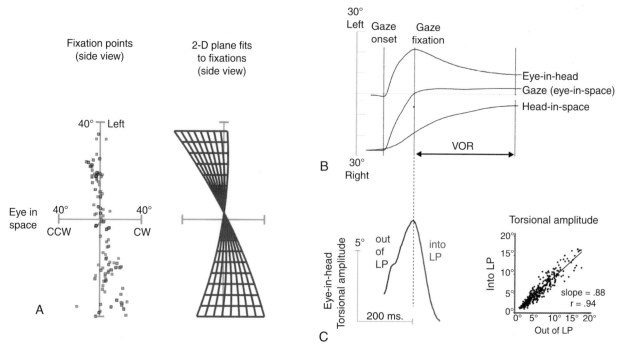

Fig. 9.2 **(A)** Three-dimensional behavior of eye-in-space, a combination of eye-in-head and head-in-space. Tips of rotation vectors are illustrated in the side view (*left*), and a plane is fit to illustrate the three-dimensional shape of these data. Unlike the eye-in-head data that fall on the Listing's plane (Fig. 9.1C), the eye-in-space data (which also incorporate head rotation) look like a twisted plane known as a Fick surface. (Modified with permission from Klier EM, Wang H, Crawford JD. Three-dimensional eye-head coordination is implemented downstream from the superior colliculus. *J Neurophysiol.* 2003;89(5):2839–2853.) **(B)** A plot of eye-in-head, eye-in-space, and head-in-space position as a function of time during a gaze shift. The gaze onset is when the eye moves in space (by a combination of eye-in-head and head-in-space rotation). Gaze fixation is when gaze (i.e., eye-in-space) is fixed on the destination. At this point, the head is still rotating in space but the eye-in-head has to counter this rotation through the vestibulo-ocular reflex (*VOR*). **(C)** During the shift of gaze (from gaze onset to gaze fixation) the eye-in-head torsion falls outside of the Listing's plane in a predictive manner to counter the torsion that occurs during the VOR. This brings the torsion back to 0. *CCW*, Counterclockwise; *CW*, clockwise; *LP*, Listing's Plane.

First, the position plane becomes a twisted surface, where one opposing pair of corners (e.g., up-left, down-right) shift in one torsional direction and the other pair (up-right, down-left) in the other torsional direction (Fig. 9.2A). The specific pattern resembles the torsion produced by a Fick Gimbal, where the vertical axis of rotation is fixed in space but the horizontal axis rotates about this (like a telescope mount). This is in part because the head behaves like a Fick Gimbal, and in part because the head is used relatively more for horizontal range and the eyes for vertical range, again acting like a Fick Gimbal. One effect of this is to minimize torsional rotation of the eye about the visual axis, thus reducing "false torsion."

Second, the torsional eye orientation in space becomes much more variable (from about ±1 degree to ±5 degrees). This is partially because head torsion is more variable, and partially because eye-in-head control gets more complicated: saccades are typically followed by head rotation, and this is accompanied by VOR movements (Fig. 9.2 B), which include torsional components. Rather than wait till the end of gaze shift to correct these, the system generates anticipatory torsional components (out of Listing's plane) in the opposite direction (Fig. 9.2C). This coordination strategy causes eye-in-head position to leave and then return to Listing's plane during each head-unrestrained gaze shift but has the important advantage (for vision) of gaze shifts ending with the system stable and torsion minimized.

All of these kinematics observations (with and without head motion) have geometric consequences for vision, which we will

return to later. But first, we will consider control mechanisms. What causes saccade axes to tile out of Listing's plane? How does the brain decide when to use or not use LL? And how are these processes coordinated?

THREE-DIMENSIONAL CONTROL MECHANISMS
Motoneurons and muscles
The extraocular muscles are arranged in anatomic coordinate system where the horizontal recti control horizontal eye rotation, whereas the other muscles (vertical recti and obliques) and their corresponding motoneuron pools in the brainstem each control a combination of vertical and torsional rotation (Fig. 9.3A, see Chapter 7 for details). If one defines torsional rotation about the visual axes, then the relative contributions of the latter muscles to vertical and torsional rotation varies with horizontal eye position, but if torsion is defined in LL coordinates as described, the arrangement is simpler: they appear to control roughly equal amounts of torsion. For example, in the right eye the directions would be superior rectus: up-counterclockwise, inferior oblique: up-clockwise, inferior rectus: down-clockwise, and superior oblique: down-counterclockwise (with torsional directions reversed in the left eye). Thus, assuming the moment that the horizontal recti control an axis of rotation parallel to Listing's plane, the brain has to co-activate a vertical rectus + oblique muscle to get pure vertical (or pure torsional) eye rotation. This is important for interpreting the

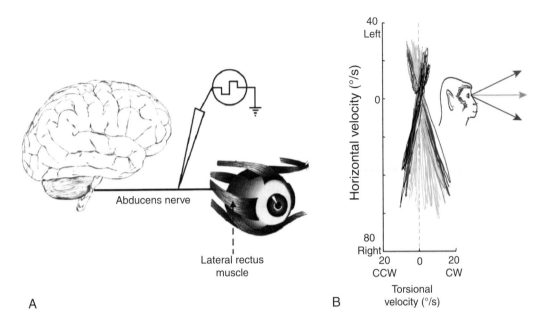

Fig. 9.3 Abducens nerve stimulation and half angle rule. (**A**) Experimental procedures used by stimulating the abducens nerve (cranial nerve VI) that innervates the lateral rectus muscle to carry brainstem neural commands. (From Klier EM, Meng H, Angelaki DE. Three-dimensional kinematics at the level of the oculomotor plant. *J Neurosci.* 2006;26(10); 2732–2737.) (**B**) Horizontal versus torsional eye velocity during abducens nerve microstimulation, resulting in changes in eye orientation pointing in different vertical positions ranging 25-degrees upward (*red*) to 25-degrees downward (*blue*). The orientation of Listing's plane is indicated by the vertical dashed line at 0-degrees torsion. *CCW*, Counterclockwise; *CW*, clockwise. (Modified with permission from Klier EM, Meng H, Angelaki DE. Three-dimensional kinematics at the level of the oculomotor plant. *J Neurosci.* 2006;26(10):2732–2737.)

complex 3D oculomotor deficits resulting from eye muscle damage, but this cannot be entirely separated from potential compensatory mechanisms in the brain (we will return to the brain further in the chapter).

A second issue surrounding the contributions of motoneurons and muscles relates to the half angle rule described previously. The 1990s were witness to a theoretical debate, with Tweed espousing the view that the oculomotor system requires a 3D noncommutative controller, whereas Raphan led the opposing view that a 2D linear controller is sufficient for saccades.[4,7,22] Over time, this debate coalesced to the question of whether the oculomotor plant itself implements the half angle rule, negating the need for the brain to compute its position-dependent axis tilts.[23,24] Klier and Angelaki (Fig. 9.3) showed that motoneurons do not encode position-dependent saccade axis tilts, suggesting that the half angle rule is implemented mechanically somehow by the oculomotor plant itself.[25] Mathematically, this means that the phasic component of motoneuron activity (the part that drives motion) does not encode angular velocity, but rather the derivative of eye orientation. This is a feature that has been implicitly or explicitly included in most 3D saccade models over the past 25 years.[24,26–28]

The next obvious question is: What in the plant is causing these tilts? Surprisingly, we do not know enough about the physics and physiology of the plant to be certain. For example, it could be that the elastic properties of tissues surrounding the eye are responsible. However, the leading candidates for this function are the eye muscle "pulleys" proposed by J. Miller and J. Demer. Based on anatomic images, it appears that tissues surrounding the eye muscles could cause them to change pulling direction as a function of eye position in a way that is consistent with the half angle rule.[29] At this time this is the accepted view, but to

conclusively close this topic it will be important to verify the anatomical evidence for pulley actions with more functional physiology.

The preceding discussion might seem to resolve the LL issue, but this would be a mistake. There are several other issues to consider. First, as we have seen, the oculomotor plant itself is a 3D controller, and the brain must select the right balance of muscle activity to give zero torsion, even for head-restrained saccades. Further, we have seen that the brain seems to use or reduce this dimensionality at will, depending on current needs of the visual system (e.g., image stabilization for the VOR vs. gaze pointing for saccades) and can generate torsional saccade components (in or out of Listing's plane) whenever required to modify, anticipate, or correct for LL (Fig. 9.2C). It is also known that LL breaks down during various brain pathologies (see next section). The upshot is that although plant mechanics seem to simplify one aspect of LL (the half angle rule), the question of how the brain chooses (or does not choose) to obey LL requires further consideration.

BRAINSTEM OCULOMOTOR COORDINATES

The "fundamental theorem" of oculomotor control, proposed by D.A. Robinson, can be simplified as follows: eye movements are driven by velocity signals that (1) drive both the phasic component of motoneuron activity (mentioned previously) to contract eye muscles and move the eye and (2) are also input to a "neural integrator" that converts these velocity signals into a position signal that maintains motoneuron/muscle activity after a movement, thus holding eye position.[30] In the case of the saccade system, the phasic signal derives from brainstem reticular formation burst neurons (Fig. 9.4B), whereas the rotational VOR signal originates in the semicircular canals themselves.

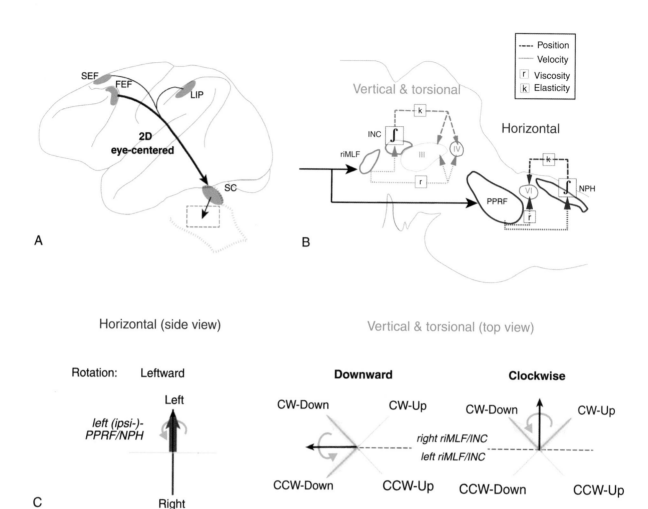

Fig. 9.4 Neural control of three-dimensional (3D) eye movement control. (**A**) Eye movement signals in areas upstream of brainstem. Cortical areas in parietal and frontal cortex, as well as the superior colliculus, encode spatial parameters of eye movement goal in two-dimensional coordinates defined in eye-centered coordinates. (**B**) This two-dimensional code is processed in the brainstem in two parallel streams, one dedicated to torsional/vertical rotations (*blue*) and one to horizontal rotations (*red*). (**B**) shows a midsagittal section through the primate brainstem revealing the anatomical locations of the components of the brainstem saccade generator. The circuit diagram is based on the Robinson[30] model of the brainstem. Motor neurons that innervate eye muscles receive a velocity command that counters the viscosity (r) and a position command that counters the eye's elasticity (k). For horizontal rotations (*red*), burst neurons in the paramedian pontine reticular formation (*PPRF*) output the velocity command (*dotted line*). This velocity command is sent to the neural integrators ($\int$) in the nucleus prepositus hypoglossi (*NPH*) outputting a position command (*dashed line*). For torsional and vertical rotations (*blue*), burst neurons are found in the rostral interstitial nucleus of the medial longitudinal fasciculus (*riMLF*), which send velocity signal to the neural integrators in the interstitial nucleus of Cajal (*INC*). This neural integrator generates the position command. (Modified with permission from Henn V, Büttner-Ennever JA, Hepp K. The primate oculomotor system. I. Motoneurons. A synthesis of anatomical, physiological, and clinical data. *Hum Neurobiol.* 1982;1[2]:77–85.) (**C**) The 3D control of the torsional, vertical, and horizontal components of gaze shifts across the midline. Each cardinal axis (*thin, colored arrows*) represents one burst neuron population, roughly corresponding to the pulling directions of the six extraocular muscles shown in Fig. 9.3A. The rotation controlled by the activation of each population is indicated by the label. The *thick colored arrows* represent activated populations for horizontal (*red*) and vertical/torsional (*blue*) rotations, with the resultant eye rotation vector shown with the *black arrow*. The activation of neurons in left (*ipsilateral*) PPRF and NPH (*thick red arrow*) results in leftward eye rotation. The concurrent activation of right and left riMLF and INC (*thick blue arrows*) results in a downward rotation and no torsional component owing to cancellation of two opposing torsional components. Simultaneous activation of two populations in right riMLF and INC results in a clockwise rotation. *CCW*, Counterclockwise; *CW*, clockwise; *FEF*, frontal eye fields; *LIP*, lateral intraparietal area; *SC*, superior colliculus; *SEF*, supplementary eye fields. (Modified with permission from Crawford JD, Vilis T. Symmetry of oculomotor burst neuron coordinates about Listing's plane. *J Neurophysiol*, 1992;68[2]:432–448.)

If saccade burst neurons encode eye orientation derivatives, this can be input directly to both a neural integrator and the type of motoneurons described previously. However, for the VOR to work properly, semicircular canal outputs would have to be compared to 3D eye orientation to compute eye position derivatives, effectively canceling the half angle axis tilts added by the eye muscles.[31]

A second issue for the brainstem is coordinate transformations (Fig. 9.4C). The brainstem oculomotor system is largely organized around coordinates similar to the semicircular canals and eye muscles.[32] This includes both saccade burst generator and the neural integrator (Fig. 9.4B). One part of the neural integrator (in the medial vestibular nucleus/nucleus prepositus hypoglossi) encodes horizontal eye position,[33] whereas four bilateral populations of neurons in the midbrain interstitial nucleus of Cajal (INC) encode directional components of position similar to those of the vertical recti/obliques.[32] Similarly, burst neurons in the paramedian pontine reticular formation (PPRF) encode horizontal saccade components, whereas the midbrain rostral interstitial nucleus of the medial longitudinal fasciculus (riMLF) possesses the remaining torsional/vertical populations.[34] Notably, in both the riMLF and INC these populations are separated so that up/clockwise and down/clockwise components are represented on the right side and up/counterclockwise and down/counterclockwise are located left of the midline.

This arrangement gives rise to a simple rule: to generate zero torsion saccades, co-activate the up or down populations across the midline (Fig. 9.4C). Thus, this has the capacity to collapse to a 2D controller for head-restrained saccades, but this relies on an assumption: The coordinate axes align with Listing's plane. For example, the vertical axis of rotation controlled by the horizontal system would need to align with Listing's plane, and the other axes would need to be arranged symmetrically about Listing's plane. Fortunately, there is evidence that this is true: For example, obliterating the riMLF leaves only horizontal saccades about a vertical axis in Listing's plane,[35] and unilateral damage to the INC results in torsional drift orthogonal to Listing's plane.[36] This is curious because the vertical axis through Listing's plane does not generally align with the vertical axes of rotation controlled by the horizontal canals and muscles. Either the physiologic actions of the muscles are not quite the same as anatomy suggests, or some neural coordinate transformations are required.

This discussion is not academic; it has important applications for understanding the symptoms of brainstem damage. Damage to the burst generator and/or neural integrator results in deficit with the physiology and theory described (Fig. 9.4). For example, damage to riMLF results in vertical saccade deficits, often accompanied by torsional offsets in eye orientation,[34,35] whereas damage to the INC results in vertical eye position drift (gaze paretic nystagmus) toward a central "null" position. This is accompanied by torsional drift (clockwise or counterclockwise, depending on the side of damage) that is initially corrected by opposite torsional saccades.[32] These nuclei are close neighbors near the midline of the midbrain; so often such deficits overlap and combine. Finally, these nuclei may have similar roles for head control, such that INC damage also causes torsional head drift that settles into a posture resembling cervical dystonia.[37,38]

HIGHER-LEVEL TRANSFORMATIONS

The cortical circuits for saccades (the frontal eye fields, the supplementary eye fields, and parietal eye fields), project to the midbrain superior colliculus (SC), which in turn provides direct anatomical input to the brainstem structures for saccades and head-unrestrained gaze shifts (Fig. 9.4A). Cortical and SC response fields show a progression

from coding visual-to-motor codes in eye-centered coordinates.[39–42] Further, in the SC these response fields are topographically organized much like the retina (Fig. 9.5A). The neural progression from this primarily topographic code to the velocity rate code in brainstem burst neurons is often called a *spatiotemporal transformation*.[43,44] However, in 3D, this transformation must accomplish two other transformations.

THE REFERENCE FRAME TRANSFORMATION

To produce accurate gaze shifts, the eye-centered SC code must be transformed into the head or body-fixed brainstem/muscle coordinates described previously.[45] This is most clearly evident during electrical stimulation of the SC, which produces saccades/gaze shifts in various directions (depending on stimulation site in the topographic map[46]). When these trajectories are rotated into eye coordinates (by the inverse of 3D eye orientation; subtracting off initial gaze position is not mathematically correct), they follow a fixed-vector pattern.[47] However, the same gaze shifts can appear to be fixed vector (for small saccades), moderately converging as a function of initial eye position (for medium-sized gaze shifts), to completely converging to one point in space for large gaze shifts (Fig. 9.5B). This is not a stimulation artifact, but rather the mathematically correct *reference frame transformation* from fixed retinal points within a sphere (see section Perceptual consequences) to the gaze shifts required for the corresponding points in external space. This demonstrates that the brain knows these properties, somehow transforming eye-centered visual codes into brainstem motor codes as a function of initial eye orientation,[47] perhaps using gaze-position "gain fields" found in the SC system.[48–50]

THE TWO-DIMENSIONAL TO THREE-DIMENSIONAL TRANSFORMATION

A second consistent property of neurons found in higher-level gaze control centers is that they do not appear to encode fixed torsional components.[51] This does not mean they encode zero torsion; they simply do not encode torsion. They simply seem to be concerned with pointing 2D gaze direction the right way. For example, SC stimulation results in head-unrestrained gaze shifts with the complex torsional patterns shown in Fig. 9.2.[52] This suggests that something downstream from the SC converts the simple 2D output of these areas into 3D commands, with or without torsion. This could occur through position-dependent modulations on the direct SC-brainstem path, or through side loops such as the medial reticular formation[53] or cerebellum.[54] In particular, the nucleus reticularis tegmenti pontis (which relays information from the SC to the cerebellum) shows modulations in neural activity that correlate with torsional corrections to small errors in LL.[55] Consistent with these ideas, damage to the cerebellum degrades LL, (i.e., leading to increased torsional variance).[56] We know even less about the neural mechanisms that modify LL (e.g., for counterroll), but there are clues that this is also an active process.[57] Such neural mechanisms ultimately determine whether LL (and its variants) are obeyed, modified, or abandoned altogether.

PERCEPTUAL CONSEQUENCES

Finally, we consider the consequences that 3D eye rotations have for vision. In principle this is a list as long as the topic of vision because the orientation of the eye determines how external stimuli project onto the retina in healthy individuals, let alone pathologic situations. However, we can highlight specific cases that are specific to the topic and have been investigated, and some of their clinical correlates.

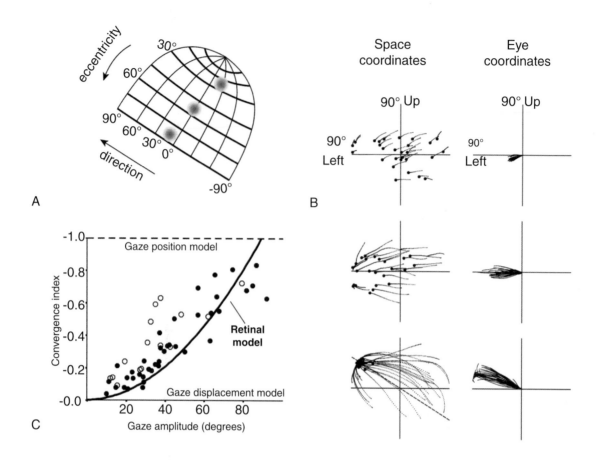

Fig. 9.5 (**A**) The superior colliculus topographic map of visual-motor space and three stimulation sites generating head-unrestrained gaze shifts of approximately 30, 60, and 90 degrees shown in **B**. (**B**) Stimulation-evoked gaze trajectories are shown in space coordinates (*left column*) and eye or retinal coordinates (*right column*). Each movement begins at the origin and proceeds in a direction and distance proportional to the gaze shift. Subtle variations in gaze displacement direction in retinal coordinates may be accounted for as minor changes in the underlying neural state superimposed on the stimulus-evoked activity. These gaze shifts were kinematically indistinguishable from natural gaze behavior. (**C**) Convergence index plot versus gaze amplitude for two monkeys (first monkey: *white circles*, second monkey: *black circles*). For details on calculating the convergence index see. The gaze displacement model predicts a fixed convergence index of 0 (*slope along the abscissa*), whereas the gaze-position model predicts a fixed convergence index of –1 (*dashed line*). The retinal model requires that convergence indices be small for small gaze amplitudes, but then increase nonlinearly for larger gaze amplitudes (*solid line*). The data favor the retinal model. (Modified with permission from Klier EM, Wang H, Crawford JD. The superior colliculus encodes gaze commands in retinal coordinates. *Nat Neurosci.* 2001;4[6]:627–632.)

MONOCULAR CONSEQUENCES

The most obvious perceptual consequence of 3D eye orientation is that torsion of the eye will cause the proximal retinal stimulus to tilt with respect to the real world (Fig. 9.6A,B). However, even vertical or horizontal rotation of the eye causes distortions of visual space (Fig. 9.6C,D), which in turn can interact with both real torsion (Fig. 9.6D, right column) or false torsion. This becomes more complex in head-unrestrained conditions (Fig. 9.2). Fortunately, internal knowledge of eye position in space could be used to decode retinal images associated from any eye orientation. As noted in the previous section (Fig. 9.5), these geometric distortions arise (and are corrected) in the gaze system,[47] and they are also compensated for the reach system.[58] It has been suggested that compensation for torsion could start as early as primary visual cortex.[59,60] Healthy humans also compensate for torsional eye rotation in visual memory,[61–63] but uncompensated torsional nystagmus can lead to vertigo.[64,65]

BINOCULAR CONSEQUENCES

The perceptual consequences of 3D eye rotation become more complex and pronounced for binocular vision, because they influence the correspondence of their two retinal images. In this sense, the binocular version of LL simplifies stereopsis (compared to random torsion) by reducing the possible "search zones" for binocular correspondence.[66] As we have seen, LL is often violated or modified, but healthy visuomotor systems appear to account for this, e.g., accounting for eye and head orientation when decoding object depth with the head tilted.[67]

These challenges will be exacerbated by any pathology that results in 3D misalignments of the two eyes.[68,69] As discussed previously, the torsional and vertical control systems are inextricably combined, so damage to these systems will tend to produce both torsional and vertical misalignments of the visual image. For example, tonic torsional offsets owing to midbrain damage are often accompanied by

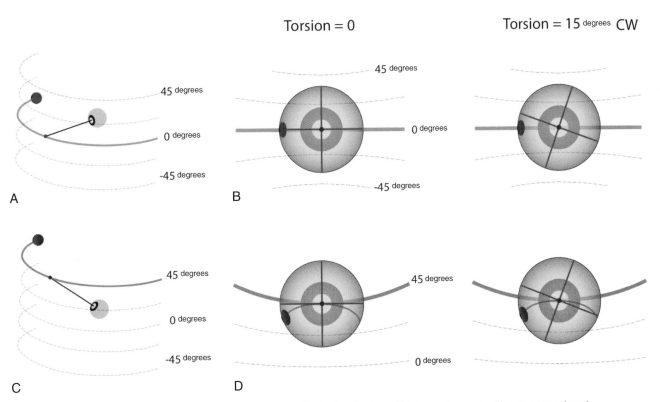

Fig. 9.6 Eye position-dependent geometry of retinal projections. (**A**) shows the eye looking at a central position (*small circle*), with the peripheral visual stimulus (*large green circle*) on the right from the perspective of the eye. The middle and right panels show the projection of this visual stimulus on the retina (*green patch*). (**B**) Close-up view of the semitransparent eye from behind while it looks toward the central stimulus. The optically inverted projections of the stimulus lines onto the retina are visible. *Red lines* represent retinal cardinal axes. When torsion is 0 (*left*) the projection falls on the cardinal axis. However, when the eye rotates torsionally (*right panel*) the projection falls off the cardinal axis. (**C**) shows the eye looking at an elevated position above the central position. Once again, there is a peripheral visual stimulus (*purple circle*) on the right from the perspective of the eyes. (**D**) This time, however, even when the eye has no torsion, because of the spherical retinal geometry, the projection of the peripheral visual stimulus falls off the cardinal retinal axis. As in **B**, the projection on the retina changes when the eyes rotate torsionally. Therefore, the perceptual system has to account for the nonlinearity in retinal projection as a function of eye orientation that arises owing to the geometry of the eyes. (Modified with permission from Klier EM, Wang H, Crawford JD. The superior colliculus encodes gaze commands in retinal coordinates. *Nat Neurosci.* 2001;4(6):627–632.)

"skew deviation" (vertical offsets of the two eyes). Additionally, given the delicate balance of muscle activations required to maintain LL (Fig. 9.4C), it should not be surprising that cranial neve palsy gives rise to acute position-dependent distortions in Listing's plane. Fortunately, it appears that some corrective mechanisms seem to partially adjust for these LL deficits over time.[70] It might be expected that these deficits grow worse in the more complex head-unrestrained situation, but little is known on this subject.

CONCLUSIONS

The topic of 3D eye rotations is complex and often difficult compared to our more intuitive grasp of object translation in external space. Fortunately, there are a few "rules of thumb" that one can offer as take-home messages. First, eye rotations are not only 3D (including torsion) but also fundamentally noncommutative, which has important implications for both oculomotor measurement and theory. Second, when the system requires all three degrees of freedom (as in the VOR and OKN), it uses them, but when it only needs to point 2D gaze, it reduces these degrees of freedom using LL or some variant. Third, the muscle versus brain debate is hopefully settled: it is now clear that oculomotor plant implements some aspects of LL (such as the half angle rule), whereas the brain possesses some control system, perhaps distributed, to enforce, modify, or violate LL as required. Finally, knowing these rules (and how they are perturbed in various pathologic situations) is important for understanding their real-world consequences for vision. However, for oculomotor scientists, important questions remain, including a fundamental understanding of the physical properties of the extraocular tissues, a detailed understanding of the neural transformations that implement LL (and its variants), and how the brain compensates for their visual consequences in normal and pathologic states.[71]

REFERENCES

1. Westheimer G, Blair SM. The ocular tilt reaction—a brainstem oculomotor routine. *Invest Ophthalmol Vis Sci.* 1975;14(11):833–839.
2. Ferman L, Collewijn H, van den Berg AV. A direct test of Listing's law—I. Human ocular torsion measured in static tertiary positions. *Vision Research.* 1987;27(6):929–938.
3. Tweed D, Cadera W, Vilis T. Computing three-dimensional eye position quaternions and eye velocity from search coil signals. *Vision Research.* 1990;30(1):97–110.
4. Tweed D, Vilis T. Implications of rotational kinematics for the oculomotor system in three dimensions. *Journal of Neurophysiology.* 1987;58(4):832–849.
5. Donders FC. Beiträge zur Lehre von den Bewegungen des menschlichen Auges. *Holländische Beiträge Anat Physiol Wiss.* 1848;1:105–145.
6. Von Helmholtz H. *Handbuch der physiologischen Optik: Mit 213 in den Text eingedruckten Holzschnitten und 11 Tafeln.* Vol. 9. Leipzig: Voss; 1867.
7. Tweed D, Vilis T. Geometric relations of eye position and velocity vectors during saccades. *Vision Research.* 1990;30(1):111–127.
8. Roelofs CO. Optokinetic nystagmus. *Documenta Ophthalmologica.* 1954;7(1):579–650.
9. Crawford JD, Vilis T. Axes of eye rotation and Listing's law during rotations of the head. *Journal of Neurophysiology.* 1991;65(3):407–423.
10. Straumann D, Zee DS, Solomon D, Lasker AG, Roberts DC. Transient torsion during and after saccades. *Vision Research.* 1995;35(23–24):3321–3334.
11. Tweed D, Vilis T. The superior colliculus and spatiotemporal translation in the saccadic system. *Neural Networks.* 1990;3(1):75–86.
12. Haslwanter T, Straumann D, Hepp K, Hess BJM, Henn V. Smooth pursuit eye movements obey Listing's law in the monkey. *Experimental Brain Research.* 1991;87(2):470–472.
13. Straumann D, Zee DS, Solomon D, Kramer PD. Validity of Listing's law during fixations, saccades, smooth pursuit eye movements, and blinks. *Experimental Brain Research.* 1996;112(1):135–146.
14. Angelaki DE, Zhou H-H, Wei M. Foveal versus full-field visual stabilization strategies for translational and rotational head movements. *Journal of Neuroscience.* 2003;23(4):1104–1108.
15. Fetter M, Tweed D, Hermann W, Wohland-Braun B, Koenig E. The influence of head position and head reorientation on the axis of eye rotation and the vestibular time constant during postrotatory nystagmus. *Experimental Brain Research.* 1992;91(1):121–128.
16. Misslisch H, Tweed D, Fetter M, Sievering D, Koenig E. Rotational kinematics of the human vestibuloocular reflex. III. Listing's law. *Journal of Neurophysiology.* 1994;72(5):2490–2502.
17. Haslwanter T, Straumann D, Hess BJM, Henn V. Static roll and pitch in the monkey: Shift and rotation of Listing's plane. *Vision Research.* 1992;32(7):1341–1348.
18. Misslisch H, Tweed D, Fetter M, Dichgans J, Vilis T. Interaction of smooth pursuit and the vestibuloocular reflex in three dimensions. *Journal of Neurophysiology.* 1996;75(6):2520–2532.
19. Mok D, Ro A, Cadera W, Crawford JD, Vilis T. Rotation of Listing's plane during vergence. *Vision Research.* 1992;32(11):2055–2064.
20. Glenn B, Vilis T. Violations of Listing's law after large eye and head gaze shifts. *Journal of Neurophysiology.* 1992;68(1):309–318.
21. Crawford JD, Ceylan MZ, Klier EM, Guitton D. Three-dimensional eye-head coordination during gaze saccades in the primate. *Journal of Neurophysiology.* 1999;81(4):1760–1782.
22. Schnabolk C, Raphan T. Modeling three-dimensional velocity-to-position transformation in oculomotor control. *Journal of Neurophysiology.* 1994;71(2):623–638.
23. Demer JL, Miller JM, Poukens V, Vinters HV, Glasgow BJ. Evidence for fibromuscular pulleys of the recti extraocular muscles. *Investigative Ophthalmology & Visual Science.* 1995;36(6):1125–1136.
24. Raphan T. Modeling control of eye orientation in three dimensions. I. Role of muscle pulleys in determining saccadic trajectory. *Journal of Neurophysiology.* 1998;79(5):2653–2667.
25. Klier EM, Meng H, Angelaki DE. Reaching the limit of the oculomotor plant: 3D kinematics after abducens nerve stimulation during the torsional vestibulo-ocular reflex. *Journal of Neuroscience.* 2012;32(38):13,237–13,243.
26. Crawford JD, Guitton D. Visual-motor transformations required for accurate and kinematically correct saccades. *Journal of Neurophysiology.* 1997;78(3):1447–1467.
27. Quaia C, Optican LM. Commutative saccadic generator is sufficient to control a 3-D ocular plant with pulleys. *Journal of Neurophysiology.* 1998;79(6):3197–3215.
28. Tweed D. Three-dimensional model of the human eye-head saccadic system. *Journal of Neurophysiology.* 1997;77(2):654–666.
29. Demer JL, Oh SY, Poukens V. Evidence for active control of rectus extraocular muscle pulleys. *Investigative Ophthalmology & Visual Science.* 2000;41(6):1280–1290.
30. Robinson DA. The use of control systems analysis in the neurophysiology of eye movements. *Annual Review of Neuroscience.* 1981;4(1):463–503.
31. Smith MA, Crawford JD. Neural control of rotational kinematics within realistic vestibuloocular coordinate systems. *Journal of Neurophysiology.* 1998;80(5):2295–2315.
32. Crawford JD, Cadera W, Vilis T. Generation of torsional and vertical eye position signals by the interstitial nucleus of Cajal. *Science.* 1991;252(5012):1551–1553.
33. Cannon SC, Robinson D. Loss of the neural integrator of the oculomotor system from brain stem lesions in monkey. *Journal of Neurophysiology.* 1987;57(5):1383–1409.
34. Henn V, Straumann D, Hess BJM, Hepp K, Vilis T, Reisine H. Generation of vertical and torsional rapid eye movement in the rostral mesencephalon: Experimental data and clinical implications. *Acta Oto-Laryngologica.* 1991;111(sup481):191–193.
35. Crawford JD, Vilis T. Symmetry of oculomotor burst neuron coordinates about Listing's plane. *Journal of Neurophysiology.* 1992;68(2):432–448.
36. Crawford JD. The oculomotor neural integrator uses a behavior-related coordinate system. *Journal of Neuroscience.* 1994;14(11):6911–6923.
37. Klier EM, Wang H, Constantin AG, Crawford JD. Midbrain control of three-dimensional head orientation. *Science.* 2002;295(5558):1314–1316.
38. Shaikh AG, Zee DS, Crawford JD, Jinnah HA. Cervical dystonia: A neural integrator disorder. *Brain.* 2016;139(10):2590–2599.
39. Bharmauria V, Sajad A, Yan X, Wang H, Crawford JD. Spatiotemporal coding in the macaque supplementary eye fields: Landmark influence in the target-to-gaze transformation. *Eneuro.* 2021;8(1).
40. Sadeh M, Sajad A, Wang H, Yan X, Crawford JD. Spatial transformations between superior colliculus visual and motor response fields during head-unrestrained gaze shifts. *European Journal of Neuroscience.* 2015;42(11):2934–2951.
41. Sajad A, Sadeh M, Keith GP, Yan X, Wang H, Crawford JD. Visual-motor transformations within frontal eye fields during head-unrestrained gaze shifts in the monkey. *Cerebral Cortex.* 2015;25(10):3932–3952.
42. Sajad A, Sadeh M, Yan X, Wang H, Crawford JD. Transition from target to gaze coding in primate frontal eye field during memory delay and memory-motor transformation. *Eneuro.* 2016;3(2).
43. Smalianchuk I, Jagadisan UK, Gandhi NJ. Instantaneous midbrain control of saccade velocity. *Journal of Neuroscience.* 2018;38(47):10,156–10,167.
44. Sparks DL, Mays LE. Signal transformations required for the generation of saccadic eye movements. *Annual Review of Neuroscience.* 1990;13(1):309–336.
45. Klier EM, Crawford JD. Human oculomotor system accounts for 3-D eye orientation in the visual-motor transformation for saccades. *Journal of Neurophysiology.* 1998;80(5):2274–2294.
46. Sparks DL, Nelson IS. Sensory and motor maps in the mammalian superior colliculus. *Trends in Neurosciences.* 1987;10(8):312–317.
47. Klier EM, Wang H, Crawford JD. The superior colliculus encodes gaze commands in retinal coordinates. *Nature Neuroscience.* 2001;4(6):627–632.
48. DeSouza JFX, Keith GP, Yan X, Blohm G, Wang H, Crawford JD. Intrinsic reference frames of superior colliculus visuomotor receptive fields during head-unrestrained gaze shifts. *Journal of Neuroscience.* 2011;31(50):18,313–18,326.
49. Smith MA, Crawford JD. Distributed population mechanism for the 3-D oculomotor reference frame transformation. *Journal of Neurophysiology.* 2005;93(3):1742–1761.
50. Van Opstal AJ, Hepp K, Suzuki Y, Henn V. Influence of eye position on activity in monkey superior colliculus. *Journal of Neurophysiology.* 1995;74(4):1593–1610.
51. Van Opstal AJ, Hepp K, Hess BJ, Straumann D, Henn V. Two rather than three-dimensional representation of saccades in monkey supeior colliculus. *Science.* 1991;252(5010):1313–1315.
52. Klier EM, Wang H, Crawford JD. Three-dimensional eye-head coordination is implemented downstream from the superior colliculus. *Journal of Neurophysiology.* 2003;89(5):2839–2853.
53. Pathmanathan JS, Presnell R, Cromer JA, Cullen KE, Waitzman DM. Spatial characteristics of neurons in the central mesencephalic reticular formation (cMRF) of head-unrestrained monkeys. *Experimental Brain Research.* 2006;168(4):455–470.
54. Quaia C, Lefèvre P, Optican LM. Model of the control of saccades by superior colliculus and cerebellum. *Journal of Neurophysiology.* 1999;82(2):999–1018.
55. Van Opstal AJ, Hepp K, Suzuki Y, Henn V. Role of monkey nucleus reticularis tegmenti pontis in the stabilization of Listing's plane. *Journal of Neuroscience.* 1996;16(22):7284–7296.
56. Straumann D, Zee DS, Solomon D. Three-dimensional kinematics of ocular drift in humans with cerebellar atrophy. *Journal of Neurophysiology.* 2000;83(3):1125–1140.
57. Crawford JD, Tweed DB, Vilis T. Static ocular counterroll is implemented through the 3-D neural integrator. *Journal of Neurophysiology.* 2003;90(4):2777–2784.
58. Blohm G, Crawford JD. Computations for geometrically accurate visually guided reaching in 3-D space. *Journal of Vision.* 2007;7(5):4.
59. Daddaoua N, Dicke PW, Thier P. Eye position information is used to compensate the consequences of ocular torsion on V1 receptive fields. *Nature Communications.* 2014;5(1):1–9.
60. Khazali MF, Ramezanpour H, Thier P. V1 neurons encode the perceptual compensation of false torsion arising from Listing's law. *Proceedings of the National Academy of Sciences.* 2020;117(31):18,799–18,809.
61. Medendorp WP, Smith MA, Tweed DB, Crawford JD. Rotational remapping in human spatial memory during eye and head motion. *Journal of Neuroscience.* 2002;22(1):RC196.
62. Murdison TS, Blohm G, Bremmer F. Saccade-induced changes in ocular torsion reveal predictive orientation perception. *Journal of Vision.* 2019;19(11):10.
63. Ruiz-Ruiz M, Martinez-Trujillo JC. Human updating of visual motion direction during head rotations. *Journal of Neurophysiology.* 2008;99(5):2558–2576.
64. Helmchen C, Rambold H, Kempermann J, Büttner-Ennever JA, Büttner U. Localizing value of torsional nystagmus in small midbrain lesions. *Neurology.* 2002;59(12):1956–1964.
65. Leigh RJ, Zee DS. *The neurology of eye movements.* Contemporary Neurology Series. Oxford: Oxford University Press; 2015.
66. Schreiber K, Crawford JD, Fetter M, Tweed D. The motor side of depth vision. *Nature.* 2001;410(6830):819–822.
67. Blohm G, Khan AZ, Ren L, Schreiber KM, Crawford JD. Depth estimation from retinal disparity requires eye and head orientation signals. *Journal of Vision.* 2008;8(16):3.
68. Bergamin O, Zee DS, Roberts DC, Landau K, Lasker AG, Straumann D. Three-dimensional Hess screen test with binocular dual search coils in a three-field magnetic system. *Investigative Ophthalmology & Visual Science.* 2001;42(3):660–667.
69. Wong AMF. *Eye Movement Disorders.* Oxford: Oxford University Press; 2008.
70. Wong AMF, Sharpe JA, Tweed D. Adaptive neural mechanism for Listing's law revealed in patients with fourth nerve palsy. *Investigative Ophthalmology & Visual Science.* 2002;43(6):1796–1803.
71. Snyder LH. Coordinate transformations for eye and arm movements in the brain. *Current Opinion in Neurobiology.* 2000;10(6):747–754.

Production and Flow of Aqueous Humor

W. Daniel Stamer, Paul L. Kaufman, and Nicholas A. Delamere

INTRODUCTION

Intraocular pressure (IOP) is an essential feature of the eye. It influences the shape and curvature of the globe, thus indirectly affecting the eye's optical performance. The pressure is the result of the continuous entry of fluid, aqueous humor, into the eye and the hydraulic resistance that restricts its exit. The value for normal IOP is often given as approximately 15 mmHg, but it is more appropriate to consider a normal range, which in humans is from 10 to 21 mmHg. This reflects individual differences and the fact that IOP is higher in the day and lower at night. This fluctuation is primarily due to aqueous humor inflow following a circadian rhythm.

The flow of aqueous humor though the anterior eye provides nutrients to the avascular trabecular meshwork (TM), cornea, and lens. The latter two are adapted for transparency and thus optical performance. The anterior and posterior chambers are filled with clear aqueous humor and are important parts of the eye's light path. In fact, the overall refractive power of the eye is influenced by the refractive index of the aqueous humor (1.33332), more specifically the refractive index difference at the cornea–aqueous humor interface, and the aqueous humor–lens interface[1-3]. As a transparent and colorless liquid, aqueous humor is different in composition from plasma. Owing to its ultra-low protein content and cell-free composition, aqueous humor has the required optical properties of light transmittance in the visible spectrum with low scatter.

Aqueous humor is formed by the ciliary processes, which are located at the posterior of the iris root. The fluid enters the posterior chamber and flows across the anterior surface of the lens. It passes through the pupil into the anterior chamber, in which there is evidence of convective mixing that follows a pattern of downward fluid movement close to the cornea, where evaporation causes the temperature to be cooler, and upward movement near the iris, where the temperature is warmer[4]. To exit the eye, a large fraction of aqueous humor fluid passes through the TM at the anterior chamber angle, then into Schlemm's canal (SC), driven by the hydrostatic pressure force of IOP. Hydrostatic pressure also causes a significant amount of fluid to exit by seeping through extracellular spaces in the iris root, ciliary muscle, and other uveal structures. This is termed unconventional outflow. The pathways of aqueous humor flow are shown schematically in Figs. 10.1 and 10.2.

Aqueous humor production is a good example of homeostasis. Whereas aqueous humor inflow is influenced by factors such as age and exercise, the rate of aqueous humor formation is remarkably stable[5]. In a study of 300 normal volunteers aged 5 to 83 years, the age-related decline in aqueous flow was found to be minor, although a detectable decline occurs in humans over 65 years of age[5-7]. There is no age-related decline in aqueous humor formation in rhesus monkeys 25 to 29 years of age (human equivalent 62–73 years) compared with those 3 to 10 years or 19 to 23 years of age[8].

STRUCTURE OF THE CILIARY BODY AND CILIARY EPITHELIUM

The ciliary body is a secretory tissue, as well as the location of the ciliary muscle and the anchor for the zonules that support the lens[9]. The surface of the ciliary body is structured in a way that provides a large surface area for fluid production. The surface that faces the aqueous humor is folded to form multiple radially oriented ridges, ciliary processes[10]. The ridges are most pronounced anteriorly in the *pars plicata* region, and less well defined in the *pars plana* region of the ciliary body near the retina. The ridges, as well as the valleys in between, are covered with a unique epithelial formation, a bilayer made of two entirely different epithelial cell types. The nonpigmented ciliary epithelium cell layer (NPE) that faces the aqueous humor is developmentally related to the neural retina. The pigmented ciliary epithelium cell layer (PE) underneath is developmentally related to the retinal pigment epithelium. As the name indicates, PE cells contain black pigment granules. Nonpigmented cells are larger and contain a greater number of mitochondria than pigmented cells, which indicates higher metabolic activity in the nonpigmented cell layer. The architecture of the ciliary epithelium is unique. The two cell types are arranged with their apical surfaces touching. Thus, the apical-basolateral orientation of the pigmented ciliary epithelium aligns with the orientation of the retinal pigment epithelium. The basolateral surface of the NPE faces the aqueous humor and displays a high degree of invagination[11]. This infolding of basolateral plasma membrane of the nonpigmented ciliary epithelium is another specialization that equips the ciliary body with a large surface area. Together, the ridges and valleys of the ciliary processes and the invaginations on the surface of each nonpigmented ciliary epithelial cell provide a huge surface for the ion transport mechanisms that power fluid production.

The ciliary epithelium bilayer is draped over an elaborate network of blood vessels that occupies the interior of the ciliary processes. In broad terms, the ciliary epithelium forms aqueous humor by modifying blood plasma in various ways. It follows that the rate of aqueous

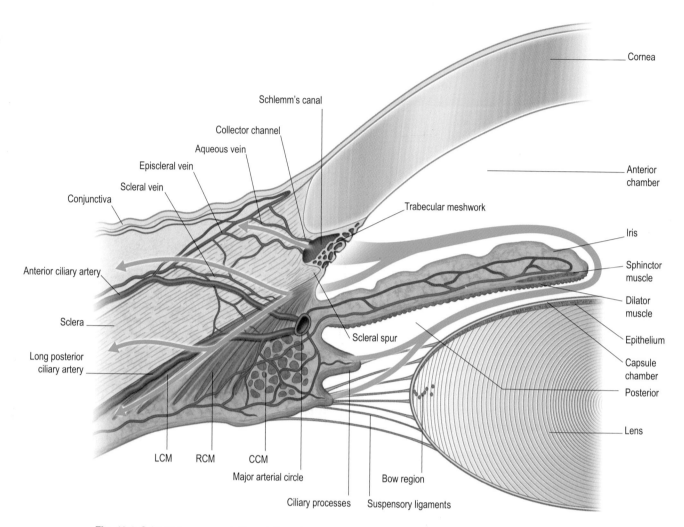

Fig. 10.1 Schematic representation of the primate anterior ocular segment. *Green arrows* indicate aqueous humor flow pathways. Aqueous humor is formed by the ciliary processes, enters the posterior chamber, flows through the pupil into the anterior chamber, and exits at the chamber angle via the conventional and unconventional routes. *CCM*, Circular ciliary muscle; *LCM*, longitudinal ciliary muscle; *RCM*, radial ciliary muscle. (From Kaufman PL, Wiedman T, Robinson JR. Cholinergics. In: Sears ML, ed. *Pharmacology of the Eye: Handbook of Experimental Pharmacology*. Berlin: Springer-Verlag; 1984. Reproduced with kind permission of Springer Science + Business Media.)

humor production is dependent, to an extent, on the rate of blood flow to the ciliary body. Importantly, blood flow is subject to regulation. Throughout the body, factors such as norepinephrine and certain prostaglandins cause blood vessels to constrict, while other factors such as nitric oxide bring about relaxation. Blood vessel diameter is governed by the balance between relaxing factors and constricting factors. Using a microcasting technique, investigators studying blood flow within the ciliary processes demonstrated vasoconstriction in eyes treated with catecholamines[12]. Freddo has suggested that blood flow in the ciliary body microvasculature is under regional control because there are reports of localized constrictions[13]. Unlike the capillaries that serve the ciliary muscle, the capillaries in the ciliary process are fenestrated and leaky. Studies using horseradish peroxidase as a tracer demonstrate the permeability of the capillaries to macromolecules, and presumably ions and water[14]. In effect, the permeability barrier is the ciliary epithelium, not the ciliary body microvasculature.

AQUEOUS HUMOR COMPOSITION

The ciliary body defines the composition of aqueous humor, as well as its rate of formation. Large macromolecules in the ciliary body stroma are unable to diffuse across the ciliary epithelium. As a consequence, the most obvious difference between the composition of aqueous humor and plasma is the low protein concentration in the aqueous humor (200 times less than plasma, Table 10.1) ([15–17] #1071, [18]). There may be slight regional differences in protein concentration. For example, in the peripheral portion of the anterior chamber, close to the TM, the protein concentration may be higher than in the more central region because of protein entry directly from the peripheral iris, as demonstrated in monkey and human eyes[19–21]. Owing to its contact with multiple specialized tissues in the anterior eye, proteomic analysis of aqueous humor biomarkers has the potential to provide insights into disease mechanisms[22]. As mentioned previously, low protein

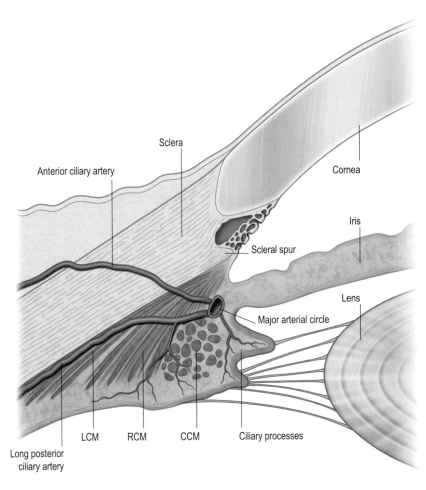

Fig. 10.2 (**A**) Blood supply to the ciliary processes. *CCM*, Circular ciliary muscle; *LCM*, longitudinal ciliary muscle; *RCM*, radial ciliary muscle. (**B**) Vascular architecture in the human ciliary body. *1*, Perforating branches of the anterior ciliary arteries; *2*, major arterial circle of iris; *3*, first vascular territory. The second vascular territory is depicted in *4a*, marginal route, and *4b*, capillary network in the center of this territory. *5*, Third vascular territory; *6* and *7*, arterioles to the ciliary muscle; *8*, recurrent choroidal arteries. (From Funk R, Rohen JW. Scanning electron microscopic study on the vasculature of the human anterior eye segment, especially with respect to the ciliary processes. *Exp Eye Res.* 1990;51(6):651–661. https://doi.org/10.1016/0014-4835(90)90049-Z.)

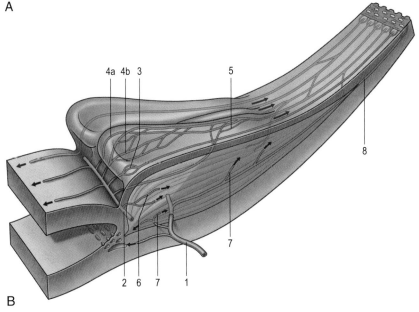

concentration makes for efficient light transmission through the aqueous humor. When the protein concentration rises much above its normal 20 mg/100 mL[23], as in uveitis, the resultant light scattering (Tyndall effect) makes the slit-lamp beam visible as it traverses the anterior chamber (a phenomenon known as "flare").

In humans and many other species, a particularly striking feature of aqueous humor composition is its high ascorbate concentration (Table 10.1). In guinea pigs the aqueous humor ascorbate concentration is almost 60 times that of plasma[24]; in humans the concentration is 20 times higher[24,25]. The high ascorbate concentration likely protects

TABLE 10.1   Composition of aqueous humor

Concentration (mmol/kg H₂O)	Rabbit			Human	
	Anterior aqueous humor	Posterior aqueous humor	Plasma	Aqueous humor	Plasma
Na⁺	138	159	143	163	146
K⁺	4.3	4.7	4.6		
Cl⁻	101	97	108	134	109
HCO₃⁻	30	34	25	20	28
Ascorbate	1.1	1.4	0.04	1.06	0.04
Lactate	9.3	9.9	10.3		
Glucose	6	6	6	3	6

Data from Macknight AD, McLaughlin CW, Peart D, Purves RD, Carré DA, Civan MM. Formation of the aqueous humor. *Clin Exp Pharmacol Physiol.* 2000;27(1–2):100–106.

the anterior ocular structures from ultraviolet light–induced oxidative damage[26,27]. In addition to being an antioxidant, ascorbate may regulate structure and function of the TM[28], and may partially absorb ultraviolet radiation[29]. Extensive and repeated oxidative stress in vivo may result in reduced TM cell adhesion, leading to TM cell loss, which is associated with glaucomatous conditions[30,31]. It is noteworthy that diurnal mammals have approximately 35 times the concentration of aqueous ascorbate compared with nocturnal mammals[32,33].

The high concentration of ascorbate in aqueous humor reflects active transport by the ciliary epithelium[34–36]. In mammalian cells, ascorbic acid, the reduced form, is transported by the sodium dependent L-ascorbic acid transporters SLC23A2 and SLC23A1, whereas the oxidized form, dehydro-ascorbic acid, is transported by the dehydro-ascorbic acid, is transported by the family of facilitated glucose transporters[37]. SLC23A2 is expressed in the PE of human donor eyes but is absent in mouse, a nocturnal species[38]. Diminished ascorbate levels in the aqueous humor have been observed in subjects with various forms of glaucoma, and a single-nucleotide polymorphism (SNP) in *SLC23A2* is associated with a higher risk of primary open-angle glaucoma (POAG)[39].

The concentration of glucose, urea, and nonprotein nitrogen is reportedly slightly lower in aqueous humor than in plasma, while there is an excess of Cl⁻ and certain amino acids[1,2,40] (Table 10.1). MicroRNAs are detectable in aqueous humor[41], likely protected by extracellular nanovesicles known as exosomes[42]. It has been suggested that these endogenous noncoding RNAs might have a role in signaling between cells, and there is interest in whether they may also serve as disease biomarkers[43–45]. Oxygen levels are low in the aqueous humor, and there are differences between pO₂ in various regions of the anterior and posterior chamber[46,47]. Lactate concentration is high in the aqueous, presumably because of glycolytic activity of the lens, cornea, and other ocular structures[23,48].

Physiology of aqueous humor formation

Kiel and colleagues[49] eloquently summarized aqueous humor formation as a three-stage process: (1) delivery of water, ions, proteins, and metabolic fuel by the ciliary circulation, (2) ultrafiltration and diffusion from the capillaries into the stroma under the influence of oncotic pressure, hydrostatic pressure, and concentration gradients, and (3) active ion transport across the ciliary epithelium followed by water movement down the resultant osmotic gradient into the posterior chamber. The hydrostatic pressure driving force for ultrafiltration across the ciliary epithelium is diminished by an opposing oncotic pressure gradient due to the relative lack of protein in aqueous humor compared with the ciliary process stroma[50]. Put simply, aqueous humor production

involves diffusion and ultrafiltration but is fundamentally an active process requiring the expenditure of metabolic energy[3]. Active transport of sodium ions into the posterior chamber by the NPE results in water movement from the stromal pool into the posterior chamber. There is general agreement that under normal conditions active secretion accounts for perhaps 80% to 90% of total aqueous humor formation[51–54]. The observation that moderate alterations in systemic blood pressure and ciliary process blood flow have relatively little effect on aqueous humor formation rate supports this notion[54,55]. Furthermore, Bill[56] noted that the hydrostatic and oncotic forces that exist across the ciliary epithelium (between the posterior aqueous humor and the ciliary body stroma) favor resorption, not ultrafiltration-mediated production, of aqueous humor. Active secretion is essentially pressure-insensitive at near-physiologic IOP. However, the ultrafiltration component of aqueous humor formation is sensitive to changes in IOP, decreasing with increasing IOP. This phenomenon is quantifiable and is termed facility of inflow, or pseudofacility, the latter because a pressure-induced decrease in inflow will appear as an increase in outflow when techniques such as tonography and constant-pressure perfusion are used to measure outflow facility ([57–62] #1072). Although measurements vary, pseudofacility in the noninflamed monkey and human eye constitute a very small percentage of total facility[60,61,63–67]. Recently it has been argued that fluid transport rates exhibited by the ciliary epithelia may not be sufficient to account for the rate of aqueous humor formation and there may be some contribution from fluid directly entering the anterior chamber across the anterior surface of the iris[68,69].

In most mammalian species, the turnover number for aqueous humor in the anterior chamber is approximately 0.01 to 0.015 per minute, that is, the rate of aqueous humor formation and drainage is approximately 1% to 1.5% of the anterior chamber volume per minute[51,60,61,70]. This is true also in the normal human eye, in which the aqueous formation rate is approximately 2.5 μL per minute[5,7,71]. Several studies have provided comprehensive theoretical analyses of the fluid mechanics of aqueous production and can be found elsewhere[3,49,68,72–76].

Aqueous humor as a secretion

If aqueous humor was formed simply by ultrafiltration of plasma, the concentrations of ions in aqueous humor would fit the predictions of a Gibbs-Donnan equilibrium, but this is not the case[1,2]. In fact, aqueous humor contains a slight excess of sodium, as active fluid secretion is powered by Na,K-ATPase in the ciliary epithelium (Table 10.1). Na,K-ATPase transports Na⁺ ions from the NPE into the posterior chamber and establishes ion gradients that support the coordinated activity of several different ion transporters and channels arranged at specific locations in the two cell layers of the bilayer (detailed further in chapter).

The architecture of the ciliary epithelium is unique[77]. The bilayer consists of the PE facing the ciliary stroma and the NPE facing the aqueous humor. The cells are extensively coupled via connexin (Cx) gap junctions, forming a syncytium-like structure. In rabbit and rat, Cx50 is found in the NPE layer while Cx43 is abundant in the region where the NPE-PE apical surfaces touch[78], although other connexins might also be expressed[79]. Neighboring cells in each layer are coupled and the two cell layers are connected to each other at their apical membranes[80]. Tight junctions are present between the apical borders of NPE cells, where they form a barrier that restricts paracellular diffusion[13,14]. It should be kept in mind that the functional properties of tight junctions, as well as gap junctions, are subject to dynamic regulation. The ciliary epithelium is a living barrier that can sense and respond to external stimuli.

The process of fluid secretion is mediated via active transport of ions across the bilayer[81]. Two enzymes abundantly present in the NPE are intimately involved in this process: Na,K-ATPase and carbonic anhydrase (CA)[11,82-87]. Na,K-ATPase is found predominantly bound to the plasma membrane of the basolateral infoldings of the NPE[11,51,83,84,88].

Primary active transport by Na,K-ATPase establishes a Na+ concentration gradient across the plasma membrane of the coupled NPE and PE cells. The NPE is particularly rich in Na,K-ATPase and is one of few cell types that expresses the α1, α2, α3, β1, and β2 isoforms[89]. The pattern of Na,K-ATPase isoform expression suggests functional differences between the *pars plana* and *pars plicata*[90]. Other ions and molecules are transported by secondary active transport mechanisms that use the Na+ gradient as a driving force. Thus, aqueous humor in humans exhibits increased levels of Na+ and C− compared with plasma[1,2,91]. The bilayered epithelium has Na+-coupled transporters for some amino acids, L-ascorbic acid, glucose transporters, and Cl−/HCO3− exchange

transporters[92,93]. Another ATPase, an H+-ATPase proton pump, has also been detected in the NPE basolateral surface[94,95], and other solute transporters have been detected by single cell–RNA sequencing analysis[96]. To maintain electroneutrality, anions must accompany the actively secreted Na+. It is thought that Cl− passes through chloride channels in the basolateral membrane and HCO3− can enter aqueous via exchange with Cl−. Gap junctions permit diffusion between the cell layers, enabling transporters in the NPE and PE to operate in a coordinated manner to pass solutes across the bilayer. The principal function of the ciliary epithelium, net transport of solutes and water in a blood to aqueous direction, is dependent on the specific localization of transporters and channels on either the stromal-facing or aqueous humor–facing surfaces of the bilayer. A simplified scheme is shown in Fig. 10.3. Based on studies in the rabbit, it has been proposed that the arrangement of transporters and channels in the anterior of the ciliary processes is different and this part of the ciliary body might absorb solutes and fluid[97]. If this is the case, stimulation of reabsorption would have the effect of reducing the rate of net aqueous humor formation, and thereby IOP.

Selective inhibition of Na+-K+-ATPase activity by cardiac glycosides (e.g., ouabain) significantly reduces the rate of aqueous humor formation and IOP in experimental animals and humans[82,98-103], consistent with the notion that active transport of Na+ is the primary driving force for the secretion of aqueous humor. Vanadate, a different Na,K-ATPase inhibitor was also found to reduce aqueous humor formation[99,104-107] although later studies suggest it might inhibit additional mechanisms[35,36,108-110]. The activity of Na,K-ATPase activity in the NPE may be subject to endogenous regulation by protein kinase signaling pathways that are activated by nitric oxide, cAMP, cytoplasmic calcium, insulin, and other factors[111-114].

The metabolically driven, ATP-dependent active transport of Na+ by Na,K-ATPase, and the accompanying movement of anions, creates

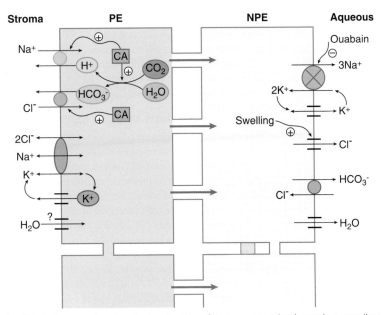

Fig. 10.3 A simplified diagram showing the localization of transport mechanisms that contribute to transepithelial solute and water movement across the ciliary epithelium during aqueous humor formation. The flow of aqueous humor occurs in the PE-to-NPE direction. Pigmented epithelium (*PE*) and nonpigmented epithelium (*NPE*) cells are coupled by gap junctions and function in the manner of a syncytium. Na,K-ATPase activity is highest at the basolateral, aqueous humor–facing, surface of the NPE. The scheme, which has been simplified for clarity, is modified from Charles W. McLaughlin CW, Zellhuber-McMillan S, Macknight ADC, Civan MM. Electron microprobe analysis of rabbit ciliary epithelium indicates enhanced secretion posteriorly and enhanced absorption anteriorly. *Am J Physiol Cell Physiol.* 2007;293:C1455-C1466. (Used with permission.)

an osmotic force that drives the osmotic movement of water across the invaginated basolateral surface of the NPE cells[115]. The theoretical basis for coupling the flow of ions and water is described elsewhere[116]. The movement of water is facilitated by water channels, aquaporins AQP1 and AQP4, in NPE cells[117–120]. AQP1 null mice have decreased IOP and aqueous humor production compared to normal[120,121]. Na^+ and Cl^- enter the bilayer via the basolateral surface of the PE cells. This involves transport by Na^+/H^+ and Cl^-/HCO_3^- exchange transporters and the Na-K-2Cl cotransporter. It follows that inhibition or activation of the various transporters and channels in the ciliary epithelium bilayer can alter the rate of formation of aqueous humor[97,122,123]. The contribution of anion transport, particularly HCO_3^-, is critical but far from straightforward because it is not the same in all species[1,2,123,124]. HCO_3^- transport is intimately linked to CA enzymes[113,114,124–126]. Transport of another anion, Cl^-, also plays an important role in the aqueous humor formation[102,127–129]. In isolated bovine eyes, the principal mechanisms responsible for aqueous humor formation are Na,K-ATPase-mediated active transport and chloride transport[102]. In rabbit preparations, the transfer of Cl^- ions is enhanced by agonists of A3 adenosine receptors[122]. A3 adenosine receptor agonists and antagonists, respectively, increase and lower IOP in mice[130]. Bestrophin-2, a protein that regulates Ca^{2+}-activated Cl^- conductance, is localized to the NPE, suggesting that it may play a role in regulating aqueous humor formation. Mice deficient in bestrophin-2 have significantly diminished IOP[131].

In bovine eyes in vitro, 4,4′-diisothiocyanatostilbene-2,2′-disulfonic acid (DIDS, an inhibitor of the Cl^-/HCO_3^- exchanger, Na-HCO_3 cotransporter, and chloride channels) and 5-nitro-2-(3-phenylpropylamino)-benzoic acid (NPPB, a chloride channel blocker) reduce aqueous humor formation by 55% and 25%, respectively[102]. In mice, topical inhibitors of Na^+H^+ exchange lower IOP[132]. Bumetanide (a specific inhibitor of Na-K-Cl cotransport) and furosemide (a nonspecific anion transport inhibitor) reduce aqueous humor formation by 35% and 45% in bovine eyes in vitro[102]. These transport inhibitors may have both direct and indirect effects on aqueous humor formation as DIDS and Na-H exchange inhibitors are known to activate protein kinase signaling pathways that change Na,K-ATPase activity[111,133]. Because the Na-K-Cl cotransporter can be stimulated by catecholamines (such as epinephrine, norepinephrine, isoproterenol, and dopamine), there was interest in Na-K-Cl inhibition as a strategy to reduce aqueous humor formation[128]. However, topical application of bumetanide to mice[132] or monkeys[134] has no effect on IOP. Because aqueous secretion is an active process, it is not surprising that metabolic inhibitors such as dinitrophenol decrease aqueous humor formation, but none of these has yet been found useful for glaucoma therapy[135].

CA is abundant in the ciliary epithelium and is present both in the cytoplasm and basolateral plasma membranes of the NPE and PE[136–140]. There are multiple CA isoenzymes, and CAII, CAIV, and Carbonic anhydrase XII (CAXII) all are known to be present in the ciliary body[141,142]. CAs catalyze the hydration of CO_2, speeding the conversion of CO_2 and H_2O to carbonic acid and its subsequent dissociation to H^+ and HCO_3^-. This provides the HCO_3^-, which is essential for the active secretion of aqueous humor. CA inhibitors (CAIs) reduce the rate of aqueous humor formation in multiple species, regardless of whether they concentrate HCO_3^- into the aqueous humor. It is likely that inhibition of CA causes a decrease in HCO_3^- anions necessary for outward transport from the NPE along with Na^+ in order to maintain electroneutrality[81]. However, CAIs reduce intracellular pH and this may inhibit Na^+-K^+-ATPase activity in the NPE[113,114,126,143,144], and decrease the driving force for Na-H exchange to import Na^+ from the stroma into the PE[125]. In the case of orally administered CAIs, there is also an impact of systemic acidosis on inhibition of aqueous humor formation[145]. CA inhibitors given systemically can reduce aqueous humor

secretion by up to 50%[48,136,137,146–153] and have been in use for clinical glaucoma therapy for over 50 years[48,145,147]. For CAIs to be effective, over 99% of the CA activity must be inhibited and it was once thought that the topical CA inhibitor penetration to the ciliary epithelium would not be able to produce the required degree of CA inhibition. Fortunately, there are now available topically effective CA inhibitors such as dorzolamide[154–158] and brinzolamide[155,159,160] that achieve substantial (albeit usually not quite as much) reduction in IOP as the earlier oral CA inhibitors but without their systemic side effects[145,158,161].

Coordination between the pigmented and nonpigmented epithelium

The NPE and PE work in a coordinated manner to form aqueous humor. The PE is specialized for solute entry while the NPE is specialized for solute exit in terms of transporter expression[162–164]. Solute and water move through the two cells in the bilayer, and Brubaker calculated that a ciliary epithelial cell transports the equivalent of 30% of its own volume every minute[5]. Clearly, the cells are at risk of swelling or shrinkage if there were to be a mismatch between the entry and exit of water that flows through the bilayer. It has been proposed that in corneal endothelium, as well as ciliary epithelium, transepithelial fluid transport might be associated with cell volume oscillation with pulsatile water entry and exit[116,164]. It is possible that certain mechanosensitive ion channels, TRPV4 and TRPV1, have a role in maintenance of cell volume homeostasis in the bilayer[165]. Jo and coworkers[166] observed swelling-induced calcium responses in NPE but not PE. TRPV4 inhibition prevented the swelling-induced calcium responses, and they were absent in TRPV4 knockout mice. Some responses to TRPV4 channel activation are thought to involve the opening of hemichannels formed by unpaired connexins[167] and there is evidence for such hemichannels at the aqueous humor–facing surface of the ciliary epithelium bilayer[168]. The TRPV4 agonist GSK1016790A reduces IOP and TRPV4 knockout mice have elevated IOP[169]. However, IOP is normal in TRPV4 knockout mice[170]. Interpretation of IOP responses is far from straightforward because TRPV4 activation has an influence on both aqueous formation and drainage. TRPV4 has a role in regulating function of the TM and SC[171–173]. In studies on the different IOP responses to systemic and topical administration of a TRPV4 antagonist, HC067047, a mechanistic link between TRPV4 and the primary cilium in TM cells has been considered important[169,170].

Blood-aqueous barrier

Tight junctions between adjacent NPE cells make the ciliary epithelium bilayer a physical barrier. The blood-aqueous barrier is a broader functional concept invoked to explain the very limited ability of large molecules such as proteins to pass from the circulation into the aqueous humor. For present purposes, the blood-aqueous barrier comprises the tight junctions of the ciliary process NPE, the inner wall endothelium of SC, the iris vasculature, and the outward directed–active transport systems of the ciliary processes[174]. Tight junctions prevent plasma protein leakage across the iridial vascular endothelium[175–177] although there may be limited diffusion into the iris stroma from the ciliary body[14]. Tight junctions in the posterior iris epithelium prevent protein diffusing from the iris to the posterior chamber[14,175,176]. The capillaries of the ciliary processes and choroid are fenestrated and thus leaky, but tight junctions in the NPE constitute an effective barrier to diffusion[23,175,176,178–187]. The endothelia of the inner wall of SC prevent retrograde movement of solutes and fluid from the canal lumen into the TM and anterior chamber[175,176,188].

Trauma, certain pathologic conditions, and some drugs, cause breakdown of the blood-aqueous barrier (Table 10.2)[174]. This allows plasma components to enter the aqueous humor. Net fluid movement

TABLE 10.2 Factors that disrupt the blood-aqueous barrier

I. Traumatic	II. Pathophysiologic	III. Pharmacologic
A. Mechanical	A. Vasodilation	A. Melanocyte-stimulating hormone
• Paracentesis	1. Histamine	B. Nitrogen mustard
• Corneal abrasion	2. Sympathectomy	C. Cholinergic drugs, especially cholinesterase inhibitors
• Blunt trauma	B. Corneal and intraocular infections	D. Plasma hyperosmolality
• Intraocular surgery	C. Intraocular inflammation	
• Stroking of the iris	D. Prostaglandins (varies with type, dose, and species)	
B. Physical	E. Anterior segment ischemia	
• Radiotherapy		
• Nuclear radiation		
C. Chemical		
• Alkali		
• Irritants (e.g., nitrogen mustard)		

Modified from Stamper RL. Aqueous humor: secretion and dynamics. In Tasman W, Jaeger EA, eds. *Clinical Ophthalmology, Vol 2.* Philadelphia: Lippincott; 1979.

from blood to aqueous increases, but so does its IOP dependence (pseudofacility)[189]. Total facility, as measured by IOP-altering techniques, cannot distinguish pseudofacility from total outflow facility (C_{tot}) and therefore erroneously records the pseudofacility component as increased C_{tot}, therefore underestimating the extent to which the outflow pathways have been compromised by the insult. Under these circumstances, increased pseudofacility provides some protection against a precipitous rise in IOP; as IOP rises, aqueous inflow by ultrafiltration is partly suppressed, blunting (but not completely suppressing) further IOP elevation[60,187]. Additionally, the inflammatory process that occurs during blood–aqueous barrier breakdown leads to a reduction in active secretion of aqueous humor, possibly via interference with active transport mechanisms[71,190]. This in turn may actually produce ocular hypotony, despite compromised conventional outflow pathways (due to plasma protein blockage of the TM). Prostaglandin release during inflammation may contribute to the hypotony by increasing aqueous outflow via the unconventional route[191–193]. When the noxious stimulus is removed, however, the ciliary body may recover before the TM, and the resulting normalization of the aqueous humor formation and unconventional outflow rates in the face of still-compromised conventional outflow pathways leads to elevated IOP, as seen from the modified Goldmann equation (Eq. 10.1):

$$IOP = [(AHF - F_u)/C_{trab}] + P_e$$

where IOP = intraocular pressure, AHF = aqueous humor formation rate, F_u = unconventional outflow, C_{trab} = facility of outflow from the anterior chamber via the TM and SC, and P_e = episcleral venous pressure (the pressure against which fluid leaving the anterior chamber via the TM and SC must drain)[194].

Active transport of organic molecules

Xenobiotic transporters evolved as part of a mechanism to clear potentially harmful organic molecules from tissues into the bloodstream for removal by the liver or kidneys. Problems arise because the transporters also carry therapeutic drugs. The aqueous humor compartment, along with other protected sites such as the brain or the placenta, excludes many organic molecules. The ciliary body transports organic molecules from aqueous humor to blood. This is a two-step process driven by multiple xenobiotic transporters that include uptake transporters OAT1,

OAT3, NADC3, and Multidrug resistance protein (MRP) 4, as well as efflux transporters MRP2, p-glycoprotein, and BCRP[195–197]. These mechanisms have exceptionally wide substrate specificity and pose challenges to ocular drug delivery because they extrude therapeutic molecules, as well as toxic molecules, from the eye[195]. For example, penicillin and other antibiotics are actively transported out of the eye. It has been known for some time that prostaglandins are actively transported out of the eye[198–201] and the prostaglandin transporter OATP2A1, also known as PGT, that operates in the ciliary epithelium is able to carry latanoprost, the prostaglandin $F_2\alpha$ analog used for glaucoma therapy[202]. The xenobiotic transport mechanisms in the ciliary epithelium bear a striking resemblance to those in the renal tubules and blood-brain barrier[203]. Because of their obvious influence on drug distribution, their transport kinetics have been extensively characterized[1,2,199,204–212]. However, more research is needed before we understand the normal day-to-day physiologic role of these, and other outwardly-directed transport mechanisms such as the sodium-iodide symporter[210]. The various efflux transporters in ocular tissues are discussed in more detail in Chapter 17.

REGULATION OF AQUEOUS HUMOR FORMATION

The rate of aqueous humor formation is not static (Box 10.1). IOP displays a circadian rhythm that is attributed to diminished production of aqueous humor during sleep[5,213–215]. The reduction of flow during sleep is roughly comparable to the reduction achieved by CAI and β-adrenergic antagonist glaucoma drugs[214]. The nighttime reduction in secretion is related, in large part, to the level of circulating catecholamines and possibly glucocorticoids[216,217]. The understanding that the rate of aqueous humor production is subject to regulation, over the years guided development of several useful IOP-lowering drugs (see Aqueous humor drainage). Circadian patterns are synchronized by the suprachiasmatic nucleus, which resets peripheral clocks by mechanisms that include adrenal glucocorticoids and sympathetic nerves[216–218]. Circadian changes of adenylate cyclase activity are detectable in the ciliary processes[219]. Autonomic regulation of the ciliary epithelium function and, to a lesser extent, blood flow within the ciliary body, influence aqueous humor formation. Sympathetic and parasympathetic nerve terminals in the ciliary body[220–223] arise from branches of the long and short posterior ciliary nerves. These nerve fibers are of both the myelinated and nonmyelinated variety. Parasympathetic fibers originate in the Edinger-Westphal nucleus of the third cranial nerve, run with the inferior division of this nerve in the orbit, and synapse in the ciliary ganglion (Fig. 10.4)[222,224]. Vasodilatory parasympathetic nerve fibers originating in the pterygopalatine ganglion are likely to release nitric oxide and vasoactive intestinal peptide (VIP) in addition to acetylcholine (see Chapter 6). Nerves displaying VIP immunoreactivity are also detected in the ciliary processes, posterior third of the ciliary muscle and around small to medium-sized blood vessels in the posterior uvea of the cat[225]. Relatively few VIP-positive fibers are found in the ciliary processes of humans and monkeys[226]. In the cat eye, nerve fibers containing pituitary adenylate cyclase–activating peptide (PACAP) are detected in the iris, ciliary body, and conjunctiva.

BOX 10.1   Aqueous humor formation

- Aqueous humor production involves diffusion and ultrafiltration but is fundamentally an active process requiring the expenditure of metabolic energy.
- β-Adrenergic antagonists, such as timolol, that lower intraocular pressure (IOP) by decreasing aqueous humor formation, continue to be a mainstay in clinical glaucoma therapy.
- IOP displays a circadian rhythm that is attributed to diminished production of aqueous humor during sleep. There can be differences between the nocturnal and diurnal effectiveness of an IOP-lowering drug.
- α2-Adrenergic agonists such as apraclonidine and brimonidine are powerful ocular hypotensive agents, lowering IOP primarily by decreasing aqueous humor formation.
- In subjects treated with drugs that decrease outflow resistance (e.g., latanoprost), it is possible to obtain additional reduction of daytime IOP by adding carbonic anhydrase isoenzymes (CAIs) and β-adrenergic antagonists that reduce aqueous humor formation.

PACAP immunoreactivity colocalizes with VIP in the sphenopalatine ganglion and with calcitonin gene–related peptide (CGRP) in the trigeminal ganglion[227]. Sympathetic fibers synapse in the superior cervical ganglion and distribute to the muscles and blood vessels of the ciliary body. Stimulation of the cervical sympathetic nerves in vervet monkeys significantly increases the rate of aqueous humor formation[228]. Numerous unmyelinated nerve fibers surround the blood vessels in the stroma of the ciliary processes. These are likely noradrenergic and control vascular tone[23].

Various investigators have studied the consequences of eliminating autonomic input, and the results illustrate a degree of complexity in the control of aqueous formation. Experimental sympathetic denervation in monkeys does not alter resting aqueous humor formation and marginally affects the aqueous humor formation response to timolol or epinephrine[229]. Studies have been done on individuals with Horner's syndrome who have an interruption of sympathetic nerve supply to the eye. In human subjects with unilateral Horner's syndrome, the rate of daytime aqueous humor formation, IOP, tonographic outflow facility, and the flow and IOP response to the β-adrenergic antagonist timolol are similar in both eyes[230]. However, eyes with Horner syndrome show a decrease in aqueous humor formation in response to epinephrine, a combined α- and β-adrenergic agonist, instead of the normal increase. The β-adrenergic agonist isoproterenol, on the other hand, increases flow during sleep in both normal and Horner's syndrome eyes but has no significant effect on flow in either during the day[231]. Chemical sympathectomy with guanethidine sulfate in glaucomatous humans lowers IOP, presumably by reducing aqueous humor production measured indirectly by tonography[232].

The rate of aqueous humor secretion is increased by VIP and PACAP, two structurally related neuropeptides. The stimulation of aqueous formation following intravenous VIP administration in

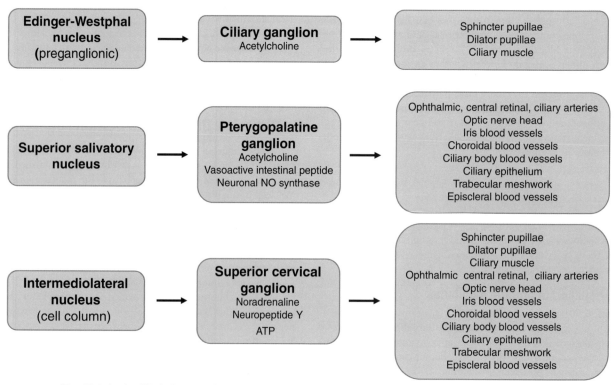

Fig. 10.4 A simplified diagram of the parasympathetic and sympathetic innervation of the eye, showing neurotransmitters and neuropeptides that are generally present in postganglionic neurons. (Modified from McDougal DH and Gamlin PD Autonomic control of the eye. 2015 *Compr. Physiol 5*:439–473.)

monkeys occurs secondary to activation of the sympathetic nervous system, while the effect of intracameral administration of VIP to the eye is a direct effect on the ciliary epithelium[233]. PACAP appears to be slightly more potent than VIP as a stimulator of aqueous humor flow in the monkey[226]. There are still unanswered questions about the role of sympathetic innervation in mediating aqueous inflow responses to pharmacologic agents, and species differences add to the challenge.

Cholinergic control of aqueous humor formation

The effects of cholinergic drugs on the rate of aqueous humor formation, its composition, and on the blood-aqueous barrier, are unclear. Overall, cholinomimetics have little effect on the volumetric rate of aqueous humor formation. In general, cholinergic drugs cause vasodilation in the anterior segment resulting in increased blood flow to the choroid, iris, ciliary processes, and ciliary muscle (see Chapter 11). However cholinergic drugs may also promote vasoconstriction in the rabbit eye[234]. Congestion in the iris and ciliary body is a well-recognized clinical side effect of topical cholinomimetics, especially the anticholinesterases[48]. The presence of flare and cells in the aqueous humor by biomicroscopy indicates that these agents can cause breakdown of the blood-aqueous barrier and perhaps frank inflammation[48]. Pilocarpine increases blood-aqueous barrier permeability to iodide[235] and inulin[236]. Cholinergic drugs may alter the aqueous humor concentration of inorganic ions[237] and the movement of certain amino acids from the blood into the aqueous humor, and may also influence the outward-directed transport systems of the ciliary processes[238,239]. Studies in vitro indicate acetylcholine and carbachol can disrupt the gap junctions that couple PE and NPE cells[240,241]. Because aqueous humor secretion requires the NPE and PE to work together in a coordinated manner, diminished coupling would be likely to contribute to inhibition of aqueous secretion. However, the cholinergic effect on aqueous humor formation appears minor and not entirely consistent across various species. Cholinergic agents or parasympathetic nerve stimulation is reported to elicit a range of responses that include increasing, decreasing, or not altering the aqueous humor formation rate[64,70,242-251]. Under certain conditions, pilocarpine may increase pseudofacility[72,252]. In short, the effects on the rate of aqueous humor formation is likely not a major factor in the drug-induced decrease in IOP that forms the basis of the therapeutic efficacy of pilocarpine in chronic glaucoma; the latter resides in its ability to decrease outflow resistance via its effect on the ciliary muscle[253] (see Aqueous humor drainage).

Adrenergic control of aqueous humor formation

There is still much to be learned regarding the precise role and receptor specificity of adrenergic mechanisms in regulating the rate of aqueous humor formation. At one time it was generally thought that long-term topical administration of epinephrine, a combined α1, α2, β1, β2-adrenergic agonist, decreased the rate of aqueous humor formation[48]. This effect was thought to be mediated by β-adrenergic receptors in the nonpigmented ciliary epithelium, via activation of a membrane adenylate cyclase[8,254,255]. This line of thinking was supported by studies with forskolin, which directly and irreversibly activates intracellular adenylate cyclase. Forskolin was found to decrease the rate of aqueous humor formation when given topically or intravitreally[256-258]. However, fluorophotometric studies show that short-term topical administration of epinephrine increases the rate of aqueous humor formation[229,259,260] as did other adrenergic agonists, including salbutamol[261], isoproterenol (isoprenaline),[231] and terbutaline[262]. These results are consistent with studies showing that β-adrenergic antagonists alter aqueous humor formation[263-265].

The ocular hypotensive action of β-antagonists led to the development of drugs that became mainstays of clinical glaucoma

therapy. Effective drugs include the nonselective β1, β2 antagonists timolol[259,261,266,267], levobunolol[268], and metipranolol[269], the nonselective β1, β2 partial agonist carteolol[270,271], and the relatively β1-selective antagonist betaxolol[272]. However, their pharmacology is not easy to explain. Adrenergic receptors in the ciliary epithelium are of the β2 subtype[273-275], but antagonists that are relatively selective for β1 receptors such as betaxolol are effective (although less potent) in suppressing aqueous humor formation[5,272,276,277]. Nevertheless, the apparent β1 efficacy may be related to a sufficiently high concentration reaching the ciliary epithelium so that nonselective blockade of β2 receptors may occur[278]. There has been some debate as to whether β-adrenergic antagonists suppress aqueous humor formation via their effect on β-adrenergic receptors in the ciliary epithelium. Some studies suggest that classical β-adrenergic receptor blockade may not be involved, and that other receptor types such as $5HT_{1A}$, may be relevant[279]. The reduced rate of aqueous humor formation during sleep[5,214,215] has been linked to the β-arrestin–mediated regulation of the β-adrenergic G-protein–coupled receptors on the ciliary epithelium. β-antagonists produce little additional reduction in aqueous humor formation during sleep[280] or in pentobarbital-anesthetized monkeys[281].

Sympathetic fibers synapse in the superior cervical ganglion and distribute to the muscles and blood vessels of the ciliary body, regulating blood flow to the ciliary process vasculature (Fig. 10.4) (see Chapter 16). Catecholaminergic and Neuropeptide Y (NPY)-ergic nerve fibers preferentially supply the vasculature and epithelium of the monkey anterior ciliary processes, suggesting that they assist in the precise regulation of aqueous humor formation[282]. Stimulation of the cervical sympathetic nerves in vervet monkeys significantly increases the rate of aqueous humor formation[228]. However, the adrenergic tone of the ciliary epithelium may be more influenced by circulating catecholamines than sympathetic innervation. Two major hormones of the adrenal gland, epinephrine and cortisol, can regulate aqueous formation[283]. Moreover, the pattern of aqueous flow in human subjects during sleep and wakefulness correlates with circulating catecholamine levels[217,284]. Autonomic regulation of the ciliary epithelium function is consistent with the observation that ciliary epithelial cells express adrenergic receptors[285]. Coupling between the NPE and PE cell layers likely allows coordination of signal transduction responses[286]. Moreover, adrenergic agents are capable of changing the activity of ion transporters and gap junctions that support fluid secretion across the bilayer[240,241,287-289]. Adrenergic drugs also may exert their effect by causing localized constriction in the arterioles that supply the ciliary processes[290,291].

Topically applied α1-adrenergic agonists and antagonists appear to have little effect on fluorophotometrically determined aqueous humor formation in the normal intact human eye[292,293]. Clonidine, which has both α1-antagonist and α2-agonist properties, decreases aqueous humor formation and ocular blood flow[262,294-296]. Therefore, epinephrine may have a dual effect on aqueous humor formation: stimulation via β-adrenoceptors, and inhibition via α2-adrenoceptors[297-299]. α2-Adrenergic agonists, such as apraclonidine and brimonidine, are powerful ocular hypotensive agents when applied topically. Drugs such as brimonidine (Alphagan), and apraclonidine (Iopidine) lower IOP primarily by decreasing aqueous humor formation[192,193,300-302], although there may be effects on unconventional outflow, and responses in sleeping subject may be different[303,304]. α2-Adrenergic agonists have been found effective when used alone, as well as with other IOP-lowering drugs in fixed combination formulations[305]. For example, a fixed combination of two inflow-reducing drugs, brimonidine and a CAI brinzolamide, was found to have an additive IOP-lowering effect compared with a prostaglandin analog alone[306].

Carbonic anhydrase inhibitor effects on aqueous humor formation

As detailed previously, the physiology of the ciliary epithelium is highly dependent on CA, and CAIs have been used for many decades to reduce the rate of aqueous humor formation and lower IOP. The use of CAIs in the treatment of glaucoma was greatly increased by the development of topically effective CAIs, such as dorzolamide[154–158] and brinzolamide[155,159,160], and the ability to use them in combination therapies with β-blockers and α2-agonists that have different mechanisms of action[307]. Thus, in subjects treated with prostaglandin analog drugs like latanoprost that increase outflow, it is possible to obtain additional reduction of daytime IOP by adding CAIs and β-adrenergic antagonists that reduce aqueous humor formation[305,308].

Other pharmacological strategies

The rate of aqueous humor formation can also be reduced by a wide variety of agents from different drug categories (Table 10.3)[300,309]. This comprises guanylate cyclase activators, natriuretic peptides[310] including atrial natriuretic peptide[311,312], neuropeptides[313], opioid receptor agonists[314], and the nitrovasodilators sodium nitroprusside[315,316], sodium azide[317], and nitroglycerin[315]. Agents that increase cyclic GMP tend to reduce aqueous humor formation. This includes nitric oxide, atrial natriuretic peptide (ANP)[311], brain natriuretic peptide (BNP), and C-type natriuretic peptide (CNP), as well as peptide analogs more suitable for topical administration[310]. It has been proposed that endogenous neuropeptides regulate fluid secretion[313] 8-Bromo cyclic GMP

also reduces the aqueous humor formation rate by 15% to 20% in the monkey[318]. Interactions between pathways are likely. For example, ANP levels are elevated in the aqueous humor of rabbits following application of kappa opioid agonists to reduce aqueous humor formation suppression[319]. Nitric oxide may be involved in mediating the IOP-lowering response to mu3 opioid agonists in rabbits[320–322].

Serotonin (5-hydroxytryptamine (5-HT)) receptors are expressed in the ciliary epithelium and 5-HT agonists have been proposed as IOP-lowering agents[323]. The serotonergic antagonist ketanserin reduces the aqueous humor formation rate in rabbits, cats, and monkeys[324]. Serotonergic receptors of a 5-HT_{1A}-like subtype are reported to exist in the iris-ciliary body of rabbits and humans[279,325,326]. It may be significant that these receptors seem to be activated by timolol and other β-blockers[279]. The 5-HT_{1A} agonist 8-OH-DPAT dose-dependently decreases IOP in normotensive rabbits during light and dark cycles[325,327]. The more selective 5-HT_{1A} agonist flesinoxan also decreases IOP in rabbits[328]. However, the precise nature of the putative 5-HT_{1A}-like receptor subtype in the ciliary epithelium is still in question. Also, IOP and aqueous flow suppression of 5-HT_{1A} receptor agonists in nonhuman primates is variable[329].

The ability of cannabinoids and endocannabinoids to reduce aqueous humor formation has received considerable interest[300,330,331]. It has been known for some time that an active component of marijuana (cannabis), Δ^9-tetrahydrocannabinol, reduces secretion of aqueous in human volunteers[332] when injected intravenously or when inhaled via marijuana smoking. In contrast, topical Δ^9-tetrahydrocannabinol has no effect on the human eye[333,334]. Studies demonstrate the presence of functional CB1 cannabinoid receptors, as well as endogenous

TABLE 10.3   Factors causing reduced aqueous humor secretion

I. General	II. Systemic	III. Local	IV. Pharmacologic	V. Surgical
A. Age	A. Artificial reduction in internal carotid arterial blood flow	A. Increased IOP (pseudo-facility)	A. β-Adrenoceptor antagonists (e.g., timolol, betaxolol, levobunolol, carteolol, metipranolol)	A. Cyclodialysis
B. Diurnal cycle	B. Diencephalic stimulation	B. Uveitis (especially iridocyclitis)	B. Carbonic anhydrase inhibitors	B. Cyclocryothermy
C. Exercise	C. Hypothermia	C. Retinal detachment	C. Nitrovasodilators; atrial natriuretic factor (route and species dependent)	C. Cyclodiathermy
	D. Acidosis	D. Retrobulbar anesthesia	D. 5-HT_{1A} antagonists (e.g., ketanserin)	D. Cyclophotocoagulation
	E. General anesthesia	E. Choroidal detachment	E. DA_2 agonists (e.g., pergolide, lergotrile, bromocriptine)	
			F. α_2-Adrenoceptor agonists (e.g., apraclonidine, brimonidine)	
			G. Opioid agonists	
			H. Δ9-Tetrahydrocannabinol (Δ9 - THC)	
			I. Metabolic inhibitors (e.g., DNP, fluoroacetamide)	
			J. Cardiac glycosides (e.g., ouabain, digoxin)	
			K. Spironolactone	
			L. Plasma hyperosmolality	
			M. cGMP	

cGMP, Cyclic guanosine monophosphate; *DA₂*, dopamine; *DNP*, dinitrophenol; *IOP*, intraocular pressure.
Modified from Stamper RL. Aqueous humor: secretion and dynamics. In Tasman W, Jaeger EA, eds. *Clinical Ophthalmology, Vol. 2*. Philadelphia: Lippincott; 1979.

cannabinoids, in the ciliary processes and TM of human and animal tissue[331,335–338]. Topical application of the cannabinoid receptor agonist, WIN-55-212-2, significantly reduces aqueous humor formation in normal and glaucomatous cynomolgus monkeys[339].

AQUEOUS HUMOR DRAINAGE

Fluid mechanics

The tissues of the anterior chamber angle of the eye normally generate resistance to aqueous humor outflow. In response to the inflow and accumulation of aqueous humor, IOP builds up to the level sufficient to drive fluid across that resistance at the same rate it is produced by the ciliary body; this is the steady-state IOP. In the glaucomatous eye, this resistance is often unusually high, causing elevated IOP. Results from four major clinical trials confirm the value of reducing IOP in patients with ocular hypertension or glaucoma to prevent the onset of glaucoma in the former case, and the progression of disease in the latter[340–343]. Understanding the factors governing normal and abnormal aqueous humor formation, aqueous humor outflow, IOP, and their interrelationships and manipulation is vital in understanding and treating glaucoma.

The factors can be mathematically represented as follows:
- F = flow (μL/min)
- F_{in} = total aqueous humor inflow: human = approximately 2.5 μL per minute[5,7,344].
- F_s = inflow from active secretion
- F_f = inflow from ultrafiltration
- F_{out} = total aqueous humor outflow
- F_{trab} = outflow via the conventional (trabecular) pathway
- F_u = outflow via the unconventional pathway (includes uveoscleral and uveovortex pathways), appears to decrease with age; with older eyes ranging from 0.3 to 1.16 μL/min and younger eyes at 1.64 μL/minute[7,345]
- P = pressure (mmHg)
- P_i = IOP: humans = 16 mmHg[346]
- P_e = episcleral venous pressure: human = approximately 9 mmHg[347–349]
- R = resistance to flow (mmHg $\times$ min/μL)
- C = facility or conductance of flow (μL/min per mmHg) = 1/R
- C_{tot} = total aqueous humor outflow facility: measurements in healthy humans 0.19 to 0.28 μL/min per mmHg[7,350–352]
- C_{trab} = facility of outflow via trabecular pathway: measurements in healthy humans range from 0.21 to 0.27 μl/min per mmHg[215,353,354]
- C_{ps} = facility of inflow, also known as pseudofacility, which reflects the decrease of aqueous humor flow in response to an increase in IOP. In healthy humans, measurement ranges from 0.06 to 0.08 μL/min per mmHg[67,353]. These values for C_{ps} are most likely overestimates: under normal circumstances in a noninflamed eye the phenomenon is negligible[66]; values for the normal monkey measured by a more precise tracer technique are <0.02 μL/min per mmHg[60,61,355].

Then (Eq. 10.2):

$$F_{in} = F_s + F_f$$

$$F_{out} = F_{trab} + F_u$$

$$C_{tot} = C_{trab} + C_{ps}$$

At steady state (Eq. 10.3):

$$F = F_{in} + F_{out}$$

The simplest hydraulic model, represented by the classic Goldmann equation, views aqueous flow as passive nonenergy-dependent bulk fluid movement down a pressure gradient, with aqueous humor leaving the eye only via the trabecular route, where $\Delta P = P_i - P_e$, so that $F = C_{trab}(P_i - P_e)$. This relationship is generally correct, but it is vastly oversimplified. For example, there is good evidence that maintaining outflow resistance is an active process that requires energy[300] such as the maintenance of contractile tone. Wiederholt et al., ($year$)[356] Moreover, because there is no complete endothelial layer covering the anterior surface of the ciliary body and no delimitation of the spaces between the trabecular beams and the spaces between the ciliary muscle bundles[175,176], fluid can pass from the chamber angle into the tissue spaces within the ciliary muscle. These spaces in turn open into the suprachoroid, from which fluid can pass through the sclera or the perivascular/perineural scleral spaces into the episcleral tissues. Some fluid is also drawn osmotically into the vortex veins by the high protein content in the blood of these vessels[357–359]. Along these uveal routes, the fluid mixes with tissue fluid from the ciliary muscle, ciliary processes, and choroid. Thus, this flow pathway may be analogous to lymphatic drainage of tissue fluid in other organs, providing an important means of ridding the eye of potentially toxic tissue metabolites[71,191]. The eye has long been considered to be devoid of lymphatics, but expression of lymphatic markers are present in the ciliary body and muscle[360], having apparent lymphatic flow[361,362]; however their contribution to aqueous humor drainage is unclear.

Flow from the anterior chamber across the TM into SC is pressure-dependent, but drainage via the unconventional pathway is virtually independent of pressure[54,60–62,363,364]. The reasons for the pressure-independence of the unconventional pathway are not entirely clear but might be consequent to the complex nature of the pressure and resistance relationships between the various fluid compartments within the soft intraocular tissues along the route[54]. For instance, pressure in the potential suprachoroidal space (Ps) is directly dependent on IOP, such that at any IOP level, Ps is considerably but constantly less than IOP[54]. Because the pressure gradient between the anterior chamber and suprachoroid is independent of IOP, bulk fluid flow between these compartments will also be IOP-independent. Intraorbital pressure is such that under normal circumstances there is always a positive pressure gradient between the suprachoroidal and intraorbital spaces[54]. Fluid and solutes, including large protein molecules, can easily exit the eye by passing through the spaces surrounding the neural or vascular scleral emissaria or through the scleral substance itself[60,61,365–367]. At very low IOP levels, the net pressure gradient across the unconventional pathways is apparently so low that unconventional drainage decreases[62].

The absence of an outflow gradient from the suprachoroid may contribute to the development of choroidal detachments seen during the ocular hypotony that sometimes follows intraocular surgery[54]. However, other investigators find unconventional outflow to be more pressure-sensitive under certain circumstances[358,368,369]. For example, unconventional outflow may become more sensitive to pressure following prostaglandin treatment[370]. Based on calculations of diffusional transport properties, there is no need for a pressure gradient to drive tracer across the sclera because it can diffuse across on its own[357]. Direct evidence for a uveovortex pathway[358] is demonstrated after perfusion of the anterior chamber with fluorescein, and finding the fluorescein concentration in the vortex veins is higher than in the general circulation. Also, flow across the sclera is pressure-dependent[368]. Uveovortex flow explains the relative insensitivity of the flow to pressure because most of the driving force is the colloidal osmotic pressure of the blood that draws the fluid into these vessels[357]. Clearly, more needs to be learned about this flow pathway. As under normal steady-state conditions, C_{ps} is low compared with C_{trab}, the hydraulics of aqueous dynamics may be reasonably approximated for clinical purposes by (Eq. 10.4):

$$F_{in} = F_{out} = C_{trab}(P_i - P_e) + F_u$$

or rearranged (Eq. 10.5):

$$P_i = P_e(F_{in} - F_u)/C_{trab}$$

Clinically significant increases in inflow occur only in situations involving breakdown of the blood-aqueous barrier. The pressure sensitivity of the ultrafiltration component of aqueous secretion blunts the tendency for IOP to rise under such conditions, that is, C_{ps} is increased. Elevated episcleral venous pressure, such as may occur with arteriovenous communications resulting from congenital malformations or trauma[48] and perhaps, as shown for the first time in one study, in POAG and normal-tension glaucoma[347], causes a nearly mmHg for every mmHg increase in IOP, consistent with the Goldmann equation. Clinically relevant reductions in IOP are produced by decreasing F_{in}

or by increasing C_{trab} and F_u. Pharmacologic agents, particularly vasodilators, also appear to exert a small, but clinically significant effect on P_e.[371]

Anatomy of the conventional outflow pathway

Depending upon age, 70% to 90% of the aqueous in humans leaves the eye through the pressure-dependent[354,363] conventional outflow pathway, which includes the TM, SC, and distal vasculature (aqueous veins, collector channels, and intrascleral venous plexus)[7,350,354]. SC and the TM reside within the internal scleral groove spanning the scleral spur to the ring of Schwalbe's line at the termination of Descemet's membrane. An anterior nonfiltering portion (also called the "insert" region) presents minimal resistance to fluid outflow and can be distinguished from a posterior filtering portion of the meshwork because it does not overlie SC and houses resident TM stem cells. The TM itself consists of three functionally and structurally different parts: the iridic and uveal part, which represents the innermost portion of the TM; the corneoscleral part, which extends between the scleral spur and the cornea; and the juxtacanalicular tissue (JCT, also called the cribriform layer), which lies adjacent to the inner wall of SC (Fig. 10.5)[372–376].

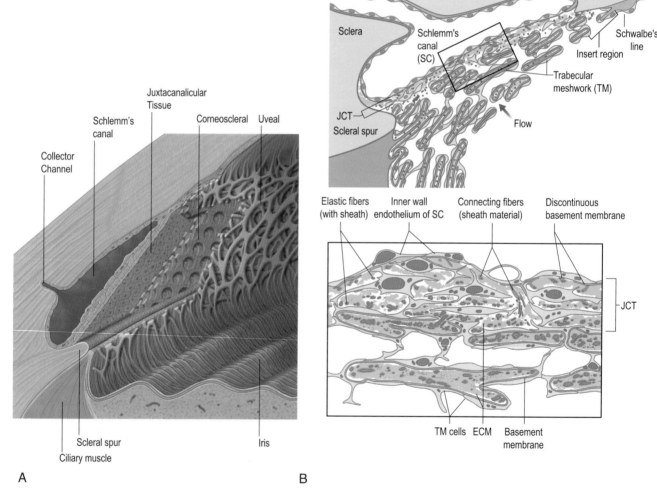

Fig. 10.5 (**A**) Three layers of trabecular meshwork (shown in *cutaway view*): uveal, corneoscleral, and juxtacanalicular tissue (JCT). (From Acott TS, Kelley MJ. Extracellular matrix in the trabecular meshwork. *Exp Eye Res.* 2008;86(4):543–561. https://doi.org/10.1016/j.exer.2008.01.013.) (**B**) Diagram of the outflow pathway and JCT (also called the cribriform region). The upper portion of the figure shows a stylized view of the TM, and the lower inset shows an expanded view of the JCT region. *ECM,* Extracellular matrix. (Funktionelle Anatomie des Nervensystems. Jonannes W. Rohen. 1978. FK Schattauerverlag. Stuttgart. New York.)

With age, the TM changes from being a long, wedge-shaped tissue to having a shorter, rhomboid shape[377]. The scleral spur appears more prominent in older eyes, with the inner TM being more compact. The trabeculae become progressively thickened and extracellular materials appear more abundant and different in appearance, by transmission electron microscopy. Some of these changes are likely a result of decreased cellularity observed in older eyes. Hence, TM cell loss declines in a linear fashion with age and is more severe in the filtration region[378,379]. These structural changes correspond to a decline in outflow facility with age[350].

The JCT is thought to be the major site of hydraulic resistance[372,373,375,376,380–382], the outermost part of the TM consisting of several layers of cells embedded in a ground substance comprising a wide variety of macromolecules, including hyaluronic acid, other glycosaminoglycans, collagen, fibronectin, and other glycoproteins presumably produced by the resident cells[383–389]. The JCT is supported by an elastic-like fiber network and fine collagen fiber bundles (Fig. 10.6)[390], extending from the anterior tendons of the longitudinal ciliary muscle bundles, and having the same orientation as the elastic-like network in the central core of the trabecular lamellae. This network is connected on the inner wall endothelium of SC by fine, bent, connecting fibrils. This elastic plexus is far more extensive in the JCT of human eyes than other species, perhaps contributing to the lack of "washout" in human eyes ex vivo[391]. Washout is the phenomenon by which outflow facility increases over time of perfusion with artificial aqueous humor. Interestingly, rodents do not appear to wash out, and also have an extensive cribriform plexus like humans[392,393]. The washout-associated increase in outflow facility in nonhuman species[394–397] correlates with the extent of physical separation between the JCT and the inner wall endothelium lining SC or, in some species, the angular aqueous plexus (anatomical equivalent of SC in many nonprimates)[398].

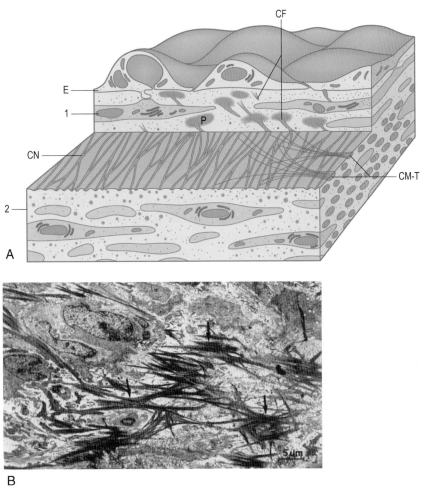

Fig. 10.6 (A) Schematic drawing of the juxtacanalicular tissue (JCT, also known as cribriform) region of the trabecular meshwork and the endothelial lining of Schlemm's canal (*E*). Note the connection between the ciliary muscle tendons (*CM-T*) and the elastic-like fiber plexus, or "cribriform plexus" (*CN*), located mainly in the region between the first and second subendothelial cell layers (*1* and *2*). The cribriform plexus is connected to the inner wall endothelium and the plaque material (*P*) by a system of fine fibrils or "connecting fibrils" (*CF*). **(B)** Electron micrograph of a tangential section through the cribriform region almost at the level between the second subendothelial cell layer and the first corneoscleral trabecular lamellas (normal eye). The cells seen in the *upper left* are subendothelial. The elastic-like fibers of the cribriform region (*arrows*) form a plexus that shows the same equatorial orientation as the network of the elastic-like fibers of the trabecular lamellas. (From Rohen JW, Futa R, Lütjen-Drecoll E. The fine structure of the cribriform meshwork in normal and glaucomatous eyes as seen in tangential sections. *Invest Ophthalmol Vis Sci.* 1981;21:574–585. Reproduced with permission from the Association for Research in Vision and Ophthalmology.)

A contributor to outflow resistance in the JCT[399–401] appears to be the inner wall itself and its discontinuous basement membrane of the inner wall endothelial cells. Separation of the basal lamina cells lining of the inner wall of SC from the underlying JCT, as seen using quick-freeze/deep-etch electron microscopy, reveals apparent flow pathways[402]. Under normal conditions, the inner wall of SC and JCT cells are likely in a contracted state (having contractile tone), which limits the routes available for fluid flow as demonstrated with gold particle infusion studies in nonhuman primates (Fig. 10.7)[403,404]. Expansion of the area available for fluid drainage increases the rate of fluid outflow[403,404]; although the accompanying loss of extracellular material does not appear to be responsible for the decrease in resistance to fluid outflow[402–404].

The inner wall of SC has two primary roles—to maintain the blood-aqueous barrier and to facilitate the movement of aqueous humor out of the eye in the basal to apical direction. To accomplish these apparently opposing tasks, SC cells are a hybrid endothelia, part blood vascular and part lymphatic[405–408]. Fluid movement across the inner SC wall endothelium is predominantly via pressure-dependent transcellular and paracellular pathways[372,409] including giant vacuole formation (Fig. 10.8) especially near collector channels[410–414]. Pore formation is often associated with the giant vacuoles, but may also be found in thin, flat regions in the inner wall[372]. Calculations of the number and size of pores and openings in the inner wall endothelium of SC are too large to

account for most of the outflow resistance[415,416]. These and other findings lead to the hypothesis that the main resistance to aqueous outflow is located internal to the endothelial lining, within the subendothelial tissue or JCT[417].

Although the pores are large, and likely contribute negligible flow resistance, they force the fluid to "funnel" through confined regions of the cribriform TM tissues nearest the pores (Fig. 10.7). Thus, their number and size can greatly influence the effective outflow resistance of the cribriform tissue[418,419]. Two studies[415,416] failed to find a correlation between outflow facility and inner wall pore density as would be expected if the funneling effect contributed to aqueous outflow resistance[357]; however, other studies report a significant linear relationship between pore density/size and outflow facility[420–422]. The best evidence of funneling is provided by a perfusion study with gold particles showing exclusion of large segments of the conventional outflow pathway and punctate decoration of SC (Fig. 10.7). Significantly, disruption of funneling by relaxing inner wall cells and JCT cells expands the JCT to increase fluid drainage with rho kinase inhibitors has been exploited therapeutically to lower outflow resistance (described in detail further in the chapter)[403,423,424].

Experimental studies of the transendothelial passage of ferritin particles in monkey eyes indicate that ferritin also traverses tortuous paracellular routes that lie between the endothelial cells of SC[425]. The functional significance of these paracellular routes for aqueous outflow is not known. However, tight junctions between endothelial cells of SC become less complex with increasing pressure, suggesting that the paracellular pathway into SC in the normal eye may be sensitive to modulation within a range of physiologically relevant pressures[409].

Active involvement of the conventional outflow pathway in IOP homeostasis

Mounting evidence portrays the TM as a living, active, and reactive organ, rather than just a passive mélange of tissue components. Long-term homeostasis in response to physical stress requires modulation by cellular constituents of the conventional outflow pathway, including the cellular lining trabecular lamellae, JCT cells, SC endothelia, and cells of the distal venous vessels. Extracellular load-bearing constituents include the extracellular matrix (ECM) of the trabecular lamellae and the cribiform elastin network, which suspend the TM between two fluid compartments (anterior chamber and SC) at different pressures. The TM likely "senses" this pressure differential by "monitoring" stretch, deformation, shear stress, etc., and strives to maintain these parameters within a homeostatic range. A visual example of the pressure gradient experienced by conventional outflow tissues is provided by the formation of giant vacuoles, where SC cells are extensively stretched into its lumen (Fig. 10.8); or the pressure-dependent narrowing of SC, which as a result increases shear stress experienced by SC endothelial cells to levels approaching arterial vessels[426]. This narrowing of the SC lumen corresponds to an expansion and stretching of the TM and its resident cells[413]. Among other mechanosensors such as ion channels[171,427–430], ATP release mechanisms[431], and caveoli[432,433], these cellular deformations activate integrins[434], which in turn mediate regulation of ECM deposition and relaxation/contractility of the cells themselves[383,435]. ECM rigidity in turn modulates cytoskeletal structures, protein expression patterns, signal transduction, and fibronectin deposition in TM cells[436,437].

IOP is not stagnant. Overlaid on the mean IOP gradient experienced by cells of the conventional outflow pathway are IOP fluctuations, primarily owing to the filling and draining of the choroid during cycles of the heartbeat, resulting in the ocular pulse[438,439]. These

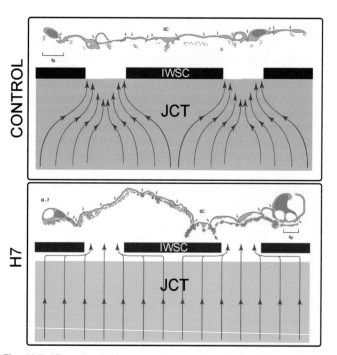

Fig. 10.7 "Funneling" of aqueous humor through the juxtacanalicular region (*JCT*) of the conventional outflow pathway. Shown are reproductions of two stretches of inner wall of Schlemm's canal (SC) (*IWSC*, 15-cells, cell-cell junctions marked by *arrows*) that display the distribution of perfused gold particles in the JCT of eyes in the absence (*upper*) or presence (*lower*) of H-7 (1-[5-isoquinoline sulfonyl]-2-methyl piperazine). Below the reproduction of control eye is a schematic showing flow distribution due to the funneling phenomenon, with inner wall cells attached to substratum. In contrast, the schematic below the H-7-treated eye shows uniform flow that results when these attachments are broken due to treatment. The location of individual gold particles is represented by *red dots*. (Bars = 4 μm.) (Modified from Overby D, Gong H, Qiu G, Freddo TF, Johnson M. The mechanism of increasing outflow facility during washout in the bovine eye. *Invest Ophthalmol Vis Sci.* 2002;43(11):3455–64. PMID: 12407156.)

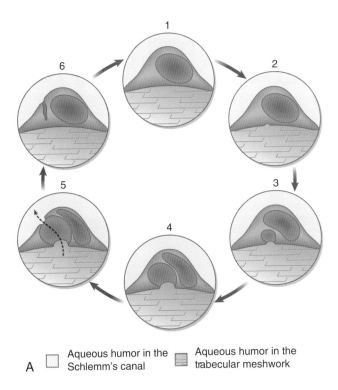

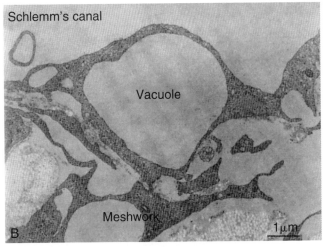

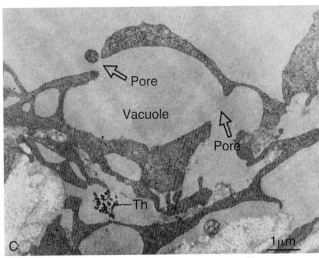

Fig. 10.8 (**A**) Theory of transcellular aqueous transport in which a series of pores and giant vacuoles opens (probably in response to transendothelial hydrostatic pressure) on the connective tissue side of the juxtacanalicular region of the trabecular meshwork (2–4). Fusion of basal and apical cell plasmalemma creates a temporary transcellular channel (5) that allows bulk flow of aqueous humor into Schlemm's canal (SC). (From Tripathi RC. Mechanism of the aqueous outflow across the trabecular wall of Schlemm's canal. *Exp Eye Res.* 1971;11:116–121.) (**B**) Transmission electron micrograph of the inner wall of SC and the adjacent subendothelial tissue showing empty spaces or "giant vacuoles" within the endothelial cells. (From Inomata H, Bill A, Smelser GK. Aqueous humor pathways through the trabecular meshwork and into Schlemm's canal in the cynomolgus monkey (Macaca irus). An electron microscopic study. *Am J Ophthalmol.* 1972;73(5):760–789.) (**C**) Serial sections of the inner wall of SC indicate that the "giant vacuoles" of the endothelial cells have openings toward the trabecular side, indicating that they are invaginations from the trabecular meshwork side. Some of the invaginations also have openings (pores) into SC. Aqueous humor can pass through the cells via the invaginations and the pores. *Th,* Thorotrast. (From Inomata H, Bill A, Smelser GK. Aqueous humor pathways through the trabecular meshwork and into Schlemm's canal in the cynomolgus monkey (Macaca irus). An electron microscopic study. *Am J Ophthalmol.* 1972;73(5):760–789.)

approximately 3-mmHg fluctuations in IOP cause the TM and inner wall of SC to oscillate (Fig. 10.9). Such TM movements can be visualized via a specialized imaging technique called phase-sensitive optical coherence tomography[440,441], and induction of ocular pulse in perfused eyes increases outflow facility[442]. Thus, the TM and inner wall of SC are constantly moving, sensing changes in IOP, and changing outflow resistance, and this movement is depressed in glaucoma[443], likely due to increased conventional outflow tissue stiffness[382,444,445].

In addition to responding to IOP-induced stretch by altering its contractile tone and ECM, TM cells secrete dozens of soluble mediators[446]. These substances appear to act in both an autocrine and paracrine fashion, some traveling with aqueous flow to impact SC cells downstream. For example, stretching of TM cells triggers the release of vascular endothelial growth factor (VEGF), which increases outflow facility owing to activation of VEGF receptor 2 in SC cells[447]. In contrast, chronic injection of antibodies against VEGF in patients with

neovascular age-related macular degeneration results in decreased outflow facility and elevated IOP[448–450].

Another paracrine signaling relationship between TM and SC involves the angiopoietin/Tie2 pathway. Here, angiopoetin-1 is expressed by TM cells and its receptor, Tie2 is expressed by SC cells. Thus, conditional knock out of angiopoetin-1 or Tie2 in adult mice results in ocular hypertension[451,452]. Alternatively, directly activating Tie2 with antibodies or indirectly activating Tie2 by inhibiting its phosphatase decreases IOP by increasing outflow facility[453]. Importantly, this phosphatase inhibitor, AKB-9778 was the first SC-selective drug to be evaluated in human clinical trials for the treatment of ocular hypertension. Although safe and significantly lowering IOP, it unfortunately failed to meet clinical end points.

The oscillatory movements owing to ocular pulse also impact SC by amplifying the shear stress experienced by SC cells during IOP elevations that narrow its lumen[454,455]. Similar to other blood vessels, shear

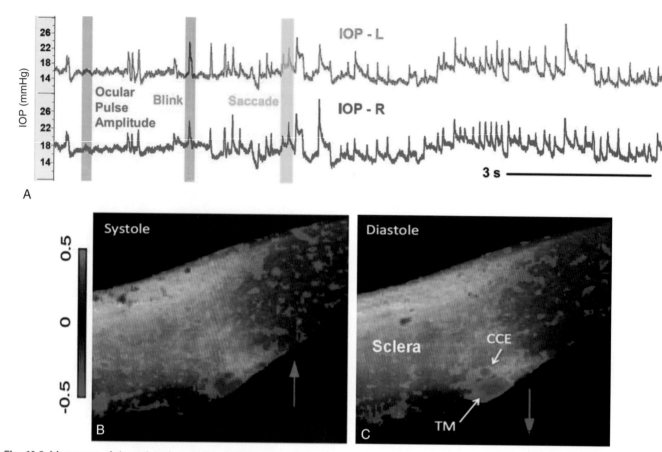

Fig. 10.9 Movement of the trabecular meshwork (TM) due to the ocular pulse. **(A)** Continuous telemetry data showing fluctuations in intraocular pressure signals from the left *(L)* and right *(R)* eyes of a nonhuman primate. *Highlighted* are verified blinks, saccades, and ocular pulse amplitude events *(red, green,* and *blue shading,* respectively). *IOP,* Intraocular pressure. **(B)** and **(C)** Color-encoded changes in instantaneous velocities owing to ocular pulse overlaid on the iridocorneal angle structures of a human eye that were obtained using phase-sensitive optical coherence tomography. The *red* color indicates tissue movement anteriorly toward the scleral surface, whereas the *blue* color indicates the tissue movement posteriorly toward the anterior chamber *(red* versus *blue arrow). CCE,* Collector channel entrances. (From Turner DC, Edmiston AM, Zohner YE, et al. Transient Intraocular Pressure Fluctuations: Source, Magnitude, Frequency, and Associated Mechanical Energy. *Invest Ophthalmol Vis Sci.* 2019;60(7):2572–2582. https://doi.org/10.1167/iovs.19-26600; Xin C, Song S, Johnstone M, Wang N, Wang RK. Quantification of Pulse-Dependent Trabecular Meshwork Motion in Normal Humans Using Phase-Sensitive OCT. *Invest Ophthalmol Vis Sci.* 2018;59(8):3675–3681. https://doi.org/10.1167/iovs.17-23579.)

stress in a narrow SC lumen results in the production of nitric oxide by endothelial nitric oxide synthase (NOS) (Fig. 10.10). Owing to its unique properties as a gas, nitric oxide can diffuse upstream of aqueous humor flow and relax JCT cells or diffuse downstream and change the permeability of SC inner wall or dilate distal veins[442,456–459]. The net effect is increased outflow facility to oppose increased IOP. Importantly, the time scale of these homeostatic effects is dynamic and rapid (milliseconds to seconds), and complement the slow homeostasis mediated by ECM turnover, which occurs over hours to days. Emphasizing the role of nitric oxide produced by SC cells in IOP homeostasis, knockout of endothelial NOS results in elevated IOP owing to decreased outflow facility, and transgenic mice overexpressing nitric oxide have lower IOP because of increased outflow facility[460,461].

Nitric oxide synthase–immunoreactive nerve fibers are present in the primate TM, especially in the cribriform region adjacent to the inner wall of SC[462]. NOS released from nerve terminals could relax JCT cells and increase outflow facility independent from the ciliary muscle. In human glaucoma eyes there are dramatic reductions in staining indicative of NOS activity in ciliary muscle, TM, and SC, compared with control eyes[463,464], that are unrelated to the use of multiple glaucoma therapies, or the severity of the disease[464]. Staining for NOS activity is

likely due to nitric oxide produced by all three subtypes of NOS: neuronal NOS in ciliary muscle and TM, inducible NOS from macrophages throughout the conventional outflow pathway, and endothelial NOS in SC. Hence, nitric oxide–mimicking nitrovasodilators, delivered systemically or locally to the eye, decrease IOP by altering outflow resistance, without apparent effects on the ciliary muscle[465,466]. Drug companies have capitalized on the impact of nitric oxide on outflow physiology by developing several nitric oxide–donating compounds[467–471], one of which (latanoprostene bunod) has been approved for use in humans[472].

Importantly, only 50% to 75% of total outflow resistance resides in the proximal part of the conventional tract in the JCT[473–475]. The remaining 25% to 50% of resistance is distal to the inner wall of SC, likely in collector channel ostia or contractile intrascleral veins[393,476,477]. Vasoconstriction at these sites likely explains clinical observations whereby surgical bypass or elimination of the JCT region of the conventional outflow pathway only lowers IOP to mid to high teens, instead of near episcleral venous pressure (EVP) (i.e., ~8 mmHg) as predicted by the Goldmann equation[478,479]. These data suggest that the distal part of the conventional tract is actively responding to removal of upstream resistance. In fact, direct evidence for distal outflow regulation are provided by studies in human and porcine anterior segments

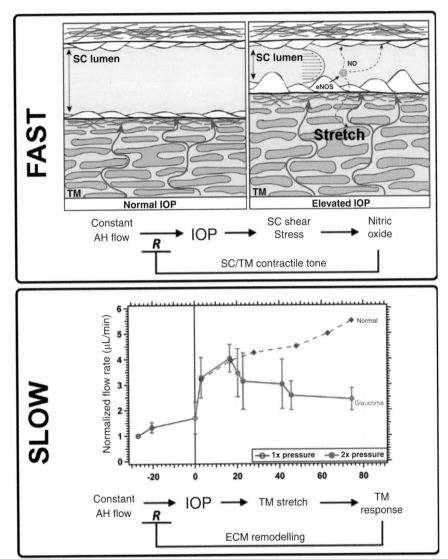

Fig. 10.10 A model for intraocular pressure (IOP)-dependent mechanosensation in the conventional outflow pathway and fast versus slow homeo-static responses. *Upper panels:* A schematic showing physical changes in the trabecular meshwork (TM) and Schlemm's canal (SC) due to increasing IOP. In addition to stretching of the tissues, the SC lumen narrows (double arrows), which increases shear stress and consequently nitric oxide (NO, *green dot*) production. NO may diffuse upstream to reach the TM or may act elsewhere on SC cells or on collector channels. Below the schematic is a diagram depicting this fast (seconds) homeostatic feedback loop where outflow resistance *(R)* determines IOP based on the magnitude of aqueous humor flow, which is typically constant for a living eye. IOP in turn defines the level of shear stress experienced by SC cells and thus NO production. NO-mediated reduction in contractile tone feeds back to reduce R, and thereby return IOP toward a homeostatic set-point. Lower panels: Graph showing flow rate for normal *(gray)* versus glaucomatous *(red)* anterior segments in organ culture calculated at normal (1× or 8.8 mmHg) and elevated (2× or 17.6 mmHg) perfusion pressures. Increasing perfusion pressure in glaucomatous eyes triggers a homeostatic response over the first several hours that eventually fails, with outflow initially increasing, then decreasing over time. In contrast, increasing pressure in normal eyes causes R to decrease and outflow to increase over time. This slow (hours to days) response is diagrammed below, showing a similar feedback loop as the fast response, however, in this case stretching of TM cells causes changes in expression of a number of proteins involved in extracellular matrix (ECM) remodeling that decreases R to normalize IOP. (From Reina-Torres E, De Ieso ML, Pasquale LR, et al. The vital role for nitric oxide in intraocular pressure homeostasis. *Prog Retin Eye Res.* 2021;83:100922. https://doi.org/10.1016/j.preteyeres.2020.100922; Raghunathan VK, Benoit J, Kasetti R, et al. Glaucomatous cell derived matrices differentially modulate non-glaucomatous trabecular meshwork cellular behavior. *Acta Biomater.* 2018;71: 444–459. https://doi.org/10.1016/j.actbio.2018.02.037.)

where the TM and inner wall of SC have been removed, but outflow facility is altered pharmacologically[458,480]. Both here in the distal region of the conventional outflow tract and proximally, endothelin-1 physiologically opposes nitric oxide to regulate vascular/trabecular tone and regulate IOP[458,481–483].

Taken together, conventional outflow tissues sense the physical, as well as the biochemical, environment in which they reside, and make modifications to their physical and conformational properties to affect their overall hydraulic conductivity and thereby allow the eye to reach a specific target pressure (discussed further in chapter). Evidence for such a homeostatic response is provided by experiments that artificially increase IOP of eyes during organ culture perfusions. In response to elevated IOP, outflow facility increases steadily over 2 to 3 days until IOP is normalized (Fig. 10.10)[383,436,484]. Responses of the TM to long-term increases in IOP can be visualized with tracer, showing that there are alterations in the distribution of preferential flow passageways[485]. This "slow" homeostatic response is likely mediated by increased ECM turnover[383]. Interestingly, homeostatic response to an elevated IOP challenge appears disrupted in glaucomatous eyes (Fig. 10.10)[486].

OBSTRUCTION OF OUTFLOW

Extracellular matrix accumulation

In glaucomatous eyes there is an increase in ECM beneath the inner wall of SC and in the cribriform region of the TM and thickening of the trabecular lamellae compared with age-matched normal controls[487–489]. In advanced cases of POAG there is additional loss of TM cells beyond that associated with normal aging[30,31]. In this condition, the inner uveal and corneoscleral lamellae appear fused together[31], and SC can be partly obliterated. Areas with more ECM are less perfused, presumably because of the higher resistance of the area[487]. The origin of the increased amounts of ECM in glaucomatous eyes is still unknown. Complicating interpretation of results, most specimens of glaucomatous eyes investigated morphologically are derived from patients who have been treated for many years with antiglaucoma drugs, which can themselves induce changes in the biology of the trabecular cells by slowing or diverting flow of aqueous humor[490].

Transforming growth factor (TGF) β2, a component of normal aqueous humor in many mammalian eyes[491–494], influences ECM production in the TM and has been implicated in IOP elevation[495,496]. Increased levels of total and active TGFβ2 are found in the aqueous humor of POAG patients compared with age-matched controls[494,497]. TGFβ2 decreases the activity of matrix metalloproteinases (MMP), and thus possibly contributes to increased ECM in the TM of glaucomatous eyes[498]. Perfusion of human anterior segments ex vivo with TGFβ2 results in decreased outflow facility and increased focal accumulation of ECM under the inner wall of SC[496]. One of these ECM proteins, cochlin, is elevated in the TM upon TGFβ2 treatment of perfused anterior segments and in glaucomatous eyes. Overexpression in cochlin results in decreased outflow facility[499,500]. In vitro treatment of cultured TM cells with TGFβ2 results in elevated production of ECM proteins such as fibronectin and plasminogen activator inhibitor (PAI-1)[495]. In addition, interactions between bone morphogenic protein (BMP), Wnt proteins, and TGFβ represent potential checkpoints to regulate TM cell function, IOP, and glaucoma pathogenesis. For instance, the expression of secreted frizzled-related protein-1 (sFRP-1) is significantly elevated in the glaucomatous TM. Accordingly, perfusion of human eyes with sFRP-1 significantly decreased outflow facility[501].

How important "extra" ECM is in increasing resistance to aqueous humor outflow (and thus increasing IOP) in open-angle glaucoma is uncertain. TM cells are highly phagocytic[502–504] and the normal turnover of ECM is fast, similar to that of a healing wound[505]. This appears to be in part for outflow resistance regulation and in part for maintenance of a patent drainage pathway for aqueous humor. Thus, the TM is in effect a self-cleaning filter, and that in most of the open-angle glaucomas, the self-cleaning (i.e., phagocytic) function is deficient or at least inadequate to cope with the amount of material present[54,506]. Phagocytosis, especially of particulate matter and red blood cells, is also carried out by resident macrophages of the TM, which are numerous[406,408,507,508]. Macrophages appear important in clearing the anterior chamber of some inflammatory debris after laser trabeculoplasty[509], or a pigment shower[506,510]. However, their role in normal housekeeping and bulk outflow of aqueous humor is currently unclear.

Combining the clogged-filter concept of glaucoma and the washout concept of perfusion-induced resistance decrease inevitably led to interest in compounds that might disrupt or remodel the structure of the TM and SC inner wall to enhance flow through the tissue and/or promote washout of normal and pathologic resistance–producing ECM (discussed further in chapter). For example, a rho kinase inhibitor was shown to prevent and reverse ECM accumulation in the JCT due to chronic glucocorticoid treatment[511]. Such compounds will likely provide insights into cellular and extracellular mechanisms governing outflow resistance in normal and glaucomatous states. Additionally, if normal or pathologic ECM required many years to accumulate to the extent that IOP became elevated, perhaps a one-time washout would provide years of normalized outflow resistance and IOP[512,513].

Cells and other particulates

Normal erythrocytes are deformable and pass easily from the anterior chamber through the tortuous pathways of the TM and the inner wall of SC[372]. However, nondeformable erythrocytes such as sickled or clastic (ghost) cells may become trapped within and obstruct the TM, elevating outflow resistance and IOP[514–516]. Similarly, macrophages that are swollen after ingesting lens proteins leaking from a hypermature cataract[517] or breakdown products from intraocular erythrocytes[518] or pigmented tumors (or the tumor cells themselves)[519] may produce JCT obstruction. Pigment liberated from the iris spontaneously (pigmentary dispersion syndrome) or iatrogenically (following laser iridotomy) may clog or otherwise alter the TM function temporarily, presumably without prior ingestion by wandering macrophages[520,521], as may zonular fragments following iatrogenic enzymatic zonulolysis[522,523] or lens capsular fragments following laser posterior capsulotomy[524,525]. Ocular amyloidosis can lead to elevated IOP as a result of blockage of the TM with amyloid particles[526].

Glaucoma secondary to hypermature cataract (phacolytic glaucoma) or uveitis has long been ascribed to JCT obstruction. In the former entity, the presence of protein-laden macrophages lining the chamber angle seems adequate to account for increased outflow resistance[517]. The uveitis-related glaucomas comprise many different entities, and the etiology of the increased outflow resistance seems less clear; postulated mechanisms include TM involvement by the primary inflammatory process, JCT obstruction by inflammatory cells, or secondary alteration of TM cellular physiology by inflammatory mediators or byproducts released elsewhere in the eye.

Small amounts of purified high-molecular-weight, soluble lens proteins[527,528] or serum itself[529], when perfused through the anterior chamber of freshly enucleated human eyes, causes an acute and marked increase in outflow resistance. Thus, it may be that specific proteins, protein subfragments, or other macromolecules are themselves capable of obstructing or altering the TM to increase outflow resistance, perhaps contributing to the elevated IOP in entities such as the phacolytic, uveitic, exfoliation[530], and hemolytic[518] glaucomas. In the living eye, serum proteins constantly diffuse out from the iris stroma into the anterior chamber, equilibrating at an approximately 1% concentration and exiting via the trabecular outflow pathway[14]. Experimental perfusion of the enucleated calf eye[531,532] or monkey eye in vivo[533] with medium containing higher serum protein concentrations than found in normal aqueous humor indeed reduces or eliminates resistance washout. Perhaps protein in the aqueous humor that passes through the TM is essential for maintenance of normal resistance either by providing resistance itself, or by signaling or modifying some property of the TM such as stimulation of focal adhesion and stress fiber formation, to enhance adhesion of TM cells to the ECM[533–535]. Hyaluronate- and chondroitin sulfate–based agents used as tissue spacers during intraocular surgery ("viscoelastic agents") may raise IOP in human eyes if not completely removed from the eye by irrigation/aspiration at the conclusion of a procedure, presumably by obstructing trabecular outflow[536,537].

PHARMACOLOGY AND REGULATION OF OUTFLOW

Cholinergic effects on conventional outflow

In primates the iris root inserts into the ciliary muscle and the uveal TM just posterior to the scleral spur, while the ciliary muscle inserts at the scleral spur and the posterior inner aspect of the TM[538]. The anterior tendons of the longitudinal portion of the ciliary muscle insert into the outer lamellated portion of the TM and into the JCT, and via elastic elements into specialized cell surface adaptations on the inner wall of SC endothelial cells (Fig. 10.6). Ciliary muscle contraction results, not only in spreading of the lamellated portion of the TM but also in an inward pulling of the cribriform elastic fiber plexus and straightening of the connecting fibrils and dilation of SC[539]. Movement of the inner wall region affects the area and configuration of the outflow pathways and thereby outflow resistance[540], which in the nonaccommodating rodent eye suggest that the initial function of longitudinal ciliary muscle fibers was to regulate trabecular outflow[539]. Voluntary accommodation (human)[541], electrical stimulation of the third cranial nerve (cat)[542], topical, intracameral, or systemically administered cholinergic agonists (monkey and human)[543,544], and, in enucleated eyes (monkey and human), pushing the lens posteriorly with a plunger through a corneal fitting[545] all decrease outflow resistance, while ganglionic blocking agents and cholinergic antagonists increase resistance[544,546–548].

Furthermore, the resistance-decreasing effect of intravenous pilocarpine in monkeys is virtually instantaneous, implying that the effect is mediated by an arterially perfused structure or structures[549]. However, not all the experimental evidence supports this strictly mechanical view of cholinergic and anticholinergic effects on TM function. For example, in monkeys, intravenous atropine rapidly reverses some, but not all of the pilocarpine-induced resistance decrease[550,551], and topical pilocarpine causes a much greater resistance decrease per diopter of induced accommodation than does systemic pilocarpine (monkey)[551] or voluntary accommodation (human)[552]. The inability of atropine to rapidly and completely reverse the pilocarpine-induced facility increase in normal eyes could be due to mechanical hysteresis of the TM[553–555]. The variation in the relative magnitude of pilocarpine-induced accommodation and resistance decrease when the drug is administered by different routes might reflect differences in bioavailability of the drug to different regions of the muscle[551]. However, following ciliary muscle disinsertion and total iris removal (but not iris removal alone), there is virtually no acute outflow resistance response to intravenous or intracameral pilocarpine and no response to topical pilocarpine[553–555]. Thus, it seems certain that the acute resistance-decreasing action of pilocarpine, and presumably other cholinomimetics, is mediated entirely by drug-induced ciliary muscle contraction, with no direct pharmacologic effect on the TM itself.

Cholinergic and nitrenergic nerve terminals that could induce contraction and relaxation of TM and scleral spur cells are present in primate TM and scleral spur. Terminals in contact with the elastic-like network of the TM and containing substance P immunoreactive fibers resemble afferent mechanoreceptor–like terminals[462]. Afferent mechanoreceptors that measure stress or strain in the connective tissue elements of the scleral spur have also been identified[556]. These findings raise the possibility that the TM may have some ability to self-regulate aqueous humor outflow; however, this has not been demonstrated experimentally.

Muscarinic receptors and contractile elements are present in the TM. The m3 muscarinic receptor transcript and m2 receptor protein is detected in human TM of cadaver eyes[557,558]. Carbachol (CARB)-induced mobilization of Ca^{2+} and phosphoinositide production in human TM cells in culture are associated with the M3 muscarinic receptor activation[559]. Smooth muscle–specific contractile proteins are present in cells within the human TM and adjacent to the outer wall of SC and the collector channels[476,560]. Isolated bovine TM strips contract isometrically in response to CARB, pilocarpine, aceclidine (ACEC), and acetylcholine and endothelin-1[561–563]. However, in the organ-cultured perfused bovine anterior segment, endothelin-1 and CARB-induced contractions result in a reduction of the outflow rate[482]. Also, low (10^{-8} to 10^{-6}M) but not high (10^{-4} to 10^{-2}M) doses of pilocarpine, ACEC, or CARB induce increased outflow facility in human perfused anterior ocular segments, devoid of ciliary muscle[564]. However, low doses of pilocarpine have no effect on outflow facility in living monkey eyes[565]; facility increases occur only at doses that also produced miosis and accommodation.

Pilocarpine-induced ciliary muscle contraction spreads the TM, perhaps with the same physiologic consequences as direct relaxation of the TM—decreased tissue density and thus decreased flow resistance due to opening of new flow pathways. Combination of threshold facility–effective doses of pilocarpine with maximal outflow facility–effective doses of H-7 (discussed further in chapter) can further enhance the outflow facility response with minimal effects on accommodation[566].

At least two different subtypes of muscarinic receptors, M2 and M3, are present in the ciliary muscle[557,567,568]. The M2 receptor shows preferential localization to the longitudinal[567], putatively more facility-relevant portion of the ciliary muscle, but to date no functional role for this subtype has been elucidated. mRNA from the M2, M3, and M5 subtypes is strongly expressed in the longitudinal and circular portions of human ciliary muscle cells and tissue[568]. The M3 subtype appears to mediate the outflow facility and accommodative responses to pilocarpine and aceclidine in monkeys[569,570]. In monkeys, the outer longitudinal region of the ciliary muscle differs ultrastructurally and histochemically from the inner reticular and circular portions[571]. Although differential distribution of muscarinic subtypes is probably not responsible for the outflow facility/accommodation dissociation occurring under certain conditions, functional dissociation might be produced by combinations of drugs from different classes.

Given the long-term use of cholinergic agonists in glaucoma therapy and the vital role of ciliary muscle tone in regulating outflow resistance, it is important to note that in the monkey, topical administration of the cholinesterase inhibitor echothiophate or the direct-acting agonist pilocarpine desensitizes the outflow facility and accommodative responses to pilocarpine, accompanied by decreased numbers of muscarinic receptors in the ciliary muscle[553–555,572–576]. Even a single dose of pilocarpine or carbachol reduces receptor number[574]. Because cholinergic drug therapy is not the mainstay of glaucoma therapy that it once was, the issues related to refractoriness to long-term therapy versus disease progression are no longer prominent areas of research.

Cholinergic effects on unconventional outflow

When the ciliary muscle contracts in response to exogenous pilocarpine (Fig. 10.11), the spaces between the muscle bundles are substantially obstructed[490,538,544]. Conversely, during atropine-induced ciliary muscle relaxation, the spaces are widened[544]. If mock aqueous humor–containing albumin labeled with iodine-125 or iodine-131 (which under resting conditions leave the anterior chamber essentially by bulk flow via the conventional and unconventional drainage routes) is perfused through the anterior chamber, autoradiographs show

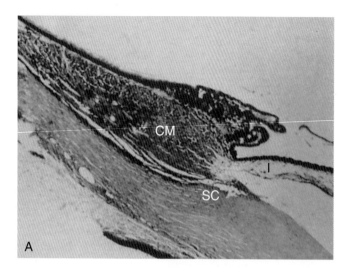

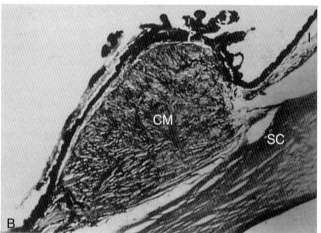

Fig. 10.11 Histologic sagittal sections through the chamber angle region of monkey eyes treated acutely with atropine (A) or pilocarpine (B) topically. After treatment with pilocarpine, the muscle moves anteriorly and inwardly, thereby expanding the trabecular lamellas and widening of Schlemm's canal (*SC*). This contraction also obliterates the spaces between the ciliary muscle (*CM*) bundles, obstructing unconventional outflow. Conversely, atropine relaxes the CM bundles. (Vervet monkey, Azan stain; original magnification ×25.) *I*, Iris. (From Lütjen-Drecoll E, Kaufman PL. Morphological changes in primate aqueous humor formation and drainage tissues after long-term treatment with antiglaucomatous drugs. *J Glaucoma.* 1993;2:316–328.)

qualitatively the distribution of the flow[59,577]. In the pilocarpinized eye, radioactivity is present in the iris stroma, the iris root, the region of SC and the surrounding sclera, and the most anterior portion of the ciliary muscle. In the atropinized eye, radioactivity is found in all these tissues, as well as throughout the entire ciliary muscle and even further posteriorly in the suprachoroid/sclera[59,577]. In other perfusion experiments quantifying unconventional drainage, pilocarpinized eyes demonstrate but a fraction of the unconventional flow in atropinized eyes[59,251,578,579]. Thus, to generalize in the primate eye, the magnitude of the pilocarpine (and presumably all cholinergic agonists) enhancement of aqueous humor drainage via the conventional route is greater than the reduction of drainage via the unconventional route, thus resulting in a reduction in IOP.

Adrenergic effects on conventional outflow

Adrenergic innervation of the primate TM is sparse and concentrated mainly in the region of the TM near the ciliary muscle tendons. No functional significance can as yet be ascribed to these terminals[580–582]. Regardless, topical and intracameral epinephrine increase outflow facility in monkey and human eyes[228,578,579,583–586]. Much work has been done attempting to define the time course, type of receptors (e.g. α, β, adenosine), and biochemical pathways (e.g., prostaglandins, cyclic adenosine monophosphate)[587] involved in these responses. Adrenergic receptor stimulation could alter intraocular, intrascleral, and extrascleral vascular tone, as well as have possible direct effects on the outflow pathways, all of which might alter IOP. These potential sites of action are not mutually exclusive, and indeed might account for much of the variability and confusion in the literature.

In surgically untouched, aniridic, and ciliary muscle disinserted monkey eyes with widely varying starting facilities, epinephrine and norepinephrine increase facility by a constant percentage of the starting facility, indicating that neither the iris nor the ciliary muscle is involved in the responses and that the drugs exert their effects on conventional outflow facility (discussed further in chapter)[588,589]. Hence, outflow facility increases in response to β-adrenergic agonists[228,260,590]. Human TM or SC endothelial cells grown on porous filter supports separate and shrink when exposed to isoproterenol or epinephrine, resulting in increased transendothelial fluid flow[591]. It appears that epinephrine effects on outflow may be due to cytoskeletal changes in TM[592]. Thus, epinephrine causes disruption of actin filaments within the TM cells, which alters their cell shape and cell-cell and cell-ECM adhesions. Consistent with this idea, cytochalasin B (a disruptor of actin filament formation) potentiates the facility-increasing effect of epinephrine[593], whereas phalloidin (a stabilizer of actin filaments) inhibits it[594].

The facility-increasing effect of epinephrine and norepinephrine is mediated by β2-adrenergic receptors on the TM cells, and the subsequent G-protein adenylate cyclase–cyclic adenosine monophosphate (AMP) cascade[74,595]. The facility-increasing effect of epinephrine is blocked by timolol[596,597] but not betaxolol[598–600], in both humans and monkeys, consistent with the hypothesis that there are no β1 receptors present in the primate TM. TM cells synthesize cyclic adenosine monophosphate (cAMP) in response to stimulation with β-adrenoceptor–selective agonists[586]. The increase in cAMP synthesis by TM cells in response to epinephrine can be blocked by timolol[586], although not by betaxolol (a β1-receptor antagonist), consistent with the hypothesis that there are only β2-receptors present in the TM. Intracameral injection of cAMP or its analogs, but not the inactive metabolite 5-AMP, lowers IOP and increases outflow facility[601,602]. The cAMP-induced facility increase is not additive to that induced by adrenergic agonists, and vice-versa[603]. Epinephrine increases facility and perfusate cAMP levels in the organ-cultured perfused human anterior segment, effects that are blocked by timolol and the selective β2-antagonist, ICI 118,551[604].

In terms of α-adrenergic receptors in the TM, the α1-agonist phenylephrine and the α2-agonist brimonidine induce contractions of TM strips in organ culture[605]. The latter finding was validated, showing that treatment of human TM cells with the α2-adrenergic receptor agonist dexmedetomidine inhibits forskolin-stimulated cAMP formation, a response that was reversed by the α2-adrenergic receptor–selective antagonists rauwolscine and atipamezole[606].

Adrenergic effects on unconventional outflow

β-Adrenergic receptors are present in the primate ciliary muscle, and their physiologic or pharmacologic stimulation relaxes the muscle[607–609]. Epinephrine, in addition to increasing conventional outflow, also increases unconventional outflow in monkeys[578,579] and humans[259,260].

The mechanism is unknown, but may be in part due to the mildly relaxant effect of epinephrine on the ciliary muscle, presumably acting via its β-adrenergic receptors[220,607–609]. Pretreatment with the cyclooxygenase inhibitor indomethacin inhibits the ocular hypotensive effect of topically applied epinephrine in humans[610] suggesting that the IOP-lowering action of epinephrine may be mediated at least in part by prostaglandins or other cyclooxygenase products[590,610].

Numerous clinical studies in humans claim that topical application of timolol, a nonselective β1-, β2-adrenergic receptor antagonist, induces no change in distance refraction[48]. However, a single topical application of 0.5% timolol may increase myopia by nearly 1 diopter, presumably by blocking the effect of endogenous ciliary muscle–relaxing sympathetic neuronal tone[611]. Indirect fluorophotometric estimates fail to demonstrate any effect of timolol on unconventional outflow[259]. However, timolol may reduce epinephrine-induced increases in unconventional outflow when the two drugs are applied concurrently[259]. These findings are consistent with the data concerning adrenergic influences on ciliary muscle contractile tone and also illustrate the importance of the ambient neuronal and pharmacologic adrenergic tone in determining the response of a target tissue to an exogenous adrenergic agent.

In addition to suppressing aqueous formation, α2-adrenergic agonists may enhance unconventional outflow. In humans apraclonidine- and brimonidine-induced IOP reductions are associated with decreased aqueous humor formation and decreased (apraclonidine) or increased (brimonidine) unconventional outflow[612,613]. Treatment of ocular hypertensive patients with brimonidine for 1 month results in a suppression of aqueous formation early on with a later increase in unconventional outflow[304]. A single topical application of either brimonidine or apraclonidine decreases IOP and aqueous flow by similar amounts in timolol-treated normal human eyes[301], suggesting that both α2-agonists act by a similar mechanism.

Bunazosin, a selective α1-adrenoceptor antagonist, can further enhance IOP lowering when used as an adjunctive therapy with latanoprost in monkeys (normotensive)[614] and humans (glaucoma)[615] or with timolol[614] by a mechanism partly owing to ciliary muscle (bovine) relaxation but independent of an effect on MMP activities in cultured monkey ciliary muscle cells[615].

Changes in conventional outflow related to the cytoskeleton and cell junctions

Agents that alter the cytoskeleton, cell junctions, contractile proteins, or ECM in cells of the JCT increase outflow facility (Box 10.2). The adhesion of cells to their neighbors, or to the ECM has multiple effects on cell shape and dynamics. Cell-cell and cell-ECM adherens junctions are complex and dynamic in nature, comprising a myriad of proteins, and are modulated by the ambient physical (pressure, shear stress) and chemical (endogenous hormonal and biochemical, exogenous

---

BOX 10.2   Cytoskeletal, cell contractility/relaxation, and cell junctional mechanisms

- Agents that alter the actin cytoskeleton and cellular contractility lower IOP by directly targeting the trabecular meshwork and decreasing outflow resistance.
- Relaxation of the trabecular meshwork and Schlemm's canal increases the area available for fluid drainage.
- Two rho kinase inhibitors, netarsudil and ripasudil, directly target conventional outflow cells to lower intraocular pressure and have been approved for human use to treat ocular hypertension.

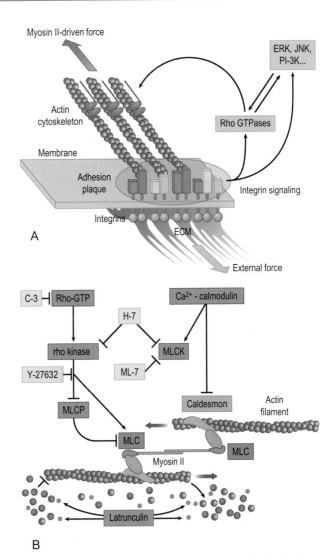

Fig. 10.12 (**A**) Focal adhesion (FA) as a mechanosensor. Focal adhesions are multimolecular complexes connecting the extracellular matrix (*ECM*) with the actin cytoskeleton. Heterodimeric transmembrane integrin receptors *(red)* bind matrix proteins via their extracellular domains, while their cytoplasmic domains are associated with a dense submembrane plaque containing more than 50 different proteins ("boxes" enclosed in the *oval* area) including structural elements, as well as signal transduction proteins such as FAK, Src, ILK, etc. The plaque, in turn, is connected to the termini of actin filament bundles. The assembly and maintenance of FA depend on local mechanical forces. This force may be generated by myosin II–driven isometric contraction of the actin cytoskeleton, or by extracellular perturbations such as matrix stretching or fluid shear stress. Force-induced assembly of the adhesion plaque leads to the activation of a variety of signaling pathways that control cell proliferation, differentiation, and survival (e.g., mean arterial pressure (MAP) kinase and phosphoinositide 3-kinase (PI-3K) pathways), as well as the organization of the cytoskeleton (e.g., Rho family GTPase pathways). Rho, in particular, is an indispensable regulator of FA assembly affecting, via its immediate targets Dia1 and ROCK, actin polymerization and myosin II–driven contractility. (Geiger B, Bershadsky A. Exploring the neighborhood: adhesion-coupled cell mechanosensors. *Cell.* 2002;110(2):139–42. https://doi.org/10.1016/s0092-8674(02)00831-0.) (**B**) Schematic drawing illustrating targets for agents known to disrupt the actin cytoskeleton to enhance outflow facility. C-3, Y-27632, and H-7 block the Rho cascade, inhibiting actomyosin contraction and disrupting actin stress fibers; H-7 and ML-7 block myosin light-chain kinase phosphorylation of the myosin light chain to interfere with actin-myosin interactions; latrunculin sequesters monomeric G-actin leading to microfilament disassembly; caldesmon negatively regulates actin-myosin interactions. (Modified with permission from the original by Alexander Bershadsky.)

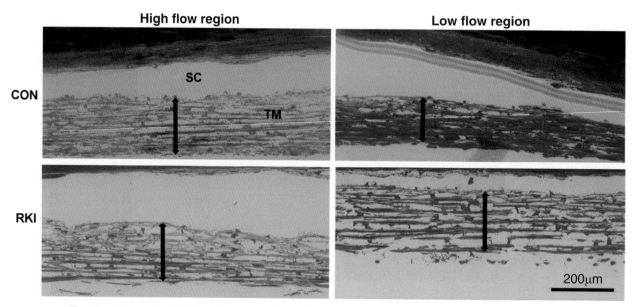

Fig. 10.13 Expansion of trabecular meshwork (*TM*) in response to perfusion with a rho kinase inhibitor (*RKI*). Enucleated human donor eye pairs were perfused under a constant pressure in the presence or absence of netarsudil, an RKI. Shown are representative light microscopic images of frontal sections of the TM in high-flow versus low-flow regions of control (*CON*) and RKI-treated eyes. TM structures were more expanded (*double arrows*) in low-flow regions versus in high-flow regions, which corresponded to a 60% increase in outflow facility. *SC*, Schlemm's canal. (Ren R, Li G, Le TD, Kopczynski C, Stamer WD, Gong H. Netarsudil increases outflow facility in human eyes through multiple mechanisms. *Invest Ophthalmol Vis Sci.* 2016;57(14):6197–6209. https://doi.org/10.1167/iovs.16-20189.)

pharmacologic) milieu. Thus, junctional complexes play a central role in monitoring the state of the cell's external environment. Importantly, actin filaments are the "backbone" of the submembrane plaque in both types of junctions (Fig. 10.12), with the coupling of actin and myosin being essential for cell contractility[616,617].

In the conventional outflow pathway, both TM and SC cells are highly contractile, similar to smooth muscle cells[456,618]. As a consequence, changes in contractile tone of the TM and/or SC cells directly affects outflow resistance by altering the dimensions or direction of flow pathways[423] (Fig. 10.13). Moreover, the amount and composition of the ECM can be modulated directly by actin-disrupting agents or indirectly by inhibition of specific protein kinase(s)[619,620]. Early studies involving anterior chamber perfusions of living monkey eyes with cytochalasins, fungal metabolites that block actin filament assembly, resulted in marked and rapid increases in total outflow facility[593,621,622]. Tracer studies demonstrate that the increase in total outflow facility is due to increased facility across the TM and inner canal wall[623]. Cytochalasin effects are not related to contraction of the ciliary muscle because the effect is similar in eyes with and without surgically disinserted ciliary muscles[355,622]. Subsequently, studies show that potent actin-disrupting agents such as marine macrolides like latrunculins, which sequester monomeric G-actin, lead to massive disassembly of filamentous actin (Fig. 10.12). Treatment of human TM cells with latrunculin A or B (LAT-A, LAT-B) results in cell rounding and retraction of the lamellipodium[624,625]. LAT-A or -B administered intracamerally or topically to living monkey eyes induces a two- to fourfold increase in outflow facility[626,627]. In organ-cultured postmortem porcine eyes or human eyes, LAT-B significantly increases outflow facility by 60% to 70%[625,628]. Single or multiple topical treatments with LAT-A and/or -B also significantly decrease IOP in monkeys[626–629].

Morphologically, the LAT-B–induced decrease in outflow resistance in monkey eyes in vivo is associated with massive "ballooning" of the JCT, leading to expansion of the space between the inner wall of SC and the trabecular collagen beams without observable separations between inner wall cells[630]. However, in postmortem human eyes, the facility increase is accompanied by increased openings between inner wall cells with only very modest rarefaction of the JCT and separation of the inner wall of SC from the JCT[628]. The utility of using LAT-B as a therapeutic was tested in a phase I trial in ocular hypertensive patients, finding that twice-a-day treatment lowered IOP by ~5 mmHg, although it was not advanced to late-stage trials[631].

Perturbation of the cellular actomyosin system by inhibition of myosin light-chain kinase (MLCK) and/or rho kinase is demonstrated with the nonselective serine-threonine kinase inhibitor H-7[625,632–635]. H-7, administered intracamerally or topically to living monkey eyes doubles outflow facility and decreases IOP[634] by directly affecting the TM[636]. In cultured anterior segments of porcine, human, or monkey eyes, H-7 also significantly increases outflow facility[625,637,638]. The H-7–induced increase in outflow facility in the live monkey eye is associated with cellular relaxation and expansion of the TM and SC (Fig. 10.7), accompanied by loss of ECM. Interestingly, the inner wall cells of SC become highly extended, yet cell-cell junctions are maintained[403,404]. A specific rho kinase inhibitor, Y-27632, induces reversible changes in cell shape and decreases in actin stress fibers, focal adhesions, and protein phosphotyrosine staining in human TM and SC cells[639,640]. In isolated bovine TM strips, Y-27632 completely blocks Ca^{2+}-independent phorbol myristate acetate or endothelin-1–induced contraction[641–643]. Rho kinase inhibitors increase outflow facility and/or decrease IOP in enucleated porcine eyes and/or living monkeys[639,640,644–648]. Morphologic studies in bovine eyes indicate that Y-27632 increases outflow facility by increasing the physical separation between the JCT and inner wall of SC, reminiscent of what is observed in eyes that washout[649]. The first clinical study testing the topical administration of a selective rho kinase inhibitor (SNJ-1656, an ophthalmic solution of Y-39983 which is 30 times more potent at Rho-associated kinase (ROCK) than Y-27632)[647] showed efficacious IOP lowering in humans[650], although ocular surface toxicity prevented further development. In parallel, another rho kinase inhibitor, K-115 (ripasudil, a derivative of fasudil) was being developed and tested in humans[651]. Subsequently, ripasudil was approved in Japan for commercial use to treat ocular hypertension in humans in 2014, the first drug that selectively targeted the conventional outflow pathway. In the United States, the rho kinase inhibitor netarsudil was approved shortly afterwards in 2017 as a result of functional data in human eyes demonstrating a unique mechanism of action in the conventional outflow pathway[423], and a series of clinical trials showing efficacy and safety in patients[652].

TM relaxation is also induced by modulating proteins, such as caldesmon, that negatively regulate actin-myosin interactions. When caldesmon is overexpressed, actin becomes uncoupled from myosin. Additionally, the exoenzyme C3 transferase disrupts actin-myosin interactions by inhibiting Rho-Guanosine-5'-triphosphate (GTP), thereby blocking the whole Rho cascade (Fig. 10.12). Adenovirus-delivered exoenzyme C3 transferase (C3-toxin) cDNA and nonmuscle caldesmon cDNA express in cultured human TM cells[653,654], and outflow facility dramatically increases in organ-cultured human or monkey eyes following overexpression of these genes[654,655]. Specific inhibition of rho kinase activity in the TM by dominant negative Rho expression also increases outflow facility in organ-cultured human anterior segments[645,646].

Uncoupling of cellular adhesions from their underlying ECM is another approach to disrupt the actin cytoskeleton, resulting in increased outflow facility. It is well established that signaling events mediated by the ECM play a critical role in maintaining tissue architecture by regulating the organization of the actin cytoskeleton and cell contacts. Hence, ECM signaling events could potentially regulate outflow facility. For example, when perfused into cultured human anterior segments, the heparin II (HepII) domain of fibronectin, an ECM protein found in the TM, increases outflow facility[656]. Presumably this domain increases outflow facility by mediating the disassembly of the actin cytoskeleton in TM cells[657] because the HepII domain plays an important role in regulating the organization of the actin cytoskeleton by acting as a ligand for members of the syndecan and integrin family of receptors[658]. As such, HepII appears to mediate effects on TM contractility through an $\alpha4\beta1$ cosignaling pathway[659].

Microtubules comprise 25-nm diameter hollow polar fibers that are densely packed near the nucleus and extend toward the cell periphery. They are not intrinsically contractile but are important for directional cell motility and, driven by specific microtubule motor proteins such as kinesins and dyneins, for cytoplasmic trafficking of vesicles and organelles. Associated proteins bind to microtubules and can affect their stability and potentially attach them to other cellular structures, including other cytoskeletal filaments. Microtubule function could affect outflow pathway events through direct cellular mechanical effects, influences on extracellular or cell membrane turnover, or secondary signaling leading to activation of the actin cytoskeleton[660]. Important for conventional outflow, microtubule disrupting agents such as ethacrynic acid, colchicine, and vinblastine increase outflow facility and cause cellular contraction in TM cells if the actin cytoskeleton is intact[661,662].

Ethacrynic acid (ECA), a sulfhydryl-reactive diuretic drug, inhibits microtubule assembly in vitro, and induces a rapid decrease in phosphotyrosine levels of focal adhesion kinase and a more subtle decrease in paxillin phosphorylation. Dephosphorylation of these proteins disrupts signaling pathways that normally maintain the stability of the actin microfilaments and cellular adhesions, indicating a close relationship between the microtubule system and the actomyosin system. This action leads both to cell shape change in culture[661,663] and to facility changes in vivo[664–667]. In enucleated human eyes, submaximal concentrations of ethacrynic acid do not produce morphologic changes in the TM, whereas higher concentrations induce separations between

TM and SC cells[666,668]. Accordingly, several derivatives of ECA significantly decrease IOP in cats and monkeys[669,670]. These ECA derivatives are more potent than ECA in terms of inducing cell shape alterations and decreasing actin stress fiber content in human TM cells[671], suggesting that microtubule disruption may reduce outflow resistance at least partially through perturbation of the actomyosin system.

General disruption of cell adhesion complexes increases outflow. Thus, perfusion of the monkey anterior chamber with calcium- and magnesium-free mock aqueous humor containing 4 to 6 mM Na_2EDTA or with calcium-free mock aqueous containing 4 mM ethylene glycol bis (aminoethylether) tetra-acetate (EGTA) dramatically increases outflow facility, which is accompanied by ultrastructural changes in which the cell-cell junctions in the TM and SC are clearly fractured, unlike H-7. Moreover, disrupted junctions were accompanied by an expansion of the JCT[672]. Effects on outflow, and presumably ultrastructure, were partially restored after removal of chelators and perfusion with normal media.

Corticosteroid effects on outflow

Glucocorticoids play a major role in the normal physiologic regulation of outflow facility and IOP. Glucocorticoid receptors are expressed in the cells of the outflow pathways[673], but corticosteroid regulation of IOP is proposed to occur via 11β-hydroxysteroid dehydrogenase (HSD)-1 expression, which is localized in the NPE[674–676]. This enzyme catalyzes the conversion of cortisone to cortisol. Levels of cortisol compared to cortisone in the aqueous humor are normally much greater than in the systemic circulation[674,675].

Long-term interactions of cortisol in the aqueous humor with glucocorticoid receptors in the TM could contribute to increasing outflow resistance in susceptible individuals[674]. In the normal population, approximately 40% of patients treated with topical or systemic corticosteroids are termed "steroid responders," and develop markedly elevated IOP after several weeks[677,678]. This contrasts to patients with POAG, in whom 90% are steroid responders, likely owing to an already dysfunctional conventional outflow pathway[677,678]. Glaucoma patients also have increased plasma levels of cortisol compared with normal individuals[679,680] and increased vascular sensitivity to glucocorticoids[681]. Oral administration of the glucocorticoid biosynthesis inhibitor metyrapone to glaucoma patients[682] or the 11β-hydroxysteroid dehydrogenase inhibitor carbenoxolone to ocular hypertensive patients[674] elicits a small, transient decline in IOP. Interestingly, a single anterior juxtascleral depot of anecortave acetate (an angiostatic cortisene used in age-related macular degeneration) is effective in lowering IOP in POAG eyes[683,684]. The mechanism of action is currently unknown, but anecortave acetate prevented IOP elevation and decreased outflow facility in a sheep model of steroid-induced ocular hypertension[685]. In this same model, ocular hypertension was reversed or prevented by a single dose of an adenovirus vector encoding a glucocorticoid response element inducing expression of human metalloproteinase-1 gene, suggesting the involvement in ECM accumulation in steroid-induced ocular hypertension[686].

The glucocorticoid dexamethasone (DEX) alters complex carbohydrate, hyaluronic acid, protein, and collagen synthesis and distribution in cells and tissues of human aqueous humor outflow systems[503,687–689]. In TM cells, DEX inhibits prostaglandin synthesis, reduces phagocytic[690,691] and extracellular protease activity, and changes gene expression[692–694]. Cortisol metabolism may be altered in cultured TM cells from patients with POAG. These cells accumulate 5β-dihydrocortisol and, to a lesser extent, 5α-dihydrocortisol, metabolites, which potentiate the facility-decreasing and IOP-increasing effects of DEX; these cells produce relatively little 3α, 5β-tetrahydrocortisol from cortisol[695]. Normal human TM cells show no accumulation of active dihydrocortisol intermediates; all cortisol is rapidly metabolized to the inactive tetrahydrocortisols. Topical application of 3α, 5β-tetrahydrocortisol decreases IOP and increases outflow facility in glaucomatous human eyes[695], and antagonizes DEX-induced cytoskeletal reorganization (see further) in normal TM cells[695,696] but has no effect on outflow facility in normotensive monkeys following intracameral injection or 10 days of topical administration[697].

Glucocorticoid glaucoma and POAG eyes both exhibit increased amounts of ECM in the TM[698]. However, the ECM that accumulates in eyes with corticosteroid-induced glaucoma differs from that seen in eyes with POAG[699]. The human anterior segment in organ culture exposed to DEX exhibits morphologic changes similar to those reported for corticosteroid glaucoma and a resulting increase in IOP and decrease in outflow facility[700]. Studies of DEX effects in cultured human TM cells show a myriad of changes, including ECM expression, growth factor/receptor expression, alterations in phagocytosis, surface binding properties, an unusual stacked arrangement of smooth and rough endoplasmic reticulum, proliferation of the Golgi apparatus, increased cell and nuclear size, and pleomorphic nuclei[701–703]. Moreover, prolonged treatment of TM cells with DEX decreases hyaluronan synthesis. Hyaluronan is an inert molecule, which may be necessary to prevent adherence of larger molecules to the JCT[702], whereas inhibition of DEX-induced overexpression of laminin or collagen using antisense oligonucleotides increases permeability of DEX-treated TM cells[704]. These and other DEX-induced alterations in several other molecules involved in the regulation of the ECM are extensively reviewed[701].

In the presence of DEX, human TM and SC cell monolayers grown on filters exhibit enhanced tight junction formation and decreased hydraulic conductivity[705,706]. There is a 2-fold increase in the number of tight junctions, a 10- to 30-fold reduction in the mean area occupied by interendothelial "gaps" or preferential flow channels, and a 3- to 5-fold increase in the expression of the junction-associated protein, ZO-1. Inhibition of ZO-1 expression abolishes the DEX-induced increase in resistance and the accompanying alteration in cell junctions and gaps. These results support the hypothesis that intercellular junctions are necessary for the development and maintenance of transendothelial flow resistance in SC and may be involved in the mechanism of increased resistance associated with glucocorticoid exposure.

Glucocorticoids also reorganize the TM cytoskeleton. Most intriguing in terms of outflow resistance are the unusual geodesic dome–like crosslinked actin networks (CLANs) formed in response to DEX treatment of TM cells and perfusion-cultured anterior segments (Fig. 10.14)[707–709]. Higher basal levels of CLANs are present in glaucomatous TM cells and tissues and a greater CLAN response to glucocorticoids occurs in glaucomatous TM cells[710]. Studies have shown that CLANs exist within TM cells in situ in both normal and glaucoma donor eyes. There may be a CLAN in all cells in glaucomatous TM in situ and in two-thirds of cells in normal TM[711]. Glucocorticoid-induced CLAN formation in TM cells involves enhanced β3-integrin signaling, possibly by an inside-out mechanism[712,713].

Myocilin and conventional outflow dysfunction

One of the most prominent genes in TM cells induced by glucocorticoids is myocilin (the protein product of the MYOC gene), which is a secreted protein of unknown function. Its progressive induction over time matches the time course of clinical steroid effects on IOP and outflow facility, and is hypothesized to play a role in glaucoma pathogenesis (see review[714]). Compared to cell neighbors, myocilin's induction by glucocorticoids is unique in TM cells, and thus is used for positive identification of TM cell isolates from complex tissues[715]. However, in a mouse model of steroid-induced ocular hypertension, both wild-type and MYOC knockout mice had equivalent and significantly elevated IOPs, suggesting that MYOC is not a contributor[716]. Moreover, overexpression of wild-type myocilin to glucocorticoid-induced levels does not elevate IOP[717].

Mutations in the MYOC gene cause ocular hypertension owing to decreased outflow facility and open-angle glaucoma[718,719]. However, MYOC mutations account for only a minor percentage (approximately 3%–4%) of patients with adult forms of POAG[720] although prevalence might be higher in juvenile open-angle glaucoma (see reviews[714,721,722]). Notwithstanding its widespread expression by different tissues, myocilin likely plays a unique role in maintaining normal outflow pathways because mutations in MYOC do not functionally affect any other tissue in the body[723–725]. Evidence suggests that myocilin's role in the TM must be redundant, as mice completely lacking MYOC have no discernable IOP phenotype. Thus, myocilin haploinsufficiency is not a critical mechanism for MYOC glaucoma[265]. In contrast, overexpression of myocilin mutants leads to decreased secretion, intracellular accumulation, TM cell death, and ocular hypertension owing to decreased outflow facility[726–728]. Thus, MYOC mutations are likely gain of function and disease-causing MYOC mutants are misfolded[729,730]. Interestingly, overexpression of mutant MYOC in living cats or in mice on some genetic backgrounds does not elevate IOP[731–733]. In addition to a mutant myocilin protein, it appears that IOP elevation is dependent on other factors or that longer duration of exposure may be required in vivo.

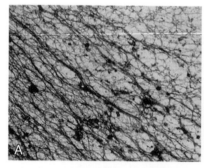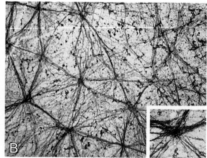

Fig. 10.14 Whole mount transmission electron micrographs of the cytoskeleton of control trabecular meshwork cells (**A**) and trabecular meshwork cells exposed to 10^{-7} M dexamethasone for 14 days (**B**). The stress fibers in the control cells are arranged in normal linear arrays, whereas dexamethasone-treated microfilaments are grouped into 90- to 120-nm bundles radiating from electron-dense vertices. (From Clark AF, Wilson K, McCartney MD, Miggans ST, Kunkle M, W Howe W. Glucocorticoid-induced formation of cross-linked actin networks in cultured human trabecular meshwork cells. *Invest Ophthalmol Vis Sci.* 1994:35(1):281–294.)

Prostaglandin effects on outflow

The unconventional outflow system likely evolved to protect the eye in several ways during inflammation (Box 10.3). Here, the TM becomes compromised by inflammation or obstructed by inflammatory debris, and the choroid is overloaded with debris and extravasated proteins that must be removed from the eye[191]. In this situation, prostaglandins are released and, as autacoids or hormones that are synthesized, released, and locally acting, induce the changes described. Because the eye has a restricted lymphatic architecture, unconventional outflow may serve as an analog to an intraocular lymphatic drainage system[54]. However, long-term exposure to prostaglandins may lead to lymphatization of the unconventional pathway (see further in this section)[734]. The low flow rate that is sufficient to remove normal levels of extravascular protein may be inadequate when protein levels are increased as in uveitis. Redirection of aqueous humor outflow from the conventional to the unconventional pathway would both rid the eye of excess proteins and maintain physiologic IOP. This could also explain the very low IOP that often accompanies uveitis; during experimental iridocyclitis in monkeys, unconventional outflow increases approximately fourfold (Table 10.4)[71].

These proinflammatory effects of prostaglandins were investigated for therapeutic possibilities. For example, there is a 60% increase in aqueous humor outflow via the unconventional pathways in monkeys after a single submaximal dose of $PGF_{2\alpha}$-1-isopropyl ester ($PGF_{2\alpha}$-IE)[345]. Following multiple submaximal doses (Table 10.5), there is more than a 100% increase in unconventional outflow[370]. In both instances, outflow is substantially redirected from the conventional to the unconventional pathway. In vitro, $PGF_{2\alpha}$ produces a weak dose-dependent relaxation of carbachol-precontracted rhesus monkey ciliary muscle strips[735]. Such relaxation may contribute to widening the intermuscular spaces in vivo[736]. However, the majority of the outflow effect resulting from $PGF_{2\alpha}$ treatment is likely due to ECM remodeling in the anterior segment characterized by an increase in MMP-1, -2, and -3 and reduction in collagen types I, II and IV, within the ciliary muscle, iris root, and periciliary body sclera[737–739]. Possibly associated with activation of the proto-oncogene c-fos[740], $PGF_{2\alpha}$ and latanoprost (13, 14-dihydro-17-phenyl-18,19,20-trinor-$PGF_{2\alpha}$-isopropyl ester) cause reductions in collagen types I, III, and IV, and fibronectin, laminin, and hyaluronan immunoreactivity in the ciliary muscle and adjacent sclera, while MMP-2 and MMP-3 are increased. Plasmin generation, an activator of MMPs is also enhanced[739,741].

$PGF_{2\alpha}$ stimulates the formation of endogenous prostaglandins via phospholipase A2 and release of arachidonic acid for prostaglandin synthesis[742]. Human ciliary muscle cells exposed to PGF_2 ethanolamine

or latanoprost for 9 days downregulate the FP receptor[743]. Long-term treatment with various subtype-selective prostaglandins results in intermuscular spaces become more organized and lined with an incomplete layer of endothelial cells, resembling lymphatic pathways[734].

Prostaglandin-induced changes in the sclera also are important in the regulation of unconventional outflow and may be used to enhance trans-scleral delivery of peptides and other high-molecular-weight substances to the posterior segment of the eye. Five days of topical treatment with $PGF_{2\alpha}$-isopropyl ester increases MMP-1, -2, and -3 in the sclera of monkeys[744]. Immunocytochemistry studies and mRNA analysis of human sclera and cultured human scleral fibroblasts show the presence of EP_1, EP_2, and FP receptor subtypes but not EP_3 and EP_4 subtypes[745]. Human scleral permeability to dextrans, measured in an Ussing chamber following exposure to $PGF_{2\alpha}$ and latanoprost acid for 1 to 3 days, increases in a dose- and time-dependent manner. This is accompanied by an increase in MMP concentration in the media, with the greatest increases in MMP-2 and -3 compared to MMP-1[746]. $PGF_{2\alpha}$ and latanoprost acid also induce increases in mRNA for MMPs and tissue inhibitors of MMPs in human scleral organ cultures[747]. MMPs alone are shown to directly increase scleral permeability of mouse eyes[748].

Mice deficient in various prostaglandin receptors delineate the role of prostanoid receptor subtypes in mediating the IOP-lowering response to clinical prostaglandin analogs. Studies in FP receptor–deficient mice show that the FP receptor is essential for the IOP-lowering response to topical latanoprost, travoprost, bimatoprost, and unoprostone[749]. Upregulation of MMP-2, -3, -9 and FP mRNA in the sclera following 7 days of topical treatment with latanoprost is also dependent

TABLE 10.4 Uveoscleral outflow on day 5 of twice-daily unilateral treatment with $PGF_{2\alpha}$

	Treated	Control	Treated/control
(a) Spontaneous IOP; approximately 235–325 min ($n = 6$)			
Albumin	0.78 ± 0.12^a	0.46 ± 0.03	1.66 ± 0.20^b
(b) IOP = 17–18 mmHg; approximately 240–335 min ($n = 2$)			
Albumin	$1.45 \pm 0.01^§$	0.62 ± 0.11	2.41 ± 0.42
(c) IOP = 17–18 mmHg; approximately 135–195 min ($n = 1$)			
Albumin	2.03	0.63	3.21
(d) All IOP time group combined ($n = 9$)			
Albumin	1.07 ± 0.17^c	0.52 ± 0.04	2.00 ± 0.24^d

IOP, Intraocular pressure; $PGF_{2\alpha}$, prostaglandin $F_{2\alpha}$.
On day 5 anterior chambers were exchanged with 2 mL of either[125]I- or[131]I-albumin. Infusion was continued at a lower rate for the balance of the indicated times. Pressures other than spontaneous were maintained by tracer flow from an elevated reservoir. Animals were then sacrificed, and the equivalent anterior chamber fluid recovered in the ocular and periocular tissues was determined. Overall, $PGF_{2\alpha}$ increased uveoscleral outflow approximately twofold compared with control eyes. Data are mean ± standard error of mean uveoscleral outflow (µL/min) for n animals, each contributing one treated and one control eye, following the ninth unilateral dose of $PGF_{2\alpha}$ on day 5; min indicates time window following $PGF_{2\alpha}$ encompassed by the measurement. Significantly different from 1.0 by the two-tailed paired t-test: $^bP < .05$; $^dP < .01$. Significantly different from contralateral control by the two-tailed two sample t-test: $^aP < .05$; $^cP < .01$.
(From Gabelt BT, Kaufman PL. Prostaglandin F2α increases uveoscleral outflow in the cynomolgus monkey. *Exp Eye Res.* 1989; 49(3):389–402. https://doi.org/10.1016/0014-4835(89)90049-3.)

BOX 10.3 Prostaglandin mechanisms

- Prostaglandin $FP_2\alpha$ analogs are the most effective IOP-lowering glaucoma drugs, exerting their ocular hypotensive effects primarily by increasing unconventional outflow, and secondarily by increasing unconventional outflow.
- Bimatoprost, latanoprost, and travoprost have similar mechanisms of action, primarily increasing unconventional outflow and secondarily increasing conventional outflow of aqueous humor in healthy adult human subjects.
- A single bimatoprost sustained release implant lowers IOP for 6 months to similar levels of topical administration in the majority of patients, with some experiencing sustained IOP-lowering for 2 years.
- Omidenepag was the first prostaglandin E2 selective agonist approved for use to treat ocular hypertension in humans and has similar mechanism of action as prostaglandin $FP_2\alpha$ analogs, working on both the unconventional and trabecular outflow pathways.

TABLE 10.5 Distribution of dextran tracer, uveoscleral outflow, protein, and intraocular pressure in control and inflamed cynomolgus monkey eyes

	Control eye (µL)	Inflamed eye (µL)	Probability[a]
Iris	1.2 ± 0.3	2.4 ± 0.3	0.07
Anterior uvea	8.5 ± 2.4	18.6 ± 4.3	0.43
Posterior uvea	0.3 ± 0.2	4.2 ± 0.8	0.006
Anterior sclera	8.4 ± 1.6	28.4 ± 4.4	0.01
Posterior sclera	1.9 ± 0.9	21.5 ± 3.9	0.006
Retina	0.1 ± 0.1	2.1 ± 0.9	0.08
Fluid[b]	0.7 ± 0.4	11.2 ± 3.4	0.03
Total	**21.0 ± 4.7**	**88.4 ± 14.7**	**0.009**
Uveoscleral outflow (µL/min)	0.7 ± 0.2	2.9 ± 0.5	0.009
AC protein (mg/mL)	0.20 ± 0.02	7.8 ± 4.0	0.006
Pre-IOP	16.7 ± 0.8	15.2 ± 1.3	0.43
Post-IOP	14.2 ± 1.6	3.0 ± 1.1	<0.001

Inflammation was induced by intravitreal injection of bovine serum albumin. Two days later, tracers were perfused through the anterior chamber and F_u was determined after 30 minutes at 15 mmHg. Uveoscleral outflow was increased in inflamed eyes up to fourfold with the 70,000 molecular weight (MW) fluoresceinated dextran. Values are mean ± standard error of mean; $n = 6$.
AC, Anterior chamber; *IOP*, intraocular pressure.
[a]Paired t-test analysis value.
[b]Includes vitreous, posterior chamber fluid, suprachoroidal fluid.
From Toris CB, Pederson JE. Aqueous humor dynamics in experimental iridocyclitis. *Invest Ophthalmol Vis Sci.* 1987;28:477. Reproduced with permission from the Association for Research in Vision and Ophthalmology.

on an intact FP receptor gene[749,750] EP receptor–deficient mice are studied in similar ways. When EP1, EP_2, and EP3 receptor–deficient mice and their wild-type background strain are treated topically with latanoprost, travoprost, bimatoprost, or unoprostone, EP3 receptors are involved in the IOP—lowering response to latanoprost, travoprost, and bimatoprost at 3 hours after drug administration—but EP1 and EP2 receptors are not[751]. This is in contrast to what is expected from in vitro receptor binding[752,753] and functional assays[753] in which FP receptor binding and functional responses (phosphoinositide turnover) are at least two orders of magnitude greater than for EP3 receptors. Also, immunohistochemistry studies show that EP2 receptors are the most abundantly expressed EP subtype in human ocular tissues[754].

EP2 selective agonists are effective in lowering IOP in monkeys[755–757]. Topical treatment with a combination of EP1, EP2, EP3, and FP receptor agonists increases the magnitude of the IOP-lowering response in monkeys when compared with FP agonist therapy alone[755]. Accordingly, the prostanoid EP2 receptor agonist butaprost increases unconventional outflow in the cynomolgus monkey[756]. Owing to these beneficial effects on IOP and outflow, pharmaceutical companies developed several EP2 receptor agonists for the treatment of glaucoma, but use in patients has been derailed mostly because of adverse ocular surface issues. However, a novel prostaglandin E2 agonist, omidenepag, was developed and demonstrates efficacy and an acceptable safety profile in clinical trials[758], which resulted in its approval in Japan for use in humans in 2018.

Although the unconventional pathway is the primary target for Prostaglandin $F_2\alpha$ analogs, they also increase conventional outflow, where prostaglandin FP receptors are also expressed[745]. Using human anterior segments in organ culture, two different prostaglandin analogs were shown to increase outflow facility over a couple of days by 40% to 65% (Bahler, et al. 2007,[759]). In normotensive humans, bimatoprost decreased tonographic outflow resistance (increased outflow facility) by 23%[760]. The transcripts and protein for MMP-1, -3, and -9, as well as TIMP2 and TIMP4, are increased by latanoprost treatment of TM cells[761,762]. Using a cell impedance assay to measure cell contractility, bimatoprost activates prostaglandin FP receptors in both TM and SC cells[763]. Thus, conventional outflow effects of prostaglandins appear to be due to both cellular relaxation and increase in ECM turnover.

After 25 years in clinical use, $PGF_{2\alpha}$ analogs remain the first line medication for POAG, owing to their dramatic effects on increasing outflow, which provides a larger reduction in IOP than any other known drug class. $PGF_{2\alpha}$ analogs and metabolites are clinically useful ocular hypotensive agents, despite some undesirable side effects (conjunctival foreign body sensation, conjunctival hyperemia, stinging pain, photophobia, increased iris pigmentation, and decreased orbital fat)[764–766]. Gene therapy approaches to overexpress prostaglandin pathway components in the anterior segment to lower IOP are being investigated so that problems with patient compliance for drug administration may be reduced. Success has been demonstrated in cat and nonhuman primate models in which IOP was decreased for 5 months following transduction with lentiviral or feline immunodeficiency vectors, respectively encoding prostaglandin pathway genes[767,768]. An alternative strategy to gene therapy is implantation of sustained delivery systems containing prostaglandins. Bimatoprost was loaded into a biodegradable implant, injected into anterior chambers of glaucoma patients, and evaluated for safety and efficacy in lowering IOP[769,770]. Clinical trial results demonstrated IOP reduction similar to bimatoprost drops that was sustained for 6 months in most subjects. Interestingly, 28% of patients experienced continuous IOP lowering two years after implantation, well after the last implant had completely reabsorbed, without need of rescue from topical glaucoma medications.

Cell volume effects on conventional outflow

Owing to the narrow passageways between cells in the JCT, changes in cell volume impact outflow facility. Thus, perfusion with increasingly hypo-osmotic media induces a progressive increase in outflow facility, which corresponds to increased cell volume, whereas hyperosmotic media causes a progressive decrease in outflow facility and decrease in cell volume of cells during anterior segment perfusions[771]. Outflow facility recovered in both scenarios only after return to perfusion with isosmotic media.

The Na-K-Cl cotransporter is a plasma membrane protein that participates in vectoral transport of Na and Cl across epithelia and also regulates intracellular volume in a variety of epithelial and nonepithelial cell types[772–775]. Changes in TM cell volume by agents that modulate Na-K-Cl cotransport activity affect outflow facility in human and calf eyes in vitro[776]. However, no change in outflow facility is observed in monkeys in vivo following administration of the Na-K-Cl inhibitor bumetanide[134], whereas oubain increased outflow facility in perfused porcine anterior segments where the conventional pathway is functionally isolated[777].

In addition to its canonical role in the transcellular movement of water across TM and SC cells, aquaporin-1 appears to also participate in establishing resting cell volume of TM cells[120,778–780]. However, aquaporin-1 deletion in mice or viral knockdown in human organ–cultured anterior segments does not influence outflow facility[781,782]. Instead, it appears that the role for aquaporin-1 in the TM is cytoprotective, enabling the rapid movement of water across its plasma membrane during times of repetitive and substantial mechanical stretching owing to ocular pulse and other dynamic processes that alter IOP (Fig. 10.9)[428].

Although chloride channels are thought to be involved in the regulation of cellular volume and intracellular chloride concentration, they do not appear to contribute significantly to the regulation of outflow facility[783,784]. However, BK channel activation increases outflow facility and decreases cell volume in perfused porcine anterior segments, suggesting that potassium efflux regulates TM cell function[785]. As well, TRPV4, a mechanosensitive calcium channel, participates in cell volume regulation of TM and SC cells and its antagonism lowers IOP by increasing outflow facility[170]. Moreover, TRPV4-deficient mice have elevated IOPs, compared with wild-type littermates[429].

Hyaluronidase and protease effects on outflow

The dynamic maintenance of ECM content, especially glycosaminoglycans (GAGs), contribute to the filtration barrier of aqueous outflow through the JCT. A quantitative biochemical profile of GAGs from normal and POAG TM suggests that there is depletion of hyaluronic acid and an accumulation of chondroitin sulfates in the POAG TM[786]. Substantial hyaluronan is present in the nonglaucomatous outflow pathway associated with the cells lining the TM beams. These findings support potential roles for this glycosaminoglycan in the regulation of the physiologic aqueous outflow resistance or in the maintenance of the outflow channels, or both[787]. Hyaluronic acid covering the surfaces of the outflow pathways might prevent adherence of molecules to ECM components within the JCT and thereby prevent clogging of the outflow pathways[540]. It is hypothesized that POAG is characterized by a decreased concentration of hyaluronic acid and increased turnover and downregulation of the hyaluronic acid receptor CD44 in the eye, which, in turn, may influence cell survival of TM cells[788]. Interestingly, intracameral infusion of hyaluronidase markedly increases facility in the bovine eye, presumably as the result of washout of acid mucopolysaccharide–rich ECM in the chamber angle tissues[789]. Effects in primates are much more variable[473,790–793]. The variations are attributed to interspecies differences, the type and source of hyaluronidase, and the conditions used for the enzymatic digestion that may have contributed to a variable and incomplete degradation of hyaluronic acid.

Another protease, α-chymotrypsin, was routinely used during intracapsular cataract surgery to lyse lens zonules, so it was examined ex vivo and in vivo for effects on outflow. In the enucleated human eye perfused at room temperature, α-chymotrypsin has little effect on facility[473]. However, effects of trypsin may be masked at low temperatures[794] and a combination of trypsin and ethylenediaminetetraacetic acid (EDTA) may have a marked effect in dissociating cultured cells not easily dissociated by either agent alone[795]. Perfusion of the anterior chamber of living monkeys with 50 U/mL α-chymotrypsin gives a large facility increase that persists for several hours even after the enzyme is removed from the infusate[796]. The facility increase induced by intracameral 0.5 mM Na$_2$EDTA is augmented and prolonged by α-chymotrypsin[796].

Exposure of porcine TM cells to growth factors such as TGF-β induces increases in MMPs such as stromelysin, gelatinase B, and collagenase, suggesting a role in the regulation of ECM turnover by TM cells[797]. However, prolonged elevation of TGFβ2, as occurs in POAG, can have the opposite effects and contribute to outflow obstruction. The importance of ECM turnover was demonstrated by perfusion of purified MMPs in organ-cultured human anterior segments, which increase outflow facility by 160% for at least 125 hours[384].

The composition of the ECM in the TM is complicated, and extensively reviewed elsewhere[798]. Presumably any of the enzymes involved in the biosynthesis or degradation of the ECM are potential targets to be manipulated for enhancing conventional outflow. Indeed, an adenosine A1 agonist alters ECM turnover by TM cells and increases conventional outflow facility. Adenosine A1 agonist treatment significantly increased MMP-2 activity and MMP-14 abundance, while decreasing fibronectin and collagen IV expression[799,800]. Adenosine levels in aqueous humor positively correlate with IOP in ocular hypertensive individuals, and could possibly serve as an endogenous modulator of IOP[801]. Indeed, an adenosine A1 agonist lowered IOP by increasing outflow facility in monkeys. As a result, this purinergic pathway was exploited therapeutically with the development of a topical adenosine A1 agonist, trabodenoson. In early clinical trials, trabodenoson effectively reduced IOP in patients with ocular hypertension, but was not advanced[802,803].

Renin-angiotensin effects on outflow

In addition to VEGF, nitric oxide, endothelin-1, and angiopoetin-1 signaling in the conventional outflow pathway, there is evidence that the eye contains a renin-angiotensin system and that it may be involved in the regulation of IOP. The presence of angiotensin-converting enzyme activities, the concentration of angiotensinogen and angiotensin-II, and the density of angiotensin-II AT1 receptors in ocular tissues and fluids are demonstrated in several species, including humans[804–809]. Oral administration of an angiotensin-II receptor type 1 antagonist[810] or an angiotensin-converting enzyme inhibitor[811,812] reduces IOP in normotensive and POAG patients. Moreover, topical application of a renin inhibitor decreases IOP in rabbits and monkeys without affecting systemic blood pressure or heart rate[813].

Multiple topical doses of an angiotensin AT1 receptor antagonist, CS-088, decreases IOP in monkey eyes with unilateral laser-induced glaucoma[814]. In humans, the oral AT1 receptor antagonist, losartan, increases outflow facility[810]. The angiotensin-converting enzyme inhibitor, captopril[812], decreases IOP and increases total outflow facility without affecting blood pressure, heart rate, or pupil diameter. Another study suggests the IOP-lowering responses to Angiotensin Converting Enzyme (ACE) inhibition is due to prostaglandin biosynthesis and increased uveoscleral outflow[815]. Angiotensin itself slightly decreases outflow facility in monkeys following intracameral injection[589].

SUMMARY

Dynamic and tightly regulated specialized processes have evolved to produce aqueous humor and deliver nutrients to the avascular tissues of the eye. Aqueous humor also serves to carry away their metabolic wastes, transmit light, and pressurize the eye. For 90% to 95% of people, IOP is maintained within a couple of millimeters of mercury over a lifetime and is established by the regulation of outflow resistance in the conventional outflow pathway. Ocular hypertension in the other 5% to 10% of people is a result of conventional outflow dysfunction and abnormally high resistance to aqueous humor outflow. If left unchecked, prolonged ocular hypertension places people at high risk for damage to the retinal ganglion cells and the optic nerve. Knowledge gained over the past 50 years about the physiologic processes that regulate the production and removal of aqueous humor have resulted in an arsenal of therapeutics that are used clinically to treat ocular hypertension in glaucoma.

REFERENCES

1. Davson H. The aqueous humor and the intraocular pressure. In: Davson H, ed. *Physiology of the Eye*. New York: Pergamon Press; 1990:3.
2. Davson H. The aqueous humour and the intraocular pressure. In: Davson H, ed. *Physiology of the Eye*. London. UK: Macmillan Education; 1990:3–95.
3. Millar C, Kaufman PL. Aqueous humor: secretion and dynamics. In: Tasman W, Jaeger EA, eds. *Duane's Foundations of Clinical Ophthalmology*. Philadelphia: Lippincott-Raven; 1995.
4. McLaren JW. Control of aqueous humor flow. In: Dartt DA, ed. *Encyclopedia of the Eye*. Oxford: Academic Press; 2010:389–397.
5. Brubaker RF. Flow of aqueous humor in humans [The Friedenwald Lecture]. *Invest Ophthalmol Vis Sci*. 1991;32(13):3145–3166.
6. Brubaker RF, Nagataki S, Townsend DJ, Burns RR, Higgins RG, Wentworth W. The effect of age on aqueous humor formation in man. *Ophthalmology*. 1981;88(3):283–288.
7. Toris CB, Yablonski ME, Wang YL, Camras CB. Aqueous humor dynamics in the aging human eye. *Am J Ophthalmol*. 1999;127(4):407–412.
8. Gabelt BT, Gottanka J, Lütjen-Drecoll E, Kaufman PL. Aqueous humor dynamics and trabecular meshwork and anterior ciliary muscle morphologic changes with age in rhesus monkeys. *Invest Ophthalmol Vis Sci*. 2003;44(5):2118–2125.
9. Bassnett S. Zinn's zonule. *Prog Retin Eye Res*. 2021;82:100902.
10. Tamm ER, Lütjen-Drecoll E. Ciliary body. *Microsc Res Tech*. 1996;33(5):390–439.
11. Usukura J, Fain GL, Bok D. [3H]ouabain localization of Na-K ATPase in the epithelium of rabbit ciliary body pars plicata. *Invest Ophthalmol Vis Sci*. 1988;29(4):606–614.
12. Funk R, Rohen JW. SEM studies on the functional morphology of the rabbit ciliary process vasculature. *Exp Eye Res*. 1987;45(4):579–595.
13. Freddo T, Gong H, Civan M. Anatomy of the ciliary body and outflow pathways. In: *Duane's Ophthalmology*. Philadelphia: Lippincott Williams & Wilkins; 2011.
14. Freddo TF. A contemporary concept of the blood-aqueous barrier. *Prog Retin Eye Res*. 2013;32:181–195.
15. DiMattio J. A comparative study of ascorbic acid entry into aqueous and vitreous humors of the rat and guinea pig. *Invest Ophthalmol Vis Sci*. 1989;30(11):2320–2331.
16. Krause U, Raunio V. Protein content of normal human aqueous humour in vivo. *Acta Ophthalmol (Copenh)*. 1969;47(1):215–221.
17. Stjernschantz J, Uusitalo R, Palkama A. The aqueous proteins of the rat in normal eye and after aqueous withdrawal. *Exp Eye Res*. 1973;16(3):215–221.
18. Fielder AR, Rahi AH. Immunoglobulins of normal aqueous humour. *Trans Ophthalmol Soc U K*. 1979;99(1):120–125.
19. Freddo TF, Bartels SP, Barsotti MF, Kamm RD. The source of proteins in the aqueous humor of the normal rabbit. *Invest Ophthalmol Vis Sci*. 1990;31(1):125–137.
20. Kolodny NH, Freddo TF, Lawrence BA, Suarez C, Bartels SP. Contrast-enhanced magnetic resonance imaging confirmation of an anterior protein pathway in normal rabbit eyes. *Invest Ophthalmol Vis Sci*. 1996;37(8):1602–1607.
21. Barsotti MF, Bartels SP, Freddo TF, Kamm RD. The source of protein in the aqueous humor of the normal monkey eye. *Invest Ophthalmol Vis Sci*. 1992;33(3):581–595.
22. Hubens WHG, Mohren RJC, Liesenborghs I, Eijssen LMT, Ramdas WD, Webers CAB, Gorgels T. The aqueous humor proteome of primary open angle glaucoma: An extensive review. *Exp Eye Res*. 2020;197:108077.
23. Caprioli J. The ciliary epithelia and aqueous humor. In: Hart WM, ed. *Adler's Physiology of the Eye, Clinical Application*. St Louis: CV Mosby; 1992:228.
24. DiMattio J. Active transport of ascorbic acid into lens epithelium of the rat. *Exp Eye Res*. 1989;49(5):873–885.
25. Delamere NA. Ascorbic acid and the eye. *Subcell Biochem*. 1996;25:313–329.
26. Reddy VN, Giblin FJ, Lin LR, Chakrapani B. The effect of aqueous humor ascorbate on ultraviolet-B-induced DNA damage in lens epithelium. *Invest Ophthalmol Vis Sci*. 1998;39(2):344–350.
27. Rose RC, Bode AM. Ocular ascorbate transport and metabolism. *Comp Biochem Physiol A Comp Physiol*. 1991;100(2):273–285.
28. Xu P, Lin Y, Porter K, Liton PB. Ascorbic acid modulation of iron homeostasis and lysosomal function in trabecular meshwork cells. *Journal of ocular pharmacology and therapeutics*. 2014;30(2-3):246–253.
29. Ringvold A. The significance of ascorbate in the aqueous humour protection against UV-A and UV-B. *Exp Eye Res*. 1996;62(3):261–264.
30. Alvarado J, Murphy C, Juster R. Trabecular meshwork cellularity in primary open-angle glaucoma and nonglaucomatous normals. *Ophthalmology*. 1984;91(6):564–579.
31. Grierson I, Howes RC. Age-related depletion of the cell population in the human trabecular meshwork. *Eye (Lond)*. 1987;1(Pt 2):204–210.
32. Koskela TK, Reiss GR, Brubaker RF, Ellefson RD. Is the high concentration of ascorbic acid in the eye an adaptation to intense solar irradiation? *Invest Ophthalmol Vis Sci*. 1989;30(10):2265–2267.
33. Reiss GR, Werness PG, Zollman PE, Brubaker RF. Ascorbic acid levels in the aqueous humor of nocturnal and diurnal mammals. *Archives of Ophthalmology*. 1986;104(5):753–755.
34. Becker B. Ascorbate transport in guinea pig eyes. *Investigative Ophthalmology & Visual Science*. 1967;6(4):410–415.
35. Socci RR, Delamere NA. Characteristics of ascorbate transport in the rabbit iris-ciliary body. *Experimental Eye Research*. 1988;46(6):853–861.
36. Socci RR, Delamere NA. The effect of vanadate upon calcium-stimulated ATPase of the rabbit iris-ciliary body. *Invest Ophthalmol Vis Sci*. 1988;29(12):1866–1870.
37. Liang WJ, Johnson D, Jarvis SM. Vitamin C transport systems of mammalian cells. *Mol Membr Biol*. 2001;18(1):87–95.
38. Ma W, Hui H, Pelegrin P, Surprenant A. Pharmacological characterization of pannexin-1 currents expressed in mammalian cells. *Journal of Pharmacology & Experimental Therapeutics*. 2009;328(2):409–418.
39. Zanon-Moreno V, Ciancotti-Olivares L, Asencio J, Sanz P, Ortega-Azorin C, Pinazo-Duran MD, Corella D. Association between a SLC23A2 gene variation, plasma vitamin C levels, and risk of glaucoma in a Mediterranean population. *Molecular vision*. 2011;17:2997–3004.
40. Duke-Elder S. The aqueous humor. In: Duje-Elder S, editor. *The Physiology of the Eye and of Vision. System of Ophthalmology*. 4. St Louis: CV Mosby; 1968:104.
41. Wecker T, Hoffmeier K, Plötner A, et al. MicroRNA profiling in aqueous humor of individual human eyes by next-generation sequencing. *Invest Ophthalmol Vis Sci*. 2016;57(4):1706–1713.
42. Dismuke WM, Challa P, Navarro I, Stamer WD, Liu Y. Human aqueous humor exosomes. *Exp Eye Res*. 2015;132:73–77.
43. Drewry MD, Challa P, Kuchtey JG, Navarro I, Helwa I, Hu Y, Mu H, Stamer WD, Kuchtey RW, Liu Y. Differentially expressed microRNAs in the aqueous humor of patients with exfoliation glaucoma or primary open-angle glaucoma. *Hum Mol Genet*. 2018;27(7):1263–1275.
44. Hubens WHG, Krauskopf J, Beckers HJM, Kleinjans JCS, Webers CAB, Gorgels T. Small RNA sequencing of aqueous humor and plasma in patients with primary open-angle glaucoma. *Invest Ophthalmol Vis Sci*. 2021;62(7):24.
45. Lerner N, Schreiber-Avissar S, Beit-Yannai E. Extracellular vesicle-mediated crosstalk between NPCE cells and TM cells result in modulation of Wnt signalling pathway and ECM remodelling. *J Cell Mol Med*. 2020;24(8):4646–4658.
46. McLaren JW, Dinslage S, Dillon JP, Roberts JE, Brubaker RF. Measuring oxygen tension in the anterior chamber of rabbits. *Invest Ophthalmol Vis Sci*. 1998;39(10):1899–1909.
47. Siegfried CJ, Shui Y-B, Holekamp NM, Bai F, Beebe DC. Oxygen distribution in the human eye: relevance to the etiology of open-angle glaucoma after vitrectomy. *Investigative ophthalmology & visual science*. 2010;51(11):5731–5738.
48. Stamper RL, Lieberman MF, Drake MV. Aqueous humor formation. In: Klein EA, ed. *Becker-Shaffers's Diagnosis and Therapy of the Glaucomas*. St. Louis: CV Mosby; 2009:8–24.
49. Kiel JW, Hollingsworth M, Rao R, Chen M, Reitsamer HA. Ciliary blood flow and aqueous humor production. *Progress in retinal and eye research*. 2011;30(1):1–17.
50. Goel M, Picciani RG, Lee RK, Bhattacharya SK. Aqueous humor dynamics: a review. *Open Ophthalmol J*. 2010;4:52–59.
51. Cole DF. Secretion of the aqueous humor. *Exp Eye Res*. 1977;25(Suppl):161.
52. Green K, Pederson JE. Contribution of secretion and filtration to aqueous humor formation. *Am J Physiol*. 1972;222(5):1218–1226.
53. Pederson JE. Fluid permeability of monkey ciliary epithelium in vivo. *Invest Ophthalmol Vis Sci*. 1982;23(2):176–180.
54. Bill A. Blood circulation and fluid dynamics in the eye. *Physiol Rev*. 1975;55(3):383–417.
55. Wilson WS, Shahidullah M, Millar C. The bovine arterially-perfused eye: an in vitro method for the study of drug mechanisms on IOP, aqueous humour formation and uveal vasculature. *Current Eye Research*. 1993;12(7):609–620.
56. Bill A. The role of ciliary blood flow and ultrafiltration in aqueous humor formation. *Exp Eye Res*. 1973;16(4):287–298.
57. Goldmann H. On pseudofacility. *Bibl Ophthalmol*. 1968;76:1–14.
58. Bárány EH. Pseudofacility and uveoscleral outflow routes: some non-technical difficulties in the determination of outflow facility rate and rate of formation of aqueous humor. In: Leydhecker W, ed. *Glaucoma Symposium*. Tutzing Castle. Basel: Karger; 1966:27.
59. Bill A. Effects of atropine and pilocarpine on aqueous humour dynamics in cynomolgus monkeys (Macaca irus). *Exp Eye Res*. 1967;6(2):120–125.
60. Bill A. Aqueous humor dynamics in monkeys (Macaca irus and Cercopithecus ethiops). *Exp Eye Res*. 1971;11(2):195–206.
61. Bill A. Effects of longstanding stepwise increments in eye pressure on the rate of aqueous humor formation in a primate (Cercopithecus ethiops). *Exp Eye Res*. 1971;12(2):184–193.
62. Bill A, Bárány EH. Gross facility, facility of conventional routes, and pseudofacility of aqueous humor outflow in the cynomolgus monkey. The reduction in aqueous humor formation rate caused by moderate increments in intraocular pressure. *Arch Ophthalmol*. 1966;75(5):665–673.
63. Brubaker RF. The measurement of pseudofacility and true facility by constant pressure perfusion in the normal rhesus monkey eye. *Invest Ophthalmol*. 1970;9(1):42–52.
64. Kupfer C. Clinical significance of pseudofacility. Sanford R. Gifford Memorial Lecture. *Am J Ophthalmol*. 1973;75(2):193–204.
65. Kupfer C, Sanderson P. Determination of pseudofacility in the eye of man. *Arch Ophthalmol*. 1968;80(2):194–196.
66. Moses RA, Grodzki Jr. WJ, Carras PL. Pseudofacility. Where did it go? *Arch Ophthalmol*. 1985;103(11):1653–1655.
67. Beneyto Martin P, Fernandez-Vila PC, Perez TM. Determination of the pseudofacility by fluorophotometry in the human eye. *Int Ophthalmol*. 1995;19(4):219–223.
68. Candia OA, Alvarez LJ. Fluid transport phenomena in ocular epithelia. *Prog Retin Eye Res*. 2008;27(2):197–212.
69. Freddo TF. Shifting the paradigm of the blood-aqueous barrier. *Exp Eye Res*. 2001;73(5):581–592.
70. Berggren L. Further studies on the effect of autonomous drugs on in vitro secretory activity of the rabbit eye ciliary processes. A. Inhibition of the pilocarpine effect by isopilocarpine, arecoline, and atropine. B. Influence of isoproterenol and norepinephrine. *Acta Ophthalmol (Copenh)*. 1970;48(2):293–302.
71. Toris CB, Pederson JE. Aqueous humor dynamics in experimental iridocyclitis. *Invest Ophthalmol Vis Sci*. 1987;28(3):477–481.
72. Bárány EH. A Mathematical formulation of intraocular pressure as dependent on secretion, ultrafiltration, bulk outflow, and osmotic reabsorption of fluid. *Invest Ophthalmol*. 1963;2:584–590.
73. Krupin T, Civan MM. Physiologic basis of aqueous humor formation. In: Ritch R, ed. *The Glaucomas*. 2nd ed. St Louis: CV Mosby; 1996.
74. Nilsson SFEB A. Physiology and neurophysiology of aqueous humor inflow and outflow. In: Kaufman PL, Mittag TW, eds. *Glaucoma*. London: Mosby-Year Book Europe Ltd; 1994:1–17.

75. Pederson JE, Green K. Aqueous humor dynamics: a mathematical approach to measurement of facility, pseudofacility, capillary pressure, active secretion and X c. *Exp Eye Res*. 1973;15(3):265–276.
76. Sacco R, Guidoboni G, Jerome JW, et al. A theoretical approach for the electrochemical characterization of ciliary epithelium. *Life (Basel, Switzerland)*. 2020;10(2):8.
77. Raviola G, Raviola E. Intercellular junctions in the ciliary epithelium. *Invest Ophthalmol Vis Sci*. 1978;17(10):958–981.
78. Wolosin JM, Schütte M, Chen S. Connexin distribution in the rabbit and rat ciliary body. A case for heterotypic epithelial gap junctions. *Invest Ophthalmol Vis Sci*. 1997;38(2):341–348.
79. Coffey KL, Krushinsky A, Green CR, Donaldson PJ. Molecular profiling and cellular localization of connexin isoforms in the rat ciliary epithelium. *Exp Eye Res*. 2002;75(1):9–21.
80. Li SK, Shan SW, Li HL, et al. Characterization and regulation of gap junctions in porcine ciliary epithelium. *Invest Ophthalmol Vis Sci*. 2018;59(8):3461–3468.
81. Macknight AD, McLaughlin CW, Peart D, Purves RD, Carré DA, Civan MM. Formation of the aqueous humor. *Clinical and Experimental Pharmacology and Physiology*. 2000;27(1-2):100–106.
82. Bonting SL, Becker B. Studies on sodium-potassium activated adenosinetriphosphatase. XIV. Inhibition of enzyme activity and aqueous humor flow in the rabbit eye after intravitreal injection of ouabain. *Invest Ophthalmol*. 1964;3:523–533.
83. Flügel C, Lütjen-Drecoll E. Presence and distribution of Na+/K+-ATPase in the ciliary epithelium of the rabbit. *Histochemistry*. 1988;88(3-6):613–621.
84. Riley MV, Kishida K. ATPases of ciliary epithelium: cellular and subcellular distribution and probable role in secretion of aqueous humor. *Exp Eye Res*. 1986;42(6):559–568.
85. Bhattacherjee P. Distribution of carbonic anhydrase in the rabbit eye as demonstrated histochemically. *Exp Eye Res*. 1971;12(3):356–359.
86. Tsukahara S, Maezawa N. Cytochemical localization of adenyl cyclase in the rabbit ciliary body. *Exp Eye Res*. 1978;26(1):99–106.
87. Wistrand PJ. Carbonic anhydrase in the anterior uvea of the rabbit. *Acta Physiol Scand*. 1951;24(2-3):145–148.
88. Dunn JJ, Lytle C, Crook RB. Immunolocalization of the Na-K-Cl cotransporter in bovine ciliary epithelium. *Invest Ophthalmol Vis Sci*. 2001;42(2):343–353.
89. Martin-Vasallo P, Ghosh S, Coca-Prados M. Expression of Na,K-ATPase alpha subunit isoforms in the human ciliary body and cultured ciliary epithelial cells. *J Cell Physiol*. 1989;141(2):243–252.
90. Ghosh S, Hernando N, Martín-Alonso JM, Martin-Vasallo P, Coca-Prados M. Expression of multiple Na+,K(+)-ATPase genes reveals a gradient of isoforms along the nonpigmented ciliary epithelium: functional implications in aqueous humor secretion. *J Cell Physiol*. 1991;149(2):184–194.
91. Do CW, Civan MM. Basis of chloride transport in ciliary epithelium. *J Membr Biol*. 2004;200(1):1–13.
92. Ma N, Siegfried C, Kubota M, et al. Expression Profiling of Ascorbic Acid-Related Transporters in Human and Mouse Eyes. *Investigative ophthalmology & visual science*. 2016;57(7):3440–3450.
93. Tsukamoto H, Mishima HK, Kurokawa T, Kiuchi Y, Sato E, Ishibashi S. Isoforms of glucose transporter in the iris-ciliary body. *Jpn J Ophthalmol*. 1995;39(3):242–247.
94. Hou Y, Delamere NA. Studies on H(+)-ATPase in cultured rabbit nonpigmented ciliary epithelium. *J Membr Biol*. 2000;173(1):67–72.
95. Wax MB, Saito I, Tenkova T, et al. Vacuolar H+-ATPase in ocular ciliary epithelium. *Proceedings of the National Academy of Sciences of the United States of America*. 1997;94(13):6752–6757.
96. Youkilis JC, Bassnett S. Single-cell RNA-sequencing analysis of the ciliary epithelium and contiguous tissues in the mouse eye. *Experimental Eye Research*. 2021;213:108811.
97. McLaughlin CW, Zellhuber-McMillan S, Macknight AD, Civan MM. Electron microprobe analysis of rabbit ciliary epithelium indicates enhanced secretion posteriorly and enhanced absorption anteriorly. *Am J Physiol Cell Physiol*. 2007;293(5):C1455–1466.
98. Hoffman BF, Bigger JTJ. Digitalis and allied cardiac glyosides. In: Gilman AG, ed. *The pharmacological basis of therapeutics*. New York: McGraw-Hill; 1990:814.
99. Podos SM, Lee PY, Severin C, Mittag T. The effect of vanadate on aqueous humor dynamics in cynomolgus monkeys. *Invest Ophthalmol Vis Sci*. 1984;25(3):359–361.
100. Riley MV. The sodium-potassium-stimulated adenosin E triphosphatase of rabbit ciliary epithelium. *Exp Eye Res*. 1964;3:76–84.
101. Becker B. Ouabain and aqueous humor dynamics in the rabbit eye. *Invest Ophthalmol*. 1963;2:325–331.
102. Shahidullah M, Wilson WS, Yap M, To CH. Effects of ion transport and channel-blocking drugs on aqueous humor formation in isolated bovine eye. *Investigative Ophthalmology & Visual Science*. 2003;44(3):1185–1191.
103. Simon KA, Bonting SL. Possible usefulness of cardiac glycosides in treatment of glaucoma. *Arch Ophthalmol*. 1962;68:227–234.
104. Krupin T, Becker B, Podos SM. Topical vanadate lowers intraocular pressure in rabbits. *Invest Ophthalmol Vis Sci*. 1980;19(11):1360–1363.
105. Lee PY, Podos SM, Howard-Williams JR, Severin CH, Rose AD, Siegel MJ. Pharmacological testing in the laser-induced monkey glaucoma model. *Curr Eye Res*. 1985;4(7):775–781.
106. Lee PY, Podos SM, Serle JB, Camras CB, Severin CH. Intraocular pressure effects of multiple doses of drugs applied to glaucomatous monkey eyes. *Arch Ophthalmol*. 1987;105(2):249–252.
107. Becker B. Vanadate and aqueous humor dynamics. Proctor Lecture. *Invest Ophthalmol Vis Sci*. 1980;19(10):1156–1165.
108. Delamere NA, Williams RN. The influence of reserpine and propranolol upon the IOP response to vanadate in the rabbit. *Invest Ophthalmol Vis Sci*. 1985;26(10):1442–1445.
109. Delamere NA, Williams RN. Modulation by vanadate of the adrenergic characteristics of the iris, ileum, and vas deferens. *Invest Ophthalmol Vis Sci*. 1986;27(9):1336–1341.
110. Mittag TW, Guo WB, Taniguchi T. Interaction of vanadate and iodate oxyanions with adenylyl cyclase of ciliary processes. *Biochem Pharmacol*. 1993;45(6):1311–1316.
111. Shahidullah M, Mandal A, Delamere NA. Responses of sodium-hydrogen exchange to nitric oxide in porcine cultured nonpigmented ciliary epithelium. *Invest Ophthalmol Vis Sci*. 2009;50(12):5851–5858.
112. Shahidullah M, Mandal A, Delamere NA. Src family kinase links insulin signaling to short term regulation of Na,K-ATPase in nonpigmented ciliary epithelium. *J Cell Physiol*. 2017;232(6):1489–1500.
113. Shahidullah M, Mandal A, Wei G, Delamere NA. Nitric oxide regulation of na, k-atpase activity in ocular ciliary epithelium involves Src family kinase. *J Cell Physiol*. 2014;229(3):343–352.
114. Shahidullah M, Mandal A, Wei G, Levin LR, Buck J, Delamere NA. Nonpigmented ciliary epithelial cells respond to acetazolamide by a soluble adenylyl cyclase mechanism. *Investigative Ophthalmology & Visual Science*. 2014;55(1):187–197.
115. Delamere NA. Ciliary body and ciliary epithelium. *Adv Organ Biol*. 2005;10:127–148.
116. Fischbarg J. Mechanism of fluid transport across corneal endothelium and other epithelial layers: a possible explanation based on cyclic cell volume regulatory changes. *The Br J Ophthalmol*. 1997;81(1):85–89.
117. Frigeri A, Gropper MA, Turck CW, Verkman AS. Immunolocalization of the mercurial-insensitive water channel and glycerol intrinsic protein in epithelial cell plasma membranes. *Proc Natl Acad Sci U S A*. 1995;92(10):4328–4331.
118. Patil RV, Han Z, Yiming M, et al. Fluid transport by human nonpigmented ciliary epithelial layers in culture: a homeostatic role for aquaporin-1. *Am J Physiol Cell Physiol*. 2001;281(4):C1139–1145.
119. Schey KL, Wang Z, Wenke JL, Qi Y. Aquaporins in the eye: expression, function, and roles in ocular disease. *Biochimica et biophysica acta*. 2014;1840(5):1513–1523.
120. Verkman AS. Role of aquaporin water channels in eye function. *Exp Eye Res*. 2003;76(2):137–143.
121. Wu J, Bell OH, Copland DA, et al. Gene therapy for glaucoma by ciliary body aquaporin 1 disruption using CRISPR-Cas9. *Mol Ther*. 2020;28(3):820–829.
122. Civan MM, Macknight AD. The ins and outs of aqueous humour secretion. *Exp Eye Res*. 2004;78(3):625–631.
123. Do CW, Civan MM. Species variation in biology and physiology of the ciliary epithelium: similarities and differences. *Exp Eye Res*. 2009;88(4):631–640.
124. Maren TH. Biochemistry of aqueous humor inflow. Glaucoma. In: Kaufman PL, Mittag TW, eds. London: Mosby-Year Book Europe Ltd; 1994:1–35.
125. McLaughlin CW, Peart D, Purves RD, et al. Effects of HCO3- on cell composition of rabbit ciliary epithelium: a new model for aqueous humor secretion. *Invest Ophthalmol Vis Sci*. 1998;39(9):1631–1641.
126. Shahidullah M, To CH, Pelis RM, Delamere NA. Studies on bicarbonate transporters and carbonic anhydrase in porcine nonpigmented ciliary epithelium. *Invest Ophthalmol Vis Sci*. 2009;50(4):1791–1800.
127. Do CW, To CH. Chloride secretion by bovine ciliary epithelium: a model of aqueous humor formation. *Invest Ophthalmol Vis Sci*. 2000;41(7):1853–1860.
128. Hochgesand DH, Dunn JJ, Crook RB. Catecholaminergic regulation of Na-K-Cl cotransport in pigmented ciliary epithelium: differences between PE and NPE. *Exp Eye Res*. 2001;72(1):1–12.
129. Jacob TJ, Civan MM. Role of ion channels in aqueous humor formation. *Am J Physiol*.1996; 271(3 Pt 1):C703–720.
130. Do CW, Civan MM. Swelling-activated chloride channels in aqueous humour formation: on the one side and the other. *Acta Physiol (Oxf)*. 2006;187(1-2):345–352.
131. Bakall B, McLaughlin P, Stanton JB, Zhang Y, Hartzell HC, Marmorstein LY, Marmorstein AD. Bestrophin-2 is involved in the generation of intraocular pressure. *Invest Ophthalmol Vis Sci*. 2008;49(4):1563–1570.
132. Avila MY, Seidler RW, Stone RA, Civan MM. Inhibitors of NHE-1 Na+/H+ exchange reduce mouse intraocular pressure. *Invest Ophthalmol Vis Sci*. 2002;43(6):1897–1902.
133. Shahidullah M, Wei G, Delamere NA. DIDS inhibits Na,K-ATPase activity in porcine nonpigmented ciliary epithelium by a Src family kinase-dependent mechanism. *Am J Physiol Cell Physiol*. 2013;305(5):C492–501.
134. Gabelt BT, Wiederholt M, Clark AF, Kaufman PL. Anterior segment physiology after bumetanide inhibition of Na-K-Cl cotransport. *Invest Ophthalmol Vis Sci*. 1997;38(9):1700–1707.
135. Kodama T, Reddy VN, Macri FJ. Pharmacological study on the effects of some ocular hypotensive drugs on aqueous humor formation in the arterially perfused enucleated rabbit eye. *Ophthalmic Res*. 1985;17(2):120–124.
136. Lütjen-Drecoll E, Lonnerholm G, Eichhorn M. Carbonic anhydrase distribution in the human and monkey eye by light and electron microscopy. *Graefes Arch Clin Exp Ophthalmol*. 1983;220(6):285–291.
137. Maren TH. Carbonic anhydrase: chemistry, physiology, and inhibition. *Physiol Rev*. 1967;47(4):595–781.
138. Maren TH. The rates of movement of Na+, Cl-, and HCO-3 from plasma to posterior chamber: effect of acetazolamide and relation to the treatment of glaucoma. *Invest Ophthalmol*. 1976;15(5):356–364.
139. Mudge GH, Weiner IM. Agents affecting volume and composition of body fluids. In: Gilman AG, ed. *The Pharmacological Basis of Therapeutics*. New York: McGraw-Hill; 1990:682.
140. Muther TF, Friedland BR. Autoradiographic localization of carbonic anhydrase in the rabbit ciliary body. *J Histochem Cytochem*. 1980;28(10):1119–1124.
141. Brechue WF, Maren TH. A comparison between the effect of topical and systemic carbonic anhydrase inhibitors on aqueous humor secretion. *Exp Eye Res*. 1993;57(1):67–78.
142. Mincione F, Scozzafava A, Supuran CT. The development of topically acting carbonic anhydrase inhibitors as anti-glaucoma agents. *Curr Top Med Chem*. 2007;7(9):849–854.
143. Wu Q, Delamere NA, Pierce Jr. W. Membrane-associated carbonic anhydrase in cultured rabbit nonpigmented ciliary epithelium. *Invest Ophthalmol Vis Sci*. 1997;38(10):2093–2102.
144. Wu Q, Pierce Jr. WM, Delamere NA. Cytoplasmic pH responses to carbonic anhydrase inhibitors in cultured rabbit nonpigmented ciliary epithelium. *J Membr Biol*. 1998;162(1):31–38.

145. Kaufman PL, Mittag TW. Medical therapy of glaucoma. In: Kaufman PL, Mittag TW, eds. *Glaucoma.* 9. London: Mosby-Year Book Europe Ltd; 1994:7.

146. Eller MG, Schoenwald RD, Dixson JA, Segarra T, Barfknecht CF. Topical carbonic anhydrase inhibitors. III: Optimization model for corneal penetration of ethoxzolamide analogues. *J Pharm Sci.* 1985;74(2):155–160.

147. Maren TH. The development of ideas concerning the role of carbonic anhydrase in the secretion of aqueous humor. Relations to the treatment of glaucoma. In: Drance SM, Neufeld AH, eds. *Glaucoma. Applied Pharmacology in Medical Treatment.* Orlando: Grune & Stratton; 1984:325.

148. Maren TH, Jankowska L, Sanyal G, Edelhauser HF. The transcorneal permeability of sulfonamide carbonic anhydrase inhibitors and their effect on aqueous humor secretion. *Exp Eye Res.* 1983;36(4):457–479.

149. Pierce Jr. WM, Sharir M, Waite KJ, Chen D, Kaysinger KK. Topically active ocular carbonic anhydrase inhibitors: novel biscarbonylamidothiadiazole sulfonamides as ocular hypotensive agents. *Proc Soc Exp Biol Med.* 1993;203(3):360–365.

150. Becker B. Decrease in intraocular pressure in man by a carbonic anhydrase inhibitor, diamox; a preliminary report. *Am J Ophthalmol.* 1954;37(1):13–15.

151. Schoenwald RD, Eller MG, Dixson JA, Barfknecht CF. Topical carbonic anhydrase inhibitors. *J Med Chem.* 1984;27(6):810–812.

152. Sugrue MF, Gautheron P, Grove J, et al. MK-927: a topically active ocular hypotensive carbonic anhydrase inhibitor. *J Ocul Pharmacol.* 1990;6(1):9–22.

153. Sugrue MF, Mallorga P, Schwam H, Baldwin JJ, Ponticello GS. A comparison of L-671,152 and MK-927, two topically effective ocular hypotensive carbonic anhydrase inhibitors, in experimental animals. *Curr Eye Res.* 1990;9(6):607–615.

154. Gunning FP, Greve EL, Bron AM, Bosc JM, Royer JG, George JL, Lesure P, Sirbat D. Two topical carbonic anhydrase inhibitors sezolamide and dorzolamide in Gelrite vehicle: a multiple-dose efficacy study. *Graefes Arch Clin Exp Ophthalmol.* 1993;231(7):384–388.

155. Herkel U, Pfeiffer N. Update on topical carbonic anhydrase inhibitors. *Curr Opin Ophthalmol.* 2001;12(2):88–93.

156. Lippa EA, Carlson LE, Ehinger B, et al. Dose response and duration of action of dorzolamide, a topical carbonic anhydrase inhibitor. *Arch Ophthalmol.* 1992;110(4):495–499.

157. Vanlandingham BD, Maus TL, Brubaker RF. The effect of dorzolamide on aqueous humor dynamics in normal human subjects during sleep. *Ophthalmology.* 1998;105(8):1537–1540.

158. Wilkerson M, Cyrlin M, Lippa EA, et al. Four-week safety and efficacy study of dorzolamide, a novel, active topical carbonic anhydrase inhibitor. *Arch Ophthalmol.* 1993;111(10):1343–1350.

159. Ingram CJ, Brubaker RF. Effect of brinzolamide and dorzolamide on aqueous humor flow in human eyes. *Am J Ophthalmol.* 1999;128(3):292–296.

160. Silver LH. Clinical efficacy and safety of brinzolamide (Azopt), a new topical carbonic anhydrase inhibitor for primary open-angle glaucoma and ocular hypertension. Brinzolamide Primary Therapy Study Group. *Am J Ophthalmol.* 1998;126(3):400–408.

161. Podos SM, Serle JB. Topically active carbonic anhydrase inhibitors for glaucoma. *Arch Ophthalmol.* 1991;109(1):38–40.

162. Edelman JL, Loo DD, Sachs G. Characterization of potassium and chloride channels in the basolateral membrane of bovine nonpigmented ciliary epithelial cells. *Invest Ophthalmol Vis Sci.* 1995;36(13):2706–2716.

163. Edelman JL, Sachs G, Adorante JS. Ion transport asymmetry and functional coupling in bovine pigmented and nonpigmented ciliary epithelial cells. *Am J Physiol.* 1994;266(5 Pt 1):C1210–1221.

164. Walker VE, Stelling JW, Miley HE, Jacob TJ. Effect of coupling on volume-regulatory response of ciliary epithelial cells suggests mechanism for secretion. *Am J Physiol.* 1999;276(6):C1432–1438.

165. Delamere NA, Shahidullah M. Ion transport regulation by TRPV4 and TRPV1 in lens and ciliary epithelium. *Front Physiol.* 2021;12:834916.

166. Jo AO, Lakk M, Frye AM, et al. Differential volume regulation and calcium signaling in two ciliary body cell types is subserved by TRPV4 channels. *Proceedings of the National Academy of Sciences.* 2016;113(14):3885.

167. Shahidullah M, Mandal A, Delamere NA. TRPV4 in porcine lens epithelium regulates hemichannel-mediated ATP release and Na-K-ATPase activity. *American Journal of Physiology - Cell Physiology.* 2012;302(12):C1751–1761.

168. Shahidullah M, Delamere NA. Connexins form functional hemichannels in porcine ciliary epithelium. *Exp Eye Res.* 2014;118(12):20–29.

169. Luo N, Conwell MD, Chen X, et al. Primary cilia signaling mediates intraocular pressure sensation. *Proceedings of the National Academy of Sciences of the United States of America.* 2014;111(35):12871–12876.

170. Ryskamp DA, Frye AM, Phuong TTT, et al. TRPV4 regulates calcium homeostasis, cytoskeletal remodeling, conventional outflow and intraocular pressure in the mammalian eye. *Sci Rep.* 2016630583-30583.

171. Lakk M, Krizaj D. TRPV4-Rho signaling drives cytoskeletal and focal adhesion remodeling in trabecular meshwork cells. *Am J Physiol Cell Physiol.* 2021;320(6):C1013–C1030.

172. Patel PD, Chen YL, Kasetti RB, et al. Impaired TRPV4-eNOS signaling in trabecular meshwork elevates intraocular pressure in glaucoma. *Proc Natl Acad Sci U S A.* 2021;118(16).

173. Yarishkin O, Baumann JM, Križaj D. Mechano-electrical transduction in trabecular meshwork involves parallel activation of TRPV4 and TREK-1 channels. *Channels (Austin, Tex.).* 2019;13(1):168–171.

174. Coca-Prados M. The blood-aqueous barrier in health and disease. *J Glaucoma.* 2014;23 (8 Suppl 1):S36–38.

175. Hogan MJ. Ciliary body and posterior chamber. In: Hogan MJ, ed. *Histology of the Human Eye.* Philadelphia: WB Saunders; 1971:260.

176. Hogan MJ. *Iris and Anterior Chamber.* Philadelphia: WB Saunders Co; 1971.

177. Sonsino J, Gong H, Wu P, Freddo TF. Co-localization of junction-associated proteins of the human blood—aqueous barrier: occludin, ZO-1 and F-actin. *Exp Eye Res.* 2002;74(1):123–129.

178. Alm A. Ocular circulation. In: Hart WM, ed. *Adler's Physiology of the Eye. Clinical Application.* St Louis: CV Mosby; 1992:198.

179. Rodriguez-Peralta L. The blood-aqueous barrier in five species. *Am J Ophthalmol.* 1975;80(4):713–725.

180. Shiose Y, Oguri M. [Electron microscopic studies on the blood-retinal barrier and the blood-aqueous barrier]. *Nippon Ganka Gakkai Zasshi.* 1969;73(9):1606–1622.

181. Smith RS. Ultrastructural studies of the blood-aqueous barrier. I. Transport of an electron-dense tracer in the iris and ciliary body of the mouse. *Am J Ophthalmol.* 1971;71(5):1066–1077.

182. Bill A. The drainage of albumin from the uvea. *Exp Eye Res.* 1964;3:179–187.

183. Uusitalo R, Stjernschantz J, Palkama A. Studies on the ultrastructure of the blood-aqueous barrier in the rabbit. *Acta Ophthalmol Suppl.* 1974;123:61–68.

184. Uusitalo R, Stjernschantz J, Palkama A. Blood-aqueous barrier in newborn and young rabbits. An electron microscopic study. *Acta Ophthalmol (Copenh).* 1976;54(1):17–26.

185. Vegge T. An epithelial blood-aqueous barrier to horseradish peroxidase in the ciliary processes of the vervet monkey (Cercopithecus aethiops). *Z Zellforsch Mikrosk Anat.* 1971;114(3):309–320.

186. Vinores SA, Van Niel E, Swerdloff JL, Campochiaro PA. Electron microscopic immunocytochemical demonstration of blood-retinal barrier breakdown in human diabetics and its association with aldose reductase in retinal vascular endothelium and retinal pigment epithelium. *Histochem J.* 1993;25(9):648–663.

187. Bill A. Capillary permeability to and extravascular dynamics of myoglobin, albumin and gammaglobulin in the uvea. *Acta Physiol Scand.* 1968;73(1):204–219.

188. Raviola G. Effects of paracentesis on the blood-aqueous barrier: An electron microscope study on macaca mulatto, using horseradish peroxidase as a tracer. *Investigative Ophthalmology & Visual Science.* 1974;13(11):828–858.

189. Masuda K, Mishima S. Effects of prostaglandins on inflow and outflow of the aqueous in rabbits. *Japn J Ophthalmol.* 1973;17:300.

190. Kaufman PL, Crawford K. Aqueous humor dynamics: how PGF2a lowers intraocular pressure. In: Bito LZ, Stjernschantz J, eds. *The Ocular Effects of Prostaglandins and Other Eicosanoids.* New York: Alan R. Liss; 1989:387.

191. Kaufman PL. The effects of prostaglandins on aqueous humor dynamics. In: Kooner KS, Zimmerman TJ, eds. *New Ophthalmic Drugs. Ophthalmological Clinics of North America.* Philadelphia: WB Saunders; 1989:141.

192. Kaufman PL, Gabelt B. Alpha2adrenergic agonist effects on aqueous humor dynamics. *J Glaucoma.* 1995;4(Suppl 1):S8–S14.

193. Kaufman PL, Gabelt BT. Presbyopia, prostaglandins and primary open angle glaucoma. In: Krieglstein GK, ed. *Glaucoma Update V. Proceedings of the Symposium of the Glaucoma Society of the International Congress of Ophthalmology in Quebec City, June 1994.* New York: Springer-Verlag; 1995:224.

194. Kaufman PL. Pressure-dependent outflow. In: Ritch R, ed. *The Glaucomas.* St Louis: CV Mosby; 1996:307.

195. Lee J, Pelis RM. Drug transport by the blood-aqueous humor barrier of the eye. *Drug Metab Dispos.* 2016;44(10):1675–1681.

196. Lee J, Shahidullah M, Hotchkiss A, Coca-Prados M, Delamere NA, Pelis RM. A renal-like organic anion transport system in the ciliary epithelium of the bovine and human eye. *Mol Pharmacol.* 2015;87(4):697–705.

197. Pelis RM, Shahidullah M, Ghosh S, et al. Localization of multidrug resistance-associated protein 2 in the nonpigmented ciliary epithelium of the Eye. *Journal of Pharmacology and Experimental Therapeutics.* 2009;329(2):479–485.

198. Schuster VL, Lu R, Coca-Prados M. The prostaglandin transporter is widely expressed in ocular tissues. *Surv Ophthalmol.* 1997;41(Suppl 2):S41–45.

199. Bito LZ. Accumulation and apparent active transport of prostaglandins by some rabbit tissues in vitro. *J Physiol.* 1972;221(2):371–387.

200. Bito LZ. Species differences in the responses of the eye to irritation and trauma: a hypothesis of divergence in ocular defense mechanisms, and the choice of experimental animals for eye research. *Exp Eye Res.* 1984;39(6):807–829.

201. Bito LZ. Prostaglandins. Old concepts and new perspectives. *Arch Ophthalmol.* 1987;105(8):1036–1039.

202. Kraft ME, Glaeser H, Mandery K, et al. The prostaglandin transporter OATP2A1 is expressed in human ocular tissues and transports the antiglaucoma prostanoid latanoprost. *Invest Ophthalmol Vis Sci.* 2010;51(5):2504–2511.

203. Schäfer AM, Meyer Zu Schwabedissen HE, Grube M. Expression and function of organic anion transporting polypeptides in the human brain: Physiological and pharmacological implications. *Pharmaceutics.* 2021;13(6).

204. Forbes M, Becker B. The transport of organic anions by the rabbit eye. II. In vivo transport of iodopyracet (Diodrast). *Am J Ophthalmol.* 1960;50:867–875.

205. Bárány EH. Inhibition by hippurate and probenecid of in vitro uptake of iodipamide and o-iodohippurate. A composite uptake system for iodipamide in choroid plexus, kidney cortex and anterior uvea of several species. *Acta Physiol Scand.* 1972;86(1):12–27.

206. Bárány EH. The liver-like anion transport system in rabbit kidney, uvea and choroid plexus. II. Efficiency of acidic drugs and other anions as inhibitors. *Acta Physiol Scand.* 1973;88(4):491–504.

207. Bárány EH. Bile acids as inhibitors of the liver-like anion transport system in the rabbit kidney, uvea and choroid plexus. *Acta Physiol Scand.* 1974;92(2):195–203.

208. Bárány EH. In vitro uptake of bile acids by choroid plexus, kidney cortex and anterior uvea. I. The iodipamide-sensitive transport systems in the rabbit. *Acta Physiol Scand.* 1975;93(2):250–268.

209. Becker B. The transport of organic anions by the rabbit eye. I. In vitro iodopyracet (Diodrast) accumulation by ciliary body-iris preparations. *Am J Ophthalmol.* 1960;50:862–867.

210. Becker B. Iodide transport by the rabbit eye. *Am J Physiol.* 1961;200:804–806.

211. Stone RA. Cholic acid accumulation by the ciliary body and by the iris of the primate eye. *Invest Ophthalmol Vis Sci.* 1979;18(8):819–826.

212. Stone RA. The transport of para-aminohippuric acid by the ciliary body and by the iris of the primate eye. *Invest Ophthalmol Vis Sci.* 1979;18(8):807–818.
213. Liu H, Fan S, Gulati V, et al. Aqueous humor dynamics during the day and night in healthy mature volunteers. *Arch Ophthalmol.* 2011;129(3):269–275.
214. Reiss GR, Lee DA, Topper JE, Brubaker RF. Aqueous humor flow during sleep. *Invest Ophthalmol Vis Sci.* 1984;25(6):776–778.
215. Sit AJ, Nau CB, McLaren JW, Johnson DH, Hodge D. Circadian variation of aqueous dynamics in young healthy adults. *Invest Ophthalmol Vis Sci.* 2008;49(4):1473–1479.
216. Chiquet C, Denis P. [The neuroanatomical and physiological bases of variations in intraocular pressure]. *J Fr Ophtalmol.* 2004;27Spec(No 2):2S11–12S18.
217. Ikegami K, Shigeyoshi Y, Masubuchi S. Circadian regulation of IOP rhythm by dual pathways of glucocorticoids and the sympathetic nervous system. *Invest Ophthalmol Vis Sci.* 2020;61(3):26.
218. Tsuchiya S, Buhr ED, Higashide T, Sugiyama K, Van Gelder RN. Light entrainment of the murine intraocular pressure circadian rhythm utilizes non-local mechanisms. *PLoS One.* 2017;12(9):e0184790.
219. Nii H, Ikeda H, Okada K, Yoshitomi T, Gregory DS. Circadian change of adenylate cyclase activity in rabbit ciliary processes. *Curr Eye Res.* 2001;23(4):248–255.
220. Ehinger B. Connections between adrenergic nerves and other tissue components in the eye. *Acta Physiol Scand.* 1966;67(1):57–64.
221. Laties AM, Jacobowitz D. A comparative study of the autonomic innervation of the eye in monkey, cat, and rabbit. *Anat Rec.* 1966;156(4):383–395.
222. McDougal DH, Gamlin PD. Autonomic control of the eye. *Comprehensive Physiology.* 2015;5(1):439–473.
223. Ruskell GL. Innervation of the anterior segment of the eye. In: Lütjen-Drecoll E, ed. *Basic Aspects of Glaucoma Research.* Stuttgart: Schattauer; 1982:49.
224. Bryson JM, Wolter JR, O'Keefe NT. Ganglion cells in the human ciliary body. *Arch Ophthalmol.* 1966;75(1):57–60.
225. Uddman R, Alumets J, Ehinger B, Hakanson R, Loren I, Sundler F. Vasoactive intestinal peptide nerves in ocular and orbital structures of the cat. *Invest Ophthalmol Vis Sci.* 1980;19(8):878–885.
226. Nilsson SFE. Neuropeptides in the autonomic nervous system influencing uveal blood flow and aqueous humour dynamics. In: Troger J, Kieselbach G, eds. *Neuropeptides in the Eye.* Kerala: Research Signpost; 2009:1.
227. Elsas T, Uddman R, Sundler F. Pituitary adenylate cyclase-activating peptide-immunoreactive nerve fibers in the cat eye. *Graefes Arch Clin Exp Ophthalmol.* 1996;234(9):573–580.
228. Bill A. Effects of norepinephrine, isoproterenol and sympathetic stimulation on aqueous humour dynamics in vervet monkeys. *Exp Eye Res.* 1970;10(1):31–46.
229. Gabelt BT, Robinson JC, Gange SJ, Kaufman PL. Superior cervical ganglionectomy in monkeys: aqueous humor dynamics and their responses to drugs. *Exp Eye Res.* 1995;60(5):575–584.
230. Wentworth WO, Brubaker RF. Aqueous humor dynamics in a series of patients with third neuron Horner's syndrome. *Am J Ophthalmol.* 1981;92(3):407–415.
231. Larson RS, Brubaker RF. Isoproterenol stimulates aqueous flow in humans with Horner's syndrome. *Invest Ophthalmol Vis Sci.* 1988;29(4):621–625.
232. Bonomi L, DiComite P. Outflow facility after guanethidine sulfate administration. *Arch Ophthalmol.* 1967;78(3):337–340.
233. Nilsson SF, Maepea O, Samuelsson M, Bill A. Effects of timolol on terbutaline- and VIP-stimulated aqueous humor flow in the cynomolgus monkey. *Curr Eye Res.* 1990;9(9):863–872.
234. Bill A, Stjernschantz J. Cholinergic vasoconstrictor effects in the rabbit eye: vasomotor effects of pentobarbital anesthesia. *Acta Physiol Scand.* 1980;108(4):419–424.
235. Becker B. The measurement of rate of aqueous flow with iodide. *Invest Ophthalmol.* 1962;1:52–58.
236. Swan K WH. A comparative study of the effects of mecholyl, doryl, pilocarpine, atropine, and epinephrine on the blood-aqueous barrier. *Am J Ophthalmol.* 1940;23:1311.
237. Bito LZ, Davson H, Levin E, Murray M, Snider N. The relationship between the concentrations of amino acids in the ocular fluids and blood plasma of dogs. *Exp Eye Res.* 1965;4(4):374–380.
238. Walinder PE. Influence of pilocarpine on iodopyracet and iodide accumulation by rabbit ciliary body-iris perparations. *Invest Ophthalmol.* 1966;5(4):378–385.
239. Walinder PE, Bill A. Aqueous flow and entry of cycloleucine into the aqueous humor of vervet monkeys (Cercopithecus ethiops). *Invest Ophthalmol.* 1969;8(4):434–445.
240. Shi XP, Zamudio AC, Candia OA, Wolosin JM. Adreno-cholinergic modulation of junctional communications between the pigmented and nonpigmented layers of the ciliary body epithelium. *Invest Ophthalmol Vis Sci.* 1996;37(6):1037–1046.
241. Stelling JW, Jacob TJ. Functional coupling in bovine ciliary epithelial cells is modulated by carbachol. *Am J Physiol.* 1997;273(6):C1876–1881.
242. Chiou GC, Liu HK, Trzeciakowski J. Studies of action mechanism of antiglaucoma drugs with a newly developed cat model. *Life Sci.* 1980;27(25-26):2445–2451.
243. Green K, Padgett D. Effect of various drugs on pseudofacility and aqueous humor formation in the rabbit eye. *Exp Eye Res.* 1979;28(2):239–246.
244. Liu HK, Chiou CY. Continuous, simultaneous, and instant display of aqueous humor dynamics with a micro-spectrophotometer and a sensitive drop counter. *Exp Eye Res.* 1981;32(5):583–592.
245. Macri FJ, Cevario SJ. The induction of aqueous humor formation by the use of Ach+eserine. *Invest Ophthalmol.* 1973;12(12):910–916.
246. Macri FJ, Cevario SJ. The dual nature of pilocarpine to stimulate or inhibit the formation of aqueous humor. *Invest Ophthalmol.* 1974;13(8):617–619.
247. Macri FJ, Cevario SJ. A possible vascular mechanism for the inhibition of aqueous humor formation by ouabain and acetazolamide. *Exp Eye Res.* 1975;20(6):563–569.
248. Nagataki S, Brubaker RF. Effect of pilocarpine on aqueous humor formation in human beings. *Arch Ophthalmol.* 1982;100(5):818–821.
249. Stjernschantz J. Effect of parasympathetic stimulation on intraocular pressure, formation of the aqueous humour and outflow facility in rabbits. *Exp Eye Res.* 1976;22(6):639–645.
250. Uusitalo R. Effect of sympathetic and parasympathetic stimulation on the secretion and outflow of aqueous humour in the rabbit eye. *Acta Physiol Scand.* 1972;86(3):315–326.
251. Bill A, Walinder P-E. The effects of pilocarpine on the dynamics of aqueous humor in a primate (Macaca irus). *Invest Ophthalmol.* 1966;5:170.
252. Gaasterland D, Kupfer C, Ross K. Studies of aqueous humor dynamics in man. IV. Effects of pilocarpine upon measurements in young normal volunteers. *Invest Ophthalmol.* 1975;14(11):848–853.
253. Erickson KA, Schroeder A. Direct effects of muscarinic agents on the outflow pathways in human eyes. *Invest Ophthalmol Vis Sci.* 2000;41(7):1743–1748.
254. Gregory D, Sears M, Bausher L, Mishima H, Mead A. Intraocular pressure and aqueous flow are decreased by cholera toxin. *Invest Ophthalmol Vis Sci.* 1981;20(3):371–381.
255. Neufeld AH, Sears ML. Cyclic-AMP in ocular tissues of the rabbit, monkey, and human. *Invest Ophthalmol.* 1974;13(6):475–477.
256. Shahidullah M, Wilson WS, Rafiq K, Sikder MH, Ferdous J, Delamere NA. Terbutaline, forskolin and cAMP reduce secretion of aqueous humour in the isolated bovine eye. *PLoS One.* 2020;15(12):e0244253.
257. Shibata T, Mishima H, Kurokawa T. Ocular pigmentation and intraocular pressure response to forskolin. *Curr Eye Res.* 1988;7(7):667–674.
258. Smith BR, Gaster RN, Leopold IH, Zeleznick LD. Forskolin, a potent adenylate cyclase activator, lowers rabbit intraocular pressure. *Arch Ophthalmol.* 1984;102(1):146–148.
259. Schenker HI, Yablonski ME, Podos SM, Linder L. Fluorophotometric study of epinephrine and timolol in human subjects. *Arch Ophthalmol.* 1981;99(7):1212–1216.
260. Townsend DJ, Brubaker RF. Immediate effect of epinephrine on aqueous formation in the normal human eye as measured by fluorophotometry. *Invest Ophthalmol Vis Sci.* 1980;19(3):256–266.
261. Coakes RL, Brubaker RF. The mechanism of timolol in lowering intraocular pressure. In the normal eye. *Arch Ophthalmol.* 1978;96(11):2045–2048.
262. Gharagozloo NZ, Larson RS, Kullerstrand LJ, Brubaker RF. Terbutaline stimulates aqueous humor flow in humans during sleep. *Arch Ophthalmol.* 1988;106(9):1218–1220.
263. Kiland JA, Gabelt BT, Kaufman PL. Studies on the mechanism of action of timolol and on the effects of suppression and redirection of aqueous flow on outflow facility. *Exp Eye Res.* 2004;78(3):639–651.
264. Novack GD. Ophthalmic beta-blockers since timolol. *Surv Ophthalmol.* 1987;31(5):307–327.
265. Zimmerman TJ. Topical ophthalmic beta blockers: a comparative review. *J Ocul Pharmacol.* 1993;9(4):373–384.
266. Dailey RA, Brubaker RF, Bourne WM. The effects of timolol maleate and acetazolamide on the rate of aqueous formation in normal human subjects. *Am J Ophthalmol.* 1982;93(2):232–237.
267. Yablonski ME, Zimmerman TJ, Waltman SR, Becker B. A fluorophotometric study of the effect of topical timolol on aqueous humor dynamics. *Exp Eye Res.* 1978;27(2):135–142.
268. Yablonski ME, Novack GD, Burke PJ, Cook DJ, Harmon G. The effect of levobunolol on aqueous humor dynamics. *Exp Eye Res.* 1987;44(1):49–54.
269. Mills KB, Wright G. A blind randomised cross-over trial comparing metipranolol 0.3% with timolol 0.25% in open-angle glaucoma: a pilot study. *Br J Ophthalmol.* 1986;70(1):39–42.
270. Henness S, Swainston Harrison T, Keating GM. Ocular carteolol: a review of its use in the management of glaucoma and ocular hypertension. *Drugs Aging.* 2007;24(6):509–528.
271. Maruyama K, Shirato S. Additive effect of dorzolamide or carteolol to latanoprost in primary open-angle glaucoma: a prospective randomized crossover trial. *J Glaucoma.* 2006;15(4):341–345.
272. Stewart RH, Kimbrough RL, Ward RL. Betaxolol vs timolol. A six-month double-blind comparison. *Arch Ophthalmol.* 1986;104(1):46–48.
273. Nathanson JA. Adrenergic regulation of intraocular pressure: identification of beta 2-adrenergic-stimulated adenylate cyclase in ciliary process epithelium. *Proc Natl Acad Sci U S A.* 1980;77(12):7420–7424.
274. Nathanson JA. Human ciliary process adrenergic receptor: pharmacological characterization. *Invest Ophthalmol Vis Sci.* 1981;21(6):798–804.
275. Sears ML. Autonomic nervous system. Adrenergic agonists. In: Sears ML, ed. *Pharmacology of the Eye. Handbook of Experimental Pharmacology.* Berlin: Springer-Verlag; 1984:193.
276. Berrospi AR, Leibowitz HM. Betaxolol. A new beta-adrenergic blocking agent for treatment of glaucoma. *Arch Ophthalmol.* 1982;100(6):943–946.
277. Berry Jr. DP, Van Buskirk EM, Shields MB. Betaxolol and timolol. A comparison of efficacy and side effects. *Arch Ophthalmol.* 1984;102(1):42–45.
278. Vuori ML, Kaila T, Iisalo E, Saari KM. Concentrations and antagonist activity of topically applied betaxolol in aqueous humour. *Acta Ophthalmol (Copenh).* 1993;71(5):677–681.
279. Osborne NN, Chidlow G. Do beta-adrenoceptors and serotonin 5-HT1A receptors have similar functions in the control of intraocular pressure in the rabbit? *Ophthalmologica.* 1996;210(5):308–314.
280. Topper JE, Brubaker RF. Effects of timolol, epinephrine, and acetazolamide on aqueous flow during sleep. *Invest Ophthalmol Vis Sci.* 1985;26(10):1315–1319.
281. Robinson JC, Kaufman PL. Dose-dependent suppression of aqueous humor formation by timolol in the cynomolgus monkey. *J Glaucoma.* 1993;2(4):251–256.
282. Rittig MG, Licht K, Funk RH. Innervation of the ciliary process vasculature and epithelium by nerve fibers containing catecholamines and neuropeptide Y. *Ophthalmic Res.* 1993;25(2):108–118.
283. Jacob E, FitzSimon JS, Brubaker RF. Combined corticosteroid and catecholamine stimulation of aqueous humor flow. *Ophthalmology.* 1996;103(8):1303–1308.
284. MacCumber MW, Ross CA, Glaser BM, Snyder SH. Endothelin: visualization of mRNAs by in situ hybridization provides evidence for local action. *Proc Natl Acad Sci U S A.* 1989;86(18):7285–7289.
285. Polansky JR, Zlock D, Brasier A, Bloom E. Adrenergic and cholinergic receptors in isolated non-pigmented ciliary epithelial cells. *Curr Eye Res.* 1985;4(4):517–522.
286. Hirata K, Nathanson MH, Sears ML. Novel paracrine signaling mechanism in the ocular ciliary epithelium. *Proc Natl Acad Sci U S A.* 1998;95(14):8381–8386.
287. Farahbakhsh NA, Cilluffo MC. Synergistic effect of adrenergic and muscarinic receptor activation on [Ca2+]i in rabbit ciliary body epithelium. *J Physiol.* 1994;477(Pt 2):215–221.

288. Ryan JS, Tao QP, Kelly ME. Adrenergic regulation of calcium-activated potassium current in cultured rabbit pigmented ciliary epithelial cells. *J Physiol*. 1998;511(Pt 1):145–157. (Pt 1).

289. Schütte M, Wolosin JM. Ca2+ mobilization and interlayer signal transfer in the heterocellular bilayered epithelium of the rabbit ciliary body. *J Physiol*. 1996;496(Pt 1): 25–37. (Pt 1).

290. Reitsamer HA, Posey M, Kiel JW. Effects of a topical alpha2 adrenergic agonist on ciliary blood flow and aqueous production in rabbits. *Exp Eye Res*. 2006;82(3):405–415.

291. Van Buskirk EM, Bacon DR, Fahrenbach WH. Ciliary vasoconstriction after topical adrenergic drugs. *Am J Ophthalmol*. 1990;109(5):511–517.

292. Lee DA, Brubaker RF. Effect of phenylephrine on aqueous humor flow. *Curr Eye Res*. 1982;2(2):89–92.

293. Lee DA, Brubaker RF, Nagataki S. Acute effect of thymoxamine on aqueous humor formation in the epinephrine-treated normal eye as measured by fluorophotometry. *Invest Ophthalmol Vis Sci*. 1983;24(2):165–168.

294. Krieglstein GK, Langham ME, Leydhecker W. The peripheral and central neural actions of clonidine in normal and glaucomatous eyes. *Invest Ophthalmol Vis Sci*. 1978;17(2): 149–158.

295. Lee DA, Topper JE, Brubaker RF. Effect of clonidine on aqueous humor flow in normal human eyes. *Exp Eye Res*. 1984;38(3):239–246.

296. Bill A, Heilmann K. Ocular effects of clonidine in cats and monkeys (Macaca irus). *Exp Eye Res*. 1975;21(5):481–488.

297. Jin Y, Verstappen A, Yorio T. Characterization of alpha 2-adrenoceptor binding sites in rabbit ciliary body membranes. *Invest Ophthalmol Vis Sci*. 1994;35(5):2500–2508.

298. Liu JH, Gallar J. In vivo cAMP level in rabbit iris-ciliary body after topical epinephrine treatment. *Curr Eye Res*. 1996;15(10):1025–1032.

299. Schutte M, Diadori A, Wang C, Wolosin JM. Comparative adrenocholinergic control of intracellular Ca2+ in the layers of the ciliary body epithelium. *Invest Ophthalmol Vis Sci*. 1996;37(1):212–220.

300. Cvenkel B, Kolko M. Current medical therapy and future trends in the management of glaucoma treatment. *J Ophthalmol*. 2020;20206138132-6138132.

301. Maus TL, Nau C, Brubaker RF. Comparison of the early effects of brimonidine and apraclonidine as topical ocular hypotensive agents. *Arch Ophthalmol*. 1999;117(5):586–591.

302. Oh DJ, Chen JL, Vajaranant TS, Dikopf MS. Brimonidine tartrate for the treatment of glaucoma. *Expert Opin Pharmacother*. 2019;20(1):115–122.

303. Fan S, Agrawal A, Gulati V, Neely DG, Toris CB. Daytime and nighttime effects of brimonidine on IOP and aqueous humor dynamics in participants with ocular hypertension. *J Glaucoma*. 2014;23(5):276–281.

304. Toris CB, Camras CB, Yablonski ME. Acute versus chronic effects of brimonidine on aqueous humor dynamics in ocular hypertensive patients. *Am J Ophthalmol*. 1999;128(1):8–14.

305. Khouri AS, Realini T, Fechtner RD. Use of fixed-dose combination drugs for the treatment of glaucoma. *Drugs Aging*. 2007;24(12):1007–1016.

306. Fechtner RD, Myers JS, Hubatsch DA, Budenz DL, DuBiner HB. Ocular hypotensive effect of fixed-combination brinzolamide/brimonidine adjunctive to a prostaglandin analog: a randomized clinical trial. *Eye*. 2016;30(10):1343–1350.

307. Stoner A, Harris A, Oddone F, et al. Topical carbonic anhydrase inhibitors and glaucoma in 2021: where do we stand? *Br J Ophthalmol*. 2021.

308. Liu JH, Medeiros FA, Slight JR, Weinreb RN. Comparing diurnal and nocturnal effects of brinzolamide and timolol on intraocular pressure in patients receiving latanoprost monotherapy. *Ophthalmology*. 2009;116(3):449–454.

309. Toris CB. Pharmacotherapies for glaucoma. *Curr Mol Med*. 2010;10(9):824–840.

310. Millar JC, Savinainen A, Josiah S, Pang IH. Effects of TAK-639, a novel topical C-type natriuretic peptide analog, on intraocular pressure and aqueous humor dynamics in mice. *Exp Eye Res*. 2019;188:107763.

311. Korenfeld MS, Becker B. Atrial natriuretic peptides. Effects on intraocular pressure, cGMP, and aqueous flow. *Invest Ophthalmol Vis Sci*. 1989;30(11):2385–2392.

312. Mittag TW, Tormay A, Ortega M, Severin C. Atrial natriuretic peptide (ANP), guanylate cyclase, and intraocular pressure in the rabbit eye. *Curr Eye Res*. 1987;6(10):1189–1196.

313. Coca-Prados M, Escribano J. New perspectives in aqueous humor secretion and in glaucoma: the ciliary body as a multifunctional neuroendocrine gland. *Prog Retin Eye Res*. 2007;26(3):239–262.

314. Rasmussen CA, Gabelt BT, Kaufman PL. Aqueous humor dynamics in monkeys in response to the kappa opioid agonist bremazocine. *Trans Am Ophthalmol Soc*. 2007;105:225–238. discussion 238-229.

315. Nathanson JA. Nitrovasodilators as a new class of ocular hypotensive agents. *J Pharmacol Exp Ther*. 1992;260(3):956–965.

316. Nathanson JA. Nitric oxide and nitrovasodilators in the eye: implications for ocular physiology and glaucoma. *J Glaucoma*. 1993;2(3):206–210.

317. Shahidullah M, Wilson WS. Atriopeptin, sodium azide and cyclic GMP reduce secretion of aqueous humour and inhibit intracellular calcium release in bovine cultured ciliary epithelium. *Br J Pharmacol*. 1999;127(6):1438–1446.

318. Kee C, Kaufman PL, Gabelt BT. Effect of 8-Br cGMP on aqueous humor dynamics in monkeys. *Invest Ophthalmol Vis Sci*. 1994;35(6):2769–2773.

319. Russell KR, Potter DE. Dynorphin modulates ocular hydrodynamics and releases atrial natriuretic peptide via activation of kappa-opioid receptors. *Exp Eye Res*. 2002;75(3):259–270.

320. Bonfiglio V, Bucolo C, Camillieri G, Drago F. Possible involvement of nitric oxide in morphine-induced miosis and reduction of intraocular pressure in rabbits. *Eur J Pharmacol*. 2006;534(1-3):227–232.

321. Dortch-Carnes J, Russell K. Morphine-stimulated nitric oxide release in rabbit aqueous humor. *Exp Eye Res*. 2007;84(1):185–190.

322. Dortch-Carnes J, Russell KR. Morphine-induced reduction of intraocular pressure and pupil diameter: role of nitric oxide. *Pharmacology*. 2006;77(1):17–24.

323. Sharif NA. Serotonin-2 receptor agonists as novel ocular hypotensive agents and their cellular and molecular mechanisms of action. *Curr Drug Targets*. 2010;11(8):978–993.

324. Chang FW, Burke JA, Potter DE. Mechanism of the ocular hypotensive action of ketanserin. *J Ocul Pharmacol*. 1985;1(2):137–147.

325. Chidlow G, Le Corre S, Osborne NN. Localization of 5-hydroxytryptamine1A and 5-hydroxytryptamine7 receptors in rabbit ocular and brain tissues. *Neuroscience*. 1998;87 (3):675–689.

326. Barnett NL, Osborne NN. The presence of serotonin (5-HT1) receptors negatively coupled to adenylate cyclase in rabbit and human iris-ciliary processes. *Exp Eye Res*. 1993;57(2):209–216.

327. Chu TC, Ogidigben MJ, Potter DE. 8OH-DPAT-Induced ocular hypotension: sites and mechanisms of action. *Exp Eye Res*. 1999;69(2):227–238.

328. Chidlow G, Cupido A, Melena J, Osborne NN. Flesinoxan, a 5-HT1A receptor agonist/ alpha 1-adrenoceptor antagonist, lowers intraocular pressure in NZW rabbits. *Curr Eye Res*. 2001;23(2):144–153.

329. Gabelt BT, Millar CJ, Kiland JA, Peterson JA, Seeman JL, Kaufman PL. Effects of serotonergic compounds on aqueous humor dynamics in monkeys. *Curr Eye Res*. 2001;23(2):120–127.

330. Cairns EA, Baldridge WH, Kelly ME. The endocannabinoid system as a therapeutic target in glaucoma. *Neural Plast*. 2016;2016:9364091.

331. Nucci C, Bari M, Spanò A, et al. Potential roles of (endo)cannabinoids in the treatment of glaucoma: from intraocular pressure control to neuroprotection. In: Nucci C, Cerulli L, Osborne NN, Bagetta G, eds. *Progress in Brain Research*. 173. Elsevier; 2008:451–464.

332. Purnell WD, Gregg JM. Delta(9)-tetrahydrocannabinol,, euphoria and intraocular pressure in man. *Ann Ophthalmol*. 1975;7(7):921–923.

333. Green K, Roth M. Ocular effects of topical administration of delta 9-tetrahydrocannabinol in man. *Arch Ophthalmol*. 1982;100(2):265–267.

334. Jay WM, Green K. Multiple-drop study of topically applied 1% delta 9-tetrahydrocannabinol in human eyes. *Arch Ophthalmol*. 1983;101(4):591–593.

335. Chen J, Matias I, Dinh T, Lu T, Venezia S, Nieves A, Woodward DF, Di Marzo V. Finding of endocannabinoids in human eye tissues: implications for glaucoma. *Biochem Biophys Res Commun*. 2005;330(4):1062–1067.

336. Porcella A, Maxia C, Gessa GL, Pani L. The synthetic cannabinoid WIN55212-2 decreases the intraocular pressure in human glaucoma resistant to conventional therapies. *Eur J Neurosci*. 2001;13(2):409–412.

337. Stamer WD, Golightly SF, Hosohata Y, Ryan EP, Porter AC, Varga E, Noecker RJ, Felder CC, Yamamura HI. Cannabinoid CB(1) receptor expression, activation and detection of endogenous ligand in trabecular meshwork and ciliary process tissues. *Eur J Pharmacol*. 2001;431(3):277–286.

338. Straiker AJ, Maguire G, Mackie K, Lindsey J. Localization of cannabinoid CB1 receptors in the human anterior eye and retina. *Invest Ophthalmol Vis Sci*. 1999;40(10):2442–2448.

339. Chien FY, Wang RF, Mittag TW, Podos SM. Effect of WIN 55212-2, a cannabinoid receptor agonist, on aqueous humor dynamics in monkeys. *Arch Ophthalmol*. 2003;121(1):87–90.

340. Collaborative Normal-Tension Glaucoma Study Group Comparison of glaucomatous progression between untreated patients with normal-tension glaucoma and patients with therapeutically reduced intraocular pressures. Collaborative Normal-Tension Glaucoma Study Group. *Am J Ophthalmol*. 1998;126(4):487–497.

341. Kass MA, Heuer DK, Higginbotham EJ, et al. The Ocular Hypertension Treatment Study: a randomized trial determines that topical ocular hypotensive medication delays or prevents the onset of primary open-angle glaucoma. *Arch Ophthalmol*. 2002;120(6): 701–713. discussion 829-730.

342. Leske MC, Heijl A, Hussein M, et al. Factors for glaucoma progression and the effect of treatment: the early manifest glaucoma trial. *Arch Ophthalmol*. 2003;121(1):48–56.

343. Wahl J. [Results of the Collaborative Initial Glaucoma Treatment Study (CIGTS)]. *Ophthalmologe*. 2005;102(3):222–226.

344. Jones RF, Maurice DM. New methods of measuring the rate of aqueous flow in man with fluorescein. *Exp Eye Res*. 1966;5(3):208–220.

345. Nilsson SF, Samuelsson M, Bill A, Stjernschantz J. Increased uveoscleral outflow as a possible mechanism of ocular hypotension caused by prostaglandin F2 alpha-1-isopropylester in the cynomolgus monkey. *Exp Eye Res*. 1989;48(5):707–716.

346. Armaly MF. On the distribution of applanation pressure. I. Statistical features and the effect of age, sex, and family history of glaucoma. *Arch Ophthalmol*. 1965;73:11–18.

347. Selbach JM, Posielek K, Steuhl KP, Kremmer S. Episcleral venous pressure in untreated primary open-angle and normal-tension glaucoma. *Ophthalmologica*. 2005;219(6):357–361.

348. Sit AJ, Ekdawi NS, Malihi M, McLaren JW. A novel method for computerized measurement of episcleral venous pressure in humans. *Exp Eye Res*. 2011;92(6):537–544.

349. Sultan M, Blondeau P. Episcleral venous pressure in younger and older subjects in the sitting and supine positions. *J Glaucoma*. 2003;12(4):370–373.

350. Croft MA, Oyen MJ, Gange SJ, Fisher MR, Kaufman PL. Aging effects on accommodation and outflow facility responses to pilocarpine in humans. *Arch Ophthalmol*. 1996;114(5):586–592.

351. Grant WM. Tonographic method for measuring the facility and rate of aqueous flow in human eyes. *Arch Ophthal*. 1950;44(2):204–214.

352. Kupfer C, Gaasterland D, Ross K. Studies of aqueous humor dynamics in man. II. Measurements in young normal subjects using acetazolamide and L-epinephrine. *Invest Ophthalmol*. 1971;10(7):523–533.

353. Kupfer C, Ross K. Studies of aqueous humor dynamics in man. I. Measurements in young normal subjects. *Invest Ophthalmol*. 1971;10(7):518–522.

354. Toris CB, Koepsell SA, Yablonski ME, Camras CB. Aqueous humor dynamics in ocular hypertensive patients. *J Glaucoma*. 2002;11(3):253–258.

355. Kaufman PL, Bill A, Bárány EH. Formation and drainage of aqueous humor following total iris removal and ciliary muscle disinsertion in the cynomolgus monkey. *Invest Ophthalmol Vis Sci*. 1977;16(3):226–229.

356. Wiederholt M, Thieme H, Stumpff F. The regulation of trabecular meshwork and ciliary muscle contractility. *Prog Retin Eye Res*. 2000;19(3):271–295.

357. Johnson M, Erickson K. Mechanisms and routes of aqueous humor drainage. In: Albert DM, Jakobiec FA, eds. *Principles and Practice of Ophthalmology*. Philadelphia: WB Saunders Co; 2000:2577.

358. Pederson JE, Gaasterland DE, MacLellan HM. Uveoscleral aqueous outflow in the rhesus monkey: importance of uveal reabsorption. *Invest Ophthalmol Vis Sci.* 1977;16(11):1008-1007.
359. Sherman SH, Green K, Laties AM. The fate of anterior chamber flurescein in the monkey eye. 1. The anterior chamber outflow pathways. *Exp Eye Res.* 1978;27(2):159–173.
360. Yücel YH, Johnston MG, Ly T, et al. Identification of lymphatics in the ciliary body of the human eye: a novel uveolymphatic outflow pathway. *Exp Eye Res.* 2009;89(5):810–819.
361. Kim M, Johnston MG, Gupta N, Moore S, Yücel YH. A model to measure lymphatic drainage from the eye. *Exp Eye Res.* 2011;93(5):586–591.
362. Tam AL, Gupta N, Zhang Z, Yücel YH. Quantum dots trace lymphatic drainage from the mouse eye. *Nanotechnology.* 2011;22(42):425101.
363. Brubaker RF. The effect of intraocular pressure on conventional outflow resistance in the enucleated human eye. *Invest Ophthalmol.* 1975;14(4):286–292.
364. Bill A. Conventional and uveo-scleral drainage of aqueous humour in the cynomolgus monkey (Macaca irus) at normal and high intraocular pressures. *Exp Eye Res.* 1966;5(1):45–54.
365. Jackson TL, Hussain A, Hodgetts A, et al. Human scleral hydraulic conductivity: age-related changes, topographical variation, and potential scleral outflow facility. *Invest Ophthalmol Vis Sci.* 2006;47(11):4942–4946.
366. Bill A. The aqueous humor drainage mechanism in the cynomolgus monkey (Macaca irus) with evidence for unconventional routes. *Invest Ophthalmol.* 1965;4(5):911–919.
367. Bill A. Movement of albumin and dextran through the sclera. *Arch Ophthalmol.* 1965;74: 248–252.
368. Kleinstein RN, Fatt I. Pressure dependency of transcleral flow. *Exp Eye Res.* 1977;24(4): 335–340.
369. Toris CB, Pederson JE. Effect of intraocular pressure on uveoscleral outflow following cyclodialysis in the monkey eye. *Invest Ophthalmol Vis Sci.* 1985;26(12):1745–1749.
370. Gabelt BT, Kaufman PL. Prostaglandin F2 alpha increases uveoscleral outflow in the cynomolgus monkey. *Exp Eye Res.* 1989;49(3):389–402.
371. Kazemi A, McLaren JW, Kopczynski CC, Heah TG, Novack GD, Sit AJ. The effects of netarsudil ophthalmic solution on aqueous humor dynamics in a randomized study in humans. *J Ocul Pharmacol Ther.* 2018;34(5):380–386.
372. Inomata H, Bill A, Smelser GK. Aqueous humor pathways through the trabecular meshwork and into Schlemm's canal in the cynomolgus monkey (Macaca irus). An electron microscopic study. *Am J Ophthalmol.* 1972;73(5):760–789.
373. Lütjen-Drecoll E. Structural factors influencing outflow facility and its changeability under drugs. A study in Macaca arctoides. *Invest Ophthalmol.* 1973;12(4):280–294.
374. Lütjen-Drecoll E, Futa R, Rohen JW. Ultrahistochemical studies on tangential sections of the trabecular meshwork in normal and glaucomatous eyes. *Invest Ophthalmol Vis Sci.* 1981;21(4):563–573.
375. Lütjen-Drecoll E, Wiendl H, Kaufman PL. Acute and chronic structural effects of pilocarpine on monkey outflow tissues. *Trans Am Ophthalmol Soc.* 1998;96:171–191. discussion. 192-175.
376. Bill A, Svedbergh B. Scanning electron microscopic studies of the trabecular meshwork and the canal of Schlemm—an attempt to localize the main resistance to outflow of aqueous humor in man. *Acta Ophthalmol (Copenh).* 1972;50(3):295–320.
377. McMenamin PG, Lee WR, Aitken DA. Age-related changes in the human outflow apparatus. *Ophthalmology.* 1986;93(2):194–209.
378. Alvarado J, Murphy C, Polansky J, Juster R. Age-related changes in trabecular meshwork cellularity. *Invest Ophthalmol Vis Sci.* 1981;21(5):714–727.
379. Miyazaki M, Segawa K, Urakawa Y. Age-related changes in the trabecular meshwork of the normal human eye. *Jpn J Ophthalmol.* 1987;31(4):558–569.
380. Ellingsen BA, Grant WM. Influence of intraocular pressure and trabeculotomy on aqueous outflow in enucleated monkey eyes. *Invest Ophthalmol.* 1971;10(9):705–709.
381. Ellingsen BA, Grant WM. Trabeculotomy and sinusotomy in enucleated human eyes. *Invest Ophthalmol.* 1972;11(1):21–28.
382. Vahabikashi A, Gelman A, Dong B, et al. Increased stiffness and flow resistance of the inner wall of Schlemm's canal in glaucomatous human eyes. *Proc Natl Acad Sci U S A.* 2019;116(52):26555–26563.
383. Bradley JM, Kelley MJ, Zhu X, Anderssohn AM, Alexander JP, Acott TS. Effects of mechanical stretching on trabecular matrix metalloproteinases. *Invest Ophthalmol Vis Sci.* 2001;42(7):1505–1513.
384. Bradley JM, Vranka J, Colvis CM, Conger DM, Alexander JP, Fisk AS, Samples JR, Acott TS. Effect of matrix metalloproteinases activity on outflow in perfused human organ culture. *Invest Ophthalmol Vis Sci.* 1998;39(13):2649–2658.
385. Hassell JR, Newsome DA, Martin GR. Isolation and characterization of the proteoglycans and collagens synthesized by cells in culture. *Vision Res.* 1981;21(1):49–53.
386. Keller KE, Bradley JM, Acott TS. Differential effects of ADAMTS-1, -4, and -5 in the trabecular meshwork. *Invest Ophthalmol Vis Sci.* 2009;50(12):5769–5777.
387. Keller KE, Bradley JM, Vranka JA, Acott TS. Segmental versican expression in the trabecular meshwork and involvement in outflow facility. *Invest Ophthalmol Vis Sci.* 2011;52(8):5049–5057.
388. Rohen JW, Schachtschabel DO, Wehrmann R. Structural changes of human and monkey trabecular meshwork following in vitro cultivation. *Graefes Arch Clin Exp Ophthalmol.* 1982;218(5):225–232.
389. Schachtshabel DO, Bigalke B, Rohen JW. Production of glycosaminoglycans by cell cultures of the trabecular meshwork of the primate eye. *Exp Eye Res.* 1977;24(1):71–80.
390. Rohen JW, Futa R, Lütjen-Drecoll E. The fine structure of the cribriform meshwork in normal and glaucomatous eyes as seen in tangential sections. *Invest Ophthalmol Vis Sci.* 1981;21(4):574–585.
391. Erickson-Lamy K, Schroeder AM, Bassett-Chu S, Epstein DL. Absence of time-dependent facility increase (washout) in the perfused enucleated human eye. *Invest Ophthalmol Vis Sci.* 1990;31(11):2384–2388.
392. Lei Y, Overby DR, Boussommier-Calleja A, Stamer WD, Ethier CR. Outflow physiology of the mouse eye: pressure dependence and washout. *Invest Ophthalmol Vis Sci.* 2011;52(3): 1865–1871.
393. Overby DR, Bertrand J, Schicht M, Paulsen F, Stamer WD, Lütjen-Drecoll E. The structure of the trabecular meshwork, its connections to the ciliary muscle, and the effect of pilocarpine on outflow facility in mice. *Invest Ophthalmol Vis Sci.* 2014;55(6):3727–3736.
394. Erickson KA, Kaufman PL. Comparative effects of three ocular perfusates on outflow facility in the cynomolgus monkey. *Curr Eye Res.* 1981;1(4):211–216.
395. Gaasterland DE, Pederson JE, MacLellan HM, Reddy VN. Rhesus monkey aqueous humor composition and a primate ocular perfusate. *Invest Ophthalmol Vis Sci.* 1979;18(11): 1139–1150.
396. Kaufman PL, True-Gabelt B, Erickson-Lamy KA. Time-dependence of perfusion outflow facility in the cynomolgus monkey. *Curr Eye Res.* 1988;7(7):721–726.
397. Bárány EH. Simultaneous measurement of changing intraocular pressure and outflow facility in the vervet monkey by constant pressure infusion. *Invest Ophthalmol.* 1964;3: 135–143.
398. Scott PA, Overby DR, Freddo TF, Gong H. Comparative studies between species that do and do not exhibit the washout effect. *Exp Eye Res.* 2007;84(3):435–443.
399. Alvarado JA, Yun AJ, Murphy CG. Juxtacanalicular tissue in primary open angle glaucoma and in nonglaucomatous normals. *Arch Ophthalmol.* 1986;104(10):1517–1528.
400. Hamard P, Valtot F, Sourdille P, Bourles-Dagonet F, Baudouin C. Confocal microscopic examination of trabecular meshwork removed during ab externo trabeculectomy. *Br J Ophthalmol.* 2002;86(9):1046–1052.
401. Murphy CG, Johnson M, Alvarado JA. Juxtacanalicular tissue in pigmentary and primary open angle glaucoma. The hydrodynamic role of pigment and other constituents. *Arch Ophthalmol.* 1992;110(12):1779–1785.
402. Gong H, Ruberti J, Overby D, Johnson M, Freddo TF. A new view of the human trabecular meshwork using quick-freeze, deep-etch electron microscopy. *Exp Eye Res.* 2002;75(3):347–358.
403. Sabanay I, Gabelt BT, Tian B, Kaufman PL, Geiger B. H-7 effects on the structure and fluid conductance of monkey trabecular meshwork. *Arch Ophthalmol.* 2000;118(7):955–962.
404. Sabanay I, Tian B, Gabelt BT, Geiger B, Kaufman PL. Functional and structural reversibility of H-7 effects on the conventional aqueous outflow pathway in monkeys. *Exp Eye Res.* 2004;78(1):137–150.
405. Kizhatil K, Ryan M, Marchant JK, Henrich S, John SW. Schlemm's canal is a unique vessel with a combination of blood vascular and lymphatic phenotypes that forms by a novel developmental process. *PLoS Biol.* 2014;12(7):e1001912.
406. Patel G, Fury W, Yang H, et al. Molecular taxonomy of human ocular outflow tissues defined by single-cell transcriptomics. *Proc Natl Acad Sci U S A.* 2020;117(23):12856–12867.
407. Ramos RF, Hoying JB, Witte MH, Daniel Stamer W. Schlemm's canal endothelia, lymphatic, or blood vasculature? *J Glaucoma.* 2007;16(4):391–405.
408. van Zyl T, Yan W, McAdams A, et al. Cell atlas of aqueous humor outflow pathways in eyes of humans and four model species provides insight into glaucoma pathogenesis. *Proc Natl Acad Sci U S A.* 2020;117(19):10339–10349.
409. Ye W, Gong H, Sit A, Johnson M, Freddo TF. Interendothelial junctions in normal human Schlemm's canal respond to changes in pressure. *Invest Ophthalmol Vis Sci.* 1997;38(12):2460–2468.
410. Grierson I, Lee WR. The fine structure of the trabecular meshwork at graded levels of intraocular pressure. (1) Pressure effects within the near-physiological range (8-30 mmHg). *Exp Eye Res.* 1975;20(6):505–521.
411. Grierson I, Lee WR. The fine structure of the trabecular meshwork at graded levels of intraocular pressure. (2) Pressures outside the physiological range (0 and 50 mmHg). *Exp Eye Res.* 1975;20(6):523–530.
412. Grierson I, Lee WR. Light microscopic quantitation of the endothelial vacuoles in Schlemm's canal. *Am J Ophthalmol.* 1977;84(2):234–246.
413. Johnstone MA, Grant WG. Pressure-dependent changes in structures of the aqueous outflow system of human and monkey eyes. *Am J Ophthalmol.* 1973;75(3):365–383.
414. Parc CE, Johnson DH, Brilakis HS. Giant vacuoles are found preferentially near collector channels. *Invest Ophthalmol Vis Sci.* 2000;41(10):2984–2990.
415. Ethier CR, Coloma FM, Sit AJ, Johnson M. Two pore types in the inner-wall endothelium of Schlemm's canal. *Invest Ophthalmol Vis Sci.* 1998;39(11):2041–2048.
416. Sit AJ, Coloma FM, Ethier CR, Johnson M. Factors affecting the pores of the inner wall endothelium of Schlemm's canal. *Invest Ophthalmol Vis Sci.* 1997;38(8):1517–1525.
417. Johnson M. What controls aqueous humour outflow resistance? *Exp Eye Res.* 2006;82:545.
418. Johnson M, Shapiro A, Ethier CR, Kamm RD. Modulation of outflow resistance by the pores of the inner wall endothelium. *Invest Ophthalmol Vis Sci.* 1992;33(5):1670–1675.
419. Overby DR, Stamer WD, Johnson M. The changing paradigm of outflow resistance generation: towards synergistic models of the JCT and inner wall endothelium. *Exp Eye Res.* 2009;88(4):656–670.
420. Allingham RR, de Kater AW, Ethier CR, Anderson PJ, Hertzmark E, Epstein DL. The relationship between pore density and outflow facility in human eyes. *Invest Ophthalmol Vis Sci.* 1992;33(5):1661–1669.
421. Ethier CR, Coloma FM. Effects of ethacrynic acid on Schlemm's canal inner wall and outflow facility in human eyes. *Invest Ophthalmol Vis Sci.* 1999;40(7):1599–1607.
422. Johnson M, Chan D, Read AT, Christensen C, Sit A, Ethier CR. The pore density in the inner wall endothelium of Schlemm's canal of glaucomatous eyes. *Invest Ophthalmol Vis Sci.* 2002;43(9):2950–2955.
423. Ren R, Li G, Le TD, Kopczynski C, Stamer WD, Gong H. Netarsudil increases outflow facility in human eyes through multiple mechanisms. *Invest Ophthalmol Vis Sci.* 2016;57 (14):6197–6209.
424. Sit AJ, Gupta D, Kazemi A, et al. Netarsudil improves trabecular outflow facility in patients with primary open angle glaucoma or ocular hypertension: A phase 2 study. *Am J Ophthalmol.* 2021;226:262–269.
425. Epstein DL, Rohen JW. Morphology of the trabecular meshwork and inner-wall endothelium after cationized ferritin perfusion in the monkey eye. *Invest Ophthalmol Vis Sci.* 1991;32(1):160–171.
426. Ethier CR, Read AT, Chan D. Biomechanics of Schlemm's canal endothelial cells: influence on F-actin architecture. *Biophys J.* 2004;87(4):2828–2837.

427. Gasull X, Ferrer E, Llobet A, et al. Cell membrane stretch modulates the high-conductance Ca2+-activated K+ channel in bovine trabecular meshwork cells. *Invest Ophthalmol Vis Sci.* 2003;44(2):706–714.
428. Baetz NW, Hoffman EA, Yool AJ, Stamer WD. Role of aquaporin-1 in trabecular meshwork cell homeostasis during mechanical strain. *Exp Eye Res.* 2009;89(1):95–100.
429. Uchida T, Shimizu S, Yamagishi R, et al. TRPV4 is activated by mechanical stimulation to induce prostaglandins release in trabecular meshwork, lowering intraocular pressure. *PLoS One.* 2021;16(10):e0258911.
430. Yarishkin O, Phuong TTT, Baumann JM, et al. Piezo1 channels mediate trabecular meshwork mechanotransduction and promote aqueous fluid outflow. *J Physiol.* 2021;599(2):571–592.
431. Li A, Banerjee J, Peterson-Yantorno K, Stamer WD, Leung CT, Civan MM. Effects of cardiotonic steroids on trabecular meshwork cells: search for mediator of ouabain-enhanced outflow facility. *Exp Eye Res.* 2012;96(1):4–12.
432. De Ieso ML, Gurley JM, McClellan ME, et al. Physiologic consequences of caveolin-1 ablation in conventional outflow endothelia. *Invest Ophthalmol Vis Sci.* 2020;61(11):32.
433. Elliott MH, Ashpole NE, Gu X, et al. Caveolin-1 modulates intraocular pressure: implications for caveolae mechanoprotection in glaucoma. *Sci Rep.* 2016;6:37127.
434. Bradley JM, Kelley MJ, Rose A, Acott TS. Signaling pathways used in trabecular matrix metalloproteinase response to mechanical stretch. *Invest Ophthalmol Vis Sci.* 2003;44(12):5174–5181.
435. Pattabiraman PP, Rao PV. Mechanistic basis of Rho GTPase-induced extracellular matrix synthesis in trabecular meshwork cells. *Am J Physiol Cell Physiol.* 2010;298(3):C749–763.
436. Acott TS, Kelley MJ, Keller KE, et al. Intraocular pressure homeostasis: maintaining balance in a high-pressure environment. *J Ocul Pharmacol Ther.* 2014;30(2-3):94–101.
437. Schlunck G, Han H, Wecker T, Kampik D, Meyer-ter-Vehn T, Grehn F. Substrate rigidity modulates cell matrix interactions and protein expression in human trabecular meshwork cells. *Invest Ophthalmol Vis Sci.* 2008;49(1):262–269.
438. Coleman DJ, Trokel S. Direct-recorded intraocular pressure variations in a human subject. *Arch Ophthalmol.* 1969;82(5):637–640.
439. Turner DC, Edmiston AM, Zohner YE, et al. Transient intraocular pressure fluctuations: source, magnitude, frequency, and associated mechanical energy. *Invest Ophthalmol Vis Sci.* 2019;60(7):2572–2582.
440. Li P, Shen TT, Johnstone M, Wang RK. Pulsatile motion of the trabecular meshwork in healthy human subjects quantified by phase-sensitive optical coherence tomography. *Biomed Opt Express.* 2013;4(10):2051–2065.
441. Xin C, Song S, Johnstone M, Wang N, Wang RK. Quantification of pulse-dependent trabecular meshwork motion in normal humans using phase-sensitive OCT. *Invest Ophthalmol Vis Sci.* 2018;59(8):3675–3681.
442. Madekurozwa M, Stamer WD, Reina-Torres E, Sherwood JM, Overby DR. The ocular pulse decreases aqueous humor outflow resistance by stimulating nitric oxide production. *Am J Physiol Cell Physiol.* 2021;320(4):C652–C665.
443. Gao K, Song S, Johnstone MA, et al. Reduced pulsatile trabecular meshwork motion in eyes with primary open angle glaucoma using phase-sensitive optical coherence tomography. *Invest Ophthalmol Vis Sci.* 2020;61(14):21.
444. Last JA, Pan T, Ding Y, et al. Elastic modulus determination of normal and glaucomatous human trabecular meshwork. *Invest Ophthalmol Vis Sci.* 2011;52(5):2147–2152.
445. Wang K, Read AT, Sulchek T, Ethier CR. Trabecular meshwork stiffness in glaucoma. *Exp Eye Res.* 2017;158:3–12.
446. Stamer WD, Acott TS. Current understanding of conventional outflow dysfunction in glaucoma. *Curr Opin Ophthalmol.* 2012;23(2):135–143.
447. Reina-Torres E, Wen JC, Liu KC, et al. VEGF as a paracrine regulator of conventional outflow facility. *Invest Ophthalmol Vis Sci.* 2017;58(3):1899–1908.
448. de Vries VA, Bassil FL, Ramdas WD. The effects of intravitreal injections on intraocular pressure and retinal nerve fiber layer: a systematic review and meta-analysis. *Scientific Reports.* 2020;10(1):13248.
449. Levin AM, Chaya CJ, Kahook MY, Wirostko BM. Intraocular pressure elevation following intravitreal anti-VEGF injections: Short- and long-term considerations. *J Glaucoma.* 2021;30(12):1019–1026.
450. Wen JC, Reina-Torres E, Sherwood JM, et al. Intravitreal anti-VEGF injections reduce aqueous outflow facility in patients with neovascular age-related macular degeneration. *Invest Ophthalmol Vis Sci.* 2017;58(3):1893–1898.
451. Kim J, Park DY, Bae H, et al. Impaired angiopoietin/Tie2 signaling compromises Schlemm's canal integrity and induces glaucoma. *J Clin Invest.* 2017;127(10):3877–3896.
452. Thomson BR, Grannonico M, Liu F, et al. Angiopoietin-1 knockout mice as a genetic model of open-angle glaucoma. *Transl Vis Sci Technol.* 2020;9(4):16.
453. Li G, Nottebaum AF, Brigell M, et al. A small molecule inhibitor of VE-PTP activates Tie2 in Schlemm's canal increasing outflow facility and reducing intraocular pressure. *Invest Ophthalmol Vis Sci.* 2020;61(14):12.
454. McDonnell F, Perkumas KM, Ashpole NE, et al. Shear stress in Schlemm's canal as a sensor of intraocular pressure. *Sci Rep.* 2020;10(1):5804.
455. Sherwood JM, Stamer WD, Overby DR. A model of the oscillatory mechanical forces in the conventional outflow pathway. *J R Soc Interface.* 2019;16(150):20180652.
456. Dismuke WM, Liang J, Overby DR, Stamer WD. Concentration-related effects of nitric oxide and endothelin-1 on human trabecular meshwork cell contractility. *Exp Eye Res.* 2014;120:28–35.
457. Ashpole NE, Overby DR, Ethier CR, Stamer WD. Shear stress-triggered nitric oxide release from Schlemm's canal cells. *Invest Ophthalmol Vis Sci.* 2014;55(12):8067–8076.
458. McDonnell F, Dismuke WM, Overby DR, Stamer WD. Pharmacological regulation of outflow resistance distal to Schlemm's canal. *Am J Physiol Cell Physiol.* 2018;315(1): C44–C51.
459. Wiederholt M, Sturm A, Lepple-Wienhues A. Relaxation of trabecular meshwork and ciliary muscle by release of nitric oxide. *Invest Ophthalmol Vis Sci.* 1994;35(5):2515–2520.
460. Song M, Li L, Lei Y, Sun X. NOS3 deletion in Cav1 deficient mice decreases drug sensitivity to a nitric oxide donor and two nitric oxide synthase inhibitors. *Invest Ophthalmol Vis Sci.* 2019;60(12):4002–4007.
461. Stamer WD, Lei Y, Boussommier-Calleja A, Overby DR, Ethier CR. eNOS, a pressure-dependent regulator of intraocular pressure. *Invest Ophthalmol Vis Sci.* 2011;52(13):9438–9444.
462. Selbach JM, Gottanka J, Wittmann M, Lütjen-Drecoll E. Efferent and afferent innervation of primate trabecular meshwork and scleral spur. *Invest Ophthalmol Vis Sci.* 2000;41(8): 2184–2191.
463. Chen Z, Gu Q, Kaufman PL, Cynader MS. Histochemical mapping of NADPH-diaphorase in monkey and human eyes. *Curr Eye Res.* 1998;17(4):370–379.
464. Nathanson JA, McKee M. Alterations of ocular nitric oxide synthase in human glaucoma. *Invest Ophthalmol Vis Sci.* 1995;36(9):1774–1784.
465. Schuman JS, Erickson K, Nathanson JA. Nitrovasodilator effects on intraocular pressure and outflow facility in monkeys. *Exp Eye Res.* 1994;58(1):99–105.
466. Wizemann AJ, Wizemann V. Organic nitrate therapy in glaucoma. *Am J Ophthalmol.* 1980;90 (1):106–109.
467. Borghi V, Bastia E, Guzzetta M, Chiroli V, Toris CB, Batugo MR, Carreiro ST, Chong WK, Gale DC, Kucera DJ, Jia L, Prasanna G, Ongini E, Krauss AH, Impagnatiello F. A novel nitric oxide releasing prostaglandin analog, NCX 125, reduces intraocular pressure in rabbit, dog, and primate models of glaucoma. *J Ocul Pharmacol Ther.* 2010;26(2):125–132.
468. Impagnatiello F, Toris CB, Batugo M, et al. Intraocular pressure-lowering activity of NCX 470, a novel nitric oxide-donating bimatoprost in preclinical models. *Invest Ophthalmol Vis Sci.* 2015;56(11):6558–6564.
469. Krauss AH, Impagnatiello F, Toris CB, et al. Ocular hypotensive activity of BOL-303259-X, a nitric oxide donating prostaglandin F2alpha agonist, in preclinical models. *Exp Eye Res.* 2011;93(3):250–255.
470. Bastia E, Toris C, Bukowski JM, et al. NCX 1741, a novel nitric oxide-donating phosphodiesterase-5 inhibitor, exerts rapid and long-lasting intraocular pressure-lowering in cynomolgus monkeys. *J Ocul Pharmacol Ther.* 2021;37(4):215–222.
471. Bastia E, Toris CB, Brambilla S, et al. NCX 667, a novel nitric oxide donor, lowers intraocular pressure in rabbits, dogs, and non-human primates and enhances TGFbeta2-induced outflow in HTM/HSC constructs. *Invest Ophthalmol Vis Sci.* 2021;62(3):17.
472. Weinreb RN, Ong T, Scassellati Sforzolini B, et al. A randomised, controlled comparison of latanoprostene bunod and latanoprost 0.005% in the treatment of ocular hypertension and open angle glaucoma: the VOYAGER study. *Br J Ophthalmol.* 2015;99(6):738–745.
473. Grant WM. Experimental aqueous perfusion in enucleated human eyes. *Arch Ophthalmol.* 1963;69:783–801.
474. Rosenquist R, Epstein D, Melamed S, Johnson M, Grant WM. Outflow resistance of enucleated human eyes at two different perfusion pressures and different extents of trabeculotomy. *Curr Eye Res.* 1989;8(12):1233–1240.
475. Schuman JS, Chang W, Wang N, de Kater AW, Allingham RR. Excimer laser effects on outflow facility and outflow pathway morphology. *Invest Ophthalmol Vis Sci.* 1999;40(8):1676–1680.
476. de Kater AW, Shahsafaei A, Epstein DL. Localization of smooth muscle and nonmuscle actin isoforms in the human aqueous outflow pathway. *Invest Ophthalmol Vis Sci.* 1992;33 (2):424–429.
477. Bentley MD, Hann CR, Fautsch MP. Anatomical variation of human collector channel orifices. *Invest Ophthalmol Vis Sci.* 2016;57(3):1153–1159.
478. Malvankar-Mehta MS, Chen YN, Iordanous Y, Wang WW, Costella J, Hutnik CM. iStent as a solo procedure for glaucoma patients: A systematic review and meta-analysis. *PLoS One.* 2015;10(5):e0128146.
479. Mosaed S, Dustin L, Minckler DS. Comparative outcomes between newer and older surgeries for glaucoma. *Trans Am Ophthalmol Soc.* 2009;107:127–133.
480. Chen S, Waxman S, Wang C, Atta S, Loewen R, Loewen NA. Dose-dependent effects of netarsudil, a Rho-kinase inhibitor, on the distal outflow tract. *Graefes Arch Clin Exp Ophthalmol.* 2020;258(6):1211–1216.
481. Waxman S, Wang C, Dang Y, et al. Structure-function changes of the porcine distal outflow tract in response to nitric oxide. *Invest Ophthalmol Vis Sci.* 2018;59(12):4886–4895.
482. Wiederholt M, Bielka S, Schweig F, Lütjen-Drecoll E, Lepple-Wienhues A. Regulation of outflow rate and resistance in the perfused anterior segment of the bovine eye. *Exp Eye Res.* 1995;61(2):223–234.
483. Zhou EH, Paolucci M, Dryja TP, et al. A compact whole-eye perfusion system to evaluate pharmacologic responses of outflow facility. *Invest Ophthalmol Vis Sci.* 2017;58(7):2991–3003.
484. Borras T, Rowlette LL, Tamm ER, Gottanka J, Epstein DL. Effects of elevated intraocular pressure on outflow facility and TIGR/MYOC expression in perfused human anterior segments. *Invest Ophthalmol Vis Sci.* 2002;43(1):33–40.
485. Vranka JA, Staverosky JA, Raghunathan V, Acott TS. Elevated pressure influences relative distribution of segmental regions of the trabecular meshwork. *Exp Eye Res.* 2020;190: 107888.
486. Raghunathan VK, Benoit J, Kasetti R, et al. Glaucomatous cell derived matrices differentially modulate non-glaucomatous trabecular meshwork cellular behavior. *Acta Biomater.* 2018;71: 444–459.
487. de Kater AW, Melamed S, Epstein DL. Patterns of aqueous humor outflow in glaucomatous and nonglaucomatous human eyes. A tracer study using cationized ferritin. *Arch Ophthalmol.* 1989;107(4):572–576.
488. Lütjen-Drecoll E, Rohen JW. Morphology of aqueous outflow pathways in normal and glaucomatous eyes. In: Ritch R, ed. *The Glaucomas.* St. Louis: CV Mosby; 1989:41.
489. Lütjen-Drecoll E, Shimizu T, Rohrbach M, Rohen JW. Quantitative analysis of 'plaque material' in the inner- and outer wall of Schlemm's canal in normal- and glaucomatous eyes. *Exp Eye Res.* 1986;42(5):443–455.
490. Lütjen-Drecoll E, Kaufman PL. Morphological changes in primate aqueous humor formation and drainage tissues after long-term treatment with antiglaucomatous drugs. *J Glaucoma.* 1993;2(4):316–328.

491. Cousins SW, McCabe MM, Danielpour D, Streilein JW. Identification of transforming growth factor-beta as an immunosuppressive factor in aqueous humor. *Invest Ophthalmol Vis Sci.* 1991;32(8):2201–2211.

492. Granstein RD, Staszewski R, Knisely TL, Zeira E, Nazareno R, Latina M, Albert DM. Aqueous humor contains transforming growth factor-beta and a small (less than 3500 daltons) inhibitor of thymocyte proliferation. *J Immunol.* 1990;144(8):3021–3027.

493. Jampel HD, Roche N, Stark WJ, Roberts AB. Transforming growth factor-beta in human aqueous humor. *Curr Eye Res.* 1990;9(10):963–969.

494. Tripathi RC, Li J, Chan WF, Tripathi BJ. Aqueous humor in glaucomatous eyes contains an increased level of TGF-beta 2. *Exp Eye Res.* 1994;59(6):723–727.

495. Fleenor DL, Shepard AR, Hellberg PE, Jacobson N, Pang IH, Clark AF. TGFbeta2-induced changes in human trabecular meshwork: implications for intraocular pressure. *Invest Ophthalmol Vis Sci.* 2006;47(1):226–234.

496. Gottanka J, Chan D, Eichhorn M, Lütjen-Drecoll E, Ethier CR. Effects of TGF-beta2 in perfused human eyes. *Invest Ophthalmol Vis Sci.* 2004;45(1):153–158.

497. Picht G, Welge-Luessen U, Grehn F, Lütjen-Drecoll E. Transforming growth factor beta 2 levels in the aqueous humor in different types of glaucoma and the relation to filtering bleb development. *Graefes Arch Clin Exp Ophthalmol.* 2001;239(3):199–207.

498. Fuchshofer R, Welge-Lussen U, Lütjen-Drecoll E. The effect of TGF-beta2 on human trabecular meshwork extracellular proteolytic system. *Exp Eye Res.* 2003;77(6):757–765.

499. Lee ES, Gabelt BT, Faralli JA, et al. COCH transgene expression in cultured human trabecular meshwork cells and its effect on outflow facility in monkey organ cultured anterior segments. *Invest Ophthalmol Vis Sci.* 2010;51(4):2060–2066.

500. Bhattacharya SK, Gabelt BT, Ruiz J, Picciani R, Kaufman PL. Cochlin expression in anterior segment organ culture models after TGFbeta2 treatment. *Invest Ophthalmol Vis Sci.* 2009;50(2):551–559.

501. Wang WH, McNatt LG, Pang IH, et al. Increased expression of the WNT antagonist sFRP-1 in glaucoma elevates intraocular pressure. *J Clin Invest.* 2008;118(3):1056–1064.

502. Grierson I, Lee WR. Erythrocyte phagocytosis in the human trabecular meshwork. *Br J Ophthalmol.* 1973;57(6):400–415.

503. Polansky JR, Wood IS, Maglio MT, Alvarado JA. Trabecular meshwork cell culture in glaucoma research: evaluation of biological activity and structural properties of human trabecular cells in vitro. *Ophthalmology.* 1984;91(6):580–595.

504. Rohen JW, Van der Zypen E. The phagocytic activity of the trabecular meshwork endothelium. An electron microscopic study of the vervet (Cercopithecus ethiops). *Albrecht Von Graefes Arch Klin Exp Ophthalmol.* 1968(175):143.

505. Acott TS, Kingsley PD, Samples JR, Van Buskirk EM. Human trabecular meshwork organ culture: morphology and glycosaminoglycan synthesis. *Invest Ophthalmol Vis Sci.* 1988;29(1):90–100.

506. Alvarado JA, Murphy CG. Outflow obstruction in pigmentary and primary open angle glaucoma. *Arch Ophthalmol.* 1992;110(12):1769–1778.

507. Camelo S, Shanley AC, Voon AS, McMenamin PG. An intravital and confocal microscopic study of the distribution of intracameral antigen in the aqueous outflow pathways and limbus of the rat eye. *Exp Eye Res.* 2004;79(4):455–464.

508. Margeta MA, Lad EM, Proia AD. CD163+ macrophages infiltrate axon bundles of postmortem optic nerves with glaucoma. *Graefes Arch Clin Exp Ophthalmol.* 2018;256(12):2449–2456.

509. Alvarado JA, Katz LJ, Trivedi S, Shifera AS. Monocyte modulation of aqueous outflow and recruitment to the trabecular meshwork following selective laser trabeculoplasty. *Arch Ophthalmol.* 2010;128(6):731–737.

510. Epstein DL, Freddo TF, Anderson PJ, Patterson MM, Bassett-Chu S. Experimental obstruction to aqueous outflow by pigment particles in living monkeys. *Invest Ophthalmol Vis Sci.* 1986;27(3):387–395.

511. Li G, Lee C, Read AT, et al. Anti-fibrotic activity of a rho-kinase inhibitor restores outflow function and intraocular pressure homeostasis. *Elife.* 2021:10.

512. Epstein DL. Open angle glaucoma. Why not a cure? [editorial]. *Arch Ophthalmol.* 1987(105):1187.

513. Kaufman PL. Medical trabeculocanalotomy in monkeys with cytochalasin B or EDTA. *Ann Ophthalmol.* 1979;11:795.

514. Campbell DG, Essigmann EM. Hemolytic ghost cell glaucoma. Further studies. *Arch Ophthalmol.* 1979;97(11):2141–2146.

515. Campbell DG, Simmons RJ, Grant WM. Ghost cells as a cause of glaucoma. *Am J Ophthalmol.* 1976;81(4):441–450.

516. Goldberg MF. The diagnosis and treatment of sickled erythrocytes in human hyphemias. *Trans Am Ophthalmol Soc.* 1978;76:481.

517. Flocks M. Phacolytic glaucoma. Clinicopathologic study of 138 cases of glaucoma associated with hypermature cataract. *Arch Ophthalmol.* 1955;54:37.

518. Fenton RH, Zimmerman LE. Hemolytic glaucoma. An unusual cause of acute open-angle secondary glaucoma. *Arch Ophthalmol.* 1963;70:236–239.

519. Yanoff M. Glaucoma mechanisms in ocular malignant melanomas. *Am J Ophthalmol.* 1970;70(6):898–904.

520. Petersen HP. Can pigmentary deposits on the trabecular meshwork increase the resistance of the aqueous outflow? *Acta Ophthalmol (Copenh).* 1969;47(3):743–749.

521. Quigley HA. Long-term follow-up of laser iridotomy. *Ophthalmology.* 1981;88(3):218–224.

522. Anderson DR. Experimental alpha chymotrypsin glaucoma studied by scanning electron microscopy. *Am J Ophthalmol.* 1971;71(2):470–476.

523. Worthen DM. Scanning electron microscopy after alpha chymotrypsin perfusion in man. *Am J Ophthalmol.* 1972;73(5):637–642.

524. Channell MM, Beckman H. Intraocular pressure changes after neodymium-YAG laser posterior capsulotomy. *Arch Ophthalmol.* 1984;102(7):1024–1026.

525. Ge J, Wand M, Chiang R, Paranhos A, Shields MB. Long-term effect of Nd:YAG laser posterior capsulotomy on intraocular pressure. *Arch Ophthalmol.* 2000;118(10):1334–1337.

526. Nelson GA, Edward DP, Wilensky JT. Ocular amyloidosis and secondary glaucoma. *Ophthalmology.* 1999;106(7):1363–1366.

527. Epstein DL. Identification of heavy molecular weight soluble lens protein in aqueous humor in phakolytic glaucoma. *Invest Ophthalmol Vis Sci.* 1978(17):398.

528. Epstein DL, Jedziniak JA, Grant WM. Obstruction of aqueous outflow by lens particles and by heavy-molecular-weight soluble lens proteins. *Invest Ophthalmol Vis Sci.* 1978;17(3):272–277.

529. Epstein DL, Hashimoto JM, Grant WM. Serum obstruction of aqueous outflow in enucleated eyes. *Am J Ophthalmol.* 1978;86(1):101–105.

530. Davanger M. On the molecular composition and physiochemical properties of the pseudoexfoliation material. *Acta Ophthalmol.* 1977(55):621.

531. Johnson M, Gong H, Freddo TF, Ritter N, Kamm R. Serum proteins and aqueous outflow resistance in bovine eyes. *Invest Ophthalmol Vis Sci.* 1993;34(13):3549–3557.

532. Sit AJ, Gong H, Ritter N, Freddo TF, Kamm R, Johnson M. The role of soluble proteins in generating aqueous outflow resistance in the bovine and human eye. *Exp Eye Res.* 1997;64(5):813–821.

533. Kee C, Gabelt BT, Gange SJ, Kaufman PL. Serum effects on aqueous outflow during anterior chamber perfusion in monkeys. *Invest Ophthalmol Vis Sci.* 1996;37(9):1840–1848.

534. Chrzanowska-Wodnicka M, Burridge K. Tyrosine phosphorylation is involved in reorganization of the actin cytoskeleton in response to serum or LPA stimulation. *J Cell Sci.* 1994;107(Pt 12):3643–3654.

535. Seufferlein T, Rozengurt E. Lysophosphatidic acid stimulates tyrosine phosphorylation of focal adhesion kinase, paxillin, and p130. Signaling pathways and cross-talk with platelet-derived growth factor. *J Biol Chem.* 1994;269(12):9345–9351.

536. Dada VK. Postoperative intraocular pressure changes with use of different viscoelastics. *Ophthal Surg.* 1994(25):540.

537. Shibasaki H, Kurome H, Hayasaka S, Noda S, Setogawa T. Viscoelastic substance in the anterior chamber elevates intraocular pressure. *Ann Ophthalmol.* 1994;26(1):10–11.

538. Rohen JW, Lütjen E, Bárány E. The relation between the ciliary muscle and the trabecular meshwork and its importance for the effect of miotics on aqueous outflow resistance. A study in two contrasting monkey species, Macaca irus and Cercopithecus aethiops. *Albrecht Von Graefes Arch Klin Exp Ophthalmol.* 1967;172(1):23–47.

539. Li G, Farsiu S, Chiu SJ, et al. Pilocarpine-induced dilation of Schlemm's canal and prevention of lumen collapse at elevated intraocular pressures in living mice visualized by OCT. *Invest Ophthalmol Vis Sci.* 2014;55(6):3737–3746.

540. Lütjen-Drecoll E. Functional morphology of the trabecular meshwork in primate eyes. *Prog Retin Eye Res.* 1999;18(1):91–119.

541. Armaly MF, Burian HM. Changes in the tonogram during accommodation. *AMA Arch Ophthalmol.* 1958;60(1):60–69.

542. Armaly MF. Studies on intraocular effects of the orbital parasympathetics. II. Effect on intraocular pressure. *AMA Arch Ophthalmol.* 1959;62(1):117–124.

543. Kaufman PL, Gabelt BT. Cholinergic mechanisms and aqueous humor dynamics. In: Drance SM, ed. *Pharmacology of Glaucoma.* Baltimore: Williams & Wilkins; 1992:64.

544. Bárány EH, Rohen JW. Localized contraction and relaxation within the ciliary muscle of the vervet monkey (Cercopithecus ethiops). In: Rohen JW, ed. *The Structure of the Eye. Second Symposium.* Stuttgart: Schattauer; 1965:287.

545. Van Buskirk EM, Grant WM. Lens depression and aqueous outflow in enucleated primate eyes. *Am J Ophthalmol.* 1973;76(5):632–640.

546. Harris LS. Cycloplegic-induced intraocular pressure elevations a study of normal and open-angle glaucomatous eyes. *Arch Ophthalmol.* 1968;79(3):242–246.

547. Bárány E, Christensen RE. Cycloplegia and outflow resistance in normal human and monkey eyes and in primary open-angle glaucoma. *Arch Ophthalmol.* 1967;77(6):757–760.

548. Schimek RA, Lieberman WJ. The influence of Cyclogyl and Neosynephrine on tonographic studies of miotic control in open-angle glaucoma. *Am J Ophthalmol.* 1961;51:781–784.

549. Bárány EH. The immediate effect on outflow resistance of intravenous pilocarpine in the vervet monkey. *Invest Ophthalmol.* 1967;6:373.

550. Bárány EH. The mode of action of pilocarpine on outflow resistance in the eye of a primate (Cercopithecus ethiops). *Invest Ophthalmol.* 1962;1:712–727.

551. Bárány EH. The mode of action of miotics on outflow resistance. A study of pilocarpine in the vervet monkey Cercopithecus ethiops. *Trans Ophthalmol Soc U K.* 1966;86:539–578.

552. Shaffer R.N. In: Newell FW, ed. Glaucoma: Transactions of the Fifth Conference. New York: Josiah Macy Jr. Foundation; 1960:234.

553. Kaufman PL, Bárány EH. Loss of acute pilocarpine effect on outflow facility following surgical disinsertion and retrodisplacement of the ciliary muscle from the scleral spur in the cynomolgus monkey. *Invest Ophthalmol.* 1976;15(10):793–807.

554. Kaufman PL, Bárány EH. Residual pilocarpine effects on outflow facility after ciliary muscle disinsertion in the synomolgus monkey. *Invest Ophthalmol.* 1976;15(7):558–561.

555. Kaufman PL, Bárány EH. Subsensitivity to pilocarpine of the aqueous outflow system in monkey eyes after topical anticholinesterase treatment. *Am J Ophthalmol.* 1976;82(6):883–891.

556. Tamm ER, Flügel C, Stefani FH, Lütjen-Drecoll E. Nerve endings with structural characteristics of mechanoreceptors in the human scleral spur. *Invest Ophthalmol Vis Sci.* 1994;35(3):1157–1166.

557. Gupta N, Drance SM, McAllister R, Prasad S, Rootman J, Cynader MS. Localization of M3 muscarinic receptor subtype and mRNA in the human eye. *Ophthalmic Res.* 1994;26(4):207–213.

558. Thieme H, Hildebrandt J, Choritz L, Strauss O, Wiederholt M. Muscarinic receptors of the M2 subtype in human and bovine trabecular meshwork. *Graefes Arch Clin Exp Ophthalmol.* 2001;239(4):310–315.

559. Shade DL, Clark AF, Pang IH. Effects of muscarinic agents on cultured human trabecular meshwork cells. *Exp Eye Res.* 1996;62(3):201–210.

560. de Kater AW, Spurr-Michaud SJ, Gipson IK. Localization of smooth muscle myosin-containing cells in the aqueous outflow pathway. *Invest Ophthalmol Vis Sci.* 1990;31(2):347–353.

561. Lepple-Wienhues A, Stahl F, Wiederholt M. Differential smooth muscle-like contractile properties of trabecular meshwork and ciliary muscle. *Exp Eye Res.* 1991;53(1):33–38.

562. Lepple-Wienhues A, Stahl F, Willner U, Schafer R, Wiederholt M. Endothelin-evoked contractions in bovine ciliary muscle and trabecular meshwork: interaction with calcium, nifedipine and nickel. *Curr Eye Res.* 1991;10(10):983–989.

563. Wiederholt M, Schafer R, Wagner U, Lepple-Wienhues A. Contractile response of the isolated trabecular meshwork and ciliary muscle to cholinergic and adrenergic agents. *Ger J Ophthalmol.* 1996;5(3):146–153.

564. Schroeder A, Erickson K. Cholinergic agonists do not increase trabecular outflow facility in the human eye. *Invest Ophthalmol Vis Sci.* 1994;(34):2054.

565. Kiland JA, Hubbard WC, Kaufman PL. Low doses of pilocarpine do not significantly increase outflow facility in the cynomolgus monkey. *Exp Eye Res.* 2000;70(5):603–609.

566. Tian B, Kaufman PL. Combined effects of H7 and pilocarpine on anterior segment physiology in monkey eyes. *Curr Eye Res.* 2007;32(6):491–500.

567. Gupta N, McAllister R, Drance SM, Rootman J, Cynader MS. Muscarinic receptor M1 and M2 subtypes in the human eye: QNB, pirenzipine, oxotremorine, and AFDX-116 in vitro autoradiography. *Br J Ophthalmol.* 1994;78(7):555–559.

568. Zhang X, Hernandez MR, Yang H, Erickson K. Expression of muscarinic receptor subtype mRNA in the human ciliary muscle. *Invest Ophthalmol Vis Sci.* 1995;36(8):1645–1657.

569. Gabelt BT, Kaufman PL. Inhibition of outflow facility and accommodative and miotic responses to pilocarpine in rhesus monkeys by muscarinic receptor subtype antagonists. *J Pharmacol Exp Ther.* 1992;263(3):1133–1139.

570. Gabelt BT, Kaufman PL. Inhibition of aceclidine-stimulated outflow facility, accommodation and miosis in rhesus monkeys by muscarinic receptor subtype antagonists. *Exp Eye Res.* 1994;58(5):623–630.

571. Flügel C, Bárány EH, Lütjen-Drecoll E. Histochemical differences within the ciliary muscle and its function in accommodation. *Exp Eye Res.* 1990;50(2):219–226.

572. Croft MA, Kaufman PL, Erickson-Lamy K, Polansky JR. Accommodation and ciliary muscle muscarinic receptors after echothiophate. *Invest Ophthalmol Vis Sci.* 1991;32(13):3288–3297.

573. Kaufman PL. Anticholinesterase-induced cholinergic subsensitivity in primate accommodative mechanism. *Am J Ophthalmol.* 1978;85(5 Pt 1):622–631.

574. Bárány E, Berrie CP, Birdsall NJ, Burgen AS, Hulme EC. The binding properties of the muscarinic receptors of the cynomolgus monkey ciliary body and the response to the induction of agonist subsensitivity. *Br J Pharmacol.* 1982;77(4):731–739.

575. Bárány EH. Pilocarpine-induced subsensitivity to carbachol and pilocarpine of ciliary muscle in vervet and cynomolgus monkeys. *Acta Ophthalmol (Copenh).* 1977;55(1):141–163.

576. Bárány EH. Muscarinic subsensitivity without receptor change in monkey ciliary muscle. *Br J Pharmacol.* 1985;84(1):193–198.

577. Bill A, Phillips I. Uveoscleral drainage of aqueous humor in human eyes. *Exp Eye Res.* 1971;21:275.

578. Bill A. Early effects of epinephrine on aqueous humor dynamics in vervet monkeys (Cercopithecus ethiops). *Exp Eye Res.* 1969;8(1):35–43.

579. Bill A. Effects of atropine on aqueous humor dynamics in the vervet monkey (Cercopithecus ethiops). *Exp Eye Res.* 1969;8(3):284–291.

580. Ehinger B. A comparative study of the adrenergic nerves to the anterior eye segment of some primates. *Z Zellforsch Mikrosk Anat.* 1971;116(2):157–177.

581. Nomura T, Smelser GK. The identification of adrenergic and cholinergic nerve endings in the trabecular meshwork. *Invest Ophthalmol.* 1974;13(7):525–532.

582. Ruskell GL. The source of nerve fibres of the trabeculae and adjacent structures in monkey eyes. *Exp Eye Res.* 1976;23(4):449–459.

583. Ballintine EJ, Garner LL. Improvement of the co-efficient of outflow in glaucomatous eyes. Prolonged local treatment with epinephrine. *Arch Ophthalmol.* 1961;66:314–317.

584. Krill AE, Newell FW, Novak M. Early and long-term effects of levo-epinephrine on ocular tension and outflow. *Am J Ophthalmol.* 1965;59:833–839.

585. Bárány EH. Topical epinephrine effects on true outflow resistance and pseudofacility in vervet monkeys studied by a new anterior chamber perfusion technique. *Invest Ophthalmol.* 1968;7(1):88–104.

586. Sears ML, Neufeld AH. Editorial: Adrenergic modulation of the outflow of aqueous humor. *Invest Ophthalmol.* 1975;14(2):83–86.

587. Camp JJ, Hann CR, Johnson DH, Tarara JE, Robb RA. Three-dimensional reconstruction of aqueous channels in human trabecular meshwork using light microscopy and confocal microscopy. *Scanning.* 1997;19(4):258–263.

588. Kaufman PL, Bárány EH. Adrenergic drug effects on aqueous outflow facility following ciliary muscle retrodisplacement in the cynomolgus monkey. *Invest Ophthalmol Vis Sci.* 1981;20(5):644–651.

589. Kaufman PL, Rentzhog L. Effect of total iridectomy on outflow facility responses to adrenergic drugs in cynomolgus monkeys. *Exp Eye Res.* 1981;33(1):65–74.

590. Anderson L, Wilson WS. Inhibition by indomethacin of the increased facility of outflow induced by adrenaline. *Exp Eye Res.* 1990;50(2):119–126.

591. Alvarado JA, Murphy CG, Franse-Carman L, Chen J, Underwood JL. Effect of beta-adrenergic agonists on paracellular width and fluid flow across outflow pathway cells. *Invest Ophthalmol Vis Sci.* 1998;39(10):1813–1822.

592. Wiederholt M. Direct involvement of trabecular meshwork in the regulation of aqueous humor outflow. *Curr Opin Ophthalmol.* 1998;9(2):46–49.

593. Robinson JC, Kaufman PL. Cytochalasin B potentiates epinephrine's outflow facility-increasing effect. *Invest Ophthalmol Vis Sci.* 1991;32(5):1614–1618.

594. Robinson JC, Kaufman PL. Phalloidin inhibits epinephrine's and cytochalasin B's facilitation of aqueous outflow. *Arch Ophthalmol.* 1994;112(12):1610–1613.

595. Wax MB, Molinoff PB, Alvarado J, Polansky J. Characterization of beta-adrenergic receptors in cultured human trabecular cells and in human trabecular meshwork. *Invest Ophthalmol Vis Sci.* 1989;30(1):51–57.

596. Cyrlin MN, Thomas JV, Epstein DL. Additive effect of epinephrine to timolol therapy in primary open angle glaucoma. *Arch Ophthalmol.* 1982;100(3):414–418.

597. Thomas JV, Epstein DL. Timolol and epinephrine in primary open angle glaucoma. Transient additive effect. *Arch Ophthalmol.* 1981;99(1):91–95.

598. Allen RC, Epstein DL. Additive effect of betaxolol and epinephrine in primary open angle glaucoma. *Arch Ophthalmol.* 1986;104(8):1178–1184.

599. Allen RC, Hertzmark E, Walker AM, Epstein DL. A double-masked comparison of betaxolol vs timolol in the treatment of open-angle glaucoma. *Am J Ophthalmol.* 1986;101(5):535–541.

600. Robinson JC, Kaufman PL. Effects and interactions of epinephrine, norepinephrine, timolol, and betaxolol on outflow facility in the cynomolgus monkey. *Am J Ophthalmol.* 1990;109(2):189–194.

601. Kaufman PL. Adenosine 3′,5′-cyclic-monophosphate and outflow facility in monkey eyes with intact and retrodisplaced ciliary muscle. *Exp Eye Res.* 1987;44(3):415–423.

602. Neufeld AH, Sears ML. Adenosine 3′,5′-monophosphate analogue increases the outflow facility of the primate eye. *Invest Ophthalmol.* 1975;14(9):688–689.

603. Neufeld AH. Influences of cyclic nucleotides on outflow facility in the vervet monkey. *Exp Eye Res.* 1978;27(4):387–397.

604. Erickson-Lamy KA, Nathanson JA. Epinephrine increases facility of outflow and cyclic AMP content in the human eye in vitro. *Invest Ophthalmol Vis Sci.* 1992;33(9):2672–2678.

605. Wiederholt M, Schäfer R, Wagner U, Lepple-Wienhues A. Contractile response of the isolated trabecular meshwork and ciliary muscle to cholinergic and adrenergic agents. *Ger J Ophthalmol.* 1996;5(3):146–153.

606. Stamer WD, Huang Y, Seftor RE, Svensson SS, Snyder RW, Regan JW. Cultured human trabecular meshwork cells express functional alpha 2A adrenergic receptors. *Invest Ophthalmol Vis Sci.* 1996;37(12):2426–2433.

607. Törnqvist G. Effect of cervical sympathetic stimulation on accommodation in monkeys. An example of a beta-adrenergic, inhibitory effect. *Acta Physiol Scand.* 1966;67(3):363–372.

608. Van Alphen GW, Robinette SL, Macri FJ. Drug effects on ciliary muscle and choroid preparations in vitro. *Arch Ophthalmol.* 1962;68:81–93.

609. Vanalphen GW, Kern R, Robinette SL. Adrenergic receptors of the intraocular muscles: comparison to cat, rabbit, and monkey. *Arch Ophthalmol.* 1965;74:253–259.

610. Camras CB, Feldman SG, Podos SM, Christensen RE, Gardner SK, Fazio DT. Inhibition of the epinephrine-induced reduction of intraocular pressure by systemic indomethacin in humans. *Am J Ophthalmol.* 1985;100(1):169–175.

611. Gilmartin B, Hogan RE, Thompson SM. The effect of Timolol Maleate on tonic accommodation, tonic vergence, and pupil diameter. *Invest Ophthalmol Vis Sci.* 1984;25(6):763–770.

612. Toris CB, Gleason ML, Camras CB, Yablonski ME. Effects of brimonidine on aqueous humor dynamics in human eyes. *Arch Ophthalmol.* 1995;113(12):1514–1517.

613. Toris CB, Tafoya ME, Camras CB, Yablonski ME. Effects of apraclonidine on aqueous humor dynamics in human eyes. *Ophthalmology.* 1995;102(3):456–461.

614. Kobayashi H, Kobayashi K, Okinami S. Efficacy of bunazosin hydrochloride 0.01% as adjunctive therapy of latanoprost or timolol. *J Glaucoma.* 2004;13(1):73–80.

615. Akaishi T, Takagi Y, Matsugi T, Ishida N, Hara H, Kashiwagi K. Effects of bunazosin hydrochloride on ciliary muscle constriction and matrix metalloproteinase activities. *J Glaucoma.* 2004;13(4):312–318.

616. Geiger B, Yehuda-Levenberg S, Bershadsky AD. Molecular interactions in the submembrane plaque of cell-cell and cell-matrix adhesions. *Acta Anat (Basel).* 1995;154(1):46–62.

617. Yamada KM, Geiger B. Molecular interactions in cell adhesion complexes. *Curr Opin Cell Biol.* 1997;9(1):76–85.

618. Zhou EH, Krishnan R, Stamer WD, et al. Mechanical responsiveness of the endothelial cell of Schlemm's canal: scope, variability and its potential role in controlling aqueous humour outflow. *J R Soc Interface.* 2012;9(71):1144–1155.

619. Liu X, Rasmussen CA, Gabelt BT, Brandt CR, Kaufman PL. Gene therapy targeting glaucoma: where are we? *Surv Ophthalmol.* 2009;54(4):472–486.

620. Tian B, Gabelt BT, Geiger B, Kaufman PL. The role of the actomyosin system in regulating trabecular fluid outflow. *Exp Eye Res.* 2009;88(4):713–717.

621. Johnstone M, Tanner D, Chau B, Kopecky K. Concentration-dependent morphologic effects of cytochalasin B in the aqueous outflow system. *Invest Ophthalmol Vis Sci.* 1980;19(7):835–841.

622. Kaufman PL, Bárány EH. Cytochalasin B reversibly increases outflow facility in the eye of the cynomolgus monkey. *Invest Ophthalmol Vis Sci.* 1977;16(1):47–53.

623. Kaufman PL, Bill A, Bárány EH. Effect of cytochalasin B on conventional drainage of aqueous humor in the cynomolgus monkey. *Exp Eye Res.* 1977:411.

624. Cai S, Liu X, Glasser A, Volberg T, Filla M, Geiger B, Polansky JR, Kaufman PL. Effect of latrunculin-A on morphology and actin-associated adhesions of cultured human trabecular meshwork cells. *Mol Vis.* 2000;6:132–143.

625. Epstein DL, Rowlette LL, Roberts BC. Acto-myosin drug effects and aqueous outflow function. *Invest Ophthalmol Vis Sci.* 1999;40(1):74–81.

626. Peterson JA, Tian B, Bershadsky AD, et al. Latrunculin-A increases outflow facility in the monkey. *Invest Ophthalmol Vis Sci.* 1999;40(5):931–941.

627. Peterson JA, Tian B, Geiger B, Kaufman PL. Effect of latrunculin-B on outflow facility in monkeys. *Exp Eye Res.* 2000;70(3):307–313.

628. Ethier CR, Read AT, Chan DW. Effects of latrunculin-B on outflow facility and trabecular meshwork structure in human eyes. *Invest Ophthalmol Vis Sci.* 2006;47(5):1991–1998.

629. Okka M, Tian B, Kaufman PL. Effect of low-dose latrunculin B on anterior segment physiologic features in the monkey eye. *Arch Ophthalmol.* 2004;122(10):1482–1488.

630. Sabanay I, Tian B, Gabelt BT, Geiger B, Kaufman PL. Latrunculin B effects on trabecular meshwork and corneal endothelial morphology in monkeys. *Exp Eye Res.* 2006;82(2):236–246.

631. Rasmussen CA, Kaufman PL, Ritch R, Haque R, Brazzell RK, Vittitow JL. Latrunculin B reduces intraocular pressure in human ocular hypertension and primary open-angle glaucoma. *Transl Vis Sci Technol.* 2014;3(5):1.

632. Liu X, Cai S, Glasser A, et al. Effect of H-7 on cultured human trabecular meshwork cells. *Mol Vis.* 2001;7:145–153.

633. Bershadsky A, Chausovsky A, Becker E, Lyubimova A, Geiger B. Involvement of microtubules in the control of adhesion-dependent signal transduction. *Curr Biol.* 1996;6(10):1279–1289.

634. Tian B, Kaufman PL, Volberg T, Gabelt BT, Geiger B. H-7 disrupts the actin cytoskeleton and increases outflow facility. *Arch Ophthalmol.* 1998;116(5):633–643.

635. Volberg T, Geiger B, Citi S, Bershadsky AD. Effect of protein kinase inhibitor H-7 on the contractility, integrity, and membrane anchorage of the microfilament system. *Cell Motil Cytoskeleton.* 1994;29(4):321–338.

636. Tian B, Gabelt BT, Peterson JA, Kiland JA, Kaufman PL. H-7 increases trabecular facility and facility after ciliary muscle disinsertion in monkeys. *Invest Ophthalmol Vis Sci.* 1999;40(1):239–242.

637. Bahler CK, Hann CR, Fautsch MP, Johnson DH. Pharmacologic disruption of Schlemm's canal cells and outflow facility in anterior segments of human eyes. *Invest Ophthalmol Vis Sci.* 2004;45(7):2246–2254.

638. Hu Y, Gabelt BT, Kaufman PL. Monkey organ-cultured anterior segments: technique and response to H-7. *Exp Eye Res.* 2006;82(6):1100–1108.

639. Honjo M, Tanihara H, Inatani M, et al. Effects of rho-associated protein kinase inhibitor Y-27632 on intraocular pressure and outflow facility. *Invest Ophthalmol Vis Sci.* 2001;42(1):137–144.

640. Rao PV, Deng PF, Kumar J, Epstein DL. Modulation of aqueous humor outflow facility by the Rho kinase-specific inhibitor Y-27632. *Invest Ophthalmol Vis Sci.* 2001;42(5):1029–1037.

641. Renieri G, Choritz L, Rosenthal R, Meissner S, Pfeiffer N, Thieme H. Effects of endothelin-1 on calcium-independent contraction of bovine trabecular meshwork. *Graefes Arch Clin Exp Ophthalmol.* 2008;246(8):1107–1115.

642. Rosenthal R, Choritz L, Schlott S, et al. Effects of ML-7 and Y-27632 on carbachol- and endothelin-1-induced contraction of bovine trabecular meshwork. *Exp Eye Res.* 2005;80(6):837–845.

643. Thieme H, Nuskovski M, Nass JU, Pleyer U, Strauss O, Wiederholt M. Mediation of calcium-independent contraction in trabecular meshwork through protein kinase C and rho-A. *Invest Ophthalmol Vis Sci.* 2000;41(13):4240–4246.

644. Honjo M, Inatani M, Kido N, Sawamura T, Yue BY, Honda Y, Tanihara H. A myosin light chain kinase inhibitor, ML-9, lowers the intraocular pressure in rabbit eyes. *Exp Eye Res.* 2002;75(2):135–142.

645. Rao PV, Deng P, Maddala R, Epstein DL, Li CY, Shimokawa H. Expression of dominant negative Rho-binding domain of Rho-kinase in organ cultured human eye anterior segments increases aqueous humor outflow. *Mol Vis.* 2005;11:288–297.

646. Rao PV, Deng P, Sasaki Y, Epstein DL. Regulation of myosin light chain phosphorylation in the trabecular meshwork: role in aqueous humour outflow facility. *Exp Eye Res.* 2005;80(2):197–206.

647. Tokushige H, Inatani M, Nemoto S, et al. Effects of topical administration of y-39983, a selective rho-associated protein kinase inhibitor, on ocular tissues in rabbits and monkeys. *Invest Ophthalmol Vis Sci.* 2007;48(7):3216–3222.

648. Waki M, Yoshida Y, Oka T, Azuma M. Reduction of intraocular pressure by topical administration of an inhibitor of the Rho-associated protein kinase. *Curr Eye Res.* 2001;22(6):470–474.

649. Lu Z, Overby DR, Scott PA, Freddo TF, Gong H. The mechanism of increasing outflow facility by rho-kinase inhibition with Y-27632 in bovine eyes. *Exp Eye Res.* 2008;86(2):271–281.

650. Tanihara H, Inatani M, Honjo M, Tokushige H, Azuma J, Araie M. Intraocular pressure-lowering effects and safety of topical administration of a selective ROCK inhibitor, SNJ-1656, in healthy volunteers. *Arch Ophthalmol.* 2008;126(3):309–315.

651. Tanihara H, Inoue T, Yamamoto T, et al. One-year clinical evaluation of 0.4% ripasudil (K-115) in patients with open-angle glaucoma and ocular hypertension. *Acta Ophthalmol.* 2016;94(1):e26–34.

652. Khouri AS, Serle JB, Bacharach J, Usner DW, Lewis RA, Braswell P, Kopczynski CC, Heah T. Rocket-4 Study Group. Once-daily netarsudil versus twice-daily timolol in patients with elevated intraocular pressure: The randomized phase 3 ROCKET-4 study. *Am J Ophthalmol.* 2019;204:97–104.

653. Grosheva I, Vittitow JL, Goichberg P, et al. Caldesmon effects on the actin cytoskeleton and cell adhesion in cultured HTM cells. *Exp Eye Res.* 2006;82(6):945–958.

654. Liu X, Hu Y, Filla MS, et al. The effect of C3 transgene expression on actin and cellular adhesions in cultured human trabecular meshwork cells and on outflow facility in organ cultured monkey eyes. *Mol Vis.* 2005;11:1112–1121.

655. Gabelt BT, Hu Y, Vittitow JL, et al. Caldesmon transgene expression disrupts focal adhesions in HTM cells and increases outflow facility in organ-cultured human and monkey anterior segments. *Exp Eye Res.* 2006;82(6):935–944.

656. Santas AJ, Bahler C, Peterson JA, et al. Effect of heparin II domain of fibronectin on aqueous outflow in cultured anterior segments of human eyes. *Invest Ophthalmol Vis Sci.* 2003;44(11):4796–4804.

657. Gonzalez Jr. JM, Faralli JA, Peters JM, Newman JR, Peters DM. Effect of heparin II domain of fibronectin on actin cytoskeleton and adherens junctions in human trabecular meshwork cells. *Invest Ophthalmol Vis Sci.* 2006;47(7):2924–2931.

658. Gonzalez Jr. JM, Hu Y, Gabelt BT, Kaufman PL, Peters DM. Identification of the active site in the heparin II domain of fibronectin that increases outflow facility in cultured monkey anterior segments. *Invest Ophthalmol Vis Sci.* 2009;50(1):235–241.

659. Schwinn MK, Gonzalez Jr. JM, Gabelt BT, Sheibani N, Kaufman PL, Peters DM. Heparin II domain of fibronectin mediates contractility through an alpha4beta1 co-signaling pathway. *Exp Cell Res.* 2010;316(9):1500–1512.

660. Tian B, Geiger B, Epstein DL, Kaufman PL. Cytoskeletal involvement in the regulation of aqueous humor outflow. *Invest Ophthalmol Vis Sci.* 2000;41(3):619–623.

661. Erickson-Lamy K, Schroeder A, Epstein DL. Ethacrynic acid induces reversible shape and cytoskeletal changes in cultured cells. *Invest Ophthalmol Vis Sci.* 1992;33(9):2631–2640.

662. Gills JP, Roberts BC, Epstein DL. Microtubule disruption leads to cellular contraction in human trabecular meshwork cells. *Invest Ophthalmol Vis Sci.* 1998;39(3):653–658.

663. O'Brien ET, Kinch M, Harding TW, Epstein DL. A mechanism for trabecular meshwork cell retraction: ethacrynic acid initiates the dephosphorylation of focal adhesion proteins. *Exp Eye Res.* 1997;65(4):471–483.

664. Croft MA, Hubbard WC, Kaufman PL. Effect of ethacrynic acid on aqueous outflow dynamics in monkeys. *Invest Ophthalmol Vis Sci.* 1994;35(3):1167–1175.

665. Epstein DL, Freddo TF, Bassett-Chu S, Chung M, Karageuzian L. Influence of ethacrynic acid on outflow facility in the monkey and calf eye. *Invest Ophthalmol Vis Sci.* 1987;28(12):2067–2075.

666. Liang LL, Epstein DL, de Kater AW, Shahsafaei A, Erickson-Lamy KA. Ethacrynic acid increases facility of outflow in the human eye in vitro. *Arch Ophthalmol.* 1992;110(1):106–109.

667. Melamed S, Kotas-Neumann R, Barak A, Epstein DL. The effect of intracamerally injected ethacrynic acid on intraocular pressure in patients with glaucoma. *Am J Ophthalmol.* 1992;113(5):508–512.

668. Johnson DH, Tschumper RC. Ethacrynic acid: outflow effects and toxicity in human trabecular meshwork in perfusion organ culture. *Curr Eye Res.* 1993;12(5):385–396.

669. Shimazaki A, Ichikawa M, Rao PV, et al. Effects of the new ethacrynic acid derivative SA9000 on intraocular pressure in cats and monkeys. *Biol Pharm Bull.* 2004;27(7):1019–1024.

670. Shimazaki A, Kirihara T, Rao PV, Tajima H, Matsugi T, Epstein DL. Effects of the new ethacrynic acid oxime derivative SA12590 on intraocular pressure in cats and monkeys. *Biol Pharm Bull.* 2007;30(8):1445–1449.

671. Rao PV, Shimazaki A, Ichikawa M, Franse-Carman L, Alvarado JA, Epstein DL. Effects of novel ethacrynic acid derivatives on human trabecular meshwork cell shape, actin cytoskeletal organization, and transcellular fluid flow. *Biol Pharm Bull.* 2005;28(12):2189–2196.

672. Bill A, Lütjen-Drecoll E, Svedbergh B. Effects of intracameral Na2EDTA and EGTA on aqueous outflow routes in the monkey eye. *Invest Ophthalmol Vis Sci.* 1980;19(5):492–504.

673. Weinreb RN, Bloom E, Baxter JD, et al. Detection of glucocorticoid receptors in cultured human trabecular cells. *Invest Ophthalmol Vis Sci.* 1981;21(3):403–407.

674. Rauz S, Cheung CM, Wood PJ, et al. Inhibition of 11beta-hydroxysteroid dehydrogenase type 1 lowers intraocular pressure in patients with ocular hypertension. *QJM.* 2003;96(7):481–490.

675. Rauz S, Walker EA, Shackleton CH, Hewison M, Murray PI, Stewart PM. Expression and putative role of 11 beta-hydroxysteroid dehydrogenase isozymes within the human eye. *Invest Ophthalmol Vis Sci.* 2001;42(9):2037–2042.

676. Stokes J, Noble J, Brett L, et al. Distribution of glucocorticoid and mineralocorticoid receptors and 11beta-hydroxysteroid dehydrogenases in human and rat ocular tissues. *Invest Ophthalmol Vis Sci.* 2000;41(7):1629–1638.

677. Armaly MF. Effect of corticosteroids on intraocular pressure and fluid dynamics. II. The effect of dexamethasone in the glaucomatous eye. *Arch Ophthalmol.* 1963;70:492–499.

678. Becker B, Bresnick G, Chevrette L, Kolker AE, Oaks MC, Cibis A. Intraocular pressure and its response to topical corticosteroids in diabetes. *Arch Ophthalmol.* 1966;76(4):477–483.

679. Schwartz B, Levene RZ. Plasma cortisol differences between normal and glaucomatous patients: before and after dexamethasone suppresion. *Arch Ophthalmol.* 1972;87(4):369–377.

680. Schwartz B, McCarty G, Rosner B. Increased plasma free cortisol in ocular hypertension and open angle glaucoma. *Arch Ophthalmol.* 1987;105(8):1060–1065.

681. Stokes J, Walker BR, Campbell JC, Seckl JR, O'Brien C, Andrew R. Altered peripheral sensitivity to glucocorticoids in primary open-angle glaucoma. *Invest Ophthalmol Vis Sci.* 2003;44(12):5163–5167.

682. Levi L, Schwartz B. Decrease of ocular pressure with oral metyrapone. A double-masked crossover trial. *Arch Ophthalmol.* 1987;105(6):777–781.

683. Prata TS, Tavares IM, Mello PA, Tamura C, Lima VC, Belfort R. Hypotensive effect of juxtascleral administration of anecortave acetate in different types of glaucoma. *J Glaucoma.* 2010;19(7):488–492.

684. Robin AL, Clark AF, Covert DW, et al. Anterior juxtascleral delivery of anecortave acetate in eyes with primary open-angle glaucoma: a pilot investigation. *Am J Ophthalmol.* 2009;147(1):45–50 e42.

685. Candia OA, Gerometta R, Millar JC, Podos SM. Suppression of corticosteroid-induced ocular hypertension in sheep by anecortave. *Arch Ophthalmol.* 2010;128(3):338–343.

686. Gerometta R, Spiga MG, Borras T, Candia OA. Treatment of sheep steroid-induced ocular hypertension with a glucocorticoid-inducible MMP1 gene therapy virus. *Invest Ophthalmol Vis Sci.* 2010;51(6):3042–3048.

687. Steely HT, Browder SL, Julian MB, Miggans ST, Wilson KL, Clark AF. The effects of dexamethasone on fibronectin expression in cultured human trabecular meshwork cells. *Invest Ophthalmol Vis Sci.* 1992;33(7):2242–2250.

688. Tripathi BJ, Millard CB, Tripathi RC. Corticosteroids induce a sialated glycoprotein (Cort-GP) in trabecular cells in vitro. *Exp Eye Res.* 1990;51(6):735–737.

689. Weinreb RN, Polansky JR, Kramer SG, Baxter JD. Acute effects of dexamethasone on intraocular pressure in glaucoma. *Invest Ophthalmol Vis Sci.* 1985;26(2):170–175.

690. Polansky JR. In vitro correlates of glucocorticoid effects on intraocular pressure. In: Krieglestein GK, ed. *Glaucoma Update IV.* Berlin: Springer-Verlag; 1991:20.

691. Shirato S, Murphy CG, Bloom E, et al. Kinetics of phagocytosis in trabecular meshwork cells. Flow cytometry and morphometry. *Invest Ophthalmol Vis Sci.* 1989;30(12):2499–2511.

692. Partridge CA, Weinstein BI, Southren AL, Gerritsen ME. Dexamethasone induces specific proteins in human trabecular meshwork cells. *Invest Ophthalmol Vis Sci.* 1989;30(8):1843–1847.

693. Polansky JR, Kurtz RM, Alvarado JA, Weinreb RN, Mitchell MD. Eicosanoid production and glucocorticoid regulatory mechanisms in cultured human trabecular meshwork cells. In: Bito LZ, Stjernschantz J, eds. *The Ocular Effects of Prostaglandins and Other Eicosanoids.* New York: Alan R. Liss; 1989:113.

694. Yun AJ, Murphy CG, Polansky JR, Newsome DA, Alvarado JA. Proteins secreted by human trabecular cells. Glucocorticoid and other effects. *Invest Ophthalmol Vis Sci.* 1989;30(9):2012–2022.

695. Southren AL, Wandel T, Gordon GG, Weinstein BI. Treatment of glaucoma with 3 alpha, 5 beta-tetrahydrocortisol: a new therapeutic modality. *J Ocul Pharmacol.* 1994;10(1):385–391.

696. Clark AF, Lane D, Wilson K, Miggans ST, McCartney MD. Inhibition of dexamethasone-induced cytoskeletal changes in cultured human trabecular meshwork cells by tetrahydrocortisol. *Invest Ophthalmol Vis Sci*. 1996;37(5):805–813.

697. Seeman J, Hubbard WC, Gabelt BT, Kaufman PK. 3Alpha,5beta-tetrahydrocortisol effect on outflow facility. *J Ocul Pharmacol Ther*. 2002;18(1):35–39.

698. Rohen JW, Linner E, Witmer R. Electron microscopic studies on the trabecular meshwork in two cases of corticosteroid-glaucoma. *Exp Eye Res*. 1973;17(1):19–31.

699. Johnson D, Gottanka J, Flügel C, Hoffmann F, Futa R, Lütjen-Drecoll E. Ultrastructural changes in the trabecular meshwork of human eyes treated with corticosteroids. *Arch Ophthalmol*. 1997;115(3):375–383.

700. Clark AF, Wilson K, de Kater AW, Allingham RR, McCartney MD. Dexamethasone-induced ocular hypertension in perfusion-cultured human eyes. *Invest Ophthalmol Vis Sci*. 1995;36(2):478–489.

701. Clark AF, Wordinger RJ. The role of steroids in outflow resistance. *Exp Eye Res*. 2009;88(4):752–759.

702. Engelbrecht-Schnur S, Siegner A, Prehm P, Lütjen-Drecoll E. Dexamethasone treatment decreases hyaluronan-formation by primate trabecular meshwork cells in vitro. *Exp Eye Res*. 1997;64(4):539–543.

703. Putney LK, Brandt JD, O'Donnell ME. Effects of dexamethasone on sodium-potassium-chloride cotransport in trabecular meshwork cells. *Invest Ophthalmol Vis Sci*. 1997;38(6):1229–1240.

704. Tane N, Dhar S, Roy S, Pinheiro A, Ohira A, Roy S. Effect of excess synthesis of extracellular matrix components by trabecular meshwork cells: possible consequence on aqueous outflow. *Exp Eye Res*. 2007;84(5):832–842.

705. O'Brien ET, Perkins SL, Roberts BC, Epstein DL. Dexamethasone inhibits trabecular cell retraction. *Exp Eye Res*. 1996;62(6):675–688.

706. Underwood JL, Murphy CG, Chen J, et al. Glucocorticoids regulate transendothelial fluid flow resistance and formation of intercellular junctions. *Am J Physiol*. 1999;277(2):C330–342.

707. Clark AF, Brotchie D, Read AT, et al. Dexamethasone alters F-actin architecture and promotes cross-linked actin network formation in human trabecular meshwork tissue. *Cell Motil Cytoskeleton*. 2005;60(2):83–95.

708. Clark AF, Wilson K, McCartney MD, Miggans ST, Kunkle M, Howe W. Glucocorticoid-induced formation of cross-linked actin networks in cultured human trabecular meshwork cells. *Invest Ophthalmol Vis Sci*. 1994;35(1):281–294.

709. Wilson K, McCartney MD, Miggans ST, Clark AF. Dexamethasone induced ultrastructural changes in cultured human trabecular meshwork cells. *Curr Eye Res*. 1993;12(9):783–793.

710. Clark AF, Miggans ST, Wilson K, Browder S, McCartney MD. Cytoskeletal changes in cultured human glaucoma trabecular meshwork cells. *J Glaucoma*. 1995;4(3):183–188.

711. Hoare MJ, Grierson I, Brotchie D, Pollock N, Cracknell K, Clark AF. Cross-linked actin networks (CLANs) in the trabecular meshwork of the normal and glaucomatous human eye in situ. *Invest Ophthalmol Vis Sci*. 2009;50(3):1255–1263.

712. Filla MS, Schwinn MK, Nosie AK, Clark RW, Peters DM. Dexamethasone-associated cross-linked actin network formation in human trabecular meshwork cells involves beta3 integrin signaling. *Invest Ophthalmol Vis Sci*. 2011;52(6):2952–2959.

713. Filla MS, Woods A, Kaufman PL, Peters DM. Beta1 and beta3 integrins cooperate to induce syndecan-4-containing cross-linked actin networks in human trabecular meshwork cells. *Invest Ophthalmol Vis Sci*. 2006;47(5):1956–1967.

714. Fingert JH, Stone EM, Sheffield VC, Alward WL. Myocilin glaucoma. *Surv Ophthalmol*. 2002;47(6):547–561.

715. Keller KE, Bhattacharya SK, Borras T, et al. Consensus recommendations for trabecular meshwork cell isolation, characterization and culture. *Exp Eye Res*. 2018;171:164–173.

716. Patel GC, Phan TN, Maddineni P, et al. Dexamethasone-induced ocular hypertension in mice: Effects of myocilin and route of administration. *Am J Pathol*. 2017;187(4):713–723.

717. Gould DB, Miceli-Libby L, Savinova OV, et al. Genetically increasing Myoc expression supports a necessary pathologic role of abnormal proteins in glaucoma. *Mol Cell Biol*. 2004;24(20):9019–9025.

718. Stone EM, Fingert JH, Alward WL, et al. Identification of a gene that causes primary open angle glaucoma. *Science*. 1997;275(5300):668–670.

719. Wilkinson CH, van der Straaten D, Craig JE, et al. Tonography demonstrates reduced facility of outflow of aqueous humor in myocilin mutation carriers. *J Glaucoma*. 2003;12(3):237–242.

720. Alward WL, Fingert JH, Coote MA, et al. Clinical features associated with mutations in the chromosome 1 open-angle glaucoma gene (GLC1A). *N Engl J Med*. 1998;338(15):1022–1027.

721. Tamm ER. Myocilin and glaucoma: facts and ideas. *Prog Retin Eye Res*. 2002;21(4):395–428.

722. Turalba AV, Chen TC. Clinical and genetic characteristics of primary juvenile-onset open-angle glaucoma (JOAG). *Semin Ophthalmol*. 2008;23(1):19–25.

723. Fingert JH, Ying L, Swiderski RE, et al. Characterization and comparison of the human and mouse GLC1A glaucoma genes. *Genome Res*. 1998;8(4):377–384.

724. Swiderski RE, Ying L, Cassell MD, Alward WL, Stone EM, Sheffield VC. Expression pattern and in situ localization of the mouse homologue of the human MYOC (GLC1A) gene in adult brain. *Brain Res Mol Brain Res*. 1999;68(1-2):64–72.

725. Taguchi M, Kanno H, Kubota R, Miwa S, Shishiba Y, Ozawa Y. Molecular cloning and expression profile of rat myocilin. *Mol Genet Metab*. 2000;70(1):75–80.

726. Senatorov V, Malyukova I, Fariss R, et al. Expression of mutated mouse myocilin induces open-angle glaucoma in transgenic mice. *J Neurosci*. 2006;26(46):11903–11914.

727. Zhou Y, Grinchuk O, Tomarev SI. Transgenic mice expressing the Tyr437His mutant of human myocilin protein develop glaucoma. *Invest Ophthalmol Vis Sci*. 2008;49(5):1932–1939.

728. Zode GS, Kuehn MH, Nishimura DY, et al. Reduction of ER stress via a chemical chaperone prevents disease phenotypes in a mouse model of primary open angle glaucoma. *J Clin Invest*. 2011;121(9):3542–3553.

729. Hill SE, Nguyen E, Donegan RK, Patterson-Orazem AC, Hazel A, Gumbart JC, Lieberman RL. Structure and misfolding of the flexible tripartite coiled-coil domain of glaucoma-associated myocilin. *Structure*. 2017;25(11):1697–1707 e1695.

730. Liu Y, Vollrath D. Reversal of mutant myocilin non-secretion and cell killing: implications for glaucoma. *Hum Mol Genet*. 2004;13(11):1193–1204.

731. Gould DB, Reedy M, Wilson LA, Smith RS, Johnson RL, John SW. Mutant myocilin nonsecretion in vivo is not sufficient to cause glaucoma. *Mol Cell Biol*. 2006;26(22):8427–8436.

732. Khare PD, Loewen N, Teo W, et al. Durable, safe, multi-gene lentiviral vector expression in feline trabecular meshwork. *Mol Ther*. 2008;16(1):97–106.

733. McDowell CM, Luan T, Zhang Z, et al. Mutant human myocilin induces strain specific differences in ocular hypertension and optic nerve damage in mice. *Exp Eye Res*. 2012;100:65–72.

734. Richter M, Krauss AH, Woodward DF, Lütjen-Drecoll E. Morphological changes in the anterior eye segment after long-term treatment with different receptor selective prostaglandin agonists and a prostamide. *Invest Ophthalmol Vis Sci*. 2003;44(10):4419–4426.

735. Poyer JF, Millar C, Kaufman PL. Prostaglandin F2 alpha effects on isolated rhesus monkey ciliary muscle. *Invest Ophthalmol Vis Sci*. 1995;36(12):2461–2465.

736. Tamm E, Rittig M, Lütjen-Drecoll E. [Electron microscopy and immunohistochemical studies of the intraocular pressure lowering effect of prostaglandin F2 alpha]. *Fortschr Ophthalmol*. 1990;87(6):623–629.

737. Lindsey JD, Kashiwagi K, Boyle D, Kashiwagi F, Firestein GS, Weinreb RN. Prostaglandins increase proMMP-1 and proMMP-3 secretion by human ciliary smooth muscle cells. *Curr Eye Res*. 1996;15(8):869–875.

738. Lindsey JD, Kashiwagi K, Kashiwagi F, Weinreb RN. Prostaglandin action on ciliary smooth muscle extracellular matrix metabolism: implications for uveoscleral outflow. *Surv Ophthalmol*. 1997;41(Suppl 2):S53–59.

739. Sagara T, Gaton DD, Lindsey JD, Gabelt BT, Kaufman PL, Weinreb RN. Topical prostaglandin F2alpha treatment reduces collagen types I, III, and IV in the monkey uveoscleral outflow pathway. *Archives of Ophthalmology*. 1999;117(6):794–801.

740. Lindsey JD, To HD, Weinreb RN. Induction of c-fos by prostaglandin F2 alpha in human ciliary smooth muscle cells. *Invest Ophthalmol Vis Sci*. 1994;35(1):242–250.

741. Ocklind A. Effect of latanoprost on the extracellular matrix of the ciliary muscle. A study on cultured cells and tissue sections. *Exp Eye Res*. 1998;67(2):179–191.

742. Yousufzai SY, Ye Z, Abdel-Latif AA. Prostaglandin F2 alpha and its analogs induce release of endogenous prostaglandins in iris and ciliary muscles isolated from cat and other mammalian species. *Exp Eye Res*. 1996;63(3):305–310.

743. Zhao X, Pearson KE, Stephan DA, Russell P. Effects of prostaglandin analogues on human ciliary muscle and trabecular meshwork cells. *Invest Ophthalmol Vis Sci*. 2003;44(5):1945–1952.

744. Weinreb RN. Enhancement of scleral macromolecular permeability with prostaglandins. *Trans Am Ophthalmol Soc*. 2001;99:319–343.

745. Anthony TL, Pierce KL, Stamer WD, Regan JW. Prostaglandin F2 alpha receptors in the human trabecular meshwork. *Invest Ophthalmol Vis Sci*. 1998;39(2):315–321.

746. Kim JW, Lindsey JD, Wang N, Weinreb RN. Increased human scleral permeability with prostaglandin exposure. *Invest Ophthalmol Vis Sci*. 2001;42(7):1514–1521.

747. Weinreb RN, Lindsey JD, Marchenko G, Marchenko N, Angert M, Strongin A. Prostaglandin FP agonists alter metalloproteinase gene expression in sclera. *Invest Ophthalmol Vis Sci*. 2004;45(12):4368–4377.

748. Lindsey JD, Crowston JG, Tran A, Morris C, Weinreb RN. Direct matrix metalloproteinase enhancement of transscleral permeability. *Invest Ophthalmol Vis Sci*. 2007;48(2):752–755.

749. Ota T, Aihara M, Narumiya S, Araie M. The effects of prostaglandin analogues on IOP in prostanoid FP-receptor-deficient mice. *Invest Ophthalmol Vis Sci*. 2005;46(11):4159–4163.

750. Crowston JG, Lindsey JD, Aihara M, Weinreb RN. Effect of latanoprost on intraocular pressure in mice lacking the prostaglandin FP receptor. *Invest Ohthalmol Vis Sci*. 2004;45(10):3555–3559.

751. Ota T, Aihara M, Saeki T, Narumiya S, Araie M. The effects of prostaglandin analogues on prostanoid EP1, EP2, and EP3 receptor-deficient mice. *Invest Ophthalmol Vis Sci*. 2006;47(8):3395–3399.

752. Abramovitz M, Adam M, Boie Y, et al. The utilization of recombinant prostanoid receptors to determine the affinities and selectivities of prostaglandins and related analogs. *Biochim Biophys Acta*. 2000;1483(2):285–293.

753. Sharif NA, Kelly CR, Crider JY, Williams GW, Xu SX. Ocular hypotensive FP prostaglandin (PG) analogs: PG receptor subtype binding affinities and selectivities, and agonist potencies at FP and other PG receptors in cultured cells. *J Ocul Pharmacol Ther*. 2003;19(6):501–515.

754. Biswas S, Bhattacherjee P, Paterson CA. Prostaglandin E2 receptor subtypes, EP1, EP2, EP3 and EP4 in human and mouse ocular tissues—a comparative immunohistochemical study. *Prostaglandins Leukot Essent Fatty Acids*. 2004;71(5):277–288.

755. Gabelt BT, Hennes EA, Bendel MA, Constant CE, Okka M, Kaufman PL. Prostaglandin subtype-selective and non-selective IOP-lowering comparison in monkeys. *J Ocul Pharmacol Ther*. 2009;25(1):1–8.

756. Nilsson SF, Drecoll E, Lütjen-Drecoll E, et al. The prostanoid EP2 receptor agonist butaprost increases uveoscleral outflow in the cynomolgus monkey. *Invest Ophthalmol Vis Sci*. 2006;47(9):4042–4049.

757. Stern FA, Bito LZ. Comparison of the hypotensive and other ocular effects of prostaglandins E2 and F2 alpha on cat and rhesus monkey eyes. *Invest Ophthalmol Vis Sci*. 1982;22(5):588–598.

758. Aihara M, Lu F, Kawata H, Iwata A, Odani-Kawabata N. Twelve-month efficacy and safety of omidenepag isopropyl, a selective EP2 agonist, in open-angle glaucoma and ocular hypertension: the RENGE study. *Jpn J Ophthalmol*. 2021;65(6):810–819.

759. Wan Z, Woodward DF, Cornell CL, et al. Bimatoprost, prostamide activity, and conventional drainage. *Invest Ophthalmol Vis Sci*. 2007;48(9):4107–4115.

760. Brubaker RF. Mechanism of action of bimatoprost (Lumigan). *Surv Ophthalmol*. 2001;45(Suppl 4):S347–351.

761. Heo JY, Ooi YH, Rhee DJ. Effect of prostaglandin analogs: Latanoprost, bimatoprost, and unoprostone on matrix metalloproteinases and their inhibitors in human trabecular meshwork endothelial cells. *Exp Eye Res*. 2020;194:108019.

762. Oh DJ, Martin JL, Williams AJ, Russell P, Birk DE, Rhee DJ. Effect of latanoprost on the expression of matrix metalloproteinases and their tissue inhibitors in human trabecular meshwork cells. *Invest Ophthalmol Vis Sci.* 2006;47(9):3887–3895.

763. Stamer WD, Piwnica D, Jolas T, et al. Cellular basis for bimatoprost effects on human conventional outflow. *Invest Ophthalmol Vis Sci.* 2010;51(10):5176–5181.

764. Camras CB, Alm A, Watson P, Stjernschantz J. Latanoprost, a prostaglandin analog, for glaucoma therapy. Efficacy and safety after 1 year of treatment in 198 patients. Latanoprost Study Groups. *Ophthalmology.* 1996;103(11):1916–1924.

765. Giuffre G. The effects of prostaglandin F2 alpha in the human eye. *Graefes Arch Clin Exp Ophthalmol.* 1985;222(3):139–141.

766. Villumsen J, Alm A. Prostaglandin F2 alpha-isopropylester eye drops: Effects in normal human eyes. *Br J Ophthalmol.* 1989;73(6):419–426.

767. Lee ES, Rasmussen CA, Filla MS, et al. Prospects for lentiviral vector mediated prostaglandin F synthase gene delivery in monkey eyes in vivo. *Curr Eye Res.* 2014;39(9):859–870.

768. Barraza RA, McLaren JW, Poeschla EM. Prostaglandin pathway gene therapy for sustained reduction of intraocular pressure. *Mol Ther.* 2010;18(3):491–501.

769. Craven ER, Walters T, Christie WC, et al. 24-Month phase I/II clinical trial of Bimatoprost Sustained-Release Implant (Bimatoprost SR) in glaucoma patients. *Drugs.* 2020;80(2):167–179.

770. Shen J, Robinson MR, Struble C, Attar M. Nonclinical pharmacokinetic and pharmacodynamic assessment of bimatoprost following a single intracameral injection of sustained-release implants. *Transl Vis Sci Technol.* 2020;9(4):20.

771. Gual A, Llobet A, Gilabert R, et al. Effects of time of storage, albumin, and osmolality changes on outflow facility (C) of bovine anterior segment in vitro. *Invest Ophthalmol Vis Sci.* 1997;38(10):2165–2171.

772. Haas M. The Na-K-Cl cotransporters. *Am J Physiol.* 1994;267(4 Pt 1):C869–885.

773. O'Donnell ME. Role of Na-K-Cl cotransport in vascular endothelial cell volume regulation. *Am J Physiol.* 1993;264(5 Pt 1):C1316–1326.

774. O'Donnell ME, Brandt JD, Curry FR. Na-K-Cl cotransport regulates intracellular volume and monolayer permeability of trabecular meshwork cells. *Am J Physiol.* 1995;268(4 Pt 1):C1067–1074.

775. O'Grady SM, Palfrey HC, Field M. Characteristics and functions of Na-K-Cl cotransport in epithelial tissues. *Am J Physiol.* 1987;253(2 Pt 1):C177–192.

776. Al-Aswad LA, Gong H, Lee D, et al. Effects of Na-K-2Cl cotransport regulators on outflow facility in calf and human eyes in vitro. *Invest Ophthalmol Vis Sci.* 1999;40(8):1695–1701.

777. Dismuke WM, Mbadugha CC, Faison D, Ellis DZ. Ouabain-induced changes in aqueous humour outflow facility and trabecular meshwork cytoskeleton. *Br J Ophthalmol.* 2009;93(1):104–109.

778. Stamer WD, Peppel K, O'Donnell ME, Roberts BC, Wu F, Epstein DL. Expression of aquaporin-1 in human trabecular meshwork cells: role in resting cell volume. *Invest Ophthalmol Vis Sci.* 2001;42(8):1803–1811.

779. Stamer WD, Seftor RE, Snyder RW, Regan JW. Cultured human trabecular meshwork cells express aquaporin-1 water channels. *Curr Eye Res.* 1995;14(12):1095–1100.

780. Stamer WD, Snyder RW, Smith BL, Agre P, Regan JW. Localization of aquaporin CHIP in the human eye: implications in the pathogenesis of glaucoma and other disorders of ocular fluid balance. *Invest Ophthalmol Vis Sci.* 1994;35(11):3867–3872.

781. Stamer WD, Chan DW, Conley SM, Coons S, Ethier CR. Aquaporin-1 expression and conventional aqueous outflow in human eyes. *Exp Eye Res.* 2008;87(4):349–355.

782. Zhang D, Vetrivel L, Verkman AS. Aquaporin deletion in mice reduces intraocular pressure and aqueous fluid production. *J Gen Physiol.* 2002;119(6):561–569.

783. Comes N, Abad E, Morales M, Borras T, Gual A, Gasull X. Identification and functional characterization of ClC-2 chloride channels in trabecular meshwork cells. *Exp Eye Res.* 2006;83(4):877–889.

784. Mitchell CH, Fleischhauer JC, Stamer WD, Peterson-Yantorno K, Civan MM. Human trabecular meshwork cell volume regulation. *Am J Physiol Cell Physiol.* 2002;283(1):C315–326.

785. Dismuke WM, Ellis DZ. Activation of the BK(Ca) channel increases outflow facility and decreases trabecular meshwork cell volume. *J Ocul Pharmacol Ther.* 2009;25(4):309–314.

786. Knepper PA, Goossens W, Palmberg PF. Glycosaminoglycan stratification of the juxtacanalicular tissue in normal and primary open-angle glaucoma. *Invest Ophthalmol Vis Sci.* 1996;37(12):2414–2425.

787. Lerner LE, Polansky JR, Howes EL, Stern R. Hyaluronan in the human trabecular meshwork. *Invest Ophthalmol Vis Sci.* 1997;38(6):1222–1228.

788. Knepper PA, Mayanil CS, Goossens W, et al. Aqueous humor in primary open-angle glaucoma contains an increased level of CD44S. *Invest Ophthalmol Vis Sci.* 2002;43(1):133–139.

789. Bárány EH, Scotchbrook S. Influence of testicular hyaluronidase on the resistance to flow through the angle of the anterior chamber. *Acta Physiol Scand.* 1954;30(2-3):240–248.

790. Francois J, Rabaey M, Neetens A. Perfusion studies on the outflow of aqueous humor in human eyes. *AMA Arch Ophthalmol.* 1956;55(2):193–204.

791. Hubbard WC, Johnson M, Gong H, et al. Intraocular pressure and outflow facility are unchanged following acute and chronic intracameral chondroitinase ABC and hyaluronidase in monkeys. *Exp Eye Res.* 1997;65(2):177–190.

792. Pedler C. The relationship of hyaluronidase to aqueous outflow resistance. *Trans Ophthalmol Soc U K.* 1956;76:51–63.

793. Peterson WS, Jocson VL. Hyaluronidase effects on aqueous outflow resistance. Quantitative and localizing studies in the rhesus monkey eye. *Am J Ophthalmol.* 1974;77(4):573–577.

794. Rees DA, Lloyd CW, Thom D. Control of grip and stick in cell adhesion through lateral relationships of membrane glycoproteins. *Nature.* 1977;267(5607):124–128.

795. Tokiwa T, Hoshika T, Shiraishi M, Sato J. Mechanism of cell dissociation with trypsin and EDTA. *Acta Med Okayama.* 1979;33(1):1–4.

796. Bill A. Effects of Na2 EDTA and alpha-chymotrypsin on aqueous humor outflow conductance in monkey eyes. *Ups J Med Sci.* 1980;85(3):311–319.

797. Alexander JP, Samples JR, Acott TS. Growth factor and cytokine modulation of trabecular meshwork matrix metalloproteinase and TIMP expression. *Curr Eye Res.* 1998;17(3):276–285.

798. Acott TS, Kelley MJ. Extracellular matrix in the trabecular meshwork. *Exp Eye Res.* 2008;86(4):543–561.

799. Li G, Torrejon KY, Unser AM, et al. Trabodenoson, an adenosine mimetic with A1 receptor selectivity lowers intraocular pressure by increasing conventional outflow facility in mice. *Invest Ophthalmol Vis Sci.* 2018;59(1):383–392.

800. Shearer TW, Crosson CE. Adenosine A1 receptor modulation of MMP-2 secretion by trabecular meshwork cells. *Invest Ophthalmol Vis Sci.* 2002;43(9):3016–3020.

801. Daines BS, Kent AR, McAleer MS, Crosson CE. Intraocular adenosine levels in normal and ocular-hypertensive patients. *J Ocul Pharmacol Ther.* 2003;19(2):113–119.

802. Laties A, Rich CC, Stoltz R, et al. A randomized phase 1 dose escalation study to evaluate safety, tolerability, and pharmacokinetics of trabodenoson in healthy adult volunteers. *J Ocul Pharmacol Ther.* 2016;32(8):548–554.

803. Myers JS, Sall KN, DuBiner H, et al. A dose-escalation study to evaluate the safety, tolerability, pharmacokinetics, and efficacy of 2 and 4 weeks of twice-daily ocular trabodenoson in adults with ocular hypertension or primary open-angle glaucoma. *J Ocul Pharmacol Ther.* 2016;32(8):555–562.

804. Danser AH, Derkx FH, Admiraal PJ, Deinum J, de Jong PT, Schalekamp MA. Angiotensin levels in the eye. *Invest Ophthalmol Vis Sci.* 1994;35:1008–1018.

805. Farahbakhsh NA. Ectonucleotidases of the rabbit ciliary body nonpigmented epithelium. *Invest Ophthalmol Vis Sci.* 2003;44(9):3952–3960.

806. Laliberte MF, Laliberte F, Alhenc-Gelas F, Chevillard C. Immunohistochemistry of angiotensin I-converting enzyme in rat eye structures involved in aqueous humor regulation. *Lab Invest.* 1988;59(2):263–270.

807. Meyer P, Flammer J, Luscher TF. Local action of the renin angiotensin system in the porcine ophthalmic circulation: effects of ACE-inhibitors and angiotensin receptor antagonists. *Invest Ophthalmol Vis Sci.* 1995;36(3):555–562.

808. Sramek SJ, Wallow IH, Tewksbury DA, Brandt CR, Poulsen GL. An ocular renin-angiotensin system. Immunohistochemistry of angiotensinogen. *Invest Ophthalmol Vis Sci.* 1992;33(5):1627–1632.

809. Wallow IH, Sramek SJ, Bindley CD, Darjatmoko SR, Gange SJ. Ocular renin angiotensin: EM immunocytochemical localization of prorenin. *Curr Eye Res.* 1993;12(10):945–950.

810. Costagliola C, Verolino M, De Rosa ML, Iaccarino G, Ciancaglini M, Mastropasqua L. Effect of oral losartan potassium administration on intraocular pressure in normotensive and glaucomatous human subjects. *Exp Eye Res.* 2000;71(2):167–171.

811. Constad WH, Fiore P, Samson C, Cinotti AA. Use of an angiotensin converting enzyme inhibitor in ocular hypertension and primary open-angle glaucoma. *Am J Ophthalmol.* 1988;105(6):674–677.

812. Costagliola C, Di Benedetto R, De Caprio L, Verde R, Mastropasqua L. Effect of oral captopril (SQ 14225) on intraocular pressure in man. *Eur J Ophthalmol.* 1995;5(1):19–25.

813. Giardina WJ, Kleinert HD, Ebert DM, Wismer CT, Chekal MA, Stein HH. Intraocular pressure lowering effects of the renin inhibitor ABBOTT-64662 diacetate in animals. *J Ocul Pharmacol.* 1990;6(2):75–83.

814. Wang RF, Podos SM, Mittag TW, Yokoyama T. Effect of CS-088, an angiotensin AT1 receptor antagonist, on intraocular pressure in glaucomatous monkey eyes. *Exp Eye Res.* 2005;80(5):629–632.

815. Lotti VJ, Pawlowski N. Prostaglandins mediate the ocular hypotensive action of the angiotensin converting enzyme inhibitor MK-422 (enalaprilat) in African green monkeys. *J Ocul Pharmacol.* 1990;6(1):1–7.

11

Ocular Circulation

Leopold Schmetterer

THE VASCULAR SYSTEM OF THE EYE

The vascular system transports oxygen and metabolites in the human body, ensures thermoregulation of the body and its organs, and is responsible for waste material removal. The driving force of blood is the heart, which pumps the blood through the body and ensures a pressure gradient from the arterial to the venous system. Blood vessels include three fundamental components: arteries, veins, and the microvasculature, including arterioles, venules, and capillaries. Within the arterioles, pulsatile flow is converted into steady flow. This comes with a pronounced drop in pressure, and as such the arterioles are the main site of vascular resistance.

The human posterior pole of the eye is nourished by two independent vascular beds that receive their inputs from branches of the ophthalmic artery (OA). The inner retina, including the retinal ganglion cells and the retinal nerve fiber layer, is supplied by the retinal circulation. The outer retina does not contain any blood vessels and is supplied by the choroid via diffusion of oxygen through the retinal pigment epithelium (RPE).

The retinal vessels get their vascular supply from the central retinal artery (CRA), which is a branch of the OA. It is located within the dural sheath of the optic nerve and enters the optic disc through the lamina cribrosa. The diameter of the CRA is in the order of 150 to 500 μm.[1-3] Hence, the CRA and its branches are functionally arterioles, constituting the primary site of vascular resistance for the retinal circulation. In the literature on ocular vasculature and blood flow, these vessels are, however, usually referred to as arteries, and the current chapter follows this terminology. The CRA branches into smaller vessels over the internal surface of the retina, which can be seen ophthalmoscopically, and finally into terminal arterioles and capillaries, which can be visualized with technologies such as optical coherence tomography angiography (OCTA) (Fig. 11.1). In 25% of humans, a cilioretinal artery can be found and mostly supports the macular region.

Retinal arteries are surrounded by a capillary-free zone that can be visualized by OCTA and adaptive optics scanning laser ophthalmoscopy (AO-SLO).[4,5] In nonhuman primates this zone is between 30 and 70 mm, depending on the eccentricity (Fig. 11.2).[6] The tissue surrounding the larger retinal branch arteries is oxygenated directly from these vessels. The system of the retinal veins shows similarities with the arterial angioarchitecture, and the central retinal vein (CRV) runs in parallel to the CRA, draining blood into the cavernous sinus. In contrast to other vascular beds, the retina does not contain precapillary sphincters. Hence, the retinal capillaries show continuous perfusion. The retinal capillary network is arranged in four layers (Fig. 11.3). The superficial plexus is located in the nerve fiber and ganglion cell layer and contains the larger retinal branch arteries and veins, as well as microvessels, including a dense capillary network. The intermediate plexus contains capillaries in a lobular arrangement

that shows considerable tortuosity.[7] They are located in the inner nuclear layer (INL) among the amacrine cells. The deep vascular bed consists mainly of capillary vessels and is located at the outermost side of the INL.[7] The radial peripapillary capillaries are located in the nerve fiber layer close to the optic nerve head (ONH),[8,9] where the nerve fiber bundles are thick and have high metabolic demand to maintain ion pumping.[10]

Depending on the eccentricity, retinal vessels have one to seven layers of smooth muscle cells. The retinal veins have a basement membrane, and the walls contain some pericytes. The capillaries of the retina show a high density of pericytes. Traditionally a ratio of 1:1 between pericytes and endothelial cells has been reported.[12] A recent study of the human retina, utilizing ultrastructural criteria, showed a 94.5% frequency of pericyte coverage on human retinal capillaries.[13] Endothelial cells are lined in parallel to the blood vessels. The blood vessels share their basement membrane with pericytes and endothelial cells (Fig. 11.4).

The choroidal circulation gets its main vascular supply from the long and short ciliary arteries and is part of the uveal system. The choroid consists of five layers, including Bruch's membrane and three vascular layers, as well as the suprachoroidea. The outermost vascular layer is Haller's layer, which includes the largest choroidal arteries and veins. Sattler's layer contains smaller arteries and veins. Anatomically there is no clear border between Haller's layer and Sattler's layer. The choriocapillaris consists of highly anastomosed capillaries and is between 7 and 10 μm thick. These capillaries are fenestrated and show a diameter that is larger than the diameter of the retinal capillaries.

The ONH has its own vascular supply that shows significant interindividual variability in humans.[14] This surface layer of the ONH is, in most humans, supplied by the CRA and part of the retinal vascular system. In cases with a cilioretinal artery, the corresponding sector of the surface layer usually gets its blood supply from this vessel. Below the surface nerve fiber layer is the prelaminar region, which spans toward the lamina cribrosa. The deeper layers are the vascular supply of the lamina cribrosa and the retrolaminar regions. All of these vascular beds receive their blood supply via the posterior ciliary arteries (PCAs) and the peripapillary choroid. In many cases the medial and lateral short PCAs form the circle of Zinn and Haller around the optic nerve, which can be seen ophthalmoscopically in some subjects (Fig. 11.5).

The vasculature of the anterior segment gets it main supply from the anterior ciliary arteries. The cornea is not vascularized in healthy humans. The limbus, however, contains a ring of vasculature that contributes to corneal oxygenation. Whereas the conjunctiva is richly vascularized, the sclera contains only a few blood vessels because of its low metabolic demand. The anterior uveal system includes the iris and the ciliary body. The principal blood supply of the iris is the major arterial circle, which enters the iris through its root. The iris blood vessels are

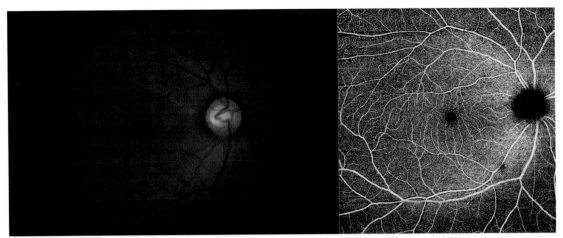

Fig. 11.1 Color fundus photography and optical coherence tomography angiography in a healthy subject, showing the retinal vasculature.

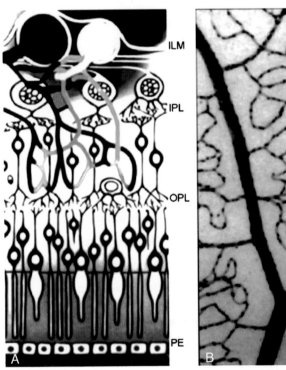
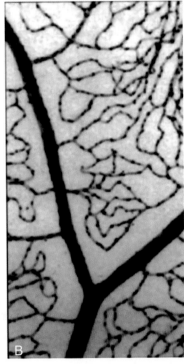

Fig. 11.2 Capillary plexus in the inner retina. (**A**) Schematic representation. (**B**) Tryptic digest of a flat-mounted monkey retina, stained with hematoxylin eosin. Note the broad capillary-free zone around the artery. *ILM*, Inner Limiting Membrane; *IPL*, Inner Plexiform Layer; *OPL*, Outer Plexiform Layer; *PE*, Pigment Epithelium. (Reproduced with permission from Pournaras CJ, Rungger-Brändle E, Riva CE, Hardarson SH, Stefansson E. Regulation of retinal blood flow in health and disease. *Prog Retin Eye Res*, 2008;27(3):284–330.)

radially oriented. The ciliary body is also supplied by the major arterial circle, which branches into the anterior parts of the ciliary processes and forms a capillary bed.

OXYGENATION AND BLOOD FLOW OF THE RETINA

There are fundamental differences in the oxygenation of the inner and outer retina. The outer retina is avascular, and the photoreceptors depend on oxygen supply from the choroid. The inner (including the two nuclear layers, the two plexiform layers, and the nerve fiber layer) retina receive oxygen mainly from the retinal vessels.[15] Oxygen profiles in the retina differ between light- and dark-adapted conditions. In the dark-adapted retina, a trough in oxygen tension (PO_2) is seen at approximately 80% retinal depth in a variety of species (Fig. 11.6). This is related to the high oxygen consumption of photoreceptor inner segments. As gradients in the PO_2 curve from both sides can be observed, both the choroidal and retinal circulation contribute to photoreceptor oxygenation, with the majority of oxygen diffusing from the choroid. In the light-adapted retina, the retinal oxygen profile looks different (Fig. 11.6). Whereas there is little change in choroidal PO_2,[16,17] the minimum PO_2 in the outer retina is higher than in the dark-adapted retina. The contribution of the retinal circulation to photoreceptor oxygenation is minimal or completely absent in the light-adapted retina.

In the inner retina the average PO_2 in the deeper region is slightly lower than in the very superficial region in dark-adapted animals.[17] This difference between the deeper region and superficial region disappears when the retina is light adapted,[17] most likely because some

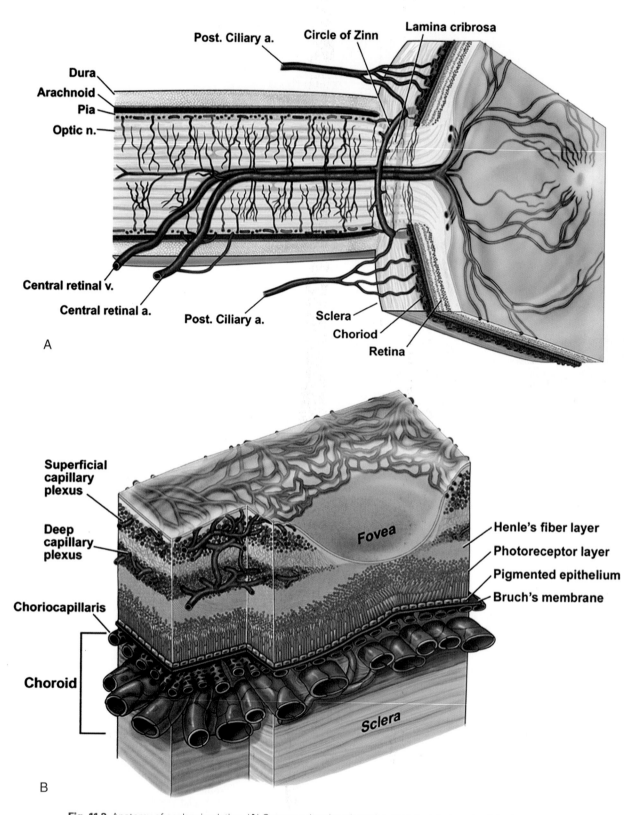

Fig. 11.3 Anatomy of ocular circulation. (**A**) Cut away drawing along the superior-inferior axis of the human eye through the optic nerve, showing the vascular supply to the retina and choroid. (**B**) Drawing showing vasculature of the retina and choroid. *a*, Artery, *v*, vein, *n*, nerve. (Reproduced with permission from Anand-Apte B, Hollyfield JG. Developmental anatomy of the retinal and choroidal vasculature, in *Encyclopedia of the Eye*, J. Besharse and D. Bok, Editors. 2009, 3061 Academic Press, Elsevier Books: London. p. 9e15.)

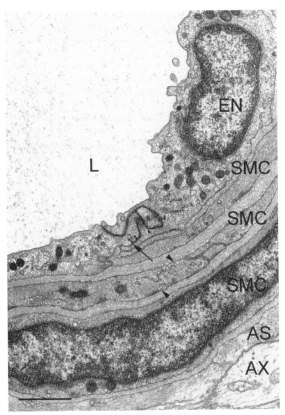

Fig. 11.4 Inner blood-retinal barrier. Electron micrograph of an artery in the inner pig retina. Tissue was fixed in the presence of tannic acid to enhance fluid filling of the intercellular endothelial cleft. The vessel wall is composed of the endothelium (*EN*) and three layers of smooth muscle cells (*SMC*), with numerous caveolae *(arrowheads)*. Astrocytic processes (*AS*) enwrap the vessel. Note high contrast in intercellular cleft and vesicular pits up to the site, where a tight junctional element is located *(arrow)*. *AX*, Axon. Bar, 1 mm. (Reproduced with permission from Pournaras CJ, Rungger-Brändle E, Riva CE, Hardarson SH, Stefansson E. Regulation of retinal blood flow in health and disease. *Prog Retin Eye Res*, 2008; 27(3): 284–330.)

choroidal O_2 diffuses from the choroid toward the inner retina during this condition. In contrast to the outer retina, inner retinal PO_2 is almost independent of the illumination level of the retina.[15] Because the oxygen consumption of the vitreous is low, vitreal PO_2 close to the retina is a good indicator of inner retinal PO_2, although this may not be true in pathologic conditions such as diabetic retinopathy (DR).

The photoreceptors also consume glucose via anaerobic glycolysis, leading to a considerable accumulation of lactate.[18] In contrast, anaerobic glycolysis is absent in the inner retina. Under light-adapted conditions, the photoreceptors are solely oxygenated by the choroid. In darkness, however, the PO_2 reaches 0 mmHg at the proximal side of the inner segments, which means a change in the gradient of PO_2 toward the inner segment. This implies that in darkness, some of the oxygen to the photoreceptors is delivered from the retinal circulation.[15] Photoreceptors consume a significant amount of oxygen that is mainly used for maintenance of the dark current and the generation of guanosine triphosphate.[19]

Akin to any other vascular bed, blood flow in the eye is determined by ocular perfusion pressure (OPP) and vascular resistance (R). As such, volumetric blood flow can be written according to the Hagen-Poiseuille equation as Q = OPP/R. R increases linearly with length of the vessel segment and the viscosity of blood and is inversely related to the fourth power of the radius of the vessel.

Retinal blood flow is characterized by a high vascular resistance and accordingly blood flow rate is low. Using noninvasive technology, the retinal blood flow rate has been measured to be approximately 40 μL/min in healthy subjects.[20-25] The diameter of larger retinal branch veins and arteries can be up to 200 μm, which makes the vessels, functionally, venules and arterioles. There is an almost linear relationship between retinal vessel diameter and retinal blood velocities in both arteries and veins,[20,22] as expected from Murray's law (Fig. 11.7). Blood velocities in retinal arteries are, however, higher than in veins, because of the equation of continuity. Blood velocities in larger retinal vessels are in the order of 6 to 25 mm/s. In the capillaries, velocities are in the range between 1 and 4 mm/s and exhibit quite significant spatial and temporal variations.[26] Recently, resistance and blood flow in the retina have been modeled using retinal vessel calibers, fractal dimension, perfusion

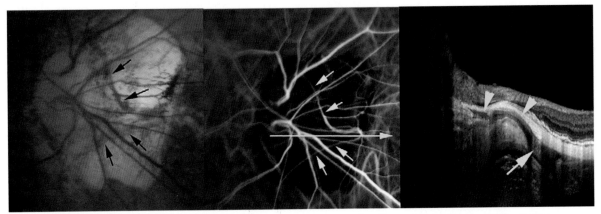

Fig. 11.5 Detection of the path from the retrobulbar short posterior ciliary artery to the Zinn-Haller ring by optical coherence tomography (OCT). *Left*: Fundus photograph of the left eye of a 55-year-old man with high myopia. A large temporal conus is observed. Blood vessels suggesting the Zinn-Haller ring are seen within the conus *(arrows)*. *Middle*, Indocyanine green angiographic finding at 1 minute after dye injection showing the temporal part of the Zinn-Haller ring with a triangular shape *(arrows)*. A lateral short posterior ciliary artery enters the Zinn-Haller ring at its most horizontally distant point. A *blue line* shows the scanned line by OCT. *Right*: Horizontal OCT scan along the *blue line* in the middle image shows that the short posterior ciliary artery enters the sclera *(arrow)* and courses toward the Zinn-Haller ring intrasclerally *(along the arrowheads)*. (Reproduced with permission from Ohno-Matsui K, Kasahara K, Moriyama M Detection of zinn-haller arterial ring in highly myopic eyes by simultaneous indocyanine green angiography and optical coherence tomography. *Am J Ophthalmol*, 2013;155(5): 920–926.e2.)

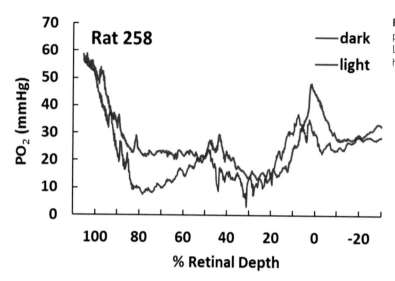

Fig. 11.6 Dark-adapted *(blue)* and light-adapted *(red)* retinal PO_2 profiles from a Long-Evans rat. (Reprinted with permission from Linsenmeier RA, Zhang HF. Retinal oxygen: from animals to humans. *Prog Retin Eye Res*, 2017;58:115–151.)

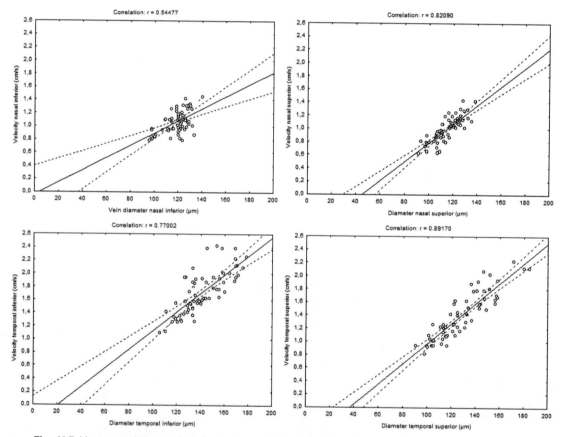

Fig. 11.7 Linear correlation analysis between mean blood velocities and vessel diameters for the largest venules in each quadrant in healthy subjects (*P* < .001 each). Data are shown separately for the nasal inferior, nasal superior, temporal inferior, and temporal superior quadrant (*n* = 64). (Reprinted from with permission from Garhofer G, Werkmeister R, Dragostinoff N, Schmetterer L. Retinal blood flow in healthy young subjects. *Invest Ophthalmol Vis Sci*, 2012; 53(2): 698–703.)

pressure, and population-based hematocrit values.[27] Retinal blood flow decreases with age, most likely owing to an age-related loss of retinal ganglion cells.[28] Oxygen extraction in retinal vessels is accordingly low. The arteriovenous oxygen difference is high, in the order of 35% to 45%.[29-33] Total retinal oxygen extraction is accordingly in the range of 2.0 to 2.5 μL (O_2)/min.[34,35] Choroidal blood flow is much higher than

retinal blood flow because the vascular resistance is low. In humans, there is no technique to measure absolute choroidal blood flow. Data in nonhuman primates indicate that the absolute flow rate is approximately 600 μL /min.[36] In humans, pulsatile ocular blood flow has been estimated as 600 to 1000 μL/min,[37-42] but the ratio between pulsatile and nonpulsatile flow is unknown. The arteriovenous O_2 difference cannot be measured in humans, but it is considered to be very small, with a value of approximately 1%, as measured in cats.[40] There is some evidence for gender differences in ocular blood flow, but the evidence for this is inconclusive.[41]

TECHNIQUES FOR MEASURING BLOOD FLOW

Measurement of blood flow in the human eye is not an easy task. Multiple techniques have been developed, but none has gained widespread clinical application for measuring blood flow.[42,43] In recent years, OCTA and laser speckle flowgraphy have gained some popularity. Some of the older historical methods will only be mentioned briefly.

Invasive technology in experimental animals
Microsphere technology

The microsphere method for measuring blood flow can be used in multiple organs, and absolute values of regional blood flow can be obtained. When microspheres are injected into the systemic circulation the number of entrapped microspheres is proportional to the blood flow through the tissues. In the eye, plastic radioactive microspheres[44,45] and fluorescent microspheres,[46,47] as well as colored microspheres, have been used.[48,49] Whereas in principle many organs can be studies simultaneously, reliable measurements of local blood flow require optimization of the size and number of microspheres. This also makes it difficult to study retina and choroid in the same experiment, because of the differences in capillary lumen. As with all other methods in experimental animal studies, care has to be taken such that the anesthesia and experimental procedures do not influence the results. This can either be directly because of the effects of the anesthetic drugs on vascular tone and/or vascular regulation, or via the fluctuations of arterial blood pressure during the course of the experiments. An obvious advantage of the microsphere method is the lack of surgical intervention. However, the animals cannot be followed longitudinally because the technique is terminal.

Hydrogen clearance

Hydrogen clearance is based on the detection of the rate of clearance of an inert gas from the tissue of interest. The technique has been used in the eye by several investigators to study perfusion in different tissues.[50–52] The technique is, however, not easily applied to the eye because the condition that the tissue is perfused uniformly in a three-dimensional (3D) volume is neither fulfilled for the choroid nor the retina. Hydrogen can either be administered via lung inhalation, intra-arterial injection or local routes. The hydrogen is detected via an intraocularly placed microelectrode that allows for the measurement of arrival and clearance of the gas. Placement of the microelectrodes can be done in proximity to either larger retinal vessels or vascularized tissue, resulting in different clearance curves. The blood flow values are usually reported in values of mL/min per 100 g tissue.

Oxygen-sensitive electrodes

Techniques that quantify oxygen can be divided into those that quantify the partial pressure of free oxygen in tissue (PO_2) and those that measure the saturation of oxygen bound to hemoglobin (SaO_2). SaO_2 and PO_2 are interrelated in a nonlinear way and can be interconverted except at conditions of very high oxygenation, when SaO_2 is almost 100%. Oxygen-sensitive electrodes work based on polarography. When a noble metal is polarized at about $-0.7\,V$ relative to a reference electrode, it becomes a cathode, where oxygen is chemically reduced.[15] This is associated with a current that is proportional to the PO_2 in the tissue. Different oxygen electrodes have been used in the vitreous humor,[53–55] the retina,[53,56,57] and the ONH.[58–60] This technique provides high spatial resolution for measuring tissue PO_2.

Noninvasive technology in humans
Dye-based angiography

Fluorescein and indocyanine green angiography are important tools for visualizing blood flow in clinics. There have been multiple approaches to quantifying retinal and choroidal blood flow based on this technique.[61–64] The most advanced technique is to combine video fluorescein angiography based on scanning laser ophthalmoscopy with digital image processing.[65,66] Early studies quantified retinal perfusion by dye dilution technique, but time resolution was low, recording images at a frame rate of 1 to 2 Hz.[67,68] Parameters obtained were arm-retina time and the arteriovenous passage time,[67,68] but only semiquantitative measurements of perfusion were obtained. More advanced approaches use arteriovenous passage time and mean dye velocity using the early phase of the angiograms.[62,69] Another approach is to directly visualize retinal capillary microcirculation in perifoveal capillaries,[70,71] providing information on the macular microcirculation. Whereas dye-based angiography still has an important role in clinical decision-making, quantification of blood flow based on the technology has lost importance. The invasive nature of dye administration and the potential risks associated with it make it difficult to apply the technology for research purposes.

Measurement of retinal vessel diameters

Measurement of retinal vessel diameter or retinal vessel caliber has been widely used as a biomarker for both ocular and systemic disease.[72–74] The technique has the advantage that it can be extracted from any high-quality fundus images. Parameters that are reported include central retinal arterial equivalent (CRAE), central retinal venular equivalent (CRVE), and arteriovenous ratio (Fig. 11.8). Several formulas for summarizing retinal vessel diameters have been proposed.[75,76] A commercial fundus camera–based system is available, specifically targeting retinal vessel caliber analysis, as well as the response of

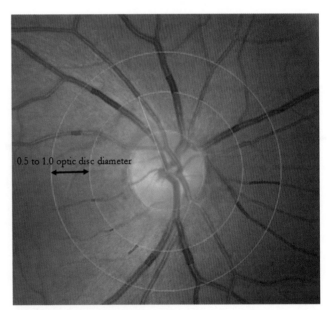

0.5 to 1.0 optic disc diameter

Fig. 11.8 Retinal fundus photograph assessed quantitatively by the IVAN software (University of Wisconsin). The measured area of retinal vascular parameters is standardized as the region from 0.5 to 1.0 disc diameters away from the disc margin. Retinal arteriolar *(red)* and venular *(blue)* calibers are summarized as central retinal artery equivalent (CRAE) and central retinal vein equivalent (CRVE), respectively, from retinal fundus photograph. CRAE and CRVE were defined based on the revised Knudtson-Parr-Hubbard formula. (Reproduced with permission from Ikram MK, Cheung CY, Lorenzi M, Klein R, Jones TLZ, Yin Wong T. Retinal vascular caliber as a biomarker for diabetes microvascular complications. *Diabetes Care* 2013;36(3):750–759) retinal vessels to flicker light stimulation.[77,78] In terms of blood flow, the information is limited, as no information on retinal blood velocity is available. In patients with systemic hypertension, for instance, CRAE is reduced, indicating arteriolar vasoconstriction, but CRVE is increased, most likely due to inflammation.[79] Whether hypertension is associated with altered volumetric blood flow based on these measurements is, however, unclear. Owing to the equation of continuity, it is, however, obvious that the ratio of retinal blood velocity between arteries and veins is shifted toward higher values, because the retina is an end organ and total arterial blood flow needs to be equal to total retinal blood flow.

Laser Doppler velocimetry

The technique is based on the optical Doppler effect. Laser light that hits moving erythrocytes is shifted in frequency, and this frequency shift is dependent on the velocity of the scatterers. The first measurements in retinal vessels were performed in the 1970s to measure the blood velocity.[80,81] As the technique does not provide any depth resolution, a continuous spectrum of Doppler shifts is detected because of the velocity profile within the vessel. The maximum Doppler shift corresponds to the maximum flow velocity in the center of the vessel. Absolute measurement of retinal blood velocity is, however, difficult because the angle between the laser beam and the retinal vessel needs to be known. One way to overcome this problem is to detect the scattered laser light in two distinct directions, a technique called bidirectional laser Doppler velocimetry.[82,83] Combining this technology with measurement of vessel diameter provided the first results for total retinal blood flow in humans.[20]

Laser Doppler flowmetry

The technique is related to laser Doppler velocimetry, but in contrast to single blood vessel, vascularized tissue is illuminated. Based on a scattering theory of light in tissue, average blood velocity, blood volume, and blood flow can be derived.[84] The technology has been used to study ONH[85] and subfoveal choroidal[86] blood flow in humans. No absolute values of blood flow can be obtained and, as such, the method is mainly suitable for measuring blood flow changes in response to stimuli. The sampling depth of laser Doppler flowmetry is difficult to determine in vivo. Studies in nonhuman primates indicate that laser Doppler flowmetry technique samples blood flow changes mainly in the superficial layers of the ONH and is less influenced by perfusion in deeper regions.[86] When the laser beam is directed toward the fovea, the signal is evidently coming from the choroidal microvasculature, because the retina lacks vessels in this region. When the laser beam is directed toward other retinal locations, the signal is also influenced largely by the choroidal perfusion.[87] Mapping of the microcirculation of the human retina can be achieved by scanning laser Doppler flowmetry based on a scanning laser ophthalmoscope.[88] Laser Doppler flowmetry has also been used by various groups in experimental animals[89–91] and much of our knowledge on blood flow regulation in the eye stems from these experiments.

Color Doppler imaging

This technique is based on the acoustical Doppler effect. It combines B-scan ultrasonography for structural imaging with velocity extraction based on the Doppler shift of the wave.[92–94] In the eye this technique is mainly used for the visualization of blood velocities in the following retrobulbar vessels: OA, PCAs, and the CRA, as well as other vessels, including retrobulbar veins (Fig. 11.9). The typical frequencies of the ultrasound probes are in the order of 5 to 10 MHz to achieve sufficient penetration. Doppler shift of the ultrasound wave does not only depend on the blood velocity but also on the Doppler angle. The direction of the sampling gate therefore needs to be adjusted based on the anatomy of the artery. Whereas this is usually achieved without problems in the CRA and the OA, it is more difficult in the PCAs. Peak systolic and end diastolic velocities (PSVs, EDVs) are extracted from the time slope of the Doppler shift. Mean flow velocity (MFV) can be calculated as the time mean of the spectral outline over a heart cycle. In addition, a resistance index (RI = [PSV − EDV]/PSV) can be calculated as a measure of vascular resistance distal to these vascular beds.

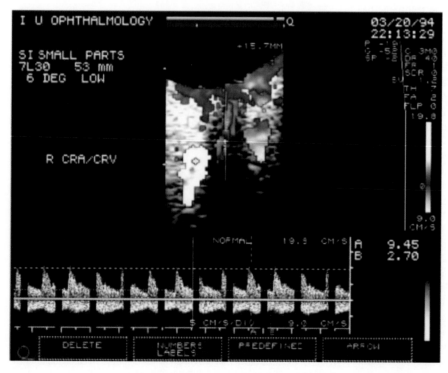

Fig. 11.9 Color Doppler image of the central retinal artery and vein taken with a 7.5-MHz linear probe (Siemens Quantum 2000 system). The Doppler shifted spectrum (time velocity curve) is displayed at the bottom of the image. *Red* and *blue* pixels represent blood movement toward and away from the transducer, respectively. (Reproduced with permission from Harris A, Chung HS, Ciulla TA, Kagemann L. Progress in measurement of ocular blood flow and relevance to our understanding of glaucoma and age-related macular degeneration. *Prog Retin Eye Res* 1999;18(5): 669–687.)

A study in healthy subjects indicates, however, that this is a poor measure of vascular resistance in the retina.[95] The technique is not capable of measuring volumetric blood flow because the resolution is not sufficient to resolve the vessel diameter with the required precision. As the ultrasound probe is put on the closed eye lid, care has to be taken such that the intraocular pressure is not increased due to the force induced on the eye.

Laser speckle flowgraphy

Laser speckle flowgraphy measures blood flow using laser speckle statistics. Laser speckles arise from reflection of coherent light at rough surfaces. The speckle pattern that appears under the illumination of laser irradiation can only be described statistically. When objects are moving, for instance, red blood cells in the blood stream, the structure of the pattern varies. The higher the variation, the higher the velocity of the scatterers. Early approaches using laser speckle flowgraphy only allowed for semiquantitative analysis of perfusion.[96] Later, instruments were developed that allow for quantification of blood flow at the posterior pole of the eye.[97–99] Nowadays several commercial systems are available.

In most systems a near infrared laser is used as a light source, coupled to a fundus camera and a digital charge–coupled device camera. The most widely used output parameter of laser speckle technology is mean blur rate (MBR), which is a measure of relative blood flow velocity and is expressed in arbitrary units (au). When a scan is started, 118 images are captured at a rate of 30 frames per second, resulting in a measurement time of 4 seconds. From the 118 acquired images, a color-coded map is calculated, which depicts the distribution of perfusion.

The system can either be used to study perfusion in vascularized tissue or to study blood flow in retinal vessels. For perfusion measurements, the ONH area is selected by positioning an ellipsoid region of interest at the ONH margin. Thereafter, larger retinal vessels are automatically detected by thresholding according to their higher blood velocities. Thus, MBR can be determined for the total ONH area, for vessel area, or for tissue area (Fig. 11.10).

There is a longstanding discussion whether the technique measures flow, velocity, or some quantity related to flow.[101] It is obvious that the speckle contrast in the tissue is not only affected by the velocity of the red blood cells but also by the number of moving scatterers. The technique has been validated in a variety of animal studies and it has been shown that measures of laser speckle flowgraphy correlate well with values obtained using either the microsphere method or the hydrogen gas clearance method.[52,102] As with laser Doppler flowmetry, the penetration depth of the technique is not completely understood. When the laser is directed toward vascularized tissue of the retina, a sum signal between retinal and choroidal blood flow is measured. Animal data indicate that the retinal contribution is in the order of 10%,[103] which is in agreement with data from laser Doppler flowmetry studies. The results may be influenced by pigmentation and, as such, results between different ethnicities may not be comparable. The majority of data with this technology

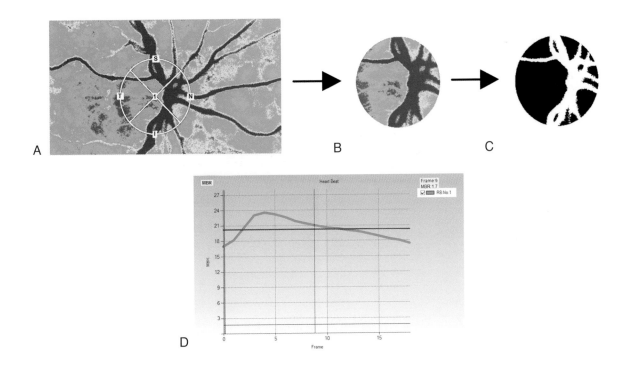

Fig. 11.10 Laser speckle flowgraphy (LSFG) scan of the optic nerve head (ONH) area. (**A**) The ONH margin is to be delineated using an ellipsoid region of interest with variable size and radii. (**B**) The selected area representing the entire optic disc is taken into account for further analysis using the "vessel extraction" function. (**C**) The vessel extraction function distinguishes between areas of visible surface vessels *(white)* and ONH tissue areas *(black)*. (**D**) Typical pulse-waveform curve *(green)* with a steep incline during the systolic phase and a flatter decline during the diastolic phase. The *red* line indicates the mean level of mean blur rate (MBR). (Reproduced with permission from Luft N, Wozniak PA, Aschinger GC, et al., Ocular blood flow measurements in healthy white subjects using laser speckle flowgraphy. *PLOS ONE* 2016;11(12):e0168190.)

have been obtained in Japan,[104,105] and recently the technique was also successfully applied in Caucasians.[100] When measurements were done in retinal vessels, the correlation with data as obtained with Doppler OCT was not good, particularly at higher arterial flow rates because of saturation effects.[106]

Doppler OCT

Doppler OCT is a functional extension of OCT.[107] The first description of this technique was realized based on a time domain–OCT system.[108] In Fourier domain–OCT, the Doppler shift of light can be quantified by analyzing the phase of the complex OCT signal.[109–111] Similarly, laser Doppler velocimetry measurement of blood velocity requires knowledge of the incident angle of the laser beam. Multibeam systems for the illumination of the retina were realized to overcome this angle ambiguity.[25,112–117] Combining these measurements with diameter measurements of retinal vessels by either using fundus photography or phase tomograms of OCT allows for measurement of total retinal blood flow.[21,25,118,119] Other approaches to overcome the angle ambiguity were also realized. The use of bidirectional Doppler cross sections perpendicular to the illumination plane allows for calculation of retinal blood flow independent of the Doppler angle.[120] Dual-plane scanning patterns have also been used to determine the

angle between blood flow and the scanning beam.[121] When using 3D Doppler data sets, en-face images can be used to extract absolute blood velocity, as well as total retinal blood flow, without knowledge of the Doppler angles (Fig. 11.11).[24,122] Another approach is to study retinal vessels at relatively high Doppler angle, which is automatically detected by autoalignment.[123] Recently it has been proposed to use the forward-scattering signal instead of the backward-scattering signal, because it is insensitive to vessel orientation.[124]

Doppler OCT has been also used to reconstruct the velocity vector field from measured phase data, allowing for the visualization of velocity profiles at retinal bifurcations (Fig. 11.12).[125] Line scanning protocols of multichannel OCT were employed to investigate venous pulsatile caliber oscillations and flow pulsatility.[126]

OCT angiography

OCTA is a technique that is closely related to Doppler OCT.[127–130] The first approach to noninvasively visualizing the vasculature in the human eye based on OCT was based on Doppler phase, as well as variance or power of the phase analysis.[131] Later, multiple algorithms and scan protocols were proposed based on logarithmic intensity and speckle contrast imaging. Split spectrum amplitude decorrelation (SSADA) improves signal to noise and bulk eye motion artifacts.[132]

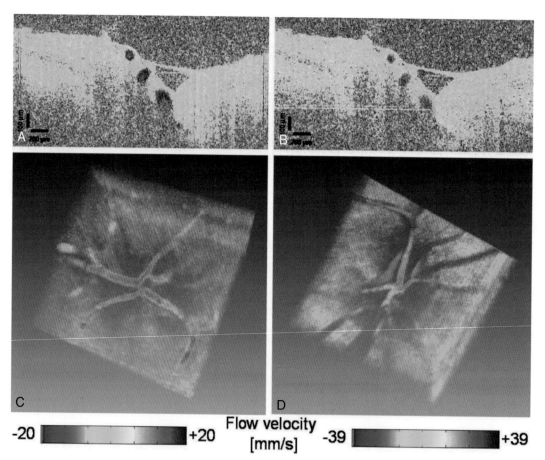

Fig. 11.11 Volumetric Doppler optical coherence tomography (OCT) imaging of retinal vasculature. (**A**) Doppler OCT B-scan image at 100 kHz close to the optic disc. (**B**) Corresponding Doppler OCT image at 200 kHz. Arterial and venous vessels in the papilla can be distinguished in *red* and *blue* color. Note that the color scale encodes the ranges of ±19.7 mm/s and ±39.5 mm/s for 100 kHz and 200 kHz, respectively. Three-dimensional renderings of volumetric data sets at 100 kHz (**C**) and 200 kHz (**D**) show the three-dimensional structure of the retinal arteries and veins branching in the optic disc. (Reproduced with permission from Baumann B, Potsaid B, Kraus MF, et al., Total retinal blood flow measurement with ultrahigh speed swept source/Fourier domain OCT. *Biomed Opt Express* 2011;2(6):1539–1552. © The Optical Society.)

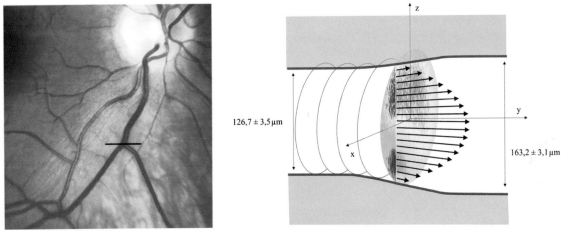

Fig. 11.12 Fundus image of a venous convergence site with the *black bar* marking the scanning position. Reconstructed velocity vector field at the scanned position of a convergence: the *red line* depicts the vessel wall geometry. (Modified with permission from Aschinger GC, Schmetterer L, Doblhoff-Dier V, et al., Blood flow velocity vector field reconstruction from dual-beam bidirectional Doppler OCT measurements in retinal veins. *Biomed Opt Express* 2015;6(5):1599–1615. © The Optical Society.)

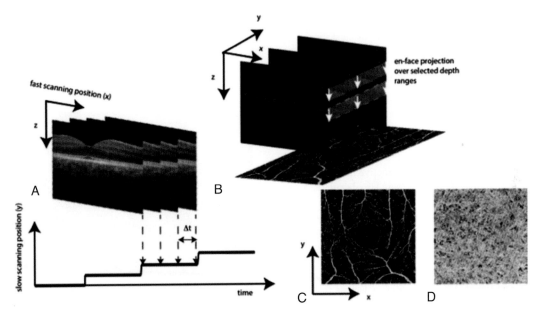

Fig. 11.13 (**A**) Recording scheme for Doppler optical coherence tomography (DOCT) angiography. (**B**) Calculated three-dimensional Doppler OCT angiography. (**C**) Taking the en-face projection visualizing the retinal vasculature. (**D**) Dense choroidal vasculature obtained by integration over dashed depth region in (**B**). (Reproduced with permission from Drexler W, Liu M, Kumar A, Kamali T, Unterhuber A, Leitgeb RA, Optical coherence tomography today: speed, contrast, and multimodality. *Journal of Biomedical Optics* 2014; 19(7): 071412)

Optical microangiography (OMAG) is another approach that includes both the amplitude and the phase of the OCT signal.[133]

Nowadays, repeated B-scans are used to detect motion contrast, thereby visualizing the ocular vasculature (Fig. 11.13). Nonmoving tissues will not produce an autocorrelation signal in repeated B-scans but moving objects produce a signal that is dependent on the blood speed. Based on this mode of function it is obvious that the technique is sensitive to eye motion and motion artifacts are common.[134] Segmentation of OCT angiograms is usually done to extract either two or three retinal vascular plexuses, as well as the choriocapillaris (Fig. 11.14).

OCTA has also been applied to the anterior segment of the eye.[135–137] The technique has several advantages over other vascular anterior segment imaging modalities including rapid image acquisition, noninvasiveness, absence of leakage, 3D visualization, and imaging in cases of corneal opacification. The technology has been used to study the vasculature of the cornea in pathologic conditions, the iris, sclera, episclera, and conjunctiva.

OCTA has recently renewed the interest of many clinicians in ocular blood flow because it is readily available as a functional extension of OCT platforms. The technology allows for the noninvasive visualization of the vasculature with unprecedented 3D resolution. This has led to the discovery of novel insights into the pathophysiology of retinal and choroidal vascular disease, and also to the standard use of the technology in clinical care. A variety of quantitative metrics have been proposed for the analysis of OCT angiograms.[138,139] The foveal avascular zone (FAZ) can be separately analyzed for each

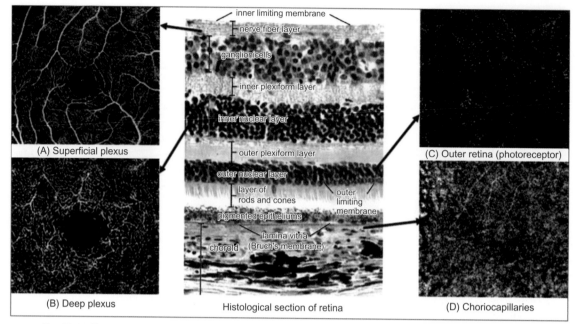

Fig. 11.14 The location of different en-face zones in relation to histology of the human retina. The four en-face zones include (**A**) the superficial plexus, the capillary network in ganglion cell layer and nerve fiber layer; (**B**) the deep plexus, a network of capillaries in the inner plexiform layer with offshoot of 55 μm; (**C**) the outer retina (photoreceptors), and (**D**) the choriocapillaries (choroid) with offshoot of 30 μm. (Reproduced with permission from Chalam KV, Sambhav K. Optical coherence tomography angiography in retinal diseases. *J Ophthalmic Vis Res* 2016;11(1):84.

capillary plexus. The vessel density is based on the skeletonized vessel map and is calculated as the ratio of vessel area to image area. A one-pixel line represents the vessel, thereby excluding the effect of vessel diameter. Perfusion density is calculated as the ratio of the binarized perfusion area to the entire imaged area. Alternative metrics such as fractal dimension[140] or complexity index[141] were also calculated from OCT angiograms.

Since the choriocapillaris is highly vascularized, the nonperfused area is usually used as an outcome measure after binarization of the image.[127] These nonperfused regions are called flow voids, flow deficits, or signal voids. The size and number of such flow voids can provide information on choroidal integrity.[142] The B-scan rate, the A-scan rate, the scan direction, and the oversampling ratio, as well as the lateral and axial resolution, need to be considered when calculating vascular metrics based on OCTA.[138,143] Magnification is another important factor to consider. The field of view is a function of axial eye length, and several approaches were published on how to correct for this.[144] This obviously has a major effect on quantification of FAZ size, which in turn affects measures such as perfusion density and vessel density.

Whenever quantitative metrics are calculated it is important to understand the area that is being analyzed. Generally, data for vessel density or perfusion density are not comparable between different OCT systems, because each vendor uses its own algorithm.[140] There is currently no consensus on an optimal approach for this problem.

Spectroscopic oximetry

Noninvasive retinal oxygen saturation measurements were first done in 1965 based on absorption profiles of hemoglobin that depend on SO_2.[145] This technique has been improved by using digital imaging[146] and automated software solutions.[147] Currently, there are two commercial systems for noninvasive spectroscopic oximetry on the market, both using a two-wavelength approach.[32,148] These two images are taken concomitantly so that the influence of eye movements is

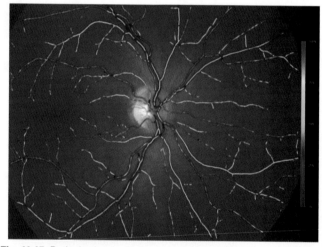

Fig. 11.15 Retinal oximetry image in a healthy subject. The color scale on the *right* shows oxygen saturation. The arterioles are generally *red*, indicating oxygen saturation in the 90%–100% range, and the venules are generally *green/yellow*, indicating oxygen saturation in the 50%–65% range. The oximeter software excludes vessels below 6 pixels (56 μm) from analysis. The variability in the measurement increases with smaller vessel diameters, and this cutoff is used to ensure high-quality data. The excluded vessel segments are labeled *gray* on the image. (Reproduced with permission from Stefánsson E, Olafsdottir OB, Eliasdottir TS, et al. Retinal oximetry: metabolic imaging for diseases of the retina and brain. *Prog Retin Eye Res* 2019;70:1–22.)

eliminated (Fig. 11.15). Validation of this technique is not easy, because of the lack of a gold standard method. One approach to study the accuracy is to compare SO_2 values obtained using oximetry in retinal arteries with systemic SO_2 values in patients with systemic hypoxemia.[149,150] The two-wavelength approach may, however, be influenced by retinal pigmentation and vessel diameter and therefore requires careful calibration.[151] Application of such calibration values to eyes from different ethnicities is, however, not possible because of differences in pigmentation levels.[146] Another factor influencing the results is blood velocity.[152] To overcome these limitations, several authors have used multiwavelength or hyperspectral approaches for retinal oximetry.[153–157] Alternatively, white light OCT can be used to study retinal SO_2,[33,158] a technique that has also been extended toward the retinal microcirculation.[159] Monte Carlo models have recently been developed that dealt with the impact of scattering, blood volume fraction, and lens yellowing[160] and will hopefully improve the reliability of this technique in the future.

REGULATION OF OCULAR BLOOD FLOW

Local metabolic control

Metabolic control of blood flow is based on the interaction between parenchymal cells and the smooth muscle cells. In the retina and the ONH, the key regulator is oxygen. During conditions of hypoxia, vasodilator signals are activated to increase retinal perfusion.[161–164] In both animals and humans, this increase in perfusion is, however, not associated with an increase in inner retinal oxygen consumption as long as the systemic PO_2 is above 35 mmHg.[40,165,166] Little is known about the mechanisms of oxygen-induced vasodilation in the retina, but nitric oxide (NO) and prostaglandins appear to be involved in this process.[167,168] During hyperoxia, strong retinal vasoconstriction is observed, which is associated with a pronounced reduction in blood flow (Fig. 11.16).[163,169–173] OCTA metrics also decrease during hyperoxia, but it needs to be kept in mind that the technique does not measure blood flow, but parameters such as vessel or perfusion density.[174–176] The vasoconstrictor response to hyperoxia involves endothelin-1, as well as the arachidonic acid metabolites thromboxane and 20-HETE.[177–180] In contrast to blood flow in the retina, perfusion in the choroid is almost independent on systemic PO_2.[181–185] This is associated with large amounts of oxygen diffusing from the choroid into the retina, increasing inner retinal PO_2.[57,186,187]

Perfusion in both the retina and the choroid is strongly dependent on partial pressure of carbon dioxide (Fig. 11.16) (PCO_2).[172,183,185,188–192] In the brain it has been demonstrated that reduced extracellular pH is mainly responsible for vasodilation in response to local changes in PCO_2.[193] In the retina this has not been confirmed, but the most likely effect is the diffusion of CO_2 across the blood-retinal barrier, which results in reduced pH in the extracellular space. Activation of

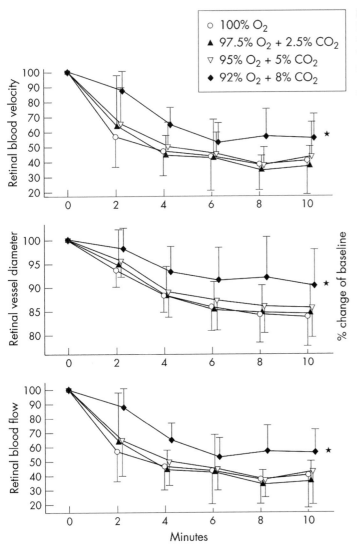

Fig. 11.16 Time course of retinal venous diameter, retinal blood velocity, and retinal blood flow during breathing of different mixtures of O_2/CO_2 in healthy subjects. Data are presented as mean (standard deviation) ($n = 12$). Asterisks indicate significant differences versus pure oxygen breathing. (Reproduced with permission from Schmetterer L, Lexer F, Findl O, Graselli U, Eichler HG, Wolzt M. The effect of inhalation of different mixtures of O2 and CO2 on ocular fundus pulsations. *Exp Eye Res* 1996;63(4):351–355.)

Legend for figure:
- ○ 100% O_2
- ▲ 97.5% O_2 + 2.5% CO_2
- ▽ 95% O_2 + 5% CO_2
- ◆ 92% O_2 + 8% CO_2

(Y-axes: Retinal blood velocity; Retinal vessel diameter; Retinal blood flow; % change of baseline. X-axis: Minutes)

acid-sensing ion channel-1A by extracellular acidosis seems to be a key mechanism in CO_2-induced vasodilation in the brain.[194] The cerebral blood flow response in the brain is dependent on nitric oxide (NO),[195,196] a mechanism that has also been confirmed for the ocular vasculature.[197]

The metabolic theory of blood flow regulation assumes that blood flow is adapted via a feedback loop in response to changes in PO_2, PCO_2, pH, and other vasoactive mediators. This may, for instance, play a role in hypoxic states, such as early diabetes when retinal blood flow increases.[35] It is, however, unlikely that such metabolic mechanisms play an important role in blood flow regulation during changes in arterial blood pressure or neuronal stimulation, because of their relatively slow mechanisms of action.

Autoregulation in response to changes in perfusion pressure

Autoregulation refers to the ability of a vascular bed to maintain its blood flow during changes in perfusion pressure.[11] In its strict sense, it refers to isolated vascular beds. Changes in vascular tone during in vivo experiments are not only due to the change in perfusion pressure but also due to potential changes in the neural or humoral input. This is unlikely to occur in the retina as the retinal vasculature lacks autonomic innervation.[198–200] In the choroid, however, the vessels are richly innervated[198] and in vivo responses to pressure stimuli are at least partially medicated via neural mechanisms.[201–203]

Another issue relates to the calculation of perfusion pressure. This is defined as the difference in arterial minus venous pressure. In the retina neither arterial nor venous pressure can be calculated noninvasively in vivo. Noninvasive plethysmographic measurements of retinal venous pressure have been performed,[204,205] but the results are dependent on cerebrospinal fluid pressure.[206,207] Hence, the vast majority of autoregulation studies have estimated OPP as mean arterial pressure (MAP) – intraocular pressure (IOP) in the supine position and as two-thirds MAP – IOP in the sitting position to account for the drop in pressure between the level of the eye and the level of the heart.[208–212] Although this may be a good approximation, there are several limitations to this approach. On the one hand the arterial tree from the heart to the eye represents a vascular resistance, which is associated with a drop in pressure. Hence, the arterial pressure at the level of the CRA will be lower than at the level of the heart. On the other hand, retinal venous pressure is slightly higher than IOP, to allow blood to exit the eyeball toward the venous circulation.[213] The same also holds true for the choroidal veins.[214] As such, the calculated OPP will always overestimate the actual OPP by a couple of mmHg. There are two principal methods to change OPP, either via modification of the arterial side or the venous side, or a combination of both. Multiple techniques have been used to study this behavior. The majority of studies investigated autoregulation either during an increase in blood pressure or an increase in IOP.

Myogenic mechanisms play a key role in autoregulation. Myogenic tone is defined as vasoconstriction that occurs in an isolated blood vessel at a constant pressure.[215] Similar to the brain, retinal arteries respond to changes in transmural pressure, which is defined as the pressure within the vessel minus outside the vessel, with development of myogenic tone.[216] When arterial blood pressure is decreased, myogenic tone is reduced and vessel diameter increases. An increase in blood pressure induces and increases myogenic tone, thereby reducing vascular diameter. These changes in vessel diameter are associated with changes in vascular resistance that keep blood flow constant within certain limits of OPP.

With increases in blood pressure, a reduction in vessel diameter helps to normalize wall tension. This concept is supported by the fact that similar phenotypic changes are seen in isolated vessels studied under pressurized conditions in vitro, but where blood flow is absent. The vascular myogenic response is intrinsic to vascular muscle cells, and experiments in cerebral vessels have shown that the mechanism is still functioning when endothelial cells are removed.[217,218] The mechanisms regulating myogenic response in brain and retina seem to be closely related.[216] When transmural pressure increases, cation channels on the surface of the vascular smooth muscle cells are activated in response to the mechanical stress.[219] This leads to cell membrane potential depolarization, which induces vasoconstriction owing to the increase in voltage-dependent Ca influx.[220–222] Transient receptor potential channels contribute to myogenic signaling in the retinal vasculature, with TRPV2 being the most important regulator.[223,224] While myogenic mechanisms in vascular smooth muscle cells are intrinsic to vascular muscle, additional factors related to endothelial-, metabolic-, neural-, and immune-related signaling, have also been identified.[215]

A schematic drawing of autoregulation in response to changes in OPP is shown in Fig. 11.17. Two examples are shown, one in which autoregulation is present over an OPP range of 40 mmHg and another in which the autoregulatory range is lower, only spanning over an OPP range of 20 mmHg. The autoregulatory range is also termed autoregulatory plateau. The lower limit of autoregulation is defined at the OPP value at which blood flow starts to decline. The OPP value at which blood flow starts to increase when OPP is increased is called the upper limit of autoregulation. This autoregulatory capacity is achieved by the adaptation of vascular tone during changes in transmural pressure, as discussed previously in this section. It is often stated that the upper and lower limit of autoregulation represent maximum vasoconstriction and maximum vasodilation, respectively. Experimental evidence, however, has shown that even below the limit of lower autoregulation, retinal vessels still exhibit flicker-induced vasodilation.[225]

Failure of autoregulatory capacity may have severe clinical consequences. When the OPP falls below the lower level of autoregulation, tissue will be at risk for ischemia and hypoxia. When the OPP exceeds the upper level of autoregulation, there is a risk of bleeding. Several common eye diseases are associated with abnormal autoregulatory ranges, which are considered to play a role in their pathophysiology.

In the retina, autoregulation has been proven in a wide variety of studies and most likely reflects myogenic blood flow regulation. During an isometric exercise–induced increase in OPP, retinal blood flow in humans stays constant until an increase in the order of 30% to 40%.[226–228] Retinal blood flow autoregulation has also been shown to occur when OPP is decreased, for instance, during an experimental increase in IOP (Fig. 11.18).[229,230]

In older textbooks it is frequently mentioned that the choroid is a strictly passive vascular bed with a linear pressure-flow relationship. This is to large degree based on animal experiments using the microsphere technology.[40] Newer studies have, however, proven that the pressure-flow relationship is nonlinear in vivo (Fig. 11.19).[89,231,232] In humans, the choroid has been shown to react to both a decrease[233,234] and an increase in OPP.[234–238] Animal studies support the concept that myogenic mechanisms play a role in this response,[231] but there is currently no study available investigating myogenic tone in choroidal arterioles. A strong modulating function of neural components to this response has been proven, which may be responsible for most of the vascular tone changes during perfusion pressure challenges.[203,239,240]

As mentioned previously, the vascular anatomy of the ONH is complex. Little is known about potential differences between the superficial and deep vascular components of the ONH in term

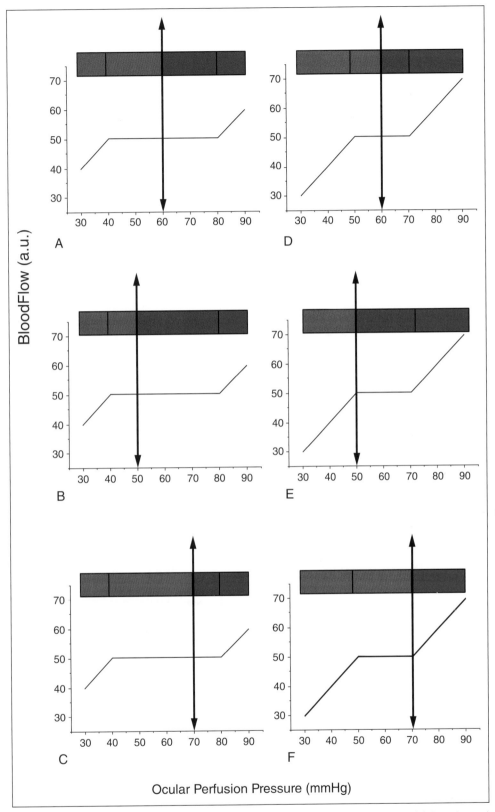

Fig. 11.17 Theoretical model of autoregulation. *Red bars* indicate the ischemic region, *pink bars* the region of autoregulatory reserve toward lower perfusion pressure, *purple bars* the region of autoregulatory reserve toward lower ocular perfusion pressure (OPP), and *blue bars* the region of hyperperfusion. (**A–C**) A person with an autoregulatory plateau of 40 mmHg. The autoregulatory reserve depends on the baseline OPP. At lower baseline OPP (**B**) the autoregulatory reserve toward lower OPPs is reduced. At higher OPP (**C**) the autoregulatory reserve toward lower OPPs is increased, but the autoregulatory reserve toward higher OPPs is reduced. (**D–F**) A person with an abnormally reduced autoregulatory plateau of 20 mmHg. When baseline OPP is 60 mmHg, (**D**) both the reserve toward higher and lower OPPs is reduced. When baseline OPP is only 50 mmHg there is no reserve toward ischemia left (**E**), whereas no reserve toward hyperperfusion is left when OPP is 70 mmHg (**F**).

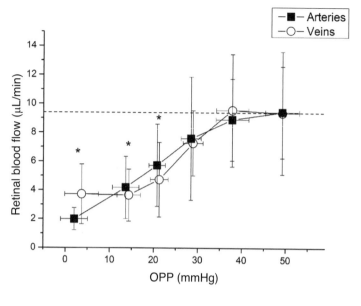

Fig. 11.18 Pressure-flow relationship for retinal arteries and veins determined by categorized ocular perfusion pressure (*OPP*) and retinal blood flow during application of the suction cup to increase intraocular pressure (IOP) in healthy subjects. Data were sorted into groups of 15 values, each according to ascending OPP. Data are presented as mean ± standard deviation (*n* = 15). *Significant changes versus baseline for retinal arteries and veins. (Reproduced with permission from Puchner S, Schmidl D, Ginner L, et al., Changes in retinal blood flow in response to an experimental increase in IOP in healthy participants as assessed with Doppler optical coherence tomography. *Invest Ophthalmol Vis Sci* 2020;61(2): 33–33.)

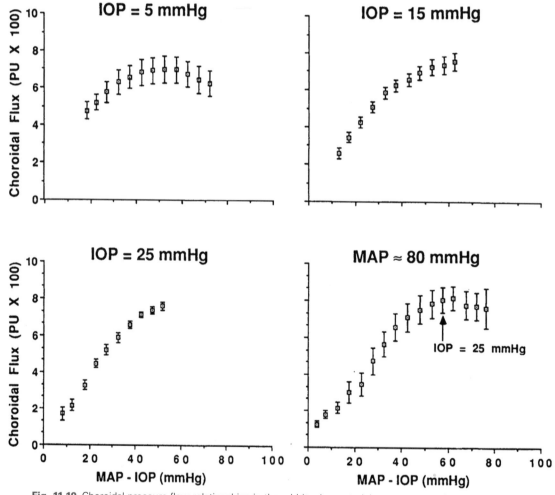

Fig. 11.19 Choroidal pressure-flow relationships in the rabbit when arterial pressure was decreased at intraocular pressures (*IOPs*) of 5, 15, and 25 mmHg, and when intraocular pressure was increased at the prevailing mean arterial pressure (≈80 mmHg). At the lowest IOP, choroidal blood flow was well maintained until the perfusion pressure fell below approximately 40 mmHg. Raising the IOP to 15 and 25 mmHg shifted the upper portion of the pressure-flow curves upward, so the curves became progressively more linear. When IOP was the manipulated variable, blood flow was pressure independent until IOP was raised above approximately 25 mmHg. *MAP*, Mean arterial pressure. (Reproduced with permission from Kiel JW, Shepherd AP. Autoregulation of choroidal blood flow in the rabbit. *Invest Ophthalmol Vis Sci* 1992;33(8):2399–2410.

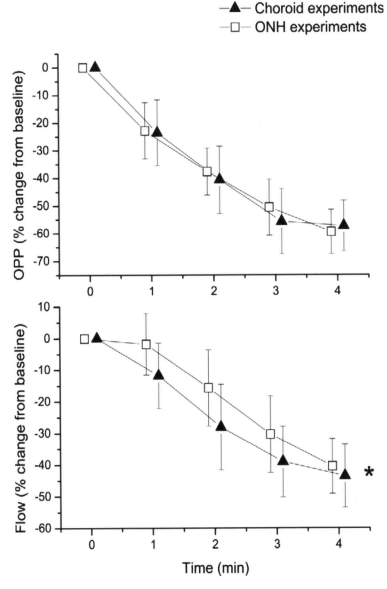

- **▲** Choroid experiments
- **□** ONH experiments

Fig. 11.20 Effect of an intraocular pressure (IOP) increase on ocular perfusion pressure (*OPP*) and flow in healthy subjects. Data are shown separately for the artificial IOP increase for choroidal (n = 24, *solid up triangles*) and optic nerve head (*ONH*) experiments (n = 24, *open squares*). Data are presented as percentage change from baseline (mean ± standard deviation). *Significant differences between the choroidal and ONH experiments. (Reproduced with permission from Schmidl D, Boltz A, Kaya S, et al., Comparison of choroidal and optic nerve head blood flow regulation during changes in ocular perfusion pressure. *Invest Ophthalmol Vis Sci* 2012;3(8):4337–4346.)

of pressure autoregulation. Most of the data on ONH autoregulation used either laser Doppler flowmetry or laser speckle flowgraphy, and therefore data are limited to the superficial vascular bed. With this technology, autoregulatory behavior was seen during an increase,[228,234,241–243] as well as a decrease,[244–247] in OPP. Two studies have compared autoregulatory changes in the ONH and choroid during standardized stimuli by either using laser speckle flowgraphy[248] or laser Doppler flowmetry[234] and found distinct differences between the two vascular beds (Fig. 11.20).

An important difference to autoregulation in the brain is that in the eye, venous pressure can become very high when IOP is high. There is now evidence from a wide array of animal and human studies that blood flow reacts differently if either the arterial or the venous pressure is modulated (Fig. 11.21).[232,249–253] In humans, the regulation of choroidal and ONH blood flow during combined changes in systemic blood pressure and IOP is dependent on the absolute values of blood pressure (BP) and IOP.[251–253] Blood flow in both vascular beds is less sensitive to changes in arterial blood pressure than in IOP. Interestingly, this finding is compatible with a myogenic mechanism

being involved. During an artificial increase in IOP, venous pressure will increase with an associated increase in the transmural pressure gradient. As mentioned earlier, the myogenic theory is based on the concept that changes in transmural pressure cause smooth muscle relaxation when OPP is lowered. Hence, ChBF may exhibit much lesser autoregulatory response during an IOP-induced drop in OPP, because it is paralleled by a decrease in perfusion pressure gradient. When OPP is changed via the arterial side, however, the full myogenic response is initiated due to the increase in transmural pressure. This concept is also supported by a study in healthy subjects in which the IOP was lowered pharmacologically with an associated increase in the autoregulatory plateau.[254]

Several studies have found that autoregulation of ocular vascular beds is altered by pharmacologic intervention. A role of NO in autoregulation of all ocular vascular beds has been shown in a wide variety of animal and human studies (Fig. 11.22).[249,255–262] Interestingly, NO synthase inhibition alters the choroidal but not the ONH pressure-flow relationship when IOP is increased, again highlighting the differences in the mechanisms between choroid and ONH.[254,261]

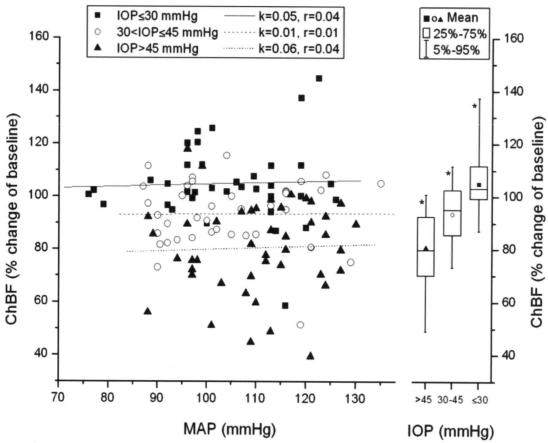

Fig. 11.21 Mean arterial pressure–choroidal blood flow (*MAP–ChBF*) relationship during combined experimental intraocular pressure (*IOP*) increase and isometric exercise using categorized data according to IOP in healthy subjects. All MAP and ChBF pairs, except baseline, were sorted into three groups according to IOP (group 1: IOP ≤30 mmHg; group 2: 30 > IOP ≤45 mmHg; group 3: IOP >45 mmHg). *Left*: regression analysis for each group, performed separately. *Right*: box-and-whisker plots, indicating mean ChBF at different IOPs independent of MAP. *Significant differences between these groups. *k*, Slope of the regression line; *r*, correlation coefficient. (Reproduced with permission from: Polska E, Simader C, Weigert G et al., Regulation of choroidal blood flow during combined changes in intraocular pressure and arterial blood pressure. *Invest Ophthalmol Vis Sci 2007*; 48(8): 3768–74.)

Modulating the endothelin system has also been proven to change the ocular pressure/flow relationship, mediated via the endothelin A receptor (Fig. 11.23).[263–266] Other factors that have been shown to modulate the autoregulatory pressure response in the eye include adenosine,[249] NMDA receptors,[249] α- and β-adrenergic blockade,[267] and calcium channel blockade.[260]

In a study of perfused and pressurized brain slices, it was postulated that astrocytes are involved in modulating myogenic tone during changes in pressure.[268] This concept is supported by rabbit experiments in which animals treated with the gliotoxic L-2-aminoadipic acid (LAA) showed reduced autoregulatory reserve in the ONH.[269]

Neurovascular coupling

When neurons are stimulated with light the retinal vessels vasodilate. This response is due to a fundamental mechanism, termed functional hyperemia, that describes the increase in blood flow when neurons are stimulated. This phenomenon has been described in detail in the brain but also occurs in the retina.[270] The increase in blood flow and vessel diameter during flicker stimulation has been described by many authors in both animals[271–279] and humans (Fig. 11.24).[280–295] This is paralleled by an increase in retinal oxygen extraction.[296,297] This relaxation can either be mediated via smooth muscle cells or via the retinal pericytes that also show contractile tone in the retina.[298,299]

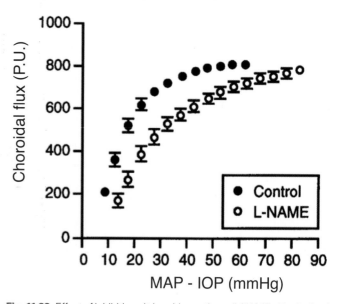

Fig. 11.22 Effect of inhibiting nitric oxide synthase (L-NAME, 10 mbg kg⁻⁴, i.v. (intravenous)). Pressure-flow curves in the rabbit choroid. L-NAME reduced group mean choroidal flow over the entire perfusion pressure range examined. *IOP*, Intraocular pressure; *i.v.*, *MAP*, mean arterial pressure. (Reproduced with permission from Kiel JW. Modulation of choroidal autoregulation in the rabbit. *Exp Eye Res* 1999;69(4):413–29.)

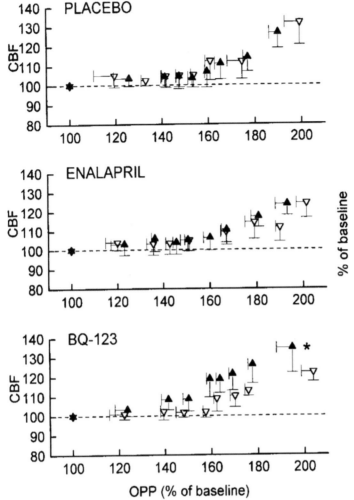

Fig. 11.23 Pressure-flow relationship between ocular perfusion pressure (*OPP*) and choroidal blood flow (*CBF*) during isometric exercise in healthy subjects. Data are shown for the angiotensin converting–enzyme inhibitor enalapril and for the endothelin receptor antagonist BQ-123. The first period of squatting was without the drug (baseline; *open triangles*). The second squatting period was during administration of placebo, BQ-123, or enalapril (*filled triangles*). The mean and the lower limits of the 95% confidence interval are shown (*n* = 12). (Reproduced with permission from Fuchsjäger-Mayrl G, Luksch A, Malec M, Polska E, Wolzt M, Schmetterer L. Role of endothelin-1 in choroidal blood flow regulation during isometric exercise in healthy humans. *Invest Ophthalmol Vis Sci* 2003;44(2):728–733.)

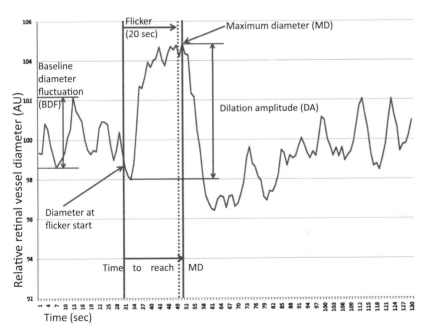

Fig. 11.24 The retinal diameter response to flicker provocation. Illustrated are changes in a retinal vessel as it is stimulated by flickering light. On the *far left*, BDF defines the fluctuation in the baseline diameter. The central section shows an increase in relative vessel diameter owing to flickering light. This response provides the MD, the DA, and the time to reach MD. The *right* side shows the responses of the vessel as it recovers. (Reproduced with permission from Heitmar R, Blann AD, Cubbidge RP, Lip GYH, Gherghel D. Continuous retinal vessel diameter measurements: the future in retinal vessel assessment? *Invest Ophthalmol Vis Sci* 2010;51(11):5833–5839.)

It has been shown that NO and prostaglandins are involved in the process of neurovascular coupling in the brain.[300,301] Results for NO have also been confirmed in the retina.[302-304] Whereas these substances are produced in neurons and directly diffuse to the vessels, another mechanism plays a key role in brain neurovascular coupling.

Astroglial cells act as intermediaries in neurovascular signaling.[305,306] According to this model, astrocytes stimulated via neurotransmitters such as glutamate promote the production of ATP in neurons (Fig. 11.25). This induces an increase in intracellular Ca^{2+}, which activates phospholipase A2 and other enzymes[307] to produce vasodilators

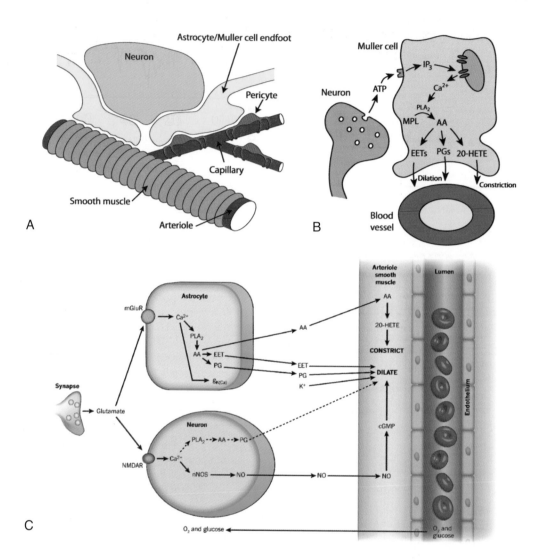

Fig. 11.25 Cellular and molecular mechanisms of neurovascular coupling. (**A**) Cells of the neurovascular unit regulate blood flow in the brain and retina. The diameters of arteries and arterioles are controlled by smooth muscle cells, while capillary diameter is controlled by pericytes. Astroglial cells in the brain and Müller glial cells in the retina surround arterioles and capillaries and their contractile cells. Signaling molecules released from neurons, and glial cell endfeet control the contractile state of smooth muscle cells and pericytes. (**B**) Signaling pathways that mediate neurovascular coupling in the brain. Glutamate released from neurons acts on NMDA receptors in neurons (NMDAR) to raise intracellular Ca^{2+} levels, causing neuronal nitric oxide synthase (nNOS) to release NO, dilating smooth muscle cells. Raised Ca^{2+} may also *(dashed line)* generate arachidonic acid (*AA*) from phospholipase A2 (*PLA2*), which is converted to prostaglandins (*PG*) that dilate vessels. Glutamate also raises Ca^{2+} levels in astrocytes by activating metabotropic glutamate receptors (mGluR), generating AA and three types of AA metabolites: PG and epoxyeicosatrienoic acids (*EETs*), which dilate vessels, and 20-hydroxy-eicosatetraenoic acid (20-HETE), which constricts vessels. (**C**) Neurovascular coupling in the retina. Adenosine triphosphate (ATP) released from neurons stimulates purinergic receptors on Müller cells, leading to the production of IP3 and the release of Ca^{2+} from internal stores. Ca^{2+} activates PLA2, which converts membrane phospholipids (MPL) to AA, which is subsequently metabolized to the vasodilators PG and EET, and to the vasoconstrictor 20-HETE. (**A** Reproduced with permission from Nippert AR, Mishra A, Newman EA. Keeping the brain well fed: The role of capillaries and arterioles in orchestrating functional hyperemia. *Neuron*, 2018;99(2):248–250. **B** and **C** Reproduced with permission from Newman EA. Glial cell regulation of neuronal activity and blood flow in the retina by release of gliotransmitters. *Philos Trans R Soc Lond B Biol Sci.* 2015;370(1672):20140195.)

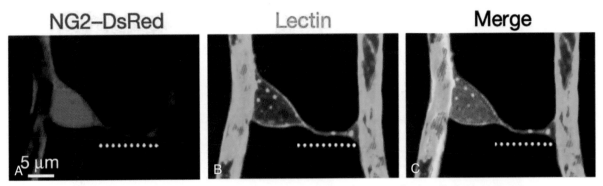

Fig. 11.26 Interpericyte tunneling nanotubes connect retinal pericytes on distal capillaries in a soma-to-process configuration. Examination of retinas from mice that express red fluorescent protein under control of the NG2 (Cspg4) promoter (NG2–DsRed) and Lectin. A: NG2-DsRed, B: Lectin, C: Merged (Reproduced with permission from Alarcon-Martinez L, Villafranca-Baughman D, Quintero H, et al., Interpericyte tunnelling nanotubes regulate neurovascular coupling. *Nature* 2020;585(7823):91–95.)

that mediate the increase in blood flow. In addition, endothelium-derived factors appear to contribute to the signaling that is responsible for functional hyperemia.[308]

In the retina, the principal glial cell is the Müller cell, which also has an important role in mediating neurovascular coupling.[309] Blockade of the neuron to glia signaling causes a pronounce reduction of the response to light stimulation, thereby highlighting the importance of this mechanism.[305] The increase in intracellular Ca^{2+} leads to a release of vasoactive substances from Müller cells that include the vasodilators prostaglandin E2 and epoxyeicosatrienoic acids, as well as the vasoconstrictor 20-hydroxy-eicosatetraenoic acid, resulting in net vasodilation under physiologic conditions. The main role of NO seems to be the regulation of production of these vasodilators in glial cells.[270]

During systemic hyperoxia, the hyperemic response in the retina is preserved in the rat,[310] but increased in humans.[311] Another potential mechanism involved in neurovascular coupling is the release of K^+ from Müller cells.[312] Nonetheless, potassium ion concentration increased in the vitreous humor close to the ONH as measured with microelectrodes during flicker stimulation in cats.[273] However, K^+ siphoning does not play a role in functional hyperemic response in the retina.[313]

Recently, nanotube-like processes that connect two pericytes with retinal capillaries systems were found to play a role in neurovascular coupling[314] in the retina (Fig. 11.26). These processes have an open-ended proximal side and a closed-ended terminal that connects the pericyte processes via gap junctions. This allows intracellular Ca^{2+} signaling to mediate communication between adjacent pericytes. Pericytes rely on the processes to control neurovascular coupling. A role for caveolin-1 in flicker-induced retinal vasodilation was also established. Caveolin-1 knockout mice show reduced response of ONH blood flow to flicker stimulation (Fig. 11.27).[315]

Endothelial factors

The endothelium plays a key role in regulating vascular tone.[316–318] Arteries, arterioles, capillaries, venules, and veins are lined with endothelial cells. Endothelial cells produce both vasodilators and vasoconstrictors that regulate blood flow. Endothelial dysfunction as observed in diseases such as diabetes alters retinal blood flow and contributes to macro- and microvascular damage.[319,320] Many mechanisms contribute to regulation of vascular tone by endothelial cells.

These can be roughly divided into two main components: release of signaling molecules that modify vascular tone[321,322] and spread of electrical signals from endothelial cells to smooth muscles.[323]

The most important endothelium-derived vasodilator is NO.[324] NO is produced from the amino acid L-arginine via three isoforms of NO synthase (NOS), NOS1, NOS2, and NOS3. NOS1 and NOS3 are constitutive, and NOS2 is inducible, playing an important role in pathologic states that are associated with alteration in the NO system. NO is a small gaseous mediator that can easily diffuse through tissue similar to oxygen. As NO cannot be stored in vivo, it only affects the cells that are in close proximity to the production site. A wide variety of studies have proven that inhibition of NO synthase reduces basal vascular tone in the ocular vasculature (Fig. 11.28).[304,325–331] NO has a wide array of functions in the vasculature of choroid and retina, as well as ONH, and appears to be involved in vascular dysregulation as observed in some diseases.[256,332–334] Other endothelium-derived vasodilators that affect vascular tone include potassium ion[273,309,335,336] and endothelium-derived hyperpolarizing factors that have not been identified so far.[337–339]

Three structurally different endothelin isoforms, endothelin-1, endothelin-2, and endothelin-3 have been identified, with endothelin-1 being one of the most potent vasoconstrictors known.[340,341] Circulating levels of endothelin-1 are low, and its main role is to act as an autocrine/paracrine mediator. Endothelin-1 is a potent endothelium-derived vasoconstrictor that controls vascular tone in many organs, including the eye.[342–351] The vascular effects of endothelin-1 are mediated by tow receptor subtypes called endothelin A and endothelin B receptors. In the eye, endothelin A receptors are localized at blood vessels, whereas endothelin B receptors are mainly found on neural and glial tissues.[352] The endothelin A mediates vasoconstriction, and stimulation of the endothelin B receptor induces vasodilation (Fig. 11.29).

Arachidonic acid metabolites control vascular tone via multiple metabolites[353,354] including prostaglandins, thromboxane A2, and prostacyclin. The majority of receptors that mediate the vasoactive actions of the arachidonic acid metabolites are present at the posterior pole of the eye.[355,356] Ocular levels of prostanoids are higher in the perinatal than in the adult eye[357] indicating an important role of prostaglandins in the regulation of blood flow in newborn animals. As such, prostanoids appear to be involved in the hypoxic processes that lead to retinopathy of prematurity.[357] In the newborn animal, prostanoids

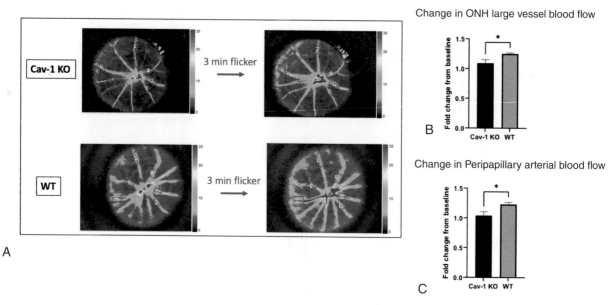

Fig. 11.27 Blood flow changes after 3 min of light flicker stimulus indicate differences in the neurovascular coupling of response of caveolin-1 knockout (*KO*) compared with wild type mice (*WT*). (**A**) Representative LSFG images taken at the optic nerve head in caveolin-1 KO and WT mice. (**B**) Caveolin-1 KO show a lesser increase in large vessel blood flow at the optic nerve head after flicker stimulus, compared with WT. (**C**) Caveolin-1 KO show a lesser increase in peripapillary arterial blood flow after flicker stimulus, compared with WT. *$P < .05$. *ONH*, Optic nerve head. (Reproduced with permission from Loo JH, Lee YS, Woon CY, et al. Loss of caveolin-1 impairs light flicker-induced neurovascular coupling at the optic nerve head. *Front Neurosci* 2021;15:764898.

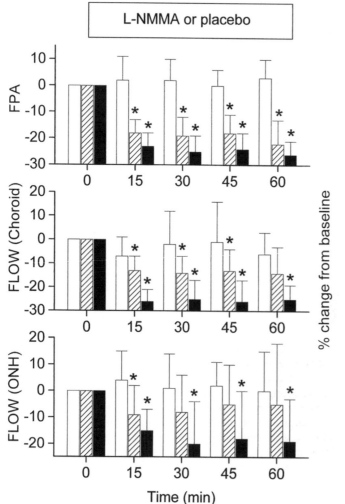

Fig. 11.28 Percent change in fundus pulsation amplitude (*FPA*); blood flow in the choroid (FLOW (choroid)), FLOW (choroid); and blood flow in the optic nerve head (*ONH*), FLOW (ONH) after administration of L-NMMA (*hatched bars*: 3 mg/kg over 5 minutes followed by 30 µg/kg per minute over 55 minutes; *solid bars*: 6 mg/kg over 5 minutes followed by 60 µg/kg per minute over 55 minutes) or placebo (*hollow bars*). Data are presented as mean ± standard deviation ($n = 12$). Asterisks indicate significant effects of L-NMMA versus baseline as calculated from the absolute values. (Reproduced with permission from Luksch A, Polak K, Beier C, et al. Effects of Systemic NO synthase inhibition on choroidal and optic nerve head blood flow in healthy subjects. *Invest Ophthalmol Vis Sci* 2000;41(10):3080–3084.)

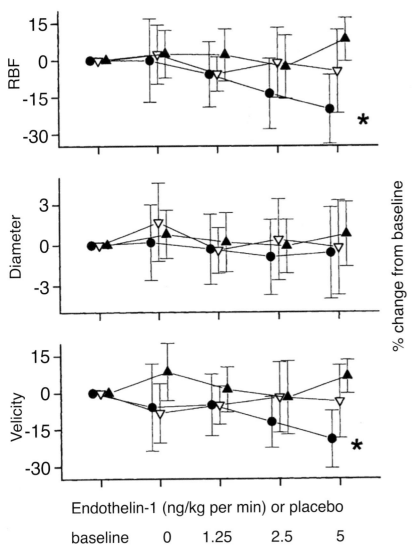

Fig. 11.29 The effect of endothelin-1 and/or the endothelin receptor antagonist BQ-123 infusion on retinal blood flow (*RBF*), retinal *VD*, Venous Diameter, and retinal blood velocity (velocity). Three study days were scheduled for each subject (*n* = 12): endothelin-1/placebo (*solid circles*), placebo/BQ-123 (*solid up triangles*), and endothelin-1/BQ-123 (*open down triangles*). Data are presented as means ± standard deviation. (Reproduced with permission from Polak K, Luksch A, Frank B, Jandrasits K, Polska E, Schmetterer L. Regulation of human retinal blood flow by endothelin-1. Exp Eye Res 2003;76(5):633–640.)

Endothelin-1 (ng/kg per min) or placebo

baseline   0   1.25   2.5   5

play a role in autoregulatory processes.[358] In adults, this effect may be less pronounced, but prostaglandin E2 is produced during an increase in perfusion pressure, partially mediating autoregulatory vasoconstriction.[358] This is, however, controversial because some studies have reported that prostaglandin E2 acts as a potent vasodilator in both the retina and the choroid.[359] Controversial data have also been reported for prostaglandin E1[360,361] and prostaglandin F2α.[362–364] Similar to other vascular beds, thromboxane is a potent vasoconstrictor.[365,366]

Shear stress regulates endothelial function, thereby influencing vascular tone.[367] In large systemic arteries, flow-mediated vasodilation is well established.[368] In smaller vessels, this phenomenon is more difficult to measure because of the lower shear stress levels owing to lower blood velocities and smaller vessel diameters. Techniques to measure flow velocity such as laser Doppler velocimetry allow for calculation of shear stress in retinal arteries based on theoretical velocity profiles.[167,369] Although Doppler OCT technologies allow for measurement of velocity profiles,[125,370,371] this technology has not yet been used to study velocity profiles. High shear stress, as caused by increased retinal blood velocities, compromise the inner blood-retinal barrier function,[372] thereby establishing a link between perfusion abnormalities and leakage as seen in diabetes.[373]

Neural control of blood flow

Owing to the rich innervation of the choroid by parasympathetic, sympathetic, and trigeminal sensory nerves, choroidal blood flow is under neural control.[203] Facial parasympathetic nerves regulate choroidal blood flow, as shown by several animal studies. Mediators such as NO, acetylcholine, and vasoactive intestinal polypeptide (VIP) all cause vasodilation in the ocular vasculature. It has, for instance, been shown that administration of VIP causes an increase in choroidal blood flow.[374] Activation of preganglionic input to the pterygopalatine ganglion by facial nerve stimulation increases choroidal blood flow.[375–377] Direct activation of the superior salivatory nucleus also induces choroidal vasodilation and an increase in blood flow.[378] Centrally mediated autonomic reflexes also play a role in the change of choroidal vascular resistance during changes in blood pressure Fig. 11.30.[379]

The choroid is also innervated by sympathetic noradrenergic nerve fibers that originate from the superior cervical ganglion.[202] The sympathetic neurotransmitter noradrenaline induces pronounced vasoconstriction in the choroid.[380] Cervical sympathetic stimulation causes an increase in choroidal vascular resistance.[378,381,382] The sympathetic input appears to exert a small vasoconstrictor tone in the choroid under basal conditions.[203] The sympathetic input into the choroid

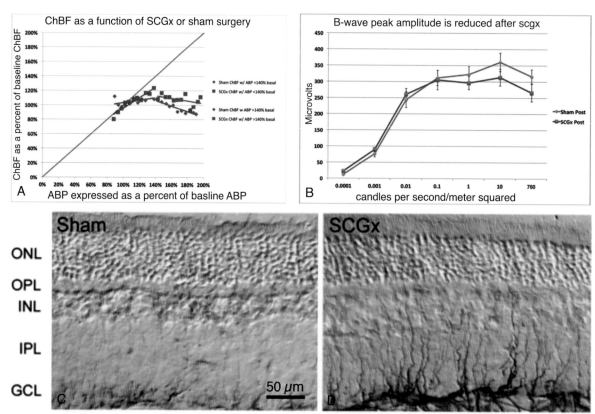

Fig. 11.30 At 2–3 months postsuperior cervical ganglion removal (*SCGx*), choroidal baroregulation during high arterial blood pressure (*ABP*) was impaired. (**A**) shows a plot of choroidal blood flow (*ChBF*) as function of ABP for sham rat eyes (*n* = 14) and superior cervical ganglion removal in rat eyes (*n* = 14). As ABP rapidly rose above baseline after L-NAME administration, ChBF in sham eyes remained relatively stable but followed ABP in superior cervical ganglion removal eyes. After ABP had stabilized at an elevated level, ChBF in superior cervical ganglion removal eyes declined toward baseline but remained elevated compared with sham eyes. The impairment in ChBF baroregulation was associated with a deficit in the flash-evoked scotopic b-wave ERG peak, which was significantly reduced for superior cervical ganglion removal eyes compared with control eyes (**B**). Additionally, Glial Fibrillary Acidic Protein (GFAP) immunolabeling of Müller cells was increased in retina by 3 weeks after superior cervical ganglion removal (**C, D**). The immunolabeled Müller cell processes in superior cervical ganglion removal eyes traversed the IPL and some extended into the INL (**C**). By contrast, in control retinas, GFAP labeling of Müller cell processes did not extend much beyond the GCL (**D**). *GCL*, Ganglion Cell Layer (GCL); *INL*, Inner Nuclear Layer (INL); *IPL*, Inner Plexiform Layer (IPL); *ONL*, Outer Nuclear Layer (ONL); *OPL*, Outer Plexiform Layer (OPL). (Reproduced with permission from Reiner A, Fitzgerald MEC, Del Mar N, Li C. Neural control of choroidal blood flow. *Prog Retin Eye Res* 2018;64:96–130.)

may also regulate choroidal vascular tone during elevated blood pressure, to keep blood flow constant.[383] This is supported by experiments showing that superior cervical ganglion removal impairs choroidal autoregulation during changes in perfusion pressure.[203] Sensory nerve fibers from the trigeminal ganglion also innervate the choroid,[198,384] and have been proposed to be involved in the thermoregulation of choroidal blood flow.[203]

Humoral control of blood flow

Adenosine is a nucleoside which is present in the entire body and exerts strong vasodilator effects.[385] Animal studies have proven that adenosine increases blood flow in newborn piglets,[386] as well as in adult cats.[387] In humans, adenosine increases retinal and choroidal blood flow.[388] The nucleoside is involved in hypoxia-induced vasodilation and retinal autoregulation in newborn animals,[389] but does not modulate the choroidal pressure/flow curve in the human choroid.[390] Recent evidence suggests that the vasoactive effect of adenosine triphosphate differs in vessels at different branching levels.[391,392]

Glucose has important vascular effects impairing endothelium-dependent relaxation.[393,394] In the eye, hyperglycemia induces vasodilator effects in the retina and the choroid.[395–398] In other vascular beds, this vasodilator effect has been attributed to changes in osmotic load.[399] Alternatively, the vasodilator responses to hyperglycemia may be linked to an increased ratio of NADH/NAD+, because of an increased rate of reduction of NAD+ to NADH.[400,401] In the eye, insulin also causes vasodilation[402,403] which is additive to glucose vasodilator action.[397] The increase in choroidal blood flow is reduced after NOS inhibition,[402] and is enhanced by coadministration of L-arginine.[404]

Altered blood flow in ocular disease
Glaucoma

Multiple cross-sectional studies have shown that glaucoma is associated with reduced retinal and ONH blood flow.[405–411] There is a longstanding discussion whether this is cause or consequence of the disease. On one hand it has been argued that a loss of retinal ganglion cells and their axons will result in decreased oxygen demand and capillaries may die as a result of this reduced need. On the other hand, theories have been formulated suggesting that ischemia may promote apoptosis of retinal ganglion cells, thereby increasing the risk of visual field loss.[412,413] Most likely both phenomena are true, because evidence has been accumulated for both mechanisms.

The first hypothesis has been supported by several recent studies indicating a strong spatial association between retinal perfusion and visual field defects (Figs. 11.31 and 11.32).[414–419] The second hypothesis is, however, nowadays supported by a wide variety of studies. Color Doppler imaging studies have shown that low blood velocities in the arteries supplying the ocular vasculature are associated with future Visual field loss does progress.[420–423] These results were confirmed by other studies using either laser Doppler flowmetry,[424] OCT angiography[425,426] or laser speckle flowgraphy (Fig. 11.33).[427,428] Moreover, there is evidence that both high and low blood pressure are risk factors for glaucoma incidence and progression.[429–431] Nocturnal hypotension is also a risk factor for visual field deterioration.[432] Additionally, cardiovascular disease has been identified an important risk factor for glaucoma progression.[433]

Evidence for altered autoregulation in glaucoma has been obtained from multiple studies. Group correlation between blood pressure or OPP and ocular hemodynamic parameters have been reported in multiple studies.[434–438] This correlation is reduced after pharmacologic reduction of IOP, in agreement with the idea that IOP has a main influence on the pressure/flow relationship in the eye.[439]

Multiple studies have reported abnormal blood flow responses to changes in OPP in glaucoma.[212] These studies can be grouped into investigations in which OPP was reduced[440,441] and those in which IOP was increased.[442,443] Evidence has also accumulated that the response to changes in OPP shows a wide variability among glaucoma patients.[241,444] A few studies did not find any difference in the

autoregulatory behavior between glaucoma patients and healthy controls, but the change in OPP induced in these studies was most likely too small to reach the lower or upper limit of autoregulation.[445–447] Abnormal autoregulation was also shown by a study investigating the variations of ONH blood flow during diurnal variations in OPP.[448]

Altered autoregulation in glaucoma is linked to pericyte dysfunction and loss of interpericyte tunneling nanotubes.[449] In addition, it has been shown that reduced ganglion cell thickness in healthy subjects is associated with both high blood pressure and abnormal blood flow autoregulation, which may make this group of subjects more susceptible to glaucomatous damage.[450] This is also compatible with findings in a nonhuman primate model indicating that abnormal autoregulation is a consequence of ganglion cell loss.[451]

A reduced hyperemic response to stimulation with diffuse luminance flicker has been consistently reported using several techniques to assess blood flow.[452–456] This is compatible with results showing an abnormal oxygenation response to flicker stimulation in glaucoma patients.[457] One study did not report a difference between flicker-evoked blood flow changes, as measured with laser speckle flowgraphy, in glaucoma patients compared with healthy controls, but the study was most likely underpowered.[458] A longitudinal study did not find an association between reduced functional hyperemia and structural progression in glaucoma patients, but again the number of included patients and the duration of follow up was too low to draw any meaningful conclusions.[459] Glaucoma has also been associated with endothelial dysfunction[460] and changes in the endothelin system.[461–464] Evidence for endothelial dysfunction has been obtained from systemic,[465–470] as well as ocular, vascular stimulation tests.[471] Dual inhibition of endothelin receptors increases ocular blood flow in patients with glaucoma.[472] In patients with pseudoexfoliation glaucoma, an accumulation of

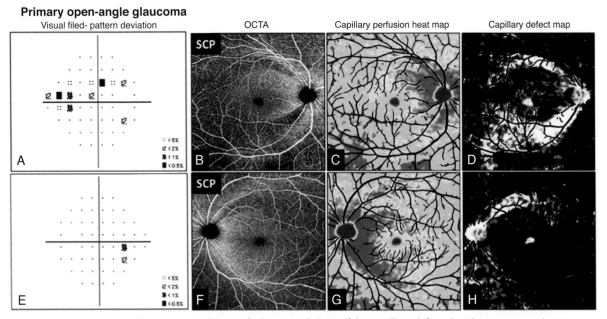

Primary open-angle glaucoma

Visual filed- pattern deviation | OCTA | Capillary perfusion heat map | Capillary defect map

Fig. 11.31 Use of normative capillary perfusion maps in quantifying capillary defects in primary open-angle glaucoma (POAG) eyes. (**A, E**) Visual fields in Primary Open-Angle Glaucoma (POAG). (**B, F**) 12 × 12-mm optical coherence tomography angiography (*OCTA*) images in POAG eyes (male, age: 38, Signal Strength Index (SSI), Superficial Capillary Plexus (SCP): 10). The original grayscale OCTA images (**B, F**) were processed to create capillary perfusion maps (**C, G**). Their comparisons with age-matched normative capillary maps (**D, H**) showed both the loci and severities of the capillary defects. (Reproduced with permission from Tan B, Sim YC, Chua J, et al., Developing a normative database for retinal perfusion using optical coherence tomography angiography. *Biomed Opt Exp* 2021;12(7):4032–4045. © The Optical Society.)

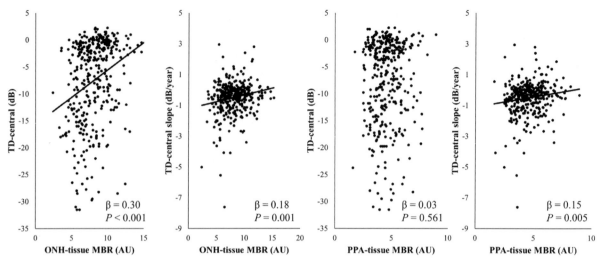

Fig. 11.32 Scatterplots showing comparisons between temporal optic nerve head (ONH)–tissue mean blur rate (MBR) and temporal peripapillary chorioretinal atrophy (PPA)–tissue MBR, total deviation (TD)–central, and TD–central slope in patients with glaucoma. Temporal ONH–tissue MBR was positively correlated with both TD–central and TD–central slope (ß = 0.30, $P < .001$; ß = 0.18, $P < .001$, respectively). Temporal PPA–tissue MBR was correlated only with TD–central slope, not with TD–central (ß = 0.15, $P < .005$; ß = 0.03, $P = .561$; respectively). *AU,* Arbitrary units. (Wong D, Chua J, Lin E, et al. Focal structure–function relationships in primary open-angle glaucoma using OCT and OCT-A measurements. *Invest Ophthalmol Vis Sci.* 2020;61(14):33–33.)

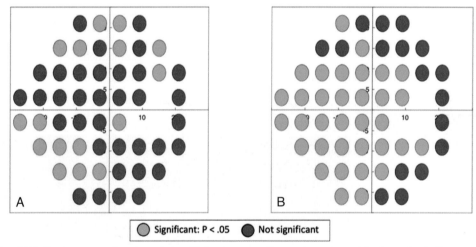

Fig. 11.33 Focal structure-function relationship in glaucoma. Factors from the multivariate mixed-effects modeling at test points from the 24-2 visual field (VF) for (**A**) focal retinal nerve fiber layer (FNL) thickness and (**B**) focal capillary perfusion density (FCL). *Green* indicates a test location in which the corresponding parameter was significantly associated with VF loss. Locations nearer fixation (0 degrees, 0 degrees) were more significantly influenced by Focal Capillary Density (FCD) than FNL thickness. Correlations for nasal VF test locations were poor for both FNL thickness and FCD. One VF test location at eccentricity (9 degrees, –3 degrees) was excluded due to the limited arc of the FNL thickness defined by the trajectories for that location. (Kiyota N, Shiga Y, Takahashi N, et al. Progression in open-angle glaucoma with myopic disc and blood flow in the optic nerve head and peripapillary chorioretinal atrophy zone. *Ophthalmol Glaucoma* 2020;3(3):202–209.)

pseudoexfoliative microfibrillar material leads to vascular endothelial dysfunction.[473]

Diabetes and diabetic retinopathy

Retinal vascular changes are well documented in diabetes and DR, including dysfunction of the blood-retinal barrier associated with the development of diabetic macular edema.[474] Other key features include vascular basement membrane thickening[475] and a progressive loss of

pericytes and vascular endothelial cells.[476] During the course of this disease, vasodegeneration occurs, which is clinically seen as vascular dropout.[477] This capillary dropout and the retinal ischemia triggers the release of growth factors including vascular endothelial growth factors (VEGF), which then leads to proliferative DR.

There are conflicting results of whether retinal blood flow is increased or decreased in early stages of DR[35,396,398,478–486] or animal models of DR.[396,487] This may be related to differences in the technology used to assess blood flow, but also due to different phenotypes. In this respect, it is important to mention that both insulin and glucose may influence the results, owing to their vasodilator actions.

OCTA has enabled the study of important aspects of vascular alterations in diabetes and DR.[488–494] Features that can be studied with OCTA include microaneurysms, neovascularization, peripheral retinal nonperfusion, and FAZ alterations, as well as quantitative changes in perfusion and vessel density. Wide-field OCTA is nowadays the preferred method to identify peripheral capillary nonperfusion (Fig. 11.34).[495–498] Interestingly, wide-field OCTA has also been shown to provide improved detection of retinal neovascularization that is not detected clinically.[499–502] Quantitative OCTA metrics predict the risk of DR progression and may therefore add to traditional risk factors in the management of DR.[503]

OCTA can also be used to study choroidal changes in diabetes. Significant loss of choriocapillaris has been described histologically,[504,505] but in vivo studies on choroidal blood flow in diabetes have been sparse.[506] Analysis of OCTA slabs has again proven that pronounced vascular changes are present in the diabetic choroid.[507–512] It has been shown that retina inflammatory processes appear to trigger endothelial cell damage in the choroid.[513] Nevertheless, the role of the choroid and its blood flow in the development and progression of DR remains poorly understood.

Diabetes is characterized by abnormal retinal and ONH vascular autoregulation.[514–517] The mechanism underlying this effect is not well characterized. Obviously, loss of perictyes,[518] as well as endothelial dysfunction, are candidates[256,519] for being involved in the loss of autoregulation. Uncoupling of gap junctions is also a candidate mechanism for disrupting the autoregulation.[520]

Functional hyperemia is reduced in the diabetic retina in a stage-dependent manner (Fig. 11.35).[521–528] Correlation between reduced blood flow responses to flicker stimulation and endothelial dysfunction has been observed in diabetes.[529,530] Interestingly, experimentally induced hyperglycemia also impacts neurovascular coupling

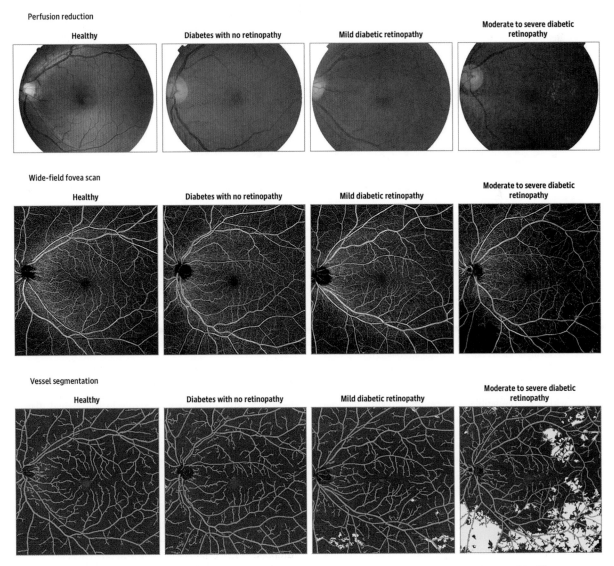

Fig. 11.34 Representative wide-field optical coherence tomography angiography images of eyes with different diabetic retinopathy severities. Larger retinal vessels are segmented in *green*, areas of nonperfusion in *yellow*. (Reproduced with permission from Tan B, Chua J, Lin E, et al. Quantitative microvascular analysis with wide-field optical coherence tomography angiography in eyes with diabetic retinopathy. *JAMA Netw Open* 2020;3(1):e1919469–e1919469.)

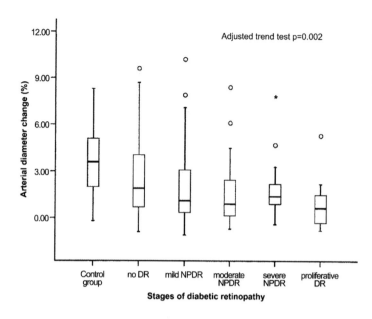

Fig. 11.35 Arterial diameter changes in response to stimulation with diffuse luminance flicker at different stages of diabetic retinopathy (DR). *NPDR*, Non-Proliferative Diabetic Retinopathy. (Reproduced with permission from Mandecka A, Dawczynski J, Blum M, et al. Influence of flickering light on the retinal vessels in diabetic patients. *Diabetes Care* 2007;30(12):3048–3052.)

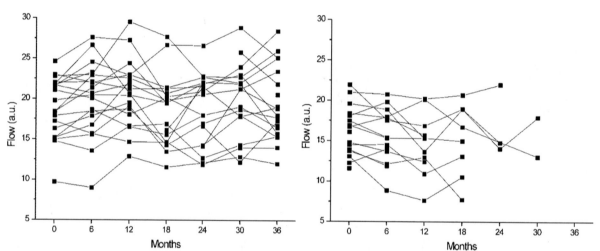

Fig. 11.36 Time course of choroidal blood flow (*FLOW*) during the 36-month observation period. *Left*, the patients with no choroidal neovascularization (CNV) in the study eye; *right*: the patients with CNV. The development of CNV was the end point, after which no further measurements were obtained. (Reproduced with permission from Boltz A, Luksch A, Wimpissinger B, et al., Choroidal blood flow and progression of age-related macular degeneration in the fellow eye in patients with unilateral choroidal neovascularization. *Invest Ophthalmol Vis Sci* 2010;51(8):4220–4225.)

in the retina,[531] which is compatible with results showing reduced flicker-induced retinal vascular reactivity in subjects with impaired glucose tolerance.[532] Abnormal retinal neurovascular coupling has also been observed in animal models of DR elucidating some of the mechanisms underlying this effect.[533–535] Upregulation of NOS2 in retinal neurons and glial cells appears to play an important role in changing neurovascular coupling in diabetes. The mechanism for the NO-induced reduction in neurovascular coupling is believed to include the blockade of production of vasoactive factors released from Müller cells.[536] This mechanism is supported by results showing that the NOS2 inhibitor aminoguanidine restores neurovascular coupling in the diabetic rat retina.[534]

Endothelial dysfunction is a key feature of diabetes[320,537,538] and can also be detected at the level of the ocular vasculature.[332,539,540] Alterations in the endothelial surface layer, specifically in the glycocalyx, also seem to play a role in the retinal distribution of red blood cells, explaining reduced blood flow in the deep capillary plexus.[541]

Age-related macular degeneration

Hypoxia and ischemia have been implicated in the pathophysiology of age-related macular degeneration to trigger angiogenesis and interplay with inflammation.[542] This is supported by studies that have associated hypoxia-inducible transcription factors (HIFs) with choroidal neovascularization (CNV).[543] As expected, choroidal blood flow is reduced in age-related macular degeneration.[480,544–548] Patients with age-related macular degeneration (AMD) also show abnormal choroidal autoregulation.[549] With increasing severity of the disease, choroidal blood flow gradually decreases.[550,551] Low choroidal blood flow has been shown to be a risk factor for the development of CNV

(Fig. 11.36).[552–554] A relationship between delayed patchy choroidal filling and pseudodrusen was also shown.[555]

Choroidal vascularity index is defined as the ratio of vascular area to the total choroidal area in OCT images.[556] Choroidal vascularity index was consistently found to be lower in AMD eyes compared with healthy eyes.[557–559] The parameter is associated with the rate of geographic atrophy enlargement in patients with AMD.[560,561]

With the introduction of OCTA, our understanding of disease progression has increased.[127] Evidence has accumulated that ischemic features of the choriocapillaris are related to the progression of early AMD, CNV, and geographic atrophy. Eyes with unilateral type 3 CNV show more pronounced choriocapillaris nonperfusion areas compared with nonexudative fellow eyes.[562] This is in agreement with other findings showing that CNV vascular complexity is correlated with choriocapillaris flow deficits adjacent to the CNV area.[563,564]

Locally there is a large overlap between areas of macular atrophy and areas of choriocapillaris dropout in AMD.[565] More importantly, abnormalities in choriocapillaris perfusion in the macular area contribute to disease progression in eyes with geographic atrophy (Fig. 11.37).[566–570] This is compatible with histologic studies showing that choriocapillaris breakdown precedes retinal degeneration.[571] In addition, choriocapillaris flow deficits predict the development and enlargement of drusen.[572]

Systemic disease

Systemic hypertension is a risk factor for major age-related eye diseases including AMD,[573] DR,[574] and glaucoma.[575] As such, it is thought that high blood pressure amplifies perfusion problems that are associated with these diseases. As expected, ONH blood flow autoregulation is altered in patients with systemic hypertension (Fig. 11.38).[576] Given the mechanisms of autoregulation as described in Fig. 11.17, one would assume that the upper limit of autoregulation will be reached earlier if the starting point is shifted toward higher levels. OCTA studies have revealed that hypertension is associated with microvascular changes in both the choroid and the retina (Fig. 11.39).[577–586].

Ocular perfusion defects have also been detected in neurodegenerative diseases of the brain. Two studies have reported that retinal venular narrowing is associated with Alzheimer's disease.[587,588] In addition, these studies investigated parameters such as fractal dimensions, tortuosity, and branching, and reported associations with the disease. One study reported reduced retinal blood flow and oxygen extractions

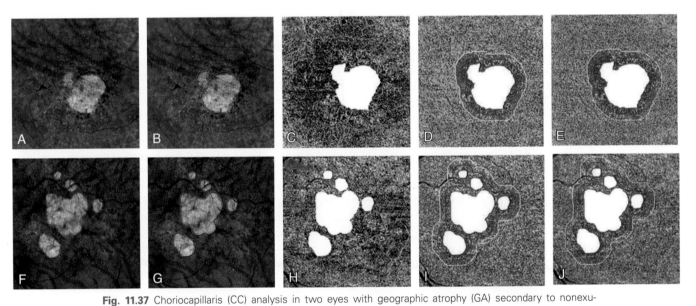

Fig. 11.37 Choriocapillaris (CC) analysis in two eyes with geographic atrophy (GA) secondary to nonexudative age-related macular degeneration, imaged using swept source optical coherence tomography angiography at the baseline visit using 6 × 6-mm scan patterns. (**A**, **F**) GA lesions identified as a bright area on en-face structure images using a custom slab from 64 μm to 400 μm under Bruch's membrane (BM) at the baseline visit from two eyes. (**B**, **G**) Manually outlined GA lesions at the baseline visits for the two eyes *(red outlines)*. (**C**, **H**) CC en-face flow images using a 15-μm thick slab with inner boundary located 4 μm under BM. The area of GA is masked as *white* and was excluded from CC analysis. (**D**, **I**) CC flow deficits (FDs) analyzed in different regions when using a global threshold method. *White*: The area of GA lesions excluded from CC FDs analysis. *R1*: CC FDs were colored coded as *red* in R1 region extending from 0 μm to 300-μm outside of GA border. *R2*: CC FDs are colored coded as *purple* in R2 region extending from >300 μm–600 μm outside of GA border. *R3*: CC FDs are colored coded as *green* in the R3 region corresponding to the total scan region minus the GA region, R1 and R2. (**E**, **J**) CC FDs analyzed in different regions when using a local threshold method (Phansalkar method with a window radius of 3 pixels = 18 μm). *White*: The area of GA lesions which were excluded from CC FDs analysis. *R1*: CC FDs are colored coded as *red* CC FDs in R1 region extending from 0 μm to 300 μm outside of GA border. *R2*: CC FDs are colored coded as *purple* in R2 region extending from >300 μm to 600 μm outside of GA border. *R3*: CC FDs are color coded as *green* in the R3 region corresponding to the total scan region minus the GA region, R1 and R2. (Reproduced with permission from Shi Y, Zhang Q, Zhou H, et al., Correlations between choriocapillaris and choroidal measurements and the growth of geographic atrophy using swept source OCT imaging. *Am J Ophthalmol* 2021;224: 321–331.)

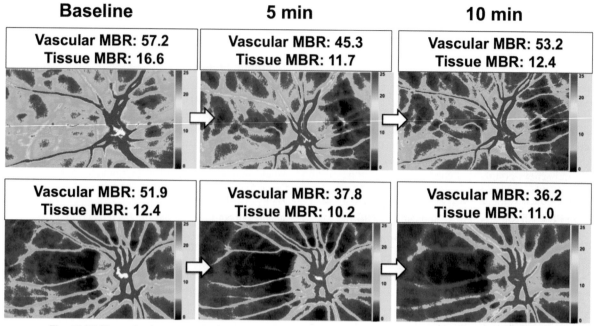

Fig. 11.38 Illustrative laser speckle flowgraphy images from subjects in control, hypertension, and hyperlipidemia groups. *Top*: Laser speckle flowgraphy color maps of optic nerve head (ONH) blood flow obtained during vitreous surgery to treat an epiretinal membrane in a 67-year-old woman without systemic disorders. The images shown were obtained at baseline and 5 and 10 min after the elevation of intraocular pressure by approximately 15 mmHg. The vascular and tissue mean blur rates (*MBRs*) are presented in the upper panels of each figure part. *Bottom*: Laser speckle flowgraphy color maps of ONH blood flow obtained in a 69-year-old woman with hypertension and hyperlipidemia during vitreous surgery to treat a macular hole. (Reproduced with permission from Hashimoto R, Sugiyama T, Ubuka M, Maeno T. Impairment of autoregulation of optic nerve head blood flow during vitreous surgery in patients with hypertension and hyperlipidemia. *Graefe's Arch Clin Exp Ophthalmol* 2017;255(11):2227–2235.)

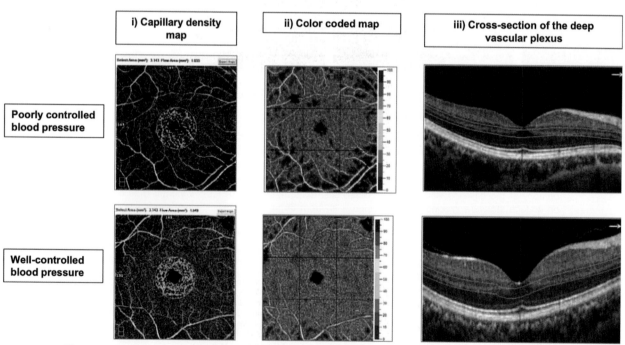

Fig. 11.39 Capillary density map of the macular region showing retinal microvasculature of participants with poorly controlled blood pressure (*less dense)* and well controlled blood pressure (*more dense)*. (1) Capillary density extracted map with a circular (diameter of 1.0 mm centered on the fovea) measurement region defined. (2) Capillary density color-coded map. *(iii)* Deep vascular plexus (slab boundary of 15- to 70-mm below the inner plexiform layer). (Reproduced with permission from Chua J, Loon Chin CW, Hong J, et al. Impact of hypertension on retinal capillary microvasculature using optical coherence tomographic angiography. *J Hypertens* 2019;37(3):572–580.)

Superficial capillary plexus   Deep capillary plexus

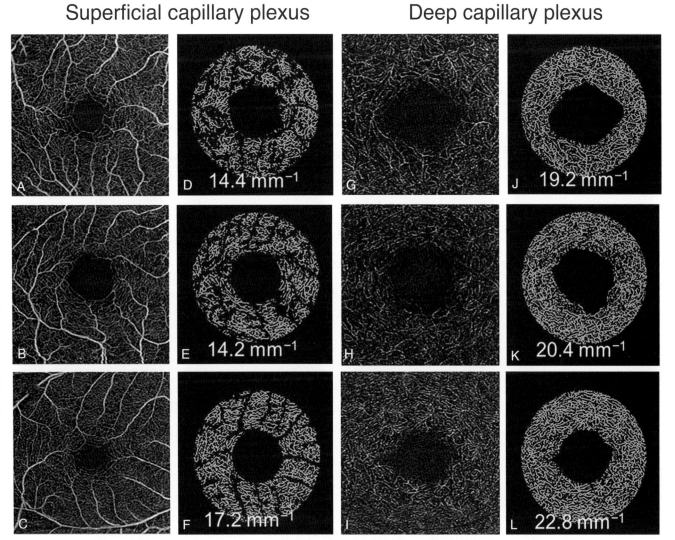

Fig. 11.40 Optical coherence tomography angiography (OCTA) images of the superficial (**A–C**) and deep (**G–I**) capillary plexuses were extracted from the OCTA machines. (**D–F, J–L**)Vessel density maps of the macular annulus region showing retinal microvasculature of participants with Alzheimer's disease (AD; **D, J**), mild cognitive impairment (MCI; **E, K**), and controls (**F, L**). AD participants showed a decrease in vessel densities in both plexuses compared with controls. MCI participants showed a decrease in vessel density only in the superficial capillary plexus and not the deep capillary plexus. (Reproduced with permission from Chua J, Hu Q, Ke M, et al. Retinal microvasculature dysfunction is associated with Alzheimer's disease and mild cognitive impairment. *Alzheimers Res Ther* 2020;12(1):161.)

in patients with Alzheimer's disease in line with OCT angiography findings.[589] In the longitudinal Rotterdam Study, however, retinal vascular features were not associated with incident dementia.[590] Multiple studies using OCTA have detected retinal microvascular changes in Alzheimer's disease and mild cognitive impairment (Fig. 11.40).[591–598] In multiple sclerosis, the pattern appears to be more complex, because increased and decreased blood flow in the retina have been indicated.[599–605] This may be related to the level of inflammation in these patients, which may cause vasodilation and counteract the state of vasoconstriction that is usually associated with neurodegenerative diseases.

REFERENCES

1. Dorner GT, Polska E, Garhöfer G, Zawinka C, Frank B, Schmetterer L. Calculation of the diameter of the central retinal artery from noninvasive measurements in humans. *Current Eye Research*. 2002:341–345.

2. Pemp B, Cherecheanu AP, Garhofer G, Schmetterer L. Calculation of central retinal artery diameters from non-invasive ocular haemodynamic measurements in type 1 diabetes patients. *Acta Ophthalmologica*. 2013:1755–3768. (Electronic).

3. Baldoncini M, Campero A, Moran G, et al. Microsurgical anatomy of the central retinal artery. *World Neurosurgery*. 2019;130:e172–e187.

4. Arthur E, Elsner AE, Sapoznik KA, Papay JA, Muller MS, Burns SA. Distances from capillaries to arterioles or venules measured using OCTA and AOSLO. *Investigative Ophthalmology & Visual Science*. 2019;60(6):1833–1844.

5. Balaratnasingam C, An D, Sakurada Y, et al. Comparisons between histology and optical coherence tomography angiography of the periarterial capillary-free zone. *American Journal of Ophthalmology*. 2018;189:55–64.

6. Okada S, Ohta Y. Microvascular architecture of the retina in the Japanese monkey (Macaca fuscata fuscata). *Anthropological Science*. 1994;102(Supplement):139–153.

7. Chan G, Balaratnasingam C, Yu PK, et al. Quantitative morphometry of perifoveal capillary networks in the human retina. *Investigative Ophthalmology & Visual Science*. 2012;53(9):5502–5514.

8. Henkind P. Radial peripapillary capillaries of the retina. I. Anatomy: human and comparative. *British Journal of Ophthalmology*. 1967;51(2):115.

9. Yu PK, Cringle SJ, Yu D-Y. Correlation between the radial peripapillary capillaries and the retinal nerve fibre layer in the normal human retina. *Experimental Eye Research*. 2014;129:83–92.

10. Snodderly DM, Weinhaus RS, Choi JC. Neural-vascular relationships in central retina of macaque monkeys (Macaca fascicularis). *The Journal of Neuroscience*. 1992;12(4):1169.

11. Pournaras CJ, Rungger-Brändle E, Riva CE, Hardarson SH, Stefansson E. Regulation of retinal blood flow in health and disease. *Prog Retin Eye Res*. 2008;27(3):284–330.

12. Lutty G.A., Bhutto I., McLeod D.S. Anatomy of the ocular vasculatures. In: Schmetterer L, Kiel JW, eds. *Ocular Blood Flow*; 20123–21.

13. Chan-Ling T, Koina ME, McColm JR, et al. Role of CD44+ stem cells in mural cell formation in the human choroid: evidence of vascular instability due to limited pericyte vv. *Investigative Ophthalmology & Visual Science*. 2011;52(1):399–410.

14. Hayreh SS. The blood supply of the optic nerve head and the evaluation of it — myth and reality. *Progress in Retinal and Eye Research*. 2001;20(5):563–593.

15. Linsenmeier RA, Zhang HF. Retinal oxygen: from animals to humans. *Prog Retin Eye Res*. 2017;58:115–151.

16. Linsenmeier RA, Braun RD. Oxygen distribution and consumption in the cat retina during normoxia and hypoxemia. *Journal of General Physiology*. 1992;99(2):177–197.

17. Braun RD, Linsenmeier RA. Retinal oxygen tension and the electroretinogram during arterial occlusion in the cat. *Investigative Ophthalmology & Visual Science*. 1995;36(3):523–541.

18. Wrinkler BS. A quantitative assessment of glucose metabolism in the isolated rat retina. In: Christen Y, Doly M, Droy-Lefaix MT, eds. *Les Seminaires Ophtalmologiques D'ipsen*. New York: Elsevier Science; 1995:78–96.

19. Haugh-Scheidt LM, Griff ER, Linsenmeier RA. Light-evoked oxygen responses in the isolated toad retina. *Experimental Eye Research*. 1995;61(1):73–81.

20. Riva CE, Grunwald JE, Sinclair SH, Petrig BL. Blood velocity and volumetric flow rate in human retinal vessels. *Investigative Ophthalmology & Visual Science*. 1985;26(8):1124–1132.

21. Doblhoff-Dier V, Schmetterer L, Vilser W, et al. Measurement of the total retinal blood flow using dual beam Fourier-domain Doppler optical coherence tomography with orthogonal detection planes. *Biomedical Optics Express*. 2014;5(2):630–642.

22. Garhofer G, Werkmeister R, Dragostinoff N, Schmetterer L. Retinal blood flow in healthy young subjects. *Invest Ophthalmol Vis Sci*. 2012;53(2):698–703.

23. Tan O, Liu G, Liang L, et al. En face Doppler total retinal blood flow measurement with 70 kHz spectral optical coherence tomography. *Journal of Biomedical Optics*. 2015;6:066004.

24. Baumann B, Potsaid B, Kraus MF, et al. Total retinal blood flow measurement with ultrahigh speed swept source/Fourier domain OCT. *Biomed Opt Express*. 2011;2(6):1539–1552.

25. Haindl R, Trasischker W, Wartak A, Baumann B, Pircher M, Hitzenberger CK. Total retinal blood flow measurement by three beam Doppler optical coherence tomography. *Biomedical Optics Express*. 2016;7(2):287–301.

26. Warner RL, Gast TJ, Sapoznik KA, Carmichael-Martins A, Burns SA. Measuring temporal and spatial variability of red blood cell velocity in human retinal vessels. *Investigative Ophthalmology & Visual Science*. 2021;62(14):29–29.

27. Pappelis K, Choritz L, Jansonius NM. Microcirculatory model predicts blood flow and autoregulation range in the human retina: in vivo investigation with laser speckle flowgraphy. *American Journal of Physiology. Heart and Circulatory Physiology*. 2020;319(6):H1253–H1273.

28. Bata AM, Fondi K, Szegedi S, et al. Age-related decline of retinal oxygen extraction in healthy subjects. *Investigative Ophthalmology & Visual Science*. 2019;60(8):3162–3169.

29. Lasta M, Palkovits S, Boltz A, et al. Reproducibility of retinal vessel oxygen saturation measurements in healthy young subjects. *Acta Ophthalmologica*. 2012;90(8):e616–e620.

30. Geirsdottir A, Palsson O, Hardarson SH, Olafsdottir OB, Kristjansdottir JV, Stefánsson E. Retinal vessel oxygen saturation in healthy individuals. *Investigative Ophthalmology & Visual Science*. 2012;53(9):5433–5442.

31. Jani PD, Mwanza JC, Billow KB, Waters AB, Moyer S, Garg S. Normative values and predictors of retinal oxygen saturation. *Retina*. 2014;34(2):394–401.

32. Stefánsson E, Olafsdottir OB, Eliasdottir TS, et al. Retinal oximetry: metabolic imaging for diseases of the retina and brain. *Prog Retin Eye Res*. 2019;70:1–22.

33. Wang J, Song W, Sadlak N, Fiorello MG, Desai M, Yi J. A baseline study of oxygen saturation in parafoveal vessels using visible light optical coherence tomography. *Frontiers in Medicine*. 2022;9:1–7.

34. Werkmeister RM, Schmidl D, Aschinger G, et al. Retinal oxygen extraction in humans. *Scientific Reports*. 2015;5(1):15763.

35. Fondi K, Wozniak PA, Howorka K, et al. Retinal oxygen extraction in individuals with type 1 diabetes with no or mild diabetic retinopathy. *Diabetologia*. 2017;60(8):1534–1540.

36. Alm A, Bill A. Ocular and optic nerve blood flow at normal and increased intraocular pressures in monkeys (Macaca irus): a study with radioactively labelled microspheres including flow determinations in brain and some other tissues. *Experimental Eye Research*. 1973;15(1):15–29.

37. Yang YC, Hulbert MF, Batterbury M, Clearkin LG. Pulsatile ocular blood flow measurements in healthy eyes: reproducibility and reference values. *Journal of Glaucoma*. 1997;6(3):175–179.

38. Silver DM, Farrell RA, Langham ME, O'Brien V, Schilder P. Estimation of pulsatile ocular blood flow from intraocular pressure. *Acta Ophthalmologica*. 1989;67(S191):25–29.

39. Berisha F, Findl O, Lasta M, Kiss B, Schmetterer L. A study comparing ocular pressure pulse and ocular fundus pulse in dependence of axial eye length and ocular volume. *Acta Ophthalmologica*. 2010;88(7):766–772.

40. Alm A, Bill A. The oxygen supply to the retina, I. Effects of changes in intraocular and arterial blood pressures, and in arterial PO2 and PCO2 on the oxygen tension in the vitreous body of the cat. *Acta Physiologica Scandinavica*. 1972;84(2):261–274.

41. Schmidl D, Schmetterer L, Garhöfer G, Popa-Cherecheanu A. Gender differences in ocular blood flow. *Current Eye Research*. 2015;40(2):201–212.

42. Schmetterer L, Garhofer G. How can blood flow Be measured? *Survey of Ophthalmology*. 2007;52(6):S134–S138.

43. Schmetterer L, Kiel JW. *Ocular blood flow*. Berlin, Heidelberg: Springer; 2012.

44. Granstam E, Granstam SO. Regulation of uveal and retinal blood flow in STZ-diabetic and non-diabetic rats; involvement of nitric oxide. *Current Eye Research*. 1999;19(4):330–337.

45. Nilsson SFE, Alm A. Determination of ocular blood flows with the microsphere method, in Ocular Blood Flow. In: Schmetterer L, Kiel J, eds. *Berlin, Heidelberg*. Berlin Heidelberg: Springer; 2012:25–47.

46. Nork TM, Kim CBY, Shanmuganayagam D, Van Lysel MS, Ver Hoeve JN, Folts JD. Measurement of regional choroidal blood flow in rabbits and monkeys using fluorescent microspheres. *Archives of Ophthalmology*. 2006;124(6):860–868.

47. Shih Y-YI, Wang L, De La Garza BH, et al. Quantitative retinal and choroidal blood flow during light, dark adaptation and flicker light stimulation in rats using fluorescent microspheres. *Current Eye Research*. 2013;38(2):292–298.

48. Wang L, Fortune B, Cull G, McElwain KM, Cioffi GA. Microspheres method for ocular blood flow measurement in rats: Size and dose optimization. *Experimental Eye Research*. 2007;84(1):108–117.

49. Told R, Wang L, Cull G, et al. Total retinal blood flow in a nonhuman primate optic nerve transection model using dual-beam bidirectional Doppler FD-OCT and microsphere method. *Investigative Ophthalmology & Visual Science*. 2016;57(3):1432–1440.

50. Yu DY, Alder VA, Cringle SJ. Measurement of blood flow in rat eyes by hydrogen clearance. *The American Journal of Physiology*. 1991;261(3):H960–H968.

51. Stefánsson E, Wagner HG, Seida M. Retinal blood flow and its autoregulation measured by intraocular hydrogen clearance. *Experimental Eye Research*. 1988;47(5):669–678.

52. Sugiyama T, Utsumi T, Azuma I, Fujii H. Measurement of optic nerve head circulation: comparison of laser speckle and hydrogen clearance methods. *Japanese Journal of Ophthalmology*. 1996;40(3):339–343.

53. Alder VA, Yu D-Y, Cringle SJ. Vitreal oxygen tension measurements in the rat eye. *Experimental Eye Research*. 1991;52(3):293–299.

54. Pournaras CJ, Tsacopoulos M, Strommer K, Gilodi N, Leuenberger PM. Experimental retinal branch vein occlusion in miniature pigs induces local tissue hypoxia and vasoproliferative microangiopathy. *Ophthalmology*. 1990;97(10):1321–1328.

55. Yu DY, Cringle SJ, Alder VA. The response of rat vitreal oxygen tension to stepwise increases in inspired percentage oxygen. *Investigative Ophthalmology & Visual Science*. 1990;31(12):2493–2499.

56. Birol G, Wang S, Budzynski E, Wangsa-Wirawan ND, Linsenmeier RA. Oxygen distribution and consumption in the macaque retina. *American Journal of Physiology. Heart and Circulatory Physiology*. 2007;293(3):H1696–H1704.

57. Pournaras CJ, Riva CE, Tsacopoulos M, Strommer K. Diffusion of O2 in the retina of anesthetized miniature pigs in normoxia and hyperoxia. *Experimental Eye Research*. 1989;49(3):347–360.

58. Ahmed J, Linsenmeier RA, Dunn R. The oxygen distribution in the prelaminar optic nerve head of the cat. *Experimental Eye Research*. 1994;59(4):457–466.

59. Cour Ml, Kiilgaard J, Eysteinsson T, et al. Optic nerve oxygen tension: effects of intraocular pressure and dorzolamide. *British Journal of Ophthalmology*. 2000;84(9):1045.

60. Pedersen DB, Stefánsson E, Kiilgaard JF, et al. Optic nerve pH and PO2: the effects of carbonic anhydrase inhibition, and metabolic and respiratory acidosis. *Acta Ophthalmologica Scandinavica*. 2006;84(4):475–480.

61. Ben-Sira I, Riva CE, Roberts W. Fluorophotometric recording of fluorescein dilution curves in human retinal vessels. *Investigative Ophthalmology & Visual Science*. 1973;12(4):310–312.

62. Jung F, Kiesewetter H, Körber N, Wolf S, Reim M, Müller G. Quantification of characteristic blood-flow parameters in the vessels of the retina with a picture analysis system for video-fluorescence angiograms: initial findings. *Graefe's Archive for Clinical and Experimental Ophthalmology*. 1983;221(3):133–136.

63. Wolf S, Arend O, Reim M. Measurement of retinal hemodynamics with scanning laser ophthalmoscopy: Reference values and variation. *Survey of Ophthalmology*. 1994;38:S95–S100.

64. Duijm HFA, Rulo AH, Astin M, Mäepea O, van den Berg TJ, Greve EL. Study of choroidal blood flow by comparison of SLO fluorescein angiography and microspheres. *Experimental Eye Research*. 1996;63(6):693–704.

65. Gabel VP, Birngruber R, Nasemann J. The scanning laser ophthalmoscope and its use as a fluorescein angiography instrument. *Fortschritte Ophthalmologie: Zeitschrift der Deutschen Ophthalmologischen Gesellschaft*. 1988:0723–8045. (Print).

66. Arend O, Wolf S, Jung F, et al. Retinal microcirculation in patients with diabetes mellitus: dynamic and morphological analysis of perifoveal capillary network. *British Journal of Ophthalmology*. 1991;75(9):514.

67. Hitchings RA, Spaeth GL. Fluorescein angiography in chronic simple and low-tension glaucoma. *British Journal of Ophthalmology*. 1977;61(2):126.

68. Riva CE, Feke GT, Ben-Sira I. Fluorescein dye-dilution technique and retinal circulation. *The American Journal of Physiology*. 1978;234(3):H315–H322.

69. Preußner PR, Richard G, Darrelmann O, Weber J, Kreissig I. Quantitative measurement of retinal blood flow in human beings by application of digital image-processing methods to television fluorescein angiograms. *Graefe's Archive for Clinical and Experimental Ophthalmology*. 1983;221(3):110–112.

70. Funatsu H, Sakata K, Harino S, Okuzawa Y, Noma H, Hori S. Tracing method in the assessment of retinal capillary blood flow velocity by fluorescein angiography with scanning laser ophthalmoscope. *Japanese Journal of Ophthalmology*. 2006;50(1):25–32.

71. Noma H, Funatsu H, Sakata K, Harino S, Mimura T, Hori S. Macular microcirculation in hypertensive patients with and without branch retinal vein occlusion. *Acta Ophthalmologica*. 2009;87(6):638–642.

72. Sun C, Wang JJ, Mackey DA, Wong TY. Retinal vascular caliber: systemic, environmental, and genetic associations. *Survey of Ophthalmology*. 2009;54(1):74–95.

73. Ikram MK, Ong YT, Cheung CY, Wong TY. Retinal vascular caliber measurements: clinical significance, current knowledge and future perspectives. *Ophthalmologica*. 2013;229(3):125–136.

74. Guo S, Yin S, Tse G, Li G, Su L, Liu T. Association between caliber of retinal vessels and cardiovascular disease: a systematic review and meta-analysis. *Current Atherosclerosis Reports*. 2020;22(4):16.

75. Knudtson MD, Lee KE, Hubbard LD, Wong TY, Klein R, Klein BEK. Revised formulas for summarizing retinal vessel diameters. *Current Eye Research*. 2003;27(3):143–149.

76. Heitmar R, Kalitzeos AA, Panesar V. Comparison of two formulas used to calculate summarized retinal vessel calibers. *Optometry and Vision Science*. 2015;92(11).
77. Garhofer G, Bek T, Boehm AG, et al. Use of the retinal vessel analyzer in ocular blood flow research. *Acta Ophthalmologica*. 2010;88(7):717–722.
78. Heitmar R, Blann AD, Cubbidge RP, Lip GYH, Gherghel D. Continuous retinal vessel diameter measurements: the future in retinal vessel assessment? *Invest Ophthalmol Vis Sci*. 2010;51(11):5833–5839.
79. Ding J, Wai KL, McGeechan K, et al. Retinal vascular caliber and the development of hypertension: a meta-analysis of individual participant data. *Journal of Hypertension*. 2014;32(2).
80. Riva C, Ross B, Benedek GB. Laser Doppler measurements of blood flow in capillary tubes and retinal arteries. *Investigative Ophthalmology*. 1972;11(11):936–944.
81. Tanaka T, Riva C, Ben-Sira I. Blood velocity measurements in human retinal vessels. *Science*. 1974;186(4166):830–831.
82. Riva CE, Feke GT, Eberli B, Benary V. Bidirectional LDV system for absolute measurement of blood speed in retinal vessels. *Applied Optics*. 1979;18(13):2301–2306.
83. Riva CE, Grunwald JE, Sinclair SH, O'Keefe K. Fundus camera based retinal LDV. *Applied Optics*. 1981;20(1):117–120.
84. Bonner RF, Nossal R. In: Shepherd AP, Öberg PA, eds. *Principles of laser Doppler flowmetry, in Laser-Doppler blood flowmetry*. Boston: Kluwer Academic Publishers; 1990:57–72.
85. Riva CE, Harino S, Petrig BL, Shonat RD. Laser Doppler flowmetry in the optic nerve. *Experimental Eye Research*. 1992;55(3):499–506.
86. Riva CE, Cranstoun SD, Grunwald JE, Petrig BL. Choroidal blood flow in the foveal region of the human ocular fundus. *Investigative Ophthalmology & Visual Science*. 1994;35(13):4273–4281.
87. Polska E, Luksch A, Ehrlich P, Sieder A, Schmetterer L. Measurements in the peripheral retina using LDF and laser interferometry are mainly influenced by the choroidal circulation. *Current Eye Research*. 2002;24(4):318–323.
88. Michelson G, Schmauss B. Two dimensional mapping of the perfusion of the retina and optic nerve head. *British Journal of Ophthalmology*. 1995;79(12):1126.
89. Kiel JW, Shepherd AP. Autoregulation of choroidal blood flow in the rabbit. *Invest Ophthalmol Vis Sci*. 1992;33(8):2399–2410.
90. Koss MC. Role of nitric oxide in maintenance of basal anterior choroidal blood flow in rats. *Investigative Ophthalmology & Visual Science*. 1998;39(3):559–564.
91. Strohmaier C, Werkmeister RM, Bogner B. A novel, microscope based, non-invasive laser Doppler flowmeter for choroidal blood flow assessment. *Experimental Eye Research*. 2011;92(6):545–551.
92. Williamson TH, Harris A. Color Doppler ultrasound imaging of the eye and orbit. *Survey of Ophthalmology*. 1996;40(4):255–267.
93. Dimitrova G, Kato S. Color Doppler imaging of retinal diseases. *Survey of Ophthalmology*. 2010;55(3):193–214.
94. Stalmans I, Vandewalle E, Anderson DR, et al. Use of colour Doppler imaging in ocular blood flow research. *Acta Ophthalmologica*. 2011;89(8):e609–e630.
95. Polska E, Kircher K, Ehrlich P, Vecsei PV, Schmetterer L. RI in central retinal artery as assessed by CDI does not correspond to retinal vascular resistance. *American Journal of Physiology. Heart and Circulatory Physiology*. 2001;280(4):H1442–H1447.
96. Briers JD, Fercher AF. Retinal blood-flow visualization by means of laser speckle photography. *Investigative Ophthalmology & Visual Science*. 1982;22(2):255–259.
97. Tamaki Y, Araie M, Kawamoto E, Eguchi S, Fujii H. Noncontact, two-dimensional measurement of retinal microcirculation using laser speckle phenomenon. *Investigative Ophthalmology & Visual Science*. 1994;35(11):3825–3834.
98. Tamaki Y, Araie M, Kawamoto E, Eguchi S, Fujii H. Non-contact, two-dimensional measurement of tissue circulation in choroid and optic nerve head using laser speckle phenomenon. *Experimental Eye Research*. 1995;60(4):373–383.
99. Sugiyama T, Araie M, Riva CE, Schmetterer L, Orgul S. Use of laser speckle flowgraphy in ocular blood flow research. *Acta Ophthalmologica*. 2010;88(7):723–729.
100. Luft N, Wozniak PA, Aschinger GC, et al. Ocular blood flow measurements in healthy white subjects using laser speckle flowgraphy. *PLOS ONE*. 2016;11(12):e0168190.
101. Briers D, Duncan DD, Hirst E, et al. Laser speckle contrast imaging: theoretical and practical limitations. *Journal of Biomedical Optics*. 2013;18(6):066018.
102. Aizawa N, Nitta F, Kunikata H, et al. Laser speckle and hydrogen gas clearance measurements of optic nerve circulation in albino and pigmented rabbits with or without optic disc atrophy. *Investigative Ophthalmology & Visual Science*. 2014;55(12):7991–7996.
103. Isono H, Kimura Y, Aoyagi K, Fujii H, Konishi N. Analysis of choroidal blood flow by laser speckle flowgraphy. *Nippon Ganka Gakkai zasshi*. 1997;101(8):684–691.
104. Kobayashi T, Shiba T, Okamoto K, Usui T, Hori Y. Characteristics of laterality in the optic nerve head microcirculation obtained by laser speckle flowgraphy in healthy subjects. *Graefe's Archive for Clinical and Experimental Ophthalmology*. 2022:1–7.
105. Enomoto N, Anraku A, Tomita G, et al. Characterization of laser speckle flowgraphy pulse waveform parameters for the evaluation of the optic nerve head and retinal circulation. *Scientific Reports*. 2021;11(1):6847.
106. Luft N, Wozniak PA, Aschinger GC, et al. Measurements of retinal perfusion using laser speckle flowgraphy and Doppler optical coherence tomography. *Investigative Ophthalmology & Visual Science*. 2016;57(13):5417–5425.
107. Leitgeb RA, Werkmeister RM, Blatter C, Schmetterer L. Doppler optical coherence tomography. *Progress in Retinal and Eye Research*. 2014;41:26–43.
108. Chen Z, Milner TE, Dave D, Nelson JS. Optical Doppler tomographic imaging of fluid flow velocity in highly scattering media. *Optics Letters*. 1997;22(1):64–66.
109. White BR, Pierce MC, Nassif N, et al. In vivo dynamic human retinal blood flow imaging using ultra-high-speed spectral domain optical Doppler tomography. *Optics Express*. 2003;11(25):3490–3497.
110. Leitgeb RA, Schmetterer L, Drexler W, Fercher A, Zawadzki R, Bajraszewski T. Real-time assessment of retinal blood flow with ultrafast acquisition by color Doppler Fourier domain optical coherence tomography. *Optics Express*. 2003;11(23):3116–3121.
111. Leitgeb RA, Schmetterer L, Hitzenberger CK, et al. Real-time measurement of in vitro flow by Fourier-domain color Doppler optical coherence tomography. *Optics Letters*. 2004;29(2):171–173.
112. Pedersen CJ, Huang D, Shure MA, Rollins AM. Measurement of absolute flow velocity vector using dual-angle, delay-encoded Doppler optical coherence tomography. *Optics Letters*. 2007;32(5):506–508.
113. Werkmeister RM, Dragostinoff N, Pircher M, et al. Bidirectional Doppler Fourier-domain optical coherence tomography for measurement of absolute flow velocities in human retinal vessels. *Optics Letters*. 2008;33(24):2967–2969.
114. Dai C, Liu X, Zhang HF, Puliafito CA, Jiao S. Absolute retinal blood flow measurement with a dual-beam doppler optical coherence tomography. *Investigative Ophthalmology & Visual Science*. 2013;54(13):7998–8003.
115. Szegedi S, Hommer N, Kallab M, et al. Repeatability and reproducibility of total retinal blood flow measurements using bi-directional doppler OCT. *Translational Vision Science & Technology*. 2020;9(7):34–34.
116. Trasischker W, Werkmeister RM, Zotter S, et al. In vitro and in vivo three-dimensional velocity vector measurement by three-beam spectral-domain Doppler optical coherence tomography. *Journal of Biomedical Optics*. 2013;18(11):116010.
117. Blatter C, Coquoz S, Grajciar, et al. Dove prism based rotating dual beam bidirectional Doppler OCT. Biomedical. *Optics Express*. 2013;4(7):1188–1203.
118. Hosseinaee Z, Tan B, Martinez A, Bizheva KK. Comparative study of optical coherence tomography angiography and phase-resolved doppler optical coherence tomography for measurement of retinal blood vessels caliber. *Translational Vision Science & Technology*. 2018;7(4):18–18.
119. Fondi K, Aschinger GC, Bata AM. Measurement of retinal vascular caliber from optical coherence tomography phase images. *Investigative Ophthalmology & Visual Science*. 2016;57(9):OCT121–OCT129.
120. Blatter C, Bower BA, Izatt JA, Tan O, Huang D. Angle independent flow assessment with bidirectional Doppler optical coherence tomography. *Optics Letters*. 2013;38(21):4433–4436.
121. Wang Y, Yusof F, Vymyslicky M. In vivo total retinal blood flow measurement by Fourier domain Doppler optical coherence tomography. *Journal of Biomedical Optics*. 2007;4:041215.
122. Tayyari F, Song YS, Yoshioka T. Variability and repeatability of quantitative, fourier-domain optical coherence tomography Doppler blood flow in young and elderly healthy subjects. *Investigative Ophthalmology & Visual Science*. 2014;55(12):7716–7725.
123. Tani T, et al. Repeatability and reproducibility of retinal blood flow measurement using a doppler optical coherence tomography flowmeter in healthy subjects. *Investigative Ophthalmology & Visual Science*. 2017;58(7):2891–2898.
124. Nam AS, Braaf B, Vakoc BJ. Using the dynamic forward scattering signal for optical coherence tomography based blood flow quantification. *Optics Letters*. 2022;47(12):3083–3086.
125. Aschinger GC, Schmetterer L, Doblhoff-Dier V, et al. Blood flow velocity vector field reconstruction from dual-beam bidirectional Doppler OCT measurements in retinal veins. *Biomed Opt Express*. 2015;6(5):1599–1615.
126. Wartak A, Beer F, Desissaire S, Baumann B, Pircher M, Hitzenberger CK. Investigating spontaneous retinal venous pulsation using Doppler optical coherence tomography. *Scientific Reports*. 2019;9(1):4237.
127. Spaide RF, Fujimoto JG, Waheed NK, Sadda SR, Staurenghi G. Optical coherence tomography angiography. *Progress in Retinal and Eye Research*. 2018;64:1–55.
128. Kashani AH, Chen CL, Gahm JK, et al. Optical coherence tomography angiography: A comprehensive review of current methods and clinical applications. *Progress in Retinal and Eye Research*. 2017;60:66–100.
129. Ang M, Tan ACS, Cheung CMG, et al. Optical coherence tomography angiography: a review of current and future clinical applications. *Graefe's Archive for Clinical and Experimental Ophthalmology*. 2018;256(2):237–245.
130. Chen C-L, Wang RK. Optical coherence tomography based angiography [Invited]. *Biomedical Optics Express*. 2017;8(2):1056–1082.
131. Makita S, Hong Y, Yamanari M, Yatagai T, Yasuno Y. Optical coherence angiography. *Optics Express*. 2006;14(17):7821–7840.
132. Jia Y, Tan O, Tokayer J, et al. Split-spectrum amplitude-decorrelation angiography with optical coherence tomography. *Optics Express*. 2012;20(4):4710–4725.
133. An L, Wang RK. In vivo volumetric imaging of vascular perfusion within human retina and choroids with optical micro-angiography. *Optics Express*. 2008;16(15):11438–11452.
134. Spaide RF, Fujimoto JG, Waheed NK. Image artifacts in optical coherence tomography angiography. *Retina*. 2015;35(11):2163–2180.
135. Ang M, Baskaran M, Werkmeister RM, et al. Anterior segment optical coherence tomography. *Progress in Retinal and Eye Research*. 2018;66:132–156.
136. Lee WD, Devarajan K, Chua J, Schmetterer L, Mehta JS, Ang M. Optical coherence tomography angiography for the anterior segment. *Eye and Vision*. 2019;6(1):4.
137. Siddiqui Y, Yin J. Anterior segment applications of optical coherence tomography angiography. *Seminars in Ophthalmology*. 2019;34(4):264–269.
138. Tan B, Sim R, Chua J, et al. Approaches to quantify optical coherence tomography angiography metrics. *Annals of Translational Medicine*. 2020;8(18):1205.
139. Yao X, Alam MN, Le D, Toslak D. Quantitative optical coherence tomography angiography: a review. *Experimental Biology and Medicine*. 2020;245(4):301–312.
140. Corvi F, Pellegrini M, Erba S, Cozzi M, Staurenghi G, Giani A. Reproducibility of vessel density, fractal dimension, and foveal avascular zone using 7 different optical coherence tomography angiography devices. *American Journal of Ophthalmology*. 2018;186:25–31.
141. Chu Z, Lin J, Gao C, et al. Quantitative assessment of the retinal microvasculature using optical coherence tomography angiography. *Journal of Biomedical Optics*. 2016;6:066008.
142. Spaide RF. Choriocapillaris flow features follow a power law distribution: implications for characterization and mechanisms of disease progression. *American Journal of Ophthalmology*. 2016;170:58–67.
143. Tan B, Chua J, Barathi VA, et al. Quantitative analysis of choriocapillaris in non-human primates using swept-source optical coherence tomography angiography (SS-OCTA). *Biomedical Optics Express*. 2019;10(1):356–371.

144. Bennett AG, Rudnicka AR, Edgar DF. Improvements on Littmann's method of determining the size of retinal features by fundus photography. *Graefe's Archive for Clinical and Experimental Ophthalmology*. 1994;232(6):361–367.
145. Hickam JB, Frayser R, RJ C. A study of retinal venous blood oxygen saturation in human subjects by photographic means. *Circulation*. 1963;27(3):375–385.
146. Beach JM, Schwenzer KJ, Srinivas S, Kim D, Tiedeman JS. Oximetry of retinal vessels by dual-wavelength imaging: calibration and influence of pigmentation. *Journal of Applied Physiology*. 1999;86(2):748–758.
147. Hardarson SH, Harris A, Karlsson RA, et al. Automatic retinal oximetry. *Investigative Ophthalmology & Visual Science*. 2006;47(11):5011–5016.
148. Shughoury A, Mathew S, Arciero J, et al. Retinal oximetry in glaucoma: investigations and findings reviewed. *Acta Ophthalmologica*. 2020;98(6):559–571.
149. Traustason S, Jensen AS, Arvidsson HS, Munch IC, Søndergaard L, Larsen M. Retinal oxygen saturation in patients with systemic hypoxemia. *Investigative Ophthalmology & Visual Science*. 2011;52(8):5064–5067.
150. Palkovits S, Lasta M, Boltz A, et al. Measurement of retinal oxygen saturation in patients with chronic obstructive pulmonary disease. *Investigative Ophthalmology & Visual Science*. 2013;54(2):1008–1013.
151. Hammer M, Vilser W, Riemer T, Schweitzer D. Retinal vessel oximetry-calibration, compensation for vessel diameter and fundus pigmentation, and reproducibility. *Journal of Biomedical Optics*. 2008;5:054015.
152. Jeppesen SK, Bek T. The retinal oxygen saturation measured by dual wavelength oximetry in larger retinal vessels is influenced by the linear velocity of the blood. *Current Eye Research*. 2019;44(1):46–52.
153. Johnson W, Wilson DW, Fink W, Humayun M, Bearman G. Snapshot hyperspectral imaging in ophthalmology. *Journal of Biomedical Optics*. 2007;1:014036.
154. Desjardins M, Sylvestre JP, Jafari R, et al. Preliminary investigation of multispectral retinal tissue oximetry mapping using a hyperspectral retinal camera. *Experimental Eye Research*. 2016;146:330–340.
155. Kaluzny J, Li H, Liu W, et al. Bayer filter snapshot hyperspectral fundus camera for human retinal imaging. *Current Eye Research*. 2017;42(4):629–635.
156. Shahidi AM, Hudson C, Tayyari F, Flanagan JG. Retinal oxygen saturation in patients with primary open-angle glaucoma using a non-flash hypespectral camera. *Current Eye Research*. 2017;42(4):557–561.
157. DePaoli DT, Tossou P, Parent M, Sauvageau D, Côté DC. Convolutional neural networks for spectroscopic analysis in retinal oximetry. *Scientific Reports*. 2019;9(1):11387.
158. Chen S, Shu X, Nesper PL, Liu W, Fawzi AA, Zhang HF. Retinal oximetry in humans using visible-light optical coherence tomography [Invited]. *Biomedical Optics Express*. 2017;8(3):1415–1429.
159. Pi S, Hormel TT, Wei X, Jia Y. Retinal capillary oximetry with visible light optical coherence tomography. *Proceedings of the National Academy of Sciences of the United States of America*. 2020;117(21):11658–11666.
160. Akitegetse C, Landry P, Robidoux J, Lapointe N, Brouard D, Sauvageau D. Monte-Carlo simulation and tissue-phantom model for validation of ocular oximetry. *Biomedical Optics Express*. 2022;13(5):2929–2946.
161. Fallon TJ, Maxwell DL, Kohner EM. Autoregulation of retinal blood flow in diabetic retinopathy measured by the blue-light entoptic technique. *Ophthalmology*. 1987;94(11):1410–1415.
162. Strenn K, Menapace R, Rainer G, Findl O, Wolzt M, Schmetterer L. Reproducibility and sensitivity of scanning laser Doppler flowmetry during graded changes in PO2. *British Journal of Ophthalmology*. 1997;81(5):360.
163. Cheng RW, Yusof F, Tsui E, et al. Relationship between retinal blood flow and arterial oxygen. *The Journal of Physiology*. 2016;594(3):625–640.
164. Rose K, Kulasekara SI, Hudson C. Intervisit repeatability of retinal blood oximetry and total retinal blood flow under varying systemic blood gas oxygen saturations. *Investigative Ophthalmology & Visual Science*. 2016;57(1):188–197.
165. Enroth-Cugell C, Goldstick TK, Linsenmeier RA. The contrast sensitivity of cat retinal ganglion cells at reduced oxygen tensions. *The Journal of Physiology*. 1980;304(1):59–81.
166. Palkovits S, Told R, Schmidl D, et al. Regulation of retinal oxygen metabolism in humans during graded hypoxia. *American Journal of Physiology. Heart and Circulatory Physiology*. 2014;307(10):H1412–H1418.
167. Nagaoka T, Sakamoto T, Mori F, Sato E, Yoshida A. The effect of nitric oxide on retinal blood flow during hypoxia in cats. *Investigative Ophthalmology & Visual Science*. 2002;43(9):3037–3044.
168. Kringelholt S, Holmgaard K, Bek T. Relaxation of porcine retinal arterioles during acute hypoxia in vitro depends on prostaglandin and NO synthesis in the perivascular retina. *Current Eye Research*. 2013;38(9):965–971.
169. Kiss B, Polska E, Dorner G, et al. Retinal blood flow during hyperoxia in humans revisited: concerted results using different measurement techniques. *Microvascular Research*. 2002;64(1):75–85.
170. Werkmeister RM, Palkovits S, Told R, et al. Response of retinal blood flow to systemic hyperoxia as measured with dual-beam bidirectional Doppler fourier-domain optical coherence tomography. *PLOS ONE*. 2012;7(9):e45876.
171. Gilmore ED, Hudson C, Preiss D, Fisher J. Retinal arteriolar diameter, blood velocity, and blood flow response to an isocapnic hyperoxic provocation. *American Journal of Physiology. Heart and Circulatory Physiology*. 2005;288(6):H2912–H2917.
172. Harris A, Anderson DR, Pillunat L, et al. Laser Doppler flowmetry measurement of changes in human optic nerve head blood flow in response to blood gas perturbations. *Journal of glaucoma*. 1996;5(4):258–265.
173. Riva CE, Pournaras CJ, Tsacopoulos M. Regulation of local oxygen tension and blood flow in the inner retina during hyperoxia. *Journal of Applied Physiology*. 1986;61(2):592–598.
174. Pechauer AD, Jia Y, Liu L, Gao SS, Jiang C, Huang D. Optical coherence tomography angiography of peripapillary retinal blood flow response to hyperoxia. *Investigative Ophthalmology & Visual Science*. 2015;56(5):3287–3291.
175. Xu H, Deng G, Jiang C, Kong X, Yu J, Sun X. Microcirculatory responses to hyperoxia in macular and peripapillary regions. *Investigative Ophthalmology & Visual Science*. 2016;57(10):4464–4468.
176. Hommer N, Kallab M, Sim YC, et al. Effect of hyperoxia and hypoxia on retinal vascular parameters assessed with optical coherence tomography angiography. *Acta Ophthalmologica*. 2021:1–8.
177. Zhu YUN, Park TS, Gidday JM. Mechanisms of hyperoxia-induced reductions in retinal blood flow in newborn pig. *Experimental Eye Research*. 1998;67(3):357–369.
178. Song Y, Nagaoka T, Yoshioka T, et al. Glial endothelin-1 regulates retinal blood flow during hyperoxia in cats. *Investigative Ophthalmology & Visual Science*. 2016;57(11):4962–4969.
179. Dallinger S, Dorner GT, Wenzel R, et al. Endothelin-1 contributes to hyperoxia-induced vasoconstriction in the human retina. *Investigative Ophthalmology & Visual Science*. 2000;41(3):864–869.
180. Takagi C, King GL, Takagi H, Lin YW, Clermont AC, Bursell SE. Endothelin-1 action via endothelin receptors is a primary mechanism modulating retinal circulatory response to hyperoxia. *Investigative Ophthalmology & Visual Science*. 1996;37(10):2099–2109.
181. Schmetterer L, Dallinger S, Findl O, Graselli U, Eichler HG, Wolzt M. A comparison between laser interferometric measurement of fundus pulsation and pneumotonometric measurement of pulsatile ocular blood flow 2. Effects of changes in pCO2 and pO2 and of isoproterenol. *Eye*. 2000;14(1):46–52.
182. Schmetterer L, Lexer F, Findl O, Graselli U, Eichler HG, Wolzt M. The effect of inhalation of different mixtures of O2 and CO2 on ocular fundus pulsations. *Exp Eye Res*. 1996;63(4):351–355.
183. Geiser MH, Riva CE, Dorner GT, Diermann U, Luksch A, Schmetterer L. Response of choroidal blood flow in the foveal region to hyperoxia and hyperoxia-hypercapnia. *Current Eye Research*. 2000;21(2):669–676.
184. Kergoat Hln, Faucher C. Effects of oxygen and carbogen breathing on choroidal hemodynamics in humans. *Investigative Ophthalmology & Visual Science*. 1999;40(12):2906–2911.
185. Gallice M, Zhou T, Aptel F, et al. Hypoxic, hypercapnic, and hyperoxic responses of the optic nerve head and subfoveal choroid blood flow in healthy humans. *Investigative Ophthalmology & Visual Science*. 2017;58(12):5460–5467.
186. Linsenmeier RA, Yancey CM. Effects of hyperoxia on the oxygen distribution in the intact cat retina. *Investigative Ophthalmology & Visual Science*. 1989;30(4):612–618.
187. Palkovits S, Lasta M, Told R, et al. Retinal oxygen metabolism during normoxia and hyperoxia in healthy subjects. *Investigative Ophthalmology & Visual Science*. 2014;55(8):4707–4713.
188. Venkataraman ST, Hudson C, Fisher JA, Flanagan JG. The impact of hypercapnia on retinal capillary blood flow assessed by scanning laser Doppler flowmetry. *Microvascular Research*. 2005;69(3):149–155.
189. Shahidi AM, Patel SR, Huang D, Tan O, Flanagan JG, Hudson C. Assessment of total retinal blood flow using Doppler Fourier Domain Optical Coherence Tomography during systemic hypercapnia and hypocapnia. *Physiological Reports*. 2014;2(7):e12046.
190. Dorner GT, Garhoefer G, Zawinka C, Kiss B, Schmetterer L. Response of retinal blood flow to CO2-breathing in humans. *European Journal of Ophthalmology*. 2002;12(6):459–466.
191. Schmetterer L, Wolzt M, Lexer F, et al. The effect of hyperoxia and hypercapnia on fundus pulsations in the macular and optic disc region in healthy young men. *Experimental Eye Research*. 1995;61(6):685–690.
192. Luksch A, Garhöfer G, Imhof A, et al. Effect of inhalation of different mixtures of O2 and CO2 on retinal blood flow. *British Journal of Ophthalmology*. 2002;86(10):1143.
193. Kontos HA, Raper AJ, Patterson JL. Analysis of vasoactivity of local pH, PCO2 and bicarbonate on pial vessels. *Stroke*. 1977;8(3):358–360.
194. Faraci FM, Taugher RJ, Lynch C, Fan R, Gupta S, Wemmie JA. Acid-sensing ion channels. *Circulation Research*. 2019;125(10):907–920.
195. Okamoto H, Hudetz AG, Roman RJ, Bosnjak ZJ, Kampine JP. Neuronal NOS-derived NO plays permissive role in cerebral blood flow response to hypercapnia. *The American Journal of Physiology*. 1997;272(1):H559–H566.
196. Iadecola C, Zhang F. Permissive and obligatory roles of NO in cerebrovascular responses to hypercapnia and acetylcholine. *The American Journal of Physiology*. 1996;271(4):R990–R1001.
197. Schmetterer L, Findl O, Strenn K, et al. Role of NO in the O2 and CO2 responsiveness of cerebral and ocular circulation in humans. *The American Journal of Physiology*. 1997;273(6):R2005–R2012.
198. McDougal DH, Gamlin PD. Autonomic control of the eye, in Comprehensive. *Physiology*. 2015:439–473.
199. Bek T. Is lack of autonomic nerves in retinal vessels a protection from electrical stimulation generated by activity in visual neurons? *Acta Ophthalmologica*. 2018;96(2):e263–e263.
200. Bergua A, Kapsreiter M, Neuhuber WL, Reitsamer HA, Schrödl F. Innervation pattern of the preocular human central retinal artery. *Experimental Eye Research*. 2013;110:142–147.
201. Klooster J, Beckers HJ, Tusscher MPT, Vrensen GF, van der Want JJ, Lamers WP. Sympathetic innervation of the rat choroid: an autoradiographic tracing and immunohistochemical study. *Ophthalmic Research*. 1996;28(1):36–43.
202. Lütjen-Drecoll E. Choroidal innervation in primate eyes. *Experimental Eye Research*. 2006;82(3):357–361.
203. Reiner A, Fitzgerald MEC, Del Mar N, Li C. Neural control of choroidal blood flow. *Prog Retin Eye Res*. 2018;64:96–130.
204. Meyer-Schwickerath R, Kleinwächter T, Firsching R, Papenfuss HD. Central retinal venous outflow pressure. *Graefe's Archive for Clinical and Experimental Ophthalmology*. 1995;233(12):783–788.
205. Stodtmeister R, Wetzk E, Herber R, Pillunat KR, Pillunat LE. Measurement of the retinal venous pressure with a new instrument in healthy subjects. *Graefe's Archive for Clinical and Experimental Ophthalmology*. 2022;260(4):1237–1244.
206. Lo L, Zhao D, Ayton L, et al. *Non-invasive measurement of intracranial pressure through application of venous ophthalmodynamometry. in 2021 43rd Annual International Conference of the IEEE Engineering in Medicine & Biology Society (EMBC)*. 2021.

207. Morgan WH, Hazelton ML, Yu D-Y. Retinal venous pulsation: expanding our understanding and use of this enigmatic phenomenon. *Progress in Retinal and Eye Research.* 2016;55:82–107.

208. Costa VP, Harris A, Anderson D, et al. Ocular perfusion pressure in glaucoma. *Acta Ophthalmologica.* 2014;92(4):e252–e266.

209. Leske MC. Ocular perfusion pressure and glaucoma: clinical trial and epidemiologic findings. *Current Opinion in Ophthalmology.* 2009;20(2):73.

210. Grover DS, Budenz DL. Ocular perfusion pressure and glaucoma. *International Ophthalmology Clinics.* 2011;51(3):19–25.

211. Schmidl D, Werkmeister R, Garhöfer G, Schmetterer L. Der okuläre perfusionsdruck und seine bedeutung für das glaukom. *Klin Monbl Augenheilkd.* 2015;232(02):141–146.

212. Schmidl D, Garhofer G, Schmetterer L. The complex interaction between ocular perfusion pressure and ocular blood flow – Relevance for glaucoma. *Experimental Eye Research.* 2011;93(2):141–155.

213. Glucksberg MR, Dunn R. Direct measurement of retinal microvascular pressures in the live, anesthetized cat. *Microvascular Research.* 1993;45(2):158–165.

214. Mäepea O. Pressures in the anterior ciliary arteries, choroidal veins and choriocapillaris. *Experimental Eye Research.* 1992;54(5):731–736.

215. Claassen JAHR, Thijssen DHJ, Panerai RB, Faraci FM. Regulation of cerebral blood flow in humans: physiology and clinical implications of autoregulation. *Physiological Reviews.* 2021;101(4):1487–1559.

216. Barabas P, Augustine J, Fernández JA, McGeown JG, McGahon MK, Curtis TM. In: Jackson WF, ed. *Chapter Seven - Ion channels and myogenic activity in retinal arterioles, in Current Topics in Membranes.* Academic Press; 2020:187–226.

217. Faraci FM, Baumbach GL, Heistad DD. Myogenic mechanisms in the cerebral circulation. Journal of hypertension. *Supplement: official journal of the International Society of Hypertension.* 1989;7(4):S61–S64.

218. Knot HJ, Nelson MT. Regulation of membrane potential and diameter by voltage-dependent K+ channels in rabbit myogenic cerebral arteries. *The American Journal of Physiology.* 1995;269(1):H348–H355.

219. Welsh DG, Morielli AD, Nelson MT, Brayden JE. Transient receptor potential channels regulate myogenic tone of resistance arteries. *Circulation Research.* 2002;90(3):248–250.

220. Wu X, Davis MJ. Characterization of stretch-activated cation current in coronary smooth muscle cells. *American Journal of Physiology. Heart and Circulatory Physiology.* 2001;280(4):H1751–H1761.

221. Kur J, Bankhead P, Scholfield CN, Curtis TM, McGeown JG. Ca2+ sparks promote myogenic tone in retinal arterioles. *British Journal of Pharmacology.* 2013;168(7):1675–1686.

222. Kur J, McGahon MK, Fernández JA, Scholfield CN, McGeown JG, Curtis TM. Role of ion channels and subcellular Ca2+ signaling in arachidonic acid–induced dilation of pressurized retinal arterioles. *Investigative Ophthalmology & Visual Science.* 2014;55(5):2893–2902.

223. McGahon MK, Fernández JA, Dash DP, et al. TRPV2 channels contribute to stretch-activated cation currents and myogenic constriction in retinal arterioles. *Investigative Ophthalmology & Visual Science.* 2016;57(13):5637–5647.

224. Thébault S. Minireview: Insights into the role of TRP channels in the retinal circulation and function. *Neuroscience Letters.* 2021;765:136285.

225. Garhöfer G, Zawinka C, Huemer KH, Schmetterer L, Dorner GT. Flicker light–induced vasodilatation in the human retina: effect of lactate and changes in mean arterial pressure. *Investigative Ophthalmology & Visual Science.* 2003;44(12):5309–5314.

226. Robinson F, Riva CE, Grunwald JE, Petrig BL, Sinclair SH. Retinal blood flow autoregulation in response to an acute increase in blood pressure. *Investigative Ophthalmology & Visual Science.* 1986;27(5):722–726.

227. Dumskyj MJ, Eriksen JE, Doré CJ, Kohner EM. Autoregulation in the human retinal circulation: assessment using isometric exercise, laser Doppler velocimetry, and computer-assisted image analysis. *Microvascular Research.* 1996;51(3):378–392.

228. Witkowska KJ, Bata AM, Calzetti G, et al. Optic nerve head and retinal blood flow regulation during isometric exercise as assessed with laser speckle flowgraphy. *PLOS ONE.* 2017;12(9):e0184772.

229. Riva CE, Grunwald JE, Petrig BL. Autoregulation of human retinal blood flow. An investigation with laser Doppler velocimetry. *Investigative Ophthalmology & Visual Science.* 1986;27(12):1706–1712.

230. Puchner S, Schmidl D, Ginner L, et al. Changes in retinal blood flow in response to an experimental increase in IOP in healthy participants as assessed with Doppler optical coherence tomography. *Invest Ophthalmol Vis Sci.* 2020;61(2):33–33.

231. Kiel JW. Choroidal myogenic autoregulation and intraocular pressure. *Experimental Eye Research.* 1994;58(5):529–543.

232. Kiel JW, van Heuven WA. Ocular perfusion pressure and choroidal blood flow in the rabbit. *Investigative Ophthalmology & Visual Science.* 1995;36(3):579–585.

233. Riva CE, Titze P, Hero M, Petrig BL. Effect of acute decreases of perfusion pressure on choroidal blood flow in humans. *Investigative Ophthalmology & Visual Science.* 1997;38(9):1752–1760.

234. Schmidl D, Boltz A, Kaya S, et al. Comparison of choroidal and optic nerve head blood flow regulation during changes in ocular perfusion pressure. *Invest Ophthalmol Vis Sci.* 2012;3(8):4337–4346.

235. Calzetti G, Fondi K, Bata AM, et al. Assessment of choroidal blood flow using laser speckle flowgraphy. *British Journal of Ophthalmology.* 2018;102(12):1679.

236. Riva CE, Titze P, Hero M, Movaffaghy A, Petrig BL. Choroidal blood flow during isometric exercises. *Investigative Ophthalmology & Visual Science.* 1997;38(11):2338–2343.

237. Lovasik JV, Kergoat H, Riva CE, Petrig BL, Geiser M. Choroidal blood flow during exercise-induced changes in the ocular perfusion pressure. *Investigative Ophthalmology & Visual Science.* 2003;44(5):2126–2132.

238. Kiss B, Dallinger S, Polak K, Findl O, Eichler HG, Schmetterer L. Ocular hemodynamics during isometric exercise. *Microvascular Research.* 2001;61(1):1–13.

239. Li C, Fitzgerald MEC, Mar ND, et al. Role of the superior salivatory nucleus in parasympathetic control of choroidal blood flow and in maintenance of retinal health. *Experimental Eye Research.* 2021;206:108541.

240. Zagvazdin Y, Fitzgerald MEC, Reiner A. Role of muscarinic cholinergic transmission in edinger-westphal nucleus-induced choroidal vasodilation in pigeon. *Experimental Eye Research.* 2000;70(3):315–327.

241. Bata AM, Fondi K, Witkowska KJ, et al. Optic nerve head blood flow regulation during changes in arterial blood pressure in patients with primary open-angle glaucoma. *Acta Ophthalmologica.* 2019;97(1):e36–e41.

242. Movaffaghy A, Chamot SR, Petrig BL, Riva CE. Blood flow in the human optic nerve head during isometric exercise. *Experimental Eye Research.* 1998;67(5):561–568.

243. Boltz A, Told R, Napora KJ, et al. Optic nerve head blood flow autoregulation during changes in arterial blood pressure in healthy young subjects. *PLOS ONE.* 2013;8(12):e82351.

244. Hashimoto R, Sugiyama T, Ubuka M, Maeno T. Autoregulation of optic nerve head blood flow induced by elevated intraocular pressure during vitreous surgery. *Current Eye Research.* 2017;42(4):625–628.

245. Iwase T, Akahori T, Yamamoto K, Ra E, Terasaki H. Evaluation of optic nerve head blood flow in response to increase of intraocular pressure. *Scientific Reports.* 2018;8(1):17235.

246. Pillunat LE, Anderson DR, Knighton RW, Joos KM, Feuer WJ. Autoregulation of human optic nerve head circulation in response to increased intraocular pressure. *Experimental Eye Research.* 1997;64(5):737–744.

247. Riva CE, Hero M, Titze P, Petrig B. Autoregulation of human optic nerve head blood flow in response to acute changes in ocular perfusion pressure. *Graefe's Archive for Clinical and Experimental Ophthalmology.* 1997;235(10):618–626.

248. Kiyota N, Shiga Y, Ichinohasama K, et al. The impact of intraocular pressure elevation on optic nerve head and choroidal blood flow. *Investigative Ophthalmology & Visual Science.* 2018;59(8):3488–3496.

249. Tani T, Nagaoka T, Nakabayashi S, Yoshioka T, Yoshida A. Autoregulation of retinal blood flow in response to decreased ocular perfusion pressure in cats: comparison of the effects of increased intraocular pressure and systemic hypotension. *Investigative Ophthalmology & Visual Science.* 2014;55(1):360–367.

250. Wang L, Cull GA, Fortune B. Optic nerve head blood flow response to reduced ocular perfusion pressure by alteration of either the blood pressure or intraocular pressure. *Current Eye Research.* 2015;40(4):359–367.

251. Boltz A, Schmidl D, Werkmeister RM, et al. Regulation of optic nerve head blood flow during combined changes in intraocular pressure and arterial blood pressure. *Journal of Cerebral Blood Flow & Metabolism.* 2013;33(12):1850–1856.

252. Polska E, Simader C, Weigert G, et al. Regulation of choroidal blood flow during combined changes in intraocular pressure and arterial blood pressure. *Investigative Ophthalmology & Visual Science.* 2007;48(8):3768–3774.

253. Popa-Cherecheanu A, Schmidl D, Werkmeister RM, Chua J, Garhöfer G, Schmetterer L. Regulation of choroidal blood flow during isometric exercise at different levels of intraocular pressure. *Investigative Ophthalmology & Visual Science.* 2019;60(1):176–182.

254. Boltz A, Schmidl D, Weigert G, et al. Effect of latanoprost on choroidal blood flow regulation in healthy subjects. *Investigative Ophthalmology & Visual Science.* 2011;52(7):4410–4415.

255. Koss MC. Functional role of nitric oxide in regulation of ocular blood flow. *European Journal of Pharmacology.* 1999;374(2):161–174.

256. Schmetterer L, Polak K. Role of nitric oxide in the control of ocular blood flow. *Progress in Retinal and Eye Research.* 2001;20(6):823–847.

257. Okuno T, Oku H, Sugiyama T, Yang Y, Ikeda T. Evidence that nitric oxide Is Involved in autoregulation in optic nerve head of rabbits. *Investigative Ophthalmology & Visual Science.* 2002;43(3):784–789.

258. Schmidl D, Boltz A, Kaya S, et al. Role of nitric oxide in optic nerve head blood flow regulation during isometric exercise in healthy humans. *Investigative Ophthalmology & Visual Science.* 2013;54:1964–1970. https://doi.org/10.1167/iovs.12-11406.

259. Orgül S, Gugleta K, Flammer J. Physiology of perfusion as it relates to the optic nerve head. *Survey of Ophthalmology.* 1999;43:S17–S26.

260. Kiel JW. Modulation of choroidal autoregulation in the rabbit. *Experimental Eye Research.* 1999;69(4):413–429.

261. Simader C, Lung S, Weigert G, et al. Role of NO in the control of choroidal blood flow during a decrease in ocular perfusion pressure. *Investigative Ophthalmology & Visual Science.* 2009;50(1):372–377.

262. Luksch A, Polska E, Imhof A, et al. Role of NO in choroidal blood flow regulation during isometric exercise in healthy humans. *Investigative Ophthalmology & Visual Science.* 2003;44(2):734–739.

263. Kiel JW. Endothelin modulation of choroidal blood flow in the rabbit. *Experimental Eye Research.* 2000;71(6):543–550.

264. Boltz A, Schmidl D, Werkmeister RM, et al. Role of endothelin-A receptors in optic nerve head red cell flux regulation during isometric exercise in healthy humans. *American Journal of Physiology. Heart and Circulatory Physiology.* 2013;304(1):H170–H174.

265. Luksch A, Wimpissinger B, Polak K, Jandrasits K, Schmetterer L. ETa-receptor blockade, but not ACE inhibition, blunts retinal vessel response during isometric exercise. *American Journal of Physiology. Heart and Circulatory Physiology.* 2006;290(4):H1693–H1698.

266. Fuchsjäger-Mayrl G, Luksch A, Malec M, Polska E, Wolzt M, Schmetterer L. Role of endothelin-1 in choroidal blood flow regulation during isometric exercise in healthy humans. *Invest Ophthalmol Vis Sci.* 2003;44(2):728–733.

267. Kiel JW, Lovell MO. Adrenergic modulation of choroidal blood flow in the rabbit. *Investigative Ophthalmology & Visual Science.* 1996;37(4):673–679.

268. Kim KJ, Iddings JA, Stern JE, et al. Astrocyte contributions to flow/pressure-evoked parenchymal arteriole vasoconstriction. *The Journal of Neuroscience.* 2015;35(21):8245.

269. Shibata M, Sugiyama T, Kurimoto T, et al. Involvement of glial cells in the autoregulation of optic nerve head blood flow in rabbits. *Investigative Ophthalmology & Visual Science.* 2012;53(7):3726–3732.

270. Attwell D, Buchan AM, Charpak S, Lauritzen M, MacVicar BA, Newman EA. Glial and neuronal control of brain blood flow. *Nature*. 2010;468(7321):232–243.

271. Riva CE, Harino S, Shonat RD, Petrig BL. Flicker evoked increase in optic nerve head blood flow in anesthetized cats. *Neuroscience Letters*. 1991;128(2):291–296.

272. Toi VV, Riva CE. Variations of blood flow at optic nerve head induced by sinusoidal flicker stimulation in cats. *The Journal of Physiology*. 1995;482(1):189–202.

273. Buerk DG, Riva CE, Cranstoun SD. Frequency and luminance-dependent blood flow and K+ ion changes during flicker stimuli in cat optic nerve head. *Investigative Ophthalmology & Visual Science*. 1995;36(11):2216–2227.

274. Wang L, Bill A. Effects of constant and flickering light on retinal metabolism in rabbits. *Acta Ophthalmologica Scandinavica*. 1997;75(3):227–231.

275. Srienc A, Kurth-Nelson Z, Newman E. Imaging retinal blood flow with laser speckle flowmetry. *Frontiers in Neuroenergetics*. 2010;2:128.

276. Kornfield TE, Newman EA. Regulation of blood flow in the retinal trilaminar vascular network. *The Journal of Neuroscience*. 2014;34(34):11504.

277. Werkmeister R, Vietauer M, Knopf C, et al. Measurement of retinal blood flow in the rat by combining Doppler Fourier-domain optical coherence tomography with fundus imaging. *Journal of Biomedical Optics*. 2014(10):106008. Journal of Biomedical Optics.

278. Albanna W, Kotliar K, Lüke JN, et al. Non-invasive evaluation of neurovascular coupling in the murine retina by dynamic retinal vessel analysis. *PLOS ONE*. 2018;13(10):e0204689.

279. Tamplin MR, Broadhurst KA, Vitale AH, Hashimoto R, Kardon RH, Grumbach IM. Measuring hyperemic response to light flicker stimulus using continuous laser speckle flowgraphy in mice. *Experimental Eye Research*. 2022;216:108952.

280. Formaz F, Riva CE, Geiser M. Diffuse luminance flicker increases retinal vessel diameter in humans. *Current Eye Research*. 1997;16(12):1252–1257.

281. Riva CE, Falsini B, Logean E. Flicker-evoked responses of human optic nerve head blood flow: luminance versus chromatic modulation. *Investigative Ophthalmology & Visual Science*. 2001;42(3):756–762.

282. Falsini B, Riva CE, Logean E. Flicker-evoked changes in human optic nerve blood flow: relationship with retinal neural activity. *Investigative Ophthalmology & Visual Science*. 2002;43(7):2309–2316.

283. Garhöfer G, Huemer KH, Zawinka C, Schmetterer L, Dorner GT. Influence of diffuse luminance flicker on choroidal and optic nerve head blood flow. *Current Eye Research*. 2002;24(2):109–113.

284. Garhöfer G, Zawinka C, Resch H, Huemer KH, Dorner GT, Schmetterer L. Diffuse luminance flicker increases blood flow in major retinal arteries and veins. *Vision Research*. 2004;44(8):833–838.

285. Polak K, Schmetterer L, Riva CE. Influence of flicker frequency on flicker-induced changes of retinal vessel diameter. *Investigative Ophthalmology & Visual Science*. 2002;43(8):2721–2726.

286. Riva CE, Logean E, Falsini B. Temporal dynamics and magnitude of the blood flow response at the optic disk in normal subjects during functional retinal flicker-stimulation. *Neuroscience Letters*. 2004;356(2):75–78.

287. Wang Y, Fawzi AA, Tan O, Zhang X, Huang D. Flicker-induced changes in retinal blood flow assessed by Doppler optical coherence tomography. *Biomedical Optics Express*. 2011;2(7):1852–1860.

288. Zhong Z, Huang G, Chui TYP, Petrig BL, Burns SA. Local flicker stimulation evokes local retinal blood velocity changes. *Journal of Vision*. 2012;12(6):3–3.

289. Son T, Wang B, Thapa D, et al. Optical coherence tomography angiography of stimulus evoked hemodynamic responses in individual retinal layers. *Biomedical Optics Express*. 2016;7(8):3151–3162.

290. Duan A, Bedggood PA, Bui BV, Metha AB. Evidence of flicker-induced functional hyperaemia in the smallest vessels of the human retinal blood supply. *PLOS ONE*. 2016;11(9):e0162621.

291. Aschinger GC, Schmetterer L, Fondi K, et al. Effect of diffuse luminance flicker light stimulation on total retinal blood flow assessed with dual-beam bidirectional Doppler OCT. *Investigative Ophthalmology & Visual Science*. 2017;58(2):1167–1178.

292. Fondi K, Bata AM, Luft N, et al. Evaluation of flicker induced hyperemia in the retina and optic nerve head measured by laser speckle flowgraphy. *PLOS ONE*. 2018;13(11):e0207525.

293. Warner RL, de Castro A, Sawides L, et al. Full-field flicker evoked changes in parafoveal retinal blood flow. *Scientific reports*. 2020;10:16051. https://doi.org/10.1038/s41598-020-73032-0.

294. Nesper PL, Lee HE, Fayed AE, Schwartz GW, Yu F, Fawzi AA. Hemodynamic response of the three macular capillary plexuses in dark adaptation and flicker stimulation using optical coherence tomography angiography. *Investigative Ophthalmology & Visual Science*. 2019;60(2):694–703.

295. Kallab M, Hammer N, Tan B, et al. Plexus-specific effect of flicker-light stimulation on the retinal microvasculature assessed with optical coherence tomography angiography. *American Journal of Physiology. Heart and Circulatory Physiology*. 2021;320(1):H23–H28.

296. Felder AE, Wanek J, Blair NP, Shahidi M. Inner retinal oxygen extraction fraction in response to light flicker stimulation in humans. *Investigative Ophthalmology & Visual Science*. 2015;56(11):6633–6637.

297. Palkovits S, Lasta M, Told R, et al. Relation of retinal blood flow and retinal oxygen extraction during stimulation with diffuse luminance flicker. *Scientific Reports*. 2015;5(1):18291.

298. Anderson DR. Glaucoma, capillaries and pericytes. 1. Blood flow regulation. *Ophthalmologica*. 1996;210(5):257–262.

299. Erdener S, Küreli G, Dalkara T. Contractile apparatus in CNS capillary pericytes. *Neurophotonics*. 2022;9(2):021904.

300. Lindauer U, Megow D, Matsuda H, Dirnagl U. Nitric oxide: a modulator, but not a mediator, of neurovascular coupling in rat somatosensory cortex. *The American Journal of Physiology*. 1999;277(2):H799–H811.

301. Lacroix A, Toussay X, Anenberg E, et al. COX-2-derived prostaglandin E2 produced by pyramidal neurons contributes to neurovascular coupling in the rodent cerebral cortex. *The Journal of Neuroscience*. 2015;35(34):11791.

302. Kondo M, Wang L, Bill A. The role of nitric oxide in hyperaemic response to flicker in the retina and optic nerve in cats. *Acta Ophthalmologica Scandinavica*. 1997;75(3):232–235.

303. Buerk DG, Riva CE, Cranstoun SD. Nitric Oxide Has a Vasodilatory Role in Cat Optic Nerve Head during Flicker Stimuli. *Microvascular Research*. 1996;52(1):13–26.

304. Dorner GT, Garhofer G, Kiss B, et al. Nitric oxide regulates retinal vascular tone in humans. *American Journal of Physiology. Heart and Circulatory Physiology*. 2003;285(2):H631–H636.

305. Metea MR, Newman EA. Glial cells dilate and constrict blood vessels: a mechanism of neurovascular coupling. *The Journal of Neuroscience*. 2006;26(11):2862.

306. Iadecola C. The neurovascular unit coming of age: a journey through neurovascular coupling in health and disease. *Neuron*. 2017;96(1):17–42.

307. Mishra A, Reynolds JP, Chen Y, Gourine AV, Rusakov DA, Attwell D. Astrocytes mediate neurovascular signaling to capillary pericytes but not to arterioles. *Nature Neuroscience*. 2016;19(12):1619–1627.

308. Chen BR, Kozberg MG, Bouchard MB, Shaik MA, Hillman EMC. A Critical role for the vascular endothelium in functional neurovascular coupling in the brain. *Journal of the American Heart Association*. 2014;3(3):e000787.

309. Metea MR, Newman EA. Signalling within the neurovascular unit in the mammalian retina. *Experimental Physiology*. 2007;92(4):635–640.

310. Mishra A, Hamid A, Newman EA. Oxygen modulation of neurovascular coupling in the retina. *Proceedings of the National Academy of Sciences of the United States of America*. 2011;108(43):17827–17831.

311. Palkovits S, Told R, Boltz A, et al. Effect of increased oxygen tension on flicker-induced vasodilatation in the human retina. *Journal of Cerebral Blood Flow & Metabolism*. 2014;34(12):1914–1918.

312. Newman EA, Frambach DA, Odette LL. Control of extracellular potassium levels by retinal glial cell K+ siphoning. *Science*. 1984;225(4667):1174–1175.

313. Metea MR, Kofuji P, Newman EA. Neurovascular coupling is not mediated by potassium siphoning from glial cells. *The Journal of Neuroscience*. 2007;27(10):2468.

314. Alarcon-Martinez L, Villafranca-Baughman D, Quintero H, et al. Interpericyte tunnelling nanotubes regulate neurovascular coupling. *Nature*. 2020;585(7823):91–95.

315. Loo JH, Lee YS, Woon CY, et al. Loss of caveolin-1 impairs light flicker-induced neurovascular coupling at the optic nerve head. *Front Neurosci*. 2021;15:764898.

316. Ashby JW, Mack JJ. Endothelial control of cerebral blood flow. *The American Journal of Pathology*. 2021;191(11):1906–1916.

317. Busse R, Fleming I. Vascular Endothelium and Blood Flow. In: Moncada S, Higgs A, eds. *The Vascular Endothelium II. Berlin, Heidelberg*. Berlin Heidelberg: Springer; 2006:43–78.

318. Haefliger IO, Meyer P, Flammer J, Lüscher TF. The vascular endothelium as a regulator of the ocular circulation: A new concept in ophthalmology? *Survey of Ophthalmology*. 1994;39(2):123–132.

319. De Vriese AS, Verbeuren TJ, Van de Voorde J, Lameire NH, Vanhoutte PM. Endothelial dysfunction in diabetes. *British Journal of Pharmacology*. 2000;130(5):963–974.

320. Shi Y, Vanhoutte PM. Macro- and microvascular endothelial dysfunction in diabetes. *Journal of Diabetes*. 2017;9(5):434–449.

321. Furchgott RF, Vanhoutte PM. Endothelium-derived relaxing and contracting factors. *FASEB Journal*. 1989;3(9):2007–2018.

322. Godo S, Shimokawa H. Endothelial functions. *Arteriosclerosis, Thrombosis & Vascular Biology*. 2017;37(9):e108–e114.

323. Aydin F, Rosenblum WI, Povlishock JT. Myoendothelial junctions in human brain arterioles. *Stroke*. 1991;22(12):1592–1597.

324. Moncada S. Nitric oxide. Journal of hypertension. *Supplement: official journal of the International Society of Hypertension*. 1994;12(10):S35–S39.

325. Donati G, Pournaras CJ, Munoz JL, Poitry S, Poitry-Yamate CL, Tsacopoulos M. Nitric oxide controls arteriolar tone in the retina of the miniature pig. *Investigative Ophthalmology & Visual Science*. 1995;36(11):2228–2237.

326. Haefliger IO, Zschauer A, Anderson DR. Relaxation of retinal pericyte contractile tone through the nitric oxide-cyclic guanosine monophosphate pathway. *Investigative Ophthalmology & Visual Science*. 1994;35(3):991–997.

327. Haefliger IO, Flammer J, Lüscher TF. Nitric oxide and endothelin-1 are important regulators of human ophthalmic artery. *Investigative Ophthalmology & Visual Science*. 1992;33(7):2340–2343.

328. Laspas P, Goloborodko E, Sniatecki JJ, et al. Role of nitric oxide synthase isoforms for ophthalmic artery reactivity in mice. *Experimental Eye Research*. 2014;127:1–8.

329. Mann RM, Riva CE, Stone RA, Barnes GE, Cranstoun SD. Nitric oxide and choroidal blood flow regulation. *Investigative Ophthalmology & Visual Science*. 1995;36(5):925–930.

330. Schmetterer L, Krejcy K, Kastner J, et al. The effect of systemic nitric oxide-synthase inhibition on ocular fundus pulsations in man. *Experimental Eye Research*. 1997;64(3):305–312.

331. Luksch A, Polak K, Beier C, et al. Effects of systemic NO synthase inhibition on choroidal and optic nerve head blood flow in healthy subjects. *Investigative Ophthalmology & Visual Science*. 2000;41(10):3080–3084.

332. Toda N, Nakanishi-Toda M. Nitric oxide: ocular blood flow, glaucoma, and diabetic retinopathy. *Progress in Retinal and Eye Research*. 2007;26(3):205–238.

333. Erdinest N, London N, Ovadia H, Levinger N. Nitric oxide interaction with the eye. *Vision (Basel)*. 2021;5(2):29.

334. Toda N, Imamura T, Okamura T. Alteration of nitric oxide-mediated blood flow regulation in diabetes mellitus. *Pharmacology & Therapeutics*. 2010;127(3):189–209.

335. Needham M, McGahon MK, Bankhead P, et al. The role of K+ and Cl− channels in the Rregulation of retinal arteriolar Ttone and blood flow. *Investigative Ophthalmology & Visual Science*. 2014;55(4):2157–2165.

336. Kur J, Newman EA, Chan-Ling T. Cellular and physiological mechanisms underlying blood flow regulation in the retina and choroid in health and disease. *Progress in Retinal and Eye Research*. 2012;31(5):377–406.

337. Delaey C, Boussery K, Breyne J, Vanheel B, Van de Voorde J. The endothelium-derived hyperpolarising factor (EDHF) in isolated bovine choroidal arteries. *Experimental Eye Research*. 2007;84(6):1067–1073.

338. Haefliger IO, Flammer J, Bény JL, Lüscher TF. Endothelium-dependent vasoactive modulation in the ophthalmic circulation. *Progress in Retinal and Eye Research*. 2001;20(2):209–225.

339. Delaey C, van de Voorde J. Regulatory mechanisms in the retinal and choroidal circulation. *Ophthalmic Research*. 2000;32(6):249–256.

340. Mateo AO, AADe ArtiÑAno. Highlights on endothelins: a review. *Pharmacological Research*. 1997;36(5):339–351.

341. Barton M, Yanagisawa M. Endothelin: 30 Years From discovery to therapy. *Hypertension*. 2019;74(6):1232–1265.

342. Granstam E, Wang L, Bill A. Vascular effects of endothelin-1 in the cat; modification by indomethacin and l-NAME. *Acta Physiologica Scandinavica*. 1993;148(2):165–176.

343. Nishimura K, Riva CE, Harino S, Reinach P, Cranstoun SD, Mita S. Effects of endothelin-1 on optic nerve head blood flow in cats. *Journal of Ocular Pharmacology & Therapeutics*. 1996;12(1):75–83.

344. Polak K, Luksch A, Frank B, Jandrasits K, Polska E, Schmetterer L. Regulation of human retinal blood flow by endothelin-1. *Exp Eye Res*. 2003;76(5):633–640.

345. Polak K, Petternel V, Luksch A, et al. Effect of endothelin and BQ123 on ocular blood flow parameters in healthy subjects. *Investigative Ophthalmology & Visual Science*. 2001;42(12):2949–2956.

346. Schmetterer L, Findl O, Strenn K, et al. Effects of endothelin-1 (ET-1) on ocular hemodynamics. *Current Eye Research*. 1997;16(7):687–692.

347. Kida T, Flammer J, Oku H, et al. Data on the involvement of endothelin-1 (ET-1) in the dysregulation of retinal veins. *Data in Brief*. 2018;21:59–62.

348. Kawamura H, Oku H, Li Q, Sakagami K, Puro DG. Endothelin-induced changes in the physiology of retinal pericytes. *Investigative Ophthalmology & Visual Science*. 2002;43(3):882–888.

349. Chakravarthy U, Gardiner TA, Anderson P, Archer DB, Trimble ER. The effect of endothelin 1 on the retinal microvascular pericyte. *Microvascular Research*. 1992;43(3):241–254.

350. Bursell SE, Clermont AC, Oren B, King GL. The in vivo effect of endothelins on retinal circulation in nondiabetic and diabetic rats. *Investigative Ophthalmology & Visual Science*. 1995;36(3):596–607.

351. Hétu S, Pouliot M, Cordahi G, Couture R, Vaucher E. Assessment of retinal and choroidal blood flow changes using laser Doppler flowmetry in rats. *Current Eye Research*. 2013;38(1):158–167.

352. MacCumber MW, D'Anna SA. Endothelin receptor-binding subtypes in the human retina and choroid. *Archives of Ophthalmology*. 1994;112(9):1231–1235.

353. Chawengsub Y, Gauthier KM, Campbell WB. Role of arachidonic acid lipoxygenase metabolites in the regulation of vascular tone. *American Journal of Physiology. Heart and Circulatory Physiology*. 2009;297(2):H495–H507.

354. Zhou Y, Khan H, Xiao J, Cheang WS. Effects of arachidonic acid metabolites on cardiovascular health and disease. *International Journal Molecular Sciences*. 2021;22(21):12029.

355. Abran D, Li DY, Varma DR, Chemtob S. Characterization and ontogeny of PGE2 and PGF2α receptors on the retinal vasculature of the pig. *Prostaglandins*. 1995;50(5):253–267.

356. Abran D, Dumont I, Hardy P. Characterization and regulation of prostaglandin E2 receptor and receptor-coupled functions in the choroidal vasculature of the pig during development. *Circulation Research*. 1997;80(4):463–472.

357. Hardy P, Dumont I, Bhattacharya M. Oxidants, nitric oxide and prostanoids in the developing ocular vasculature: a basis for ischemic retinopathy. *Cardiovascular Research*. 2000;47(3):489–509.

358. Hardy P, Abran D, Li DY, Fernandez H, Varma DR, Chemtob S. Free radicals in retinal and choroidal blood flow autoregulation in the piglet: interaction with prostaglandins. *Investigative Ophthalmology & Visual Science*. 1994;35(2):580–591.

359. Mori A, Saito M, Sakamoto K, Narita M, Nakahara T, Ishii K. Stimulation of prostanoid IP and EP2 receptors dilates retinal arterioles and increases retinal and choroidal blood flow in rats. *European Journal of Pharmacology*. 2007;570(1):135–141.

360. Kitanishi K, Harino S, Suzuki M, Okamoto N, Reinach P. Liposomal prostaglandin E1 enhances optic nerve head blood flow in cats. *Journal of Ocular Pharmacology & Therapeutics*. 2001;17(2):115–122.

361. Pournaras C, Tsacopoulos M, Chapuis P. Studies on the role of prostaglandins in the regulation of retinal blood flow. *Experimental Eye Research*. 1978;26(6):687–697.

362. Astin M, Stjernschantz J, Selén G. Role of nitric oxide in PGF2α-induced ocular hyperemia. *Experimental Eye Research*. 1994;59(4):401–408.

363. Stjernschantz J, Selén G, Astin M, Resul B. Microvascular effects of selective prostaglandin analogues in the eye with special reference to latanoprost and glaucoma treatment. *Progress in Retinal and Eye Research*. 2000;19(4):459–496.

364. Ohkubo H, Chiba S. Responses of isolated canine ophthalmic and ciliary arteries to vasoactive substances. *Japanese Journal of Ophthalmology*. 1987;31(4):627–634.

365. Faraci FM, Williams JK, Breese KR, Armstrong ML, Heistad DD. Atherosclerosis potentiates constrictor responses of cerebral and ocular blood vessels to thromboxane in monkeys. *Stroke*. 1989;20(2):242–247.

366. Torring MS, Aalkjaer C, Bek T. Constriction of porcine retinal arterioles induced by endothelin-1 and the thromboxane analogue U46619 in vitro decreases with increasing vascular branching level. *Acta Ophthalmologica*. 2014;92(3):232–237.

367. Bilotta J, Abramov I. Orientation and direction tuning of goldfish ganglion cells. *Visual Neuroscience*. 1989;2(1):3–13.

368. Thijssen DHJ, Black MA, Pyke KE. Assessment of flow-mediated dilation in humans: a methodological and physiological guideline. *American Journal of Physiology. Heart and Circulatory Physiology*. 2011;300(1):H2–H12.

369. Nagaoka T, Yoshida A. Noninvasive evaluation of wall shear stress on retinal microcirculation in humans. *Investigative Ophthalmology & Visual Science*. 2006;47(3):1113–1119.

370. Yazdanfar S, Rollins AM, Izatt JA. In vivo imaging of human retinal flow dynamics by color Doppler optical coherence tomography. *Archives of Ophthalmology*. 2003;121(2):235–239.

371. Logean E, Schmetterer LF, Riva CE. Optical Doppler velocimetry at various retinal vessel depths by variation of thesource coherence length. *Applied Optics*. 2000;39(16):2858–2862.

372. Molins B, Mora A, Romero-Vázquez S, et al. Shear stress modulates inner blood retinal barrier phenotype. *Experimental Eye Research*. 2019;187:107751.

373. Cunha-Vaz J. Mechanisms of retinal fluid accumulation and blood-retinal barrier breakdown. *Developments in Ophthalmology*. 2016;58:11–20.

374. Nilsson SFE, Bill A. Vasoactive intestinal polypeptide (VIP): effects in the eye and on regional blood flows. *Acta Physiologica Scandinavica*. 1984;121(4):385–392.

375. Stjernschantz J, Bill A. Vasomotor effects of facial nerve stimulation: noncholinergic vasodilation in the eye. *Acta Physiologica Scandinavica*. 1980;109(1):45–50.

376. Nilsson SFE, Linder J, Bill A. Characteristics of uveal vasodilation produced by facial nerve stimulation in monkeys, cats and rabbits. *Experimental Eye Research*. 1985;40(6):841–852.

377. Nilsson SFE. The significance of nitric oxide for parasympathetic vasodilation in the eye and other orbital tissues in the cat. *Experimental Eye Research*. 2000;70(1):61–72.

378. Steinle JJ, Krizsan-Agbas D, Smith PG. Regional regulation of choroidal blood flow by autonomic innervation in the rat. *American Journal of Physiology. Regulatory, Integrative & Comparative Physiology*. 2000;279(1):R202–R209.

379. Reiner A, Del Mar N, Zagvazdin Y, Li C, Fitzgerald MEC. Age-related impairment in choroidal blood flow compensation for arterial blood pressure fluctuation in pigeons. *Investigative Ophthalmology & Visual Science*. 2011;52(10):7238–7247.

380. Gherezghiher T, Okubo H, Koss MC. Choroidal and ciliary body blood flow analysis: Application of laser Doppler flowmetry in experimental animals. *Experimental Eye Research*. 1991;53(2):151–156.

381. Riva CE, Cranstoun SD, Mann RM, Barnes GE. Local choroidal blood flow in the cat by laser Doppler flowmetry. *Investigative Ophthalmology & Visual Science*. 1994;35(2):608–618.

382. Alm A. The effect of sympathetic stimulation on blood flow through the uvea, retina and optic nerve in monkeys (Macaca irus). *Experimental Eye Research*. 1977;25(1):19–24.

383. Bill A. Some aspects of the ocular circulation. Friedenwald lecture. *Investigative Ophthalmology & Visual Science*. 1985;26(4):410–424.

384. Corvetti G, Pignocchino P, Sisto Daneo L. Distribution and development of substance P immunoreactive axons in the chick cornea and uvea. *Basic and applied histochemistry*. 1988;32(1):187–192.

385. Zhang Y, Wernly B, Cao X, Mustafa SJ, Tang Y, Zhou Z. Adenosine and adenosine receptor-mediated action in coronary microcirculation. *Basic Research in Cardiology*. 2021;116(1):22.

386. Gidday JM, Park TS. Microcirculatory responses to adenosine in the newborn pig retina. *Pediatric Research*. 1993;33(6):620–627.

387. Portellos M, Riva CE, Cranstoun SD, Petrig BL, Brucker AJ. Effects of adenosine on ocular blood flow. *Investigative Ophthalmology & Visual Science*. 1995;36(9):1904–1909.

388. Polska E, Ehrlich P, Luksch A, Fuchsjäger-Mayrl G, Schmetterer L. Effects of adenosine on intraocular pressure, optic nerve head blood flow, and choroidal blood flow in healthy humans. *Investigative Ophthalmology & Visual Science*. 2003;44(7):3110–3114.

389. Gidday JM, Park TS. Adenosine-mediated autoregulation of retinal arteriolar tone in the piglet. *Investigative Ophthalmology & Visual Science*. 1993;34(9):2713–2719.

390. Schmidl D, Weigert G, Dorner GT, et al. Role of adenosine in the control of choroidal blood flow during changes in ocular perfusion pressure. *Investigative Ophthalmology & Visual Science*. 2011;52(8):6035–6039.

391. Dons-Jensen A, Petersen L, Bøtker HE, Bek T. The diameter of retinal arterioles is unaffected by intravascular administration of the adenosine a2A receptor agonist regadenoson in normal persons. *Biomedicine Hub*. 2019;4(2):1–10.

392. Ernst C, Aalkjær C, Bek T. ATP induced calcium signaling activity in perivascular cells differ at different vascular branch levels in the porcine retina. *Microvascular Research*. 2022;139:104256.

393. Guo X, Liu WL, Chen LW, Guo ZG. High glucose impairs endothelium-dependent relaxation in rabbit aorta. *Acta pharmacologica Sinica*. 2000;21(2):169–173.

394. Kito K, Tanabe K, Sakata K, et al. Endothelium-dependent vasodilation in the cerebral arterioles of rats deteriorates during acute hyperglycemia and then is restored by reducing the glucose level. *Journal of Anesthesia*. 2018;32(4):531–538.

395. Sullivan PM, Davies GE, Caldwell G, Morris AC, Kohner EM. Retinal blood flow during hyperglycemia. A laser Doppler velocimetry study. *Investigative Ophthalmology & Visual Science*. 1990;31(10):2041–2045.

396. Bursell SE, Clermont AC, Kinsley BT, Simonson DC, Aiello LM, Wolpert HA. Retinal blood flow changes in patients with insulin-dependent diabetes mellitus and no diabetic retinopathy. *Investigative Ophthalmology & Visual Science*. 1996;37(5):886–897.

397. Luksch A, Polak K, Matulla B, et al. Glucose and insulin exert additive ocular and renal vasodilator effects on healthy humans. *Diabetologia*. 2001;44(1):95–103.

398. Pemp B, Polska E, Garhofer G, Bayerle-Eder M, Kautzky-Willer A, Schmetterer L. Retinal blood flow in type 1 diabetic patients with no or mild diabetic retinopathy during euglycemic clamp. *Diabetes Care*. 2010;33(9):2038–2042.

399. Hoffman RP, Hausberg M, Sinkey CA, Anderson EA. Hyperglycemia without hyperinsulinemia produces both sympathetic neural activation and vasodilation in normal humans. *Journal of Diabetes and its Complications*. 1999;13(1):17–22.

400. Williamson JR, Chang K, Frangos M, et al. Hyperglycemic pseudohypoxia and diabetic complications. *Diabetes*. 1993;42(6):801–813.

401. Ido Y, Chang K, Woolsey TA, Williamson JR. NADH: sensor of blood flow need in brain, muscle, and other tissues. *FASEB Journal*. 2001;15(8):1419–1421.

402. Schmetterer L, Müller M, Fasching P, et al. Renal and ocular hemodynamic effects of insulin. *Diabetes*. 1997;46(11):1868–1874.

403. Polak K, Dallinger S, Polska E, et al. Effects of insulin on retinal and pulsatile choroidal blood flow in humans. *Archives of Ophthalmology*. 2000;118(1):55–59.

404. Dallinger S, Sieder A, Strametz J, Bayerle-Eder M, Wolzt M, Schmetterer L. Vasodilator effects of l-arginine are stereospecific and augmented by insulin in humans. *American Journal of Physiology. Endocrinology & Metabolism*. 2003;284(6):E1106–E1111.

405. Yoshioka T, Song Y, Kawai M, et al. Retinal blood flow reduction in normal-tension glaucoma with single-hemifield damage by Doppler optical coherence tomography. *British Journal of Ophthalmology*. 2021;105(1):124.

406. Inada E, Philbin DM, Machaj V, et al. Histamine antagonists and d-tubocurarine-induced hypotension in cardiac surgical patients. *Clinical Pharmacology & Therapeutics*. 1986;40(5):575–580.

407. Hwang JC, Konduru R, Zhang X, et al. Relationship among visual field, blood flow, and neural structure measurements in glaucoma. *Investigative Ophthalmology & Visual Science*. 2012;53(6):3020–3026.

408. Deokule S, Vizzeri G, Boehm A, Bowd C, Weinreb RN. Association of visual field severity and parapapillary retinal blood flow open-angle glaucoma. *Journal of Glaucoma*. 2010;19(5):293–298.

409. Yamada Y, Higashide T, Udagawa S, et al. The relationship between interocular asymmetry of visual field defects and optic nerve head blood flow in patients with glaucoma. *Journal of Glaucoma*. 2019;28(3):231–237.

410. Resch H, Schmidl D, Hommer A, et al. Correlation of optic disc morphology and ocular perfusion parameters in patients with primary open angle glaucoma. *Acta Ophthalmologica*. 2011;89(7):e544–e549.

411. Jeon SJ, Jung KI, Park CK, Park HYL. Macular blood flow and pattern electroretinogram in normal tension glaucoma. *Journal of Clinical Medicine*. 2022;11(7):1790.

412. Osborne NN, Ugarte M, Chao M, et al. Neuroprotection in relation to retinal ischemia and relevance to glaucoma. *Survey of Ophthalmology*. 1999;43:S102–S128.

413. Cherecheanu AP, Garhofer G, Schmidl D, Werkmeister R, Schmetterer L. Ocular perfusion pressure and ocular blood flow in glaucoma. *Current Opinion in Pharmacology*. 2013;13(1):36–42.

414. Tan B, Sim YC, Chua J, et al. Developing a normative database for retinal perfusion using optical coherence tomography angiography. *Biomed Opt Exp*. 2021;12(7):4032–4045.

415. Wong D, Chua J, Lin E, et al. Focal structure–function relationships in primary open-angle glaucoma using OCT and OCT-A measurements. *Invest Ophthalmol Vis Sci*. 2020;61(14):33–33.

416. Yaoeda K, Shirakashi M, Fukushima A, et al. Relationship between optic nerve head microcirculation and visual field loss in glaucoma. *Acta Ophthalmologica Scandinavica*. 2003;81(3):253–259.

417. Wong D, Chua J, Tan B, et al. Combining OCT and OCTA for focal structure–function modeling in early primary open-angle glaucoma. *Investigative Ophthalmology & Visual Science*. 2021;62(15):8–8.

418. Kallab M, Hommer N, Schlatter A, et al. Combining vascular and nerve fiber layer thickness measurements to model glaucomatous focal visual field loss. *Annals of the New York Academy of Sciences*. 2022;1511(1):133–141.

419. Calzetti G, Mursch-Edlmayr AS, Bata AM, et al. Measuring optic nerve head perfusion to monitor glaucoma: a study on structure–function relationships using laser speckle flowgraphy. *Acta Ophthalmologica*. 2022;100(1):e181–e191.

420. Satilmis MÜc Orgül S, Doubler B, Flammer J. Rate of progression of glaucoma correlates with retrobulbar circulation and intraocular pressure. *American Journal of Ophthalmology*. 2003;135(5):664–669.

421. Galassi F, Sodi A, Ucci F, Renieri G, Pieri B, Baccini M. Ocular hemodynamics and glaucoma prognosis: a color Doppler imaging study. *Archives of Ophthalmology*. 2003;121(12):1711–1715.

422. Zeitz O, Galambos P, Wagenfeld L, et al. Glaucoma progression is associated with decreased blood flow velocities in the short posterior ciliary artery. *British Journal of Ophthalmology*. 2006;90(10):1245.

423. Siesky B, Harris A, Carr J, et al. Reductions in retrobulbar and retinal capillary blood flow strongly correlate with changes in optic nerve head and retinal morphology over 4 years in open-angle glaucoma patients of african descent compared with patients of european descent. *Journal of Glaucoma*. 2016;25(9):750–757.

424. Zink JM, Grunwald JE, Piltz-Seymour J, Staii A, Dupont J. Association between lower optic nerve laser Doppler blood volume measurements and glaucomatous visual field progression. *British Journal of Ophthalmology*. 2003;87(12):1487.

425. Jeon SJ, Shin DY, Park HYL, Park CK. Association of retinal blood flow with progression of visual field in glaucoma. *Scientific Reports*. 2019;9(1):16813.

426. Wang YM, Shen R, Lin TPH. Optical coherence tomography angiography metrics predict normal tension glaucoma progression. *Acta Ophthalmologica*. 2022

427. Kiyota N, Shiga Y, Omodaka K, Pak K, Nakazawa T. Time-course changes in optic nerve head blood flow and retinal nerve fiber layer thickness in eyes with open-angle glaucoma. *Ophthalmology*. 2021;128(5):663–671.

428. Kiyota N, Shiga Y, Omodaka K, Nakazawa T. The relationship between choroidal blood flow and glaucoma progression in a Japanese study population. *Japanese Journal of Ophthalmology*. 2022

429. Leeman M, Kestelyn P. Glaucoma and blood pressure. *Hypertension*. 2019;73(5):944–950.

430. Costa VP, Arcieri ES, Harris A. Blood pressure and glaucoma. *British Journal of Ophthalmology*. 2009;93(10):1276.

431. Skrzypecki J, Ufnal M, Szaflik JP, Filipiak KJ. Blood pressure and glaucoma: At the crossroads between cardiology and ophthalmology. *Cardiology. Journal*. 2019;26(1):8–12.

432. Charlson ME, de Moraes CG, Link A, et al. Nocturnal systemic hypotension increases the risk of glaucoma progression. *Ophthalmology*. 2014;121(10):2004–2012.

433. Marshall H, Mullany S, Qassim A, et al. Cardiovascular disease predicts structural and functional progression in early glaucoma. *Ophthalmology*. 2021;128(1):58–69.

434. Marjanović I, Marjanović M, Martinez A, Marković V, Božić M, Stojanov V. Relationship between blood pressure and retrobulbar blood flow in dipper and nondipper primary open-angle glaucoma patients. *Eur J Ophthalmol*. 2016;26(6):588–593.

435. Fuchsjäger-Mayrl G, Wally B, Georgopoulos M, et al. Ocular blood flow and systemic blood pressure in patients with primary open-angle glaucoma and ocular hypertension. *Investigative Ophthalmology & Visual Science*. 2004;45(3):834–839.

436. Garhöfer G, Fuchsjäger-Mayrl G, Vass C, Pemp B, Hommer A, Schmetterer L. Retrobulbar blood flow velocities in open angle glaucoma and their association with mean arterial blood pressure. *Investigative Ophthalmology & Visual Science*. 2010;51(12):6652–6657.

437. Gherghel D, Orgül S, Gugleta K, Gekkieva M, Flammer J. Relationship between ocular perfusion pressure and retrobulbar blood flow in patients with glaucoma with progressive damage. *American Journal of Ophthalmology*. 2000;130(5):597–605.

438. Plange N, Kaup M, Remky A, Arend KO. Prolonged retinal arteriovenous passage time is correlated to ocular perfusion pressure in normal tension glaucoma. *Graefe's Archive for Clinical and Experimental Ophthalmology*. 2008;246(8):1147–1152.

439. Fuchsjäger-Mayrl G, Georgopoulos M, Hommer A, et al. Effect of dorzolamide and timolol on ocular pressure: blood flow relationship in patients with primary open-angle glaucoma and ocular hypertension. *Investigative Ophthalmology & Visual Science*. 2010;51(3):1289–1296.

440. Quaranta L, Manni G, Donato F, Bucci MG. The effect of increased intraocular pressure on pulsatile ocular blood flow in low tension glaucoma. *Survey of Ophthalmology*. 1994;38:S177–S182.

441. Grunwald JE, Riva CE, Stone RA, Keates EU, Petrig BL. Retinal autoregulation in open-angle glaucoma. *Ophthalmology*. 1984;91(12):1690–1694.

442. Galambos P, Vafiadis J, Vilchez SE, et al. Compromised autoregulatory control of ocular hemodynamics in glaucoma patients after postural change. *Ophthalmology*. 2006;113(10):1832–1836.

443. Evans DW, Harris A, Garrett M, Chung HS, Kagemann L. Glaucoma patients demonstrate faulty autoregulation of ocular blood flow during posture change. *British Journal of Ophthalmology*. 1999;83(7):809.

444. Feke GT, Pasquale LR. Retinal blood flow response to posture change in glaucoma patients compared with healthy subjects. *Ophthalmology*. 2008;115(2):246–252.

445. Weigert G, Findl O, Luksch A, et al. Effects of moderate changes in intraocular pressure on ocular hemodynamics in patients with primary open-angle glaucoma and healthy controls. *Ophthalmology*. 2005;112(8):1337–1342.

446. Pournaras CJ, Riva CE, Bresson-Dumont H, De Gottrau P, Bechetoille A. Regulation of optic nerve head blood flow in normal tension glaucoma patients. *European Journal of Ophthalmology*. 2004;14(3):226–235.

447. Mursch-Edlmayr AS, Luft N, Podkowinski D, Ring M, Schmetterer L, Bolz M. Differences in optic nerve head blood flow regulation in normal tension glaucoma patients and healthy controls as assessed with laser speckle flowgraphy during the water drinking test. *Journal of Glaucoma*. 2019;28(7):649–654.

448. Sehi M, Flanagan JG, Zeng L, Cook RJ, Trope GE. Anterior optic nerve capillary blood flow response to diurnal variation of mean ocular perfusion pressure in early untreated primary open-angle glaucoma. *Investigative Ophthalmology & Visual Science*. 2005;46(12):4581–4587.

449. Alarcon-Martinez L, Shiga Y, Villafranca-Baughman D, et al. Pericyte dysfunction and loss of interpericyte tunneling nanotubes promote neurovascular deficits in glaucoma. *Proceedings of the National Academy of Sciences of the United States of America*. 2022;119(7):e2110329119.

450. Pappelis K, Jansonius NM. U-shaped effect of blood pressure on structural OCT metrics and retinal perfusion in ophthalmologically healthy subjects. *Investigative Ophthalmology & Visual Science*. 2021;62(12):5–5.

451. Cull G, Told R, Burgoyne CF, Thompson S, Fortune B, Wang L. Compromised optic nerve blood flow and autoregulation secondary to neural degeneration. *Investigative Ophthalmology & Visual Science*. 2015;56(12):7286–7292.

452. Riva CE, Salgarello T, Logean E, Colotto A, Galan EM, Falsini B. Flicker-Evoked Response Measured at the Optic Disc Rim Is Reduced in Ocular Hypertension and Early Glaucoma. *Investigative Ophthalmology & Visual Science*. 2004;45(10):3662–3668.

453. Garhöfer G, Zawinka C, Resch H, Huemer KH, Schmetterer L, Dorner GT. Response of retinal vessel diameters to flicker stimulation in patients with early open angle glaucoma. *Journal of Glaucoma*. 2004;13(4):340–344.

454. Gugleta K, Kochkorov A, Waldmann N, et al. Dynamics of retinal vessel response to flicker light in glaucoma patients and ocular hypertensives. *Graefe's Archive for Clinical and Experimental Ophthalmology*. 2012;250(4):589–594.

455. Gugleta K, Waldmann N, Polunina A, et al. Retinal neurovascular coupling in patients with glaucoma and ocular hypertension and its association with the level of glaucomatous damage. *Graefe's Archive for Clinical and Experimental Ophthalmology*. 2013;251(6):1577–1585.

456. Mroczkowska S, Benavente-Perez A, Negi A, Sung V, Patel SR, Gherghel D. Primary open-angle glaucoma vs normal-tension glaucoma: the vascular perspective. *JAMA Ophthalmology*. 2013;131(1):36–43.

457. Al Zoubi H, Riemer T, Simon R, et al. Optic disc blood perfusion and oxygenation in glaucoma. *Graefe's Archive for Clinical and Experimental Ophthalmology*. 2022

458. Mursch-Edlmayr AS, Pickl L, Calzetti G, et al. Comparison of neurovascular coupling between normal tension glaucoma patients and healthy individuals with laser speckle flowgraphy. *Current Eye Research*. 2020;45(11):1438–1442.

459. Waldmann NP, Kochkorov A, Polunina A, Orgül S, Gugleta K. The prognostic value of retinal vessel analysis in primary open-angle glaucoma. *Acta Ophthalmologica*. 2016;94(6):e474–e480.

460. Resch H, Garhofer G, Fuchsjäger-Mayrl G, Hommer A, Schmetterer L. Endothelial dysfunction in glaucoma. *Acta Ophthalmologica*. 2009;87(1):4–12.

461. Chauhan BC. Endothelin and its potential role in glaucoma. *Canadian Journal of Ophthalmology*. 2008;43(3):356–360.

462. Prasanna G, Krishnamoorthy R, Yorio T. Endothelin, astrocytes and glaucoma. *Experimental Eye Research*. 2011;93(2):170–177.

463. Shoshani YZ, Harris A, Shoja MM, et al. Endothelin and its suspected role in the pathogenesis and possible treatment of glaucoma. *Current Eye Research*. 2012;37(1):1–11.

464. Yorio T, Krishnamoorthy R, Prasanna G. Endothelin: is it a contributor to glaucoma pathophysiology? *Journal of Glaucoma*. 2002;11(3):259–270.

465. Henry E, Newby DE, Webb DJ, O'Brien C. Peripheral endothelial dysfunction in normal pressure glaucoma. *Investigative Ophthalmology & Visual Science*. 1999;40(8):1710–1714.

466. Buckley C, Hadoke PWF, Henry E, O'Brien C. Systemic vascular endothelial cell dysfunction in normal pressure glaucoma. *British Journal of Ophthalmology*. 2002;86(2):227.
467. Bukhari SMI, Kiu KY, Thambiraja R, Sulong S, Rasool AHG, Liza-Sharmini AT. Microvascular endothelial function and severity of primary open angle glaucoma. *Eye*. 2016;30(12):1579–1587.
468. Cellini M, Strobbe E, Gizzi C, Balducci N, Toschi PG, Campos EC. Endothelin-1 plasma levels and vascular endothelial dysfunction in primary open angle glaucoma. *Life Sciences*. 2012;91(13):699–702.
469. Su W-W, Cheng ST, Ho WJ, Tsay PK, Wu SC, Chang SHL. Glaucoma Is associated with peripheral vascular endothelial dysfunction. *Ophthalmology*. 2008;115(7):1173–1178. e1.
470. Bojic L, Rogosic V, Markovic D, Rogosic LV, Glavas D. Brachial flow—mediated dilation and carotid intima—media thickness in glaucoma patients. *BMC Ophthalmology*. 2022;22(1):275.
471. Polak K, Luksch A, Berisha F, Fuchsjaeger-Mayrl G, Dallinger S, Schmetterer L. Altered nitric oxide system in patients with open-angle glaucoma. *Archives of Ophthalmology*. 2007;125(4):494–498.
472. Resch H, Karl K, Weigert G, et al. Effect of dual endothelin receptor blockade on ocular blood flow in patients with glaucoma and healthy subjects. *Investigative Ophthalmology & Visual Science*. 2009;50(1):358–363.
473. Bourouki E, Oikonomou E, Moschos M, et al. Pseudoexfoliative glaucoma, endothelial dysfunction, and arterial stiffness: the role of circulating apoptotic endothelial microparticles. *Journal of Glaucoma*. 2019;28(8):749–755.
474. Bhagat N, Grigorian RA, Tutela A, Zarbin MA. Diabetic macular edema: pathogenesis and treatment. *Survey of Ophthalmology*. 2009;54(1):1–32.
475. Roy S, Ha J, Trudeau K, Beglova E. Vascular basement membrane thickening in diabetic retinopathy. *Current Eye Research*. 2010;35(12):1045–1056.
476. Simó R, Stitt AW, Gardner TW. Neurodegeneration in diabetic retinopathy: does it really matter? *Diabetologia*. 2018;61(9):1902–1912.
477. Tonade D, Liu H, Kern TS. Photoreceptor cells produce inflammatory mediators that contribute to endothelial cell death in diabetes. *Investigative Ophthalmology & Visual Science*. 2016;57(10):4264–4271.
478. Khuu LA, Tayyari F, Sivak JM, et al. Aqueous humor endothelin-1 and total retinal blood flow in patients with non-proliferative diabetic retinopathy. *Eye*. 2017;31(10):1443–1450.
479. Patel V, Rassam S, Newsom R, Wiek J, Kohner E. Retinal blood flow in diabetic retinopathy. *BMJ*. 1992;305(6855):678–683.
480. Pemp B, Schmetterer L. Ocular blood flow in diabetes and age-related macular degeneration. *Canadian Journal of Ophthalmology*. 2008;43(3):295–301.
481. Ludovico J, Bernardes R, Pires I, Figueira J, Lobo C, Cunha-Vaz J. Alterations of retinal capillary blood flow in preclinical retinopathy in subjects with type 2 diabetes. *Graefe's Archive for Clinical and Experimental Ophthalmology*. 2003;241(3):181–186.
482. Kohner EM, Hamilton AM, Saunders SJ, Sutcliffe BA, Bulpitt CJ. The retinal blood flow in diabetes. *Diabetologia*. 1975;11(1):27–33.
483. Kohner EM. The problems of retinal blood flow in diabetes. *Diabetes*. 1976;25(2 SUPPL):839–844.
484. Burgansky-Eliash Z, Barak A, Barash H, et al. Increased retinal blood flow velocity in patients with early diabetes mellitus. *Retina*. 2012;32(1):112–119.
485. Omae T, Nagaoka T, Yoshida A. Relationship between retinal blood flow and serum adiponectin concentrations in patients with type 2 diabetes mellitus. *Investigative Ophthalmology & Visual Science*. 2015;56(6):4143–4149.
486. Findl O, Dallinger S, Rami B, et al. Ocular haemodynamics and colour contrast sensitivity in patients with type 1 diabetes. *British Journal of Ophthalmology*. 2000;84(5):493.
487. Muir ER, Rentería RC, Duong TQ. Reduced ocular blood flow as an early indicator of diabetic retinopathy in a mouse model of diabetes. *Investigative Ophthalmology & Visual Science*. 2012;53(10):6488–6494.
488. Borrelli E, Battista M, Sacconi R, Querques G, Bandello F. Optical coherence tomography angiography in diabetes. *Asia-Pacific Journal of Ophthalmology*. 2021;10(1):20–25.
489. Boned-Murillo A, Albertos-Arranz H, Diaz-Barreda MD, et al. Optical coherence tomography angiography in diabetic patients: a systematic review. *Biomedicines*. 2022;10(1):88.
490. Chua J, Sim R, Tan B, et al. Optical coherence tomography angiography in diabetes and diabetic retinopathy. *Journal of Clinical Medicine*. 2020;9(6):1723.
491. Lee J, Rosen R. Optical coherence tomography angiography in diabetes. *Current Diabetes Reports*. 2016;16(12):123.
492. Johannesen SK, Viken JN, Vergmann AS, Grauslund J. Optical coherence tomography angiography and microvascular changes in diabetic retinopathy: a systematic review. *Acta Ophthalmologica*. 2019;97(1):7–14.
493. Tey KY, Teo K, Tan ACS, et al. Optical coherence tomography angiography in diabetic retinopathy: a review of current applications. *Eye and Vision*. 2019;6(1):37.
494. Kannenkeril D, Nolde JM, Kiuchi MG, et al. Retinal capillary damage Is already evident in patients with hypertension and prediabetes and associated with HbA1c levels in the nondiabetic range. *Diabetes Care*. 2022;45(6):1472–1475.
495. Hirano T, Kakihara S, Toriyama Y, Nittala MG, Murata T, Sadda S. Wide-field en face swept-source optical coherence tomography angiography using extended field imaging in diabetic retinopathy. *British Journal of Ophthalmology*. 2018;102(9):1199.
496. Zhang Q, Rezaei KA, Saraf SS, Chu Z, Wang F, Wang RK. Ultra-wide optical coherence tomography angiography in diabetic retinopathy. *Quantitative Imaging in Medicine & Surgery*. 2018;8(8):743–753.
497. Tan B, Chua J, Lin E, et al. Quantitative microvascular analysis with wide-field optical coherence tomography angiography in eyes with diabetic retinopathy. *JAMA Netw Open*. 2020;3(1):e1919469–e1919469.
498. Guo Y, Camino A, Wang J, Huang D, Hwang TS, Jia Y. MEDnet, a neural network for automated detection of avascular area in OCT angiography. *Biomedical Optics Express*. 2018;9(11):5147–5158.
499. You QS, Guo Y, Wang J, et al. Detection of clinically unsuspected retinal neovascularization with wide-field optical coherence tomography angiography. *Retina*. 2020;40(5):891–897.
500. Khalid H, Schwartz R, Nicholson L, et al. Widefield optical coherence tomography angiography for early detection and objective evaluation of proliferative diabetic retinopathy. *British Journal of Ophthalmology*. 2021;105(1):118.
501. Vaz-Pereira S, Morais-Sarmento T, Engelbert M. Update on optical coherence tomography and optical coherence tomography angiography imaging in proliferative diabetic retinopathy. *Diagnostics (Basel)*. 2021;11(10):1869.
502. Lu ES, Cui Y, Le R, et al. Detection of neovascularisation in the vitreoretinal interface slab using widefield swept-source optical coherence tomography angiography in diabetic retinopathy. *British Journal of Ophthalmology*. 2022;106(4):534.
503. Sun Z, Tang F, Wong R, et al. OCT angiography metrics predict progression of diabetic retinopathy and development of diabetic macular edema: a prospective study. *Ophthalmology*. 2019;126(12):1675–1684.
504. Johnson MA, Lutty GA, McLeod DS, et al. Ocular structure and function in an aged monkey with spontaneous diabetes mellitus. *Experimental Eye Research*. 2005;80(1):37–42.
505. Lutty GA. Diabetic choroidopathy. *Vision Research*. 2017;139:161–167.
506. Nagaoka T, Kitaya N, Sugawara R, et al. Alteration of choroidal circulation in the foveal region in patients with type 2 diabetes. *British Journal of Ophthalmology*. 2004;88(8):1060.
507. Dodo Y, Suzuma K, Ishihara K, et al. Clinical relevance of reduced decorrelation signals in the diabetic inner choroid on optical coherence tomography angiography. *Scientific Reports*. 2017;7(1):5227.
508. Li L, Almansoob S, Zhang P, Zhou YD, Tan Y, Gao L. Quantitative analysis of retinal and choroid capillary ischaemia using optical coherence tomography angiography in type 2 diabetes. *Acta Ophthalmologica*. 2019;97(3):240–246.
509. Tan B, Lim NA, Tan R, et al. Combining retinal and choroidal microvascular metrics improves discriminative power for diabetic retinopathy. *British Journal of Ophthalmology*. 2022:1–7.
510. Wang W, Guo X, Chen Y, et al. Choriocapillaris perfusion assessed using swept source optical coherence tomographic angiography and the severity of diabetic retinopathy. *British Journal of Ophthalmology*. 2022:320163.
511. Wang W, Cheng W, Yang S, Chen Y, Zhu Z, Huang W. Choriocapillaris flow deficit and the risk of referable diabetic retinopathy: a longitudinal SS-OCTA study. *British Journal of Ophthalmology*. 2022:320704.
512. Liu T, Lin W, Shi G, et al. Retinal and choroidal vascular perfusion and thickness measurement in diabetic retinopathy Ppatients by the swept-source optical coherence tomography angiography. *Frontiers in Medicine*. 2022;9
513. Brinks J, van Dijk EHC, Klaassen I, et al. Exploring the choroidal vascular labyrinth and its molecular and structural roles in health and disease. *Progress in Retinal and Eye Research*. 2022;87:100994.
514. Sinclair SH, Grunwald JE, Riva CE, Braunstein SN, Nichols CW, Schwartz SS. Retinal vascular autoregulation in diabetes mellitus. *Ophthalmology*. 1982;89(7):748–750.
515. Rassam S, Patel V, Kohner E. The effect of experimental hypertension on retinal vascular autoregulation in humans: a mechanism for the progression of diabetic retinopathy. *Experimental Physiology*. 1995;80(1):53–68.
516. Mehlsen J, Jeppesen P, Erlandsen M, Poulsen PL, Bek T. Lack of effect of short-term treatment with Amlodipine and Lisinopril on retinal autoregulation in normotensive patients with type 1 diabetes and mild diabetic retinopathy. *Acta Ophthalmologica*. 2011;89(8):764–768.
517. Hashimoto R, Sugiyama T, Masahara H, Sakamoto M, Ubuka M, Maeno T. Impaired autoregulation of blood flow at the optic nerve head during vitrectomy in patients with type 2 diabetes. *American Journal of Ophthalmology*. 2017;181:125–133.
518. Trost A, Bruckner D, Rivera FJ, Reitsamer HA. Pericytes in the retina. In: Birbrair A, ed. *Pericyte Biology in Different Organs*. Cham: Springer International Publishing; 2019:1–26.
519. Wong VHY, Vingrys AJ, Jobling AI, Bui BV. Susceptibility of streptozotocin-induced diabetic rat retinal function and ocular blood flow to acute intraocular pressure challenge. *Investigative Ophthalmology & Visual Science*. 2013;54(3):2133–2141.
520. Shibata M, Oku H, Sugiyama T, et al. Disruption of gap junctions may be involved in impairment of autoregulation in optic nerve head blood flow of diabetic rabbits. *Investigative Ophthalmology & Visual Science*. 2011;52(5):2153–2159.
521. Garhöfer G, Zawinka C, Resch H, Kothy P, Schmetterer L, Dorner GT. Reduced response of retinal vessel diameters to flicker stimulation in patients with diabetes. *British Journal of Ophthalmology*. 2004;88(7):887.
522. Nguyen TT, Kawasaki R, Wang JJ, et al. Flicker light–induced retinal vasodilation in diabetes and diabetic retinopathy. *Diabetes Care*. 2009;32(11):2075–2080.
523. Lecleire-Collet A, Audo I, Aout M, et al. Evaluation of retinal function and flicker light-induced retinal vascular response in normotensive patients with diabetes without retinopathy. *Investigative Ophthalmology & Visual Science*. 2011;52(6):2861–2867.
524. Sörensen BM, Houben AJHM, Berendschot TTJM, et al. Prediabetes and type 2 diabetes are associated with generalized microvascular dysfunction. *Circulation*. 2016;134(18): 1339–1352.
525. Mandecka A, Dawczynski J, Blum M, et al. Influence of flickering light on the retinal vessels in diabetic patients. *Diabetes Care*. 2007;30(12):3048–3052.
526. Pemp B, Garhofer G, Weigert G, et al. Reduced retinal vessel response to flicker stimulation but not to exogenous nitric oxide in type 1 diabetes. *Investigative Ophthalmology & Visual Science*. 2009;50(9):4029–4032.
527. Lasta M, Pemp B, Schmidl D, et al. Neurovascular dysfunction precedes neural dysfunction in the retina of patients with Type 1 diabetes. *Investigative Ophthalmology & Visual Science*. 2013;54(1):842–847.
528. Garhöfer G, Chua J, Tan B, Wong D, Schmidl D, Schmetterer L. Retinal neurovascular coupling in diabetes. *Journal of Clinical Medicine*. 2020;9(9):2829.
529. Pemp B, Weigert G, Karl K, et al. Correlation of flicker-induced and flow-mediated vasodilatation in patients with endothelial dysfunction and healthy volunteers. *Diabetes Care*. 2009;32(8):1536–1541.

530. Schirutschke H, Kochan J, Haink K, et al. Comparative study of microvascular function: Forearm blood flow versus dynamic retinal vessel analysis. *Clinical Physiology & Functional Imaging*. 2021;41(1):42–50.
531. Dorner GT, Garhöfer G, Huemer KH, Riva CE, Wolzt M, Schmetterer L. Hyperglycemia affects flicker-induced vasodilation in the retina of healthy subjects. *Vision Research*. 2003;43(13):1495–1500.
532. Patel SR, Bellary S, Qin L, Balanos GM, McIntyre D, Gherghel D. Abnormal retinal vascular reactivity in individuals with impaired glucose tolerance: a preliminary study. *Investigative Ophthalmology & Visual Science*. 2012;53(9):5102–5108.
533. Hanaguri J, Yokota H, Watanabe M, et al. Retinal blood flow dysregulation precedes neural retinal dysfunction in type 2 diabetic mice. *Scientific Reports*. 2021;11(1):18401.
534. Mishra A, Newman E. Aminoguanidine reverses the loss of functional hyperemia in a rat model of diabetic retinopathy. *Frontiers in Neuroenergetics*. 2012;3
535. Mishra A, Newman EA. Inhibition of inducible nitric oxide synthase reverses the loss of functional hyperemia in diabetic retinopathy. *Glia*. 2010;58(16):1996–2004.
536. Nippert AR, Newman EA. Regulation of blood flow in diabetic retinopathy. *Visual Neuroscience*. 2020;37:E004.
537. Schiekofer S, Balletshofer B, Andrassy M, Bierhaus A, Nawroth PP. Endothelial dysfunction in diabetes mellitus. Seminars in thrombosis and hemostasis. Seventh Avenue, New: Copyright© 2000 by Thieme Medical Publishers. *Inc*. 2000;333
538. Triggle CR, Ding H. A review of endothelial dysfunction in diabetes: a focus on the contribution of a dysfunctional eNOS. *Journal of the American Society of Hypertension*. 2010;4(3):102–115.
539. Schmetterer L, Findl O, Fasching P, et al. Nitric oxide and ocular blood flow in patients with IDDM. *Diabetes*. 1997;46(4):653–658.
540. Wright WS, Eshaq RS, Lee M, Kaur G, Harris NR. Retinal physiology and circulation: effect of diabetes. *Comprehensive Physiology*. 2020:933–974.
541. Harris NR, Leskova W, Kaur G, Eshaq RS, Carter PR. Blood flow distribution and the endothelial surface layer in the diabetic retina. *Biorheology*. 2019;56:181–189.
542. Bressler SB. Introduction: understanding the role of angiogenesis and antiangiogenic agents in age-related macular degeneration. *Ophthalmology*. 2009;116(10):S1–S7.
543. Mammadzada P, Corredoira PM, André H. The role of hypoxia-inducible factors in neovascular age-related macular degeneration: a gene therapy perspective. *Cellular and Molecular Life Sciences*. 2020;77(5):819–833.
544. Grunwald JE, Hariprasad SM, DuPont J, et al. Foveolar choroidal blood flow in age-related macular degeneration. *Investigative Ophthalmology & Visual Science*. 1998;39(2):385–390.
545. Metelitsina TI, Grunwald JE, DuPont JC, Ying GS. Effect of systemic hypertension on foveolar choroidal blood flow in age related macular degeneration. *British Journal of Ophthalmology*. 2006;90(3):342.
546. Chen S-J, Cheng C, Lee A, et al. Pulsatile ocular blood flow in asymmetric exudative age related macular degeneration. *British Journal of Ophthalmology*. 2001;85(12):1411.
547. Üretmen Ö, Akkin C, Erakgün T, Killi R. Color Doppler imaging of choroidal circulation in patients with asymmetric age-related macular degeneration. *Ophthalmologica*. 2003;217(2):137–142.
548. Ciulla TA, Harris A, Kagemann L, et al. Choroidal perfusion perturbations in non-neovascular age related macular degeneration. *British Journal of Ophthalmology*. 2002;86(2):209.
549. Metelitsina TI, Grunwald JE, DuPont JC, Ying GS. Effect of isometric exercise on choroidal blood flow in patients with age-related macular degeneration. *British Journal of Ophthalmology*. 2010;94(12):1629.
550. Berenberg TL, Metelitsina TI, Madow B, et al. The association between drusen extent and foveolar choroidal blood flow in age-related maculare degeneration. *Retina*. 2012;32(1):25–31.
551. Grunwald JE, Metelitsina TI, Dupont JC, Ying GS, Maguire MG. Reduced foveolar choroidal blood flow in eyes with increasing AMD severity. *Investigative Ophthalmology & Visual Science*. 2005;46(3):1033–1038.
552. Metelitsina TI, Grunwald JE, DuPont JC, Ying GS, Brucker AJ, Dunaief JL. Foveolar choroidal circulation and choroidal neovascularization in age-related macular degeneration. *Investigative Ophthalmology & Visual Science*. 2008;49(1):358–363.
553. Boltz A, Luksch A, Wimpissinger B, et al. Choroidal blood flow and progression of age-related macular degeneration in the fellow eye in patients with unilateral choroidal neovascularization. *Invest Ophthalmol Vis Sci*. 2010;51(8):4220–4225.
554. Xu W, Grunwald JE, Metelitsina TI, et al. Association of risk factors for choroidal neovascularization in age-related macular degeneration with decreased foveolar choroidal circulation. *American Journal of Ophthalmology*. 2010;150(1):40–47.
555. Zhou Q, Daniel E, Grunwald JE, et al. Association between pseudodrusen and delayed patchy choroidal filling in the comparison of age-related macular degeneration treatments trials. *Acta Ophthalmologica*. 2017;95(6):e518–e520.
556. Betzler BK, Ding J, Wei X, et al. Choroidal vascularity index: a step towards software as a medical device. *British Journal of Ophthalmology*. 2022;106(2):149.
557. Koh LHL, Agrawal R, Khandelwal N, Charan LS, Chhablani J. Choroidal vascular changes in age-related macular degeneration. *Acta Ophthalmologica*. 2017;95(7):e597–e601.
558. Wei X, Ting DSW, Ng WY, Khandelwal N, Agrawal R, Cheung CMG. Choroidal vascularity index: a novel optical coherence tomography based parameter in patients with exudative age-related macular degeneration. *Retina*. 2017;37(6):1120–1125.
559. Keenan TD, Klein B, Agrón E, Chew EY, Cukras CA, Wong WT. Choroidal thickness and vascularity vary with disease severity and subretinal drusenoid deposit presence in nonadvanced age-related macular degeneration. *Retina*. 2020;40(4):632–642.
560. Giannaccare G, Pellegrini M, Sebastiani S, et al. Choroidal vascularity index quantification in geographic atrophy using binarization of enhanced-depth imaging optical coherence tomographic scans. *Retina*. 2020;40(5):960–965.
561. Sacconi R, Battista M, Borrelli E, et al. Choroidal vascularity index is associated with geographic atrophy progression. *Retina*. 2022;42(2):381–387.
562. Borrelli E, Souied EH, Freund KB, et al. Reduced choriocapillaris flow in eyes with type 3 neovascularization and age-related macular degeneration. *Retina*. 2018;38(10):1968–1976.
563. Alagorie AR, Verma A, Nassisi M, et al. Quantitative assessment of choriocapillaris flow deficits surrounding choroidal neovascular membranes. *Retina*. 2020;40(11):2106–2112.
564. Nesper PL, Ong JX, Fawzi AA. Exploring the relationship between multilayered choroidal neovascularization and choriocapillaris flow deficits in AMD. *Investigative Ophthalmology & Visual Science*. 2021;62(3):12–12.
565. Takasago Y, Shiragami C, Kobayashi M, et al. Macular atrophy findings by optical coherence tomography angiography compared with fundus autofluorescence in treated exudation age-related macular degeneration. *Retina*. 2019;39(2):296–302.
566. Shi Y, Zhang Q, Zhou H, et al. Correlations between choriocapillaris and choroidal measurements and the growth of geographic atrophy using swept source OCT imaging. *Am J Ophthalmol*. 2021;224:321–331.
567. You QS, Camino A, Wang J, et al. Geographic atrophy progression is associated with choriocapillaris flow deficits measured with optical coherence tomographic angiography. *Investigative Ophthalmology & Visual Science*. 2021;62(15):28–28.
568. Corvi F, Corradetti G, Tiosano L, McLaughlin JA, Lee TK, Sadda SR. Topography of choriocapillaris flow deficit predicts development of neovascularization or atrophy in age-related macular degeneration. *Graefe's Archive for Clinical and Experimental Ophthalmology*. 2021;259(10):2887–2895.
569. Corradetti G, Tiosano L, Nassisi M, et al. Scotopic microperimetric sensitivity and inner choroid flow deficits as predictors of progression to nascent geographic atrophy. *British Journal of Ophthalmology*. 2021;105(11):1584.
570. Corvi F, Tiosano L, Corradetti G, et al. Choriocapillaris flow deficits as a risk factor for progression of age-related macular degeneration. *Retina*. 2021;41(4):686–693.
571. Biesemeier A, Taubitz T, Julien S, Yoeruek E, Schraermeyer U. Choriocapillaris breakdown precedes retinal degeneration in age-related macular degeneration. *Neurobiology of Aging*. 2014;35(11):2562–2573.
572. Nassisi M, Tepelus T, Nittala MG, Sadda SR. Choriocapillaris flow impairment predicts the development and enlargement of drusen. *Graefe's Archive for Clinical and Experimental Ophthalmology*. 2019;257(10):2079–2085.
573. Katsi VK, Marketou ME, Vrachatis DA, et al. Essential hypertension in the pathogenesis of age-related macular degeneration: a review of the current evidence. *Journal of Hypertension*. 2015;33(12):2382–2388.
574. Yamazaki D, Hitomi H, Nishiyama A. Hypertension with diabetes mellitus complications. *Hypertension Research*. 2018;41(3):147–156.
575. Nislawati R, Zainal ATF, Ismail A, Waspodo N, Kasim F, Gunawan AMAK. Role of hypertension as a risk factor for open-angle glaucoma: a systematic review and meta-analysis. *BMJ Open Ophthalmology*. 2021;6(1):e000798.
576. Hashimoto R, Sugiyama T, Ubuka M, Maeno T. Impairment of autoregulation of optic nerve head blood flow during vitreous surgery in patients with hypertension and hyperlipidemia. *Graefes Arch Clin Exp Ophthalmol*. 2017;255(11):2227–2235.
577. Zeng R, Garg I, Bannai D, et al. Retinal microvasculature and vasoreactivity changes in hypertension using optical coherence tomography-angiography. *Graefe's Archive for Clinical and Experimental Ophthalmology*. 2022:1–11.
578. Tan W, Yao X, Le TT, Tan B, Schmetterer L, Chua J. The new era of retinal imaging in hypertensive patients. *Asia-Pacific Journal of Ophthalmology*. 2022;11(2):149–159.
579. Tan W, Yao X, Le TT, et al. The application of optical coherence tomography angiography in systemic hypertension: a meta-analysis. *Frontiers in Medicine*. 2021;8:1–15.
580. Anjos R, Ferreira A, Barkoudah E, Claggett B, Pinto LA, Miguel A. Application of optical coherence tomography angiography macular analysis for systemic hypertension. A systematic review and meta-analysis. *American Journal of Hypertension*. 2021;35(4):356–364.
581. Nolde JM, Frost S, Kannenkeril D, et al. Capillary vascular density in the retina of hypertensive patients is associated with a non-dipping pattern independent of mean ambulatory blood pressure. *Journal of Hypertension*. 2021;39(9):1826–1834.
582. Monteiro-Henriques I, Rocha-Sousa A, Barbosa-Breda J. Optical coherence tomography angiography changes in cardiovascular systemic diseases and risk factors: A Review. *Acta Ophthalmologica*. 2022;100(1):e1–e15.
583. Chua J, Le TT, Tan B, et al. Choriocapillaris microvasculature dysfunction in systemic hypertension. *Scientific Reports*. 2021;11(1):4603.
584. Sun C, Ladores C, Hong J, et al. Systemic hypertension associated retinal microvascular changes can be detected with optical coherence tomography angiography. *Scientific Reports*. 2020;10(1):9580.
585. Chua J, Chin CWL, Tan B, et al. Impact of systemic vascular risk factors on the choriocapillaris using optical coherence tomography angiography in patients with systemic hypertension. *Scientific Reports*. 2019;9(1):5819.
586. Chua J, Loon Chin CW, Hong J, et al. Impact of hypertension on retinal capillary microvasculature using optical coherence tomographic angiography. *J Hypertens*. 2019;37(3):572–580.
587. Frost S, Kanagasingam Y, Sohrabi H, et al. Retinal vascular biomarkers for early detection and monitoring of Alzheimer's disease. *Translational Psychiatry*. 2013;3(2):e233–e233.
588. Cheung CY-l, Ong YT, Ikram MK, et al. Microvascular network alterations in the retina of patients with Alzheimer's disease. *Alzheimer's & Dementia: The Journal of the Alzheimer's Association*. 2014;10(2):135–142.
589. Szegedi S, et al. Anatomical and functional changes in the retina in patients with Alzheimer's disease and mild cognitive impairment. *Acta Ophthalmologica*. 2020;98(7):e914–e921.
590. Schrijvers EMC, Buitendijk GHS, Ikram MK, et al. Retinopathy and risk of dementia. *The Rotterdam Study*. 2012;79(4):365–370.
591. Yeh T-C, Kuo C-T, Chou Y-B. Retinal microvascular changes in mild cognitive impairment and Alzheimer's disease: a systematic review, meta-analysis, and meta-regression. *Frontiers in Aging Neuroscience*. 2022;14:1–17.
592. Chalkias E, Chalkias IN, Bakirtzis C, et al. Differentiating degenerative from vascular dementia with the help of optical coherence tomography angiography biomarkers. *Healthcare (Basel)*. 2022;10(3):539.

593. Jin Q, Lei Y, Wang R, Wu H, Ji K, Ling L. A systematic review and meta-analysis of retinal microvascular features in Alzheimer's disease. Frontiers in Aging. *Neuroscience.* 2021;13:1–11.

594. Zabel P, Kaluzny JJ, Zabel K, et al. Quantitative assessment of retinal thickness and vessel density using optical coherence tomography angiography in patients with Alzheimer's disease and glaucoma. *PLOS ONE.* 2021;16(3):e0248284.

595. Rifai OM, McGrory S, Robbins CB, et al. The application of optical coherence tomography angiography in Alzheimer's disease: a systematic review. *Alzheimer's & Dementia.* 2021;13(1):e12149.

596. Wang X, Zhao Q, Tao R, et al. Decreased retinal vascular density in Alzheimer's disease (AD) and mild cognitive impairment (MCI): an optical coherence tomography angiography (OCTA) study. Frontiers in Aging. *Neuroscience.* 2021;12

597. Chua J, Hu Q, Ke M, et al. Retinal microvasculature dysfunction is associated with Alzheimer's disease and mild cognitive impairment. *Alzheimers Res Ther.* 2020;12(1):161.

598. Wu J, Zhang X, Azhati G, Li T, Xu G, Liu F. Retinal microvascular attenuation in mental cognitive impairment and Alzheimer's disease by optical coherence tomography angiography. *Acta Ophthalmologica.* 2020;98(6):e781–e787.

599. Wang L, Kwakyi O, Nguyen J, et al. Microvascular blood flow velocities measured with a retinal function imager: inter-eye correlations in healthy controls and an exploration in multiple sclerosis. *Eye and Vision.* 2018;5(1):29.

600. Kallab M, Hommer N, Schlatter A, et al. Retinal oxygen metabolism and haemodynamics in patients with multiple sclerosis and history of optic neuritis. *Frontiers in Neuroscience.* 2021;15

601. Chen Q, Fang M, Miri S, et al. Retinal microvascular and neuronal function in patients with multiple sclerosis: 2-year follow-up. *Multiple Sclerosis and Related Disorders.* 2021;56

602. Svrčinová T, Hok P, Šínová I, et al. Changes in oxygen saturation and the retinal nerve fibre layer in patients with optic neuritis associated with multiple sclerosis in a 6-month follow-up. *Acta Ophthalmologica.* 2020;98(8):841–847.

603. Liu Y, Delgado S, Jiang H, et al. Retinal tissue perfusion in patients with multiple sclerosis. *Current Eye Research.* 2019;44(10):1091–1097.

604. Wang X, Jia Y, Spain R, et al. Optical coherence tomography angiography of optic nerve head and parafovea in multiple sclerosis. *British Journal of Ophthalmology.* 2014;98(10):1368.

605. Akarsu C, Tan FU, Kendi T. Color Doppler imaging in optic neuritis with multiple sclerosis. *Graefe's Archive for Clinical and Experimental Ophthalmology.* 2004;242(12):990–994.

Metabolic Interactions Between Neurons and Glial Cells

Rupali Vohra and Miriam Kolko

Introduction

The predominant function of the retina is to transmit light impulse–converted nerve signals from the retina to the brain, thereby forming an interpreted image. Light waves initially enter the outer part of the eye (cornea, pupil, lens, and vitreous) to reach the retina. In the retina, the waves are converted into nerve signals mediated by the photoreceptor cells in the outer retina. These cells synapse with bipolar cells, spanning from the outer plexiform layer to the inner plexiform layer of the retina. In the inner retina, bipolar cells synapse with retinal ganglion cells, which transfer nerve signals through its axons that form the optic nerve, to the lateral geniculate nucleus of the brain, and then to the visual cortex. Thus, neuronal interactions are crucial for facilitating visual function.

To ensure neuroprotection of the innermost neurons, the most abundant retinal glial cells, Müller glia, offer several protective properties (Fig. 12.1). Müller glia are located between retinal vessels and neurons and provide a buffering capacity by taking up excessive glutamate from the synapses to prevent excitotoxic damage of neurons, in particular retinal ganglion cells.[1,2] These excess amounts of glutamate are taken up primarily by the vast representation of the glutamate transporter, excitatory amino acid transporter (EAAT) 1, on the cell surface.[3–5] Once entering the Müller glia, the enzyme glutamine synthetase (GS) detoxifies glutamate and ammonia into glutamine, which can be shuttled back to neurons. Alternatively, glutamate may also be used as an energy substrate within the Müller glia mitochondria.[6,7] Energy for excitatory glutamatergic synaptic transmission in the mammalian retina, as elsewhere in the central nervous system (CNS), is most commonly provided by the metabolism of blood-borne glucose. In fact, retinal preparations become synaptically silent as a result of glucose depletion.[8] From an ultrastructural point of view, the remarkable concentration of mitochondria in synaptic terminals of axons indicates that glutamatergic synapses have high capacity for oxygen consumption and are major users of metabolic energy.[9–11]

Metabolic energy may be provided actively by transformation and transfer of energy substrates directly from Müller glia to neurons or indirectly by Müller glia regulation of retinal blood flow. Müller glia are an integrated part of the blood-retinal barrier (BRB) and offer structural support of the retina, in particular the retinal ganglion cells and their axons.[12] Owing to the close relation to the retinal blood vessels, Müller glia are also responsible for controlling transfer of energy substrates and other molecules to and from retinal neurons and the blood supply.[2,13] Additionally, Müller glia play a prominent role in regulating the actual supply of these molecules by neurovascular coupling, in which Müller glia dilate or constrict the vasculature supporting the inner retina.[14]

The vasculature of both the retina and brain can autoregulate, meaning that blood flow changes in response to neuronal activity (see Chapter 11). Glial cells, such as the Müller glia, sense neuronal activity and alter blood flow accordingly by communicating directly with the inner retinal vasculature. Thus, stimulation of retinal whole-mounts by light or direct glial stimulation has been shown to lead to either vasoconstriction or vasodilation of inner retinal blood vessels.[15] In particular, these vascular caliber changes were found to be associated with increases in intracellular calcium within the retinal glia. Therefore, like their counterparts in the brain, retinal glia induce caliber changes in capillaries in response to neuronal activity.

Glia also communicate with each other via increases in intracellular calcium in the form of a calcium wave propagating from one astrocyte to another via gap junctions or by releasing bursts of extracellular adenosine triphosphate (ATP).[16,17] Studies in retinal whole-mounts have shown that transmitters released from neurons induce transient elevations in intracellular calcium in glia.[16] Mechanical, chemical, and light stimulation can evoke increases in intracellular calcium in both astrocytes and Müller glia that propagate to neighboring glia as a "wave."[16] Extracellular ATP evokes large increases in intracellular calcium in both astrocytes and Müller glia, which subsequently causes these cells to release ATP extracellularly in response to stimulation. The source of the calcium elevations in retinal glia is thought to be primarily from intracellular calcium stores, although there are also a number of calcium permeable channels, pumps, and exchangers that can mediate calcium influx to the glia from the environment.

The functional significance of ATP release and the subsequent elevation in intracellular calcium within retinal glia is twofold: direct modulation of neurons and alteration of vessel caliber.

Many types of retinal neurons are known to express ATP receptors (called P2 receptors), including photoreceptors, amacrine cells, and retinal ganglion cells.[18–21] Moreover, photoreceptor function is modulated by extracellular ATP.[19] Therefore, it is possible that the release of ATP extracellularly by glia could in turn modulate a variety of neuronal cell types from photoreceptors to retinal ganglion cells. With respect to glial-dependent modulation of vessel caliber, increases in intracellular calcium in cortical astrocyte endfeet are linked to marked vasodilation in the adjacent arteriole, suggesting a relationship between astrocytes and the vasculature within different regions of the CNS in response to an increase in neural activity.[22,23]

Thus, glia play a crucial role not only in maintaining normal neuronal function but also in ensuring adequate retinal blood flow. Similarly, the function of glial cells can be affected by alterations in blood flow, which is known to change during systemic stress or disease.[15,24,25]

In addition to regulating blood flow and transferring various substrates, Müller glia also produce and secrete various neurotrophic factors that support neuronal survival, e.g., neutrophins, brain-derived neurotrophic factor (BDNF), ciliary neurotrophic factor (CNTF) and glial cell–derived neurotrophic factor (GDNF).[26,27] Coculture studies of

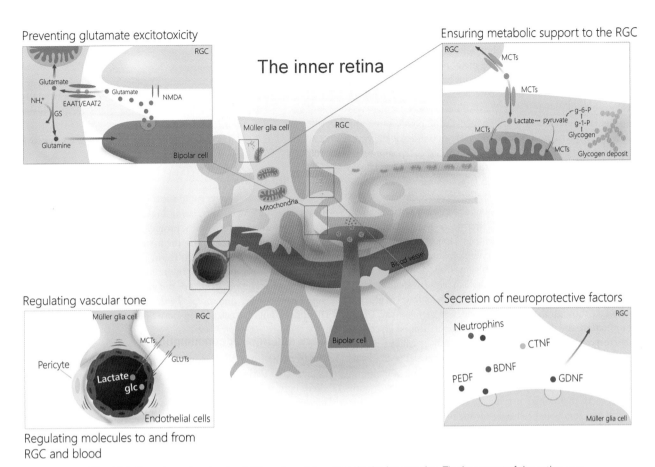

Fig. 12.1 Overview of protective Müller glia cell functions in the inner retina. The inner part of the retina consists of a triad of cells, the retinal ganglion cell (*RGC*), bipolar cell, and Müller glia. The Müller glia contributes to inner retinal homeostasis and function by preventing glutamate excitotoxicity, ensuring metabolic support to surrounding neurons, regulating vascular tone, and secreting neuroprotective factors. *BDNF*, brain-derived neurotrophic factor; *CNTF*, ciliary neurotrophic factor; *EAAT*, excitatory amino acid transporter; *GDNF*, glial-derived neurotrophic factor; *GLC*, glucose; *MCT*, monocarboxylate transporter; *NMDA*, N-methyl-D-aspartate; *PEDF*, Pigment epithelium-derived factor.

Müller glia and retinal ganglion cells have also verified that the mere presence of Müller glia ensures retinal ganglion cell survival by regulating various processes. These processes include neurite formation,[28] and protection against high glucose exposure,[29] glutamate excitotoxicity, and nitric oxide (NO) neurotoxicity,[30] which further highlights that Müller glia are crucial for inner retinal function.

A recent coculture study further established that the protective effect of Müller cells on retinal ganglion cell survival was abolished once Müller cell mitochondria were inhibited, indicating that Müller cell energy metabolism is important in providing the protection of retinal ganglion cells.[31] Overall, dysfunctional glial cells, especially Müller cells, are likely to be a trigger for neuronal death due to altered energy metabolism and/or mitochondrial function leading to disrupted retinal function.

RETINAL ENERGY METABOLISM

The general energy substrates consist of carbohydrates, lipids, and amino acids, where the carbohydrates in the form of glucose are attributed to being the most prevalent energy source for the retina. The first step in glucose metabolism is by glycolysis, where two ATP molecules and two pyruvate or lactate molecules are produced. In 1972, Krebs et al.[32] established that the eye, and especially the retina, is highly glycolytic and that lactate release from the eye exceeds that from the brain.

This is supported by reported elevated retinal lactate levels between 5 and 50 mmol/L[33–37] compared with only 1 to 2 mmol/L in the peripheral blood of healthy humans.[38] In particular, the Müller glia contribute to this high glycolytic rate with a favorable conversion of glucose into lactate rather than pyruvate,[39–41] despite sufficient oxygen availability, a phenomenon known as the Warburg effect.

Recent studies have suggested that Müller glia may shift from glycolysis to oxidative phosphorylation during excessive stress, such as hypoglycemia and oxidative stress,[5,42] indicating that mitochondrial metabolism in Müller glia may be equally important as glycolysis. In addition to producing pyruvate or lactate as the end product of glycolysis, nicotinamide adenine dinucleotide (NAD+) is also produced. NAD+ production is essential to facilitate well-functioning mitochondria, as it cofactors multiple steps in the tricarboxylic acid cycle (TCA), by which the majority of ATP is yielded.

Although electrophysiological evidence shows that neurotransmission through the inner retina is supported by glycolysis,[8] there is currently no clear experimental evidence showing that synaptic activity of pre- and postsynaptic retinal neurons is directly sustained by glucose. However, indirect evidence is suggested from the classical work of Lowry et al.[43] on the distribution of enzymes of glucose metabolism determined from pure samples of each retinal layer from monkey and rabbit. A brief introductory overview of this particular paper is given further as it provides invaluable insight into the contribution of Müller glia to overall retinal function and energy metabolism.

All enzymes of glycolysis are in the cytoplasm rather than in the mitochondria. To initiate glycolysis, hexokinase irreversibly phosphorylates glucose to glucose-6-phosphate (G6P). The distribution of hexokinase was confined to the layer containing inner segments of photoreceptors, the inner synaptic layer and to the innermost retinal layer bordering the vitreous. The second step in glycolysis is the conversion of G6P to fructose-6P by glucose-phosphate isomerase. The distribution of this enzyme was largely confined to the inner and outer synaptic layers. Phosphofructokinase, the third enzyme in glycolysis, irreversibly phosphorylates fructose-6P to fructose-1,6diP, and its distribution was confined to both synaptic layers and the innermost retinal layer. The ninth enzyme in glycolysis, phosphoglyceromutase, converts 3-phosphoglycerate to 2-phosphoglycerate, and its distribution was similar to that of phosphofructokinase.

In tissues with adequate oxygen supply, pyruvate formation is the 11th and final step of glycolysis. The metabolism of pyruvate for energy production consumes oxygen and completes the breakdown of glucose to CO_2 and water through the process of oxidative metabolism. Upon careful examination, the distribution of the aforementioned glycolytic enzymes corresponds to the morphologic position of Müller glia in situ. Müller glia extend radially through all of the retinal layers from the photoreceptor inner segments to the inner limiting membrane bordering the vitreous, and they extend fine filaments laterally in both synaptic layers. As mentioned previously, they also form an additional physical and functional cell layer for the diffusion of substances from the blood to neurons. Kuwabara and Cogan[44,45] undertook the first comprehensive histochemical study to identify Müller glia as the primary glucose-utilizing cells in the retina. However, Müller glia are also known to utilize lactate. In fact, they have a preferred metabolism of lactate, even when glucose is present[46,47] (see Fig. 12.8). This was thought to occur in order to spare glucose for neurons, but retinal ganglion cells in culture have also been shown to metabolize lactate before glucose.[48] However, the notion of preferential lactate metabolism in the presence of glucose is still controversial and needs to be validated by in vivo studies. Müller glia have been shown to switch their metabolic state from glycolysis to oxidative phosphorylation during stress.[7] Certain cells, including neurons, are known to release lactate during stress, thus Müller glia uptake of lactate for oxidative phosphorylation may provide a rapid metabolic production of ATP by passing glucose breakdown to pyruvate, which involves more steps.[46,47]

Regardless of how the energy consumption of the retina (or other parts of the CNS) is altered locally to meet changing demands, it is important to know from a neurophysiological point of view which cell types and what cellular events are associated with local changes in blood flow, metabolism, and tissue oxygenation.

RETINAL OXYGEN DISTRIBUTION AND CONSUMPTION

Under normal conditions, O_2 is the limiting factor in retinal metabolism. Oxygen is used by mitochondria and their distribution is important for understanding locations of high O_2 demand. The O_2 consumption (QO_2) of the retinal pigment epithelial (RPE) cells is about 20% of that of the retina per mg protein.[49] Mitochondria are densely observed in the inner segments (IS) of photoreceptors. Cones have more mitochondria than rods.[50,51] Mitochondria are also found in each rod spherule and cone pedicle. In the inner retina, the inner plexiform layer has a larger number of mitochondria than the nuclear layers.[52]

The human retina has a complex vascular supply system to ensure adequate oxygenation. The inner retina is nourished by the retinal circulation, while the outer retina is supplied by the choroidal vasculature.[53] Just as in the brain, the retina has a continuous demand for oxygen and, as such, a lack of oxygen supply will be associated with hypoxia leading to retinal disease.[54]

Using dual-beam bidirectional Doppler optical coherence tomography, the total retinal blood flow was $44.3 \pm 9.0 \mu L/min$ at baseline and decreased to $18.7 \pm 4.2 \mu L/min$ during 100% oxygen breathing, resulting in a pronounced decrease in retinal oxygen extraction from $2.33 \pm 0.51 \mu L(O_2)/min$ to $0.88 \pm 0.14 \mu L(O_2)/min$ during breathing of 100% oxygen, a known hyperoxic state.[55]

The inner retina

The distribution of oxygen tension (Po_2) close to the vitreoretinal interface is heterogeneous, being higher close to the arteriolar wall.[56] Preretinal and transretinal Po_2 profiles indicate that O_2 diffusion from the arterioles affects the Po_2 in the juxta-arteriolar areas (Fig. 12.2).[56,57] O_2 reaches the vitreous by diffusion from the retinal circulation. In contrast, far from the vessels, the preretinal Po_2 remains constant and the average preretinal Po_2 from the vitreal side is similar to that measured in the inner retina.[56,58,59] In the inner retina, Po_2 averages about 20 mmHg, but up to 60 mmHg close to the arteriolar wall.[56,60,61]

Dark and light O_2 consumption

Inner retinal oxygen consumption has been shown to be the same in light and darkness,[62] indicating no influence of light adaptation as there is in the outer retina. In the inner retina, retinal ganglion cells have much higher firing rates if a stimulus is presented repeatedly than if the same amount of light is delivered as a steady background. Consequently, one would expect the inner retina to use more energy when a stimulus is flickering. Indeed, there is, in response to a flickering stimulus, a higher lactate production in the inner retina of rabbit than during darkness or steady illumination[8] and a higher deoxy-D-glucose uptake in monkey retina.[63]

The outer retina

Transretinal Po_2 measurements have provided data about the O_2 supply to the photoreceptors and their QO_2. Po_2 profiles made in cat,[64,65] pig,[56] and monkey[66] indicate that oxygen diffuses from the inner retina and from the choroid toward the middle of the retina, i.e., the outer plexiform layer (OPL). The choroidal circulation supplies about 90% of the photoreceptor's O_2 use.[60]

Photoreceptor QO_2 in darkness

In the dark-adapted retina, photoreceptor QO_2 (Q_{OR}) depends strongly on choriocapillary Po_2 in cat and monkey.[60,67] In the IS of photoreceptors the local value of QO_2 is about five times higher than in the outer segments (OS). A similar range for QO_2 in the outer retina was obtained in rat, rabbit, and pig retinas.[8,33,68] In both cat and monkey, the average value of Po_2 in the choriocapillaries is about 50 mmHg, and the corresponding average value of QO_2 in the outer retina is 4 to 5 mL $O_2/100 g^{-1}$ per min^{-1}.[60,67]

The average Po_2 value in cat was 5 mmHg; the minimum was frequently indistinguishable from zero in the dark, as predicted by Dollery et al.[60,69] The amount of oxygen consumed is an indirect measure of ATP synthesis and thus of ATP utilization. The ATP produced in the dark fuels many cellular processes, mainly the Na^+/K^+-ATPase in the IS, which extrudes a large amount of sodium that enters through the light-dependent channels in the OS.[8,70] An additional process is the turnover of Cyclic guanosine monophosphate (cGMP) that holds these channels open.[8,71]

As noted previously, there is no evidence about whether individual rods and cones use different amounts of O_2. Cones in the primate fovea appear to use slightly less O_2 than the parafoveal photoreceptors.[66,67]

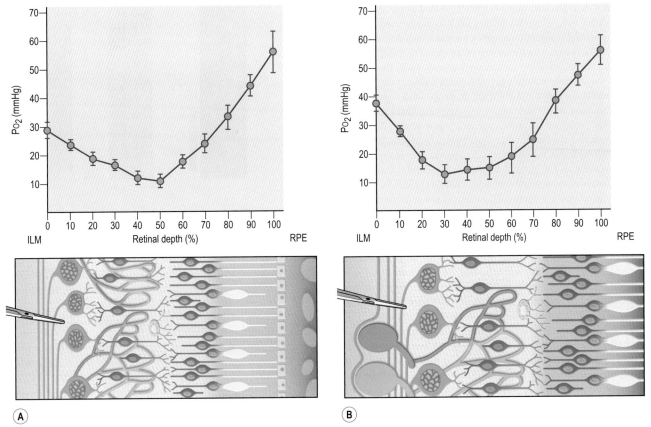

Fig. 12.2 Transretinal oxygen partial pressure (Po_2) profiles recorded in intravascular (**A**) and juxta-arteriolar (**B**) retinal areas in minipigs. The intraretinal values indicate a progressive decrease of the tissue Po_2 from both the vitreoretinal interface (internal limiting membrane, *ILM*) and the pigment epithelium toward the middle of the retina, with the minimum mean value recorded at 40% and 50% retinal depth. At the vitreoretinal interface, the higher Po_2 suggests that oxygen diffusing from the larger vessels reaches the inner retina. Each point is the mean ± standard error of 13 measurements. The drawings indicate the pathway of the microelectrode through the retina. *RPE*, Retinal pigment epithelium. (Modified from Pournaras CJ. Retinal oxygen distribution. Its role in the physiopathology of vasoproliferative microangiopathies. *Retina.* 1995;15(4):332–347.)

Photoreceptor QO_2 in light

QO_2 in the outer retina is lower in steady light than in darkness in various animals investigated.[8,60,66,72] The activity of the Na^+/K^+-ATPase decreases in light, but the turnover of cGMP increases,[73,74] so the decrease in Q_{OR} is not as great as the decrease in the pump rate. The maximum size of the overall change appears to be species dependent.

THE ROLE OF GLYCOLYSIS UNDERLYING RETINAL FUNCTION: FROM WHOLE RETINA TO ITS PARTS

Visualization of dynamic functional activity in the retina is an *indirect* measurement of neuronal activity. It is important to appreciate that any dynamic "functional imaging" of the CNS, for example, functional magnetic resonance imaging (fMRI) or positron emission tomography (PET) imaging, measures local changes in brain metabolism and physiology that are associated with neuronal activity. Therefore, examining and evaluating retinal function necessarily involves understanding the energy metabolism of this particular tissue.

The significance of glucose and its metabolism through the glycolytic pathway in mammalian retina is attested by the measured high rate of aerobic glycolysis in vitro (high capacity for oxygen consumption),[50,75] its susceptibility to iodoacetate, a strong Pasteur effect (inhibition of glucose utilization),[32,50,76,77] and the aerobic and anaerobic production of lactate.[76,78,79]

The adult retina, as is the case for every CNS region, depends on an uninterrupted supply of blood-borne glucose. Under normal conditions, glucose is virtually the main substrate supporting the intense energy metabolism required to maintain retinal function, (e.g., normal electrical responsiveness to light and neurotransmission).[8,79,80] Lactate generated from either anaerobic glycolysis or glycogenolysis within the retina has recently been proposed as another important energy source during synaptic transmission.[39,48,81,82] but its uptake and metabolism by retinal cells has yet to be demonstrated in vivo. Nevertheless, a recent study found significantly lower peripheral blood lactate levels in glaucoma patients with well-defined retinal neurodegeneration, implying that diminished or dysfunctional lactate turnover may contribute to obscured retinal health.[83]

The distribution of key enzymes in glucose metabolism through the individual neuronal and synaptic retinal layers and the dehydrogenases for several of the intermediate stages of glucose degradation in retina have been documented in a series of pioneering histochemical work.[6,43,44,84,85]

Metabolic studies have demonstrated that Müller glia both in situ and when acutely isolated, preferentially and massively take up and phosphorylate glucose, part of which is stored as glycogen.[46,86,87] Further evidence to confirm this finding has been performed in vivo.[88]

More supporting evidence comes from the use of iodoacetate, a well-known glycolytic poison which exerts its effect when the transformation of glucose is committed to proceed through glycolysis. In the 1950s, it was shown that intravenous delivery of sodium iodoacetate in rabbit, monkey, and cat abolished the electrical response of the visual pathway to illumination within minutes, with a resulting histologic picture similar to that presented in human retinitis pigmentosa.[89] This led to the speculation that the initial effect must be on visual cells,[90] although Warburg suggested that the different cell types in the retina may not contribute equally to the general biochemical picture.[89] Indeed, this suggestion has been unambiguously supported by the differential suppression of the component waves of the extracellular electroretinogram (ERG).[91,92] However, beyond this evidence, the identity of the retinal cell types taking up iodoacetate remains unknown. Recently this was explored using synchrotron-based x-ray fluorescence of iodoacetate at the cellular level in situ (Fig. 12.3). The fluorescence map (Fig. 12.3A) generated from the dark-adapted retina (Fig. 12.3B) showed that iodoacetate was taken up specifically by Müller glia and not by retinal neurons, including photoreceptors, indicating that the effect of iodoacetate on neurons is not direct but secondary to inhibiting glycolysis in glia (Poitry-Yamate *unpublished data*). Together, these results suggest a key role played by Müller glia in transporting glucose from the blood into the retina. Müller glia have also been shown to take up lactate, which is then metabolized and used as an additional energy source.[46] In addition, Müller glia secrete lactate, which can be taken up and processed by surrounding neurons, e.g., photoreceptors and retinal ganglion cells.[48,93]

Acutely isolated mammalian photoreceptors produce $^{14}CO_2$ from $^{14}C(U)$-glucose,[39] whereas photoreceptor OS produce both lactate from glucose and $^{14}CO_2$ from $^{14}C(U)$-glucose.[94] The results have been interpreted as indicating that both glycolysis and the pentose phosphate pathway contribute to photoreceptor function. Given that only one in six carbons from $^{14}C(U)$-glucose is converted to $^{14}CO_2$ through the pentose phosphate pathway, and the abundance of photoreceptor mitochondria, $^{14}CO_2$ is likely to reflect the rate of mitochondrial respiration.[39]

Photoreceptors of some species do not express Gpi 1, the enzyme catalyzing the isomerization of glucose-6-phosphate to fructose-6-phosphate,[95] leaving the phosphate pentose pathway as the only possible downstream path, with a gain of two NADPH molecules potentially serving as a reducing agent for reduction of retinaldehyde.

A number of studies of glucose metabolism have been undertaken in intact retinal tissue or with acutely isolated cell models in vertebrate/mammalian retina.[39,86–88,94,96] Of these, one is unique in studying not only glucose metabolism but also metabolic compartmentation: the cell model of acutely isolated Müller glia still attached to photoreceptors (termed "the cell complex") shown in Fig. 12.4 and further discussed in sections Biochemical specialization of glial cells, Functional neuronal activity and division of metabolic labor, and Experimental models of retinal metabolism and function, in this chapter. This study confirmed not only the previous work by Kuwabara and Cogan, but showed for the first time in a mammalian preparation of the CNS tissue that glial cells *transform rather than simply transfer* the primary energy substrate glucose, and supply neurons with a glucose-derived metabolite.[39,97,98]

Cell culture models of transformed rat Müller glia, human RPE, and transformed mouse photoreceptor cells and retinal ganglion cells were all found to produce lactate, aerobically and anaerobically, in the presence of 5 mM glucose.[99] This may not be surprising as culturing techniques influence cell metabolism and function. The composition of culturing medium may be a key underlying factor to explain

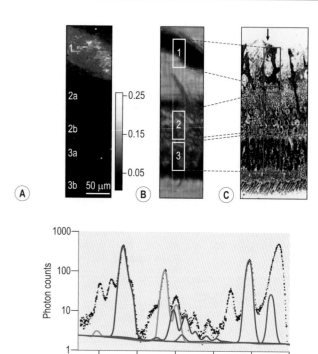

Fig. 12.3 The glycolytic poison iodoacetate is localized to Müller glia and not to retinal neurons: indirect evidence of which cell type depends directly on glucose metabolism. (**A**) Synchrotron radiation–based hard x-ray fluorescence map (90-μm height × 20-μm width) of the period table element iodine from iodoacetate *(orange)* subsequent to scanning the retina from the inner *(top)* to outer *(bottom)* layers. Iodoacetate was localized in the retina to Region 1 comprising the endfeet of Müller glia. The metabolic experiment consisted of dark-adapting the tissue prior to a 50-minute exposure ex vivo to bicarbonate buffered Ringer's physiological solution carrying iodoaceate and D-glucose. Note that iodoacetate inactivates the glyceraldehyde-3-phosphate dehydrogenase reaction and therefore inhibits the sixth step in glycolysis. (**B**) Phase contrast image of the retina from which the fluorescence map shown in (**A**) was obtained. Region 1, Müller glial endfeet; Region 2a, inner plexiform layer; Region 2b, inner nuclear layer; Region 3a, photoreceptor layer; Region 3b, photoreceptor segments. (**C**) Reference, methyl blue–stained coronal section used for identifying individual retinal layers. (**D**) X-ray fluorescence energy emission spectra from Region 1. An La energy emission at 3.9 keV is specific to iodine from iodoacetate *(blue trace)*. The y-axis expresses the number of fluorescence photons emitted from iodine subsequent to exposing the preparation to synchrotron light.

why cells are predominantly glycolytic, irrespective of cell type.[100] However, the production of lactate by these cells did not significantly differ with the addition of 10 mM lactate.[99] In general, lactate production and its release into the extracellular space as a lactate anion plus a proton (H^+) creates an extracellular pH gradient, i.e., increased proton concentration and consequently pH values become less than 7.4. Depending on the magnitude, direction, and time course of the extracellular pH gradient, lactate may accumulate extracellularly, or alternatively, lactate may be taken up on a proton-linked monocarboxylate transporter.[101] In this context, both cultured retinal ganglion cells and freshly isolated retinas from mice have revealed lactate uptake and metabolism.[48,102] In addition, metabolic studies using gas-chromatography mass spectrometry have shown preferential uptake and metabolism of lactate in Müller glia and retinal ganglion cells, even in the presence of glucose.[46–48] Taken together, these cells may

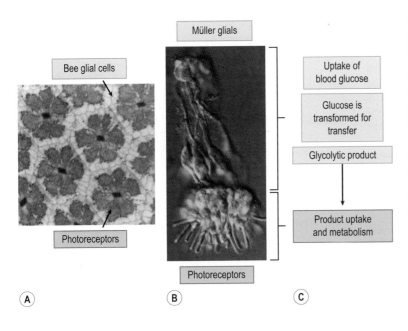

Fig. 12.4 Acutely isolated cell models for exploring retinal function, metabolism, and the trafficking of metabolites between glial cells and photoreceptor neurons. (**A**) Honeybee drone, illustrating its crystalline-like structure of six photoreceptors that form a rosette surrounded by glia. The outline of the extracellular space between glia is seen as web-like. The compartmentation of glycolysis to glia and of oxidative metabolism to photoreceptors renders this CNS model unique for studying neuron-glial interactions. (From Tsacopoulos M, Evêquoz-Mercier V, Perrottet P, Buchner E. Honeybee retinal glial cells transform glucose and supply the neurons with metabolic substrate. *Proc Natl Acad Sci USA*. 1998;85(22):8727–8731. https://doi.org/10.1073/pnas.85.22.8727.) (**B**) Mammalian Müller glia still attached to photoreceptors (cell complex) after their acute isolation and purification from guinea pig. Prominent glial endfeet are oriented at top. The distal ends of Müller glia are hidden by photoreceptor cell bodies. (Modified from Poitry-Yamate CL, Poitry S, Tsacopoulos M. Lactate released by Muller glial cells is metabolized by photoreceptors from mammalian retina. *J Neurosci*. 1995;15(7):5179–5191. https://doi.org/10.1523/JNEUROSCI.15-07-05179.1995. Copyright 1995 by Society for Neuroscience.) (**C**) In both models, glia take up exogenous glucose and transform it to a glycolytic product *(green)*, which in turn is released extracellularly, then taken up and metabolized by the photoreceptors *(blue)*.

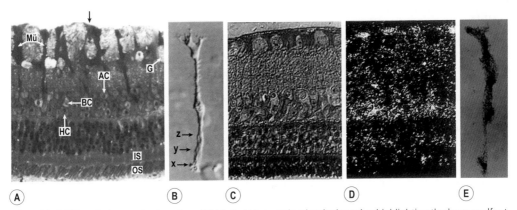

Fig. 12.5 Müller glia in vertebrate retina. (**A**) Methyl blue–stained retinal section highlighting the large endfeet and radial structure of Müller glia (*Mü*) through the thickness of the retina. Laminar organization of this tissue allows for clear identification of nuclear and synaptic layers. *Arrow at top* indicates direction of light hitting the retina; * indicates synaptic layers. Müller glia endfeet form the vitreoretinal interface. *G*, ganglion cell; *AC*, amacrine cell; *BC*, bipolar cell; *HC*, horizontal cell; *IS* and *OS*, inner and outer segments of photoreceptors. (**B**) Müller glia after acute isolation and purification; approximately to scale with Müller glia shown in (**A**). The descending radial process (z), radial strands (y), and terminal angular buttons (x) of the Müller glia are landmarks of that part of the Müller glia in contact with the outer synaptic layer, and the cell body and inner segments of photoreceptor, respectively. (Poitry-Yamate CL, Poitry S, Tsacopoulos M. Lactate released by Müller glial cells is metabolized by photoreceptors from mammalian retina. *J Neurosci*. 1995;15(7):5179–5191. https://doi.org/10.1523/JNEUROSCI.15-07-05179.1995. Copyright 1995 by Society for Neuroscience.) (**C**) Phase contrast image of retinal cells from guinea pig in situ, oriented as in (**A**). Note that individual cell types can be distinguished using the section in (**A**). (Poitry-Yamate C, Tsacopoulos M. Glial (Müller) cells take up and phosphorylate [3H]2-deoxy-d-glucose in a mammalian retina. *Neurosci Lett*. 1991;122(2):241–244. https://doi.org/10.1016/0304-3940(91)90868-T.) (**D**) High-resolution ³H-DG-6P autoradiogram of retinal preparation shown in (**C**). The silver grains shown in *white* were determined by high pressure liquid chromatography and correspond to ³H-DG-6P. (**E**) High-resolution ³H-DG-6P autoradiogram of a single Müller glia similar to that shown in (**B**), illustrating homogeneity of phosphorylated DG intracellulary extending about 120 μm starting from the endfoot *(at top)* to the distal end of the cell *(at bottom)*. Autoradiograms in (**D**) and (**E**) provide evidence that Müller glia, in situ and when acutely isolated, take up and phosphorylate the sugar analog deoxy-ᴅ-glucose.

act as buffers of lactate in the extracellular environment, thereby securing adequate pH levels.

BIOCHEMICAL SPECIALIZATION OF GLIAL CELLS

As previously outlined, Müller glia (also termed radial fibers or sustentacular cells of Heinrich Müller) are the major glial cell type in vertebrate retina. Structurally, Müller glia are elongated, possess a prominent specialized region called endfeet at the inner limiting membrane, and are vertically oriented with respect to the retinal layers (Fig. 12.5). As Müller glia extend through the synaptic and nuclear layers of the retina from the inner to outer limiting membranes, they are in intimate apposition to every neuron cell type. Müller glia also serve as an additional physical and functional cell layer to the diffusion of substances into and out of the extracellular space, the vitreous, the subretinal space, and retinal vascular supply. Histochemical evidence has shown that glycogen synthesis, glycogenolysis, and anaerobic glycolysis are localized to Müller glia in situ.[44] This was confirmed and quantitated in living, intact, dark-adapted retina using biochemical and autoradiographic methodologies,[86,87] and provided strong experimental evidence for the working hypothesis of all retinal cell types, that is, that Müller glia play a major role beyond the blood-retinal barriers in transporting glucose from the blood into the neural retina. However, once in the neural retina, it remains to be shown along the entire radial length of Müller glia whether the distribution of transporters related to energy substrate uptake and release are tailored to this cell's own metabolic needs, yet adapted to the function and metabolic needs of their immediate neuronal environment.

Two functional and biochemical specializations unique to Müller glia are their capacity to inactivate the excitatory neurotransmitter glutamate[103,104] and inhibitory neurotransmitters GABA and glycine.[105–107] They are the exclusive and/or predominant cellular site of:

1. GS activity for the synthesis and release of glutamine, a precursor for photoreceptor neurotransmitter resynthesis[108]; and
2. carbonic anhydrase for the conversion of water and CO_2 of neuron origin to bicarbonate, an enzymatic activity implicated in the regulation of intracellular and extracellular pH and volume.[109,110]

ROLE OF GLYCOGEN

As an endogenous source of glucose-6-phosphate, glycogen, as well as glycogen phosphorylase, is exclusively localized to the cytoplasm of Müller glia in situ in a variety of mammalian species.[111] This important finding suggests that Müller glia can effectively mobilize this energy store, but it remains unclear whether it is for the purpose of meeting their own energy needs[87] or, alternatively, partly those of the surrounding neurons in the form of lactate generated via glycogenolysis.[39] One isoform of glycogen phosphorylase is expressed in cone photoreceptors (brain type), and another isoform (muscle type) is expressed in the inner plexiform synaptic layers of primate retina.[96] So, although glycogen metabolism in Müller glia is established, the function of Müller glia glycogen is still far from clear. The prevailing view is that glycogen plays the role of an *emergency* retinal carbohydrate reservoir supporting neuron function when glucose delivery is compromised, such as during retinal ischemia.[46] This contrasts with another view that Müller glia glycogen is mobilized as an immediate and accessible energy store under normal physiologic conditions (Fig. 12.6), such as changes in illumination, that is, light and darkness, and which are linked to the direct effects of altering photoreceptor function.[39,112] In addition, glycogenolysis can be stimulated in the retina by neurotransmitters increasing Cyclic adenosine monophosphate (cAMP), such as vasoactive intestinal peptide, which are contained in and released from amacrine cells.[113] In the context of cAMP, lactate has also been shown to play a role. Hence, lactate acts as a ligand of the Hydroxycarboxylic acid receptor 1 (HCAR1), which induces a Gi-mediated pathway that results in decreased cAMP.[114] In turn, this leads to reduced glycogenolysis, thereby triggering the cells to utilize lactate prior to glucose stored as glycogen, thereby potentially sparing glucose for neurons. Glycogen is also localized in neurons of the cat retina, particularly of the rod-driven pathway, the rod-driven components of which are selectively sensitive to prolonged hypoglycemia,[115] but whether this glycogen is mobilized is not presently known.

FUNCTIONAL NEURONAL ACTIVITY AND DIVISION OF METABOLIC LABOR

A continuous supply of blood-borne glucose is vital to maintaining retinal function but does not necessarily dictate that all retinal cells (both neurons and glia) take up and metabolize this energy substrate as

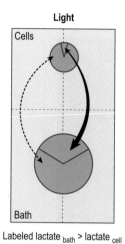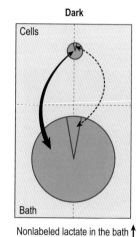

■ Radiolabeled lactate from ^{14}C-glucose
■ Nonlabeled lactate from glycogen

Fig. 12.6 Lactate released by Müller glia is formed from exogenous radiolabeled glucose in the light-adapted cell complex but from glycogen in the dark-adapted cell complex. The preparation shown in Fig. 12.4B was maintained either in darkness or light before exposure to uniformly radiolabeled glucose ([14]C(U) glucose) with the aim of determining the contribution of glucose and glycogen to the production of lactate when modulating photoreceptor metabolism and neurotransmitter release. It is known that: (1) photoreceptors release neurotransmitter glutamate and that their metabolism is increased in darkness; and (2) glutamate release stimulates glycolysis and production of lactate. The results shown are simplified and drawn as a pie to reflect changes both inside the cells *(top)* and in the surrounding bath *(bottom)*. Pie size represents the total pool size of lactate, (i.e., radiolabeled + nonradiolabeled lactate). The size of the wedge represents the specific activity of lactate, so the larger the wedge, the larger is the contribution of exogenous glucose to the formation of lactate. The direction of the *solid arrow* in the *left* panel indicates that the amount of radiolabeled lactate *(pink)* in the bathing solution was much greater than that inside the preparation. This is only possible when lactate is produced from ^{14}C-glucose and is released earlier than nonradiolabeled lactate formed from glycogen. In the *right* panel, the direction of the *solid arrow* indicates that the amount of nonradiolabeled lactate *(blue)* in the surrounding bath greatly increased. This is only possible when glycogen (gly) in glia is mobilized to produce additional, unlabeled lactate.

is generally believed. Indeed, the conventional view of glucose metabolism in CNS is that glucose is the principal substrate for oxidative metabolism in both cell types, i.e., neurons and glia.[116] The experimental evidence described in the previous sections is a major departure from this view and raises three highly controversial and still unresolved questions about the brain and about the generality of the findings in retina to other parts of the CNS:

1. Is glucose, the major brain energy substrate, taken up in a cell type–specific manner?
2. Does glycolysis predominate in one particular cell type, physiologic condition, or brain region and oxidative metabolism of glucose in another? and
3. Does coupling of metabolic and physiologic changes to changes in neuronal activity involve the transformation of blood glucose by glial cells and do they supply neurons with glucose-derived metabolite(s)?

Underlying these issues is the idea of a predominant division of metabolic labor between neurons and glia. In other words, energy substrate production and substrate use are partitioned in a relatively cell-specific

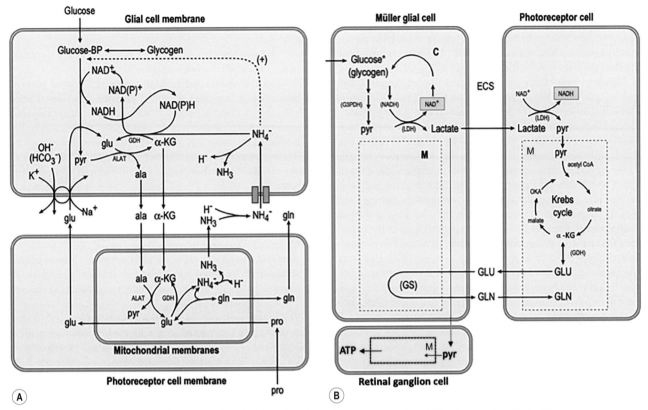

Fig. 12.7 Proposed scheme of retinal function, from bee to mammals, highlighting metabolite trafficking between glial cells and photoreceptors. The honeybee drone model is shown in (**A**), and the mammalian models are shown in (**B**). Both models display relative metabolic compartmentation: glycolysis to glia and oxidative metabolism to photoreceptor neurons. Commonalities of the models include production of a glycolytic product, i.e., lactate or alanine, their release extracellularly, and uptake by photoreceptors; maintenance of the redox potential in glia, i.e., NADH/NAD ratio; and photoreceptor release of glutamate that acts to stimulate glial glycolysis. Glutamate is thus a chemical signal that turns the nourishing of neurons by glia into a function, instead of a passive process. In (**B**), the cytosol is indicated as **C**; mitochondria are indicated as **M**. *α-Kg*, α-Ketoglutaric acid; *ALA*, alanine; *ALAT*, alanine aminotransferase; *ATP*, adenosine triphosphate; *C*, cytosol; *ECS*, extracellular space; *GAPDH*, glyceraldehyde-3-phosphate dehydrogenase; *GDH*, glutamate dehydrogenase; *GLN*, glutamine; *GLU*, glutamate; *GS*, glutamine synthetase; *K*, Kalium (potassium); *LDH*, lactate dehydrogenase; *M*, mitochondria; *Na*, Natrium (sodium); *NAD*, nicotinamide adenine dinucleotide; *OXA*, Oxaloacetate; *PRO*, proline; *PYR*, pyruvate.

manner. This working hypothesis, summarized in Fig. 12.7, was developed and tested in retina in the mid-1990s in insect and mammal, and has seen a revival in the recent decade, particularly with regards to the recognition that the coordinated action of glial cells and neurons extends to energy metabolism throughout the CNS.

As will be developed in the next sections, the major theme is that glial cells *transform rather than simply transfer* the primary energy substrate glucose, and supply activated neurons with a glucose-derived metabolite, i.e., lactate and/or alanine. In this regard, the vertebrate retina has proven to be a CNS model of choice because its laminar organization of metabolism and blood flow lends itself to the study of compartmentation by virtue of its structure. It should, however, be recognized that the high specialization of this nervous tissue, (e.g., phototransduction and high energy metabolism), makes it different from other regions of the CNS and any comparisons must be made with caution. Moreover, the retina has two barriers, the retinal capillary endothelial cells of the inner BRB, and the RPE comprising the outer BRB, which is located between the photoreceptors and choroid. Thus, their expression and distribution of glucose transporters[117] and glycolysis will inevitably determine whether one, or alternatively both, of these barriers is the rate-limiting step for glucose delivery to the neuroretina.

CELLULAR COMPARTMENTATION OF ENERGY SUBSTRATES OTHER THAN GLUCOSE

As mentioned earlier in the chapter, one distinctive property of the mammalian retina is its large production of endogenous lactate in the presence and absence of oxygen.[32] The production of lactate is a normal function of retinal tissue and can effectively replace glucose in oxygenated Ringer's solution in maintaining retinal oxidative metabolism and photoreceptor function.[79] It was only in the mid-1990s that this phenomenon was explored at the cellular level[87] and when the idea was launched that energy metabolism underlying retinal function in mammals was relatively compartmentalized and moreover orchestrated between glial cells and neurons.[39]

The use of high-resolution light microscopic autoradiography of [3]H-2DG in the dark-adapted retina in situ, coupled with high-performance liquid chromatography (HPLC) for the identification of silver grains in autoradiograms[86] showed that glucose is not taken up by the majority of retinal cells but preferentially taken up and phosphorylated by the Müller glia (Fig. 12.5C,D), leaving the question as to the identification of the energy substrate used by neurons. Using a cell model of acutely isolated Müller glia, the metabolic fate of glucose-6-phosphate and the identity of metabolites released by these cells was first assessed by Poitry-Yamate and

Tsacopoulos.[87] The experimental results of that study raised the hypothesis that lactate, synthesized and released in situ by a retinal cell type with high glycolytic capacity, may be transferred to and metabolized by photoreceptors that possess a high respiratory capacity. This working hypothesis was tested in the acutely isolated retinal model of the cell complex (see Fig. 12.3B) comprising Müller glia still attached to photoreceptors, and in which the effect of altering illumination on glucose metabolism was quantitated.[39] A major finding of that study showed that lactate *formation* versus lactate *use* was cell type–dependent. As already discussed in section Biochemical specialization of glial cells, sources of this glial lactate were from exogenous glucose, or alternatively, from endogenous glycogen (Fig. 12.6). The functional role for the release into the extracellular space of lactate and H+ by Müller glia during either glycolysis or glycogenolysis is expected to prevent intracellular acidification and maintain the regeneration of NAD+ for glycolysis to proceed. Lactate and other glucose-derived metabolites released from the Müller glia would participate in the regeneration of the excitatory neurotransmitter glutamate, released by photoreceptors in darkness.[39] Similar to photoreceptor cells, retinal ganglion cells also take up and metabolize lactate.[48] Moreover, activation of the lactate receptor, HCAR1, has been shown to increase mitochondrial function measured by oxygen consumption rates in Müller glia, implying that lactate may act as a metabolic regulatory molecule in the retina.[47]

Within a larger framework, the current debate in the neuroscientific community is whether in other parts of the CNS, a net production and extracellular release by glial cells of glucose/glycogen-derived lactate provides sufficient fuel for activated neurons in vivo. Nuclear magnetic resonance (NMR) studies on brain function and energy metabolism have provided indirect support of a lactate flux from glia to neurons as providing the coupling mechanism between increased fluxes of the glucose carbon into the glycolytic pathway in glia, and into the oxidative pathway in neurons, in the form of lactate, during glutamatergic/excitatory synaptic transmission.[118]

Unraveling the current debate surrounding the glial (astrocyte)-neuron–lactate shuttle hypothesis[119,120] in the CNS at large is a key step toward: (1) understanding the regulation of retinal and cerebral energy metabolism during neuronal activity; and (2) interpreting [18]fluorodeoxyglucose (FDG)-positron emission tomography (PET) and fMRI images in both clinical medicine and fundamental neuroscience, and for which there is accumulating evidence for the central importance of glial cells in brain imaging signals.[121]

EXPERIMENTAL MODELS OF RETINAL METABOLISM AND FUNCTION

The most comprehensive model in vivo of metabolism and function in the inner and outer retina is the cat eye, followed by that of the rabbit. Niemeyer et al.[122,123] have quantitated the effects of controlled, stepwise, and transient changes in arterial supply of glucose on retinal and optic nerve function at multiple levels of retinal information processing (e.g., light-evoked electrical signals of the ERG b-wave and light-independent retinal field potentials of negative polarity) in the arterially perfused enucleated eye of the cat, and have verified directly these in vitro findings in anesthetized cats under insulin-induced glucose clamping.[124] Although the entire body of work by this group cannot be justly summarized here, Niemeyer and colleagues made a number of important observations that have current clinical and fundamental relevance in understanding retinal function as related to metabolism:

1. Electrophysiological measurements of the ERG b-wave, the scotopic threshold response (STR), and optic nerve action potentials indicate an exquisite, immediate, and reversible sensitivity of the inner retina to changes in the supply of glucose between approximately 1 and 10 mmol/L glucose.

2. In contrast to the cone-driven, light-evoked signals, the rod-driven, light-evoked signals increased or decreased in parallel to changes in glucose.

3. Blood-borne insulin enhanced the reduction in b-wave amplitude at low (1–2 mM) glucose concentrations.

4. Glycogen is distributed in Müller glia and central perivascular astrocytes. It is present in retinal ganglion cells, on-off amacrine cells, and rod bipolar cells of the rod pathway, but entirely absent in cone and rod photoreceptors[115] under conditions in which the ERG is affected by changes in plasma glucose concentrations.

These studies raise a number of interesting questions about retinal energy metabolism with regard to insulin-induced hypoglycemia and diabetes:

1. Can glycogen reserves in the retina in vivo serve as glucose equivalents during hypoglycemia, as has been shown recently for brain?[125]

2. Does impaired glucose sensing, (i.e., hypoglycemia unawareness in the brain), also affect the retina?

3. If retinal glycogen metabolism and content are insulin or glucose-sensitive, do increased retinal concentrations of glucose result in a lowered glycemic threshold of counter-regulation, as observed in chronic hypoglycemia?

The experiments carried out by Ames and colleagues[8,75] using isolated cat retinas maintained in a miniaturized heart-lung apparatus characterized the energy requirements of retinal function by monitoring retinal lactate production and oxygen consumption.[8] Finally, Linsenmeier and colleagues[60,126] have devoted a great deal of effort to studying the distribution and consumption of oxygen throughout the inner and outer retina in anesthetized cats during systemic normoxia and hypoxia and, more recently, retinal pH changes during hypoxemia, hyperglycemia, and anaerobic glycolysis. Other important contributions on energy metabolism in the retina have been studies carried out in monkey and miniature pigs in vivo,[127,128] and in rabbit[50] and rat in vitro.[79,129]

Complementary to laser Doppler flow measurements[55,130–132] and oxygen electrode measurements in anesthetized pig,[56,133] exciting developments using blood-oxygen level–dependent functional magnetic resonance imaging (BOLD fMRI) and intravascular contrast agents in the intact eye of the cat[134–136] provide significant promise for noninvasive, real-time visualization of retinal function, structure, blood flow, and oxygenation in health and disease, for example, in diabetic retinopathy. Multiple MRI contrast mechanisms presently permit laminar spatial visualization of the retina, corresponding to the inner and outer retina and choroid microvasculature.[137]

METABOLIC INTERACTIONS BETWEEN VERTEBRATE PHOTORECEPTORS AND MÜLLER GLIA

In the retina of the guinea pig[39] (see Figs. 12.4 and 12.5), analogous experimental findings supported the concept of metabolic compartmentation (see Fig. 12.7B). Four conclusions were drawn from that study and are summarized in Fig. 12.8:

1. Müller glia massively produced lactate from radiolabeled glucose, most of which was found extracellularly in the corresponding cell bath (Fig. 12.8A,B: blue bars).

2. The effects of altering illumination of the cell complex (thereby specifically altering photoreceptor function and metabolism) affect the production, release and/or uptake of glucose/glycogen-derived lactate in Müller glia (Fig. 12.8A,B: purple and green bars).

3. From numerical calculations, the "missing lactate" in the bath of the cell complex (vertical arrow in Fig. 12.8B) matched the expected production of [14]CO_2 by photoreceptor oxidative metabolism (see

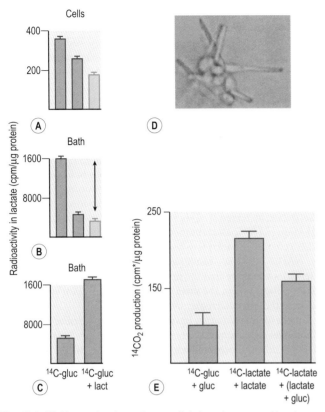

Fig. 12.8 Glial lactate is released extracellularly and consumed by photoreceptors in mammalian retina. Metabolic trafficking between neurons and glia was explored using three cell models: purified populations of acutely isolated Müller glia (Fig. 12.5B), acutely isolated photoreceptors (**D**), and the acutely isolated cell complex (Fig. 12.4B) from guinea pig retina. The effect of altering illumination of the cell complex (*purple*: maintained in light vs. *green*: maintained in darkness) was the strategy used to specifically alter photoreceptor function and metabolism. Darkness increases photoreceptor metabolism and the release of neurotransmitter glutamate. Retinal glia are not directly affected by light. Müller glia alone massively produced lactate from uniformly radiolabeled glucose, most of which was released into the extracellular space, as shown by the *blue* columns in (**A**) and (**B**). The effects of altering illumination of the cell complex, particularly in darkness, lowered significantly the amount of radiolabeled lactate in the corresponding bath (**B**, *second* and *third columns*) compared with the bath of Müller glia alone (**B**, *first column*). This "missing lactate" matched the expected production of $^{14}CO_2$ by photoreceptor oxidative metabolism. As expected, this "missing lactate" was also antagonized by the addition of unlabeled lactate to the cell complex bath (**C**), indicating that lactate released extracellularly by glia was consumed. Finally, (**E**) shows the amount of $^{14}CO_2$ produced by the cells in (**D**) as a function of three different substrate mixtures. The conclusion drawn was that glial lactate was preferentially consumed by photoreceptors, even in the presence of millimolar concentrations of glucose. Overall, the effects of altering illumination of the cell complex affected the production, release and or uptake of glucose-derived glial lactate. (Modified from Poitry-Yamate CL, Poitry S and Tsacopoulos M. Lactate released by Muller glial cells is metabolized by photoreceptors from mammalian retina. *J Neurosci.* 1995;15(7):5179–5191. https://doi.org/10.1523/JNEUROSCI.15-07-05179.1995. Copyright 1995 by Society for Neuroscience.)

Box 12.1) and was antagonized by the addition of unlabeled lactate (Fig. 12.8C).

4. Glial-derived lactate is preferentially consumed by purified populations of acutely isolated photoreceptors (Fig. 12.8D), even in the presence of millimolar concentrations of glucose (Fig. 12.8E).

These results showed that a *relative* compartmentation of substrate *formation* to the glial cells and substrate *use* to the photoreceptor neurons previously established in bee retina can be generalized to mammals (see Fig. 12.7). Such compartmentation may underlie the need for a continuous trafficking of lactate/alanine from glia to neurons (see also section Functional neuronal activity and division of metabolic labor). It should be noted that guinea pig photoreceptors have in fact been shown to take up and phosphorylate glucose,[39] but when challenged with either one alone or a combination of both, lactate has been shown to be a preferred substrate, as evaluated by $^{14}CO_2$ produced (Fig. 12.8E). Lastly, the presence of photoreceptors, thus the model of Müller glia still attached to photoreceptors, has been found to modify, in a light/dark-dependent manner, either the synthesis, release, or metabolic fate of glucose-derived metabolites, i.e., lactate and glutamine, in the Müller glia.[39]

To summarize, neuroretina can serve as an important CNS model in which one can assess the use of energy fuel in terms of function. Neurons and glia thus divide metabolic labor in a way that is vital to function.

METABOLIC INTERACTION BETWEEN PHOTORECEPTORS AND RETINAL PIGMENT EPITHELIAL

The retinal RPE forms part of the choroidal blood/outer retinal barrier, facing the outer photoreceptor segments on its apical membrane side, Bruch's membrane on its basolateral membrane side and plays an essential role in maintaining photoreceptor excitability and sensitivity and in the reisomerization of all-*trans*-retinal after photon absorption.[138] In rod outer segments (ROS), all-*trans*-retinal is transformed to all-*trans*-retinol by retinol dehydrogenase using NADPH. NADPH is restored in ROS by the pentose phosphate pathway utilizing high amounts of glucose supplied by choriocapillaries. The retinal formed is transported to PE cells where regeneration of 11-*cis*-retinal occurs (see Chapter 13).

The RPE apical membrane is separated from the neuroretina by the subretinal space, which serves to mediate the transport of metabolic intermediates, ions, and water between the choroid and the retina. Considering the vascular sources of fuel substrate, the choroidal microcirculation is one source of glucose for photoreceptor OS. However, it is presently unclear whether glucose crosses the RPE on glucose transporters GLUT1 and GLUT3[139] or if it is consumed and transformed through the glycolytic pathway to lactate for transfer and, to a lesser extent, oxidized through the Kreb's cycle.[49] This is a relevant point as RPE cells depend on glucose as their primary energy substrate.[140,141] The expression of the monocarboxylate transporter MCT3 on the RPE basolateral side for the efflux of lactate from RPE to the choroidal microcirculation and the expression of MCT1 on the apical side for the transport of lactate and water from the retina to choroid[101] (see Chapter 13) suggest that lactate is not used by RPE cells, at least when glucose is nonlimiting.[140,141] Thus, if RPE cells synthesize and release glucose-derived lactate in vivo, as has been demonstrated in acutely isolated RPE[21] and in cultured RPE,[99] any lactate leaving the eye, as determined by either choroidal venous drainage or femoral artery–choroidal vein differences,[33] is a twofold contribution (neuroretina and RPE). Presently, the contributions from these two sources have not been quantitated, nor has their contribution to the amount of secreted lactate to the choroidal vein. These unknowns need to be considered when critically evaluating the astrocyte-neuron–lactate shuttle hypothesis that aerobic glycolysis in glia increases in response to activation of neurotransmitter glutamate systems and the neuronal oxidation of glial lactate.[142,143] In the eye, *endogenous* lactate production does not appear to be linked only to energy metabolism: the cotransport of H^+ and lactate with water in the direction from retina to choroid plays a role in volume regulation, and thereby retinal adhesion.[82,144]

METABOLIC FACTORS IN THE REGULATION OF RETINAL BLOOD FLOW

In a series of original papers on the metabolic factors involved in the regulation of retinal blood flow in monkey and miniature pigs, it was proposed that an extravascular, intraretinal acidosis was a key step in the process leading to retinal arteriolar vasodilation, either by hypercapnia, hypoxia, ischemia, or release of ATP.[14,127,145–148] Moreover, it was speculated that this acidosis can provoke the release of a substance from the periarteriolar glial cells, which in turn would act on the smooth muscle cells of the arteriolar wall. In this case, that the retinal arteriolar tone may be controlled by factors such as K^+, lactate, ATP, and NO released from the retinal tissue surrounding the arterioles was tested in the miniature pig.[149,150] Of these factors, intraretinal lactate and NO, both of which can be synthesized from glucose in Müller glia, were found to either mediate acute hypoxia–induced vasodilation or basal retinal arteriolar tone (e.g., for review, see Pournaras et al.[151]).

Further experimental evidence supporting the role of extracellular lactate as a dynamic vasoactive signal was provided by studying freshly isolated rat retinal microvessels using a combination of patch-clamp technique, fluorescence imaging, and time-lapse photography.[152] In that study, lactate exposure was associated with an intracellular rise of calcium in pericytes, cell contraction, and lumen constriction when energy supplies were adequate. Hypoxia, on the other hand, switched lactate's effect from vasocontraction to vasorelaxation. This dual vasoactive capability may provide an efficient mechanism to match microvascular function to local metabolic needs. Another mechanism is through lactate-mediated activation of HCAR1, which promotes angiogenesis.[153]

In minipigs, preretinal microinjections of L-lactate (0.5 mol/L, pH 2 and 7.4) close to the retinal arterioles produced a local, segmental, and reversible arteriolar dilation, whereas D-lactate had no effect. This effect was not pH-dependent or mediated by prostaglandins. However, both systemic and sublingual administration of L-lactate (0.1 mol/L, pH 2) had no effect on retinal arteriolar diameter,[149] suggesting that exposure to endothelial cells of the arterioles to lactate was not sufficient to trigger a vasomotor response. These authors concluded that to induce vasodilation, lactate had to reach the vascular smooth muscle cells from the vitreoretinal side, raising the hypothesis that intraretinal lactate is a mediator of acute hypoxia–induced vasodilation.

Intravenous administration of sodium lactate has been reported to increase retinal blood flow at steady state or during flicker stimulation.[154,155] High-dose lactate reduced flicker response, whereas low-dose lactate increased it. This is most likely related to the fact that high-dose lactate leads to pronounced prevasodilation and a reduced flicker response, whereas low-dose lactate shifts the ratio of cytosolic-free NADH to NAD^+, resulting in increased flicker response. Both observations indicate that the ratio of cytosolic-free NADH to NAD^+ plays a critical role in the maintenance of retinal vascular tone (also known as the "pseudohypoxia hypothesis").[154]

Uptake of intravenous or intravitreal lactate by vascular endothelial cells or glial cells via monocarboxylate transporters[156,157] causes retinal arteriolar dilation, predominantly via stimulation of NO synthase[158] and subsequent activation of guanylate cyclase. In turn, guanylate cyclase/cGMP signaling triggers opening of K_{ATP} channels for vasodilation. This process suggests that lactate either mediates the release of endothelial vasoactive substances (i.e., NO) or interferes with the metabolism and release of vasoactive substances by cells surrounding the arterioles (i.e., glial cells).

Vasodilation of retinal arterioles in minipigs induced by juxta-arteriolar administration of L-lactate was also observed during continuous intravenous infusion of L-NAME, inhibiting endothelial-derived NO. In contrast, juxta-arteriolar L-NAME microinjection that inhibited nitric oxide synthase (NOS) within the neuronal/glial cells significantly suppressed the vasodilatory effect of L-lactate. Those findings suggested that, in vivo, neuronal/glial cells are the major source of NO mediating the retinal arteriolar vasodilatation response to lactate in minipigs (Fig. 12.9).[159]

METABOLIC PATHWAY LEADING TO NITRIC OXIDE RELEASE

The diffusible and nonpolar gas NO is synthesized from L-arginine by NOS. One function of NO is as an endothelium-derived releasing factor that controls vascular tone. Acutely isolated mammalian retinal Müller glia were shown to synthesize the NO precursor L-arginine from glucose, as well as the key requisite amino acids—fumarate and aspartate—through which arginine is synthesized.[150] Moreover, NOS has been shown to be localized to Müller glia using NADH diaphorase histochemistry and NOS immunocytochemistry.[160,161] Hence, the conversion of L-arginine and oxygen into NO and L-citrulline through the enzymatic action of NOS highlights the role of glia in the generation and release of extravascular, intraretinal, and periarteriolar NO, for either target neurons or in promoting arteriolar vasodilation and/or controlling the basal dilating arteriolar tone.

Support for this hypothesis in vivo in the inner retina of the miniature pig are the following findings:

1. An increasing NO gradient from the vitreous toward the inner retina is measurable using an NO microprobe. This gradient is reversibly modulated by light, and light flicker stimulation of the dark-adapted retina induces a reversible increase of NO.[150]

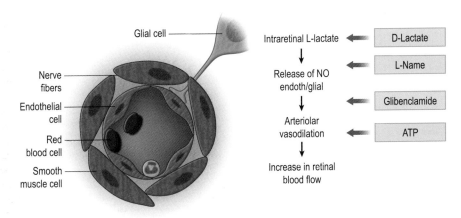

Fig. 12.9 Components of the blood vessel wall hypothesized to play a role in arteriolar vasodilation and retinal blood flow. Endothelial cells and smooth muscle cells are two major components of retinal arteries and arterioles. The retinal glial cells send their endfeet processes out and over the vascular wall. The putative regulatory role of lactate is shown in the schema. Retinal arteriolar tone is controlled by the dynamic vasoactive signals lactate and nitric oxide (NO). Intraretinal L-lactate, but not D-lactate, causes a pH-independent dilation of retinal arterioles. Juxta-arteriolar application, but not intravenous delivery, of L-NAME, an inhibitor of NO synthase, suppresses the vasodilatory effect of L-lactate, suggesting a glial rather than an endothelial source of NO. The L-lactate-induced vasodilatory response is mediated by stimulation of NO synthase and subsequent activation of smooth muscle guanylyl cyclase, leading to the opening of glibenclamide-sensitive K_{ATP} channels in smooth muscle. The regulation of arterial smooth muscle membrane potential through activation or inhibition of K^+ channel activity provides an important mechanism to dilate or constrict arteries or arterioles. Local changes in retinal arteriolar diameter in response to intraretinal vasoactive metabolites such as ATP link the regulation of retinal blood flow to the metabolic needs of the surrounding retinal tissue. *ATP*, Adenosine triphosphate.

2. Focal microinjection, but not intravenous infusion, of the NO-synthase inhibitor nitro-L-arginine leads to a segmental and reversible arteriolar vasoconstriction of 45%.[150] Intravenous[154] and intravitreal administration of L-arginine also increases retinal blood flow, but it remains to be shown that this effect is related to an increase of NO production.

3. In vivo, neuronal/glial cells are the major source of NO mediating the retinal arteriolar vasodilation response to lactate in minipigs.[159]

Local factors released by neurons and perivascular glial cells appear to be involved in the regulation of the vascular tone of the retinal resistance vessels, through the interaction of myogenic and metabolic mechanisms. These factors may be ionic, molecular, or related to arterial blood gas modifications. They affect the arteriolar tone and thus regulate the retinal vasomotor responses, relaxing or contracting the tone. NO and prostacyclin (PGI$_2$) are probable relaxing factors, whereas the contracting factors include endothelin-1 (ET-1), angiotensin II, and cyclo-oxygenase (COX) products such as thromboxane-A2 (TXA$_2$) and prostaglandin H$_2$ (PGH$_2$).[151]

What may be the role of extracellular lactate in the contraction and relaxation of the vessel wall according to the metabolic needs of the tissue? Lactate could either mediate the release of endothelial vasoactive substances (i.e., NO) or, alternatively, lactate could interfere with the metabolism of cells surrounding the arterioles, namely glial cells and neurons, leading either to release of vasoactive substances (NO, prostaglandins [PGs]) or activation of retinal endothelin receptors.

The close interaction between PG and NO metabolic pathways could ensure that when one process is inhibited, the other may rapidly compensate for the deficiency and maintain blood flow constant. However, whether this interaction is a major component of the control of vasomotion and autoregulation in the inner retina remains to be shown.

Impairment of structure and function of the neural tissue and endothelium is the cause of abnormal retinal blood flow regulation observed during the evolution of ischemic microangiopathies.[151] However, impaired metabolism may underlie alterations of both neural structure and function. This raises the question of whether impaired glycolysis leads to a decrease in preretinal lactate, which in turn affects the NO pathway. Equally as important is the transport of glucose to neural cells, which is compromised in ischemia and/or by alterations of the retinal-blood barrier, both of which are functional triggers leading to neovascularization and formation of macular edema.

In this regard, the expression of hypoxia-related vascular endothelial growth factor (VEGF), known as the major inducer of angiogenesis, correlates in a temporal and spatial manner with the formation of new vessels and retinal-blood barrier alterations. Insights into the multiple pathways controlling retinal blood flow, tissue oxygenation, and metabolism should offer new therapeutic strategies to restore retinal blood flow and prevent damage observed during the evolution of ischemic microangiopathies.

ACKNOWLEDGMENTS

The authors thank Carole Poitry-Yamate and Constantin J. Pounaras for their contribution to the chapter.

REFERENCES

1. Bringmann A, Grosche A, Pannicke T, Reichenbach A. GABA and glutamate uptake and metabolism in retinal glial (Müller) cells. *Front Endocrinol.* 2013;4:48.
2. Reichenbach A, Bringmann A. New functions of Müller cells. *Glia.* 2013;61(5):651–678.
3. Rauen T, Rothstein JD, Wassle H. Differential expression of three glutamate transporter subtypes in the rat retina. *Cell Tissue Res.* 1996;286(3):325–336.
4. Rauen T, Taylor WR, Kuhlbrodt K, Wiessner M. High-affinity glutamate transporters in the rat retina: a major role of the glial glutamate transporter GLAST-1 in transmitter clearance. *Cell Tissue Res.* 1998;291(1):19–31.
5. Toft-Kehler AK, Skytt DM, Poulsen KA, et al. Limited energy supply in Müller cells alters glutamate uptake. *Neurochem Res.* 2014;39(5):941–949.
6. Ola MS, Hosoya KI, LaNoue KF. Regulation of glutamate metabolism by hydrocortisone and branched chain keto acids in cultured rat retinal Müller cells (TR-MUL). *Neurochem Int.* 2011;59(5):656–663.
7. Toft-Kehler AK, Skytt DM, Svare A, et al. Mitochondrial function in Müller cells—Does it matter? *Mitochondrion.* 2017;36:43–51.
8. Ames A, Li YY, Heher EC, Kimble CR. Energy metabolism of rabbit retina as related to function: high cost of Na+ transport. *J Neurosci.* 1992;12(3):840–853.
9. Germer A, Biedermann B, Wolburg H, et al. Distribution of mitochondria within Müller cells—I. Correlation with retinal vascularization in different mammalian species. *J Neurocytol.* 1998;27(5):329–345.
10. Carelli V, Ross-Cisneros FN, Sadun AA. Mitochondrial dysfunction as a cause of optic neuropathies. *Prog Retin Eye Res.* 2004;23(1):53–89.
11. Osborne NN, Olmo-Aguado Sdel. Maintenance of retinal ganglion cell mitochondrial functions as a neuroprotective strategy in glaucoma. *Curr Opin Pharmacol.* 2013;13(1):16–22.
12. Tout S, Chan-Ling T, Holländer H, Stone J. The role of Müller cells in the formation of the blood-retinal barrier. *Neuroscience.* 1993;55(1):291–301.
13. Reichenbach A., Bringmann A. *Müller Cells in the Healthy and Diseased Retina.* Published online; 2009:35-214. Available at: 10.1007/978-1-4419-1672-3_2
14. Kur J, Newman EA. Purinergic control of vascular tone in the retina: Purinergic control of vascular tone in the retina. *J Physiol.* 2014;592(3):491–504.
15. Metea MR, Newman EA. Signalling within the neurovascular unit in the mammalian retina. *Exp Physiol.* 2007;92(4):635–640.
16. Newman EA, Zahs KR. Calcium waves in retinal glial cells. *Science.* 1997;275(5301):844–847.
17. Haydon PG, Carmignoto G. Astrocyte control of synaptic transmission and neurovascular coupling. *Physiol Rev.* 2006;86(3):1009–1031.
18. Puthussery T, Yee P, Vingrys AJ, Fletcher EL. Evidence for the involvement of purinergic P2X receptors in outer retinal processing. *European J Neurosci.* 2006;24(1):7–19.
19. Puthussery T, Fletcher EL. Neuronal expression of P2X3 purinoceptors in the rat retina. *Neuroscience.* 2007;146(1):403–414.
20. Puthussery T, Fletcher EL. P2X2 receptors on ganglion and amacrine cells in cone pathways of the rat retina. *J Comp Neurol.* 2006;496(5):595–609.
21. Puthussery T, Fletcher EL. Synaptic localization of P2X7 receptors in the rat retina. *J Comp Neurol.* 2004;472(1):13–23.
22. Takano T, Tian GF, Peng W, et al. Astrocyte-mediated control of cerebral blood flow. *Nat Neurosci.* 2006;9(2):260–267.
23. Zonta M, Angulo MC, Gobbo S, et al. Neuron-to-astrocyte signaling is central to the dynamic control of brain microcirculation. *Nat Neurosci.* 2003;6(1):43–50.
24. Mulligan SJ, MacVicar BA. Calcium transients in astrocyte endfeet cause cerebrovascular constrictions. *Nature.* 2004;431(7005):195–199.
25. Metea MR, Newman EA. Glial cells dilate and constrict blood vessels: a mechanism of neurovascular coupling. *J Neurosci.* 2006;26(11):2862–2870.
26. Bringmann A, Iandiev I, Pannicke T, et al. Cellular signaling and factors involved in Müller cell gliosis: neuroprotective and detrimental effects. *Prog Retin Eye Res.* 2009;28(6):423–451.
27. Ruzafa N, Pereiro X, Lepper MF, Hauck SM, Vecino E. A proteomics approach to identify candidate proteins secreted by Müller glia that protect ganglion cells in the retina. *Proteomics.* 2018;18(11):e1700321.
28. Ruzafa N, Vecino E. Effect of Müller cells on the survival and neuritogenesis in retinal ganglion cells. *Archivos De La Sociedad Española De Oftalmología.* 2015;90(11):522–526.
29. Matteucci A, Gaddini L, Villa M, et al. Neuroprotection by rat Müller glia against high glucose-induced neurodegeneration through a mechanism involving ERK1/2 activation. *Exp Eye Res.* 2014;125:20–29.
30. Kawasaki A, Otori Y, Barnstable CJ. Müller cell protection of rat retinal ganglion cells from glutamate and nitric oxide neurotoxicity. *Invest Ophth Vis Sci.* 2000;41(11):3444–3450.
31. Skytt DM, Toft-Kehler AK, Brndstrup CT, et al. Glia-neuron interactions in the retina can be studied in cocultures of Müller cells and retinal ganglion Cells. *Biomed Res Int.* 2016;2016(11):1087647-10.
32. Krebs HA. The Pasteur effect and the relations between respiration and fermentation. *Essays Biochem.* 1972;8:1–34.
33. Wang L, Kondo M, Bill A. Glucose metabolism in cat outer retina. Effects of light and hyperoxia. *Invest Ophth Vis Sci.* 1997;38(1):48–55.
34. Wang L, Tornquist P, Bill A. Glucose metabolism in pig outer retina in light and darkness. *Acta Physiol Scand.* 1997;160(1):75–81.
35. Wang L, Tornquist P, Bill A. Glucose metabolism of the inner retina in pigs in darkness and light. *Acta Physiol Scand.* 1997;160(1):71–74.
36. Adler AJ, Southwick RE. Distribution of glucose and lactate in the interphotoreceptor matrix. *Ophthalmic Res.* 1992;24(4):243–252.
37. Berkowitz BA, Bansal N, Wilson CA. Non-invasive measurement of steady-state vitreous lactate concentration. *NMR Biomed.* 1994;7(6):263–268.
38. Goodwin ML, Harris JE, Hernandez A, Gladden LB. Blood lactate measurements and analysis during exercise: a guide for clinicians. *J Diabetes Sci Technology.* 2007;1(4):558–569.
39. Poitry-Yamate CL, Poitry S, Tsacopoulos M. Lactate released by Müller glial cells is metabolized by photoreceptors from mammalian retina. *J Neurosci.* 1995;15(7 Pt 2):5179–5191.
40. Winkler BS, Arnold MJ, Brassell MA, Puro DG. Energy metabolism in human retinal Müller cells. *Invest Ophth Vis Sci.* 2000;41(10):3183–3190.
41. Winkler BS, Sauer MW, Starnes CA. Modulation of the Pasteur effect in retinal cells: implications for understanding compensatory metabolic mechanisms. *Exp Eye Res.* 2003;76(6):715–723.
42. Toft-Kehler AK, Gurubaran IS, Desler C, Rasmussen LJ, Skytt DM, Kolko M. Oxidative stress-induced dysfunction of Müller cells during starvation. *Invest Ophth Vis Sci.* 2016;57(6):2721–2728.
43. Lowry OH, Roberts NR, Schulz DW, Clow JE, Clark JR. Quantitative histochemistry of retina. *J Biol Chem.* 1961;236(10):2813–2820.
44. Kuwabara T, Cogan DG. Retinal glycogen. *Arch Ophthalmol-chic.* 1961;66:680–688.
45. Cogan DG, Kuwabara T. Tetrazolium studies on the retina: II. Substrate dependent patterns. *J Histochem Cytochem.* 1959;7(5):334–341.
46. Vohra R, Aldana BI, Skytt DM, et al. Essential roles of lactate in Müller cell survival and function. *Mol Neurobiol.* 2018;55(12):9108–9121.
47. Vohra R, Aldana BI, Waagepetersen H, Bergersen LH, Kolko M. Dual properties of lactate in Müller cells: The effect of GPR81 activation. *Invest Ophth Vis Sci.* 2019;60(4):999–1008.
48. Vohra R, Aldana BI, Bulli G, et al. Lactate-mediated protection of retinal ganglion cells. *J Mol Biol.* 2019;431(9):1878–1888.
49. Glocklin VC, Potts AM. The metabolism of retinal pigment cell epithelium. II. Respiration and glycolysis. *Invest Ophth Visual.* 1965;4:226–234.
50. Cohen LH, Noell WK. Glucose catabolism of rabbit retina before and after development of visual function. *J Neurochem.* 1960;5:253–276.
51. Hoang QV, Linsenmeier RA, Chung CK, Curcio CA. Photoreceptor inner segments in monkey and human retina: Mitochondrial density, optics, and regional variation. *Visual Neurosci.* 2002;19(4):395–407.
52. Kageyama GH, Wong-Riley MT. The histochemical localization of cytochrome oxidase in the retina and lateral geniculate nucleus of the ferret, cat, and monkey, with particular reference to retinal mosaics and ON/OFF-center visual channels. *J Neurosci Official J Soc Neurosci.* 1984;4(10):2445–2459.
53. Wangsa-Wirawan ND, Linsenmeier RA. Retinal oxygen: Fundamental and clinical aspects. *Arch Ophthalmol-chic.* 2003;121(4):547–557.
54. Cringle SJ, Yu DY. Oxygen supply and consumption in the retina: implications for studies of retinopathy of prematurity. *Doc Ophthalmol.* 2010;120(1):99–109.
55. Werkmeister RM, Schmidl D, Aschinger G, et al. Retinal oxygen extraction in humans. *Sci Rep.* 2015;5(1):15763.
56. Pournaras CJ, Riva CE, Tsacopoulos M, Strommer K. Diffusion of O2 in the retina of anesthetized miniature pigs in normoxia and hyperoxia. *Exp Eye Res.* 1989;49(3):347–360.
57. Pournaras CJ. Retinal oxygen distribution. Its role in the physiopathology of vasoproliferative microangiopathies. *Retin Phila Pa.* 1995;15(4):332–347.
58. Pournaras CJ, Miller JW, Gragoudas ES, et al. Systemic hyperoxia decreases vascular endothelial growth factor gene expression in ischemic primate retina. *Arch Ophthalmol.* 1997;115(12):1553–1558.
59. Alder VA, Cringle SJ. The effect of the retinal circulation on vitreal oxygen tension. *Curr Eye Res.* 2009;4(2):121–130.
60. Linsenmeier RA, Braun RD. Oxygen distribution and consumption in the cat retina during normoxia and hypoxemia. *J Gen Physiology.* 1992;99(2):177–197.
61. Riva CE, Pournaras CJ, Tsacopoulos M. Regulation of local oxygen tension and blood flow in the inner retina during hyperoxia. *J Appl Physiol.* 1986;61(2):592–598.
62. Braun RD, Linsenmeier RA. Retinal oxygen tension and the electroretinogram during arterial occlusion in the cat. *Invest Ophth Vis Sci.* 1995;36(3):523–541.
63. Bill A, Sperber GO. Aspects of oxygen and glucose consumption in the retina: effects of high intraocular pressure and light. *Graefes Archive Clin Exp Ophthalmol.* 1990;228(1):124–127.
64. Alder VA, Cringle SJ, Constable IJ. The retinal oxygen profile in cats. *Invest Ophth Vis Sci.* 1983;24(1):30–36.
65. Linsenmeier RA. Effects of light and darkness on oxygen distribution and consumption in the cat retina. *J Gen Physiology.* 1986;88(4):521–542.
66. Yu DY, Cringle SJ, Su EN. Intraretinal Oxygen Distribution in the Monkey Retina and the Response to Systemic Hyperoxia. *Invest Ophth Vis Sci.* 2005;46(12):4728–4733.
67. Birol G, Wang S, Budzynski E, Wangsa-Wirawan ND, Linsenmeier RA. Oxygen distribution and consumption in the macaque retina. *Am J Physio Heart Circ Physiol.* 2007;293(3):H1696–H1704.
68. Medrano CJ, Fox DA. Oxygen consumption in the rat outer and inner retina: Light- and pharmacologically-induced inhibition. *Exp Eye Res.* 1995;61(3):273–284.
69. Dollery CT, Bulpitt CJ, Kohner EM. Oxygen supply to the retina from the retinal and choroidal circulations at normal and increased arterial oxygen tensions. *Invest Ophth Visual.* 1969;8(6):588–594.
70. Haugh-Scheidt LM, Griff ER, Linsenmeier RA. Light-evoked oxygen responses in the isolated toad retina. *Exp Eye Res.* 1995;61(1):73–81.
71. Haugh-Scheidt LM, Linsenmeier RA, Griff ER. Oxygen consumption in the isolated toad retina. *Exp Eye Res.* 1995;61(1):63–72.
72. Ahmed J, Braun RD, Dunn R, Linsenmeier RA. Oxygen distribution in the macaque retina. *Invest Ophth Vis Sci.* 1993;34(3):516–521.
73. Ames A, Walseth TF, Heyman RA, Barad M, Graeff RM, Goldberg ND. Light-induced increases in cGMP metabolic flux correspond with electrical responses of photoreceptors. *J Biol Chem.* 1986;261(28):13034–13042.
74. Goldberg ND, Ames AA, Gander JE, Walseth TF. Magnitude of increase in retinal cGMP metabolic flux determined by 18O incorporation into nucleotide alpha-phosphoryls corresponds with intensity of photic stimulation. *J Biol Chem.* 1983;258(15):9213–9219.
75. Ames A, Nesbett FB. In vitro retina as an experimental model of the central nervous system. *J Neurochem.* 1981;37(4):867–877.
76. Futterman S, Kinoshita JH. Metabolism of the retina. I. Respiration of cattle retina. *J Biological Chem.* 1959;234(4):723–726.

77. Racker E. History of the Pasteur effect and its pathobiology. *Mol Cell Biochem*. 1974;5(1-2):17–23.
78. Matschinsky FM. Energy metabolism of the microscopic structures of the cochlea, the retina, and the cerebellum. *Adv Biochem Psychoph*. 1970;2:217–243.
79. Winkler BS. Glycolytic and oxidative metabolism in relation to retinal function. *J Gen Physiol*. 1981;77(6):667–692.
80. Niemeyer G. The function of the retina in the perfused eye. *Doc Ophthalmol*. 1975;39(1):53–116.
81. Vohra R, Kolko M. Neuroprotection of the inner retina: Müller cells and lactate. *Neural Regen Res*. 2018;13(10):1741–1742.
82. Vohra R, Kolko M. Lactate: more than merely a metabolic waste product in the inner retina. *Mol Neurobiol*. 2020;57(4):2021–2037.
83. Vohra R, Dalgaard LM, Vibaek J, et al. Potential metabolic markers in glaucoma and their regulation in response to hypoxia. *Acta Ophthalmol*. 2019;94:592.
84. Kuwabara T, Cogan DG, Futterman S, Kinoshita JH. Dehydrogenases in the retina and Müller's fibers. *J Histochem Cytochem*. 1959;7(1):67–68.
85. Rueda EM, Johnson JE, Giddabasappa A, et al. The cellular and compartmental profile of mouse retinal glycolysis, tricarboxylic acid cycle, oxidative phosphorylation, and ~P transferring kinases. *Mol Vis*. 2016;22:847–885.
86. Poitry-Yamate C, Tsacopoulos M. Glial (Müller) cells take up and phosphorylate [3H]2-deoxy-d-glucose in a mammalian retina. *Neurosci Lett*. 1991;122(2):241–244.
87. Poitry-Yamate CL, Tsacopoulos M. Glucose metabolism in freshly isolated Müller glial cells from a mammalian retina. *J Comp Neurol*. 1992;320(2):257–266.
88. Wilson DJ. 2-Deoxy-d-glucose uptake in the inner retina: an in vivo study in the normal rat and following photoreceptor degeneration. *T Am Ophthal Soc*. 2002;100:353–364.
89. Graymore C, Tansley K. Iodoacetate poisoning of the rat retina. I. Production of retinal degeneration. *Br J Ophthalmol*. 1959;43(3):177–185.
90. Graymore CN. Biochemistry of the retina. *Am J Medical Sci*. 1966;252(3):379.
91. Dick E, Miller RF. Extracellular K+ activity changes related to electroretinogram components. I. Amphibian (I-type) retinas. *J Gen Physiology*. 1985;85(6):885–909.
92. Lachapelle P, Benoit J, Guité P, Tran CN, Molotchnikoff S. The effect of iodoacetic acid on the electroretinogram and oscillatory potentials in rabbits. *Doc Ophthalmol*. 1990;75(1):7–14.
93. Hurley JB, Lindsay KJ, Du J. Glucose, lactate, and shuttling of metabolites in vertebrate retinas. *J Neurosci Res*. 2015;93(7):1079–1092.
94. Hsu SC, Molday RS. Glucose metabolism in photoreceptor outer segments. Its role in phototransduction and in NADPH-requiring reactions. *J Biol Chem*. 1994;269(27):17954–17959.
95. Archer SN, Ahuja P, Caffé R, et al. Absence of phosphoglucose isomerase-1 in retinal photoreceptor, pigment epithelium and Müller cells. *Eur J Neurosci*. 2004;19(11):2923–2930.
96. Nihira M, Anderson K, Gorin FA, Burns MS. Primate rod and cone photoreceptors may differ in glucose accessibility. *Invest Ophth Vis Sci*. 1995;36(7):1259–1270.
97. Tsacopoulos M, Magistretti P. Metabolic coupling between glia and neurons. *J Neurosci*. 1996;16(3):877–885.
98. Tsacopoulos M, Poitry-Yamate CL, MacLeish PR, Poitry S. Trafficking of molecules and metabolic signals in the retina. *Prog Retin Eye Res*. 1998;17(3):429–442.
99. Winkler BS, Starnes CA, Sauer MW, Firouzgan Z, Chen SC. Cultured retinal neuronal cells and Müller cells both show net production of lactate. *Neurochem Int*. 2004;45(2-3):311–320.
100. Hertz L. The astrocyte-neuron lactate shuttle: a challenge of a challenge. *J Cereb Blood Flow Metab*. 2004;24(11):1241–1248.
101. Halestrap AP, Price NT. The proton-linked monocarboxylate transporter (MCT) family: structure, function and regulation. *Biochem J*. 1999;343(2):281–299.
102. Vohra R, Sanz-Morello B, Tams ALM, et al. Prevention of cell death by activation of hydroxycarboxylic acid receptor 1 (GPR81) in retinal explants. *Cells*. 2022;11(13):2098.
103. Sarthy VP, Pignataro L, Pannicke T, et al. Glutamate transport by retinal Müller cells in glutamate/aspartate transporter-knockout mice. *Glia*. 2005;49(2):184–196.
104. Brew H, Attwell D. Electrogenic glutamate uptake is a major current carrier in the membrane of axolotl retinal glial cells. *Nature*. 1987;327(6124):707–709.
105. Biedermann B, Bringmann A, Reichenbach A. High-affinity GABA uptake in retinal glial (Müller) cells of the guinea pig: Electrophysiological characterization, immunohistochemical localization, and modeling of efficiency. *Glia*. 2002;39(3):217–228.
106. Gadea A, López E, Hernández-Cruz A, López-Colomé AM. Role of Ca2+ and calmodulin-dependent enzymes in the regulation of glycine transport in Müller glia. *J Neurochem*. 2002;80(4):634–645.
107. Sarthy PV. The uptake of [3h] γ-aminobutyric acid by isolated glial (Müller) cells from the mouse retina. *J Neurosci Methods*. 1982;5(1-2):77–82.
108. Derouiche A, Rauen T. Coincidence of L-glutamate/L-aspartate transporter (GLAST) and glutamine synthetase (GS) immunoreactions in retinal glia: Evidence for coupling of GLAST and GS in transmitter clearance. *J Neurosci Res*. 1995;42(1):131–143.
109. Linser PJ, Sorrentino M, Moscona AA. Cellular compartmentalization of carbonic anhydrase-C and glutamine synthetase in developing and mature mouse neural retina. *Dev Brain Res*. 1984;13(1):65–71.
110. Nagelhus EA, Mathiisen TM, Bateman AC, et al. Carbonic anhydrase XIV is enriched in specific membrane domains of retinal pigment epithelium, Müller cells, and astrocytes. *Proc National Acad Sci*. 2005;102(22):8030–8035.
111. Pfeiffer-Guglielmi B, Francke M, Reichenbach A, Fleckenstein B, Jung G, Hamprecht B. Glycogen phosphorylase isozyme pattern in mammalian retinal Müller (glial) cells and in astrocytes of retina and optic nerve. *Glia*. 2005;49(1):84–95.
112. Coffe V, Carbajal RC, Salceda R. Glycogen metabolism in the rat retina. *J Neurochem*. 2004;88(4):885–890.
113. Schorderet M, Hof P, Magistretti PJ. The effects of VIP on cyclic AMP and glycogen levels in vertebrate retina. *Peptides*. 1984;5(2):295–298.
114. Lauritzen KH, Morland C, Puchades M, et al. Lactate receptor sites link neurotransmission, neurovascular coupling, and brain energy metabolism. *Cereb Cortex*. 2014;24(10):2784–2795.
115. Rungger-Brändle E, Kolb H, Niemeyer G. Histochemical demonstration of glycogen in neurons of the cat retina. *Invest Ophth Vis Sci*. 1996;37(5):702–715.
116. Wong-Riley M. Energy metabolism of the visual system. *Eye Brain*. 2010;2:99–116.
117. Kumagai AK. Glucose transport in brain and retina: implications in the management and complications of diabetes. *Diabetes Metab Res Rev*. 1999;15(4):261–273.
118. Matthews PM. Neuroenergetics: relevance in functional brain imaging. *Brain*. 2002;125(10):2365–2367.
119. Magistretti PJ, Pellerin L. Astrocytes couple synaptic activity to glucose utilization in the brain. *News Physiol Sci*. 1999;14(5):177–182.
120. Magistretti PJ, Pellerin L. [Functional brain imaging: role metabolic coupling between astrocytes and neurons]. *Rev Méd Suisse Romande*. 2000;120(9):739–742.
121. Raichle ME. Functional brain imaging and human brain function. *J Neurosci*. 2003;23(10):3959–3962.
122. Niemeyer G, Steinberg RH. Differential effects of pCO2 and pH on the ERG and light peak of the perfused cat eye. *Vision Res*. 1984;24(3):275–280.
123. Macaluso C, Onoe S, Niemeyer G. Changes in glucose level affect rod function more than cone function in the isolated, perfused cat eye. *Invest Ophth Vis Sci*. 1992;33(10):2798–2808.
124. Niemeyer G. Glucose concentration and retinal function. *Clin Neurosci N Y*. 1997;4(6):327–335.
125. Gruetter R. Glycogen: The forgotten cerebral energy store. *J Neurosci Res*. 2003;74(2):179–183.
126. Padnick-Silver L, Linsenmeier RA. Quantification of in vivo anaerobic metabolism in the normal cat retina through intraretinal pH measurements. *Visual Neurosci*. 2002;19(6):793–806. https://doi.org/10.1017/s095252380219609x.
127. Tsacopoulos M, Levy S. Intraretinal acid-base studies using pH glass microelectrodes: Effect of respiratory and metabolic acidosis and alkalosis on inner-retinal pH. *Exp Eye Res*. 1976;23(5):495–504.
128. Tsacopoulos M, Baker R, Levy S. Oxygen transport to tissue—II. *Adv Exp Med Biol*. 1976;75:413–416.
129. Bui BV, Kalloniatis M, Vingrys AJ. The contribution of glycolytic and oxidative pathways to retinal photoreceptor function. *Invest Ophth Vis Sci*. 2003;44(6):2708–2715.
130. Riva CE, Pournaras CJ, Poitry-Yamate CL, Petrig BL. Rhythmic changes in velocity, volume, and flow of blood in the optic nerve head tissue. *Microvasc Res*. 1990;40(1):36–45.
131. Riva CE, Harino S, Shonat RD, Petrig BL. Flicker evoked increase in optic nerve head blood flow in anesthetized cats. *Neurosci Lett*. 1991;128(2):291–296.
132. Riva CE, Grunwald JE, Petrig BL. Autoregulation of human retinal blood flow. An investigation with laser Doppler velocimetry. *Invest Ophth Vis Sci*. 1986;27(12):1706–1712.
133. Petropoulos IK, Pournaras CJ. Effect of indomethacin on the hypercapnia-associated vasodilation of the optic nerve head vessels: an experimental study in miniature pigs. *Ophthalmic Res*. 2005;37(2):59–66.
134. Duong TQ, Ngan SC, Ugurbil K, Kim SG. Functional magnetic resonance imaging of the retina. *Invest Ophth Vis Sci*. 2002;43(4):1176–1181.
135. Shen Q, Cheng H, Pardue MT, et al. Magnetic resonance imaging of tissue and vascular layers in the cat retina. *J Magn Reson Imaging*. 2006;23(4):465–472.
136. Duong TQ, Pardue MT, Thulé PM, et al. Layer-specific anatomical, physiological and functional MRI of the retina. *Nmr Biomed*. 2008;21(9):978–996.
137. Cheng H, Nair G, Walker TA, et al. Structural and functional MRI reveals multiple retinal layers. *Proc National Acad Sci*. 2006;103(46):17525–17530.
138. Strauss O. The retinal pigment epithelium in visual function. *Physiol Rev*. 2005;85(3):845–881.
139. Bergersen L, Jóhannsson E, Veruki ML, et al. Cellular and subcellular expression of monocarboxylate transporters in the pigment epithelium and retina of the rat. *Neuroscience*. 1999;90(1):319–331.
140. Wood JPM, Chidlow G, Graham M, Osborne NN. Energy substrate requirements of rat retinal pigmented epithelial cells in culture: relative importance of glucose, amino acids, and monocarboxylates. *Invest Ophth Vis Sci*. 2004;45(4):1272–1280.
141. Wood JPM, Chidlow G, Graham M, Osborne NN. Energy substrate requirements for survival of rat retinal cells in culture: the importance of glucose and monocarboxylates. *J Neurochem*. 2005;93(3):686–697.
142. Dienel GA. Brain lactate metabolism: the discoveries and the controversies. *J Cereb Blood Flow Metabol*. 2012;32(7):1107–1138.
143. Dienel GA, Cruz NF. Nutrition during brain activation: does cell-to-cell lactate shuttling contribute significantly to sweet and sour food for thought? *Neurochem Int*. 2004;45(2-3):321–351.
144. Zeuthen T, Hamann S, la Cour M. Cotransport of H+, lactate and H2O by membrane proteins in retinal pigment epithelium of bullfrog. *J Physiol*. 1996;497(1):3–17.
145. Tsacopoulos M, Baker R, David NJ, Strauss J. The effect of arterial PCO2 on inner-retinal oxygen consumption rate in monkeys. *Invest Ophth Visual*. 1973;12(6):456–460.
146. Bardy M, Tsacopoulos M. [Metabolic changes in the retina after experimental microembolism in the miniature pig (author's transl)]. *Klin Monbl Augenheilkd*. 1978;172(4):451–460.
147. Tsacopoulos M. [Role of metabolic factors in the regulation of retinal blood minute volume]. *Adv Ophthalmol*. 1979;39:233–273.
148. Ernst C, Jensen PS, Aalkjaer C, Bek T. Differential effects of intra- and extravascular ATP on the diameter of porcine vessels at different branching levels ex vivo. *Invest Ophth Vis Sci*. 2020;61(12):8.
149. Brazitikos PD, Pournaras CJ, Munoz JL, Tsacopoulos M. Microinjection of L-lactate in the preretinal vitreous induces segmental vasodilation in the inner retina of miniature pigs. *Invest Ophth Vis Sci*. 1993;34(5):1744–1752.

150. Donati G, Pournaras CJ, Munoz JL, Poitry S, Poitry-Yamate CL, Tsacopoulos M. Nitric oxide controls arteriolar tone in the retina of the miniature pig. *Invest Ophth Vis Sci*. 1995; 36(11):2228–2237.

151. Pournaras CJ, Rungger-Brändle E, Riva CE, Hardarson SH, Stefansson E. Regulation of retinal blood flow in health and disease. *Prog Retin Eye Res*. 2008;27(3):284–330.

152. Yamanishi S, Katsumura K, Kobayashi T, Puro DG. Extracellular lactate as a dynamic vasoactive signal in the rat retinal microvasculature. *Am J Physiol Heart Circ Physiol*. 2006; 290(3):H925–34.

153. Morland C, Andersson KA, Haugen OP, et al. Exercise induces cerebral VEGF and angiogenesis via the lactate receptor HCAR1. *Nat Commun*. 2017;8(1):15557.

154. Garhöfer G, Resch H, Lung S, Weigert G, Schmetterer L. Intravenous administration of l-arginine increases retinal and choroidal blood flow. *Am J Ophthalmol*. 2005;140(1):69–76.

155. Ido Y, Chang K, Williamson JR. NADH augments blood flow in physiologically activated retina and visual cortex. *P Natl Acad Sci USA*. 2004;101(2):653–658.

156. Poole RC, Halestrap AP. Transport of lactate and other monocarboxylates across mammalian plasma membranes. *Am J Physiol*. 1993;264(4):C761–C782.

157. Gerhart DZ, Leino RL, Drewes LR. Distribution of monocarboxylate transporters MCT1 and MCT2 in rat retina. *Neurosci*. 1999;92(1):367–375.

158. Hein TW, Xu W, Kuo L. Dilation of retinal arterioles in response to lactate: role of nitric oxide, guanylyl cyclase, and ATP-sensitive potassium channels. *Invest Ophth Vis Sci*. 2006; 47(2):693–699.

159. Mendrinos E, Petropoulos IK, Mangioris G, Papadopoulou DN, Stangos AN, Pournaras CJ. Lactate-induced retinal arteriolar vasodilation implicates neuronal nitric oxide synthesis in minipigs. *Invest Ophth Vis Sci*. 2008;49(11):5060–5066.

160. Liepe BA, Stone C, Koistinaho J, Copenhagen DR. Nitric oxide synthase in Müller cells and neurons of salamander and fish retina. *J Neurosci*. 1994;14(12):7641–7654.

161. Kim IB, Lee EJ, Kim KY, et al. Immunocytochemical localization of nitric oxide synthase in the mammalian retina. *Neurosci Lett*. 1999;267(3):193–196.

The Function of the Retinal Pigment Epithelium

Catherine Bowes Rickman and Olaf Strauss

Introduction

The retinal pigment epithelium (RPE) is a monolayer of pigmented cells located between the light-sensitive photoreceptor outer segments and the fenestrated endothelium of the choriocapillaris. On both sides, specialized extracellular matrices enable a close interaction of the RPE with its adjacent tissues. On the basolateral side, the multilayered Bruch's membrane combines barrier function and selective transport matrix as part of the blood retina barrier. On the apical side of the RPE, the interphotoreceptor matrix provides an interface for interaction between the photoreceptor outer segments and the RPE.[1] In humans, every RPE cell interacts with a mean of 23 photoreceptors with variations between macular and peripheral cells.[2] Through these interactions, the RPE forms a functional unit with the photoreceptors[3-5] (Fig. 13.1). The formation of this functional unit affects embryonic development, with the RPE and neural retina depending on each other for their differentiation, as well as for maturation and maintenance.[6] This is evidenced by the effect of mutations in genes expressed in the RPE that lead to primary photoreceptor degeneration and mutations in genes expressed in photoreceptors that lead to primary RPE degenerations. As an integral component of this functional unit the RPE fulfills a multitude of tasks that are essential for visual function. The failure of any one of these functions leads to retinal degeneration.

ABSORPTION OF LIGHT

The pigmented RPE covers the inner wall of the bulbus and absorbs scattered light to improve optical quality by removing stray photons of light.[7] In the human eye, light is focused by a lens onto the central part of the retina (macula) leading to accumulation of potentially excessive high-energy light that is absorbed by melanin granules within melanosomes in the RPE protecting the photoreceptors. This causes a temperature increase in the RPE that is then dissipated by choroidal blood flow.[8] The relative blood perfusion of the choriocapillaris is very high, higher than that of the kidney.[9,10] Despite this, only small amounts of oxygen are extracted by the adjacent tissues and venous blood from the choroid, which has an oxygen saturation of more than 90%. This functional arrangement produces an excess of oxygen in combination with a large density of light energy, leading to a risk of photo-oxidative damage owing to production of reactive oxygen species.[11,12] As a consequence, the RPE is protected by various lines of defense against this toxicity.[13] In addition to melanin in the RPE, there are carotenoids, lutein, and zeaxanthin, in the neural retina that absorb light energy. In addition, ascorbate, α-tocopherol and β-carotene, and glutathione are nonenzymatic antioxidants, and melanin itself can function as an antioxidant. This is further augmented by the natural ability of RPE cells to repair damaged DNA, lipids, and proteins.[14]

TRANSEPITHELIAL TRANSPORT

The RPE forms the outer blood-retinal barrier. The RPE is, by its electrophysiological parameters, a tight epithelium in which the paracellular resistance is at least 10 times larger than that of the transcellular resistance.[15,16] This barrier is formed by two types of connections on the lateral domains of adjacent RPE, apical zonulae occludens (tight junctions) and zonulae adherentes (adherens junctions), which form a barrier that regulates transepithelial diffusion through the paracellular spaces.[17] This barrier function is also important for the immune privilege of the eye (see further in chapter). Owing to this tight barrier function, the complete exchange of molecules and ions between the blood stream and the photoreceptor side relies on transepithelial transport through the RPE.

Transport from the blood side to the photoreceptor side

The transport from the blood to the photoreceptor side consists mainly of transport of nutrients such as glucose, omega-3 (ω3) fatty acids, and retinal.

For glucose transport, the RPE contains an abundance of the glucose transporters GLUT1 and GLUT3 in both the apical and the basolateral membrane.[18,19] GLUT3 mediates the basal transport, whereas GLUT1 is responsible for inducible glucose transport that adapts to different metabolic demands.[20]

All-trans retinol (vitamin A) is taken up from the blood stream via a receptor-mediated process involving a serum retinol binding protein/transthyretin complex. Retinol is converted to all-trans retinyl ester and then directly enters the visual cycle (see further in chapter).

Docosahexaenoic acid (DHA) is a polyunsaturated ω-3 fatty acid (22:6ω3) that is a major structural lipid of retinal photoreceptor outer segment membranes and is essential for outer segment renewal, but it cannot be synthesized by the photoreceptors.[21-24] DHA is synthesized in the liver from the precursor linolenic acid and transported to the eye in the blood bound to plasma proteins.[25] The RPE preferentially takes up DHA via the sodium-dependent lyso-phosphatidylcholine transporter, Mfsd2a, in a concentration-dependent manner.[26]

Transport from the retinal side to the blood side

The retina is one of the most energy-demanding tissues, due primarily to the photoreceptors that are among the most metabolically active cells. This results in the production of large amounts of water and accumulation of lactic acid. Additional water is moved toward the retina by intraocular pressure from the vitreous. Water cannot pass through the RPE via the paracellular route because the RPE is a tight epithelium. Therefore, water and lactic acid are eliminated from the subretinal space by active transcellular transport by the RPE.[27-29]

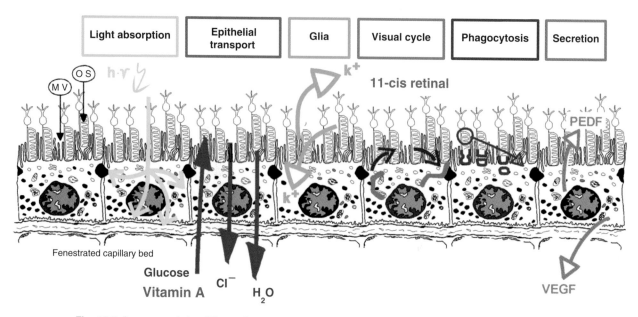

Fig. 13.1 Summary of the different functions of the retinal pigment epithelium by which a functional unit between photoreceptors is formed. (MV = microvilli; OS = outer segments; PEGF = pigment epithelium derived growth factor; VEGF = vascular endothelial growth factor *MV*, microvilli; *OS*, outer segements; *PEGF*, pigment epithelium derived growth factor; *VEGF*, vascular endothelial growth factor. (Modified from Strauss O. The retinal pigment epithelium in visual function. *Physiol Rev.* 2005;85(3):845-881.)

The transport of water is driven by an active transport of Cl⁻ from the retina though the RPE to the blood side (Fig. 13.2).[15,29–31] The energy for this process is supplied by the apically located Na^+/K^+-ATPase, which uses ATP to transport Na^+ out of the RPE in exchange for transport of K^+ into the cytosol of the RPE. The K^+ ions are recycled across the apical membrane through inward rectifier potassium channels, which provide the large K^+-conductance of the apical membrane. This recycling keeps the K^+ gradient across the apical membrane small to support the activity of the Na^+/K^+-ATPase. On the apical membrane a $Na^+/2Cl^-/K^+$-cotransporter uses the Na^+ gradient across the apical membrane to transport K^+ and Cl^- into the cytosol of the RPE. Since K^+ moves back through inward rectifier channels to the subretinal space, the $Na^+/2Cl^-/K^+$-cotransporter accumulates Cl^- in the intracellular space of the RPE cells (40–60 mM).[32] This high Cl^- concentration provides a driving force for Cl^- to leave the cell. The basolateral membrane displays a large conductance for Cl^- through which Cl^- leaves the cell from the intracellular space to the blood side. This is the last step of transepithelial Cl^- transport from the subretinal space to the blood side, resulting in a basolateral negative transepithelial potential between –6 and –15 mV.[27] Voltage-gated ClC-2 Cl^- channels appear to provide a major part of the basolateral Cl^- conductance.[33] Other channels providing basolateral Cl^- conductance are Cl^- channels linked to intracellular second-messenger systems. Cl^- transport can be increased by rises in intracellular free Ca^{2+} [34] or by increases in cytosolic cAMP concentration[35] resulting from either activation of Ca^{2+}-dependent Cl^- channels or cAMP-dependently regulated Cl^- channels.

Large subretinal concentrations of lactic acid are formed by the high metabolic activity of the retina and removed by the RPE (Fig. 13.2B).[18,36] This lactic acid transport requires a tight regulation of the intracellular pH.[37,38] Lactic acid is removed from the subretinal space by the monocarboxylate transporter 1 (MCT1),[39] which transports H^+ in cotransport with lactic acid (in concentrations that can be as high as 19 mM). This transport is driven by the activity of the Na^+/H^+-exchanger that eliminates H^+ from cytosol of the RPE cells using the gradient for Na^+ provided by the activity of the Na^+/K^+-ATPase.[40]

Across the basolateral membrane, lactic acid leaves the cell via the activity of another monocarboxylate transporter, MCT3, which is also an H^+/lactic acid cotransporter. Intracellular pH is stabilized by the transport of bicarbonate (HCO_3^-).[37,38] HCO_3^- is transported into the cell across the apical membrane by the $Na^+/2HCO_3^-$-cotransporter which uses the Na^+ gradient established by the Na^+/K^+-ATPase. HCO_3^- leaves the RPE cell across the basolateral membrane by the activity of the Cl^-/HCO_3^- exchanger.[41]

Production of metabolic water and accumulation of lactic acid are linked. Therefore, transport of water and pH regulation are also coupled.[36] An increase in the transport of lactic acid leads to intracellular acidification that inhibits the transport activity of the $Cl^-/HCO3^-$ exchanger.[29] Since the Cl^-/HCO_3^- exchanger transports Cl^- in the opposite direction from the Cl^- channels, it decreases the Cl^- transport efficiency in resting conditions. The inhibition of the $Cl^-/HCO3^-$ exchanger, thus, increases the transepithelial transport of Cl^- and water. This is further increased by the ClC-2 channels, which are activated by a decrease in extracellular pH. Extracellular acidification can result from the increased transport of lactic acid by the MCT3 in the basolateral membrane (Box 13.1).

CAPACITIVE COMPENSATION OF FAST CHANGES IN THE ION COMPOSITION IN THE SUBRETINAL SPACE

In the dark, cGMP-gated cation channels in photoreceptor outer segments generate an inward current of Na^+ and Ca^{2+} that is counterbalanced by a K^+ outward current at the inner segments.[44] In the light, cGMP-gated cation channels close and the K^+ current is decreased, resulting in a decrease of the K^+ concentration in the subretinal space from 5 to 2 mM. The decrease of the Na^+ conductance in the light in outer segments leads to an increase in the subretinal Na^+ concentration. In addition, illumination of the retina also causes an increase in the subretinal volume. Both light-induced changes

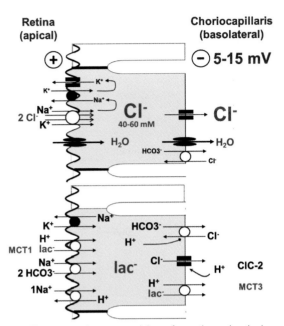

Fig. 13.2 Transport of water and ions from the subretinal space to the blood. *Upper panel*: Using the energy of ATP hydrolysis the Na⁺/K⁺-ATPase establishes a gradient for Na⁺ which drives the uptake of Na⁺, K⁺ and Cl⁻ by the Na⁺/K⁺/2Cl⁻-cotransporter. K⁺ recycles across the apical membrane through inward rectifier K⁺ channels. The concerted transport activity of the three transport proteins results in the accumulation of Cl in the cytosol of the RPE. Cl⁻ leaves the cell through a variety of basolateral Cl⁻ channels. The net transport of Cl⁻ results in a basolateral negative transepithelial potential. The transport of Cl⁻ as osmolytes drives a transcellular transport of water through aquaporin water channels located in both the apical and the basolateral membrane. *Lower panel*: Lactate (lac⁻) is taken up from subretinal space via the activity of the monocarboxylate transporter-1 (*MCT1*) and accumulated in the cell. The driving force for this transport is large because the activity of retinal neurons produces large amounts of lactic acid (concentration in the subretinal space can be as high as 19mM). Lactate leaves the cell through the basolateral membrane via the activity of the MCT3 transporter. The required pH regulation occurs at the apical membrane by the activity of sodium-dependent transporters: Na⁺/H⁺ exchanger and the Na⁺/HCO3⁻-cotransporter that use the sodium gradient of the Na⁺/K⁺-ATPase. At the basolateral membrane, pH regulation occurs by the activity of Cl⁻-dependent transport proteins, which use the large intracellular Cl⁻ activity using a Cl⁻/HCO3⁻ exchanger and the Cl⁻ channel ClC-2.

are compensated for the moment they occur, by modulation of ion transport by the RPE.[4,45-47]

Compensation for changes in the K⁺ concentration and in extracellular volume are both linked to the potassium transport.[27] The apical membrane of the RPE displays a large K⁺ conductance. Decrease in the subretinal K⁺ concentration leads to hyperpolarization of the apical membrane that corresponds to the c-wave in the electroretinogram. The decrease in the potassium concentration decreases the activity of the Na⁺/K⁺/2Cl⁻-cotransporter, which subsequently decreases the intracellular Cl⁻ activity and hyperpolarizes the basolateral membrane.[31] On an electroretinogram this can be seen as the delayed hyperpolarization. The hyperpolarization of the apical membrane activates inward rectifier K⁺ channels that generate an efflux of K⁺ into the subretinal space to compensate for the light-induced decrease in the subretinal K⁺ concentration. At the same time, the apical hyperpolarization decreases the activity of the Na⁺/HCO3⁻-cotransporter that is an electrogenic transporter by its stoichiometry. The subsequent intracellular acidification increases the transepithelial Cl⁻ and water transport as described earlier.

The light-induced increase in subretinal Na⁺ concentration is compensated for by the activity of the Na⁺/K⁺/2Cl⁻-cotransporter and by the Na⁺/H⁺ exchanger.[48,49] The Na⁺/K⁺-ATPase takes up Na⁺ to compensate for the increase in the subretinal Na⁺ concentration during the transition from light to dark. This task appears to be the reason for its localization in the apical membrane of the RPE.[50]

VISUAL CYCLE

The visual cycle is initiated in photoreceptor outer segments by a photon reacting with rhodopsin, consisting of a G-coupled receptor opsin (rods) or cone opsin (cones) and the light-detecting chromophore, 11-cis retinal, which is photo-isomerized to all-trans retinal.[51] To maintain visual function, regeneration of 11-cis retinal from all-trans retinal occurs through a complex process initiated in the photoreceptors that is completed in the RPE (Fig. 13.3).[3,52-56] All-trans retinal leaves the disc membrane as N-retinylidene-phosphatidylethanolamine (N-retinylidene-PE), the Schiff base adduct of retinal and PE, by the importer activity of the ATP-binding cassette protein (ABC) transporter, ABCA4 (also known as ABCR or the rim protein),[57,58] which flips N-retinylidene-PE across the photoreceptor disc membrane. Following dissociation from N-retinylidene-PE, all-trans retinal is reduced to all-trans retinol by retinol dehydrogenase (RDH).[59] All-trans retinol diffuses across the interphotoreceptor matrix chaperoned by the interphotoreceptor retinoid binding protein (IRBP) into the RPE.[60,61] In the cytosol of the RPE, it binds to the cellular retinol binding protein (CRBP). All-trans retinol is esterified by lecithin:retinol transferase (LRAT) to all-trans retinyl esters. These may be stored as retinosomes[62] or converted to 11-cis retinol by RPE65,[63] and oxidized by 11-cis retinol dehydrogenase (11cRDH or RDH5) back to 11-cis retinal.chaperoned by cellular retinaldehyde binding protein (CRALBP). The 11-cis retinal diffuses across the IPM with IRBP into photoreceptor outer segments where it completes the cycle by recombining with opsin. Cones have an additional cone-specific visual cycle involving Müller cells.[64]

Since the visual cycle maintains the excitability of the photoreceptors, it needs to be adapted to the different photoreceptor activities between light and dark.[65] In the light, there is a fast turnover of retinal, whereas in the dark the turnover occurs much more slowly. Retinal that is not needed in the state of a slower turnover must be quickly available for the transition from dark to light, and vice versa. The different retinal binding proteins represent connected pools for retinal. In the transition from dark to light, IRPB represents the first pool that

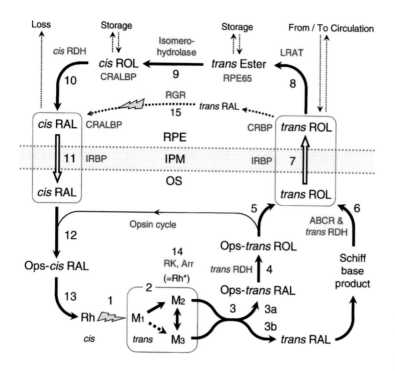

Fig. 13.3 Visual cycle: biochemical cycle of retinoid processing. The process of vision is started by the conformational change of the chromophore of rhodopsin from 11-cis retinal (*cis RAL*) to all-trans retinal (*trans RAL*). trans RAL is re-isomerized to 11-cis in the retinal pigment epithelium (*RPE*). The first step in this cycle is the reduction of trans RAL to all-trans retinol (trans ROL). trans ROL leaves the photoreceptor and binds to interstitial retinal binding protein (*IRPB*), and is transported to the RPE. Inside the RPE, trans ROL binds to cellular retinol binding protein (*CRBP*) and enters the re-isomerization pathway. The reaction is catalyzed by a protein complex consisting of lecithin retinol acyltransferase (*LRAT*), retinal pigment epithelium–specific protein 65 kDa (*RPE65*), and 11-cis retinol dehydrogenase (*RDH5*). The reaction product, cis RAL, binds to cellular retinaldehyde binding protein (*CRALBP*) and leaves the cell where it binds to IRPB again to be transported to the photoreceptors. This schematic illustrates the biochemical sequence of events in the retinoid cycle using the numbering convention of Lamb and Pugh from which this figure is taken,[56] starting in the rod outer segment with (1) photo-activation, (2) protein re-arrangement, (3) hydrolysis of Schiff base bond, (4) reduction of aldehyde, (5) release of trans ROL, (6) flippase, (7) transport across interphotoreceptor matrix (IPM) and within RPE, (8) esterification, (9) isomerization, (10) oxidation of alcohol, (11) transport within RPE and across IPM, (12) noncovalent binding, (13) Schiff base formation, (14a) phosphorylation, (14b) arrestin binding, and (15) photo-isomerization. *RDH*, Retinol dehydrogenase; *Rho*, rhodopsin; *SER*, smooth endoplasmic reticulum. (From Lamb TD, Pugh EN Jr. Dark adaptation and the retinoid cycle of vision. *Prog Retin Eye Res.* 2004;23(3):307–380.)

delivers retinal.[60] This pool cannot be depleted because it refills retinal from the pool of CRALBP proteins. CRALBP in turn can recruit retinal from RPE65. Thus, with increasing light intensity retinal can be recruited from the different pools, and in the transition from light to darkness retinal can be stored. IRBP can carry larger amounts of retinal in the dark than in the light. Another key function is the modulation of the RPE65 function.[66] In the light, RPE65 is palmitoylated and bound to intracellular membranes. In this configuration, RPE65 predominantly catalyzes the re-isomerization of all-trans retinol to 11-cis retinol. In the dark, RPE65 is water soluble and freely diffusible in the cytosol and in this configuration, RPE65 may function as a retinal store, although there is some question about the physiologic relevance of the form (Box 13.2).[67]

PHAGOCYTOSIS OF PHOTORECEPTOR OUTER SEGMENTS

The focus of high levels of light energy onto the retina and increased formation of reactive oxygen species by photo-oxidation constantly expose photoreceptor outer segments to toxic compounds, leading to outer segment damage. To maintain the excitability of the photoreceptors, outer segment discs are renewed at the connecting cilium every day[75,76] as evaginations of the ciliary membrane.[77] The damaged distal tips of the photoreceptor outer segments are shed and phagocytosed by the RPE through interactions with the interdigitated apical RPE microvilli.[78–81] The process of outer segment disc renewal and shedding and phagocytosis by the RPE is tightly coordinated to maintain the proper length of the outer segments. Coordination of phagocytosis is a receptor-mediated multistep process leading to the efficient degradation of the internalized photoreceptor outer segments (POS). Rod outer segment disc shedding is regulated in a circadian manner at light onset.[80,82–84] Every 11 days the equivalent of a whole length of a photoreceptor outer segment is renewed

BOX 13.2   Diseases caused by genetic defects in the retinal pigment epithelium

The regeneration of the visual pigment in the retinal pigment epithelium (RPE) involves a complex cascade of steps and a variety of molecules. Mutations in these molecules can cause retinal diseases. Mutations in RPE65 can cause the severe congenital blinding disease Leber's congenital amaurosis (LCA). Mutations in the RLBP1 gene and its product, CRALBP, have been identified in patients with autosomal recessive retinitis punctata albescens, a tape to retinal degeneration.[68–70]

Clinically these diseases manifest with different degrees of visual loss. They include congenital blindness (LCA), and slow loss of central vision with peripheral visual field remaining intact throughout life (Stargardt's disease). Other forms are night blindness with progressive loss of the peripheral visual field progressing to blindness at an adult age. Some are forms of retinitis pigmentosa, a class of diseases involving progressive degeneration of the retina, typically starting in the midperiphery and advancing toward the macula and fovea.[68–70] The first proof-of-concept gene augmentation therapy was for the treatment of LCA caused by *RPE65* mutations and was performed in a dog model.[71] This led to the first US Food and Drug Administration (FDA) approval of a gene therapy, voretigene neparvovec-rzyl (Luxturna), for an inherited disease, in 2017.[72–74]

Rod outer segment phagocytosis by the RPE consists of recognition, binding, internalization, and degradation of the ingested outer segment (Fig. 13.4). The first step in phagocytosis is recognition, a receptor-mediated process involving the integrin αvβ5, which interacts with phosphatidylserine of rod OS (outer segment) plasma membranes.[84] This binding initiates a signal cascade in the RPE involving the activation of focal adhesion kinase (FAK).[85] This process serves two functions. One leads to phosphorylation of the TAM receptor tyrosine

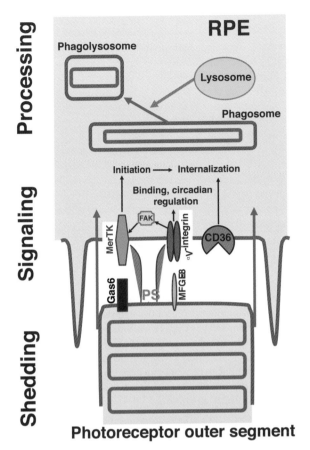

Processing

RPE

Phagolysosome

Lysosome

Phagosome

Signaling

Initiation ⟶ Internalization

Binding, circadian
regulation

FAK

MerTK

αv-integrin

CD36

Gas6

PS

MFGE8

Shedding

Photoreceptor outer segment

Fig. 13.4 Photoreceptor outer membranes phagocytosis. With onset of light, the distal tips of the photoreceptor outer segments are shed from photoreceptors and phagocytosed by the retinal pigment epithelium (*RPE*). The first step consists of recognition through the receptor-mediated binding of αv-integrin, which enables the initiation of the cascade regulating phagocytosis. This cascade is initiated by the activation of the MerTK receptor. Internalization of the shed photoreceptor outer segments is activated by CD36. *αv-integrin*, Vitronectin binding integrin; *CD36*, macrophage phagocytosis receptor; *FAK*, focal adhesion kinase; *MerTK*, c-mer tyrosine kinase receptor.

regulates secretion. The RPE secretes pigment epithelium–derived factor (PEDF), which aids in maintenance of the structural integrity of photoreceptors by protecting against hypoxia- and glutamate-induced apoptosis; ciliary neurotrophic factor (CNTF), which protects against photoreceptor cell death; and members of the fibroblast growth factor family.[105] The RPE secretes vascular endothelial growth factor (VEGF) and tissue inhibitors of matrix metalloproteases (TIMPs) to stabilize the choriocapillaris.[106] TIMPs function in stabilizing the extracellular matrix and preventing neovascularization.[107] In short, the regulation of secretion is embedded in a network of paracrine and autocrine stimulation.[108,109] There are a variety of receptors on the RPE to coordinate secretion with neighboring tissues and these are activated by factors including insulin-like growth factor-1 (IGF-1), tumor necrosis factor-α (TNFα), VEGF, and glutamate. The secretion of ATP by the RPE is involved in autocrine regulation of phagocytosis.[110,111]

ACTIVE IMMUNE BARRIER

As described previously, the RPE maintains the outer blood-retinal barrier, including a tight barrier between the circulation and the retina. Concomitantly, the RPE forms an interface between the retina and the blood with its basolateral membrane.[112] The RPE establishes a structure that helps to maintain the immune privilege of the retina by formation of the combination of a barrier and interface.[113] The RPE forms part of a unique type of immune barrier that can be defined as an "educational gate" composed of a fenestrated endothelium and an epithelium, the RPE, that establishes the functional barrier.[114] This "educational gate" in the outer retina is formed by the fenestrated endothelium of the choriocapillaris, the extracellular matrix, Bruch's membrane, and the RPE itself. The physical barrier results from the functional properties of the tight junctions and their specialized composition of tight-junction proteins, the claudins and occludin.[112,114] However, the RPE does not only form a physical barrier because it can interact with the immune system that is present in the circulation. The interaction is based on secretion of immune modulators by the RPE in response to the immunogenic

kinase, MerTK, another receptor that is involved in the regulation of phagocytosis. The second function leads to the circadian regulation of phagocytosis. MerTK triggers the process of internalization of POS[86–88] after binding to v-integrin. Protein S and Gas6 both function as bona fide TAM receptor ligands in vivo.[89] The downstream cascade initiated after activation of MerTK involves the generation of inositol-1,4,5-triphosphate and an increase of cytosolic free Ca²⁺ as second messenger. The ligand, CD36, is also required to activate the OS internalization process of the RPE (Box 13.3).[90]

SECRETION

The RPE can secret a large variety of growth factors, cytokines, and immune modulators.[102,103] This function serves to maintain the structural integrity of photoreceptors,[104] to maintain the fenestrae on the side of choriocapillaris facing the RPE and to actively interact with the immune system[5] (Fig. 13.5). The intracellular regulation of the secretion involves voltage-dependent L-type Ca^{2+} channels of the neuroendocrine subtype (Cav1.3), which are regulated by tyrosine kinases such as pp60c-src and fibroblast growth factor receptors tyrosine kinases. In this way, activation of tyrosine kinases by growth factors

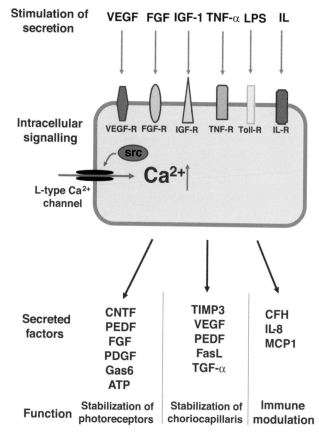

Stimulation of secretion: VEGF FGF IGF-1 TNF-α LPS IL

Intracellular signalling: VEGF-R FGF-R IGF-R TNF-R Toll-R IL-R

src

$Ca^{2+}\uparrow$

L-type Ca²⁺ channel

Secreted factors: CNTF PEDF FGF PDGF Gas6 ATP | TIMP3 VEGF PEDF FasL TGF-α | CFH IL-8 MCP1

Function: Stabilization of photoreceptors | Stabilization of choriocapillaris | Immune modulation

Fig. 13.5 Secretion by the retinal pigment epithelium (RPE). The secretion of different factors serves to maintain the structural integrity of the neighboring tissues and to modulate the immune system, which helps to establish the immune privilege of the eye. To establish communication between the RPE and the surrounding tissues, the RPE is equipped with a large variety of receptors. The secretion itself is mainly regulated by a neuroendocrine voltage-dependent Ca²⁺ channel (L-type Ca²⁺ channel).[103] This Ca²⁺ channel is regulated by src-kinase, which is activated by different receptors of mediators leading to higher secretion rates. This schematic shows the major receptor types[109] from which several different receptors are expressed (e.g., VEGF-R includes VEGFR-1, VEGFR-2, VEGFR-3). The factors indicated represent the major family (e.g., VEGF includes VEGF-A, VEGF-C). Furthermore, as it can be concluded from the figure, the secretion itself is not only regulated in a paracrine manner, but also in an autocrine manner. Factors: ATP, Adenosine triphosphate; CFH, complement factor H; CNTF, ciliary neurotrophic factor; FasL, CD95 apoptosis receptor ligand; FGF, fibroblast growth factor; Gas6, growth arrest protein 6; IL, interleukin; IGF-1, insulin-like growth factor-1; LPS, lipopolysaccharides; PEDF, pigment epithelium–derived factor; PDGF, platelet-derived growth factor; TIMP3, tissue inhibitor of metalloproteinase 3; VEGF, vascular endothelial growth factor; TGFβ, transforming growth factor-β; TNFα, tumor necrosis factor alpha. Receptors: FGF-R, fibroblast growth factor receptor; IGF-R, insulin-like growth factor receptor; IL-R, interleukin receptor; MCP-1, monocyte chemotactic protein 1; TNF-R, tumor necrosis factor receptor; Toll-R, toll-like receptors; VEGF-R, vascular endothelial growth factor receptor. Intracellular signaling: L-type Ca²⁺ channel, voltage-dependent L-type Ca²⁺ channel; src, src-type intracellular tyrosine kinase.

activity of immune cells or the complement system in the plasma.[113] In this way, the RPE senses the activities of local immune reactions and can specifically react to those immune reactions. Under physiologic conditions, the RPE acts as an immune inhibitor, but this can change into immune activation in the disease state. In this case, the RPE can open its barrier and let immune cells pass into the retinal space. The immune modulation is achieved by secretion of immune active

peptides.[109] Among them are the immune inhibitory factor transforming growth factor-β (TGFβ), the interleukin-1 (IL1) antagonist IL1-RA or the soluble receptor for transforming growth factor-α (TNFα) that neutralizes TNα by immobilization. Furthermore, the complement system is under inhibitory control through secretion of the inhibitory factor complement factor H (CFH) or through expression of surface inhibitors of the complement system. The secretion or release of these immune inhibitory factors can be stimulated by pro-inflammatory cytokines that bind RPE receptors including toll-like receptors, receptors for TNFα, and interleukins (ILs), and also major histocompatibility complexes (MHCs) (Box 13.4).[109]

REFERENCES

1. Hageman GS, Johnson LV. Structure, composition and function of the retinal interphotoreceptor matrix. *Prog Retinal Res.* 1991;10:207–249.
2. Gao H, Hollyfield JG. Aging of the human retina. Differential loss of neurons and retinal pigment epithelial cells. *Invest Ophthalmol Vis Sci.* 1992;33(1):1–17.
3. Bok D. The retinal pigment epithelium: a versatile partner in vision. *J Cell Sci Suppl.* 1993; 17:189–195.
4. Steinberg RH. Interactions between the retinal pigment epithelium and the neural retina. *Doc Ophthalmol.* 1985;60(4):327–346.
5. Strauss O. The retinal pigment epithelium in visual function. *Physiol Rev.* 2005;85(3): 845–881.
6. Marmorstein AD, Finnemann SC, Bonilha VL, Rodriguez-Boulan E. Morphogenesis of the retinal pigment epithelium: toward understanding retinal degenerative diseases. *Ann N Y Acad Sci.* Oct 23 1998;857:1–12.
7. Schmidt SY, Peisch RD. Melanin concentration in normal human retinal pigment epithelium. Regional variation and age-related reduction. *Invest Ophthalmol Vis Sci.* 1986; 27(7):1063–1067.
8. Parver LM, Auker C, Carpenter DO. Choroidal blood flow as a heat dissipating mechanism in the macula. *Am J Ophthalmol.* 1980;89(5):641–646.
9. Alm A, Bill A. Blood flow and oxygen extraction in the cat uvea at normal and high intraocular pressures. *Acta Physiol Scand.* 1970;80(1):19–28.
10. Alm A, Bill A. The oxygen supply to the retina. I. Effects of changes in intraocular and arterial blood pressures, and in arterial P O2 and P CO2 on the oxygen tension in the vitreous body of the cat. *Acta Physiol Scand.* 1972;84(2):261–274.
11. Boulton M. In: Marmor MF, Wolfensberger TJ, eds. *The role of melanin in the RPE., in The retinal pigment epithelium.* Oxford: Oxford University Press; 1998.68-65.
12. Boulton M, Dayhaw-Barker P. The role of the retinal pigment epithelium: topographical variation and ageing changes. *Eye.* 2001;15:384–389.
13. Boulton M, Moriarty P, Jarvis-Evans J, Marcyniuk B. Regional variation and age-related changes of lysosomal enzymes in the human retinal pigment epithelium. *Br J Ophthalmol.* Feb 1994;78(2):125–129.
14. Winkler BS, Boulton ME, Gottsch JD, Sternberg P. Oxidative damage and age-related macular degeneration. *Molecular vision.* Nov 3 1999;5:32.
15. Miller SS, Steinberg RH. Active transport of ions across frog retinal pigment epithelium. *Exp Eye Res.* 1977;25(3):235–248.
16. Miller SS, Steinberg RH. Passive ionic properties of frog retinal pigment epithelium. *J Membr Biol.* 1977;36(4):337–372.
17. Fine BS. Limiting membranes of the sensory retina and pigment epithelium. An electron microscopic study. *Arch Ophthalmol.* 1961;66:847–860.
18. Adler AJ, Southwick RE. Distribution of glucose and lactate in the interphotoreceptor matrix. *Ophthalmic Res.* 1992;24(4):243–252.
19. Ban Y, Rizzolo LJ. Regulation of glucose transporters during development of the retinal pigment epithelium. *Brain Res Dev Brain Res.* 2000;121(1):89–95.
20. Kim DI, Lim SK, Park MJ, Han HJ, Kim GY, Park SH. The involvement of phosphatidylinositol 3-kinase /Akt signaling in high glucose-induced downregulation

of GLUT-1 expression in ARPE cells. *Life Sci.* Jan 23 2007;80(7):626–632. https://doi.org/10.1016/j.lfs.2006.10.026.
21. Bibb C, Young RW. Renewal of fatty acids in the membranes of visual cell outer segments. *J Cell Biol.* 1974;61(2):327–343.
22. Anderson RE, O'Brien PJ, Wiegand RD, Koutz CA, Stinson AM. Conservation of docosahexaenoic acid in the retina. *Adv Exp Med Biol.* 1992;318:285–294.
23. Bazan NG, Gordon WC, Rodriguez de Turco EB. Docosahexaenoic acid uptake and metabolism in photoreceptors: retinal conservation by an efficient retinal pigment epithelial cell-mediated recycling process. *Neurobiology of Essential Fatty Acids.* 1992:295–306.
24. Bazan NG, Rodriguez de Turco EB, Gordon WC. Pathways for the uptake and conservation of docosahexaenoic acid in photoreceptors and synapses: biochemical and autoradiographic studies. *Can J Physiol Pharmacol.* 1993;71(9):690–698.
25. SanGiovanni JP, Chew EY. The role of omega-3 long-chain polyunsaturated fatty acids in health and disease of the retina. *Prog Retin Eye Res.* 2005;24(1):87–138.
26. Wong BH, Chan JP, Cazenave-Gassiot A, et al. Mfsd2a Is a Transporter for the Essential omega-3 Fatty Acid Docosahexaenoic Acid (DHA) in Eye and Is Important for Photoreceptor Cell Development. *J Biol Chem.* May 13 2016;291(20):10501–10514. https://doi.org/10.1074/jbc.M116.721340.
27. Dornonville de la Cour M. Ion transport in the retinal pigment epithelium. A study with double barrelled ion-selective microelectrodes. *Acta Ophthalmol Suppl.* 1993;209:1–32.
28. Philp NJ, Wang D, Yoon H, Hjelmeland LM. Polarized expression of monocarboxylate transporters in human retinal pigment epithelium and ARPE-19 cells. *Invest Ophthalmol Vis Sci.* Apr 2003;44(4):1716–1721. https://doi.org/10.1167/iovs.02-0287.
29. Hughes BA, Gallemore RP, Miller SS. In: Marmor MF, Wolfensberger TJ, eds. *Transport mechanisms in the retinal pigment epithelium, in The retinal pigment epithelium.* New York, Oxford: Oxford University Press; 1998:103–134.
30. La Cour M. Cl- transport in frog retinal pigment epithelium. *Exp Eye Res.* 1992;54(6):921–931.
31. Adorante JS, Miller SS. Potassium-dependent volume regulation in retinal pigment epithelium is mediated by Na,K,Cl cotransport. *J Gen Physiol.* 1990;96(6):1153–1176.
32. Wiederholt M, Zadunaisky JA. Decrease of intracellular chloride activity by furosemide in frog retinal pigment epithelium. *Curr Eye Res.* 1984;3(4):673–675.
33. Bosl MR, et al. Male germ cells and photoreceptors, both dependent on close cell-cell interactions, degenerate upon ClC-2 Cl(-) channel disruption. *Embo J.* 2001;20(6):1289–1299.
34. Rymer J, Miller SS, Edelman JL. Epinephrine-induced increases in [Ca2+](in) and KCl-coupled fluid absorption in bovine RPE. *Invest Ophthalmol Vis Sci.* 2001;42(8):1921–1929.
35. Hughes BA, Segawa Y. cAMP-activated chloride currents in amphibian retinal pigment epithelial cells. *J Physiol.* 1993;466:749–766.
36. Edelman JL, Lin H, Miller SS. Potassium-induced chloride secretion across the frog retinal pigment epithelium. *Am J Physiol.* 1994;266(4 Pt 1):C957–C966.
37. la Cour M. Kinetic properties and Na+ dependence of rheogenic Na(+)-HCO3- co-transport in frog retinal pigment epithelium. *J Physiol.* 1991;439:59–72.
38. la Cour M, Lin H, Kenyon E, Miller SS. Lactate transport in freshly isolated human fetal retinal pigment epithelium. *Invest Ophthalmol Vis Sci.* Feb 1994;35(2):434–442.
39. Bergersen L, et al. Cellular and subcellular expression of monocarboxylate transporters in the pigment epithelium and retina of the rat. *Neuroscience.* 1999;90(1):319–331.
40. Keller SK, et al. Regulation of intracellular pH in cultured bovine retinal pigment epithelial cells. *Pflugers Arch.* 1988;411(1):47–52.
41. Keller SK, Jentsch TJ, Koch M, Wiederholt M. Interactions of pH and K+ conductance in cultured bovine retinal pigment epithelial cells. *Am J Physiol.* Jan 1986;250(1 Pt 1):C124–C137.
42. Marmor MF, Maack T. Enhancement of retinal adhesion and subretinal fluid resorption by acetazolamide. *Invest Ophthalmol Vis Sci.* 1982;23(1):121–124.
43. Machemer R. Proliferative vitreoretinopathy (PVR): a personal account of its pathogenesis and treatment. Proctor lecture. *Invest Ophthalmol Vis Sci.* 1988;29(12):1771–1783.
44. Kaupp UB, Seifert R. Cyclic nucleotide-gated ion channels. *Physiol Rev.* 2002;82(3):769–824.
45. Bialek S, Miller SS. K+ and Cl- transport mechanisms in bovine pigment epithelium that could modulate subretinal space volume and composition. *J Physiol.* 1994;475(3):401–417.
46. Edelman JL, Lin H, Miller SS. Acidification stimulates chloride and fluid absorption across frog retinal pigment epithelium. *Am J Physiol.* 1994;266(4 Pt 1):C946–C956. doi:10.1038/ng0397-236.
47. Joseph DP, Miller SS. Apical and basal membrane ion transport mechanisms in bovine retinal pigment epithelium. *J Physiol.* 1991;435:439–463.
48. Ames 3rd A, Li YY, Heher EC, Kimble CR. Energy metabolism of rabbit retina as related to function: high cost of Na+ transport. *J Neurosci.* Mar 1992;12(3):840–853.
49. Hodson S, Armstrong I, Wigham C. Regulation of the retinal interphotoreceptor matrix Na by the retinal pigment epithelium during the light response. *Experientia.* 1994;50(5):438–441.
50. Griff ER, Shirao Y, Steinberg RH. Ba2+ unmasks K+ modulation of the Na+-K+ pump in the frog retinal pigment epithelium. *J Gen Physiol.* 1985;86(6):853–876.
51. Wald G. Molecular basis of visual excitation. *Science.* 1968;162(3850):230–239.
52. McBee JK, Palczewski K, Baehr W, Pepperberg DR. Confronting complexity: the interlink of phototransduction and retinoid metabolism in the vertebrate retina. *Prog Retin Eye Res.* Jul 2001;20(4):469–529.
53. Thompson DA, Gal A. Genetic defects in vitamin A metabolism of the retinal pigment epithelium. *Dev Ophthalmol.* 2003;37:141–154.
54. Bachr W, Wu SM, Bird AC, Palczewski K. The retinoid cycle and retina disease. *Vis Res.* 2003;43:2957–2958.
55. Besch D, Jägle H, Scholl HPN, Seeliger MW, Zrenner E. Inherited multifocal RPE-diseases: mechanisms for local dysfunction in global retinoid cycle defects. *Vis Res.* 2003;43:3095–3108.
56. Lamb TD, Pugh Jr. EN. Dark adaptation and the retinoid cycle of vision. *Prog Retin Eye Res.* 2004;23(3):307–380.
57. Quazi F, Lenevich S, Molday RS. ABCA4 is an N-retinylidene-phosphatidylethanolamine and phosphatidylethanolamine importer. *Nat Commun.* 2012;3:925.
58. Allikmets R, Singh N, Sun H, et al. A photoreceptor cell-specific ATP-binding transporter gene (ABCR) is mutated in recessive Stargardt macular dystrophy. *Nat Genet.* Mar 1997;15(3):236–246. https://doi.org/10.1038/ng0397-236.
59. Rattner A, Smallwood PM, Nathans J. Identification and characterization of all-trans-retinol dehydrogenase from photoreceptor outer segments, the visual cycle enzyme that reduces all-trans-retinal to all-trans-retinol. *J Biol Chem.* 2000;275(15):11034–11043.
60. Gonzalez-Fernandez F. Evolution of the visual cycle: the role of retinoid-binding proteins. *J Endocrinol.* 2002;175(1):75–88.
61. Okajima TI, Pepperberg DR, Ripps H, Wiggert B, Chader GJ. Interphotoreceptor retinoid-binding protein: role in delivery of retinol to the pigment epithelium. *Exp Eye Res.* Oct 1989;49(4):629–644.
62. Imanishi Y, Gerke V, Palczewski K. Retinosomes: new insights into intracellular managing of hydrophobic substances in lipid bodies. *J Cell Biol.* 2004;166(4):447–453.
63. Jin M, Li S, Moghrabi WN, Sun H, Travis GH. Rpe65 is the retinoid isomerase in bovine retinal pigment epithelium. *Cell.* Aug 12 2005;122(3):449–459. doi:S0092-8674(05)00696-3 [pii] 10.1016/j.cell.2005.06.042.
64. Wang JS, Kefalov VJ. The cone-specific visual cycle. *Prog Retin Eye Res.* 2011;30(2):115–128.
65. Lamb TD, Pugh Jr. EN. Phototransduction, dark adaptation, and rhodopsin regeneration the proctor lecture. *Invest Ophthalmol Vis Sci.* 2006;47(12):5137–5152.
66. Xue L, Gollapalli DR, Maiti P, Jahng WJ, Rando RR. A palmitoylation switch mechanism in the regulation of the visual cycle. *Cell.* Jun 11 2004;117(6):761–771.
67. Kiser PD. Retinal pigment epithelium 65 kDa protein (RPE65): An update. *Prog Retin Eye Res.* 2021:101013.
68. Goodwin P. Hereditary retinal disease. *Curr Opin Ophthalmol.* 2008;19(3):255–262.
69. Thompson DA, Gal A. Vitamin A metabolism in the retinal pigment epithelium: genes, mutations, and diseases. *Prog Retin Eye Res.* 2003;22(5):683–703.
70. Travis GH, Golczak M, Moise AR, Palczewski K. Diseases caused by defects in the visual cycle: retinoids as potential therapeutic agents. *Annu Rev Pharmacol Toxicol.* 2007;47:469–512. https://doi.org/10.1146/annurev.pharmtox.47.120505.105225.
71. Acland GM, et al. Gene therapy restores vision in a canine model of childhood blindness. *Nat Genet.* 2001;28(1):92–95.
72. Cideciyan AV. Leber congenital amaurosis due to RPE65 mutations and its treatment with gene therapy. *Prog Retin Eye Res.* 2010;29(5):398–427.
73. Patel U, Boucher M, de Leseleuc L, Visintini S. Voretigene Neparvovec: An Emerging Gene Therapy for the Treatment of Inherited Blindness. *CADTH Issues in Emerging Health Technologies.* 2016:1–11.
74. Bainbridge JW, et al. Effect of gene therapy on visual function in Leber's congenital amaurosis. *N Engl J Med.* 2008;358(21):2231–2239.
75. Young RW. The renewal of photoreceptor cell outer segments. *J Cell Biol.* 1967;33(1):61–72.
76. Young RW, Bok D. Participation of the retinal pigment epithelium in the rod outer segment renewal process. *J Cell Biol.* 1969;42(2):392–403.
77. Spencer WJ, Lewis TR, Pearring JN, Arshavsky VY. Photoreceptor Discs: Built Like Ectosomes. *Trends Cell Biol.* Nov 2020;30(11):904–915. https://doi.org/10.1016/j.tcb.2020.08.005.
78. Bok D, Hall MO. The role of the pigment epithelium in the etiology of inherited retinal dystrophy in the rat. *J Cell Biol.* 1971;49(3):664–682.
79. Custer NV, Bok D. Pigment epithelium-photoreceptor interactions in the normal and dystrophic rat retina. *Exp Eye Res.* 1975;21(2):153–166.
80. LaVail MM. Rod outer segment disk shedding in rat retina: relationship to cyclic lighting. *Science.* 1976;194(4269):1071–1074.
81. Kevany BM, Palczewski K. Phagocytosis of retinal rod and cone photoreceptors. *Physiology (Bethesda).* 2010;25(1):8–15.
82. Besharse JC, Defoe DM. In: Marmor MF, Wolfensberger TJ, eds. *Role of the retinal pigment epithelium in photoreceptor membrane turnover., in The retinal pigment epithelium.* Oxford: Oxford University Press; 1998:152–172.
83. Besharse JC, Hollyfield JG. Turnover of mouse photoreceptor outer segments in constant light and darkness. *Invest Ophthalmol Vis Sci.* 1979;18(10):1019–1024.
84. Nandrot EF, Kim Y, Brodie SE, Huang X, Sheppard D, Finnemann SC. Loss of Synchronized Retinal Phagocytosis and Age-related Blindness in Mice Lacking {alpha}v{beta}5 Integrin. *J Exp Med.* Dec 20 2004;200(12):1539–1545.
85. Finnemann SC. Focal adhesion kinase signaling promotes phagocytosis of integrin-bound photoreceptors. *Embo J.* 2003;22(16):4143–4154.
86. D'Cruz PM, Yasumura D, Weir J, et al. Mutation of the receptor tyrosine kinase gene Mertk in the retinal dystrophic RCS rat. *Hum Mol Genet.* Mar 1 2000;9(4):645–651.
87. Feng W, et al. Mertk triggers uptake of photoreceptor outer segments during phagocytosis by cultured retinal pigment epithelial cells. *J Biol Chem.* 2002;277(19):17016–17022.
88. Gal A, et al. Mutations in MERTK, the human orthologue of the RCS rat retinal dystrophy gene, cause retinitis pigmentosa. *Nat Genet.* 2000;26(3):270–271.
89. Burstyn-Cohen T, Lew ED, Traves PG, Burrola PG, Hash JC, Lemke G. Genetic dissection of TAM receptor-ligand interaction in retinal pigment epithelial cell phagocytosis. *Neuron.* Dec 20 2012;76(6):1123–1132. https://doi.org/10.1016/j.neuron.2012.10.015.
90. Finnemann SC, Silverstein RL. Differential roles of CD36 and alphavbeta5 integrin in photoreceptor phagocytosis by the retinal pigment epithelium. *J Exp Med.* 2001;194(9):1289–1298.
91. Wong WL, Su X, Li X, et al. Global prevalence of age-related macular degeneration and disease burden projection for 2020 and 2040: a systematic review and meta-analysis. *Lancet Glob Health..* Feb 2014;2(2):e106–e116. https://doi.org/10.1016/S2214-109X(13)70145-1.
92. Lim LS, et al. Age-related macular degeneration. *Lancet.* 2012;379(9827):1728–1738.
93. Klein R, et al. The epidemiology of age-related macular degeneration. *Am J Ophthalmol.* 2004;137(3):486–495.
94. Fleckenstein M, et al. The Progression of Geographic Atrophy Secondary to Age-Related Macular Degeneration. *Ophthalmology.* 2018;125(3):369–390.
95. Holz FG, et al. Geographic atrophy: clinical features and potential therapeutic approaches. *Ophthalmology.* 2014;121(5):1079–1091.

96. Wang J, et al. ATAC-Seq analysis reveals a widespread decrease of chromatin accessibility in age-related macular degeneration. *Nat Commun.* 2018;9(1):1364.

97. Fritsche, L.G., et al., *Seven new loci associated with age-related macular degeneration.* Nat Genet, 2013. 45(4): p. 433-9, 439e1-2.

98. Fritsche LG, et al. A large genome-wide association study of age-related macular degeneration highlights contributions of rare and common variants. *Nat Genet.* 2016;48(2):134–143.

99. Pappas CM, et al. Protective chromosome 1q32 haplotypes mitigate risk for age-related macular degeneration associated with the CFH-CFHR5 and ARMS2/HTRA1 loci. *Hum Genomics.* 2021;15(1):60.

100. Anderson DH, et al. A role for local inflammation in the formation of drusen in the aging eye. *Am J Ophthalmol.* 2002;134(3):411–431.

101. Anderson DH, Radeke MJ, Gallo NB, et al. The pivotal role of the complement system in aging and age-related macular degeneration: hypothesis re-visited. *Progress in retinal and eye research.* Mar 2010;29(2):95–112.

102. Wimmers S, Karl MO, Strauss O. Ion channels in the RPE. *Prog Retin Eye Res.* 2007;26(3):263–301.

103. Rosenthal R, Strauss O. Ca2+-channels in the RPE. *Adv Exp Med Biol.* 2002;514:225–235.

104. Bazan NG. Neurotrophins induce neuroprotective signaling in the retinal pigment epithelial cell by activating the synthesis of the anti-inflammatory and anti-apoptotic neuroprotectin D1. *Adv Exp Med Biol.* 2008;613:39–44.

105. Walsh N, Valter K, Stone J. Cellular and subcellular patterns of expression of bFGF and CNTF in the normal and light stressed adult rat retina. *Exp Eye Res.* 2001;72(5):495–501.

106. Ruiz A, Brett P, Bok D. TIMP-3 is expressed in the human retinal pigment epithelium. *Biochem Biophys Res Commun.* 1996;226(2):467–474.

107. Anand-Apte B, et al. Inhibition of angiogenesis by tissue inhibitor of metalloproteinase-3. *Invest Ophthalmol Vis Sci.* 1997;38(5):817–823.

108. Schlingemann RO. Role of growth factors and the wound healing response in age-related macular degeneration. *Graefes Arch Clin Exp Ophthalmol.* 2004;242(1):91–101.

109. Holtkamp GM, Kijlstra A, Peek R, de Vos AF. Retinal pigment epithelium-immune system interactions: cytokine production and cytokine-induced changes. *Prog Retin Eye Res.* Jan 2001;20(1):29–48. https://doi:S1350946200000173 [pii].

110. Besharse JC, Spratt G. Excitatory amino acids and rod photoreceptor disc shedding: analysis using specific agonists. *Exp Eye Res.* 1988;47(4):609–620.

111. Mitchell CH. Release of ATP by a human retinal pigment epithelial cell line: potential for autocrine stimulation through subretinal space. *J Physiol.* 2001;534(Pt 1):193–202.

112. Fields MA, Del Priore LV, Adelman RA, Rizzolo LJ. Interactions of the choroid, Bruch's membrane, retinal pigment epithelium, and neurosensory retina collaborate to form the outer blood-retinal-barrier. *Prog Retin Eye Res.* May 2020;76:100803. https://doi.org/10.1016/j.preteyeres.2019.100803.

113. Streilein JW. Ocular immune privilege: therapeutic opportunities from an experiment of nature. *Nat Rev Immunol.* 2003;3(11):879–889.

114. Shechter R, London A, Schwartz M. Orchestrated leukocyte recruitment to immune-privileged sites: absolute barriers versus educational gates. *Nat Rev Immunol.* 2013;13(3):206–218.

115. Zamiri P, Sugita S, Streilein JW. Immunosuppressive properties of the pigmented epithelial cells and the subretinal space. *Chem Immunol Allergy.* 2007;92:86–93.

116. Binder S, Stanzel BV, Krebs I, Glittenberg C. Transplantation of the RPE in AMD. *Progress in retinal and eye research.* Sep 2007;26(5):516–554. http://doi.org/10.1016/j.preteyeres.2007.02.002.

117. Allocca M, Tessitore A, Cotugno G, Auricchio A. AAV-mediated gene transfer for retinal diseases. *Expert Opin Biol Ther.* Dec 2006;6(12):1279–1294. http://doi.org/10.1517/14712598.6.12.1279.

Functions of the Orbit and Eyelids

Gregory J. Griepentrog and Mark J. Lucarelli

Introduction

The cranium protects the brain and provides scaffolding for facial structures. During primate evolution, the orbits were enlarged and reoriented toward the front of the face.[1] This, along with the gradual flattening of the face, allowed for improved binocular vision owing to overlapping visual fields. Along with morphologic skull changes, facial mimetic musculature evolved in primates as a means of close-proximity nonvocal communication.[2] It is in this context that the function of the eyelids to protect, lubricate, and cleanse the ocular surface is most fully appreciated. This chapter examines anatomy of the eyelids, orbits, and related facial structures.

ORBITAL ANATOMY AND FUNCTION

Orbit osteology

Derived from cranial neural crest cells, the bony orbit consists of seven individual bones combining into four walls that surround the globe, extraocular muscles, nerves, fat, and blood vessels. The orbital bones include the sphenoid (greater and lesser wings), frontal, ethmoid, maxillary, zygomatic, palatine, and lacrimal bones. Posteriorly approaching the apex, this four-sided pyramid becomes three-sided with the gradual merger of the medial wall and orbital floor after the floor is cut off by the inferior orbital fissure. The adult orbit has a volume of 25 to 30 mL, with the globe filling approximately 7 mL or 25% of the space.[3] The orbit depth as measured from the center of the orbital margin to the apex is approximately 45 mm. The widest diameter of the orbit occurs 1 cm behind the orbital rim. The lateral walls of the orbit are oriented 90 degrees from one another and run approximately 40 to 45 mm, while the medial walls are parallel to one another (Fig. 14.1). Owing to this bony orientation, the eyes tend to diverge, and thus are tonically held in adduction by the medial rectus muscles to achieve ocular alignment.

The orbital rim provides a hard tissue shield to surround and protect the eye. It is a thick discontinuous spiral that begins medially at the anterior lacrimal (maxillary bone) crest and coils to end at the posterior lacrimal (lacrimal bone) crest (Fig. 14.2). The lacrimal fossa, which contains the lacrimal excretory sac, lies between these two crests. Formed by the zygomatic bone and the zygomatic process of the frontal bone, the lateral orbital rim is the strongest and thickest portion of the rim. Although the posteriorly directed concavity of the lateral orbital rim allows for a wide visual field, it also makes the eye prone to injury from objects approaching from a lateral direction. The superior orbital rim is formed by the frontal bone. Medially,

the superior rim contains the supraorbital notch through which the supraorbital nerve and artery pass. In some individuals, a supraorbital foramen replaces the notch.[4] The infraorbital nerve and artery exit through the infraorbital foramen approximately 4 to 6 mm below the inferior orbital rim medially.

The orbital roof is comprised of the orbital plate of the frontal bone along with a minor contribution from the lesser wing of the sphenoid, posteriorly. The frontal bone is the strongest component of the craniofacial skeleton, withstanding between 800 and 2200 pounds of force (363 and 998 kilograms) before fracturing.[5] This is equivalent to the force achieved in a frontal collision at 30 mph (48 kilometers per hour) for an unrestrained adult passenger. Orbital roof "blow-in" fractures may be associated with a number of ocular and neurologic injuries including proptosis, ptosis, optic nerve contusion, and orbital hematoma, as well as contusive and hemorrhagic injuries to the ipsilateral frontal and parietal lobes.[6] Important bony landmarks of the orbital roof include the lacrimal gland fossa temporally and the trochlear fossa; a small depression 3 to 5 mm behind the orbital rim anteromedially. Here resides the fibrocartilaginous trochlea through which the superior oblique tendon passes.

The frontal sinus begins to develop between 1 and 2 years of age through invagination of the frontal bone by frontoethmoidal air cells. The filling of air or pneumatization of the sinus begins at about 5 to 8 years old and continues into adulthood.[7] Therefore, there is a relative absence of frontal sinusitis in very young children. Yet, orbital complications from frontal sinusitis such as orbital cellulitis and abscess may occur between the ages of 5 and 10 years.[8] It has been hypothesized that direct extension through the relatively thin orbital roof in children or congenital bony dehiscences (gaps) posterior to the trochlear and supraorbital notch may account for these findings.[9]

The lateral wall is comprised of the zygomatic bone anteriorly and the greater wing of the sphenoid posteriorly. The vertically oriented zygomaticosphenoidal suture represents the thinnest portion of the lateral wall and is a convenient breaking point during lateral orbitotomy. The posterior boundaries of the wall are marked by superior and inferior orbital fissures. The frontosphenoidal suture forms the boundary between the lateral wall and orbital roof. About one-third of individuals have a meningeal foramen just superior to this suture that transmits the recurrent meningeal artery (a branch of the external carotid system) to form an anastomosis with the lacrimal artery (a branch of the internal carotid system). This collateral system has potential importance if the primary internal carotid vascular supply becomes compromised. An important bony prominence of the lateral wall is Whitnall's lateral tubercle, a small, rounded protuberance of the zygomatic bone

3 to 4 mm inside of the lateral orbital wall and approximately 11 mm below the frontozygomatic suture.[10,11]

Fractures to the lateral wall may result from blunt trauma to the zygomatic bone and lateral orbital rim. Owing to its multiple bony articulations, fractures of the zygoma may disrupt the wider anatomy and are often referred to as zygomaticomaxillary complex fractures or ZMC fractures (Fig. 14.3). Clinical signs include lateral canthal dystopia (inferior displacement of the lateral canthal angle), cheek depression, and trismus (difficulty opening the mouth owing to spasm of the masticatory muscles or impingement of the coronoid process of the mandible). Hypoesthesia may be noted at the lateral midface from disrupted branches of the zygomaticotemporal and zygomaticofacial neurovascular bundles (V1 branches traveling through the zygomatic bone), as well as in the distribution of the infraorbital nerve (V2 branch).

The orbital floor consists of the maxillary bone, the zygoma anterolaterally, and the palatine bone posteriorly. It is triangular and extends from the maxillary-ethmoid buttress (the relatively dense bone strut at the union of the orbital floor and medial wall) to the inferior orbital fissure. The shortest of the walls, it travels posteriorly from the rim 35 to 40 mm and ends before the orbital apex at the pterygopalatine fossa. The infraorbital neurovascular bundle passes in the infraorbital groove and infraorbital canal of the orbital floor as it travels toward the infraorbital foramen. The floor remains strong laterally but thins posteromedially with expansion of the maxillary sinus. This thinned maxillary bone is where the floor usually fractures during trauma and is also a convenient site to initiate an inferior wall decompression. The infraorbital nerve is often contused during an orbital floor fracture but is rarely severed, thus, initial hypoesthesia in the V2 distribution will commonly resolve over several months' time.

The medial wall consists of the maxillary, lacrimal, and ethmoid bones, as well as the lesser wing of the sphenoid bone. The two medial walls are parallel to one another and extend 45 to 50 mm from the anterior lacrimal crest to the orbital apex. The lamina papyracea of the ethmoid bone is an extremely thin portion of bone that has a honeycombed structure. Giving support to the medial wall, the multiple bullae that form this structure develop secondarily to pneumatization of the ethmoid bone. This helps to explain why the medial wall fractures less often than the thicker orbital floor. Landmarks important to the orbital surgeon include the anterior and posterior ethmoidal foramina that reside at the frontoethmoidal suture and convey respective branches of the ophthalmic artery and nasociliary nerve. The anterior ethmoidal foramen is located approximately 24 mm posterior to the anterior lacrimal crest and the posterior ethmoidal foramen 36 mm posterior to the rim. The orbital foramen is located approximately 6 mm behind the posterior ethmoidal foramen. The frontoethmoidal suture may also be used surgically to approximate the level of the floor of the anterior cranial fossa.

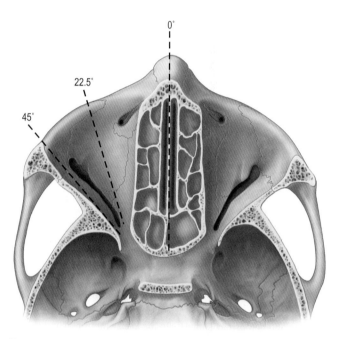

Fig. 14.1 Horizontal section through orbits. Medial walls are nearly parallel, and lateral walls diverge 45 degrees from midline. ((Copyright: Virginia Cantarella). Salmon, JF. Kanski's Clinical Ophthalmology: A Systematic Approach, 9th ed. 2019. Elsevier.)

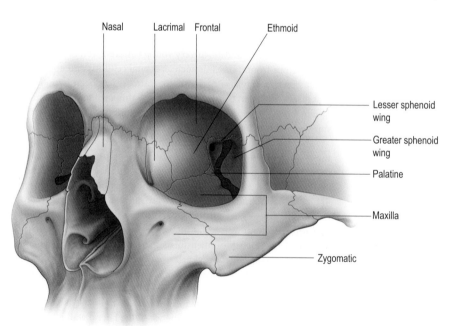

Fig. 14.2 Osteology of the orbital bones and orbital apex. (Copyright: Virginia Cantarella).

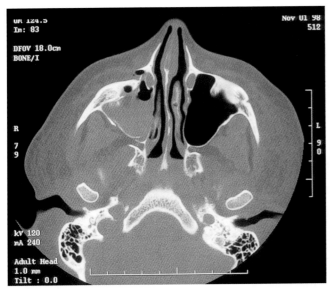

Fig. 14.3 Axial section of CT scan revealing a right zygomatic fracture as a part a zygomaticomaxillary complex (ZMC) fracture.

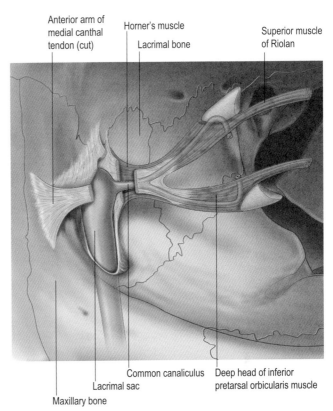

Fig. 14.4 Lacrimal drainage system, superficial anatomy. (Modified from Dutton JJ. *Atlas of Clinical and Surgical Orbital Anatomy*. Philadelphia: WB Saunders; 1994.)

Providing support for the inferomedial wall and helping to maintain globe position is the thickened region of bone known as the inferomedial strut. The strut is constructed using elements of multiple orbital and facial bones including the maxillary bone, ethmoid bone, and palatine bone posteriorly.[12,13] Preservation of the anterior portion of the inferomedial strut during orbital decompression has been shown to reduce the incidence of postoperative globe dystopia.[14]

As previously mentioned, the lacrimal sac fossa lies between the anterior (maxillary bone) crest and posterior (lacrimal bone) crest of the orbital rim (Fig. 14.4). The relative contribution of these two bones may vary. The lacrimal bone at the lacrimal sac fossa has a mean thickness of 106 μm, which allows easy penetration during dacryocystorhinostomy surgery (surgical procedure to restore the normal flow of tears into the nose from the lacrimal sac by bypassing the nasolacrimal duct).[15] The maxillary bone is considerably denser than the lacrimal bone and may require the surgeon to create a more posterior osteotomy during dacryocystorhinostomy. The nasolacrimal canal directs the nasolacrimal duct to the inferior meatus of the nose under the inferior turbinate.

The orbital apex

Many important neural and vascular structures pass through the orbit apex including cranial nerves (CNs) II through VI, the origins of all the extraocular muscles except the inferior oblique, and arterial and venous blood supplies (Fig. 14.5 & Box 14.1). Pathology in this crucial location of the orbit may lead to the orbital apex syndrome with characteristic hallmarks of visual loss from optic neuropathy and ophthalmoplegia.[16]

The optic foramen conveys the optic nerve and ophthalmic artery from the optic canal into the orbit. The canal is housed in the lesser wing of the sphenoid bone with a contribution from the inferomedial optic strut. It runs 8 to 10 mm in length and is 5 to 6 mm in diameter. The optic canal and foramen attain adult dimensions by 3 years and are symmetric in most persons. A canal/foramen that is larger in diameter by at least 1 mm than the contralateral side may be considered abnormal.

The superior orbital fissure is located just lateral to the optic canal. Approximately 20 to 22 mm in length, the fissure divides the lesser and greater wings of the sphenoid bone. The superior ophthalmic vein, as well as the lacrimal, trochlear, and frontal nerves, passes through the superolateral portion of the fissure outside the annulus of Zinn, a fibrous ring formed by the common origins of the rectus muscles. The annulus is further subdivided by the oculomotor foramen through which the superior and inferior divisions of the oculomotor nerve, the abducens nerve, the nasociliary nerve (a terminal sensory branch of the ophthalmic division of the trigeminal nerve), and sympathetic fibers all pass.[17,18] Also passing through the annulus of Zinn are the optic nerve and ophthalmic artery. As the extraocular rectus muscles proceed forward to their insertions on the globe, they form a conoid enclosure known as the intraconal space. This compartment is useful radiologically (Fig. 14.6). Intraconal pathology of the fat, vessels, and optic nerve sheath complex may be distinguished from extraconal pathology of the lacrimal gland, bony orbit, and remaining extraconal fat.[19,20]

The inferior orbital fissure divides the greater wing of the sphenoid laterally from the maxillary bone of the orbital floor inferomedially. The fissure measures approximately 20 mm in length. It communicates with the pterygopalatine fossa, which rests behind the maxillary sinus. Traveling through the fissure are the maxillary division of the trigeminal nerve, branches from the sphenopalatine ganglion, and the inferior ophthalmic vein. Branching away from the fissure and entering the infraorbital groove and canal are the infraorbital (V2) and the terminal branch of the internal maxillary artery.

Orbital soft tissues
Periorbital fascia

The periorbital fascia is a single interconnecting network emanating from the periosteal lining of the orbital walls, globe (Tenon's capsule), and extraocular muscles (Figs. 14.7 & 14.8).[21] There are also check

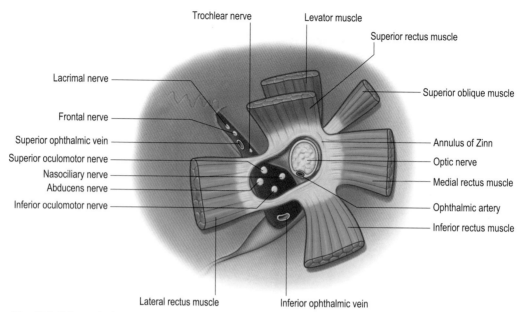

Fig. 14.5 Schematic drawing of the annulus of Zinn and orbital apex. (Modified from Lemke BN, Lucarelli MJ. Anatomy of the ocular adnexa, orbit, and related facial structures. In: Nesi FA, Lisman RD, Levine MR, eds. *Smith's Ophthalmic Plastic and Reconstructive Surgery.* 2nd ed. St. Louis: Mosby; 1998.)

BOX 14.1 Orbital Apex

- Passing through the optic foramen: optic nerve, ophthalmic artery, and sympathetic fibers.
- Passing through the superior orbital fissure: oculomotor nerve, trochlear nerve, abducens nerve, the ophthalmic division of the trigeminal nerve (frontalis, lacrimal, and nasociliary nerves), sympathetic fibers, and the superior ophthalmic vein.
- Passing through the annulus of Zinn: optic nerve, ophthalmic artery, oculomotor nerve, abducens nerve, nasociliary nerve, and sympathetic fibers.
- Passing through the inferior orbital fissure: maxillary division of the trigeminal nerve, branches from the sphenopalatine ganglion, and the inferior ophthalmic vein.

ligament extensions from the extraocular muscle fascia that attach to the bony orbit, as well as sheaths that extend between the rectus muscles. The periorbita is firmly attached at the suture lines, foramina, fissures, arcus marginalis, and the posterior lacrimal crest. Elsewhere, it is loosely attached to the bone, which creates a potential space for accumulation of blood, pus, or tumor growth. It is most firmly attached along the arcus marginalis. The orbital septum is a thin, multilayered extension of the periorbita and is the anterior soft tissue boundary of the orbit. It functions as a physical barrier to pathogens and contributes to the normal posterior position of the orbital fat pads. In the upper eyelid, the fibrous lamellae of the orbital septum gradually blends with those of the levator aponeurosis on average 3.4 mm above the superior tarsal border (with a range of 2–5 mm).[22] In the lower eyelid, the septum inserts onto the inferior border of the tarsus after joining with the inferior retractors 4 to 5 mm below the tarsus.[23] Laterally the septum fuses with the lateral canthal tendon and attaches 2 to 3 mm posterior to the rim at the lateral orbital tubercle (Whitnall's tubercle). Medially the septum splits and inserts onto the anterior and posterior lacrimal crest. Finally, it is anchored anteriorly to the orbicularis muscle by multiple fibrous attachments.[24]

Tenon's capsule, or fascia bulbi, is a fibroelastic membrane that extends anteriorly from the dural sheath to encircle the globe and

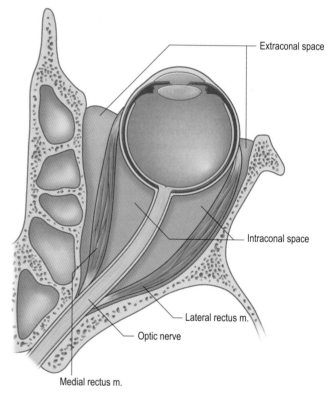

Fig. 14.6 Schematic drawing of the compartments of the orbital space. (Modified from Muller-Forell WS. *Imaging of Orbital and Visual Pathway Pathology.* Springer-Verlag; 2002. Reproduced by kind permission of Springer Science + Business Media.)

fuse with the conjunctiva just behind the limbus.[25] Posteriorly it separates orbital fat from the globe and muscles. Openings within the fascia allow passage of the extraocular muscles, which are in turn surrounded by their own muscular fascia. Anteriorly the muscular fascia thickens and connects with the orbital wall to form the

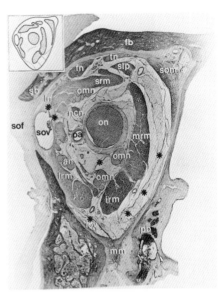

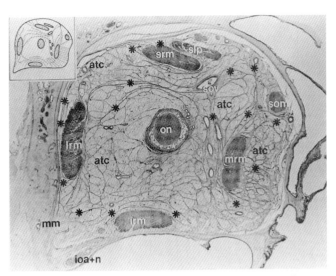

Fig. 14.7 A view 18.4 mm from back of globe. Vertical diameter 1.5 cm; transversal diameter 1.1 cm; magnification approximately 11×. The following artifacts are present in this section: *inside muscle cone* several holes in adipose tissue are seen; *outside the cone* adipose tissue is torn off from frontal and trochlear nerves, superior levator palpebrae/superior rectus complex, medial and inferior recti muscles, and medial orbital wall. *fb,* frontal bone; *sb,* sphenoid bone; *sof,* superior orbital fissure; *mm,* Müller's muscle; *pb,* palatine bone; *on,* optic nerve; *fn,* frontal nerve; *ln,* lacrimal nerve; *ncn;* nasociliary nerve; *tn,* trochlear nerve; *an,* abducens nerve; *omn,* oculomotor nerve; *oa,* ophthalmic artery; *sov,* superior ophthalmic vein; *iov,* inferior ophthalmic vein; *slp,* superior levator palpebrae muscle; *srm,* superior rectus muscle; *lrm,* lateral rectus muscle; *irm,* inferior rectus muscle; *mrm,* medial rectus muscle; *som,* superior oblique muscle; *asterisks (*),* connective tissue septa. (Reproduced from Koorneef L. *Spatial Aspect of Orbital Musculo-Fibrous Tissue in Man: A New Anatomical and Histological Approach.* Amsterdam: Swets en Zeitlinger B.V; 1976.)

check ligament of the extraocular muscles, preventing overaction of the muscle from which they extend.[26] The strongest of these is the lateral check ligament that inserts on the lateral orbital tubercle, while the medial rectus check ligament inserts behind the posterior lacrimal crest.[27]

Orbital fat
Orbital fat provides cushioned support for the globe and other intraocular structures. Eyelid fat pads are the anterior projections of the orbital fat. Changes in orbital fat, along with extraocular muscle expansion, play a significant role in the development of thyroid eye disease (TED), through abnormal activation of orbital fibroblasts with abnormal production of extracellular matrix proteins.[28] In addition, overexpression of insulin-like growth factor-1 receptor (IGF-1R) and interaction with thyrotropin receptor (TSH-R) lead to an increased production of proinflammatory cytokines, interleukin-2 (IL2), tumor necrosis factor-α (TNFα), and IL8. Orbital fat and extraocular muscle volume expansion may result in soft tissue swelling, proptosis, lid retraction (with characteristic temporal flare), strabismus (usually due to muscle fibrosis), and compressive optic neuropathy.[29,30] Treatments such as teprotumumab, a human monoclonal immunoglobulin, have been directed toward binding and blocking signal transduction of the IGF-1R (insulin-like growth factor-1 receptor) and IGF-1R/TSH-R complex on orbital fibroblasts, resulting in reduced proptosis, diplopia, and inflammation in patients with active TED.[28]

Fig. 14.8 An orbital view 1.4 mm posterior to the globe. Vertical diameter, 2.4 cm; transversal diameter, 2.7 cm; magnification approximately 3.5×. Note artifacts in superior, medial, and inferolateral areas. *on,* optic nerve; *sov,* superior ophthalmic vein; *slp,* superior levator palpebrae muscle; *srm,* superior rectus muscle; *lrm,* lateral rectus muscle; *irm,* inferior rectus muscle; *mrm,* medial rectus muscle; *som,* superior oblique muscle; *asterisks (*),* connective tissue septa; *atc,* adipose tissue compartment; *ioa + n,* infraorbital artery and nerve; *mm,* Müller's muscle. (Reproduced from Koorneef L. *Spatial Aspect of Orbital Musculo-Fibrous Tissue in Man: A New Anatomical and Histological Approach.* Amsterdam: Swets en Zeitlinger B.V; 1976.)

Orbital nerves
Entering the orbit are the optic (CN II), oculomotor (CN III), trochlear (CN IV), abducens (CN VI), the first and second divisions of the trigeminal (CN V), parasympathetic, and sympathetic nerves. The trigeminal nerve will be discussed in the eyelid portion of this chapter whereas the extraocular muscles are discussed in Chapter 7.

Composed of approximately 1.2 million nerve fibers, the optic nerve is an extension of the central nervous system. It has supportive neuroglial cells and is surrounded by the three layers of the meninges: the dura mater, the arachnoid layer, and the pia mater. Cerebrospinal fluid flows freely within the space between the arachnoid and pia. The nerve arises from the ganglion cell layer of the retina. These axons converge at the optic nerve head, which is approximately 1.5 mm in diameter. As the nerve exits the globe at the lamina cribrosa and enters the orbit, its diameter increases to 3.5 mm owing to the addition of the myelin sheath. The intraorbital portion of the nerve runs approximately 25 mm, although the distance from the globe to the optic foramen is 18 mm. This extra slack allows freedom of movement of the globe and a certain degree of proptosis. When excessively stretched, the nerve may exert tension on the globe—seen radiologically as "globe tenting"—which may result in vision loss owing to compromise of the nerves' vascular supply.[31] The intracanalicular portion of the nerve is tethered within the bone, making it susceptible to damage from blunt trauma.[32,33] The intracranial portion of the optic nerve runs approximately 15 mm just medial to the internal carotid artery, ending at the optic chiasm.

Motor innervation of the orbit involves the oculomotor (CN III), trochlear (CN IV), and abducens nerves (CN VI) (Fig. 14.9). The oculomotor nerve innervates the superior, inferior, and medial recti; the inferior oblique; and the levator palpebrae superioris muscles. Additionally, parasympathetic fibers travel within the inferior division of the nerve. The nerve exits the brainstem medially and travels through the superolateral portion of the cavernous sinus while

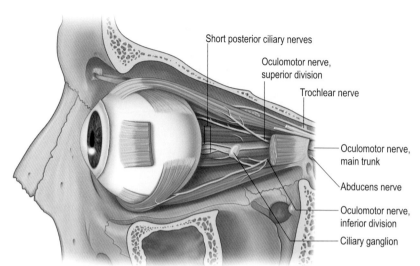

Fig. 14.9 Lateral orbital view and major orbital motor nerves. (Modified from Dutton JJ. *Atlas of Clinical and Surgical Orbital Anatomy*. Philadelphia: WB Saunders; 1994.)

dividing into a superior and inferior division. Both branches enter the orbit through the oculomotor foramen within the annulus of Zinn. The superior branch enters the underside of the superior rectus, on its way to innervate the overlying levator palpebrae superioris muscle. The inferior branch of the oculomotor nerve travels beneath the optic nerve and supplies innervation to the medial and inferior rectus, as well as the inferior oblique.

Studies in both monkeys and humans have revealed that parasympathetic fibers, issued from cells of the pterygopalatine ganglion, pass into the orbit.[34] Nilsson et al.[35] showed that parasympathetic fibers responsible for uveal vasodilation travel to the eye from the facial nerve via the pterygopalatine ganglion. As previously mentioned, a small bundle of parasympathetic fibers destined for the ciliary ganglion travel within the inferior division of the oculomotor nerve. Included within this parasympathetic bundle are pupillomotor fibers. During orbital floor repair, damage to these fibers may result in postoperative mydriasis.[36]

The trochlear nerve is the only CN to exit dorsally from the midbrain, crossing the midline to emerge adjacent to the superior cerebellar peduncle. It travels within the wall of the cavernous sinus and enters the orbit via the superior orbital fissure *outside* of the annulus of Zinn. It is the only extraocular CN that travels extraconally within the orbit. It crosses medially over the origin of the superior rectus and levator palpebrae superioris and enters the superior oblique muscle. The long intracranial course of the trochlear nerve makes it particularly vulnerable to closed head trauma.[37]

The abducens nerve exits between the pons and the medulla in one or multiple trunks.[38] The nerve ascends through the subarachnoid space, then climbs along the bony clivus before passing through Dorello's canal into the posterior cavernous sinus. Unlike the oculomotor and trochlear nerves, the abducens nerve is not located in the lateral wall of the cavernous sinus. Instead, it travels within the body of the sinus with the internal carotid artery. It enters the orbit through the oculomotor foramen and inserts onto the inner surface of the lateral rectus at approximately one-third the distance from the muscle origin to its insertion.

Sympathetic fibers, originating in the superior cervical ganglion, travel along the internal carotid artery through the cavernous sinus and into the orbit along the ophthalmic artery. Fibers have also been shown to travel with the abducens and ophthalmic (V1) division of the trigeminal nerve.[17] While in the orbit, some of the sympathetic fibers pass through the ciliary ganglion without synapsing. Orbital sympathetics allow for pupillary dilation of the iris dilator muscle, function of the smooth muscle of the eyelid (Müller's muscle), and vasoconstriction.

Vascular anatomy

Arterial supply

The arterial supply to the orbit is an anastomotic network with contributions from the internal and external carotid circulation. Most of the arterial supply of the eye and orbit is provided through the ophthalmic artery, the first intracranial branch of the internal carotid artery (Fig. 14.10). The most important branch of the external carotid artery regarding orbital supply is the internal maxillary artery.

The ophthalmic artery branches off from the internal carotid artery just before the latter artery exits the cavernous sinus. It travels with the optic nerve within the inferolateral portion of a common dural sheath, and gradually bends medially, at which point branching of the artery occurs.[39,40] There is a great deal of variability in the order of branching vessels originating from the ophthalmic artery. In general, the first branch is the central retinal artery. Originating at the level of the orbital apex and eventually supplying the outer layers of the retina, the central retinal artery travels lateral or inferior to the optic nerve and penetrates the nerve at 5 to 16 mm posterior to the globe (average 10 mm).[41,42] Also arising near the medial bend of the ophthalmic artery are the lateral and medial posterior ciliary arteries that branch and give rise to 15 to 20 short posterior ciliary arteries as well as the two long posterior ciliary arteries. The short posterior ciliary arteries supply the optic nerve head and choroid, while the long posterior ciliary arteries travel within scleral canals anteriorly to supply the ciliary muscle, anterior choroid, and iris.

Other intraorbital structures supplied by the ophthalmic artery include the extraocular muscles and lacrimal gland. There are two main muscular branches that supply the extraocular muscles: the medial and lateral branches. The medial muscular branch supplies the medial rectus, inferior rectus, and inferior oblique muscles, while the lateral branch supplies the levator palpebrae superioris, superior rectus, superior oblique, and lateral rectus muscles. The vessels run along the muscle belly or medial surface of the muscle. Each rectus muscle artery branches into two anterior ciliary arteries, except for the lateral rectus muscular artery, which terminates into one anterior ciliary artery. The anterior ciliary arteries anastomose with the long posterior ciliary arteries to supply the globe. Simultaneous surgery on three rectus muscles or two muscles in patients with poor vascular supply may result in anterior segment ischemia, characterized by corneal edema

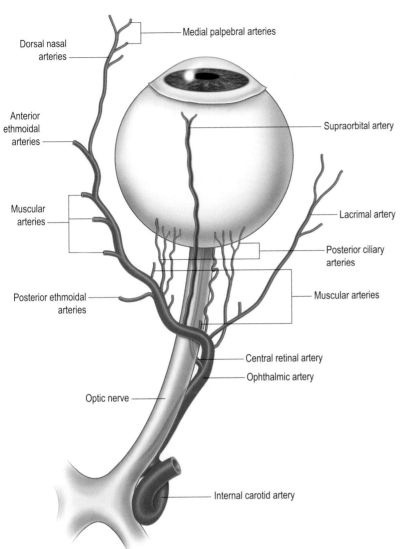

Dorsal nasal arteries

Medial palpebral arteries

Anterior ethmoidal arteries

Muscular arteries

Posterior ethmoidal arteries

Optic nerve

Supraorbital artery

Lacrimal artery

Posterior ciliary arteries

Muscular arteries

Central retinal artery

Ophthalmic artery

Internal carotid artery

Fig. 14.10 Typical branching pattern of the ophthalmic artery. (Modified from Lemke BN, Lucarelli MJ. Anatomy of the ocular adnexa, orbit, and related facial structures. In: Nesi FA, Lisman RD, Levine MR, eds. *Smith's Ophthalmic Plastic and Reconstructive Surgery*. 2nd ed. St. Louis: Mosby; 1998.)

and a mild anterior uveitis.[43] The lacrimal artery travels superolaterally in the orbit to reach the posterior surface of the lacrimal gland. It also gives off the zygomaticotemporal, zygomaticofacial, and the lateral palpebral arterial branches. The latter branch supplies the lateral portion of the arcades of the upper and lower eyelids. Portions of the lacrimal artery anastomose with the middle meningeal artery through branches of the recurrent meningeal artery and temporal arteries.

The posterior and anterior ethmoidal arteries course medially from the ophthalmic artery. While traveling at the level of the frontoethmoidal suture, they exit the orbit through the posterior ethmoid foramen and anterior ethmoid foramen, respectively. They supply the ethmoid and frontal sinus mucosa, as well as the frontal dura.

The supraorbital artery comes off from a more distal portion of the ophthalmic artery, exits through the supraorbital foramen or notch, and supplies mainly the eyebrow, forehead, and medial portion of the eyelids. The anterior continuation of the ophthalmic artery is the nasofrontal artery. Just posterior to the trochlea, the nasofrontal artery divides into the supratrochlear artery, which supplies the medial forehead and scalp, and the dorsal nasal artery. The dorsal nasal artery and its branches, the medial palpebral arteries, supply the medial eyelids and nose.

The two terminal branches of the external carotid artery are the maxillary and superficial temporal arteries. The maxillary artery branches off from the external carotid artery just behind the neck of the mandible an average of 25.7 mm (range 24.86–27.47 mm) below the condyle.[44] It passes deep to the mandible and enters the pterygopalatine fossa through the infratemporal fossa.[45] Among its branches are the middle meningeal and infraorbital arteries. The middle meningeal artery, which has been previously discussed, may anastomose with the lacrimal artery via the recurrent meningeal artery. Rarely, it may provide the majority of orbital blood in patients with ipsilateral carotid stenosis or congenital atresia (lack of patency) of the ophthalmic artery.[46] Branches from the infraorbital artery supply the inferior rectus and inferior oblique muscles, the lacrimal sac, orbital fat, upper cheek, and lower eyelid.[42] The superficial temporal artery supplies the forehead and may anastomose with the supraorbital and supratrochlear arteries of the internal carotid circulation.

Venous drainage

Venous drainage of the orbit consists of a valveless anastomotic system with multiple tributaries that drain anteriorly to the facial veins or posteriorly into the cavernous sinus or pterygoid plexus. The major venous branches of the orbit are the superior and inferior ophthalmic veins. The superior ophthalmic vein is formed at the confluence of the angular, supraorbital, and supratrochlear veins. It travels posteriorly along the roof of the orbit, before diving into the muscle cone where it picks up venous drainage from the globe through the superior vortex and ciliary veins. The superior ophthalmic vein then drains into the cavernous sinus after passing through the superior orbital fissure. The inferior orbital vein is responsible for venous drainage of the inferior orbit. It collects venous blood from the inferior extraocular muscles and inferior vortex veins and drains into both the cavernous sinus and pterygoid plexus. Some of the venous blood from the surrounding periorbita drains through a system of anterior facial veins. These typically drain directly into the external jugular vein.

Orbital lymphatic drainage

The goal of identifying the orbital lymphatic drainage system has been pursued in both human and animal studies.[47–49] Traditionally thought to be absent in the orbit, the more recent use of selective lymphatic markers has identified lymphatics in at least some areas of the human orbit.[50,51] Using CD-34 and D2-40 monoclonal antibodies, specific for blood vessel endothelium and a protein on lymphatic endothelium, respectively, lymphatics were confirmed in human lacrimal gland and optic nerve dura.[51] Additional work has revealed orbital lymphatic vessels in the orbital fat and extrinsic oculomotor muscles.[52]

FACIAL AND EYELID ANATOMY AND FUNCTION

The eyebrow and forehead

The eyebrow plays an important role in facial expressions. Eyebrow position and contour are maintained by a group of muscles innervated by the temporal branch of the facial nerve (CN VII). The muscles of the eyebrow and forehead may be divided into superficial (frontalis, procerus, orbicularis oculi), intermediate (depressor supercilii), and deep (corrugator supercilii) groups.[53] (Fig. 14.11). The skin of the brow and accompanying subcutaneous fibroadipose are the thickest layers on the face.

The main elevators of the eyebrows and forehead are the paired frontalis muscles. Recruitment of the vertically oriented frontalis may be used to compensate in cases of eyelid ptosis. The frontalis muscle interdigitates with the remaining superficial forehead muscles including the orbicularis oculi, which surrounds the anterior orbit. The orbicularis may be conceptually divided into three topographic regions: the orbital, preseptal, and pretarsal. The orbital portion of the muscle is responsible for forced eyelid closure and is an important depressor of the eyebrow and forehead. The pretarsal portion of the muscle is responsible for spontaneous blinking. The procerus muscle arises from the nasal bones and upper lateral cartilages and inserts into eyebrow skin medially. It depresses the glabella to form horizontal skin folds.

The depressor supercilii muscle originates on the frontal process of the maxillary bone and inserts into the dermis of the medial eyebrow.[54] During this course, it travels over the origin of the corrugator muscle. The bilateral corrugator supercilii muscles (transverse head and deep head) lie deep to the frontalis muscle and travel from their insertion on the superomedial orbital margin to insert into the muscle and skin of the respective medial eyebrow. Contraction of the corrugator draws the eyebrow medially and inferiorly resulting in vertical glabellar rhytids (wrinkles).

The midface

Our understanding of the anatomy of the midface and its dynamic relationship with other periocular structures has advanced considerably during the past 30 years. The midface extends from the upper lip to the inferior orbital rim. The facial soft tissue layers include skin, subcutaneous fat, superficial fascia (superficial musculoaponeurotic system [SMAS]), mimetic muscles, deep facial fascia, and a plane containing the parotid duct, buccal fat pad, and facial nerve.

The SMAS was first described in the parotid and cheek area by Mitz and Peyronie (Fig. 14.12 & Box 14.2).[55] Multiple fibrous extensions from the SMAS to the skin are thought to distribute muscular contractions that aid in facial expression. Initially described as dividing the parotid and cheek fat into two layers, it has subsequently been shown to lie 11 to 13 mm deep to the skin at the midcheek and invest the zygomaticus major, zygomaticus minor, and levator labii

Fig. 14.11 Forehead muscles. *FM*, frontalis muscle; *PM*, procerus muscle, *DSM*, depressor supercilii muscle, *CSM-O*, corrugator supercilii muscle—oblique head; *CSM-T*, corrugator supercilii muscle—transverse head. (J. Peter Rubin, Peter C. Neligan, Plastic Surgery – E-Book: Volume 2: *Aesthetic Surgery*, 4th ed. Elsevier Health Sciences, 2017.)

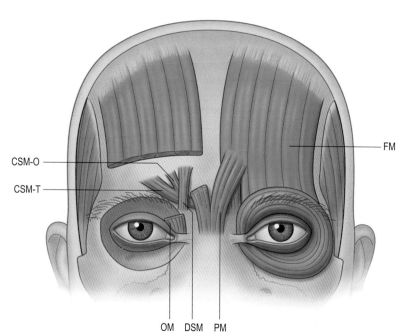

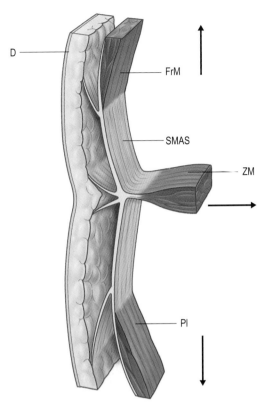

Fig. 14.12 Schematic view of the superficial musculoaponeurotic system (*SMAS*) showing relation to frontalis muscle (*FrM*), zygomatic muscle (*Zm*), dermis (*D*), and platysma (*Pl*). (From Mitz V, Peyronie M. The superficial musculo-aponeurotic system (SMAS) in the parotid and cheek area. *Plast Reconstr Surg.* 1976;58:80–88.)

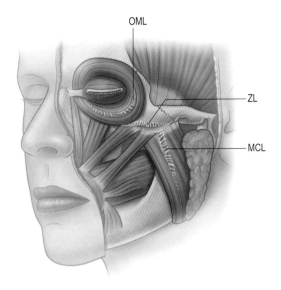

Fig. 14.13 Ligamentous support of the midface. *MCL*, Masseteric cutaneous ligaments; *OL*, orbitomalar ligament; *ZL*, zygomatic ligaments. (From Lucarelli MJ, Khwarg SI, Lemke BN, Kozel JS, Dortzbach RK. The anatomy of midfacial ptosis. *Ophthalmic Plast Reconstr Surg.* 2000;16(1):7-22.)

BOX 14.2 Key Midfacial Support Components

- The superficial musculoaponeurotic system (SMAS) is an aponeurotic system that is contiguous with the occipitalis, frontalis, orbicularis, and platysma.
- Fibrous extensions from SMAS to the skin may help to transmit facial muscular contractions.
- Midface bony attachments: zygomatic ligaments and orbitomalar ligaments; attenuation of these ligaments contributes to midfacial ptosis.

---

superioris.[56] It is continuous with the platysma in the lower face and the frontalis in the upper face, as well as the anterior and posterior fascia of the orbicularis oculi muscle.[57,58] The facial nerve courses beneath the SMAS.

The SMAS has a number of bony attachments. Shortly after its initial description, the SMAS was recognized as an important structure in facial rhytidectomy (face-lift).[59] In the midface, the zygomatic ligaments and orbitomalar ligaments have been characterized (Fig. 14.13).[60,61] The mandibular ligaments have been described in the lower face. The orbitomalar ligament has been characterized to provide major osseocutaneous midfacial support owing to its steadfast lateral component found approximately 5 mm lateral to the lateral orbital rim.[62] Work by Lucarelli and colleagues showed that attenuation of the zygomatic, masseteric cutaneous, and orbitomalar ligament is associated with age-related midfacial ptosis (Fig. 14.14).[62] Others have recently referred to the orbitomalar ligament as the orbital retaining ligament.[63]

The facial mimetic muscles are arranged into lamella. Freilinger et al.[64] have categorized in detail the mimetic muscle into four distinct layers. A superficial layer consists of the orbicularis oculi, zygomatic minor, and depressor anguli oris. The second layer contains the platysma, depressor labii inferioris, the levator labii superioris alaeque nasi, and zygomatic major muscles. The third layer consists of the levator labii superioris and orbicularis oris. Finally, the deepest layer consists of the mentalis, the levator anguli oris, and the buccinator. Branches of the facial nerve supply the first three layers of muscles from the underside, while the deepest layer is innervated from the outer surface.

Paralysis of the facial nerve may have profound effects on facial symmetry and corneal protection. Idiopathic facial nerve palsy, or Bell's palsy, is estimated to have an incidence of 25 cases per 100,000 (Box 14.3).[65] The differential diagnosis of facial palsy includes infectious (Ramsey Hunt, herpes zoster/Lyme disease), neoplastic (facial nerve neuroma or hemangioma, acoustic neuroma, meningioma, metastatic), inflammatory (Wegener's granulomatosis, sarcoidosis), traumatic (basilar skull fracture, temporal bone trauma, parotid injury), and congenital etiologies. Lagophthalmos (inability to close the eyelid fully) and a poor blink may lead to corneal exposure. Intensive lubrication, patching, lid taping, and use of a moisture chamber may be adequate therapies to prevent complications of corneal exposure. More severe cases may require surgery (e.g., upper lid weight or eyelid closure from a tarsorrhaphy or, occasionally, midface lifting).[66,67]

The eyelid

The eyelid margin

The eyelid margin may be divided into anterior and posterior lamella. The anterior lamella is composed of skin, muscle, and associated glands, while the posterior lamella consists of the tarsal plate, conjunctiva, and associated glands (Fig. 14.15). The two lamella may be separated from one another along the gray line, a terminal extension of the orbicularis known as the muscle of Riolan. This portion of the muscle has been hypothesized to keep the eyelid edges in close approximation to the

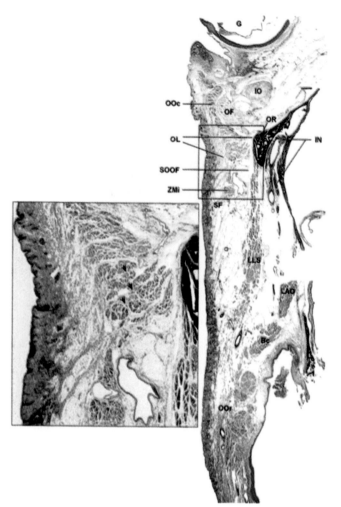

Fig. 14.14 Merged sections through central lower eyelid extending to the oral commissure from specimen with midfacial ptosis (Masson trichrome staining). The globe (*G*), inferior oblique (*IO*), and orbital fat (*OF*) are visible superiorly. The orbitomalar ligament (*OL*) extends off the orbital rim (*OR*) and passes through the orbicularis oculi muscle (*OOc*) to the dermis. The nasolabial fold (*NLF*) is seen inferiorly. The subcutaneous fat (*SF*) can be seen anterior to the OOc and zygomatic minor (*ZMi*) muscles. The suborbicularis oculi fat (*SOOF*) rests posterior to the orbicularis oculi muscle and surrounds the proximal portion of the levator labii superioris muscle (*LLS*). Note the continuity of the inferior SOOF and the SF. The infraorbital nerve (*IN*) and accompanying vessel can be seen traversing the SOOF deep to the LLS muscle. The LLS muscle extends into the upper lip. The levator anguli oris (*LAO*) arises from the maxilla inferior to the infraorbital foramen. The orbicularis oris (*OOr*) and buccinator (*Bc*) are visible in the inferior portion of the specimen. The inset details the orbitomalar ligament *(arrowheads)* traversing the OOc muscle. (From Lucarelli MJ, Khwarg SI, Lemke BN, Kozel JS, Dortzbach RK. The anatomy of midfacial ptosis. *Ophthalmic Plast Reconstr Surg.* 2000;16(1):7–22.)

BOX 14.3   Idiopathic Facial Nerve Palsy

- Incidence of approximately 25 cases per 100,000 persons.
- Must be differentiated from infectious, inflammatory, neoplastic, traumatic, and congenital etiologies.
- May lead to corneal exposure and ulceration.
- Mild exposure may require intensive lubrication, patching, or lid taping.
- Severe exposure may require surgical correction (temporary or permanent tarsorrhaphy or implantation of a gold weight).

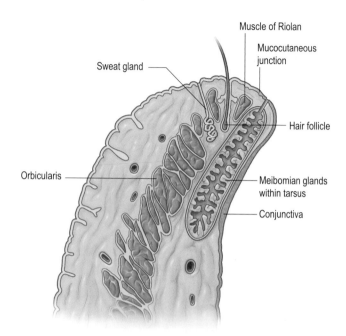

Fig. 14.15 Sagittal section of the eyelid margin. (From Lemke BN, Lucarelli MJ: Anatomy of the ocular adnexa, orbit, and related facial structures. In: Nesi FA, Lisman RD, Levine MR, eds. *Smith's Ophthalmic Plastic and Reconstructive Surgery.* 2nd ed. St. Louis: Mosby; 1998.)

surface of the globe, as well as help expel glandular contents during blinking.[68,69] The cilia serve to protect the globe from large airborne particles. They are also highly sensitive to touch and elicit the blink reflex when stimulated.

The anterior lamella functions as a single anatomic unit. The eyelid skin is the thinnest in the body, due in part to a relative thinning of dermis and absence of a subcutaneous fat layer. In adults, the palpebral fissure measures 9 to 12 mm vertically, while the horizontal distance between the medial and lateral commissures measures approximately 30 mm. The lower eyelid rests at or up to 1.5 mm above the inferior limbus whereas the upper eyelid rests at approximately 1.5 to 2.0 mm below the superior limbus.[41] The highest point of the upper eyelid rests just nasal to the central pupillary axis.

The orbicularis muscle is located beneath the eyelid skin. The pretarsal portion of the muscle originates from the anterior and posterior arms of the medial canthal ligament. The deep head of the muscle (Horner's muscle) inserts onto the posterior lacrimal crest and lacrimal fascia, whereas the anterior head attaches to the anterior lacrimal crest (see Fig. 14.4). The muscle therefore surrounds the lacrimal sac, and during contraction assists the lacrimal pump mechanism.[70] Laterally, the pretarsal orbicularis muscle inserts into the lateral canthal tendon.

Glands of the anterior lamella include the glands of Zeis and Moll. The Zeis glands are sebaceous glands whereas the tubular glands of Moll are apocrine sweat glands. The Zeis glands empty into the cilial follicular infundibulum while the tubular glands of Moll are located in between the lash follicles.

The posterior lamella of the eyelid consists of the tarsal plate, meibomian glands, and conjunctiva. The tarsal plates are composed of collagens (types I and III collagen), as well as components more typical of cartilage (aggrecan, chondroitins 4 and 6 sulfate).[71] They provide rigidity and allow for dynamic movement of the eyelids. The height of the upper tarsus measures approximately 10 mm centrally, while the height of the lower tarsus measures on average 3 to 4 mm.[72] Medially and laterally, both the upper and lower tarsal plates taper to become the medial and lateral canthal tendons. As previously described, the medial canthal tendon splits into anterior and posterior heads that attach to the anterior lacrimal crest and posterior lacrimal crest, respectively. The lateral canthal tendon inserts at Whitnall's lateral tubercle, a small, rounded protuberance of the zygomatic bone a few millimeters inside of the lateral orbital wall. Laxity of the canthal tendon may lead to ectropion (turning outward of the eyelid) and may require an eyelid-tightening procedure by shortening and reattaching the lateral canthal tendon. Whitnall's lateral tubercle is also an insertion site for the lateral horn of the levator aponeurosis, the inferior (Lockwood's) and superior (Whitnall's) transverse ligament, the deep pretarsal orbicularis, and the expansion of the superior rectus muscle sheath.[11,73]

The tarsal plates of both the upper and lower eyelids contain the sebaceous meibomian glands. There are approximately 25 in the upper eyelid and 20 in the lower eyelid.[22] The glands secrete the lipid layer (outer layer) of the tear film, which helps prevent evaporation of the tears. In the setting of meibomian gland dysfunction, the relative absence of the lipid layer may result in dry eyes.[74] Chronic inflammation of the glands or meibomitis may lead to dysplastic hair follicles that curve toward the globe, known as distichiasis.[75] Treatment for distichiasis (misdirected lashes from the meibomian gland orifices) or trichiasis (misdirection of normal eyelash follicles) may include cryotherapy, argon laser, electrolysis, trephination, and other lid-modifying modalities.[76–78]

Tightly bound to the posterior aspect of the tarsal plates is the palpebral conjunctiva. It consists of a nonkeratinized stratified columnar epithelium overlying loose connective tissue known as substantia propria. The accessory glands of Wolfring, located in the tarsal conjunctiva, and Krause, located in conjunctival fornix, help to produce the aqueous layer of the tear film. This middle layer of the tear film is tightly bound to the hydrophilic mucin layer (inner layer) produced from conjunctival goblet cells. Mucocutaneous disorders such as ocular cicatricial pemphigoid, Stevens-Johnson syndrome, and bullous pemphigoid may lead to destruction of goblet cells and their progenitor stem cells, leading to severe chronic inflammation with scarring and conjunctival contraction.[79]

The inferior and superior puncta provide entrance to the lacrimal excretory system. The lower eyelid punctum is approximately 10 mm from the lacrimal tear sac with the upper punctum 8 mm from the sac. The puncta are normally oriented toward the tear lake.

EYELID MUSCULATURE

The major protractor of the eyelids is the orbicularis muscle, which may be divided into the orbital, preseptal, and pretarsal components. The orbicularis myofibers have the smallest diameter of any skeletal muscle and, although they vary somewhat in length, are overall relatively short.[80] The variability in myofiber length may help to explain the variety of complex eyelid movements including blinking, winking, and spasm.

The main retractor of the upper eyelid is the levator palpebrae superioris (Fig. 14.16).[81] Assistance is also provided by the superior tarsal muscle (Müller's muscle), which is supplied by sympathetic innervation. The levator is divided into muscular and aponeurotic

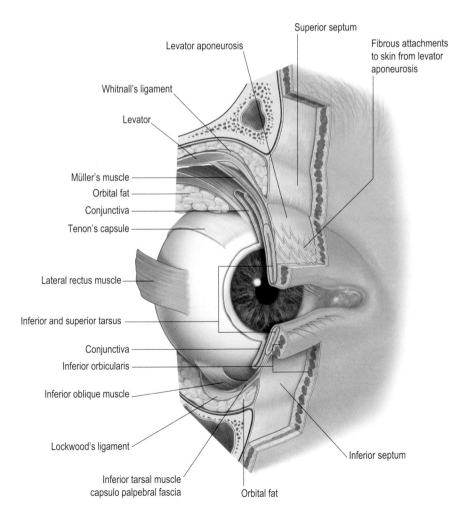

Fig. 14.16 Oblique section through the upper and lower eyelids. (Baert AL, Sartor K, Wibke S. Müller-Forell, Imaging of Orbital and Visual Pathway Pathology. 1st ed. Berlin Heidelberg: Springer-Verlag; 2002.)

portions. The muscular portion of the levator measures approximately 36 mm in length and lies just above the superior rectus.[82] The two muscles can be separated easily except along the medial borders, where they are bound by a fascial sheath. As the muscle moves anteriorly in the orbit, it begins to widen, eventually joining Whitnall's ligament, a transverse fibrous condensation just posterior to the superior orbital rim.[10] Whitnall's ligament provides structural support to the upper eyelids. It has been suggested that it acts as either a fulcrum or swinging suspender for the levator.[13,83] After passing Whitnall's ligament, the levator muscle transitions into the fibrous levator aponeurosis. The aponeurosis courses another 14 to 20 mm to insert onto the inferior third of the anterior surface of the tarsus. An anterior portion of the aponeurosis sends fine attachments to the upper eyelid skin as well as multiple elastic fiber insertions of the levator muscle complex that includes the levator aponeurosis, the conjoined fascia, the lid crease area, and Müller's muscle tendon.[84] The upper eyelid crease is formed by attachments to the skin.

The smooth superior tarsal muscle of Müller arises from the underside of the levator muscle approximately 15 mm above the superior tarsal border and inserts at the upper border of the tarsus.[85] This sympathetically innervated muscle provides approximately 2 mm of upper eyelid lift. Interruption of this innervation may result in Horner's blepharoptosis (oculosympathetic paresis). Approximately 2 mm of ptosis along with miosis and occasional unilateral anhidrosis is highly suggestive of Horner's syndrome due to an interruption of the sympathetic system. The vascular arterial arcade is found between the levator aponeurosis and Müller's muscle. This serves as a useful surgical landmark to identify the underlying Müller's muscle.

The lower eyelid retractors are palpebral extensions from the inferior rectus muscle and are utilized, along with the rectus muscle, during down-gaze.[86] This muscular extension splits to surround the inferior oblique muscle as it travels anterior in the orbit. The outer division or capsulopalpebral fascia is analogous to the levator palpebrae superioris, while the inner division, which is composed of smooth muscle fibers, is analogous to Müller's muscle.[23] The two layers are typically not distinct during surgical dissection. The lower eyelid retractors have three distinct insertions. Anteriorly, the capsulopalpebral fascia fuses with the orbital septum 4 mm inferior to the tarsus. A middle layer of inferior tarsal muscle (the capsulopalpebral fascia and smooth muscle) fibers terminates a few millimeters inferior to the tarsus. Finally, a posterior layer of retractors inserts on Tenon's fascia.

Medial and lateral canthal anatomy has been described in significant detail.[87,88] The medial canthal region consists not only of the medial canthal tendon, but also of support structures including Horner's muscle, the medial rectus capsulopalpebral fascia, the medial horn of the levator aponeurosis, supporting ligaments, as well as contributions from the lower eyelid retractors, pretarsal part of the orbicularis oculi muscle, and Lockwood's ligament. This composite structure may also be referred to as the medial retinaculum.[87] The lateral canthal region consists of a bifurcated structure of the orbital septum (septal band: anterior limb) and a ligament (tarsoligamentous band: posterior limb), leading some groups to refer to this structure as not simply the lateral canthal tendon, but instead a lateral canthal band.[88]

Blinking

Spontaneous blinking occurs every 3 to 8 seconds with an average of 12 blinks per minute. During the normal blink cycle, eyelid closure is a result of activity *and* co-inhibition of two groups of muscles: the protractors of the eyelids (the orbicularis oculi, corrugator, and procerus muscles), and the voluntary retractors of the eyelids (the levator palpebra superioris and frontalis muscles), respectively. The pretarsal

---

portion of the orbicularis muscle is thought to be responsible for spontaneous blinking.

Blinking assists in the maintenance of a normal ocular tear surface. A blink initiates a cycle of secretion, dispersal, evaporation, and drainage of tears.[89] Closure of the eyelids occludes the puncta, thus preventing fluid regurgitation. At the same time the canaliculi and sac are compressed, which forces fluid down the nasolacrimal duct. When the eyelid opens, both the puncta and canalicular system open, creating a partial vacuum that sucks in tears from the ocular surface. Closure of the eyelids also stimulates the expression of the aqueous tear layer from the lacrimal and accessory lacrimal glands.

During delayed blinking, the normal tear cycle is altered. This may result in dry eye or secondary reflexive tearing. Seen in a variety of clinical scenarios including reading, older age, and in patients with Parkinson's disease, delayed blinking results in decreased tear expression, increased tear evaporation, and potentially decreased tear drainage.[90]

Benign essential blepharospasm (BEB) is a bilateral, involuntary, spasmodic forced eyelid closure with accompanying brow depression in the absence of any other ocular or adnexal cause (Box 14.4). Most cases of BEB are considered sporadic; about 20% to 30% of cases have a family history.[91] It may initially begin with simply an increased blink rate. Blepharospasm may also be secondary to ocular surface disease or neurodegenerative diseases such as Parkinson's.[92] BEB affects women more often than men, and typically presents during the fifth to seventh decades of life.[93]

During BEB, the normal activation/inhibition pathways (possibly related to basal ganglia damage and abnormalities in dopaminergic pathways) are disrupted, resulting in sustained activation of the protractors with sustained inhibition of the retractors.[94] Repeated botulinum toxin type A (Botox) approximately every 3 months is the treatment of choice for many patients with BEB. The neurotoxin, which is produced from *Clostridium botulinum*, inhibits the release of acetylcholine (ACh) and may be used to temporarily paralyze the eyelid protractors.[95]

Eyelid fat

Bounded by the orbital septum anteriorly and the levator muscle/aponeurosis posteriorly, there are two upper eyelid fat pads separated by the trochlea and superior oblique tendon. The most medial fat pad takes on a fibrous white appearance, whereas the central preaponeurotic fat pad is yellow, due to a high level of free-radical scavenging carotenoids.[96] The fatty acid levels found in the fat are similar in samples throughout the orbit, despite these color variations. Orbital fats are typically unsaturated. Some of these fatty acids include oleic acid (18:1) and linoleic acid (18:2), among others. The preponderance of unsaturated fats may provide a lubricating surface with advantages for ocular motility. Laterally, the pink and firm lacrimal gland should not be confused with eyelid fat during surgery. The lower eyelid contains three fat pads that are enclosed in fibrous compartments: medial, central, and lateral.

Eyelid vasculature

The eyelids are highly vascularized with contributions from both the external and internal carotid systems. The external carotid system supplies the eyelid through branches from the facial artery, superficial temporal artery, infraorbital artery (via the maxillary artery), and superficial temporal artery (Fig. 14.17). The facial artery arises from the external carotid artery just below the angle of the jaw and travels superomedially along the nasolabial fold. As it approaches the medial canthus it becomes the angular artery. The artery runs approximately 5 to 6 mm medial to the medial canthus. External dacryocystorhinostomy incisions should be positioned to avoid damage to the artery. The artery perforates the orbital septum to anastomose with branches of the ophthalmic artery. The superficial temporal artery supplies the forehead and may anastomose with the supraorbital and supratrochlear arteries of the internal carotid circulation. The maxillary artery and its branches were discussed in the orbital section.

The main arterial supply of the upper eyelids is supplied by four arterial arcades: the marginal, peripheral, superficial orbital, and deep orbital arcades.[97] In the upper and lower eyelids, the marginal arcades lie anterior to the tarsus approximately 2 to 4 mm from the eyelid margin. Anastomoses between the supratrochlear, lacrimal, and angular arteries compose the superior arcade, while anastomoses from the infraorbital, angular, and zygomaticofacial arteries form the inferior arcade. During tarsal sharing procedures such as free tarsoconjunctival grafts or tarsoconjunctival flaps (e.g., Hughes procedure), proper care should be taken to maintain vascular supply to both eyelids.

Arising from the confluence of the frontal and supraorbital veins, the facial vein is the main venous drainage pathway of the eyelids. It

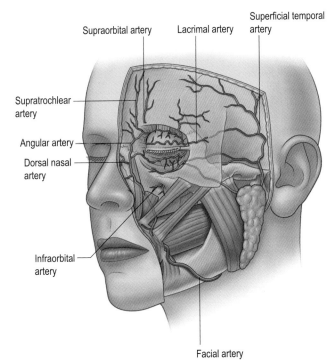

Fig. 14.17 Superficial facial arteries in the ocular region. (Modified from Lemke BN, Lucarelli MJ. Anatomy of the ocular adnexa, orbit, and related facial structures. In: Nesi FA, Lisman RD, Levine MR, eds. *Smith's Ophthalmic Plastic and Reconstructive Surgery*. 2nd ed. St. Louis: Mosby; 1998.)

starts as the angular vein 6 to 8 mm medial to the medial canthus and travels roughly with the facial artery, ending at the external jugular vein. A minor proportion of the facial venous drainage passes posteriorly through veins that empty into cavernous sinus and pterygoid plexus, as discussed earlier.

Eyelid lymphatics

Lymphoscintigraphy of Cynomolgus monkey eyelids has revealed discrete lymphatic drainage pathways for the upper and lower eyelids and a dual pathway for the central upper eyelid.[98,99] More recent work from fresh fetus cadavers reveals three layers of lymphatic plexuses: a superficial or preorbicularis muscle plexus, a pretarsal or postorbicularis muscle plexus, and a deep or post-tarsal plexus.[100] The lateral and medial portions of the upper and lower eyelids drain to the superficial preauricular and submandibular lymph nodes, respectively. This drainage continues through the deep cervical nodes.

Eyelid innervation

The eyelids and periocular structures are innervated by the oculomotor nerve (CN III), facial nerve (CN VII), trigeminal nerve (CN V), and sympathetic fibers.

The facial nerve supplies most of the motor innervation to the face. After passing through the parotid gland the nerve divides into five divisions: temporal, zygomatic, buccal, mandibular, and cervical nerves. There is a great deal of overlap of regions innervated by the nerve. In general, the temporal branch innervates the frontalis muscle while the zygomatic, temporal, and buccal divisions innervate the orbicularis oculi. Motor innervation to the levator palpebrae is provided by the superior division of the oculomotor nerve. Sympathetic fibers innervate the underlying Müller's muscle. The exact course of these sympathetic fibers is controversial.

Sensory innervation to the face is supplied by the trigeminal nerve. The nerve is composed of the ophthalmic (V1), maxillary (V2), and mandibular divisions (V3), of which the ophthalmic and maxillary divisions provide sensory innervation to the periorbita (Fig. 14.18).

The ophthalmic (V1) division enters the orbit through the superior orbital fissure after dividing into three branches: the lacrimal, frontal, and nasociliary nerves. The frontal and lacrimal nerves enter the orbit in the superolateral portion of the superior ophthalmic fissure outside of the annulus of Zinn. A superior division of the lacrimal nerve supplies sensation to the nearby conjunctiva, the lateral upper eyelid, and the lacrimal gland. An inferior division of the nerve anastomoses with the zygomaticotemporal branch of the maxillary trigeminal nerve and is joined by parasympathetic secretory fibers destined for the lacrimal gland.

While traveling just below the periorbita in the anterior orbit, the frontal nerve divides into the supraorbital and supratrochlear divisions. The supratrochlear nerve innervates the glabellar skin, medial upper eyelid, and lower forehead. The supraorbital nerve typically divides into a superficial (medial) division that supplies the anterior margin of the scalp and forehead skin, and a deep (lateral) division that provides sensation to the frontoparietal scalp (Fig. 14.19). Damage to this deep (lateral) division during a forehead lift may result in a large area of scalp numbness and paresthesia.

The nasociliary branch of the ophthalmic trigeminal nerve passes through the annulus of Zinn and travels within the intraconal space. It gives off a small sensory branch to the ciliary ganglion and long ciliary nerves to the globe, before dividing into the ethmoid and infratrochlear end branches. The long ciliary nerves innervate the iris, cornea, and ciliary muscle. The ethmoid branch provides sensation to the nasal mucosa and skin on the anterior tip of the nose. A small unilateral

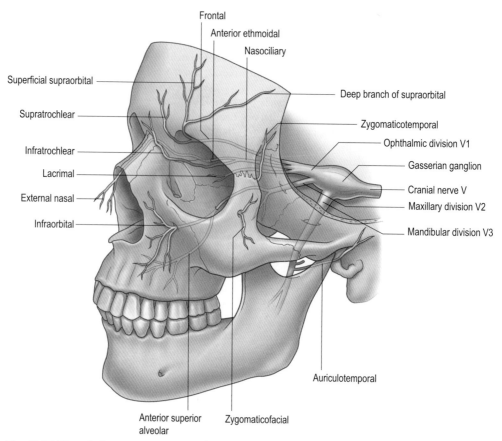

Fig. 14.18 Trigeminal nerve pathways. (Modified from Lemke BN, Lucarelli MJ. Anatomy of the ocular adnexa, orbit, and related facial structures. In: Nesi FA, Lisman RD, Levine MR, eds. *Smith's Ophthalmic Plastic and Reconstructive Surgery*. 2nd ed. St. Louis; Mosby; 1998.)

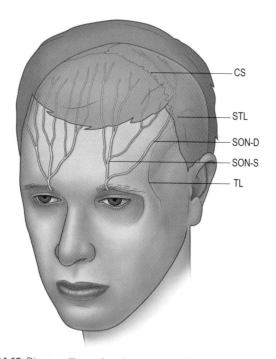

Fig. 14.19 Diagram illustrating the courses of the deep (*SON-D*) and the superficial (*SON-S*) divisions of the supraorbital nerve trunk. *CS* (coronal suture), *STL* (superior temporal fusion line), *TL* (temporal fusion line). (Modified from Knize, DM. A study of the supraorbital nerve. *Plast Reconstr Surg*. 1995;96:564–569.)

vesicular rupture of herpes zoster on the tip of the nose is known as Hutchinson's sign and is associated with an increased risk of herpes zoster ophthalmicus.

The maxillary (V2) division of the trigeminal nerve exits the middle cranial fossa at the foramen rotundum and passes through the lateral wall of the cavernous sinus and pterygopalatine fossa to enter the inferior orbital fissure. Within the pterygopalatine fossa, it also gives rise to the zygomatic, sphenopalatine, and posterior superior alveolar branches. The infraorbital nerve is the terminal branch of the maxillary nerve, which enters the infraorbital groove approximately 30 mm posterior to the orbital rim. The zygomatic nerve divides into the zygomaticofacial and zygomaticotemporal nerves, which provide innervation to the lateral cheek and lateral brow, respectively. Parasympathetic secretory fibers join the zygomaticotemporal nerve prior to joining the lacrimal nerve en route to the lacrimal gland.

REFERENCES

1. Langdon JH. *The human strategy: an evolutionary perspective on human anatomy*. Oxford: Oxford University Press; 2005.
2. Burrows AM. The facial expression musculature in primates and its evolutionary significance. *Bioessays*. 2008;30(3):212–225.
3. Zide BM, Jelks GW. *Surgical anatomy of the orbit*. New York: Lippincott Williams & Wilkins; 1985.
4. Webster RC. Supraorbital and supratrochlear notches and foramina: anatomical variations and surgical relevance. *Laryngoscope*. 1986;96:311–315.
5. Nahum AM. The biomechanics of maxillofacial trauma. *Clin Plast Surg*. 1975;2:59–64.
6. Karesh JW, Kelman SE, Chirico PA, et al. Orbital roof "blow-in" fractures. *Ophthal Plast Reconstr Surg*. 1991;7(2):77–83.
7. Lee D, Brody R, Har-El G. Frontal sinus outflow anatomy. *Am J Rhinol*. 1997;11(4):283–285.

8. Goldberg AN, Oroszlan G, Anderson TD. Complications of frontal sinusitis and their management. *Otolaryngol Clin North Am*. 2001;34(1):211–225.
9. Garcia CE, Cunningham MJ, Clary RA, et al. The etiologic role of frontal sinusitis in pediatric orbital abscesses. *Am J Otolaryngol*. 1993;14:449–452.
10. Whitnall SE. On a tubercle on the malar bone, and on the lateral attachments of the tarsal plates. *J Anat Physiol*. 1911;45:426–432.
11. Whitnall SE. On a ligament acting as a check to the action of the levator palpebrae superioris. *J Anat Phys*. 1910;14:131.
12. Kim JW, Goldberg RA, Shorr N. The inferomedial orbital strut: an anatomic and radiographic study. *Ophthal Plast Reconstr Surg*. 2002;18(5):355–364.
13. Goldberg RA, Wu JC, Jesmanowicz A, Hyde JS. Eyelid anatomy revisited. Dynamic high-resolution magnetic resonance images of Whitnall's ligament and upper eyelid structures with the use of a surface coil. *Arch Ophthalmol*. 1992;110(11):1598–1600.
14. Goldberg RA, Shorr N, Cohen MS. The medical orbital strut in the prevention of postdecompression dystopia in dysthyroid ophthalmopathy. *Ophthal Plast Reconstr Surg*. 1992;8(1):32–34.
15. Hartikainen J, Aho HJ, Seppa H, et al. Lacrimal bone thickness at the lacrimal sac fossa. *Ophthalmic Surg Lasers*. 1996;27:679–684.
16. Yeh S, Foroozan R. Orbital apex syndrome. *Curr Opin Ophthalmol*. 2004;15(6):490–498.
17. Lyon DB, Lemke BN, Wallow I, Dortzbach RK. Sympathetic nerve anatomy in the cavernous sinus and retrobulbar orbit of the cynomolgous monkey. *Ophthal Plast Reconstr Surg*. 1992;8:1–12.
18. Monard M, Tcherekayev V, deTribolet N. The superior orbital fissure: a microanatomical study. *Neurosurgery*. 1994;35:1087–1093.
19. Aviv RI, Casselman J. Orbital imaging: Part 1. Normal anatomy. *Clin Radiol*. 2005;60(3): 279–287.
20. Aviv RI, Casselman J. Orbital imaging: Part 2. Intraorbital pathology. *Clin Radiol*. 2005;60(3): 288–307.
21. Koornneef L. *Details of the orbital connective tissue system in the adult. Spatial aspect of orbital musculo-fibrous tissue in man*. New York: Swets & Zweitlinger,; 1977.
22. Meyer DR, Linberg JV, Wobig JL, et al. Anatomy of the orbital septum and associated eyelid connective tissues. *Ophthal Plast Reconstr Surg*. 1991;7:104.
23. Hawes MJ, Dortzbach RK. The microscopic anatomy of the lower eyelid retractors. *Arch Ophthalmol*. 1982;100:1313–1318.
24. Anderson RL, Beard C. The levator aponeurosis attachments and their clinical significance. *Arch Ophthalmol*. 1977;95:1437–1441.
25. Kakizaki H, Takahashi Y, Nakano T, Asamoto K, Ikeda H, Ichinose A, Iwaki M, Selva D, Leibovitch I. Anatomy of Tenons capsule. *Clin Exp Ophthalmol*. 2012;40(6):611–616.
26. Hargiss JL. Surgical anatomy of the eyelids. *Trans Pacif Coast Otolaryngol Soc*. 1963;44:193–202.
27. Fink WH. An anatomical study of the check mechanism of the vertical muscles of the eye. *Trans Am Ophthalmol Soc*. 1956;54:193–213.
28. Douglas RS, Kahaly GJ, Patel A, Sile S, Thompson EHZ, Perdok R, Fleming JC, Fowler BT, Marcocci C, Marinò M, Antonelli A, Dailey R, Harris GJ, Eckstein A, Schiffman J, Tang R, Nelson C, Salvi M, Wester S, Sherman JW, Vescio T, Holt RJ, Smith TJ. Teprotumumab for the treatment of active thyroid eye disease. *N Engl J Med*. 2020;382(4):341–352.
29. Garrity JA, Bahn RS. Pathogenesis of graves ophthalmopathy: implications for prediction, prevention, and treatment. *Am J Ophthalmol*. 2006;142:147–153.
30. Kazim M, Goldberg RA, Smith TJ. Insights into the pathogenesis of thyroid-associated orbitopathy: evolving rationale for therapy. *Arch Ophthalmol*. 2002;120(3):380–386.
31. Dalley RW, Robertson WD, Rootman J. Globe tenting: a sign of increased orbital tension. *Am J Neuroradiol*. 1989;10:181–186.
32. Sarkies N. Traumatic optic neuropathy. *Eye*. 2004;18:1122–1125.
33. Anderson RL, Panje WR, Gross CE. Optic nerve blindness following blunt forehead trauma. *Ophthalmology*. 1982;89:445–455.
34. Ruskell GL. The orbital branches of the pterygopalatine ganglion and their relationship with the internal carotid nerve branches in primates. *J Anat*. 1970;106:323–339.
35. Nilsson SF, Linder J, Bill A. Characteristics of uveal vasodilation produced by facial nerve stimulation in monkeys, cats, and rabbits. *Exp Eye Res*. 1985;40(6):841–852.
36. Hornblass A. Pupillary dilation in fractures of the floor of the orbit. *Ophthalmic Surg*. 1979;10:44–46.
37. Mansour AM, Reinecke RD. Central trochlear palsy. *Surv Ophthalmol*. 1986;30:279–297.
38. Lyon DB, Lemke BN, Wallow I, Dortzbach RK. Sympathetic nerve anatomy in the cavernous sinus and retrobulbar orbit of the cynomolgous monkey. *Ophthal Plast Reconstr Surg*. 1992;8:1–12.
39. Lang H, Kageyama I. The ophthalmic artery and its branches, measurements, and clinical importance. *Surg Radiol Anat*. 1990;12:83–90.
40. Bergen MP. A literature review of the vascular system in the human orbit. *Acta Morphol Neerl Scan*. 1981;19:273–305.
41. Dutton JJ. *Atlas of clinical and surgical orbital anatomy*. Philadelphia: WB Saunders; 1994.
42. Singh S, Dass R. The central artery of the retina. *Br J Ophthalmol*. 1960;44:193–212.
43. Saunders RA, Bluestein EC, Wilson ME, et al. Anterior segment ischemia after strabismus surgery. *Surv Ophthalmol*. 1994;38:456–466.
44. Orbay H, Kerem M, Ünlü RE, et al. Maxillary artery: anatomical landmarks and relationship with the mandibular subcondyle. *Plast Reconst Surg*. 2007;120:1865–1870.
45. Pearson BW, Mackenzie RG, Goodman WS. The anatomical basis of transantral ligation of the maxillary artery in severe epistaxis. *Laryngoscope*. 1969;79:969–984.
46. Lemke BN, Lucarelli MJ. Anatomy of the ocular adnexa, orbit, and related facial structures. In: Nesi FA, Lisman RD, eds. *Smith's ophthalmic plastic and reconstructive surgery*. St Louis: CV Mosby; 1998.
47. McGetrick JJ, Wilson DG, Dortzbach RK, Kaufman PL, Lemke BN. A search for lymphatic drainage of the monkey orbit. *Arch Ophthalmol*. 1989;107:255–260.
48. Gausas RE, Gonnering RS, Lemke BN, Dortzbach RK, Sherman DD. Identification of human orbital lymphatics. *Ophthal Plast Reconst Surg*. 1999;15(4):252–259.
49. Sherman DD, Gonnering RS, Wallow IHL, et al. Identification of orbital lymphatics: enzyme histochemical light microscopic and electron microscopic studies. *Ophthal Plast Reconstr Surg*. 1993;9(3):153–169.
50. Dickinson AJ, Gausas RE. Orbital lymphatics: do they exist? *Eye*. 2006;20:1145–1148.
51. Gausas RE. Advances in applied anatomy of the eyelid and orbit. *Curr Opin Ophthalmol*. 2004;15:422–425.
52. Damasceno R.W.F., Barbosa J.A.P., Cortez L.R.C., et al. Orbital lymphatic vessels: immunohistochemical detection in the lacrimal gland, optic nerve, fat tissue, and extrinsic oculomotor muscles. Arq Bras Oftalmol; 84(3):209-213.
53. Daniel RK, Landon B. Endoscopic forehead lift: anatomic basis. *Aesthetic Surg J*. 1997;17:97–104.
54. Cook BE, Lucarelli MJ, Lemke BN. Depressor supercilii muscle: anatomy, histology, and cosmetic implications. *Ophthal Plast Reconstr Surg*. 2001;17(6):411–414.
55. Mitz V, Peyronie M. The superficial musculo-aponeurotic system (SMAS) in the parotid and cheek area. *Plast Reconstr Surg*. 1976;58:80–88.
56. Rose J.G., Lucarelli M.J., Lemke B.N. Radiologic measurement of the subcutaneous depth of the SMAS in the midface. In *Proceedings of American Society of Ophthalmic Plastic and Reconstructive Surgery*. Orlando, FL; Oct 18–19, 2002.
57. Wassef M. Superficial fascial and muscular layers in the face and neck: a histologic study. *Aesthetic Plast Surg*. 1987;11:171–176.
58. Thaller SR, Kim S, Patterson H, et al. The submuscular aponeurotic system (SMAS): a histologic and comparative anatomy evaluation. *Plast Reconstr Surg*. 1990;86(4):690–696.
59. Jost G, Lamouche G. SMAS in rhytidectomy. *Aesthetic Plast Surg*. 1982;6:69–74.
60. Furnas DW. The retaining ligaments of the cheek. *Past Reconstr Surg*. 1989;83(1):11–16.
61. Kikkawa DO, Lemke BN, Dortzbach RK. Relations of the superficial musculoaponeurotic system to the orbit and characterization of the orbitomalar ligament. *Ophthal Plast Reconstr Surg*. 1996;12:77–88.
62. Lucarelli MJ, Khwarg SI, Lemke BN, et al. The anatomy of midfacial ptosis. *Ophthal Plast Reconstr Surg*. 2000;16(1):7–22.
63. Muzaffar AR, Mendelson BC, Adams Jr. WP. Surgical anatomy of the ligamentous attachments of the lower lid and lateral canthus. *Plast Reconstr Surg*. 2002;110(3):873–884.
64. Freilinger G, Gruber H, Happak W, et al. Surgical anatomy of the mimic muscle system and the facial nerve: importance for reconstructive and aesthetic surgery. *Plast Reconst Surg*. 1987;80(5):686–690.
65. Katusic S.K., Beard C.M., Wiederholt W.C. et al. *Incidence, clinical features, and prognosis in Bell's palsy*, Rochester, Minnesota, 1968–1982.
66. Rahman I, Sadiq SA. Ophthalmic management of facial nerve palsy: a review. *Surv Ophthalmol*. 2007;52(2):121–144.
67. Graziani C, Panico C, Botti G, Collin RJ. Subperiosteal midface lift: its role in static lower eyelid reconstruction after chronic facial nerve palsy. *Orbit*. 2011;30(3):140–144.
68. Whitnall SE. *The anatomy of the human orbit and accessory organs of vision*. 2nd edn. New York: Oxford University Press; 1932.
69. Lipham WJ, Tawfik HA, Dutton JJ. A histologic analysis and three-dimensional reconstruction of the muscle of Riolan. *Ophthal Plast Reconstr Surg*. 2002;18(2):93–98.
70. Becker BB. Tricompartment model of the lacrimal pump mechanism. *Ophthalmology*. 1992;99:1139–1145.
71. Milz S, Neufang J, Higashiyama I, et al. An immunohistochemical study of the extracellular matrix of the tarsal plate in the upper eyelid in human beings. *J Anat*. 2005;206:37–45.
72. Wesley RE, McCord CD, Jones NA. Height of the tarsus of the lower eyelid. *Am J Ophthalmol*. 1980;90(1):102–105.
73. Jones LT. A new concept of the orbital fascia and rectus muscle sheaths and its surgical implications. *Trans Am Acad Ophthalmol Otolaryngol*. 1968;72:755–764.
74. Mathers WD. Ocular evaporation in meibomian gland dysfunction and dry eye. *Ophthalmology*. 1993;100(3):347–351.
75. Scheie HG, Albert DM. Distichiasis and trichiasis: origin and management. *Am J Ophthalmol*. 1966;61:718–720.
76. Frueh BR. Treatment of distichiasis with cryotherapy. *Ophthalmic Surg*. 1981;12(2):100–103.
77. Bartley GB, Lowry JC. Argon laser treatment of trichiasis. *Am J Ophthalmol*. 1992;113(1): 71–74.
78. McCracken MS, Kikkawa DO, Vasani SN. Treatment of trichiasis and distichiasis by eyelash trephination. *Ophthal Plast Reconstr Surg*. 2006;22(5):349–351.
79. Foster CS. Cicatricial pemphigoid. *Trans Am Ophthalmol Soc*. 1986;84:527–563.
80. Lander T, Wirtschafter JD, McLoon LK. Orbicularis oculi muscle fibers are relatively short and heterogeneous in length. *Invest Ophthalmol Vis Sci*. 1996;37(9):1732–1739.
81. Ng SK, Chan W, Marcet MM, Kakizaki H, Selva D. Levator palpebrae superioris: an anatomical update. *Orbit*. 2013;32(1):76–84.
82. Lemke BN, Stasior OG, Rosenberg PN. The surgical relations of the levator palpebrae superioris muscle. *Ophthal Plast Reconstr Surg*. 1988;4(1):25–30.
83. Anderson RL, Dixon RS. The role of Whitnall's ligament in ptosis surgery. *Arch Ophthalmol*. 1979;97:705.
84. Stasior GO, Lemke BN, Wallow IH, et al. Levator aponeurosis elastic fiber network. *Ophthal Plast Reconstr Surg*. 1993;9(1):1–10.
85. Kuwabara T, Cogan DG, Johnson CC. Structure of the muscles of the upper eyelid. *Arch Ophthalmol*. 1975;93:1189–1197.
86. Kakizaki H, Malhotra R, Madge SN, Selva D. Lower eyelid anatomy: an update. *Ann Plast Surg*. 2009;63(3):344–351.
87. Kang H, Takahashi Y, Nakano T, Asamoto K, Ikeda H, Kakizaki H. Medial canthal support structures: the medial retinaculum: a review. *Ann Plast Surg*. 2017;74(4):508–514.
88. Kang H, Takahashi Y, Ichinose A, Nakano T, Asamoto K, Ikeda H, Iwaki M, Kakizaki H. Lateral canthal anatomy: a review. *Orbit*. 2012;31(4):279–285.
89. Doane MG. Blinking and the mechanics of the lacrimal drainage system. *Ophthalmology*. 1981;88(8):844–851.
90. Sahlin S, Laurell CG, Chen E, et al. Lacrimal drainage capacity, age and blink rate. *Orbit*. 1998;17:155–159.

91. Dong H, Luo Y, Fan S, Yin B, Weng C, Peng B. Screening gene mutations in Chinese patients with benign essential blepharospasm. *Front Neurol.* 2020;10:1387.
92. Mauriello JA, Carbonaro P, Dhillon S, et al. Drug-associated facial dyskinesias: a study of 238 patients. *J Neuroophthalmol.* 1998;18(2):153–157.
93. Frueh B, Callahan A, Dortzbach RK, et al. A profile of patients with intractable blepharospasm. *Trans Sect Ophthalmol Am Acad Ophthalmol Otolaryngol.* 1976;81:591–594.
94. Evinger C. Benign essential blepharospasm is a disorder of neuroplasticity: lessons from animal models. *J Neuroophthalmol.* 2015;35:374–379.
95. Dutton JJ, Buckley EG. Long-term results and complications of botulinum A toxin in the treatment of blepharospasm. *Ophthalmology.* 1988;95:1529–1534.
96. Sires BS, Saari JC, Garwin GG, et al. The color difference in orbital fat. *Arch Ophthalmol.* 2001;119(6):868–871.
97. Kawai K, Imanishi N, Nakajima Y, et al. Arterial anatomical features of the upper palpebra. *Plast Reconstr Surg.* 2004;113(2):479–484.
98. Cook Jr BE, Lucarelli MJ, Lemke BN, et al. Eyelid Lymphatics I: Histochemical comparisons between the monkey and human. *Ophthal Plast Reconstr Surg.* 2002;18(1):18–23.
99. Cook Jr BE, Lucarelli MJ, Lemke BN, et al. Eyelid Lymphatics II: A search for drainage patterns in the monkey and correlations with human lymphatics. *Ophthal Plast Reconstr Surg.* 2002;18(2):99–106.
100. Knize DM. A study of the supraorbital nerve. *Plast Reconst Surg.* 1995;96(3):564–569.

15

Formation and Function of the Tear Film

Darlene A. Dartt

TEAR FILM OVERVIEW

The tear film overlays the ocular surface, which is comprised of the corneal and conjunctival epithelia and provides the interface between these epithelia and the external environment. The tear film is essential for the health and protection of the ocular surface and for clear vision, as the tear film is the first refractive surface of the eye.[1]

Tears produced by the ocular surface epithelia and adnexa are distributed throughout the cul-de-sac. Using ocular coherence tomography, the thickness of the precorneal tear film was measured as $3.4 + 2.6\,\mu m$,[2] agreeing with previous measurements using less accurate techniques.[3–7]

The tear film is an exceedingly complex mixture of secretions from multiple tissues and epithelia (Fig. 15.1) and consists of two layers (Fig. 15.2). Not a layer, but a component that interacts with the tear film, is the glycocalyx, which extends from the superficial layer of the ocular surface epithelium. The first layer of the tear film consists of two components. The first is mucus that covers the glycocalyx and mixes with the aqueous components. The second layer is the outermost layer that contains lipids. Production and function of main tear film components are distinct and will be presented separately.

Tear secretion by all ocular adnexa and ocular surface epithelia must be coordinated. For the mucoaqueous layer, secretion is predominantly regulated by neural reflexes. Stimulation of sensory nerves in cornea and conjunctiva activates a complex neural reflex. Briefly, the ascending portion includes the corneal and conjunctival sensory nerves, the trigeminal ganglion, then the trigeminal brainstem complex nucleus, and the superior salivatory nucleus. The descending parasympathetic pathway runs from the parasympathetic nucleus of the facial nerve to the pterygopalatine ganglion, and the post-ganglionic parasympathetic nerves that travel to the lacrimal gland (Fig. 15.3). The descending sympathetic pathway travels through the superior cervical ganglion and the post-ganglionic sympathetic nerves innervate the lacrimal gland. Activation of this reflex stimulates the lacrimal gland and conjunctival goblet cells to cause mucus, protein, and fluid secretion. For the lipid layer, the blink itself regulates release of presecreted meibomian gland lipids stored in the meibomian gland duct. When the eyelids retract, a thin film of lipid overspreads the underlying mucoaqueous layer.

Tear secretion is balanced by drainage and evaporation. Tears on the ocular surface are drained through lacrimal puncta into the lacrimal drainage system. Drainage of tears can be regulated by neural reflexes from the ocular surface that cause vasodilation and vasoconstriction of the cavernous sinus blood supply of the drainage duct (Fig. 15.4). Both vasoconstriction and vasodilation cause a change in geometry of the lumen that decreases drainage.[8] Evaporation depends on the amount of time the tear film is exposed between blinks and temperature, humidity, wind speed, and composition of the tear film. The remainder of the chapter focuses on regulation of tear secretion.

GLYCOCALYX

Structure

The glycocalyx is a network of polysaccharides that project from cellular surfaces. In corneal and conjunctival epithelia, the glycocalyx can be found on the apical portion of the microvilli that project from the apical plasma membrane of the superficial cell layer (Fig. 15.2). Mucins are a critical component of the glycocalyx. Mucins consist of a protein core of amino acids linked by *O*-glycosylation to carbohydrate sidechains of varying length and complexity. Mucins are classified by the nomenclature MUC1–21 and are divided into secreted and membrane-spanning categories (Fig. 15.5). Membrane-spanning mucins consist of a short intracellular tail, a membrane-spanning domain, and a large, extended extracellular domain that forms the glycocalyx. Secreted mucins are either gel-forming or small soluble. Gel-forming mucins are large molecules (20–40 million Da) secreted by exocytosis from goblet cells. Small soluble mucins are secreted by the lacrimal gland.

The ocular surface contains the membrane-spanning mucins MUC1, MUC4, and MUC16.[9] These mucins are produced by stratified squamous cells of the cornea and conjunctiva and are stored in small, clear secretory vesicles in the cytoplasm (Fig. 15.1). Fusion of secretory vesicles with the plasma membrane inserts these molecules into the plasma membrane. Mucin molecules are localized to the tips of the squamous cell microplicae and extend up to 500 nm above the plasma membrane.[10] These mucins form a distinct glycocalyx by extending far above the other glycoconjugates such as the proteoglycans (heparan sulfate and chondroitin sulfate) and gangliosides that are richly present in the glycocalyx. In addition, the galactosyl residues on the mucins in the glycocalyx are crosslinked by the multimeric lectin galectin-3. This interaction is important for the maintenance of the epithelial barrier and the prevention of cellular damage.

There is limited information on the regulation of membrane-spanning mucin synthesis and secretion. Regulation of secretion would be by the regulation of insertion of mucins into plasma membranes or by control of ectodomain shedding, whereby matrix metalloproteinases (MMPs) cleave the mucin and release the extracellular, active domain of the protein into the extracellular space. In immortalized stratified corneal-limbal cells, tumor necrosis factor induced the ectodomain shedding of MUC1, MUC4, and MUC16, whereas MMP-7 and neutrophil elastase induced the shedding of MUC16 only.[11] These compounds that caused shedding are elevated in the tears of dry eye patients and thus may cause the increase in Rose-Bengal staining found in dry eye and associated with loss of MUC16 (Box 15.1).

Function on the ocular surface

The membrane-spanning mucins function to hydrate the ocular surface and serve as a barrier to pathogens. Membrane-spanning mucins

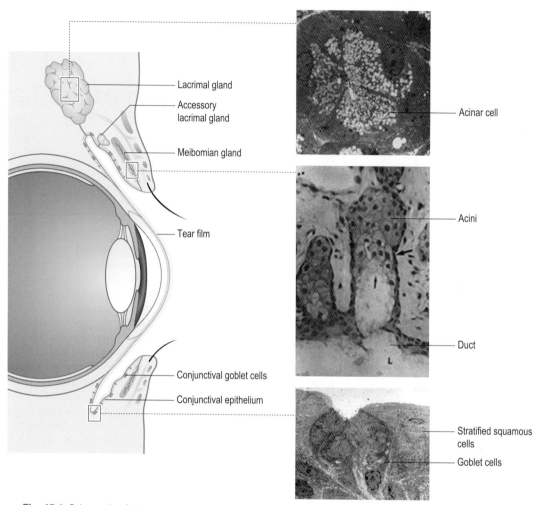

Fig. 15.1 Schematic of the glands and epithelia that secrete tears. The ocular surface epithelia are in *beige* and the lacrimal glands are in *pink*, and their contribution to the tear film is in *blue*. An electron micrograph of conjunctival goblet cells is in the *bottom inset*. An electron micrograph of a lacrimal gland acinus is shown in the *top inset*. An electron micrograph of a meibomian gland acinus with its attached duct is shown in the *middle inset*. (Modified from Dartt DA. The lacrimal gland and dry eye diseases. In: Levin LA, Albert DA, eds. *Ocular Disease: Mechanism and Management*. Amsterdam: Elsevier; 2008. Copyright Elsevier 2010.)

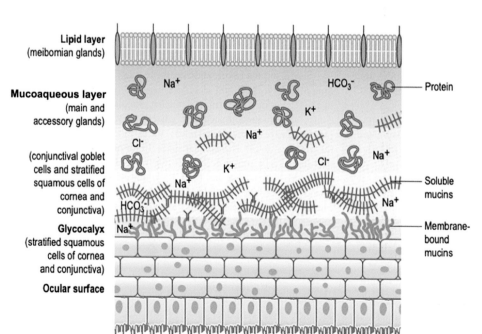

Fig. 15.2 Schematic of the tear film. The outer lipid layer is secreted by meibomian glands. The inner layer contains electrolytes, water, proteins, and small soluble mucins produced by lacrimal glands and conjunctival epithelium, as well as gel-forming mucin (MUC5AC), proteins, electrolytes, and water secreted by conjunctival goblet cells. The glycocalyx is comprised of membrane-bound mucins produced by stratified squamous cells of the corneal and conjunctival epithelial cells. The tear film overlies the ocular surface. (Modified from Hodges RR, Dartt DA. Regulatory pathways in lacrimal gland epithelium. *Int Rev Cytol*. 2003;231:129–196. Copyright Elsevier 2003.)

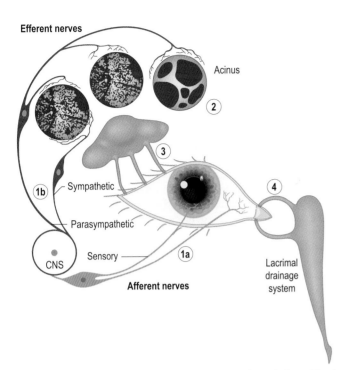

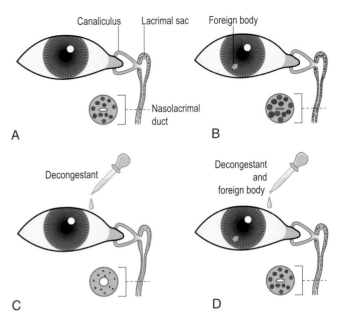

Fig. 15.3 Schematic of afferent and efferent neural regulation of lacrimal gland secretion. Schematic of the neural regulation of lacrimal gland electrolyte, water, and protein secretion. Lacrimal gland secretion is stimulated by the sensory nerves in the cornea or conjunctiva, which, in turn, activate the efferent parasympathetic and sympathetic nerves that innervate the acini of the lacrimal gland. Lacrimal gland fluid flows onto the ocular surface through the lacrimal gland excretory ducts and is drained from the eye via the lacrimal drainage system. *CNS*, Central nervous system; *PG*, pterygopalatine ganglion; *SC*, superior cervical ganglion; *TG*, trigeminal ganglion. (Modified from Dartt DA. The lacrimal gland and dry eye diseases. In: Levin LA, Albert DA, eds. *Ocular Disease: Mechanism and Management*. Amsterdam: Elsevier; 2008.)

Fig. 15.4 Schematic anatomic model of the state of the cavernous body and lacrimal passage. **(A)** The lumen of the nasolacrimal duct under resting conditions. **(B)** A foreign body in the eye causes activation of nerves in the cavernous body causing vasodilation of the blood vessels and a narrowing of the lumen that results in decreased tear drainage. **(C)** Placement of decongestant of the ocular surface causes vasoconstriction of the blood vessels of the cavernous body, and opening of the lumen of the nasolacrimal duct, and surprisingly a decrease in drainage. **(D)** Vasoconstriction caused by the foreign body and vasodilation by the topical congestant prevent a change in the shape of the lumen and in the drainage of tears. (Modified from Ayub M, Thale AB, Hedderich J, Tillmann BN, Paulsen FP. The cavernous body of the human efferent tear ducts contributes to regulation of tear outflow. *Invest Ophthalmol Vis Sci*. 2003 Nov;44(11):4900–4907. Reproduced from the Association for Research in Vision and Ophthalmology.)

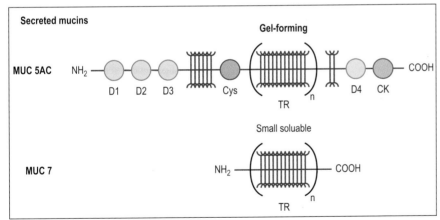

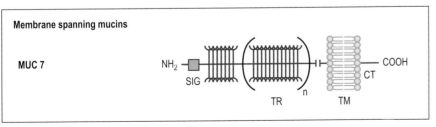

Fig. 15.5 Structural motifs of the secreted and membrane-spanning mucins (MUC). MUC5AC consists of four cysteine-rich D domains (D1–D4) for disulfide crosslinking and flank a region of variable number tandem repeats (*TRs*). MUC7 is monomeric and has a variable number of TRs. The membrane-spanning mucins have a peptide signal sequence (*SIG*) domain, a variable number of TRs, a site for cleavage of the extracellular domain, a transmembrane domain (*TM*) for insertion of the molecule into membranes, and a carboxyterminus (*CT*) that is the intracellular domain. *CK*, cysteine knot. (Modified from Gipson IK, Argueso P. Role of mucins in the function of the corneal and conjunctival epithelia. *Int Rev Cytol*. 2003. 231:1–49. Copyright Elsevier 2003.)

are considered to be dysadhesive, allowing the goblet cell mucus (see section Mucus production) to move over the ocular surface. The carbohydrate side-chains hold water at the surface of the apical cell membranes. The function of individual membrane-spanning mucins remains unclear.

Membrane-spanning mucins appear to be altered in dry eye. MUC16 protein levels were decreased in conjunctival epithelium and increased in tears of patients with Sjögren's syndrome.[12,13] MUC1 splice variants also play a role in dry eye.[14] Human cornea and conjunctiva contain five previously identified MUC1 splice variants and a new splice variant. These splice variants have unique changes that could affect their ectodomain shedding, signaling properties of the intracellular domain, and water retention, lubrication, and barrier properties of the extracellular domains. When the type of MUC1 splice variant was determined in dry eye patients (both evaporative dry eye and Sjögren's syndrome), compared with control patients, there was a reduced frequency of MUC1/A variant and an increase in MUC1/B variant in the dry eye patients.[14,15]

MUCOUS PRODUCTION

Structure

Mucus produced by the conjunctiva consists of MUC5AC, proteins, electrolytes, and water synthesized and secreted by the goblet and stratified squamous cells of the corneal and conjunctival epithelia. The backbone of mucus is the gel-forming mucin, MUC5AC, synthesized and secreted by conjunctival goblet cells. MUC5AC is encoded by one of the largest genes known, producing a protein of about 600 kDa. The protein backbone of MUC5AC consists of four D domains (cysteine-rich domains) (Fig. 15.5) that flank a tandem repeat sequence in which amino acids in the protein backbone are O-glycosylated and linked to carbohydrate side-chains. The D domains provide sites for disulfide bonds crosslinking multiple MUC5AC molecules, which forms the framework of the mucus. Also contained in the mucous layer are shed ectodomains of membrane-spanning mucins, membrane-spanning mucins secreted by a soluble pathway, other proteins synthesized and secreted by goblet cells, and electrolytes and water secreted by goblet and stratified squamous cells.

Conjunctival goblet cells

Goblet cells are interspersed among stratified squamous cells of the conjunctiva (see Fig. 15.1). Goblet cells occur in clusters in rat and mouse, but singly in rabbit and humans.[16–18] In all species studied, goblet cells are unevenly distributed over the conjunctiva.

Goblet cells are identified by the large accumulation of mucin granules in the apex (see Fig. 15.1). Secretory products can be visualized using Alcian blue–periodic acid stain, the lectins *Ulex europaeus* agglutinin I (UEA-I) or *Helix pomatia* agglutinin (HPA), or antibodies

to MUC5AC. MUC5AC is synthesized in the endoplasmic reticulum, and carbohydrate side-chains are added in the Golgi apparatus. The mature proteins are stored in secretory granules. Upon stimulation, secretory granules fuse with each other and the apical membrane and release secretory product into the tear film. Upon cell stimulation the entire complement of granules is released.[19] The amount of secretion is controlled by regulating the number of cells that are activated by a given stimulus.

Regulation of goblet cell mucin production
Overview

Mucin production is regulated by controlling the rate of mucin synthesis, rate of mucin secretion, and the number of goblet cells present in the conjunctiva. The rate of mucin synthesis has yet to be studied in conjunctival goblet cells. Thus, the remainder of this section focuses on regulation of secretion and proliferation. Under physiologic conditions in health, goblet cells secrete mucus in response to the challenges from the environment to maintain homeostasis. In disease, goblet cell mucous secretion can be overproduced, as in ocular allergy, or underproduced, as in dry eye. As goblet cell secretion is tightly regulated, goblet cells and their secretion can be returned to homeostasis.

Regulation of goblet cell secretion in health

Nerves are the primary regulators of conjunctival goblet cell secretion under physiologic conditions. The conjunctiva is innervated by afferent sensory nerves and efferent sympathetic and parasympathetic nerves. Sensory nerves end as free nerve endings between the stratified squamous cells. The parasympathetic and sympathetic nerve endings also surround the middle of the goblet cells at the level of the most basal secretory granules (Fig. 15.6). Stimulation of the sensory nerves in the cornea by a neural reflex induces goblet cell secretion via the efferent nerves. Goblet cells have receptors for neurotransmitters from both parasympathetic and sympathetic nerves. Parasympathetic nerves release both acetylcholine (Ach) and vasoactive intestinal peptide (VIP). Muscarinic receptors of the muscarinic 3 acetylcholine receptor (M_3AchR) and M_2AchR subtypes are located on the goblet cells at the middle near the efferent nerve endings (Fig. 15.6).[20,21] VIP receptors of the VIPAC2 receptor subtype are located in the same area as M_3AchR.[21] Sympathetic nerves release norepinephrine and NPY. Several subtypes of both α_1- and β-adrenergic receptors are present on goblet cells.[20] It appears that parasympathetic nerves using Ach and VIP are the primary stimuli of goblet cell secretion. The function of the sympathetic nerves remains unstudied.

Components of the signaling pathways used by Ach and VIP have been delineated.[21] Cholinergic agonists use M_3AchR and M_2AchR to stimulate goblet cell secretion.[22] Cholinergic agonists presumably use the $G_{\alpha q/11}$ subtype of G protein that activates phospholipase C to break down phosphatidylinositol 4,5 bisphosphate to produce inositol 1,4,5 trisphosphate (IP_3) and diacylglycerol. IP_3 would then release intracellular Ca^{2+} by binding to its receptors on the endoplasmic reticulum. Based on a variety of experiments, cholinergic agonists are known to increase the intracellular $[Ca^{2+}]$ to stimulate secretion.[23,24]

The diacylglycerol released with IP_3 activates protein kinase C (PKC). Nine PKC isoforms are present in conjunctival goblet cells, and phorbol esters, activators of PKC isoforms, stimulate goblet cell secretion.[23] Although a role for PKC isoforms in secretion could not be substantiated,[23] it is likely that cholinergic agonists use PKC isoforms to stimulate secretion, as PKC inhibitors block a distal step in the signaling pathway, the activation of extracellular regulated kinase (ERK1/2)[25] (Fig. 15.7).

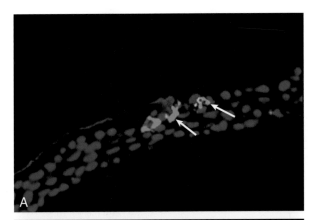

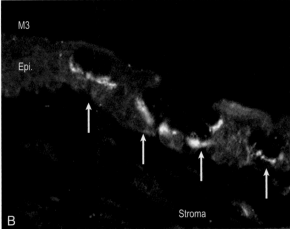

Fig. 15.6 Immunofluorescence micrographs of parasympathetic nerves and M$_3$Ach receptors in rat conjunctiva. (**A**) The parasympathetic neurotransmitter vasoactive intestinal peptide (VIP) is shown in *green*. The lectin *Ulex europeaus* is shown in *red* and indicates the location of goblet cells. The goblet cell body is subjacent to the secretory granules. The cell nuclei are shown in *blue*. (Reprinted with permission from Diebold Y, Ríos JD, Hodges RR, Rawe I, Dartt DA. Presence of nerves and their receptors in mouse and human conjunctival goblet cells. *Invest Ophthalmol Vis Sci.* 2001;42(10):2270–2282.) (**B**) The M$_3$AchR is shown. The *dark areas* indicate the goblet cell secretory granules. *Arrows* indicate cell bodies of goblet cells. *EPi*, epithelium. (Reprinted with permission from Ríos JD, Zoukhri D, Rawe IM, Hodges RR, Zieske JD, Dartt DA. Immunolocalization of muscarinic and VIP receptor subtypes and their role in stimulating goblet cell secretion. *Invest Ophthalmol Vis Sci.* 1999;40(6):1102–1111. Reproduced from the Association for Research in Vision and Ophthalmology.)

Cholinergic agonists are known to activate the epidermal growth factor (EGF) signaling pathway. In goblet cells, cholinergic agonists activate the nonreceptor tyrosine kinases Pyk2 and p60Src.[22] These kinases transactivate (phosphorylate) the EGF receptor. This transactivation is usually mediated by ectodomain shedding by MMP, causing the release of the extracellular, active domain of one member of the EGF family of growth factors, but this ectodomain shedding has yet to be tested in goblet cells. The released growth factor would bind to the EGF receptor inducing two receptors to associate and be autophosphorylated. This attracts the adapter proteins Shc and Grb2 that are phosphorylated, activating the guanine nucleotide exchange factor, SOS, to increase Ras activity. Ras activates MAPK kinase kinase (Raf) that phosphorylates MAPK kinase (MEK) that phosphorylates ERK1/2. In both rat and human goblet cells, cholinergic agonists

increase intracellular [Ca^{2+}] and activate PKC to stimulate goblet cell secretion by activating Pyk2 and p60Src to transactivate the EGF receptor, inducing the signaling cascade that activates extracellular signal-regulated kinase 1/2 (ERK1/2) (Fig. 15.7).[22,25,26]

There are several non-neural agonists that stimulate goblet cell secretion. These agonists include the specialized proresolving mediators (SPMs) that are biosynthesized from omega-6 and omega-3 fatty acids. They also include ATP, which stimulates goblet cell secretion via purinergic receptors (P) of the P2X$_7$ and P2Y$_2$ subtypes,[27] and the neurotrophin family of growth factors, of which nerve growth factor (NGF) and brain-derived neurotrophic factor (BDNF) stimulate secretion.[28] The SPMs include the lipoxins (LXA$_4$),[29] D-series resolvins (RvD1–2),[30,31] E-series resolvins (RvE1),[32] and maresins (MaR1).[33] In conjunctival goblet cells, these mediators use specific G protein–coupled receptors; activate phospholipase C, D, and/or A$_2$; increase intracellular [Ca^{2+}]; activate PKA (selected mediators); transactivate epidermal growth factor receptor (EGFR) (selected mediators); and stimulate secretion.

The action of the purinergic receptor, P2X$_7$, was studied by patch-clamp analysis in freshly isolated tissue,[34] whereas all the other agonists that were studied were by biochemical and cell biologic methods in cultured cells in health and disease.

Regulation of goblet cell secretion in disease

In health, goblet cell secretion is regulated by nerves and SPMs responding to the environment to secrete enough mucus to protect the ocular surface. Both a decrease and an increase in goblet cell secretion leads to disease. Diseases such as allergic conjunctivitis and dry eye increase and decrease secretion, respectively, with destabilization of the tear film causing symptoms in both. In allergy, autacoids such as histamine and proinflammatory mediators such as leukotrienes and prostaglandins, through their receptors present on goblet cells, causing an overproduction of mucus. SPMs can block this overproduction by phosphorylating the proinflammatory receptors and counter-regulating their actions. This returns the tear film back to homeostasis.

The P2X$_7$ receptor plays a role in dry eye disease. Patch-clamp analysis indicated that hyperosmolarity, as occurs in dry eye, activates the ATP-sensitive potassium channels (K$_{ATP}$), nonspecific cation channels (NSCs), voltage-gated calcium channels, and P2X$_7$ channels all found on goblet cells, and in that order.[34] These channels, either by themselves or by interacting with efferent nerve neurotransmitters, cause mucous secretion through exocytosis and resolve dry eye by replenishing the mucous layer. Activation of the P2X$_7$ receptors by ATP released from dying cells can also cause goblet cell death that contributes to chronic dry eye. Thus, changing the balance of action of P2X$_7$ receptors can either resolve or exacerbate dry eye disease. The finding of voltage-sensitive channels in the goblet cells suggests that their role should be re-evaluated in the action of neural agonists and SPMs.

Regulation of goblet cell proliferation

The amount of goblet cell mucin on the ocular surface can also be modulated by controlling goblet cell proliferation. Serum, which contains a variety of growth factors, stimulates proliferation of cultured conjunctival goblet cells, both human and rat.[35] EGF, transforming growth factor (TGFα), and heparin binding–EGF (HB-EGF), but not heregulin, stimulate proliferation.[35] EGF, TGFα, and HB-EGF bind to the EGF receptor (EGFR or erb-B1), EGF binds to erb-B4, and heregulin binds to erb-B3 and erb-B4. That EGF, TGFα, and HB-EGF are equipotent in stimulating conjunctival goblet cell proliferation suggests that EGFR and erb-B4 are the primary receptors used.[35]

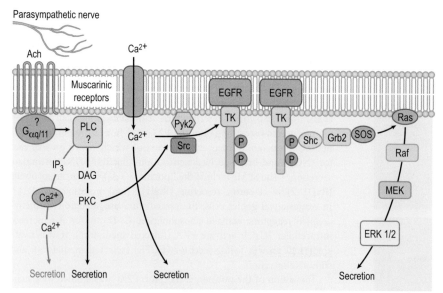

Fig. 15.7 Signaling pathways used by cholinergic agonists to stimulate conjunctival goblet cell secretion—the pathway is described in the text. *Ach*, Acetylcholine; *DAG*, diacylglycerol; *EGFR*, epidermal growth factor receptor; *ERK 1/2*, extracellular regulated kinase; *Gαq/11*, G protein alpha q/11; *IP3*, inositol 1,4,5 trisphosphate; *MEK*, mitogen activated protein kinase kinase; *P*, phosphorylation; *PKC*, protein kinase C; *PLC*, phospholipase C; *SOS*, guanine nucleotide exchange factor; *TK*, tyrosine kinase. (Modified from Dartt DA. Regulation of mucin and fluid secretion by conjunctival epithelial cells. *Prog Ret Eye Res.* 2002;21:555–576.)

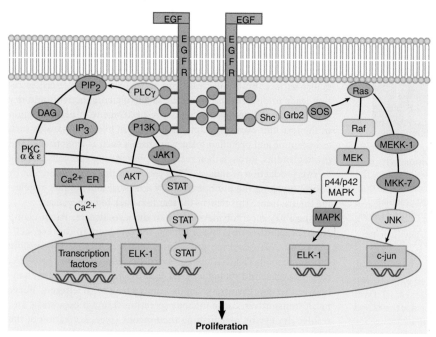

Fig. 15.8 Schematic of epidermal growth factor (*EGF*)–dependent signaling pathways. Potential signaling pathways that can be used by EGF to stimulate cell proliferation. *Ach*, Acetylcholine; *DAG*, diacylglycerol; *EGF*, epidermal growth factor; *EGFR*, epidermal growth factor receptor; *ER*, endoplasmic reticulum; *ERK 1/2*, extracellular regulated kinase; *IP3*, inositol 1,4,5 trisphosphate; *P*, phosphorylation; *JNK*, Jun-N terminal kinase; *MAPK*, mitogen activated protein kinase; *MEKK-1*, mitogen activated protein kinase kinase kinase; *p44/p42* goes with *MAPK, PIP2*, phosphatidylinositol 4,5 bisphosphate; *PI3K*, phosphoinositide 3-kinase; *PKC*, protein kinase C; *PLCγ*, phospholipase C gamma; *SOS*, guanine nucleotide exchange factor; *TK*, tyrosine kinase.

EGF was used as the prototype of the EGF family. EGF increases the activation of EGFR in rat conjunctival goblet cells and activates ERK1/2 (also known as p44/p42 mitogen-activated protein kinase [MAPK]) (Fig. 15.8) causing its biphasic translocation to the nucleus.[36] The slower sustained second peak response is responsible for cell proliferation, but the role of the rapid transient first peak is not known. Activation of PKC isoforms also mediates EGF-stimulated goblet cell proliferation (Fig. 15.8). In rat and human goblet cells, EGF uses PKCα and PKCε to stimulate conjunctival goblet cell proliferation.

The experiments on proliferation were performed in cell culture. These findings may not apply to goblet cells in vivo, because the conjunctival epithelium architecture, including polarized goblet cells linked with each other and stratified squamous cells by tight junctions, is lacking in culture. Experiments on cell proliferation in tissues are challenging but critical to perform.

Regulation of conjunctival electrolyte and water secretion

The electrolyte and water composition of the external environment has an important effect on release of mucins from secretory granules. Both the stratified squamous and goblet cells of the conjunctiva express ion and water transport proteins and appear to secrete electrolytes and water. Mucin, electrolyte, and water secretion may not be coordinated as the stimuli of mucin secretion appear to differ from those of electrolyte and water secretion.

The conjunctival epithelium secretes Cl^- and absorbs Na^+ with the ratio of 1.5 to 1 causing a net secretion of fluid into the tear film.[37] Interestingly, both absorption and secretion occur within the same cell in the conjunctiva. The ion transport proteins are distributed evenly in all areas of the conjunctiva, suggesting that the entire conjunctiva participates in fluid secretion.

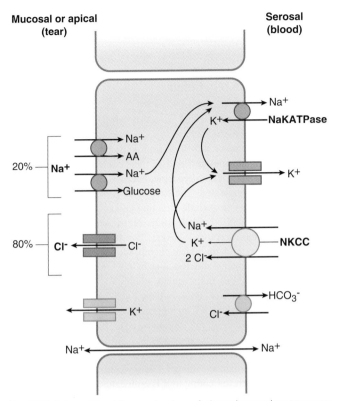

Mucosal or apical (tear)

Serosal (blood)

Fig. 15.9 Schematic of the mechanism of electrolyte and water secretion by conjunctival epithelial cells – a description of the process is found in the text. *Cl⁻*, Chloride; *HCO3⁻*, bicarbonate; *K⁺*, potassium; *Na⁺*, sodium; *NaKATPase*, sodium—potassium adenosine triphosphatase; *NKCC*, Na⁺-K⁺-2Cl⁻ cotransporter. (Modified from Dartt DA. Regulation of mucin and fluid secretion by conjunctival epithelial cells. *Prog Ret Eye Res.* 2002;21:555–576.)

The driving force for conjunctival fluid secretion is the basolaterally located Na^+K^+-ATPase (NKA) that extrudes three Na^+ ions for the influx of two K^+ ions and generates a negative intracellular voltage (Fig. 15.9). Also on the basolateral side is the Na^+-K^+-$2Cl^-$ cotransporter (NKCC1). The Cl^-/HCO_3^- exchangers take up Cl^- into the cell. Cl^- is secreted from the apical side of the cell through a variety of Cl^- channels. K^+ is also secreted from the apical side with Na^+ moving through the paracellular pathway to the apical side. The net effect is isotonic secretion of Na^+, K^+, and Cl^- into the tears.[38]

Na^+ is absorbed across the apical membrane into the cell by the Na^+-dependent glucose cotransporter. The Na^+ that enters the cell on the apical side is extruded on the basolateral side by the NKA. The Na^+ influx mechanism can also be used to transport amino acids into the cell.[39]

Fluid secretion by the conjunctiva can be stimulated, contributing to the volume of the tear film and ensuring proper hydration of mucins as they are released from the secretory granules. Increasing the intracellular $[Ca^{2+}]$ or the cellular level of cAMP causes Cl^- secretion.[40,41] The β-adrenergic agonist epinephrine stimulates secretion via cAMP. Increasing cellular cAMP levels activate PKA, which stimulates both Cl^- secretion and Na^+ absorption by activating K^+ channels in the basolateral membrane to hyperpolarize the cell. Hyperpolarization stimulates Na^+ influx (into the cell) and Cl^- efflux (into tears) across the apical membrane. PKA also stimulates apical Cl^- channels. Because there is a higher rate of Cl^- secretion relative to Na^+ absorption, water moves into tears in the basolateral to apical direction. In addition, Na^+ moves paracellularly to produce an isotonic NaCl secretion into tears. Water moves through water channels known as aquaporins (AQP).

AQP5 is expressed in the apical membrane and AQP3 in the lateral membrane of conjunctival epithelial cells.

Activation of the purinergic receptor $P2Y_2$ by uridine triphosphate (UTP) and ATP also stimulates electrolyte and water secretion from the conjunctiva. $P2Y_2$ receptors increase intracellular $[Ca^{2+}]$.[42]

Mucous function on the ocular surface

The major roles of the conjunctiva are to contribute to tear production by secreting electrolytes and water, modify composition of the tear film by secreting mucins, absorb various organic compounds found in tears (including ophthalmic therapeutics), and contribute to resistance of the eye to infection by providing protection against microorganisms.[43] Mucins serve as wetting agents that keep the apical epithelia hydrated. Finally, conjunctival cells release paracrine signaling agents, such as growth factors that affect ocular surface properties.

AQUEOUS PRODUCTION

Overview

The main lacrimal gland is the major producer of the electrolytes, water, and protein portion (volume) of the mucoaqueous layer of the tear film. Other ocular surface epithelia also contribute to the volume of the tear film, most notably the conjunctiva (discussed in the section Regulation of conjunctival electrolyte and water secretion), accessory lacrimal glands, and to a small extent corneal epithelium. Accessory lacrimal glands, which are similar to the main gland, are imbedded in the conjunctiva. Function of the accessory lacrimal glands has not been extensively investigated as they are difficult to study in isolation. Results to date, however, indicate that these glands are similar in structure and function to the main lacrimal gland. This section focuses on the main lacrimal gland, which is referred to as the lacrimal gland.

Lacrimal gland structure

The lacrimal gland is comprised of acini that drain into progressively larger tubules or ducts that coalesce into one or more excretory ducts. Acini are made up of basal myoepithelial cells that surround an inner layer of columnar secretory cells known as acinar cells (see Fig. 15.1). The stellate-shaped myoepithelial cells contract in response to the purinergic agonists UTP and ATP and the parasympathomimetic agonist carbachol,[44] as well as the hormone oxytocin, which is known to work in the mammary gland myoepithelial cells.[45] In the lacrimal gland, these cells contribute to the repair of acinar cells, but their role in secretion remains unknown. Acinar cells comprise about 80% of the gland and are organized in clusters. In cross-section, an acinus contains a ring of pyramid-shaped acinar cells that are joined at the junction of the apical and lateral membranes by tight junctions. The tight junctions polarize the cells and ensure unidirectional secretion of electrolytes, water, and protein, the secretory product of the lacrimal gland.

The lacrimal gland ducts are lined with one or two layers of cuboidal duct cells that make up 10% to 12% of the gland. Similarly to acinar cells, duct cells are joined at the apical side by tight junctions and secrete water, electrolytes, and protein, modifying the primary lacrimal gland fluid secreted by the acinar cells.

The lacrimal gland also contains a population of lymphocytes, plasma cells, mast cells, and macrophages. The plasma cells express immunoglobulins. IgA is a major immunoglobulin, which is taken up into the lacrimal gland acinar cells, where it binds with intracellular secretory components to form secretory IgA. Secretory IgA is secreted into the lacrimal gland fluid and ultimately into the tear fluid. Tear secretory IgA is an important component of the mucosal immune system.

Parasympathetic nerves

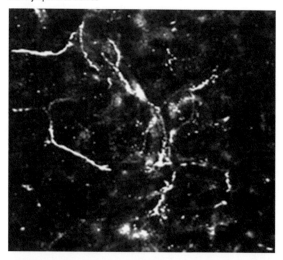

Sympathetic nerves

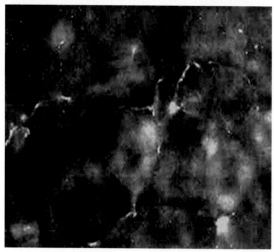

Fig. 15.10 Immunofluorescence micrographs of the distribution of parasympathetic and sympathetic nerves in the lacrimal gland. *Top panel:* anti-vasoactive intestinal peptide demonstrates location of parasympathetic nerves. *Bottom panel:* anti-tyrosine hydroxylase indicates sympathetic nerves.

Lacrimal gland innervation

The lacrimal branch of the trigeminal nerves carries sensory stimuli from the lacrimal gland and forms the afferent innervation of the gland. The efferent innervation of the gland consists of parasympathetic and sympathetic nerves. The parasympathetic nerve endings predominate, surrounding most acini (Fig. 15.10). Sympathetic innervation is less dense, although this is species dependent. Sensory nerves are the most sparsely located.

Afferent sensory nerves from the ocular surface activate the efferent parasympathetic nerves to stimulate lacrimal gland secretion. A complex neural reflex through the CNS, as described in the section Tear film overview and Fig. 15.3, forms the predominant stimulus of lacrimal gland secretion and allows the gland to protect the ocular surface by responding to environmental stimuli.

Parasympathetic nerves release the neurotransmitters Ach and VIP that activate receptors on the myoepithelial, acinar, and duct cells. M_3AchR is the only cholinergic muscarinic receptor in the lacrimal gland. The VIP receptor VIPAC1 is on acinar cells and

VIPAC2 on myoepithelial cells. Sympathetic nerves release the neurotransmitters norepinephrine and neuropeptide Y (NPY). Norepinephrine activates α_{1D}-adrenergic and β-adrenergic receptors located on acinar cells.

Protein secretion regulation

Types of protein secretion

The majority of lacrimal gland secretory proteins are secreted by exocytosis. Secretory proteins are stored in secretory granules. Upon the appropriate stimulus, secretory granule membranes fuse with the apical plasma membranes and release their contents into the lumen. This secretion is known as merocrine, because only a small percentage of granules are released. The exocytotic process is controlled by trafficking effectors that include targeting and specificity factors such as SNAREs (soluble N-ethylmaleimide [NEM] sensitive factor [NSF] attachment protein receptors [SNAPs]) that function in bringing the secretory granules and the apical membrane together for release of cargo secretory proteins and Ras-like in rat brain (Rabs). Rabs are small Ras-like GTPases that regulate membrane trafficking and are active when bound to GTP. Rabs, notably Rab3D and Rab27 isoforms, recruit proteins necessary for membrane fusion and vesicle maturity. Transport factors such as microtubules, actin filaments, and motor proteins are also involved in exocytosis.[46]

Proteins such as secretory IgA are secreted by a combination of transcytosis and ectodomain shedding.[47] Transcytosis is a complex trafficking process in which the compound is endocytosed at the basolateral membrane, transported across the cell in a series of endomembrane components, and secreted at the apical membrane. Secretory IgA and the EGF family of growth factors are secreted by ectodomain shedding.

The signaling pathways used by neurotransmitters to stimulate lacrimal gland secretion were correlated to exocytosis, not to transcytosis or ectodomain shedding. Thus, the following section on signaling pathways focuses on exocytosis. They were performed in vitro in freshly isolated lacrimal gland acini. Electrolyte and water (fluid) secretion needs to be measured in vivo and is discussed in the section Regulation of electrolyte and water secretion.

Cholinergic agonists

The cholinergic agonist Ach binds to M_3AchR on lacrimal gland acinar cells and stimulates the $G\alpha_{q/11}$ subtype of G protein that activates phospholipase $C\beta$ (Fig. 15.11). Phospholipase $C\beta$ breaks down the membrane phospholipid, phosphatidylinositol bisphosphate, into IP_3 and diacyglycerol. IP_3 binds to its receptor on the endoplasmic reticulum and releases Ca^{2+} increasing the intracellular $[Ca^{2+}]$. The depletion of intracellular Ca^{2+} stores leads to Ca^{2+} influx across the plasma membrane, known as capacitative Ca^{2+} influx. This influx sustains the Ca^{2+} increase and replenishes the stores. The interaction of the endoplasmic reticulum protein, STIM1, and the plasma membrane protein, Orai, form the Ca^{2+} influx channel. The increase in intracellular Ca^{2+} stimulates exocytosis by activating target proteins involved in the release process.

The diacylglycerol produced with IP_3 activates the PKC isoforms $PKC\alpha$, $PKC\delta$, and $PKC\epsilon$ to stimulate protein secretion. PKC stimulates secretion by phosphorylating unknown substrate proteins involved in exocytosis.[48]

Cholinergic agonists also activate inhibitory pathways that attenuate secretion. Cholinergic agonists activate Pyk2 and p60Src that cause a Ca^{2+}-dependent activation of ERK1/2 (also known as MAPK) (Fig. 15.12). The step in the pathway that activates Ras is unknown; however, the Ras/Raf/MEK pathway leads to activation (phosphorylation) of ERK1/2. Activated ERK1/2 decreases cholinergic agonist-stimulated secretion.

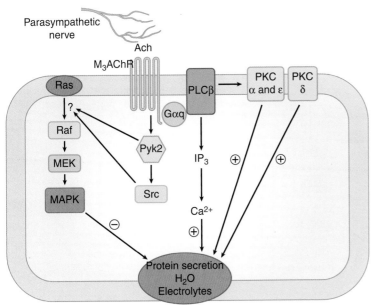

Fig. 15.11 Schematic of parasympathetic signaling pathway—the pathway is described in the text. *Ach*, Acetylcholine; *Gαq*, G protein alpha q; *IP3*, inositol 1,4,5 trisphosphate; *M3AChR*, type 3 muscarinic acetylcholine receptor; *MAPK*, mitogen-activated protein kinase; *MEK*, mitogen activated protein kinase kinase; *PKC*, protein kinase C; *PLC*, phospholipase C.

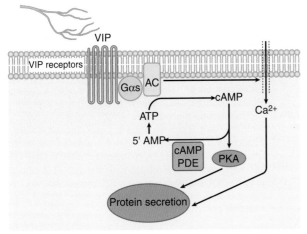

Fig. 15.12 Schematic of vasoactive intestinal peptide (*VIP*) signaling pathway—the pathway is described in the text. *5′ AMP*, 5′ Adenosine monophosphate; *Gαs*, G protein alpha s; *AC*, adenylyl cyclase; *ATP*, adenosine triphosphate; *cAMP*, cyclic adenosine monophosphate; *PDE*, phosphodiesterase; *PKA*, protein kinase A.

A second pathway activated by cholinergic agonists that attenuates secretion is the phospholipase D pathway, which breaks down phosphatidylcholine to phosphatidic acid and choline. Phosphatidic acid can be metabolized to diacylglycerol and, through PKC, stimulates ERK1/2 to attenuate secretion. Even though cholinergic agonists activate inhibitory pathways, their ultimate effect is to stimulate secretion.[49]

Vasoactive Intestinal Peptide

VIP released from parasympathetic nerves activates a separate pathway from cholinergic agonists. VIP binds to VIPAC1 and VPAC2 to activate the G protein $G\alpha_s$ that stimulates adenylyl cyclase (Fig. 15.12).[50] Adenylyl cyclase produces cAMP from ATP, and cAMP activates PKA that phosphorylates target proteins in the exocytotic machinery. VIP also increases intracellular $[Ca^{2+}]$.[50] Together, increased levels of cAMP and Ca^{2+} induce protein secretion.

VIP also interacts with ERK1/2. Unlike cholinergic agonists, VIP inhibits ERK1/2. VIP inhibition of ERK1/2 plays a critical role in the interaction of the VIP pathway, with those stimulated by cholinergic and α_1-adrenergic agonists described subsequently.[51]

α_1-Adrenergic agonists

The sympathetic neurotransmitter norepinephrine binds to α_{1D}-AR on the acinar cells (Fig. 15.13). To stimulate protein secretion, α_1-adrenergic agonists activate endothelial nitric oxide synthase (eNOS) colocalized with caveolin on the basolateral membranes of acinar cells. eNOS produces nitric oxide (NO) that activates soluble guanylate cyclase.[52] Guanylate cyclase produces cGMP from GTP. cGMP stimulates secretion by phosphorylating target proteins in the exocytotic machinery.

α_1-Adrenergic agonists also give a small increase in intracellular Ca^{2+} that could interact with cGMP to stimulate secretion.[53] The mechanism by which α_1-adrenergic agonists activate eNOS in the lacrimal gland is not known.

α_1-Adrenergic agonists also activate PKC isoforms. The effector enzyme that produces diacylglycerol is not known but it is not phospholipase C or D. Diacylglycerol activates PKCε to stimulate secretion.[53] Unlike cholinergic agonists that activate PKCα and PKCδ that stimulate secretion, when α_1-adrenergic agonists activate these PKC isoforms, they inhibit secretion.[54]

α_1-Adrenergic agonists also activate the ERK1/2 inhibitory pathway (Fig. 15.13).[55] The mechanism by which α_1-adrenergic agonists activate ERK1/2 is different from that used by cholinergic agonists. α_1-Adrenergic agonists activate an MMP, A Disintegrin and Metalloprotease 17 (ADAM17), which cleaves the membrane-spanning growth factor EGF, releasing its extracellular domain.[56] The extracellular domain contains the active EGF-binding domain that binds to the EGFR causing it to dimerize. The EGFR dimer autophosphorylates through the signaling pathway described in section Mucous production and activates ERK1/2 to attenuate secretion. Although α_1-adrenergic agonists activate inhibitory pathways, the overall action of these agonists is to stimulate secretion.

The neurotransmitters released from the efferent nerves can interact with each other at the level of the signaling pathways they induce. Activation of parasympathetic nerves alone or both parasympathetic

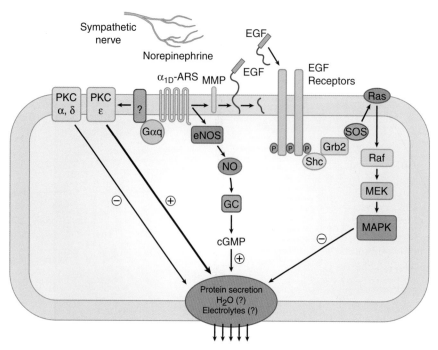

Fig. 15.13 Schematic of α_{1D}-adrenergic signaling pathway—the pathway is described in the text. α_{1D}-ARS, α_{1D}-adrenergic receptors; *Ach*, Acetylcholine; $G\alpha q$, G protein alpha q; *GC*, guanylate cyclase; *eNOS*, endothelial nitric oxide synthase; *EGF*, epidermal growth factor; *IP3*, inositol 1,4,5 trisphosphate; M_3AchR, type 3 muscarinic acetylcholine receptor; *MAPK*, mitogen-activated protein kinase; *MMP*, matrix metalloproteinase; *NO*, nitric oxide; *PKC*, protein kinase C.

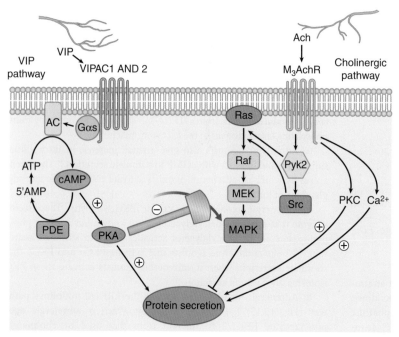

Fig. 15.14 Schematic of the interaction between Ca^{2+}/protein kinase C (PKC) and cyclic adenosine monophosphate (cAMP)-dependent signaling pathways. *5'AMP*, 5' Adenosine monophosphate; *AC*, adenyl cyclase; *Ach*, acetylcholine; *ATP*, adenosine triphosphate; *eNOS*, endothelial nitric oxide synthase; $G\alpha q$, G protein alpha q; $G\alpha s$, G protein alpha s; *IP3*, inositol 1,4,5 trisphosphate; M_3AchR, type 3 muscarinic acetylcholine receptor; *MAPK*, mitogen-activated protein kinase; *NO*, nitric oxide; *PDE*, phosphodiesterase; *PLC*, phospholipase C; *PKA*, protein kinase A; *PKC*, protein kinase C; *MEK*, mitogen activated protein kinase kinase; *VIP*, vasoactive intestinal peptide.

and sympathetic nerves releases two or more neurotransmitters that cause secretion differently to one agonist alone. Release of cholinergic and α_1-adrenergic agonists stimulates secretion that is additive, as these agonists activate separate and different signaling pathways.[53] Release of VIP with cholinergic or α_1-adrenergic agonists causes secretion that is synergistic or potentiated.[57] The potentiation is caused by VIP inhibition of ERK1/2 that prevents activation of ERK1/2 by cholinergic and α_1-adrenergic agonists (Fig. 15.14). When ERK1/2 activation is blocked, it cannot inhibit secretion and the secretory response is increased.[51]

Epidermal Growth Factor

Addition of exogenous EGF (the 6 kDa EGF) gives a small stimulation of protein secretion. EGF uses IP_3, $PKC\alpha$, and $PKC\delta$ to stimulate lacrimal gland secretion.[58]

Purinergic agonists

P1, P2X, and P2Y receptors are present and functional in lacrimal gland cells. P1 receptors are adenosine receptors and the adenosine (A) $_1$, $_{2A}$, and $_{2B}$ receptors are present in the lacrimal gland.[59] Adenosine stimulates protein secretion through A_1 and A_{2B} receptors and additionally interacts with the M_3AchR-stimulated pathway to potentiate secretion.

Of the seven P2X receptors, all except $P2X_5$ were shown in lacrimal gland acinar cells.[59] Use of specific P2X receptor agonists and examination of the other characteristics of the P2X receptors found that activation of $P2X_3$ and $P2X_7$ receptors increased intracellular $[Ca^{2+}]$ and stimulated protein secretion. $P2X_7$ receptor–stimulated pathways interact with both parasympathetic and sympathetic pathways. For cholinergic agonists, acetylcholine released from parasympathetic nerves interacts with M_3AChR receptors on the acinar cells to stimulate secretion and on the nerve endings to release ATP. The released ATP interacts with the $P2X_7$ receptors to stimulate secretion. When added together, these agonists potentiate the intracellular $[Ca^{2+}]$, but secretion was additive. $P2X_7$ receptors also interact with the a_{1D}-adrenergic agonists of the sympathetic pathway. When intracellular $[Ca^{2+}]$ was measured, the addition of both agonists together was additive and inhibitors of one receptor blocked the action of the other. This interaction did not occur for protein secretion. The interaction between $P2X_3$ receptors and neural pathways has yet to be published.

Of the seven P2Y[59] receptors, only three are present in the lacrimal gland acini, $P2Y_1$, $_{11}$, and $_{13}$. These receptors have not been investigated in detail, but an agonist of $P2Y_1$ and $_{11}$ is effective in increasing intracellular $[Ca^{2+}]$.

P2 receptors are present on myoepithelial cells. For the P2X receptors, only $P2X_7$ is present, but it does not behave as a typical $P2X_7$ receptor. Instead, $P2X_7$ has characteristics of P2Y receptors including activating phospholipase C. For P2Y receptors, $P2Y_1$, $_{11}$, and $_{13}$ are present. Furthermore, UTP activates, predominantly, P2Y receptors and causes the largest increase in intracellular $[Ca^{2+}]$ and contraction compared with ATP. Thus the actions of P2X receptors predominate in the lacrimal gland acini and P2Y in myoepithelial cells.[44]

Regulation of electrolyte and water secretion
Mechanism of acinar electrolyte and water secretion
Electrolyte and water secretion are driven by the basolateral NKA that produces energy to drive the efflux of Na^+ and influx of K^+ across the basolateral membrane into the acinar cell against their electrochemical gradients (Fig. 15.15). The Na^+/H^+ (NHE) and Cl^-/HCO_3^- (AE) exchangers and the Na^+-K^+-$2Cl^-$ symporter (NKCC1) use the energy of the favorable inward Na^+ gradient to drive Cl^- influx across the basolateral membrane. This Cl^- influx establishes a favorable gradient for Cl^- efflux across the apical membrane through Cl^- selective channels into the acinar lumen, generating a lumen negative transepithelial potential difference. This potential difference drives the flux of Na^+ from the basal to apical side of the cell through the paracellular pathway. K^+ selective channels allow the K^+ to recycle across the basolateral membrane so that acini can produce a Na^+-Cl^- rich fluid.

Mechanism of ductal electrolyte and water secretion
Isolated ducts from the acinar cells[60] were used to investigate electrolyte and water secretion. Duct cells secrete about 30% of the lacrimal gland fluid. These cells use mechanisms similar to those used by acini to secrete fluid, with a few exceptions. First the K^+ channels are placed with Cl^- channels in the apical rather than basolateral membranes to produce a K^+-Cl^-–rich fluid (Fig. 15.6) Those channels include the K^+-Cl^- symporter KCC1, intermediate conductance calcium-activated K^+ channel ($IK_{Ca}1$), cystic fibrosis transmembrane conductance regulator (CFTR) Cl^- channel, and CIC3 Cl^- channel.

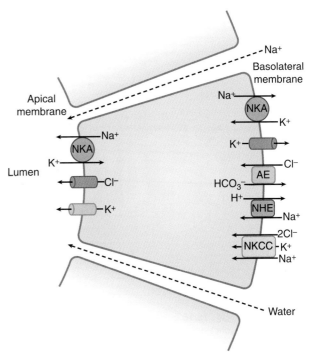

Fig. 15.15 Mechanism of electrolyte and water secretion by lacrimal gland acinar cells—see text for description. *AE,* Anion exchanger or Cl^-/HCO_3^- exchanger; *NHE,* Na^+/H^+ exchanger; *NKA,* Na^+K^+-ATPase; *NKCC,* $Na^+K^+2Cl^-$ cotransporter. (Modified from Selvam S, Thomas PB, Gukasyan HJ, et al. Transepithelial bioelectrical properties of rabbit acinar cell monolayers on polyester membrane scaffolds. *Am J Physiol Cell Physiol.* 2007;293(4):C1412–C1419. Used with permission.)

Neural activation of electrolyte and water secretion
Fluid secretion from lacrimal gland acini is difficult to study because of the architecture of the acinus. Use of in vivo methods permitted the observation that the parasympathetic agonists Ach and VIP each stimulate electrolyte and water secretion.[61] Cholinergic agonists cause fluid secretion by activating apical Cl^- and K^+ channels and basolateral Na^+/H^+ exchangers, and increase the translocation of the NKA from the cytoplasm to the basolateral membranes. VIP stimulates fluid secretion by cAMP activating the Ca^{2+}-dependent BK potassium channel (BK K^+) channel in the basolateral membrane. However, the mechanisms by which cholinergic agonists and VIP stimulate fluid secretion have not been thoroughly investigated.

In contrast to acinar cells, mechanisms of duct cell electrolyte and water secretion stimulated by neurotransmitters can be investigated in detail.[60] As in acinar cells, both increases in intracellular Ca^{2+} signaling and cytosolic levels of cAMP stimulate fluid secretion, but each uses different ionic channels (Fig. 15.16). Cholinergic agonists increase the intracellular $[Ca^{2+}]$ that activates NHE and AE on the basolateral membrane to drive Na^+ and Cl^- into the duct cell cytoplasm. NKCC and NKA, also on the basolateral membrane, couple influx of Na^+, K^+, and Cl^-. The increase in intracellular $[Ca^{2+}]$ then activates apical IK_{Ca}^{2+} and CIC3 to move K^+ and Cl^- into the lumen. A rise in cellular cAMP activates the apical CFTR channel to secrete Cl^- into the lumen. Cl^- movement into the lumen is the main driver of ductal fluid secretion. The overall action of the basolateral and apical ion transporters produces an osmotic gradient that passively drives water into the lumen. The role of aquaporins and Na^+ in ductal fluid secretion has yet to be published.

Lacrimal gland fluid composition
Lacrimal gland fluid is isotonic, and in human and rabbit it is 300 mOsm. The electrolyte composition is similar to plasma except

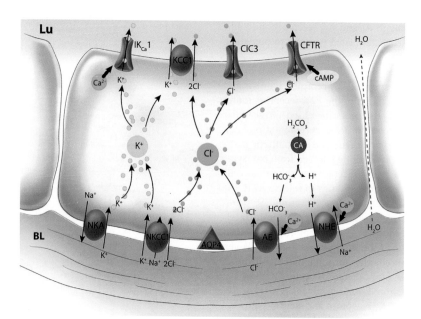

Fig. 15.16 Schematic model of intracellular mechanisms underlying electrolyte secretion in lacrimal gland duct epithelial cells. Summarized actions of depicted ion channels and transporters of duct epithelial cells result in intraluminal flux of Cl⁻ and K⁺. *AE*, Anion exchanger or Cl⁻/HCO3⁻ exchanger; *AQP4*, aquaporin 4; *BL*, basolateral side; *CA*, carbo-anhydrase; *ClC3*, chloride channel type 3; *CFTR*, cystic fibrosis transmembrane conductance regulator; *IKCa1*, intermediate conductance Ca²⁺-activated K⁺ channel; *KCC1*, K⁺/Cl⁻ cotransporter type 1; *Lu*, luminal side; *NHE*, Na⁺/H⁺ exchanger; *NKA*, Na⁺K⁺-ATPase; *NKCC1*, Na⁺K⁺2Cl⁻ cotransporter type 1. (Reprinted from Tóth-Molnár E, Ding C. New insight into lacrimal gland function: Role of the duct epithelium in tear secretion. *Ocul Surf*. 2020;18(4):595–603.)

that it has a decreased [Na⁺] and increased [Cl⁻] and [K⁺]. The lacrimal gland also secretes a myriad of proteins.[62] The most extensively studied are lysozyme, lactoferrin, secretory IgA, and lipocalin. Other minor proteins secreted include EGF and other growth factors; lacritin, a protein unique to the lacrimal gland; and surfactant proteins A–D.[63] Many proteins are antibacterial and function in the defense of the ocular surface. Lacritin is selectively expressed in the lacrimal gland, cornea, conjunctival goblet cells, and meibomian glands.[64] It is secreted by the lacrimal gland onto the ocular surface, where it is a growth factor for the ocular surface tissues and also stimulates tear secretion.

Aqueous function

The aqueous layer has multiple functions critical to the health and defense of the ocular surface from the environment. The electrolyte composition of the aqueous layer is critical to the health of the ocular surface, as small changes in osmolarity or electrolyte composition leads to aqueous deficiency dry eye. Multiple causes can alter lacrimal gland secretion leading to aqueous deficiency dry eye and damage to the ocular surface (see Box 15.2). The proteins in the aqueous layer protect the ocular surface from bacterial infection and alter corneal and conjunctival function. Reflex secretion of the aqueous layers helps to wash away noxious substances and particulates into the drainage duct. The buffer system of the fluid helps to protect against changes in pH.

LIPID LAYER

Structure of meibomian glands and mechanism of lipid production

The lipid layer is secreted by the meibomian glands, modified sebaceous glands that line the upper and lower eyelids in a single row.[65,66] A single meibomian gland consists of multiple acini that secrete into small ducts. These ducts converge to form a common duct that exits

---

BOX 15.2   Conditions associated with aqueous deficiency dry eye

- Primary lacrimal gland deficiencies, including age-related dry eye, congenital alacrima, and familial dysautonomia.
- Secondary lacrimal gland deficiencies, including Sjögren's syndrome, lacrimal gland infiltration, lymphoma, AIDS, graft versus host disease, lacrimal gland ablation, and lacrimal gland denervation.
- Obstruction of the lacrimal gland ducts from trachoma; cicatricial pemphigoid and mucous membrane pemphigoid; erythema multiforme; and chemical and thermal burns.
- Reflex hyposecretion from reflex sensory block during contact lens wear, diabetes, and neurotrophic keratitis.
- Reflex hyposecretion from reflex motor block after cranial nerve VII damage, multiple neuromatosis, and exposure to certain systemic drugs.

(Modified from 2007 Report of the International Dry Eye Workshop. *Ocul Surf*. 2007;5(2):80.)

---

onto the eyelid near the mucocutaneous junction (Fig. 15.1). The acini are surrounded on the basal side by nerves and blood vessels. The cells in the acini are arranged in a specific order that reflects their function such that the outer basal cell layer consists of undifferentiated, flattened cells. As these cells mature, they move inward to the center of the acinus and concomitant with this inward migration is continuing synthesis of lipids. Meibomian gland lipids are stored in vesicles. As the cells move closer to the center, they contain increasingly more lipid secretory vesicles reflecting continued lipid synthesis. Upon the appropriate stimulus (unknown), the cells in the acinus center burst, releasing the entire cell contents in their secretory granule lipids and other components of the cell into the duct system. This releases the entire cell contents and is known as holocrine secretion. The secreted cells are replaced by proliferation of the basal cells.[67]

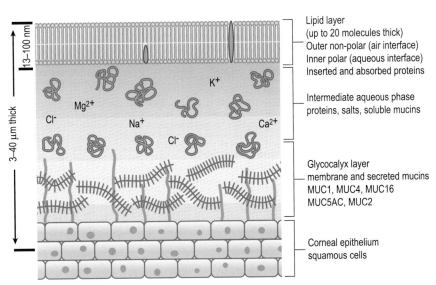

Fig. 15.17 Schematic diagram of the tear film showing a new concept for the structure of the lipid layer. (Modified from Butovich IA, Millar TJ, Ham BM. Understanding and analyzing meibomian lipids—a review. *Curr Eye Res.* 2008;33(5):405–420.)

Labels on figure:
- Lipid layer (up to 20 molecules thick)
- Outer non-polar (air interface)
- Inner polar (aqueous interface)
- Inserted and absorbed proteins
- Intermediate aqueous phase proteins, salts, soluble mucins
- Glycocalyx layer membrane and secreted mucins MUC1, MUC4, MUC16 MUC5AC, MUC2
- Corneal epithelium squamous cells
- 13–100 nm
- 3–40 μm thick
- K^+, Mg^{2+}, Cl^-, Na^+, Cl^-, Ca^{2+}

Thus, the secretory product contains a complex mixture of lipids and proteins and is termed meibum. The synthesized lipids are the major component of meibum, with the minor lipid classes probably reflecting the cellular membrane lipids. Meibum is a mixture of non-polar lipids (wax esters, cholesterol, and cholesterol esters) and polar lipids (mainly phospholipids) and is liquid at lid temperature.

The secreted lipid is stored in the duct system that terminates in orifices with a muscular cuff, which open onto the lid.[66] Meibum is released onto the ocular surface in small amounts with each blink, forming a casual reservoir with about 30 times more lipid than needed for each blink. With the up-phase of each blink, the upper lid draws oil from the lid reservoir and spreads it over the anterior tear film surface. With the down-phase, the lipid film is returned to the marginal reservoir as the lid closes.[66] The lipids mix only slightly with the lipid reservoir as it folds up as an intact sheet, providing a gradual turnover of the lipids in the tear film.

Butovich et al.[68] have proposed that proteins and mucins contribute to the lipid layer so that the proteins, which contain hydrophobic, hydrophilic, and charged portions, can unfold and form a variety of shapes depending upon the local milieu (Fig. 15.17). The proteins could extend across the lipid layer, suggesting a complex mixture of islands of proteins, mucins, and lipids, similar to that of lung surfactant. More recently, Tsitova and Lin[69] found that proteins from the mucoaqueous layer can associate with the lipid layer, but Georgiev et al.[70] suggest that in the healthy tear film, proteins only transiently associate with the lipid layer, but are unlikely to penetrate in depth. Although the lipid layer is well studied, multiple controversies remain based on the complexity of the fluid and limited amounts of meibum to study.

Regulation of meibum secretion

Neural regulation

Meibomian glands are richly innervated by sensory, sympathetic, and parasympathetic nerves.[71] The sensory nerves contain substance P and calcitonin gene–related peptide (CGRP). The sympathetic fibers use catecholamines and NPY as neurotransmitters. Parasympathetic nerves are immunopositive for cholinergic neurotransmitters, VIP, and NO. However, the role of nerves in meibomian gland function is unknown.

Hormonal regulation

The meibomian glands have both androgen and estrogen receptors. Androgens regulate lipid secretion by controlling lipid synthesis.

Meibomian acinar cells have nuclear androgen receptors[72] and the ratio of androgens and estrogens is critical for controlling lipid synthesis.[73] Stimulating androgen receptors increases gene transcription for enzymes associated with fatty acid and cholesterol synthetic pathways and hence stimulate lipid production. Androgen deficiency is associated with meibomian gland dysfunction. Immortalized human meibomian gland epithelial cells (acinar cells) were developed that will allow investigation of the cellular mechanism of neural and hormonal regulation of meibomian gland secretion.[74]

Function

The composition of meibum collected from normal and dry eye patients differs less than the changes between collection from the lids and lipid extracts from contact lenses, suggesting that the tear film lipid layer is quite robust to alterations in its constituents. Only a small number of the lipid layer components, most likely the polar lipids, can significantly impact its performance in either health or disease.[70] Thus, the lipid layer is relatively stable.

The lipid layer simultaneously performs multiple functions. The meibomian gland secretion forms a hydrophobic barrier to prevent

---

BOX 15.3 Meibomian gland diseases causing evaporative dry eye

- Reduced number of glands in congenital deficiency and acquired disease.
- Replacement of glands in distichiasis and distichiasis lymphedema syndrome.
- Hypersecretory gland dysfunction in meibomian seborrhea.
- Hyposecretory gland dysfunction in retinoid therapy.
- Obstructive disease from primary or secondary causes, of focal or diffuse nature, that is simple or cicatricial or can be atrophic or inflammatory.
- Primary or secondary due to the local diseases, anterior blepharitis.
- Primary or secondary due to systemic disease such as acne rosacea, seborrheic dermatitis, and atopy.
- Primary or secondary due to systemic toxicity from 13-*cis* retinoic acid, polychlorinated biphenyls, and epinephrine.
- Cicatricial disease from chemical burns, trachoma, pemphigoid, erythema multiforme, acne rosacea, vernal keratoconjunctivitis, or atopic keratoconjunctivitis.

(Modified from 2007 Report of the International Dry Eye Workshop. *Ocul Surf.* 2007;5(2):82.)

tear overflow onto the lids and sebum from the skin from entering the tear film.[75] The mucocutaneous junction itself separates the tear-wettable conjunctiva from the oil-wettable eyelid skin, preventing overgrowth in both directions.[76] The meibum forms a water-tight seal of the apposed lid margins during sleep.[65,66] The tear lipids also provide a barrier to reduce mucoaqueous tear evaporation during eyelid opening, render optimal viscoelasticity to the air/tear surface, and aid in lubrication for the eyelids during blinking. Lipids enhance the stability of the tear film and provide a smooth optical surface for the cornea at the air/lipid interface. The lipid layer is also antibacterial due to the disruptive action of the long-chain fatty acid chains on bacterial cell membrane integrity.[70] A decrease or an alteration in meibomian gland secretion leads to evaporative dry eye. There are multiple ways in which meibomian gland function can be altered to cause evaporative dry eye (Box. 15.3) and damage the ocular surface.

REFERENCES

1. Cotlier E. *The Lens.* St. Louis: CV Mosby; 1975.
2. Wang J, Aquavella J, Palakuru J, Chung S, Feng C. Relationships between central tear film thickness and tear menisci of the upper and lower eyelids. *Invest Ophthalmol Vis Sci.* 2006;47(10):4349–4355.
3. Chen HB, Yamabayashi S, Ou B, Tanaka Y, Ohno S, Tsukahara S. Structure and composition of rat precorneal tear film. A study by an in vivo cryofixation. *Invest Ophthalmol Vis Sci.* 1997;38(2):381–387.
4. Ehlers N. The precorneal film. Biomicroscopical, histological and chemical investigations. *Acta Ophthalmol Suppl.* 1965(SUPPL 81):81–134.
5. King-Smith PE, Fink BA, Fogt N, Nichols KK, Hill RM, Wilson GS. The thickness of the human precorneal tear film: evidence from reflection spectra. *Invest Ophthalmol Vis Sci.* 2000;41(11):3348–3359.
6. Mishima S. Some physiological aspects of the precorneal tear film. *Arch Ophthalmol.* 1965;73:233–241.
7. Wang J, Fonn D, Simpson TL, Jones L. Precorneal and pre- and postlens tear film thickness measured indirectly with optical coherence tomography. *Invest Ophthalmol Vis Sci.* 2003;44(6):2524–2528.
8. Ayub M, Thale AB, Hedderich J, Tillmann BN, Paulsen FP. The cavernous body of the human efferent tear ducts contributes to regulation of tear outflow. *Invest Ophthalmol Vis Sci.* 2003;44(11):4900–4907.
9. Gipson IK, Argueso P. Role of mucins in the function of the corneal and conjunctival epithelia. *Int Rev Cytol.* 2003;231:1–49.
10. Argueso P. Disrupted glycocalyx as a source of ocular surface biomarkers. *Eye Contact Lens.* 2020;46(Suppl 2):S53–S56.
11. Blalock TD, Spurr-Michaud SJ, Tisdale AS, Gipson IK. Release of membrane-associated mucins from ocular surface epithelia. *Invest Ophthalmol Vis Sci.* 2008;49(5):1864–1871.
12. Danjo Y, Watanabe H, Tisdale AS, et al. Alteration of mucin in human conjunctival epithelia in dry eye. *Invest Ophthalmol Vis Sci.* 1998;39(13):2602–2609.
13. Caffery B, Joyce E, Heynen M, et al. MUC16 Expression in Sjogren's syndrome, KCS, and control subjects. *Mol Vis.* 2008;14:2547–2555.
14. Imbert Y, Darling DS, Jumblatt MM, et al. MUC1 splice variants in human ocular surface tissues: possible differences between dry eye patients and normal controls. *Exp Eye Res.* 2006;83(3):493–501.
15. Imbert Y, Foulks GN, Brennan MD, et al. MUC1 and estrogen receptor alpha gene polymorphisms in dry eye patients. *Exp Eye Res.* 2008
16. Tseng SC, Hirst LW, Farazdaghi M, Green WR. Goblet cell density and vascularization during conjunctival transdifferentiation. *Invest Ophthalmol Vis Sci.* 1984;25(10):1168–1176.
17. Kessing SV. Investigations of the conjunctival mucin. (Quantitative studies of the goblet cells of conjunctiva). (Preliminary report). *Acta Ophthalmol (Copenh).* 1966;44(3):439–453.
18. Srinivasan B, Worgul B, Iwamoto T, Merriam G. The conjunctiva epithelium:II. Histochemical and ultrastructural studies on human and rat conjunctiva. *Ophthalmic Res.* 1977;9:65–79.
19. Puro DG. Role of ion channels in the functional response of conjunctival goblet cells to dry eye. *Am J Physiol Cell Physiol.* 2018;315(2):C236–246.
20. Diebold Y, Rios JD, Hodges RR, Rawe I, Dartt DA. Presence of nerves and their receptors in mouse and human conjunctival goblet cells. *Invest Ophthalmol Vis Sci.* 2001;42(10):2270–2282.
21. Rios JD, Zoukhri D, Rawe IM, Hodges RR, Zieske JD, Dartt DA. Immunolocalization of muscarinic and VIP receptor subtypes and their role in stimulating goblet cell secretion. *Invest Ophthalmol Vis Sci.* 1999;40(6):1102–1111.
22. Kanno H, Horikawa Y, Hodges RR, et al. Cholinergic agonists transactivate EGFR and stimulate MAPK to induce goblet cell secretion. *Am J Physiol Cell Physiol.* 2003;284(4):C988–998.
23. Dartt DA, Rios JD, Kanno H, et al. Regulation of conjunctival goblet cell secretion by Ca(2+) and protein kinase C. *Exp Eye Res.* 2000;71(6):619–628.
24. Jumblatt J, Jumblatt M. Detection and quantification of conjunctival mucins. *Adv Exp Med Biol.* 1998;438:239–246.
25. Hodges RR, Horikawa Y, Rios JD, Shatos MA, Dartt DA. Effect of protein kinase C and Ca(2+) on p42/p44 MAPK, Pyk2, and Src activation in rat conjunctival goblet cells. *Exp Eye Res.* 2007;85(6):836–844.
26. Horikawa Y, Shatos MA, Hodges RR, et al. Activation of mitogen-activated protein kinase by cholinergic agonists and EGF in human compared with rat cultured conjunctival goblet cells. *Invest Ophthalmol Vis Sci.* 2003;44(6):2535–2544.
27. Jumblatt JE, Jumblatt MM. Regulation of ocular mucin secretion by P2Y2 nucleotide receptors in rabbit and human conjunctiva. *Exp Eye Res.* 1998;67(3):341–346.
28. Rios JD, Ghinelli E, Gu J, Hodges RR, Dartt DA. Role of neurotrophins and neurotrophin receptors in rat conjunctival goblet cell secretion and proliferation. *Invest Ophthalmol Vis Sci.* 2007;48(4):1543–1551.
29. Hodges RR, Li D, Shatos MA, et al. Lipoxin A4 activates ALX/FPR2 receptor to regulate conjunctival goblet cell secretion. *Mucosal Immunol.* 2017;10(1):46–57.
30. Lippestad M, Hodges RR, Utheim TP, Serhan CN, Dartt DA. Resolvin D1 increases mucin secretion in cultured rat conjunctival goblet cells via multiple signaling pathways. *Invest Ophthalmol Vis Sci.* 2017;58(11):4530–4544.
31. Botten N, Hodges RR, Li D, et al. Resolvin D2 elevates cAMP to increase intracellular [Ca(2+)] and stimulate secretion from conjunctival goblet cells. *FASEB J.* 2019;33(7):8468–8478.
32. Lippestad M, Hodges RR, Utheim TP, Serhan CN, Dartt DA. Signaling pathways activated by resolvin E1 to stimulate mucin secretion and increase intracellular Ca(2+) in cultured rat conjunctival goblet cells. *Exp Eye Res.* 2018;173:64–72.
33. Olsen MV, Lyngstadaas AV, Bair JA, et al. Maresin 1, a specialized proresolving mediator, stimulates intracellular [Ca(2+)] and secretion in conjunctival goblet cells. *J Cell Physiol.* 2021;236(1):340–353.
34. Puro DG. Impact of P2X(7) Purinoceptors on goblet cell function: Implications for dry eye. *Int J Mol Sci.* 2021;22(13).
35. Gu J, Chen L, Shatos MA, et al. Presence of EGF growth factor ligands and their effects on cultured rat conjunctival goblet cell proliferation. *Exp Eye Res.* 2008;86(2):322–334.
36. Shatos MA, Gu J, Hodges RR, Lashkari K, Dartt DA. ERK/p44p42 mitogen-activated protein kinase mediates EGF-stimulated proliferation of conjunctival goblet cells in culture. *Invest Ophthalmol Vis Sci.* 2008;49(8):3351–3359.
37. Hosoya K, Horibe Y, Kim KJ, Lee VH. Na(+)-dependent L-arginine transport in the pigmented rabbit conjunctiva. *Exp Eye Res.* 1997;65(4):547–553.
38. Turner HC, Alvarez LJ, Candia OA. Identification and localization of acid-base transporters in the conjunctival epithelium. *Exp Eye Res.* 2001;72(5):519–531.
39. Turner HC, Alvarez LJ, Bildin VN, Candia OA. Immunolocalization of Na-K-ATPase, Na-K-Cl and Na-glucose cotransporters in the conjunctival epithelium. *Curr Eye Res.* 2000;21(5):843–850.
40. Kompella UB, Kim KJ, Shiue MH, Lee VH. Cyclic AMP modulation of active ion transport in the pigmented rabbit conjunctiva. *J Ocul Pharmacol Ther.* 1996;12(3):281–287.
41. Shiue MH, Kim KJ, Lee VH. Modulation of chloride secretion across the pigmented rabbit conjunctiva. *Exp Eye Res.* 1998;66(3):275–282.
42. Li Y, Kuang K, Yerxa B, Wen Q, Rosskothen H, Fischbarg J. Rabbit conjunctival epithelium transports fluid, and P2Y2(2) receptor agonists stimulate Cl(-) and fluid secretion. *Am J Physiol Cell Physiol.* 2001;281(2):C595–602.
43. Candia O, Alvarea L. Overview of electrolyte and fluid transport across the conjunctiva. In: Dartt D, ed. *Encyclopedia of the Eye.* London: Elsevier; 2009.
44. García-Posadas L, Hodges RR, Utheim TP, et al. Lacrimal gland myoepithelial cells are altered in a mouse model of dry eye disease. *Am J Pathol.* 2020;190(10):2067–2079.
45. Gárriz A, Aubry S, Wattiaux G, et al. Role of the phospholipase c pathway and calcium mobilization in oxytocin-induced contraction of lacrimal gland myoepithelial cells. *Invest Ophthalmol Vis Sci.* 2021;62(14):25.
46. Wu K, Jerdeva GV, da Costa SR, Sou E, Schechter JE, Hamm-Alvarez SF. Molecular mechanisms of lacrimal acinar secretory vesicle exocytosis. *Exp Eye Res.* 2006;83(1):84–96.
47. Evans E, Zhang W, Jerdeva G, et al. Direct interaction between Rab3D and the polymeric immunoglobulin receptor and trafficking through regulated secretory vesicles in lacrimal gland acinar cells. *Am J Physiol Cell Physiol.* 2008;294(3):C662–674.
48. Zoukhri D, Hodges RR, Sergheraert C, Dartt DA. Cholinergic-induced Ca2+ elevation in rat lacrimal gland acini is negatively modulated by PKCdelta and PKCepsilon. *Invest Ophthalmol Vis Sci.* 2000;41(2):386–392.
49. Zoukhri D, Dartt DA. Cholinergic activation of phospholipase D in lacrimal gland acini is independent of protein kinase C and calcium. *Am J Physiol.* 1995;268(3 Pt 1):C713–720.
50. Hodges RR, Zoukhri D, Sergheraert C, Zieske JD, Dartt DA. Identification of vasoactive intestinal peptide receptor subtypes in the lacrimal gland and their signal-transducing components. *Invest Ophthalmol Vis Sci.* 1997;38(3):610–619.
51. Funaki C, Hodges RR, Dartt DA. Role of cAMP inhibition of p44/p42 mitogen-activated protein kinase in potentiation of protein secretion in rat lacrimal gland. *Am J Physiol Cell Physiol.* 2007;293(5):C1551–1560.
52. Hodges RR, Shatos MA, Tarko RS, Vrouvlianis J, Gu J, Dartt DA. Nitric oxide and cGMP mediate alpha1D-adrenergic receptor-Stimulated protein secretion and p42/p44 MAPK activation in rat lacrimal gland. *Invest Ophthalmol Vis Sci.* 2005;46(8):2781–2789.
53. Hodges RR, Dicker DM, Rose PE, Dartt DA. Alpha 1-adrenergic and cholinergic agonists use separate signal transduction pathways in lacrimal gland. *Am J Physiol.* 1992;262 (6 Pt 1):G1087–1096.
54. Zoukhri D, Hodges RR, Sergheraert C, Toker A, Dartt DA. Lacrimal gland PKC isoforms are differentially involved in agonist-induced protein secretion. *Am J Physiol.* 1997;272 (1 Pt 1):C263–269.
55. Ota I, Zoukhri D, Hodges RR, et al. Alpha 1-adrenergic and cholinergic agonists activate MAPK by separate mechanisms to inhibit secretion in lacrimal gland. *Am J Physiol Cell Physiol.* 2003;284(1):C168–178.
56. Chen L, Hodges RR, Funaki C, et al. Effects of alpha1D-adrenergic receptors on shedding of biologically active EGF in freshly isolated lacrimal gland epithelial cells. *Am J Physiol Cell Physiol.* 2006;291(5):C946–956.
57. Dartt DA, Baker AK, Vaillant C, Rose PE. Vasoactive intestinal polypeptide stimulation of protein secretion from rat lacrimal gland acini. *Am J Physiol.* 1984;247(5 Pt 1):G502–509.
58. Tepavcevic V, Hodges RR, Zoukhri D, Dartt DA. Signal transduction pathways used by EGF to stimulate protein secretion in rat lacrimal gland. *Invest Ophthalmol Vis Sci.* 2003;44(3):1075–1081.

59. Hodges RR, Dartt DA. Signaling pathways of purinergic receptors and their interactions with cholinergic and adrenergic pathways in the lacrimal gland. *J Ocul Pharmacol Ther.* 2016;32(8):490–497.

60. Tóth-Molnár E, Ding C. New insight into lacrimal gland function: Role of the duct epithelium in tear secretion. *Ocul Surf.* 2020;18(4):595–603.

61. Dartt DA, Moller M, Poulsen JH. Lacrimal gland electrolyte and water secretion in the rabbit: localization and role of (Na+ + K+)-activated ATPase. *J Physiol.* 1981;321:557–569.

62. Dartt DA, Hodges RR, Zoukhri D. Tears and their secretion. In: Fischbarg J, editor. *Advances in Organ Biology: The Biology of the Eye.* Volume No. 10. London: Elsevier; 2006.

63. McKown RL, Wang N, Raab RW, et al. Lacritin and other new proteins of the lacrimal functional unit. *Exp Eye Res.* 2008

64. McKown RL, Wang N, Raab RW, et al. Lacritin and other new proteins of the lacrimal functional unit. *Exp Eye Res.* 2009;88(5):848–858.

65. McCulley JP, Shine WE. Meibomian gland function and the tear lipid layer. *Ocul Surf.* 2003;1(3):97–106.

66. Foulks GN, Bron AJ. Meibomian gland dysfunction: a clinical scheme for description, diagnosis, classification, and grading. *Ocul Surf.* 2003;1(3):107–126.

67. Olami Y, Zajicek G, Cogan M, Gnessin H, Pe'er J. Turnover and migration of meibomian gland cells in rats' eyelids. *Ophthalmic Res.* 2001;33(3):170–175.

68. Butovich IA, Millar TJ, Ham BM. Understanding and analyzing meibomian lipids—a review. *Curr Eye Res.* 2008;33(5):405–420.

69. Svitova TF, Lin MC. Evaporation retardation by model tear-lipid films: The roles of film aging, compositions and interfacial rheological properties. *Colloids Surf B Biointerfaces.* 2021;197:111392.

70. Georgiev GA, Eftimov P, Yokoi N. Structure-function relationship of tear film lipid layer: A contemporary perspective. *Exp Eye Res.* 2017;163:17–28.

71. Seifert P, Spitznas M. Immunocytochemical and ultrastructural evaluation of the distribution of nervous tissue and neuropeptides in the meibomian gland. *Graefes Arch Clin Exp Ophthalmol.* 1996;234(10):648–656.

72. Sullivan DA, Sullivan BD, Ullman MD, et al. Androgen influence on the meibomian gland. *Invest Ophthalmol Vis Sci.* 2000;41(12):3732–3742.

73. Suzuki T, Schirra F, Richards SM, Jensen RV, Sullivan DA. Estrogen and progesterone control of gene expression in the mouse meibomian gland. *Invest Ophthalmol Vis Sci.* 2008;49(5):1797–1808.

74. Kam WR, Sullivan DA. Neurotransmitter influence on human meibomian gland epithelial cells. *Invest Ophthalmol Vis Sci.* 2011;52(12):8543–8548.

75. Nicolaides N, Kaitaranta JK, Rawdah TN, Macy JI, Boswell 3rd FM, Smith RE. Meibomian gland studies: comparison of steer and human lipids. *Invest Ophthalmol Vis Sci.* 1981;20(4):522–536.

76. Norn M. Meibomian orifices and Marx's line. Studied by triple vital staining. *Acta Ophthalmol (Copenh).* 1985;63(6):698–700.

16

Sensory Innervation of the Eye

Juana Gallar and M. Carmen Acosta

Introduction

Somatosensory innervation of the eye is provided by the peripheral axons of a small number of primary sensory neurons located in the trigeminal ganglion (TG). Most sensory axons enter the eyeball through the long and short ciliary nerves and reach all ocular tissues with the exception of the lens and the retina. Ocular innervation is particularly rich in the cornea, although all tissues of the anterior segment of the eye have an abundant sensory supply. Ocular sensory nerve fibers are functionally heterogeneous and include low mechanoreceptor, mechano- and polymodal nociceptor, and cold thermoreceptor types of sensory units responding to a variety of physical and chemical stimuli. Impulse activity originated at peripheral sensory nerve fibers innervating the eye reaches second-order neurons located at the trigeminal nucleus caudalis in the lower brainstem, from where sensory information travels to relay stations in the contralateral posterior thalamic nucleus and finally reaches the brain cortex.

Pain is the main sensation elicited by stimulation of ocular sensory nerves, although tactile sensations are evoked at the conjunctiva and feelings of cold are also evoked by mild cooling of the ocular surface. After repeated noxious stimulation or tissue injury, ocular polymodal nociceptors become sensitized and cause sustained pain and hyperalgesia. They also contribute to local inflammation through the antidromic release of peptide neurotransmitters stored in their peripheral endings (the "neurogenic inflammation"). Intact sensory nerve endings, particularly in the corneal epithelium, are subjected to a continuous remodeling. Ocular sensory nerves damaged by accidental or surgical injury or as a consequence of pathologic processes may also experience long-lasting changes of their excitability, giving rise to ocular dysesthesia and neuropathic pain referred to the eye.

Sensations originated at the ocular surface can be explored by esthesiometry. The cornea has an overall higher sensitivity than the conjunctiva. Sensitivity of the ocular surface is reduced by age and by a variety of pathologic processes that affect sensory innervation, such as herpetic keratitis, some types of corneal trauma and postinfectious conditions, certain hereditary corneal dystrophies, and anterior segment or vitreoretinal surgery. Although the principal eye diseases leading to impaired vision—such as retinal pathologies, chronic open-angle glaucoma, or cataract—course without pain, pain is a cardinal symptom of inflammatory and traumatic disturbances of the anterior segment of the eye. These include postsurgical conditions that may lead to ocular neuropathic pain, that is, pain caused by injury or disease of the ocular somatosensory system, either in the peripheral nerves or the central structures involved in ocular sensitivity. Dry eye, a multi-etiological condition that leads to the alteration of the ocular surface and its innervation, is the most common cause of ocular discomfort and pain.

ANATOMY OF OCULAR SENSORY NERVES

Origin of the ocular sensory nerves

Trigeminal ganglion neurons

The sensory innervation of the eye is provided by primary sensory neurons (most of them of small or medium size), clustered in the ophthalmic (medial) region of the ipsilateral TG. Ocular sensory neurons represent about 1.5% of the total number of neurons of the TG, most of them devoted to the cornea.[1] Trigeminal neurons are pseudounipolar and their axons divide into a peripheral branch that projects to the peripheral target tissues and a central myelinated branch that enters the brainstem to reach the trigeminal sensory complex. Based on the size and the presence (or absence) of a myelin sheath in the peripheral axons, corneal TG neurons can be classified as myelinated and unmyelinated (20% and 80% in the mouse, respectively).[1,2] The physiologic significance of myelin content is reflected in the conduction velocity of the peripheral axons (see further).

Most TG neurons innervating the eyeball contain several neuropeptides typical of primary sensory neurons, including calcitonin gene–related peptide (CGRP, present in about 50% of corneal neurons), the tachykinin substance P (present in about 20%), cholecystokinin, somatostatin, opioid peptides, pituitary adenylate cyclase–activating peptide (PACAP), vasoactive intestinal peptide (VIP), galanin, and neuropeptide Y (NPY), as well as neuronal nitric oxide synthase (nNOS).[1,3–8]

The ophthalmic nerve and its branches

The peripheral axonal branch of most ocular sensory neurons in humans exits the TG running with the ophthalmic division of trigeminal nerve (fifth cranial nerve), which traverses the superior orbital fissure and then branches into the nasociliary, the frontal, and the lacrimal nerves (Fig. 16.1). The nasociliary nerve gives several sensory branches: (1) two long ciliary nerves that reach the eyeball and pierce the sclera, constituting the major somatosensory output of the eye; (2) the infratrochlear nerve that innervates the medial aspect of lids, nose, and lacrimal sac; (3) the external nasal nerve that innervates the skin of the nose, the ala nasi and the nasal vestibule; and (4) a communicating branch to the ciliary ganglion. The ciliary ganglion is a parasympathetic ganglion located within the orbit that sends 5 to 10 short ciliary nerves carrying parasympathetic postganglionic axons, postganglionic sympathetic axons originating at the superior cervical ganglion, and the trigeminal sensory nerve axons arriving through the communicating branch of the nasociliary nerve. These mixed, short ciliary nerves enter the eyeball around the optic nerve. The second branch of the ophthalmic nerve is the frontal nerve, which bifurcates

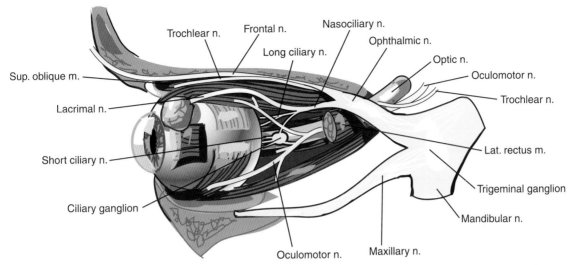

Fig. 16.1 Innervation of the eye. Medial view of the orbit showing the sensory and autonomic nerves directed to the eye. The ophthalmic branch of the trigeminal ganglion gives the nasociliary nerve that sends long and short ciliary nerves to the eyeball, the last through the ciliary ganglion. The trigeminal maxillary branch gives the infraorbital nerve that innervates part of the eye and the lower lid. Sympathetic fibers from the superior cervical ganglion, traveling within the carotid plexus and parasympathetic branches of the ciliary and the pterygopalatine ganglia join the short ciliary nerves. (Steven D. Waldman, Corey W. Waldman, Chapter 53 - Pain of Ocular and Periocular Origin, from Steven D. Waldman, *Pain Management*, 2nd Edition, W.B. Saunders, 2011.)

into the supraorbital nerve to innervate the upper eyelid and the frontal sinus, and the supratrochlear nerve that provides innervation to the forehead and the upper eyelid. Finally, the third branch of the ophthalmic nerve is the lacrimal nerve, which also incorporates postganglionic parasympathetic nerve fibers from the pterygopalatine ganglion and innervates the lacrimal gland and some areas of the conjunctiva and the skin of the upper lid.

A minor part of the sensory axons arising from the eye is conveyed together with the innervation of the conjunctiva and the lower eyelid skin, by the infraorbital nerve, a branch of the maxillary nerve, which in turn constitutes the second major branch of the TG (Fig. 16.1).

Trigeminal sensory axons end in the epithelia, connective tissue, and blood vessels of the lids, orbit, extraocular muscles, ciliary body, choroid, iris, scleral spur, sclera, cornea, and conjunctiva—the retina and lens being the only ocular tissues not receiving direct trigeminal sensory innervation.

Distribution of sensory nerve fibers within the eye

After penetrating the sclera around the optic nerve at the posterior eye pole, long and short ciliary nerves containing a mixture of sensory, sympathetic, and parasympathetic axons form a ring around the optic nerve, keeping the lamina cribrosa devoid of innervation. From there, ciliary nerve fascicles travel anteriorly toward the cornea within the suprachoroidal space, giving a few collaterals that provide the sparse innervation of the posterior part of the eye. Along their trajectory to the front of the eye, these nerve fiber bundles undergo repetitive branching. Some of the resulting nerve fibers innervate the sclera itself, especially the episcleral portion; others leave the sclera to enter the choroid, while most nerve filaments continue to innervate the ciliary body, the iris, and the cornea. Most of them finally form a series of ring meshworks of nerve fibers at the limbus—the so-called limbal or pericorneal plexuses.

Nerve filaments entering the choroid are composed of sensory, sympathetic, and parasympathetic axons, and branch extensively forming a dense network in which individual parasympathetic ganglion cells are also found.[9]

Limbal plexus nerves supply the sensory and autonomic innervation of the limbal vessels, the trabecular meshwork, and the scleral spur. Nerve bundles also form a circumferential plexus at the root of the iris that gives origin to the iridal innervation. Finally, a variable number of nerve trunks arising from the limbal plexus enter the corneal stroma (corneal stromal nerves). The cornea receives a significant portion of the ocular innervation, presenting a nerve density that is estimated to be 300–400 times higher than that of the human fingers or the teeth.[4,10]

The majority of the nerves directed to the eye are composed of thin, unmyelinated nerve fibers often incompletely surrounded by Remak (nonmyelinating) Schwann cells, while less than 30% present a myelin sheath provided by myelinating Schwann cells. Ocular nerves branch extensively, and most of them terminate as free nerve endings showing small enlargements (varicosities) along their terminal course. In addition, some encapsulated nerve endings similar to Krause and Meissner bodies have been observed in the choroid, in particular near the ciliary body[11,12] and the iris,[13] and in the episclera and chamber angle but not in the cornea.[14]

Architecture of corneal sensory nerves

The corneal innervation is anatomically organized in four levels from the penetrating stromal nerve trunks up to the intraepithelial nerve terminals (Fig. 16.2A).

Corneal stromal nerves

The anatomy of nerve trunks radially entering the corneal stroma is quite similar among mammals, varying only in their number (6–8 in rat, 15–40 in cat or dog, about 60 in human).[15–17] Stromal nerves

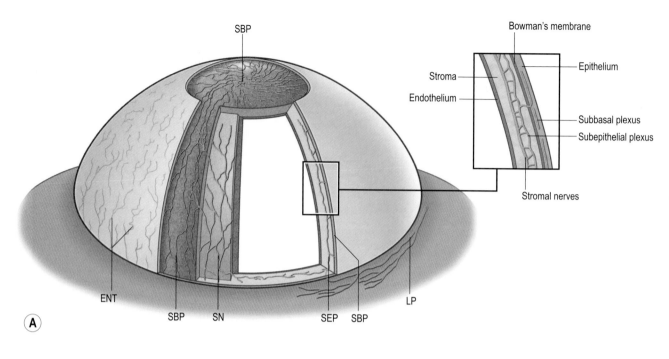

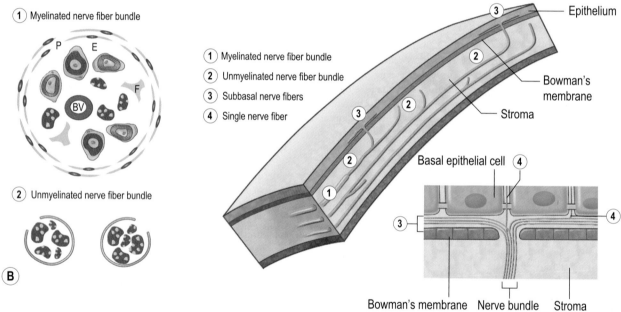

Fig. 16.2 Schematic representation of corneal innervation. (**A**) Distribution of nerves in the cornea. From the limbal plexus (*LP*), stromal nerve trunks (*SN*) penetrate the stroma radially and divide dichotomously to form the subepithelial plexus (*SEP*). Branches of this plexus ascend toward the epithelium, traverse Bowman's layer and the basal lamina of the epithelium, and form the sub-basal plexus (*SBP*) between the basal cells of the epithelium and its basal lamina, where nerve branches run horizontally as families of long parallel nerves with a common origin (leashes), which in turn give rise to intraepithelial nerve terminals (*ENT*). (**B**) Characteristics of nerve fibers in the peripheral and central cornea. Nerve fascicles with both unmyelinated and thin myelinated axons (1) penetrate the stroma and immediately lose the myelin and blood vessels. Thus, only unmyelinated axons are found throughout the corneal stroma (2). Subepithelial nerves ascend to form the sub-basal nerve plexus (3) from which individual axons (4) ascend vertically toward the corneal surface, with axons terminating at various levels of the corneal epithelium *BV*, blood vessel; *E*, epineurium; *F*, fibroblast; *P*, perineurium.

branch immediately after entering the cornea and run within the stroma as ribbon-like filaments enclosed by a basal lamina and Schwann cells. Stromal nerve trunks are composed of both unmyelinated and thinly myelinated (Aδ) axons[1,18] (Fig. 16.2B), although myelinated axons (about 20–30% of the nerve fibers) lose their myelin sheath within a millimeter after penetrating the stroma. Similarly, nerve fascicles also lose the intrinsic blood vessels once in the stroma, which contributes to the transparency of the cornea.[16,17]

The branches of the stromal nerve arborization anastomose extensively, forming the anterior stromal nerve plexus, a dense and complex network of intersecting small- and medium-sized nerve bundles and individual axons with no preferred orientation laying in the anterior corneal stroma, at different depths depending on the species but being the densest in the anterior third of the stroma (Fig. 16.3A,B).[19] In contrast, the posterior half of the human stroma and the corneal endothelium are devoid of sensory nerve fibers.

In addition to the stromal nerve innervation, a few small nerve fascicles originating at the limbal plexus and at the conjunctiva superficially enter the peripheral cornea to innervate the perilimbal and peripheral corneal zones.[16]

Subepithelial nerve plexus

In humans and higher mammals, the most superficial layer of the anterior stromal nerve plexus, located in a narrow strip of stroma immediately beneath Bowman's layer, is especially dense and is referred to as the corneal subepithelial nerve plexus, its nerve density generally higher in the peripheral than in the central cornea.[19] Two anatomically distinct types of nerve bundles are distinguished in the subepithelial plexus. One forms a highly anastomotic meshwork made of single axons and thin nerve fascicles located immediately beneath Bowman's layer without penetrating it, toward the corneal epithelium. The second type consists of about 400–500 medium-sized, curvilinear bundles that penetrate Bowman's layer and the epithelium basal membrane, mainly in the peripheral and intermediate cornea. These bundles shed the Schwann cell coating, bend at a 90-degree angle, and divide, each into 2 to 20 thinner nerve fascicles that continue into the corneal epithelium as the sub-basal nerve plexus (Fig. 16.2A,B; Fig. 16.3A,C,D).[17] A relatively low number of stromal nerves penetrate Bowman's layer in the central cornea, which receives most of its innervation from long sub-basal nerves that enter the peripheral corneal epithelium directly from the limbal plexus.[19] Remak Schwann cells cover nerve axons within the stroma until the nerve bundles traverse the epithelium basal membrane. Once in the epithelium, nerve axons are no longer covered by glial cells[20] (Fig. 16.2.B).

Despite their considerable branching, most stromal and subepithelial nerve bundles pass uninterrupted through the stroma to reach the corneal epithelium and apparently do not provide functional innervation to stromal tissue. However, a small proportion of corneal nerve fibers appear to travel downward to terminate in the stroma as expanded structures resembling free nerve endings or in close relation with stromal keratocytes and resident immune cells.[21,22]

Sub-basal nerve plexus

The sub-basal nerve plexus in humans is formed by 5000 to 7000 nerve fascicles inside an area of about 90 mm². A sub-basal nerve bundle gives several side branches, each containing three to seven individual axons. Thus, the total number of axons in the sub-basal plexus is estimated to vary between 20,000 and 44,000.[4]

The sub-basal nerve axons may travel up to 6 mm between the basal epithelial cells and their basal lamina, roughly parallel to one another. The arrangement of a stromal nerve bundle branching into multiple, parallel daughter nerve fascicles constitutes a unique neuroanatomical structure characteristic of the cornea and is termed an *epithelial leash*.[10,19] Epithelial leashes are constituted by up to 40 individual unmyelinated straight and beaded nerve fibers of variable diameter (0.05–2.5 microns).[23] Nerve fibers in adjacent leashes interconnect repeatedly such that they are no longer recognizable as individual leashes, forming, finally, a relatively homogeneous nerve plexus. In vivo confocal microscopy (IVCM) has shown that the sub-basal nerve plexus often forms a whorl-like spiral pattern of nerve fibers, the center of which

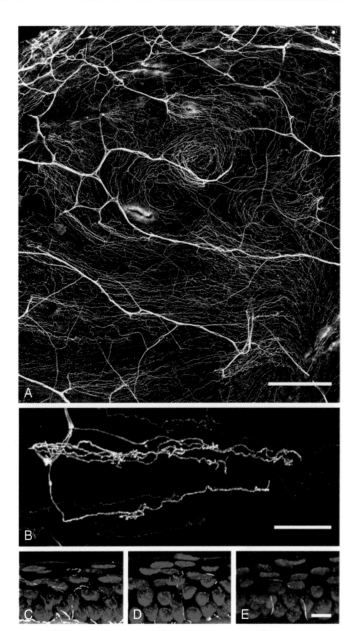

Fig. 16.3 Corneal innervation. (**A**) Architecture of the intrastromal and sub-basal nerves of the mouse cornea. Nerve trunks enter from the limbus into the stroma where they ramify, giving rise to a moderately dense subepithelial plexus whose nerves penetrate the basal lamina of the epithelium to form a dense sub-basal plexus. This confocal image of a whole mount C57BL/6J mouse cornea stained with anti-β tubulin III antibody depicts two sub-basal whorl areas. (**B**) Confocal image of the cornea of an anesthetized TRPM8-EYFP mice showing a nerve leash at the sub-basal plexus. From the stroma, a nerve penetrates through the basal lamina of the corneal epithelium and forms the leash, the nerve fibers of which run parallel for a long distance within the epithelium basal cell layer. (**C–E**) Sub-basal nerves give rise to nerve terminals that ascend through the corneal epithelium cells. According to their branching complex (**C**), ramified (**D**) and simple (**E**) nerve terminals are identified. Corneal sections 15 μm thick stained with anti-β tubulin III antibody depict the different types of nerve endings ascending within the epithelium cells, whose blue, fluorescent nuclei are stained with Hoechst 33342. Scale bars: A, 250 μm; B, 100 μm; C–E, 10 μm. (A, C–E: Modified from Frutos-Rincón L, Gómez-Sánchez JA, Íñigo-Portugués A, Acosta MC, Gallar J. An experimental model of neuro-immune interactions in the eye: corneal sensory nerves and resident dendritic cells. Published online 2022).

is called the "vortex" (Fig. 16.3A).[24] In humans it is located 2 to 3 millimeters inferior and nasal to the corneal apex. Many mammal species including mouse, rat, guineapig, cat, dog, and macaque also present this centripetal spiral whorl-like nerve pattern. Most species have only one spiral whereas multiple spirals are present in the mouse cornea (Fig. 16.3A).[25–27] The mechanisms that govern the formation and maintenance of this spiral pattern remain unknown. Basal corneal epithelial cells and sub-basal nerves appear to migrate centripetally in tandem during development and in the adult.[28,29] Thus it is possible that basal epithelial cells derived from limbal stem cells migrate centripetally in a whorl-like fashion toward the corneal apex in response to a chemotropic guidance, electromagnetic cues, population pressures, and/or preferential desquamation of epithelial cells in the central cornea. The sub-basal nerves that occupy the narrow intercellular spaces between these migrating cells would be pulled along their trajectory.[20,30] An alternate possibility is that sub-basal nerves would develop first their whorl-like orientation, providing in turn a structural scaffolding that directs epithelial cell migration, or it may be that both nerves and epithelial cells follow the same cues, either when moving at the same time or at different times during development.[28,31–33]

Intraepithelial nerve terminals

From the sub-basal nerves running horizontally through the basal epithelium, single fibers split off and turn 90 degrees vertically as a profusion of thin, short, and beaded terminal axons ascending between the epithelial cells, often with a modest amount of additional branching, up to the more superficial layers of the corneal epithelium (Fig. 16.3C–E). Depending on their branching pattern, intraepithelial nerve terminals are described as simple, ramifying, or complex (Fig. 16.3C–E).[4,26,34] Some nerve terminals do not branch after leaving the sub-basal nerves and end as free nerve endings within the outermost cell layer of the corneal epithelium, being classified as simple intraepithelial nerve terminals. Ramifying nerve terminals branch between the wing and squamous cell layers of the epithelium into three to four parallel nerve fibers traveling for up to 100 μm. Complex nerve terminals branch profusely within the wing cell layer of the epithelium, forming clusters of fibers that end both between the wing and squamous cell layers. All three types of intraepithelial fibers end as free nerve endings, appearing as prominent, bulbous terminal expansions that appear morphologically homogeneous when visualized using optical or electron microscopy, although immunocytochemical staining reveals differences in the expression of neuropeptides and other neurotransmitters, suggesting a functional heterogeneity.[4] At the ultrastructural level, corneal nerve endings contain abundant small clear vesicles, perhaps filled with excitatory amino acids, and large, dense-cored vesicles containing neuropeptides such as calcitonin gene–related peptide (CGRP), substance P, and other peptides. They also contain mitochondria, glycogen particles, neurotubules, and neurofilaments.[3,4,35] The nerve terminals are located throughout all layers of the corneal epithelium, extending up to a few microns of the corneal surface. Occasionally, epithelial cell membranes facing the nerve terminals show invaginations that may eventually completely surround the nerve ending.[4,32,34] This intimate relationship raises the possibility of bidirectional exchange of diffusible substances between both structures. Epithelial cells may also function as substitute glial cells for intraepithelial axons, phagocytizing distal axon fragments within hours after corneal nerve lesion.[20,30] The intimate contacts also allow nerve endings to detect changes in epithelial cell shape or volume, such as those produced by ocular surface desiccation or swelling, thus contributing to corneal sensitivity.

The innervation density of the corneal epithelium is probably the highest of any surface epithelium. Although the actual number of corneal nerve endings remains a matter of speculation, considering that each sub-basal nerve fiber gives at least 10 to 20 intraepithelial nerve terminals, it is reasonable to speculate that the human central cornea contains approximately 3500 to 7000 nerve terminals/mm². This rich innervation provides the cornea with a highly sensitive detection system, and it has been hypothesized that injury of a single epithelial cell may be sufficient to trigger pain perception.[32] Nerve terminal density, and thus corneal sensitivity, is higher in the central cornea and decreases progressively when moving toward the periphery. Similarly, corneal sensitivity and nerve density decrease progressively as a function of age and in several ocular pathologies, including systemic metabolic diseases such as diabetes, and ocular viral, parasitic, and bacterial infections (Table 16.1).[36–40]

An individual stromal axon entering at the corneoscleral limbus undergoes repetitive branching and eventually travels across as much as three-quarters of the cornea before terminating.[27] As a result, individual receptive fields of corneal sensory fibers range in size from less than 1 mm² to as much as 50 mm² and may cover up to 25% of the corneal surface. The extensive branching also explains the significant overlapping of receptive fields found in electrophysiological studies of single corneal nerve fibers.

Morphology of conjunctiva and lid margin sensory innervation

Compared with the cornea, little is known about the sensory innervation of the conjunctiva and eyelid margins. Sensory innervation of the conjunctiva and lid margin is provided by the supratrochlear, infratrochlear, supraorbital, and lacrimal nerves (all of them branches of the ophthalmic nerve), and the infraorbital nerve (branch of the maxillary nerve). Nerve bundles innervating the conjunctiva are thin myelinated and unmyelinated axons containing CGRP and/or substance P and terminating as free nerve endings located around the stromal blood and lymph vessels.[41–46] Some nerve endings locate in the conjunctival epithelium or around the acini of meibomian glands.[44,45,47–49] Myelinated axons terminating at the limbal conjunctiva as structures resembling Krause nerve endings have been described in the human eye. They are distributed in all the bulbar conjunctiva but are more abundant around the limbus.[14,50]

The lid margin is innervated by free nerve endings, mostly located within the epithelial cells at the mucocutaneous junction, as well as by abundant structures similar to the Merkel disc endings and Meissner corpuscles described in the skin.[43] Similarly to the hairy skin, the lid margin is also innervated by myelinated axons ending as lanceolate terminals associated with clusters of Merkel cells, encapsulated Ruffini endings and/or with the base of eyelashes.[43] These are specialized structures associated to low-threshold mechanoreceptors that may provide extreme mechanical sensitivity of the eyelid margin, where protective reflex blink responses are evoked even by mechanical stimuli of very low intensity.[51]

Central sensory pathways
Trigeminal brainstem nuclear complex

Sensory information from the eye is carried by TG neurons to the ventral portion of the ipsilateral trigeminal brainstem nuclear complex (TBNC), to activate ocular sensory second-order neurons located at several levels of TBNC. Most second-order neurons receiving input from TG neurons innervating the cornea are found in the intermediate zone between interpolaris and caudalis subnuclei (Vi/Vc), in laminae I and II of the subnucleus caudalis/upper cervical spinal cord (Vc/C1), and in the adjacent bulbar lateral reticular formation (Fig. 16.4). Additionally, few trigeminal neurons innervating ocular and periocular tissues project to the principal nucleus of the TBNC, and a very

TABLE 16.1 Causes of reduced or enhanced corneal sensitivity

Reduced sensitivity

Genetic diseases	• Familial corneal hypoesthesia • Congenital corneal anesthesia (CCA) • CCA associated with trigeminal hypoesthesia and neurologic disorders (Moebius syndrome; hereditary sensory and autonomic neuropathies type III — Riley-Day syndrome —, and type IV type V — congenital insensitivity to pain —; cerebellar ataxia, etc.) • CCA associated with somatic disorders (Goldenhar-Gorlin syndrome — oculo-auriculo-vertebral dysplasia —; ectodermal dysplasia, etc.) • CCA associated with multiple endocrine neoplasia 2b (prominent corneal nerves) • CCA associated with other genetic ocular alterations (corneal dystrophies, epithelial basement dystrophy, microsomia, etc.)
Other systemic diseases	• Diabetes • CNS disturbances (infarctions, tumors, and other space-occupying lesions) • Leprosy • Neurosarcoidosis • Orbital tumors and inflammations (occasionally)
Eye surgery	• Long cataract incisions • Refractive surgery • Keratoplasty • Retinal surgery (especially circular buckling operations) • Extensive cyclophotocoagulation • Orbital surgery damaging sensory pathways to the eye • Lid speculum damage (occasionally)
Infections	• Ocular zoster • Other herpetic infections • Large bacterial ulcers • Acanthamoeba keratitis (initially hypersensitive)
Drugs	• Topical anesthetics (abuse) • Topical beta-blockers • Topical nonsteroidal anti-inflammatory drugs (NSAIDs) • Cocaine abuse
Other conditions	• Chemical or thermal corneal burns • Ocular surface disease/dry eye in some cases • Contact lens wear • Neurosurgical procedures (acoustic neuroma, trigeminal neuralgia, etc.) • Aging

Enhanced sensitivity or irritation sensations

Diseases of the ocular surface	• Dry eye with conjunctival or corneal epithelial lesions (sensitivity to air conditioning, contact lenses, cigarette smoke, etc.) or unstable tear fluid (lid function, pinguecula, stitches) • Recurrent erosion or map-dot-fingerprint corneal dystrophy, exposure to toxic chemicals
Acute or chronic inflammation of the ocular surface	• Inflammatory dry eye in Sjögren's syndrome, rheumatoid arthritis, graft-versus-host disease • Conjunctivalization of the cornea, pterygium • Postrefractive surgery pain (occasionally) • Acute acanthamoeba infection • Corneal ulcers and inflammations (acute stage)

Modified from Belmonte C, Tervo TM. Pain in and around the eye. In: McMahon S, Koltzenburg M, eds. *Wall and Melzack's Textbook of Pain.* Philadelphia, PA: Elsevier; 2006:887–901.

sparse number are confined to a few locations along the ventral border of the pars oralis and interpolaris of the spinal trigeminal nucleus.[52–58]

A similar pattern has been described for the central connections of TG neurons innervating the eyelid and the lacrimal glands.[55,59–61]

The different areas of the TBNC are interconnected through a dense fiber system. Its functional significance is not fully understood, but it seems to contribute to protective mechanisms integrated at the brainstem and driven by ocular sensory input, as is the case of reflex blinking.[62–64]

Ocular representation at higher levels of the central nervous system

Most ocular second-order neurons project to different places in the central nervous system including brainstem regions as the superior salivatory/facial motor nucleus and the contralateral thalamus, although very little is known still about the central sensory pathway involved in ocular sensations.[65–67] Neurons receiving corneal information have been identified in the most posterior and medial areas of the somatosensory thalamus,[68] which in terms of somatotopy correspond to the

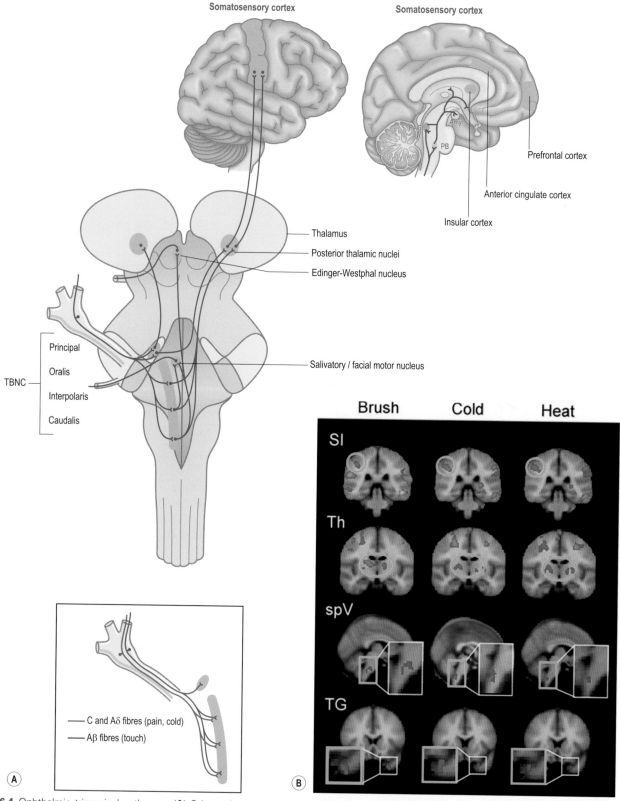

Fig. 16.4 Ophthalmic trigeminal pathways. (**A**) Schematic representation of the trigeminal brainstem nuclear complex (*TBNC*), composed of the principal nucleus, located in the mesencephalon, and the spinal nucleus, subdivided into subnucleus oralis, interpolaris, and caudalis. TBNC projects to the contralateral thalamus, and from there to the primary somatosensory cortex, and the insular, cingulate, and prefrontal cortex, responsible for sensory-discriminative processing. TBNC projections also reach other areas of the brain involved in the processing of affective and modulatory aspects of ocular pain such as the periaqueductal gray (PAG), the parabrachial area (PB), the lateral and posterior hypothalamus, and the amygdala (Amy). Trigeminal projections to the salivatory/facial motor nucleus, and to the Edinger-Westphal nucleus are also represented. *Inset:* Distribution of thick myelinated mechanosensory fibers and thin (thermosensitive and nociceptive) fibers within the TBNC. (**B**) MRI images showing the activation by noxious stimulation of the trigeminal sensory pathway. *TG,* Trigeminal ganglion; *spV,* spinal trigeminal nucleus; *Th,* thalamus; *SI,* primary somatosensory cortex. (From Becerra L, Morris S, Bazes S, et al. Trigeminal neuropathic pain alters responses in CNS circuits to mechanical (brush) and thermal (cold and heat) stimuli. *J Neurosci.* 2006;26(42):10646–10657. https://doi.org/10.1523/JNEUROSCI.2305-06.2006. Copyright 2006 Society for Neuroscience.)

representation of the trigeminal ophthalmic branch.[69,70] These thalamic neurons project in turn to primary (SI) and secondary (SII) somatosensory cortical areas responsible for pain sensations and reactions. Nonvisual sensory input from the eye is represented in contralateral cortical SI areas 3b and 1 (Fig. 16.4), located together with those that represent nose, ear, and scalp.[71–73]

Some ocular second-order neurons at the Vi/Vc transition and the VcC1 region project to the parabrachial area, which is in turn connected with the insular, cingulate, and prefrontal cortex and the amygdala, hypothalamus, and periaqueductal gray matter. These projections provide the neural substrate for the affective components of sensations evoked by eye stimulation, as well as for the involvement of the autonomic nervous system in ocular pain.[74–76]

DEVELOPMENT, REMODELING AND REGENERATION OF CORNEAL INNERVATION

Development of corneal nerves

The cornea lacks sensory innervation until the fifth gestational month, when corneal nerve endings appear. During development, sensory axons first form the nerve ring around the cornea (the limbal nerve plexus) and subsequently axons grow radially into the corneal tissue (Fig. 16.5A).[34,77] The molecular signals controlling ocular nerve growth remain unknown, although several guidance molecules may regulate the process. Nerve growth factor (NGF; one of the neurotrophic factors released by corneal epithelial cells, keratocytes, and bone marrow-derived cells present in the cornea) influences the development and survival of corneal nerves.[78–81] The human cornea also expresses other neurotrophins as brain-derived neurotrophic factor (BDNF), and neurotrophins-3 (NT-3) and 4 (NT-4).[78] Regulators of cell movement and migration also contribute to guide the trigeminal axons during development. These regulators include Slits, netrins, ephrins, and semaphorins and their respective receptors: Roundabout (ROBO), UNC/DCC, Eph receptors, and neuropilins.[82] Some members of the semaphorin family, in particular the so-called immune semaphorins, are expressed in corneal epithelium and regulate corneal nerve development by exerting different roles. Semaphorins promote axon outgrowth and also mediate, together with other nerve guidance molecules as Slit2, the initial repulsion of trigeminal sensory axons from the cornea, thus inducing the proper formation of the pericorneal nerve ring meshwork, and also contribute to the positioning of a subset of axonal projections in the choroid fissure that form a ventral plexus from which the iris innervation is later supplied.[82–87] Upon completion of the pericorneal nerve ring, sensory nerves enter the cornea as bundles, at uniformly spaced sites around its entire circumference, and begin to extend radially inside the cornea, first innervating its periphery and then the entire stromal surface. The depth at which nerves enter the corneal stroma correlates with the area of the cornea that they will innervate, so that the deepest stromal nerves innervate almost the entire corneal surface, whereas the more superficial nerves that enter the stroma nearest to the epithelium mainly supply the periphery.[31]

The uniform separation between corneal nerve bundles during embryogenesis seems to be due to the release of neurorepulsive factors from pioneering growth cones as they leave the limbal nerve ring and enter the corneal stroma, keeping nerve bundles growing relatively straight toward the center of the cornea as centripetal radii and separated one from another. Semaphorin 3A, a secreted semaphorin expressed in the developing lens and cornea, and its receptors neuropilin11 and plexin-A4 present in trigeminal nerve sprouts, are key regulators of trigeminal axon branching in the cornea.[82,88–90] While guiding nerve growth, semaphorins may also contribute to keeping the cornea avascular. Semaphorins repel angioblasts and vascular endothelial cells during development.[85] The extension or radial innervation within the cornea is produced by bifurcation of nerve fascicles in successive, concentric zones, thus suggesting that the position and orientation of intracorneal nerves is determined by the intracorneal milieu[28] and the migration of epithelial cells.[31] However, sub-basal nerve arrangement in a swirl pattern seems to precede the centripetal epithelial cell migration to form the central cornea.[89] Stromal composition and neurotrophic factors released from corneal epithelium also participate in the regulation of nerve density and orientation of corneal nerves during development.[91,92]

Dynamic remodeling of adult corneal innervation

Corneal nerves are subjected to a remodeling in the adult cornea throughout life. Deep stromal nerve fiber bundles maintain a relatively constant position and configuration within the cornea, whereas the corneal sub-basal nerve plexus, and especially intraepithelial nerve terminals, experience an extensive rearrangement (Fig. 16.5B; Box 16.1). Time-lapse IVCM examination of living human eyes reveals that the human sub-basal corneal nerve plexus is a dynamic structure with a slow but continuous centripetal movement (5–15 microns/day) that changes the whorl-centered plexus in a 6-week period.[93] Intraepithelial nerve endings are subjected to more prominent morphofunctional changes; their continuous remodeling follows the long-term sub-basal nerve reconfiguration.[94] Glial cells do not appear to be involved, as there are no Schwann cells within the epithelium. The possibility exists that the continuous shedding of corneal epithelial cells strongly influences the rearrangement and dynamics of epithelial nerve terminals.

Reorganization of differentiating corneal epithelial cells migrating up to the most superficial layers of the corneal epithelium induces changes in intraepithelial nerve ending architecture that occur continuously and can be appreciated from one day to the next.[94,95] The molecular mechanisms responsible for this continuous rearrangement of corneal nerves are unknown. Adult corneal sensory nerves retain the ability to respond to semaphorins, which promote nerve sprouting both in transected and intact nerves,[90,96,97] suggesting the semaphorins as drug targets to improve corneal nerve regeneration.[98]

Changes of corneal sensory innervation with aging

In several mammalian species, corneal nerve terminal density decreases with age,[25,99] and this may be the basis of the decreased corneal sensitivity and the altered tearing regulation reported in the elderly.[100–103] Although corneal nerves may have uncompromised morphology and function throughout life, it is common for them to be subject to degenerative processes typical of aging. The availability of transgenic and knock-in mice allows the visualization of nerves in the transparent corneal tissue in living animals and ex vivo corneas, to study corneal nerve remodeling with age. The sub-basal plexus is fully developed in 3- to 4-month-old mice and starts disorganizing at 9 months. In old mice (18–24 months old), there is a reduction of sub-basal and intraepithelial nerve density, and an increased tortuosity and profound disorientation of sub-basal leashes that affect both the CGRP-positive axons (presumably nociceptors) and Transient receptor potential cation channel melastatin subfamily member 8 (TRPM8)-positive axons (presumably cold thermoreceptors). The proportion of straight and beaded nerve fibers of sub-basal leashes is also altered in aged animals, where most fibers are straight. Similarly, there are changes with age in the proportion of the different morphologic types of intraepithelial nerve endings, with simple intraepithelial nerve endings being abundant and complex nerve endings being very sparse in older animals.[40,104]

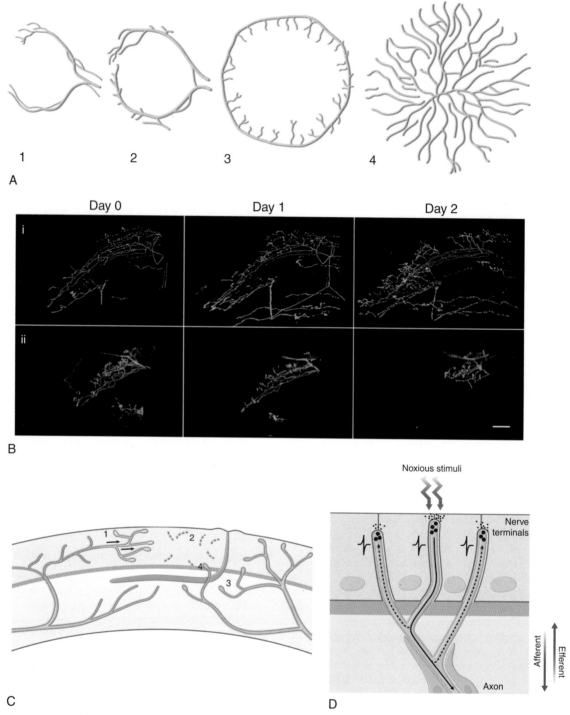

Fig. 16.5 Development, remodeling and regeneration of corneal sensory nerves. (**A**) Schematic representation of corneal sensory nerve growth during development, in the chick cornea. Growing trigeminal sensory axons avoid the cornea and extend dorsally and ventrally (**1**), forming a pericorneal nerve ring at E8 (**2**). Upon completion of this ring, sensory nerves begin to enter the cornea radially, first innervating its periphery at E9–E10 (**3**), and finally its entire surface at E15 (**4**). (**B**) Continuous remodeling of nerves in the healthy cornea. Remodeling of TRPM8+ sub-basal leashes and their intraepithelial terminals occurring within 1 week in the mouse cornea. Green fluorescence constitutively expressed by TRPM8+ nerve fibers and three-dimensional rendering reconstruction of sub-basal leashes *(red)* and nerve terminals *(gray)*. Nerves increasing (**i**) and decreasing (**ii**) their length over time are present in the same cornea. *Arrowheads* indicate the penetration point of a stromal nerve to form the sub-basal leash. (**C**) Schematic representation of the changes taking place in corneal sensory axons following injury. Sprouts of intact nerves (**1**) invade the injured area while the distal end of axotomized fibers degenerate (**2**). Central stumps of lesioned nerves form neuroma endings (**3**) from which sprouts begin to invade the denervated area (**4**), initiating the recovery of corneal sensitivity. (**D**) Schematic representation of afferent and efferent functions of polymodal nociceptors. Stimulation of a section of the peripheral branches of a polymodal nociceptor fiber by a noxious substance directly depolarizes the nerve endings affected by the stimulus. This depolarization generates action potentials that travel centripetally *(continuous arrow)*, and also cause the local release of neuropeptides *(dots)* contained in sensory nerve terminals, which contribute to local inflammation. Action potentials traveling centrally also antidromically invade *(interrupted arrows)* unstimulated neighboring branches. These then become depolarized and release neuropeptides in an area of the tissue that was not directly affected by the stimulus, thus extending inflammation (neurogenic inflammation). B, From Íñigo-Portugués et al., unpublished results. C, D, Modified from Belmonte C, Aracil A, Acosta MC, Luna C, Gallar J. Nerves and sensations from the eye surface. *Ocul Surf.* 2004;2(4):248–253. https://doi.org/10.1016/S1542-0124(12)70112-X.)

Regeneration of injured corneal nerves

Like other peripheral nerves, adult corneal nerves retain the ability to regenerate following injury. After damage or transection, the morphology and functional properties of corneal nerves change substantially. Their morphologic and functional recovery depends on the extension, depth, and type of injury.[105–107] After nerve transection, nerve processes distal to the site of lesion degenerate, whereas central stumps start to regenerate, finally producing a nerve pattern rather different from the original corneal nerve architecture.[108,109] The regenerative process takes place in several stages (Fig. 16.5C). When corneal nerves are cut, the denervated area is first invaded by sprouts of adjacent, intact nerve fibers. Later, the central stump of injured axons starts to regenerate, forming microneuroma-like structures from which newly formed sprouts begin to develop, while the early branches from intact fibers begin to degenerate.[4,108] Morphologic and functional changes in regenerating neurons may be due to the interruption of the uptake of signal molecules produced by corneal cells such as NGF. The absence of these molecules, usually centripetally transported along the parent axon to the neuron's soma to regulate gene expression, causes morphologic and functional changes in regenerating neurons.[110] Regeneration of corneal nerves after refractive vision correction surgeries or corneal transplant depends on the depth of ablation, considering whether or not it affects the stromal nerves. Whereas the fibers of the sub-basal plexus regenerate in months, especially from the sub-basal nerves external to the injury, the stromal nerves hardly regenerate and seem to stop at the edge of the injury. This is the reason why many corneal transplants completely lack stromal nerves, or these are limited to the peripheral area of the graft.

Corneal nerves are also negatively affected by many systemic and local diseases inducing neuropathies. Images suggestive of corneal nerve regeneration as the presence of neuroma-like structures and increased nerve tortuosity are common in herpes virus keratitis, diabetes, and dry eye.[111–113] A highly prevalent systemic disease altering corneal nerve morphology and function is diabetes, in which corneal nerve density and sensitivity are reduced.[114–116] In diabetic patients, the appearance of sub-basal nerves resembles the characteristics of intraepidermal small fiber neuropathy. Therefore, IVCM of corneal nerves could be used as a biomarker for the follow-up of diabetic neuropathy.[117]

FUNCTIONAL CHARACTERISTICS OF OCULAR SENSORY INNERVATION

Most available data on the sensory neurons innervating the eye have been obtained by recording the electrical activity from the peripheral axons (innervating the cornea and the bulbar conjunctiva) or from the nerve terminals at the cornea of the primary sensory neurons located at the ophthalmic region of the TG. Knowledge is less abundant about the functional characteristics of the ocular trigeminal neurons, studied by recording the activity of TG neurons in situ or in tissue culture, or on the second-order ocular neurons located in the TBNC. Moving up the somatosensory pathway, knowledge about the somatosensory neurons that innervate the eye is even more scarce. These sensory neurons have been functionally classified depending on their response to different modalities of stimuli (mechanical, thermal, and chemical) (Fig. 16.5).

Trigeminal ganglion neurons

Sensory neurons innervating the cornea

Mechanonociceptors. Around 15% to 20% of the nerve fibers innervating the cornea respond only to mechanical forces and are classified as mechanonociceptors.[118,119] Their mechanical threshold is about 10 times lower than in the skin, possibly because corneal nerve terminals are more accessible to the stimulus, owing to its proximity to the surface of a nonkeratinized epithelium.

Corneal mechanonociceptors are medium-sized TG neurons whose peripheral axons are thinly myelinated and have conduction velocities in the Aδ range. They end as simple or sparsely ramified nerve terminals located in the uppermost cell layers of the corneal epithelium.[120] The receptive fields are generally round and of medium size, covering about 10% of the corneal surface (Fig. 16.6). The ability of mechanonociceptors to respond to mechanical stimulation is mediated by the mechanically sensitive ion channel Piezo2, expressed in the soma and peripheral nerve endings of corneal mechanonociceptor neurons.[18,121] Their response to mechanical stimulation is phasic, firing only a few nerve impulses in response to both brief or sustained mechanical stimuli (Fig. 16.7Ai). Therefore, they probably serve mainly to signal the presence of noxious mechanical stimuli (touching of the corneal surface, foreign bodies, etc.), and are presumably responsible for the acute, sharp sensation of pain produced by sudden mechanical insults.

Polymodal nociceptors. More than 60% of the sensory neurons innervating the cornea and the bulbar conjunctiva are activated by stimuli of intensity within the noxious or near noxious range, including mechanical forces, heat, intense cold, exogenous chemical irritants, and a large variety of endogenous molecules released by injured corneal tissue and by resident and migrating immune cells participating in the inflammation response.[22] Accordingly, they were named polymodal nociceptors (Figs 16.6 & 16.7A,B).[118,122,123] Most of polymodal nociceptor neurons are small and medium-sized TG neurons that express the transducing channel TRPV1 and have unmyelinated (C) axons, while a small portion, depending on species, have thin, myelinated (Aδ) nerve fibers. Most corneal polymodal nociceptors and their axons in the cornea are peptidergic and express CGRP, and about two-thirds of them also contain substance P.[2,7,124] They end as simple single-nerve terminals in the sub-basal plexus and the medium corneal epithelium layers, or as ramifying nerve terminals within the squamous cell layers.[26,120,125] Their receptive fields are round or oval, usually large, often covering up to one-quarter or more of the cornea, and may extend several millimeters beyond the cornea onto the adjacent limbus and sclera (Fig. 16.6). The large size and extensive overlapping of adjacent receptive fields of polymodal nociceptors, coupled with convergent mechanisms in the central nervous system, explain why stimuli of the corneal surface are poorly localized. Corneal polymodal nociceptors have tonic responses to the stimulation, with a continuous, irregular discharge of nerve impulses at a frequency roughly proportional to the magnitude of the stimulus, persisting as long as the stimulus is maintained and codifying its intensity and duration. Occasionally, the nerve impulse discharge overpasses the duration of the stimulus (postdischarge). Polymodal nociceptors respond to mechanical, chemical (local pH reduction), and heat (over 39–40°C) stimuli (Fig. 16.7Aii,iii). About half of them also develop a low-frequency response to corneal temperature reductions below 29°C.[118,122,123,126,127] A large number of endogenous chemicals

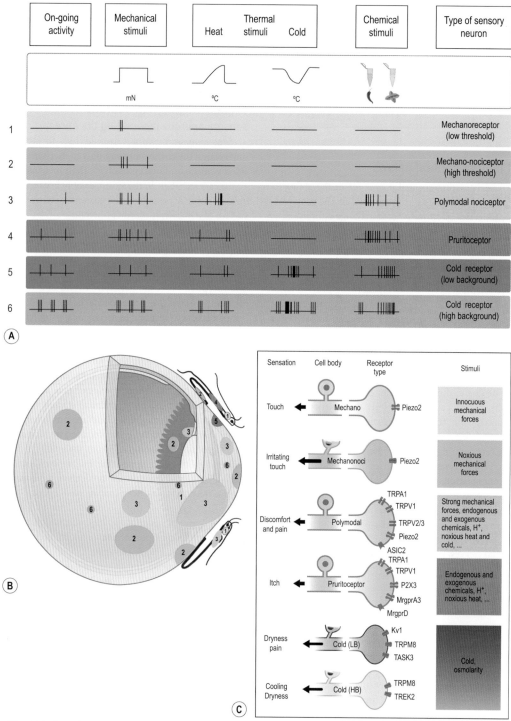

Fig. 16.6 Functional characteristics of ocular sensory fibers. (**A**) The presence of ongoing activity at rest and impulse discharges in response to different stimuli are represented for each functional type of sensory receptor innervating the eye. (**B**) Diagram of the eyeball and eyelids showing the distribution, size, and location on the ocular surface, the ciliary body, the iris, the palpebral and bulbar conjunctiva, and the lid border of the receptive fields of mechanosensory, polymodal, and cold sensory fibers innervating the eye. (**C**) Schematic representation of the peripheral nerve endings of various modality-specific primary sensory neurons, and the putative membrane ion channels involved in the detection and transduction of the different stimuli. (A, B, Modified from Belmonte C, Garcia-Hirschfeld J, Gallar J. Neurobiology of ocular pain. *Prog Retin Eye Res.* 1997;16(1):117–156; Belmonte C, Acosta MC, Gallar J. Neural basis of sensation in intact and injured corneas. *Exp Eye Res.* 2004;78(3):513–525; Frutos-Rincón L, Gómez-Sánchez JA, Íñigo-Portugués A, Acosta MC, Gallar J. An experimental model of neuro-immune interactions in the eye: corneal sensory nerves and resident dendritic cells. *Int J Mol Sci* 2022;23(6):2997. C, Modified from Belmonte C, Viana F. Molecular and cellular limits to somatosensory specificity. *Mol Pain.* 2008;4; Belmonte C, Acosta MC, Merayo-Lloves J, Gallar J. What causes eye pain? *Curr Ophthalmol Rep.* 2015;3(2):111–121; Comes N, Gasull X, Callejo G. Proton sensing on the ocular surface: Implications in eye pain. *Front Pharmacol.* 2021;12:773871)

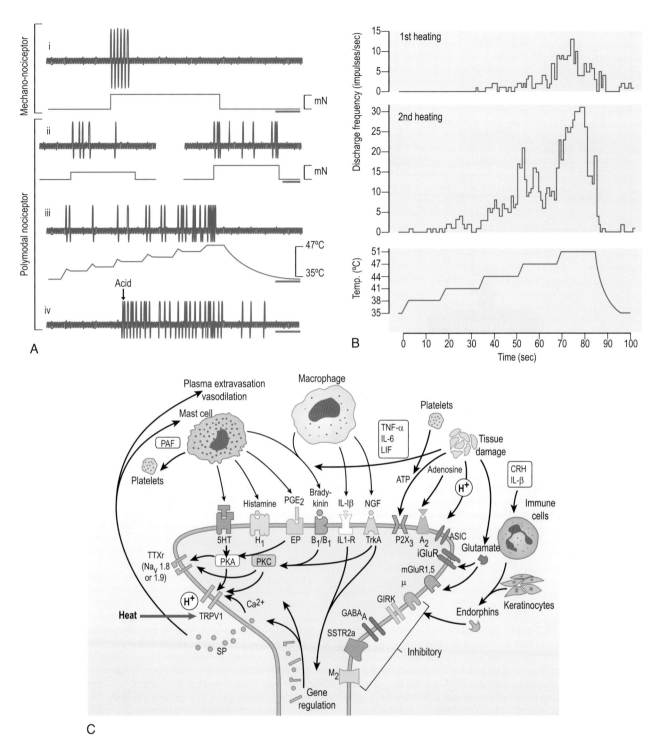

Fig. 16.7 Response characteristics of corneal sensory fibers in basal conditions and under inflammation. (**A**) Response to different types of stimuli of mechano- and polymodal nociceptors. (**i**) Transient (phasic) discharge evoked by a sustained mechanical indentation in a corneal mechanonociceptor fiber. (**ii**) Response of a polymodal nociceptor fiber to mechanical indentations of increasing amplitude (80 and 150 μm). (**iii**) Activation of a polymodal nociceptor fiber by stepwise heating (from 35°C to 47°C) of the corneal surface. (**iv**) Response of a polymodal nociceptor fiber to application of a drop of 10 mM acetic acid *(arrow)* on the corneal receptive field. The upper traces depict nerve impulse recordings and lower traces the stimulus waveform. (**B**) Sensitization of corneal polymodal nociceptors. Frequency histograms of the impulse discharge evoked by two identical stepwise heating cycles of the corneal surface separated by a 3-min interval, showing the lowered threshold and enhanced impulse firing in response to the second heating cycle. (**C**) Membrane receptor mechanisms and signaling pathways underlying activation and sensitization of polymodal nociceptive afferents by inflammatory mediators released after tissue injury. In turn, neuropeptides released by activated nociceptors contribute to local inflammation (neurogenic inflammation).

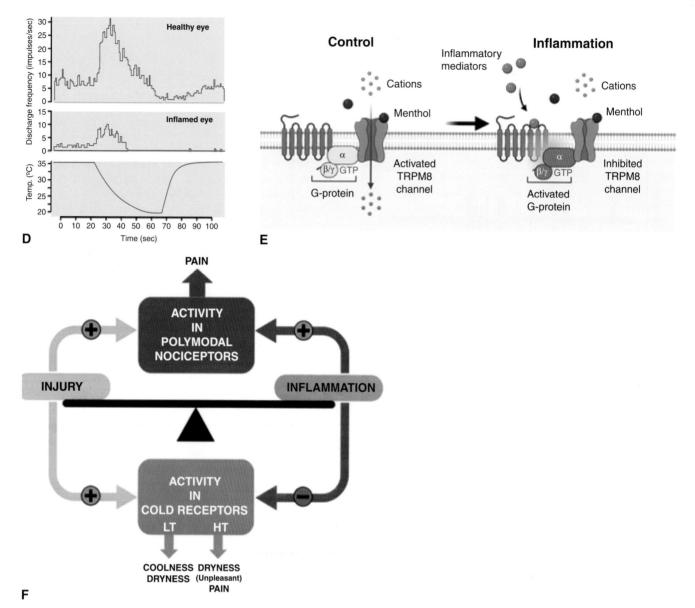

Fig. 16.7, cont'd (D) Inhibition of corneal cold thermoreceptors. Frequency histograms of the impulse discharge evoked by two identical cooling ramps (from 34°C to 20°C) applied to the cornea of a healthy eye and a UV-inflamed eye, showing the reduced impulse firing of the cold thermoreceptor fiber under inflammation. **(E)** Membrane receptor mechanism underlying the regulation of TRPM8 activity by G proteins in cold thermoreceptors. In healthy eyes, TRPM8 is pre-bound to Gαq. The channel has low activity at of 34°C and opens when the temperature drops and/or in the presence of menthol, allowing ions to pass through and increasing the firing frequency of the cold thermoreceptor fiber. Inflammatory mediators released by damaged tissue bind to a G protein–coupled receptor and activates Gαq, which inhibits the response of TRPM8 to cooling and menthol, thus decreasing firing activity of the cold thermoreceptor fiber. **(F)** Schematic representation of the influence of inflammation and injury on the activity of sensory neurons innervating the ocular surface (polymodal nociceptors, high background–low threshold cold thermoreceptors—LT, and low background–high threshold cold thermoreceptors—HT) as the cause of inflammatory pain, dryness sensations and neuropathic pain. The yellow shadow indicates the activated state of the G proteins. (A, From Belmonte C, Gallar J. The primary nociceptive neuron: A nerve cell with many functions. In: Rowe M, ed. *Somatosensory Processing: From Single Neuron to Brain Imaging.* Philadelphia, PA: Gordon & Breach Science Publisher; 2000:27–49. B, Modified from Belmonte C, Giraldez F. Responses of cat corneal sensory receptors to mechanical and thermal stimulation. *J Physiol.* 1981;321(1):355–368. https://doi.org/10.1113/JPHYSIOL.1981.SP013989. C, Modified from Meyer R, Ringkamp M, Campbell J, Raja S. Peripheral mechanisms of cutaneous nociception. In: McMahon S, Koltzenbrug M, eds. *Wall and Melzack's Textbook of Pain.* 5th ed. Philadelphia, PA: Elsevier; 2006:3–34. D, Modified from Acosta MC, Luna C, Quirce S, Belmonte C, Gallar J. Corneal sensory nerve activity in an experimental model of UV keratitis. *Investig Ophthalmol Vis Sci.* 2014;55(6):3403–3412. https://doi.org/10.1167/iovs.13-13774. E, Based on Zhang X, Mak S, Li L, et al. Direct inhibition of the cold-activated TRPM8 ion channel by Gαq. *Nat Cell Biol.* 2012;14(8):851–858. https://doi.org/10.1038/ncb2529. F, From Belmonte C, Acosta MC, Merayo-Lloves J, Gallar J. What causes eye pain? *Curr Ophthalmol Rep.* 2015;3(2):111–121. https://doi.org/10.1007/s40135-015-0073-9.)

(inflammatory mediators) also activate polymodal nociceptors (see section Inflammation). Their ability to respond to different modalities of stimuli depends on their expression of different membrane transduction molecules (Fig. 16.6C). These include various members of the TRP (transient receptor potential) ion channels superfamily: (1) TRPV1 (transient receptor potential vanilloid type 1 ion channel), a heat-activated transducing channel that integrates the responses to injury and inflammation by its ability to be also activated by protons, several endogenous mediators, and external chemical irritants; (2) TRPA1, considered a chemoreceptor for environmental irritants and inflammation agents that is opened by exogenous irritant chemicals, natural toxins, bacterial LPS, pruritogenic agents, and noxious cold temperatures; and (3) TRPV2 (transient receptor potential vanilloid type 2 ion channel) and TRPV3 (transient receptor potential vanilloid type 3 ion channel), which are opened by high temperatures.[125,128-134] Corneal polymodal neurons also express several members of the Acid-sensing ion channel (ASIC) family, which open in response to protons and endogenous mediators, and P2X channels opened by ATP, and presumably the mechanosensory channel Piezo2.[18,121,135,136]

Cold thermoreceptors. About 10% to 15% of corneal nerve fibers discharge spontaneously at the resting temperature of the corneal surface (around 34°C). They increase their firing rate as soon as this temperature is decreased (which occurs, for example, during evaporation of the corneal surface tear film, or after application of cold solutions or air jets onto the cornea) and are transiently silenced upon warming.[119,123,134,137-140] Corneal cold thermoreceptors have small receptive fields (around 1 mm diameter) located all over the corneal surface but more abundant in the peripheral cornea (Fig. 16.6). Cold thermoreceptor axons end as richly branched complex nerve endings superficially located within the corneal epithelium, and are less frequently simple and ramifying nerve endings.[26,40,120] Their sensitivity to cold is due to the expression of the cold-sensing channel TRPM8.[141-144]

Depending on the level of expression of TRPM8 channels, two types of corneal cold thermoreceptors are present in the cornea of young and adult animals (Fig. 16.6C).[40,123,134] About 60% of cold-sensitive neurons innervating the cornea and their peripheral nerve endings express abundant TRPM8 channels. They exhibit a high firing rate at the resting temperature of the ocular surface and are able to detect small corneal temperature decreases (≤0.5°C),[145] which is the reason they are called high background activity–low threshold (HB-LT) cold thermoreceptors. The frequency of action potentials generated by HB-LT cold thermoreceptors encode the static temperature of the cornea, although they respond with a high frequency peak response to sudden temperature changes. HB-LT cold thermoreceptors also detect changes in osmolarity, increasing their firing rate when exposed to moderate hyperosmolarity (around 340–360 mOsm/L) and reducing their firing activity in the presence of hyposmolar solutions. The response to osmolarity changes also depends on TRPM8 channel.[142,143] Under normal conditions, the activity of cold thermoreceptors is driven by the temperature reduction produced by tear film evaporation, as well as by the subsequent changes in tear film osmolarity.

Other cold thermoreceptor neurons show a weaker TRPM8 expression both in their somata and corneal nerve endings. Functionally, they correspond to a subpopulation of cold thermoreceptors with low firing rate at the background temperature of the cornea that require large temperature decreases to be activated (about –4°C) and encode a wide range of corneal temperature decreases, being named low background activity–high threshold (LB-HT) cold thermoreceptors.[123,134]

HB-LT cold thermoreceptors are recruited by small corneal temperature reductions, which are perceived as a sensation of freshness and cooling although with a variable irritative component. LB-HT cold thermoreceptors need more intense cooling of the cornea to be

activated, being probably responsible for the unpleasant irritation and dryness sensations.[127,146] In addition to evoking sensations, the information on corneal cooling and tear osmolarity changes provided to the central nervous system by cold thermoreceptors is used to regulate basal tearing and blinking rate.[142,143]

Sensory neurons innervating the sclera, iris, ciliary body, conjunctiva, and lid margin

The functional properties of the sensory neurons innervating other parts of the eye globe, as well as the conjunctiva and lid margin, have not been studied in great detail yet. However, the same main functional classes of sensory afferents as in the cornea, i.e., mechanonociceptors, polymodal nociceptors, and cold receptors, have been identified in the sclera,[123,147-149] iris and ciliary body,[13,147,150] and the bulbar conjunctiva (Fig. 16.6).[122,149,151-153] Mechanosensitive and polymodal nociceptor fibers of the sclera, uvea, and cornea are readily activated by externally applied pressure but only transiently by sudden increases of intraocular pressure up to 100 mmHg,[147] which explains the absence of pain in most forms of glaucoma. However, a combination of high intraocular pressure with inflammation, as occurs in congestive glaucoma, possibly causes nociceptor sensitization and a more sustained nociceptive inflow from ocular polymodal nociceptors to the brain, producing the intense pain characteristic for this disease. However, a small number of myelinated low-threshold mechanosensory nerve fibers responding to moderate changes of intraocular pressure and to mechanical stimulation have been functionally identified in the corneoscleral limbus and the lid margin.[147,149,153] They may correspond to axons of the encapsulated nerve endings found in the chamber angle and scleral spur that may be associated with neural regulation of the intraocular pressure,[154,155] and to the specialized structures associated with low-threshold mechanoreceptors present in the limbus and lid margin[43] that are activated by airborne particles, as well as by blinking and contact lens wear.

Whereas almost all corneal polymodal nociceptor fibers are peptidergic, the conjunctiva contains both peptidergic and nonpeptidergic polymodal nociceptor fibers. Next-generation sequencing techniques have allowed the distinguishing in the conjunctiva of two main types of nonpeptidergic nociceptor fibers that are involved in mechanical pain and nonhistaminergic itch (expressing the oncogene-like MAS-related G protein–coupled receptor member D, MrgprD, innervating mostly the lid wiper), and in the conventional histaminergic itch (MAS-related G protein–coupled receptor member A3, MrgprA3, innervating the nasal and temporal conjunctiva). These pruritoceptors are not present in the cornea (Figure 16.6).[156]

Cold-sensitive nerve fibers with response properties similar to cold thermoreceptors present in the cornea are also found in the conjunctiva, especially in the bulbar conjunctiva, where their stimulation evokes pure cold sensations.[157] Cold thermoreceptor nerve fibers also innervate the iris and the posterior sclera (Fig, 16.6). Cold receptor endings in these locations are not exposed to environmental temperature changes but are close to blood vessels and may serve to detect choroidal and retinal blood flow changes, thus contributing to reflex blood flow regulation rather than to the production of conscious thermal sensations or basal tearing and blinking regulation.[142,143,148,158]

Central pathways
Trigeminal brainstem nuclear complex
TG neurons innervating the eye and periocular tissues send the central projection of their axons to second-order neurons located at different levels of the TBNC. Most of them terminate at the lower part of the complex, the transition between the interpolaris and caudalis subnuclei (Vi/Vc), and the transition between the subnucleus

caudalis and the cervical spinal cord (Vc/C1). Only a few TG neurons terminate at the upper part of TBNC, that is, the principal nucleus (Vp) and the subnucleus oralis (Vo). A modality-specific distribution of corneal neurons within the TBNC has been proposed: Vi/Vc neurons respond to all modalities of stimuli and are related to the control of blinking and tearing, whereas those within the superficial laminae of Vc/C1 area respond only to heat and chemical irritation, which suggests that the input to this region is restricted to TG polymodal nociceptor neurons.[54,67,68,159] TG neurons innervating the eye lids and meibomian glands project over second-order neurons following a similar pattern.[55,61,160,161]

Second-order neurons of the Vi/Vc transition have large receptive fields that cover almost the entire ocular surface. They encode mechanical, cold, heat, and chemical stimuli in the innocuous and noxious range, are sensible to changes in the level of moistness of the ocular surface, and become desensitized upon repeated stimulation.[67,162–165] Some of them are also activated by intense light,[166] probably those receiving projections of the small subset of photosensitive TG neurons containing melanopsin.[167] These second-order ocular neurons project to the thalamus and to several brainstem regions as the superior salivatory or facial motor nucleus—depending on their peripheral input,[65–67] and the accessory oculomotor nucleus (Fig. 16.4A).[168] Their role in sensory-discriminative processing of ocular sensations seems minor, although Vi/Vc neurons participate in several trigeminal-evoked blink reflexes (initiated by mechanical stimulation, acidic or hyperosmolar solutions applied onto the ocular surface, bright light, etc.) in which afferent information from the ocular surface projects from the Vi/Vc to the superior salivatory nucleus and facial motor nucleus, responsible for the control of lacrimation and lid closing respectively.[64,169,170] Likewise, a population of neurons specifically inhibited by wetting and excited by drying and cooling of the ocular surface may be involved in reflex tearing and fluid homeostasis of the ocular surface.[67,162] We can speculate that these neurons receive at least part of their input originated at the peripheral cold fibers innervating eye surface tissues, whose sensory input is used to maintain basal lacrimation rate.[142]

Second-order neurons of the Vc/C1 region also encode mechanical, cold, heat, and chemical stimuli in the noxious range, and bright light. Their receptive fields cover part of the ocular surface and the neighbor lid skin and are sensitized by repeated stimulation. Some of ocular Vc/C1 neurons also receive input from the dura mater, which suggests that they contribute to the development of headache.[171,172] Vc/C1 ocular neurons project to the sensory thalamus, and also to the facial motor nucleus, the parabrachial nucleus, the amygdala, and the hypothalamus.[62,68,163,164,173]

Little is known about neurons at Vp and Vo regions of the TBNC activated by stimulation of the periocular skin and the ocular surface, whose properties and contribution to ocular functions have not been yet established.[174,175] Nevertheless, the development of aberrant "salt and pepper" ocular sensations in stroke patients with damaged lateral pons and medulla suggests a role for the Vp/Vo region in ocular sensory processing.[176]

Thalamus and brain cortex

Going up along the ocular surface sensory pathway, studies are even scarcer, and no systematic mapping of the eye and periocular tissues has been yet performed. Neurons of the Vc/C1 region project to the posterior thalamus nucleus (see section Ocular representation at higher levels of the central nervous system), whose neurons project, in turn, to the amygdala and insular cortex rather than to the somatosensory cortex.[76] So, it seems that very little information reaches the somatosensory cortex. In fact, early studies reported the absence of sensation

evoked by electrical stimulation of the primary somatosensory cortex,[177] an area that receives projections mainly from the somatosensory thalamus. It was assumed for decades that the surface of the eye was very poorly represented at the primary and secondary somatosensory cortex, until a recent case study using brain imaging pointed to the primary sensory cortex as a structure involved in ocular pain perception in humans (Fig. 16.4B).[73,178] Supporting this, several studies in animals have reported the activation of primary somatosensory cortex neurons by mechanical stimulation of the cornea and periorbital tissues,[71,72] and their differential response to noxious and non-noxious stimulation of the ocular surface.[179]

However, there is evidence of the contribution to ocular sensory processing of various areas of the brain that are considered to be involved in the affective and behavioral aspects of sensory processing and, especially, in pain. This includes the anterior cingulate cortex, definite areas of the prefrontal cortex, and the insular cortex, whose electrical stimulation evokes pain and tingling sensations on the face and periocular area (Fig. 16.4B).[180] This may explain our low capacity to evaluate with precision the sensory-discriminative aspects of the stimuli acting on the ocular surface, and why they are usually experienced as irritation or pain, with an intense and negative affective component and evoking nocifensive behaviors. The central processing of sensory information originating at the ocular surface evokes unique sensations, unmatched in other areas of the body, including those innervated by the TG. Whereas mechanical stimuli evoke clear tactile and cold sensations when applied to the skin, including the face skin, in the cornea they evoke sensations defined as gritty eyes, irritation, or pain.

In summary, sensory information initiated by the activation of sensory nerve endings at the eye surface and periocular tissues is processed by the central nervous system and leads to pain perception and affect, while evoking protective behavioral responses. First, the trigeminal primary sensory neurons detect the noxious stimulus acting over the ocular surface and send this information to TBNC neurons that, in turn, engage autonomic and motor brainstem circuits responsible for protective reflex responses (tearing, blinking). These brainstem-integrated reflexes reduce or avoid the exposure to the acting stimulus while the information is sent to upper levels of the central nervous system following two different pathways. In one of these pathways, ocular information is processed at the parabrachial area and then the hypothalamus and the amygdala, which in turn project to the insular, anterior cingulate, and prefrontal cortex, areas belonging to the brain circuits involved in the affective-motivational dimension of pain. Ocular information is processed in parallel by a second pathway where the sensory thalamus and the somatosensory cortex analyze the sensory-discriminative components. Altogether, brain processing will evaluate the sensory-discriminative and affective-motivational components of the multidimensional pain perception, leading to the ocular pain perception itself, to the activation of descending pathways of pain modulation, and to complex adaptive behaviors derived from recalling our previous experience and understanding the context (see section Sensations arising from the eye).

TROPHIC EFFECTS OF OCULAR PRIMARY SENSORY NEURONS

As well as their role in signaling external or internal stimuli, ocular sensory neurons play an important role in the trophic maintenance of their innervated tissues, an effect that is particularly prominent in the cornea. Impairment of corneal sensory innervation causes a number of functional disturbances and the development of epithelial defects and recurrent ulcers (neurotrophic keratitis), which leads finally to loss of corneal transparency. Any condition that may damage corneal innervation (including cornea, lens and retina surgeries, infections, drug treatments, trauma, contact lens wear, genetic ocular and systemic diseases, and other systemic or ocular diseases) results in corneas with reduced sensitivity and altered healing capabilities,[4,181-185] increased epithelial permeability,[186] punctate staining following instillation of fluorescein or Rose-Bengal, poor healing of corneal ulcers, and, finally, reduced transparency. In patients with decreased corneal sensitivity, small epithelial defects expressive of an altered innervation may be seen in the cornea or the conjunctiva, usually in the areas not covered by the lids and, therefore, continuously exposed to the environment.

Many molecules may act as regulators that stimulate migration, proliferation, differentiation, and adhesion of corneal epithelial cells during wound healing. These include growth factors and cytokines (the epidermal growth factor family, basic fibroblast growth factors, transforming growth factors α and β, platelet-derived growth factor, insulin-like growth factor, keratinocyte growth factors, tumor necrosis factor-α, and several interleukins such as IL1, IL6, and IL10) that are present in the cornea and are activated as part of the wound healing process. This is also modulated by other effectors such as neuropeptides (CGRP, SP, cholecystokinin, etc.), ATP (released immediately after injury and acting through P2Y and P2X receptors), Toll-like receptor 4, protein kinases associated to Rho-GTPases, and the extracellular matrix components.[187-190] Upon activation by the adequate stimuli, corneal sensory neurons generate action potentials that are conveyed to the central nervous system and also invade all axon branches of the neuron (Fig. 16.5D). This electrical depolarization of all the axon nerve endings releases neuropeptides locally, in particular SP and CGRP, that either by themselves or in combination with other growth factors present in the cornea and/or in corneal nerves (e.g., insulin-like growth factor, epidermal growth factor, PACAP, cholecystokinin, gastrin, NGF, etc.) appear to be important agents in maintaining corneal epithelial integrity and promoting wound healing in the normal cornea.[4,5,7,182,191-195] Therefore, any situation that leads to a partial or total loss of the corneal innervation leads to a reduced activity of corneal nerves and subsequent trophic problems of the corneal tissue.

However, ocular tissues produce several growth factors necessary for the development, remodeling, and regeneration of corneal nerves. Growth and neurotrophic factors such as glial cell line–derived neurotrophic factors (GCNF), BDNF, opioid growth factor (OGF), ciliary neurotrophic factor (CNTF), pigment epithelium–derived factor (PEDF), vascular endothelial growth factor (VEGF), semaphorin A7, NGF, and NT-3 and NT-4 have been found in the cornea (produced by either the cellular components of the cornea or by its resident immune cells) and possibly participate in the maintenance of corneal innervation (Box 16.2).[4,78,182,196-201]

BOX 16.2 Symbiosis between ocular tissues and sensory neurons

Ocular tissues and their sensory nerves maintain a symbiotic, dynamic interdependence. Sensory neurons innervating the eye exert a well-known trophic effect on target ocular structures. Long-standing clinical observations show that accidental or surgical lesion of the trigeminal nerve leads to the appearance of severe lesions in the cornea (keratitis neuroparalytica). Conversely, ocular tissues strongly contribute to the development, remodeling, and survival of their sensory and autonomic innervations.

MORPHOLOGIC AND FUNCTIONAL ALTERATIONS OF OCULAR SENSORY INNERVATION BY INJURY, INFLAMMATION, AND AGING

Any aggression of the ocular tissues may modify the activity of the sensory neurons innervating the eye. Ocular surgery (photorefractive corneal surgery, keratoplasty, cataract and retina surgery, etc.) and inflammatory conditions with or without infection may lead to ocular nerve damage and dysfunction. Although nerve injury and tissue inflammation do not normally occur in isolation, many ocular surface insults produce inflammation and nerve lesion in different proportions. In some of these conditions the lesion component predominates (e.g., after surgery) whereas in others the inflammation predominates, and there are also conditions that begin as an inflammatory process that leads to permanent morphologic and functional changes in the sensory neuron cell bodies and their peripheral nerve terminals. The changes in the activity of the sensory neurons innervating the eye are the result of both the direct action of the aggressive stimulus and the subsequent reaction by the ocular tissue and the immune system, which may explain why even when only one of the eyes has been affected, changes appear in the activity of the nerves of both eyes.[202]

Inflammation

Any harmful stimuli acting on the corneal, scleral, uveal, or conjunctival tissues will set in motion a series of protective mechanisms that include the activation of nociceptive nerves and the initiation of the inflammatory response. The inflammatory response is started by resident immune cells present in ocular tissues and stimulated by the local release of inflammatory mediators (including H^+ and K^+ ions, adenosine and ATP, nitric oxide, serotonin, histamine, platelet-activating factor, bradykinin, prostaglandins, leukotrienes, thromboxane, proinflammatory cytokines such as interleukins, macrophage inflammatory protein-1a, tumor necrosis factor-α, and neurotrophins such as NGF and GDNF, among others) by damaged cells, as well as by resident and invasive cells of the immune system attracted to the injured area.[22,110,124,203-207] These inflammatory mediators attract and activate immune cells, and also act directly on the sensory nerve terminals, either activating them or modifying their responsiveness. Thus, the direct action of noxious or potentially noxious stimuli will induce impulse firing of ocular nociceptors leading to immediate pain and aversive motor responses. The inflammatory reaction developed by tissue aggression will also induce changes in the activity of sensory nerves, which are different depending on the functional type of sensory nerve. Overall, nociceptive nerves increase their excitability (leading to the "peripheral sensitization")[131,132,208,209] and cold thermoreceptor nerves decrease their excitability.[131,132] Sensitization of nociceptors is characterized by an increase of their ongoing firing activity in the absence of stimulation (which may explain the presence of spontaneous pain after injury or inflammation of the eye), as well as by their enhanced response to noxious and non-noxious stimuli, which leads to the development symptoms as hyperalgesia (increased pain from a stimulus that usually provokes pain) and allodynia (pain evoked by a stimulus that does not usually provoke pain), respectively. The increased excitability of sensitized nociceptors is due to the effects of inflammatory mediators on ion channels responsible of the detection and transduction of stimuli (i.e., the channels that convert the stimulus into a membrane depolarization, including TRPV1, TRPA1, ASICs, etc.), the modulation of nerve ending depolarization (i.e., the channels that change the resting potential and regulate the general excitability of nerve endings, including several types of K^+, Ca^{2+}, and hyperpolarization-activated, cyclic nucleotide-gated (HCN) channels, among others), and/or the conduction to the central nervous system of the generated action potentials (i.e., Na$^+$ and K$^+$ voltage-gated ion channels). These effects of inflammatory mediators are exerted either directly on the ion channels or binding other G-protein–coupled membrane receptors that activate intracellular signal pathways that, in turn, modify the ion channel activity (Fig. 16.7C).

On the contrary, the ongoing activity and the response of cold thermoreceptors to cold stimulation and the TRPM8 agonist menthol is reduced during inflammation. This reduced activity and responsiveness of cold thermoreceptor nerves is due to the binding of inflammatory mediators to G-protein–coupled receptors, leading to GDP/GTP exchange and activation of a Ga$_q$ subunit that forms a constitutive complex with the cold-transducing channel TRPM8. Ga$_q$ activation causes the inhibition of TRPM8, reducing its permeability to ion channels and consequently decreasing the spontaneous and stimulus-evoked firing of cold nerve fibers (Fig. 16.7D).[131,132,210]

These changes in the sensory nerve activity, namely sensitization of nociceptors and the imbalance of nociceptors and cold thermoreceptor activity induced by inflammatory mediators, may explain the spontaneous pain sensations and the increased sensitivity experienced when the ocular tissues are inflamed (Box 16.3).[146,211] Drugs that interfere with the formation and/or release of inflammatory mediators, such as the nonsteroidal anti-inflammatory drugs (NSAIDs) that inhibit the production of prostaglandins, not only decrease local inflammation but also reduce sensitization of ocular nociceptors,[212,213] which explains the well-known analgesic effect of these drugs on postsurgical ocular pain.[214,215]

In addition to signaling damage, ocular nerves also contribute to the local response to injury. Nerve impulses evoked by noxious stimuli in a nociceptor fiber also travel antidromically to the nonstimulated peripheral branches of the axon (see Fig. 16.5D).[140,216] Depolarization of nerve endings evokes the release of the neuropeptides they contain, especially CGRP and substance P (SP).[110,217,218] When released by endings, CGRP and SP contribute to the local inflammatory response inducing vasodilation, plasma extravasation, and cytokine release, thus amplifying the inflammatory effect of the endogenous mediators. This "neurogenic inflammation" caused by activation of sensory nerves in response to a noxious insult affects both the injured and the neighbor noninjured areas innervated by branches of the activated nerves, which may explain the extension of inflammation to distant, intact tissues (conjunctiva, iris, ciliary body, etc.) and probably contributes to the contralateral eye effects.[110,202,217]

Sensitization of nociceptors and inhibition of cold thermoreceptors develops within a few minutes after tissue insult and normally persists as long as the inflammation remains. During long-lasting inflammatory processes, as in chronic dry eye, more permanent changes take place in the cell bodies and peripheral terminals of nociceptor neurons, including the modified expression of membrane receptors and

ion channels present in both structures (see section Chronic ocular surface dryness). The increased impulse activity of ocular nociceptive fibers during inflammation constitutes an altered sensory message sent to the second-order ocular neurons located at the brainstem, which exhibit sensitized responses to stimulation of the ocular surface days after development of an experimental inflammation.[219] This "central sensitization" contributes to the hyperalgesia experienced in ocular inflammation. Although the mechanisms underlying ocular central sensitization are not well known, it can be assumed that they are similar to those of other territories innervated by dorsal root ganglia. Therefore, central sensitization may be due in part to the chronic increase of nerve impulses transmitted from the eye to the second-order ocular neurons, as well as to functional changes in the synapses between the TG neurons and the TBNC neurons. The development of these functional changes involve the nervous and the immune systems. They are induced by the altered activity of peripheral ocular nerves, the subsequent abnormal activity of local brainstem neurons and interneurons, as well as the microglia, and the altered descending control from higher levels of the central nervous system, which altogether lead to permanent alterations of the connection pattern of ocular neurons (see also section Nerve injury).[220–222]

Nerve injury

Ocular nerve injury is mainly produced by ocular surgery (such as keratoplasty, photorefractive corneal surgery, cataract surgery, etc.) or trauma, although it can also be a consequence of ocular and systemic chronic conditions. The changes experienced by sensory nerves after injury is the basis of so-called neuropathic pain. Therefore, pain generated by functional disturbances consecutive to nerve injury at any level along the ocular somatosensory pathway is called ocular neuropathic pain. Ocular neuropathic pain can be classified as peripheral (when nerve damage triggering the neuropathic process occurred in the peripheral nervous system, i.e., the ocular TG neurons and/or their central or peripheral projections to the eye) or central (when nerve damage triggering the process occurred at the central nervous system, i.e., at the synapses between TG neurons and the second-order neurons or beyond). Additionally, ocular neuropathic pain can be classified as traumatic, infectious, metabolic, degenerative, or toxic, according to the agent originating nerve damage.

After nerve injury, the distal part of damaged axons degenerates and the central stumps start to regenerate. The denervated area is invaded by outgrowths of adjacent, noninjured nerve fibers and by sprouts of the injured axons, which are sometimes entrapped by scar tissue and form microneuromas (see also section Changes of corneal sensory innervation with aging).[223] The denervated area would have reduced or even total loss of ocular sensitivity, which can persist for months and even years after injury[181,224–226] and is due to the total absence of active nerve endings within the denervated region.[227–230] Simultaneously with the reduced or absent sensitivity inside the denervated area, there are also sensitivity changes in the surrounding areas, as a consequence of the functional changes experienced by the regenerating axons (see further in section).

Injury of ocular trigeminal neurons and their axons elicits a cellular response from these neurons that is necessary to regenerate the injured axons and depends on the extent and location of injury, in which Schwann cells also participate. Superficial lesions restricted to the corneal epithelium (i.e., affecting only the intraepithelial nerve endings and the sub-basal nerve fibers, all void of Schwann cells) do not affect TG neuron gene expression. However, injuries affecting intrastromal nerves (where axons are covered by nonmyelinating Schwann cells) or the ciliary nerves (where axons are covered by either myelinating or nonmyelinating Schwann cells) trigger in the trigeminal neurons the

---

BOX 16.3 Ocular nociceptive nerve fibers

Sensitization of nociceptive nerve fibers innervating the eye is the basis of persistent pain developing after ocular injury or inflammation. It also accounts for the development of primary hyperalgesia (enhanced pain evoked by noxious stimulation) and allodynia (pain sensations evoked by non-noxious stimuli) in the inflamed eye. Sensitization of ocular nociceptors explains, for instance, the development of sustained pain after the iris has been touched accidentally during ocular surgery or after argon laser pulse application to the posterior uvea, and is possibly also the reason for the intense sustained ocular pain experienced in acute angle–closure glaucoma, in which uveal inflammation probably induces sensitization of nociceptors, increasing their excitability.

immediate expression of protooncogene c-jun and further changes in their expression of transcription factors, neuropeptides, and ion channels, modifying the neuron phenotype.[1,231–233] The expression of ligand-gated and voltage-gated channels (especially an increase of sodium channel expression, sometimes accompanied by a decrease of potassium channel expression)[234,235] in injured neurons leads to ectopic discharges and abnormal responsiveness to natural stimuli of the growing neurites of regenerating nociceptors and cold thermoreceptors.[227,228,230,236,237] After corneal injury, there is a great increase in the expression of voltage-gated channels supporting nerve impulse generation, which accumulate abnormally at certain points along the nerve terminal branches and generate spontaneous firing in absence of stimulation,[113,202,227–230,238] leading to spontaneous and persistent ocular pain and unpleasant dryness sensations, as is the case of the abnormal sensations experienced after photorefractive surgery.[239] Besides the spontaneous firing, injured ocular neurons present abnormal responsiveness to stimulation. This is because the regenerating nerve terminals have many voltage-gated channels but instead lack those channels (TRPV1, TRPA1, ASIC, TRPM8, etc., see section Sensory neurons innervating the cornea) necessary for sensing and transducing the stimuli. Until the full recovery of the transducing channels in regenerated nerve terminals, their response to stimulation is reduced, which explains the coexistence of spontaneous pain and hypoesthesia (reduced sensitivity) after ocular nerve injury. The time course of transducing channel recovery in humans is unknown, although in mice TRPV1 and Piezo2 channels begin to reappear in the regenerating polymodal nociceptor terminals at 1 month after photorefractive keratectomy.[229]

Chronic ocular surface dryness

In dry eye disease (DED), there are numerous morphologic and functional changes of ocular innervation (Box 16.4). On the one hand, these changes in ocular sensory nerves induce symptoms such as unpleasant sensations of different intensities, ranging from dryness or ocular discomfort to lacerating and burning pain. On the other hand, the abnormal nerve functioning causes alterations in tissue trophism and in the regulation of tear production and blinking, which in turn contributes to aggravating DED symptoms and signs. In other words, sensory innervation is altered by chronic eye dryness and also contributes to DED pathogenesis.

Reduction of the ocular surface moistness either by reduced tearing or increased tear evaporation represents a stressful situation for the corneal epithelium exposed to a hyperosmotic tear film and the environment. As a response to this stress, corneal epithelial cells and immune resident cells produce local inflammatory mediators, and local inflammation occurs,[240] leading to sensitization of nociceptive nerve terminals and development of discomfort and pain sensations. When dryness becomes chronic, it also leads to corneal nerve damage and, consequently, the morpho-functional changes of the sensory nerves during chronic eye dryness resemble both those produced during inflammation and those produced by nerve injury (see also sections Inflammation and Nerve injury). The eyelid movement causes a great mechanical tension on the ocular surface when the tear film is thin and does not lubricate well. Together with chronic inflammation, this movement damages the epithelium and the intraepithelial nerve terminals, and eventually the sub-basal nerve fibers, triggering the mechanisms of nerve degeneration and regeneration. In clinical practice, these degeneration and regeneration processes are evidenced by signs such as the reduction in the density and branching of the sub-basal plexus nerve fibers, and the increase in their tortuosity when explored by IVCM.[241–243] They are also evidenced clinically by a reduction in corneal sensitivity to stimulation (shown by increased sensation thresholds) that often occurs simultaneously with hyperalgesia and spontaneous pain

---

BOX 16.4 Dry eye

The most common reason for superficial eye discomfort is possibly "dry eye disease," also termed "ocular surface disease." This is a common multi-etiological condition in which ocular surface inflammation and damage, altered tear film stability and neurosensory abnormalities compromise the ocular surface, producing dot-like microlesions in conjunctival and corneal epithelia, suggestive of neurotrophic defects.

BOX 16.5 Alterations of ocular sensitivity

Until recently, most alterations of ocular sensitivity were associated with ocular inflammatory processes (that cause hypersensitivity, sustained pain, itching, etc.) or were the consequence of surgical procedures directed to preserve or recover vision (such as keratoplasty, cataract removal, vitreo-retinal surgery, etc., usually producing ocular hypoesthesia). Nowadays, reduced sensitivity and in particular dysesthesias (abnormal sensations) are increasingly associated with lifestyle (use of screens, pollution, air conditioning, etc.) and the growing number of ocular interventions, in particular corneal refractive surgery.

---

sensations and is aggravated by tear film instability.[102,244–249] Most of the alterations of ocular surface sensitivity in chronic eye dryness are due to functional changes in corneal nerves that resemble those seen in injured nerves (Box 16.5). There is an increased excitability of corneal nerves consecutive to the increased activity and expression of sodium channels.[113,250] This results in an increased spontaneous firing of cold thermoreceptors that leads not only to dryness sensations but also to dysregulation of protective mechanisms driven by thermal sensory input such as tearing and blinking, contributing to increasing and perpetuating ocular surface disturbances.

SENSATIONS ARISING FROM THE EYE

Methods for testing ocular surface sensitivity

Until the development of the Cochet-Bonnet esthesiometer in the 1960s, the clinical exploration of ocular surface sensitivity was performed using a wisp of cotton applied gently on the cornea or the conjunctiva, expecting to evoke a blink reflex and asking the patient about the experienced sensation. A more quantitative approach was the use of modified von Frey filaments,[251] a series of nylon threads of different lengths and diameters that exert on the cornea a force that is proportional to the diameter and inversely proportional to the length of the thread. Based on this principle the Cochet-Bonnet esthesiometer was developed,[252] an instrument composed of a single nylon filament of adjustable length that was the first esthesiometer that allowed the quantification of the sensitivity threshold to mechanical stimulation of the ocular surface. After subsequent modifications to the instrument and even new designs,[253–255] the Cochet-Bonnet esthesiometer has continued to be the most widely used to detect changes in corneal sensitivity in healthy and pathologic conditions.

A disadvantage of the Cochet-Bonnet and other contact esthesiometers is the risk of tissue injury, especially in hypesthesic corneas. To prevent this risk, several noncontact esthesiometers were developed in the 1990s[256–260] and have even been updated since. These instruments were based on the application of air jets at room temperature exerting different pressures on the cornea. An improvement of noncontact esthesiometers was the development of the Belmonte gas esthesiometer[261] that, unlike the previous ones, allows the exploration of the mechanical, as well as the thermal and chemical, sensitivity of the ocular surface, enabling the selective stimulation of the different types of sensory receptors innervating the ocular surface (see section Sensory neurons innervating the cornea).[127] This instrument, and its subsequent modifications, allows adjustment of the gas flow in order to apply a controlled pressure over the ocular surface (which, in turn, allows evaluation of the mechanical sensitivity threshold), as well as adjustment of the temperature of the gas, thus producing either cold or hot thermal stimulation and allowing the evaluation of thermal sensitivity thresholds.[262,263] Also, the gas used can be a mixture of air with CO_2 at variable concentrations to test chemical sensitivity. When CO_2 in the gas jet combines with water at the ocular surface, they form carbonic acid, decreasing local pH proportionally to the CO_2 concentration and causing a chemical stimulation.[126,127,261,264] Gas esthesiometry has allowed the definition of normal values of mechanical, chemical, and thermal sensitivity in relation to age, sex, iris color, pregnancy, and so on in healthy subjects, as well as their changes related to contact lens wearing, surgery, ocular surface pathologies (such as dry eye, infectious and noninfectious keratitis or keratoconjunctivitis, etc.) or systemic diseases such as diabetes or fibromyalgia.[102,103,116,265–270]

Both contact and noncontact esthesiometers are used, fundamentally, to measure the sensation threshold, that is, the smallest stimulus sufficient to evoke a sensation. According to this, ocular surface sensitivity is high when sensation threshold values are low (i.e., when low-intensity stimuli are perceived), and, vice versa, high sensation threshold values indicate a low sensitivity.

Classical contact esthesiometry studies showed that corneal sensitivity is higher in the center than in the peripheral cornea,[100,252,271] a difference that was initially associated with the varying density of innervation, although the correlation between both parameters is controversial.[17,272,273] There are several factors that affect corneal sensitivity in healthy individuals. Throughout the day, corneal sensitivity decreases during the night and increases during the daylight hours, a variation that has been attributed to changes in corneal thickness.[265,274] Corneal sensitivity is decreased during pregnancy and menstruation, probably owing to corneal edema associated with the hormonal status.[275–277] Corneal sensitivity threshold values, measured with either contact or noncontact esthesiometers, are lower in individuals with blue irises, although the difference could be due to a central mechanism because nerve activity and sensitivity thresholds of ocular nerves are similar in animals with light-colored and dark-colored irises.[103,278–280]

Corneal sensitivity and sensations evoked at the ocular surface

Although pioneering studies on corneal sensitivity proposed that different sensory modalities (touch, heat, cold, and pain) could be evoked upon selective stimulation of the cornea,[281] most classical psychophysical studies concluded that pain was the only sensation that can be evoked from the cornea independently of the applied stimulus.[251,282–284] This controversy continued for decades, owing to the absence of a method that would allow truly selective stimulation of the cornea, applying stimuli of controlled intensity and modality to selectively recruit the different functional types of corneal sensory nerves. The use of the Belmonte's gas esthesiometer in healthy humans evidenced that sensations evoked by corneal stimulation with mechanical forces, heating, or acidification of tear film always include a component of irritation. This is unsurprising because all these stimuli activate polymodal nociceptors.[127,157] Mechanical stimuli applied to the cornea evoke sensations that are not described as tactile but as sensations of foreign body, gritty eyes, and so on. On the contrary, low-intensity mechanical stimuli applied to the conjunctiva are felt as nonirritating,[103,157,283–285]

suggesting the innervation of this tissue by low-threshold mechanoreceptors. Besides, application of mild or moderate cold stimuli to the cornea or the conjunctiva evokes almost exclusively a cooling sensation that becomes irritating only when more pronounced temperature reductions are applied (Fig. 16.8).[127,157,283] This is because mild and moderate cooling of the ocular surface increases the activity of HB-LT cold thermoreceptor nerves (evoking sensations of freshness and cooling), whereas intense cooling activates LB-HT cold thermoreceptors and polymodal nociceptors (evoking sensations of irritation and dryness).[127,146,286,287] Therefore, the distinct quality of the conscious sensations evoked by a stimulus applied on the cornea or conjunctiva appears to be primarily determined by the variable recruitment of mechanonociceptor, polymodal nociceptor, HBLT and LBHT cold thermoreceptor, and low threshold mechanoreceptor neurons innervating these structures, in which variable responses are induced by selective stimulation. However, the contribution of the little-known processing of this sensory input by the central nervous system cannot be ruled out. Indeed, recent results suggest that although ocular trigeminal neurons (except polymodal nociceptor neurons) are preferentially activated by a single stimulus modality, ocular neurons in the primary somatosensory cortex are activated by multiple stimulus modalities.[179] The presence of these multimodal neurons could explain the unique sensations experienced on the ocular surface.

Corneal sensitivity under ocular and systemic conditions that alter corneal nerves

A large variety of conditions producing ocular inflammation or nerve injury change the activity of the sensory neurons (see section Trophic effects of ocular primary sensory neurons for details), thus evoking sensations of discomfort, dryness, irritation, or pain, depending on the degree and type of insult.[211] The imbalance between the increased activity of sensitized nociceptors and the decrease activity of cold thermoreceptors during ocular inflammation (Fig. 16.7.F) lead to development of spontaneous pain and the enhanced response to noxious stimuli (hyperalgesia).[131,132,202,211] Even when the inflammation is unilateral, the activity of sensory nerves of both eyes is altered leading to sensitivity changes in both eyes, although to a lesser degree in the contralateral eye.[202,288]

After nerve injury (produced by trauma, ocular surgery, corneal infections, or ocular and systemic diseases causing nerve damage such as diabetes or chronic tear deficiency), there is no nerve activity at the affected area, and the spontaneous and stimulus-evoked activity of corneal nociceptors and cold thermoreceptors regenerating around the injury is increased.[113,202,227,229,230] This leads to reduced (hypoesthesia) or absent sensitivity to stimulation (anesthesia) while experiencing pain and unpleasant dryness sensations.[39,102,116,249,266,268,269,289,290] The abnormal firing of corneal nerve fibers regenerating after damage (Fig. 16.9), similar to the ectopic activity in the sensory nerve stump of amputated body extremities that is interpreted as aberrant sensations from the lost limb (the "phantom limb"), may be read erroneously as ocular dryness by the brain even when tear production is normal (Fig. 16.10).[146,211,239] Unlike the sensory disturbances caused by inflammation, which usually disappear when the inflammation resolves, the alterations in sensitivity induced by nerve injury are long-lasting. In many cases they can take months to recover (as is usually the case after photorefractive surgery) or never return to normal.[224–226,291]

In brief, the altered nerve activity after nerve damage leads patients to experience sensations of dryness and pain while they have low sensitivity to stimulation. This situation also occurs in other circumstances, for instance, during aging and contact lens wearing. Corneal sensitivity is also decreased in contact lens users, depending on the type of lens

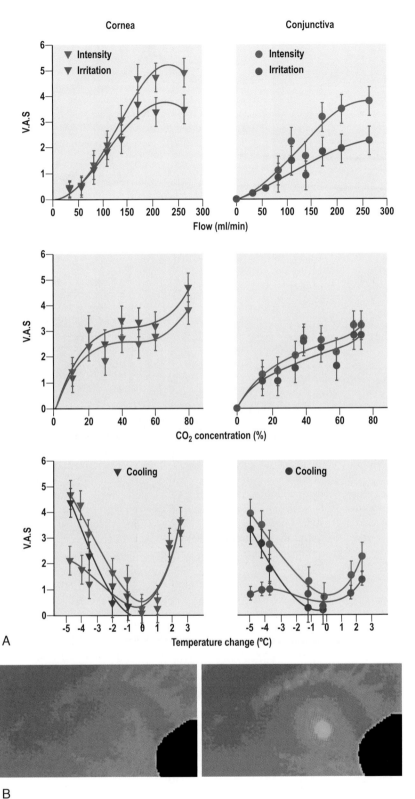

Fig. 16.8 Sensations evoked by selective stimulation of the cornea and conjunctiva. (**A**) Subjective score given to the intensity and the irritation components of the sensation evoked by selective mechanical, chemical, and thermal stimuli on the cornea *(triangles)* and the conjunctiva *(circles)* with the Belmonte gas esthesiometer. Sensation parameters are expressed in arbitrary units marked on a visual analog scale *(VAS)* ranging from 0 (no sensation) to 10 (maximal value of the parameter). For thermal stimulation, VAS scores for the cooling component of the sensation have also been represented. (**B**) Thermographic images recorded during application of a gas pulse at neutral temperature for selective mechanical stimulation *(left)* and at 29°C *(right)* for cold stimulation of the cornea. (A, From Acosta MC, Tan ME, Belmonte C, Gallar J. Sensations evoked by selective mechanical, chemical, and thermal stimulation of the conjunctiva and cornea. *Investig Ophthalmol Vis Sci.* 2001;42(9):2063–2067. Reproduced from Association for Research in Vision and Ophthalmology. B, From Acosta MC. Corneal sensitivity to mechanical, chemical and thermal stimuli: correlation with the electrical activity of nociceptors. PhD dissertation. Universidad Miguel Hernández de Elche, Spain; 1999.)

and time of wearing.[292-300] The sensory changes may result from adaptation of mechanosensitive nerves to the presence of the continuous stimulus exerted by the contact lens over the cornea, conjunctiva, and lid border, and to the sensitization of nociceptive nerves by the presence of hyperosmolarity and/or the release of inflammatory mediators induced by contact lens wear, although changes subsequent to corneal nerve damage cannot be ruled out.[301] The absence of mechanical

adaptation and the local inflammation induced by the lens wearing may explain why contact lens users experience dryness and discomfort sensations, and are at risk of developing DED.[302-306]

Elderly people commonly experience unpleasant dry eye sensations that are sometimes explained by a reduction in tear production, but in other cases are present with normal or increased tears, (e.g., epiphora).[211,287,307] The altered activity of LB-HT cold thermoreceptor

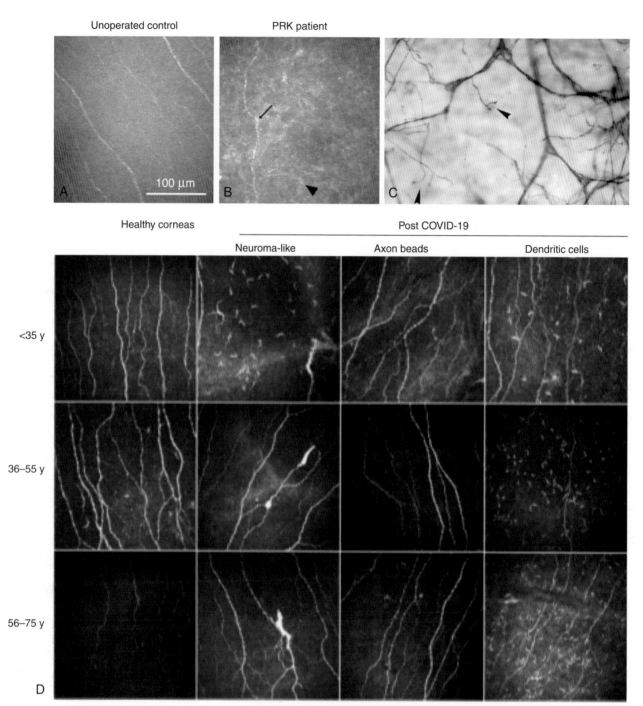

Fig. 16.9 Disturbances of corneal innervation following refractive surgery and infections. (**A,B**) In vivo confocal microscopy images of human corneal nerves. (**A**) Sub-basal leashes in an intact cornea (**B**) Appearance of a sub-basal nerve fiber *(arrow)* 3 years after photorefractive keratectomy *(PRK)*, to illustrate incomplete nerve recovery and the persistence of haze signs *(arrowhead)*. (**C**) Regenerating stromal nerve fibers in the rabbit cornea after PRK. Acetylcholinesterase-stained corneal nerves 1 month after surgery, showing abundant regenerating leashes, sometimes with "growth cone-like" endings *(arrowheads)* (**D**) In vivo confocal microscopy images of corneas of healthy subjects and patients that have overcome SARS-CoV-2 infection, showing typical morphologic signs of small fiber neuropathy such as beaded nerve fibers and neuroma-like images. Also notice the increased number of dendritic cells in COVID-19 patients, especially in the youngest. (A, Modified from Müller LJ, Marfurt CF, Kruse F, Tervo TMT. Corneal nerves: Structure, contents and function. *Exp Eye Res.* 2003;76(5):521–542. https://doi.org/10.1016/S0014-4835(03)00050-2. B, From Tervo T, Moilanen J. In vivo confocal microscopy for evaluation of wound healing following corneal refractive surgery. *Prog Retin Eye Res.* 2003;22(3):339–358. https://doi.org/10.1016/S1350-9462(02)00064-2. D, Modified from Barros A, Queiruga-Piñeiro J, Lozano-Sanroma J, et al. Small fiber neuropathy in the cornea of Covid-19 patients associated with the generation of ocular surface disease. *Ocul Surf.* 2022;23:40–48. https://doi.org/10.1016/J.JTOS.2021.10.010.)

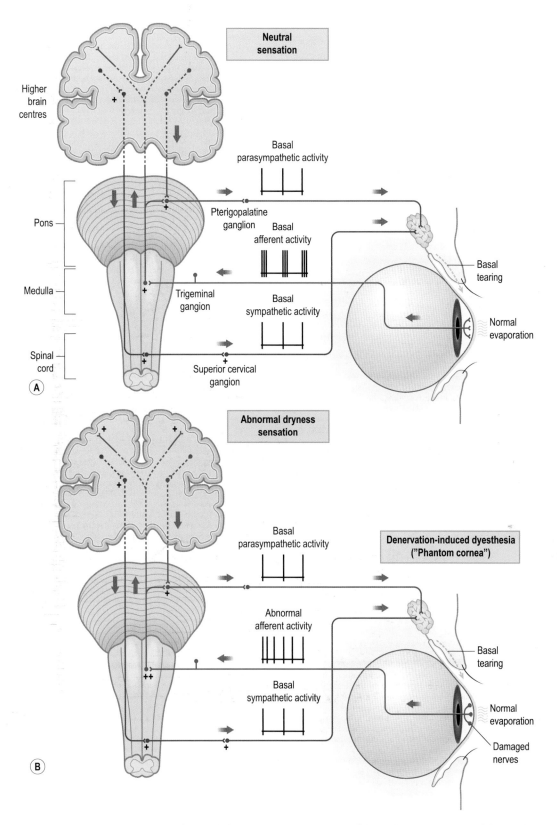

Fig. 16.10 Corneal sensations and tear secretion before and after corneal nerve damage. Schematic representation of the mechanisms involved in ocular sensations and lacrimal secretion. (**A**) Basal tearing is maintained by a low-frequency ongoing impulse activity of corneal sensory nerves. This activates efferent parasympathetic, and perhaps also sympathetic, pathways in the central nervous system, thus stimulating the basal tear secretion. However, ongoing sensory activity is too low to produce conscious sensations of ocular dryness. (**B**) When corneal nerves are injured and during aging, severed axons generate ectopic impulse discharges that reach the brain and evoke abnormal dryness sensations despite a normal tear production being present. (Modified from Belmonte C. Eye dryness sensations after refractive surgery: Impaired tear secretion or "phantom" cornea? *J Refract Surg.* 2007;23(6):598–602; Belmonte C, Gallar J. Cold thermoreceptors, unexpected players in tear production and ocular dryness sensations. *Invest Ophthalmol Vis Sci.* 2011;52(6):3888–3892.)

fibers has been described in aged mice, in which the cooling threshold is reduced and the fibers are then activated at the normal corneal temperature.[40] This would be the basis of the dryness dysesthesia experienced by elder individuals.[211] Classical studies using contact esthesiometers showed a decreased sensitivity to mechanical stimulation with age, especially from the age of 60 years, later confirmed also for chemical stimulation using the gas esthesiometer.[103,308,309] The decline of ocular surface sensitivity with age is associated with a reduction of corneal nerve density and length, and with an increase of sub-basal nerve tortuosity and the presence of neuroma-like images, features that resemble nerve regeneration after injury.[40,310–313]

REFERENCES

1. De Felipe C, Gonzalez GG, Gallar J, Belmonte C. Quantification and immunocytochemical characteristics of trigeminal ganglion neurons projecting to the cornea: Effect of corneal wounding. *Eur J Pain*. 1999;3(1):31–39.
2. Belmonte C, Garcia-Hirschfeld J, Gallar J. Neurobiology of ocular pain. *Prog Retin Eye Res*. 1997;16(1):117–156.
3. Tervo T, Tervo K, Eranko L. Ocular neuropeptides. *Med Biol*. 1982;60(2):53–60.
4. Müller LJ, Marfurt CF, Kruse F, Tervo TMT. Corneal nerves: Structure, contents and function. *Exp Eye Res*. 2003;76(5):521–542.
5. Gonzalez-Coto AF, Alonso-Ron C, Alcalde I, et al. Expression of cholecystokinin, gastrin, and their receptors in the mouse cornea. *Investig Ophthalmol Vis Sci*. 2014;55(3):1965–1975.
6. Troger J, Kieselbach G, Teuchner B, et al. Peptidergic nerves in the eye, their source and potential pathophysiological relevance. *Brain Res Rev*. 2007;53(1):39–62.
7. He J, Bazan HEP. Neuroanatomy and Neurochemistry of Mouse Cornea. *Invest Ophthalmol Vis Sci*. 2016;57(2):664–674.
8. He J, Pham TL, Bazan HEP. Neuroanatomy and neurochemistry of rat cornea: Changes with age. *Ocul Surf*. 2021;20(December 2020):86–94.
9. Lütjen-Drecoll E. Choroidal innervation in primate eyes. *Exp Eye Res*. 2006;82(3):357–361.
10. Rózsa AJ, Beuerman RW. Density and organization of free nerve endings in the corneal epithelium of the rabbit. *Pain*. 1982;14(2):105–120.
11. Kurus E. [A system of ganglion cells in the human choroid]. *Klin Monbl Augenheilkd Augenarztl Fortbild*. 1955;127(2):198–206.
12. Castro-Correia J. Inervacao de coroideia. In: *Anales del Instituto Barraquer*. Instituto Barraquer; 1961:487–518.
13. Mintenig GM, Sanchez-Vives MV, Martin C, Gual A, Belmonte C. Sensory receptors in the anterior uvea of the cat's eye: An in vitro study. *Investig Ophthalmol Vis Sci*. 1995;36(8):1615–1624.
14. Lawrenson JG, Ruskell GL. The structure of corpuscular nerve endings in the limbal conjunctiva of the human eye. *J Anat*. 1991;177:75–84.
15. Sasaoka A, Ishimoto I, Kuwayama Y, et al. Overall distribution of substance P nerves in the rat cornea and their three-dimensional profiles. *Investig Ophthalmol Vis Sci*. 1984;25(3):351–356.
16. Zander E, Weddell G. Observations on the innervation of the cornea. *J Anat*. 1951;85(1):68–99.
17. Müller LJ, Pels L, Vrensen GFJM. Ultrastructural organization of human corneal nerves. *Investig Ophthalmol Vis Sci*. 1996;37(4):476–488.
18. Bron R, Wood RJ, Brock JA, Ivanusic JJ. Piezo2 expression in corneal afferent neurons. *J Comp Neurol*. 2014;522(13):2967–2979.
19. Marfurt CF, Cox J, Deek S, Dvorscak L. Anatomy of the human corneal innervation. *Exp Eye Res*. 2010;90(4):478–492.
20. Stepp MA, Tadvalkar G, Hakh R, Pal-Ghosh S. Corneal epithelial cells function as surrogate Schwann cells for their sensory nerves. *Glia*. 2017;65(6):851–863.
21. Seyed-Razavi Y, Chinnery HR, McMenamin PG. A novel association between resident tissue macrophages and nerves in the peripheral stroma of the murine cornea. *Investig Ophthalmol Vis Sci*. 2014;55(3):1313–1320.
22. Frutos-Rincón L, Gómez-Sánchez JA, Íñigo-Portugués A, Acosta MC, Gallar J. An experimental model of neuro-immune interactions in the eye: corneal sensory nerves and resident dendritic cells. *Int J Mol Sci*. 2022;23(6):2997.
23. Ueda S, del Cerro M, LoCascio JA, Aquavella JV. Peptidergic and catecholaminergic fibers in the human corneal epithelium: An immunohistochemical and electron microscopic study. *Acta Ophthalmol*. 1989;67(192 S):80–90.
24. Patel DV, McGhee CNJ. Mapping of the normal human corneal sub-Basal nerve plexus by in vivo laser scanning confocal microscopy. *Invest Ophthalmol Vis Sci*. 2005;46(12):4485–4488.
25. Dvorscak L, Marfurt CF. Age-related changes in rat corneal epithelial nerve density. *Investig Ophthalmol Vis Sci*. 2008;49(3):910–916.
26. Ivanusic JJ, Wood RJ, Brock JA. Sensory and sympathetic innervation of the mouse and guinea pig corneal epithelium. *J Comp Neurol*. 2013;521(4):877–893.
27. Marfurt C, Anokwute MC, Fetcko K, et al. Comparative anatomy of the mammalian corneal subbasal nerve plexus. *Investig Ophthalmol Vis Sci*. 2019;60(15):4972–4984.
28. Bee JA, Hay RA, Lamb EM, Devore JJ, Conrad GW. Positional specificity of corneal nerves during development. *Investig Ophthalmol Vis Sci*. 1986;27(1):38–43.
29. Thoft RA, Friend J. The X, Y, Z hypothesis of corneal epithelial maintenance. *Investig Ophthalmol Vis Sci*. 1983;24(10):1442–1443.
30. Auran JD, Koester CJ, Kleiman NJ, et al. Scanning slit confocal microscopic observation of cell morphology and movement within the normal human anterior cornea. *Ophthalmology*. 1995;102(1):33–41.
31. Riley NC, Lwigale PY, Conrad GW. Specificity of corneal nerve positions during embryogenesis. *Mol Vis*. 2001;7:297–304.
32. Marfurt C. Nervous control of the cornea. In: Burnstock G, Sillito A, eds. *Nervous Control of the Eye*. Reading, UK: Harwood Academic; 2000:41–92.
33. Nagasaki T, Zhao J. Centripetal movement of corneal epithelial cells in the normal adult mouse. *Investig Ophthalmology Vis Sci*. 2003;44(2):558.
34. Marfurt C. Corneal nerves anatomy. In: Dartt D, ed. *Encyclopedia of the Eye*. Elsevier; 2009.
35. Tervo T, Joó F, Huikuri KT, Toth I, Palkama A. Fine structure of sensory nerves in the rat cornea: an experimental nerve degeneration study. *Pain*. 1979;6(1):57–70.
36. Cillà S De, Ranno S, Carini E, et al. Corneal subbasal nerves changes in patients with diabetic retinopathy: An in vivo confocal study. *Investig Opthalmology Vis Sci*. 2009;50(11):5155.
37. Kurbanyan K, Hoesl LM, Schrems WA, Hamrah P. Corneal nerve alterations in acute Acanthamoeba and fungal keratitis: an in vivo confocal microscopy study. *Eye (Lond)*. 2012;26(1):126–132.
38. Hamrah P, Cruzat A, Dastjerdi MH, et al. Unilateral herpes zoster ophthalmicus results in bilateral corneal nerve alteration: an in vivo confocal microscopy study. *Ophthalmology*. 2013;120(1):40–47.
39. Barros A, Queiruga-Piñeiro J, Lozano-Sanroma J, et al. Small fiber neuropathy in the cornea of Covid-19 patients associated with the generation of ocular surface disease. *Ocul Surf*. 2022;23:40–48.
40. Alcalde I, Íñigo-Portugués A, González-González O, et al. Morphological and functional changes in TRPM8-expressing corneal cold thermoreceptor neurons during aging and their impact on tearing in mice. *J Comp Neurol*. 2018;526(11):1859–1874.
41. ten Tusscher MPM, Klooster J, van der Want JJL, Lamers WPMA, Vrensen GFJM. The allocation of nerve fibres to the anterior eye segment and peripheral ganglia of rats. I. The sensory innervation. *Brain Res*. 1989;494(1):95–104.
42. Oppenheimer DR, Palmer E, Weddell G. Nerve endings in the conjunctiva. *J Anat*. 1958;92(3):321–352.
43. Munger BL, Halata Z. The sensorineural apparatus of the human eyelid. *Am J Anat*. 1984;170(2):181–204.
44. Luhtala J, Uusitalo H. The distribution and origin of substance P immunoreactive nerve fibres in the rat conjunctiva. *Exp Eye Res*. 1991;53(5):641–646.
45. Elsås T, Edvinsson L, Sundler F, Uddman R. Neuronal pathways to the rat conjunctiva revealed by retrograde tracing and immunocytochemistry. *Exp Eye Res*. 1994;58(1):117–126.
46. Dartt DA, McCarthy DM, Mercer HJ, Kessler TL, Chung EH, Zieske JD. Localization of nerves adjacent to goblet cells in rat conjunctiva. *Curr Eye Res*. 1995;14(11):993–1000.
47. Van Der Werf F, Baljet B, Prins M, Ruskell GL, Otto JA. Innervation of the palpebral conjunctiva and the superior tarsal muscle in the cynomolgous monkey: A retrograde fluorescent tracing study. *J Anat*. 1996;189(2):285–292.
48. Luhtala J, Palkama A, Uusitalo H. Calcitonin gene-related peptide immunoreactive nerve fibers in the rat conjunctiva. *Investig Ophthalmol Vis Sci*. 1991;32(3):640–645.
49. Chung CW, Tigges M, Stone RA. Peptidergic innervation of the primate meibomian gland. *Investig Ophthalmol Vis Sci*. 1996;37(1):238–245.
50. Al-Aqaba MA, Dhillon VK, Mohammed I, Said DG, Dua HS. Corneal nerves in health and disease. *Prog Retin Eye Res*. 2019;73(May):100762.
51. Lowther GE, Hill RM. Sensitivity threshold of the lower lid margin in the course of adaptation to contact lenses. *Am J Optom Arch Am Acad Optom*. 1968;45(9):587–594.
52. Marfurt CF. The central projections of trigeminal primary afferent neurons in the cat as determined by the tranganglionic transport of horseradish peroxidase. *J Comp Neurol*. 1981;203(4):785–798.
53. Martinez S, Belmonte C. C-Fos expression in trigeminal nucleus neurons after chemical irritation of the cornea: reduction by selective blockade of nociceptor chemosensitivity. *Exp brain Res*. 1996;109(1):56–62.
54. Meng ID, Hu JW, Bereiter DA. Parabrachial area and nucleus raphe magnus inhibition of corneal units in rostral and caudal portions of trigeminal subnucleus caudalis in the rat. *Pain*. 2000;87(3):241–251.
55. Panneton WM, Burton H. Corneal and periocular representation within the trigeminal sensory complex in the cat studied with transganglionic transport of horseradish peroxidase. *J Comp Neurol*. 1981;199(3):327–344.
56. Marfurt CF, Del Toro DR. Corneal sensory pathway in the rat: a horseradish peroxidase tracing study. *J Comp Neurol*. 1987;261(3):450–459.
57. Marfurt CF, Echtenkamp SF. Central projections and trigeminal ganglion location of corneal afferent neurons in the monkey, Macaca fascicularis. *J Comp Neurol*. 1988;272(3):370–382.
58. Panneton WM, Hsu H, Gan Q. Distinct central representations for sensory fibers innervating either the conjunctiva or cornea of the rat. *Exp Eye Res*. 2010;90(3):388–396.
59. Simons E, Smith PG. Sensory and autonomic innervation of the rat eyelid: Neuronal origins and peptide phenotypes. *J Chem Neuroanat*. 1994;7(1–2):35–47.
60. Baljet B, VanderWerf F. Connections between the lacrimal gland and sensory trigeminal neurons: a WGA/HRP study in the cynomolgous monkey. *J Anat*. 2005;206(3):257–263.
61. Kirch W, Horneber M, Tamm E. Characterization of Meibomian gland innervation in the cynomolgus monkey (Macaca fascicularis). *Anat Embryol (Berl)*. 1996;193(4):365–375.
62. Hirata H, Okamoto K, Bereiter DA. GABAA receptor activation modulates corneal unit activity in rostral and caudal portions of trigeminal subnucleus caudalis. *J Neurophysiol*. 2003;90(5):2837–2849.
63. Warren S, May PJ. Morphology and connections of intratrigeminal cells and axons in the macaque monkey. *Front Neuroanat*. 2013;7(May):11.
64. Henriquez VM, Evinger C. The three-neuron corneal reflex circuit and modulation of second-order corneal responsive neurons. *Exp Brain Res*. 2007;179(4):691–702.
65. Pellegrini JJ, Horn AKE, Evinger C. The trigeminally evoked blink reflex - I. Neuronal circuits. *Exp Brain Res*. 1995;107(2):166–180.

66. Tóth IE, Boldogkoi Z, Medveczky I, Palkovits M. Lacrimal preganglionic neurons form a subdivision of the superior salivatory nucleus of rat: Transneuronal labelling by pseudorabies virus. *J Auton Nerv Syst.* 1999;77(1):45–54.
67. Hirata H, Okamoto K, Tashiro A, Bereiter DA. A novel class of neurons at the trigeminal subnucleus interpolaris/caudalis transition region monitors ocular surface fluid status and modulates tear production. *J Neurosci.* 2004;24(17):4224–4232.
68. Hirata H, Takeshita S, Hu JW, Bereiter DA. Cornea-responsive medullary dorsal horn neurons: Modulation by local opoids and projections to thalamus and brain stem. *J Neurophysiol.* 2000;84(2):1050–1061.
69. Rausell E, Jones EG. Chemically distinct compartments of the thalamic VPM nucleus in monkeys relay principal and spinal trigeminal pathways to different layers of the somatosensory cortex. *J Neurosci.* 1991;11(1):226–237.
70. Noseda R, Monconduit L, Constandil L, Chalus M, Villanueva L. Central nervous system networks involved in the processing of meningeal and cutaneous inputs from the ophthalmic branch of the trigeminal nerve in the rat. *Cephalalgia.* 2008;28(8):813–824.
71. Dreyer DA, Loe PR, Metz CB, Whitsel BL. Representation of head and face in postcentral gyrus of the macaque. *J Neurophysiol.* 1975;38(3):714–733.
72. Nelson RJ, Sur M, Felleman DJ, Kaas JH. Representations of the body surface in postcentral parietal cortex of Macaca fascicularis. *J Comp Neurol.* 1980;192(4):611–643.
73. Moulton EA, Becerra L, Rosenthal P, Borsook D. An approach to localizing corneal pain representation in human primary somatosensory cortex. *PLoS One.* 2012;7(9):30–32.
74. Aicher SA, Hermes SM, Hegarty DM. Corneal afferents differentially target thalamic- and parabrachial-projecting neurons in spinal trigeminal nucleus caudalis. *Neuroscience.* 2013;232:182–193.
75. Bernard JF, Bester H, Besson JM. Involvement of the spino-parabrachio -amygdaloid and -hypothalamic pathways in the autonomic and affective emotional aspects of pain. *Prog Brain Res.* 1996;107:243–255.
76. Gauriau C, Bernard JF. A comparative reappraisal of projections from the superficial laminae of the dorsal horn in the rat: The forebrain. *J Comp Neurol.* 2004;468(1):24–56.
77. Bee JA. The development and pattern of innervation of the avian cornea. *Dev Biol.* 1982;92(1):5–15.
78. You L, Kruse FE, Völcker HE. Neurotrophic factors in the human cornea. *Investig Ophthalmol Vis Sci.* 2000;41(3):692–702.
79. Sarkar J, Chaudhary S, Jassim SH, et al. CD11B+GR1+ myeloid cells secrete NGF and promote trigeminal ganglion neurite growth: Implications for corneal nerve regeneration. *Investig Ophthalmol Vis Sci.* 2013;54(9):5920–5936.
80. Mastropasqua L, Massaro-Giordano G, Nubile M, Sacchetti M. Understanding the pathogenesis of neurotrophic keratitis: the role of corneal nerves. *J Cell Physiol.* 2017; 232(4):717–724.
81. Jamali A, Kenyon B, Ortiz G, et al. Plasmacytoid dendritic cells in the eye. *Prog Retin Eye Res.* 2021:80.
82. Kubilus JK, Linsenmayer TF. Developmental guidance of embryonic corneal innervation: Roles of Semaphorin3A and Slit2. *Dev Biol.* 2010;344(1):172–184.
83. Lwigale PY, Bronner-Fraser M. Lens-derived Semaphorin3A regulates sensory innervation of the cornea. *Dev Biol.* 2007;306(2):750–759.
84. Kirby ML, Diab IM, Mattio TG. Development of adrenergic innervation of the iris and fluorescent ganglion cells in the choroid of the chick eye. *Anat Rec.* 1978;191(3):311–319.
85. Guttmann-Raviv N, Shraga-Heled N, Varshavsky A, Guimaraes-Sternberg C, Kessler O, Neufeld G. Semaphorin-3A and semaphorin-3F work together to repel endothelial cells and to inhibit their survival by induction of apoptosis. *J Biol Chem.* 2007;282(36): 26294–26305.
86. Okuno T, Nakatsuji Y, Kumanogoh A. The role of immune semaphorins in multiple sclerosis. *FEBS Lett.* 2011;585(23):3829–3835.
87. Takamatsu H, Kumanogoh A. Diverse roles for semaphorin-plexin signaling in the immune system. *Trends Immunol.* 2012;33(3):127–135.
88. Ko JA, Mizuno Y, Yanai R, ichiro Chikama T, Sonoda KH. Expression of semaphorin 3A and its receptors during mouse corneal development. *Biochem Biophys Res Commun.* 2010;403(3–4):305–309.
89. Mckenna CC, Lwigale PY. Innervation of the mouse cornea during development. *Investig Ophthalmol Vis Sci.* 2011;52(1):30–35.
90. Bouheraoua N, Fouquet S, Marcos-Almaraz MT, Karagogeos D, Laroche L, Chédotal A. Genetic analysis of the organization, development, and plasticity of corneal innervation in mice. *J Neurosci.* 2019;39(7):1150–1168.
91. Chan KY, Jarvelainen M, Chang JH, Edenfield MJ. A cryodamage model for studying corneal nerve regeneration. *Investig Ophthalmol Vis Sci.* 1990;31(10):2008–2021.
92. Leiper LJ, Ou J, Walczysko P, et al. Control of patterns of corneal innervation by Pax6. *Invest Ophthalmol Vis Sci.* 2009;50(3):1122–1128.
93. Patel DV, McGhee CNJ. In vivo laser scanning confocal microscopy confirms that the human corneal sub-basal nerve plexus is a highly dynamic structure. *Investig Ophthalmol Vis Sci.* 2008;49(8):3409–3412.
94. Íñigo-Portugués A, Exposito G, Gallar J, Belmonte C, Meseguer V. Remodeling of corneal cold sensory nerve fibers in the adult living mouse. *Invest Ophthalmol Vis Sci.* 2017;58(8):1021–1021.
95. Harris LW, Purves D. Rapid remodeling of sensory endings in the corneas of living mice. *J Neurosci.* 1989;9(6):2210–2214.
96. Tanelian DL, Barry MA, Johnston SA, Le T, Smith GM. Semaphorin III can repulse and inhibit adult sensory afferents in vivo. *Nat Med.* 1997;3(12):1398–1401.
97. Zhang M, Zhou Q, Luo Y, Nguyen T, Rosenblatt MI, Guaiquil VH. Semaphorin3A induces nerve regeneration in the adult cornea-a switch from its repulsive role in development. *PLoS One.* 2018;13:1.
98. Omoto M, Yoshida S, Miyashita H, et al. The semaphorin 3A inhibitor SM-345431 accelerates peripheral nerve regeneration and sensitivity in a murine corneal transplantation model. *PLoS One.* 2012;7(11).
99. Erie JC, McLaren JW, Hodge DO, Bourne WM. The effect of age on the corneal subbasal nerve plexus. *Cornea.* 2005;24(6):705–709.
100. Boberg-Ans J. On the corneal sensitivity. *Acta Ophthalmol.* 1956;34(3):149–162.
101. Millodot M. The influence of age on the sensitivity of the cornea. *Invest Ophthalmol Vis Sci.* 1977;16(3):240–242.
102. Bourcier T, Acosta MC, Borderie V, et al. Decreased corneal sensitivity in patients with dry eye. *Investig Ophthalmol Vis Sci.* 2005;46(7):2341–2345.
103. Acosta MC, Alfaro ML, Borrás F, Belmonte C, Gallar J. Influence of age, gender and iris color on mechanical and chemical sensitivity of the cornea and conjunctiva. *Exp Eye Res.* 2006;83(4):932–938.
104. Bouheraoua N, Fouquet S, Marcos-Almaraz MT, Karagogeos D, Laroche L, Chédotal A. Genetic analysis of the organization, development, and plasticity of corneal innervation in mice. *J Neurosci.* 2019;39(7):1150–1168.
105. Pajoohesh-Ganji A, Pal-Ghosh S, Tadvalkar G, Kyne BM, Saban DR, Stepp MA. Partial denervation of sub-basal axons persists following debridement wounds to the mouse cornea. *Lab Investig.* 2015;95(11):1305–1318.
106. Pal-Ghosh S, Tadvalkar G, Stepp MA. Alterations in corneal sensory nerves during homeostasis, aging, and after injury in mice lacking the heparan sulfate proteoglycan syndecan-1. *Investig Ophthalmol Vis Sci.* 2017;58(12):4959–4975.
107. McKay TB, Seyed-Razavi Y, Ghezzi CE, et al. Corneal pain and experimental model development. *Prog Retin Eye Res.* 2019;71(March 2018):88–113.
108. Rozsa AJ, Guss RB, Beuerman RW. Neural remodelling following experimental surgery of the rabbit cornea. *Investig Ophthalmol Vis Sci.* 1983;24(8):1033–1051.
109. Yu CQ, Rosenblatt MI. Transgenic corneal neurofluorescence in mice: A new model for in vivo investigation of nerve structure and regeneration. *Investig Ophthalmol Vis Sci.* 2007;48(4):1535–1542.
110. Belmonte C, Acosta MC, Gallar J. Neural basis of sensation in intact and injured corneas. *Exp Eye Res.* 2004;78(3):513–525.
111. Al-Aqaba MA, Faraj L, Fares U, Otri AM, Dua HS. The morphologic characteristics of corneal nerves in advanced keratoconus as evaluated by acetylcholinesterase technique. *Am J Ophthalmol.* 2011;152(3):364–376. e1.
112. Chirapapaisan C, Muller RT, Sahin A, et al. Effect of herpes simplex keratitis scar location on bilateral corneal nerve alterations: An in vivo confocal microscopy study. *Br J Ophthalmol.* 2022 Mar;106(3):319–325.
113. Kovács I, Luna C, Quirce S, et al. Abnormal activity of corneal cold thermoreceptors underlies the unpleasant sensations in dry eye disease. *Pain.* 2016;157(2):399–417.
114. Rosenberg ME, Tervo TM, Immonen IJ, Müller LJ, Grönhagen-Riska C, Vesaluoma MH. Corneal structure and sensitivity in type 1 diabetes mellitus. *Invest Ophthalmol Vis Sci.* 2000;41(10):2915–2921.
115. Tavakoli M, Kallinikos PA, Efron N, Boulton AJM, Malik RA. Corneal sensitivity is reduced and relates to the severity of neuropathy in patients with diabetes. *Diabetes Care.* 2007;30(7):1895–1897.
116. Neira-Zalentein W, Holopainen JM, Tervo TMT, et al. Corneal sensitivity in diabetic patients subjected to retinal laser photocoagulation. *Investig Ophthalmol Vis Sci.* 2011;52(8):6043–6049.
117. Petropoulos IN, Ponirakis G, Ferdousi M, et al. Corneal Confocal Microscopy: A Biomarker for Diabetic Peripheral Neuropathy. *Clin Ther.* 2021;43(9):1457–1475.
118. Belmonte C, Gallar J, Pozo MA, Rebollo I. Excitation by irritant chemical substances of sensory afferent units in the cat's cornea. *J Physiol.* 1991;437(1):709–725.
119. MacIver MB, Tanelian DL. Structural and functional specialization of A delta and C fiber free nerve endings innervating rabbit corneal epithelium. *J Neurosci.* 1993;13(10): 4511–4524.
120. Alamri AS, Wood RJ, Ivanusic JJ, Brock JA. The neurochemistry and morphology of functionally identified corneal polymodal nociceptors and cold thermoreceptors. *PLoS One.* 2018;13(3):e0195108.
121. Fernández-Trillo J, Florez-Paz D, Íñigo-Portugués A, et al. Piezo2 mediates low-threshold mechanically evoked pain in the cornea. *J Neurosci.* 2020;40(47):8976–8993.
122. Belmonte C, Giraldez F. Responses of cat corneal sensory receptors to mechanical and thermal stimulation. *J Physiol.* 1981;321(1):355–368.
123. Gallar J, Pozo MA, Tuckett RP, Belmonte C. Response of sensory units with unmyelinated fibres to mechanical, thermal and chemical stimulation of the cat's cornea. *J Physiol.* 1993;468(1):609–622.
124. Belmonte C, Aracil A, Acosta MC, Luna C, Gallar J. Nerves and sensations from the eye surface. *Ocul Surf.* 2004;2(4):248–253.
125. Alamri A, Bron R, Brock JA, Ivanusic JJ. Transient receptor potential cation channel subfamily V member 1 expressing corneal sensory neurons can be subdivided into at least three subpopulations. *Front Neuroanat.* 2015;9(June).
126. Chen X, Gallar J, Pozo MA, Baeza M, Belmonte C. CO2 stimulation of the cornea: a comparison between human sensation and nerve activity in polymodal nociceptive afferents of the cat. *Eur J Neurosci.* 1995;7(6):1154–1163.
127. Acosta MC, Belmonte C, Gallar J. Sensory experiences in humans and single-unit activity in cats evoked by polymodal stimulation of the cornea. *J Physiol.* 2001;534(2):511–525.
128. Caterina MJ, Schumacher MA, Tominaga M, Rosen TA, Levine JD, Julius D. The capsaicin receptor: a heat-activated ion channel in the pain pathway. *Nature.* 1997;389(6653): 816–824.
129. Julius D, Basbaum AI. Molecular mechanisms of nociception. *Nature.* 2001;413(6852): 203–210.
130. Belmonte C, Viana F. Molecular and cellular limits to somatosensory specificity. *Mol Pain.* 2008:4.
131. Acosta MC, Luna C, Quirce S, Belmonte C, Gallar J. Changes in sensory activity of ocular surface sensory nerves during allergic keratoconjunctivitis. *Pain.* 2013;154(11): 2353–2362.
132. Acosta MC, Luna C, Quirce S, Belmonte C, Gallar J. Corneal sensory nerve activity in an experimental model of UV keratitis. *Investig Ophthalmol Vis Sci.* 2014;55(6):3403–3412.
133. Meseguer V, Alpizar YA, Luis E, et al. TRPA1 channels mediate acute neurogenic inflammation and pain produced by bacterial endotoxins. *Nat Commun.* 2014:5.

134. González-González O, Bech F, Gallar J, Merayo-Lloves J, Belmonte C. Functional properties of sensory nerve terminals of the mouse cornea. *Investig Ophthalmol Vis Sci.* 2017;58(1):404–415.

135. Callejo G, Castellanos A, Castany M, et al. Acid-sensing ion channels detect moderate acidifications to induce ocular pain. *Pain.* 2015;156(3):483–495.

136. Comes N, Gasull X, Callejo G. Proton sensing on the ocular surface: Implications in eye pain. *Front Pharmacol.* 2021;12:773871.

137. Tanelian DL, Beuerman RW. Responses of rabbit corneal nociceptors to mechanical and thermal stimulation. *Exp Neurol.* 1984;84(1):165–178.

138. Carr RW, Pianova S, Fernandez J, Fallon JB, Belmonte C, Brock JA. Effects of heating and cooling on nerve terminal impulses recorded from cold-sensitive receptors in the guinea-pig cornea. *J Gen Physiol.* 2003;121(5):427–439.

139. Brock J, Acosta MC, Al Abed A, Pianova S, Belmonte C. Barium ions inhibit the dynamic response of guinea-pig corneal cold receptors to heating but not to cooling. *J Physiol.* 2006;575(2):573–581.

140. Brock JA, McLachlan EM, Belmonte C. Tetrodotoxin-resistant impulses in single nociceptor nerve terminals in guinea-pig cornea. *J Physiol.* 1998;512(Pt 1):211–217.

141. McKemy DD, Neuhausser WM, Julius D. Identification of a cold receptor reveals a general role for TRP channels in thermosensation. *Nature.* 2002;416(6876):52–58.

142. Parra A, Madrid R, Echevarria D, et al. Ocular surface wetness is regulated by TRPM8-dependent cold thermoreceptors of the cornea. *Nat Med.* 2010;16(12):1396–1399.

143. Quallo T, Vastani N, Horridge E, et al. TRPM8 is a neuronal osmosensor that regulates eye blinking in mice. *Nat Commun.* 2015:6.

144. Peier AM, Moqrich A, Hergarden AC, et al. A TRP channel that senses cold stimuli and menthol. *Cell.* 2002;108(5):705–715.

145. Diaz-Tahoces A, Velasco E, García CL, et al. Coding of small temperature changes by high-background cold thermosensitive trigeminal neurons innervating the ocular surface. *Invest Ophthalmol Vis Sci.* 2018;59(9):155–155.

146. Belmonte C, Acosta MC, Merayo-Lloves J, Gallar J. What causes eye pain? *Curr Ophthalmol Rep.* 2015;3(2):111–121.

147. Zuazo A, Ibañez J, Belmonte C. Sensory nerve responses elicited by experimental ocular hypertension. *Exp Eye Res.* 1986;43(5):759–769.

148. Gallar J, Acosta MC, Belmonte C. Activation of scleral cold thermoreceptors by temperature and blood flow changes. *Investig Ophthalmol Vis Sci.* 2003;44(2):697–705.

149. Gallar J. Caracterización electrofisiológica de los receptores sonsoriales del ojo del gato. PhD Dissertation. Universidad de Alicante, Spain; 1991.

150. Tower SS. Unit for sensory reception in cornea. *J Neurophysiol.* 1940;3(6):486–500.

151. Aracil A., Belmonte C., Gallar J. Functional types of conjunctival primary sensory neurons. *Invest Ophthalmol Vis Sci.* 2001;42(4): S662-S662.

152. Gallar J, Santiago B, Acosta MC, Belmonte C. In vivo functional characterization of trigeminal neurons innervating the eye and periocular tissues. *Invest Ophthalmol Vis Sci.* 2014;55(13):3645–3645.

153. Santiago B, Diaz-Tahoces A, Gallar J, Belmonte C, Acosta MC. Somatotopic organization of the different functional types of trigeminal ganglion neurons innervating the ocular surface and periocular tissues. *Invest Ophthalmol Vis Sci.* 2017;58(8):1020–1020.

154. Belmonte C, Simon J, Gallego A. Effects of intraocular pressure changes on the afferent activity of ciliary nerves. *Exp Eye Res.* 1971;12(3):342–355.

155. Tamm ER, Flugel C, Stefani FH, Lutjen-Drecoll E. Nerve endings with structural characteristics of mechanoreceptors in the human scleral spur. *Investig Ophthalmol Vis Sci.* 1994;35(3):1157–1166.

156. Huang CC, Yang W, Guo C, et al. Anatomical and functional dichotomy of ocular itch and pain. *Nat Med.* 2018;24(8):1268–1276.

157. Acosta MC, Tan ME, Belmonte C, Gallar J. Sensations evoked by selective mechanical, chemical, and thermal stimulation of the conjunctiva and cornea. *Investig Ophthalmol Vis Sci.* 2001;42(9):2063–2067.

158. Heppelmann B, Gallar J, Trost B, Schmidt RF, Belmonte C. Three-dimensional reconstruction of scleral cold thermoreceptors of the cat eye. *J Comp Neurol.* 2001;441(2):148–154.

159. Pozo MÁ, Cerveró F. Neurons in the rat spinal trigeminal complex driven by corneal nociceptors: receptive-field properties and effects of noxious stimulation of the cornea. *J Neurophysiol.* 1993;70:2370–2378.

160. May PJ, Porter JD. The distribution of primary afferent terminals from the eyelids of macaque monkeys. *Exp Brain Res.* 1998;123(4):368–381.

161. Gong S, Zhou Q, LeDoux MS. Blink-related sensorimotor anatomy in the rat. *Anat Embryol (Berl).* 2003;207(3):193–208.

162. Kurose M, Meng ID. Corneal dry-responsive neurons in the spinal trigeminal nucleus respond to innocuous cooling in the rat. *J Neurophysiol.* 2013;109(10):2517–2522.

163. Meng ID, Hu JW, Benetti AP, Bereiter DA. Encoding of corneal input in two distinct regions of the spinal trigeminal nucleus in the rat: Cutaneous receptive field properties, responses to thermal and chemical stimulation, modulation by diffuse noxious inhibitory controls, and projections to the parabrachial area. *J Neurophysiol.* 1997;77(1):43–56.

164. Meng ID, Hu JW, Bereiter DA. Differential effects of morphine on corneal-responsive neurons in rostral versus caudal regions of spinal trigeminal nucleus in the rat. *J Neurophysiol.* 1998;79(5):2593–2602.

165. Hirata H, Hu JW, Bereiter DA. Responses of medullary dorsal horn neurons to corneal stimulation by CO2 pulses in the rat. *J Neurophysiol.* 1999;82(5):2092–2107.

166. Okamoto K, Tashiro A, Chang Z, Bereiter DA. Bright light activates a trigeminal nociceptive pathway. *Pain.* 2010;149(2):235–242.

167. Matynia A, Nguyen E, Sun X, et al. Peripheral sensory neurons expressing melanopsin respond to light. *Front Neural Circuits.* 2016;10(Aug).

168. Tanaka T, Kuchiiwa S, Izumi H. Parasympathetic mediated pupillary dilation elicited by lingual nerve stimulation in cats. *Invest Ophthalmol Vis Sci.* 2005;46(11):4267–4274.

169. Okamoto K, Tashiro A, Thompson R, Nishida Y, Bereiter DA. Trigeminal interpolaris/caudalis transition neurons mediate reflex lacrimation evoked by bright light in the rat. *Eur J Neurosci.* 2012;36(11):3492–3499.

170. Rahman M, Okamoto K, Thompson R, Bereiter DA. Trigeminal pathways for hypertonic saline- and light-evoked corneal reflexes. *Neuroscience.* 2014;277:716–723.

171. Ebersberger A, Ringkamp M, Reeh PW, Handwerker HO. Recordings from brain stem neurons responding to chemical stimulation of the subarachnoid space. *J Neurophysiol.* 1997;77(6):3122–3133.

172. Schepelmann K, Ebersberger A, Pawlak M, Oppmann M, Messlinger K. Response properties of trigeminal brain stem neurons with input from dura mater encephali in the rat. *Neuroscience.* 1999;90(2):543–554.

173. Malick A, Strassman AM, Burstein R. Trigeminohypothalamic and reticulohypothalamic tract neurons in the upper cervical spinal cord and caudal medulla of the rat. *J Neurophysiol.* 2000;84(4):2078–2112.

174. Kerr FW, Kruger L, Schwassmann HO, Stern R. Somatotopic organization of mechanoreceptor units in the trigeminal nuclear complex of the macaque. *J Comp Neurol.* 1968;134(2):127–144.

175. Greenwood LF, Sessle BJ. Inputs to trigeminal brain stem neurones from facial, oral, tooth pulp and pharyngolaryngeal tissues: II. Role of trigeminal nucleus caudalis in modulating responses to innocuous and noxious stimuli. *Brain Res.* 1976;117(2):227–238.

176. Chen WH, Chui C, Lin HS, Yin HL. Salt-and-pepper eye pain and brainstem stroke. *Clin Neurol Neurosurg.* 2012;114(7):972–975.

177. Penfield W, Boldrey E. Somatic motor and sensory representation in the cerebral cortex of man as studied by electrical stimulation. *Brain.* 1937;60(4):389–443.

178. Becerra L, Morris S, Bazes S, et al. Trigeminal neuropathic pain alters responses in CNS circuits to mechanical (brush) and thermal (cold and heat) stimuli. *J Neurosci.* 2006;26(42):10646–10657.

179. Gallar J, Velasco E, Zaforas M, Acosta MC, Aguilar J. Thalamic and somatosensory cortex neurons innervating the ocular surface are multimodal. *Invest Ophthalmol Vis Sci.* 2022;63(7):1975–1975.

180. Mazzola L, Isnard J, Mauguière F. Somatosensory and pain responses to stimulation of the second somatosensory area (SII) in humans. A comparison with SI and insular responses. *Cereb Cortex.* 2006;16(7):960–968.

181. Tervo T, Moilanen J. In vivo confocal microscopy for evaluation of wound healing following corneal refractive surgery. *Prog Retin Eye Res.* 2003;22(3):339–358.

182. Bonini S, Rama P, Olzi D, Lambiase A. Neurotrophic keratitis. *Eye (Lond).* 2003;17(8):989–995.

183. Clarke MP, Sullivan TJ, Kobayashi J, Rootman DS, Cherry PMH. Familial congenital corneal anaesthesia. *Aust N Z J Ophthalmol.* 1992;20(3):207–210.

184. Klintworth GK. The molecular genetics of the corneal dystrophies—current status. *Front Biosci.* 2003:8.

185. Liesegang TJ. Varicella-zoster virus eye disease. *Cornea.* 1999;18(5):511–531.

186. Beuerman RW, Schimmelpfennig B. Sensory denervation of the rabbit cornea affects epithelial properties. *Exp Neurol.* 1980;69(1):196–201.

187. Lee A, Derricks K, Minns M, et al. Hypoxia-induced changes in Ca(2+) mobilization and protein phosphorylation implicated in impaired wound healing. *Am J Physiol Cell Physiol.* 2014;306(10).

188. Eslani M, Movahedan A, Afsharkhamseh N, Sroussi H, Djalilian AR. The role of toll-like receptor 4 in corneal epithelial wound healing. *Invest Ophthalmol Vis Sci.* 2014;55(9):6108–6115.

189. Kim A, Matthew Petroll W. Microtubule regulation of corneal fibroblast morphology and mechanical activity in 3-D culture. *Exp Eye Res.* 2007;85(4):546–556.

190. Ljubimov AV, Saghizadeh M. Progress in corneal wound healing. *Prog Retin Eye Res.* 2015;49:17–45.

191. Gallar J, Pozo MA, Rebollo I, Belmonte C. Effects of capsaicin on corneal wound healing. *Investig Ophthalmol Vis Sci.* 1990;31(10):1968–1974.

192. Garcia-Hirschfeld J, Lopez-Briones LG, Belmonte C. Neurotrophic influences on corneal epithelial cells. *Exp Eye Res.* 1994;59(5):597–605.

193. Tan MH, Bryars J, Moore J. Use of nerve growth factor to treat congenital neurotrophic corneal ulceration. *Cornea.* 2006;25(3):352–355.

194. Imanishi J, Kamiyama K, Iguchi I, Kita M, Sotozono C, Kinoshita S. Growth factors: Importance in wound healing and maintenance of transparency of the cornea. *Prog Retin Eye Res.* 2000;19(1):113–129.

195. Lambiase A, Manni L, Bonini S, Rama P, Micera A, Aloe L. Nerve growth factor promotes corneal healing: structural, biochemical, and molecular analyses of rat and human corneas. *Invest Ophthalmol Vis Sci.* 2000;41(5):1063–1069.

196. De Castro F, Silos-Santiago I, López de Armentia M, Barbacid M, Belmonte C. Corneal innervation and sensitivity to noxious stimuli in trkA knockout mice. *Eur J Neurosci.* 1998;10(1):146–152.

197. Shaheen BS, Bakir M, Jain S. Corneal nerves in health and disease. *Surv Ophthalmol.* 2014;59(3):263–285.

198. Jamali A, Lopez M, Sendra V, Harris D, Hamrha P. Plasmacytoid dendritic cells demonstrate vital neuro-protective properties in the cornea and induce corneal nerve regeneration. *Invest Ophthalmol Vis Sci.* 2015;56:4355.

199. Kruse FE, Tseng SC. Growth factors modulate clonal growth and differentiation of cultured rabbit limbal and corneal epithelium. *Invest Ophthalmol Vis Sci.* 1993;34(6):1963–1976.

200. Yin J, Huang J, Chen C, Gao N, Wang F, Fu-Shin XY. Corneal Complications in streptozocin-induced type I diabetic rats. *Investig Ophthalmol Vis Sci.* 2011;52(9):6589–6596.

201. Gao N, Yan C, Lee P, Sun H, Yu FS. Dendritic cell dysfunction and diabetic sensory neuropathy in the cornea. *J Clin Invest.* 2016;126(5):1998–2011.

202. Luna C, Quirce S, Aracil-Marco A, Belmonte C, Gallar J, Acosta MC. Unilateral Corneal Insult Also Alters Sensory Nerve Activity in the Contralateral Eye. *Front Med.* 2021;8:767967.

203. Basbaum AI, Bautista DM, Scherrer G, Julius D. Cellular and molecular mechanisms of pain. *Cell.* 2009;139(2):267–284.

204. Binshtok AM, Wang H, Zimmermann K, et al. Nociceptors are interleukin-1beta sensors. *J Neurosci.* 2008;28(52):14062–14073.

205. Gold MS, Gebhart GF. Nociceptor sensitization in pain pathogenesis. *Nat Med.* 2010;16(11):1248–1257.
206. Pethö G, Reeh PW. Sensory and signaling mechanisms of bradykinin, eicosanoids, platelet-activating factor, and nitric oxide in peripheral nociceptors. *Physiol Rev.* 2012;92(4): 1699–1775.
207. Stevenson W, Chauhan SK, Dana R. Dry eye disease: an immune-mediated ocular surface disorder. *Arch Ophthalmol (Chicago, Ill 1960).* 2012;130(1):90–100.
208. Bessou P, Perl ER. Response of cutaneous sensory units with unmyelinated fibers to noxious stimuli. *J Neurophysiol.* 1969;32(6):1025–1043.
209. Reeh PW, Bayer J, Kocher L, Handwerker HO. Sensitization of nociceptive cutaneous nerve fibers from the rat's tail by noxious mechanical stimulation. *Exp Brain Res.* 1987;65(3): 505–512.
210. Zhang X, Mak S, Li L, et al. Direct inhibition of the cold-activated TRPM8 ion channel by Gαq. *Nat Cell Biol.* 2012;14(8):851–858.
211. Belmonte C. Pain, Dryness, and Itch Sensations in Eye Surface Disorders Are Defined by a Balance between Inflammation and Sensory Nerve Injury. *Cornea.* 2019;38:S11–S24.
212. Chen X, Gallar J, Belmonte C. Reduction by antiinflammatory drugs of the response of corneal sensory nerve fibers to chemical irritation. *Investig Ophthalmol Vis Sci.* 1997;38(10):1944–1953.
213. Acosta MC, Luna C, Graff G, et al. Comparative effects of the nonsteroidal anti-inflammatory drug nepafenac on corneal sensory nerve fibers responding to chemical irritation. *Investig Ophthalmol Vis Sci.* 2007;48(1):182–188.
214. Stein R, Stein HA, Cheskes A, Symons S. Photorefractive keratectomy and postoperative pain. *Am J Ophthalmol.* 1994;117(3):403–405.
215. Acosta MC, Berenguer-Ruiz L, García-Gálvez A, Perea-Tortosa D, Gallar J, Belmonte C. Changes in mechanical, chemical, and thermal sensitivity of the cornea after topical application of nonsteroidal anti-inflammatory drugs. *Invest Ophthalmol Vis Sci.* 2005;46(1):282–286.
216. Weidner C, Schmidt R, Schmelz M, Torebjörk HE, Handwerker HO. Action potential conduction in the terminal arborisation of nociceptive C-fibre afferents. *J Physiol.* 2003;547(Pt 3):931–940.
217. Lasagni Vitar RM, Rama P, Ferrari G. The two-faced effects of nerves and neuropeptides in corneal diseases. *Prog Retin Eye Res.* 2022;86:100974.
218. Belmonte C, Gallar J. The primary nociceptive neuron: A nerve cell with many functions. In: Rowe M, ed. *Somatosensory Processing: From Single Neuron to Brain Imaging.* Philadelphia, PA: Gordon & Breach Science Publisher; 2000:27–49.
219. Bereiter DA, Okamoto K, Tashiro A, Hirata H. Endotoxin-induced uveitis causes long-term changes in trigeminal subnucleus caudalis neurons. *J Neurophysiol.* 2005;94(6):3815–3825.
220. Von Hehn CA, Baron R, Woolf CJ. Deconstructing the neuropathic pain phenotype to reveal neural mechanisms. *Neuron.* 2012;73(4):638–652.
221. Grace PM, Hutchinson MR, Maier SF, Watkins LR. Pathological pain and the neuroimmune interface. *Nat Rev Immunol.* 2014;14(4):217–231.
222. Baron R, Hans G, Dickenson AH. Peripheral input and its importance for central sensitization. *Ann Neurol.* 2013;74(5):630–636.
223. Beuerman RW, Rózsa AJ. Collateral sprouts are replaced by regenerating neurites in the wounded corneal epithelium. *Neurosci Lett.* 1984;44(1):99–104.
224. Campos M, Hertzog L, Garbus JJ, McDonnell PJ. Corneal sensitivity after photorefractive keratectomy. *Am J Ophthalmol.* 1992;114(1):51–54.
225. Gallar J, Acosta MC, Moilanen JAO, Holopainen JM, Belmonte C, Tervo TMT. Recovery of corneal sensitivity to mechanical and chemical stimulation after laser in situ keratomileusis. *J Refract Surg.* 2004;20(3):229–235.
226. Rao GN, John T, Ishida N, Aquavella JV. Recovery of corneal sensitivity in grafts following penetrating keratoplasty. *Ophthalmology.* 1985;92(10):1408–1411.
227. Gallar J, Acosta MC, Gutiérrez AR, Belmonte C. Impulse activity in corneal sensory nerve fibers after photorefractive keratectomy. *Investig Ophthalmol Vis Sci.* 2007;48(9):4033–4037.
228. McLaughlin CR, Acosta MC, Luna C, et al. Regeneration of functional nerves within full thickness collagen-phosphorylcholine corneal substitute implants in guinea pigs. *Biomaterials.* 2010;31(10):2770–2778.
229. Bech F, González-González O, Artime E, et al. Functional and morphologic alterations in mechanical, polymodal, and cold sensory nerve fibers of the cornea following photorefractive keratectomy. *Investig Ophthalmol Vis Sci.* 2018;59(6):2281–2292.
230. Luna C, Mizerska K, Quirce S, et al. Sodium channel blockers modulate abnormal activity of regenerating nociceptive corneal nerves after surgical lesion. *Investig Ophthalmol Vis Sci.* 2021;62(1).
231. Byun YS, Mok JW, Chung SH, Kim HS, Joo CK. Ocular surface inflammation induces de novo expression of substance P in the trigeminal primary afferents with large cell bodies. *Sci Reports.* 2020;10(1):1–11. *2020 101.*
232. Sullivan C, Lee J, Bushey W, et al. Evidence for a phenotypic switch in corneal afferents after lacrimal gland excision. *Exp Eye Res.* 2022;218:109005.
233. De Felipe C, Belmonte C. c-Jun expression after axptomy of corneal trigeminal ganglion neurons is dependent on the site of injury. *Eur J Neurosci.* 1999;11(3):899–906.
234. Black JA, Waxman SG. Molecular identities of two tetrodotoxin-resistant sodium channels in corneal axons. *Exp Eye Res.* 2002;75(2):193–199.
235. Waxman SG, Dib-Hajj S, Cummins TR, Black JA. Sodium channels and pain. *Proc Natl Acad Sci U S A.* 1999;96(14):7635–7639.
236. Matzner O, Devor M. Hyperexcitability at sites of nerve injury depends on voltage-sensitive Na+ channels. *J Neurophysiol.* 1994;72(1):349–359.
237. Rivera L, Gallar J, Pozo MA, Belmonte C. Responses of nerve fibres of the rat saphenous nerve neuroma to mechanical and chemical stimulation: An in vitro study. *J Physiol.* 2000;527(2):305–313.
238. Masuoka T, Gallar J, Belmonte C. Inhibitory effect of amitriptyline on the impulse activity of cold thermoreceptor terminals of intact and tear-deficient Guinea pig corneas. *J Ocul Pharmacol Ther.* 2018;34(1-2):195–203.
239. Belmonte C. Eye dryness sensations after refractive surgery: Impaired tear secretion or "phantom" cornea? *J Refract Surg.* 2007;23(6):598–602.
240. Bron AJ, de Paiva CS, Chauhan SK, et al. TFOS DEWS II pathophysiology report. *Ocul Surf.* 2017;15(3):438–510.
241. Tuisku IS, Konttinen YT, Konttinen LM, Tervo TM. Alterations in corneal sensitivity and nerve morphology in patients with primary Sjögren's syndrome. *Exp Eye Res.* 2008;86(6):879–885.
242. Labbé A, Liang Q, Wang Z, et al. Corneal nerve structure and function in patients with non-sjogren dry eye: clinical correlations. *Invest Ophthalmol Vis Sci.* 2013;54(8): 5144–5150.
243. Tuominen ISJ, Konttinen YT, Vesaluoma MH, Moilanen JAO, Helintö M, Tervo TMT. Corneal innervation and morphology in primary Sjögren's syndrome. *Invest Ophthalmol Vis Sci.* 2003;44(6):2545–2549.
244. De Paiva CS, Pflugfelder SC. Corneal epitheliopathy of dry eye induces hyperesthesia to mechanical air jet stimulation. *Am J Ophthalmol.* 2004;137(1):109–115.
245. Versura P, Frigato M, Cellini M, Mulè R, Malavolta N, Campos EC. Diagnostic performance of tear function tests in Sjogren's syndrome patients. *Eye (Lond).* 2007;21(2):229–237.
246. Situ P, Simpson TL, Fonn D, Jones LW. Conjunctival and corneal pneumatic sensitivity is associated with signs and symptoms of ocular dryness. *Investig Ophthalmol Vis Sci.* 2008;49(7):2971–2976.
247. Vehof J, Kozareva D, Hysi PG, et al. Relationship between dry eye symptoms and pain sensitivity. *JAMA Ophthalmol.* 2013;131(10):1304–1308.
248. Begley C, Simpson T, Liu H, et al. Quantitative analysis of tear film fluorescence and discomfort during tear film instability and thinning. *Invest Ophthalmol Vis Sci.* 2013;54(4):2645–2653.
249. Benítez-Del-Castillo JM, Acosta MC, Wassfi MA, et al. Relation between corneal innervation with confocal microscopy and corneal sensitivity with noncontact esthesiometry in patients with dry eye. *Investig Ophthalmol Vis Sci.* 2007;48(1):173–181.
250. Mecum NE, Russell R, Lee J, Sullivan C, Meng ID. Optogenetic inhibition of Nav1.8 expressing corneal afferents reduces persistent dry eye pain. *Invest Ophthalmol Vis Sci.* 2021;62(14):15.
251. Von Frey M. Beiträge sur Sinnesphysiologie der Haut. *Sächsischen Akademie Der Wissenschaften Zu Leipzig. Math-Phys Cl.* Sächsischen Akademie Der Wissenschaften Zu Leipzig; 1895:166–184.
252. Cochet P, Bonnet R. L'esthésie cornéenne. *Clin Ophthalmol.* 1960;4:3–27.
253. Larson WL. Electro-mechanical corneal aesthesiometer. *Br J Ophthalmol.* 1970;54(5):342–347.
254. Beuerman RW, McCulley JP. Comparative clinical assessment of corneal sensation with a new aesthesiometer. *Am J Ophthalmol.* 1978;86(6):812–815.
255. Draeger J. *Corneal Sensitivity. Measurement and Clinical Importance.* Berlin: Springer-Verlag; 1984.
256. Zaidman G, Weinstein C, Weinstein S, Drozdenko R. A new corneal microaesthesiometer. *Invest Ophthalmol Vis Sci.* 1988;29(4):454.
257. Kohlhaas M, Draeger J, Schmitz N, Bohm A, Bosse I, Hechler B. [Physical and aerodynamic airflow relations of the air stream of the Micro-Air aesthesiometer]. *Klin Monbl Augenheilkd.* 1994;205(4):218–225.
258. Murphy PJ, Patel S, Marshall J. A new non-contact corneal aesthesiometer (NCCA). *Ophthalmic Physiol Opt.* 1996;16(2):101–107.
259. Vega JA, Simpson TL, Fonn D. A noncontact pneumatic esthesiometer for measurement of ocular sensitivity: A preliminary report. *Cornea.* 1999;18(6):675–681.
260. Weinstein S, Drozdenko R, Weinstein C. A new device for corneal esthesiometry. Clinical significance and application. *Clin Eye Vis Care.* 1992;4(3):123–128.
261. Belmonte C, Acosta MC, Schmelz M, Gallar J. Measurement of corneal sensitivity to mechanical and chemical stimulation with a CO2 esthesiometer. *Investig Ophthalmol Vis Sci.* 1999;40(2):513–519.
262. Stapleton F, Tan ME, Papas EB, et al. Corneal and conjunctival sensitivity to air stimuli. *Br J Ophthalmol.* 2004;88(12):1547–1551.
263. Golebiowski B, Papas E, Stapleton F. Assessing the sensory function of the ocular surface: implications of use of a non-contact air jet aesthesiometer versus the Cochet-Bonnet aesthesiometer. *Exp Eye Res.* 2011;92(5):408–413.
264. Tesón M, Calonge M, Fernández I, Stern ME, González-García MJ. Characterization by belmonte's gas esthesiometer of mechanical, chemical, and thermal corneal sensitivity thresholds in a normal population. *Investig Ophthalmol Vis Sci.* 2012;53(6):3154–3160.
265. Du Toit R, Vega JA, Fonn D, Simpson T. Diurnal variation of corneal sensitivity and thickness. *Cornea.* 2003;22(3):205–209.
266. Murphy PJ, Patel S, Kong N, Ryder REJ, Marshall J. Noninvasive assessment of corneal sensitivity in young and elderly diabetic and nondiabetic subjects. *Investig Ophthalmol Vis Sci.* 2004;45(6):1737–1742.
267. Golebiowski B, Papas Eb, Stapleton F. Factors affecting corneal and conjunctival sensitivity measurement. *Optom Vis Sci.* 2008;85(4):E241–E246.
268. Gallar J, Morales C, Freire V. Carmen Acosta M, Belmonte C, Duran JA. Decreased corneal sensitivity and tear production in fibromyalgia. *Investig Ophthalmol Vis Sci.* 2009;50(9):4129–4134.
269. Gallar J, Tervo TMT, Neira W, et al. Selective changes in human corneal sensation associated with herpes simplex virus keratitis. *Investig Ophthalmol Vis Sci.* 2010;51(9): 4516–4522.
270. Situ P, Simpson TL. Interaction of corneal nociceptive stimulation and lacrimal secretion. *Invest Ophthalmol Vis Sci.* 2010;51(11):5640–5645.
271. Millodot M. Objective measurement of corneal sensitivity. *Acta Ophthalmol.* 1973;51(3):325–334.
272. Patel DV, Tavakoli M, Craig JP, Efron N, McGhee CNJ. Corneal sensitivity and slit scanning in vivo confocal microscopy of the subbasal nerve plexus of the normal central and peripheral human cornea. *Cornea.* 2009;28(7):735–740.
273. Chan-Ling T. Sensitivity and neural organization of the cat cornea. *Invest Ophthalmol Vis Sci.* 1989;30(6):1075–1082.
274. Millodot M. Diurnal variation of corneal sensitivity. *Br J Ophthalmol.* 1972;56(11): 844–847.

275. Millodot M, Lamont A. Influence of menstruation on corneal sensitivity. *Br J Ophthalmol.* 1974;58(8):752–756.
276. Millodot M. The influence of age on the sensitivity of the cornea. *Invest Ophthalmol Vis Sci.* 1977;16(3):240–242.
277. Riss B, Binder S, Riss P, Kemeter P. Corneal sensitivity during the menstrual cycle. *Br J Ophthalmol.* 1982;66(2):123–126.
278. Millodot M. Do blue-eyed people have more sensitive corneas than brown-eyed people? *Nature.* 1975;255(5504):151–152.
279. Millodot M. Corneal sensitivity in people with the same and with different iris color. *Invest Ophthalmol.* 1976;15(10):861–862.
280. Millodot M. Corneal sensitivity in albinos. *J Pediatr Ophthalmol Strabismus.* 1978;15(5):300–302.
281. Lele PP, Weddell G. The relationship between neurohistology and corneal sensibility. *Brain.* 1956;79(1):119–154.
282. Kenshalo DR. Comparison of thermal sensitivity of the forehead, lip, conjunctiva and cornea. *J Appl Physiol.* 1960;15:987–991.
283. Beuerman RW, Maurice DM, Tanelian DL. Thermal stimulation of the cornea. In: Anderson D, Matthews B, eds. *Pain in the Trigeminal Region.* Elsevier; 1977:422–423.
284. Beuerman RW, Tanelian DL. Corneal pain evoked by thermal stimulation. *Pain.* 1979;7(1):1–14.
285. Feng Y, Simpson TL. Nociceptive sensation and sensitivity evoked from human cornea and conjunctiva stimulated by CO2. *Investig Ophthalmol Vis Sci.* 2003;44(2):529–532.
286. Belmonte C, Gallar J. Cold thermoreceptors, unexpected players in tear production and ocular dryness sensations. *Invest Ophthalmol Vis Sci.* 2011;52(6):3888–3892.
287. Belmonte C, Nichols JJ, Cox SM, et al. TFOS DEWS II pain and sensation report. *Ocul Surf.* 2017;15(3):404–437.
288. Ursea R, Feng MT, Zhou M, Lien V, Loeb R. Pain perception in sequential cataract surgery: comparison of first and second procedures. *J Cataract Refract Surg.* 2011;37(6):1009–1014.
289. Rosenberg ME, Tervo TMT, Gallar J, et al. Corneal morphology and sensitivity in lattice dystrophy type II (familial amyloidosis, Finnish type). *Invest Ophthalmol Vis Sci.* 2001;42(3):634–641.
290. Dienes L, Kiss HJ, Perényi K; et al. Corneal sensitivity and dry eye symptoms in patients with keratoconus. *PLoS One.* 2015;10(10).
291. Belmonte C, Tervo TM. Pain in and around the eye. In: McMahon S, Koltzenburg M, eds. *Wall and Melzack's Textbook of Pain.* Philadelphia, PA: Elsevier; 2006:887–901.
292. Polse KA. Etiology of corneal sensitivity changes accompanying contact lens wear. *Invest Ophthalmol Vis Sci.* 1978;17(12):1202–1206.
293. Millodot M. Does the long term wear of contact lenses produce a loss of corneal sensitivity? *Experientia.* 1977;33(11):1475–1476.
294. Tanelian DL, Beuerman RW. Recovery of corneal sensation following hard contact lens wear and the implication for adaptation. *Investig Ophthalmol Vis Sci.* 1980;19(11):1391–1394.
295. Murphy PJ, Patel S, Marshall J. The effect of long-term, daily contact lens wear on corneal sensitivity. *Cornea.* 2001;20(3):264–269.
296. Situ P, Simpson TL, Jones LW, Fonn D. Effects of silicone hydrogel contact lens wear on ocular surface sensitivity to tactile, pneumatic mechanical, and chemical stimulation. *Invest Ophthalmol Vis Sci.* 2010;51(12):6111–6117.
297. Lum E, Golebiowski B, Gunn R, Babhoota M, Swarbrick H. Corneal sensitivity with contact lenses of different mechanical properties. *Optom Vis Sci.* 2013;90(9):954–960.
298. Millodot M, Henson DB, Oleary DJ. Measurement of corneal sensitivity and thickness with PMMA and gas-permeable contact lenses. *Am J Optom Physiol Opt.* 1979;56(10):628–632.
299. Bergenske PD, Polse KA. The effect of rigid gas permeable lenses on corneal sensitivity. *J Am Optom Assoc.* 1987;58(3):212–215.
300. Patel SV, McLaren JW, Hodge DO, Bourne WM. Confocal microscopy in vivo in corneas of long-term contact lens wearers. *Invest Ophthalmol Vis Sci.* 2002;43(4):995–1003.
301. Stapleton F, Marfurt C, Golebiowski B, et al. The TFOS International Workshop on Contact Lens Discomfort: report of the subcommittee on neurobiology. *Invest Ophthalmol Vis Sci.* 2013;54(11).
302. Chen J, Simpson TL. A role of corneal mechanical adaptation in contact lens-related dry eye symptoms. *Investig Ophthalmol Vis Sci.* 2011;52(3):1200–1205.
303. Muntz A, Subbaraman LN, Sorbara L, Jones L. Tear exchange and contact lenses: A review. *J Optom.* 2015;8(1):2–11.
304. Stapleton F, Alves M, Bunya VY, et al. TFOS DEWS II Epidemiology Report. *Ocul Surf.* 2017;15(3):334–365.
305. Craig JP, Nichols KK, Akpek EK, et al. TFOS DEWS II Definition and Classification Report. *Ocul Surf.* 2017;15(3):276–283.
306. Wolffsohn JS, Arita R, Chalmers R, et al. TFOS DEWS II Diagnostic Methodology report. *Ocul Surf.* 2017;15(3):539–574.
307. De Paiva CS. Effects of aging in dry eye. *Int Ophthalmol Clin.* 2017;57(2):47–64.
308. Jalavisto E, Orma E, Tawast M. Ageing and relation between stimulus intensity and duration in corneal sensibility. *Acta Physiol Scand.* 1951;23(2–3):224–233.
309. Millodot M, Owens H. The influence of age on the fragility of the cornea. *Acta Ophthalmol.* 1984;62(5):819–824.
310. Grupcheva CN, Wong T, Riley AF, McGhee CNJ. Assessing the sub-basal nerve plexus of the living healthy human cornea by in vivo confocal microscopy. *Clin Experiment Ophthalmol.* 2002;30(3):187–190.
311. Marco B, Alessandro R, Philippe F, Fabio B, Paolo R, Giulio F. The effect of aging on nerve morphology and substance p expression in mouse and human corneas. *Invest Ophthalmol Vis Sci.* 2018;59(13):5329–5335.
312. De Silva MEH, Hill LJ, Downie LE, Chinnery HR. The effects of aging on corneal and ocular surface homeostasis in mice. *Invest Ophthalmol Vis Sci.* 2019;60(7):2705–2715.
313. Chirapapaisan C, Thongsuwan S, Chirapapaisan N, Chonpimai P, Veeraburinon A. Characteristics of corneal subbasal nerves in different age groups: An in vivo confocal microscopic analysis. *Clin Ophthalmol.* 2021;15:3563–3572.

17

Outward-Directed Transport

Eva Ramsay, Laura Hellinen, Heidi Kidron, Tetsuya Terasaki, and Arto Urtti

Introduction

Several barriers protect the eye from exogenous compounds that may exert toxic reactions in the eye. These barriers can be classified anatomically into three groups. First, the eye is protected from the air and lacrimal fluid by the tight epithelial barriers of the cornea and conjunctiva. Second, the tight tissue barriers in the iris and ciliary body form the blood-aqueous barrier (BAB) between the blood circulation and aqueous humor. Third, blood-retinal barriers (BRBs) (inner barrier: retinal capillaries; outer barrier: retinal pigment epithelium [RPE]) regulate molecular transfer between the neural retina and systemic blood circulation. The entire barrier function of these tissues includes several key components: (1) a physical barrier formed by tight intercellular junctions, (2) the metabolism of xenobiotics, and (3) transport activity (inward and outward transport).

In this chapter, ocular outward transport is discussed in the context of pharmacology, toxicology, and pathophysiology. Outward transport shuttles compounds from the eye to the lacrimal fluid and systemic blood circulation. This action is accomplished mostly by efflux transporters that actively transport compounds from the intracellular space to the extracellular environment. In the context of outward transport from the eye, those efflux transporters located at the barriers between the eye and lacrimal fluid or eye and blood circulation are the most interesting ones.

The most anterior ocular barrier consists of the epithelia of the cornea and conjunctiva that line the lacrimal fluid (Fig. 17.1). Outward transport in these tissues protects the eye from compounds in the lacrimal fluid. In the case of drug administration, the outward transport must compete with inward passive diffusion and inward active transport, thereby leading to relative changes, but not necessarily complete block of drug transport from the lacrimal fluid into the eye. The final outcome of such competition depends on the physicochemical properties of the drug (affecting passive diffusion and transport) and the expression of relevant transporters in the cornea and conjunctiva.[1] Thus, ocular absorption of topically applied drugs depends on the barrier properties of the corneal and conjunctival epithelia and expression of transporters. It should be noted that conjunctival permeability of small molecules is about nine times higher than their permeation in the cornea.[2] Overall, transcorneal bioavailability of topically applied small-molecule drugs in the aqueous humor is approximately 0.1% to 5%, whereas biologics have negligible absorption to the cornea. Ocular bioavailability across conjunctiva has not been quantitated, but the transconjunctival route tends to be more important for hydrophilic compounds with poor corneal permeability.[3]

The BRB regulates molecular transfer between the posterior eye segment and the systemic circulation. The BRB is composed of retinal vascular endothelium (inner BRB) and retinal-pigmented epithelium (outer BRB).[1] The inner BRB is composed of a tight monolayer of endothelial cells, and the outer BRB is composed of retinal pigmented epithelial cells that form a monolayer with tight junctions.

Bruch's membrane and the choroid are relatively leaky tissues providing a negligible barrier compared with the RPE. In general, the BRB allows the permeation of small molecules with adequate lipophilicity, but restricts serious permeation of proteins and protein-bound drugs in the plasma.[4,5] Likewise, the BRB limits the elimination of large molecules from the vitreous, prolonging the vitreal half-lives of injected biologics, such as vascular endothelial growth factor inhibitors, for up to several days.[4] On the contrary, small molecules, capable of permeating the BRB, are rapidly eliminated from the vitreous with half-lives of a few hours. Outward transport in the BRB may limit retinal access of systemically circulating compounds, whereas it may accelerate elimination of vitreal compounds from the eye, thereby reducing retinal exposure to the exogenous substances.

This chapter comprises a discussion on the efflux transporters on the ocular surface (cornea, conjunctiva) and the BRB (retinal capillaries, RPE). Information about the biologic and pharmacologic roles of efflux transporters in the eye is still emerging and changing. This chapter provides an update of current knowledge about the expression and functionality of the efflux transporters in the eye. The main focus will be on outward transport in the cornea and BRB, as they have been investigated more than the conjunctiva and BAB.

EFFLUX TRANSPORTERS

The efflux transporters are transmembrane proteins that are expressed in the liver and kidney, where they contribute to the pharmacokinetics of various drugs and their metabolites.[6] In physiologic barriers such as the intestine, blood-brain barrier (BBB), and placenta, the efflux transporters protect the body from harmful xenobiotics and excrete endogenous metabolites.[7] Additionally, cancer cells often overexpress efflux transporters to provide protection from anticancer agents. In fact, P-glycoprotein (P-gp) was initially found through its ability to provide drug resistance in colchicine-selected Chinese hamster ovary cells.[8] P-gp was later called multidrug resistance protein 1 (MDR1), based on its involvement in the resistance toward a broad range of anticancer drugs such as paclitaxel and doxorubicin. Breast cancer resistance protein (BCRP) and the multidrug resistance–associated proteins (MRPs) were also initially found through their involvement in multidrug resistance in cancer cells, which is reflected in their persisting unofficial nomenclature. The efflux transporters belong to the ATP-binding cassette (ABC) family of transporters, which in humans contains 48 members, divided into 7 subfamilies, A–G. Not all the transporters are involved in drug transport; however, the most important ones involved in drug transport are listed in Table 17.1. In the eye, efflux transporters have been found at several barrier tissues—for example, the cornea and BRB.[1]

The ABC transporters share the same structure, consisting of two transmembrane domains and two cytoplasmic adenosine triphosphate (ATP) -binding domains (Table 17.2; Fig. 17.2A). The

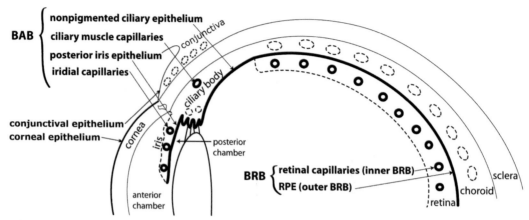

Fig. 17.1 Tissue barriers of the eye. *BAB*, Blood-aqueous barrier; *BRB*, blood-retinal barrier; *RPE*, retinal pigment epithelium.

TABLE 17.1 Efflux transporters with pharmacokinetic impact

Gene name	Protein name	Uniprot ID	Example drug substrates
ABCB1	P-gp, MDR1	P08183	Erythromycin, methotrexate, ciprofloxacin
ABCC1	MRP1	P33527	Methotrexate
ABCC2	MRP2	Q92887	Erythromycin, methotrexate
ABCC3	MRP3	O15438	Methotrexate
ABCC4	MRP4	O15439	Methotrexate, ganciclovir
ABCC5	MRP5	O15440	Acyclovir, latanoprost
ABCG2	BCRP	Q9UNQ0	Ciprofloxacin, methotrexate

ABC, ATP-binding cassette; *BCRP*, Breast cancer resistance protein; *MDR1*, multidrug resistance protein 1; *MRP*, multidrug resistance–associated protein; *P-gp*, P-glycoprotein.

TABLE 17.2 ABC transporter family and members identified in human ocular tissues

Family	Function	Members	Ocular tissue
ABCA	Cholesterol and lipid transport	ABCA4	Retina
ABCB	Transport peptides, toxins etc.	P-glycoprotein	BRB, BAB
ABCC	Mainly ion transport	MRP1	Cornea, BAB, BRB
		MRP2	Cornea, BAB
		MRP3	Cornea
		MRP4	Cornea, BAB, BRB
		MRP5	Cornea, BRB
ABCD	Peroxisomal transport		
ABCE/ ABCF	No transport function, only ATP-binding domain		
ABCG	Transport ions, lipids, toxins, etc.	BCRP	Cornea, BAB Retina

ABC, ATP-binding cassette; *BAB*, blood-aqueous barrier; *BCRP*, breast cancer resistance protein; *BRB*, blood-retinal barrier.

energy from ATP is used to drive the transport of substrates over the membrane against the concentration gradient (i.e., from lower concentration toward higher concentration). The transmembrane domain containing the substrate cavity consists of 12 transmembrane helices. Some efflux transporters contain five additional transmembrane helices forming an N-terminal transmembrane domain, with a largely unknown function (Fig. 17.2B). Other ABC transporters are so-called half-transporters, where the peptide chain only forms one ATP-binding domain and six transmembrane helices. In the ABCG family, the order of the ATP-binding domain and the transmembrane helices is reversed (Fig. 17.2C). Two of these half-transporters need to dimerize to form a functional unit.

METHODS OF STUDYING TRANSPORTERS

Transporters can be investigated in terms of structure, substrate specificity, expression, localization, and functionality. Most data on transporter structure, substrates, and general functionality are available in the general biologic and medical literature. In this section, we briefly summarize some methods that are relevant for understanding the expression and functions of efflux proteins in outward-directed transport in the eye.

Proteomic analysis

Historically, expression of proteins in the eye has been widely studied with western blots, but modern mass spectrometry–based methods of proteomics can provide much more complete information on protein expression, including in the eye. As transporter proteins regulate substrate movement across the plasma membrane of the cells, identification and quantification of the proteins facilitates understanding of ocular physiology and pharmacology.[9] Global proteomics, comprehensive untargeted protein identification using mass spectrometry, has been used to reveal transporter and relevant protein profiles in the RPE cells,[10] whereas quantitative targeted proteomics, a precise protein quantification, has been used to determine the amounts of transporter proteins in the RPE using liquid chromatography tandem mass spectrometry.[11] As transmembrane domains of transporter proteins are water insoluble, peptides with specific amino acid sequences of transporter protein are usually selected from water-soluble extracellular domains. Efflux transporter protein expression may vary under

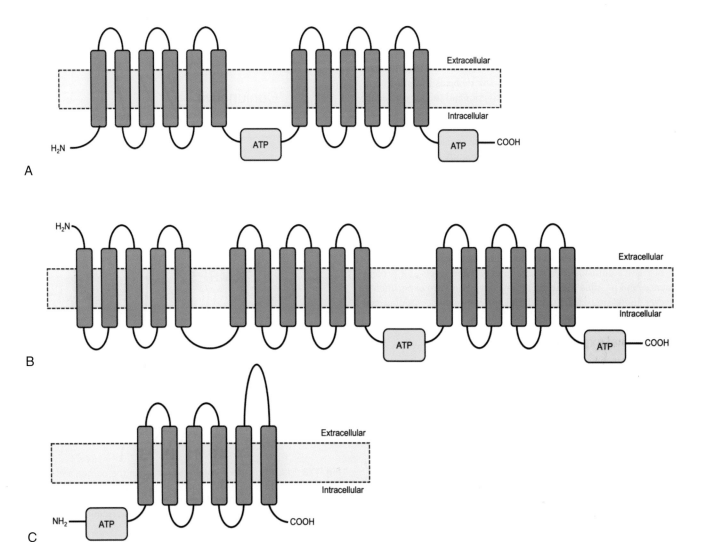

Fig. 17.2 Schematic structures of ATP-binding cassette (ABC) transporters. (**A**) Protein with 12 transmembrane heli-ces and 2 cytoplasmic adenosine triphosphate (ATP)–binding sites. (**B**) Protein with five additional transmembrane helices. (**C**) "Reverse" half-transporters with six transmembrane helices and single ATP-binding site. The N- and C- terminus of the peptide chain is indicated with an amino group (NH2) and a carboxyl group (COOH), respectively.

different conditions, such as oxidative stress and inflammation.[12] A combination of phospho-proteomic analysis of phosphorylated pro-teins and quantitative targeted proteomics is also a useful methodology, providing fundamental insights into the cellular mechanisms of the functional changes of efflux transporters.[13,14] Overall, proteomic tech-niques are useful for generating data on transporter expression in the ocular barriers, as exemplified in the case of RPE cells.[10] However, such data are not available yet for the cornea, conjunctiva, or BAB.

Overexpressing cells

The function of efflux transporters is often studied at a cellular level in overexpression systems because this approach enables the study of a specific transporter in a controlled environment. Dissecting the specific role of a single efflux transporter type can be difficult because substrate specificities of efflux transporters are relatively wide and often overlap. The pharmacologic impact of the transporter in overexpressed cell sys-tems cannot be reliably assessed because the transporter amount does not necessarily correspond to the in vivo situation and many other transporters with overlapping substrate specificity may contribute in vivo. The intact cells may not be appropriate for efflux transporter stud-ies if the substrate has poor transcellular permeability or the cell does

not express relevant uptake transporters because the compound usu-ally needs to enter the cells before binding to the efflux transporters.[15] Instead, ATP-dependent substrate transport by individual efflux trans-porters can be studied in inverted cell membrane vesicles. Assays mea-suring only the ATPase activity of the efflux transporters are not ideal, as the transporters have a basal ATPase activity, and not all substrates or inhibitors significantly change ATP consumption. Detection of the accumulated substrate in the vesicles is more accurate.

Ocular cell and tissue models

Expression and function of efflux transporters have been investigated in cell lines and primary cells. It is important to note that cell lines may differ significantly from their in vivo counterparts, thus leading to potentially misleading conclusions. For example, the widely used human corneal epithelial (HCE) cell line overexpressed several efflux transporters at mRNA compared with normal human corneal epithe-lial cells that expressed only BCRP, MRP1, and MRP5.[16] Moreover, transcriptomic analysis revealed major differences in the protein expression patterns of differentiated HCE cell line and normal human cornea.[17] In contrast, the widely used human RPE cell line ARPE-19 showed similar expression of efflux transporters as primary human

RPE cells,[11] but another cell line (D407) showed a very different expression pattern.[18] Overall, cell model and cell culture conditions must be carefully selected to avoid misleading conclusions about efflux transport of compounds in vivo.[19,20]

Isolated tissues such as the cornea and RPE are often used to characterize molecular transport in the eye. The rabbit is the most commonly used species in ocular pharmacokinetics and the most relevant species for in vitro to in vivo translation, but the differences or similarity in transporter protein expression between rabbit and human is not known. Porcine and bovine tissues have also been used in permeation studies in vitro. Ussing chambers enable the study of directionality, which can be used to assess the impact of efflux transport on overall net transfer of compounds in the barrier. An example is a study with bovine RPE-choroid, which shows the importance of maintaining and controlling tissue viability.[21] Data on protein expression and transport in vitro can be further extended toward in vivo predictions by using pharmacokinetic models.[1,14] In vivo translation is not straightforward because there are several confounding factors such as contribution of passive diffusion, differences in expression levels and protein sequence, and possible tissue alterations during in vitro experiments. However, increasing experimental data and improving computational capacity enhance the value of such predictions.

In vivo animal experiments

Kinetic ocular in vivo studies are performed with rabbits. In general, the rabbit is considered a relevant model that provides a reasonable human translation of pharmacokinetics in terms of topical and intravitreal drug administration.[22] However, the validity of the rabbit model for efflux transporter functions is still unclear. It is difficult to dissect the functions of efflux transport from the overall pharmacokinetics that are affected by various factors. Some approaches from BBB studies could be applicable also in the ocular context. These approaches include prediction of $K_{p,uu,brain}$ (i.e., the steady state unbound drug concentration ratio between blood and the brain). This is based on the pharmacokinetic model, with an efflux transporter expression level per surface area of BBB ($\mu mol/cm^2$), an intrinsic efflux rate of drug per transporter protein ($\mu L/[min \times \mu mol$ of transporter protein]), and the passive diffusion rate of drug per surface area of BBB ($\mu L/[min \times cm^2]$).[23]

CORNEAL OUTWARD TRANSPORT

The cornea serves as a barrier to harmful substances and drug molecules owing to the tight multilayered epithelium, but also because of the presence of efflux transporters. Fig. 17.3 illustrates the efflux transporters that are known to be expressed in the human and rabbit cornea. The protein expression levels have been determined in primary cells or tissues using western blot or immunohistochemical staining, but absolute and relative protein expression data are lacking still.

The impact of corneal efflux transporters in drug delivery has been studied mainly in rabbits, using either excised cornea or in vivo models.[1] The P-gp substrate, rhodamine 123, had a more than twofold larger basolateral-to-apical permeability in an isolated rabbit cornea compared with the opposite apical-to-basolateral permeability.[24] Additionally, the directionality was inhibited by the P-gp inhibitor, verapamil. Comparable results were seen in rabbit in vivo using a single-dose infusion method, in which a small well was placed on top of the cornea containing the P-gp substrate, erythromycin.[25] The bioavailability of erythromycin in the anterior chamber was increased by up to fourfold in the presence of P-gp inhibitors.

Erythromycin was shown also to be a substrate of the MRP2 efflux transporter.[26,27] The aqueous humor bioavailability of erythromycin increased by 2.5- to 4-fold in the presence of P-gp and MRP inhibitors,

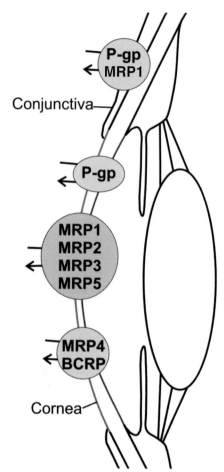

Fig. 17.3 Efflux transport protein expressed in the cornea and conjunctiva. *Purple:* expressed only in rabbit; *pink:* expressed both in rabbit and human; *turquoise:* expressed only in human.[16,23,26,27,32,34–39] *BCRP,* Breast cancer resistance protein; *MRP,* multidrug resistance–associated protein; *P-gp,* P-glycoprotein.

using the single-dose infusion method in rabbits.[25] The involvement of MRP2 in erythromycin transport was also studied in excised rabbit cornea.[28] The efflux protein P-gp was first inhibited by verapamil and then the remaining MRP2 efflux transport was inhibited by MK571, resulting in a similar permeability of erythromycin in both directions.

Functionally active MRP1 and MRP5 efflux transporters were shown in an uptake assay with isolated rabbit cornea. Concentration differences were seen for 5(6)-carboxy-2',7'-dichlorofluorescein (CDCF) substrate in the presence of an MRP1 and MRP5 inhibitor, probenecid.[28] CDCF is a polar substrate produced intracellularly by hydrolysis of CDCF diacetate (CDCFDA), and it cannot exit the cell without efflux transporters. Probenecid, an inhibitor of MRP2, affected efflux of CDCF from the cells.[29,30] The presence of MRP2 and MRP5 activity in the rabbit cornea was supported by an in vivo study in which the bioavailability of acyclovir was increased 2.2-fold in the presence of the MRP2 and MRP5 inhibitor, MK571.[31]

MRP3 expression was observed in the rabbit cornea, but no activity was detected for MRP3 and BCRP after the use of methotrexate as a substrate.[24] MRP4 activity was not detected in the rabbit cornea, using adefovir in the presence of an indomethacin inhibitor.[28] However, in the human cornea, a variant of MRP4 caused lower intraocular pressure after latanoprost treatment.[32]

Species-dependent expression of efflux transporters is important to consider when trying to translate functionality studies into clinical settings (Fig. 17.3). For example, the function of P-gp has been studied in rabbits, but the transporter is not expressed in the human cornea.[24,33,34] Conversely, the clinically relevant efflux transporters, MRP4 and BCRP, are present in the human cornea but not in the rabbit.[16,24,28,35]

The role of corneal efflux transporters in topical drug delivery is most likely modest due to the high drug concentrations used clinically. However, it was predicted[1] that corneal efflux transporters have a high impact on the aqueous humor bioavailability of drugs at applied concentrations of 0.1% to 1% if the drug has low passive permeability and high efflux transporter affinity. Drugs released from pharmaceutical suspensions and controlled release devices might be more prone to efflux transport, owing to lower drug concentrations in the tear fluid and inside the corneal epithelial cells; however, many other factors may influence the overall clinical impact of efflux transporters.

BLOOD-RETINAL BARRIER OUTWARD TRANSPORT

The BRB consists of retinal capillary endothelium that forms the inner BRB and the RPE that forms the outer BRB (Fig. 17.4). The outer BRB has an important role in outward transport from the eye as permeation across the RPE is the main elimination route for low-molecular-weight

drugs from the vitreous.[41] Both inner and outer BRB contain several efflux proteins that may contribute to their barrier function and outward transport from the eye.[1]

The majority of the expression data regarding efflux transporters in the BRB have been generated with cultured cell lines, either primary or stem cell–derived RPE cells.[1] Owing to the wide range of assay procedures and cell sources, the expression data from different research sites are partly conflicting.[1] However, the expression of some efflux proteins, including P-gp, has been confirmed in the human BRB (Fig. 17.4). Although the BRB consists of two distinct tissues, the functional evaluation in vivo cannot distinguish these barriers from each other, and the specific localization of the efflux proteins needs to be evaluated with immunohistochemistry. In addition, because many influx and efflux transporter substrates overlap, the role of a single transporter is difficult to estimate in vivo or in cell models displaying several transporters.

P-glycoprotein (ABCB1)

P-gp has been detected on both sides of human RPE.[42] In the case of the inner BRB (the retinal vasculature), expression has not been verified in humans, although expression of the protein has been shown in rodents and rabbits.[43–46] A recent positron-emission tomography (PET) scan

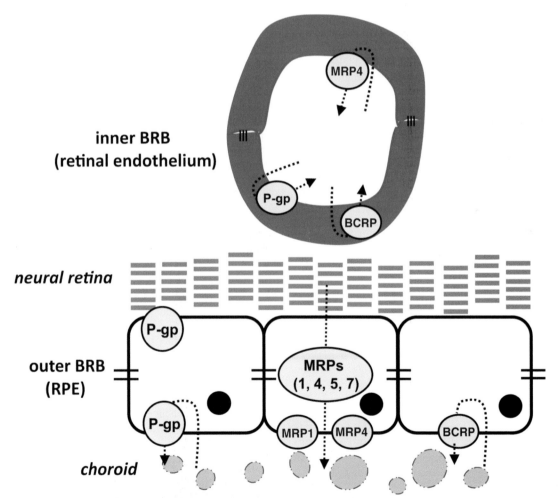

Fig. 17.4 Transporter protein expression in the blood-retinal barrier (*BRB*). Expression in human tissue or primary human cultures with *green*, expression in other species (rabbit, mouse, or pig) with *yellow*. In the case of cultured human retinal pigment epithelium (*RPE*) cells, specific location to apical or basolateral membranes is not displayed. The inward P-glycoprotein (*P-gp*) function is not confirmed in vivo, as the studies have shown outward net transport (see text for details). *BCRP*, Breast cancer resistance protein; *MRP*, multidrug resistance–associated protein; *P-gp*, P-glycoprotein.

study in humans showed that systemically administered P-gp substrate, verapamil, had significantly higher retinal distribution during P-gp inhibition (1.5-fold), confirming P-gp function in the human BRB.[47] However, the clinical significance of P-gp in the BRB compared with the BBB seems to be lower, as the retinal distribution of verapamil was higher ($V_T = 1.03\,mL/g$) compared with the brain ($V_T = 0.72\,mL/g$) and the inhibition had a lower effect on the retinal (1.5-fold) than the brain distribution (3.8-fold).[47,48] A similar conclusion was drawn in a mouse study describing increased entry rate of verapamil after P-gp inhibition (1.5-fold) and in P-gp knockout mice (1.3-fold).[43] However, the relative increase in the entry rate in the BRB was less than in the BBB, where P-gp inhibition increased verapamil entry 5.6 to 9.7 times.[43]

Breast cancer resistance protein (ABCG2)

BCRP expression has not been confirmed in normal human BRB tissue—an immunohistochemistry study showed that BCRP was not expressed in the large blood vessels ($>20\,\mu m$) of the human retina[35] and the protein was not detected in the primary human RPE cells with a proteomics-based quantitation.[10,11] However, the expression in the inner BRB is evident in rodents,[43,46,49] but there are discrepancies in the literature regarding expression in the inner BRB—both negative[43] and positive[50] expression in the outer BRB have been reported. In porcine BRB, high BCRP abundance in the inner BRB was shown with quantitative proteomics.[51] In a rodent study, the retinal entry of the BCRP substrate, mitoxantrone, was similar in wild-type (WT) animals with or without BCRP inhibitor treatment and also in WT compared with BCRP knockout animals. This suggests that BCRP has a lesser role in the BRB than in the BBB, where significant differences in the mitoxantrone transport were observed in knockout and WT animals during BCRP inhibition.[43] Although the expression pattern in the human BRB has not been confirmed, a recent PET scan study with a P-gp/BCRP dual substrate, tariquidar, suggested that the human BRB has a functioning BCRP. The retinal distribution of systemically administered tariquidar in subjects carrying a fully functioning ABCG2 allele (c.421CC) was unaltered during P-gp inhibition, whereas subjects with c.421CA genotype, resulting in lower BCRP abundance and function, had significantly higher retinal distribution of tariquidar during P-gp inhibition (1.4-fold).[52] This finding also suggests that the carriers of c.421C>A. SNP may be more susceptible to transporter-mediated drug-drug interactions in the BRB.

Multidrug resistance–associated proteins (ABCC)

The expression of MRPs has not been confirmed in human tissue at the protein level, even though the MRP members 1, 4, 5, and 7 were detected in human RPE cultures.[10,11,53] The specific localization of the MRP members may vary depending on the cell culture model—apical enrichment[53] and expression on both cell surfaces, including the lateral membrane,[10] have been reported for MRP1. There are also discrepancies regarding the specific localization of MRPs in rodents—MRP1 and MRP4 were detected in the basal membrane of the mouse RPE and reported to be absent in the inner BRB,[43] whereas in another study MRP4 was detected in the luminal side of the inner BRB in mice.[46] In an immunohistochemistry study of human tissue, MRP1 and MRP5 were not detected in any regions of the retina.[35] However, blood-ocular permeation of the MRP substrate, fluorescein, was clearly higher in an outward (10^{-5} cm/s) than inward direction (10^{-7}–10^{-6} cm/s) in monkeys and humans, indicating MRP activity in the BRB.[54,55] An ex vivo study using isolated porcine RPE-choroid also showed that high fluorescein directionality in a retina-to-choroid direction (11.3-fold) was equalized in the presence of the MRP inhibitor, probenecid, indicating MRP function in the basal surface of the RPE.[56] Further, MRP activity in the BRB was similar to that in the BBB in a rodent study, evident by

increased retinal entry of zidovudine when the MRP inhibitor, MK571, was coadministered.[43]

Taken together, several efflux proteins are present in the BRB, contributing as a functional component. However, there is still uncertainty regarding efflux protein localization in humans. Further, functional studies have implied less clinical significance of P-gp and BCRP in the BRB than in the BBB, but that MRPs seem to have similar roles in BRB and BBB efflux. The quantitative expression of ABC transporters in human primary RPE cells supports this finding, as MRPs have clearly higher abundance in primary RPE cells than P-gp and BCRP.[10,11] However, passive diffusion is estimated to be the main permeation mechanism across the blood-ocular barriers for the majority of compounds. Simple models of ocular kinetics based on physicochemical descriptors for passive diffusion were able to successfully predict the drug transfer between the vitreous and systemic circulation of compound sets of 10 to 40 compounds.[5,21] The lack of significant outliers in those data sets indicates that strong directionality (i.e., active transport) was absent. The efflux proteins may, however, effectively restrict drug access into the RPE, which itself is an important drug target in many retinal diseases.[1]

OTHER OCULAR BARRIERS

Blood-aqueous barrier

The BAB is a complex system of tissue lining between the blood circulation and the extravascular space in the iris, ciliary body, and aqueous humor (Fig. 17.1). It is composed of the capillary endothelia of the iris and the ciliary muscle vessels, the epithelial cell layers of the ciliary body (nonpigmented epithelium), and the posterior iris. The epithelium of the ciliary body also comprises the pigmented epithelium. Fenestrated vessels of the ciliary body are not part of the BAB. The complexity of the BAB and similar activity of the BRB complicate mechanistic studies of the functions of the BAB, as it is difficult to separate the roles of the components of the BAB and BRB from each other.

Efflux transporters in the nonpigmented epithelium have been proposed to limit access of molecules to the aqueous humor. Efflux transporters pump compounds from the aqueous humor to the space between the nonpigmented epithelium and the pigmented epithelium for further transfer to the blood stream.[1,37] Studies with competing P-gp ligand, verapamil, and P-gp knockdown rats indicate that P-gp is active in the BAB, reducing access of systemic drugs into the aqueous humor. The reduction is less pronounced than in the BBB, but more significant than in the BRB.

Several other efflux transporters (MRP1, MRP2, MRP4, BCRP) have been identified in the human iris and ciliary body using western blot and immunohistochemistry.[37] Directional transport experiments in vivo in rabbits[56] and ex vivo with isolated bovine ciliary body[58] support functional MRP-mediated outward-directed transport in the BAB. More details about efflux and influx transporters in the BAB can be found in a recent review.[1]

Conjunctiva

The conjunctival epithelium is a barrier on the ocular surface, but active transport processes in this tissue have been rarely studied because, unlike the cornea, the conjunctiva is not directly involved in vision. The conjunctiva has been explored as a route of ocular drug delivery, although the quantitative role of this route in vivo is still unclear. A recent comparison of a large number of drugs indicates that the ex vivo conjunctiva is leakier than the isolated cornea.[2] Some evidence of outward-directed transport in the conjunctiva is also available—the

MDR1 substrates, verapamil and propranolol, showed between two- and ninefold higher transport in the basolateral-to-apical direction than in the opposite direction in excised rabbit conjunctiva.[38,39]

TRANSPORTER GENETICS AND IMPLICATIONS IN OCULAR DISEASES

Genetic variation in efflux transporters is implicated in many ocular diseases (Boxes 17.1–17.4; Table 17.3). In addition, genetic variation in transporters can affect the pharmacokinetics and pharmacodynamics of substrate drugs. For instance, a common polymorphism in BCRP (rs2231142) is well known to affect drug plasma levels and is associated with adverse effects (e.g., for statins).[65] Much less is known of the impact of transporter genetics on ocular pharmacokinetics and pharmacodynamics. Additionally, studies in carriers of genetic variants with altered transport activity can reveal the impact of specific

BOX 17.1 ABCA4 and retinal degeneration

ABCA4 mutations are directly related to retinal degeneration.[67] The degree of ABCA4 functional loss leads to different diseases, such as Stargardt disease, age-related macular degeneration, and retinitis pigmentosa. The deficiency in the efflux protein leads to accumulation of toxic end products derived from rhodopsin in photoreceptors. Subsequently, the shed photoreceptor outer segments poison the RPE, eventually causing photoreceptor death and loss of vision.

RPE, Retinal pigment epithelium.

BOX 17.2 MRP6 and pseudoxanthoma elasticum (PXE)

Mutations in MRP6 cause pseudoxanthoma elasticum syndrome, which is defined by the calcification and fragmentation of elastic fibers. Clinical signs in the eye primarily involve lesions and breaks in the Bruch's membrane in the retina. MRP6 is present in the liver and kidney, whereas expression in the retina is low.[59] ATP is an endogenous substrate of MRP6,[60] but other putative substrates are still unknown.

BOX 17.3 ALDP and adrenoleukodystrophy

Adrenoleukodystrophy protein (ALDP) is a peroxisome transporter that mediates the efflux of very long chain fatty acids (VLCFA) from the cytosol into peroxisomes for degradation. Mutations decreasing the activity of ABCD1 lead to intracellular accumulation of VLCFA, causing adrenoleukodystrophy—a variable-onset X-linked recessive disease characterized by adrenal deficiency and neuronal deficits. Ocular manifestations include progressive vision loss, optic nerve hypoplasia, exotropia, esotropia, retinal ganglionic atrophy, cataracts, and altered macular pigment.

BOX 17.4 Sterol homeostasis

Many ATP-binding cassette (ABC) transporters are involved in maintaining sterol homeostasis, and mutations in these genes can cause several disorders. Mutations in either Sterolin-1 or Sterolin-2, which form a heterodimer, lead to sitosterolemia, a rare autosomal recessive lipid metabolism disorder in which xanthelasmas around the eyes can be observed. Furthermore, the involvement of cholesterol efflux regulatory protein (CERP) in cholesterol metabolism has been implicated in both age-related macular degeneration and glaucoma.[61]

TABLE 17.3 Efflux transporters causing ocular diseases

Gene name	Protein name	Uniprot ID	Endogenous substrate	Tissue expression
ABCA1	CERP	O95477	Cholesterol, lipids	Widely expressed
ABCA4	ABCA4, ABCR	P78363	Retinal-phosphatidyl-ethanolamine conjugates	Photoreceptors
ABCC6	MRP6	O95255	Adenosine triphosphate	Liver, kidney, retina
ABCD1	ALDP	P33897	Very long chain fatty acids	Widely expressed
ABCG5	Sterolin-1	Q9H222	Cholesterol	Liver, intestine
ABCG8	Sterolin-2	Q9H221	Cholesterol	Liver, intestine

ALDP, Adrenoleukodystrophy protein; *CERP*, cholesterol efflux regulatory protein; *MRP*, multidrug resistance–associated protein.

BOX 17.5 Multidrug resistance

Overexpression of efflux transporters such as P-gp, BCRP, and MRPs enables cancer cells to develop multidrug resistance, which is a predominant factor behind failure of chemotherapy. Overexpression of efflux proteins is observed in several types of ocular cancers, such as retinoblastoma and uveal melanoma,[62,63] but it can also affect the treatment of other ocular diseases such as noninfectious uveitis.[64]

BCRP, Breast cancer resistance protein; *MRP*, multidrug resistance–associated protein; *P-gp*, P-glycoprotein.

transporters in vivo, which is otherwise hard to determine due to a lack of transporter-specific substrates and inhibitors. Recently, the involvement of both P-gp and BCRP in limiting tariquidar distribution over the BRB was demonstrated in carriers of the common BCRP polymorphism (rs2231142) causing low transport activity.[52] Variants of both MRP4 (rs11568658) and P-gp (rs1045642) were associated with altered responses after latanoprost treatment of glaucoma.[32,66] However, a similar association was not found for several other variants of P-gp and MRP4 after latanoprost or other prostaglandin analog treatments.

PHARMACOLOGIC IMPACT OF OUTWARD TRANSPORT

The pharmacologic impact of outward-directed transport in the eye is still unclear. Sorting out the role of efflux transport is not a trivial task as several confounding factors are involved. Firm conclusions are often hampered by overlapping substrate specificity among efflux proteins, species- and model-dependent differences in transporter expression, species-dependent substrate affinity, and the confounding roles of influx transport and passive diffusion (Box 17.5).

Several studies have demonstrated the influence of efflux transport on ocular drug absorption after eyedrop instillation. These data suggest that efflux transport can modulate ocular drug absorption across the cornea to some extent. These effects are dependent on drug doses, as well as affinity to and expression of efflux transporters. Overall, the highest impact of efflux transport is expected at low doses of substrates with high affinity to efflux transporters. In the case of intravitreal injections, there is no evidence indicating that outward transport would have significant influence on intravitreal drug clearance. However, efflux transporters in the BRB have been shown to affect drug distribution from the systemic circulation into the eye. Current data suggest that these pharmacokinetic effects are less pronounced than those in tighter BBBs, but particularly significant effects on the concentrations and drug responses may be expected in the retinal capillaries and RPE itself, the cellular components of the BRB.

FUTURE ASPECTS

Outward-directed transport is an important component in the protective functions of the eye. Its role is emerging in terms of disease association, genetics, physiology, and pharmacology. New analytical methods will play a crucial role in future research on outward-directed transport. For example, PET studies have been useful in finding out the functional role of efflux transport in the human BRB in vivo. Improving imaging capabilities will certainly shed more light on the role of outward-directed transport in humans. Furthermore, improved mass spectrometry techniques will facilitate proteomics analyses of ocular tissue barriers, providing information about transporter expression in animals and humans. Finally, computational data integration and simulation will be helpful in building systematic understanding of the functions and impact of outward-directed transport in the eye.

REFERENCES

1. Vellonen KS, Hellinen L, Mannermaa E, Ruponen M, Urtti A, Kidron H. Expression, activity and pharmacokinetic impact of ocular transporters. *Adv Drug Deliv Rev*. 2018;126:3–22.
2. Ramsay E, del Amo E, Toropainen E, et al. Corneal and conjunctival drug permeability: systematic comparison and pharmacokinetic impact in the eye. *Eur J Pharm Sci*. 2018;119:83–89.
3. Ahmed I, Patton TF. Importance of the noncorneal route in topical ophthalmic drug delivery. *Invest Ophthalmol Vis Sci*. 1985;26:584–587.
4. Maurice DM, Mishima S. Ocular pharmacokinetics. In: Sears ML, ed. *Handbook of Experimental Pharmacology, Pharmacology of the Eye*. New York: Springer Verlag; 1984:16–119.
5. Kati-Sisko Vellonen Esa-Matti, Soini Eva M, del Amo Veli-Pekka, Ranta Arto. Urtti: Prediction of ocular drug distribution from systemic blood circulation. *Mol Pharmaceut*. 2016;13:2906–2911.
6. International Transporter Consortium Giacomini KM, Huang SM, Tweedie DJ, Benet LZ, et al. Membrane transporters in drug development. *Nat Rev Drug Discov*. 2010 Mar;9(3):215–236.
7. Nigam SK. What do drug transporters really do? *Nat Rev Drug Discov*. 2015 Jan;14(1):29–44.
8. Juliano Rudolph L, Ling Victor. "A surface glycoprotein modulating drug permeability in Chinese hamster ovary cell mutants.". *Biochimica et biophysica acta*. 1976;455(1):152–162.
9. Bludau I, Aebersold R. Proteomic and interactomic insights into the molecular basis of cell functional diversity. *Nat Rev Mol Cell Biol*. 2020;21:327–340.
10. Hellinen L, Sato K, Reinisalo M, et al. Quantitative protein expression in the human retinal pigment epithelium: comparison between apical and basolateral plasma membranes with emphasis on transporters. *Invest Ophthalmol Vis Sci*. 2019;60:5022–5034.
11. Pelkonen L, Sato K, Reinisalo M, et al. LC-MS/MS based quantitation of ABC and SLC transporter proteins in plasma membranes of cultured primary human retinal pigment epithelium cells and immortalized ARPE19 cell line. *Mol Pharmaceut*. 2017;14:605–613. 2017.
12. Miller DS. Regulation of ABC transporters at the blood-brain barrier. *Clin Pharmacol Ther*. 2015;97(4):395–403.
13. Hoshi Y, Uchida Y, Tachikawa M, et al. Oxidative stress-induced activation of Abl and Src kinases rapidly induces P-glycoprotein internalization via phosphorylation of caveolin-1 on tyrosine-14, decreasing cortisol efflux at the blood-brain barrier. *J Cereb Blood Flow Metab*. 2020;40:420–436.
14. Uchida Y, Ohtsuki S, Terasaki T. Pharmacoproteomics-based reconstruction of in vivo P-glycoprotein function at blood-brain barrier and brain distribution of substrate verapamil in pentylenetetrazole-kindled epilepsy, spontaneous epilepsy, and phenytoin treatment models. *Drug Metab Dispos*. 2014;42:1719–1726.
15. Brouwer KL, Keppler D, Hoffmaster KA, et al. International Transporter Consortium. In vitro methods to support transporter evaluation in drug discovery and development. *Clin Pharmacol Ther*. 2013 Jul;94(1):95–112.
16. Vellonen KS, Mannermaa E, Turner H, et al. Effluxing ABC transporters in human corneal epithelium. *J Pharm Sci*. 2010;99:1087–1098.
17. Greco D, Vellonen KS, Turner H, et al. Differential gene expression analysis between human corneal epithelium and stratified epithelium generated in vitro by SV40 immortalized cells. *Mol Vis*. 2010;16:2109–2120.
18. Mannermaa E, Vellonen KS, Ryhänen T, et al. Efflux protein expression in human retinal pigment epithelium cell lines. *Pharm Res*. 2009;26:1785–1791.
19. Mannermaa E, Reinisalo M, Ranta VP, et al. Filter cultured ARPE-19 cells as outer blood – retina barrier model. *Eur J Pharm Sci*. 2010;40:289–297.
20. Vellonen KS, Malinen M, Mannermaa E, et al. A critical assessment of in vitro tissue models for ADME and drug delivery. *J Control Rel*. 2014;190:94–114.
21. Pitkänen L, Ranta VP, Moilanen H, et al. Permeability of retinal pigment epithelium: effects of permeant molecular weight and lipophilicity. *Invest Ophthalmol Vis Sci*. 2005 Feb;46(2) 641–6.
22. Del Amo, E.M., Vellonen, K.S., Kidron, H. and Urtti, A. Intravitreal clearance and volume of distribution of compounds in rabbits: In silico prediction and pharmacokinetic simulations for drug development. European journal of pharmaceutics and biopharmaceutic. *95(Pt B)*. 2015:215–226.
23. Huttunen K, Terasaki T, Urtti A, Montaser A, Uchida Y. Pharmacoproteomics of brain barrier transporters and substrate design for the brain targeted drug delivery. *Pharm. Res*. 2022 Mar 7
24. Verstraelen J. Reichl. Expression analysis of MDR1, BCRP and MRP3 transporter proteins in different in vitro and ex vivo cornea models for drug absorption studies. *Int. J. Pharm*. 2013;441:765–775.
25. Dey S, Gunda S, Mitra AK. Pharmacokinetics of erythromycin in rabbit corneas after single-dose infusion: role of P-glycoprotein as a barrier to in vivo ocular drug absorption. *J Pharmacol Exp Ther*. 2004;311:246–255.
26. Hariharan S, Gunda S, Mishra GP, Pal D, Mitra AK. Enhanced corneal absorption of erythromycin by modulating P-glycoprotein and MRP mediated efflux with corticosteroids. *Pharm. Res*. 2009;26:1270–1282.
27. Karla PK, Pal D, Mitra AK. Molecular evidence and functional expression of multidrug resistance associated protein (MRP) in rabbit corneal epithelial cells. *Exp Eye Res*. 2007;84:53–60.
28. Verstraelen J, Reichl S. Multidrug resistance-associated protein (MRP1, 2, 4 and 5) expression in human corneal cell culture models and animal corneal tissue. *Mol. Pharm*. 2014;11:2160–2171.
29. Heredi-Szabo K, Kis E, Molnar E, Gyorfi A, Krajcsi P. Characterization of 5(6)-carboxy-2',7'-dichlorofluorescein transport by MRP2 and utilization of this substrate as a fluorescent surrogate for LTC4. *J. Biomol. Screen*. 2008;13:295–300.
30. Zamek-Gliszczynski MJ, Xiong H, Patel NJ, Turncliff RZ, Pollack GM, Brouwer KLR. Pharmacokinetics of 5(and 6)-carboxy-2',7'-dichlorofluorescein and its diacetatepromoiety in the liver. *J. Pharmacol. Exp. Ther*. 2003;304:801–809.
31. Karla PK, Quinn TL, Herndon BL, Thomas P, Pal D, Mitra A. Expression of multidrug resistance associated protein 5 (MRP5) on cornea and its role in drug efflux. *J Ocul Pharmacol Ther*. 2009;25:121–132.
32. Gao LC, Wang D, Liu FQ, et al. Influence of PTGS1, PTGFR, and MRP4 genetic variants on intraocular pressure response to latanoprost in Chinese primary open-angle glaucoma patients. *Eur J Clin Pharmacol*. 2015 Jan;71(1):43–50.
33. Dey D, Patel J, Anand BS, et al. Molecular evidence and functional expression of P-glycoprotein (MDR1) in human and rabbit cornea and corneal epithelial cell lines. *Invest Ophthalmol Vis Sci*. 2003;44:2909–2918.
34. Becker U, Ehrhardt C, Daum N, et al. Expression of ABC-transporters in human corneal tissue and the transformed cell line, HCE-T. *J Ocul Pharmacol Ther*. 2007;23:172–181.
35. Dahlin A, Geier E, Stocker SL, Cropp CD, et al. Gene expression profiling of transporters in the solute carrier and ATP-binding cassette superfamilies in human eye substructures. *Molecular pharmaceutics*. 2013;10(2):650–663.
36. Kawazu K, Yamada K, Nakamura N, Ota A. Characterization of cyclosporin A transport in cultured rabbit corneal epithelial cells: P-glycoprotein transport activity and binding to cyclophilin. *Invest Ophthalmol Vis Sci*. 1999;40:1738–1744.
37. Pelis MR, Shahidullah M, Ghosh S, Coca-Prados M, Wright SH, Delamere NA. Localization of multidrug resistance-associated protein 2 in the nonpigmented ciliary epithelium of the eye. *J. Pharmacol. Exp. Ther*. 2009;329:479–485.
38. Saha P, Yang JJ, Lee VH. Existence of a p-glycoprotein drug efflux pump in cultured rabbit conjunctival epithelial cells. *Invest. Ophthalmol. Vis. Sci*. 1998;39:1221–1226.
39. Yang JJ, Kim KJ, Lee VH. Role of P-glycoprotein in restricting propranolol transport in cultured rabbit conjunctival epithelial cell layers. *Pharm. Res*. 2000;17:533–538.
40. Yang JJ, Ann DK, Kannan R, Lee VH. Multidrug resistance protein 1 (MRP1) in rabbit conjunctival epithelial cells: its effect on drug efflux and its regulation by adenoviral infection. *Pharm. Res*. 2007;24:1490–1500.
41. Ramsay E, Hagstrom M, Vellonen KS, et al. Role of retinal pigment epithelium permeability in drug transfer between posterior eye segment and systemic blood circulation. *European journal of pharmaceutics and biopharmaceutics*. 2019;143:18–23.
42. Kennedy BG, Mangini NJ. P-glycoprotein expression in human retinal pigment epithelium. *Molecular vision*. 2002;8:422–430.
43. Chapy H, Saubamea B, Tournier N, et al. Blood-brain and retinal barriers show dissimilar ABC transporter impacts and concealed effect of P-glycoprotein on a novel verapamil influx carrier. *British journal of pharmacology*. 2016;173(3):497–510.
44. Hosoya K, Makihara A, Tsujikawa Y, et al. Roles of inner blood-retinal barrier organic anion transporter 3 in the vitreous/retina-to-blood efflux transport of p-aminohippuric acid, benzylpenicillin, and 6-mercaptopurine. *J Pharmacol Exp Ther*. 2009 Apr;329(1):87–93.
45. Pascual-Pasto G, Olaciregui NG, Opezzo JAW, et al. Increased delivery of chemotherapy to the vitreous by inhibition of the blood-retinal barrier. *J Control Release*. 2017 Oct 28;264:34–44.
46. Tagami M, Kusuhara S, Honda S, et al. Expression of ATP-binding cassette transporters at the inner blood-retinal barrier in a neonatal mouse model of oxygen-induced retinopathy. *Brain research*. 2009;1283:186–193.
47. Bauer M, Karch R, Tournier N, et al. Assessment of P-glycoprotein transport activity at the human blood-retinal barrier with (R)-11C-verapamil PET. *J Nucl Med*. 2017;58(4):678–681.
48. Bauer M, Karch R, Zeitlinger M, et al. Approaching complete inhibition of P-glycoprotein at the human blood-brain barrier: an (R)-[11C]verapamil PET study. *Journal of Cerebral Blood Flow and Metabolism*. 2015;35(5):743–746.
49. Asashima T, Hori S, Ohtsuki S, et al. ATP-binding cassette transporter G2 mediates the efflux of phototoxins on the luminal membrane of retinal capillary endothelial cells. *Pharmaceutical Research*. 2006;23(6):1235–1242.

50. Gnana-Prakasam JP, Reddy SK, Veeranan-Karmegam R, et al. Polarized distribution of heme transporters in retinal pigment epithelium and their regulation in the iron-overload disease hemochromatosis. *Investigative ophthalmology & visual science*. 2011;52(12):9279–9286.

51. Zhang Z, Uchida Y, Hirano S., et al. Inner Blood-Retinal Barrier Dominantly Expresses Breast Cancer Resistance Protein: Comparative Quantitative Targeted Absolute Proteomics Study of CNS Barriers in Pig. Mol Pharm. 2017 Nov 6;14(11):3729–3738.

52. El Biali M, Karch R, Philippe C, et al. ABCB1 and ABCG2 together limit the distribution of ABCB1/ABCG2 substrates to the human retina and the ABCG2 single nucleotide polymorphism Q141K (c.421C> A) may lead to increased drug exposure. *Front Pharmacol*. 2021 Jun 16;12:698966.

53. Juuti-Uusitalo K, Vaajasaari H, Ryhanen T, et al. Efflux protein expression in human stem cell-derived retinal pigment epithelial cells. *PloS one*. 2012;7(1):e30089.

54. Oguro Y, Tsukahara Y, Saito I., et al. Estimation of the permeability of the blood-retinal barrier in normal individuals. *Invest Ophthalmol Vis Sci*. 1985 Jul;26(7):969-76.

55. Blair NP, Rusin MM. Blood-retinal barrier permeability to carboxyfluorescein and fluorescein in monkeys. Graefes Arch Clin Exp Ophthalmol. 1986;224(5):419–22.

56. Steuer H, Jaworski A, Elger B, et al. Functional characterization and comparison of the outer blood-retina barrier and the blood-brain barrier. *Investigative ophthalmology & visual science*. 2005;46(3):1047–1053.

57. Kondo M, Araie M. Movement of carboxyfluorescein across the isolated rabbit iris-ciliary body. *Curr. Eye Res*. 1994;13:251–255.

58. Lee J, Shahidullah M, Hotchkiss A, et al. A renal-like organic anion transport system in the ciliary epithelium of the bovine and human eye. *Mol. Pharmacol*. 2015;87:697–705.

59. Bergen AA, Plomp AS, Schuurman EJ, et al. Mutations in ABCC6 cause pseudoxanthoma elasticum. *Nat Genet*. 2000;25:228–2231.

60. Jansen RS, Duijst S, Mahakena S, et al. ABCC6-mediated ATP secretion by the liver is the main source of the mineralization inhibitor inorganic pyrophosphate in the systemic circulation-brief report. *Arterioscler Thromb Vasc Biol*. 2014;34:1985e9.

61. Jacobo-Albavera L, Domínguez-Pérez M, Medina-Leyte DJ, et al. The role of the ATP-binding cassette A1 (ABCA1) in human disease. *Int J Mol Sci*. 2021;22(4):1593.

62. Baggetto LG, Gambrelle J, Dayan G, et al. Major cytogenetic aberrations and typical multidrug resistance phenotype of uveal melanoma: current views and new therapeutic prospects. *Cancer Treat Rev*. 2005 Aug;31(5):361–379.

63. Shukla S, Srivastava A, Kumar S, et al. Expression of multidrug resistance proteins in retinoblastoma. *Int J Ophthalmol*. 2017;10(11):1655–1661.

64. Tagirasa R, Rana K, Kaza H, et al. Role of multidrug resistance proteins in nonresponders to immunomodulatory therapy for noninfectious uveitis. *Transl Vis Sci Technol*. 2020 Apr 18;9(5):12.

65. Niemi M. Transporter pharmacogenetics and statin toxicity. *Clin Pharmacol Ther*. 2010; 87:130–133.

66. Liu H, Yang ZK, Li Y, et al. ABCB1 variants confer susceptibility to primary open-angle glaucoma and predict individual differences to latanoprost treatment. *Biomed Pharmacother*. 2016 May;80:115–120.

67. Strauss O. The retinal pigment epithelium in visual function. *Physiol Rev*. 2005 Jul;85(3):845–81.

18

Biochemical Cascade of Phototransduction

Theodore G. Wensel

OVERVIEW

Phototransduction is the series of biochemical events that leads from photon capture by a photoreceptor cell to its hyperpolarization and slowing of neurotransmitter release at the synapse.[1-10] This overall process includes an activation phase and a recovery phase. While the fundamental mechanisms of phototransduction are constant over a wide range of light intensities and very similar in rods and cones, the quantitative features differ strikingly depending on the level of ambient light (see Chapters 19, 20) and the cell type. Although we know more about the biochemistry of phototransduction than we do about any other neuronal signaling pathway, numerous mysteries remain.

LOCATION AND COMPARTMENTALIZATION OF RODS AND CONES

Rod and cone photoreceptors are densely packed in the outermost layer of the neural retina, stretching from their synapses in the outer plexiform layer to their most distal tips, which are embedded in the membrane processes of the retinal pigmented epithelium (RPE) (Fig. 18.1). Photoreceptors are long, thin cells with their long axes aligned along the radii of the eye to maximize light collection. Efficient phototransduction depends upon the organization of photoreceptors into distinct membrane compartments (Figs. 18.1–18.3). Absorption of light and the biochemical cascade of phototransduction are restricted to the outer segment, which is an elongated membrane compartment that is separated from the rest of the cell by a thin connecting cilium or ciliary transition zone. The cilium consists of a bundle of nine microtubule doublets surrounded by a very thin layer of cytoplasm and a plasma membrane. Immediately adjacent is the inner segment, the site of active biosynthesis and oxidative metabolism. Although small molecules and proteins can diffuse along the connecting cilium between the inner and outer segments, this process generally occurs on a slower time scale than that of a light response.[11] This intercompartment transport plays an important role in producing the molecules necessary for phototransduction and modulating their levels, but it does not contribute directly to the phototransduction cascade. Although cytoplasmic diffusion is limited by the constriction at the connecting cilium, this constriction does not pose a major barrier to the propagation of electrical changes along the plasma membrane. Therefore, changes in membrane potential can be passively communicated from the outer segment to the synaptic terminal at the other end of the cell, where they control neurotransmitter release and transmit the signal to higher-order neurons.

The phototransduction cascade takes place in the outer segments. There are two membrane systems in rods (Figs. 18.3 and 18.4). The disc membranes, which can be thought of as flattened sealed vesicles, are stacked up along the long axis of the outer segment and make up the vast majority of membrane surface in the cells. The plasma membrane surrounds the discs and the cytoplasm (Figs. 18.1e, 18.3, 18.4) and forms the interface between the cell and the extracellular space. Although there are proteins linking these two membranes in the outer segment, there does not appear to be flow of lipid or transmembrane proteins between them. In contrast, cones have a single membrane that forms multiple invaginations that resemble discs but are not sealed and are continuous with the plasma membrane. A cone-like relationship between plasma membrane and nascent discs appears to be present at the base of rod outer segments.[12-15]

The components of phototransduction, discussed in detail further in this section, are primarily localized in the outer segments, and are mostly peripheral or integral membrane proteins. The disc and plasma membranes have distinct protein and lipid compositions.

DARK-ADAPTED RODS

The most information at the molecular level is available for the dim light responses of dark-adapted rods (see Chapters 19, 20). The cells in this state can respond with amazingly high efficiency to single photon capture events.[16] It is useful conceptually to begin with the resting dark state and then consider the chain of events set in motion when a photon is absorbed.

The resting dark-adapted state
The membrane potential
The following treatment is meant to outline the electrophysiology of rods and cones in biochemical terms; for more details, see Chapters 19 and 20. In the dark, rods have a resting membrane potential of about −40 mV.[17] The negative value means that there is more positive charge on the outside of the plasma membrane than on the inside. In most resting neurons, the potential is closer to −70 mV, so rods are considered to be relatively depolarized compared with other cells or, as we shall see, compared with fully light-activated rods. In rods, as in other neurons, the source of membrane potential is the inequality of ion concentrations on either side of the plasma membrane generated by the Na⁺/K⁺-ATPase.[18-21] This protein uses the energy released upon ATP hydrolysis to pump sodium ions out of the cell and potassium ions into the cell, and in rods it is found in the plasma membrane of the inner segment (see Chapter 19). In most neurons, potassium channels are the

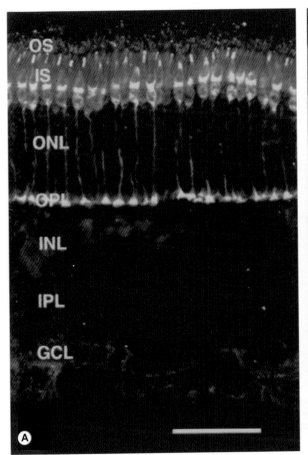

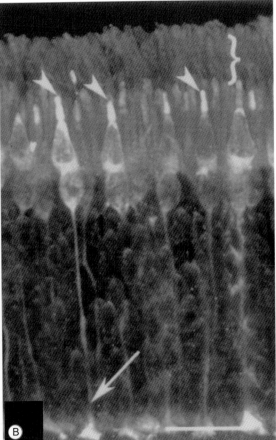

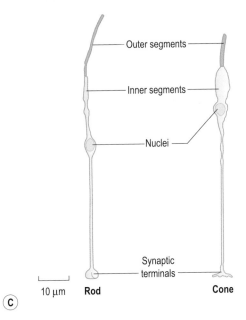

Fig. 18.1 Immunofluorescence image of mammalian rods and cones. (**A**) Low magnification (scale bar, 50 μm), showing photoreceptor positions with respect to other retinal layers. *OS*, Photoreceptor outer segments; *IS*, photoreceptor inner segments; *ONL*, outer nuclear layer (photoreceptor nuclei); *OPL*, outer plexiform layer (photoreceptor synapses and processes of bipolar and horizontal cells); *INL*, inner nuclear layer (nuclei of inner retinal neurons); *IPL*, inner plexiform layer (inner retinal synapses and processes); *GCL*, ganglion cell layers (cell bodies of retinal ganglion cells). Scale bar, 50 μm. (**B**) Higher magnification showing photoreceptors. The antibody used for immunofluorescence staining is specific for RGS9-1, whose concentration is 10-fold higher in cones than in rods. *Arrow*, cone axon; *arrowheads*, cone outer segments; *bracket*, rod outer segments. Scale bar, 20 μm. (Cowan CW, Fariss RN, Sokal I, Palczewski K, Wensel TG. High expression levels in cones of RGS9, the predominant GTPase accelerating protein of rods. *Proc Natl Acad Sci USA.* 1998;95(9):5351–5356. Copyright (1998) National Academy of Sciences, U.S.A.) (**C**) Schematic diagram of rods and cones and their compartments with sizes and shapes based on a fluorescence micrograph of human retina.

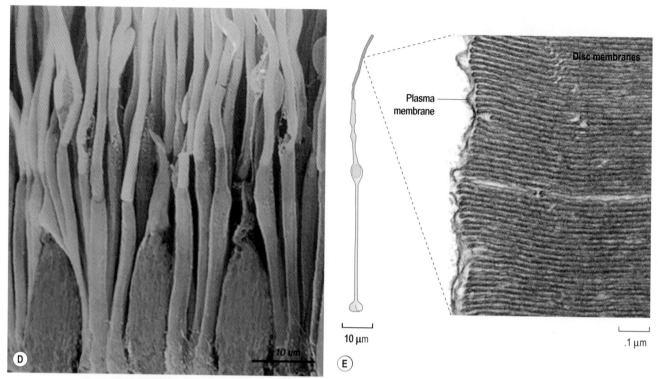

Fig. 18.1, cont'd (**D**) Scanning electron micrograph of rods and cones in primate retina. (Reproduced with permission from Dr. Ralph C Eagle (webvision.med.utah.edu/imageswv/scanEMphoto.jpg)). (**E**) Magnified region of rod outer segment from transmission electron micrograph, showing the tightly packed disc membranes, and their relationship to the plasma membrane. (Reproduced with permission from Dr. Ralph C Eagle (webvision.med.utah.edu/imageswv/scanEMphoto.jpg).)

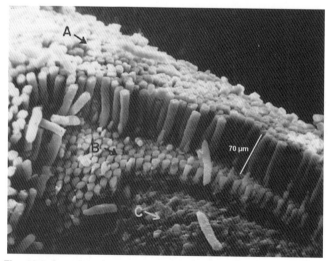

Fig. 18.2 Scanning electron micrograph of bull frog outer segments. A, outer segments; B, inner segments; C, outer nuclear layer. (From Bownds D, Brodie AE. Light-sensitive swelling of isolated frog rod outer segments as an in vitro assay for visual transduction and dark adaptation. *J Gen Physiol* 1975;66(4):407-425.)

predominant conductance at resting potentials, and these allow potassium ions to flow out of the cell down their concentration gradient. Because these channels pass a specific cation, but no anions, a net positive charge accumulates on the outside of the membrane and a net negative charge accumulates on the inside of the membrane. This charge accumulation occurs until the electrical energy stored in the charge separation equals the energy stored in the potassium gradient, the relationship described by the Nernst equation, described in detail in many textbooks. Strictly speaking, this equation only works when the membrane in question contains only a single type of channel permeable to only a single type of ion. In reality, there are always additional minor sources of conductance (other channels and transporters), so that the resting potential is modified by these to give the typical resting value of about −70 mV to −90 mV for excitable cells.

The dark current and the cyclic GMP–gated channel

Rods also have a negative resting membrane potential, but its magnitude is less than in many other neurons because the effects of potassium channels in the inner segment are balanced by a major additional channel current in the outer segment. The lower negative resting potential, or partially depolarized state, of rods is due to the cyclic GMP (cGMP)–gated cation channel (see Chapter 19), also known as the cyclic nucleotide–gated (CNG channel), or light-sensitive channel or phototransduction channel (see Chapter 19). This multisubunit channel[22] only passes cations, but does not discriminate strictly among different cations, allowing Na^+, K^+, and Ca^{2+} to pass. Among physiologically important cations, it has the highest permeability to Ca^{2+}; however, the much higher concentration of Na^+ outside the cell (>140 mM, compared with ~1.5 mM for Ca^{2+}) makes Na^+ the primary carrier of the current through the CNG channel in the dark. Because it tends to dissipate the gradient of charge, by allowing positive charge to enter the cell, the open CNG channel causes the cells to be partially depolarized. Put another way, because there are substantial inward sodium currents in the outer segment to balance outward potassium currents in the inner segment, the resting potential is moved away from the potassium "equilibrium" or Nernst potential of approximately −90 mV, and toward the sodium "equilibrium" or Nernst potential of approximately +60 mV. Because there is net flux of cations out of the inner

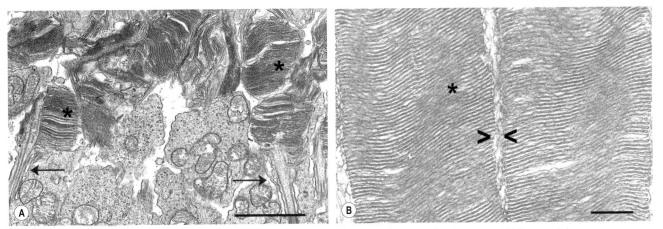

Fig. 18.3 Electron micrographs showing postnatal development of outer retina in mouse. (**A**) Postnatal day 10; **B**) 5 weeks postnatal. Scale bar in A, 2.5 μ, in B, 0.4 μm. *, Rod outer segment discs; *arrows*, connecting cilia; *arrowheads*, plasma membrane separating individual rods.

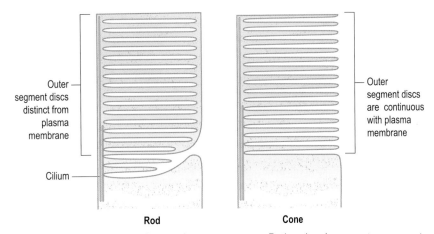

Fig. 18.4 Schematic representation of base of outer segments. Both rod and cone outer segments are connected to the inner segments via the connecting cilium, or ciliary transition zone. Membrane topologies of rods and cones are similar near the base, with both rod and cones showing disc-like membranes as invaginations of the plasma membrane. Along the outer segment axis moving from the inner segment toward the distal tips, the rod discs become sealed compartments, completely surrounded by, but distinct from, the plasma membrane, whereas the cone disc and plasma membranes are continuous, with the plasma membranes, and their interior is continuous with the extracellular space.

segment plasma membrane and a net flux of cations into the outer segment plasma membrane, as well as electrical conductance between the inner and outer segments, a complete circuit is made that is known as the circulating current or dark current.

Ca²⁺ and the exchanger

The CNG channel also has an influence on the concentration of Ca^{2+}, which plays an important role in signaling and regulation in rods and cones, as in other cells. An Na^+/Ca^{2+}, K^+ exchanger protein, NCKX2,[23] uses the energy stored in the Na^+ gradient across the plasma membrane to push Ca^{2+} ions outside the cell against their concentration gradient (see Chapter 19). In the absence of any inward flux of Ca^{2+}, this mechanism would lower the Ca^{2+} concentration in the outer segment cytoplasm to about 10 nM. In the dark, there is an inward leak of Ca^{2+} through the CNG channel, so the resting level of Ca^{2+} is a few hundred nanomolar.

Even though in the dark more channels are open than at any other time, because cGMP levels are at their highest, the percentage of open channels is small; most of the channels are closed even in the dark (see Chapter 19). One reason for this situation is that binding of more than one cGMP is necessary to give each channel a high probability of opening, (i.e., the response of the channel to cGMP is nonlinear and shows positive cooperativity). The other reason is that the dark concentration of cGMP is well below the concentration of cGMP at which channel opening probability is 50%, a number that reflects the affinity of cGMP for the channel subunits, as well as the positive cooperativity. Because the dark cGMP concentration is at the low end of the dose-response curve for the channel (therefore, very far from saturation), even a small change in cytoplasmic concentration of cGMP can be immediately sensed as a change in the number of open channels and therefore of the dark current (Fig. 18.5).

Control of [cGMP] by guanylate cyclase and PDE6

The resting, or dark, level of cGMP is determined by the balance between the activity of the enzyme, guanylate cyclase (GC) that synthesizes cGMP[24–26] and the cGMP phosphodiesterase, PDE6,[27–30] that

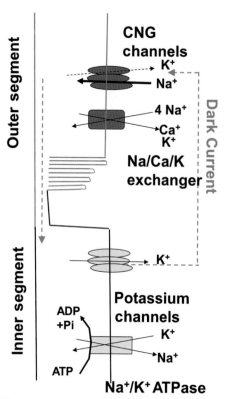

Fig. 18.5 Major components of circulating dark current of rod cells.

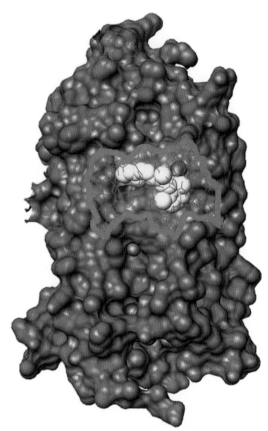

Fig. 18.6 Surface rendering of rhodopsin crystal structure with cut-out of retinal binding pocket *(red)* to show 11-*cis* retinal chromophore *(yellow spacefill)*. PDB (Protein Data Bank) coordinates, 1U19. (From Okada T, Sugihara M, Bondar AN, Elstner M, Entel P, Buss V. The retinal conformation and its environment in rhodopsin in light of a new 2.2A crystal structure. *J Mol Biol* 2004;342(2):571-583.)

degrades cGMP. Both of these have much lower activity in the dark than they do in the light. When fully activated, PDE6 is one of the most efficient enzymes known, and the most active of any of the PDE superfamily of cyclic nucleotide phosphodiesterases. The maximal turnover at saturating cGMP concentrations, k_{cat}, has been reported to be between $1000\,s^{-1}$ and $7000\,s^{-1}$, and the Michaelis constant, the cGMP concentration at which activity is half-maximal, is about 40 μM. Thus, the enzymatic efficiency, k_{cat}/K_m, is in the range of $2.5 \times 10^7\,M^{-1}s^{-1}$ to $1.75 \times 10^8\,M^{-1}s^{-1}$, implying that PDE6 operates near the diffusion limit. PDE6 requires two kinds of metal ions for activity. Mg^{2+} binds reversibly along with cGMP, and Zn^{2+} is permanently bound to high affinity sites essential for catalysis.[31] The other key players in photoactivation are also in quiescent states under dark conditions. The mechanisms for regulation of these enzymes by light are discussed further in this section. GC uses GTP as a substrate and produces cGMP and inorganic pyrophosphate as products. Inorganic pyrophosphate is rapidly broken down by the enzyme inorganic pyrophosphatase,[32] which is found at higher levels in rod outer segments than in any other cell type in which it has been measured. GC is a transmembrane protein that is thought to exist in photoreceptor membranes as a dimer, with each dimer bound to the calcium-binding protein, GC-activating protein (GCAP).[33-35] PDE6 is a heterotetrameric peripheral membrane protein consisting of two large catalytic subunits, PDE6α and PDE6β, as well as two smaller identical inhibitory PDE6γ subunits. High resolution structures have been determined by cryo-electron microscopy.[36,37] The catalytic subunits are subject to the set of post-translational modifications associated with isoprenylation, as described further, so the enzyme is bound to the surface of the disc membranes. The PDE6α and PDE6β subunits found in rods are similar in structure to one another, whereas in cones, two identical PDE6α' subunits are found. PDE6 catalytic subunits are related in sequence to a large family of cyclic nucleotide phosphodiesterases, the PDE superfamily.[38] These share sequence similarity in their catalytic domains, where the PDE6 isoforms most closely resemble in structure the PDE5 isoforms, which are the targets of sildenafil citrate (Viagra) and other drugs used to treat erectile dysfunction. In addition to the catalytic domains, PDE6 catalytic subunits each contain two GAF domains, one of which contains a noncatalytic binding site for cGMP. Because the total concentration of cGMP-binding GAF domains in the outer segments is about 50 μM, most of the cGMP in the cell is bound to PDE6. The physiologic function of these noncatalytic sites is unclear, but their occupancy is coupled to binding of the catalytic subunits by the inhibitory PDE6γ subunit.[39-41] It is the PDE6γ subunit that interacts most extensively with the activated form of the G-protein, as described further.

Rhodopsin

In the dark, the photon receptor rhodopsin[3,42-44] is in its inactive state[45-47] with an inverse agonist, 11-*cis* retinal, covalently attached to its active site (Figs. 18.6–18.8). Ligands that activate receptors are called agonists, those that block the action of agonists are called antagonists, and those that actually reduce receptor activity below the level it has in the absence of any ligand are called inverse agonists. Rhodopsin has seven membrane-spanning helices and is a part of the G-protein–coupled receptor (GPCR) superfamily of signal transducing receptors. Like other GPCRs, its activity consists of its ability to catalyze the activation of a heterotrimeric G-protein. This is the activity of rhodopsin that is inhibited by the chromophore and inverse agonist 11-*cis* retinal. The

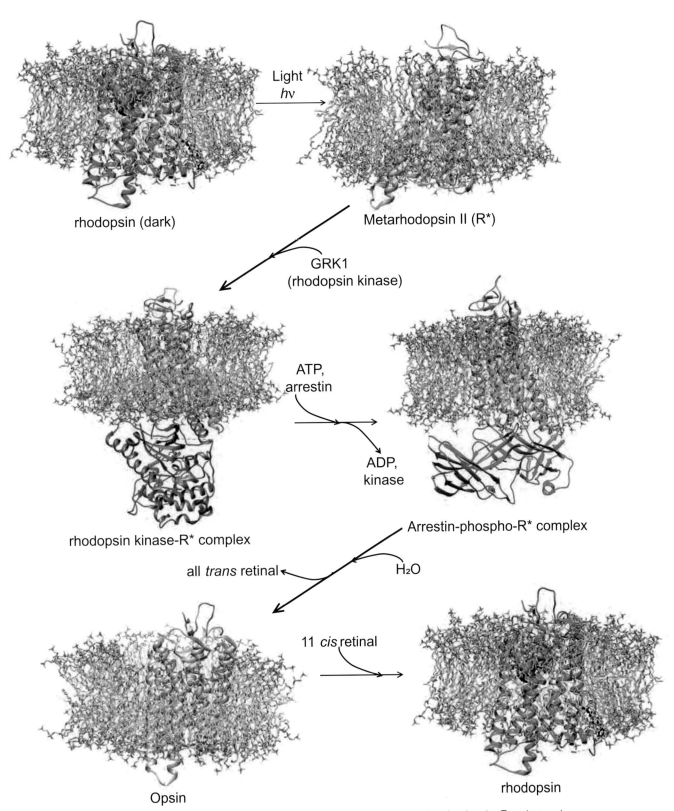

Fig. 18.7 Photoactivation, inactivation, and regeneration of rhodopsin in the visual cycle. *Top*, photon absorption photoisomerizes 11-*cis* retinal, attached to rhodopsin via Schiff-base linkage to Lys296 (*left*), to the all-*trans* form, generating through a series of photochemical intermediates, the catalytically active form, metarhodopsin II (MII or R*; *right*). *Middle*, rhodopsin kinase, GRK1, binds to R*, and catalyzes phosphorylation at multiple sites (*left*). Phosphorylated R* binds tightly to arrestin (*right*), inhibiting R* binding by transducin, G_t. *Bottom*, all-*trans* retinal is released via hydrolysis, leading to release of arrestin and dephosphorylation and formation of opsin (*left*), and finally, regeneration of rhodopsin by incorporation of 11-*cis* retinal. Structures from PDB (Protein Data Bank) files: phospholipid membrane, 6clz,[126] rhodopsin, 1gzm,[127] metarhodopsin II and MII-G_t complex 6oy9,[128] Opsin 5te3,[129] MII-GRK1 complex 7mt9,[130] MII-arrestin complex 1zwj.[131]

apo-form of rhodopsin without a ligand, known as opsin, has much higher G-protein–activating activity than rhodopsin does, a fact that becomes important at high light levels but is relatively unimportant in the dark-adapted state. Rhodopsin is present at very high concentrations in the disc membrane (and somewhat lower concentrations in the plasma membrane), so that about one-third the surface area of the discs is occupied by rhodopsin, and the other two-thirds is occupied by phospholipids, cholesterol, and other minor lipids. Rhodopsin is subject to post-translational modifications that are important for its function. N-linked carbohydrates are found on the domain of rhodopsin that faces the inside of the discs and the extracellular solution, and they appear to be important for proper transport of rhodopsin from its site of synthesis in the inner segment to the outer segment membranes. Two palmitoyl groups are attached via thio-ester linkages to two adjacent cysteine residues near its carboxyl terminus, which tether the polypeptide chain to the cytoplasmic surface of the disc membrane forming a fourth cytoplasmic loop. In addition, the aldehyde moiety of 11-*cis* retinal and all-*trans* retinal is not bound to rhodopsin as a free aldehyde, but rather a covalent Schiff's base linkage is formed between 11-*cis* retinal and lysine residue 296 in the transmembrane domain of rhodopsin (Fig. 18.8).

The rhodopsin sequence contains 348 amino acid residues. Whereas mutations at only four different positions are found in patients with the disease congenital stationary night blindness (CSNB, see Box 18.1), there are over 100 amino acid positions that are found mutated in patients with the blinding disease autosomal dominant retinitis pigmentosa (ADRP, see Box 18.4). Therefore, the molecule is not only so sensitive to light that it can become activated by one photon of light, it is also remarkably sensitive to its amino acid composition.

BOX 18.1   Congenital stationary night blindness

Congenital stationary night blindness (CSNB) comprises a group of genetically and clinically heterogeneous nonprogressive retinal disorders that are mainly caused by defects in rod photoreceptor signal transduction and transmission. Mutations in genes coding for proteins of the phototransduction cascade (RHO, GNAT1, PDE6B, RHOK, SAG, and RDH5) or genes associated with the transmission of the signals from the photoreceptors to bipolar cells (NYX, GRM6, CANCA1F, and CABP4) can lead to this disease.

Night blindness and reduced or absent dark adaptation are typical and early signs of various forms of retinal dystrophies. Forms differ in inheritance pattern (autosomal dominant, autosomal recessive, or X-linked), electroretinograms (ERG; presence or absence of a-wave), refractive error (presence or absence of myopia), and fundus appearance. All patients with CSNB have severely reduced rod ERG amplitudes and many have modestly reduced cone ERG amplitudes (Fig. 18.9). Rod sensitivity in patients is decreased by 100 Å~ to 1000 Å~ compared with normals. Almost all have cone responses with a normal peak implicit time (time interval between the light flash and subsequent peak of b-wave).

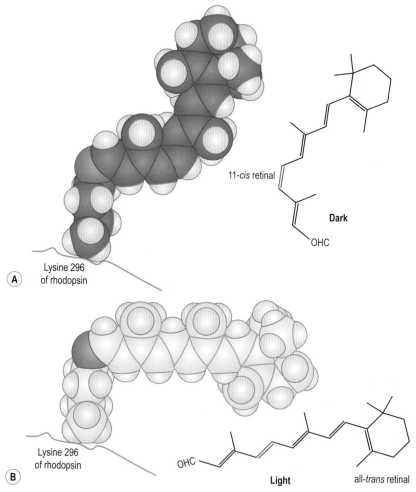

11-*cis* retinal

Dark

OHC

Lysine 296 of rhodopsin

(A)

Lysine 296 of rhodopsin

(B)

OHC

Light

all-*trans* retinal

Fig. 18.8 (**A**) Molecular structure, in space-filling representation, of 11-*cis* retinal in rhodopsin. The *lower left* depicts the side-chain of lysine 296, with the Schiff's base nitrogen shown in *blue*. Carbon atoms are shown in *red*, and hydrogens in *white*. (**B**) Molecular structure, in space-filling representation, of all-*trans* retinal in rhodopsin. The *lower left* depicts the side-chain of lysine 296, with the Schiff's base nitrogen shown in *blue*. Carbon atoms are shown in *yellow*, and hydrogens in *white*.

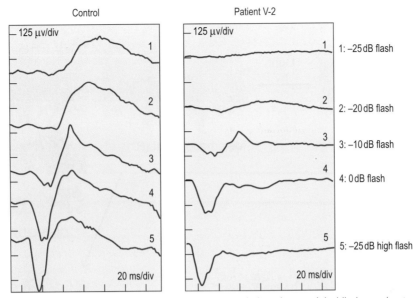

Fig. 18.9 Electroretinograms (ERGs) of a patient with congenital stationary night blindness due to rhodopsin A295V show altered signaling. The ERG represents the massed potential changes across the retina in response to light. The early negative deflection is the a-wave, derived from hyperpolarization of the photoreceptors. The later positive deflection is the b-wave, largely derived from depolarization of ON (depolarizing in response to light) bipolar cells, which receive inputs from the photoreceptors. Scotopic ERGs of a representative control subject *(left)* and a patient *(right)*. Intensities represented are 1, 0.01; 2, 0.03; 3, 0.03; 4, 1.0; 5, 3.0 cds s m⁻². The rod response is severely diminished in the patient. (From Zeitz C, Gross AK, Leifert D, Kloeckener-Gruissem B, McAlear SD, Lemke J, et al. Identification and functional characterization of a novel rhodopsin mutation associated with autosomal dominant CSNB. *Invest Ophthalmol Vis Sci* 2008;49(9):4105-4114.)

G-protein, G_t

Like rhodopsin, the rod phototransduction G-protein, known as transducin[48-52] or G_t (Fig. 18.10), is also found in an inactive state in the dark. For a G-protein, this means that it has GDP, rather than GTP, bound to its α subunit, $G_{t\alpha}$, and exists in a heterotrimeric form, $G_{t\alpha\beta\gamma}$. The G-protein associates with the disc membranes by virtue of its covalently attached lipids.[53,54] A heterogeneous mixture of saturated and unsaturated 12- and 14-carbon fatty acids is found attached to the amino terminal glycine residue of $G_{t\alpha\beta\gamma}$,[55-57] linked through an amide bond. This reaction occurs during protein translation and is important for G-protein localization in the outer segment.[58] There is a 15-carbon isoprenyl group, farnesyl, attached to the carboxyl terminus of the γ subunit[59,60] through a thio-ether linkage. This sort of isoprenylation is found in other phototransduction proteins; in each case it occurs at a cysteine residue four residues from the carboxyl terminus of the initial translation product. The final three residues are cleaved by the action of a protease,[61] and the hydrophobicity conferred by the isoprenyl group is enhanced by the methyl esterification of the carboxyl group on what has been converted into a C-terminal cysteine residue. A prenyl-binding protein, sometimes referred to as PDEδ, binds to the isoprenyl group and acts as a chaperone to help deliver the enzyme in stable form to the outer segment.[62,63]

Importance of lipid milieu

The lipids of the disc membrane play an important role in assembling the phototransduction machinery[64] and providing the proteins a stage on which to act. Rhodopsin and GC are transmembrane proteins, and G_t and PDE6 (Figs. 18.10 and 18.11) are peripheral membrane proteins, attached to the membrane by covalently attached lipids. GCAPs are also covalently lipidated by fatty acids on their amino termini, and another phototransduction protein, rhodopsin kinase, is isoprenylated (discussed further in section). The transmembrane CNG channel is found only in the plasma membrane, not in the discs. Experiments with purified proteins have shown that the proper assembly of these proteins on the disc membrane is essential for efficient interactions among them. Rhodopsin diffuses rather rapidly within the lipids of the disc membrane,[65-69] so that many encounters between it and the G-protein occur every second, even in the dark. Rod outer segment (ROS) membranes have an unusual lipid composition, with a high content of polyunsaturated fatty acids. Close to 40% of the fatty acyl groups of ROS phospholipids are the ω-3 fatty acid, docosahexaenoic acid (DHA or 22:6), which has 22 carbons and 6 double bonds,[70] and DHA can only be synthesized in the body if essential ω-3 fatty acids are consumed in the diet. Cholesterol and cholesteryl esters make up only 10% to 15% of total outer segment lipids but play an important role in establishing the lipid environment in which phototransduction reactions occur.[69]

The activation phase of a light response

Photoisomerization of rhodopsin

Phototransduction begins with absorption of light by rhodopsin (Figs. 18.6–18.8). Rhodopsin has a broad absorption spectrum with a wavelength of peak absorbance close to 500 nm in the green portion of the visible spectrum (discussed further in section). The probability of capture by rhodopsin of a photon of green light passing through the retina is fairly high (~50% for 20 μm long human rods and ~89% for 60 μm long toad rods) due to the large number of discs (~1000) through which the photon must pass and the high concentration of rhodopsin in each rod. When rhodopsin absorbs light, the probability that it will undergo a structural transition, or photoisomerization, is extraordinarily high: 65%.[71] This is one of the most efficient photochemical reactions known, and this efficiency helps explain

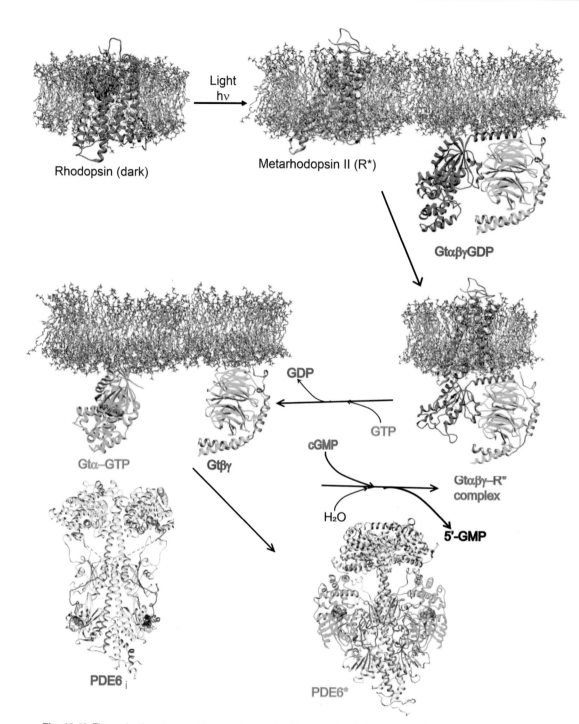

Fig. 18.10 The activation phase of the guanine nucleotide cascade of vision. Formation of catalytically active R* (MII) species *(top)* increases binding of the transducin heterotrimer, Gtαβγ-GDP. Upon binding to R*, *(middle, right)* transducin releases GDP from the Gtα subunit, leading to binding of GTP, release of separate Gtα-GTP and Gtβγ subunits *(middle, left)*. Gtα-GTP binding to the inactive form of PDE6 *(bottom, left)*, relieves inhibition of the large catalytic PDE6 subunits by the PDE6γ and leads to catalysis of cGMP hydrolysis at a rate near the diffusion limit *(bottom, right)*. Structures as in Fig. 18.6 and: MII-G_t complex, 6oy9,[128] G_{tα}-GTPγS, 1tnd,[132] G_α-GDP, 1tag,[133] G_{tβγ}, 1TBG,[134] inactive PDE6, Gulati 6mzb,[37] activated PDE6-G_{tα}-GTPγS 7jsn.[36]

the exquisite sensitivity of rod cells to a single photon of light. The bound 11-*cis* retinal chromophore is responsible for the light absorption (polypeptides do not absorb visible light unless they are bound to some chromophoric ligand). In its excited state induced by the light absorption, 11-*cis* retinal undergoes a photoisomerization at the bond between carbon 11 and carbon 12 in its structure from 11-*cis* to all-*trans* retinal (Fig. 18.8). The rearrangement of bonds causes a dramatic change in the structure of retinal, with the new all-*trans* form representing a straightening out of a kinked molecule. This molecule no longer acts as an inverse agonist locking the opsin protein in an inactive state, but now acts instead as an agonist, or activator of opsin, stimulating it to activate G-proteins.

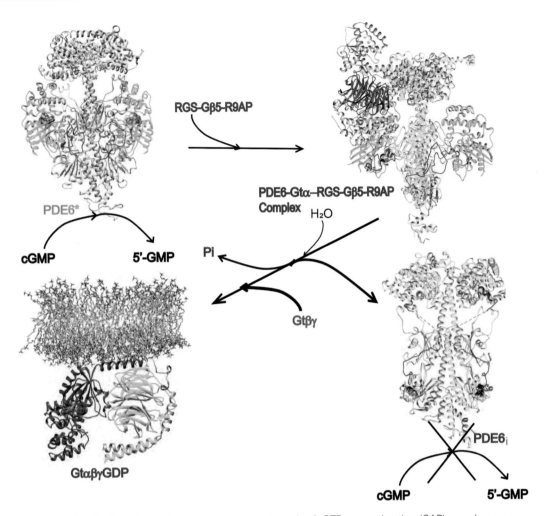

Fig. 18.11 Inactivation phase of guanine nucleotide cascade. A GTPase-accelerating (GAP) complex, comprising RGS9-1, $G_{\beta 5L}$, and membrane anchor, R9AP, binds to the $G_{t\alpha}$-GTP-PDE6 complex and accelerates the hydrolysis of GTP, resulting in inactivation of the complex and ultimate re-association of $G_{t\alpha}$-GDP with $G_{t\beta\gamma}$ (*lower left*). PDE6 returns to its inactive state (*lower right*). These events and those of Fig. 18.9, occur at the surface of the disc membranes, which are not shown because their geometric relationships to the PDE6-containing complexes are not known. Structure of GAP complex depicted by alignments of activated PDE6-$G_{t\alpha}$–GTPγS 7jsn,[36] RGS9-domain-$G_{t\alpha}$-PDEγ complex 1fqj,[135] and RGS9-Gβ5 complex. 2PBI.[136]

The retinal chromophore, covalently attached via a Schiff's base linkage to a lysine residue at amino acid position 296 on rhodopsin (see previously), induces structural changes in the protein upon photoisomerization. After photoisomerization of the chromophore, the protein undergoes a series of conformational changes in the arrangement of its helices to accommodate this event. In other words, when retinal stretches out into the all-*trans* shape, it pushes part of the protein out of the way. These conformational changes ultimately lead to formation of metarhodopsin II, a significantly different structure than dark rhodopsin (Fig. 18.7). The intermediate conformations of photolyzed rhodopsin can be monitored by high speed and/or low temperature spectroscopy, including UV-visible absorbance, infrared, Raman, and fluorescence spectroscopies.[72–74] These and other studies have shown that upon light activation, rhodopsin first changes to bathorhodopsin, lumirhodopsin, metarhodopsin I (MI) and metarhodopsin II (MII or R*, the form that activates transducin), and ultimately metarhodopsin III (MIII) before the all-*trans* chromophore becomes hydrolyzed, leaving the apoprotein opsin. At physiologic temperatures, almost immediately upon photoactivation MI and MII establish a dynamic equilibrium, which can be monitored by the differences in their absorbance spectra. It is MII rather than MI that preferentially binds to and activates the G-protein.

G-protein activation

The key functional difference between rhodopsin and metarhodopsin II is in their interactions with the G-protein transducin (G_t). MII binds to the G-protein much more tightly than does rhodopsin and serves as an efficient catalyst for the activation of G_t. G-protein activation occurs about 10 million times faster at high MII concentrations than it does in the dark.[75] The G-protein binds to MII when it is bound to GDP, but rapidly releases the bound GDP (Fig. 18.9). This GDP release is the slow step (~once per 10,000 s) for G-protein activation in the dark but occurs very rapidly when G_t is bound to MII. Once GDP is released, the millimolar concentrations of GTP in the cell ensure rapid binding of GTP. Once GTP is bound to the $G_{t\alpha}$ subunit, the G-protein is in its active state. The activated $G_{t\alpha}$-GTP complex has much lower affinity for both the $G_{\beta\gamma}$ subunits and for MII than do either the nucleotide-free state or the GDP-bound state of $G_{t\alpha}$. One MII molecule can activate many G-proteins in a catalytic fashion at a rate exceeding 150 per second in mammalian rods.

PDE6 activation

When $G_{t\alpha}$ loses its affinity for MII and $G_{t\beta\gamma}$ upon binding GTP, it also gains greatly enhanced affinity for the cGMP phosphodiesterase, PDE6.[29,76] When $G_{t\alpha}$-GTP is bound, the catalytic activity of PDE6 goes up about 1000-fold. This dramatic increase in enzymatic activity means that cytoplasmic levels of cGMP begin to fall rapidly in the vicinity of activated PDE6. Fully activated PDE6 is one of the most efficient enzymes known, with a catalytic efficiency, k_{cat}/K_m, of about $4 \times 10^8 M^{-1}s^{-1}$. This high catalytic efficiency means that nearly every time a cGMP molecule collides by diffusion with an activated PDE6 molecule, it will be hydrolyzed to form 5'-GMP. If 350 PDE6 molecules are fully activated in a single primate rod cell, they can hydrolyze most of its cGMP in one-tenth of a second.

Channel closing

Individual cGMP molecules are constantly dissociating from and binding to their sites on the CNG channel, even in the dark (see Chapter 19). Thus, each CNG channel samples the cGMP concentration in the adjacent cytoplasm once every few milliseconds. For practical purposes, the channels respond immediately to the decline in cGMP in the cytoplasm, and they do this with a very steep concentration dependence, because of the cooperativity noted previously. Closing of channels reduces the flow of Na^+ ions into the cell, reducing the dark current and making the membrane potential more negative (i.e., hyperpolarized). Simultaneously, the flux of Ca^{2+} into the cell is also reduced[77] and its concentration diminished by the action of the Na^+/Ca^{2+} exchanger discussed previously.

Slowing of neurotransmitter release

Communication of rods with downstream bipolar cells is the release of the neurotransmitter, glutamate. High levels of glutamate release by rods signal total darkness to bipolar cells, and reductions in the levels of glutamate release signal absorption of light. This change results from the hyperpolarization of the cell membrane, which is passively propagated along the plasma membrane from outer segment to synaptic terminal. Because rod cells are relatively short compared to neurons with long axons, active propagation of the signal by action potentials is not needed to communicate potential changes at the outer segment to the synapse.

The recovery phase

The biochemical changes that occur during activation contain within them the seeds of destruction for the activated state; they set the stage for the recovery phase. It is simplest to consider this process, which is rather more complex than activation, in terms of recovery from activation by a single dim flash of light, after which no more MII formation occurs.

Rhodopsin phosphorylation, retinoid recycling, and regeneration

Because of the catalytic activity of MII, as long as MII survives intact downstream signaling will continue, and cGMP will be subject to rapid degradation. There are multiple mechanisms for inactivating MII, but the fastest-acting and most important one appears to be phosphorylation by rhodopsin kinase,[78] RK or RK1 (Fig. 18.12). Like the G-protein, RK preferentially recognizes the activated form of rhodopsin, MII. RK uses ATP to attach phosphate groups to serine residues in the carboxyl-terminal tail of rhodopsin. Up to eight phosphates may be added, and if any of the key residues are missing, MII inactivation kinetics are slowed.[79,80] Phosphorylation of MII reduces its affinity for the G-protein and slows the activation of the G-protein. RK is a member of a family of kinases specific for activated forms of G-protein–coupled receptors, which includes a kinase found only in cones (but not found in all species with cones), RK7.[81,82] RK1 associates with the disc membranes via a covalently attached farnesyl group[83,84] and RK7 via a geranylgeranyl group. The greater hydrophobicity of the 20-carbon geranylgeranyl group compared with 15-carbon farnesyl moiety may enhance the efficiency of interactions between RK7 and photoexcited cone pigments.

On a slower time scale than that of phosphorylation, photoexcited rhodopsin also undergoes loss of covalently attached all-*trans* retinal. The conformational change accompanying *cis-trans* isomerizations and light activation renders the Schiff's base between lysine 296 and retinal accessible to water, so that unlike the dark form of rhodopsin, MII is subject to Schiff's base hydrolysis and release of all-*trans* retinal from its binding pocket. All-*trans* retinal, like other aldehydes, is a chemically reactive species that can associate with proteins in the disc membrane, including rhodopsin, and form new Schiff's base linkages to amino groups from protein lysine residues or from phosphatidylethanolamine in the lipid phase into which it segregates. The conjugate between phosphatidylethanolamine and all-*trans* retinal, sometimes referred to as APE, is the precursor of a compound known as A2E (Fig. 18.14), which accumulates in animals and human patients deficient in the product of the Stargardt disease gene ABCA4[85,86] (or ABCR, see Box 18.2). Evidence for a nonexchangeable ADP in the first nucleotide binding domain belongs to a

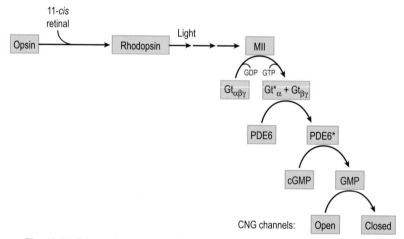

Fig. 18.12 Schematic representation of phototransduction activation cascade.

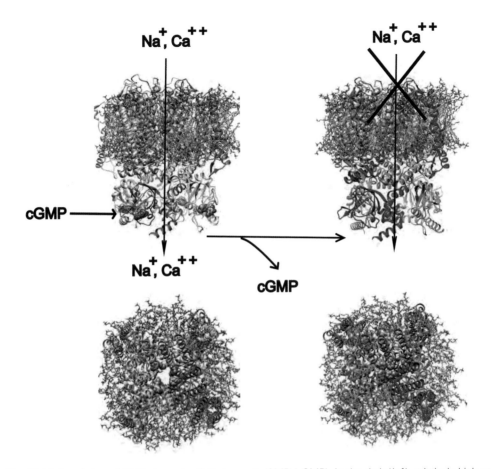

Fig. 18.13 Regulation of CNG channel activity by cyclic GMP (cGMP). In the dark (*left*), relatively high concentrations of cGMP lead to opening of the channel, which is embedded in the plasma membrane, and an inward dark current, carried predominantly by sodium ions, and to a lesser but important extent by calcium ions. Light leads to PDE6 activation, lowering of cytoplasmic concentrations of cGMP, closure of channels, and a reduction in the dark current (*right*). *Top* panels show views of the channel parallel to the plasma membrane surface, and the *bottom* panels show views from the outside of the cell.

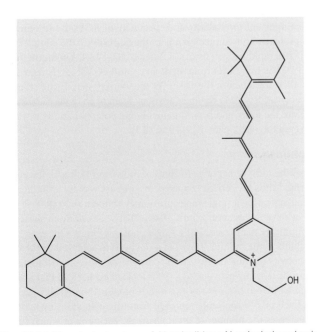

Fig. 18.14 Chemical structure of N-retinylidene-N-retinylethanolamine (A2E).

BOX 18.2   Stargardt disease

Stargardt disease is an autosomal recessive form of juvenile macular degeneration with variable progression and severity. It is caused by mutations in the ABCR (ABCA4) gene on chromosome 1 which encodes a retina-specific ATP-binding cassette transporter protein, in the rims of rod and cone outer segment discs, proposed to serve as a flippase protein for phospholipids conjugated to all-*trans* retinal. Mutations in this gene have also been attributed to some cases of cone-rod dystrophy, retinitis pigmentosa, and age-related macular degeneration. Pathologic features of Stargardt include accumulation of fluorescent lipofuscin pigments in the retinal pigmented epithelium (RPE) cells and retinal degeneration.

An important fluorophore in lipofuscin is the bis-retinoid pyridinium salt N-retinylidene-N-retinylethanolamine (A2E) formed by the condensation of all-*trans* retinaldehyde with phosphatidylethanolamine. Significant accumulation of A2E is seen in the RPE of patients with Stargardt disease (Eagle et al.,[137] Birnbach et al.,[138]). A2E has several potential cytotoxic effects on RPE cells, including destabilization of membranes, release of apoptotic proteins from mitochondria, sensitization of cells to blue light damage, and impaired degradation of phospholipids from phagocytosed outer segments.

family of ATP-binding cassette transmembrane transporters, which includes multidrug resistance proteins and lipid flippases. A proposed function for ABCA4 is the transbilayer transport of APE. The aldehyde all-*trans* retinal must be converted to its alcohol form before being transported to the RPE for recycling into 11-*cis* retinal (see Chapter 13). This reduction reaction is catalyzed by one or more dehydrogenase enzymes, known as retinol dehydrogenases, all of which use NADPH as the reducing agent.

Opsin, whether phosphorylated or not, can bind 11-*cis* retinal, supplied by the retinoid cycle in the RPE, to regenerate rhodopsin in its dark state. Phosphorylated rhodopsin does not bind arrestin (see further) with high affinity and can be dephosphorylated by the action of protein phosphatase 2 A (PP2A). Because rhodopsin with 11-*cis* retinal bound does not activate RK, rhodopsin in the dark is predominantly in a nonphosphorylated state.

Arrestin binding

Phosphorylation of rhodopsin by RK is not, in itself, sufficient for shutting off the activity of MII completely. A key additional step is binding of the capping protein, arrestin.[87,88] When MII is multiply phosphorylated, arrestin binds very tightly and blocks further binding and activation of G_t (Fig. 18.13). This MII is unable to propagate phototransduction due to steric hindrance of the G_t binding site. Eventually, all-*trans* retinal will be removed by hydrolysis of the Schiff's base linkage and dissociation from the protein, yielding opsin, from which arrestin will dissociate, and phosphates will be removed by a phosphoprotein phosphatase. This latter series of reactions occurs on a much longer time scale than the recovery from a dim flash excitation, as does regeneration of rhodopsin by binding of 11-*cis* retinal to opsin (see discussion of dark adaptation further in Chapter 20). Arrestin is a 48 kDa protein also known as 48 K or S-antigen due to its involvement in experimentally induced autoimmune uveitis.

[cGMP] restoration by guanylate cyclase activation

On an even faster time scale than MII activation,[89,90] changes in GC activity occur via a calcium feedback mechanism,[91] and these serve to halt the lowering of cytoplasmic [cGMP] and eventually restore it to dark levels. The calcium feedback consists of a lowering of cytoplasmic $[Ca^{2+}]$ that in turn activates Gc.[92] The mechanism by which $[Ca^{2+}]$ is lowered is simply that the Na^+/Ca^{2+} exchanger continues to pump Ca^{2+} out of the cell while the leak of Ca^{2+} into the cell through the CNG channels is reduced or blocked when the channels close (see Chapter 19). Changes in $[Ca^{2+}]$ work through calcium-binding proteins[93] known as GCAPs, members of the calmodulin superfamily of calcium-binding proteins. They bind to GC and keep its activity low when they have calcium bound but dramatically enhance its activity when $[Ca^{2+}]$ becomes low. Ca^{2+} inhibition of the GCAP-GC complex is also cooperative, so that the dependence of GC activity is very steeply dependent on Ca^{2+} concentration. This cooperativity allows very rapid changes in GC activity in response to changes in CNG channel current. GC activation through Ca^{2+} feedback begins to balance the activation of PDE6 in less than 100 ms after a dim flash (in mice) and eventually restores [cGMP] to the resting dark level.

The retinal photoreceptor GC isoforms[94] are members of a family of transmembrane or particulate GCs, some of which, unlike the photoreceptor isoforms, are receptors for peptides or other extracellular ligands. Transmembrane GC enzymes are found in membranes as dimers. Each GC polypeptide has a glycosylated extracellular domain, which participates in dimer formation, a single transmembrane alpha-helix, and intracellular domains. The intracellular domains include a kinase homology domain, a dimerization domain, the catalytic domain, which is responsible for the production of cGMP, and a C-terminal

domain, which may mediate interactions with proteins at the cytoplasmic surface of the membrane. The GCAP proteins, which have fatty acids attached to their amino termini, remain bound to GC even at low concentrations of intracellular Ca^{2+}. Binding of Ca^{2+} changes their conformation in such a way as to allow dramatic stimulation of the activity of GC.

There are two isoforms each of GC and GCAPs in human photoreceptors and most mammals. The importance of GC1 (also known as GCE or retGC1 or ROS-GC1) in human phototransduction is underscored by mutations in the gene (GUCY2D) encoding this protein, which causes Leber's congenital amaurosis (LCA) in human patients.[95,96] The importance of GCAP1 is underscored by the association of mutations in GCAP1 with autosomal dominant cone dystrophy.[97] In mice, a double-knockout of the GCAP1 and GCAP2 genes, which are in close proximity on the chromosome, leads to dark-adapted rod flash responses that are much slower and larger in amplitude than those in wildtype rods. Transgenic expression of GCAP2 only partially rescues this phenotype, whereas GCAP1 expression appears to provide complete rescue if expression levels are sufficient.[98]

G-protein and PDE6 inactivation by RGS9-1

Even after MII has been quenched by phosphorylation and arrestin binding, signaling continues as long as GTP remains bound to the G-protein, so that PDE6 remains in an activated state. The dark GDP state of $G_{t\alpha}$ is restored through hydrolysis of the bound GTP. Once phosphate is released, it causes a conformational transformation in $G_{t\alpha}$ that restores its affinity for $G_{t\beta\gamma}$ and dramatically lowers its affinity for PDE6. PDE6 then returns to its dark inactive state. This GTP hydrolysis step is the slowest step[99,100] in rod vision (time constant of about 200 ms in mammals and about 2 s in amphibians) and is regulated by a complex of proteins that act as GTPase-accelerating proteins (GAPs). The core of this complex is RGS9-1,[101,102] a member of the regulator of G-protein signaling (RGS) family of GAPs found only in photoreceptor cells. It is always bound to two obligate subunits $G_{\beta5L}$, and a transmembrane anchor protein R9AP. $G_{\beta5L}$[103,104] is a member of the G-protein β subunit family, but its function is distinct from the other four members, which bind very tightly to G-protein γ subunits and help G-protein α subunits couple to receptors. Rather, $G_{\beta5L}$, binds tightly to a G-γ-like domain,[105] or GGL domain, found in the R7 family of RGS proteins. $G_{\beta5L}$ binding is important for stability and specificity of RGS9-1 and other R7 RGS proteins. This complex binds to the $G_{t\alpha}$-GTP-PDE6 complex and stimulates rapid hydrolysis of GTP by $G_{t\alpha}$ (Fig. 18.11), with the result that PDE6 activity falls to its dark levels and cGMP levels recover to what they were before the flash. As the slowest step in the recovery phase concludes, CNG channels are once again open to the same extent as before the flash, and both the membrane potential and $[Ca^{2+}]$ have recovered too (see Chapter 19) (Box 18.3).

Amplification

One of the most remarkable features of rod vision is that all the events described thus far can be triggered in a robust way by an individual photon activating a single molecule of MII within a rod cell. Rod cells thus achieve the quantum limit of sensitivity, the ability to sense and communicate the presence of a single photon of light. One reason for this ability is the multiple stages of amplification achieved by the catalytic activity of phototransduction components. A single MII molecule can produce many activated $G_{t\alpha}$-GTP molecules. Each of these, when bound to PDE6, can destroy thousands of cGMP molecules per second. Each cGMP molecule removed from the cytoplasm by hydrolysis decreases the number of open channels, each one of which passes nearly 2000 positively charged ions per second. Moreover, the cooperativity of the channel means that a 10% change in [cGMP] yields a

BOX 18.3 **Bradyopsia**

Patients with bradyopsia, or slow vision, show a prolonged response suppression in electroretinogram recordings.

Bradyopsia is a recently discovered rare genetic disorder of the retina characterized by an inability to rapidly shut off the phototransduction cascade following the stimulation of the photoreceptors by a photon of light. Patients present with symptoms of photophobia, problems adjusting to bright light, and difficulties seeing moving objects; they often complain that they cannot play ball sports such as soccer, as they cannot see the ball in motion.[139] The mutation in these patients is in the RGS9 (regulator of G-protein signaling 9) gene, the product of which is involved in the deactivation of photoreceptor responses (Fig. 18.11), or in the gene encoding R9AP, the RGS9-1 anchor protein, whose presence is essential to prevent degradation of RGS9-1. The discovery of bradyopsia and its molecular basis provides a fascinating insight into the ever-expanding role of medical genetics and animal models of human disease.

When the RGS9 gene was first discovered as one encoding a key player in phototransduction, it was recognized as a candidate gene for human retinal disease. However, sequencing of DNA from numerous patients with hereditary retinal degenerations uncovered polymorphisms in the RGS9 gene, but none with any disease association.[139,140] Results from mice engineered to have a genetic defect in their RGS9 gene revealed that homozygotes suffered not from retinal degeneration, but from slowed recovery from light responses in rod and cone photoreceptors. R9AP knockout mice had retinal phenotypes almost identical to those of RGS9 knockouts. These findings led researchers at the Massachusetts Eye and Ear Infirmary to search through patient records and the ophthalmological literature for patients whose ERG results resembled those of the knockout mice. This work, combined with DNA sequencing, led to the discovery of this previously uncharacterized disease.[141]

nearly 30% change in the number of open channels. Depending on the species and their rod geometry, the overall gain in terms of numbers of ions blocked per rhodopsin photoisomerized is between 5×10^5 and 10^7.[106] These staggering numbers would seem to make it obvious why a single photon can be detected, but there is one problem that always accompanies amplification: noise is amplified along with the signal. Ultimately, reliable detection depends not just on a strong signal, but on a high signal-to-noise ratio. There are many sources of noise in the phototransduction cascade, and detailed studies suggest that many of the features of the phototransduction cascade and the molecules that mediate it have evolved to minimize noise. Individual rods produce false single photon–like signals with a frequency of about once every 160 seconds, making it difficult for us to discriminate real light from darkness at intensity levels below that needed to induce single photon responses with this frequency.

Responses to saturating light levels

When light levels exceed that needed to photoisomerize 1 rhodopsin in every 10,000 (0.01%), nearly all the cGMP in the cell is hydrolyzed, pushing the concentration to near zero, and all the channels close, completely shutting off the dark current. Beyond this intensity, increasing the light intensity only accelerates the kinetics of the rising phase and prolongs the time in saturation. As described in Chapter 19, following a flash of saturating intensity, further rod responses cannot be elicited until several seconds later when the cell has recovered from the initial response. Over a fairly wide range of intensities, the time from the flash to recovery of the dark current to a criterion level (e.g., 90% or 50%) varies linearly with the logarithm of the flash intensity,[107] indicating a single exponential process, characterized by a "dominant time constant."[108] This time constant corresponds to the slowest step in the transduction cascade over that intensity range. Results from transgenic mice with increased levels of the RGS9-1 GAP complex[99] have revealed that the levels of this complex and, therefore, the kinetics of GTP hydrolysis by $G_{t\alpha}$, determine the timing of the slow step in rod photoresponse recovery, and the time resolution of rod dim light vision.

Adaptation to changing levels of ambient lighting

In the presence of even a fairly dim background light, the responses of rods to increments in intensity are attenuated and accelerated relative to those obtained in completely dark-adapted conditions (see Chapter 20). This desensitizing effect becomes more pronounced as the intensity of the background light increases. These changes are referred to as light adaptation. The changes are reversible upon return to darkness, with the return of sensitivity occurring over a time scale of minutes, proceeding through both fast and slow phases. This restoration of sensitivity is referred to as dark adaptation. The slow phase of dark adaptation is usually attributed to the regeneration of rhodopsin from opsin that has been formed by prolonged exposure to bright light, that is, the rebinding of 11-*cis* retinal to the pool of apoprotein formed in bright background light. Light adaptation can be observed on a time scale of seconds, and, while it is not completely understood, it appears to result from changes at several steps in the phototransduction cascade. The most important of these is simply an acceleration of cGMP hydrolysis and synthesis caused by PDE6 activation and low-$[Ca^{2+}]$–induced GC activation. Because these reactions are already proceeding at a fast clip due to the background light, further increases in light elicit lower amplitude responses, but these occur more rapidly. In addition, the low $[Ca^{2+}]$ present under these conditions may modulate the activity of rhodopsin kinase, the CNG channel, and the RGS9-1 GAP complex.

Turnover of guanine nucleotides

While light greatly accelerates the turnover of guanine nucleotides in photoreceptors, even in the dark there is a very high rate of flux through cycles of synthesis and hydrolysis.[109] Each PDE6 molecule may have only 0.1% or so of its maximal enzymatic activity in the dark; however, the high concentration of PDE6 (on the order of 20 µM) and its high enzymatic efficiency means that the entire cellular pool of cGMP in a mammalian rod is hydrolyzed at a rate of about once every two and one-half seconds. This hydrolytic flux is balanced by continual cGMP synthesis catalyzed by Gc to achieve a constant steady-state level of cGMP in the dark. This dark cycling through cGMP consumes high amounts of GTP, which must be continually replenished by energy metabolism. To that end photoreceptors can use both aerobic respiration by dense concentrations of mitochondria in the region of the inner segment proximal to the outer segment, and glycolysis, the enzymes of which are found in both the outer and inner segments. GTP is produced from GDP and inorganic phosphate, Pi, in the citric acid cycle by the action of succinate dehydrogenase, from GDP and ATP by the action nucleoside diphosphate kinase, and from two molecules of GDP by the action of a GDP phosphotransferase.[110] This apparent futile cycling accompanied by squandering of cellular energy sources may seem wasteful. However, it likely contributes to the speed of phototransduction, and its cost in terms of ATP use is dwarfed by the needs of the Na^+/K^+-ATPase pump in the inner segment.

Mitochondria are also important for generation of reducing equivalents, in the form of NADPH, needed for reduction to retinol of all-*trans* retinaldehyde, generated following rhodopsin photoisomerization, and of excess 11-*cis* retinaldehyde, both of which can be toxic. More details of energy metabolism in the retina and RPE can be found in a recent review.[111]

COMPARISON OF CONES AND RODS

Similarities and differences of phototransduction molecules

Many of the phototransduction molecules of rods have homologs that perform similar functions in cones. The cone pigments are very similar in structure to rhodopsin but have different absorption spectra and different photophysical properties (Fig. 18.15). The thermal isomerization rates of cone pigments are higher than those for rhodopsin,[112] as are the rates of spontaneous dissociation of 11-*cis* retinal.[113] The evolution of different absorption spectra,[114] known as spectral tuning, for the color pigments and rhodopsin arises owing to varying amino acid side-chains in and near the chromophore binding pocket. Pioneering work[115] by George Wald (for which he shared the Nobel Prize in Physiology or Medicine in 1967[116]), Ruth Hubbard,[46] and others showed that rod cells are most sensitive to green light (absorbance maximum around 498 nm), and are not sensitive in the red (wavelengths longer than 640 nm). Many studies have addressed the molecular mechanism of spectral tuning, and it has been determined that the protonation state of the Schiff's base, as well as the polarity of the amino acids adjacent to it, dictate whether the absorption spectrum of the photoreceptor is shifted to the blue (short wavelengths) or to the red (long wavelengths) (Fig. 18.15).[117-122]

The G-protein subunits of rods and cones are distinct but closely related. Cone $G_{\alpha t}$ is known as $G_{\alpha t2}$ or cone transducin and is 81% identical to rod transducin. Rod transducin's β subunit is $G_{\beta 1}$, whereas cone transducin uses $G_{\beta 3}$, which has 83% sequence identity. The rod $G_{\gamma 1}$ and cone $G_{\gamma 8}$ subunits are less than 40% identical; both undergo proteolytic cleavage of three residues, farnesylation, and methyl esterification at their C-termini.

Unlike rods, in which there are two related but distinct PDE6 catalytic subunits, PDE6$_\beta$ and PDE6$_\alpha$, cones contain a single PDE6$_{\alpha'}$ subunit, which forms a homodimer that together with two copies of cone-specific PDE6$_{\gamma C}$ forms the holoenzyme heterotetramer. The CNG channel has cone-specific α and β subunits. Both rod rhodopsin kinase, GRK-1 and a cone-specific rhodopsin kinase, GRK-7 are found in cones, and there is a cone-specific form of arrestin. The RGS9-1-$G_{\beta 5}$-R9AP complex is identical in composition in cones (except that some of the $G_{\beta 5}$ is a shorter splice variant not found in rods) but is present at 10-fold higher levels in cones than in rods[102,123] to allow the fast kinetics described in the next section.

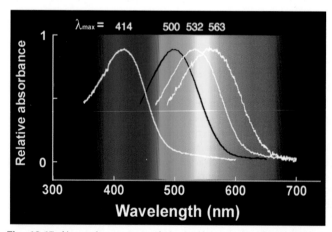

Fig. 18.15 Absorption spectra of rhodopsin and the red-sensitive (L, 563 nm), green-sensitive (M, 532 nm), and blue-sensitive (S, 414 nm) cone pigments. (Courtesy of Dr. Masahiro Kono.)

Physiological differences

Cones are much less sensitive than rods, they have much faster kinetics, and they are nearly impossible to saturate even in bright sunlight. The reasons for these differences are currently the subject of research in numerous laboratories and remain controversial. However, most current data point away from the reactions of the activation phase. The quantum sensitivity of the cone pigments is very similar to that of rhodopsin, as is their efficiency at activating the G-protein. The cone PDE6 has similar kinetic properties to those of the rod isoform, and the CNG channels have similar responsiveness to cGMP. Rather, most research points toward faster mechanisms for shutting off the response as the major sources for differences in kinetics and sensitivity between rods and cones. These include, possibly, faster phosphorylation of the activated cone pigments, compared with MII phosphorylation,[124,125] faster dissociation of all-*trans* retinal, and faster G-protein GTP hydrolysis, driven by 10-fold higher concentrations of the RGS9-1-Gβ5-R9AP GAP complex in cones than in rods. Low activity (poor G-protein activation) of bleached pigment (opsin-like apoprotein or phosphorylated and arrestin-capped forms) may also play a role in preventing saturation of cones.

PHOTOTRANSDUCTION AND DISEASE

The major classes of disease resulting from defects in phototransduction include retinal degeneration, night blindness, color blindness, and achromatopsia. Of these, each of the heritable diseases, except for X-linked color blindness, is quite rare, but in total these conditions affect many thousands of patients who suffer various degrees of visual impairment.

Retinal degeneration and night blindness

Retinal degeneration is a progressive loss of visual function, usually accompanied by death of both rod and cone photoreceptor cells, and can lead to severe visual impairment and complete blindness. Such conditions are classified under a variety of names according to the appearance of the retina and pathology of the disease. Hereditary degenerative disorders, including retinitis pigmentosa, can arise from mutations in genes encoding photoreceptor proteins, as well as from mutations in many other nonphototransduction genes (see Box 18.4). Many such mutations have been identified in humans and animals, and lists of these can be accessed on the web site for the Retinal Information Network: http://www.sph.uth.tmc.edu/Retnet/ or the site for the Ocular Molecular Genetics Institute: http://eyegene.meei.harvard.edu/. Among the phototransduction proteins discussed in this chapter, retinal degeneration has been linked to defects in the genes encoding rhodopsin, PDE6, CG, CNG channel, and GCAPs. CSNB, an absence or severe deficiency in rod vision, (referred to as "stationary" because it does not progress) has been linked to genes encoding rhodopsin, the transducin (G-protein) α subunit, RK, and arrestin (Box 18.4).

WHAT WE DON'T KNOW

Although the basic biochemistry of the major events in phototransduction is fairly well understood, most of the structural and mechanistic details remain to be determined. Although some hints are available, we do not know exactly how MII activates the G-protein or how the G-protein activates PDE6. Many of the biochemical events are mediated by large, membrane-attached multiprotein complexes, but we do not know how these are organized. For example, during the rate limiting step of vision, G-protein GTP hydrolysis, a minimum of eight different polypeptides, ($G_{t\alpha}$, PDEα, PDEβ, 2 PDEγ, RGS9-1,

BOX 18.4 Retinitis pigmentosa

Retinitis pigmentosa (RP) is a progressive rod-cone dystrophy that presents with progressive field loss and eventual visual activity decline. The worldwide prevalence of RP is 1 in 3500 individuals.[142]

Typical symptoms include night blindness followed by decreasing visual fields, leading to tunnel vision and eventually blindness. Clinical hallmarks include gradual increased bone-spiculed pigmentation, attenuation of retinal vasculature, waxy disc pallor, as well as diminished, abnormal, or absent electroretinograph (ERG) responses. Typically, symptoms start in early teenage years, and severe visual impairment occurs by the ages of 40 to 50 years. There are early-onset forms of RP, with the underlying genetic cause proving to be a useful predictor of the severity of the disease. The earliest of symptoms, measurable before visible onset of the disease, are abnormal light-evoked ERGs.[143] The autosomal dominant (ADRP) form is less prevalent and less severe than the recessive form and has been linked to a variety of genes involved in phototransduction or rod cell function. The most prevalent mutation in human ADRP patients, in which Pro23 is replaced by His (P34H) in the rhodopsin gene, has been identified in approximately 15% of ADRP families in the United States. A comprehensive list of genes causing RP and other retinopathies can be found at the RetNet website (https://sph.uth.edu/retnet/). In addition to simple forms of RP, there are syndromes involving pleiotropic effects. The most frequent form of syndromic RP is Usher syndrome. This disease presents as early-onset hearing loss followed by development of RP in the teenage years.[144]

BOX 18.5 Cone-specific disease

Whereas retinitis pigmentosa and congenital stationary night blindness are thought of as diseases that primarily or initially affect the rods, there are additional hereditary visual disorders that primarily target cones. These include color blindness (see Chapter 19), achromatopsia (see Chapter 19), cone- or cone/rod dystrophies, and inherited forms of macular dystrophy. Numerous genes have been implicated in these genes, and these include some cone-specific phototransduction genes, including cone pigment genes, cyclic nucleotide–gated channel subunit genes, a gene encoding cone-specific G-protein, guanylate cyclase–activating protein (GCAP) genes, and genes encoding potassium and calcium channels. In addition to ABCA4, discussed in the text, a gene encoding a fatty acid elongase, ELOV4, has been implicated in Stargardt-like macular dystrophy.

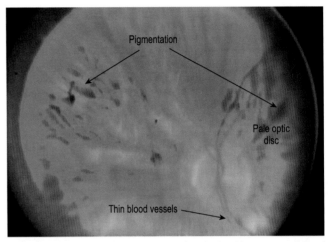

Fig. 18.16 Fundus photograph taken of patient with autosomal dominant retinitis pigmentosa. Note the pale optic disc, presence of pigmentation and narrowed blood vessels (where indicated). (Courtesy of Dr. Leo P. Semes.)

Gβ5, R9AP) are present, and we have no idea how they are arranged on the surface of the disc membrane. The multisubunit CNG channel, and Na/Ca exchanger are associated with one another in the plasma membrane and tightly attached to proteins in the disc rims, but the structures of these complexes are also unknown. Rhodopsin can form ordered rows of dimers in isolated disc membranes, but the physiologic roles of these arrays and of the dimers themselves remain controversial. These structural questions remain an active area of current research.

There are also many remaining questions about the inactivation phase of the light response and about the events of light and dark adaptation. For example, the active lifetime of MII molecules seems to be under much more stringent control than would be expected for an excited species whose inactivation occurs by way of a randomly timed event such as phosphorylation or any other chemical reaction. Modeling studies suggest that multiple sequential chemical changes are needed to explain what is known as the reproducibility of the single photon responses. Studies of the kinetics of rhodopsin phosphorylation have mostly been carried out at very high levels of MII formation under conditions very far from single photon responses; so how MII phosphorylation proceeds at very low light intensities and how it is influenced by $[Ca^{2+}]$ remain controversial topics for further research. Certain features of long-term light adaptation are still without a molecular explanation.

There is only a partial understanding of how the levels of the phototransduction proteins are regulated. This is despite the fact that it has been known for years that the levels of many of them are remarkably constant under a given set of conditions but can vary in response to genetic defects or metabolic stress. Our understanding of how the phototransduction proteins are selectively transported to the outer segments from their sites of synthesis in the inner segment, and how they are kept there, is still at a rudimentary stage. In recent years, there has been much interest in the migration during prolonged bright illumination of the G-protein transducin from the outer to the inner segment, and the movement of arrestin, under the same conditions,

from the inner to the outer segment. The mechanisms by which these dramatic changes are achieved, and their physiologic significance, are still under study.

One of the most important remaining areas of inquiry has to do with the connection between phototransduction and disease. Although defects in phototransduction components are known to lead to retinal degeneration, the molecular mechanisms by which cell death occurs are very poorly understood. It will be very important to understand these mechanisms in order to develop new therapeutic interventions and to discover common pathways that might someday lead to therapies that could be applied to a number of different degenerative disorders (Box 18.5).

WHERE THE FIELD IS HEADED

The study of phototransduction is quite satisfying because each new piece of information can be fitted into an overall scheme that is very comprehensive. It is like working on a jigsaw puzzle that is one-third to one-half finished. Each new piece of the puzzle can often fit into the emerging picture and immediately reveals something new about the scene. The field at present is shifting: from the activation phase, the mechanisms of which are fairly well understood, to the recovery phase, which holds more mysteries; from rods, whose properties make them easier to study, to cones, which present greater challenges;

from the functions of proteins in the outer segments to understanding how they are transported and maintained there and how they are organized; from functioning of normal photoreceptors to how their malfunctioning leads to disease. There will be many exciting opportunities for discovery in these areas in the coming years.

REFERENCES

1. Chabre M. Trigger and amplification mechanisms in visual phototransduction. *Annu Rev Biophys Biophys Chem.* 1985;14:331–360.
2. Schwartz EA. Phototransduction in vertebrate rods. *Annu Rev Neurosci.* 1985;8:339–367.
3. Hargrave PA, McDowell JH. Rhodopsin and phototransduction: a model system for G protein-linked receptors. *Faseb J.* 1992;6(6):2323–2331.
4. Arshavsky VY, Lamb TD, Pugh EN Jr. G proteins and phototransduction. *Annu Rev Physiol.* 2002;64:153–187.
5. Burns ME, Arshavsky VY. Beyond counting photons: trials and trends in vertebrate visual transduction. *Neuron.* 2005;48(3):387–401.
6. Chen CK. The vertebrate phototransduction cascade: amplification and termination mechanisms. *Rev Physiol Biochem Pharmacol.* 2005;154:101–121.
7. Stryer L. Cyclic GMP cascade of vision. *Annu Rev Neurosci.* 1986;9:87–119.
8. Baylor DA. Photoreceptor signals and vision. Proctor lecture. *Invest Ophthalmol Vis Sci.* 1987;28(1):34–49.
9. Schnapf JL, Baylor DA. How photoreceptor cells respond to light. *Sci Am.* 1987;256(4):40–47.
10. Stryer L. Molecular mechanism of visual excitation. *Harvey Lect.* 1991;87:129–143.
11. Young RW. Passage of newly formed protein through the connecting cilium of retina rods in the frog. *J Ultrastruct Res.* 1968;23(5):462–473.
12. Volland S, Hughes LC, Kong C, Burgess BL, Linberg KA, Luna G, et al. Three-dimensional organization of nascent rod outer segment disk membranes. *Proc Natl Acad Sci U S A.* 2015;112(48):14870–14875.
13. Burgoyne T, Meschede IP, Burden JJ, Bailly M, Seabra MC, Futter CE. Rod disc renewal occurs by evagination of the ciliary plasma membrane that makes cadherin-based contacts with the inner segment. *Proc Natl Acad Sci U S A.* 2015;112(52):15922–15927.
14. Ding JD, Salinas RY, Arshavsky VY. Discs of mammalian rod photoreceptors form through the membrane evagination mechanism. *J Cell Biol.* 2015;211(3):495–502.
15. Peters KR, Palade GE, Schneider BG, Papermaster DS. Fine structure of a periciliary ridge complex of frog retinal rod cells revealed by ultrahigh resolution scanning electron microscopy. *J Cell Biol.* 1983;96(1):265–276.
16. Baylor DA, Lamb TD, Yau KW. Responses of retinal rods to single photons. *J Physiol (Lond).* 1979;288:613–634.
17. Schneeweis DM, Schnapf JL. Photovoltage of rods and cones in the macaque retina. *Science.* 1995;268(5213):1053–1056.
18. Pirahanchi Y, Jessu R, Aeddula NR. *Physiology, Sodium Potassium Pump. StatPearls.* Treasure Island (FL): StatPearls Publishing LLC; 2021.
19. Ames A 3rd, Li YY, Heher EC, Kimble CR. Energy metabolism of rabbit retina as related to function: high cost of Na+ transport. *J Neurosci.* 1992;12(3):840–853.
20. Pech IV, Stahl WL. Immunocytochemical localization of NA+, K+-ATPase in primary cultures of rat retina. *Neurochem Res.* 1994;9(6):757–769.
21. Plössl K, Royer M, Bernklau S, et al. Retinoschisin is linked to retinal Na/K-ATPase signaling and localization. *Mol Biol Cell.* 2017;28(16):2178–2189.
22. Warren R, Molday RS. Regulation of the rod photoreceptor cyclic nucleotide-gated channel. *Adv Exp Med Biol.* 2002;514:205–223.
23. Schnetkamp PP. The SLC24 Na+/Ca2+-K+ exchanger family: vision and beyond. *Pflugers Arch.* 2004;447(5):683–688.
24. Koch KW. Purification and identification of photoreceptor guanylate cyclase. *J Biol Chem.* 1991;266(13):8634–8637.
25. Shyjan AW, de Sauvage FJ, Gillett NA, Goeddel DV, Lowe DG. Molecular cloning of a retina-specific membrane guanylyl cyclase. *Neuron.* 1992;9(4):727–737.
26. Dizhoor AM, Lowe DG, Olshevskaya EV, Laura RP, Hurley JB. The human photoreceptor membrane guanylyl cyclase, RetGC, is present in outer segments and is regulated by calcium and a soluble activator. *Neuron.* 1994;12(6):1345–1352.
27. Miki N, Baraban JM, Keirns JJ, Boyce JJ, Bitensky MW. Purification and properties of the light-activated cyclic nucleotide phosphodiesterase of rod outer segments. *J Biol Chem.* 1975;250(16):6320–6327.
28. Yee R, Liebman PA. Light-activated phosphodiesterase of the rod outer segment. Kinetics and parameters of activation and deactivation. *J Biol Chem.* 1978;253(24):8902–8909.
29. Wensel TG. The light-regulated cGMP phosphodiesterase of vertebrate photoreceptors: Structure and mechanism of activation by Gtα. In: Dickey BF, Birnbaumer L, eds. *GTPases in Biology II.* Berlin: Springer-Verlag; 1993:213–223.
30. Cote RH. Photoreceptor phosphodiesterase (PDE6): activation and inactivation mechanisms during visual transduction in rods and cones. *Pflugers Arch.* 2021;473(9):1377–1391.
31. He F, Seryshev AB, Cowan CW, Wensel TG. Multiple zinc binding sites in retinal rod cGMP phosphodiesterase, PDE6alpha beta. *J Biol Chem.* 2000;275(27):20572–20577.
32. Yang Z, Wensel TG. Inorganic pyrophosphatase from bovine retinal rod outer segments. *J Biol Chem.* 1992;267(34):24634–24640.
33. Baehr W, Palczewski K. Guanylate cyclase-activating proteins and retina disease. *Subcell Biochem.* 2007;45:71–91.
34. Palczewski K, Sokal I, Baehr W. Guanylate cyclase-activating proteins: structure, function, and diversity. *Biochem Biophys Res Commun.* 2004;322(4):1123–1130.
35. Koch KW, Duda T, Sharma RK. Photoreceptor specific guanylate cyclases in vertebrate phototransduction. *Mol Cell Biochem.* 2002;230(1-2):97–106.
36. Gao Y, Eskici G, Ramachandran S, et al. Structure of the visual signaling complex between transducin and phosphodiesterase 6. *Mol Cell.* 2020;80(2):237–245. e4.
37. Gulati S, Palczewski K, Engel A, Stahlberg H, Kovacik L. Cryo-EM structure of phosphodiesterase 6 reveals insights into the allosteric regulation of type I phosphodiesterases. *Sci Adv.* 2019;5(2):eaav4322.
38. Conti M, Beavo J. Biochemistry and physiology of cyclic nucleotide phosphodiesterases: essential components in cyclic nucleotide signaling. *Annu Rev Biochem.* 2007;76:481–511.
39. Mou H, Cote RH. The catalytic and GAF domains of the rod cGMP phosphodiesterase (PDE6) heterodimer are regulated by distinct regions of its inhibitory gamma subunit. *J Biol Chem.* 2001;276(29):27527–27534.
40. Yamazaki M, Li N, Bondarenko VA, Yamazaki RK, Baehr W, Yamazaki A. Binding of cGMP to GAF domains in amphibian rod photoreceptor cGMP phosphodiesterase (PDE). Identification of GAF domains in PDE alphabeta subunits and distinct domains in the PDE gamma subunit involved in stimulation of cGMP binding to GAF domains. *J Biol Chem.* 2002;277(43):40675–40686.
41. Cote RH. Cyclic guanosine 5'-monophosphate binding to regulatory GAF domains of photoreceptor phosphodiesterase. *Methods Mol Biol.* 2005;307:141–154.
42. Palczewski K, Kumasaka T, Hori T, et al. Crystal structure of rhodopsin: A G protein-coupled receptor. *Science.* 2000;289(5480):739–745.
43. Palczewski K, Hofmann KP, Baehr W. Rhodopsin--advances and perspectives. *Vision Res.* 2006;46(27):4425–4426.
44. Nathans J. Rhodopsin: structure, function, and genetics. *Biochemistry.* 1992;31(21):4923–4931.
45. Wald G, Brown PK. Human rhodopsin. *Science.* 1958;127(3292):222–226.
46. Hubbard R, Wald G. Cis-trans isomers of vitamin A and retinene in vision. *Science.* 1952;115(2977).
47. Wald G. The chemistry of rod vision. *Science.* 1951;113(2933):287–291.
48. Fung BK, Hurley JB, Stryer L. Flow of information in the light-triggered cyclic nucleotide cascade of vision. *Proc Natl Acad Sci U S A.* 1981;78(1):152–156.
49. Stryer L. Transducin and the cyclic GMP phosphodiesterase: amplifier proteins in vision. *Cold Spring Harb Symp Quant Biol.* 1983;48(Pt 2):841–852.
50. Baehr W, E.A. M, Swanson RJ, Applebury ML. Characterization of bovine rod outer segment G protein. *J Biol Chem.* 1982;257:6452–6460.
51. Kuhn H, Bennett N, Michel-Villaz M, Chabre M. Interactions between photoexcited rhodopsin and GTP-binding protein: kinetic and stoichiometric analyses from light-scattering changes. *Proc Natl Acad Sci U S A.* 1981;78(11):6873–6877.
52. Liebman PA, Pugh EN Jr. Gain, speed and sensitivity of GTP binding vs PDE activation in visual excitation. *Vision Res.* 1982;22:1475–1480.
53. Bigay J, Faurobert E, Franco M, Chabre M. Roles of lipid modifications of transducin subunits in their GDP-dependent association and membrane binding. *Biochemistry.* 1994;33(47):14081–14090.
54. Zhang Z, Melia TJ, He F, et al. How a G protein binds a membrane. *J Biol Chem.* 2004;279(32):33937–33945.
55. Neubert TA, Johnson RS, Hurley JB, Walsh KA. The rod transducin alpha subunit amino terminus is heterogeneously fatty acylated. *J Biol Chem.* 1992;267(26):18274–18277.
56. Yang Z, Wensel TG. N-myristoylation of the rod outer segment G protein, transducin, in cultured retinas. *J Biol Chem.* 1992;267(32):23197–23201.
57. Kokame K, Fukada Y, Yoshizawa T, Takao T, Shimonishi Y. Lipid modification at the N terminus of photoreceptor G-protein alpha-subunit. *Nature.* 1992;359(6397):749–752.
58. Kerov V, Rubin WW, Natochin M, Melling NA, Burns ME, Artemyev NO. N-terminal fatty acylation of transducin profoundly influences its localization and the kinetics of photoresponse in rods. *J Neurosci.* 2007;27(38):10270–10277.
59. Fukada Y, Takao T, Ohguro H, Yoshizawa T, Akino T, Shimonishi Y. Farnesylated gamma-subunit of photoreceptor G protein indispensable for GTP-binding. *Nature.* 1990;346:658–660.
60. Lai RK, Perez-Sala D, Canada FJ, Rando RR. The gamma subunit of transducin is farnesylated. *Proc Natl Acad Sci U S A.* 1990;87(19):7673–7677.
61. Cheng H, Parish CA, Gilbert BA, Rando RR. A novel endoprotease responsible for the specific cleavage of transducin gamma subunit. *Biochemistry.* 1995;34(51):16662–16671.
62. Baehr W. Membrane protein transport in photoreceptors: the function of PDEδ: the Proctor lecture. *Invest Ophthalmol Vis Sci.* 2014;55(12):8653–8666.
63. Zhang Z, He F, Constantine R, et al. Domain organization and conformational plasticity of the G protein effector, PDE6. *J Biol Chem.* 2015;290(28):17131–17132.
64. Wensel TG. Signal transducing membrane complexes of photoreceptor outer segments. *Vision Res.* 2008;48(20):2052–2061.
65. Cone RA. Rotational diffusion of rhodopsin in the visual receptor membrane. *Nat New Biol.* 1972;236(63):39–43.
66. Poo M, Cone RA. Lateral diffusion of rhodopsin in the photoreceptor membrane. *Nature.* 1974;247(441):438–441.
67. Wey CL, Cone RA, Edidin MA. Lateral diffusion of rhodopsin in photoreceptor cells measured by fluorescence photobleaching and recovery. *Biophys J.* 1981;33(2):225–232.
68. Liebman PA, Weiner HL, Drzymala RE. Lateral diffusion of visual pigment in rod disk membranes. *Methods Enzymol.* 1982;81:660–668.
69. Wang Q, Zhang X, Zhang L, et al. Activation-dependent hindrance of photoreceptor G protein diffusion by lipid microdomains. *J Biol Chem.* 2008;283(44):30015–30024.
70. Nielsen JC, Maude MB, Hughes H, Anderson RE. Rabbit photoreceptor outer segments contain high levels of docosapentaenoic acid. *Invest Ophthalmol Vis Sci.* 1986;27(2):261–264.
71. Kim JE, Tauber MJ, Mathies RA. Wavelength dependent cis-trans isomerization in vision. *Biochemistry.* 2001;40(46):13774–13778.
72. Applebury ML. Dynamic processes of visual transduction. *Vision Res.* 1984;24(11):1445–1454.

73. Imai H, Mizukami T, Imamoto Y, Shichida Y. Direct observation of the thermal equilibria among lumirhodopsin, metarhodopsin I, and metarhodopsin II in chicken rhodopsin. *Biochemistry*. 1994;33(47):14351–14358.

74. Lewis JW, van Kuijk FJ, Thorgeirsson TE, Kliger DS. Photolysis intermediates of human rhodopsin. *Biochemistry*. 1991;30(48):11372–11376.

75. Ramdas L, Disher RM, Wensel TG. Nucleotide exchange and cGMP phosphodiesterase activation by pertussis toxin inactivated transducin. *Biochemistry*. 1991;30(50):11637–11645.

76. Malinski JA, Wensel TG. Membrane stimulation of cGMP phosphodiesterase activation by transducin: comparison of phospholipid bilayers to rod outer segment membranes. *Biochemistry*. 1992;31(39):9502–9512.

77. Yau KW, Nakatani K. Light-induced reduction of cytoplasmic free calcium in retinal rod outer segment. *Nature*. 1985;313(6003):579–582.

78. Maeda T, Imanishi Y, Palczewski K. Rhodopsin phosphorylation: 30 years later. *Prog Retin Eye Res*. 2003;22(4):417–434.

79. Doan T, Mendez A, Detwiler PB, Chen J, Rieke F. Multiple phosphorylation sites confer reproducibility of the rod's single-photon responses. *Science*. 2006;313(5786):530–533.

80. Mendez A, Burns ME, Roca A, et al. Rapid and reproducible deactivation of rhodopsin requires multiple phosphorylation sites. *Neuron*. 2000;28(1):153–164.

81. Zhao X, Yokoyama K, Whitten ME, Huang J, Gelb MH, Palczewski K. A novel form of rhodopsin kinase from chicken retina and pineal gland. *FEBS Lett*. 1999;454(1-2):115–121.

82. Hisatomi O, Matsuda S, Satoh T, Kotaka S, Imanishi Y, Tokunaga F. A novel subtype of G-protein-coupled receptor kinase, GRK7, in teleost cone photoreceptors. *FEBS Lett*. 1998;424(3):159–164.

83. Anant JS, Fung BK. In vivo farnesylation of rat rhodopsin kinase. *Biochem Biophys Res Commun*. 1992;183(2):468–473.

84. Inglese J, Glickman JF, Lorenz W, Caron MG, Lefkowitz RJ. Isoprenylation of a protein kinase. Requirement of farnesylation/alpha-carboxyl methylation for full enzymatic activity of rhodopsin kinase. *J Biol Chem*. 1992;267(3):1422–1425.

85. Molday RS. ATP-binding cassette transporter ABCA4: molecular properties and role in vision and macular degeneration. *J Bioenerg Biomembr*. 2007;39(5-6):507–517.

86. Ahn J, Beharry S, Molday LL, Molday RS. Functional interaction between the two halves of the photoreceptor-specific ATP binding cassette protein ABCR (ABCA4). Evidence for a non-exchangeable ADP in the first nucleotide binding domain. *J Biol Chem*. 2003;278(41):39600–39608.

87. Gurevich VV, Gurevich EV, Cleghorn WM. Arrestins as multi-functional signaling adaptors. *Handb Exp Pharmacol*. 2008;186:15–37.

88. Palczewski K. Structure and functions of arrestins. *Protein Sci*. 1994;3(9):1355–1361.

89. Mendez A, Burns ME, Sokal I, et al. Role of guanylate cyclase-activating proteins (GCAPs) in setting the flash sensitivity of rod photoreceptors. *Proc Natl Acad Sci U S A*. 2001;98(17):9948–9953.

90. Burns ME, Mendez A, Chen J, Baylor DA. Dynamics of cyclic GMP synthesis in retinal rods. *Neuron*. 2002;36(1):81–91.

91. Dizhoor AM, Peshenko IV. Regulation of retinal membrane guanylyl cyclase (RetGC) by negative calcium feedback and RD3 protein. *Pflugers Arch*. 2021;473(9):1393–1410.

92. Koch KW, Stryer L. Highly cooperative feedback control of retinal rod guanylate cyclase by calcium ions. *Nature*. 1988;334(6177):64–66.

93. Gorczyca WA, Gray-Keller MP, Detwiler PB, Palczewski K. Purification and physiological evaluation of a guanylate cyclase activating protein from retinal rods. *Proc Natl Acad Sci U S A*. 1994;91(9):4014–4018.

94. Sokal I, Alekseev A, Palczewski K. Photoreceptor guanylate cyclase variants: cGMP production under control. *Acta Biochim Pol*. 2003;50(4):1075–1095.

95. Perrault I, Rozet JM, Calvas P, et al. Retinal-specific guanylate cyclase gene mutations in Leber's congenital amaurosis. *Nat Genet*. 1996;14(4):461–464.

96. Duda T, Koch KW. Retinal diseases linked with photoreceptor guanylate cyclase. *Mol Cell Biochem*. 2002;230(1-2):129–138.

97. Payne AM, Downes SM, Bessant DA, et al. A mutation in guanylate cyclase activator 1A (GUCA1A) in an autosomal dominant cone dystrophy pedigree mapping to a new locus on chromosome 6p21.1. *Hum Mol Genet*. 1998;7(2):273–277.

98. Howes KA, Pennesi ME, Sokal I, et al. GCAP1 rescues rod photoreceptor response in GCAP1/GCAP2 knockout mice. *Embo J*. 2002;21(7):1545–1554.

99. Krispel CM, Chen D, Melling N, et al. RGS expression rate-limits recovery of rod photoresponses. *Neuron*. 2006;51(3):409–416.

100. Pugh EN Jr. RGS expression level precisely regulates the duration of rod photoresponses. *Neuron*. 2006;51(4):391–393.

101. He W, Cowan CW, Wensel TG. RGS9, a GTPase accelerator for phototransduction. *Neuron*. 1998;20(1):95–102.

102. Cowan CW, Fariss RN, Sokal I, Palczewski K, Wensel TG. High expression levels in cones of RGS9, the predominant GTPase accelerating protein of rods. *Proc Natl Acad Sci USA*. 1998;95(9):5351–5356.

103. Watson AJ, Aragay AM, Slepak VZ, Simon MI. A novel form of the G protein beta subunit Gbeta5 is specifically expressed in the vertebrate retina. *J Biol Chem*. 1996;271:28154–28160.

104. Makino ER, Handy JW, Li T, Arshavsky VY. The GTPase activating factor for transducin in rod photoreceptors is the complex between RGS9 and type 5 G protein beta subunit. *Proc Natl Acad Sci U S A*. 1999;96(5):1947–1952.

105. Snow BE, Krumins AM, Brothers GM, et al. A G protein gamma subunit-like domain shared between RGS11 and other RGS proteins specifies binding to Gbeta5 subunits. *Proc Natl Acad Sci U S A*. 1998;95(22):13307–13312.

106. Rodiek RW. *The First Steps in Seeing*. Sunderland, MA: Sinauer Associates, Inc; 1998.

107. Pepperberg DR, Cornwall MC, Kahlert M, et al. Light-dependent delay in the falling phase of the retinal rod photoresponse. *Vis Neurosci*. 1992;8(1):9–18.

108. Nikonov S, Engheta N, Pugh EN Jr. Kinetics of recovery of the dark-adapted salamander rod photoresponse. *J Gen Physiol*. 1998;111(1):7–37.

109. Ames A 3rd, Walseth TF, Heyman RA, Barad M, Graeff RM, Goldberg ND. Light-induced increases in cGMP metabolic flux correspond with electrical responses of photoreceptors. *J Biol Chem*. 1986;261(28):13034–13042.

110. Panico J, Parkes JH, Liebman PA. The effect of GDP on rod outer segment G-protein interactions. *J Biol Chem*. 1990;265(31):18922–18927.

111. Hurley JB. Retina Metabolism and Metabolism in the Pigmented Epithelium: A Busy Intersection. *Annu Rev Vis Sci*. 2021;7:665–692.

112. Sampath AP, Baylor DA. Molecular mechanism of spontaneous pigment activation in retinal cones. *Biophys J*. 2002;83(1):184–193.

113. Kefalov VJ, Estevez ME, Kono M, et al. Breaking the covalent bond--a pigment property that contributes to desensitization in cones. *Neuron*. 2005;46(6):879–890.

114. Lamb TD. Evolution of the genes mediating phototransduction in rod and cone photoreceptors. *Prog Retin Eye Res*. 2019:100823.

115. Wald G, Brown PK. The molar extinction of rhodopsin. *J Gen Physiol*. 1953;37:189–200.

116. Wald G. Molecular basis of visual excitation. *Science*. 1968;162:230–239.

117. Fasick JI, Lee N, Oprian DD. Spectral tuning in the human blue cone pigment. *Biochemistry*. 1999;38(36):11593–11596.

118. Kochendoerfer GG, Lin SW, Sakmar TP, Mathies RA. How color visual pigments are tuned. *Trends Biochem Sci*. 1999;24(8):300–305.

119. Lin SW, Kochendoerfer GG, Carroll KS, Wang D, Mathies RA, Sakmar TP. Mechanisms of spectral tuning in blue cone visual pigments. Visible and raman spectroscopy of blue-shifted rhodopsin mutants. *J Biol Chem*. 1998;273(38):24583–24591.

120. Fasick JI, Applebury ML, Oprian DD. Spectral tuning in the mammalian short-wavelength sensitive cone pigments. *Biochemistry*. 2002;41(21):6860–6865.

121. Merbs SL, Nathans J. Role of hydroxyl-bearing amino acids in differentially tuning the absorption spectra of the human red and green cone pigments. *Photochem Photobiol*. 1993;58(5):706–710.

122. Fasick JI, Robinson PR. Spectral-tuning mechanisms of marine mammal rhodopsins and correlations with foraging depth. *Vis Neurosci*. 2000;17(5):781–788.

123. Zhang X, Wensel TG, Kraft TW. GTPase regulators and photoresponses in cones of the eastern chipmunk. *J Neurosci*. 2003;23(4):1287–1297.

124. Tachibanaki S, Tsushima S, Kawamura S. Low amplification and fast visual pigment phosphorylation as mechanisms characterizing cone photoresponses. *Proc Natl Acad Sci U S A*. 2001;98(24):14044–14049.

125. Tachibanaki S, Arinobu D, Shimauchi-Matsukawa Y, Tsushima S, Kawamura S. Highly effective phosphorylation by G protein-coupled receptor kinase 7 of light-activated visual pigment in cones. *Proc Natl Acad Sci U S A*. 2005;102(26):9329–9334.

126. Marcink TC, Simoncic JA, An B, et al. MT1-MMP Binds membranes by opposite tips of its beta propeller to position it for pericellular proteolysis. *Structure*. 2019;27(2):281–292. e6.

127. Li J, Edwards PC, Burghammer M, Villa C, Schertler GF. Structure of bovine rhodopsin in a trigonal crystal form. *J Mol Biol*. 2004;343(5):1409–1438.

128. Gao Y, Hu H, Ramachandran S, Erickson JW, Cerione RA, Skiniotis G. Structures of the rhodopsin-transducin complex: Insights into G-protein activation. *Mol Cell*. 2019;75(4):781–790. e3.

129. Gulati S, Jastrzebska B, Banerjee S, et al. Photocyclic behavior of rhodopsin induced by an atypical isomerization mechanism. *Proc Natl Acad Sci U S A*. 2017;114(13):E2608–E2615.

130. Chen Q, Plasencia M, Li Z, et al. Structures of rhodopsin in complex with G-protein-coupled receptor kinase 1. *Nature*. 2021;595(7868):600–605.

131. Kang Y, Zhou XE, Gao X, et al. Crystal structure of rhodopsin bound to arrestin by femtosecond X-ray laser. *Nature*. 2015;523(7562):561–567.

132. Noel JP, Hamm HE, Sigler PB. The 2.2 A crystal structure of transducin-alpha complexed with GTP gamma S [see comments]. *Nature*. 1993;366(6456):654–663.

133. Lambright DG, Noel JP, Hamm HE, Sigler PB. Structural determinants for activation of the alpha-subunit of a heterotrimeric G protein [see comments]. *Nature*. 1994;369(6482):621–628.

134. Sondek J, Bohm A, Lambright DG, Hamm HE, Sigler PB. Crystal structure of a G_A protein βγ dimer at 2.1 A resolution. *Nature*. 1996;379:369–374.

135. Slep KC, Kercher MA, He W, Cowan CW, Wensel TG, Sigler PB. Structural determinants for regulation of phosphodiesterase by a G protein at 2.0 A. *Nature*. 2001;409(6823):1071–1077.

136. Cheever ML, Snyder JT, Gershburg S, Siderovski DP, Harden TK, Sondek J. Crystal structure of the multifunctional Gbeta5-RGS9 complex. *Nat Struct Mol Biol*. 2008;15(2):155–162.

137. Eagle RC Jr, Lucier AC, Bernardino VB Jr, Yanoff M. Retinal pigment epithelial abnormalities in fundus flavimaculatus: a light and electron microscopic study. *Ophthalmology*. 1980;87(12):1189–1200.

138. Birnbach CD, Jarvelainen M, Possin DE, Milam AH. Histopathology and immuno-cytochemistry of the neurosensory retina in fundus flavimaculatus. *Ophthalmology*. 1994;101(7):1211–1219.

139. Hartong DT, Pott JW, Kooijman AC. Six patients with bradyopsia (slow vision): clinical features and course of the disease. *Ophthalmology*. 2007;114(12):2323–2331.

140. Hagstrom SA, Zhang K, Baehr W, et al. Comprehensive mutation screen in the RGS9 gene in 558 patients with inherited retinal degenerations. *Invest Ophthal Vis Sci*. 2001;42:S646.

141. Nishiguchi KM, Sandberg MA, Kooijman AC, et al. Defects in RGS9 or its anchor protein R9AP in patients with slow photoreceptor deactivation. *Nature*. 2004;427(6969):75–78.

142. Weleber RG. Inherited and orphan retinal diseases: phenotypes, genotypes, and probable treatment groups. *Retina*. 2005;25(8 Suppl):S4–S7.

143. Dryja TP, McGee TL, Reichel E, et al. A point mutation of the rhodopsin gene in one form of retinitis pigmentosa. *Nature*. 1990;343(6256):364–366.

144. Keats BJ, Savas S. Genetic heterogeneity in Usher syndrome. *Am J Med Genet A*. 2004;130A(1):13–16.

19

Photoresponses of Rods and Cones

Peter R. MacLeish and Clint L. Makino

Retinal rods and cones are highly specialized neurons that transform light into an electrical signal (see Chapter 18) and provide the sensory input for vision. In contrast to most neurons, rods and cones maintain a relatively depolarized membrane potential at rest (in darkness), and when stimulated (by light) they decrease Na$^+$ entry by closing ion channels. The resultant hyperpolarization closes Ca^{2+} channels at the synapse, and the ensuing fall in intracellular Ca^{2+} reduces an ongoing vesicular release of the neurotransmitter glutamate onto second-order neurons. This chapter describes the signaling properties of rods and cones that subserve vision in dim and bright light, respectively. An overview of the voltage changes induced by light will be followed by a description of the properties of the photocurrent and then an explanation of how voltage-gated inner segment conductances shape the final voltage response. For readers interested in the underlying molecular designs and mechanisms, summaries on ion channels and exchangers are included. Although the retinal photoreceptors of all vertebrates operate similarly, there are some qualitative, as well as quantitative, differences. Therefore, wherever possible, we will focus on primate photoreceptors.

PHOTOVOLTAGE RESPONSE TO FLASHES

In darkness, rods and cones maintain a membrane potential near −40 mV.[1] When stimulated by flashes, rods and cones do not "fire" action potentials but instead respond with slow graded hyperpolarizations (Fig. 19.1)[2] that in some cells exceed 25 mV (e.g.,[3]). The hyperpolarization then spreads passively to the synapse. In comparing rod and cone responses, the latter are considerably faster and require many more photons. Photoisomerization of 75 rhodopsins gives rise to a half-maximal response in rods, whereas in cones it takes close to 1000 photoisomerizations (estimated from [1,4]).

The amplitude of the single photon response in rods is about a millivolt, a few percent of the maximal response.[1,3,5] The time to a peak of approximately 200 ms is relatively slow, considering that Olympic sprinter Usain Bolt covered more than two meters in the same time span. The recovery to baseline is even slower and may take over a second for completion. The slow time course of the single photon response provided compelling evidence for an internal second messenger(s) and for amplification steps in the signaling pathway. The duration can be specified as an integration time, calculated by dividing the response integral by the peak amplitude. For rods, the integration time of the quantal response is several hundred milliseconds. Although cones are less sensitive than rods, they too "respond" to single photons, but the amplitude of their quantal response is much smaller and does not emerge from the baseline noise.[1] The cone response is faster, with a time to peak of 30 ms and integration time of only 25 ms. These values are approximate because responses of foveal cones are slower than those in the periphery, and responses of blue cones are slightly slower than those of red and green cones.[4,6–8] Response kinetics and sensitivity are intimately linked, and the relationship is discussed further in the chapter. The waveforms of rod and cone flash responses change with flash strength. Responses peak sooner and the initial recovery is faster as the flash strength increases, but with responses greater than half maximal, recovery stalls to a plateau before the final recovery. In cones, the recovery overshoots the baseline before the final recovery, whereas in rods, the plateau slowly returns to baseline without an overshoot.

Background light attenuates the response to a flash as the cells adapt (for discussions of the underlying mechanisms, see Chapters 18 and 20). The dim flash response reduces in size twofold during exposure for several tens of seconds to backgrounds producing approximately 150 photoisomerizations per second in rods and approximately 8700 photoisomerizations per second in cones.[6] Background light quickens flash responses in rods but has little effect on response kinetics in cones (ignoring the rod component of the response in cones communicated electrotonically, see Chapter 22).

PHOTOCURRENT RESPONSE TO FLASHES

The photon response derives from a decrease in the number of open cyclic nucleotide-gated (CNG) channels that changes the flow of ions across the plasma membrane and shifts the transmembrane potential to more negative voltages. CNG channels are located exclusively in the outer segments of rods and cones. In darkness, a small fraction of the channels are in the open state, allowing an influx of cations. The intracellular concentration of Na$^+$ is low, whereas that of K$^+$ is high relative to the extracellular space, owing to the action of Na$^+$/K$^+$-ATPases in the inner segment. Thus, Na$^+$ and also some Ca^{2+} ions flow in through the CNG channels in the outer segment. K$^+$ ions flow out through leak and voltage-gated ion channels in the inner segment to complete the electrical circuit, which is referred to as the "dark" or circulating current (Fig. 19.2). Light absorbed by a visual pigment molecule in the outer segment closes CNG channels in an annulus of plasma membrane surrounding the site of photon absorption on the disk membrane.[9–11]

When two photons are absorbed, it is unlikely that both absorptions occur in close proximity, so the response to each photon is generated independently and they summate. In other words, dim flashes lie within a linear operating range, wherein the response simply scales with the flash strength. However, with increasing numbers of photon absorptions, local effects begin to overlap, so fewer channels are closed per photon absorbed. With enough photons, all of the channels are closed, and the rod response is maximal (Fig. 19.3). Hence, the normalized response grows with flash strength according to a saturating exponential function[10]:

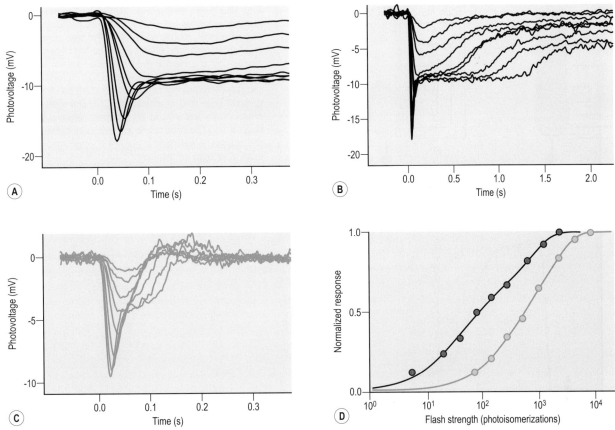

Fig. 19.1 Slower voltage responses in a rod (**A**, **B** on two different time scales) than in a cone (**C**) to flashes. Photovoltage is the change in membrane potential induced by a flash, given at time zero. (**D**) The stimulus-response relation of the cone *(green circles)* is to the right of that of the rod *(black circles)*, reflecting the lower sensitivity of the cone. Each response has been divided by the maximal, saturating response for that cell. (Panels A and B from Schneeweis DM, Schnapf JL. Photovoltage of rods and cones in the macaque retina. *Science.* 1995;268:1053–1056. Reprinted with permission from AAAS, copyright 1995; Panels C and D – Schnapf JL, University of California at San Francisco & David Schneeweis, Deputy Scientific Director, National Eye Institute, NIH.)

$$r/r_{max} = 1 - \exp(-k_f i) \qquad \textbf{(Eq. 19.1)}$$

where r is the photocurrent response amplitude, r_{max} is the amplitude of the maximal saturating response, i is flash strength, k_f is a constant equal to $\ln(2)/i_{0.5}$, and $i_{0.5}$ is the flash strength giving rise to a half-maximal response. The $i_{0.5}$ for rods produces 30 to 70 photoisomerizations on average,[12–14] whereas that for cones produces approximately 10 times as many photoisomerizations.[15]

As is the case with photovoltage, photocurrent responses speed up with flash strength, although the effect is less pronounced in cones.[12,15] Responses are faster in cones than in rods (note the difference in time scales in Fig. 19.3A,C) and have a marked undershoot (although the undershoot is controversial, compare [16,17]). However, the photovoltage and photocurrent responses of rods and cones are not mirror images of each other. At least for red and green cones, the photovoltage response peaks slightly sooner than the photocurrent response, even for dim flashes. For rods, the dim flash photovoltage response peaks at about the same time as the photocurrent response, but the recovery is faster for the latter. In both rods and cones, there is a "nose" in the photovoltage response to brighter flashes (Fig. 19.1 A,C) that is absent from the photocurrent response (Fig. 19.3 A,C).[3,6] The basis for the nose is described further.

Once the flash is bright enough to close all the CNG channels, more light cannot produce a larger response, but instead, the duration of the photocurrent response increments with the natural logarithm of the flash strength (Fig. 19.3D). The basis for this behavior is that a single molecular process, namely the shutoff of transducin ([18]; see Chapter 18), which has a stochastic, exponential time course,[19,20] dominates the recovery from phototransduction activation in rods. The slope of the saturation function or "Pepperberg Plot" yields the dominant time constant of about approximately 0.2 s[21] (a similar value has been reported by many others for murine rods). The rate limiting step(s) in the recovery of the cone response has not been firmly established, but pigment quench is likely to contribute[22] because transducin shutoff may be an order of magnitude faster than in rods.[16,17]

MODULATION OF THE FLASH RESPONSE BY BICARBONATE

Bicarbonate is ubiquitous in the body and serves important roles in acid-base regulation and in providing a means to rid the body of metabolic CO_2 waste. In rods and cones, bicarbonate enlarges the dark current and accelerates flash response recovery[10,12,23–25] by stimulating the membrane guanylate cyclases in a Ca^{2+}-dependent fashion.[26] Rods and

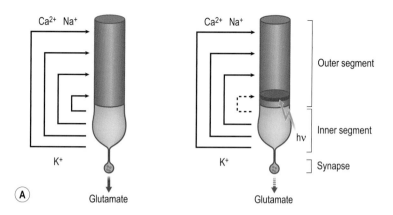

Fig. 19.2 The dark current. (**A**) Light suppresses the entry of Na⁺ and a lesser amount of Ca²⁺ into the outer segment in a ring of plasma membrane around the disc containing photoexcited rhodopsin (*darkened band*). The rod hyperpolarizes, which closes Ca²⁺ channels at the synapse and attenuates the release of neurotransmitter. (**B**) The inward Na⁺ current in this rod, plotted downward by convention, was −13.3 pA. A saturating flash, given at time zero, closes all the CNG channels and completely shuts down the inward Na⁺ current. After a while, channels reopen and the membrane current is restored. For simplicity, the change in membrane current is often measured as photocurrent, shown on the *right*.

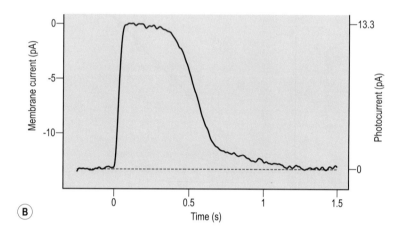

cones take up bicarbonate through anion channels and transporters located at their synapses.[27–30] Red and green cones, but not blue cones and rods, also synthesize bicarbonate internally because they express carbonic anhydrase.[31] Bicarbonate diffuses throughout the cell, eventually exiting from the outer segments by way of a bicarbonate/chloride exchanger.[26,30,32]

DETECTION OF SINGLE PHOTONS

Rods count single photons.[33] To do so, they must minimize noise and generate highly amplified, reproducible quantal responses. Amplification is achieved by cascading several enzymatic reactions (see Chapter 18). Each chemical reaction takes time, hence the decrement in the dark current after photon absorption is delayed by a few milliseconds. Then the photocurrent response rises to a peak amplitude of 0.1 to 1 pA (this wide range is likely due to issues associated with experimental measurement and to species differences) approximately 200 ms later, reflecting the suppression of the dark current by a few percent.[12,13,34] With the cascade working as fast as it can, the size of the response is determined by when shutoff and recovery processes kick in. In rods, hundreds of CNG channels are closed during the single photon response. Na⁺ ions traverse the channel at a rate of approximately 10^4 per second (reviewed in [35]), so one photon blocks the entry of a million Na⁺ ions. Responses to brighter flashes in rods and in cones appear with a shorter delay and rise more steeply because many more photoexcited rhodopsin molecules are activating the phototransduction machinery. In cones, the "single photon response" shuts off in 50 ms or less at a time when it has only reached an amplitude of a few tens of fA.[15,17]

It is imperative that single photon responses do not vary in size or duration because if they did, the rod would be unable to distinguish one large, slow quantal response from two or more small, brief quantal responses occurring close together in time. When stimulated by dim flashes, the rod does not respond the same way every time, but most of the unpredictability arises from the Poisson distribution of photon absorptions, rather than from single photon response variability. Whenever the rod does respond, the amplitude is quantized (Fig. 19.4A). The coefficient of variation of the rod response, defined as the quotient of the standard deviation divided by the mean amplitude, has a low value of approximately 0.2.[33,36–38]

In darkness, rods exhibit two physiologic kinds of electrical fluctuations in the current baseline: discrete noise and continuous noise (Fig. 19.4B).[12,39] Discrete noise is produced by thermal isomerizations of rhodopsin. Although rhodopsin has a half-life of approximately 400 years at body temperature,[12] a rod contains so many copies (around a hundred million) that one spontaneously activates every couple of minutes. Continuous noise springs mainly from the spontaneous activity of phosphodiesterase (PDE)[40] and is much more prevalent than discrete events but typically has a lower amplitude. The continuous noise amplitude distribution is approximately Gaussian, so occasionally there is a single photon response-like event. However, such events are inconsequential because they take place 10 times less frequently than the thermal isomerizations of rhodopsin. Although blue cone pigment may be even more thermally stable than rhodopsin, red and green cone visual pigments are far less stable.[15,41–43] Regardless, the overabundance of continuous noise, arising from gating transitions of the CNG channel, as well as from spontaneous activations of transducin and/or PDE, coupled with the low gain of phototransduction, preclude photon counting in cones.[44]

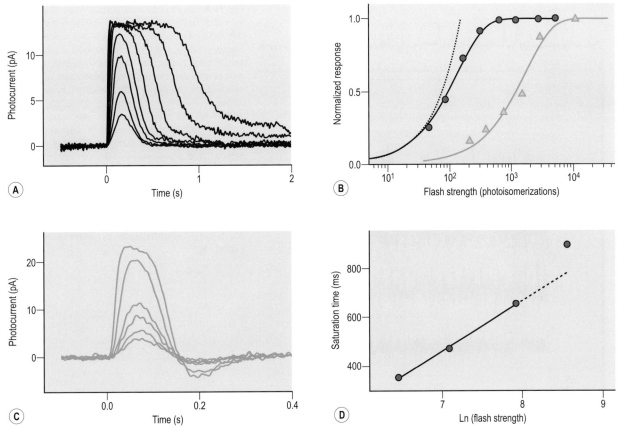

Fig. 19.3 Current responses of a human rod (**A**) and a cone (**C**) to flashes. (**B**) The stimulus-response relations of the rod (*black circles*) and cone *(green triangles)* follow Eq. 19.1 *(black and green lines)*. The dotted line shows a linear relation on semilogarithmic coordinates for comparison. (**D**) Saturation times for the rod in (**A**), measured from midflash to 25% recovery. The line passing through the initial points has a slope of 205 ms and has been extended with a *dashed line*. (Panel A from Kraft TW, Schneeweis DM, Schnapf JL. Visual transduction in human rod photoreceptors. *J Physiol (Lond)*. 1993;464:747–765. Reproduced with permission from Blackwell Publishing. Panel B contains results from Kraft TW, Schneeweis DM, Schnapf JL. Visual transduction in human rod photoreceptors. *J Physiol (Lond)*. 1993;464:747–765, and unpublished results from T.W. Kraft, University of Alabama. Panel C from Kraft TW, Neitz J, Neitz M. Spectra of human L cones. *Vis Res*. 1998;38:3663–3670. Panel D courtesy of Timothy W. Kraft (University of Alabama), Julie L. Schnapf (University of California at San Francisco) and David Schneeweis (Deputy Scientific Director, National Eye Institute, NIH).)

Thermal isomerizations of rhodopsin confound the detection of very dim light because responses to real photons cannot be distinguished from "responses" to virtual ones. To guard against false alarms, the visual system relies on coincidence detection. A single photon response in one rod does not suffice for vision; a few rods in a small cluster within the retina must each generate a single photon response within a certain period of time before a flash is "seen."[45] The temporal requirement is specified by the integration time of the response. Thus, shortening the integration time reduces false alarms but detracts from sensitivity of the system. This consideration also applies when rods and cones respond to steps of light. The integration time for rods is approximately 300 ms,[12,13,34] whereas for cones it is approximately 20 ms (segment preceding undershoot[15]).

Clearly, rods are well suited for single photon detection. Oddly though, rods sometimes generate single photon responses that are truly aberrant.[12,46] For reasons unknown, one photoexcited rhodopsin out of several hundred fails to shut off properly[47,48] and gives rise to a twofold larger than average response that can last for a very, very long time (Fig. 19.5). Aberrant response durations are exponentially distributed with a mean value of about 4 s, but some last for tens of seconds. Aberrant responses have little impact on photon counting owing to their rarity and are not "seen" because the visual system requires several rods signaling the presence of a photon. However, they do improve sensitivity to steady light and by prolonging the recovery after exposure to bright light (flashes and steps), they leave rods vulnerable to saturation (see Box 19.1).

PHOTOCURRENT RESPONSE TO STEADY LIGHT

The rod response to dim, steady light summates individual single photon responses.[12] But with brighter light, adaptation within the outer segment causes the step responses to fall short of the amplitude expected from a simple saturation behavior ([34,49,50]; see Chapter 20). Midrange responses droop as additional adaptational mechanisms with a slower time course reduce the cascade gain and cause the stimulus-response relation to rise even more gently (Fig. 19.6). Light producing about 100 to 600 photoisomerizations per second decreases the dark current in darkness by 50% in rods of various primates.[12,34,51] In contrast, the peak of the cone response to steps does almost obey simple saturation.[15] A hundred milliseconds in the light later, however,

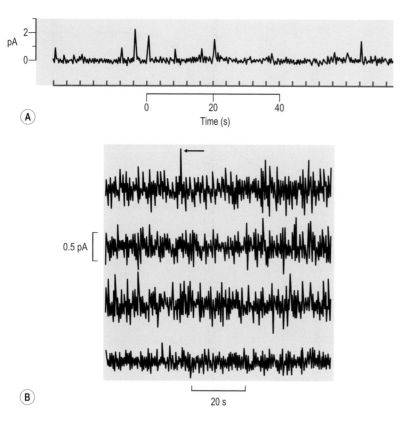

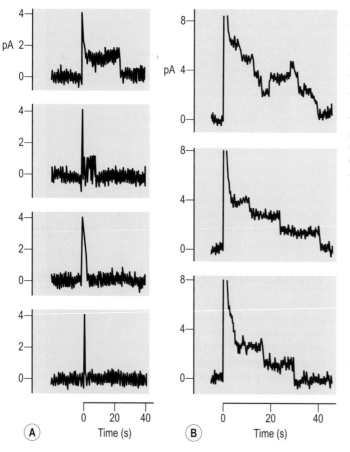

Fig. 19.4 Single photon responses of a primate rod. (**A**) With very dim flashes *(upward tick marks in the lower trace for the flash monitor)*, a response is not present in every trial because sometimes no photon gets absorbed. Other trials produce responses the amplitudes of which are multiples of the unitary response, dependent upon the number of photons absorbed. (**B**) Discrete noise events (e.g., *arrow in top trace*), resembling single photon responses, appear sporadically in darkness after spontaneous activations of individual rhodopsins. In addition, a continuous, lower amplitude noise component arises from basal PDE activity *(top three traces)*. Both noise components disappear in bright light after closure of all of the CNG channels *(bottom trace)*, leaving only the instrumental noise in the recording. (From Baylor DA, Nunn BJ, Schnapf JL. The photocurrent, noise and spectral sensitivity of rods of the monkey *Macaca fascicularis*. J Physiol (Lond). 1984; 357:575–607. Reproduced by permission of Blackwell Publishing.)

Fig. 19.5 Aberrant responses in rods. (**A**) In the four responses to a flash eliciting about 250 photoisomerizations, an aberrant response component can be seen at late times in the top three traces. The appearance of an aberrant response after a flash, as well as its duration, is random. The aberrant response in the top trace persists for more than 20 s. The second trace does not initially contain an aberrant response. Then one appears and recovers, only to reappear before shutting off permanently. (**B**) In these three responses to a flash over 10 times brighter than that in (**A**), multiple individual aberrant responses add together to create protracted, stair-cased recoveries. The peaks of the responses are not shown. (From Baylor DA, Nunn BJ, Schnapf JL. The photocurrent, noise and spectral sensitivity of rods of the monkey *Macaca fascicularis*. J Physiol (Lond). 1984;357:575–607. Reproduced by permission of Blackwell Publishing.)

BOX 19.1 Diseases caused by hyperactive signaling

Excessive phototransduction cascade activity in photoreceptors can interfere with vision and lead to retinal disease (reviewed in [60]). For example, mutations that interfere with the normal shutoff of rhodopsin by targeting rhodopsin kinase (see Chapter 18) can cause a form of night blindness known as Oguchi disease. Mutant mouse rods lacking rhodopsin kinase generate aberrant single photon responses like those shown in Fig. 19.5 for every rhodopsin isomerization. Cones are only mildly affected in the disease,[61] because they express a second type of rhodopsin kinase.[62,63] Patients with defects in the nuclear receptor NR2E3 develop enhanced S cone syndrome in which there is a higher prevalence of blue cones in the retina at the expense of red and green cones.[64] Very interestingly, the blue cones in these patients fail to express either type of rhodopsin kinase. Hence, flash responses of their blue cones (but not red or green cones) take an abnormally long time to recover.[16]

Mutations in arrestin, the protein normally responsible for quenching photoexcited rhodopsin's activity, can also cause Oguchi disease (see Chapter 18). Flash responses from rods of mutant, arrestin knockout mice are very prolonged (Fig. 19.8). Since longer lasting responses enhance absolute sensitivity, it might at first seem surprising that the mutations in either rhodopsin kinase or arrestin should lead to night blindness. The problem is that the mutant rods saturate at very low light levels and then take an inordinately long period of time and much dimmer conditions to recover from saturation. In theory, Oguchi patients with rhodopsin kinase or arrestin mutations might actually see better than normal persons under the dimmest conditions when given adequate time for dark adaptation. Photopic vision is largely spared because cones express a unique arrestin.[65,66]

Mutations in either RGS9 or R9AP can sabotage the timely shutoff of transducin (see Chapter 18). Because these two proteins are used in rods and cones, there is night blindness and a problem with daytime vision. The ability of cones to light adapt enables them to escape saturation, so photopic vision is still possible. But long-lasting photoresponses translate into a disturbing persistence in sensation, and the person has difficulty following moving objects and adjusting to luminance changes, a condition termed bradyopsia.[67]

Genetic defects in RPE65, the isomerase that converts all-*trans* to 11-*cis* retinal (see Chapter 13), can prevent the de novo synthesis of rhodopsin. The persistent presence of catalytically active apo-opsin (rhodopsin lacking 11-*cis* retinal is essentially equivalent to bleached rhodopsin) gives rise to Leber congenital amaurosis, an especially severe form of retinal degeneration. RPE65 knockout mouse rods exist in an inescapable state of light adaptation, with greatly attenuated dark current and smaller, faster flash responses (Fig. 19.9).

considered to be purely photopic,[54] and it seems likely that human rods share that capacity.

Light that is bright enough to bleach a significant fraction of visual pigment causes rods to behave for a period as if they were being exposed to a virtual, "equivalent light" that lingers after the light is removed (reviewed in[55]). Rods adapt to the equivalent light with a reduction in dark current and accelerated flash response kinetics, as well as a profound loss of flash sensitivity exceeding that expected from the decrease in photon capture (e.g.,[56]). It turns out that bleached rhodopsin constitutively activates the phototransduction cascade. Although the activity of a single bleached rhodopsin is minuscule, the summated activity of hundreds of millions of bleached rhodopsin molecules is substantial. The equivalent light fades as visual pigment regenerates (see Chapter 13 and Box 19.1). Dark current after full bleach recovers halfway in 15 min and is fully restored in approximately 25 min.[51] Cones are not impaired in this way by bleaching[15,57]; their bleached pigment seems to be inactive (although the situation is not yet clear for bleached blue cone pigment, compare[58]). That means that when very bright light is turned on, cones may saturate, but they actually manage to recover circulating current during the exposure as loss of some of their visual pigment by bleaching lowers the ongoing rate of photon capture. Even after extensive bleaching, cones regain their full dark current and the reduction in sensitivity scales in proportion to the loss in photon capture.[15,57,59] In the intact eye, cone pigment regeneration is faster than in rods, with full sensitivity returning after complete bleach within minutes. Therefore, whereas cones lack the absolute sensitivity of rods, they are better equipped to rapidly adapt over a wide range of brighter light intensities.

ACTION SPECTRA OF RODS AND CONES

Rods and cones respond to a wide range of wavelengths (Fig. 19.10), their action spectra being determined by the spectral absorptions of the visual pigment they express. For a given number of photons, the response amplitude varies with wavelength because the probability of absorption by the visual pigment varies with wavelength. The response itself to a photoisomerization is independent of wavelength. Rods respond maximally to a wavelength of approximately 493 nm (blue-green light).[12,13] There are three types of cones, commonly referred to as blue, green, and red with maxima near 430 nm (violet light), 530 nm (green light), and 560 nm (greenish-orange light), respectively ([68,69] but see Box 19.2) (Fig. 19.11). Since these cone names do not correspond to the colors of the maxima in every case, many prefer the designations short-wavelength sensitive or S, middle-wavelength sensitive or M, and long-wavelength sensitive or L.

CNG CHANNEL AND SODIUM/POTASSIUM/CALCIUM EXCHANGER

Ions move across the outer segment plasma membrane by two principal means: a CNG channel and a sodium/potassium/calcium exchanger. CNG channels are heterotetramers consisting of CNGA1 and CNGB1 subunits (Fig. 19.12) in a ratio of 3:1 in rods[71–73] and CNGA3 and CNGB3 subunits in a ratio of 3:1 in cones[74], (see Box 19.3). Although CNG channels are members of the same superfamily as voltage-gated K$^+$ channels, they are only mildly voltage-dependent in their gating (reviewed in [75]). Instead, CNG channels in rods and cones are directly gated by cGMP.[76,77] Cyclic AMP also works, but with a fiftyfold higher $K_{0.5}$, reflecting the reduced affinity of the channel for cAMP and the reduced efficacy in opening once cAMP has bound.[78] Whereas other ligand-gated ion channels in the body desensitize in the continued presence of

cone responses begin to droop as they too adapt. For dim steps, the droop reduces the amplitude to less than half that at the peak. The initial droop is typically larger and faster in cones than in rods.

In steady light, incremental flashes give rise to responses in rods that are smaller (Fig. 19.7) and recover more rapidly than in darkness, another manifestation of light adaptation ([12–14,34,49,50]; see Chapter 20). Flash response kinetics change very little with background light in primate cones, differing in this respect from cones of cold-blooded vertebrates.[15] Light producing a few hundred photoisomerizations per second reduces flash sensitivity to half its value in darkness in rods,[12,13,34,51] where the value increases slowly over time in the light.[52,53] Adaptation is powerful in cones, for which 10,000 or more photoisomerizations per second reduce sensitivity twofold.[6,15] Mammalian rods were thought to adapt over several log units of background light intensity before saturating.[34,49,50] However, recent studies found that mouse rods slowly adapt over tens of minutes to light levels previously

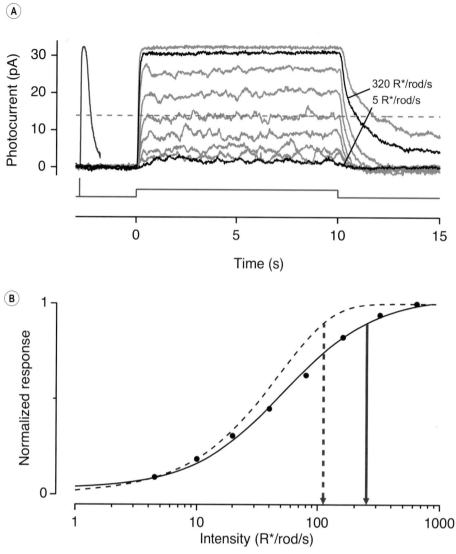

Fig. 19.6 Adaptation of a primate rod to steady light. (**A**) The response to a saturating flash is shown with the red trace. The Poisson nature of light absorption causes bumpiness in the responses to dim steps despite averaging. Midrange responses droop as the rod adapts. At the two highest intensities, both the droop and the bumpiness are compressed as the rod saturates so the traces become smoother. (**B**) In the response vs intensity relations for 12 primate rods measured after 9-10 seconds of light exposure, the continuous, vertical, red line shows the intensity eliciting a 90% maximal response. The dashed line plots the saturating exponential that would obtain in the absence of adaptation: $r/r_{max} = 1-exp(-k_s \, I)$, where k_s is a constant and I is the intensity of the step. The vertical, dashed red line indicates that the intensity that would elicit a response that is 90% maximal would be shifted to the left. Thus, lacking adaptation, rods would saturate at a lower intensity. (From Grimes WN, Baudin J, Azevedo AW, Rieke F. Range, routing and kinetics of rod signaling in primate retina. *eLife*. 2018;7:e38281. https://doi.org/10.7554/eLife.38281. Modified under Creative Commons CC0 https://creativecommons.org/share-your-work/public-domain/cc0/.)

their ligand, the CNG channel does not have any intrinsic mechanisms of desensitization and thus steadily monitors the [cGMP] in darkness.[78–80] Channel sensitivity is subject to modulation under different conditions, for example, during light adaptation by calmodulin or a similar calcium-binding protein (see Chapter 20), by phosphorylation and by diacylglycerol.

The rod CNG channel allows many different cations to pass: Ca^{2+}, Mg^{2+}, Na^+, and even K^+. Permeability is greatest for Ca^{2+}, but under normal conditions, Na^+ carries approximately 80% of the current while Ca^{2+} carries 15% to 20%[81,82] because the extracellular concentration of Na^+ is 10 times higher than that of Ca^{2+}. Mg^{2+} influx comprises a few percent of the dark current. The proportion of current carried by Ca^{2+} is twice greater through the cone channel because of its higher Ca^{2+} to Na^+ permeability ratio.[83,84] Nevertheless, divalents are critical to the physiology of both rods and cones (see further in section and Chapters 18 and 20).

For fast responsivity to increases in [cGMP], it would be advantageous for the CNG channel to avidly bind cGMP. However, the channel would release cGMP too slowly and fail to detect decreases in cGMP rapidly. As a compromise, the channel has a fairly high K_m for cGMP (i.e., moderately low sensitivity), of the order of $10\,\mu M$.[76,77] The channel subunits work together in such a way that cGMP binding affinity increases, with each binding of cGMP causing channel opening to be steeply dependent on ligand concentration (Fig. 19.12D). Cooperativity is one of Nature's ways of building a biologic switch.

Cyclic GMP binding stabilizes the open state of the channel, so by the law of microscopic reversibility, cGMP unbinds best from the closed state. Therefore, to be constantly vigilant for a decrease in [cGMP], the channel reverts incessantly to the closed state (reviewed in [35]). The channel can then respond to changes in [cGMP] on a time scale that is considerably faster than the photoresponse. However, flickering makes the channel extremely noisy (Fig. 19.12E). To minimize the noise, the rod channel detains Ca^{2+} and Mg^{2+} during their passage through the pore. As long as divalents reside in the pore, no other ions can pass and the conductance of the CNG channel drops by two orders of magnitude from about 25 pS to 100 fS.[85] Divalent block is weaker in cones, which contributes to greater noisiness of the cone (see previously). Given that channel conductance is low and that the channel is relatively insensitive to cGMP, rods must express a lot of channels (a few hundred per μm^2) to maintain a reasonable dark current. The arrangement averages channel noise across many channels, but it also puts the cell at risk. Normally, the free [cGMP] in darkness is only a few micromolar and a small percentage of channels are open. Should the cell synthesize too much cGMP, the number of open channels could increase by well over an order of magnitude to flood the cell with lethal levels of Ca^{2+} and possibly even annihilate the transmembrane ion gradients.

For the purposes of photon counting, it would be desirable for the light-induced decrease in dark current to be proportional to the number of channels closed. But CNG channel closure hyperpolarizes the

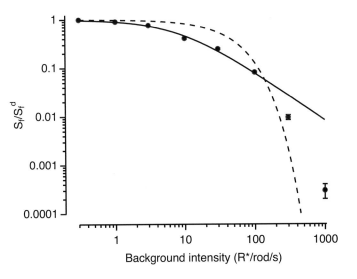

Fig. 19.7 Loss in incremental flash sensitivity with background light. In the absence of adaptation, relative flash sensitivity, $S_f/S_f d$, defined as response amplitude divided by flash strength for responses in the linear range normalized by its value in darkness, would drop off along a saturating exponential function (*dashed line*). Instead, rods exhibit Weber-Fechner behavior: $S_f/S_f^d = (1 + I/I_0)^{-1}$ where I_0 is the background intensity that reduces S_f/S_f^d to 0.5, over much of their range. Rods sacrifice some sensitivity at lower background intensities (*symbols below dashed line*) in order to maintain sensitivity at intensities that would otherwise be saturating (*symbols above the dashed line*). At high background intensities, rods deviate from Weber-Fechner behavior and begin to approach saturation. (From Grimes WN, Baudin J, Azevedo AW, Rieke F. Range, routing and kinetics of rod signaling in primate retina. *eLife*. 2018;7:e38281. https://doi.org/10.7554/eLife.38281. Modified under Creative Commons CC0 https://creativecommons.org/share-your-work/public-domain/cc0/.)

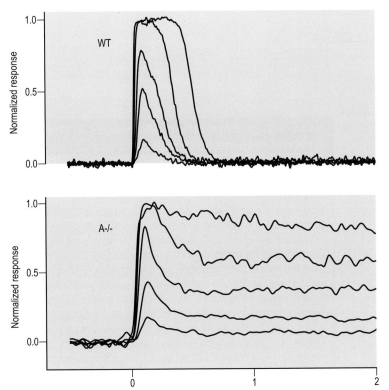

Fig. 19.8 Murine model for Oguchi disease. Flash responses from a mutant rod lacking arrestin (A-/-, *bottom*) recover a hundred times more slowly than wild type (*WT, top*) rod responses. (From Makino CL, Flannery JG, Chen J, Dodd RL. Effects of photoresponse prolongation on retinal rods of transgenic mice. In: Williams TP, Thistle AB, eds. *Photostasis and Related Phenomena*. Plenum Press; 1998. Modified with kind permission from Springer Science and Business Media.)

rod, and Ohm's law dictates an increase in current flowing through each of the remaining open channels. However, two mechanisms conspire against such a linear, Ohmic relationship between current and voltage. First, hyperpolarization enhances divalent block by increasing the driving force on Ca^{2+} and Mg^{2+} to enter the channel pore.[86,87] Second, gating of the CNG channel is slightly voltage-dependent, so hyperpolarization tends to close the channel. The net effect is that over the physiologic range of membrane potentials, the inward current is nearly constant (Fig. 19.13). The CNG channel in cones is also outwardly rectifying over the physiologic range of voltages, but to a lesser extent than the rod channel.[77] So, in brighter light, as the cone becomes more hyperpolarized, the increased driving force sends more Na^+ and Ca^{2+} ions through the remaining open channels. Cones are not concerned with single photons and are more interested in dynamic range. The reduced effect of closing channels at hyperpolarized potentials may contribute to their remarkable capacity to operate over a wide range of intensities. Another consequence is that the photocurrent in cones will not isolate events occurring in the outer segment and can be influenced by voltage changes induced by external sources (see Chapters 21 and 22).

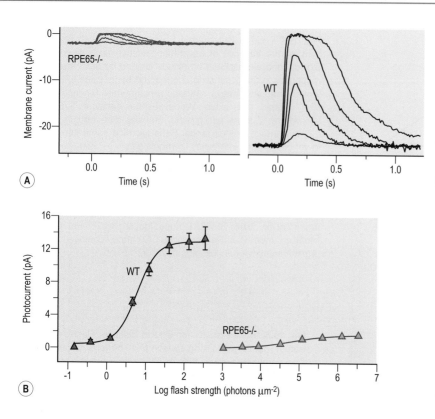

Fig. 19.9 Murine model for Leber congenital amaurosis. (**A**) The outer segment membrane current and averaged flash responses of mutant rods lacking RPE65 (n=3) are smaller than those of wild type (*WT*) rods (n=4). Mutant rods also generate flash responses with faster kinetics. (**B**) On average, the mutant rods (n=16) are 10,000 times less sensitive than WT rods (n=32). (From Woodruff ML, Wang Z, Chung HY. Redmond TM, Fain GL, Lem J. Spontaneous activity of opsin apoprotein is a cause of Leber congenital amaurosis. *Nat Genet.* 2003;35:158–164. Reprinted by permission from Macmillan Publishers Ltd, copyright 2003.)

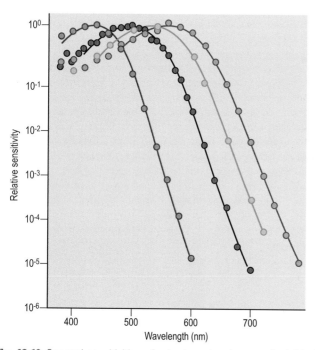

Fig. 19.10 Spectral sensitivities of primate rod and cones. Rod *(black symbols)*, green cone *(green symbols)*, and red cone *(red symbols)* spectra are from human.[13,69] The blue cone spectrum *(blue symbols)* is from a macaque monkey,[68] whose color vision is very similar to that of humans.

inhibitors include the Na+ channel blocking amiloride, the Ca2+-activated K+ channel blocker dequalinium, the local anesthetic tetracaine, and the snake venom peptide, pseudechetoxin (reviewed in [88]). Interestingly, nanomolar levels of retinoids lower the apparent affinity of the CNG channel for cGMP, yet do not seem to interfere with dark adaptation.

Ca2+ is removed from the outer segment by special sodium/potassium/calcium exchangers: sodium/potassium/calcium exchanger 1 (encoded by *SLC24A1* or *NCKX1*) in rods, and sodium/potassium/calcium exchanger 2 (encoded by *SLC24A2* or *NCKX2*) (Fig. 19.14A) and sodium/potassium/calcium exchanger 4 (encoded by *SLC24A4* or *NCKX4*) in cones (reviewed in [93,94]). Sodium/potassium/calcium exchanger 1 forms a dimer in rods that physically couples to the

L-cis diltiazem is a potent and reversible inhibitor of the CNG channel. *D-cis* diltiazem blocks Ca2+ channels and is often prescribed as a vasodilator to treat hypertension. Because Ca2+ channels and CNG channels are sensitive to different enantiomers, the photocurrents are little affected by the vasodilator. Other CNG channel

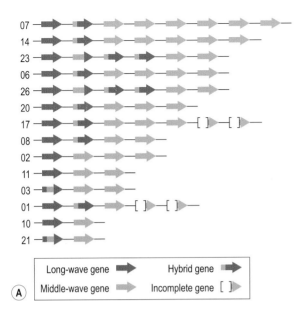

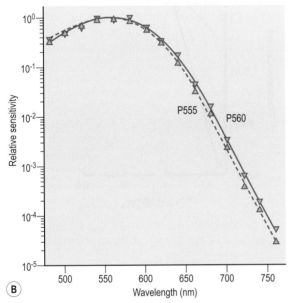

Fig. 19.11 Genetic basis for heterogeneity in human color vision. (**A**) X-chromosome arrays of "red" (long-wave) and "green" (middle-wave) pigment genes are diverse, as shown by this small sample of male subjects with normal color vision. (Modified from Neitz M, Neitz J, Grishok A. Polymorphism in the number of genes encoding long-wavelength sensitive cone pigments among males with normal color vision. *Vis Res.* 1995;35:2395–2407.) (**B**) Red cone pigment variants of two individuals with spectral sensitivity maxima at 555 nm and 560 nm. (Modified from Kraft TW, Neitz J, Neitz M. Spectra of human L cones. *Vis Res.* 1998;38:3663–3670.)

CNGA1 subunit of the CNG channel, roughly two exchangers per channel. Sodium/potassium/calcium exchanger 2 also forms a dimer that is capable of binding CNGA3, but exchanger/channel complexes have not yet been proven to occur in cones. Little is known about sodium/potassium/calcium exchanger 4 structure at this time. Although there may be some exchangers at the cone synapse, the exchangers in rods are located exclusively in the outer segment. The exchangers in photoreceptors differ from sodium/calcium exchangers

found elsewhere in the body in that they couple the removal of Ca^{2+} to the entry of four Na^+ ions and the extrusion of one K^+ ion. By taking advantage of the K^+ gradient, as well as sending four Na^+ inside rather than three, photoreceptors could potentially take internal Ca^{2+} down to 0.2 nM, a level hundreds of times lower than that reachable by sodium/calcium exchangers[95]:

$$[Ca]_i = \frac{[Ca]_o[Na]_i^4[K]_o \exp(V_mF/RT)}{[Na]_o^4[K]_i}$$

(Eq. 19.2)

where V_m is the membrane potential, F is Faraday's constant, R is Boltzmann's constant, and T is absolute temperature. In reality, internal Ca^{2+} never gets that low, possibly because the exchanger inactivates. Since there is a net movement of charge, the action of the exchanger comprises a small percentage of the dark current. After closure of all the CNG channels by a saturating flash, to a first approximation, Ca^{2+} falls exponentially in the rod outer segment with a time constant between 40 and 90 ms (Fig. 19.14B).[34,38] In cones, the combined properties of two exchangers and the cone CNG channel support a higher Ca^{2+} flux and faster light-induced changes in Ca^{2+} concentration.

ROLE OF INNER SEGMENT CONDUCTANCES

Closure of CNG channels in response to light hyperpolarizes rods and cones toward the equilibrium potential for K^+; however, the transmembrane voltage is subject to modification by a variety of conductances located on the inner segment, cell body, and synaptic terminal (reviewed in[98]). A net, inward current increases in magnitude as the transmembrane potential becomes more negative. The effect of these conductances, referred to collectively as inner segment conductances, is readily apparent from a comparison of the photocurrents to the photovoltages for either a rod or a cone (Figs. 19.1, 19.3, and 19.15). For dim flashes, the inner segment conductances are little affected, so the time courses of the voltage responses are similar to those of the current responses.[3,6,12,15] But for bright flashes, the time courses differ; there is a prominent "nose" in the voltage response, whereas there is no such nose in the current response.

Overall, the inner segment conductances tend to return the membrane potential to the resting value. Such an action helps ensure that the membrane potential remains within the dynamic range of neurotransmitter release and prevents regenerative spiking (e.g.,[99-102]). Large depolarizations that might arise from activation of voltage-dependent Ca^{2+} currents, particularly in small compartments, are thwarted by voltage- and Ca^{2+}-activated K^+ currents. Large hyperpolarizations that might arise, for example, from the electrogenic Na^+K^+-ATPase, are counteracted by a nonspecific cationic current activated at voltages more negative than the resting potential. Changes in these various currents at different voltages within the normal operating range of rods and cones occur slowly with respect to the photocurrent, and therefore act to high-pass filter the response to bright light (Fig. 19.15). A third role is to control the entry of Ca^{2+}, which in turn regulates transmitter release and other cellular activities. The intracellular concentrations of Ca^{2+} and other ions may also mediate effects in the cell beyond vesicular release. Five currents—three voltage-gated and two Ca^{2+}-activated—are described next.

Delayed rectifier potassium current, I_{KV}

The channels underlying I_{KV} activate at $V_m = -70$ mV in rods[103] and at $V_m = -50$ mV for monkey cones.[104,105] The outward flow of K^+ ions

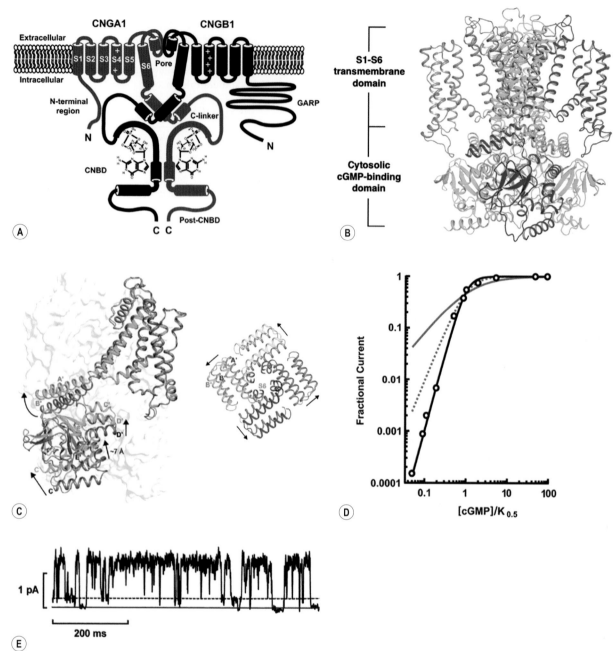

Fig. 19.12 Cyclic nucleotide-gated (CNG) channel. (**A**) The channel consists of four subunits, two of which are shown in this schematic diagram. Each subunit has six transmembrane segments, a pore-forming domain between helices 5 and 6 and a cyclic nucleotide-binding domain (*CNBD*) on the carboxy terminus. Helix 4 contains positively charged lysine residues and functions as a voltage sensor. The carboxy and amino termini are located intracellularly. The amino terminus of the CNGB1 subunit contains a large glutamic acid-rich protein (*GARP*) segment. (Courtesy of W.N. Zagotta.) (**B**) The cryo-EM structure of a human CNG channel composed of four CNGA1 subunits was solved to 2.64Å, in side view. Each subunit is shown in a different color. (**C**) Upon binding of a cyclic GMP (*yellow, blue, and red stick structure, bottom left*), the CNBD moves upward toward the membrane. The C' segment of the C linker swings helix A'-turn-helix B' up and outward, spreading the S6 helices apart, which then opens the conduction pore. Side view of one subunit is shown on the *left*, superimposed on the global structure. On the *right* is a down view of the gating ring formed by the helix A'-turn-helix B' segments of the four subunits, each shown in a different color. Positions of segments in the closed state are shown in *gray*. (Panels **B** and **C** are adapted from Xue J, Han Y, Zeng W, Wang Y, Jiang Y. Structural mechanisms of gating and selectivity of human rod CNGA1 channel. *Neuron*. 2021;109:1302–1313.) (**D**) CNG channel opening is steeply dependent on [cGMP]. Lines show Hill functions: fractional current = $[cGMP]^n/([cGMP]^n + K_{0.5}^n)$, where $K_{0.5}$ is the concentration of cGMP that opens half of the channels and n is the Hill coefficient taking values of 1 (*gray, continuous line*), 2 (*gray, dashed line*), and 3 (*black line*). Hill coefficients greater than 1 indicate cooperativity. (Courtesy of A.L. Zimmerman and D.A. Baylor.) (**E**) A single CNG channel in a patch of membrane excised from a salamander rod flickers between an open state, a second open state of lower conductance (*dashed line*), and a closed state (*horizontal line*). The "fuzziness" of the trace above the dashed line represents extremely brief transitions out of the open state that were unresolved by the recording. The activity was recorded in symmetric salt solutions containing low concentrations of divalent cations and 5 μM cGMP on the intracellular face with a voltage of +70 mV applied to the membrane. (From Taylor WR, Baylor DA. Conductance and kinetics of single cGMP-activated channels in salamander rod outer segments. *J Physiol (Lond)*. 1995:483:567–582. Adapted with permission from Blackwell Publishing, copyright 1995.)

BOX 19.3 Color blindness due to a channelopathy

Rod monochromacy is an autosomal recessive condition presenting with achromatopsia, poor visual acuity, photophobia, nystagmus, and modest degeneration of the cones (reviewed in [89–91]). It is rare, affecting fewer than 1 in 30,000 persons, although the prevalence is as high as 1 in 10 amongst the native population of Pingelap (see [92] for an interesting account). In most cases, the condition is a channelopathy, caused by mutations in CNGA3 and/or CNGB3 channel subunits that disable phototransduction in cones. Homozygous, compound heterozygous, and even triallelic cases have been documented. Interestingly, there is a greater tendency for CNGA3 involvement in Chinese, Israeli, and Palestinian patients, whereas CNGB3 mutations are more common in Europe and in the USA (and almost exclusively in Pingelap). A slowly progressive cone dystrophy occurs in at least some patients. Rods continue to function because they express distinct cyclic nucleotide-gated (CNG) channel subunits. Gene therapy trials aimed at replacing the defective component have demonstrated improved cone function in animal models, and clinical trials are now underway.

Failure to express the rod CNG channel is far more devastating and causes autosomal recessive retinitis pigmentosa in which rods degenerate over months, followed by a secondary loss of cones, so there is complete blindness rather than just night blindness (reviewed in [89]). Mutations can occur in either the CNGA1 subunit or in the CNGB1 subunit.

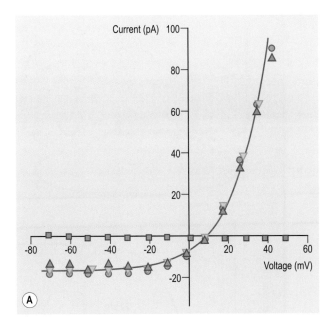

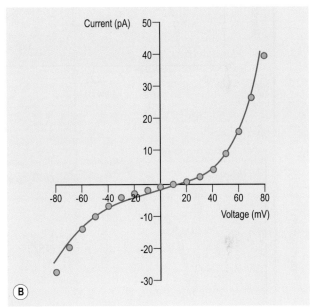

Fig. 19.13 Outward rectification of the current-to-voltage relations of cyclic nucleotide-gated (CNG) channels in rods (**A**) and cones (**B**). Physiologically relevant voltages range from about –40 to –65 mV. The *purple squares* in **A** represent measurements made during exposure to light that closed all of the CNG channels. *Triangles* and *circles* are from three determinations made in darkness. (Panel A from Baylor DA, Nunn BJ. Electrical properties of the light-sensitive conductance of rods of the salamander *Ambystoma tigrinum. J Physiol (Lond).* 1986;371:115–145. Adapted with permission from Blackwell Publishing, copyright 1986. Panel B from Haynes L, Yau K-W. Cyclic GMP-sensitive conductance in outer segment membrane of catfish cones. *Nature.* 1985;317:61–64. Modified with permission from Macmillan Publishers Ltd, copyright 1985.)

through I_{KV} together with a leak current constitute the inner segment leg of the circulating current and help to set the membrane potential of the photoreceptor in darkness. I_{KV} channels close slowly when the photoreceptor hyperpolarizes (Figs. 19.16 and 19.17). In so doing, they limit the light-induced hyperpolarization and may contribute to the nose in the response to brighter flashes and steps (see Box 19.4). This current is blocked by extracellular tetraethyl ammonium ions.

Hyperpolarization-activated current, I_H

A cationic conductance appears at potentials negative to –50 mV[104,105] (Fig. 19.18). It has a reversal potential of –30 to –40 mV, reflecting its permeability to K^+, Na^+, and even Ca^{2+}. I_H turns on slowly and tends to counteract closure of the CNG channels in the outer segment by allowing the entry of Na^+ and depolarizing the photoreceptor. It therefore has an effect similar to closure of I_{KV} channels but comes into play with brighter flashes, since it is active at more negative potentials. However, the gradual building of I_H upon hyperpolarization precludes it from greatly affecting the initial rising phase of the photoresponse. It is primarily responsible for quickening the initial photovoltage response recovery at its peak and creating the "nose[109]." The channels are formed from HCN1 subunits[110] that share structural similarities with CNG channel subunits (reviewed in [75]). As is the case with CNG channels, HCN1 channels are gated by cyclic nucleotides that shift the I_H current-to-voltage relation slightly to the right (i.e., to voltages a few mV less negative).

Voltage-activated calcium current, I_{Ca}

The major calcium conductance in rods and cones is the "long-lasting" or L-type channel, $Ca_V1.4$, composed of α_{1F}, $\alpha_2\delta_4$, and β_2 subunits (reviewed in [98,111,112]). But the calcium channels in rods and cones are heterogeneous; there are 20 splice variants of α_{1F} and 2 splice variants of β_2 present in photoreceptor synapses. In addition, two other isoforms of the pore-forming α_1 subunit are expressed: α_{1C} and α_{1D}, to form $Ca_V1.2$ and $Ca_V1.3$, respectively.

The various channels differ in their voltage dependence and Ca^{2+}-dependent inactivation. Ca^{2+} channels are found on somata and synaptic terminals, the latter localization mediating synaptic transmission in rods and cones (see Box 19.5). Studies on isolated salamander rods report an activation potential of around –45 mV,

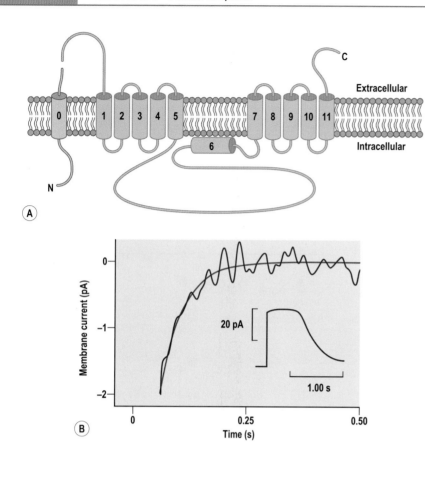

Fig. 19.14 Calcium exchange. (**A**) The sodium/potassium/calcium exchanger 1 in rods and 2 in cones have an extracellular C terminus.[96,97] A leader sequence (red) is cleaved off prior to localization of the exchanger to the outer segment plasma membrane. (**B**) A bright flash given to a rod at time zero, which closes all of the cyclic nucleotide-gated (CNG) channels very suddenly, reveals a residual current owing to the electrogenic removal of Ca^{2+} by the sodium/potassium/calcium exchanger 1 (red trace, inset: flash response in its entirety). The exchange current declines (exponential fit, blue trace) in this rod with a time constant of 59 ms, as the internal Ca^{2+} drops to a minimum. (From Field GD, Rieke F. Mechanisms regulating variability of the single photon responses of mammalian rod photoreceptors. Neuron. 2002;35:733–747.)

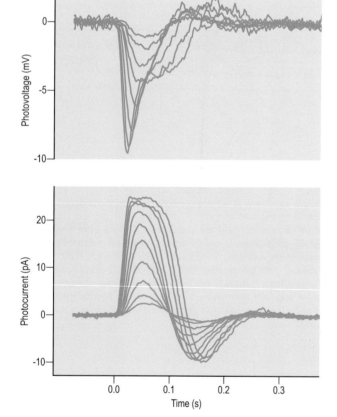

Fig. 19.15 Differences in the current and voltage response waveforms. The photovoltages and photocurrents were recorded from different cones at 37°C. In the top panel (from Fig. 19.1C), flashes deflect the transmembrane potential from its resting level of −43 mV, whereas in the lower panel, flashes decrease the dark current from a value in darkness of −24.9 pA. (Lower panel from Baylor DA, Nunn BJ, Schnapf JL. Spectral sensitivity of cones of the monkey Macaca fascicularis. J Physiol (Lond). 1987;390:145–160. Modified with permission from Blackwell Publishing, copyright 1987.)

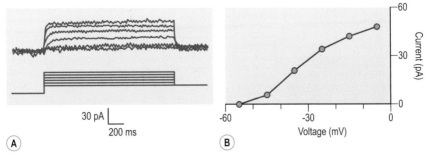

Fig. 19.16 Voltage-dependent K+ current. (**A**) I_{KV} turns on slowly in response to voltage steps from a holding potential of –105 mV to command voltages ranging from –55 mV to –5 mV at 33–36°C. The I_{KV} was isolated pharmacologically and by careful selection of the ionic composition of the bath and pipette solutions in voltage clamp experiments on monkey cone inner segments. (**B**) At steady state the current-to-voltage relations of I_{KV} indicate an outward current at potentials less negative than –60 mV in this cell. (From Yagi T, MacLeish PR. Ionic conductances of monkey solitary cone inner segments. *J Neurophysiol.* 1994;71:656–665. Used with permission from the American Physiological Society.)

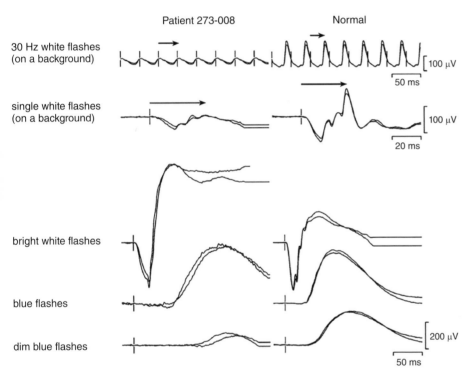

Fig. 19.17 Full field electroretinograms (ERGs, see Chapter 24) from a patient who was homozygous for a 1348T>G mutation in *KCNV2*, resulting in a Trp450Gly substitution in the pore domain of the voltage-gated potassium channel, and from an age-matched control. Depressed responses with delays (increased implicit time, *arrows*) in response to flicker (30 Hz) and flashes superposed on a rod-adapting background reveal impaired cone function in the patient. Rod dominant responses to bright white flashes under dark-adapted conditions and rod responses to blue flashes were larger than normal with longer implicit times, but for dim blue flashes, responses from the patient were small. Thus, the disease gives rise to a steeper than normal stimulus-response function for the positive-going b-wave. (From Thiagalingam S, McGee TL, Weleber RG, et al. Novel mutations in the *KCNV2* gene in patients with cone dystrophy and a supernormal rod electroretinogram. *Ophthalmic Genet.* 2007;28:135–142, with permission from Taylor & Francis Ltd, www.tandfonline.com.)

BOX 19.4   Cone-rod dystrophy caused by an inner segment channelopathy

An autosomal recessive condition in humans called cone dystrophy with supernormal rod responses has been described[106]; electroretinogram findings are summarized in Fig. 19.17. Genetic studies of patients and their families found mutations in the *KCNV2* gene[107] on chromosome 9p24 that codes for a voltage-gated potassium channel subunit ($K_V8.2$) that is expressed on the inner segments of rods and cones. A total of 95 mutations has been identified to date (reviewed in [108]). Current through this potassium channel is thought to play a role in setting the resting potential and kinetics of the light responses in photoreceptors. Retinal imaging and the slow progression of disease in some patients indicate that besides playing an acute role in shaping the light response, inner segment conductances are also critical for cell viability and function in human photoreceptors that normally have a lifespan of many decades.

which is, paradoxically, close to the membrane potential in the dark. The activation potential for Ca^{2+} channels in primate rods and cones is more reasonable, close to –60 mV, leaving a wide operating range of voltage for modifying Ca^{2+} entry in response to light (Fig. 19.19). The Ca^{2+} channels in rods and cones react promptly to voltage changes and are noninactivating, a property that is well suited for a high rate of sustained vesicular neurotransmitter release in darkness. The α_{1F} subunit may be regulated by PKA phosphorylation with a different effect in rods and in cones, and through interactions with two Ca^{2+}-binding proteins, calmodulin and CaBP4, that compete for binding to the carboxy terminus. Extracellular protons, Zn^{2+}, and retinoids inhibit I_{Ca}, while intracellular Cl^- enhances it. The channels are blocked by diltiazem, verapamil, and dihydropyridines such as nifedipine and nimodipine and are activated by Bay K 8644.[101,113]

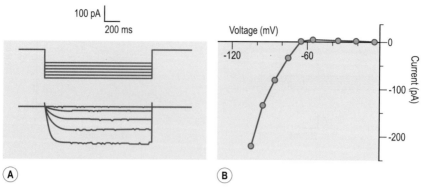

Fig. 19.18 Slow development of an inwardly rectifying current (I_H) with hyperpolarization. (**A**) Stepping the membrane potential of an isolated monkey cone under voltage clamp from −5 mV to values between −55 and −105 mV turns on an inward current over a period of approximately 100 ms at 33–36°C. Currents other than I_H were blocked pharmacologically and by manipulating the ionic composition of the bathing solutions, or were subtracted from the records. (**B**) The current-to-voltage relations of I_H at steady state indicate an inward current at negative potentials. Under physiologic conditions with proper ionic solutions and cyclic nucleotide concentrations, I_H activates at slightly less negative potentials. Nevertheless, I_H remains negligible at the dark resting potential. (From Yagi T, MacLeish PR. Ionic conductances of monkey solitary cone inner segments. *J Neurophysiol.* 1994;71:656–665. Used with permission from the American Physiological Society.)

BOX 19.5   Night blindness resulting from a defective calcium channel

Patients with incomplete Schubert-Bornschein congenital stationary night blindness (icCSNB or CSNB2A) and those with Åland Island eye disease (Forsius-Eriksson ocular albinism) present with varying degrees of photophobia, nyctalopia, refractive error, nystagmus, strabismus, and disturbances in color vision, and an "electronegative" electroretinogram (ERG) (reviewed in [111,112,114]). The initial negative a-wave reflecting phototransduction in rods is present, but the later, positive b-wave due to postreceptoral cell activity is attenuated or missing (e.g., Fig. 19.20A), indicating transmission failure at the rod synapse. Depression of the 30 Hz flicker cone ERG and the ON-OFF ERG indicate that both ON and OFF cone pathways are severely impaired. Most cases are X-linked, resulting from genetic defects in *CACNA1F*, which encodes the pore-forming α_{1F} subunit of the L-type calcium channel $Ca_V1.4$ in the synapses of rods and cones.[115,116] Over 260 disease-causing mutations have been documented,[117] some of which are shown in Fig. 19.20B. Female carriers are typically asymptomatic due to X-inactivation, but clinical abnormalities do sometimes occur (e.g.,[118,119]).

Besides icCSNB and Åland Island eye disease, mutations have also been found in cases of X-linked progressive cone-rod dystrophy (CORDX3) (see https://web.sph.uth.edu/RetNet/). The wide spectrum of presentations, ranging from little or no nyctalopia in half the patients to more incapacitating symptoms with progressive retinal degeneration, has led to discussion about disease classification and nomenclature. Night blindness is incomplete, probably owing to differences in the expression of splice variants, alternative subunits, and/or modifier proteins, and because gap junctions afford parallel albeit less efficient rod signaling through the cone neural circuitry (reviewed in [98,112]). Transmission at the cone synapse is affected, but maintained nonetheless because cones also express other α_1 isoforms.

Autosomal recessive forms of icCSNB and cone/cone-rod dystrophy can be caused by mutations in *CABP4* or *CACNA2D4*, which encode a calcium-binding protein that complexes with calcium channels and the $\alpha_2\delta_4$ subunit of the Cav1.4 channel, respectively.

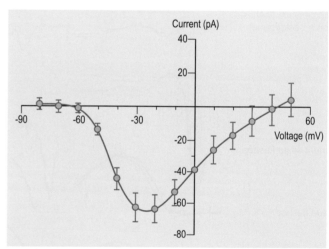

Fig. 19.19 Current-to-voltage relations for I_{Ca}. Measurements were made in porcine rods with Ba^{2+} to minimize interference from other currents. The physiological voltage range controls nearly the full span of I_{Ca}. (From Cia D, Bordais A, Varela C, et al. Voltage-gated channels and calcium homeostasis in mammalian rod photoreceptors. *J Neurophysiol.* 2005;93:1468–1475. Used with permission from the American Physiological Society.)

Calcium-activated potassium current, $I_{K(Ca)}$

Two currents in rods and cones are activated by a rise in intracellular Ca^{2+}: the Ca^{2+}-activated anion current and the Ca^{2+}-activated K^+ current.[103] The latter shows the N-shaped current-to-voltage relationship characteristic of other calcium-activated currents. The magnitude of the outward current is reduced by charybdotoxin,[28,120] indicating the involvement of big potassium (BK, also called MaxiK, Slo1, or $K_{Ca}1.1$) channels. Although $I_{K(Ca)}$ is sizable in rods at positive voltages, the current is minimal within the physiologic range and absent in cones. For that matter, $I_{K(Ca)}$ does not

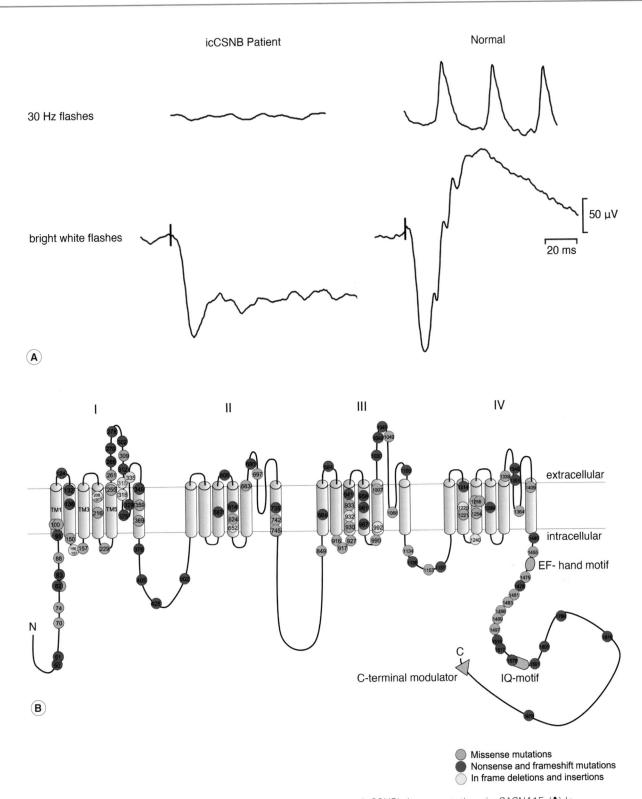

Fig. 19.20 Incomplete congenital stationary night blindness (icCSNB) due to mutations in *CACNA1F*. (**A**) In the electroretinogram (ERG) from a patient, the response to 30 Hz flicker was reduced due to a defect in cone signaling. In the rod dominant response to a bright white flash, the negative-going a-wave was followed by a very minor, positive-going b-wave, forming the "electronegative" ERG. (Modified from Jiang X, Mahroo OA. Negative electroretinograms: Genetic and acquired causes, diagnostic approaches and physiological insights. *Eye*. 2021;35:2419–2437.) (**B**) Partial spectrum of mutations in *CACNA1F*. There are four repeating domains of six transmembrane segments in the α_{1F}-subunit. The S4 segment in each domain is a voltage sensor. Residues comprising the dihydropyridine binding site are present within repeats III and IV. Disease-causing mutations (*red, yellow and green circles*) are found in each of the four repeats. (Modified from Zeitz C, Robson AG, Audo I. Congenital stationary night blindness: An analysis and update of genotype-phenotype correlations and pathogenic mechanisms. *Prog Retin Eye Res*. 2015;45:58–110.)

appear to be expressed in primate cones at all.[104,105] $I_{K(Ca)}$ may therefore serve as a safety net, capable of moving V_m toward the equilibrium potential for K^+ to guard against large depolarizations that would flood the rod interior with Ca^{2+}. Cones rely on other currents to fulfill that function.

Calcium-activated anion current, $I_{Cl(Ca)}$

Both rods and cones express a robust Ca^{2+}-activated anion current.[28,101,103–105] The main permeant anion is Cl^-, and given an equilibrium potential near $-20\,mV$ in rods[121] and $-46\,mV$ in cones,[122] $I_{Cl(Ca)}$ helps to set and stabilize the resting potential. Experimentally, the current is observed most prominently as a tail current following a step of voltage that opens Ca^{2+} channels and allows Ca^{2+} to enter the

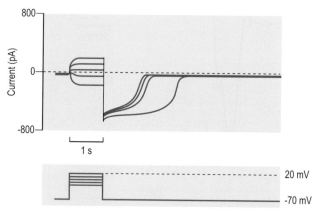

Fig. 19.21 Ca^{2+}-activated Cl^- conductance. Depolarizations of salamander rods from $-70\,mV$ to voltages between -20 and $+20\,mV$ at $10\,mV$ intervals evoke an anionic current with a reversal potential near $0\,mV$, the equilibrium potential for Cl^- under the nonphysiologic conditions of these experiments. The depolarization increases intracellular Ca^{2+}, so upon return of the membrane potential to $-70\,mV$, $I_{Cl\,(Ca)}$ gives rise to an enormous tail current. Ca^{2+} currents have been subtracted and other currents blocked to isolate $I_{Cl\,(Ca)}$. Tail currents do not appear if the cell is bathed in a Ca^{2+}-free solution. Recordings were made near 10°C. (From MacLeish PR, Nurse CA. Ion channel compartments in photoreceptors: Evidence from salamander rods with intact and ablated terminals. *J Neurophysiol.* 2007;98:86–95. Modified with permission from the American Physiological Society.)

cytoplasm (Fig. 19.21). The time course of the tail current reflects the time course of the restoration of free Ca^{2+} to basal levels. In the case of rods, the Ca^{2+}-activated Cl^- conductance is highly targeted to the synaptic terminal. Its strategic location near the site of transmitter release raises the possibility of local control over I_{Ca} by a direct effect of Cl^- on the Ca^{2+} channel itself[123] and by altering the membrane potential at the release site, thereby indirectly affecting Ca^{2+} channel gating. Given the sizes of the pedicle and spherule and their separation from the soma by a thin fiber, the membrane potential in the terminal region could differ from that in the soma. After hyperpolarizations lasting hundreds of milliseconds, the absence of Cl^- efflux through $I_{Cl(Ca)}$ would prime Ca^{2+} channels and shift their activation potentials to lower voltages. This mechanism could hasten the recovery after bright flashes and sensitize the synapse to bright steady light being turned off.

The approximate contribution of each inner segment conductance to the photovoltage response is summarized in Fig. 19.22. Rapid closure of CNG channels hyperpolarizes the photoreceptor and slowly shuts down an outward current (I_{KV}) at voltages slightly more negative than the resting potential and activates an inward current at even more negative voltages (I_H) to carve out the nose in the response to a bright flash. Ca^{2+}-activated Cl^- currents may sharpen the voltage response at the synapse. Ultimately, the light-induced cessation of Ca^{2+}-mediated synaptic release gets dampened and proceeds over a faster time course.

Electrotonic coupling

In addition to inner segment conductances, the membrane potentials of rods and cones are influenced by neighboring cells via cell-cell coupling and synaptic feedback.[4–6,124,125] Single photon responses from rods induce a voltage response in cones but with an amplitude that is eight times smaller. Time to peak is about twice faster because the network behaves as a high-pass filter. A consequence of coupling between rods and cones and between cones of different spectral types is that if the spot of light falling on the retina is large, the size and shape of the response in a given cone will depend on wavelength. In addition, modulation by horizontal cells confers an antagonistic center-surround receptive field. These effects are described in greater detail in Chapter 22.

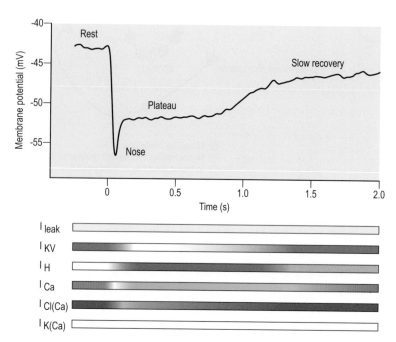

Fig. 19.22 Influence of inner segment conductances on the photovoltage response to a bright flash in a rod. I_{leak}, Leak current; I_{KV}, delayed rectifier potassium current; I_H, hyperpolarization-activated current; I_{Ca}, voltage-activated calcium current; $I_{Cl(Ca)}$, calcium-activated anion current; $I_{K(Ca)}$, calcium-activated potassium current.

SUMMARY

Rods and cones divide the intensity range for vision. Rods attain the ultimate in sensitivity by adeptly counting single photons. Their sensitivity is limited only by photon capture. To achieve high sensitivity, they sacrifice rapidity in their response kinetics and dynamic range. The photocurrent response to single photons generated in the outer segment is delayed, peaks in 200 ms, and has an integration time of 300 ms. Since cones are not concerned with dim light, their photocurrent response to single photons is an order of magnitude smaller, time to peak is several times shorter, and integration time is reduced over tenfold. It is important that cones do not saturate, so their operating range not only shifts to the higher light intensities, but also stretches out compared to rods, and accommodations have been made to prevent bleaching from doing more than reducing photon capture. Higher intensities allow a point in visual space to be encoded by multiple receptors so that information about color may be extracted. Fast cone responses improve on temporal resolution. Inner segment conductances in rods and cones set the resting membrane potential, speed up the kinetics of the photovoltage response near its peak, and modulate intracellular Ca^{2+}. Certain heritable diseases may target rods, cones, or both, depending upon their particular patterns of gene expression.

ACKNOWLEDGMENTS

We thank numerous colleagues for figures and discussions. Supported by R01 EY031702 (CLM) and by the endowed George H.W. and Barbara P. Bush Chair of Neuroscience (PRM).

REFERENCES

1. Schneeweis DM, Schnapf JL. Photovoltage of rods and cones in the macaque retina. *Science.* 1995;268:1053–1056.
2. Tomita T. Electrophysiological study of the mechanisms subserving color coding in the fish retina. *Cold Spring Harb Symp Quant Biol.* 1965;30:559–566.
3. Schneeweis DM, Schnapf JL. Noise and light adaptation in rods of the macaque monkey. *Vis Neurosci.* 2000;17:659–666.
4. Hornstein EP, Verweij J, Schnapf JL. Electrical coupling between red and green cones in primate retina. *Nat Neurosci.* 2004;7:745–750.
5. Hornstein EP, Verweij J, Li PH, Schnapf JL. Gap-junctional coupling and absolute sensitivity of photoreceptors in macaque retina. *J Neurosci.* 2005;25:11201–11209.
6. Schneeweis DM, Schnapf JL. The photovoltage of macaque cone photoreceptors: Adaptation, noise, and kinetics. *J Neurosci.* 1999;19:1203–1216.
7. Sinha R, Hoon M, Baudin J, Okawa H, Wong ROL, Rieke F. Cellular and circuit mechanisms shaping the perceptual properties of the primate fovea. *Cell.* 2017;168:413–426.
8. Baudin J, Angueyra JM, Sinha R, Rieke F. S-cone photoreceptors in the primate retina are functionally distinct from L and M cones. *eLife.* 2019;8:e39166.
9. McNaughton PA, Yau K-W, Lamb TD. Spread of activation and desensitisation in rod outer segments. *Nature.* 1980;283:85–87.
10. Lamb TD, McNaughton PA, Yau K-W. Spatial spread of activation and background desensitization in toad rod outer segments. *J Physiol (Lond).* 1981;319:463–496.
11. Matthews G. Spread of the light response along the rod outer segment: An estimate from patch-clamp recordings. *Vision Res.* 1986;26:535–541.
12. Baylor DA, Nunn BJ, Schnapf JL. The photocurrent, noise and spectral sensitivity of rods of the monkey *Macaca fascicularis. J Physiol (Lond).* 1984;357:575–607.
13. Kraft TW, Schneeweis DM, Schnapf JL. Visual transduction in human rod photoreceptors. *J Physiol (Lond).* 1993;464:747–765.
14. Pepperberg DR, Birch DG, Hood DC. Photoresponses of human rods in vivo derived from paired-flash electroretinograms. *Vis Neurosci.* 1997;14:73–82.
15. Schnapf JL, Nunn BJ, Meister M, Baylor DA. Visual transduction in cones of the monkey *Macaca fascicularis. J Physiol (Lond).* 1990;427:681–713.
16. Cideciyan AV, Jacobson SG, Gupta N, et al. Cone deactivation kinetics and GRK1/GRK7 expression in enhanced S cone syndrome caused by mutations in NR2E3. *Invest Ophthalmol Vis Sci.* 2003;44:1268–1274.
17. Friedburg C, Allen CP, Mason PJ, Lamb TD. Contribution of cone photoreceptors and post-receptoral mechanisms to the human photopic electroretinogram. *J Physiol (Lond).* 2004;556:819–834.
18. Krispel CM, Chen D, Melling N, et al. RGS expression rate-limits recovery of rod photoresponses. *Neuron.* 2006;51:409–416.
19. Pepperberg DR, Cornwall MC, Kahlert M, et al. Light-dependent delay in the falling phase of the retinal rod photoresponse. *Vis Neurosci.* 1992;8:9–18.
20. Nikonov S, Engheta N, Pugh EN Jr. Kinetics of recovery of the dark-adapted salamander rod photoresponse. *J Gen Physiol.* 1998;111:7–37.
21. Birch DG, Hood DC, Nusinowitz S, Pepperberg DR. Abnormal activation and inactivation mechanisms of rod transduction in patients with autosomal dominant retinitis pigmentosa and the Pro-23-His mutation. *Invest Ophthalmol Vis Sci.* 1995;36:1603–1614.
22. Matthews HR, Sampath AP. Photopigment quenching is Ca^{2+} dependent and controls response duration in salamander L-cone photoreceptors. *J Gen Physiol.* 2010;135:355–366.
23. Lamb TD. Effects of temperature changes on toad rod photocurrents. *J Physiol (Lond).* 1984;346:557–578.
24. Donner K, Hemilä S, Kalamkarov G, Koskelainen A, Shevchenko T. Rod phototransduction modulated by bicarbonate in the frog retina: Roles of carbonic anhydrase and bicarbonate exchange. *J Physiol (Lond).* 1990;426:297–316.
25. Koskelainen A, Donner K, Lerber T, Hemilä S. pH regulation in frog cones studied by mass receptor photoresponses from the isolated retina. *Vision Res.* 1993;33:2181–2188.
26. Duda T, Wen X-H, Isayama T, Sharma RK, Makino CL. Bicarbonate modulates photoreceptor guanylate cyclase (ROS-GC) catalytic activity. *J Biol Chem.* 2015;290:11052–11060.
27. Bok D, Galbraith G, Lopez I, et al. Blindness and auditory impairment caused by loss of the sodium bicarbonate cotransporter NBC3. *Nat Genet.* 2003;34:313–319.
28. MacLeish PR, Nurse CA. Ion channel compartments in photoreceptors: Evidence from salamander rods with intact and ablated terminals. *J Neurophysiol.* 2007;98:86–95.
29. Kao L, Kurtz LM, Shao X, et al. Severe neurologic impairment in mice with targeted disruption of the electrogenic sodium bicarbonate cotransporter NBCe2 (*Slc4a5* gene). *J Biol Chem.* 2011;286:32,563–32,574.
30. Makino CL, Duda T, Pertzev A, et al. Modes of accessing bicarbonate for the regulation of membrane guanylate cyclase (ROS-GC) in retinal rods and cones. *eNeuro.* 2019;6:e0393–18.2019.
31. Nork TM, McCormick SA, Chao GM, Odom JV. Distribution of carbonic anhydrase among human photoreceptors. *Invest Ophthalmol Vis Sci.* 1990;31:1451–1458.
32. Koskelainen A, Donner K, Kalamkarov G, Hemilä S. Changes in the light-sensitive current of salamander rods upon manipulation of putative pH-regulating mechanisms in the inner and outer segment. *Vision Res.* 1994;34:983–994.
33. Baylor DA, Lamb TD, Yau K-W. Responses of retinal rods to single photons. *J Physiol (Lond).* 1979;288:613–634.
34. Tamura T, Nakatani K, Yau K-W. Calcium feedback and sensitivity regulation in primate rods. *J Gen Physiol.* 1991;98:95–130.
35. Yau K-W, Baylor DA. Cyclic GMP-activated conductances of retinal photoreceptor cells. *Annu Rev Neurosci.* 1989;12:289–327.
36. Rieke F, Baylor DA. Origin of reproducibility in the responses of retinal rods to single photons. *Biophys J.* 1998;75:1836–1857.
37. Whitlock GC, Lamb TD. Variability in the time course of single photon responses from toad rods: Termination of rhodopsin's activity. *Neuron.* 1999;23:337–351.
38. Field GD, Rieke F. Mechanisms regulating variability of the single photon responses of mammalian rod photoreceptors. *Neuron.* 2002;35:733–747.
39. Baylor DA, Matthews G, Yau K-W. Two components of electrical dark noise in toad retinal rod outer segments. *J Physiol (Lond).* 1980;309:591–621.
40. Rieke F, Baylor DA. Origin and functional impact of dark noise in retinal cones. *Neuron.* 2000;26:181–186.
41. Luo D-G, Yue WWS, Ala-Laurila P, Yau K-W. Activation of visual pigments by light and heat. *Science.* 2011;332:1307–1312.
42. Lamb TD, Simon EJ. Analysis of electrical noise in turtle cones. *J Physiol (Lond).* 1977;272:435–468.
43. Rieke F, Baylor DA. Molecular origin of continuous dark noise in rod photoreceptors. *Biophys J.* 1996;71:2553–2572.
44. Angueyra JM, Rieke F. Origin and effect of phototransduction noise in primate cone photoreceptors. *Nat Neurosci.* 2013;16:1692–1700.
45. Hecht S, Schlaer S, Pirenne MH. Energy, quanta and vision. *J Gen Physiol.* 1942;25:819–840.
46. Kraft TW, Schnapf JL. Aberrant photon responses in rods of the macaque monkey. *Vis Neurosci.* 1998;15:153–159.
47. Chen J, Makino CL, Peachey NS, Baylor DA, Simon MI. Mechanisms of rhodopsin inactivation in vivo as revealed by a COOH-terminal truncation mutant. *Science.* 1995;267:374–377.
48. Chen C-K, Burns ME, Spencer M, et al. Abnormal photoresponses and light-induced apoptosis in rods lacking rhodopsin kinase. *Proc Natl Acad Sci USA.* 1999;96:3718–3722.
49. Tamura T, Nakatani K, Yau K-W. Light adaptation in cat retinal rods. *Science.* 1989;245:755–758.
50. Nakatani K, Tamura T, Yau K-W. Light adaptation in retinal rods of the rabbit and two other nonprimate mammals. *J Gen Physiol.* 1991;97:413–435.
51. Thomas MM, Lamb TD. Light adaptation and dark adaptation of human rod photoreceptors measured from the a-wave of the electroretinogram. *J Physiol (Lond).* 1999;518:479–496.

52. Calvert PD, Govardovskii VI, Arshavsky VY, Makino CL. Two temporal phases of light adaptation in retinal rods. *J Gen Physiol.* 2002;119:129–145.
53. Krispel CM, Chen C-K, Simon MI, Burns ME. Novel form of adaptation in mouse retinal rods speeds recovery of phototransduction. *J Gen Physiol.* 2003;122:703–712.
54. Tikidji-Hamburyan A, Reinhard K, Storchi R, et al. Rods progressively escape saturation to drive visual responses in daylight conditions. *Nat Commun.* 2017;8:1813.
55. Lamb TD, Pugh EN Jr. Dark adaptation and the retinoid cycle of vision. *Prog Retin Eye Res.* 2004;23:307–380.
56. Jones GJ, Cornwall MC, Fain GL. Equivalence of background and bleaching desensitization in isolated rod photoreceptors of the larval tiger salamander. *J Gen Physiol.* 1996;108:333–340.
57. Paupoo AAV, Mahroo OAR, Friedburg C, Lamb TD. Human cone photoreceptor responses measured by the electroretinogram a-wave during and after exposure to intense illumination. *J Physiol (Lond).* 2000;529:469–482.
58. Nikonov SS, Kholodenko R, Lem J, Pugh EN Jr. Physiological features of the S- and M-cone photoreceptors of wild-type mice from single-cell recordings. *J Gen Physiol.* 2006;127:359–374.
59. Kenkre JS, Moran NA, Lamb TD, Mahroo OAR. Extremely rapid recovery of human cone circulating current at the extinction of bleaching exposures. *J Physiol (Lond).* 2005;567:95–112.
60. Paskowitz DM, LaVail MM, Duncan JL. Light and inherited retinal degeneration. *Br J Ophthalmol.* 2006;90:1060–1066.
61. Cideciyan AV, Zhao X, Nielsen L, Khani SC, Jacobson SG, Palczewski K. Null mutation in the rhodopsin kinase gene slows recovery kinetics of rod and cone phototransduction in man. *Proc Natl Acad Sci USA.* 1998;95:328–333.
62. Weiss ER, Ducceschi MH, Horner TJ, Li A, Craft CM, Osawa S. Species-specific differences in expression of G-protein-coupled receptor kinase (GRK) 7 and GRK1 in mammalian cone photoreceptor cells: Implications for cone cell phototransduction. *J Neurosci.* 2001;21: 9175–9184.
63. Chen C-K, Zhang K, Church-Kopish J, et al. Characterization of human GRK7 as a potential cone opsin kinase. *Mol Vis.* 2001;7:305–313.
64. Haider NB, Jacobson SG, Cideciyan AV, et al. Mutation of a nuclear receptor gene, *NR2E3*, causes enhanced S cone syndrome, a disorder of retinal cell fate. *Nat Genet.* 2000;24:127–131.
65. Craft CM, Whitmore DH, Wiechmann AF. Cone arrestin identified by targeting expression of a functional family. *J Biol Chem.* 1994;269:4613–4619.
66. Sakuma H, Inana G, Murakami A, Higashide T, McLaren MJ. Immunolocalization of X-arrestin in human cone photoreceptors. *FEBS Lett.* 1996;382:105–110.
67. Nishiguchi KM, Sandberg MA, Kooijman AC, et al. Defects in RGS9 or its anchor protein R9AP in patients with slow photoreceptor deactivation. *Nature.* 2004;427:75–78.
68. Baylor DA, Nunn BJ, Schnapf JL. Spectral sensitivity of cones of the monkey *Macaca fascicularis. J Physiol (Lond).* 1987;390:145–160.
69. Schnapf JL, Kraft TW, Baylor DA. Spectral sensitivity of human cone photoreceptors. *Nature.* 1987;325:439–441.
70. Hofmann L, Palczewski K. Advances in understanding the molecular basis of the first steps in color vision. *Prog Ret Eye Res.* 2015;49:46–66.
71. Weitz D, Ficek N, Kremmer E, Bauer PJ, Kaupp UB. Subunit stoichiometry of the CNG channel of rod photoreceptors. *Neuron.* 2002;36:881–889.
72. Zheng J, Trudeau MC, Zagotta WN. Rod cyclic nucleotide-gated channels have a stoichiometry of three CNGA1 subunits and one CNGB1 subunit. *Neuron.* 2002;36:891–896.
73. Zhong H, Molday LL, Molday RS, Yau K-W. The heteromeric cyclic nucleotide-gated channel adopts a 3A:1B stoichiometry. *Nature.* 2002;420:193–198.
74. Zheng X, Hu Z, Li H, Yang J. Structure of the human cone photoreceptor cyclic nucleotide-gated channel. *Nat Struct Mol Biol.* 2022;29:40–46.
75. James ZM, Zagotta WN. Structural insights into the mechanisms of CNBD channel function. *J Gen Physiol.* 2018;150:225–244.
76. Fesenko EE, Kolesnikov SS, Lyubarsky AL. Induction by cyclic GMP of cationic conductance in plasma membrane of retinal rod outer segment. *Nature.* 1985;313:310–313.
77. Haynes L, Yau K-W. Cyclic GMP-sensitive conductance in outer segment membrane of catfish cones. *Nature.* 1985;317:61–64.
78. Tanaka JC, Eccleston JF, Furman RE. Photoreceptor channel activation by nucleotide derivatives. *Biochemistry.* 1989;28:2776–2784.
79. Karpen JW, Zimmerman AL, Stryer L, Baylor DA. Molecular mechanics of the cyclic-GMP-activated channel of retinal rods. *Cold Spring Harb Symp Quant Biol.* 1988;53: 325–332.
80. Watanabe S-I, Matthews G. Cyclic GMP-activated channels of rod photoreceptors show neither fast nor slow desensitization. *Vis Neurosci.* 1990;4:481–487.
81. Nakatani K, Yau K-W. Calcium and magnesium fluxes across the plasma membrane of the toad rod outer segment. *J Physiol (Lond).* 1988;395:695–729.
82. Ohyama T, Hackos DH, Frings S, Hagen V, Kaupp UB, Korenbrot JI. Fraction of the dark current carried by Ca^{2+} through cGMP-gated ion channels of intact rod and cone photoreceptors. *J Gen Physiol.* 2000;116:735–754.
83. Frings S, Seifert R, Godde M, Kaupp UB. Profoundly different calcium permeation and blockage determine the specific function of distinct cyclic nucleotide-gated channels. *Neuron.* 1995;15:169–179.
84. Picones A, Korenbrot JI. Permeability and interaction of Ca^{2+} with cGMP-gated ion channels differ in retinal rod and cone photoreceptors. *Biophys J.* 1995;69:120–127.
85. Bodoia RD, Detwiler PB. Patch-clamp recordings of the light-sensitive dark noise in retinal rods from the lizard and frog. *J Physiol (Lond).* 1985;367:183–216.
86. Zimmerman AL, Baylor DA. Cyclic GMP-sensitive conductance of retinal rods consists of aqueous pores. *Nature.* 1986;321:70–72.
87. Matthews G. Comparison of the light-sensitive and cyclic GMP-sensitive conductances of the rod photoreceptor: Noise characteristics. *J Neurosci.* 1986;6:2521–2526.
88. Brown RL, Strassmaier T, Brady JD, Karpen JW. The pharmacology of cyclic nucleotide-gated channels: Emerging from the darkness. *Curr Pharmaceut Des.* 2006;12:3597–3613.
89. Michalakis S, Becirovic E, Biel M. Retinal cyclic nucleotide-gated channels: From pathophysiology to therapy. *Int J Mol Sci.* 2018;19:749.
90. El Moussawi Z, Boueiri M, Al-Haddad C. Gene therapy in color vision deficiency: A review. *Int Ophthalmol.* 2021;41:1917–1927.
91. Michalakis S, Gerhardt M, Rudolph G, Priglinger S, Priglinger C. Achromatopsia: Genetics and gene therapy. *Mol Diagn Ther.* 2022;26:51–59.
92. Sachs OW. *The Island of the Colorblind.* New York: Vintage Books; 1997.
93. Vinberg F, Chen J, Kefalov VJ. Regulation of calcium homeostasis in the outer segments of rod and cone photoreceptors. *Prog Ret Eye Res.* 2018;67:87–101.
94. Hassan MT, Lytton J. Potassium-dependent sodium-calcium exchanger (NCKX) isoforms and neuronal function. *Cell Calcium.* 2020;86:102135.
95. Cervetto L, Lagnado L, Perry RJ, Robinson DW, McNaughton PA. Extrusion of calcium from rod outer segments is driven by both sodium and potassium gradients. *Nature.* 1989;337:740–743.
96. Cai X, Zhang K, Lytton J. A novel topology and redox regulation of the rat brain K^+-dependent Na^+/Ca^{2+} exchanger, NCKX2. *J Biol Chem.* 2002;277:48923–48930.
97. Kinjo TG, Szerencsei RT, Winkfein RJ, Kang KJ, Schnetkamp PPM. Topology of the retinal cone NCKX2 Na/Ca-K exchanger. *Biochemistry.* 2003;42:2485–2491.
98. Van Hook MJ, Nawy S, Thoreson WB. Voltage- and calcium-gated ion channels of neurons in the vertebrate retina. *Prog Ret Eye Res.* 2019;72:100760.
99. Fain GL, Quandt FN, Gerschenfeld HM. Calcium-dependent regenerative responses in rods. *Nature.* 1977;269:707–710.
100. Burkhardt DA, Gottesman J, Thoreson WB. Prolonged depolarization in turtle cones evoked by current injection and stimulation of the receptive field surround. *J Physiol (Lond).* 1988;407:329–348.
101. Maricq AV, Korenbrot JI. Calcium and calcium-dependent chloride currents generate action potentials in solitary cone photoreceptors. *Neuron.* 1988;1:503–515.
102. Kawai F, Horiguchi M, Suzuki H, Miyachi E. Na^+ action potentials in human photoreceptors. *Neuron.* 2001;30:451–458.
103. Bader CR, Bertrand D, Schwartz EA. Voltage-activated and calcium-activated currents studied in solitary rod inner segments from the salamander retina. *J Physiol (Lond).* 1982;331:253–284.
104. Hestrin S. The properties and function of inward rectification in rod photoreceptors of the tiger salamander. *J Physiol (Lond).* 1987;390:319–333.
105. Yagi T, MacLeish PR. Ionic conductances of monkey solitary cone inner segments. *J Neurophysiol.* 1994;71:656–665.
106. Gouras P, Eggers HM, MacKay CJ. Cone dystrophy, nyctalopia, and supernormal rod responses. A new retinal degeneration. *Arch Ophthalmol.* 1983;101:718–724.
107. Wu H, Cowing JA, Michaelides M, et al. Mutations in the gene *KCNV2* encoding a voltage-gated potassium channel subunit cause "cone dystrophy with supernormal rod electroretinogram" in humans. *Am J Hum Genet.* 2006;79:574–579.
108. De Guimaraes TAC, Georgiou M, Robson AG, Michaelides M. *KCNV2* retinopathy: Clinical features, molecular genetics and directions for future therapy. *Ophthalmic Genet.* 2020;41:208–215.
109. Barrow AJ, Wu SM. Low-conductance HCN_1 ion channels augment the frequency response of rod and cone photoreceptors. *J Neurosci.* 2009;29:5841–5853.
110. Demontis GC, Moroni A, Gravante B, et al. Functional characterisation and subcellular localisation of HCN1 channels in rabbit retinal rod photoreceptors. *J Physiol (Lond).* 2002;542:89–97.
111. Waldner DM, Bech-Hansen NT, Stell WK. Channeling vision: $Ca_V1.4$—A critical link in retinal signal transmission. *Biomed Res Internatl.* 2018:7272630.
112. Koschak A, Fernandez-Quintero ML, Heigl T, Ruzza M, Seitter H, Zanetti L. Cav 1.4 dysfunction and congenital stationary night blindness type 2. *Pflügers Arch.* 2021;473: 1437–1454.
113. Cia D, Bordais A, Varela C, et al. Voltage-gated channels and calcium homeostasis in mammalian rod photoreceptors. *J Neurophysiol.* 2005;93:1468–1475.
114. Zeitz C, Robson AG, Audo I. Congenital stationary night blindness: An analysis and update of genotype-phenotype correlations and pathogenic mechanisms. *Prog Retin Eye Res.* 2015;45:58–110.
115. Bech-Hansen NT, Naylor MJ, Maybaum TA, et al. Loss-of-function mutations in a calcium-channel α_1-subunit gene in Xp11.23 cause incomplete X-linked congenital stationary night blindness. *Nat Genet.* 1998;19:264–267.
116. Strom TM, Nyakatura G, Apfelstedt-Sylla E, et al. An L-type calcium-channel gene mutated in incomplete X-linked congenital stationary night blindness. *Nat Genet.* 1998;19:260–263.
117. Mahmood U, Méjécase C, Ali SMA, Moosajee M, Kozak I. A novel splice-site variant in *CACNA1F* causes a phenotype synonymous with Åland Island eye disease and incomplete congenital stationary night blindness. *Genes.* 2021;12:171.
118. Michalakis S, Shaltiel L, Sothilingam V, et al. Mosaic synaptopathy and functional defects in Cav1.4 heterozygous mice and human carriers of CSNB2. *Hum Mol Genet.* 2017;26:466.
119. Kimchi A, Meiner V, Silverstein S, et al. An Ashkenazi Jewish founder mutation in *CACNA1F* causes retinal phenotype in both hemizygous males and heterozygous female carriers. *Ophthalmic Genet.* 2019;40:443–448.
120. Xu JW, Slaughter MM. Large-conductance calcium-activated potassium channels facilitate transmitter release in salamander rod synapse. *J Neurosci.* 2005;25:7660–7668.
121. Thoreson WB, Stella SL Jr, Bryson EJ, Clements J, Witkovsky P. D2-like dopamine receptors promote interactions between calcium and chloride channels that diminish rod synaptic transfer in the salamander retina. *Vis Neurosci.* 2002;19:235–247.
122. Thoreson WB, Bryson EJ. Chloride equilibrium potential in salamander cones. *BMC Neurosci.* 2004;5:53.
123. Thoreson WB, Bryson EJ, Rabl K. Reciprocal interactions between calcium and chloride in rod photoreceptors. *J Neurophysiol.* 2003;90:1747–1753.
124. Verweij J, Hornstein EP, Schnapf JL. Surround antagonism in macaque cone photoreceptors. *J Neurosci.* 2003;23:10249–10257.
125. O'Brien JJ, Chen X, MacLeish PR, O'Brien J, Massey SC. Photoreceptor coupling mediated by connexin36 in the primate retina. *J Neurosci.* 2012;32:4675–4687.

20

Light Adaptation in Photoreceptors

Trevor D. Lamb and Vladimir J. Kefalov

VISION FROM STARLIGHT TO SUNLIGHT

The human visual system operates effectively over an enormously wide range of intensities, of at least a billion-fold, from around 10^{-4} cd m^{-2} under starlight conditions to around 10^5 cd m^{-2} under intense sunlight. Changes in pupil area account for only about 1 log unit of this 9 log-unit range, since the pupil diameter changes from a maximum of 8 mm to a minimum of 2.5 mm, corresponding to about a 10-fold reduction in area. Instead, the great bulk of the operational range is achieved by the combination of, first, a switch between the scotopic (rod-based) and photopic (cone-based) pathways in our duplex visual system and, second, the ability of each of these photoreceptor systems to operate over a range of 5 log units (100,000-fold) or more.

Light adaptation versus dark adaptation

This ability of the visual system (or of any of its component parts, such as a photoreceptor) to adjust its performance to the ambient level of illumination is known as "light adaptation." This adjustment typically occurs very rapidly (within seconds), whether the light intensity is increasing or decreasing. The term "dark adaptation" is reserved for the special case of recovery in darkness, following exposure of the eye to extremely bright and/or prolonged illumination that activates (and thereby bleaches) a substantial fraction of the visual pigment, rhodopsin, or its cone equivalent. Dark adaptation occurs slowly, and full recovery of the scotopic visual system after a very large bleach can take as much as an hour.

Light adaptation and the changes that accompany it are beneficial to the possessor of the eye. At very low intensities, visual sensitivity is increased to the utmost possible, so that the rod photoreceptors reliably signal the arrival of individual photons, and the scotopic visual system operates in a photon-counting mode. This ability of the scotopic system to operate at incredibly low intensities is enhanced by two deliberate trade-offs that permit more reliable detection of small signals in the presence of noise: first, reduced spatial resolution (i.e., increased spatial summation), and second, reduced time resolution (i.e., increased temporal integration). Similar trade-offs are used in the photopic system, so that as the ambient illumination decreases from daylight levels toward twilight levels, one's spatial and temporal resolution deteriorate, making it very difficult to play fast ballgames when the light fades.

In contrast, the changes that characterize dark adaptation are disadvantageous. To be effectively blind to dim stimuli for some considerable time after intense light exposure, cannot in any way be useful to an organism. Indeed, for our ancestors (as well as ourselves) entering a cave from bright sunshine is likely to have been quite dangerous, given that visual sensitivity is greatly reduced for tens of minutes. Why should such an apparently unsatisfactory situation have persisted? One possibility is that this slowness of recovery represents an inevitable "cost" of the evolutionary changes that were needed to enable the scotopic system to signal individual photon hits. Another possible explanation is that a slow rod dark adaptation and the underlying slow rod visual pigment regeneration prevent excessive accumulation of light damage and oxidative stress to the rods during the day.

Purposes of light adaptation

A photoreceptor that did not adapt to the ambient light intensity would have a very narrow operating range of only 100-fold span of light responsiveness: low intensities would provide negligible response, whereas high intensities would saturate the cell. Accordingly, photoreceptor light adaptation can be viewed as a means for extending the operating range of the cell.

The purpose of light adaptation can be viewed more generally as being to permit the visual system (or any neuron within it) to provide the best possible performance at that particular level of illumination; however, in this context it is not always clear what constitutes "best". For example, it is difficult for us to specify the time course of response that is best at any given level of illumination. A brief response is likely to provide a better reaction time for the organism, but it may result in very poor sensitivity; conversely, allowing the response to integrate for a longer period will provide greater sensitivity, but may result in a very poor reaction time.

In setting the best performance of a photoreceptor, one crucial task is to endow the cell with very high sensitivity at low light levels yet prevent it from saturating at higher light levels. Light adaptation accomplishes this by reducing the cell's sensitivity to light as the background light level increases; however, this task needs to be performed in a manner that avoids excessive reduction in sensitivity. Cone photoreceptors excel in this capacity and are able to avoid saturation no matter how intense the steady light becomes, and to continue to signal contrast effectively. Rods, on the other hand, are only able to adjust their sensitivity over a relatively narrow range of intensities, before they are driven into saturation, thereby becoming completely unresponsive. One advantage of this saturation of the rods, however, is that it substantially reduces the metabolic demand of the rods for maintaining their transduction current and synaptic transmission at intensities at which the cones are already functional.

In addition to the very important function of optimizing the photoreceptor's sensitivity over a broad range of light intensities, there are two other ways in which photoreceptor light adaptation optimizes the cell's response. First, as will be explained below, when Eq. 20.1 is presented, Weber Law light adaptation permits automatic extraction of the contrast in the visual scene, independent of the absolute level of illumination. Second, light adaptation provides real-time adjustment of the time course of the response to an incremental flash of light in a manner that is presumed to be optimal for the visual system, although, as explained before, we are not yet able to quantify optimality in this regard.

PERFORMANCE OF THE PHOTOPIC AND SCOTOPIC DIVISIONS OF THE VISUAL SYSTEM

Photopic vision: the cone system is the workhorse of vision

For humans, the photopic cone system can be considered the "workhorse" of vision because it is operational under almost all of the conditions that we experience (in the 21st century). Thus, it is the photopic system that underlies our sense of vision at all light levels apart from the exceptionally low intensities experienced in moonlit and starlit conditions. Under moonlight levels of illumination, our scotopic and photopic systems are both functional over an intensity range that is termed "mesopic." To determine whether you are using your photopic system under twilight or nighttime conditions, there is a simple test: if you are able to detect any color in the scene, then your cones are active; if you cannot, then it is likely that only your rods are active. As the ambient intensity increases at dawn, the photopic system remains functional, up to the brightest sunlit conditions that we ever experience.

Despite their enormous importance to our vision, cones make up only about 5% of the population of photoreceptors. The low density of cone photoreceptors in the peripheral retina is quite adequate for our peripheral vision, even in daytime, as we require only relatively low spatial acuity in the periphery. Although the great majority of peripheral photoreceptors are rods, they are not in fact used under most of the circumstances that we think of as vision—instead, they are only used at exceedingly low ambient lighting levels. The reason for having a very high density of rods is to be able to capture every available photon under starlight conditions.

The responses of cones are rapid and moderately sensitive

One of the greatest advantages of cones over rods is their much faster speed of response. Our rods, even when they are light adapted, have responses that are much too slow to allow us to function visually at the speeds that are required to escape predators and to capture prey. Cones, instead, are specialized to permit extremely rapid signaling of visual stimuli to the brain.

Cones are often described as being far less sensitive than rods, but this view is misleading, especially when considered in terms of the rapidly changing visual stimuli that the cones are specialized for signaling. Although a cone may exhibit a *peak* sensitivity to a brief flash of light that is perhaps 30-fold lower than in a rod, the sensitivity to rapidly fluctuating stimuli is considerably *higher* in cones than in rods; thus, the slow response of the rod makes it very insensitive to rapidly changing stimuli. When calculated in terms of the efficacy of activation in the G-protein cascade of phototransduction, the "amplification" in cones and rods appears to be essentially indistinguishable. The observed difference in sensitivity measured at the peak of the response to a flash instead stems from a difference in the speed of response inactivation.

Comparison of photopic and scotopic light adaptation

A classical result comparing light adaptation in the photopic and scotopic divisions of the visual system is illustrated in Fig. 20.1A, from the work of Stiles.[1] The threshold of a human subject for the detection of a flash is plotted against background intensity in double logarithmic coordinates. In this panel, the stimulus conditions provided a rod-based scotopic sensitivity that was only about 30× better than the cone-based photopic sensitivity—thus, the parafoveal region was tested with a small diameter yellow/green test flash (1 degree diameter, 60 ms, 580 nm) on a green background. The measurements are well described by Weber law curves, in both the scotopic (*blue trace*) and photopic (*red trace*) regions; see Eq. 20.1 below. However, the "dark light" that is described shortly is over 10,000× (4.1 log units) higher in the cone system than the rod system.

Scotopic vision: the rod system provides specialization for night vision

Light adaptation is examined under conditions that optimized detection by the scotopic (rather than photopic) system using the blue symbols of Fig. 20.1B. To achieve scotopic dominance, the test stimulus was presented in the peripheral retina, and comprised a large area, long duration green flash (9 degrees diameter, 200 ms, 520 nm) on a red background. The measurements are from Fig. 3 of Aguilar and Stiles[2] and their troland values have been converted using a factor of $K = 8.6$ photoisomerizations s^{-1} per troland.

For comparison, the red symbols plot the desensitization of primate rod photoreceptors, obtained from Fig. 9A and Table III in Tamura et al.[3] Their measurements of sensitivity have been converted to desensitization by taking the reciprocal; in addition, the symbols have been shifted vertically to provide a good fit to the psychophysical data in the high-intensity range.

The crucial difference between the blue and red symbols is that the overall scotopic visual system begins desensitizing at intensities around 1000 times lower than those required to begin desensitizing the rod photoreceptors. Thus, a considerable region at the lowest end of scotopic light adaptation is *post*receptoral, rather than being internal to the rods. Because the postreceptoral scotopic system is able to integrate photon signals from large numbers of rod photoreceptors, and thereby gain increased sensitivity, it needs to begin desensitizing at much lower background intensities to avoid saturation. As a result, the rod photoreceptors maintain their maximal sensitivity for several log units of the lowest-intensity regimen (up to approximately 10 isomerizations s^{-1}) over which the visual system exhibits gradual desensitization.

When the background intensity is reduced from relatively high scotopic intensities (moving from *right to left* along the x-axis in Fig. 20.1B) the desensitization of the rods, and of the scotopic visual system, steadily falls. However, below the intensities indicated by the *red and blue arrows*, the desensitization of first the rods and second the visual system fails to continue falling, as if the respective mechanism were experiencing a phenomenon equivalent to light. Accordingly, the arrowed intensities for the rods and for the scotopic visual system have been referred to as "equivalent background intensities," or "dark light." Clearly, the equivalent background for the scotopic system (around 0.016 photoisomerizations s^{-1}) is more than 1000× lower than the equivalent background intensity for the rods (around 50 isomerizations s^{-1}).

Each of the curves in Fig. 20.1 plots desensitization according to Weber's law, although the curves in Fig. 20.1B additionally include saturation at high intensities, as described by the equation:

$$\frac{Desens}{Desens_{D}} = \{1 + (I/I_0)\} \exp(I/I_{sat}) \qquad \textbf{(Eq. 20.1)}$$

where *Desens* is desensitization, $Desens_{D}$ is its dark-adapted value, and I is the background intensity. The first term on the right expresses Weber's law, where I_0 is the equivalent background intensity mentioned previously. This first term indicates that at low background intensities (when $I << I_0$) the desensitization approaches a constant level (its dark-adapted value, $Desens_{D}$), whereas for brighter backgrounds (when $I >> I_0$) the desensitization increases linearly with background intensity.

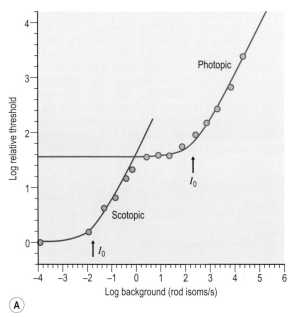

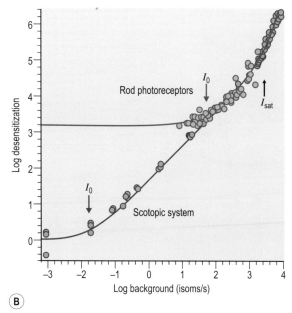

Fig. 20.1 Light adaptation of the photopic (cone) and scotopic (rod) divisions of the human visual system. Both panels plot psychophysical threshold as a function of background intensity in double logarithmic coordinates. (**A**) Scotopic and photopic thresholds for a test flash that was only about 30× more sensitive to the scotopic system. Data are from Stiles, converted to isomerizations s^{-1} in the rods, horizontally, and to threshold relative to the dark-adapted scotopic value, vertically. (**B**) *Blue symbols* are for conditions that optimized scotopic detection; data from Aguilar and Stiles. *Red symbols* are suction pipette measurements from isolated rod photoreceptors of monkeys (*Macaca fascicularis*), shifted vertically to align with the *blue symbols* in the upper intensity range; data from Tamua et al. All curves plot Weber's law; see text. (Panel A data from Stiles WS. Color vision: the approach through increment-threshold sensitivity. *Proc Natl Acad Sci USA.* 1959;45(1):100–114. Panel B data from Aguilar M, Stiles WS. Saturation of the rod mechanism of the retina at high levels of stimulation. *Optica Acta.* 1954;1:59–65 and Tamura T, Nakatani K, Yau K-W. Calcium feedback and sensitivity regulation in primate rods. *J Gen Physiol.* 1991;98(1):95–130.

At higher scotopic intensities, both the rods and the overall scotopic system exhibit saturation, characterized by a steep rise in desensitization with increasing background intensity. This behavior is described by the second term on the right in Eq. 20.1, where I_{sat} is termed the saturation intensity. It is almost certain that saturation of the overall scotopic system results directly from saturation of the rods. Thus, for the *blue and red curves* in Fig. 20.1B, the same value of saturation intensity, $I_{sat} = 2500$ photoisomerizations s^{-1} (*black arrow*), has been used. In contrast, the dark light is enormously different between the two curves, with $I_0 = 0.016$ and 50 photoisomerizations s^{-1}, respectively, for the psychophysical data (*blue arrow*) and the rod photoreceptor data (*red arrow*).

The span of intensities from I_0 (the dark light) to I_{sat} (the saturation intensity) represents the Weber region, and in this range of background intensities the desensitization is directly proportional to background intensity. The reciprocal of desensitization is the sensitivity, $S = 1/Desens$, and hence within the Weber region the sensitivity declines inversely with background intensity, i.e., $S \propto 1/I$.

Because the contrast in a visual stimulus is likewise inversely proportional to background intensity (i.e., contrast = $\Delta I/I$), this Weber region is characterized by a fixed level of contrast sensitivity, that is, a given level of contrast elicits a fixed size of response. Hence, an important feature of Weber law light adaptation is that it provides automatic extraction of visual contrast.

Fig. 20.1B shows that for the overall scotopic system the Weber region covers a very wide range, of at least 5 log units (i.e., over 100,000-fold).

LIGHT ADAPTATION OF THE ELECTRICAL RESPONSES OF CONES AND RODS

In the presence of background illumination, it is not only the overall visual system that adapts—the rod and cone photoreceptors themselves display light adaptation, characterized by desensitization and acceleration of their electrical response to an incremental flash.

However, for rods, such adaptation occurs over only a restricted range of intensities before saturation sets in. Thus, the *red* data in Fig. 20.1B show that the Weber region for mammalian rods encompasses only 1 to 2 log units of intensity before saturation; for the larger rods of lower vertebrates the Weber region may encompass a slightly wider range of about 3 log units.

In contrast, cone photoreceptors undergo light adaptation over an enormously wide range of intensities, and they manage to escape saturation no matter how intense the steady light. In the overall photopic visual system it is likely that the observed adaptation results primarily from these changes at the level of the cones, rather than through post-receptoral processing.

Saturation of the electrical response in rods and its avoidance in cones

The response of a salamander rod to the onset of steady illumination at different intensities is illustrated in Fig. 20.2. At the beginning of the step of light, the rod's response begins rising according to the prediction from the time integral of the flash response (noisy traces). But under normal conditions (*upper panel*) the response very soon

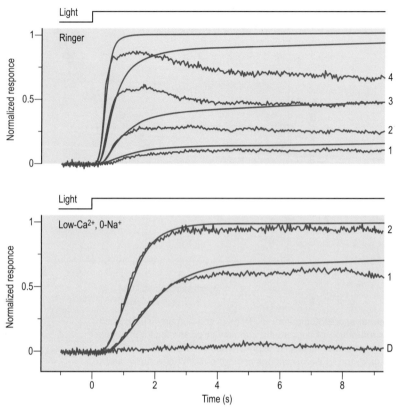

Fig. 20.2 Responses of a salamander rod to onset of steps of light of different intensity. *Upper panel:* under control conditions (Ringer solution). *Lower panel:* in the presence of Ca²⁺-clamping solution. The step intensities increased by factors of approximately 4 for traces labeled 1–4; *D,* darkness. The smooth curves are predictions obtained by integrating the measured dim-flash response (not shown) and represent the step responses that are predicted in the absence of any adaptation. (From Fain GL, Lamb TD, Matthews HR, Murphy RLW. Cytoplasmic calcium as the messenger for light adaptation in salamander rods. *J Physiol.* 1989;416:215.243.)

deviates, falling well below the linear prediction. Characteristically, the response to such a step of light typically exhibits an early peak followed by a sag? This deviation from the simplest linear prediction is a crucial aspect of light adaptation—if this deviation did not occur, then the rod would be driven into saturation by lights of very low intensity. Saturation can readily be induced by exposing the rod to a solution that clamps the cytoplasmic calcium concentration *(lower panel)*; the measured responses then follow the predictions of the theoretical curves, and a very low intensity *(labeled 2)* saturates the rod. This result shows that at least a part of the rod's ability to continue operating in backgrounds of moderate intensity is a consequence of changes in cytoplasmic calcium concentration; the molecular mechanisms that contribute to this will be discussed in section Molecular basis of photoreceptor light adaptation.

However, at higher background intensities, the circulating current in the normal rod becomes completely suppressed. Thus, for the *upper panel* of Fig. 20.2, intensities higher than that labeled 4 (not shown) cause the response simply to rise to its maximum level, corresponding to the closure of all cGMP-gated channels in the outer segment, with the consequence that incremental stimuli are unable to elicit any incremental response, and the cell's response is "saturated." Typically, such saturation sets in exponentially with increasing background intensity, as described earlier by the second term on the right of Eq. 20.1

Cone photoreceptors exhibit even more pronounced "sag" from an initial peak when steady background illumination is turned on. An example is illustrated for modest steady intensities in the early region of the traces in Fig. 20.3. The phenomenon is extremely robust in cones and, no matter how high the light intensity, the cone photoresponse always recovers to a reasonable operating level, even if it is transiently driven into saturation at the onset of intense illumination.

Desensitization and acceleration of the photoreceptor's electrical response

In addition to showing the transient nature of the responses elicited by the onset of backgrounds in cones, the main purpose of Fig. 20.3 is to illustrate the desensitization of the responses to incremental flashes that is elicited by these backgrounds.

The traces illustrate the responses of a cone photoreceptor to an identical set of flashes presented under three different conditions. In Fig. 20.3A the flashes (*a–f,* of progressively greater intensity) are presented in darkness. In Fig. 20.3B the same flashes are presented on a dim steady background, and in Fig. 20.3C they are presented on a brighter background. In the presence of background illumination, the responses to dim flashes are smaller. For example, for the second flash intensity, *b,* the response amplitude becomes markedly smaller from panel (A) to panel (B) to panel (C) of Fig. 20.3. In other words, backgrounds of increasing intensity progressively desensitized the cone's incremental response. Such behavior is very characteristic of photoreceptors (both cones and rods).

The changes in the dim-flash response elicited by backgrounds of different intensity are shown in Fig. 20.4A. The largest trace is the response to a dim flash presented under fully dark-adapted conditions, whereas the other traces are for the same flash presented on backgrounds of progressively brighter intensity. (In fact, to maintain responses of measurable amplitudes, the flash intensities were increased in the presence of backgrounds, and the traces actually plot response divided by flash intensity, i.e., response sensitivity.)

The traces in Fig. 20.4A demonstrate that the effect of increasing background intensity is both to desensitize and to accelerate the response to an incremental dim flash. This behavior of cones is very similar to that exhibited by rods, as illustrated in Fig. 20.4B.

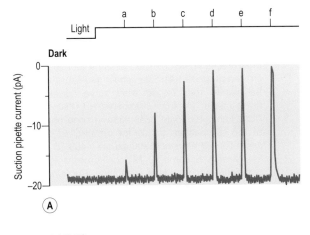

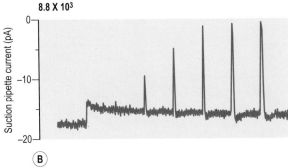

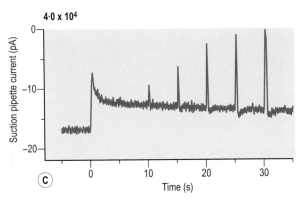

Fig. 20.3 Circulating current of a salamander cone in response to flashes and steps of illumination. Timing of illumination is indicated by the marker trace at the top; flashes *a–f* increased in intensity by factors of ~4 and were the same intensity in each of panels (**A–C**). In panel (**A**) these flashes were presented in darkness; in panels (**B**) and (**C**) the same flashes were presented on steady backgrounds that had been switched on at time zero; the background in (**C**) was approximately 4 times brighter than in (**B**). (From Matthews HR, Fain GL, Murphy RLW, Lamb TD. Light adaptation in cone photoreceptors of the salamander: a role for cytoplasmic calcium concentration. *J Physiol.* 1990;420:447–469.)

Unaltered rising phase but accelerated recovery

For the incremental flash responses of the rod illustrated in Fig. 20.4B, the vertical scale has been adjusted to take account of changes in the level of circulating current remaining in the presence of the different background intensities. Thus, rather than plotting raw sensitivity (response per photoisomerization), as is done in Fig. 20.4A for the cone, Fig. 20.4B for the rod instead plots the fractional response (i.e., the incremental response as a fraction of the circulating current at that

background) per photoisomerization. This has been done to provide a direct measure of the level of activation of the guanine nucleotide–binding protein (G-protein) cascade of phototransduction; thus, it can be shown that the level of cascade activation is best measured by the fractional channel opening, which in turn is measured by the incremental response expressed as a fraction of the existing circulating current.

When plotted in this manner, the incremental responses in Fig. 20.4B demonstrate the remarkable property that the onset phase of the response is invariant, (i.e., the traces for different background intensities exhibit a common rise at early times), indicated by the smooth *black trace*. This behavior indicates that the amplification parameter describing the activation steps in phototransduction is unaltered during light adaptation; in other words, light adaptation causes no change in the efficacy of the activation steps in phototransduction. Instead, what light adaptation does is to cause a marked speeding-up of the shut-off steps in the transduction cascade. The molecular identity of the steps that are accelerated is considered in section Molecular basis of photoreceptor light adaptation.

Dependence of sensitivity on background intensity: Weber's law

By plotting the peak amplitude of each of the traces in Fig. 20.4A as a function of the background intensity on which it was measured, one obtains a sensitivity versus background plot of the kind illustrated in Fig. 20.5.

The results plotted in Fig. 20.5 were obtained over an extremely wide range of background intensities by Burkhardt,[4] using a laser source of illumination. Importantly, the preparation was the intact eyecup (of the turtle), so that the photoreceptors remained in contact with the retinal pigment epithelium (RPE) and thereby experienced normal regeneration of visual pigment, so that physiologic results could be obtained even at very high background intensities.

For background intensities from 10^3 to 10^{11} photons μm^{-2} s^{-1}, the relationship between log sensitivity and log background intensity is a straight line with a slope of −1; in other words, over roughly 8 log units of background, the turtle cone's sensitivity declines inversely with background intensity. The curve plotted near the points in Fig. 20.5 represents Weber's law, described by:

$$\frac{S}{S_D} = \frac{1}{1 + (I/I_0)} \qquad \text{(Eq. 20.2)}$$

where S is flash sensitivity, S_D is its dark-adapted value, I is the background intensity, and I_0 is the half-desensitizing intensity, also known as the dark-adapted equivalent background intensity. This is the same equation as used in Fig. 20.1B for light adaptation of human rods, although without the saturation term (and in coordinates of sensitivity rather than its reciprocal). The good fit of the Weber law expression shows, very importantly, that cone photoreceptors in the intact eyecup are able to completely avoid saturation, even at enormously high intensities of steady illumination. This feature represents a crucial distinction between the properties of cones and rods. As illustrated earlier in Fig. 20.2, the circulating current of rods is shut off at quite low background intensities so that the rods become unresponsive to superimposed stimuli in the presence of background illumination of moderate intensity.

In the same set of experiments, Burkhardt[4] measured the intensity at which 90% of the pigment was in the bleached state, and found this to be around 10^6 photons μm^{-2} s^{-1}. Hence, for all intensities above that level, the observed Weber law behavior can be accounted for in terms of pigment bleaching. For each additional 10-fold increase in intensity there will be a 10-fold reduction in the amount of pigment

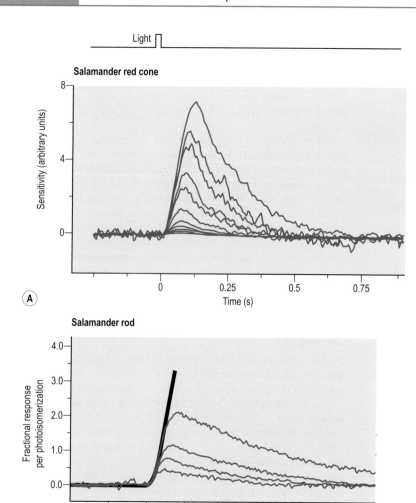

Fig. 20.4 Incremental responses of cone and rod photoreceptors to test flashes presented on backgrounds of progressively higher intensity. In each panel, the largest trace is for a dim flash presented in darkness, while the other traces correspond to the same test flash presented on backgrounds. (**A**) Salamander red-sensitive cone. (**B**) Salamander rod. *Smooth black curve* indicates common rising phase. (A, from Matthews HR, Fain GL, Murphy RLW, Lamb TD. Light adaptation in cone photoreceptors of the salamander: a role for cytoplasmic calcium concentration. *J Physiol.* 1990;420:447–469. B, from Pugh EN, Nikonov S, Lamb TD. Molecular mechanisms of vertebrate photoreceptor light adaptation. *Curr Opin Neurobiol.* 1999;9(4):410–418.)

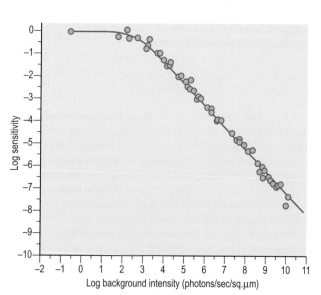

Fig. 20.5 Cone sensitivity as a function of background intensity. Results are plotted in double logarithmic coordinates and were obtained from intracellular measurements averaged from 15 cones in the turtle eyecup preparation. These experiments monitored step sensitivity rather than the more conventional flash sensitivity. The smooth curve plots Weber's law, given by Eq. 20.2. (Reproduced with permission from Nikonov S, Lamb TD, Pugh EN. The role of steady phosphodiesterase activity in the kinetics and sensitivity of the light-adapted salamander rod photoresponse. *J Gen Physiol.* 2000;116(6):795–824.)

remaining available to absorb light, and hence there will necessarily be a 10-fold reduction in sensitivity in the absence of any other change of parameters of transduction in the outer segment. In other words, if the photoreceptor is able to avoid saturation up to intensities that cause substantial bleaches, then it will be able to exhibit Weber law desensitization at all higher intensities purely by means of pigment bleaching. Cones are able to function up to this critical intensity, whereas rods saturate at much lower intensities.

Extremely rapid recovery of human cone photocurrent

Experiments on photoreceptors at high intensities must be undertaken in a preparation in which the retina is in contact with the retinal pigment epithelium (as was the case in the experiments previously described on turtle cones), so that visual pigment is regenerated. Thus, it is not possible to investigate cone responses at high intensities using single-cell or isolated retina preparations. Instead, to assess the performance of human cones at high background intensities, one is essentially restricted to experiments measuring the electroretinogram (ERG) in the intact eye.

Fig. 20.6 illustrates results from an experiment designed to measure the kinetics of recovery of the circulating current of human cone photoreceptors upon extinction of steady illumination that bleached 90% of the visual pigment. The traces show recordings of the human photopic ERG *a*-wave, which monitors the massed response primarily of the cone photoreceptors.

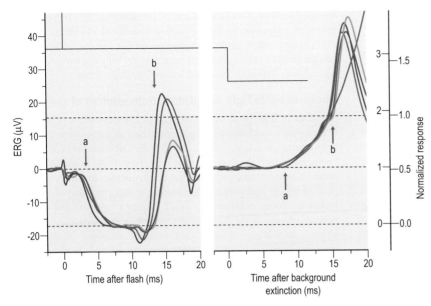

Fig. 20.6 Extremely rapid recovery of human cone photocurrent upon extinction of intense illumination, measured with the electroretinogram (*ERG*). The *left panel* shows the response to a bright flash superimposed on the intense steady background, while the *right panel* shows the response obtained at the extinction of that background. *Dashed horizontal lines* represent the following levels of cone circulating current (*from bottom*): zero level, steady level during intense background, dark level, as indicated by the two normalized scales on the *right*. See text for details. (From Kenkre JS, Moran NA, Lamb TD, Mahroo OAR. Extremely rapid recovery of human cone circulating current at the extinction of bleaching exposures. *J Physiol.* 2005;567(1):95–112.)

TABLE 20.1   Shut-off time constants estimated for primate cones and mouse rods

	τ_R	τ_E	τ_{Ca}	$\tau_{cG} = 1/\beta$ (Intense)		
	ms	ms	ms	ms	Preparation	Reference
Cone		18			Human electroretinogram (ERG)	6
	5	13	4		Human ERG	5
	3	9	3	4	Monkey retina	7
	3	10	3	6	Human ERG	8
Rod	70	200			Mouse suction pipette	9

Estimates for the shut-off time constants, τ_R, τ_E, τ_{Ca}, and τ_{cG}, obtained from recent experiments. It is not usually possible to determine which of the two time constants τ_R and τ_E is which; however, in the case of the mouse rod results, this identification was made using other experiments. Note that the turnover time for cyclic GMP, τ_{cG}, represents the value applicable during very intense illumination; under dark-adapted conditions, when the light-stimulated activity of the phosphodiesterase (PDE) is much lower, this time constant will be much longer.

The four *colored traces* plot ERG responses from two subjects, at two different flash intensities, while the light stimulus is monitored by the *black trace* at the top. The *left panel* is for an intense flash presented on the intense steady background, while the *right panel* is for extinction of that background. The "ON" *a*-wave and *b*-wave elicited by the bright flash are indicated by the *red arrows*, while the "OFF" *a*-wave and *b*-wave elicited by extinction of the background are indicated by the *blue arrows*. The *b*-wave is roughly similar in the two cases and arises from postreceptoral activity. The OFF *a*-wave represents recovery of the cone circulating current and begins around 7 ms after the intense background is turned off.

Fig. 20.6 shows two very important results relating to human cone responses in the presence of extremely bright illumination. First, the amplitude of the ON *a*-wave in the *left panel* shows that the steady cone circulating current remains at roughly 50% of its original level in darkness. Second, the early time at which the OFF *a*-wave in the *right panel* begins rising (indicated by the *blue arrow* at ~7 ms) shows that the cone circulating current begins recovering extremely rapidly.

Thus, although little change occurs for the first 7 ms, thereafter a substantial upward response occurs until about 15 ms after extinction of the background; at this point the *a*-wave is obscured by spike-like

activity of the *b*-wave. There is compelling evidence that the *a*-wave traces for these subjects monitor the recovery of the cone circulating current. On this basis, the cone circulating current is essentially fully recovered within about 15 ms after extinction of illumination so intense that it bleaches 90% of the cone pigment. This is extremely rapid recovery. The section Molecular basis of photoreceptor light adaptation considers the speed of the phototransduction shut-off reactions responsible for generating this rapid recovery, and the smooth curve near the measured traces in the *right-hand panel* of Fig. 20.6 was calculated from the model presented there, using the short time constants listed in Table 20.1.

Extremely rapid recovery of cone circulating current, as inferred from the results of Fig. 20.6, is required to account for classical experiments on the flicker fusion frequency of human subjects. Even at quite low photopic intensities, human subjects are able to detect square-wave flicker at a frequency of around 50 Hz using peripheral vision. But at higher intensities the flicker fusion frequency increases, to 100 Hz or more; at this frequency the illumination is being switched on and off for durations of 5 ms each. Thus, for the flicker to be detectable, some degree of recovery of cone circulating current must have occurred within 5 ms. Hence, human flicker sensitivity is broadly consistent with the time course inferred from Fig. 20.6.

MOLECULAR BASIS OF PHOTORECEPTOR LIGHT ADAPTATION

The phototransduction cascade

For a full description of the biochemistry of phototransduction, see Chapter 18. Fig. 20.7 presents a simplified schematic of these steps, emphasizing the shut-off reactions using *red arrows*. The lifetimes (or turnover times) of the important shut-off steps are: τ_R, the lifetime of activated rhodopsin; τ_E, the lifetime of activated transducin/phosphodiesterase (PDE); $\tau_{cG} = 1/\beta$, the turnover time of cyclic GMP; and τ_{Ca}, the turnover time of cytoplasmic free Ca^{2+}.

In summary, activation and recovery occur as follows. Light (of intensity *I*) activates the visual pigment, and the activated pigment (R*) is inactivated with a time constant τ_R. R* catalyzes activation of the guanine nucleotide–binding G-protein transducin to G*, which then binds to phosphodiesterase (E) to form the activated G*–E* complex (indicated E*), which has a lifetime τ_E. The activated E* catalyzes hydrolysis of cGMP (cG) with a rate constant β. The increase in β is proportional to steady intensity *I* with a scaling factor set by the product of the R* and E* lifetimes, that is, $\beta = \beta_{Dark} + (A/n_{cG}) \tau_R \tau_E I$ (see[11]). cGMP formation is catalyzed by guanylyl cyclase (GC) under the regulation of Ca^{2+}-sensitive GC–activating proteins (GCAPs). When present, cG causes the opening of ion channels (chans) in the plasma membrane, admitting Ca^{2+} ions. Cytoplasmic Ca^{2+} has a powerful negative feedback action via GCAPs onto the rate α of cGMP synthesis. Ca^{2+} ions are removed from the cytoplasm with a turnover time for free Ca^{2+} concentration of τ_{Ca}. Finally, and very slowly, visual pigment (R) is re-formed by delivery of 11-*cis* retinaldehyde (11-*cis* RAL) from the retinal pigment epithelium.

The mechanisms that contribute to light adaptation in photoreceptors (i.e., to the alteration in response properties of the photoreceptors upon exposure to background illumination) are closely associated with the mechanisms of response recovery (see Chapter 18). These mechanisms of adaptation can be classified broadly as (1) those that are calcium-dependent, and (2) those that do not involve calcium. Both categories play major roles and here the less well-known category of noncalcium-dependent mechanisms will be treated first.

Photoreceptor light adaptation independent of calcium

There are at least three classes of noncalcium-dependent phenomena that represent mechanisms of light adaptation in photoreceptors, where light adaptation is interpreted as an alteration of response properties in comparison with the dark-adapted state. First, there is response compression, whereby the reduced level of circulating current in the presence of steady background illumination reduces the size of the flash response. Cones substantially avoid response compression through powerful feedback mechanisms that maintain the circulating current. Second, there is pigment depletion, which is relevant to cones at high intensity; however, it is never relevant to rods, because they are driven into saturation by even very low levels of bleached pigment (see section Dark adaptation of the rods: very slow recovery from bleaching). Third, there is a direct effect of PDE activation, which is now considered.

Accelerated turnover of cGMP

In darkness, the activity of the PDE is relatively low, so that the turnover rate of cGMP hydrolysis (denoted β) is low and the turnover time for cGMP ($\tau_{cGMP} = 1/\beta$) is long. Under dark-adapted conditions, τ_{cGMP} is around 1 s in amphibian rods and around 200 ms in mammalian rods. The magnitude of this parameter has a major effect on both the sensitivity and the kinetics of the photoreceptor's response to a flash. Thus, when the PDE activity increases in steady illumination, the shorter turnover time for cGMP contributes both to desensitization and to acceleration of the photoresponse.

To provide an intuitive understanding of this mechanism, it is helpful to consider what we have referred to previously as the "bathtub analogy."[11] Imagine a container of water, such as a tall cylinder, and let the height of water in the cylinder represent the level (concentration) of cGMP in the outer segment. The rate at which water runs out of the cylinder through a drain-hole at the base is proportional both to the height of water and to the size of the opening, representing the cGMP level and the PDE activity, β, respectively. Likewise, the rate at which water flows into the cylinder through a tap at the top represents the activity of GC, α. When a steady state is reached, the height of water will equal the rate of influx divided by the size of the drain-hole, (i.e., cGMP = α/β). Importantly, whenever the water level is perturbed from this steady-state level (e.g., upon a brief opening of an additional drain-hole), the level will re-equilibrate with a time constant $\tau_{cGMP} = 1/\beta$ (provided that the rate of influx through the tap remains constant). Hence, if the drain-hole is small (and the inflow via the tap correspondingly small), then any perturbation in water level elicited by a transient additional outflow will be corrected only slowly; if the drain-hole is large (and the influx correspondingly large), then any perturbation will be rapidly corrected. Furthermore, although perhaps less intuitively, it can be shown that for a noninstantaneous perturbation, corresponding to the normal flash response, not only will the kinetics of recovery be faster, but also the peak will be smaller.

Hence the effect of the increased PDE activity during steady illumination is both to accelerate the response kinetics and to reduce the peak amplitude to an incremental flash. Calculations show that in amphibian rods the 20-fold increase in β during steady illumination provides the primary mechanism underlying the measured shortening of time-to-peak and the decrease in flash sensitivity.[11]

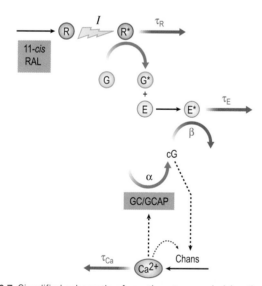

Fig. 20.7 Simplified schematic of reaction steps underlying the recovery steps in phototransduction. See text for details. (From Lamb TD, Pugh EN. Avoidance of saturation in human cones is explained by very rapid inactivation reactions and pigment bleaching. *Invest Ophthalmol Vis Sci.* 2006;47;e3714.Reproduced from Association for Research in Vision and Ophthalmology.)

Calcium-dependent mechanisms of rapid light adaptation: resensitization through prevention of saturation

When cGMP-gated ion channels in the outer segment are closed in response to light, the cytoplasmic concentration of calcium drops (see Chapter 19). This drop in Ca^{2+} concentration is vitally important to light adaptation, although it is crucial to emphasize that it does not cause the desensitization that characterizes photoreceptor light adaptation. Quite the contrary: the drop in Ca^{2+} concentration actually rescues the rod from the saturation that would otherwise be induced by light, and thereby prevents the onset of massive desensitization at relatively low intensities of background illumination. Thus, the light-induced drop in Ca^{2+} acts to increase the rod's sensitivity above the drastically reduced level that would occur either if the Ca^{2+} concentration did not alter or if the rod's calcium-dependent mechanisms were inoperative.

Powerful negative feedback loop mediated by calcium

Calcium is the cytoplasmic messenger for a very powerful negative feedback loop that tends to stabilize the photoreceptor's circulating current. If ever the Ca^{2+} concentration drops (e.g., in response to light, or as a result of some other perturbation) then, as described in Chapters 18 and 19 and further here, a number of changes occur very rapidly. These changes are stimulated by the unbinding of Ca^{2+} from at least three classes of calcium-sensitive proteins: (1) GCAPs (GCAPs 1 and 2), which activate GC; (2) recoverin, which regulates the lifetime of activated R*; and (3) a protein that modulates the opening of cGMP-gated channels—in rods this is calmodulin and in fish cones this function is accomplished by CNG-modulin. Calcium's action via each of these pathways leads to the opening of cGMP-gated channels, thereby increasing the circulating current and admitting Ca^{2+} ions from the extracellular medium. This influx of Ca^{2+} ions tends to counteract the initial reduction in Ca^{2+} concentration, thereby completing a negative feedback loop.

Each of these molecular mechanisms involved in the calcium negative feedback loop contributes toward extending the cell's operational range of light intensities by helping to prevent saturation of the circulating current. Thus, each of these three molecular mechanisms assists in *rescuing* the photoreceptor from saturation and hence *increasing*, rather than decreasing, the sensitivity compared with the case that would exist if the mechanism were absent. Each of the three mechanisms is most effective over a particular range of calcium levels, and hence over a particular range of light intensities. The most powerful of the three (at least in rods) is the GCAP activation of GC. Interestingly, rods and cones share the same calcium feedback components, including GCAP1/2 and recoverin, but GCAP3 is expressed exclusively in cones, and may therefore contribute to the more efficient light adaptation in cones.

Because the various components of the calcium negative feedback loop act quite rapidly, they contribute not only to determining the photoreceptor's sensitivity in the presence of background illumination, but also to determining the kinetics of its response to an incremental flash presented on the background. The importance of altered Ca^{2+} concentration in setting the incremental flash response kinetics can be demonstrated by incorporating a calcium buffer (such as BAPTA) into the outer segment. Fig. 20.8A shows that although the flash response begins rising exactly as in control conditions, it does not recover as rapidly and instead rises to a substantially larger and later peak with slower final recovery. The three calcium-sensitive molecular pathways will now be described.

Guanylyl cyclase activation

In response to a drop in calcium concentration, Ca^{2+} will unbind from the GCAP proteins (GCAP1 and GCAP2), thereby activating GC and stimulating the production of cGMP at a greatly increased rate, leading to the opening of cGMP-gated channels.

The cyclase activity increases roughly as the fourth power of the drop in Ca^{2+} concentration, and furthermore (as for the other two routes considered below) the number of channels open increases approximately as the cube of the cGMP concentration. Because of the cascading of two such steep dependencies, any small fractional change in Ca^{2+} concentration stimulates a large and opposite fractional change in channel opening; that is, the fractional change in channel opening

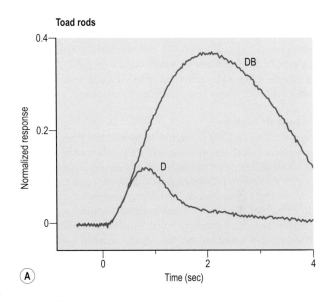

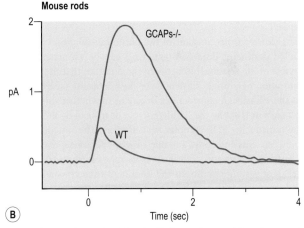

Fig. 20.8 Comparison of calcium buffering and guanylyl cyclase–activating proteins (GCAPs) knockout on the rod's dim-flash response. Both panels plot suction pipette recordings from single rods. (**A**) Salamander rod response to a flash in darkness (*D*) and to the same flash after incorporation of the calcium buffer BAPTA (*DB*). (Reproduced with permission from Van Hateren JH, Lamb TD. The photocurrent response of human cones is fast and monophasic. *BMC Neurosci.* 2006;7:34.) (**B**) Mouse rod single-photon responses, for wild type (*WT*) and GCAPs knockout (GCAPs –/–) animals. (A, from Torre V, Matthews HR, Lamb TD. Role of calcium in regulating the cyclic GMP cascade of phototransduction in retinal rods. *Proc Natl Acad Sci USA.* 1986;83:7109–7113. B, from Burns ME, Mendez A, Chen J, Baylor DA. Dynamics of cyclic GMP synthesis in retinal rods. *Neuron.* 2002;36(1):81–91.)

is opposite in sign to, and up to 12× the magnitude of, the originating fractional change in Ca^{2+} concentration. As a result, this molecular mechanism is the most potent of the three that contribute to the calcium negative feedback loop and hence to setting the adaptational state in rods. It is especially dominant at relatively bright background intensities, corresponding to low Ca^{2+} concentrations, and is therefore the most important in extending the rod's operating range to high intensities.

The role of the GCAP/GC component of the Ca^{2+} feedback loop in setting the waveform of the incremental flash response is illustrated in Fig. 20.8B, where averaged responses are shown for rods from wild type (WT) and GCAPs knockout mice. In a manner very similar to that seen in amphibian rods containing the calcium buffer BAPTA, the response in the GCAP knockout case begins rising exactly as for the control (WT) case, but it does not recover as soon, so that the response continues rising and reaches a larger and later peak. Analysis of rod physiology in GCAP1-deficient mice indicates that GCAP1 is the early sensor protein that stimulates GC1 early in the response and thus limits its amplitude, followed by activation of GCAP2 that adds stimulation of both GC1 and 2 to speed-up photoreceptor recovery.[12]

Shortened R* lifetime

Activated rhodopsin (R*) is inactivated by multiple phosphorylation steps mediated by rhodopsin kinase (GRK1) followed by binding of arrestin (for details, see Chapter 18). It is generally assumed that the decline in R* activity follows exponential kinetics and can therefore be described by a characteristic lifetime, τ_R; however, it is worth bearing in mind that there is no direct evidence for this assumption. It was established by Kawamura[13] that GRK1's phosphorylation of R* is calcium dependent and that the effect is mediated by the calcium-binding protein recoverin (termed S-modulin in frog). The molecular mechanism of this dependence is not entirely clear, but some evidence suggests that the calcium-bound form of recoverin binds to GRK1, thereby preventing it from interacting with R*. In any case, it is proposed that a reduction in Ca^{2+} concentration leads to a shortened R* lifetime, τ_R.

The slowest time constant in the phototransduction cascade (the so-called dominant time constant, τ_{dom}) can be estimated from the steepness of the relationship between the duration that the rod is held in saturation by a bright flash and the flash intensity (see[14]). Over the years there has been considerable debate as to whether this dominant time constant is set by the R* lifetime, τ_R, or instead by the lifetime τ_E of the transducin- PDE complex (the effector). The situation may differ between rods and cones and may also be species dependent. But in mouse rods, Burns and colleagues have now clearly established that under dark resting conditions the dominant time constant is that of transducin-PDE, with $\tau_E \approx 200$ ms, while the R* lifetime is shorter, with $\tau_R \leq 80$ ms[9] (see Table 20.1). In this scenario, where the R* lifetime is shorter than the transducin-PDE lifetime, then further light-induced shortening of τ_R is likely to have very little effect on the response kinetics, but it will instead cause a reduction in sensitivity, because fewer molecules of transducin will be activated during the R* lifetime.

Although it remains difficult to establish the effectiveness of any individual mechanism in an intact photoreceptor with a functional calcium feedback loop, it appears that in rods the recoverin-mediated reduction in R* lifetime plays a moderate role, especially at relatively low background intensities.

Channel reactivation

In response to a drop in calcium concentration, Ca^{2+} unbinds from calmodulin (in the case of the rods), leading to a lowered dissociation constant ($K_{1/2}$) for the binding of cGMP to the channels. The effect of the lowered $K_{1/2}$ is that any given concentration of cGMP will cause the opening of a larger fraction of the cGMP-gated channels, leading to an increase in circulating current and an influx of more calcium. However, the potency of this effect is low in rods, and the mechanism contributes only weakly to rod adaptation. In contrast, cone channels possess a more powerful regulatory mechanism, mediated by a different calcium-sensitive protein[15] (see Chapter 19). Whereas in zebrafish cones, channel modulation is accomplished by CNG-modulin,[16] the mammalian homolog of this protein, EML1, does not seem to be involved in regulating cone channel conductance and the identity of the mammalian cone calcium regulator is still unknown.

Molecular basis of the cone's incredibly rapid recovery from light exposure

The speed of recovery of human cones from prolonged intense illumination is extremely rapid (section Molecular basis of photoreceptor light adaptation), and the time constants of the various shut-off reactions shown in the schematic of Fig. 20.7 have been estimated in a number of studies of primate cones using intact preparations. In the case of monkey cones, the parameters were extracted via theoretical modeling of results obtained from intracellular recordings of horizontal cells in the retina-RPE-choroid preparation. In the case of human cones, the parameters were extracted via theoretical modeling of ERG results, including those of the kind illustrated in Fig. 20.6. The shut-off reactions have been found to be extremely rapid, and the parameters that have been reported are summarized in Table 20.1.

The collected estimates in Table 20.1 are consistent with the notion that all four of the shut-off time constants in human cones are extremely short, with three of the time constants around 5 ms or less, and one around 10 to 15 ms. Hence the shut-off time constants for both the activated visual pigment (R*) and the activated G-protein/PDE (E*), τ_R and τ_E, are around 20-fold shorter in human cones than in mouse rods, where values of approximately 70 and approximately 200 ms have been reported. It has been discovered that disruption of a molecular step involved in shut-off of phototransduction can lead to slowed light adaptation in cones (see Box 20.1).

Cone avoidance of saturation

A theoretical analysis[10] has shown that the ability of mammalian cones to avoid saturation is explicable in terms of the combination of these two 20-fold shorter time constants, together with the bleaching of cone visual pigment.

In human rod photoreceptors *in vivo*, the circulating current is halved at a steady intensity of approximately 70 scotopic trolands or $600\,R^* \text{ s}^{-1}$,[20] with complete saturation occurring at approximately 1000 scotopic trolands ($\sim 10^4\,R^* \text{ s}^{-1}$) (see also Fig. 20.1B). On the assumption that the gain of activation in transduction is the same in human cones as in human rods, then the two very short cone time constants would elevate the intensities required for half- and full-saturation by approximately 400×, to levels of approximately 240,000 and approximately $4 \times 10^6\,R^* \text{ s}^{-1}$ in human cones. An additional factor is that the cGMP-gated channels of mammalian cones show increased cGMP binding affinity when Ca^{2+} falls,[15] thus further increasing the R* rate required for saturation.

How do these estimated rates of isomerization compare with the maximum rate at which the cone visual pigment can be bleached during steady illumination? At steady state, the rate of photoisomerization equals the rate of pigment regeneration, which is set by the delivery of 11-*cis* retinal to opsin. For human L/M cones, the maximal rate of regeneration has been measured as approximately 45% min^{-1}, or 0.75% s^{-1}. If the outer segment contains approximately 40 million pigment molecules, then the maximal rate of

BOX 20.1   Altered light adaptation when phototransduction shut off is disrupted

Changes in light adaptation performance as a result of retinal disease are uncommon—any disturbance of the phototransduction cascade tends to cause major disruption of signaling rather than a subtle change in adaptation. For example, Oguchi disease, which impairs the shut off of the transduction cascade (through mutations in either rhodopsin kinase or arrestin), leads to symptoms resembling stationary night blindness.

It has been discovered that altered light-adaptation behavior can result from impairment of the reactions that inactivate the light-activated PDE (PDE6). Thus, mutations in the *RGS9-1* or *R9AP* genes have been shown to affect light adaptation,[17,18] although in a manner that may appear counter-intuitive.[19]

Patients with mutations in the *RGS9-1* or *R9AP* report difficulty in adapting to sudden changes in photopic luminance and experience difficulty seeing moving objects, especially at low contrast. This stationary condition has been termed bradyopsia (slow vision).[17,18] This slowness is expected, because disruption of the PDE shut-off process should lead to an extended time course of the photoreceptor response to illumination.

Paradoxically, at low light levels the responses of cones lacking *RGS9-1* are actually faster than those of normal cones.[19] When a second effect of PDE is taken into consideration, this result turns out to be exactly as predicted. Not only is the PDE involved in shutting off the light response by hydrolyzing cyclic GMP, but it is also involved in light adaptation and in response acceleration by shortening the "turnover time" for cyclic GMP.[11] Thus, with RGS9-1 absent, there is more PDE active at low light levels, and hence a shorter turnover time for cyclic GMP and thereby a "more adapted" state than in the normal case. Accordingly, although these patients will have slower than normal vision at high lighting levels, they will have faster than normal vision (i.e., apparent light adaptation) at dim lighting levels.

photoisomerization during intense steady light will be approximately 300,000 R* s⁻¹. This rate simply cannot be exceeded in the steady state because a higher initial rate of isomerization would deplete the available pigment thereby lowering the rate.

Hence, from the numbers in the preceding paragraphs, the rate of photoisomerization required to saturate the human cone current exceeds the highest rate of isomerization of cone pigment molecules (~300,000 R* s⁻¹) that can be elicited by a steady light of arbitrarily high intensity. Therefore, the human cone photoreceptor cannot be saturated by *steady* lights, no matter how bright they are. This does not mean that the cone can never be saturated; if an intense light is presented from dark-adapted conditions (when the cone initially has a full complement of visual pigment), then it will transiently be driven into saturation until bleaching reduces the amount of visual pigment to a suitably low level.

The extremely rapid rate of cone pigment regeneration mentioned earlier requires a very efficient supply with 11-*cis* retinal visual chromophore. Work over the past decade has demonstrated that for cones this is achieved by the combined action of two separate mechanisms—a common rod and cone pathway involving recycling chromophore through the RPE, and another, cone-specific, pathway that involves the Müller glial cells in the retina.[21] The combined action of these two chromophore recycling pathways enables the rapid pigment regeneration and dark adaptation of cones, in contrast to the significantly slower dark adaptation of the rods that is driven exclusively by chromophore supplied by the RPE.

Modeling of human cone light adaptation

A computational model of human cone light adaptation has been developed[22] that puts factors of the kind described in the preceding section into a comprehensive theoretical/numerical model. The molecular description that they use is closely similar to that illustrated in Fig. 20.7, including pigment bleaching, and they express the system as a set of differential equations. Their simulations confirm that human cones will indeed not saturate with steady intensities of any level and predict that the sensitivity will conform to Weber's law over a very wide range of background intensities.

SLOW CHANGES IN RODS: LIGHT ADAPTATION OR DARK ADAPTATION?

In addition to the conventional features of rod photoreceptor light adaptation that occur extremely rapidly (on a subsecond time scale), other changes have been reported to occur over a time frame of minutes of exposure in response to lights that saturate the cell's response. Because the effects of these changes are very slow and can only be observed in darkness when the adapting exposure is extinguished, there is a semantic issue as to whether these phenomena should be thought of as light adaptation or as dark adaptation.

Light-induced change in the dominant time constant

Exposure of mouse rods to a just-saturating intensity of around 1000 photoisomerizations s⁻¹ for 1 min or more leads to a persistent speeding of the bright-flash response upon extinction of the background.[23] The change does not involve any reduction in the activation phase of transduction, but instead involves a reduction in the dominant time constant of response recovery; typically, the dominant time constant τ_{dom} drops from around 200 ms under dark-adapted conditions to around 100 ms immediately after extinction of the saturating light. This adaptational effect develops relatively slowly, building up over 60 s or so, and it requires a rhodopsin bleach level of around 2% for full effect. The effect is relatively long-lasting, declining with a time constant of around 80 s.

The molecular mechanism giving rise to this adaptational effect is not known, although some evidence suggests that it corresponds to a reduction in lifetime of the activated transducin-PDE complex. If so, it represents a phenomenon distinct from the actions of dimmer adapting lights.

Light-induced translocation of proteins

Light-induced translocation of transducin, recoverin, and arrestin in photoreceptors is considered in Chapter 18 and will briefly be mentioned here. Movements of protein are elicited only at quite high intensities (generally in the saturating range), and they occur over a time scale of many minutes. In mouse rods, intensities above 3000 photoisomerizations s⁻¹ for 30 min (which bleach a substantial fraction of the rhodopsin) trigger the movement of transducin from the outer segment to the inner segment, whereas slightly lower intensities of 1000 photoisomerizations s⁻¹ or more trigger the movement of arrestin in the opposite direction; recoverin also leaves the outer segment in bright light.

Protein movements of these kinds can eventually affect the adaptational state of rods, allowing them to generate responses in photopic light conditions.[24] In a series of elegant experiments, Sampath and colleagues[25] demonstrated that the gradual rod escape from saturation is driven by the movement of transducin away from the rod outer segments. The resulting reduction in the amplification of the signal effectively dampens the rod response and facilitates escape

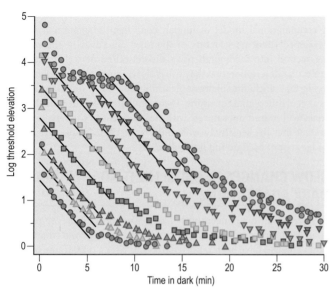

Fig. 20.9 Human psychophysical dark adaptation. Recovery of log threshold elevation in a normal human observer is plotted as a function of time in darkness, after a wide range of bleaching exposures (from 0.5% to 98%). *Parallel black lines* represent component S2, with a slope of −0.24 decades min⁻¹ (see text). The lateral shift between the lines is consistent with the rate-limited delivery of 11-*cis* retinal from the RPE to opsin in the outer segments. (From Lamb TD, Pugh EN. Phototransduction, dark adaptation, and rhodopsin regeneration. The Proctor Lecture. *Invest Ophthalmol Vis Sci*. 2006;47(12):5138–5152. Reproduced from Association for Research in Vision and Ophthalmology.)

BOX 20.2 Diseases exhibiting slowed dark adaptation

A variety of diseases lead to slowed dark adaptation, and the great majority of these do so by affecting reactions of the retinoid cycle, and thereby reducing the effective concentration of 11-*cis* retinal in the retinal pigment epithelium.[29]

Mild cases of systemic vitamin A deficiency (VAD) lead to a slowing of the S2 component of dark adaptation, yet without any alteration in the final fully dark-adapted visual threshold.[32] This occurs because all the bleached opsin is able (eventually) to recombine with retinoid—the recombination is simply slowed. In these mild cases, supplementation with vitamin A can lead to a rapid and complete recovery of dark adaptation, showing that no other pathology was present. With more pronounced or extended deficiency, the final visual threshold becomes elevated, and eventually the photoreceptors may degenerate.

Fundus albipunctatus typically results from mutation of the 11-*cis* retinol dehydrogenase *RDH5* gene. The S2 component of rod dark adaptation is greatly slowed, but (as in VAD) the final visual thresholds are entirely normal.[33]

Sorsby fundus dystrophy is caused by a mutation in *TIMP3*, a metalloproteinase of the matrix in Bruch's membrane. All the features of this disease are consistent with the slowing of dark adaptation being caused by ocular VAD.[32]

Bothnia dystrophy is one of a group of rare diseases that involve mutations in CRALBP, the chaperone protein for 11-*cis* retinal. In these patients, loss of CRALBP leads to enormously slowed dark adaptation.[34]

BOX 20.3 Slowed dark adaptation as an early indicator of age-related maculopathy

The speed of dark adaptation is slowed in age-related maculopathy (ARM).[35–37] Thus, the slope of the S2 component of recovery is noticeably lower in patients with early ARM than in healthy subjects of similar age. Characteristic changes in ARM include a thickening of Bruch's membrane and the deposition of neutral lipids. Hence, the likely explanation for the slowing of dark adaptation in ARM is that the transport of vitamin A from the choroidal circulation is hindered, so that the RPE/retina becomes vitamin A deficient, i.e., that there is ocular vitamin A deficiency.

As a result, measurement of the slowing of dark adaptation is likely to provide a valuable and noninvasive bioassay, both as a diagnostic tool for predicting the likelihood of onset of macular degeneration, and as a means of assessing the efficacy of treatments of the disease.

from saturation after minutes in photopic light. These results also help explain the long-known gradual shift in the functional properties of skate rods in the presence of steady bright light.[26]

DARK ADAPTATION OF THE RODS: VERY SLOW RECOVERY FROM BLEACHING

After our eye has been exposed to very intense illumination, our visual threshold is greatly elevated and may take tens of minutes to recover fully.[27] Comparable effects can be also measured at the level of the rod bipolar cells[28] or the rod photoreceptors.[20] The slow recovery of sensitivity is referred to as "dark adaptation" or "bleaching adaptation," but this use of the term "adaptation" is misleading. Adaptation normally refers to beneficial adjustments, yet the changes that persist after extinction of intense illumination are distinctly disadvantageous—thus, there can be no advantage in having one's vision greatly compromised following exposure to intense light.

The recovery of visual threshold for a human subject is plotted in Fig. 20.9, following the cessation of nine light exposures that bleached from 0.5% to 98% of the rhodopsin.[29,30] For a bleach of 20%, the visual threshold was initially elevated by 3.5 log units. This indicates that the elevation of threshold is out of all proportion to the fraction of pigment remaining unbleached; even though 80% of the rhodopsin remained functional, the threshold was raised 3000-fold. Instead, there is now overwhelming evidence that the phenomenon arises from the presence within the outer segment of unregenerated opsin (i.e., the presence of the protein part of the visual pigment prior to its recombination with the regenerated 11-*cis* retinal).

Remarkably, the recovery of scotopic (rod-mediated) threshold exhibits a region of common slope across all the bleach levels, as indicated by the parallel black lines in Fig. 20.9. This region is termed the

S2 component of recovery and has a slope $\Psi_{S2} = -0.24$ log unit min⁻¹ that is characteristic of dark adaptation recovery in normal (young adult) human eyes. Also characteristic is the nature of the rightward shift of the recovery traces as a function of increasing bleach level—the form of this shift is as expected for a rate-limited (zero-order) recovery process, as distinct from an exponential (first-order) recovery process.

From a detailed analysis of results of this kind, in combination with knowledge of the retinoid cycle, Lamb and Pugh[31] developed a cellular model that can account for human dark adaptation behavior. They postulated (1) that the presence of opsin (without chromophore) gives rise to a phenomenon closely equivalent to light, through activation of the G-protein cascade of transduction, and (2) that the elimination of opsin via its reconversion to rhodopsin follows rate-limited kinetics because of a limitation in the supply of 11-*cis* retinal that results from the diffusion of this substance from a pool in the RPE.

Application of this cellular model has provided an accurate account of: (1) the regeneration of visual pigment in humans and other mammals, measured by retinal densitometry; (2) normal human dark adaptation behavior (as in Fig. 20.9); and (3) the slowed regeneration of pigment and the slowed dark adaptation that is characteristic of a number of diseases that affect the photoreceptors and/or RPE (see Boxes 20.2 and 20.3).[31]

REFERENCES

1. Stiles WS. Color vision: the approach through increment-threshold sensitivity. *Proc Natl Acad Sci USA.* 1959;45(1):100–114.
2. Aguilar M, Stiles WS. Saturation of the rod mechanism of the retina at high levels of stimulation. *Optica Acta.* 1954;1:59–65.
3. Tamura T, Nakatani K, Yau K-W. Calcium feedback and sensitivity regulation in primate rods. *J Gen Physiol.* 1991;98(1):95–130.
4. Burkhardt DA. Light adaptation and photopigment bleaching in cone photoreceptors in situ in the retina of the turtle. *J Neurosci.* 1994;14(3):1091–1105.
5. Friedburg C, Allen CP, Mason PJ, Lamb TD. Contribution of cone photoreceptors and post-receptoral mechanisms to the human photopic electroretinogram. *J Physiol Lond.* 2004;556(3):819–834.
6. Kenkre JS, Moran NA, Lamb TD, Mahroo OAR. Extremely rapid recovery of human cone circulating current at the extinction of bleaching exposures. *J Physiol Lond.* 2005; 567(1):95–112.
7. Van Hateren H. A cellular and molecular model of response kinetics and adaptation in primate cones and horizontal cells. *J Vision.* 2005;5(4):331–347.
8. Van Hateren JH, Lamb TD. The photocurrent response of human cones is fast and monophasic. *BMC Neurosci.* 2006;7:34.
9. Krispel CM, Chen D, Melling N, et al. RGS expression rate-limits recovery of rod photoresponses. *Neuron.* 2006;51(4):409–416.
10. Lamb TD, Pugh EN. Avoidance of saturation in human cones is explained by very rapid inactivation reactions and pigment bleaching. *Invest Ophth Vis Sci.* 2006;47:e 3714.
11. Nikonov S, Lamb TD, Pugh EN. The role of steady phosphodiesterase activity in the kinetics and sensitivity of the light-adapted salamander rod photoresponse. *J Gen Physiol.* 2000;116(6):795–824.
12. Makino CL, Wen XH, Olshevskaya EV, Peshenko IV, Savchenko AB, Dizhoor AM. Enzymatic relay mechanism stimulates cyclic GMP synthesis in rod photoresponse: biochemical and physiological study in guanylyl cyclase activating protein 1 knockout mice. *PLoS One.* 2012;7(10):e47637.
13. Kawamura S. Rhodopsin phosphorylation as a mechanism of cyclic GMP phosphodiesterase regulation by S-modulin. *Nature.* 1993;362(6423):855–857.
14. Pepperberg DR, Cornwall MC, Kahlert M, et al. Light-dependent delay in the falling phase of the retinal rod photoresponse. *Visual Neurosci.* 1992;8(1):9–18.
15. Rebrik TI, Korenbrot JI. In intact mammalian photoreceptors, Ca²⁺-dependent modulation of cGMP-gated ion channels is detectable in cones but not in rods. *J Gen Physiol.* 2004;123(1):63–75.
16. Rebrik TI, Botchkina I, Arshavsky VY, Craft CM, Korenbrot JI. CNG-modulin: a novel Ca-dependent modulator of ligand sensitivity in cone photoreceptor cGMP-gated ion channels. *J Neurosci.* 2012;32(9):3142–3153.
17. Nishiguchi KM, Sandberg MA, Kooijman AC, et al. Defects in RGS9 or its anchor protein R9AP in patients with slow photoreceptor deactivation. *Nature.* 2004;427(6969):75–78.
18. Hartong DT, Pott JWR, Kooijman AC. Six patients with bradyopsia (slow vision) – clinical features and course of the disease. *Ophthalmology.* 2007;114(12):2323–2331.
19. Stockman A, Smithson HE, Webster AR, et al. The loss of the PDE6 deactivating enzyme, RGS9, results in precocious light adaptation at low light levels. *J Vision.* 2008;8(1).
20. Thomas MM, Lamb TD. Light adaptation and dark adaptation of human rod photoreceptors measured from the a-wave of the electroretinogram. *J Physiol Lond.* 1999; 518(2):479–496.
21. Wang JS, Kefalov VJ. The cone-specific visual cycle. *Prog Retin Eye Res.* 2011;30(2):115–128.
22. Van Hateren JH, Snippe HP. Simulating human cones from mid-mesopic up to high-photopic luminances. *J Vision.* 2007;7(4):1.
23. Krispel CM, Chen CK, Simon MI, Burns ME. Prolonged photoresponses and defective adaptation in rods of G beta 5(-/-) mice. *J Neurosci.* 2003;23(18):6965–6971.
24. Tikidji-Hamburyan A, Reinhard K, Storchi R, et al. Rods progressively escape saturation to drive visual responses in daylight conditions. *Nat Commun.* 2017;8(1):1813.
25. Frederiksen R, Morshedian A, Tripathy SA, Xu T, Travis GH, Fain GL, Sampath AP. Rod Photoreceptors avoid saturation in bright light by the movement of the G protein transducin. *J Neurosci.* 2021;41(15):3320–3330.
26. Ripps H, Dowling JE. Structural features and adaptive properties of photoreceptors in the skate retina. *J Exp Zool Suppl.* 1990;5:46–54.
27. Stiles WS, Crawford BH. Equivalent adaptational levels in localized retinal areas. *Report of a Joint Discussion on Vision.* London: Cambridge University Press; 1932:194–211. (Reprinted in Stiles WS. *Mechanisms of Colour Vision.* London: Academic Press; 1978.)
28. Cameron AM, Mahroo OAR, Lamb TD. Dark adaptation of human rod bipolar cells measured from the b-wave of the scotopic electroretinogram. *J Physiol Lond.* 2006;575(2):507–526.
29. Lamb TD, Pugh EN. Phototransduction, dark adaptation, and rhodopsin regeneration. The Proctor Lecture. *Invest Ophth Vis Sci.* 2006;47(12):5138–5152.
30. Pugh EN. Rushton's paradox: rod dark adaptation after flash photolysis. *J Physiol Lond.* 1975;248(2):413–431.
31. Lamb TD, Pugh EN. Dark adaptation and the retinoid cycle of vision. *Prog Retin Eye Res.* 2004;23(3):307–380.
32. Cideciyan AV, Pugh EN, Lamb TD, Huang YJ, Jacobson SG. Plateaux during dark adaptation in Sorsby's fundus dystrophy and vitamin A deficiency. *Invest Ophth Vis Sci.* 1997;38(9):1786–1794.
33. Cideciyan AV, Haeseleer F, Fariss RN, et al. Rod and cone visual cycle consequences of a null mutation in the 11-cis-retinol dehydrogenase gene in man. *Visual Neurosci.* 2000;17(5):667–678.
34. Burstedt MSI, Sandgren O, Golovleva I, Wachtmeister L. Retinal function in Bothnia dystrophy. An electrophysiological study. *Vision Res.* 2003;43(24):2559–2571.
35. Steinmetz RL, Haimovici R, Jubb C, Fitzke FW, Bird AC. Symptomatic abnormalities of dark adaptation in patients with age-related Bruch's membrane change. *Br J Ophthalmol.* 1993;77(9):549–554.
36. Owsley C, Jackson GR, White M, Feist R, Edwards D. Delays in rod-mediated dark adaptation in early age-related maculopathy. *Ophthalmology.* 2001;108(7):1196–1202.
37. Owsley C, McGwin G, Jackson GR, Kallies K, Clark M. Cone- and rod-mediated dark adaptation impairment in age-related maculopathy. *Ophthalmology.* 2007;114(9): 1728–1735.

21

The Synaptic Organization of the Retina

Robert E. Marc and Bryan W. Jones

The basic architecture, signal flow, and neurochemistry of signaling through the vertebrate retina is well understood: photoreceptors, bipolar cells (BCs), and retinal ganglion cells (RGCs) are all thought to be glutamatergic neurons[1] and the fundamental synaptic chain that serves vision is photoreceptor → BC → RGC. Detailed signaling network topologies and synaptic mechanisms are far from complete for any retinal network,[2] but new technologies are rapidly fleshing out key network motifs and molecular mechanisms. For example, RGCs express different mixtures of ionotropic glutamate receptors (iGluRs) and each receptor can be composed of many different subunits, leading to a vast array of possible functional varieties.[1] At a larger scale, network topologies are too numerous to resolve with current physiologic or pharmacologic data.[3] Each RGC contacts many different amacrine cells (ACs) and a full description of the inputs to any given RGC does not yet exist.[4] Physiology can screen only a limited parameter space for any cell. Even so, new systems of connectivity have emerged from connectomics data that can guide physiologic analyses. Pharmacology remains a fluid field with many incomplete tools, and an immense diversity of neurotransmitter receptor subunit combinations, modulators, and downstream effectors remains to be screened for any cell type. Morphology, augmented by immunochemistry and physiology, remains the core tool in discovering new details of retinal organization. Nothing has been as powerful as transmission electron microscopy for discovering retinal networks. Mammalian night (scotopic) vision is a prime example. Its unique pathways were described by Helga Kolb and E.V. Famiglietti Jr. using electron microscopy. Subsequent physiological analyses[5] provided clarification of how the network functions but would not have yielded the correct network architecture. Further complexities of the rod pathway have been discovered by anatomical studies,[6-8] including the fact that the network rewires in retinal degenerations (Box 21.1).[9-11] In the past decade, new high-throughput electron imaging has provided new information about retinal circuitry.[3,12] The extensive advances in the molecular bases of retinal development[13] and new findings in neuroplasticity[14] are beyond the scope of this chapter. However, many powerful new tools have revealed connections we have long considered as static or hard-wired in the retina display many of the same molecular attributes as plastic pathways in brain.

The basic signal flow in retina is overlaid on a well-studied cell architecture (Fig. 21.1). Retinal ON and OFF BC polarities are generated in the outer plexiform layer and mapped onto the inner plexiform layer (IPL) into largely separated zones. The distal sublamina a receives inputs from OFF BCs and therein the dendrites of OFF RGCs collect signals via BC synapses. The proximal sublamina b receives inputs from ON BCs and therein the dendrites of OFF RGCs collect signals via BC synapses. ON-OFF RGCs thus collect inputs from both sublayers. A key variation on this simple notion of the IPL comes from nonmammalian retinas in which many cone BCs show synaptic swellings throughout the IPL, implying that ON BCs could multiplex some of their signals into sublamina a. Combinations of electrophysiology, dye injection, and computational transmission electron microscopy have now shown that mammalian cone ON BCs provide a nominal en passant input to unusual cells (e.g., dopaminergic axonal cells [AxCs]) that arborize in sublamina a, yet show distinct ON responses. This sophistication indicates that the primary sublamination of the IPL, although profound and important for segmenting signal flow to the brain, does not prevent the emergence of exceptions, as we will note further.

KINDS OF NEURONS

The retina is a thin, multilayered tissue sheet—an image screen—containing three developmentally distinct, interconnected cell groups that form signal-processing networks:

Class 1, sensory neuroepithelium (SNE): photoreceptors and BCs

Class 2, multipolar neurons: RGCs, ACs, and AxCs

Class 3, gliaform neurons; horizontal cells (HCs)

These three cell groups comprise over 60 to 70 distinct classes of cells in mammals (Jones et al., 2008)[15-17] and well over 100 to 120 in most nonmammalian retinas,[2] all assembled into multiple pathways into the brain.

The Sensory Neuroepithelium (SNE) phenotype

The SNE phenotype includes photoreceptors and BCs. These cells are polarized neuroepithelia with apical ciliary-dendritic and basal axonal-exocytotic poles.[18] They form the first stage of synaptic gain in the glutamatergic photoreceptor → BC → RGC → CNS vertical chain. This aggregates photoreceptor signals into BC receptive fields and amplifies their signals. The basal ends of the BCs form the IPL. There are at least 12 kinds of BCs in mammals[15,19] and BCs delimit different functional zones in the IPL, suggesting nearly 1 micron precision in lamination. Both photoreceptors and BCs use high fusion–rate synaptic ribbons as their output elements, fueled by hundreds to thousands of nearby vesicles. The retina is the only known tissue in which SNE cells are arrayed in a serial chain.

As summarized in Fig. 21.2, most mammals possess three classes of photoreceptors: rods expressing rhodopsin 1 (RH1) visual pigments, blue cones expressing short wave–system 1 (SWS1) visual pigments, and green cones expressing long wave–system green (LWSG) visual pigments.[20] Conversely, the most visually advanced and diverse vertebrate classes (teleost fish, avians, reptiles) possess up to seven known classes of photoreceptors (RH1 rods; SWS1 UV/violet cones; SWS2 blue cones; LWSR and RH2 green members of double cones; and LWSR and RH2 green single cones).[21]

Similarly, the diversity of BCs in mammalians is lower (10–13) than nonmammalians (>20). This reduced diversity is a result of the Jurassic collapse of the mammalian visual system, when over half of the visual pigment genes, half of the neuronal classes, and almost two-thirds of the photoreceptor classes were abandoned to exploit nocturnal niches. In addition, the disproportionate proliferation of rods in the mammalian retina was accompanied by the loss of mixed rod-cone BCs in mammals and their replacement with pure rod BCs. How this occurred is unknown, but it could not have been due to an absolute selectivity of rod BCs for rods, as they will readily make contacts with cones when rods are lost in retinal degenerations.[9] As we will see, the mammalian retina has exploited a re-entrant use of synapses to enhance scotopic vision. The relationship between BCs and photoreceptors is still unclear, but there is both anatomical and molecular evidence that BCs were initially photoreceptors. For example, many nonmammalians possess BC Landolt clubs, which are apical extensions extending from a BC primary cilium, extending past the outer plexiform layer into the outer nuclear layer and containing packets of outer segment–like membranes. Whether they are photosensitive has never been determined. Further, SWS1 blue cones and cone BCs share some SWS1 cis-regulatory sequences.[22]

The multipolar neuron phenotype

The multipolar neuron phenotype (Jones et al., 2008) includes ACs, AxCs, and RGCs. Multipolar neurons can be further divided into axon-bearing (RGCs, AxCs) and axonless cells (ACs). Mammals display around 30 kinds of ACs.[16] The 15 to 20 kinds of mammalian RGCs[2,17] are classical projection neurons. RGCs are postsynaptic at their dendrites and presynaptic at their axon terminals in CNS projections. So far, all are presumed to be glutamatergic. ACs are local circuit neurons similar to periglomerular cells in the olfactory bulb. ACs lack classical axons and often have both presynaptic and postsynaptic contacts on their dendrites, although some ACs partition inputs and outputs into different parts of their dendritic arbors. Most ACs are GABAergic and the remainder are glycinergic.[23] Several classes of ACs are dual transmitter cells, expressing both acetylcholine and GABA; serotonin and GABA (in nonmammalians); or peptides and GABA or glycine.[1] In between are the AxCs, also known as polyaxonal cells and intraretinal RGCs, which have distinct axons that project within the retina.[24–26] One dramatic example of the AxC phenotype is the TH1 dopaminergic AxC.[27] This cell releases dopamine at unknown but probably axonal sites and likely glutamate at others (Jones et al., 2008), similar to nigrostriatal neurons.[28] Some polyaxonal cells are GABAergic. There is no evidence for a glycinergic AxC. Multipolar neurons are characterized by numerous neurites branching in the plane of the retina, most collecting signals from BCs. Multipolar neurons are among the earliest to develop in the retina and quickly define the borders of the IPL and its stratifications. Multipolar neurons all manifest somewhat classical "gray"-like synapses, generally with small clusters of less than 200 vesicles.

The gliaform cell phenotype

This phenotype contains the HCs, the somas and processes of which are restricted to the outer plexiform layer. Although HCs are multipolar and neuron-like, and may display axons, they do not spike. Further, they express many glial features such as intermediate filament expression and very slow voltage responses. Further, HCs produce high levels of glutathione and make direct contact with capillary endothelial cells in some species, suggesting they play homeostatic roles similar to glia. Even so, HCs clearly mediate a powerful network function, collecting large patches of photoreceptor input via AMPA receptors and providing a wide-field, slow signal antagonistic to the vertical channel. The mechanism of HC antagonism remains a matter of uncertainty and debate. HCs do make conventional-appearing synapses onto neuronal processes in the outer plexiform layer, and in fishes these synapses are made onto dendrites of glycinergic interplexiform cells, a form of AxC.[29] However, these are so sparse in all species and contain so few vesicles that they cannot be the source of the large, sustained opponent surrounds of retinal neurons that HCs generate. HCs must use some other mechanism. The phylogenetics of HCs has been thoroughly reviewed.[30] HCs in mammals are postsynaptic to cones at their somatic dendrites. One class of HCs common in mammals (foveal type I in primates, type A in rabbits and cats, and absent in rodents) contacts cones alone. A second class of HCs (extrafoveal type I in primates, type B in rabbit and cats, and the only known HC in rodents) displays axons several hundred microns long that branch profusely and form massive arborizations contacting hundreds to thousands of rods. Another class of primate HC (type II) has axon terminals contacting cones and rods. Importantly, the axon of HCs appears to be electrically inactive, and these somatic and terminal regions are believed to act independently. HCs also appear to be early-developing pioneer cells that define the outer plexiform layer. After the RGCs and HCs define the layout of the inner and outer plexiform layers respectively, photoreceptors and BCs mature and search for connections.

Novel cells

Ramon y Cajal's extensive analysis of retinal neuronal includes a number of unusual cell morphs yet to be analyzed by modern techniques. Indeed, it is likely that many of the cells he saw were never published. Recently, two candidate novel cell classes have been described. Della Santina et al. (2016)[31] used visualization of the fluorescent protein cerulean driven by the OFF BC promoter VsX1 to discover a set of monopolar interneurons that resemble the proximal axonal part of a BC but lack dendrites. These cells are termed glutamatergic monopolar interneurons (GluMIs) and are obviously part of the BC lineage.

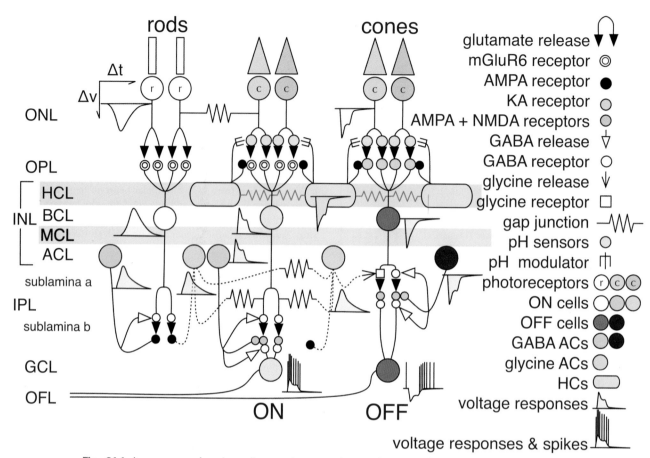

Fig. 21.1 A summary of major cell superclasses and synaptic connections in the mammalian retina. Photoreceptors include rods *(white)* and cones *(green, blue)* that hyperpolarize in response to light. All photoreceptors are glutamatergic and drive horizontal cell (*HC*) AMPA receptors on HCs, ON bipolar cell (*BC*) mGluR6 receptors, and OFF BC KA or AMPA receptors. All BCs are glutamatergic and drive either predominantly AMPA receptors on rod pathway interneurons or various mixtures of AMPA and N-methyl-D-aspartate receptor (NMDA) receptors on cone pathway amacrine cells (*ACs*) and retinal ganglion cells (*RGCs*). Homocellular gap junctions are formed between like pairs of cells (HCs, certain ACs) and heterocellular gap junctions are formed between different cells pairs (rods and green long wave–system [LWS] cones; glycinergic rod ACs and ON cone BCs; some ACs and certain RGCs). There are two major feedback paths. There is a putative HC → cone feedback path mediated by a pH-sensitive process. AC → BC feedback is primarily GABAergic, as is AC → RGC feedforward. Mammalian rod pathways are unique and not shared by any other vertebrate class. Rod BC signals are collected by a glycinergic rod AC that mediates a re-entrant bifurcation into cone ON BC channels via gap junctions and cone OFF BC channels via glycinergic synapses. The outflow from the retina is largely split into ON RGC channels that spike in response to light increments and OFF RGC channels that spike in response to light decrements. The retina is precisely laminated into cellular and synaptic zones distal-to-proximal, starting with the outer nuclear layer (*ONL*), the outer plexiform layer (*OPL*), the inner nuclear layer (*INL*), the inner plexiform layer (*IPL*), the retinal ganglion cell layer (*RGCL*), and the optic fiber layer (*OFL*). The INL is subdivided into the horizontal cell layer (*HCL*), bipolar cell layer (*BCL*), Müller cell layer (*MCL*), and amacrine cell layer (*ACL*). The IPL is subdivided into sublamina a that receives the output of OFF BCs and sublamina b that receives the output of ON BCs.

They target RGCs and are driven by ACs. Another BC-like neuron has been described by Young et al.[32] and termed a *Campana cell*. Its soma is embedded in the AC layer, but it is clearly bipolar in morphology. Pharmacologic analysis of its light responses suggest that it is driven by both rods and cones, generating largely typical ON responses via mGluR6-like mechanisms, but there may be ON BC inputs on its axonal field as well. The cells are very sparse but appear to drive RGCs.

True glia and vasculature

The neurons of the retina are embedded in an array of vertical Müller glia that span the entire neural retina, forming one-third to one-half of the retinal mass and generating high-resistance junctional seals at the distal and proximal limits of the retina. Most mammalian retinas are vascularized in three capillary beds: at the RGC-IPL border, the AC-IPL border, and the outer plexiform layer. Squirrels (Sciurids) display two beds (at the RGC-IPL and AC-IPL layer borders) and rabbits (Lagomorphs) have none at all, similar to all other nonmammalian vertebrates. The RGC layer of many vascularized species also displays classical astrocytes, although their roles remain unclear. In brain, astrocytes carry out some of the operations attributed to retinal Müller glia, including transport of spillover K⁺ and glutamate, and glucose supply via vascular > glial cell > neuron transcellular transport. Why and how most vertebrate retinas function without vasculature remains uncertain, but it is likely that Müller glia act

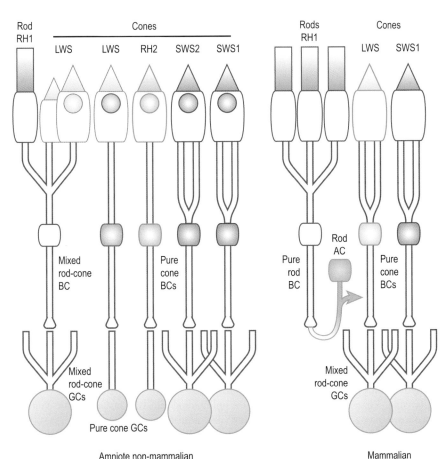

Fig. 21.2 Photoreceptor cohorts and connections in vertebrates. Nonmammalians display multiple pigment classes and cone types. There are five pigment classes and seven photoreceptor types for a fresh water turtle, including rods (comprising less than 10% of the photoreceptors) expressing class RH1 rhodopsins, three kinds of long wave–system (*LWS*) cones (short members of double cones, long members of double cones with orange oil droplets, single cones with rod oil droplets), single cones expressing RH2 green cone pigments and a yellow oil droplet, single cones expressing short wave–system 2 (*SWS2*) blue cone pigments and a UV-opaque clear oil droplet, and single cones expressing SWS1 UV cone pigments and a UV-transparent clear oil droplet. The connection patterns for nonmammalians are mixed rod-cone bipolar cells (*BCs*) and pure cone BCs, leading to mixed rod-cone retinal ganglion cells (*RGCs*) and pure cone RGCs. Mammals display three pigment classes (one rod and two cone), two cone color types in nonprimates and three color types in primates, including RH1 rods, SWS1 cones, and LWS cones. The LWS cone class forms one green type in most mammals, and red (*LWSR*) and green (*LWSG*) chromatypes in primates. The main connection rules for mammalians are pure rod BCs and pure cone BCs, with only cone BCs driving RGCs, with rod amacrine cells (*ACs; cyan*) providing the re-entrant crossover.

as a surrogate vascular system with the added ability to accumulate large glycogen stores (like hepatocytes) as part of a glucose-skeleton homeostasis. The segregation of retinal astrocytes away from the IPL remains a mystery.

BASIC SYNAPTIC COMMUNICATION

With the discovery of the signaling mechanisms of the neuromuscular junction decades ago,[33] one might have thought that the archetypal synaptic format had been discovered. Yet it has become clear, especially in the retina, that every kind of synapse is subtly different, with diverse physics, topologies, and molecular mechanisms leading to very different forms of synapses, most of which do not follow the single presynaptic "bouton" → single postsynaptic target pattern of brain. Further, the arrangement of these systems into synaptic chains in retina is unlike any other known network, including olfactory bulb. In retina, the first stage of synaptic signaling is a direct SNE → SNE synapse (Fig. 21.1): photoreceptor → BC. No other instance of this topology has been discovered in any organism. There are at least six modes of presynaptic-postsynaptic pairing in retina.

Photoreceptor ribbon synapses: small-volume multitarget signaling

It is thought that all photoreceptor signaling is glutamatergic, but sporadic indications of cholinergic physiology and molecular markers have been found in many nonmammalians.[1] Glutamate release from photoreceptors is effected by high rates of vesicle fusion at active sites on either side of a large synaptic ribbon[34] positioned close to the presynaptic membrane. The presynaptic zone is a protrusion or ridge with

vesicle fusion sites positioned on the slopes of the ridge (see Fig. 21.4). The releasable vesicle pool is so large that photoreceptors and BCs are capable of maintaining continuous glutamate release in response to steady depolarizations.[35] This, among other things, distinguishes photoreceptors and BCs from ACs, which have very small presynaptic vesicle clusters. Although the mechanism is unclear, photoreceptor ribbons accelerate vesicle release and replenishment significantly but are not absolutely required for signaling.[36]

Various vertebrate rods and cones differ greatly in the number of ribbons and postsynaptic targets arrayed within the presynaptic terminals. For example, most mammalian and teleost fish rods have small grape-like presynaptic spherules approximately 3 μm in diameter with a small entrance aperture leading to an enclosed extracellular invagination or vestibule in which thin postsynaptic dendrites are contained (Fig. 21.3). Importantly, glial processes are excluded from the interior of the spherule and any glutamate release must diffuse out of the spherule to reach the Müller glia. However, mammalian rods express the EAAT5 glutamate transporter[1] and likely regulate their own intrasynaptic glutamate levels. Each spherule contains one or two synaptic ribbons and a few postsynaptic targets.[37] In fishes, the postsynaptic targets are the dendrites of roughly five kinds of mixed rod-cone BCs[38] and one kind of rod HC.[31] Thus each ribbon serves no less than six different types of postsynaptic targets. In mammals, only two targets are common: the dendrites of one kind of rod BC and the axon terminals of HCs. There are some instances of sparse OFF BC contact in mammals, but this seems to vary with species and may be an evolutionary relict with variable expression rather than a major signaling pathway.[39-41] In sum, rod spherules form a sparse-ribbon → small-volume, sparse-target architecture.

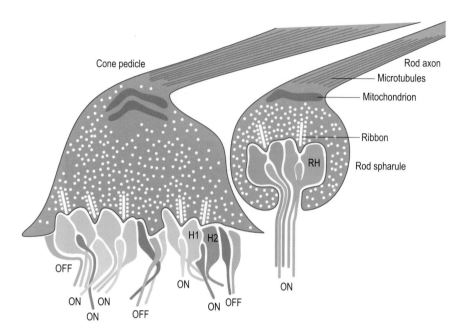

Fig. 21.3 Basic organization of mammalian photoreceptor synaptic terminals. Primate cone terminals contain many ribbons, mitochondria clustered at the head of the pedicle and thousands of synaptic vesicles (*white dots*), some of which form organized zones near the plasma membrane opposite an array of cone-specific postsynaptic processes including type H1 and H2 horizontal cells (HCs) as lateral invaginating elements (primate H1 cells tend to avoid short wave–system 1 (SWS1) cones, whereas H2 cells contact all cones). Cone ON bipolar cells (BCs) tend to center their dendrites between the lateral HC processes at varying distances from the synaptic ribbon, forming so-called invaginating and semi-invaginating contacts. Most cone OFF BCs position their dendrites outside the HC processes at so-called flat contacts. It is thought that most of these express KA receptors. Some occasional OFF BC processes invaginate, and they may express AMPA receptors.

Cones and rod terminals in some nonmammalians (e.g., urodele amphibians) adopt a different topology, with the presynaptic ending expanding to form a foot-piece or pedicle some 3 to 5 μm wide. This may be shaped either like a cupola (fishes), the broadly concave interior of which admits some 50 to 100 or more fine dendrites served by roughly 12 synaptic ribbon sites,[42] or like a true pediment (e.g., primate cones), the shallow concavity of which is studded with up to 50 ribbon sites[43] (Fig. 21.3). Cone pedicles in primates target at least 10 different kinds of BCs and at least two kinds of HCs. Mouse cone pedicles are smaller but still target 11 kinds of BCs[19] and one kind of HC. In sum, *cone pedicles form a multiribbon → small-volume, multitarget architecture* (Fig. 21.4).

BC ribbon synapses: semiprecise target signaling

As with photoreceptors, BC signaling is generally considered glutamatergic,[1] but sporadic exceptions exist. In mammals (especially primates) and amphibians, some BCs contain biomarkers of GABA-related metabolism. In contrast to photoreceptors, BC synaptic endings are topological spheroids, usually multiple (depending on BC type), with dozens to hundreds of ribbons abutting the surface. BCs form no invaginations, so there is no restricted volume into which glutamate is injected by vesicle fusion. In most cases each ribbon is directly apposed to a pair of postsynaptic targets, usually ACs. This is termed a *dyad*, and although monads, triads, and tetrads do occur, dyads dominate. Large BC terminals such as those found in teleost fishes can drive up to 200 distinct processes. Mammalian BCs drive many fewer targets and most BCs have elaborate, branched terminals with connecting neurites often as small as 100 nm. In contrast to photoreceptors, the targets of BCs are focal. BC terminals are largely fully encapsulated by neuronal processes at their release sites to which they are presynaptic or postsynaptic, with rarely direct contact between the terminal and Müller glia near the synaptic release zone. This means that any glutamate that escapes from the synaptic cleft may travel some distance before glial glutamate transporters can clear it. Thus the potential for glutamate overflow at BC synapses is substantial. This may be particularly important for the activation of NMDA receptors, as they are suspected to be displaced from primary AMPA receptors. Thus, *BCs form multiribbon → semiprecise target architectures* (Fig. 21.4).

AC and AxC conventional fast synapses: precise presynaptic → postsynaptic signaling

ACs and AxCs are the only retinal cells that make synaptic contacts resembling CNS "gray"-like, nonribbon conventional synapses. ACs target BCs, RGCs, or other ACs. The targets of most AxCs are not well known but appear likely to be ACs and RGCs. Although each AC may make many hundreds of synapses, each synapse contacts only one postsynaptic target, similar to classical multipolar neurons in CNS and spinal cord.[44] The dominant fast transmitters of AC systems are GABA and glycine, with GABAergic neurons making up half to two-thirds of the AC population, depending on species.[1] Additional transmitters such as acetylcholine, peptides, or serotonin (in non-mammalians) are also associated with GABAergic (in most cases) or glycinergic systems.[1,45] Acetylcholine (ACh) is a fast excitatory transmitter that is found in paramorphic starburst ACs in mammals and also uses conventional synapses.[1] However, we know of no distinguishing anatomical differences between GABA- and ACh-utilizing synapses in retina.

AC, AxC, and efferent slow transmitter synapses: large-volume signaling

Dopamine (and possibly norepinephrine/epinephrin), as well as peptides in retina, appear to be released by a nonfocal, Ca²⁺-dependent vesicular system[46] without any clear postsynaptic associations. Dopamine and the other slow transmitters likely act via volume conduction[47] and modulate a range of cellular responses largely via G-protein–coupled receptors (GPCRs). In nonmammalians, efferent systems from the CNS target ACs with fast neurotransmitter synapses, especially GABA.[4] In mammals, all known efferents appear to release either histamine or serotonin, likely as volume signaling systems.[48]

HC noncanonical signaling

HCs generate potent large-field, slow surround signals in retinal RGCs and BCs, and even in nonmammalian cone photoreceptors.[49–51] There is evidence for feedforward signaling via the cone → HC → BC path,[52] feedback signaling via the cone → HC → cone → BC path,[53,54] and, now, the rod → HC → rod.[55] The efficacy and sustained nature of the feedback signal is such that no known vesicular mechanism could maintain

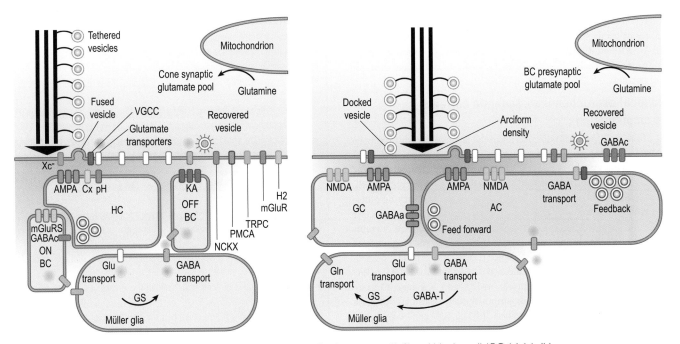

Fig. 21.4 A detailed schematic of synaptic organization at cone (*left*) and bipolar cell (*BC*) (*right*) ribbon synapses. Each synaptic ribbon is a pentalaminar structure in cross-section, in reality a disc- or lozenge-shaped solid with its two broad faces serving as attachment sites for tethered vesicles and its small paramembrane face attached to a dense structure known as the arciform density. Ribbons serve as the major site for the "readily releasable" pools of synaptic vesicles for continuous glutamate transmission, and facilitate high-speed formation of docked vesicles. Upon depolarization of the presynaptic membrane, voltage-gated calcium channels (VGCC, *black barrels*) open, allowing docked vesicles to fuse and release glutamate into the synaptic cleft. At some distance from the ribbon, endocytosis mediates vesicle recovery. BC ribbons tend to be shorter than photoreceptor ribbons. Cytoplasmic glutamate (*orange*) is formed glutamine via mitochondrial phosphate–activated glutaminase and loaded into vesicles via vGlut vesicular transporters. Glutamate release by vesicle fusion diffuses away from the release site (*shaded orange*) and is cleared by both presynaptic and distant Müller glia glutamate transporters (*white barrels*). Müller glia synthesize glutamine from glutamate via glutamine synthetase (*GS*) and exports glutamine via transporters (*gray barrels*). Similarly, neurons import glutamine via transporters. Vertebrate photoreceptors also express presynaptic cystine-glutamate (Xc-) exchangers (*orange barrels*) the function of which is unknown. Glutamate released by cones activates ON BCs via mGluR6 receptors (*light blue barrels*), horizontal cells (*HCs*) via α-amino-3-hydroxy-5-methyl-4-isoxazolepropionic acid (*AMPA*) receptors (*dark blue barrels*), and OFF BCs via either AMPA or kainate (*KA*) receptors (*bright blue barrels*). HCs are positioned at the highest glutamate concentration zone and OFF BCs at the lowest. Glutamate released by BCs activates amacrine cells (*ACs*) and retinal ganglion cells (RGCs) via AMPA receptors (*dark blue barrels*) and NMDA receptors (*green barrels*). Feedback at photoreceptors appears to be mediated by either focal connexin (*yellow barrel*) or a pH modulator (*magenta barrel*) close to the photoreceptor VGCC. Feedforward from HCs to BCs may be GABAergic in some species and mediated by GABAC receptors (*dark red barrels*). Feedback at BCs is mediated by vesicular GABA (*red shading*) release from ACs targeting largely GABAC receptors. Feedforward from ACs to BCs is mediated by largely by GABAA receptors (*bright red barrels*). ACs and mammalian Müller glia also have GABA transporters that clear the synaptic space. GABA is converted via the GABA-transaminase (*GABA-T*) complex to glutamate in glia. Cone synaptic terminals also have a number of other proteins including Na-Ca exchangers (*NCKX*), plasma membrane Ca transporters (*PMCA*), transient receptor potential channels (*TRPC*), metabotropic glutamate receptors (*mGluR*), and possibly histamine receptors (*H2*). BC terminals may share some of these features.

it (other than a ribbon-style synapse). Vesicular HC synapses are very rare and small.[30] Several models of noncanonical signaling have been proposed, including synaptic pH regulation,[56] hemijunction-mediated ephaptic signaling,[57] and even transporter-mediated signaling. Some of these will be discussed in detail further in the chapter, but this unusual functionality is further evidence that HCs are not classical neurons.

Coupling types and coupling patterns
Although gap junctional coupling was first discovered between HCs, only in the last decade has it become clear that intercellular coupling is pervasive in retina.[58] There are two simple classes of coupling:

homocellular and heterocellular (between like and different classes of cells). The participant connexins in each case are likely to be homotypic or heterotypic (similar or dissimilar connexin types). The strength of coupling is associated with the size of the junctions, as they represent summed parallel conductances, and with functional modulation by various signaling pathways. Activated dopamine D1 receptors decrease conductances between coupled HCs[46,59] and coupled ACs,[60] and dopamine D2 receptors modulate rod-cone coupling. The significance of coupling is clear in certain cases, such as the ability of HCs to spatially integrate signals over large fields (>1 mm diameter) or the crossover of rod signals into cones via heterocellular rod-cone and rod AC–cone BC coupling. Recently, heterocellular coupling between ACs and RGCs (AC::RGC) has been analyzed by ultrastructural connectomics[61] and reveals that the most common forms involve OFF AC::OFF RGC and ON AC::ON RGC. Extensive coupling occurs among sets of cone BCs[62] in which each class of BCs displays a unique set of partners.

Fast focal neurochemistry, synaptic currents, and amplification

One of the most powerful discoveries of the last two decades has been the diversity of the primary fast neurotransmitter receptors of the vertebrate nervous system. Again, the primary signaling channel of retina is the vertical glutamatergic chain from photoreceptors to brain.[1] Rods, cones, and BCs encode their voltage responses as time-varying glutamate release. The targets of photoreceptors and BCs, in turn, decode time-varying extracellular glutamate levels as time-varying currents with glutamate receptors. There are two major classes of glutamate receptors: ionotropic and metabotropic (iGluRs and mGluRs, respectively). The iGluRs are separable into two distinct families: the AMPA/KA receptors and NMDA receptors. AMPA and KA receptors are related but pharmacologically and compositionally distinct. Four basic classes of glutamate receptor subunits (GluR1, 2, 3, 4) can be recruited to form a tetrameric AMPA receptor. Similarly, five basic classes of KA receptors (GluR5, 6, 7, and KA1, 2) can be assembled into tetrameric KA receptors. With some exceptions, these receptor assemblies can have nearly any stoichiometry. NMDA receptors are a distinct group of iGluRs in several ways. First, they have an obligate tetrameric subunit composition. Second, they are coincidence detectors that require dual activations by glutamate and by a glycine-like endogenous agonist. There is substantial evidence that this co-ligand may be D-serine released from Müller glia.[63] Finally, the mGluRs represent a complex collection of GPCRs whose functions are far from clear.

Different classes of neurons express different types or different combinations of receptors and, in the end, the glutamate receptor profile of a cell appears diagnostic for its class. Mammalian BCs are unique in expressing either mGluR6, KA, or AMPA receptors as their glutamate decoding system. But immunochemical and mRNA expression analysis suggest that these associations are not so precise, as iGluR subunit expression occurs in nominally mGluR6-driven cells.[64] HCs predominantly express AMPA receptors but show no NMDA-mediated responses. Finally, ACs and RGCs resemble CNS neurons in expressing AMPA receptors augmented by varying amounts of NMDA receptors.

The key glutamate receptor systems of retina operate on the principle of cation permeation.[1] When activated, iGluRs generate increased channel conductances and carry inward currents carried mostly by Na^+ and Ca^{2+}. Thus the canonical iGluR AMPA, KA, and NMDA families of receptors are nominally *sign-conserving* (>) depolarizing systems that "copy" the polarity of the presynaptic source voltage input in the postsynaptic target. The facts that many inputs converge on one postsynaptic cell; that small presynaptic voltages can modulate the release of many vesicles (in SNE cells); and that glutamate gates large postsynaptic conductance changes to cations with a positive reversal potential means that such synapses have high gain. Signals from photoreceptor to brain are successively amplified by a chain of glutamate synapses.

The group III mGluR6 system is unique and in retina is expressed by ON BCs (Box 21.2). No known multipolar neuron in the CNS uses this receptor as its primary signaling modality. As a classical GPCR, with Goα as its cognate G-protein,[65] the binding of glutamate triggers a cascade of signals that leads ultimately to the *closure* of cation channels on BC dendrites, thus moving the BC membrane potential closer to the K^+ equilibrium potential. Thus mGluR6 receptors are nominally

---

BOX 21.2   Glutamate excitotoxicity

Glutamate excitotoxicity has been invoked as a mechanism in retinal diseases. The evidence is mixed and controversial. On balance:

- Elevations of vitreal glutamate in glaucoma have not been validated.
- Glaucoma-mediated loss of retinal ganglion cells (RGCs) does not match known excitotoxic patterns.
- Starburst amacrine cells (Acs) are the most glutamate-sensitive cells in the retina but there are no established AC losses in primate glaucoma.
- NMDA receptor antagonists appear neuroprotective in ocular hypertension models of glaucoma but the mechanism of NMDA neuroprotection may be indirect:
  - Retinal RGC death in glaucoma likely involves Ca^{+2}-mediated apoptosis.[121-126]
  - NMDA antagonists (like many drugs) will decrease Ca^{+2} loads in neurons.
  - Weak NMDA antagonists likely have no lasting role in glaucoma therapeutics.
- Glutamate is likely a major player in retinal damage in diabetes and ischemic insults.
- Neuroprotection is difficult to achieve in those cases as it involves AMPA receptors.
- Excitotoxicity in hypoxic retina is likely initiated by reverse transport of glutamate by BCs.
- Competitive, nontranslocated transporter ligands may be safer ocular neuroprotectants.

---

sign-inverting (>i) hyperpolarizing systems that invert the polarity of the input in the postsynaptic target. The modulation of a strong cation current renders the mGluR6 mechanism high gain in spite of its inverted polarity.

The differential expression of iGluRs and mGluR6 in BCs creates the two fundamental signal-processing channels of the retina: OFF and ON BCs, respectively.[1] Unknown mechanisms regulate the expression of glutamate receptors in BCs. In general, BCs that express iGluRs such as KA or AMPA receptors do not express *functional* mGluR6 receptor display, and *vice versa*. However, there is evidence that BCs expressing mGluR6 also express low levels of iGluR protein, but there is yet no evidence that such iGluR subunits contribute to an electrically detectable signaling event.[64]

There are additional mGluRs expressed in retina, including the group I mGluR1 and mGluR5 and group III mGluR 4, 7, and 8, all largely expressed in varying patterns in the IPL.[66] Their roles are thought to be associated with presynaptic glutamate feedback.

Global neurochemistry and modulation

There are a number of alternative neurochemical mechanisms that appear to operate on a larger spatial scale than conventional synapses. The most thoroughly described, although incompletely understood, is the dopamine.[46] In mammalian retinas, dopaminergic neurons are largely AxCs that arborize primarily in the distalmost layer of the IPL, appear to receive direct inputs from BCs, and have predominantly ON-type responses.[67] The exact sites of dopamine release are not known, although these cells clearly have small accumulations of synaptic vesicles distributed sparsely in their processes. Data from many species suggest that dopamine acts largely via volume conduction,[47] that is, dopamine diffuses throughout the retina and targets high-affinity type D1 and D2 receptors distributed on almost every class of cell, including Müller cells. Indeed, every species seems to show evidence of dopaminergic modulation in the outer plexiform layer.[68] Actions triggered by D1 receptors include the uncoupling of HCs,[69] the uncoupling of rod-driven glycinergic ACs,[60] and enhanced spike speeds[70] (faster waveforms). All of these are consistent with the process of converting the retina from a scotopic to a photopic state. Dopaminergic neurons are thought to also contain a fast transmitter. Previous evidence in the mouse suggested that they were GABAergic, but other studies support the possibility that they are glutamatergic.

A similar role is posited for the rapidly diffusing neuroactive gas nitric oxide (NO). A variety of retinal cells are posited to produce NO via the neuronal NO synthase (nNOS) pathway, activated by binding of Ca-activated calmodulin.[71] Thus synaptic currents with high Ca permeability (e.g., those mediated by NMDA receptors) can turn on nNOS, which catalyzes the oxidation of one of the guanido nitrogens of arginine to NO. NO appears to have the capacity to diffuse through transcellular regimes (how far is in debate) and activate soluble guanyl cyclases to produce cGMP. Acting via cGMP-dependent protein kinase G or directly on cyclic nucleotide–gated cation channels, cGMP can drive a number of modulatory actions. One site of action is thought to be the heterocellular coupling of ON cone BCs and glycinergic rod ACs, and increased cGMP appears to uncouple this network, again a light-adaptive action. While many cells appear to be able to produce NO, the best-known architecture for NOS-containing neurons is a wide-field GABAergic AC.[72]

Many retinas contain a number of neuropeptides as cotransmitters, largely in wide-field GABAergic ACs with cone BC inputs. These peptides include somatostatin, substance P, and neurotensin, with many more in nonmammalians, such as enkephalins.[45] This is probably the least understood neurochemical aspect of the retina. In general, it is thought that peptides act via specific peptide receptor GPCRs to modulate various ion channels. However, very little research on retinal peptides has been carried out in recent years.

Modulation by transporters

An important part of every signaling process is termination. Given the ability of glutamate to activate excitotoxic processes, the expression of high-affinity sodium-glutamate transporters by Müller glia likely represents the last line of defense.[1] A molecule of glutamate must have already left the synaptic cleft by diffusion to encounter glial glutamate transporters. However, both photoreceptors and BCs express glutamate transporters, presumably near the sites of synaptic release,[1] and these likely play a major role in determining the temporal dynamics of extracellular glutamate levels, although this has been difficult to quantify. Even so, every fast transmitter has a corresponding presynaptic transporter mechanism. Numerous studies support the roles of transporters in signal termination; however, the precise localization of transporters has not been achieved.

Signal processing

The roles of synaptic networks are to convert graded sensory photoreceptor potentials into patterns of action potentials for long-range transmission to the CNS, and perform spatial, temporal, and spectral signal processing on the input signals of the photoreceptors. This latter action converts the retinal image into the parallel signaling behaviors of 15 to 20 different classes of retinal RGCs in mammals. The concept of signal processing, as derived from electrical engineering, is particularly powerful.[50] Each kind of synapse, each kind of cell, and each topology of network is invoked in various ways to generate the kinds of "filters" through which the visual scene must be encoded. The physiologic analysis of retina in the 1970s (especially as carried out by Naka) represented a sea-change in thinking—a move away from Sherringtonian concepts of spinal excitation, inhibition, and circuits (loops) and toward engineering notions of polarity, inversion, networks, and filters.

Sign-conserving (>) and sign-inverting (>i, >m) transfers

The behavior of a photoreceptor is neither excitatory nor inhibitory. Photoreceptors encode time-varying changes in light intensity with fairly faithful (although nonlinear) time-varying changes in voltage. As glutamatergic neurons, one would normally think of them as "excitatory" in brain, but a more robust concept is derived by looking at the behaviors of target neurons. HCs (driven by AMPA receptors) and OFF BCs (driven by AMPA or KA receptors) merely copy the polarity of presynaptic photoreceptors (Fig. 21.1). When light hyperpolarizes photoreceptors, this decreases the rate of synaptic glutamate release and (in conjunction with glutamate transport) leads to a decrease in synaptic glutamate levels. Because AMPA and KA receptors are iGluRs, decreased synaptic glutamate means that AMPA and KA receptor–gated currents will decrease, and the HCs and OFF BCs will hyperpolarize. Conversely, when a fly navigates across the visual field, local darkening will depolarize some photoreceptors and the HCs and OFF BCs will follow. Thus photoreceptor → HC and OFF BC signaling is termed *sign-conserving* (>). In addition, iGluRs typically mediate high-gain responses (i.e., strong amplification), and over modest voltage ranges this amplification is symmetric and polarity-invariant. ON BCs behave in a totally different manner. In mammals, all ON BCs express functional mGluR6 receptors that activate a cation channel when unbound and close it upon binding of glutamate. Thus, when photoreceptors decrease their glutamate release, this leads to decreased mGluR6 receptor binding and the opening of cation channels and depolarization of ON BCs (See Box 21.3) (Fig. 21.1). This is an explicit, high-gain, metabotropic sign-inverting (>m) synaptic transfer.

BOX 21.3 Retinal remodeling in retinal degenerations

- Primary photoreceptor or retinal pigment epithelium (RPE) degenerations deafferent the neural inner retina.
- The neural retina responds by remodeling in phases, first by subtle changes in neuronal structure and gene expression and later by large-scale reorganization.
- In *Phase 1*, expression of a primary insult activates photoreceptor and glial stress signals.
- In *Phase 2*, ablation of the sensory retina via complete photoreceptor loss or cone-sparing rod loss triggers revision in downstream neurons.
- Total photoreceptor loss triggers wholesale bipolar cell remodeling.
- Cone-sparing degenerations trigger BCs reprogramming, downregulating mGluR6 expression and upregulating iGluR expression.
- Loss of cone triggers *Phase 3*: a protracted period of global remodeling, including
  - neuronal cell death
  - neuronal and glial migration
  - elaboration of new neurites and synapses
  - rewiring of retinal circuits
  - glial hypertrophy and the evolution of a fibrotic glial seal
  - elevated expression of alpha-synuclein as in CNS neurodegenerations.
- In advanced disease, glia and neurons may enter the choroid and emigrate from the retina.
- Retinal remodeling represents the pathologic invocation of plasticity mechanisms.
- Remodeling likely abrogates or attenuates many cellular and bionic rescue strategies.
- Survivor neurons are stable, active cells.
- It may be possible to influence their emergent rewiring and migration habits.

Nonmammalians display a twist on this mechanism that perhaps reveals the evolutionary history of mammalian ON BCs. The apparent homolog of the ancestral mammalian rod BC exists in the retinas of modern fishes as the mixed rod-cone BC. This cell has unusual behavior in that it has different reversal potentials and conductance changes for different stimuli. Scotopic lights that activate rods generate ON responses that display a positive reversal potential (like a cation) and an increase in conductance (like a channel opening). This is very like mammalian rod and cone ON BCs, and indeed it appears to have the same pharmacology: 2-amino-4-phosphonobutyrate (AP4) is an agonist at mGluR6 receptors[73] and blocks rod ON BCs responses in fishes. However, upon light adaptation, fish ON BCs change their behaviors. In response to photopic lights that activate cones, the "ON" reversal potential moves to very negative values (like an anion) and the cells display a decrease in conductance (like a channel closure). In fact, the cone-driven ON responses of fish BCs are mediated by an anion channel coupled to a glutamate transporter.[74,75] Thus, in photopic "dark," glutamate release activates the transporter and its coupled chloride current, leading to hyperpolarization of the BC. Thus the fish cone → ON BC synapse is sign-inverting, but not metabotropic. The degree of its amplification is also unknown.

In the IPL, BC → AC and RGC signaling is all mediated by AMPA or AMPA + NMDA receptors.[76,77] Thus all BC output synapses are sign-conserving (Fig. 21.1). The bulk of AC → BC, AC, or RGC signaling is either GABAergic or glycinergic via increased anion conductances.[73] Thus these synapses are characteristically sign-inverting (>i). GABAergic and glycinergic transmission is also usually very low gain, often because the reversal potential is very close to the membrane potential and/or the total conductance change experienced by a target cell leads to a tremendous decrease in total cell input resistance, thus decreasing signal efficacy. In any case, it takes a significant amount of inhibition to control glutamate synapses. Some inhibitory mechanisms involve the metabotropic GABAB receptor, which is a GPCR that can lead to a tremendous increase in potassium currents, but can also show paradoxical excitation.[73] Because potassium currents are usually outward (positive current flowing outward), GABAB can produce a strong and long-lasting inhibition near threshold. Different GABA receptors tend to be expressed at different sites (ionotropic GABAA on ACs and BCs, ionotropic GABAC on BCs), but the distribution of GABAB receptors is less well understood.

Synaptic chains and polarity

The effect of cascading synapses through various pathways can be estimated in terms of polarity and gain. For example, although the mechanisms of HC feedback or feedforward are poorly understood and perhaps multimodal,[78,79] the efficacy of HC signaling is not in doubt. As first established in fish retinas, currents injected into HCs have stereotyped actions on different RGCs. The net pathway from HCs to ON RGCs is sign-conserving. The net pathway from HCs to ON RGCs is sign-conserving. From a signal-processing perspective, this means that the polysynaptic chain from a given HC, somehow reaching a BC and thence to an ON RGC, must contain either no sign-inverting elements or an even number of them. The path to an OFF RGC must contain an odd number of sign-inverting elements. This poses fundamental constraints on where and how signals flow in the retina and can be used as a model for network investigations. Similarly, we know that there are chains of two and three serial ACs in the IPL of most retinas.[4] Although there are no network models that use such chains, the minimum architecture for such a chain is BC → AC → AC → BC or RGC. If the AC outputs are sign-inverting, the net transfer of the chain is > >i >i > (sign-conserving). Importantly, the low gain of GABAergic and glycinergic synapses prevents such chains

from being runaway excitations.[4,80] What roles might such networks play? In nonmammalians, the bulk of GABAergic ACs also receive some form of GABAergic input, as evidenced by their pharmacology. It was presumed that similar networks existed in mammals, but some authors argue[81] that in rabbit the only synaptic crossover networks are glycine → GABA. In fact, most OFF to ON rod-cone crossover channels involve glycine → GABA pairs.

Feedback, feedforward, and nested feedback/feedforward

Designing analog operational amplifier networks is very similar to evolving a retina: every stage of forward amplification needs feedback control.[82] In retina, sign-inverting GABAergic mechanisms are used as feedback and feedforward control systems. Feedback is the most powerful way to set synaptic gain, improve signal-to-noise ratios, and improve synaptic bandpass. The underlying mathematics of feedback have been widely discussed.[73,83] On the other hand, feedforward is an effective way to generate strong antagonistic mechanisms in target cells. These architectures are clearly at play in the retina, but we have only a hazy idea of their importance. For example, blocking GABAergic inhibition converts directionally selective RGCs into nonselective cells, but has little effect on the center-surround organization of other RGCs, despite the abundance of GABAergic synapses in the IPL. Thus it is hard to generalize function from anatomy. Conversely, it is impossible to understand function without anatomy.

Caveats

Three major problems have emerged in understanding how GABAergic (or any classical inhibitory transmitter) works in retina. The first is the chloride reversal potential. We have a very poor idea of which way GABA receptor–gated anion currents will flow: inward or outward. Small retinal cells may have the ability to adjust intracellular chloride levels with various ion transport systems. The KCC2 system (K-Cl cotransporter) tends to export Cl whereas the NKCC system (Na-K-Cl cotransporter) tends to import it.[52] If intracellular Cl is locally high, opening an anion channel may evoke an outward negative current and depolarize the cell. However, most studies of GABAC receptors at the synaptic terminals of retinal BCs support the view that it is inhibitory.[1] A second problem is temporal delay. Imagine a cell responding to a light input with a sinusoidal voltage. Then imagine a surrounding cell giving a similar response and providing feedback with a sign-inverting polarity. If the feedback was delayed so that the phase is shifted by 180 degrees, the "inhibitory" local surround would sum with the center response. There is much evidence to suggest that simple AC → BC inhibitory feedback cannot explain all BC responses.[84] Finally, it has been long assumed that BCs were effectively isopotential, and that simple lumped-parameter calculations would suffice to model their network functions. However, reconstructions of BCs in mammals[3] suggest that the isopotentiality assumption is not correct and that complex local information processing can occur at the synaptic terminal without any evidence of that filtering appearing at the BC soma.

NETWORKS

Center-surround organization

The long-standing view of any BC or RGC receptive field is that it has antagonistic center-surround organization. Where does the surround come from? Anatomically, the vast number of AC synapses at the BC synaptic terminal, as well as evidence of GABAC receptor function, suggested that ACs should have a powerful surround effect.[4] Conversely, direct current injection into nonmammalian HCs clearly shows an

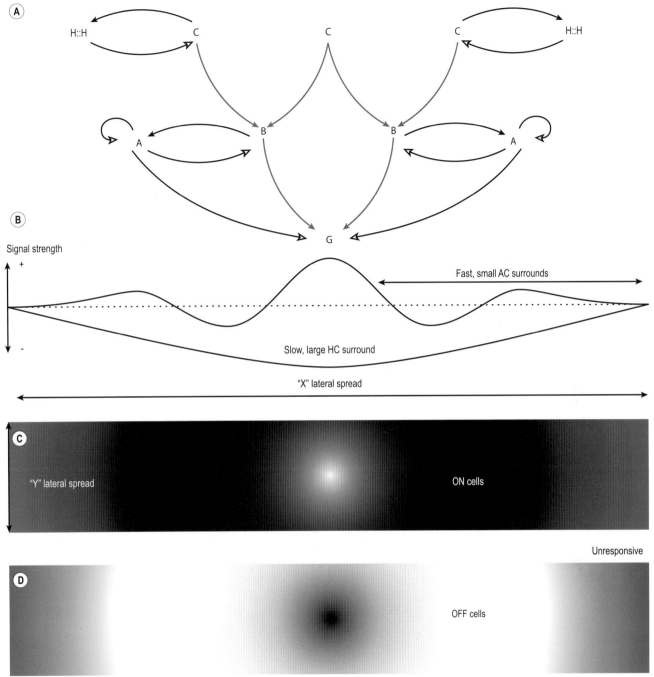

Fig. 21.5 The synaptic flow that forms retinal ganglion cell (RGC) receptive fields. (Panel A) Cone signals (C) converge on bipolar cells (BCs) (B) which then converge on RGCs (G), creating (Panel B) the canonical receptive field center, represented by a peak in the signal strength form the RGC. The coupled horizontal cell (HC) layer (H:H) forms the large, slow antagonistic surround, while narrower amacrine cells (ACs) (A) form fast, small surrounds with damp oscillatory wings. The horizontal cells (HCs) dominate sustained signaling, so typical receptive field maps of the light required to excite cells represent BC+HC contributions. For ON cells (Panel C), a spot of bright light will excite, while flanking regions of darkness will excite. For OFF cells (Panel D), a spot of darkness will excite, while flanking regions of light excite. The *red zones* indicate regions outside the field where neither excites.

effective, low frequency–dominated, sustained path from HCs to RGCs (Fig. 21.5). Reconciling the mechanism has been problematic but is likely simple. HCs and ACs function on very different time and space scales. HCs are slow, sustained (beyond the capacity of any normal neuron), and have immense receptive fields owing to strong coupling by gap junctions. Thus the presence of very large antagonistic surrounds in RGCs is likely driven through HCs. Experiments using fast pH buffers such

as HEPES block these surrounds. Conversely, GABAergic drugs have no effect on these large surrounds (in mammals). So what about ACs and all those synapses? Why do they not create the large surrounds of RGCs? First, ACs have much smaller receptive fields than HCs and their range of action will thus be smaller. Second, many ACs themselves show antagonistic center-surround organization, likely owing to AC >i AC chains.[85,86] Third, ACs are very fast and their actions at the BC terminal likely have more to do with feedback stabilization of synaptic gain than creating large, slow, antagonistic surrounds. ACs work in a highly time-and-space–restricted domain.

A more sophisticated network analysis suggests that some RGC classes can potentially inhibit different classes of surrounding RGCs via heterocellular coupling.[61] In this scenario, a single class of RGCs forms gap junctions with a few classes of costratifying GABAergic ACs which then fan out to inhibit many different classes of RGCs in the same patch of retina. When that RGC is activated by its BC drive, fast spikes can then invade the coupled ACs and inhibit a halo of different RGC classes. Heterocellular coupling may also facilitate spike synchrony among local groups of the same class of RGCs, which may be essential for upstream visual processing by providing high-coincidence spikes. In development or even in remodeling, spike coincidence appears to play a role in stabilizing retinal RGC synapses onto central targets.[87]

The functional role of coupling among patches of cone BCs[62] in the generation of RGC receptive fields is much less clear especially since coupling appears to be a mixture of in-class and cross-class targeting. Even so, all cone BCs appear to display coupling with neighboring cone BCs of the same stratum, suggesting it is a fundamental process in generating receptive field structure, perhaps by noise smoothing.

Mammalian rod pathways—evolution of a new amplification scheme

As we have described earlier, the synaptic chains that drive RGCs in all retinas are grouped into ON and OFF pathways. In nonmammalians, rod and cone pathways both use this direct chain to target the CNS. Thus rod signals undergo two-stage amplification before being encoded as a spike train: rods >m ON BCs, rods > OFF BCs, and BCs > RGCs. In mammals, a new amplification scheme evolved using cone BCs as the output stages, with rod BCs and glycinergic (gly) rod ACs as interneurons. Mammalian rod BCs are homologous to non-mammalian mixed rod-cone BCs, but have lost both cone inputs and the ability to target RGC dendrites. Nevertheless, six possible rod networks arising from three primary pathways (Fig. 21.6) exist in mammals, here grouped by amplification.

Three-stage amplification:

(1) rods >m ON rod BCs > gly rod ACs::ON cone BCs > ON RGCs
(2) rods >m ON rod BCs > gly rod ACs >i OFF cone BCs > OFF RGCs

Two-stage amplification:

(3) rods::cones >m ON cone BCs > ON RGCs
(4) rods::cones > OFF cone BCs > OFF RGCs
(5) rods > OFF cone BCs > OFF RGCs (sparse and species variable)
(6) rods >m ON cone BCs > ON RGCs (sparse)[41]

Thus, rod vision is parsed into ranges served by different networks: (1) the gly rod AC network with two arms of three-stage amplification for threshold scotopic vision and (2) the rod::cone → cone BC → RGC two-stage amplification for high brightness (moonlit) scotopic vision. Additional rod > cone BC contacts have been shown in some mammals,[39,40] but whether these additional pathways are structural errors in evolution or functional is not certain, as their incidences vary across mammalian species.[41]

The rod circuit is all the more complex for the involvement of GABAergic ACs, also known as S1 and S2 classes.[6] These γ rod ACs

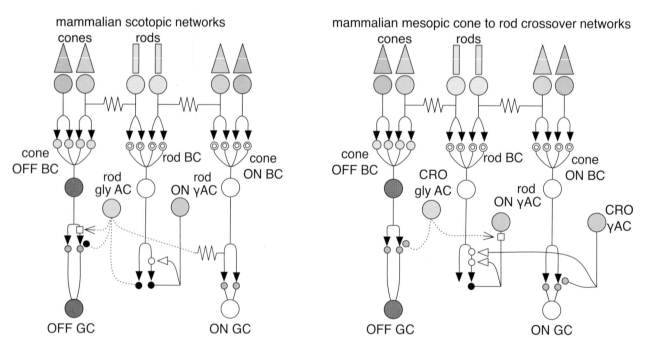

Fig. 21.6 The synaptologies of the mammalian scotopic and mesopic crossover networks. Rod signals predominantly reach retinal ganglion cells (RGCs) by three pathways. The main dark-adapted pathway flows from rods → rod BCs → glycinergic rod amacrine cells (ACs), which then redistribute the signal back into the cone bipolar cell (BC) channels via gap junctions (ON BCs) or glycinergic synapses (OFF BCs), and thence to RGCs. The second, less sensitive path is via rod:cone gap junctions. A rarer path, not found in all mammals, is the occasional sampling of rod signals by OFF BCs. Fast switching between rod and cone networks is mediated by AC chains. ON cone pathways inhibit rod pathways via crossover γACs (CRO) that capture ON cone BC input and directly inhibit rod BCs. OFF cone pathways inhibit rod paths via CRO gly ACs that capture OFF cone BC input and drive (via inverting synapses) the rod γAC network in the distal inner plexiform layer. This dual inversion allows OFF cone BCs to also inhibit rod BCs.

have dendritic arbors 1 mm in diameter and contact over 1000 rod BCs with reciprocal feedback synapses, with S2 cells providing twice the number of feedback synapses as S1.[7] This feedback likely further speeds the initially sluggish rod threshold response.

Rod-cone crossover networks

Mammalian vision engages a fast, winner-take-all switch between highly sensitive rod photoreceptor–based scotopic vision and cone photoreceptor–based photopic brightness and color vision. This switch deals with extensive environmental overlaps and confusion between rod- and cone-dominated lighting conditions. The nature of this switch remained enigmatic until the advent of ultrastructural connectomics.[88] Extensive cross-channel inhibition between cone and rod BC networks provides a fast, synaptic basis whereby dominant cone signals can inhibit rod BCs via monosynaptic ON cone BC > AC >i rod BC and disynaptic OFF cone BC > AC >i AC >i rod BC paths; and dominant rod signals can inhibit cone BCs by rod BC > AC >i ON cone BC and rod BC > AC >i AC >i OFF BC motifs, and other more sophisticated networks. Importantly, these are essentially copies of the basic BC > AC >i BC motif of lateral inhibition used by all BC networks (Fig. 21.7). Although sparse, Lauritzen et al.[88] showed by graph theory analysis that they are not random events.

Directionality—AC surrounds from afar

Although the roles of ACs in forming the center-surround features of sustained RGCs are complex, their primacy in encoding motion is established (Fig. 21.8). In some mammals, directionally selective (DS) RGCs respond to targets moving in a preferred direction but remain silent when targets move in the opposite, "null" direction.[89–91] DS RGCs have two classes: ON-OFF and ON RGCs. These networks engage BCs and perhaps several different AC inputs, including the ON and OFF subtypes[90] of starburst GABAergic/cholinergic ACs and other GABAergic ACs.[25,92] OFF starburst ACs hyperpolarize to light and are driven by OFF cone BCs. ON starburst cells have somas displaced to the RGC layer depolarize to light pulses and are driven by ON cone BC inputs. Each class stratifies with and synapses on dendrites of DS RGCs. The precise classes of other γ ACs in DS RGC networks are not known, but the functional roles of GABAergic inhibition are emerging. At least one GABAergic AC inhibits the starburst ACs, and others inhibit DS RGCs. Thus, as stimuli come from the preferred side, a combination of excitatory glutamatergic BC and cholinergic starburst AC signals converge on the RGC in advance of GABAergic inhibition. The excitatory gain is likely enhanced by the BC > starburst AC > RGC chain, which should have greater gain than a direct BC > RGC transfer. In the null direction, a strong GABA signal reaches the DS RGC in advance of the excitatory input and prevents it from reaching spike threshold. GABAA receptor antagonists block this strong inhibition and convert DS RGCs into nondirectional cells.[89] The inhibition seems so strong (almost like veto synapses in cerebellum) that the BC > starburst AC > RGC circuit cannot break through. In fact, that may be the raison d'etre for starburst ACs: to break through any residual inhibition in the preferred direction as GABA inhibition is strong *even in the preferred direction*. This is likely an archetype for all AC circuits, in which spatial properties, timing, and convergence of multiple cell classes select for fine grain features such as edges, texture, or flicker. However, new findings in the primate retina[93] show that ON-OFF DS RGCs have input

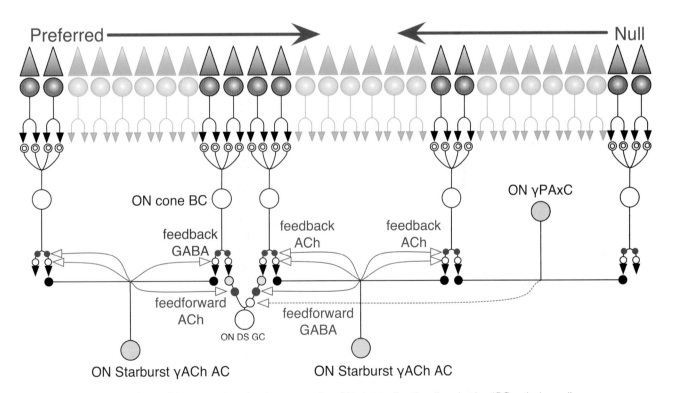

Fig. 21.7 A possible synaptology for the mammalian ON-center directionally selective (*DS*) retinal ganglion cell (RGC) network. ON DS RGCs collect glutamatergic excitatory signals from ON cone bipolar cells (*BCs*) and cholinergic excitatory signals from ON starburst amacrine cells (*ACs*). This amplifies the center response. ON starburst ACs also provide both cholinergic and GABAergic feedback onto BCs. However, additional axonal cell (*AxC*) GABAergic inputs exist input in the DS strata of the inner plexiform layer. Such cells may receive inputs in the surround on one side and send axons (*dotted*) to target distant DS RGC dendrites. Thus stimuli approaching from the left will excite and those from the right will inhibit. *ACh*, Acetylcholine.

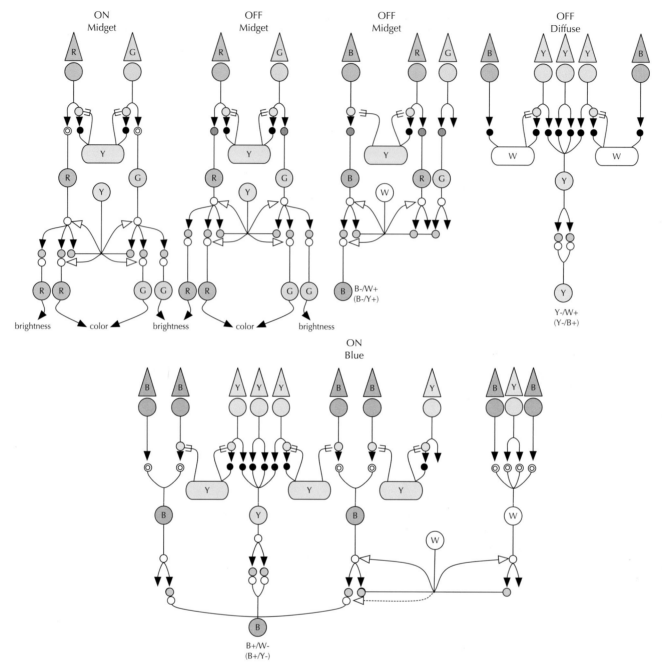

Fig. 21.8 Possible color channel synaptologies for the primate retina. Midget pathways arise from midget bipolar cells (BCs) that contact only one cone and midget retinal ganglion cells (RGCs) that contact only one BC. This creates pure red (*R*) or green (*G*) center RGCs in both ON and OFF channels. But the use of these signals is likely determined in part by the projection of their axons to appropriate thalamic and ultimately to cortical brightness- and color-coding pools via *parallel channels*. However the surround information from horizontal cells (HCs) and amacrine cells (ACs) collect from both R and G channels, generating "yellow" (*Y*) surrounds. RGCs that are R/Y will generate net R/G percepts *(shown in parenthesis)*, with similar outcomes for the three other possible R and G channels. OFF midget blue channels are likely antagonists by "yellow" H1 HCs and either Y or "white" (*W*) ACs that collect from all classes of cone BCs. RGCs that are B/W will generate net B/Y percepts *(shown in parenthesis)*, with similar outcomes for the three other possible R and G channels. It is also possible that diffuse BCs that contact all long wave–system (LWS) cones (summarized as Y cones) may have surrounds from "white" H2 HCs (either by feedback as shown or feedforward) that generate Y–/W+ fields leading to Y–/B+ percepts. Finally, the best-known B pathway involves BCs selective for short wave–system 1 (SWS1) B cones. The RGCs that collect these signals are small bistratified cells with ON B BC inputs in sublamina b and Y selective OFF BC inputs in sublamina a. There are at least three possible -Y channels: H1 HC feedforward to B cones, direct OFF BC inputs from LWS-selective BCs, and W opponent inputs from nonselective ACs. The inability of GABA antagonists to block Y opponency in these cells suggests that the HC network dominates.

from starburst ACs and polyaxonal cells as described previously, and that these cells themselves show complex directional bias. Moreover, some BCs show directional biases in their axonal terminal signals, likely arising from starburst ACs and perhaps via cholinergic drive.[94,95] In rabbit retina, the primary BC class that receives input from starburst ACs is also coupled preferentially to its own class.[62]

Primate color coding

Humans and old-world primates have cone mosaics with sparse blue (B, SWS1) cone arrays[96] surrounded by randomly distributed red cones and green cones (R, LWSR; G, LWSG). Most mammals possess dichromatic vision via B and G cone opponencies. Complete trichromatic vision has two opponent processes[97]: (1) blue/yellow (B/Y) opponency (in which the Y signal is the sum of R and G cones signals)[98,99]; and (2) red/green (R/G) opponency. Both pose conceptual problems. The R and G pigment genes are tandem head-to-tail LWS arrays on the X chromosome.[20,97] LWS cones can express only one pigment, either LWSR or LWSG, creating either R or G cones[100,101] and this may be the *only* gene product that discriminates R and G cones. This suggests that the connectivity of R and G systems is probabilistic. Even so, R/G opponency is robust in trichromatic primates.

R/G opponency

In the foveola, each midget BC contacts only one cone and each midget RGC contacts only one midget BC. Thus four types of center/surround R/G color opponency emerge (Fig. 21.8).[102] If the behavior of a single foveal R cone is not confounded by R::G coupling, a midget BC > midget RGC chain should manifest a pure R or G center. Thus all midget RGCs should be color opponent (Fig. 21.8), because their surrounds, whether derived from HCs or ACs, should be "yellower" than both: always greener than R cones or redder than G cones. HCs do not show any spectral selectivity for R or G cones and sum their inputs.[103] It was once posited that the RGC surrounds were pure (pure R versus pure G) via selective contact of opponent BCs by ACs. However, electron microscopy shows this is not so[104]—the AC-driven surrounds of midget RGCs encode mixtures of R and G cones. Even so, some midget RGCs show nearly pure opponent surrounds,[105–107] perhaps because of the patchiness of R and G cone distributions[108] and the small size of midget RGC surrounds. Thus there is much more to be understood about midget RGC networks, for example, why broad yellow-sensitive (Y) HC surrounds do not dominate midget BCs, as they do for B/Y opponent RGCs. Newer syntheses have emerged in part from single-cone psychophysics in which neighboring foveolar cones generate predominately achromatic percepts and only rarely chromatic percepts.[109] Further analysis implies no specificity in HC interactions.[110] These conflicting views are partly resolved by considering the collection of midget RGCs as multiple classes of parallel channels.[111,112]

B/Y opponency

RGCs that convey blue signals are thought to be of two varieties: large and small bistratified B+/Y– RGCs,[99,102] both of which receive B cone ON BC synapses in sublamina b and Y inputs from diffuse OFF BCs in sublamina a (Fig. 21.8). Although it was thought that B/Y centers and surrounds overlapped tremendously, recent data suggest that the Y surround originates from HCs via HC >i cone feedback and is much larger.[53] Recent anatomical evidence suggests the existence of a midget B cone OFF BC pathway in monkey[113] and a diffuse B cone OFF BC in rabbit.[114] Further, melanopsin RGCs are putative B–/Y+ RGCs with large receptive fields. As an aside, the various classes of RGCs that express melanopsin clearly overlap RGC functions that are image forming.[115] Which cells carry "the" blue signal remains uncertain, as

human patients lacking the mGluR6 receptor (and thus lacking ON BC signaling) apparently have quite excellent photopic sensitivity and no color deficits.

How retinal disease revises retinal networks

It was once thought that retinal networks were laid down once and for all in development by a process independent of sensory experience, but that is clearly incorrect. No less correct is the idea that during the process of photoreceptor deconstruction and death the neural retina remains normal. Many studies show that retina behaves much like CNS in response to challenges such as oxidative stress, denervation, and trauma by remodeling its synaptic connectivity and reprogramming neural signaling rules. For example, the loss of photoreceptors in retinitis pigmentosa leads to the retraction of BC dendrites and the evolution of new axon-like structures; the generation of abundant new processes from retinal neurons of all kinds; the formation of new synaptic zones in the form of microneuromas; the switch from mGluR6 to iGluR expression in former ON rod BCs; and the ultimate death of many neurons.[9,116] These changes challenge many strategies to restore vision by genetic, molecular, cellular, and bionic schemes. But beyond that, they demonstrate two very important concepts. First, synaptic communication is likely never static and signaling mechanisms are stabilized by active mechanisms. Second, the rules used by any neuron to decide which glutamate (or other) receptors to express are not well known. We are only beginning to map the regulators that control the decision to choose mGluR6 initially,[117] much less choose AMPA or KA receptors in response to reprogramming, or even the key adhesion molecules controlling network stabilization.[118]

REFERENCES

1. Marc RE. Retinal Neurotransmitters. In: Chalupa LM, Werner J, eds. *The Visual Neurosciences*. Cambridge, MA: MIT Press; 2004:315–330.
2. Marc RE, Cameron DA. A molecular phenotype atlas of the zebrafish retina. *J Neurocytol.* 2002;30:593–654.
3. Anderson JR, Jones BW, Yang J-H, Shaw MV, Watt CB, Koshevoy P, Spaltenstein J, Jurrus E, UV K, Whitaker R, Mastronarde D, Tasdizen T, Marc RE. A computational framework for ultrastructural mapping of neural circuitry. *PLoS Biol.* 2009;7:e1000074.
4. Marc RE, Liu W. Fundamental GABAergic amacrine cell circuitries in the retina: nested feedback, concatenated inhibition, and axosomatic synapses. *J Comp Neurol.* 2000;425: 560–582.
5. Deans MR, Volgyi B, Goodenough DA, Bloomfield SA, Paul DL. Connexin36 is essential for transmission of rod-mediated visual signals in the mammalian retina. *Neuron.* 2002;36:703–712.
6. Vaney DI. Morphological identification of serotonin-accumulating neurons in the living retina. *Science.* 1986;233:444–446.
7. Li W, Zhang J, Massey SC. Coupling pattern of S1 and S2 amacrine cells in the rabbit retina. *Vis Neurosci.* 2002;19:119–131.
8. Mills SL, O'Brien JJ, Li W, O'Brien J, Massey SC. Rod pathways in the mammalian retina use connexin 36. *J Comp Neurol.* 2001;436:336–350.
9. Marc RE, Jones BW, Watt CB, Strettoi E. Neural remodeling in retinal degeneration. *Prog Ret Eye Res.* 2003;22:607–655.
10. Pfeiffer RL, Anderson JR, Dahal J, Garcia JC, Yang JH, Sigulinsky CL, Rapp K, Emrich DP, Watt CB, Johnstun HA, Houser AR, Marc RE, Jones BW. A pathoconnectome of early neurodegeneration: Network changes in retinal degeneration. *Exp Eye Res. Oct.* 2020;199:108196.
11. Pfeiffer RL, Marc RE, Jones BW. Persistent remodeling and neurodegeneration in late-stage retinal degeneration. *Prog Retin Eye Res.* 2020;74:100771.
12. Marc RE, Jones BW, Watt CB, Anderson JR, Sigulinsky C, Lauritzen S. Retinal connectomics: towards complete, accurate networks. *Prog Retin Eye Res.* 2013;37:141–162.
13. Diacou R, Nandigrami P, Fiser A, Liu W, Ashery-Padan R, Cvekl A. Cell fate decisions, transcription factors and signaling during early retinal development. *Prog Retin Eye Res.* 2022;91:101093.
14. Strettoi E, Di Marco B, Orsini N, Napoli D. Retinal Plasticity. *Int J Mol Sci.* 2022;23: 1138–1153.
15. MacNeil MA, Heussy JK, Dacheux RF, Raviola E, Masland RH. The population of bipolar cells in the rabbit retina. *J Comp Neurol.* 2004;472:73–86.
16. MacNeil MA, Heussy JK, Dacheux RF, Raviola E, Masland RH. The shapes and numbers of amacrine cells: matching of photofilled with Golgi-stained cells in the rabbit retina and comparison with other mammalian species. *J Comp Neurol.* 1999;413:305–326.
17. Rockhill RL, Daly FJ, MacNeil MA, Brown SP, Masland RH. The diversity of ganglion cells in a mammalian retina. *J Neurosci.* 2002;22:3831–3843.

18. Morgan JL, Dhingra A, Vardi N, Wong RO. Axons and dendrites originate from neuroepithelial-like processes of retinal bipolar cells. *Nat Neurosci.* 2006;9:85–92.
19. Wässle H, Puller C, Muller F, Haverkamp S. Cone contacts, mosaics, and territories of bipolar cells in the mouse retina. *J Neurosci.* 2009;29:106–117.
20. Nathans J. The evolution and physiology of human color vision: insights from molecular genetic studies of visual pigments. *Neuron.* 1999;24:299–312.
21. Loew ER, Govardovskii VI. Photoreceptors and visual pigments in the red-eared turtle, Trachemys scripta elegans. *Vis Neurosci.* 2001;18:753–757.
22. Chiu M, Nathans J. Blue cones and cone bipolar cells share transcriptional specificity as determined by expression of human blue visual pigment-derived transgenes. *J Neurosci.* 1994;14:3426–3436.
23. Kalloniatis M, Marc RE, Murry RF. Amino acid signatures in the primate retina. *J Neurosci.* 1996;16:6807–6829.
24. Völgyi B, Xin D, Amarillo Y, Bloomfield SA. Morphology and physiology of the polyaxonal amacrine cells in the rabbit retina. *J Comp Neurol.* 2001;440:109–125.
25. Famiglietti EV. Polyaxonal amacrine cells of rabbit retina: PA2, PA3, and PA4 cells. Light and electron microscopic studies with a functional interpretation. *J Comp Neurol.* 1992;316:422–446.
26. Famiglietti EV. Synaptic organization of starburst amacrine cells in rabbit retina: analysis of serial thin sections by electron microscopy and graphic reconstruction. *J Comp Neurol.* 1991;309:40–70.
27. Dacey DM. The dopaminergic amacrine cell. *J Comp Neurol.* 1990;301:461–489.
28. Descarries, L, Bérubé-Carrière, N, Riada, M, Dal Boc, G, Mendez, JA, Trudeauc, L-E, 2007. Glutamate in dopamine neurons: Synaptic versus diffuse transmission. Brain Res Rev. 2008;58(2):290-302.29.
29. Marc RE, Liu WL. Horizontal cell synapses onto glycine-accumulating interplexiform cells. *Nature.* 1984;312:266–269.
30. Perlman I, Kolb H, Nelson R. Anatomy, circuitry, and physiology of vertebrate horizontal cells. In: Chalupa LM, Werner J, eds. *The Visual Neurosciences.* Cambridge, MA: MIT Press; 2004:369–394.
31. Della Santina L, Kuo SP, Yoshimatsu T, Okawa H, Suzuki SC, Hoon M, Tsuboyama K, Reike F, Wong ROL. Glutamatergic monopolar interneurons provide a novel pathway of excitation in the mouse retina. *Curr Biol.* 2016;26:2070–2077.
32. Young BK, Ramakrishnan C, Ganjawala T, Wang P, Deisseroth K, Tian N. An uncommon neuronal class conveys visual signals from rods and cones to retinal ganglion cells. *Proc Natl Acad Sci USA.* 2021;118e2104884118.
33. Katz B, Miledi R. A study of synaptic transmission in the absence of nerve impulses. *J Physiol.* 1967;192:407–436.
34. Bailey ME, Matthews DA, Riley BP, Albrecht BE, Kostrzewa M, Hicks AA, Harris R, Muller U, Darlison MG, Johnson KJ. Genomic mapping and evolution of human GABA(A) receptor subunit gene clusters. *Mammalian Genome.* 1999;10:839–843.
35. Thoreson WB. Transmission at rod and cone ribbon synapses in the retina. *Pflugers Arch.* 2021;473:1469–1491.
36. Mesnard CS, Barta CL, Sladek AL, Zenisek D, Thoreson WB. Eliminating synaptic ribbons from rods and cones halves the releasable vesicle pool and slows down replenishment. *Int J Mol Sci.* 2023;24(2):1561.
37. Migdale K, Herr S, Klug K, Ahmad K, Linberg K, Sterling P, Schein S. Two ribbon synaptic units in rod photoreceptors of macaque, human, and cat. *J Comp Neurol.* 2003;455:100–112.
38. Ishida AT, Stell WK, Lightfoot DO. Rod and cone inputs to bipolar cells in goldfish retina. *J Comp Neurol.* 1980;191:315–335.
39. Tsukamoto Y, Morigiwa K, Ishii M, Takao M, Iwatsuki K, Nakanishi S, Fukuda Y. A novel connection between rods and ON cone bipolar cells revealed by ectopic metabotropic glutamate receptor 7 (mGluR7) in mGluR6-deficient mouse retinas. *J Neurosci.* 2007;27: 6261–6267.
40. Li W, Keung JW, Massey SC. Direct synaptic connections between rods and OFF cone bipolar cells in the rabbit retina. *J Comp Neurol.* 2004;474:1–12.
41. Protti DA, Flores-Herr N, Li W, Massey SC, Wassle H. Light signaling in scotopic conditions in the rabbit, mouse and rat retina: A physiological and anatomical study. *J Neurophysiol.* 2005;93:3479–3488.
42. Stell WK. Horizontal cell axons and axon terminals in goldfish retina. *J Comp Neurol.* 1975;159:503–519.
43. Wässle H. Decomposing a cone's output (Parallel processing). In: Masland RH, Albright T, eds. *The Senses: A Comprehensive Reference.* Amsterdam: Elsevier; 2008.
44. Dowling JE, Boycott BB. Organization of the primate retina: electron microscopy. *Proc R Soc Lond B Biol Sci.* 1966;166:80–111.
45. Brecha NC. Peptide and peptide receptor expression in function in the vertebrate retina. In: Chalupa LM, Werner J, eds. *The Visual Neurosciences.* Cambridge, MA: MIT Press; 2004:334–354.
46. Witkovsky P. Dopamine and retinal function. *Doc Ophthalmol.* 2004;108:17–39.
47. Witkovsky P, Nicholson C, Rice ME, Bohmaker K, Meller E. Extracellular dopamine concentration in the retina of the clawed frog, Xenopus laevis. *Proc Nat Acad Sci USA.* 1993;90:5667–5671.
48. Gastinger MJ, O'Brien JJ, Larsen NB, Marshak DW. Histamine immunoreactive axons in the macaque retina. *Invest Ophthalmol Vis Sci.* 1999;40:487–495.
49. Baylor DA, Fuortes MGF, O'Bryan PM. Receptive fields of cones in the retina of the turtle. *J Physiol.* 1971;214:265–294.
50. Naka K. Functional organization of catfish retina. *Journal of Neurophysiology.* 1977;40:26–43.
51. Naka K-I, Witkovsky P. Dogfish ganglion cell discharge resulting from extrinsic polarization of the horizontal cells. *J Physiol.* 1972;223:449–460.
52. Vardi N, Zhang L-L, Payne JA, Sterling P. Evidence that different cation chloride cotransporters in retinal neurons allow opposite responses to GABA. *The J Neurosci.* 2000; 20:7657–7663.
53. Field GD, Sher A, Gauthier JL, Greschner M, Shlens J, Litke AM, Chichilnisky EJ. Spatial properties and functional organization of small bistratified ganglion cells in primate retina. *J. Neurosci.*. 2007;27:13261–13272.
54. McMahon MJ, Packer OS, Dacey DM. The classical receptive field surround of primate parasol ganglion cells is mediated primarily by a non-GABAergic pathway. *J Neurosci.* 2004;24:3736–3745.
55. Thoreson WB, Babai N, Bartoletti TM. Feedback from horizontal cells to rod photoreceptors in vertebrate retina. *J Neurosci.* 2008;28:5691–5695.
56. Davenport CM, Detwiler PB, Dacey DM. Effects of pH Buffering on horizontal and ganglion cell Light responses in primate retina: Evidence for the proton hypothesis of surround formation. *J. Neurosci.*. 2008;28:456–464.
57. Kamermans M, Fahrenfort I. Ephaptic interactions within a chemical synapse: hemichannel-mediated ephaptic inhibition in the retina. *Current Opinion in Neurobiology.* 2004;14:531–541.
58. Massey SC.In: Masland RH, Albright T, eds. *Circuit Functions of Gap Junctions in the Mammalian Retina.* The Senses. Academic Press; 2008:457–472.
59. Hampson EC, Weiler R, Vaney DI. pH-gated dopaminergic modulation of horizontal cell gap junctions in mammalian retina. *Proc Royal Soc London - Series B: Biological Sciences.* 1994;255:67–72.
60. Mills SL, Massey SC. Differential properties of two gap junctional pathways made by AII amacrine cells. *Nature.* 1995;377:734–737.
61. Marc RE, Sigulinsky CL, Pfeiffer RL, Emrich D, Anderson JR, Jones BW. Heterocellular coupling Between amacrine cells and ganglion Cells. *Front Neural Circuits.* 2018;12:90.
62. Sigulinsky CL, Anderson JR, Kerzner E, Rapp CN, Pfeiffer RL, Rodman TM, Emrich DP, Rapp KD, Nelson NT, Lauritzen JS, Meyer M, Marc RE, Jones BW. Network architecture of gap junctional coupling among parallel processing channels in the mammalian retina. *J Neurosci.* 2020;40:4483–4511.
63. Gustafson EC, Stevens ER, Wolosker H, Miller RF. Endogenous D-serine contributes to NMDA-receptor-mediated light-evoked responses in the vertebrate retina. *J Neurophysiol.* 2007;98:122–130.
64. Hanna MC, Calkins DJ. Expression of genes encoding glutamate receptors and transporters in rod and cone bipolar cells of the primate retina determined by single-cell polymerase chain reaction. *Mol Vis.* 2007;13:2194–2208.
65. Dhingra A, Lyubarsky A, Jiang M, Pugh ENJ, Birnbaumer L, Sterling P, Vardi N. The light response of ON bipolar neurons requires Gαo. *J Neurosci.* 2000;20:9053–9058.
66. Quraishi S, Gayet J, Morgans CW, Duvoisin R. Distribution of group-III metabotropic glutamate receptors in the retina. *J Comp Neurol.* 2007;501:931–943.
67. Zhang D-Q, Zhou T-R, McMahon DG. Functional heterogeneity of retinal dopaminergic neurons underlying their multiple roles in vision. *J Neurosci.* 2007;27:692–699.
68. Goel M, Mangel SC. Dopamine-mediated circadian and light/dark-adaptive modulation of chemical and electrical synapses in the outer retina. *Front Cell Neurosci.* 2021;15647–541.
69. Piccolino M, Neyton J, Gerschenfeld HM. Decrease of gap junction permeability induced by dopamine and cyclic adenosine 3':5' monophosphate in horizontal cells of turtle retina. *J Neurosci.* 1984;4:2477.
70. Vaquero CF, Pignatelli A, Partida GJ, Ishida AT. A dopamine- and protein kinase A-dependent mechanism for network adaptation in retinal ganglion cells. *J Neurosci.* 2001;21:8624–8635.
71. Eldred WD, Blute TA. Imaging of nitric oxide in the retina. *Vision Res.* 2005;45:3469–3486.
72. Vaney DI. Retinal amacrine cells. In: Chalupa LM, Werner J, eds. *The Visual Neurosciences.* Cambridge, MA: MIT Press; 2004:395–409.
73. Slaughter MM. Inhibition in the Retina. In: Chalupa LM, Werner J, eds. *The Visual Neurosciences.* Cambridge, MA: MIT Press; 2004:355–368.
74. Grant GB, Dowling JE. On bipolar cell responses in the teleost retina are generated by two distinct mechanisms. *Journal of Neurophysiology.* 1996;76:3842–3849.
75. Grant GB, Dowling JE. A glutamate-activated chloride current in cone-driven ON bipolar cells of the white perch retina. *J Neurosci.* 1995;15:3852–3862.
76. Marc R. Mapping glutamatergic drive in the vertebrate retina with a channel-permeant organic cation. *J Comp Neurol.* 1999;407:47–64.
77. Marc R. Kainate activation of horizontal, bipolar, amacrine, and ganglion cells in the rabbit retina. *J Comp Neurol.* 1999;407:65–76.
78. Diamond JS. Inhibitory interneurons in the retina: Types, circuitry, and function. *Annu Rev Vis Sci.* 2017;3:1–24.
79. Barnes S. Visual processing: When two synaptic strata are better than one. *Curr Biol.* 2022;32:R129–R131.
80. Zhang J, Jung CS, Slaughter MM. Serial inhibitory synapses in retina. *Vis Neurosci.* 1997;14:553–563.
81. Hsueh HA, Molnar A, Werblin FS. Amacrine-to-amacrine cell inhibition in the rabbit retina. *J Neurophysiol.* 2008;100:2077–2088.
82. Marmarelis PZ, Marmarelis VZ. *Analysis of Physiological Systems, Computers in Biology and Medicine.* New York: Springer; 1978.
83. Critz SD, Marc RE. Glutamate antagonists that block hyperpolarizing bipolar cells increase the release of dopamine from turtle retina. *Vis Neurosci.* 1992;9:271–278.
84. Zhang A-J, Wu SM. Receptive fields of retinal bipolar cells are mediated by heterogeneous synaptic circuitry. *J Neurosci.* 2009;29:789–797.
85. Wilson M, Vaney DI. Amacrine cells. In: Masland RH, Albright T, eds. *The Senses: A Comprehensive Reference.* Amsterdam: Elsevier; 2008:361–367.
86. Bloomfield SA, Xin D. Surround inhibition of mammalian AII amacrine cells is generated in the proximal retina. *J Physiology.* 2000;523(Pt 3):771–783.
87. Munz M, Gobert D, Schohl A, Poquérusse J, Podgorski K, Spratt P, Ruthazer ES. Rapid Hebbian axonal remodeling mediated by visual stimulation. *Science.* 2014;344:904–909.
88. Lauritzen JS, Anderson JR, Jones BW, Watt CB, Mohammed S, Hoang J, Marc RE. ON cone bipolar cell axonal synapses in the OFF inner plexiform layer of the rabbit retina. *J Comp Neurol.* 2012;521:977–1000.
89. Wyatt HJ, Daw NW. Directionally sensitive ganglion cells in the rabbit retina: specificity for stimulus direction, size, and speed. *J Neurophysiol.* 1975;38:613–626.
90. Dacheux RF, Chimento MF, Amthor FR. Synaptic input to the on-off directionally selective ganglion cell in the rabbit retina. *J Comp Neurol.* 2003;456:267–278.
91. Kittila CA, Massey SC. Pharmacology of directionally selective ganglion cells in the rabbit retina. *J Neurophysiol.* 1997;77:675–689.

92. Grzywacz NM, Amthor FR, Merwine DK. Necessity of acetylcholine for retinal directionally selective responses to drifting gratings in rabbit. *J Physiol*. 1998;512:575–581.

93. Kim YJ, Peterson BB, Crook JD, Joo HR, Wu J, Puller C, Robinson FR, Gamlin PD, Yau K-W, Viana F, Troy JB, Smith RG, Packer OS, Detwiler PB, Dacey DM. Origins of direction selectivity in the primate retina. *Nat Commun*. 2022;13:2862.

94. Hellmer CB, Hall LM, Bohl JM, Sharpe ZJ, Smith RG, Ichinose T. Cholinergic feedback to bipolar cells contributes to motion detection in the mouse retina. *Cell Rep*. 2021;37:110106.

95. Matsumoto A, Agbariah W, Nolte SS, Andrawos R, Levi H, Sabbah S, Yonehara K. Direction selectivity in retinal bipolar cell axon terminals. *Neuron*. 2021;109:2928–2942. e8.

96. Marc RE. Chromatic patterns of cone photoreceptors. 1976 Glenn A. Fry Award Lecture. *Am J Optometry & Physiological Optics*. 1977;54:212–225.

97. Carroll J, Jacobs GH. Mammalian photopigments. In: Masland RH, Albright T, eds. *The Senses: A Comprehensive Reference*. Amsterdam: Elsevier; 2008:247–268.

98. Kaplan E. The P, M and K streams of the primate visual system: What do they do for vision?. In: Masland RH, Albright T, eds. *The Senses: A Comprehensive Reference*. Amsterdam: Elsevier; 2008:369–381.

99. Lee BB. Blue-ON Cells. In: Masland RH, Albright T, eds. *The Senses: A Comprehensive Reference*. Amsterdam: Elsevier; 2008:433–438.

100. Wang Y, Smallwood PM, Cowan M, Blesh D, Lawler A, Nathans J. Mutually exclusive expression of human red and green visual pigment-reporter transgenes occurs at high frequency in murine cone photoreceptors. *Proc Nat Acad Sci USA*. 1999;96:5251–5256.

101. Smallwood PM, Wang Y, Nathans J. Role of a locus control region in the mutually exclusive expression of human red and green cone pigment genes. *Proc Nat Acad Sci USA*. 2002;99:1008–1011.

102. Dacey DM. Parallel pathways for spectral coding in primate retina. *Annu. Rev. Neurosci*. 2000;23:743–775.

103. Dacey DM, Lee BB, Stafford DK, Pokorny J, Smith VC. Horizontal cells of the primate retina: cone specificity without spectral opponency. *Science*. 1996;271:656–659.

104. Calkins DJ, Sterling P. Absence of spectrally specific lateral inputs to midget ganglion cells in primate retina. *Nature*. 1996;381:613–615.

105. Sun H, Smithson HE, Zaidi Q, Lee BB. Specificity of cone inputs to macaque retinal ganglion cells. *J Neurophysiol*. 2006;95:837–849.

106. Reid RC, Shapley RM. Space and time maps of cone photoreceptor signals in macaque lateral geniculate nucleus. *J Neurosci*. 2002;22:6158–6175.

107. Reid RC, Shapley RM. Spatial structure of cone inputs to receptive fields in primate lateral geniculate nucleus. *Nature*. 1992;356:716–718.

108. Hofer H, Carroll J, Neitz J, Neitz M, Williams DR. Organization of the human trichromatic cone mosaic. *J Neurosci*. 2005;25:9669–9679.

109. Sabesan R, Schmidt BP, Tuten WS, Roorda A. The elementary representation of spatial and color vision in the human retina. *Sci Adv*. 2016;2:e1600797.

110. Tuten WS, Harmening WM, Sabesan R, Roorda A, Sincich LC. Spatiochromatic interactions between individual cone photoreceptors in the human retina. *J Neurosci*. 2017;37:9498–9509.

111. Patterson SS, Neitz M, Neitz J. Reconciling color vision models with midget ganglion cell receptive fields. *Front Neurosci*. 2019;13:865.

112. Rezeanu D, Neitz M, Neitz J. How we see black and white: The role of midget ganglion cells. *Front Neuroanat*. 2022;16:944762.

113. Klug K, Herr S, Ngo IT, Sterling P, Schein S. Macaque retina contains an S-cone OFF midget pathway. *J Neurosci*. 2003;23:9881–9887.

114. Liu P-C, Chiao C-C. Morphologic identification of the OFF-Type blue cone bipolar cell in the rabbit retina. *Invest. Ophthalmol. Vis. Sci.*. 2007;48:3388–3395.

115. Sondereker KB, Stabio ME, Renna JM. Crosstalk: The diversity of melanopsin ganglion cell types has begun to challenge the canonical divide between image-forming and non-image-forming vision. *J Comp Neurol*. 2020;528:2044–2067.

116. Marc RE, Jones BW, Anderson JR, Kinard K, Marshak DW, Wilson JH, Wensel T, Lucas RJ. Neural reprogramming in retinal degeneration. *Invest Ophthalmol Vis Sci*. 2007;48:3364–3371.

117. Furukawa T, Ueno A, Omori Y. Molecular mechanisms underlying selective synapse formation of vertebrate retinal photoreceptor cells. *Cell Mol Life Sci*. 2020;77:1251–1266.

118. Cao Y, Wang Y, Dunn HA, Orlandi C, Shultz N, Kamasawa N, Fitzpatrick D, Li W, Zeitz C, Hauswirth W, Martemyanov KA. Interplay between cell-adhesion molecules governs synaptic wiring of cone photoreceptors. *Proc Natl Acad Sci U S A*. 2020;117:23914–23924.

119. Zeitz C, Forster U, Neidhardt J, Feil S, Kälin S, Leifert D, Flor PJ, Berger W. Night blindness-associated mutations in the ligand-binding, cysteine-rich, and intracellular domains of the metabotropic glutamate receptor 6 abolish protein trafficking. *Hum Mutat*. 2007;28:771–780.

120. Mauck MC, Salzwedel A, Kuchenbecker J, Pawela C, Garcia J, Hyde J, Hudetz A, Connor TB, Neitz J, Neitz M. Probing neural circuitry for blue-yellow color vision using high resolution functional magnetic resonance imaging. *Invest Ophthalmol Vis Sci*. 2008;49:3251.

121. Almasieh M, Wilson AM, Morquette B, Cueva Vargas JL, Di Polo A. The molecular basis of retinal ganglion cell death in glaucoma. *Prog Retin Eye Res*. 2012;31:152–181.

122. Chen H, Liu X, Tian N. Subtype-dependent postnatal development of direction- and orientation-selective retinal ganglion cells in mice. *J Neurophysiol*. 2014;112:2092–2101.

123. Jones BW, Kondo M, Terasaki H, Watt CB, Rapp K, Anderson J, Lin Y, Shaw MV, Yang JH, Marc RE. Retinal remodeling in the Tg P347L rabbit, a large-eye model of retinal degeneration. *J Comp Neurol*. 2011;519:2713–2733.

124. Seki M, Lipton SA. Targeting excitotoxic/free radical signaling pathways for therapeutic intervention in glaucoma. *Prog Brain Res*. 2008;173:495–510.

125. Tian N. Visual experience and maturation of retinal synaptic pathways. *Vision Res*. 2004;44:3307–3316.

126. Tian N, Copenhagen D. Plasticity of retinal circuitry. In: Masland RH, Albright T, eds. *The Senses: A Comprehensive Reference*. Amsterdam: Elsevier; 2008:473–490.

22

Signal Processing in the Outer Retina

Nicholas C. Brecha, Arlene A. Hirano, and Steven Barnes

INTRODUCTION

Rod and cone photoreceptors transduce light, and they operate over different levels of illumination and chromatic ranges. In the vertebrate retina, there is a single type of rod and up to four types of cones. Light-evoked signals in rods and cones are transmitted to bipolar and horizontal cells at the first synapse in the visual system, and these signals subsequently diverge into multiple bipolar cell channels that terminate on amacrine and ganglion cells in the inner retina. Ganglion cells in turn project their axons via the optic nerve to terminate in numerous visual nuclei in the brain. The major retinal cell classes were recognized over 125 years ago (see Ramón y Cajal, 1894)[1] and they have been defined in all vertebrates, from primitive fish to humans.[2,3]

Photoreceptors are electrically coupled and the coupling influences both photoreceptor signaling and downstream bipolar cell pathways. Photoreceptors form excitatory, glutamate-mediated chemical synapses with both bipolar and horizontal cells. Glutamate release from photoreceptors is vesicular and graded in a smooth manner, and the rate of release of glutamate is high in the dark and low in the light. Bipolar cells are classified into two major subtypes, depolarizing (or ON-type) and hyperpolarizing (or OFF-type) based on their response to a centered light stimulus, respectively.[4,5] Bipolar cells defined in mammalian retinas consist of a single rod type and 8 to 13 cone types based on their axonal and dendritic features, connectivity in the outer and inner retina,[6,7] and transcriptomics.[8] Bipolar cells provide excitatory glutamatergic output to amacrine and ganglion cells, and they have distinct functional properties, including center-surround antagonism and color opponency.[9] Horizontal cells, consisting of one or two types in the mammalian retina, are electrically coupled, and their dendrites innervate cone synaptic terminals, called pedicles, whereas their axon terminals innervate rod synaptic terminals, called spherules.[10] Horizontal cells mediate feedback to photoreceptors by modulation of photoreceptor voltage-gated calcium (Cav) channels, as well as feedforward signaling to bipolar cells.[11] Horizontal cells regulate the synaptic gain of the photoreceptor output synapse and generate center-surround antagonistic receptive fields that underlie contrast enhancement and color opponency in visual image processing.[11]

The networks formed by outer retinal neurons mediate early visual image processing that includes optimizing light sensitivity, chromatic discrimination, and spatiotemporal resolution of the visual image. These early visual signal components are conveyed by multiple bipolar cell channels to the inner retina,[7,9,12,13] which further process the features of the visual scene before it is conveyed to the central nervous system.

PHOTORECEPTORS

Photoreceptors are coupled in networks

Electrical coupling and gap junctions between photoreceptors are well established in all vertebrate retinas.[14-22] Coupling results in a mixing of photoreceptor signals, which average and reduce the variability of photoreceptor responses, increasing signal-to-noise ratios and the discrimination of objects.[20,23,24]

In mammalian retina, photoreceptor coupling is predominantly rod-to-cone and cone-to-cone coupling.[15,16,20,24,25] Electron microscopic studies showed cone and rod terminal gap junctions in multiple mammalian retinas.[18,19,21,26] In monkey retina, there is coupling between cones with the same and different spectral sensitivities,[24] and in ground squirrel retina, coupling occurs between cones of the same spectral type.[27] Whereas extensive rod-to-rod coupling is present in nonmammalian retinas,[17,28-30] it is not as well established in mammalian retinas,[16,21,26] with few reports of rod-to-rod coupling conductances and small size gap junctions between rods in mouse, guinea pig, and monkey retinas.[15,21,31,32]

Electrical coupling is mediated by gap junctional proteins called connexins (Cx), which span the extracellular space to form a channel between two adjacent plasma membranes.[33] In mammals, including humans, photoreceptor gap junctions are formed by connexin 36 (Cx36),[16,34-38] which is mainly localized to cone pedicle telodendria[16,38] (Fig. 22.1). Cx36 is present in mouse rods based on single-cell RNA sequencing and in situ hybridization analyses that show Cx36 mRNA, as well as Cx36 immunoreactivity at rod-to-cone junctions at the ultrastructural level.[16] Failure to detect electrical coupling when Cx36 is genetically deleted from mouse rods or cones, or from both, is also evidence that Cx36 mediates electrical coupling between photoreceptors[16,39] (Fig. 22.1). Furthermore, deletion of cone Cx36 disrupts rod-to-rod electrical coupling, indicating that rods couple to cones and not rods.[16] These findings indicate that rod-to-rod coupling is indirect in the mouse retina[16] and support a rod-cone network model based on tracer spread from cones to rods of one cone coupled to approximately 30 rods,[16] matching closely an electron microscopic study that reports approximately 30 rods converge onto a single cone.[21]

Rod gap junction coupling is regulated by ambient light levels with the highest conductance at night and the lowest during the day,[40] consistent with light and circadian clock regulation of photoreceptor coupling.[31,41-43] Additionally, electrical coupling conductance is eliminated by saturating light exposure during either subjective day or night.[40] Light regulation of gap junction coupling is mediated by dopamine, which inhibits the gap junction conductance through dopamine D_2-type receptors expressed by photoreceptors.[44,45] Therefore in low light (scotopic/mesopic), when levels of dopamine are at their minimum,[46] coupling between rods and cones is more prevalent, and in higher light conditions (photopic), with higher levels of dopamine, gap junction coupling is reduced, isolating rod and cone responses.[31]

Photoreceptor electrical coupling is dynamic and improves the signal-to-noise ratio over the photoreceptor operating range.[23,47] Under low illumination the spatial spread of rod signals and averaging of those signals within the rod network increases the signal-to-noise ratio

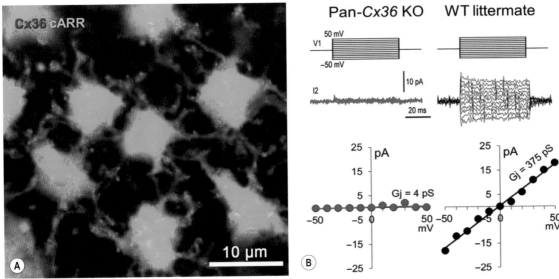

Fig. 22.1 (**A**) Connexin36 (Cx36, *red*) immunoreactive puncta on mouse cone pedicles identified by cone arrestin (cARR, *green*) immunostaining in a whole-mount mouse retina. Cx36 immunoreactive puncta are mainly localized to cone telodendria (*green processes*). Scale bar *lower right*, 10 μm. (**B**) Simultaneous voltage clamp recordings of rod-cone pairs obtained in pan-Cx36 knockout (*KO*) retinas *(red traces)* and wild-type (*WT*) control littermates *(black traces)*. Transjunctional current traces in the partner photoreceptor (in response to 50 ms voltage steps, 10 mV increments from −50 to +50 mV in driver photoreceptor) showed almost no conductance in the KO as opposed to a 375 pS conductance in the WT littermate. (Modified from Jin N, Zhang Z, Keung J, et al. Molecular and functional architecture of the mouse photoreceptor network. *Sci Adv* 2020;6(28):eaba7232. https://doi.org/10.1126/sciadv.aba7232)

and reduces rod response variability,[15,31,32] which increases detectability of very dim images.[48] Increased signal-to-noise ratio with cone-to-cone coupling is reported to improve discrimination of objects[23] and increase the range of cone sensitivity by mixing light signals from different cone types.[24,32] Rod-to-cone coupling also broadens the operating range and sensitivity of cones in mesopic light levels by transmitting the rod signal into the cones.[15,16,20]

Rod-to-cone electrical coupling is the first step of a secondary rod signaling pathway to the inner retina that operates in mesopic levels.[49,50] The rod signal is carried from rods to cones via gap junction coupling,[16,21] and the photoreceptor signal is subsequently conveyed to the inner retina by cone bipolar cells. Rod signaling pathways to the inner retina are discussed in more detail in a later section of this chapter.

Photoreceptors send synaptic output to bipolar and horizontal cells

In all vertebrate retinas, the excitatory amino acid neurotransmitter, glutamate, is the photoreceptor neurotransmitter. Glutamate is released continuously at photoreceptor ribbon synapses in darkness and release is reduced in a graded fashion with increasing light levels.[51] Glutamate release is mediated by the graded depolarization of photoreceptors and the activation of dihydropyridine-sensitive voltage-gated Cav1.4 channels at synaptic vesicle release sites near the synaptic ribbon.[52–54] Mutations in Cav1.4 channels in humans are responsible for congenital stationary night blindness type 2 (CSNB2).[53,55]

Photoreceptors form synaptic connections with rod and cone bipolar cells, and horizontal cells in the outer plexiform layer (OPL) at the first synapse in the visual system. Rod bipolar cells and ON-cone bipolar cells are characterized by an invaginating dendrite that ends within the photoreceptor terminal near the synaptic ribbon (Fig. 22.2). Within the photoreceptor terminal, the invaginating bipolar cell dendrite and horizontal cell processes near the synaptic ribbon is commonly referred to as a synaptic triad.[10] The OFF-cone bipolar cell dendritic

tips are aligned along the base of the cone pedicle, and in general a cone pedicle is innervated by the dendrites of multiple cone bipolar subtypes.[10,56] The complexity of the bipolar and horizontal cell contacts and the localization of the glutamate and γ-aminobutyric acid (GABA) transmitter receptors within the synaptic complex is illustrated for the monkey cone pedicle.[57] Within the pedicle region, metabotropic glutamate receptors (mGluRs) are expressed by the invaginating ON-bipolar cell dendrite, and ionotropic glutamate receptors are expressed by the horizontal cell dendrites. Beneath the primate cone pedicle (Fig. 22.2) is a layer of ionotropic glutamate receptor–expressing OFF-bipolar cell processes and two layers of ionotropic glutamate receptor–expressing horizontal cell processes, sandwiching bipolar cell dendrites bearing ionotropic GABAA receptors.[57]

Photoreceptor signaling to rod bipolar and ON-cone bipolar cells

Light reduces photoreceptor glutamate release onto rod bipolar and ON-cone bipolar cells, and these cells depolarize owing to a sign-inverting metabotropic glutamate receptor (mGluR)[58–60] (Fig. 22.3). The reduction in mGluR6 activation with light results in the opening of transient receptor potential, M1 isoform (TRPM1) ion channels to produce depolarization via the flux of nonselective cations.[61–63] The rapid activation and high amplification of this signaling arises from a complex of mGluR6, G-proteins, GTPase-activating proteins, GPR179, and scaffolding proteins.[287] Mutations in genes encoding nyctalopin (NYX), TRPM1, mGluR6 (GRM6), and other proteins in this signaling complex results in the "no b-wave" (nob) phenotype and underlies congenital stationary night blindness type 1 (CSNB1).[55,64–66]

Photoreceptor signaling to OFF-cone bipolar cells

Light reduces photoreceptor glutamate release onto OFF-cone bipolar cells, and these cells hyperpolarize by the closure of the ionotropic glutamate receptors of kainate (KA) and α-amino-3-hydroxy-5-methyl-4-isoxazolepropionic acid (AMPA) subtypes. KA-evoked currents

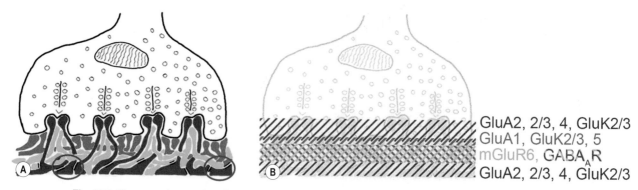

GluA2, 2/3, 4, GluK2/3
GluA1, GluK2/3, 5
mGluR6, GABA$_A$R
GluA2, 2/3, 4, GluK2/3

Fig. 22.2 The synaptic complex of mammalian cone pedicles. (**A**) Schematic view of the primate cone pedicle with the dendrites of horizontal cells (*red*), ON-cone bipolar cells (*green*), and OFF-cone bipolar cells (*blue*) cells. Desmosome-like junctions are indicated by the *black double lines* (*blue circles*) where AMPA receptor subunits (GluA) and kainate receptor subunits (GluKs) are localized.[57,78,283] (**B**) Drawing of the cone pedicle and the laminated expression of mGluR6, ionotropic GluA/GluKs and GABAA receptors. *GluA*, AMPA receptor subunit; *GluK*, kainate receptor subunit; *GABAAR*, GABAA receptor. (Modified from Haverkamp S, Grünert U, Wässle H. The cone pedicle, a complex synapse in the retina. *Neuron* 2000;27:85–95. https://doi.org/10.1016/s0896-6273(00)00011-8.)

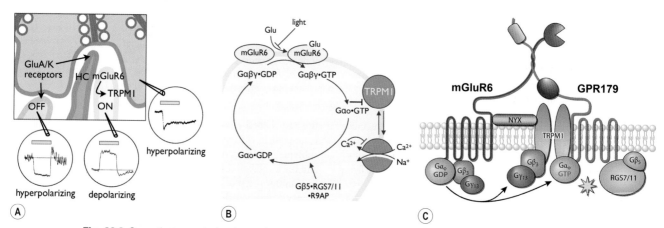

Fig. 22.3 Synaptic transmission from photoreceptors to ON- and OFF-bipolar cells and horizontal cells. (**A**) Rod and cone photoreceptors transduce light signals into a regulated release of glutamate at ribbon synapses. All photoreceptors respond to light by hyperpolarization, as do horizontal cells (HC) and OFF-bipolar cells (*pink*), which express AMPA and KA glutamate receptors (*GluA* and *GluK*). In contrast, ON-bipolar cells (*blue*) depolarize in response to light, a mechanism involving mGluR6 and TRPM1 channels. (**B**) The G-protein signaling cascade activated by mGluR6 responds to light-induced reduction of glutamate release from photoreceptors with a reduction in mGluR6 activation, resulting in TRPM1 channels opening and cell depolarization. (**C**) Components of the ON-bipolar cell signaling cascade complex. Mutations in cascade components result in a "no b-wave" electroretinogram (ERG) phenotype. (A, B modified from Morgans CW, Brown RL, Duvoisin RM. TRPM1: the endpoint of the mGluR6 signal transduction cascade in retinal ON-bipolar cells. *Bioessays* 2010;32:609–614, https://doi.org/10.1002/bies.200900198; and B from Martemyanov KA, Sampath AP. The transduction cascade in retinal ON-Bipolar cells: Signal processing and disease. *Annu Rev Vis Sci* 2017;3:25–51.)

have slower kinetics and recover more slowly from desensitization, whereas AMPA-activated currents have fast kinetics and desensitize and recover quickly from desensitization.[67] The response properties of OFF-cone bipolar cell subtypes are shaped by different, species-specific combinations of AMPA and KA receptors.[68–74] For example, in mouse retina, one OFF-cone bipolar cell type expresses AMPA receptors, others express KA receptors, while still others express both AMPA and KA receptors.[73] The differential expression and activation of KA receptors underlie differences in the OFF-cone bipolar cell temporal responses to light in mouse and monkey retina.[68,71,73,74] In contrast, in ground squirrel retina, there is a segregation of AMPA and KA receptors to different OFF-cone bipolar types, which accounts for differences in their temporal response properties.[69,70,72]

Photoreceptor signaling to horizontal cells

Horizontal cells are tonically depolarized in darkness by photoreceptor glutamate release and they hyperpolarize in response to light.[75,76] For horizontal cells, this sign-conserving response occurs primarily through AMPA receptors and to a lesser degree via KA receptors.[77–82] In primate retina, both H1 and H2 horizontal cell types express AMPA receptors on dendritic endings and at desmosome-like junctions with other horizontal cells,[57,78] but H2s, that preferentially synapse with S-cones, lack KA receptors at these synapses.[83] The preponderance of A-type horizontal cell dendrites express AMPA receptors and a smaller fraction have KA receptors; in contrast, B-type horizontal cell dendrites show a complementary distribution with a greater fraction of KA receptors than AMPA receptors.[83,84] Additionally, horizontal cell axons exhibit AMPA receptors on their terminals.[85] The differential expression of the AMPA and KA receptors suggests that the two horizontal cell types process signals with different temporal response properties.

INTERPLEXIFORM CELLS

Interplexiform cells modulate retinal neurons

Interplexiform cells, which form a sparsely occurring amacrine cell population in all vertebrate retinas,[86-88] synthesize and release dopamine with increasing light levels.[46,88,89] Interplexiform cell bodies are in the inner nuclear layer (INL) and they give rise to a widespread network of processes in the inner plexiform layer (IPL) and in most vertebrates, sparsely occurring processes that ramify in the OPL. Dopamine is released from dopaminergic processes extrasynaptically, and dopamine diffuses throughout the retina to act in a paracrine manner on all retinal cell classes.[45,90,91] Dopamine acts via two families of G-protein–coupled receptors, D_1 and D_2,[92] which are selectively expressed by multiple retinal cell types.[44,45,93,94] For example, dopamine regulates photoreceptor coupling[16,31,41,95] by activation of D_2 receptors, and bipolar[96] and horizontal cell coupling by activation of D_1 receptors.[97-99]

Dopamine exerts modulatory effects on a large number of ion channel types. Among these actions in mammals, dopamine acts at horizontal cell D_1 receptors to modulate Cav channels[98,100] and at ON-cone bipolar cells to modulate voltage-gated Na channels.[101,102] Acting at D_2/D_4 receptors, dopamine modulates mouse photoreceptor Cav and hyperpolarization-activated cyclic nucleotide-gated channels.[44,103-106] The influence of dopamine on outer retinal neuronal signaling pathways is indicative of the importance that dopamine and other neuroactive peptides[107] and molecules such as nitric oxide[108,109] have on the modulation of outer retina cell networks and early visual image processing.

HORIZONTAL CELLS

Horizontal cells are inhibitory interneurons

Horizontal cells are the only population of inhibitory interneurons in the outer retina. They have large receptive fields[110-112] owing to their expansive lateral processes in the OPL that collect inputs from numerous photoreceptors, and to their extensive electrical coupling with neighboring horizontal cells.[33,113] Given these properties, horizontal cells have a global role in outer retinal signal processing,[11] including generating antagonistic center-surround receptive fields[5,14] and providing synaptic gain control of photoreceptor output at the local level.[114-116]

In nonmammalian vertebrates, there are from two to as many as five horizontal cell subtypes, and they are characterized by their selective innervation of rods and different spectral cone types.[112,117-120] In most mammals there are two horizontal cell types, characterized by dendritic processes and a large axon terminal system that innervate photoreceptors, and dendritic or axonal processes that form connections with bipolar cell dendrites.[10,115,121-124] Different nomenclatures are used for mammalian horizontal cells. Most common are A-type and B-type, which correspond to H2 and H1, respectively, in primates. Mice and rats have only a B-type horizontal cell.[125]

A-type horizontal cell dendrites innervate cone pedicles and are without axons. B-type horizontal cell dendrites innervate cone pedicles, and they have an extensive axon terminal system that innervates rod spherules (Fig. 22.4).[121,123,124,126] The axon terminal system is generally considered to be electrically isolated from the B-type cell body,[127-130] although axons may carry signals between the cell body and the axon terminal, allowing blending of rod and cone signals, albeit in an unusual unidirectional manner.[130]

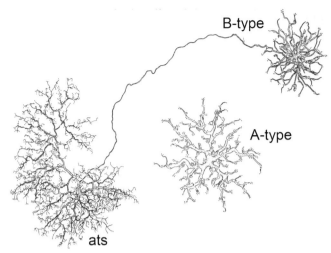

Fig. 22.4 Morphologies of the two types of horizontal cells typical of mammalian retina. The A-type shows stout dendrites with terminals that insert into cone pedicles, and this cell type does not have an axon. The B-type also shows a corona of dendrites, and their terminals that innervate cone pedicles. The B-type has a long fine axon that ends in a highly branched axon terminal system (*ats*) that innervates thousands of rod spherules. Scale bar, 100 μm. (Modified from Boycott BB, Peichl L, Wässle H. Morphological types of horizontal cell in the retina of the domestic cat. *Proc R Soc Lond B Biol Sci* 1978;203:229–245. https://doi.org/10.1098/rspb.1978.010)

Horizontal cells form coupled networks

Extensive electrical coupling between horizontal cells is well established[33,113] with coupling of homologous horizontal cell types to form separate networks.[99,131,132] In addition, the axon terminal system of B-type horizontal cells couple independently,[85] forming a third network. The electrical spread of horizontal cell signals across the horizontal cell network and the degree of coupling is dynamically modulated by dopamine, retinoic acid, and light.[97,99,132-134] There is reduced coupling in long-term, complete dark-adapted (scotopic), and full light-adapted (photopic) conditions; in contrast, low to intermediate light (mesopic) levels when rod signaling is dominant produce the greatest degree of horizontal cell coupling.[132,135,136] In monkey retina, receptive field sizes and the extent of coupling are also largest in dark-adapted conditions with reduced sizes in mesopic and photopic conditions.[99] Tracer coupling and receptive field mapping confirm the relationship between tracer spread and receptive field size as a function of background light intensity in both horizontal cell types in the rabbit retina.[33,132] This means that antagonistic surrounds formed by horizontal cells are broad under dim light conditions and narrow in bright light, properties that would differentially influence the bipolar cell receptive field properties and contrast sensitivity conveyed to the inner retina.

Mammalian horizontal cell gap junctions are formed by connexins that are distinct from photoreceptor connexins.[137,138] In rabbit retina, A-type and B-type horizontal cell dendrites are coupled by Cx50, and the B-type axon terminal system is coupled by Cx57.[139,140] In mouse retina, which only has B-type horizontal cells, both the dendrites and axonal terminals are coupled by Cx57[141]; in addition, Cx50 is found in axons, and infrequently at the same location as Cx57, indicating the likely presence of two molecularly different gap junctions.[142] The deletion of Cx57 in mouse eliminated cell coupling and reduced horizontal cell receptive field sizes, which is consistent with gap junctions contributing to the size of horizontal cell receptive fields.[137,143]

Horizontal cell synaptic output is mediated by GABA

Horizontal cells are a primary source of GABA in the vertebrate outer retina[144–149] based on GABA immunostaining, and in some vertebrates, the localization of the GABA synthetic enzymes (GAD65 and GAD67) and the vesicular GABA transporter (VGAT), which concentrates GABA into synaptic vesicles.[146,150–154] Horizontal cells express GABAA receptors,[155–159] including ρ-subunit–containing GABAA receptors at the dendritic tips and axonal terminals.[157,158] Horizontal cell feedforward targets bipolar cells, which show GABAA receptors on their dendrites within the OPL.[57,115,160–162] Differential chloride gradients are found in ON- and OFF-bipolar cell dendrites due to the action of Na-K-Cl cotransporter 1 (NKCC1) or K-Cl cotransporter 2 (KCC2) and this would underlie the polarity of their antagonistic surrounds via feedforward inhibition.[163–166] The prominent expression of extrasynaptic GABAA receptor subunits, such as α6 in horizontal cells and bipolar cell dendrites, indicate that tonically active GABA-induced currents play a role in signaling in the OPL.[157,167,168]

Horizontal cell responses initiate center-surround antagonistic receptive fields

The most comprehensively characterized synaptic pathway from horizontal cells mediates inhibitory feedback to photoreceptors. In the dark, horizontal cells have a relatively positive resting membrane potential (−40 mV to −30 mV) and respond to white light with graded hyperpolarization, concurrent with the reduction of glutamate release from photoreceptors. Consistent across all vertebrate retinas are the large receptive fields of horizontal cells, providing feedback signals that subtract from those originating from the narrow receptive fields of photoreceptors[5,14,110,169] (Fig. 22.5). The horizontal cell–modulated photoreceptor responses transmitted to bipolar cells contribute, together with inhibitory signals from amacrine cells, to the center-surround antagonistic receptive fields of both ON- and OFF-bipolar cells.[5,14,169–172] The molecular, cellular, and synaptic mechanisms mediating this interaction remain under investigation.[115,116,157,158,173–178]

Horizontal cell feedback is mediated within the photoreceptor synaptic triad between horizontal cell dendrites and the photoreceptor terminal. Surround-induced horizontal cell hyperpolarization increases Cav1.4 currents in cones[116,179] (Fig. 22.5), and this produces a higher rate of glutamate release, depolarizing the OFF-bipolar cells and hyperpolarizing the ON-bipolar cells. Several mechanisms that produce this inhibitory feedback are supported by evidence obtained in fish and amphibian retinas, including (1) horizontal cell release of GABA directly onto photoreceptors,[180–182] (2) ephaptic coupling, wherein the current entering horizontal cell glutamate receptor channels and hemichannels alters the potential in the synaptic cleft,[174,183,184] and (3) elevation of the pH in the synaptic cleft when horizontal cells hyperpolarize,[170,173,175–178,185] all cellular mechanisms that could mediate increasing Cav1.4 channel current in photoreceptors when horizontal cells hyperpolarize.[186] These different mechanisms of feedback may be dominant in different species, under different conditions, and over separate temporal ranges.

In mammalian retina, horizontal cell to photoreceptor feedback signaling favors the third mechanism. Although most models of mammalian horizontal cells do not include photoreceptor feedback responses due directly to GABA receptors, there is a report of this in mouse retina.[187] Cx hemichannels that mediate ephaptic coupling in fish[174,177,184] are not present in the mammalian synaptic cleft.[141,142] Whereas pannexin hemichannels participate in horizontal feedback in

zebrafish,[177,185] in mouse retina there is very sparse pannexin immunostaining on some horizontal cell invaginating tips,[188] where it would have to be localized to support an ephaptic mechanism.

However, there is a twist. Horizontal cells do release GABA, but they respond autaptically to their own release of GABA, and the presence of GABA is sustained, likely owing in part to the lack of GABA uptake transporters in mammalian horizontal cells.[157,168,189,190] Owing to the high permeability of bicarbonate in GABAA receptors.[157,175,191] the horizontal cell membrane potential can change the pH in the synaptic cleft via the voltage-induced driving force on bicarbonate efflux (Fig. 22.6). Hyperpolarization that accompanies a large spot or annular light stimulus causes an increase in cleft pH that increases cone Cav channel activation followed by increased glutamate release.[157] Sodium-proton exchangers (NHEs) also have a role in acidifying the synaptic cleft,[176,178] an effect typically induced by neuronal depolarization. This inhibitory feedback mechanism in the photoreceptor synaptic cleft acts rapidly to regulate glutamate release in a manner that maintains optimal synaptic gain at each local synaptic site, in addition to when more global actions, such as surround illumination, broadly alter horizontal cell membrane potential.

As noted previously, mammalian horizontal cells are GABAergic: they immunostain for GABA and show immunostaining for the vesicular and SNARE proteins required for GABA release.[168] Horizontal cells also express several GABAA receptor subunits that mediate an autaptic response to GABA.[157,190] In mouse and rat retina, horizontal cells strongly express ρ-subunit–containing GABAA receptors at the tips of their processes in the photoreceptor synaptic clefts,[157,158,168] such that when the GABA release is eliminated by genetically mediated VGAT deletion in mouse horizontal cells, and the autaptic reception of their own GABA release is halted, feedback inhibition of cones is eliminated[157,192] (Fig. 22.7).

Horizontal cells also feed inhibition forward to bipolar cells

Horizontal cell feedforward was implied by the presence of horizontal cell synaptic contacts on bipolar cell dendrites,[17,122,193–195] suggesting another pathway by which horizontal cells provide antagonistic surround inhibition to bipolar cells. Horizontal synaptic contacts are common in mudpuppy retina[17,193] and have been described in rabbit and human retina.[122,194,195] In cat and mouse OPL, horizontal cell processes and bipolar cell dendrites form junctions and, although lacking synaptic vesicles, are a possible site of synaptic transmission.[18,115] In mammals, GABAA receptors are localized to bipolar cell dendrites.[57,82,115,160,161,196] In mouse retina, horizontal cell dendritic varicosities are located about 1 μm under the base of the cone pedicles in apposition with bipolar cell dendrites expressing GABAA receptor subunits and other horizontal cell processes, suggesting possible postsynaptic sites that mediate GABA's action[115] (Fig. 22.8). In contrast to the local signal at the horizontal cell dendritic tips, which provides the synaptic gain signal that optimizes individual photoreceptor release of glutamate onto bipolar cells, the GABAergic signals from horizontal cells at these dendritic varicosities are hypothesized to carry global signals from the horizontal cell and contribute to the antagonistic surrounds in bipolar cells.

Feedforward signaling contributes to bipolar cell surround inhibition in salamander based on electrophysiological recordings[169,197–201] and chloride imaging of mouse ON-bipolar cell dendrites.[163] Electrophysiological evidence supporting horizontal cell feedforward signaling has not been observed frequently in mammals.[167] One difficulty involves the extensive GABAA receptor inputs to bipolar cells at their axon terminals from amacrine cells,[202–205] and this strong inhibitory input tends to make detection of smaller, more slowly changing

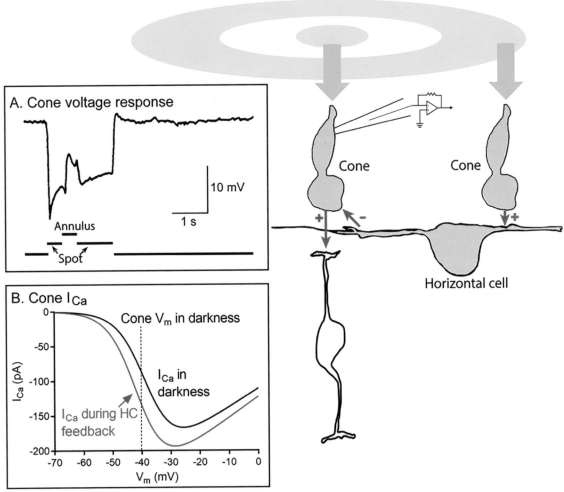

Fig. 22.5 A mechanism of horizontal cell feedback in producing bipolar cell center-surround antagonistic receptive fields. (**A**) The voltage response of a turtle cone to a small spot of light (100 μm diameter) and an added annulus (400/2200 μm inner/outer diameter). The spot produces hyperpolarization of the cone membrane potential, which begins to decay due to the opening of hyperpolarization-activated cyclic nucleotide–gated channels. The large annulus recruits the receptive field surround of the cone, generated by the large receptive field of horizontal cells, which feeds back to the central cone and antagonizes the center response, producing a pronounced relative depolarization during the annulus. (**B**) The depolarization is caused by the greater hyperpolarization of the horizontal cell due to its large receptive field being illuminated, and this voltage change disinhibits the cone Cav1.4 channels in the cones. Here the larger calcium current depolarizes the cone and may be assisted by Ca-activated Cl channel currents in the cone.[285,286] The drawing shows the sign-preserving (+) synaptic connection of a cone to the OFF-cone bipolar cell in the center of this bipolar cell's receptive field. The cone at the *far right*, within the annulus of the receptive field, feeds sign-preserving input to a horizontal cell, which summates inputs from hundreds of cones in all regions of the receptive field. At a sign-inverting feedback synaptic synapse, the horizontal cell signals inhibitory (–) output to the cone in the center of the receptive field. *HC*, horizontal cell. (From Thoreson WB, Dacey DM. Diverse cell types, circuits, and mechanisms for color vision in the vertebrate retina. *Physiol Rev* 2019:99;1527–1573 based on an earlier report, Burkhardt DA, Gottesman J, Thoreson WB. Prolonged depolarization in turtle cones evoked by current injection and stimulation of the receptive field surround. *J Physiol* 1988;407:329–348.)

horizontal cell GABAergic inputs at the dendrites of bipolar cells complicated to isolate for study.

Horizontal cells play key roles in chromatic visual processing

The first stage of color processing in vertebrate retinas, following the transduction of light stimuli by cones having chromatically distinct sensitivities, first reported in goldfish, is mediated by horizontal cell feedback to cones that generates color-opponent pathways.[120,206] Mammalian and nonmammalian vertebrates show many similarities in this processing, but there are important differences. In nonmammalian retinas, there is a rich variety of photoreceptor types, including retinas with double cones and cones with oil droplets[207–211] that mediate chromatic sensitivity. In turtles and fish, the chromatic spectrum is sampled by cones with peak chromatic absorption wavelengths ranging from around 350 nm (UV range) to nearly 700 nm (far red range), twice the range found in mammals. Their color tuning occurs through a cascaded system of color-opponent pathways using horizontal cell antagonistic feedback signaling to cones of different chromatic sensitivity.[120,206] Red cones signal to one class of horizontal cells,[120,212]

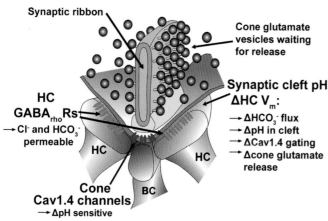

Fig. 22.6 The photoreceptor synaptic invagination and features of the GABA-pH hybrid model of inhibitory feedback. Schematic of a photoreceptor synaptic terminal with the synaptic ribbon, bipolar cell (*BC*) dendrite, and horizontal cell (*HC*) tips in the synaptic invagination. The Cav1.4 channels *(blue oval pairs)* are shown localized on the photoreceptor presynaptic membrane and the ρ-subunit–containing GABA receptors *(orange ovals)* are shown lining the HC tips. Since the ρ-subunit–containing GABAA receptors are bicarbonate (HCO_3^-) permeable, any change in the HC membrane potential alters the driving force on the efflux of this common pH modulator and changes the pH of the synaptic cleft. This in turn shifts the activation of photoreceptor Cav1.4 channels via surface charge screening and results in altered glutamate release. In the dark, when photoreceptors are depolarized, the high rate of glutamate release maintains HC depolarization, and there is a low driving force on bicarbonate efflux resulting in relative cleft acidification due to the ongoing high levels of acidity from the depolarized neurons in the vicinity. Light hyperpolarizes the photoreceptor, decreasing glutamate release and hyperpolarizing the HC, which leads to an increased driving force on and greater efflux of bicarbonate. Bicarbonate tends to alkalinize the synaptic cleft, which increases photoreceptor Cav1.4 activation, thus serving as a negative feedback system that opposes changes in glutamate release.[157] (Original illustration by Margery Fain from Fain GL. Sensory transduction. Second edn, 2020; Oxford, UK: Oxford University Press.)

accounting for a monochromatic luminosity (L) signal in L-type cone horizontal cells,[76,127–129,213] and this is fed back to green cones, which in turn synapse with horizontal cells that show red-green color opponency, generating the first type of spectrally sensitive, or chromaticity signal, in C-type cone horizontal cells.[117,213] This signal is fed back to blue cones, the output of which goes to a further horizontal cell type that shows blue-green antagonism. In zebrafish another cone type with UV sensitivity also contributes to sequential analysis, with additional feedback pathways being implemented to generate chromatic antagonism.[208,214]

Mammals have a single rod with sensitivity in the medium-wavelength (M, green) range of the chromatic spectrum, and two or three cone types with different chromatic sensitivities in the long-wavelength region (L, red), medium-wavelength region (M, green) range, and short-wavelength regions (S, blue or UV).[215] Circuitry for chromatic antagonism in dichromat mammalian retinas uses green M-cones and UV or blue S-cones that signal in varying ratios to a single horizontal cell type, which feed back to both cone types.[216] This results in a spectrum of variably tuned M- and S-cone signals, dependent on the density of cone horizontal cell inputs, providing varying degrees of chromatic tuning.[215] In ventral M-cone–poor regions of mouse retina, rod input, which has a peak sensitivity near that of M-cones, appears to be used to generate color opponency.[217,218]

In some mammals, including trichromat primates, L-cones and M-cones signal to the same horizontal cell type, which similarly feeds back to both cone types, leading to bipolar cells with variably tuned L- and M-cone opponent signals forwarded to bipolar cells.[219] In this scheme, the relative weighting of L- and M-cone inputs to the receptive field center and the mixed (L + M or yellow) antagonistic surround of the bipolar cell recipients is determined variably by how many L- and M-cones make input to the particular horizontal cell that is the source of negative feedback (Fig. 22.9).

In trichromat primates, L- and M-cones, and some S-cones, synapse with H1 horizontal cell dendrites, but S-cones preferentially contact H2 horizontal cells, which also receive minor input from L- and M-cones.[126,220–222] The S-cone signal, following mixed chromatic feedback from horizontal cells, is then passed on directly via dedicated cone bipolar cells to the ON sublamina of the IPL, contacting the dendrites of small bistratified ganglion cells.[223,224] In monkey retina, another bipolar cell type carrying mixed L- and M-cone (or yellow) signals, terminates on the dendrites of the same bistratified ganglion cell in the OFF sublamina[225] (Fig. 22.10). Together the blue ON-bipolar cell and the yellow OFF-bipolar cell contacting the dendrites of their ganglion cell target form an effective antagonistic interaction producing antagonistic blue-yellow chromatic sensitivity interaction without a major role for horizontal cells, as the surrounds cancel out.[223,225,226] There are additional color-opponent pathways in nonprimate and primate retinas.[215]

Horizontal cells influence ganglion cell responses

Contributions of horizontal cells to ganglion cell antagonistic surrounds have been established with simultaneous recordings of horizontal cells and ganglion cells in fish[227,228] and rabbit.[229,230] More recently, the impact of horizontal cell activity on ganglion cell response properties and receptive field structure has been demonstrated by experimentally silencing horizontal cell responsivity in mouse retina. Selective ablation of horizontal cells with targeted diphtheria toxin,[231] as well as genetic deletion of AMPA receptors in horizontal cells that eliminate their responses to light,[232] leads to pronounced changes to some ganglion cell receptive field structures, reducing surround inhibition and altering spatial frequency tuning. A silencing approach using expression of pharmacologically selective actuator module-glycine receptors (PSAM-GlyR),[233] which shunts the horizontal cell membrane potential with chloride conductance, produces a reduction of transient ganglion cell excitatory inputs and enhanced ON- but suppressed OFF-ganglion cell responses,[234] Compared with a simple concept of center-surround antagonism, these experimental models reveal detailed and specific components of the role horizontal cells play in forming responses of different types of ganglion cells. Remaining features of surround antagonism in ganglion cells are mediated by other lateral inhibitory systems, such as those operating in the inner retina through amacrine cell inhibition.[235]

BIPOLAR CELLS

Bipolar cells carry separate information streams from the outer to the inner retina

Bipolar cells carry the light signals in parallel visual pathways to the inner retina[7,9,13] and convey numerous visual image features, including ON- and OFF-center responsiveness, transient and sustained light responses, spatial and temporal resolution, chromatic discrimination, and local motion origin.[9,203,236,237] The functional diversity of bipolar cell responses arises from both excitatory and inhibitory inputs from

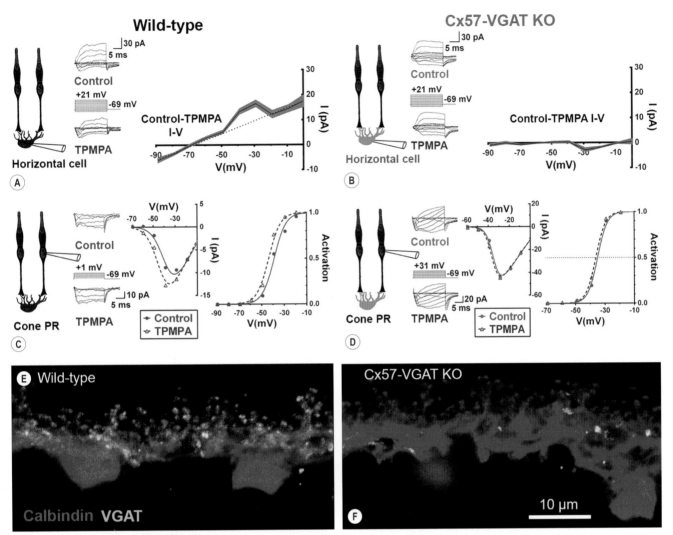

Fig. 22.7 Membrane biophysics of horizontal cell ρ-subunit–containing GABAA receptor conductance and the requirement of GABA release for feedback signaling. By taking advantage of horizontal cells being the only retinal neuron to express Cx57, an iCre mouse line with Cre recombinase expression controlled by Cx57 regulatory elements, was used to selectively eliminate VGAT, the vesicular GABA transporter that loads synaptic vesicles with GABA.[192] **(A)** Recordings of voltage-clamped wild-type (*WT*) mouse horizontal cell GABA-activated currents, in control and with (1,2,5,6-tetrahydropyridine-4-yl) methylphosphinic acid (TPMPA), an antagonist that blocks ρ-subunit–containing GABAA receptors. The current-voltage (I-V) relations of TPMPA-subtracted currents are mostly linear. **(B)** Same as in **(A)**, carried out in Cx57-VGAT knockout (*KO*) mouse horizontal cells, whose synaptic vesicles do not load GABA.[192] TPMPA had no effect on the currents owing to a lack of tonic GABA levels in the VGAT KO and showing that TPMPA-blocked currents in the WT are from horizontal cell autaptic reception of GABA. **(C)** Cone photoreceptor (*PR*) Cav channel currents in WT show altered current amplitudes in control and in presence of TPMPA. Activation curves showed that the Cav channel activation was shifted negative by about 5 mV in the presence of TPMPA. **(D)** Same protocol as in **(C)** but in a cone in the Cx57-VGAT KO showing that the Cav channel I-V relations and activation midpoints were unaffected by TPMPA in cones when horizontal cells were unable to release GABA. **(E,F)** The presence and absence of VGAT immunostaining *(cyan)* at horizontal cell processes *(red)* is shown in WT and the VGAT KO retinas, respectively. Residual VGAT staining remains visible in interplexiform cell fibers. Scale bar, 10 μm. (Modified from Grove JCR, Hirano AA, de Los Santos J, et al. Novel hybrid action of GABA mediates inhibitory feedback in the mammalian retina. *PLoS Biol* 2019;17:e3000200. https://doi.org/10.1371/journal.pbio.3000200 (2019).)

photoreceptors and horizontal cells in the outer retina, and the inhibitory inputs from amacrine cells in the inner retina.[203]

Rod and cone bipolar cell subtypes have distinct morphologic features (Fig. 22.11) and light response properties. In the best characterized mammalian retinas, including the mouse and monkey, there is one morphologic rod bipolar cell type and 8 to 13 cone bipolar cell types.[8,56,238–242] A general functional feature found across all vertebrates is the segregation of the ON- and OFF-bipolar cell light responses in the OPL. As described earlier, ON-bipolar cell dendrites invaginate rod and cone terminals and OFF-bipolar cell dendrites predominantly make basal or flat contacts at the base of cone pedicles.[10,123] There is mixing of the rod and cone input to bipolar cells in the vertebrate retina.[56,209,243–245] In nonmammalian retinas, there is little segregation of bipolar cell contacts with rods and cones, with mixed rod and cone

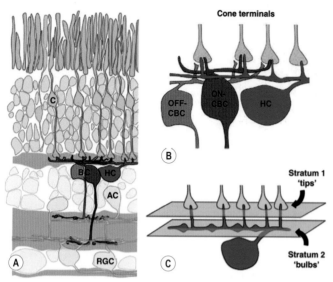

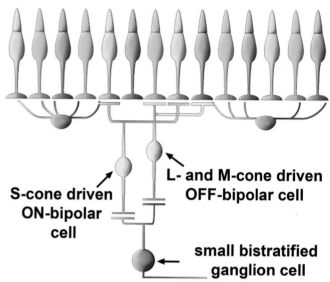

Fig. 22.8 Feedback to cones and feedforward to bipolar cells are mediated by two synaptic strata for horizontal cell output. (**A**) Organization of mouse retina showing cone photoreceptors (C), horizontal cells (*HC*), bipolar cells (*BC*), amacrine cells (*AC*) and retinal ganglion cells (*RGC*). (**B**) Classic representation of processes of horizontal cells, and ON- and OFF-cone bipolar (*ON-CBC; OFF-CBC*) cells making their synaptic contacts with cone terminals. (**C**) Relative positioning of the two strata of horizontal cell output. Stratum 1 is the classic localization of the tips of horizontal cell processes that receive cone input and return feedback output within the cone synaptic cleft or invagination. Dendrites of ON-CBCs also invaginate the cone here, receiving feedback-modulated input from cones. Stratum 2 is the location of the *en passant* swellings of horizontal cell dendrites that are in apposition to bipolar cell dendrites expressing GABAA receptor subunits. (From Behrens C, Yadav SC, Korympidou MM, et al. Retinal horizontal cells use different synaptic sites for global feedforward and local feedback signaling. *Curr Biol* 2022;32:545–558.e5. https://doi.org/10.1016/j.cub.2021.11.055)

Fig. 22.10 Primate blue-yellow opponency is provided by separate and dedicated bipolar cell pathways terminating on the small bistratified ganglion cell type dendrites in the ON and OFF sublamina of the inner plexiform layer, respectively. Blue S-cone–driven ON-bipolar cells synapse in the ON sublamina, driving the ON-ganglion cell receptive field center response, while the yellow (L + M) OFF-bipolar cells synapse in the OFF sublamina, driving the receptive field OFF response. (Modified from Thoreson WB, Dacey DM. Diverse cell types, circuits, and mechanisms for color vision in the vertebrate retina. *Physiol Rev* 2019;99:1527–1573.)

bipolar cell types,[17,244,246–248] and in mouse and rabbit retina the majority of rod bipolar cells receive some cone photoreceptor input,[56,242,245,249] and conversely, some OFF-cone bipolar cell types receive rod photoreceptor input (Fig. 22.11).[21,56,245]

In both nonmammalian and mammalian retinas, the majority of cone bipolar cells have diffuse dendritic fields and contact numerous M- and L-cones in their dendritic field.[6,56,238,250] The primate midget ON- and OFF-bipolar cells are special cases, as they contact single cones in the central retina and two to three cones in peripheral retina.[238,239] The midget bipolar cell pathway is specialized for red and green color opponency and high spatial resolution.[251–253] Another example of cone bipolar cell specialization are the ON- and OFF-S-cone–selective bipolar cells characterized by dendrites that selectively contact S-cones,[254–256] and these bipolar cells participate in chromatic coding.[257]

Bipolar cells differ most notably in the stratification of their axonal terminals to narrow laminae of the IPL.[56,238–241] These laminae are functionally distinct and integrate the excitatory bipolar cell output with inhibitory amacrine cell inputs.[203,258,259] OFF-cone bipolar cells terminate in the distal half of the IPL, and rod and ON-cone bipolar cells terminate in the proximal half of the IPL[6,204,260] (Fig. 22.11). A further refinement is a narrow band of ON-bipolar cell en passant synapses adjacent to the INL, nominally in the OFF sublamina of the IPL, which contact intrinsically photosensitive retinal ganglion cells (ipRGCs) and dopaminergic amacrine cells.[261,262] Like photoreceptors, bipolar cells release glutamate from ribbon synapses to provide an excitatory glutamatergic synaptic input/drive to amacrine and ganglion cells in the inner retina. Additionally, bipolar cells form gap junctions between homologous bipolar cell types in the IPL.[201,263–265]

Bipolar cell responses are shaped by both the photoreceptor light response and horizontal cell feedback and feedforward to photoreceptor and bipolar cell dendrites. The kinetics of the photoreceptor signal

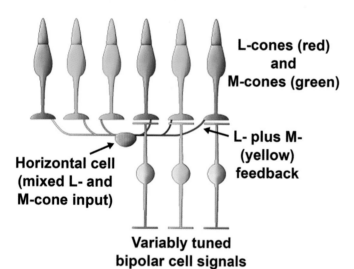

Fig. 22.9 General mammalian scheme for color-opponent signaling. In this example, which exemplifies red-green opponency but can also be a model for green-blue antagonism, cone bipolar cells receive input from L-cones *(red)* and M-cones *(green)* that have received horizontal cell feedback signals composed of mixed L- and M-cone inputs. (Modified from Thoreson WB, Dacey DM. Diverse cell types, circuits, and mechanisms for color vision in the vertebrate retina. *Physiol Rev* 2019;99:1527–1573.)

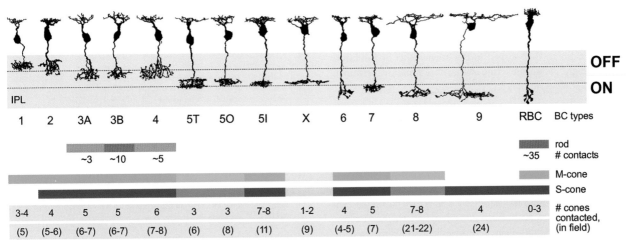

		~3		**~10**		**~5**								**~35**	# contacts
3-4	4	5	5	6	3	3	7-8	1-2	4	5	7-8		4	0-3	# cones contacted, (in field)
(5)	(5-6)	(6-7)	(6-7)	(7-8)	(6)	(8)	(11)	(9)	(4-5)	(7)	(21-22)		(24)		

Fig. 22.11 Bipolar cells in the mouse retina. Bipolar cell types in the mouse retina vary in the morphology and chromatic sensitivity of the photoreceptors they contact. The axon terminals stratify in different layers of the inner plexiform layer (*IPL*). The distal IPL corresponds to the OFF-sublamina and the proximal IPL to the ON sublamina. The dotted lines in the IPL correspond to the position of OFF and ON cholinergic amacrine cell processes.[289,290] The number and cone type–specific input, as well as rod input, is denoted below. *BC*, Bipolar cell; *RBC*, rod bipolar cell. (Modified from Behrens C, Schubert T, Haverkamp S, Euler T, Berens P. Connectivity map of bipolar cells and photoreceptors in the mouse retina. *Elife*. 2016:5:e20041. https://doi.org/10.7554/eLife.20041 (2016).)

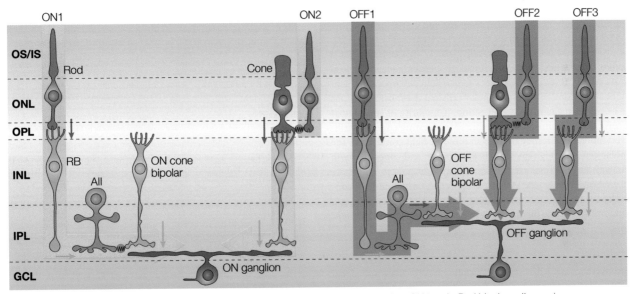

Fig. 22.12 Multiple rod pathways through the mammalian (mouse) retina. ON1 path: Rod bipolar cells receive input, mostly from rods (*red arrow* denoting sign-inverting chemical synapse) but also from cones, and make excitatory glutamatergic synapses (*green arrow*, sign-conserving synapse) onto AII amacrine cells, which in turn make gap junctions onto ON-cone bipolar cells (*orange squiggle form*). The ON-cone bipolar cells then synapse onto ON-ganglion cells. ON2 path: Rods also make gap junctions onto cones (*orange squiggle form*), and the cones then carry rod signals to ON-cone bipolar cells. OFF1 path: Rod bipolar cells make excitatory synapses onto AII amacrine cells, which make inhibitory glycinergic synapses (*red arrow*) onto OFF-cone bipolar cells. These in turn synapse onto OFF-ganglion cells. OFF2 path: Rods make gap-junctional contacts onto cones, which carry rod signals through OFF-cone bipolar cells to OFF ganglion cells. OFF3 path: Finally, some OFF-bipolar cells receive input from both rods and cones. The IPL has an upper layer (OFF sublamina) containing terminations of OFF-bipolar cells and dendrites of OFF-ganglion cells, and a lower layer (ON sublamina) containing ON-bipolar cell terminals and ON-ganglion cell dendrites. *GCL*, Ganglion cell layer; *INL*, inner nuclear layer; *IPL*, inner plexiform layer; *IS*, inner segments of photoreceptors; *ONL*, outer nuclear layer; *OPL*, outer plexiform layer; *OS*, outer segments of photoreceptors. (From Wässle H. Parallel processing in the mammalian retina. *Nat Rev Neurosci* 2004;5:747–757.)

is influenced by the distance of the photoreceptor synaptic release sites to the glutamate receptors on ON-bipolar cell dendrites and to the OFF-bipolar cell dendrites. The OFF-bipolar cell dendrites receive a slower and more diffuse glutamatergic signal than the ON-bipolar cell dendrites.[9,266] The kinetics of bipolar cell response are also determined by the complement of glutamate receptors expressed by bipolar cells: ON-bipolar cells hyperpolarize through the activation of mGluR6,[58–60] whereas OFF-bipolar cells depolarize through the faster, KA ionotropic glutamate receptors.[68,71–74] Bipolar cell dendrites are influenced also by GABA, acting at tonic GABAA receptors[167,168] with GABA being hyperpolarizing or depolarizing, depending on dendritic Cl levels.[163,267] The bipolar cell signal is further shaped in the inner retina by inhibitory GABAergic and glycinergic amacrine cells, whose processes terminate on bipolar cell axonal terminals.[202–204,235]

Cone bipolar cells and cone signal pathways

Cone bipolar cells have sustained or temporal light responses that shape retinal ganglion cell responses.[7,13,202,203,236,268] Their light response properties are segregated across the IPL, with bipolar cell types that stratify near the edges of the IPL show sustained light responses[248,259,269] and cone bipolar cells that stratify near the ON/OFF border in the center of the IPL responding more transiently.[9,216] The transient bipolar cells with the fastest responses also spike,[258] consistent with their expression of Nav channels.[270–272] Additionally, receptive field size varies systematically across the IPL, with OFF-bipolar cells having larger receptive fields than ON-bipolar cells.[203]

Rods have a dedicated rod bipolar cell pathway and secondary rod pathways that piggyback on cone bipolar cell pathways

A primary rod-to-rod bipolar cell pathway is consistently reported in the mammalian retina. There are, in addition, bipolar cells with both rod and cone input[56,209,243–245] that convey the rod signal to the inner retina.

The primary rod-to-rod bipolar cell pathway in mammals has a remarkable consistency in its functional properties and anatomical organization.[273–275] Rods are highly sensitive to light and operate in scotopic light conditions.[15,276,277] Rod bipolar cells are the most numerous bipolar cell type in the mammalian retina. A majority of rod bipolar cells receive direct, if minor, cone input,[56,245] suggesting cones contribute to rod bipolar cell responsiveness in mesopic light conditions. The rod bipolar cell is highly typical in its appearance and connectivity in the IPL, with large axonal varicosities that form excitatory glutamate ribbon synapses mainly with AII amacrine cells,[274] which in turn conveys the rod signal to ON-cone bipolar cells via sign-conserving gap junctions and OFF-cone bipolar and ganglion cells via glycinergic synaptic input[13,278] (Fig. 22.12 ON1).

A second rod pathway described in mouse, rabbit, and monkey retina[13,50,56,249] (Fig. 22.12 ON2, OFF2) arises from rod input to cones through rod-to-cone gap junction coupling.[16,18,19,21] The rod signal enters ON- and OFF-cone bipolar cells, which in turn contact amacrine and ganglion cells.[13,33,49] The secondary rod pathway is operative in mesopic light conditions. This rod signaling pathway is functionally more prominent in mouse and rabbit retina[49,50] compared with monkey retina.[275] A tertiary rod pathway consists of direct rod synaptic contacts with three types of OFF-cone bipolar cells (Fig. 22.11; types 3 A, 3B, 4) whose dendrites contact the base of rod terminals[21,56,279,280,283] (Fig. 22.12 OFF3). This rod pathway is operative in mesopic light conditions.[281] This third pathway provides for the fast transfer of rod signals to the inner retina, in comparison to the slower mGluR6-mediated ON-rod bipolar cell response.[281,282,286]

REFERENCES

1. Ramón y Cajal S. *The Structure of the Retina*. Springfield, IL: C. C. Thomas; 1972.
2. Fain GL. Lamprey vision: photoreceptors and organization of the retina. *Semin Cell Dev Biol*. 2020;106:5–11.
3. Polyak SL. *The retina; the anatomy and the histology of the retina in man, ape, and monkey, including the consideration of visual functions, the history of physiological optics, and the histological laboratory technique*. Chicago, IL: The University of Chicago press; 1941.
4. Kaneko A. Physiological and morphological identification of horizontal, bipolar and amacrine cells in goldfish retina. *J Physiol*. 1970;207:623–633.
5. Werblin FS, Dowling JE. Organization of the retina of the mudpuppy, Necturus maculosus. II. Intracellular recording. *J Neurophysiol*. 1969;32:339–355.
6. Wässle H, Puller C, Müller F, Haverkamp S. Cone contacts, mosaics, and territories of bipolar cells in the mouse retina. *J Neurosci*. 2009;29:106–117.
7. Masland RH. The neuronal organization of the retina. *Neuron*. 2012;76:266–280.
8. Shekhar K, Lapan SW, Whitney IE, et al. Comprehensive classification of retinal bipolar neurons by single-cell transcriptomics. *Cell*. 2016;166:1308–1323.
9. Euler T, Haverkamp S, Schubert T, Baden T. Retinal bipolar cells: elementary building blocks of vision. *Nat Rev Neurosci*. 2014;15:507–519.
10. Dowling JE, Boycott BB. Organization of the primate retina: electron microscopy. *Proc R Soc Lond B Biol Sci*. 1966;166:80–111.
11. Thoreson WB, Mangel SC. Lateral interactions in the outer retina. *Prog Retin Eye Res*. 2012;31:407–441.
12. Baden T, Berens P, Franke K, Román Rosón M, Bethge M, Euler T. The functional diversity of retinal ganglion cells in the mouse. *Nature*. 2016;529:345–350.
13. Wässle H. Parallel processing in the mammalian retina. *Nat Rev Neurosci*. 2004;5:747–757.
14. Baylor DA, Fuortes MG, O'Bryan PM. Receptive fields of cones in the retina of the turtle. *J Physiol*. 1971;214:265–294.
15. Hornstein EP, Verweij J, Li PH, Schnapf JL. Gap-junctional coupling and absolute sensitivity of photoreceptors in macaque retina. *J Neurosci*. 2005;25:11201–11209.
16. Jin N, Zhang Z, Keung J, et al. Molecular and functional architecture of the mouse photoreceptor network. *Sci Adv*. 2020;6(28):eaba7232.
17. Lasansky A. Organization of the outer synaptic layer in the retina of the larval tiger salamander. *Philos Trans R Soc Lond B Biol Sci*. 1973;265:471–489.
18. Kolb H. The organization of the outer plexiform layer in the retina of the cat: electron microscopic observations. *J Neurocytol*. 1977;6:131–153.
19. Raviola E, Gilula NB. Gap junctions between photoreceptor cells in the vertebrate retina. *Proc Natl Acad Sci U S A*. 1973;70:1677–1681.
20. Schneeweis DM, Schnapf JL. Photovoltage of rods and cones in the macaque retina. *Science*. 1995;268:1053–1056.
21. Tsukamoto Y, Morigiwa K, Ueda M, Sterling P. Microcircuits for night vision in mouse retina. *J Neurosci*. 2001;21:8616–8623.
22. Wu SM, Yang XL. Electrical coupling between rods and cones in the tiger salamander retina. *Proc Natl Acad Sci U S A*. 1988;85:275–278.
23. DeVries SH, Qi X, Smith R, Makous W, Sterling P. Electrical coupling between mammalian cones. *Curr Biol*. 2002;12:1900–1907.
24. Hornstein EP, Verweij J, Schnapf JL. Electrical coupling between red and green cones in primate retina. *Nat Neurosci*. 2004;7:745–750.
25. Nelson R. Cat cones have rod input: a comparison of the response properties of cones and horizontal cell bodies in the retina of the cat. *J Comp Neurol*. 1977;172:109–135.
26. Smith RG, Freed MA, Sterling P. Microcircuitry of the dark-adapted cat retina: functional architecture of the rod-cone network. *J Neurosci*. 1986;6:3505–3517.
27. Li W, DeVries SH. Separate blue and green cone networks in the mammalian retina. *Nat Neurosci*. 2004;7:751–756.
28. Attwell D, Wilson M, Wu SM. A quantitative analysis of interactions between photoreceptors in the salamander (Ambystoma) retina. *J Physiol*. 1984;352:703–737.
29. Schwartz EA. Rod-rod interaction in the retina of the turtle. *J Physiol*. 1975;246:617–638.
30. Zhang J, Wu SM. Physiological properties of rod photoreceptor electrical coupling in the tiger salamander retina. *J Physiol*. 2005;564:849–862.
31. Jin NG, Chuang AZ, Masson PJ, Ribelayga CP. Rod electrical coupling is controlled by a circadian clock and dopamine in mouse retina. *J Physiol*. 2015;593:1601–1631.
32. Li PH, Verweij J, Long JH, Schnapf JL. Gap-junctional coupling of mammalian rod photoreceptors and its effect on visual detection. *J Neurosci*. 2012;32:3552–3562.
33. Bloomfield SA, Völgyi B. The diverse functional roles and regulation of neuronal gap junctions in the retina. *Nat Rev Neurosci*. 2009;10:495–506.
34. Deans MR, Völgyi B, Goodenough DA, Bloomfield SA, Paul DL. Connexin36 is essential for transmission of rod-mediated visual signals in the mammalian retina. *Neuron*. 2002;36:703–712.
35. Feigenspan A, Janssen-Bienhold U, Hormuzdi S, et al. Expression of connexin36 in cone pedicles and OFF-cone bipolar cells of the mouse retina. *J Neurosci*. 2004;24:3325–3334.
36. Kántor O, et al. Characterization of connexin36 gap junctions in the human outer retina. *Brain Struct Funct*. 2016;221:2963–2984.
37. Lee EJ, Han JW, Kim HJ, et al. The immunocytochemical localization of connexin 36 at rod and cone gap junctions in the guinea pig retina. *Eur J Neurosci*. 2003;18:2925–2934.
38. O'Brien JJ, Chen X, Macleish PR, O'Brien J, Massey SC. Photoreceptor coupling mediated by connexin36 in the primate retina. *J Neurosci*. 2012;32:4675–4687.
39. Asteriti S, Gargini C, Cangiano L. Connexin 36 expression is required for electrical coupling between mouse rods and cones. *Vis Neurosci*. 2017;34:E006.
40. Jin NG, Ribelayga CP. Direct evidence for daily plasticity of electrical coupling between rod photoreceptors in the mammalian retina. *J Neurosci*. 2016;36:178–184.
41. Li H, Zhang Z, Blackburn MR, Wang SW, Ribelayga CP, O'Brien J. Adenosine and dopamine receptors coregulate photoreceptor coupling via gap junction phosphorylation in mouse retina. *J Neurosci*. 2013;33:3135–3150.
42. Ribelayga C, Cao Y, Mangel SC. The circadian clock in the retina controls rod-cone coupling. *Neuron*. 2008;59:790–801.
43. Ribelayga C, Mangel SC. Identification of a circadian clock-controlled neural pathway in the rabbit retina. *PLoS One*. 2010;5:e11020.
44. Cohen AI, Todd RD, Harmon S, O'Malley KL. Photoreceptors of mouse retinas possess D4 receptors coupled to adenylate cyclase. *Proc Natl Acad Sci U S A*. 1992;89:12093–12097.
45. Nguyen-Legros J, Versaux-Botteri C, Vernier P. Dopamine receptor localization in the mammalian retina. *Mol Neurobiol*. 1999;19:181–204.
46. Pérez-Fernández V, Milosavljevic N, Allen AE, et al. Rod photoreceptor activation alone defines the release of dopamine in the retina. *Curr Biol*. 2019;29:763–774.

47. Lamb TD, Simon EJ. The relation between intercellular coupling and electrical noise in turtle photoreceptors. *J Physiol.* 1976;263:257–286.
48. Field GD, Sampath AP, Rieke F. Retinal processing near absolute threshold: from behavior to mechanism. *Annu Rev Physiol.* 2005;67:491–514.
49. DeVries SH, Baylor DA. An alternative pathway for signal flow from rod photoreceptors to ganglion cells in mammalian retina. *Proc Natl Acad Sci U S A.* 1995;92:10658–10662.
50. Völgyi B, Deans MR, Paul DL, Bloomfield SA. Convergence and segregation of the multiple rod pathways in mammalian retina. *J Neurosci.* 2004;24:11182–11192.
51. Thoreson WB. Transmission at rod and cone ribbon synapses in the retina. *Pflugers Arch.* 2021;473:1469–1491.
52. Barnes S, Kelly ME. Calcium channels at the photoreceptor synapse. *Adv Exp Med Biol.* 2002;514:465–476.
53. Mansergh F, Orton NC, Vessey JP, et al. Mutation of the calcium channel gene Cacna1f disrupts calcium signaling, synaptic transmission and cellular organization in mouse retina. *Hum Mol Genet.* 2005;14:3035–3046.
54. Thoreson WB, Rabl K, Townes-Anderson E, Heidelberger R. A highly Ca2+-sensitive pool of vesicles contributes to linearity at the rod photoreceptor ribbon synapse. *Neuron.* 2004;42:595–605.
55. Zeitz C, Robson AG, Audo I. Congenital stationary night blindness: an analysis and update of genotype-phenotype correlations and pathogenic mechanisms. *Prog Retin Eye Res.* 2015;45:58–110.
56. Haverkamp S, Grünert U, Wässle H. The cone pedicle, a complex synapse in the retina. *Neuron.* 2000;27:85–95.
57. Haverkamp S, Grünert U, Wässle H. The synaptic architecture of AMPA receptors at the cone pedicle of the primate retina. *J Neurosci.* 2001;21:2488–2500.
58. Puller C, de Sevilla Müller LP, Janssen-Bienhold U, Haverkamp S. ZO-1 and the spatial organization of gap junctions and glutamate receptors in the outer plexiform layer of the mammalian retina. *J Neurosci.* 2009;29:6266–6275.
59. Behrens C, Schubert T, Haverkamp S, Euler T, Berens P. Connectivity map of bipolar cells and photoreceptors in the mouse retina. *Elife.* 2016:5:e20041.
60. Martemyanov KA, Sampath AP. The transduction cascade in retinal ON-Bipolar cells: Signal processing and disease. *Annu Rev Vis Sci.* 2017;3:25–51.
61. Nomura A, Shigenmoto R, Nakamura Y, Okamoto N, Mizuno N, Nakanishi S. Developmentally regulated postsynaptic localization of a metabotropic glutamate receptor in rat rod bipolar cells. *Cell.* 1994;77:361–369.
62. Schneider FM, Mohr F, Behrendt M, Oberwinkler J. Properties and functions of TRPM1 channels in the dendritic tips of retinal ON-bipolar cells. *Eur J Cell Biol.* 2015;94:420–427.
63. Koike C, Obara T, Uriu Y, et al. TRPM1 is a component of the retinal ON bipolar cell transduction channel in the mGluR6 cascade. *Proc Natl Acad Sci U S A.* 2010;107:332–337.
64. Morgans CW, Zhang J, Jeffrey BG, et al. TRPM1 is required for the depolarizing light response in retinal ON-bipolar cells. *Proc Natl Acad Sci U S A.* 2009;106:19174–19178.
65. Shen Y, Heimel JA, Kamermans M, Peachey N, Gregg RG, Nawy S. A transient receptor potential-like channel mediates synaptic transmission in rod bipolar cells. *J Neurosci.* 2009;29:6088–6093.
66. Chang B, Heckenlively JR, Bayley PR, et al. The nob2 mouse, a null mutation in Cacna1f: anatomical and functional abnormalities in the outer retina and their consequences on ganglion cell visual responses. *Vis Neurosci.* 2006;23:11–24.
67. McCall MA, Gregg RG. Comparisons of structural and functional abnormalities in mouse b-wave mutants. *J Physiol.* 2008;586:4385–4392.
68. Pardue MT, Peachey NS. Mouse b-wave mutants. *Doc Ophthalmol.* 2014;128:77–89.
69. Hansen KB, Wollmuth LP, Bowie D, et al. Structure, function, and pharmacology of glutamate receptor ion channels. *Pharmacol Rev.* 2021;73:298–487.
70. Borghuis BG, Looger LL, Tomita S, Demb JB. Kainate receptors mediate signaling in both transient and sustained OFF bipolar cell pathways in mouse retina. *J Neurosci.* 2014;34:6128–6139.
71. DeVries SH. Bipolar cells use kainate and AMPA receptors to filter visual information into separate channels. *Neuron.* 2000;28:847–856.
72. DeVries SH, Schwartz EA. Kainate receptors mediate synaptic transmission between cones and 'Off' bipolar cells in a mammalian retina. *Nature.* 1999;397:157–160.
73. Ichinose T, Hellmer CB. Differential signalling and glutamate receptor compositions in the OFF bipolar cell types in the mouse retina. *J Physiol.* 2016;594:883–894.
74. Lindstrom SH, Ryan DG, Shi J, DeVries SH. Kainate receptor subunit diversity underlying response diversity in retinal off bipolar cells. *J Physiol.* 2014;592:1457–1477.
75. Puller C, Ivanova E, Euler T, Haverkamp S, Schubert T. OFF bipolar cells express distinct types of dendritic glutamate receptors in the mouse retina. *Neuroscience.* 2013;243:136–148.
76. Puthussery T, Percival KA, Venkataramani S, Gayet-Primo J, Grünert U, Taylor WR. Kainate receptors mediate synaptic input to transient and sustained OFF visual pathways in primate retina. *J Neurosci.* 2014;34:7611–7621.
77. Niemeyer G, Gouras P. Rod and cone signals in S-potentials of the isolated perfused cat eye. *Vision Res.* 1973;13:1603–1612.
78. Svaetichin G, Macnichol Jr. EF. Retinal mechanisms for chromatic and achromatic vision. *Ann N Y Acad Sci.* 1959;74:385–404.
79. Hack I, Frech M, Dick O, Peichl L, Brandstätter JH. Heterogeneous distribution of AMPA glutamate receptor subunits at the photoreceptor synapses of rodent retina. *Eur J Neurosci.* 2001;13:15–24.
80. Massey SC, Miller RF. Excitatory amino acid receptors of rod- and cone-driven horizontal cells in the rabbit retina. *J Neurophysiol.* 1987;57:645–659.
81. Qin P, Pourcho RG. Immunocytochemical localization of kainate-selective glutamate receptor subunits GluR5, GluR6, and GluR7 in the cat retina. *Brain Res.* 2001;890:211–221.
82. Shen W, Finnegan SG, Slaughter MM. Glutamate receptor subtypes in human retinal horizontal cells. *Vis Neurosci.* 2004;21:89–95.
83. Vardi N, Morigiwa K, Wang TL, Shi YJ, Sterling P. Neurochemistry of the mammalian cone 'synaptic complex'. *Vision Res.* 1998;38:1359–1369.
84. Haverkamp S, Grünert U, Wässle H. Localization of kainate receptors at the cone pedicles of the primate retina. *J Comp Neurol.* 2001;436:471–486.
85. Deng Q, Wang L, Dong W, He S. Lateral components in the cone terminals of the rabbit retina: horizontal cell origin and glutamate receptor expression. *J Comp Neurol.* 2006;496:698–705.
86. Pan F, Massey SC. Rod and cone input to horizontal cells in the rabbit retina. *J Comp Neurol.* 2007;500:815–831.
87. Boycott BB, Dowling JE, Fisher SK, Kolb H, Laties AM. Interplexiform cells of the mammalian retina and their comparison with catecholamine-containing retinal cells. *Proc R Soc Lond B Biol Sci.* 1975;191:353–368.
88. Witkovsky P, Schutte M. The organization of dopaminergic neurons in vertebrate retinas. *Vis Neurosci.* 1991;7:113–124.
89. Witkovsky P. Dopamine and retinal function. *Doc Ophthalmol.* 2004;108:17–40.
90. Iuvone PM, Tosini G, Pozdeyev N, Haque R, Klein DC, Chaurasia SS. Circadian clocks, clock networks, arylalkylamine N-acetyltransferase, and melatonin in the retina. *Prog Retin Eye Res.* 2005;24:433–456.
91. Hirasawa H, Contini M, Raviola E. Extrasynaptic release of GABA and dopamine by retinal dopaminergic neurons. *Philos Trans R Soc Lond B Biol Sci.* 2015;370
92. Puopolo M, Hochstetler SE, Gustincich S, Wightman RM, Raviola E. Extrasynaptic release of dopamine in a retinal neuron: activity dependence and transmitter modulation. *Neuron.* 2001;30:211–225.
93. Seeman P, Van Tol HH. Dopamine receptor pharmacology. *Trends Pharmacol Sci.* 1994;15: 264–270.
94. Farshi P, Fyk-Kolodziej B, Krolewski DM, Walker PD, Ichinose T. Dopamine D1 receptor expression is bipolar cell type-specific in the mouse retina. *J Comp Neurol.* 2016;524: 2059–2079.
95. Veruki ML, Wässle H. Immunohistochemical localization of dopamine D1 receptors in rat retina. *Eur J Neurosci.* 1996;8:2286–2297.
96. Ribelayga C, Wang Y, Mangel SC. Dopamine mediates circadian clock regulation of rod and cone input to fish retinal horizontal cells. *J Physiol.* 2002;544:801–816.
97. Hellmer CB, Bohl JM, Hall LM, Koehler CC, Ichinose T. Dopaminergic modulation of signal processing in a subset of retinal bipolar cells. *Front Cell Neurosci.* 2020;14:253.
98. He S, Weiler R, Vaney DI. Endogenous dopaminergic regulation of horizontal cell coupling in the mammalian retina. *J Comp Neurol.* 2000;418:33–40.
99. Pflug R, Nelson R, Huber S, Reitsamer H. Modulation of horizontal cell function by dopaminergic ligands in mammalian retina. *Vision Res.* 2008;48:1383–1390.
100. Zhang AJ, Jacoby R, Wu SM. Light- and dopamine-regulated receptive field plasticity in primate horizontal cells. *J Comp Neurol.* 2011;519:2125–2134.
101. Liu X, Grove JC, Hirano AA, Brecha NC, Barnes S. Dopamine D1 receptor modulation of calcium channel currents in horizontal cells of mouse retina. *J Neurophysiol.* 2016;116: 686–697.
102. Ichinose T, Lukasiewicz PD. Ambient light regulates sodium channel activity to dynamically control retinal signaling. *J Neurosci.* 2007;27:4756–4764.
103. Smith BJ, Cote PD, Tremblay F. D1 dopamine receptors modulate cone ON bipolar cell Nav channels to control daily rhythms in photopic vision. *Chronobiol Int.* 2015;32:48–58.
104. Akopian A, Witkovsky P. D2 dopamine receptor-mediated inhibition of a hyperpolarization-activated current in rod photoreceptors. *J Neurophysiol.* 1996;76:1828–1835.
105. Demontis GC, et al. Functional characterisation and subcellular localisation of HCN1 channels in rabbit retinal rod photoreceptors. *J Physiol.* 2002;542:89–97.
106. Kawai F, Horiguchi M, Miyachi E. Dopamine modulates the voltage response of human rod photoreceptors by inhibiting the h current. *Invest Ophthalmol Vis Sci.* 2011;52: 4113–4117.
107. Stella Jr. SL, Thoreson WB. Differential modulation of rod and cone calcium currents in tiger salamander retina by D2 dopamine receptors and cAMP. *Eur J Neurosci.* 2000;12: 3537–3548.
108. Brecha N. A review of retinal neurotransmitters: Histochemical and biochemical studies. In: (Emson PC, ed). *Chemical Neuroanatomy.* Raven Press; 1983:85–129.
109. Cudeiro J, Rivadulla C. Sight and insight--on the physiological role of nitric oxide in the visual system. *Trends Neurosci.* 1999;22:109–116.
110. Kurenny DE, Barnes S. Proton modulation of M-like potassium current (IKx) in rod photoreceptors. *Neurosci Lett.* 1994;170:225–228.
111. Naka KI, Rushton WA. S-potentials from luminosity units in the retina of fish (Cyprinidae). *J Physiol.* 1966;185:587–599.
112. Steinberg RH. Rod and cone contributions to S-potentials from the cat retina. *Vision Res.* 1969;9:1319–1329.
113. Zhang AJ, Zhang J, Wu SM. Electrical coupling, receptive fields, and relative rod/cone inputs of horizontal cells in the tiger salamander retina. *J Comp Neurol.* 2006;499:422–431.
114. Witkovsky P, Owen WG, Woodworth M. Gap junctions among the perikarya, dendrites, and axon terminals of the luminosity-type horizontal cell of the turtle retina. *J Comp Neurol.* 1983;216:359–368.
115. Barnes S, Merchant V, Mahmud F. Modulation of transmission gain by protons at the photoreceptor output synapse. *Proc Natl Acad Sci U S A.* 1993;90:10081–10085.
116. Behrens C, Yadav SC, Korympidou MM, et al. Retinal horizontal cells use different synaptic sites for global feedforward and local feedback signaling. *Curr Biol.* 2022;32:545–558.e5.
117. Verweij J, Kamermans M, Spekreijse H. Horizontal cells feed back to cones by shifting the cone calcium-current activation range. *Vision Res.* 1996;36:3943–3953.
118. Connaughton VP, Nelson R. Spectral responses in zebrafish horizontal cells include a tetraphasic response and a novel UV-dominated triphasic response. *J Neurophysiol.* 2010;104:2407–2422.
119. Li YN, Matsui JI, Dowling JE. Specificity of the horizontal cell-photoreceptor connections in the zebrafish (Danio rerio) retina. *J Comp Neurol.* 2009;516:442–453.
120. Song PI, Matsui JI, Dowling JE. Morphological types and connectivity of horizontal cells found in the adult zebrafish (Danio rerio) retina. *J Comp Neurol.* 2008;506:328–338.
121. Stell WK, Lightfoot DO. Color-specific interconnections of cones and horizontal cells in the retina of the goldfish. *J Comp Neurol.* 1975;159:473–502.
122. Boycott BB, Peichl L, Wässle H. Morphological types of horizontal cell in the retina of the domestic cat. *Proc R Soc Lond B Biol Sci.* 1978;203:229–245.

123. Fisher SK, Boycott BB. Synaptic connections made by horizontal cells within the outer plexiform layer of the retina of the cat and the rabbit. *Proc R Soc Lond B Biol Sci.* 1974;186:317–331.

124. Kolb H. Organization of the outer plexiform layer of the primate retina: electron microscopy of Golgi-impregnated cells. *Philos Trans R Soc Lond B Biol Sci.* 1970;258:261–283.

125. Wässle H, Boycott BB, Peichl L. Receptor contacts of horizontal cells in the retina of the domestic cat. *Proc R Soc Lond B Biol Sci.* 1978;203:247–267.

126. Peichl L, González-Soriano J. Morphological types of horizontal cell in rodent retinae: a comparison of rat, mouse, gerbil, and guinea pig. *Vis Neurosci.* 1994;11:501–517.

127. Wässle H, Boycott BB, Röhrenbeck J. Horizontal cells in the monkey retina: Cone connections and dendritic network. *Eur J Neurosci.* 1989;1:421–435.

128. Bloomfield SA, Miller RF. A physiological and morphological study of the horizontal cell types of the rabbit retina. *J Comp Neurol.* 1982;208:288–303.

129. Dacheux RF, Raviola E. Horizontal cells in the retina of the rabbit. *J Neurosci.* 1982;2:1486–1493.

130. Nelson R, von Litzow A, Kolb H, Gouras P. Horizontal cells in cat retina with independent dendritic systems. *Science.* 1975;189:137–139.

131. Trümpler J, et al. Rod and cone contributions to horizontal cell light responses in the mouse retina. *J Neurosci.* 2008;28:6818–6825.

132. Vaney DI. The coupling pattern of axon-bearing horizontal cells in the mammalian retina. *Proc Biol Sci.* 1993;252:93–101.

133. Xin D, Bloomfield SA. Dark- and light-induced changes in coupling between horizontal cells in mammalian retina. *J Comp Neurol.* 1999;405:75–87.

134. Baldridge WH, Ball AK. Background illumination reduces horizontal cell receptive-field size in both normal and 6-hydroxydopamine-lesioned goldfish retinas. *Vis Neurosci.* 1991;7:441–450.

135. Weiler R, Pottek M, He S, Vaney DI. Modulation of coupling between retinal horizontal cells by retinoic acid and endogenous dopamine. *Brain Res Brain Res Rev.* 2000;32:121–129.

136. Lankheet MJ, Rowe MH, Van Wezel RJ, van de Grind WA. Spatial and temporal properties of cat horizontal cells after prolonged dark adaptation. *Vision Res.* 1996;36:3955–3967.

137. Reitsamer HA, Pflug R, Franz M, Huber S. Dopaminergic modulation of horizontal-cell-axon-terminal receptive field size in the mammalian retina. *Vision Res.* 2006;46:467–474.

138. Hombach S, et al. Functional expression of connexin57 in horizontal cells of the mouse retina. *Eur J Neurosci.* 2004;19:2633–2640.

139. O'Brien J, Nguyen HB, Mills SL. Cone photoreceptors in bass retina use two connexins to mediate electrical coupling. *J Neurosci.* 2004;24:5632–5642.

140. O'Brien JJ, Li W, Pan F, Keung J, O'Brien J, Massey SC. Coupling between A-type horizontal cells is mediated by connexin 50 gap junctions in the rabbit retina. *J Neurosci.* 2006;26:11624–11636.

141. Pan F, Keung J, Kim IB, et al. Connexin 57 is expressed by the axon terminal network of B-type horizontal cells in the rabbit retina. *J Comp Neurol.* 2012;520:2256–2274.

142. Janssen-Bienhold U, Trümpler J, Hilgen G, et al. Connexin57 is expressed in dendro-dendritic and axo-axonal gap junctions of mouse horizontal cells and its distribution is modulated by light. *J Comp Neurol.* 2009;513:363–374.

143. Dorgau B, et al. Connexin50 couples axon terminals of mouse horizontal cells by homotypic gap junctions. *J Comp Neurol.* 2015;523:2062–2081.

144. Shelley J, Dedek K, Schubert T, et al. Horizontal cell receptive fields are reduced in connexin57-deficient mice. *Eur J Neurosci.* 2006;23:3176–3186.

145. Chun MH, Wässle H. GABA-like immunoreactivity in the cat retina: electron microscopy. *J Comp Neurol.* 1989;279:55–67.

146. Grünert U, Wässle H. GABA-like immunoreactivity in the macaque monkey retina: a light and electron microscopic study. *J Comp Neurol.* 1990;297:509–524.

147. Guo C, Hirano AA, Stella Jr. SL, Bitzer M, Brecha NC. Guinea pig horizontal cells express GABA, the GABA-synthesizing enzyme GAD 65, and the GABA vesicular transporter. *J Comp Neurol.* 2010;518:1647–1669.

148. Studholme KM, Yazulla S. Localization of GABA and glycine in goldfish retina by electron microscopic postembedding immunocytochemistry: improved visualization of synaptic structures with LR white resin. *J Neurocytol.* 1988;17:859–870.

149. Mosinger JL, Yazulla S, Studholme KM. GABA-like immunoreactivity in the vertebrate retina: a species comparison. *Exp Eye Res.* 1986;42:631–644.

150. Zhang J, Zhang AJ, Wu SM. Immunocytochemical analysis of GABA-positive and calretinin-positive horizontal cells in the tiger salamander retina. *J Comp Neurol.* 2006;499:432–441.

151. Cueva JG, Haverkamp S, Reimer RJ, Edwards R, Wässle H, Brecha NC. Vesicular gamma-aminobutyric acid transporter expression in amacrine and horizontal cells. *J Comp Neurol.* 2002;445:227–237.

152. Jellali A, Stussi-Garaud C, Gasnier B, et al. Cellular localization of the vesicular inhibitory amino acid transporter in the mouse and human retina. *J Comp Neurol.* 2002;449:76–87.

153. Johnson MA, Vardi N. Regional differences in GABA and GAD immunoreactivity in rabbit horizontal cells. *Vis Neurosci.* 1998;15:743–753.

154. Lee H, Brecha NC. Immunocytochemical evidence for SNARE protein-dependent transmitter release from guinea pig horizontal cells. *Eur J Neurosci.* 2010;31:1388–1401.

155. Vardi N, Kaufman DL, Sterling P. Horizontal cells in cat and monkey retina express different isoforms of glutamic acid decarboxylase. *Vis Neurosci.* 1994;11:135–142.

156. Blanco R, Vaquero CF, de la Villa P. The effects of GABA and glycine on horizontal cells of the rabbit retina. *Vision Res.* 1996;36:3987–3995.

157. Feigenspan A, Weiler R. Electrophysiological properties of mouse horizontal cell GABAA receptors. *J Neurophysiol.* 2004;92:2789–2801.

158. Grove JCR, Hirano AA, de Los Santos J, et al. Novel hybrid action of GABA mediates inhibitory feedback in the mammalian retina. *PLoS Biol.* 2019;17:e3000200.

159. Kemmler R, Schultz K, Dedek K, Euler T, Schubert T. Differential regulation of cone calcium signals by different horizontal cell feedback mechanisms in the mouse retina. *J Neurosci.* 2014;34:11826–11843.

160. Qian H, Dowling JE. Novel GABA responses from rod-driven retinal horizontal cells. *Nature.* 1993;361:162–164.

161. Greferath U, Grünert U, Müller F, Wässle H. Localization of GABAA receptors in the rabbit retina. *Cell Tissue Res.* 1994;276:295–307.

162. Hoon M, et al. Neurotransmission plays contrasting roles in the maturation of inhibitory synapses on axons and dendrites of retinal bipolar cells. *Proc Natl Acad Sci U S A.* 2015;112:12840–12845.

163. Vardi N, Sterling P. Subcellular localization of GABAA receptor on bipolar cells in macaque and human retina. *Vision Res.* 1994;34:1235–1246.

164. Duebel J, Haverkamp S, Schleich W, et al. Two-photon imaging reveals somatodendritic chloride gradient in retinal ON-type bipolar cells expressing the biosensor Clomeleon. *Neuron.* 2006;49:81–94.

165. Satoh H, Kaneda M, Kaneko A. Intracellular chloride concentration is higher in rod bipolar cells than in cone bipolar cells of the mouse retina. *Neurosci Lett.* 2001;310:161–164.

166. Varela C, Blanco R, De la Villa P. Depolarizing effect of GABA in rod bipolar cells of the mouse retina. *Vision Res.* 2005;45:2659–2667.

167. Yin C, Ishii T, Kaneda M. Two types of Cl transporters contribute to the regulation of intracellular Cl concentrations in ON- and OFF-type bipolar cells in the mouse retina. *Neuroscience.* 2020;440:267–276.

168. Chaffiol A, Ishii M, Cao Y, Mangel SC. Dopamine regulation of GABAA receptors contributes to light/dark modulation of the ON-cone bipolar cell receptive field surround in the retina. *Curr Biol.* 2017;27:2600–2609 e2604.

169. Hirano AA, Liu X, Boulter J, et al. Vesicular release of GABA by mammalian horizontal cells mediates inhibitory output to photoreceptors. *Front Cell Neurosci.* 2020;14:600777.

170. Marchiafava PL. Horizontal cells influence membrane potential of bipolar cells in the retina of the turtle. *Nature.* 1978;275:141–142.

171. Barnes S, Deschenes MC. Contribution of Ca and Ca-activated Cl channels to regenerative depolarization and membrane bistability of cone photoreceptors. *J Neurophysiol.* 1992;68:745–755.

172. Wen X, Thoreson WB. Contributions of glutamate transporters and Ca(2+)-activated Cl(-) currents to feedback from horizontal cells to cone photoreceptors. *Exp Eye Res.* 2019;189:107847.

173. Babai N, Thoreson WB. Horizontal cell feedback regulates calcium currents and intra-cellular calcium levels in rod photoreceptors of salamander and mouse retina. *J Physiol.* 2009;587:2353–2364.

174. Dacey D, Packer OS, Diller L, Brainard D, Peterson B, Lee B. Center surround receptive field structure of cone bipolar cells in primate retina. *Vision Res.* 2000;40:1801–1811.

175. Werblin FS. Lateral interactions at inner plexiform layer of vertebrate retina: antagonistic responses to change. *Science.* 1972;175:1008–1010.

176. Hirasawa H, Kaneko A. pH changes in the invaginating synaptic cleft mediate feedback from horizontal cells to cone photoreceptors by modulating Ca2+ channels. *J Gen Physiol.* 2003;122:657–671.

177. Kamermans M, Fahrenfort I, Schultz K, Janssen-Bienhold U, Sjoerdsma T, Weiler R. Hemichannel-mediated inhibition in the outer retina. *Science.* 2001;292:1178–1180.

178. Liu X, Hirano AA, Sun X, Brecha NC, Barnes S. Calcium channels in rat horizontal cells regulate feedback inhibition of photoreceptors through an unconventional GABA- and pH-sensitive mechanism. *J Physiol.* 2013;591:3309–3324.

179. Vessey JP, Stratis AK, Daniels BA, et al. Proton-mediated feedback inhibition of presynaptic calcium channels at the cone photoreceptor synapse. *J Neurosci.* 2005;25:4108–4117.

180. Vroman R, Klaassen LJ, Howlett MH, et al. Extracellular ATP hydrolysis inhibits synaptic transmission by increasing pH buffering in the synaptic cleft. *PLoS Biol.* 2014;12:e1001864.

181. Warren TJ, Van Hook MJ, Supuran CT, Thoreson WB. Sources of protons and a role for bicarbonate in inhibitory feedback from horizontal cells to cones in Ambystoma tigrinum retina. *J Physiol.* 2016;594:6661–6677.

182. Verweij J, Hornstein EP, Schnapf JL. Surround antagonism in macaque cone photoreceptors. *J Neurosci.* 2003;23:10249–10257.

183. Murakami M, Shimoda Y, Nakatani K, Miyachi E, Watanabe S. GABA-mediated negative feedback from horizontal cells to cones in carp retina. *Jpn J Physiol.* 1982;32:911–926.

184. Tatsukawa T, Hirasawa H, Kaneko A, Kaneda M. GABA-mediated component in the feedback response of turtle retinal cones. *Vis Neurosci.* 2005;22:317–324.

185. Wu SM. Input-output relations of the feedback synapse between horizontal cells and cones in the tiger salamander retina. *J Neurophysiol.* 1991;65:1197–1206.

186. Byzov AL, Shura-Bura TM. Electrical feedback mechanism in the processing of signals in the outer plexiform layer of the retina. *Vision Res.* 1986;26:33–44.

187. Klaassen LJ, de Graaff W, van Asselt JB, Klooster J, Kamermans M. Specific connectivity between photoreceptors and horizontal cells in the zebrafish retina. *J Neurophysiol.* 2016;116:2799–2814.

188. Cenedese V, de Graaff W, Csikós T, Poovayya M, Zoidl G, Kamermans M. Pannexin 1 is critically involved in feedback from horizontal cells to cones. *Front Mol Neurosci.* 2017;10:403.

189. Barnes S, Grove JCR, McHugh CF, Hirano AA, Brecha NC. Horizontal cell feedback to cone photoreceptors in mammalian retina: Novel insights from the GABA-pH hybrid model. *Front Cell Neurosci.* 2020;14:595064.

190. Deniz S, Wersinger E, Picaud S, Roux MJ. Evidence for functional GABAA but not GABAC receptors in mouse cone photoreceptors. *Vis Neurosci.* 2019;36:E005.

191. Kranz K, Dorgau B, Pottek M, et al. Expression of Pannexin1 in the outer plexiform layer of the mouse retina and physiological impact of its knockout. *J Comp Neurol.* 2013;521:1119–1135.

192. Brecha NC, Weigmann C. Expression of GAT-1, a high-affinity gamma-aminobutyric acid plasma membrane transporter in the rat retina. *J Comp Neurol.* 1994;345:602–611.

193. Kamermans M, Werblin F. GABA-mediated positive autofeedback loop controls horizontal cell kinetics in tiger salamander retina. *J Neurosci.* 1992;12:2451–2463.

194. Bormann J, Hamill OP, Sakmann B. Mechanism of anion permeation through channels gated by glycine and gamma-aminobutyric acid in mouse cultured spinal neurones. *J Physiol.* 1987;385:243–286.

195. Hirano AA, Liu X, Boulter J, et al. Targeted deletion of vesicular GABA transporter from retinal horizontal cells eliminates feedback modulation of photoreceptor calcium channels. *eNeuro.* 2016;3:ENEURO.0148-15.2016.

196. Dowling JE, Werblin FS. Organization of retina of the mudpuppy, Necturus maculosus. I. Synaptic structure. *J Neurophysiol.* 1969;32:315–338.
197. Dowling JE, Brown JE, Major D. Synapses of horizontal cells in rabbit and cat retinas. *Science.* 1966;153:1639–1641.
198. Linberg KA, Fisher SK. Ultrastructural evidence that horizontal cell axon terminals are presynaptic in the human retina. *J Comp Neurol.* 1988;268:281–297.
199. Shields CR, Tran MN, Wong RO, Lukasiewicz PD. Distinct ionotropic GABA receptors mediate presynaptic and postsynaptic inhibition in retinal bipolar cells. *J Neurosci.* 2000;20:2673–2682.
200. Fahey PK, Burkhardt DA. Center-surround organization in bipolar cells: symmetry for opposing contrasts. *Vis Neurosci.* 2003;20:1–10.
201. Hare WA, Owen WG. Effects of 2-amino-4-phosphonobutyric acid on cells in the distal layers of the tiger salamander's retina. *J Physiol.* 1992;445:741–757.
202. Miller RF, Dacheux RF. Synaptic organization and ionic basis of on and off channels in mudpuppy retina. I. Intracellular analysis of chloride-sensitive electrogenic properties of receptors, horizontal cells, bipolar cells, and amacrine cells. *J Gen Physiol.* 1976;67:639–659.
203. Yang XL, Wu SM. Feedforward lateral inhibition in retinal bipolar cells: input-output relation of the horizontal cell-depolarizing bipolar cell synapse. *Proc Natl Acad Sci U S A.* 1991;88:3310–3313.
204. Zhang AJ, Wu SM. Receptive fields of retinal bipolar cells are mediated by heterogeneous synaptic circuitry. *J Neurosci.* 2009;29:789–797.
205. Euler T, Masland RH. Light-evoked responses of bipolar cells in a mammalian retina. *J Neurophysiol.* 2000;83:1817–1829.
206. Franke K, et al. Inhibition decorrelates visual feature representations in the inner retina. *Nature.* 2017;542:439–444.
207. Hartveit E. Functional organization of cone bipolar cells in the rat retina. *J Neurophysiol.* 1997;77:1716–1730.
208. Ichinose T, Lukasiewicz PD. Inner and outer retinal pathways both contribute to surround inhibition of salamander ganglion cells. *J Physiol.* 2005;565:517–535.
209. Stell WK, Lightfoot DO, Wheeler TG, Leeper HF. Goldfish retina: functional polarization of cone horizontal cell dendrites and synapses. *Science.* 1975;190:989–990.
210. Gunther A, et al. Double cones and the diverse connectivity of photoreceptors and bipolar cells in an avian retina. *J Neurosci.* 2021;41:5015–5028.
211. Kraaij DA, Kamermans M, Spekreijse H. Spectral sensitivity of the feedback signal from horizontal cells to cones in goldfish retina. *Vis Neurosci.* 1998;15:799–808.
212. Li YN, Tsujimura T, Kawamura S, Dowling JE. Bipolar cell-photoreceptor connectivity in the zebrafish (Danio rerio) retina. *J Comp Neurol.* 2012;520:3786–3802.
213. Loew ER, Govardovskii VI. Photoreceptors and visual pigments in the red-eared turtle, Trachemys scripta elegans. *Vis Neurosci.* 2001;18:753–757.
214. Pedler C, Boyle M. Multiple oil droplets in the photoreceptors of the pigeon. *Vision Res.* 1969;9:525–528.
215. Yazulla S. Cone input to horizontal cells in the turtle retina. *Vision Res.* 1976;16:727–735.
216. Naka KI, Rushton WA. S-potentials from colour units in the retina of fish (Cyprinidae). *J Physiol.* 1966;185:536–555.
217. Kamermans M, van Dijk BW, Spekreijse H. Color opponency in cone-driven horizontal cells in carp retina. Aspecific pathways between cones and horizontal cells. *J Gen Physiol.* 1991;97:819–843.
218. Thoreson WB, Dacey DM. Diverse cell types, circuits, and mechanisms for color vision in the vertebrate retina. *Physiol Rev.* 2019;99:1527–1573.
219. Baden T, et al. A tale of two retinal domains: near-optimal sampling of achromatic contrasts in natural scenes through asymmetric photoreceptor distribution. *Neuron.* 2013;80:1206–1217.
220. Joesch M, Meister M. A neuronal circuit for colour vision based on rod-cone opponency. *Nature.* 2016;532:236–239.
221. Szatko KP, Korympidou MM, Ran Y, et al. Neural circuits in the mouse retina support color vision in the upper visual field. *Nat Commun.* 2020;11:3481.
222. Crook JD, Manookin MB, Packer OS, Dacey DM. Horizontal cell feedback without cone type-selective inhibition mediates "red-green" color opponency in midget ganglion cells of the primate retina. *J Neurosci.* 2011;31:1762–1772.
223. Ahnelt P, Kolb H. Horizontal cells and cone photoreceptors in human retina: a Golgi-electron microscopic study of spectral connectivity. *J Comp Neurol.* 1994;343:406–427.
224. Dacey DM, Lee BB, Stafford DK, Pokorny J, Smith VC. Horizontal cells of the primate retina: cone specificity without spectral opponency. *Science.* 1996;271:656–659.
225. Wässle H, Dacey DM, Haun T, Haverkamp S, Grünert U, Boycott BB. The mosaic of horizontal cells in the macaque monkey retina: with a comment on biplexiform ganglion cells. *Vis Neurosci.* 2000;17:591–608.
226. Dacey DM, Lee BB. The 'blue-on' opponent pathway in primate retina originates from a distinct bistratified ganglion cell type. *Nature.* 1994;367:731–735.
227. Patterson SS, Kuchenbecker JA, Anderson JR, Neitz M, Neitz J. A color vision circuit for non-image-forming vision in the primate retina. *Curr Biol.* 2020;30:1269–1274 e1262.
228. Crook JD, et al. Parallel ON and OFF cone bipolar inputs establish spatially coextensive receptive field structure of blue-yellow ganglion cells in primate retina. *J Neurosci.* 2009;29:8372–8387.
229. Puller C, Haverkamp S, Neitz M, Neitz J. Synaptic elements for GABAergic feed-forward signaling between HII horizontal cells and blue cone bipolar cells are enriched beneath primate S-cones. *PLoS One.* 2014;9:e88963.
230. Naka KI, Nye PW. Role of horizontal cells in organization of the catfish retinal receptive field. *J Neurophysiol.* 1971;34:785–801.
231. Naka KI, Witkovsky P. Dogfish ganglion cell discharge resulting from extrinsic polarization of the horizontal cells. *J Physiol.* 1972;223:449–460. 7.
232. Mangel SC. Analysis of the horizontal cell contribution to the receptive field surround of ganglion cells in the rabbit retina. *J Physiol.* 1991;442:211–234.
233. Mangel SC, Miller RF. Horizontal cells contribute to the receptive field surround of ganglion cells in the rabbit retina. *Brain Res.* 1987;414:182–186.
234. Chaya T, Matsumoto A, Sugita Y, et al. Versatile functional roles of horizontal cells in the retinal circuit. *Sci Rep.* 2017;7:5540.
235. Ströh S, Puller C, Swirski S, et al. Eliminating glutamatergic input onto horizontal cells changes the dynamic range and receptive field organization of mouse retinal ganglion cells. *J Neurosci.* 2018;38:2015–2028.
236. Magnus CJ, Lee PH, Bonaventura J, et al. Ultrapotent chemogenetics for research and potential clinical applications. *Science.* 2019;364.
237. Strauss S, Korympidou MM, Ran Y, et al. Center-surround interactions underlie bipolar cell motion sensitivity in the mouse retina. *Nat Commun.* 2022;13(1):5574.
238. Drinnenberg A, Franke F, Morikawa RK, et al. How diverse retinal functions arise from feedback at the first visual synapse. *Neuron.* 2018;99:117–134 e111.
239. Lukasiewicz PD. Synaptic mechanisms that shape visual signaling at the inner retina. *Prog Brain Res.* 2005;147:205–218.
240. Wu SM, Gao F, Maple BR. Functional architecture of synapses in the inner retina: segregation of visual signals by stratification of bipolar cell axon terminals. *J Neurosci.* 2000;20:4462–4470.
241. Famiglietti Jr. EV. 'Starburst' amacrine cells and cholinergic neurons: mirror-symmetric on and off amacrine cells of rabbit retina. *Brain Res.* 1983;261:138–144.
242. Tauchi M, Masland RH. The shape and arrangement of the cholinergic neurons in the rabbit retina. *Proc R Soc Lond B Biol Sci.* 1984;223:101–119.
243. Boycott BB, Wässle H. Morphological classification of bipolar cells of the primate retina. *Eur J Neurosci.* 1991;3:1069–1088.
244. Grünert U, Martin PR. Cell types and cell circuits in human and non-human primate retina. *Prog Retin Eye Res.* 2020:100844.
245. Helmstaedter M, Briggman KL, Turaga SC, Jain V, Seung HS, Denk W. Connectomic reconstruction of the inner plexiform layer in the mouse retina. *Nature.* 2013;500: 168–174.
246. MacNeil MA, Heussy JK, Dacheux RF, Raviola E, Masland RH. The population of bipolar cells in the rabbit retina. *J Comp Neurol.* 2004;472:73–86.
247. Puller C, Ondreka K, Haverkamp S. Bipolar cells of the ground squirrel retina. *J Comp Neurol.* 2011;519:759–774.
248. Hensley SH, Yang XL, Wu SM. Relative contribution of rod and cone inputs to bipolar cells and ganglion cells in the tiger salamander retina. *J Neurophysiol.* 1993;69:2086–2098.
249. Ishida AT, Stell WK, Lightfoot DO. Rod and cone inputs to bipolar cells in goldfish retina. *J Comp Neurol.* 1980;191:315–335.
250. Pang JJ, Gao F, Lem J, Bramblett DE, Paul DL, Wu SM. Direct rod input to cone BCs and direct cone input to rod BCs challenge the traditional view of mammalian BC circuitry. *Proc Natl Acad Sci U S A.* 2010;107:395–400.
251. Ammermüller J, Kolb H. The organization of the turtle inner retina. I. ON- and OFF-center pathways. *J Comp Neurol.* 1995;358:1–34.
252. Connaughton VP, Graham D, Nelson R. Identification and morphological classification of horizontal, bipolar, and amacrine cells within the zebrafish retina. *J Comp Neurol.* 2004;477:371–385.
253. Pang JJ, Gao F, Wu SM. Stratum-by-stratum projection of light response attributes by retinal bipolar cells of Ambystoma. *J Physiol.* 2004;558:249–262.
254. Whitaker CM, Nobles G, Ishibashi M, Massey SC. Rod and cone connections with bipolar cells in the rabbit retina. *Front Cell Neurosci.* 2021;15:662329.
255. Dunn FA, Wong RO. Diverse strategies engaged in establishing stereotypic wiring patterns among neurons sharing a common input at the visual system's first synapse. *J Neurosci.* 2012;32:10306–10317.
256. De Monasterio FM, Gouras P. Functional properties of ganglion cells of the rhesus monkey retina. *J Physiol.* 1975;251:167–195.
257. Rossi EA, Roorda A. The relationship between visual resolution and cone spacing in the human fovea. *Nat Neurosci.* 2010;13:156–157.
258. Wool LE, Crook JD, Troy JB, Packer OS, Zaidi Q, Dacey DM. Nonselective wiring accounts for red-green opponency in midget ganglion cells of the primate retina. *J Neurosci.* 2018;38:1520–1540.
259. Klug K, Herr S, Ngo IT, Sterling P, Schein S. Macaque retina contains an S-cone OFF midget pathway. *J Neurosci.* 2003;23:9881–9887.
260. Mariani AP. Bipolar cells in monkey retina selective for the cones likely to be blue-sensitive. *Nature.* 1984;308:184–186.
261. Wässle H, Grünert U, Martin PR, Boycott BB. Immunocytochemical characterization and spatial distribution of midget bipolar cells in the macaque monkey retina. *Vision Res.* 1994;34:561–579.
262. Puller C, Haverkamp S. Bipolar cell pathways for color vision in non-primate dichromats. *Vis Neurosci.* 2011;28:51–60.
263. Baden T, Berens P, Bethge M, Euler T. Spikes in mammalian bipolar cells support temporal layering of the inner retina. *Curr Biol.* 2013;23:48–52.
264. Roska B, Werblin F. Vertical interactions across ten parallel, stacked representations in the mammalian retina. *Nature.* 2001;410:583–587.
265. Famiglietti Jr. EV, Kaneko A, Tachibana M. Neuronal architecture of on and off pathways to ganglion cells in carp retina. *Science.* 1977;198:1267–1269.
266. Dumitrescu ON, Pucci FG, Wong KY, Berson DM. Ectopic retinal ON bipolar cell synapses in the OFF inner plexiform layer: contacts with dopaminergic amacrine cells and melanopsin ganglion cells. *J Comp Neurol.* 2009;517:226–244.
267. Hoshi H, Liu WL, Massey SC, Mills SL. ON inputs to the OFF layer: bipolar cells that breakthe stratification rules of the retina. *J Neurosci.* 2009;29:8875–8883.
268. Kujiraoka T, Saito T. Electrical coupling between bipolar cells in carp retina. *Proc Natl Acad Sci U S A.* 1986;83:4063–4066.
269. Marc RE, Liu WL, Muller JF. Gap junctions in the inner plexiform layer of the goldfish retina. *Vision Res.* 1988;28:9–24.
270. Sigulinsky CL, Anderson JR, Kerzner E, et al. Network architecture of gap junctional coupling among parallel processing channels in the mammalian retina. *J Neurosci.* 2020;40:4483–4511.

271. DeVries SH, Li W, Saszik S. Parallel processing in two transmitter microenvironments at the cone photoreceptor synapse. *Neuron.* 2006;50:735–748.

272. Vardi N, Zhang LL, Payne JA, Sterling P. Evidence that different cation chloride cotransporters in retinal neurons allow opposite responses to GABA. *J Neurosci.* 2000;20:7657–7663.

273. Awatramani GB, Slaughter MM. Origin of transient and sustained responses in ganglion cells of the retina. *J Neurosci.* 2000;20:7087–7095.

274. Borghuis BG, Marvin JS, Looger LL, Demb JB. Two-photon imaging of nonlinear glutamate release dynamics at bipolar cell synapses in the mouse retina. *J Neurosci.* 2013;33:10972–10985.

275. Ichinose T, Shields CR, Lukasiewicz PD. Sodium channels in transient retinal bipolar cells enhance visual responses in ganglion cells. *J Neurosci.* 2005;25:1856–1865.

276. Puthussery T, Venkataramani S, Gayet-Primo J, Smith RG, Taylor WR. NaV1.1 channels in axon initial segments of bipolar cells augment input to magnocellular visual pathways in the primate retina. *J Neurosci.* 2013;33:16045–16059.

277. Saszik S, DeVries SH. A mammalian retinal bipolar cell uses both graded changes in membrane voltage and all-or-nothing Na+ spikes to encode light. *J Neurosci.* 2012;32:297–307.

278. Bloomfield SA, Dacheux RF. Rod vision: pathways and processing in the mammalian retina. *Prog Retin Eye Res.* 2001;20:351–384.

279. Dacheux RF, Raviola E. The rod pathway in the rabbit retina: a depolarizing bipolar and amacrine cell. *J Neurosci.* 1986;6:331–345.

280. Grimes WN, Baudin J, Azevedo AW, Rieke F. Range, routing and kinetics of rod signaling in primate retina. *Elife.* 2018;7

281. Field GD, Rieke F. Nonlinear signal transfer from mouse rods to bipolar cells and implications for visual sensitivity. *Neuron.* 2002;34:773–785.

282. Sampath AP, Rieke F. Selective transmission of single photon responses by saturation at the rod-to-rod bipolar synapse. *Neuron.* 2004;41:431–443.

283. Demb JB, Singer JH. Intrinsic properties and functional circuitry of the AII amacrine cell. *Vis Neurosci.* 2012;29:51–60.

284. Pang JJ, Gao F, Paul DL, Wu SM. Rod, M-cone and M/S-cone inputs to hyperpolarizing bipolar cells in the mouse retina. *J Physiol.* 2012;590:845–854.

285. Tsukamoto Y, Omi N. Some OFF bipolar cell types make contact with both rods and cones in macaque and mouse retinas. *Front Neuroanat.* 2014;8:105.

286. Soucy E, Wang Y, Nirenberg S, Nathans J, Meister M. A novel signaling pathway from rod photoreceptors to ganglion cells in mammalian retina. *Neuron.* 1998;21:481–493.

287. Li W, Chen S, DeVries SH. A fast rod photoreceptor signaling pathway in the mammalian retina. *Nat Neurosci.* 2010;13:414–416.

288. Morgans CW, Brown RL, Duvoisin RM. TRPM1: the endpoint of the mGluR6 signal transduction cascade in retinal ON-bipolar cells. *Bioessays.* 2010;32:609–614.

289. Burkhardt DA, Gottesman J, Thoreson WB. Prolonged depolarization in turtle cones evoked by current injection and stimulation of the receptive field surround. *J Physiol.* 1988;407:329–348.

290. Fain GL. *Sensory transduction.* Second edn. Oxford, UK: Oxford University Press; 2020.

23

Visual Processing in the Inner Retina

Gregory W. Schwartz and Thomas Euler

The bulk of the retina's computing hardware is located in the inner retina. Here, dozens of neural circuits allow the retina to detect subtle changes in brightness, contrast, color, and other, more complex visual features, including oriented edges, motion direction, and object motion. All of these circuits adapt seamlessly over the enormous range of light levels and contrasts in natural scenes (reviewed in refs[1–3]). In this chapter, our focus is on the mouse, which is currently one of the best-studied nonprimate mammalian model systems in vision research.[4] As evolutionary pressures drive visual systems to adapt to a species' ecological niche (reviewed in ref[3]), mice, like other species, feature retinal specializations that are not found in, for example, primates, and we point out where such differences occur. However, given that the fundamental bauplan of the vertebrate retina is surprisingly well conserved,[3] most of the computational principles and neural mechanisms we describe in this chapter apply to other species (Fig. 23.1).

THE PLAYERS IN THE INNER RETINA

At first glance, the organization of the retina may seem simple (Fig. 23.1A). Along an excitatory "vertical" pathway, photoreceptor signals are relayed by the bipolar cells (BCs) from the outer retina to the retinal ganglion cells (RGCs) in the inner retina (reviewed in ref[5]). The RGCs are the eye's output neurons; their axons form the optic nerve, which projects to tens of visual centers,[6,7] and are the sole conduits for all the visual information required by the rest of the brain. Synaptic transmission along this vertical pathway is modulated by laterally organized interneurons—at the photoreceptor-BC synapse by horizontal cells (see Chapter 22), and at the BC-RGC synapse by amacrine cells (ACs) (reviewed in refs[8,9]). This deceptively simple scheme is complicated by a rich diversity of cell types that form the many parallel circuits. In mouse, for example, the three different photoreceptor types (rods, M-cones, and S-cones; see Chapter 19) are contacted by 14 different BCs,[10–12] which distribute their signals to approximately 45 different RGC types,[13–15] each carrying a distinct representation of the visual world (reviewed in refs[16–18]). Moreover, the inner retina of the mouse features at least 63 types of AC,[19] highlighting the computational importance of inner retinal circuits.

Bipolar cells

BCs are the sole forward connection between the outer and inner retina. Like photoreceptors, they employ ribbon synapses to release glutamate and hence provide the excitatory drive to the inner retinal circuits (reviewed in ref[5]). Among the retinal cell classes with more than a few types, BCs are probably the best understood class in terms of type classification and function. In the mouse, anatomical,[11,12,20] genetic,[21] and functional data[22] converge on a set of 14 distinct types, plus an unusual dendrite-lacking BC type.[23]

The dendrites of BCs receive synaptic input from photoreceptor axon terminals in the outer plexiform layer. One traditionally distinguishes between a single type of rod bipolar cell (RBC) and several types of cone bipolar cells (CBCs), depending on the photoreceptor subclass contacted. However, this is not clear-cut, as RBCs may also contact cones—in mice, more than half of them do[12]—and some types of OFF CBCs additionally contact rods.[12,24,25] Although the signaling in RBCs and CBCs is quite distinct, these pathways are intimately intertwined (see further). In addition, some CBC types make selective contacts with a single spectral type of cone[17,26,27] and hence carry chromatic signals (see Chapters 22 and 34).

In addition to the photoreceptor types contacted, the responses of the different BC types are shaped by a number of mechanisms. For instance, the polarity of a BC's light response depends primarily on the kind of postsynaptic glutamate receptor (GluR) it expresses.[28–30] As photoreceptors release glutamate in darkness (see Chapter 19), the presence of sign-inverting metabotropic GluRs renders BCs responsive to light increments (ON BCs), whereas expression of sign-preserving ionotropic GluRs result in responses to light decrements (OFF BCs). Moreover, the specific GluR type expressed by OFF BCs contributes to tuning the temporal profile of the cells' light responses.[31–33] In general, OFF CBCs respond more quickly to luminance changes[34] and adapt more rapidly to changes in contrast[35] than their ON CBC counterparts. Finally, BC output is critically shaped by synaptic interactions with ACs at the BC axon terminal in the inner plexiform layer (IPL), as will be discussed in detail next.

Amacrine cells

With more than 60 types as suggested by mouse transcriptomic data,[19] ACs are the most diverse class of retinal neurons (reviewed in refs[8,36]). At the same time, the function of fewer than a dozen of them is currently well understood, making them the greatest challenge in fully understanding retinal information processing (reviewed in ref[37]).

ACs are roughly divided into narrow-field cells with arbor diameters of around 100 μm and less, and wide-field cells, whose arbors can span across several millimeters. Amacrine cells receive synaptic input from BCs and other ACs and provide synaptic output to BCs, ACs, and RGCs. Despite their name (amacrine ~ axonless), not all ACs lack an axon, especially the largest ones, which in fact have multiple axons (polyaxonal ACs[38,39]). Nevertheless, most ACs use their dendrites for both receiving synaptic input and making output synapses (dendritic processing, see further; reviewed in refs[40,41]). Because of this dual function, we will refer to the processes of axon-lacking ACs as neurites.

Many ACs are "bilingual"—they release two types of signaling molecules, like many interneurons in the brain (reviewed in ref[42]). The first one that is released is GABA or glycine, thus a fast, inhibitory transmitter. In mammals, most narrow-field ACs are glycinergic,

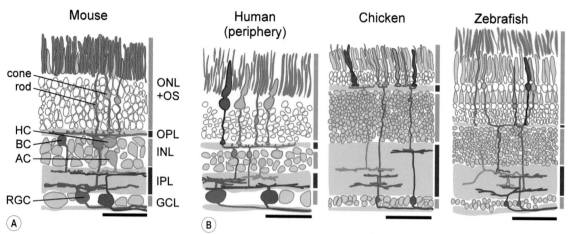

Fig. 23.1 The retinal bauplan is well conserved across vertebrates. (**A**) Cross-section of a mouse retina, with the five neuron classes indicated. Rod and cone photoreceptors and their light-sensitive outer segments (*OS*) are located in the outer nuclear layer (*ONL*); their axon terminals contact horizontal cells (*HC*) and bipolar cells (*BCs*) in the outer plexiform layer (*OPL*). BC and amacrine cell (*AC*) somata reside in the inner nuclear layer (*INL*); their neurites dive into the inner plexiform layer (*IPL*), where they interconnect with each other and the dendrites of retinal ganglion cells (*RGC*). (**B**) Cross-sections of other vertebrate retinas. Note that the cross-section of the human (primate) retina (*left*) depicts the periphery; for details on the foveal in the central primate retina, see Chapter 21. Cone photoreceptor colors indicate spectral preference: *blue* or *lilac* (short, S), *green* (medium wavelength, M), and *red* (long, L); note that lilac-colored cones in chicken and zebrafish, as well as the blue-colored cone in mouse, are sensitive to UV light. *GCL*, Ganglion cell layer. Scale bars: 50 μm. (**A** and **B** modified from Fig. 1A in Baden T, Euler T, Berens P. Understanding the retinal basis of vision across species. *Nat Rev Neurosci.* 2020;21:5–20.)

whereas most wide-field ACs are GABAergic. The second one can be a transmitter but is typically a slower-acting neuromodulator (reviewed in ref[8]). How and where these transmitters are released depends on the AC type. For instance, VGluT3 (vesicular glutamate transporter type 3) ACs, which are involved in motion detection, release glycine and glutamate from synapses in distinct partitions of their neuritic arbors.[43] In contrast, dopaminergic ACs, which play a key role in adjusting the retina's light sensitivity,[44] co-release GABA and dopamine, with the ratio of these molecules varying between vesicles and synaptic location.[45] Starburst ACs, which are central to the circuit that computes direction selectivity (reviewed in ref[46]), corelease GABA and acetylcholine likely from different vesicle pools,[47,48] with GABA relaying local inhibition and acetylcholine perhaps acting on several spatial scales.[49,50]

Retinal ganglion cells

Finally, RGCs pool many synaptic inputs from BCs and ACs impinging on their dendritic arbor and convert the resulting signal into a spike train in the optic nerve. A few RGC types strongly express the visual pigment melanopsin,[51] which renders these cells intrinsically photosensitive (ipRGCs) and enables them to provide critical input for photoentrainment of the biologic clock[52,53] (see Chapter 26). Whether these strongly melanopsin-positive cells also contribute to image-forming vision is still a matter of debate (reviewed in ref[54]). In mice, evidence from functional, anatomical, and genetic studies[13–15,55] jointly point at a total set of at least 45 types of RGCs (see also http://rgctypes.org/).

Each type of RGC can be thought of as the end point of a retinal circuit that extracts and encodes a representation of distinct visual features (reviewed in refs[18,56]). The RGCs with the smallest dendritic arbors encode the finest spatial details; here, at the extreme, are the midget RGCs in the primate fovea (reviewed in refs[57,58]), which make private-line connections between a single cone (via a single BC) and the brain (with receptive field centers of ~1/60 degrees visual angle[59]). In mice, which lack a fovea and midget cells, the representations with the highest spatial resolution (~3 degrees visual angle) are likely implemented by the "high-definition" cells

(HD RGCs[60]). Among the largest RGCs are the alpha cells, a group of RGC types that differ in response polarity and transience.[61] As they are strongly driven by RBCs and pool over a large retinal area, they remain responsive even at the limit of vision when photons are sparse.[62,63] Notably, at least one of these alpha cells, the transient OFF alpha RGC, performs other functions at higher light levels. It responds to approaching dark objects,[64] potentially warning the animal of approaching predators,[65] and it can signal image recurrence associated with saccadic eye movements.[66] Other visual features encoded by different RGCs (some of which are detailed in the next section) include motion direction,[46] which can support image stabilization,[67] object motion,[68] contrast,[69,70] color,[71] and orientation.[72]

THE PLAYING FIELD

The playing field is the IPL, where the axon terminals of BCs, the neurites of ACs, and the dendrites of RGCs interconnect. The IPL is organized in a laminar fashion (Fig. 23.1), for example, OFF responses dominate the distal portion of the IPL (toward the AC somata), ON responses the proximal portion (toward the RGC somata), and the fastest, most transient responses are clustered roughly toward the IPL center.[73] This organization is implemented by different BC and AC types stratifying at distinct IPL depths, where they provide specific combinations of functional output, which, in turn, can be picked up by an RGC that selectively targets those IPL depth(s) with its dendrites.[74] The key computational units of the IPL are (1) the BC axon terminal, (2) the AC dendrites, and (3) the RGC dendritic arbors, all of which can perform a wide range of complex nonlinear computations using a similarly broad spectrum of cellular mechanisms.

Bipolar cell axon terminals

The terminals of BCs receive massive feedforward and/or feedback inhibition often from multiple AC types, critically shaping a BC's direct photoreceptor input signal (see Chapter 22) and, hence, its glutamatergic output (reviewed in ref[5], see also Box 23.1). The GABAergic AC input tunes the temporal properties of the BC output depending on the postsynaptic receptor types (e.g., GABAA vs. GABAC[75–77]). Moreover, in concert with glycinergic inhibition, GABAergic AC input forms the BC's antagonistic center-surround receptive field.[22,78] In fact, AC input can drive a BC's response alone, which can be demonstrated by presenting an annular stimulus in a BC's antagonistic receptive field (RF) surround while leaving out its RF center (i.e., the direct photoreceptor input[22]). Thus, BC output always also reflects AC activity.[79]

Glutamate release from BCs is further modulated by several mechanisms. For example, the biophysical properties of the ribbon synapse render BC output sensitive to the recent history of its activity. Retinal contrast adaptation, for instance, partially relies on the availability and priming state of synaptic vesicles at the BC ribbon synapse.[79–81] Next, the ion channel complement present in axon and axon terminal varies between BC types, enabling some BCs to generate spikes (reviewed in ref[82]), which further extends their temporal signaling capabilities.[83,84] Finally, many of the neuromodulators released by ACs can fine-tune BC output. It has been shown, for example, that dopamine,[85] neuropeptide Y,[86] and endocannabinoids[87,88] modulate voltage-gated Ca^{2+} and/or K^+ channels in BC terminals (Box 23.1).

BOX 23.1

Vertical pathway, lateral interactions, and computational units. The transformation of the photoreceptor signal by bipolar cells (BCs) is often approximated in simple linear-nonlinear (LN) models. Here, the sum of all linear operations within the BC is combined into a single representation (impulse response). Convolution of this impulse response with a stimulus, followed by the passing of the result through a "static nonlinearity," yields a prediction of the cell's output to that stimulus. In the figure, we illustrate how elements of such LN models (center) may be mapped onto a BC's dendrite, soma, axon, and axon terminals; the respective synaptic sites in the circuit are depicted to the sides (left: input from photoreceptors and output to retinal ganglion cells [RGCs]; right: lateral interactions with horizontal cells (HCs) and amacrine cells (ACs). Note that colors mark linear operations (black), nonlinear operations (red), and time-dependent processes (blue).

In step (1), the synaptic input the BC receives at its dendrites is temporally filtered (i.e., by the neurotransmitter receptors, the passive soma + axon). In step (2), the signal from the axon is integrated at the axon terminals with local processes, including AC input, electrical gap-junctional coupling, and active channels (here approximated by a single LN element). Step (3) accounts for the potential presence of spiking activity. The result of step (2) (together with step (3), if included) is the activation of voltage-gated Ca^{2+} channels in the terminals. In step (4), the Ca^{2+} entering the terminal is subject to buffering, diffusion, and extrusion by pumps. As a result, bulk Ca^{2+} within the terminal imposes another low-pass filter onto BC activity before triggering the release of glutamate-filled vesicles. Depending on the vesicle-supply state of the synaptic ribbon, release can be highly nonlinear or roughly linear. Notably, BC synaptic release not only affects RGCs, but can also elicit input from ACs (step [5]), which may act through direct (reciprocal) or indirect (via a series of ACs) neurotransmission, and/or through neuromodulators.

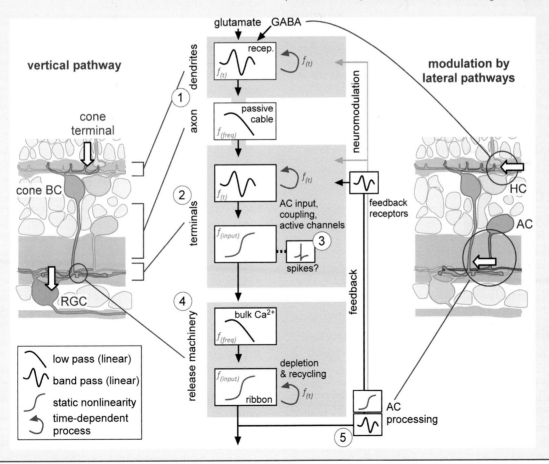

(Modified from Box 2 in Euler T, Haverkamp S, Schubert T, Baden T. Retinal bipolar cells: elementary building blocks of vision. *Nat Rev Neurosci.* 2014;15:507–519; for more details see original publication.)

Amacrine cell dendritic compartments

The dendritic arbor of ACs is often functionally partitioned, for example, through a differential distribution of input and output synapses. This partitioning dramatically varies between AC types and does not necessarily correlate with arbor size. For instance, A17 cells, which belong to the wide-field ACs, feature more than 100 regularly spaced varicosities on their neurites with each varicosity providing independent inhibitory feedback to a single RBC axon terminal.[89,90] In contrast, in the similar-sized starburst ACs, each primary neurite is roughly divided into a proximal input and distal output zone, implementing a "detector" for motion direction.[91,92] Narrow-field ACs such as the A2[93] and the A8[94] often act as vertical "conducts" by relaying signals between different depths of the IPL.[95]

Dendritic and axonal integration in retinal ganglion cells

The dendrites of RGCs integrate excitatory and inhibitory synaptic input from distinct combinations of BCs and ACs.[11] How the RGC's output signal is computed from this input depends on morphologic features, such as branching pattern, dendritic thickness, and segment length,[96] as well as on the complement and distribution of ion channels, including not only voltage-gated Na^+, K^+, and Ca^{2+} channels but also Ca^{2+}-activated K^+ channels or hyperpolarization-activated cyclic nucleotide–gated (HCN) channels.[97–99] These properties vary strongly between RGC types and impact dendritic integration.[100] For instance, small-diameter dendritic segments with high axial resistance, on one hand, can result in shorter propagation distances of dendritic signals and, hence, more independent arbor regions.[96,101] On the other hand, expression of active Na^+ channels along the dendrite may enhance signal propagation and enable backpropagation of somatic spikes.[102] Still, predicting how specific combinations of dendritic geometry and active channel densities affect dendritic integration is challenging.[101] The final step in tuning a RGC's output is the axon hillock, where cell type–specific combinations of active channels[103–106] convert the voltage signal into a train of action potentials. Differences in the number and type of Na^+ channels at the axon hillock can exert important influences on spike generation.[105,107,108] Taken together, RGCs themselves can perform nonlinear computations and therefore contribute to the functional properties of "their" information channel to higher visual centers.

EXAMPLE CIRCUITS

The players of the inner retina can come together in countless configurations to support different visual computations, and many of these retinal circuits remain to be discovered. In the following sections, we describe five retinal circuits for which we have some clarity about which players are essential and the way in which they work together to achieve a particular computation. More details and additional circuits can be found.[1]

Color polarity switching

Color vision (see Chapter 34) starts in the retina. Here, color-opponent circuits begin with BCs that sample selectively from spectrally different cone types and culminate in RGCs, the response polarity of which depends on wavelength (e.g., blue ON-yellow OFF[109]). The trichromatic (blue, green, red) visual system in humans is a relatively recent adaptation in primate evolution, resulting from a gene duplication that created separate green (medium wavelength, M) and red (long-wavelength, L) opsins,[110] although trichromatic and tetrachromatic vision are evolutionarily ancient in nonmammals.[71] Thus, human color vision is built from the ancient blue-yellow (short-wavelength,

S, vs. M/L) opponent circuit and the separate, more recent green-red (M vs. L) circuit.[111,112]

Most nonprimate mammals, such as mice, rabbits, and ground squirrels, have only S- and M-cone opsins, and they serve as models for human S vs. M color-opponent circuits. Whether color-opponent perception requires both RGC response polarities (S_{ON}/M_{OFF} and S_{OFF}/M_{ON}) remains controversial[113]; nonetheless, different RGC types with each color opponent S/M polarity have been found in ground squirrels,[114] rabbits,[115] and nonhuman primates.[116] S_{ON} responses in RGCs have a straightforward anatomical substrate in S-cone–selective ON CBCs, which are well conserved across all of these species, as well as mice.[26,27,115,117] S_{OFF} responses, however, are more difficult to explain, because there does not appear to be an S-cone–selective OFF CBC in mice,[12] ground squirrels,[118] or primates,[119] and its existence in rabbits remains unresolved.[115]

The solution to the question of how to build an S_{OFF} RGC is to invert the S_{ON} signal with an AC. A landmark study identified a narrow-field S_{ON}/M_{OFF} AC in the ground squirrel retina that is likely to receive its excitatory input from S_{ON} CBCs and provide glycinergic inhibition to S_{OFF}/M_{ON} RGCs.[120] Thus the RGC is hyperpolarized by this inhibitory input for S_{ON} or M_{OFF} and depolarized by disinhibition for S_{OFF} or M_{ON}. Pharmacology experiments suggested that a similar circuit exists in the rabbit, but the respective AC has not yet been found[115]; circuit mechanisms of the S_{OFF}/M_{ON} RGCs in primate retina have not been investigated.[109] Similar to the role of other narrow-field ACs in "crossover" inhibition between ON and OFF BC pathways,[95] this color-inversion circuit represents a "vertical" computation that acts within a narrow region of the visual field to process information between BC channels.

Circuits for night vision

Rod photoreceptors enable night (scotopic) vision. Their phototransduction cascade (see Chapter 18) and synaptic release kinetics are optimized to catch and signal when photons are scarce.[2,121–123] At light levels below around 100 P*s^{-1} (photoisomerization per second; mesopic range) per rod, the retina switches from cone- to rod-dominated signaling. There is, however, evidence that rods remain light sensitive and contribute to daylight (photopic) vision.[124]

Rod signals can reach the RGCs via different pathways.[125] In the primary rod pathway (Fig. 23.2A), the aforementioned RBCs rarely connect to RGCs directly; instead, this pathway feeds into the CBC circuits.[126] This piggyback arrangement allows sharing of the same feature-extracting hardware in the inner retina during night and day. Specifically, RBCs possess their "own" AC, the A2,[93] which relays RBC signals to the axon terminals of OFF CBCs via inhibitory glycinergic synapses in the distal IPL, and of ON CBCs via gap junctions (electrical synapses) in the proximal IPL (reviewed in ref[127]). By inverting the RBC signal in the distal but not the proximal IPL, the A2 connectivity ensures that signals reach OFF and ON CBCs, respectively, with the proper polarity. Interestingly, at daytime, A2 ACs are repurposed to serve a circuit that detects approaching dark shapes,[64,128] illustrating how intimately retinal circuits are entwined. In addition to the RBC-A2 mediated pathway, rod signals can also reach CBCs via electrical rod-cone coupling (Fig. 23.2A;[129]); this secondary rod pathway has been shown to exist in many species, including primate[130] and mice.[131] Finally, as some OFF CBC types contact rods in addition to cones, rod signals can enter the OFF CBC circuits directly, forming a tertiary rod pathway.[12,24] Recently, a further pathway has been discovered—some RGC types may receive direct glycinergic A2 input to their somata.[132]

In addition to intrinsic rod properties, it is the tremendous convergence of up to thousands of rods per RGC (Fig. 23.2B) that yields high amplification and reduction of noise in the primary rod pathway,

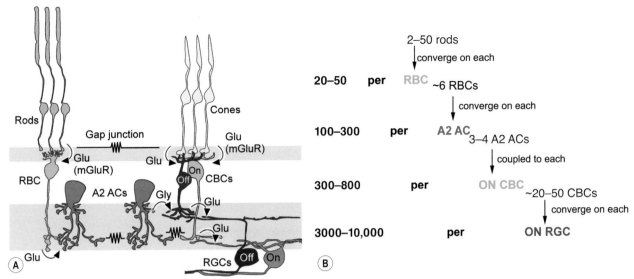

Fig. 23.2 The rod pathways. (**A**) Signal flow along the primary and secondary rod pathway; for details, see text. (**B**) Convergence of rod signals onto ON retinal ganglion cells (RGCs). Each level lists the convergence from the cells at the previous level and the total rod convergence. *AC*, Amacrine cell; *CBC*, cone bipolar cell; *Glu*, glutamate; *Gly*, glycine; *mGluR*, metabotropic glutamate receptor; *RBC*, rod bipolar cell. (**A**. own drawing; **B**, modified from Schwartz GW, Chapter 1 - Photon detection, Schwartz GW, Retinal Computation, Academic Press, 2021;2–24.)

allowing it to signal at starlight.[133,134] In addition, rod signals are differentially processed by distinct retinal circuits, making visually guided behavior at the limit of vision possible. For instance, some RGC channels are extremely light sensitive but noisy (high false-positive rate), whereas others signal more reliably at the cost of sensitivity (high false-negative rate).[62,63,135]

Object motion sensitivity

Motion is ubiquitous in most visual environments, and different types of motion, like those of predators and prey, carry special behavioral significance. An animals' own movements also cause motion on its retina, hence it is critical to distinguish self-motion from that of external objects. The computation that identifies object motion amidst a background of global motion begins in the retina, where a set of object motion–sensitive (OMS) RGC circuits (Fig. 23.3A) effectively subtract global motion and respond selectively to moving objects[68] Fig. 23.3B).

The OMS circuit was first identified in the salamander retina.[136] It relies on wide-field ACs that capture signals from the receptive field (RF) surround and provide inhibitory input to BC axon terminals in the RF center, thereby canceling BC excitation for global motion covering both the RF center and surround. Despite its name, the OMS circuit does not rely on an explicit representation of motion in the RF center or surround. Instead, it uses nonlinear BC subunits to respond to *any* spatiotemporal contrast. Thus, the requirement for global motion cancellation is that contrast edges in the RF center and surround move at the same time regardless of their size, contrast, direction, or other details.[137]

Without advanced genetic tools, it has been difficult to associate specific retinal neurons with OMS circuits in salamander or rabbit retinas, so researchers have turned to the OMS RGCs in mice.[138] The first piece of evidence about the components of the mouse OMS circuit was that it relied on spiking ACs because it was blocked by the voltage-gated Na+ channel antagonist Tetrodotoxin (TTX).[138] Initially, OMS was identified in what was thought to be a single, genetically identified RGC type,[138] but it was later shown to be present in at least several other RGC types, depending on the kind of stimuli used.[60] A GABAergic wide-field AC type called TH (tyrosine hydroxylase) 2 was identified as a component of one OMS circuit

in the mouse.[139] However, unlike the spiking ACs implicated in the original study, TH2 cells do not fire action potentials and are unaffected by TTX.[139] Excitation to OMS RGCs may be provided by both BCs and a glutamatergic AC called VG3.[140,141] Because the OMS circuit is based on circuit motifs that are common in the retina (Fig. 23.3A), and nonlinear subunits in the RF center[142] and surround,[143] it is possible that variations of this computation occur in parallel, upstream of multiple RGC types.[18] It is conceivable that OMS is multiplexed with other retinal computations at the level of RGCs. Recent work in salamander has identified RGCs that are both OMS and direction selective (DS).[144]

Direction selectivity

Another important property of visual motion is its direction, and therefore it is not surprising that DS neurons are found across species and at different levels of the visual system, including the retina (reviewed in refs[46,145]) (Fig. 23.4). Nearly 60 years ago, Barlow and Levick studied the rabbit retina and found DS RGCs—so-called DSGCs—that spiked vigorously when an object moved in a specific direction across the cell's RF[146] (Fig. 23.4A2). Since then, many researchers have investigated DS circuits and mechanisms, particularly in rabbits and mice, making it one of the most studied and best understood retinal computations (reviewed in refs[147–150]).

Based on their response polarity and function, DSGCs fall into two groups. ON-OFF DS cells respond both to the leading and trailing edge of a bright bar moving on a dark background, whereas ON DS cells respond only to the leading edge. In addition, a single type of OFF DSGC may exist (discussed in ref[14]). ON-OFF DSGCs are sensitive to motion contrast and therefore signal local motion[151]; they send their axons to the dorsal lateral geniculate nucleus and the superior colliculus.[152,153] In contrast, ON DSGCs signal global motion,[154] send projections to nuclei of the accessory optic system, and are involved in controlling eye movement for gaze stabilization.[155,156] Both groups can be further subdivided by their preferred motion direction[157]: ON-OFF DSGCs prefer one of four directions (approximately anterior, posterior, superior, or inferior), whereas ON DSGCs prefer one of three directions (roughly aligned with the ocular muscles). This

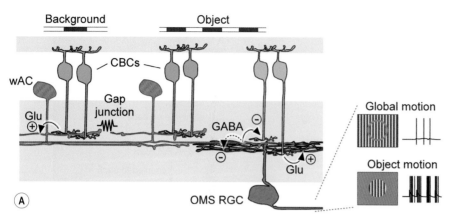

Fig. 23.3 Object motion–sensitive (*OMS*) circuits. (**A**) Schematic of circuit that implements the OMS computation.; for details, see text. (**B**) Spike rasters from OMS RGCs in rabbit and salamander responding to differential *(top)*, global *(middle)*, and local *(bottom)* motion. *CBC*, Cone bipolar cell; *Glu*, glutamate; *RGC*, retinal ganglion cell; *wAC*, wide-field amacrine cell. (**A**, own drawing; **B**, modified from Fig. 2 in Olveczky BP, Baccus SA, Meister M. Segregation of object and background motion in the retina. *Nature*. 2003;423:401–408.)

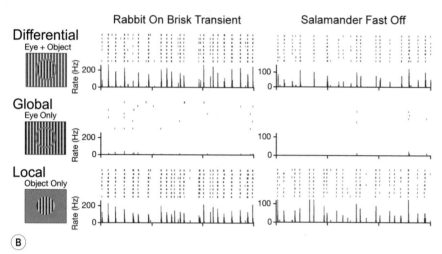

said, it is important to note that directional preference varies topographically across the retina and is aligned with optic flow fields, suggesting that the different DSGC types jointly encode specific directions of motion in space.[158]

As retinal direction selectivity is very robust, it is not surprising that several mechanisms are involved in this computation (reviewed in refs[46,145]). Some mechanisms act in parallel; some may be recruited depending on the stimulus context, for example, in the presence of noise.[159] DS RGCs receive excitatory input from different sets of CBCs and GABAergic inhibition, as well as from cholinergic excitation from so-called starburst ACs[160] (SACs; Fig. 23.4A). The role of SACs in direction selectivity was revealed by the finding that eliminating them from the circuitry strongly impairs DS tuning of DSGCs.[161] Indeed, SACs compute direction of motion in their neurites[91] (Fig. 23.4B,C), likely by a combination of intrinsic mechanisms[162,163] and asymmetries in synaptic connectivity with CBCs and among neighboring SACs.[92,164,165] SACs provide DSGCs with directionally tuned inhibitory input[166,167] that is spatially offset[168] (Fig. 23.4D,E). Recently, it has been shown also that the cholinergic output of SACs supports the DS tuning of the postsynaptic RGC.[50,169] Whether the glutamatergic input from CBCs to DSGCs contributes to direction selectivity is still a matter of debate.[170,171] Finally, the morphology and intrinsic properties of the DSGCs themselves sharpen the cells' DS spiking output.[172–175]

Orientation selectivity

Largely due to the Nobel prize-winning work of Hubel and Wiesel,[176] orientation selectivity is one of the best-known visual computations;

however, it is usually associated with cortex. In fact, at almost the same time as Hubel and Wiesel's work in cortex, orientation-selective (OS) cells were discovered in the retina of pigeons[177] and rabbits[178] (Fig. 23.5B,C). In the following decades, rabbit became the premier species for the study of retinal OS circuits. Researchers used pharmacology to identify a role for GABAergic ACs in the OS circuit[179,180] and found several types of OS ACs.[181,182]

When OS RGCs were found in mice, it became clear that they fell into at least two types: ON OS RGCs, which had OS inhibition from (unknown) ACs but also OS excitation through a variety of different mechanisms,[183] and OFF OS RGCs, the OS mechanism of which did not seem to rely on excitatory or inhibitory synapses[184] (Fig. 23.5A). Our focus here will be on the OFF OS circuit, where a specific AC type has been implicated. For in-depth reviews of both OS circuits, (see refs[72,185]).

Most RGCs inherit their feature selectivity from the interplay of their excitatory and inhibitory synaptic inputs, as described previously for the DS circuit. Therefore, it was surprising when experiments revealed that OFF OS RGCs in mice had non-OS inhibition and almost no measurable excitation in response to the same drifting grating stimuli that elicited strong OS spike responses. Instead, these RGCs inherited OS through electrical synapses via gap junctions with ACs. Anatomical tracing experiments revealed the specific AC type responsible, which is indeed OS due to its highly asymmetric morphology.[184] Notably, this "comet" AC type had previously been identified by electron microscopic reconstructions in mouse,[11] and it has counterparts in rabbit[186,187] and fish.[188]

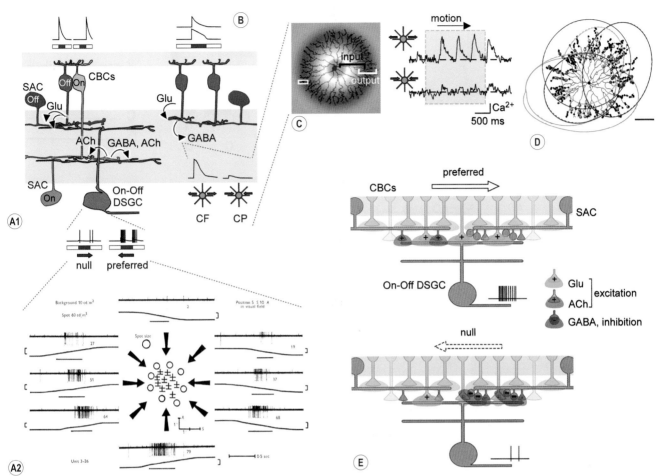

Fig. 23.4 Retinal direction selectivity. (**A1**) Simplified synaptic wiring of the retina direction-selective (*DS*) circuit: ON and OFF starburst amacrine cells (*SACs*) receive glutamatergic input from ON and OFF CBCs, respectively. Next, SACs release GABA onto DS retinal ganglion cells (*DSGCs; and other SACs, not shown*) and acetylcholine (*ACh*) onto bipolar cells (*BCs*) and DSGCs. (**A2**) Spiking activity of a DSGC recorded in rabbit retina and responding to a spot moving in eight directions. (**B**) Diverse mechanisms contribute to SACs generating directionally tuned dendritic output (for details, see text); here, one mechanism is depicted: Asymmetrical input by temporally distinct BC types along the SAC dendrite[92,165] (but see ref[164]). (**C**) SAC (*left*) with synaptic input and output zones indicated, and Ca²⁺ responses in distal dendrites (*rectangle*) to centrifugal (CF) and centripetal (CP) motion. (**D**) Asymmetric synaptic wiring between an SAC (*black*) and neighboring, postsynaptic DSGCs from electron microscopy (EM) data.[168] Synapses are color-coded by the preferred direction of the DSGCs, whose dendritic arbors are hinted by color-coded ellipses. (**E**) Illustration of synaptic input to DSGCs for preferred (*top*) and null (*bottom*) direction motion (ON circuit omitted for simplicity). Glutamatergic excitation (*green*) from CBCs and ACh-mediated excitation (*magenta*) from SACs dominate the DSGC input during preferred direction motion. Note that SACs on the *left* (preferred) side lack inhibitory connections to the DSGC. Motion in null direction evokes GABAergic inhibition (*red*) from spatially offset SACs selectively connected to the right (null) side of the DSGC, vetoing CBC input. Scale bar in (**D**) = 50 μm. (**A**, **B**: own drawings; **A2** modified from Fig. 1 in Barlow HB, Hill RM, Levick WR. Retinal ganglion cells responding selectively to direction and speed of image motion in the rabbit. *J Physiol.* 1964;173:377–407; panels **C, E** modified from Fig. 5 in Borst A, Euler T. Seeing things in motion: models, circuits, and mechanisms. *Neuron.* 2011;71:974–994; panel **D** modified from Fig. 4A in Briggman KL, Helmstaedter M, Denk W. Wiring specificity in the direction-selectivity circuit of the retina. *Nature.* 2011;471:183–188.)

CONCLUSIONS

The retina occupies a special place in neuroscience; its circuits are complex enough that they have revealed computational principles that apply throughout the central nervous system (CNS), yet it is approachable as an intact preparation with access to the full input (patterns of light) and output (RGC spikes).[189] In addition, our knowledge of cell types is more advanced in the retina than perhaps in any other part of the mammalian CNS.[13–15,19,21,55] For these reasons, research on visual processing in the inner retina has become a model for efforts to link intracellular, synaptic, and circuit motifs to neural computation. Prominent examples in which inner retinal research has led the field include the plasticity and information-processing roles of gap junctions,[190] the integration of functional and connectomic information to reveal selective wiring in the DS circuit,[168] and the dynamics of modulation of transmitter release in BCs.[191–193]

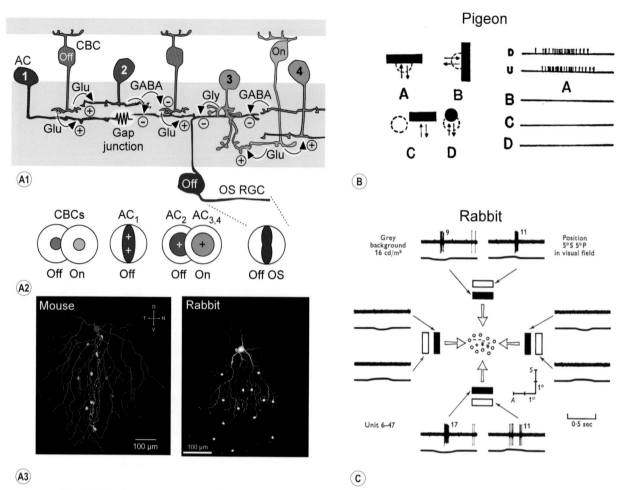

Fig. 23.5 Retinal orientation selectivity. (**A1**) Simplified synaptic wiring of a retinal orientation-selective (*OS*) circuit in mouse. (**A2**) Top-down view depicting the receptive field shapes of the cells in (**A1**). (**A3**) OFF OS retinal ganglion cells (*RGCs*) and electrically coupled amacrine cells (*ACs*). For the mouse example *(left)* the RGC is *magenta* and the ACs are *cyan*. (**B**) Example of a pigeon RGC responding to oriented bars as spots moving downward (*D*) and upward (*U*) as depicted on the *left*. (**C**) Example of rabbit RGC responding to oriented bars along with its estimated receptive field *(center)*. *CBC*, Cone bipolar cell; *Glu*, glutamate; *Gly*, glycine. (**A1 and A2**: From Schwartz, G. (2021). Retinal Computation (Elsevier Science).; **A3** used with permission from a figure in Schwartz G. *Retinal Computation*. Amsterdam: Elsevier Science; 2021; panel **B** used with permission from Fig. 2 in Maturana HR, Frenk S. Directional movement and horizontal edge detectors in the pigeon retina. *Science*. 1963;142: 977–979; **C** Adapted from Fig. 1 Schwartz, G. (2021). Retinal Computation (Elsevier Science).)

Despite these successes, significant challenges lie ahead. As mentioned in this chapter, we have only begun to scratch the surface of the complexity of AC circuits. Functions of the overwhelming majority of AC types remain unknown, including both the function of fast inhibitory transmitters (GABA and glycine) in most AC circuits and the vast array of slower-acting neuromodulators. Although the last decade has witnessed great advances in our knowledge of feature selectivity in RGCs, there remain substantially more known RGC types than specific visual features for which selectivity has been discovered.[18] A promising trend for the future of retinal computation research is the careful measurement of natural scene statistics[194] and their use as visual stimuli to discover new forms of feature selectivity.[195] Indeed, visual circuits evolved to meet particular behavioral demands, so understanding the visual behavioral repertoire of the animals we study may inspire new ideas about the feature selectivity of their neurons. Discovery of neural computations based on the statistics of the natural world and neuroethology may become another area of neuroscience in which the retina can lead the way.

REFERENCES

1. Schwartz G. *Retinal Computation*. Amsterdam: Elsevier Science; 2021.
2. Rodieck RW. *The first steps in seeing*. Sunderland, MA: Sinauer Associates; 1998.
3. Baden T, Euler T, Berens P. Understanding the retinal basis of vision across species. *Nat. Rev. Neurosci.* 2020;21:5–20.
4. Huberman AD, Niell CM. What can mice tell us about how vision works? *Trends Neurosci.* 2011;34:464–473.
5. Euler T, Haverkamp S, Schubert T, Baden T. Retinal bipolar cells: elementary building blocks of vision. *Nature Reviews Neuroscience*. 2014;15:507–519.
6. Martersteck EM, Hirokawa KE, Evarts M, Bernard A, Duan X, Li Y, Ng L, Oh SW, Ouellette B, Royall JJ, et al. Diverse central projection patterns of retinal ganglion cells. *Cell Rep.* 2017;18:2058–2072.
7. Morin LP, Studholme KM. Retinofugal projections in the mouse. *J. Comp. Neurol.* 2014;522:3733–3753.
8. Diamond JS. Inhibitory interneurons in the retina: types, circuitry, and function. *Annu Rev Vis Sci.* 2017;3:1–24.
9. Franke K, Baden T. General features of inhibition in the inner retina. *J. Physiol.* 2017;595: 5507–5515.
10. Wässle H, Puller C, Müller F, Haverkamp S. Cone contacts, mosaics, and territories of bipolar cells in the mouse retina. *J. Neurosci.* 2009;29:106–117.
11. Helmstaedter M, Briggman KL, Turaga SC, Jain V, Seung HS, Denk W. Connectomic reconstruction of the inner plexiform layer in the mouse retina. *Nature*. 2013;500:168–174.

12. Behrens C, Schubert T, Haverkamp S, Euler T, Berens P. Connectivity map of bipolar cells and photoreceptors in the mouse retina. *Elife*. 2016:5.

13. Goetz J, Jessen ZF, Jacobi A, Mani A, Cooler S, Greer D, Kadri S, Segal J, Shekhar K, Sanes J, et al. Unified classification of mouse retinal ganglion cells using function, morphology, and gene expression. *bioRxiv*. 2021:447922 2021.06.10.

14. Baden T, Berens P, Franke K, Román Rosón M, Bethge M, Euler T. The functional diversity of retinal ganglion cells in the mouse. *Nature*. 2016;529:345–350.

15. Bae JA, Alexander Bae J, Mu S, Kim JS, Turner NL, Tartavull I, Kemnitz N, Jordan CS, Norton AD, Silversmith WM, et al. Digital museum of retinal ganglion cells with dense anatomy and physiology. *Cell*. 2018;173:1293–1306.e19.

16. Sanes JR, Masland RH. The types of retinal ganglion cells: current status and implications for neuronal classification. *Annu. Rev. Neurosci*. 2015;38:221–246.

17. Wässle H, Boycott BB. Functional architecture of the mammalian retina. *Physiol. Rev*. 1991;71:447–480.

18. Schwartz GW, Swygart D. Circuits for Feature Selectivity in the Inner Retina. In *The Senses: A Comprehensive Reference*. Amsterdam: Elsevier Science Direct; 2008:275–292.

19. Yan W, Laboulaye MA, Tran NM, Whitney IE, Benhar I, Sanes JR. Mouse retinal cell atlas: Molecular identification of over sixty amacrine cell types. *J. Neurosci*. 2020;40:5177–5195.

20. Ghosh KK, Bujan S, Haverkamp S, Feigenspan A, Wässle H. Types of bipolar cells in the mouse retina. *J. Comp. Neurol*. 2004;469:70–82.

21. Shekhar K, Lapan SW, Whitney IE, Tran NM, Macosko EZ, Kowalczyk M, Adiconis X, Levin JZ, Nemesh J, Goldman M, et al. Comprehensive classification of retinal bipolar neurons by single-cell transcriptomics. *Cell*. 2016;166:1308–1323.e30.

22. Franke K, Berens P, Schubert T, Bethge M, Euler T, Baden T. Inhibition decorrelates visual feature representations in the inner retina. *Nature*. 2017;542:439–444.

23. Della Santina L, Kuo SP, Yoshimatsu T, Okawa H, Suzuki SC, Hoon M, Tsuboyama K, Rieke F, Wong ROL. Glutamatergic monopolar interneurons provide a novel pathway of excitation in the mouse retina. *Curr. Biol*. 2016;26:2070–2077.

24. Hack I, Peichl L, Brandstätter JH. An alternative pathway for rod signals in the rodent retina: rod photoreceptors, cone bipolar cells, and the localization of glutamate receptors. *Proc. Natl. Acad. Sci. U. S. A*. 1999;96:14130–14135.

25. Tsukamoto Y, Omi N. Some OFF bipolar cell types make contact with both rods and cones in macaque and mouse retinas. *Front. Neuroanat*. 2014;8:105.

26. Breuninger T, Puller C, Haverkamp S, Euler T. Chromatic bipolar cell pathways in the mouse retina. *J. Neurosci*. 2011;31:6504–6517.

27. Li W, DeVries SH. Bipolar cell pathways for color and luminance vision in a dichromatic mammalian retina. *Nat. Neurosci*. 2006;9:669–675.

28. Nomura A, Shigemoto R, Nakamura Y, Okamoto N, Mizuno N, Nakanishi S. Developmentally regulated postsynaptic localization of a metabotropic glutamate receptor in rat rod bipolar cells. *Cell*. 1994;77:361–369.

29. Vardi N, Duvoisin R, Wu G, Sterling P. Localization of mGluR6 to dendrites of ON bipolar cells in primate retina. *J. Comp. Neurol*. 2000;423:402–412.

30. Masu M, Iwakabe H, Tagawa Y, Miyoshi T, Yamashita M, Fukuda Y, Sasaki H, Hiroi K, Nakamura Y, Shigemoto R. Specific deficit of the ON response in visual transmission by targeted disruption of the mGluR6 gene. *Cell*. 1995;80:757–765.

31. Puller C, Ivanova E, Euler T, Haverkamp S, Schubert T. OFF bipolar cells express distinct types of dendritic glutamate receptors in the mouse retina. *Neuroscience*. 2013;243:136–148.

32. DeVries SH. Bipolar cells use kainate and AMPA receptors to filter visual information into separate channels. *Neuron*. 2000;28:847–856.

33. Lindstrom SH, Ryan DG, Shi J, DeVries SH. Kainate receptor subunit diversity underlying response diversity in retinal off bipolar cells. *J. Physiol*. 2014;592:1457–1477.

34. Burkhardt DA. Contrast processing by ON and OFF bipolar cells. *Vis. Neurosci*. 2011;28:69–75.

35. Rieke F. Temporal contrast adaptation in salamander bipolar cells. *J. Neurosci*. 2001;21:9445–9454.

36. MacNeil MA, Masland RH. Extreme diversity among amacrine cells: implications for function. *Neuron*. 1998;20:971–982.

37. Masland RH. The tasks of amacrine cells. *Vis. Neurosci*. 2012;29:3–9.

38. Lin B, Masland RH. Populations of wide-field amacrine cells in the mouse retina. *J. Comp. Neurol*. 2006;499:797–809.

39. Greschner M, Field GD, Li PH, Schiff ML, Gauthier JL, Ahn D, Sher A, Litke AM, Chichilnisky EJ. A polyaxonal amacrine cell population in the primate retina. *Journal of Neuroscience*. 2014;34:3597–3606.

40. Euler T, Denk W. Dendritic processing. *Curr. Opin. Neurobiol*. 2001;11:415–422.

41. Branco T, Häusser M. The single dendritic branch as a fundamental functional unit in the nervous system. *Curr. Opin. Neurobiol*. 2010;20:494–502.

42. Hnasko TS, Edwards RH. Neurotransmitter corelease: mechanism and physiological role. *Annu. Rev. Physiol*. 2012;74:225–243.

43. Tien N-W, Kim T, Kerschensteiner D. Target-specific glycinergic transmission from VGluT3-expressing amacrine cells shapes suppressive contrast responses in the retina. *Cell Rep*. 2016;15:1369–1375.

44. Roy S, Field GD. Dopaminergic modulation of retinal processing from starlight to sunlight. *J. Pharmacol. Sci*. 2019;140:86–93.

45. Hirasawa H, Betensky RA, Raviola E. Corelease of dopamine and GABA by a retinal dopaminergic neuron. *J. Neurosci*. 2012;32:13281–13291.

46. Mauss AS, Vlasits A, Borst A, Feller M. Visual circuits for direction selectivity. *Annu. Rev. Neurosci*. 2017;40:211–230.

47. Lee S, Kim K, Zhou ZJ. Role of ACh-GABA cotransmission in detecting image motion and motion direction. *Neuron*. 2010;68:1159–1172.

48. O'Malley DM, Sandell JH, Masland RH. Co-release of acetylcholine and GABA by the starburst amacrine cells. *J. Neurosci*. 1992;12:1394–1408.

49. Schmidt M, Humphrey MF, Wässle H. Action and localization of acetylcholine in the cat retina. *J. Neurophysiol*. 1987;58:997–1015.

50. Sethuramanujam S, Matsumoto A, deRosenroll G, Murphy-Baum B, Grosman C, McIntosh JM, Jing M, Li Y, Berson D, Yonehara K, et al. Rapid multi-directed cholinergic transmission in the central nervous system. *Nat. Commun*. 2021;12:1–13.

51. Provencio I, Jiang G, De Grip WJ, Hayes WP, Rollag MD. Melanopsin: an opsin in melanophores, brain, and eye. *Proc. Natl. Acad. Sci. U. S. A*. 1998;95:340–345.

52. Berson DM, Dunn FA, Takao M. Phototransduction by retinal ganglion cells that set the circadian clock. *Science*. 2002;295:1070–1073.

53. Freedman MS, Lucas RJ, Soni B, von Schantz M, Muñoz M, David-Gray Z, Foster R. Regulation of mammalian circadian behavior by non-rod, non-cone, ocular photoreceptors. *Science*. 1999;284:502–504.

54. Lucas RJ, Allen AE, Milosavljevic N, Storchi R, Woelders T. Can we see with melanopsin? *Annu Rev Vis Sci*. 2020;6:453–468.

55. Tran NM, Shekhar K, Whitney IE, Jacobi A, Benhar I, Hong G, Yan W, Adiconis X, Arnold ME, Lee JM, et al. Single-cell profiles of retinal ganglion cells differing in resilience to injury reveal neuroprotective genes. *Neuron*. 2019;104:1039–1055.e12.

56. Gollisch T, Meister M. Eye smarter than scientists believed: neural computations in circuits of the retina. *Neuron*. 2010;65:150–164.

57. Kolb H, Marshak D. The midget pathways of the primate retina. *Doc. Ophthalmol*. 2003;106:67–81.

58. Kolb H, Nelson RF, Ahnelt PK, Ortuño-Lizarán I, Cuenca N. The architecture of the human fovea. In: Kolb H, Fernandez E, Nelson R, eds. *Webvision: The Organization of the Retina and Visual System*. Salt Lake City, UT: University of Utah Health Sciences Center); 2020.

59. Westheimer G. The optics of the eye and visual acuity. *International Ophthalmology Clinics*. 1978;18:9–20.

60. Jacoby J, Schwartz GW. Three small-receptive-field ganglion cells in the mouse retina are distinctly tuned to size, speed, and object motion. *J. Neurosci*. 2017;37:610–625.

61. Krieger B, Qiao M, Rousso DL, Sanes JR, Meister M. Four alpha ganglion cell types in mouse retina: Function, structure, and molecular signatures. *PLoS One*. 2017;12:e0180091.

62. Smeds L, Takeshita D, Turunen T, Tiihonen J, Westö J, Martyniuk N, Seppänen A, Ala-Laurila P. Paradoxical rules of spike train decoding revealed at the sensitivity limit of vision. *Neuron*. 2019;104:576–587.e11.

63. Ala-Laurila P, Rieke F. Coincidence detection of single-photon responses in the inner retina at the sensitivity limit of vision. *Curr. Biol*. 2014;24:2888–2898.

64. Münch TA, da Silveira RA, Siegert S, Viney TJ, Awatramani GB, Roska B. Approach sensitivity in the retina processed by a multifunctional neural circuit. *Nat. Neurosci*. 2009;12:1308–1316.

65. Wang F, Li E, De L, Wu Q, Zhang Y. OFF-transient alpha RGCs mediate looming triggered innate defensive response. *Curr. Biol*. 2021;31:2263–2273.e3.

66. Krishnamoorthy V, Weick M, Gollisch T. Sensitivity to image recurrence across eye-movement-like image transitions through local serial inhibition in the retina. *Elife*. 2017:6.

67. Dhande OS, Estevez ME, Quattrochi LE, El-Danaf RN, Nguyen PL, Berson DM, Huberman AD. Genetic dissection of retinal inputs to brainstem nuclei controlling image stabilization. *Journal of Neuroscience*. 2013;33:17797–17813.

68. Olveczky BP, Baccus SA, Meister M. Segregation of object and background motion in the retina. *Nature*. 2003;423:401–408.

69. Homann J, Freed MA. A mammalian retinal ganglion cell implements a neuronal computation that maximizes the SNR of its postsynaptic currents. *J. Neurosci*. 2017;37:1468–1478.

70. Jacoby J, Schwartz GW. Typology and circuitry of suppressed-by-contrast retinal ganglion cells. *Front. Cell. Neurosci*. 2018;12:269.

71. Baden T, Osorio D. The retinal basis of vertebrate color vision. *Annu Rev Vis Sci*. 2019;5:177–200.

72. Antinucci P, Hindges R. Orientation-selective retinal circuits in vertebrates. *Front. Neural Circuits*. 2018;12:11.

73. Baden T, Berens P, Bethge M, Euler T. Spikes in mammalian bipolar cells support temporal layering of the inner retina. *Curr. Biol*. 2013;23:48–52.

74. Roska B, Werblin F. Vertical interactions across ten parallel, stacked representations in the mammalian retina. *Nature*. 2001;410:583–587.

75. Eggers ED, McCall MA, Lukasiewicz PD. Presynaptic inhibition differentially shapes transmission in distinct circuits in the mouse retina. *J. Physiol*. 2007;582:569–582.

76. Euler T, Wässle H. Different contributions of GABAA and GABAC receptors to rod and cone bipolar cells in a rat retinal slice preparation. *J. Neurophysiol*. 1998;79:1384–1395.

77. Euler T, Masland RH. Light-evoked responses of bipolar cells in a mammalian retina. *J. Neurophysiol*. 2000;83:1817–1829.

78. Eggers ED, Lukasiewicz PD. Multiple pathways of inhibition shape bipolar cell responses in the retina. *Vis. Neurosci*. 2011;28:95–108.

79. Nikolaev A, Leung K-M, Odermatt B, Lagnado L. Synaptic mechanisms of adaptation and sensitization in the retina. *Nat. Neurosci*. 2013;16:934–941.

80. Ozuysal Y, Baccus SA. Linking the computational structure of variance adaptation to biophysical mechanisms. *Neuron*. 2012;73:1002–1015.

81. Manookin MB, Demb JB. Presynaptic mechanism for slow contrast adaptation in mammalian retinal ganglion cells. *Neuron*. 2006;50:453–464.

82. Baden T, Euler T, Weckström M, Lagnado L. Spikes and ribbon synapses in early vision. *Trends Neurosci*. 2013;36:480–488.

83. Baden T, Esposti F, Nikolaev A, Lagnado L. Spikes in retinal bipolar cells phase-lock to visual stimuli with millisecond precision. *Curr. Biol*. 2011;21:1859–1869.

84. Puthussery T, Venkataramani S, Gayet-Primo J, Smith RG, Taylor WR. NaV1.1 channels in axon initial segments of bipolar cells augment input to magnocellular visual pathways in the primate retina. *J. Neurosci*. 2013;33:16045–16059.

85. Esposti F, Johnston J, Rosa JM, Leung K-M, Lagnado L. Olfactory stimulation selectively modulates the OFF pathway in the retina of zebrafish. *Neuron*. 2013;79:97–110.

86. D'Angelo I, Brecha NC. Y2 receptor expression and inhibition of voltage-dependent Ca2+ influx into rod bipolar cell terminals. *Neuroscience*. 2004;125:1039–1049.

87. Middleton TP, Huang JY, Protti DA. Cannabinoids modulate light signaling in ON-sustained retinal ganglion cells of the mouse. *Front. Neural Circuits*. 2019;13:37.

88. Wang X-H, Wu Y, Yang X-F, Miao Y, Zhang C-Q, Dong L-D, Yang X-L, Wang Z. Cannabinoid CB1 receptor signaling dichotomously modulates inhibitory and excitatory synaptic transmission in rat inner retina. *Brain Struct. Funct*. 2016;221:301–316.

89. Chávez AE, Diamond JS. Diverse mechanisms underlie glycinergic feedback transmission onto rod bipolar cells in rat retina. *J. Neurosci.* 2008;28:7919–7928.
90. Grimes WN, Zhang J, Graydon CW, Kachar B, Diamond JS. Retinal parallel processors: more than 100 independent microcircuits operate within a single interneuron. *Neuron.* 2010;65:873–885.
91. Euler T, Detwiler PB, Denk W. Directionally selective calcium signals in dendrites of starburst amacrine cells. *Nature.* 2002;418:845–852.
92. Vlasits AL, Morrie RD, Tran-Van-Minh A, Bleckert A, Gainer CF, DiGregorio DA, Feller MB. A role for synaptic input distribution in a dendritic computation of motion direction in the retina. *Neuron.* 2016;89:1317–1330.
93. Famiglietti Jr EV, Kolb H. A bistratified amacrine cell and synaptic circuitry in the inner plexiform layer of the retina. *Brain Res.* 1975;84:293–300.
94. Lee SCS, Meyer A, Schubert T, Hüser L, Dedek K, Haverkamp S. Morphology and connectivity of the small bistratified A8 amacrine cell in the mouse retina. *J. Comp. Neurol.* 2015;523:1529–1547.
95. Molnar A, Hsueh H-A, Roska B, Werblin FS. Crossover inhibition in the retina: circuitry that compensates for nonlinear rectifying synaptic transmission. *J. Comput. Neurosci.* 2009;27:569–590.
96. Koch C, Poggio T, Torre V. Retinal ganglion cells: a functional interpretation of dendritic morphology. *Philos. Trans. R. Soc. Lond. B Biol. Sci.* 1982;298:227–263.
97. Rheaume BA, Jereen A, Bolisetty M, Sajid MS, Yang Y, Renna K, Sun L, Robson P, Trakhtenberg EF. Single cell transcriptome profiling of retinal ganglion cells identifies cellular subtypes. *Nat. Commun.* 2018;9:2759.
98. Van Hook MJ, Nawy S, Thoreson WB. Voltage- and calcium-gated ion channels of neurons in the vertebrate retina. *Progress in Retinal and Eye Research.* 2019;72:100760.
99. Margolis DJ, Gartland AJ, Euler T, Detwiler PB. Dendritic calcium signaling in ON and OFF mouse retinal ganglion cells. *J. Neurosci.* 2010;30:7127–7138.
100. Tran-Van-Minh A, Cazé RD, Abrahamsson T, Cathala L, Gutkin BS, DiGregorio DA. Contribution of sublinear and supralinear dendritic integration to neuronal computations. *Front. Cell. Neurosci.* 2015;9:67.
101. Ran Y, Huang Z, Baden T, Schubert T, Baayen H, Berens P, Franke K, Euler T. Type-specific dendritic integration in mouse retinal ganglion cells. *Nat. Commun.* 2020;11:2101.
102. Velte TJ, Masland RH. Action potentials in the dendrites of retinal ganglion cells. *J. Neurophysiol.* 1999;81:1412–1417.
103. Kim KJ, Rieke F. Slow Na inactivation and variance adaptation in salamander retinal ganglion cells. *The Journal of Neuroscience.* 2003;23:1506–1516.
104. Mobbs P, Everett K, Cook A. Signal shaping by voltage-gated currents in retinal ganglion cells. *Brain Res.* 1992;574:217–223.
105. Raghuram V, Werginz P, Fried SI. Scaling of the AIS and somatodendritic compartments in α S RGCs. *Front. Cell. Neurosci.* 2019;13:436.
106. O'Brien BJ, Isayama T, Richardson R, Berson DM. Intrinsic physiological properties of cat retinal ganglion cells. *The Journal of Physiology.* 2002;538:787–802.
107. Werginz P, Raghuram V, Fried SI. The relationship between morphological properties and thresholds to extracellular electric stimulation in α RGCs. *J. Neural Eng.* 2020;17:045015.
108. Wienbar S, Schwartz GW. Differences in spike generation instead of synaptic inputs determine the feature selectivity of two retinal cell types. *bioRxiv.* 2021:464988 2021.10.19.
109. Dacey DM, Packer OS. Colour coding in the primate retina: diverse cell types and cone-specific circuitry. *Curr. Opin. Neurobiol.* 2003;13:421–427.
110. Mollon JD, Bowmaker JK, Jacobs GH. Variations of colour vision in a New World primate can be explained by polymorphism of retinal photopigments. *Proc. R. Soc. Lond. B Biol. Sci.* 1984;222:373–399.
111. Marshak DW, Mills SL. Short-wavelength cone-opponent retinal ganglion cells in mammals. *Vis. Neurosci.* 2014;31:165–175.
112. Martin PR, Lee BB, White AJ, Solomon SG, Rüttiger L. Chromatic sensitivity of ganglion cells in the peripheral primate retina. *Nature.* 2001;410:933–936.
113. Stockman A, Brainard DH. Color vision mechanisms. *The Optical Society of America handbook of optics.* 2010;311–11.
114. Sher A, DeVries SH. A non-canonical pathway for mammalian blue-green color vision. *Nat. Neurosci.* 2012;15:952–953.
115. Mills SL, Tian L-M, Hoshi H, Whitaker CM, Massey SC. Three distinct blue-green color pathways in a mammalian retina. *J. Neurosci.* 2014;34:1760–1768.
116. Dacey DM, Peterson BB, Robinson FR, Gamlin PD. Fireworks in the primate retina: in vitro photodynamics reveals diverse LGN-projecting ganglion cell types. *Neuron.* 2003;37:15–27.
117. Ghosh KK, Grünert U. Synaptic input to small bistratified (blue-ON) ganglion cells in the retina of a new world monkey, the marmoset Callithrix jacchus. *J. Comp. Neurol.* 1999;413:417–428.
118. Light AC, Zhu Y, Shi J, Saszik S, Lindstrom S, Davidson L, Li X, Chiodo VA, Hauswirth WW, Li W, et al. Organizational motifs for ground squirrel cone bipolar cells. *J. Comp. Neurol.* 2012;520:2864–2887.
119. Grünert U, Martin PR. Cell types and cell circuits in human and non-human primate retina. *Prog. Retin. Eye Res.* 2020:100844.
120. Chen S, Li W. A color-coding amacrine cell may provide a blue-off signal in a mammalian retina. *Nat. Neurosci.* 2012;15:954–956.
121. Schnapf JL, Copenhagen DR. Differences in the kinetics of rod and cone synaptic transmission. *Nature.* 1982;296:862–864.
122. Baylor DA, Hodgkin AL. Detection and resolution of visual stimuli by turtle photoreceptors. *J. Physiol.* 1973;234:163–198.
123. Donner K. Noise and the absolute thresholds of cone and rod vision. *Vision Res.* 1992;32:853–866.
124. Tikidji-Hamburyan A, Reinhard K, Storchi R, Dietter J, Seitter H, Davis KE, Idrees S, Mutter M, Walmsley L, Bedford RA, et al. Rods progressively escape saturation to drive visual responses in daylight conditions. *Nat. Commun.* 2017;8:1813.
125. Stockman A, Sharpe LT, Rüther K, Nordby K. Two signals in the human rod visual system: a model based on electrophysiological data. *Vis. Neurosci.* 1995;12:951–970.
126. Dacheux RF, Raviola E. The rod pathway in the rabbit retina: a depolarizing bipolar and amacrine cell. *J. Neurosci.* 1986;6:331–345.
127. Bloomfield SA, Dacheux RF. Rod vision: pathways and processing in the mammalian retina. *Prog. Retin. Eye Res.* 2001;20:351–384.
128. Oesch N, Diamond J. A night vision neuron gets a day job. *Nat. Neurosci.* 2009;12: 1209–1211.
129. Raviola E, Gilula NB. Gap junctions between photoreceptor cells in the vertebrate retina. *Proc. Natl. Acad. Sci. U. S. A.* 1973;70:1677–1681.
130. Wässle H, Grüunert U, Chun M-N, Boycott BB. The rod pathway of the macaque monkey retina: identification of AII-amacrine cells with antibodies against calretinin. *Journal of Comparative Neurology.* 1995;361:537–551.
131. Tsukamoto Y, Morigiwa K, Ueda M, Sterling P. Microcircuits for night vision in mouse retina. *J. Neurosci.* 2001;21:8616–8623.
132. Grimes WN, Sedlacek M, Musgrove M, Nath A, Tian H, Hoon M, Rieke F, Singer JH, Diamond JS. Dendro-somatic synaptic inputs to ganglion cells contradict receptive field and connectivity conventions in the mammalian retina. *Curr. Biol.* 2022;32:315–328.e4.
133. Taylor WR, Smith RG. Transmission of scotopic signals from the rod to rod-bipolar cell in the mammalian retina. *Vision Res.* 2004;44:3269–3276.
134. Smith RG, Freed MA, Sterling P. Microcircuitry of the dark-adapted cat retina: functional architecture of the rod-cone network. *J. Neurosci.* 1986;6:3505–3517.
135. Takeshita D, Smeds L, Ala-Laurila P. Processing of single-photon responses in the mammalian On and Off retinal pathways at the sensitivity limit of vision. *Philos. Trans. R. Soc. Lond. B Biol. Sci.* 2017:372.
136. Baccus SA, Olveczky BP, Manu M, Meister M. A retinal circuit that computes object motion. *J. Neurosci.* 2008;28:6807–6817.
137. Schwartz GW, Swygart D. Object motion sensitivity. In Retinal Computation. Amsterdam: Elsevier Science; 2021;230–244.
138. Zhang Y, Kim I-J, Sanes JR, Meister M. The most numerous ganglion cell type of the mouse retina is a selective feature detector. *Proc. Natl. Acad. Sci. U. S. A.* 2012;109:E2391–8.
139. Kim T, Kerschensteiner D. Inhibitory control of feature selectivity in an object motion sensitive circuit of the retina. *Cell Rep.* 2017;19:1343–1350.
140. Krishnaswamy A, Yamagata M, Duan X, Hong YK, Sanes JR. Sidekick 2 directs formation of a retinal circuit that detects differential motion. *Nature.* 2015;524:466–470.
141. Kim T, Soto F, Kerschensteiner D. An excitatory amacrine cell detects object motion and provides feature-selective input to ganglion cells in the mouse retina. *Elife.* 2015:4.
142. Schwartz GW, Okawa H, Dunn FA, Morgan JL, Kerschensteiner D, Wong RO, Rieke F. The spatial structure of a nonlinear receptive field. *Nat. Neurosci.* 2012;15:1572–1580.
143. Takeshita D, Gollisch T. Nonlinear spatial integration in the receptive field surround of retinal ganglion cells. *J. Neurosci.* 2014;34:7548–7561.
144. Kühn NK, Gollisch T. Joint encoding of object motion and motion direction in the salamander retina. *J. Neurosci.* 2016;36:12203–12216.
145. Borst A, Euler T. Seeing things in motion: models, circuits, and mechanisms. *Neuron.* 2011;71:974–994.
146. Barlow HB, Hill RM. Selective sensitivity to direction of movement in ganglion cells of the rabbit retina. *Science.* 1963;139:412–414.
147. Demb JB. Cellular mechanisms for direction selectivity in the retina. *Neuron.* 2007;55: 179–186.
148. Vaney DI, Sivyer B, Taylor WR. Direction selectivity in the retina: symmetry and asymmetry in structure and function. *Nat. Rev. Neurosci.* 2012;13:194–208.
149. Rasmussen R, Yonehara K. Contributions of retinal direction selectivity to central visual processing. *Curr. Biol.* 2020;30:R897–R903.
150. Wei W. Neural mechanisms of motion processing in the mammalian retina. *Annu Rev Vis Sci.* 2018;4:165–192.
151. Chiao C-C, Masland RH. Contextual tuning of direction-selective retinal ganglion cells. *Nat. Neurosci.* 2003;6:1251–1252.
152. Huberman AD, Wei W, Elstrott J, Stafford BK, Feller MB, Barres BA. Genetic identification of an On-Off direction-selective retinal ganglion cell subtype reveals a layer-specific subcortical map of posterior motion. *Neuron.* 2009;62:327–334.
153. Rivlin-Etzion M, Zhou K, Wei W, Elstrott J, Nguyen PL, Barres BA, Huberman AD, Feller MB. Transgenic mice reveal unexpected diversity of on-off direction-selective retinal ganglion cell subtypes and brain structures involved in motion processing. *J. Neurosci.* 2011;31:8760–8769.
154. Wyatt HJ, Daw NW. Directionally sensitive ganglion cells in the rabbit retina: specificity for stimulus direction, size, and speed. *J. Neurophysiol.* 1975;38:613–626.
155. Yonehara K, Ishikane H, Sakuta H, Shintani T, Nakamura-Yonehara K, Kamiji NL, Usui S, Noda M. Identification of retinal ganglion cells and their projections involved in central transmission of information about upward and downward image motion. *PLoS ONE.* 2009;4:e4320.
156. Berson DM. Retinal Ganglion Cell Types and Their Central Projections. In The Senses: A Comprehensive Reference, Amsterdam: Elsevier Science Direct; 2008:491–519.
157. Oyster CW, Barlow HB. Direction-selective units in rabbit retina: distribution of preferred directions. *Science.* 1967;155:841–842.
158. Sabbah S, Gemmer JA, Bhatia-Lin A, Manoff G, Castro G, Siegel JK, Jeffery N, Berson DM. A retinal code for motion along the gravitational and body axes. *Nature.* 2017;546:492–497.
159. Chen Q, Pei Z, Koren D, Wei W. Stimulus-dependent recruitment of lateral inhibition underlies retinal direction selectivity. *Elife.* 2016:5.
160. Famiglietti Jr EV. "Starburst" amacrine cells and cholinergic neurons: mirror-symmetric on and off amacrine cells of rabbit retina. *Brain Res.* 1983;261:138–144.
161. Yoshida K, Watanabe D, Ishikane H, Tachibana M, Pastan I, Nakanishi S. A key role of starburst amacrine cells in originating retinal directional selectivity and optokinetic eye movement. *Neuron.* 2001;30:771–780.
162. Tukker JJ, Taylor WR, Smith RG. Direction selectivity in a model of the starburst amacrine cell. *Vis. Neurosci.* 2004;21:611–625.
163. Hausselt SE, Euler T, Detwiler PB, Denk W. A dendrite-autonomous mechanism for direction selectivity in retinal starburst amacrine cells. *PLoS Biol.* 2007;5:e185.

164. Ding H, Smith RG, Poleg-Polsky A, Diamond JS, Briggman KL. Species-specific wiring for direction selectivity in the mammalian retina. *Nature.* 2016;535:105–110.
165. Kim JS, Greene MJ, Zlateski A, Lee K, Richardson M, Turaga SC, Purcaro M, Balkam M, Robinson A, Behabadi BF, et al. Space–time wiring specificity supports direction selectivity in the retina. *Nature.* 2014;509:331–336.
166. Borg-Graham LJ. The computation of directional selectivity in the retina occurs presynaptic to the ganglion cell. *Nat. Neurosci.* 2001;4:176–183.
167. Taylor WR, Vaney DI. Diverse synaptic mechanisms generate direction selectivity in the rabbit retina. *J. Neurosci.* 2002;22:7712–7720.
168. Briggman KL, Helmstaedter M, Denk W. Wiring specificity in the direction-selectivity circuit of the retina. *Nature.* 2011;471:183–188.
169. Sethuramanujam S, McLaughlin AJ, deRosenroll G, Hoggarth A, Schwab DJ, Awatramani GB. A central role for mixed acetylcholine/GABA transmission in direction coding in the retina. *Neuron.* 2016;90:1243–1256.
170. Matsumoto A, Agbariah W, Nolte SS, Andrawos R, Levi H, Sabbah S, Yonehara K. Synapse-specific direction selectivity in retinal bipolar cell axon terminals. *Neuron.* 2021;109(18):2928–2942.
171. Yonehara K, Farrow K, Ghanem A, Hillier D, Balint K, Teixeira M, Jüttner J, Noda M, Neve RL, Conzelmann K-K, et al. The first stage of cardinal direction selectivity is localized to the dendrites of retinal ganglion cells. *Neuron.* 2013;79:1078–1085.
172. Schachter MJ, Oesch N, Smith RG, Taylor WR. Dendritic spikes amplify the synaptic signal to enhance detection of motion in a simulation of the direction-selective ganglion cell. *PLoS Comput. Biol.* 2010:6.
173. Oesch N, Euler T, Taylor WR. Direction-selective dendritic action potentials in rabbit retina. *Neuron.* 2005;47:739–750.
174. Sivyer B, Williams SR. Direction selectivity is computed by active dendritic integration in retinal ganglion cells. *Nat. Neurosci.* 2013;16:1848–1856.
175. Trenholm S, Johnson K, Li X, Smith RG, Awatramani GB. Parallel mechanisms encode direction in the retina. *Neuron.* 2011;71:683–694.
176. Hubel DH, Wiesel TN. Receptive fields, binocular interaction and functional architecture in the cat's visual cortex. *J. Physiol.* 1962;160:106–154.
177. Maturana HR, Frenk S. Directional movement and horizontal edge detectors in the pigeon retina. *Science.* 1963;142:977–979.
178. Levick WR. Receptive fields and trigger features of ganglion cells in the visual streak of the rabbit's retina. *J. Physiol.* 1967;188:285–307.
179. Caldwell JH, Daw NW, Wyatt HJ. Effects of picrotoxin and strychnine on rabbit retinal ganglion cells: lateral interactions for cells with more complex receptive fields. *J. Physiol.* 1978;276:277–298.
180. Venkataramani S, Taylor WR. Synaptic mechanisms generating orientation selectivity in the ON pathway of the rabbit retina. *J. Neurosci.* 2016;36:3336–3349.
181. Bloomfield SA. Orientation-sensitive amacrine and ganglion cells in the rabbit retina. *J. Neurophysiol.* 1994;71:1672–1691.
182. Murphy-Baum BL, Taylor WR. The synaptic and morphological basis of orientation selectivity in a polyaxonal amacrine cell of the rabbit retina. *J. Neurosci.* 2015;35:13336–13350.
183. Nath A, Schwartz GW. Cardinal orientation selectivity is represented by two distinct ganglion cell types in mouse retina. *J. Neurosci.* 2016;36:3208–3221.
184. Nath A, Schwartz GW. Electrical synapses convey orientation selectivity in the mouse retina. *Nat. Commun.* 2017;8:2025.
185. Schwartz, G.W. Orientation selectivity. In: Retinal Computation. Amsterdam: Elsevier Science; 2021; 185.
186. Famiglietti EV. *Structural organization and development of dorsally-directed (vertical) asymmetrical amacrine cells in rabbit retina. Neurobiology of the Inner Retina.* Springer Berlin Heidelberg; 1989:169–180.
187. Hoshi H, Mills SL. Components and properties of the G3 ganglion cell circuit in the rabbit retina. *J. Comp. Neurol.* 2009;513:69–82.
188. Wagner HJ, Wagner E. Amacrine cells in the retina of a teleost fish, the roach (Rutilus rutilus): a Golgi study on differentiation and layering. *Philos. Trans. R. Soc. Lond. B Biol. Sci.* 1988;321:263–324.
189. Dowling JE. *The Retina: An Approachable Part of the Brain.* Cambridge, MA: Harvard University Press; 1987.
190. Bloomfield SA, Völgyi B. The diverse functional roles and regulation of neuronal gap junctions in the retina. *Nat. Rev. Neurosci.* 2009;10:495–506.
191. Schröder C, Klindt D, Strauss S, Franke K, Bethge M, Euler T, Berens P. System identification with biophysical constraints: a circuit model of the inner retina. In: Systems H, Larochelle M, Ranzato R, Hadsell MF, Balcan Lin H, eds. *Advances in Neural Information Processing.* (Red Hook: NY: Curran Associates, Inc.); 2020:15439–15450.
192. Oesterle J, Behrens C, Schröder C, Hermann T, Euler T, Franke K, Smith RG, Zeck G, Berens P. Bayesian inference for biophysical neuron models enables stimulus optimization for retinal neuroprosthetics. *Elife.* 2020:9.
193. Schröder C, James B, Lagnado L, Berens P. Approximate Bayesian inference for a mechanistic model of vesicle release at a ribbon synapse. In: Systems H, Wallach H, Larochelle A, Beygelzimer F, Alché-Buc E, Fox Garnett R, eds. *Advances in Neural Information Processing.* Red Hook, NY: Curran Associates, Inc; 2019:7070–7080.
194. Qiu Y, Zhao Z, Klindt D, Kautzky M, Szatko KP, Schaeffel F, Rifai K, Franke K, Busse L, Euler T. Natural environment statistics in the upper and lower visual field are reflected in mouse retinal specializations. *Curr. Biol.* 2021;31:3233–3247.e6.
195. Tanaka H, Nayebi A, Maheswaranathan N, McIntosh L, Baccus SA, Ganguli S. From deep learning to mechanistic understanding in neuroscience: the structure of retinal prediction. *Adv Neural Inf Process Syst.* 2019;2019(32):8537–8547.

24

Electroretinogram

Laura J. Frishman

INTRODUCTION

The electroretinogram (ERG) is a useful tool for objective, noninvasive assessment of retinal function both in the clinic and the laboratory. It is a mass electrical potential that represents the summed response of all the cells in the retina to a change in illumination. Recordings can be made in vivo under physiologic or nearly physiologic conditions using electrodes placed on the corneal surface. For standard recordings in the clinic,[1] ERGs such as those illustrated in Fig. 24.1 are recorded from alert subjects who are asked not to blink or to move their eyes. Anesthesia, selected for having minimal effects on retinal function, may be required for recordings from some very young human subjects, and is generally used for recordings in animals. The positive and negative waves of the ERG reflect the summed activity of overlapping positive and negative component potentials that originate from different stages of retinal processing. The choice of stimulus conditions and method of analysis will help to determine which of the various retinal cells and circuits are generating the response. Information about retinal function provided by the ERG is useful for diagnosing and characterizing retinal diseases, monitoring disease progression, and evaluating the effectiveness of therapeutic interventions.

Much of the basic research on the origins, pathophysiology, and treatment of retinal diseases that occur in humans has been carried out in animal models. The ERG provides a simple objective approach for assessing retinal function in animals. It has been of particular benefit in studies of mouse, rat, other species, various models of retinal disease, and retinal drug toxicity.[2] The ERG also has been very useful for characterizing changes in retinal function that occur as a consequence of genetic alterations in mice, in other animal models for human disease, and in humans themselves, that affect the generation, transmission, and processing of visual signals.[3,4] This chapter provides information on retinal origins and interpretation of the ERG, with emphasis on advances in our understanding of the ERG that have occurred through pharmacologic dissection studies in macaque monkeys, whose retinas are similar to those of humans. The similarity of the waveforms of flash ERGs of humans and macaques can be seen in Fig. 24.2. The chapter also will examine origins of the mouse ERG and consider similarities and differences between mouse and primate ERG. Although the focus of this chapter is on primate and rodent retinas, it is important to note that the ERG is a valuable tool for assessing retinal function of all classes of vertebrates. This includes amphibians and fish, in which classical studies of the retina were carried out (for a review, see Dowling[8]) and in which current studies continue to improve our understanding of retinal function under normal, genetically altered,[9] and pathologic conditions.

This chapter provides useful background information for interpreting the ERG but does not provide a comprehensive review of the characteristics of ERGs associated with retinal disorders encountered in the clinic. A guide to electrodiagnostic procedures[10] and the more comprehensive texts of Heckenlively and Arden[11] and Lam[12] are useful resources for learning more about clinical applications.

GENERATION OF THE ELECTRORETINOGRAM

Radial current flow

The ERG is an extracellular potential that arises from currents that flow through the retina as a result of neuronal signaling and, for some slower ERG waves, potassium (K^+) currents in glial cells. Local changes in the membrane conductance of activated cells give rise to inward or outward ion currents, and cause currents to flow in the extracellular space (ECS) around the cells, creating extracellular potentials. Although all retinal cell types can contribute to ERGs recorded at the cornea, the contribution of a particular type may be large, or hardly noticeable in the recorded waveform, depending upon several factors detailed further in the chapter.

The orientation of a cell type in the retina is a major factor in determining the extent to which its activity will contribute to the ERG. A schematic drawing of the mammalian retina with the various cell types labeled can be found in Chapter 21 (Figs. 21.1 and 21.2). When activated synchronously by a change in illumination, retinal neurons that are radially oriented with respect to the cornea, i.e., the photoreceptors and bipolar cells, make larger contributions to the major waves of the ERG than the more laterally oriented cells and their processes (i.e., the horizontal and amacrine cells). The major waves at light onset are, as marked in Figs. 24.1 and 24.2, initial negative-going a-waves (mainly from photoreceptors), which are followed by positive-going b-waves, mainly generated by ON (depolarizing) bipolar cells. For longer-duration flashes (Fig. 24.2, *bottom row*), the light-adapted ERG includes the b-wave at light onset, and another positive-going wave, the d-wave, at light offset, with major contribution from OFF (hyperpolarizing) bipolar cells. Currents that leave retinal cells and enter the ECS at one retinal depth (the current source) will leave the ECS to re-enter the cells at another (the current sink), creating a current dipole. These retinal currents also travel through the vitreous humor to the cornea, where the ERG can be recorded noninvasively, as well as through the extraocular tissue, sclera, choroid, and high resistance of the retinal pigment epithelium (RPE), before returning to the retina. Local ERGs can be recorded near the retinal generators using intraretinal microelectrodes in animals, while simultaneously recording the global ERG elsewhere in the current path, for example, from the corneal surface, or using an electrode in the vitreous humor, with a reference electrode behind the eye.[13,14] Historically, such recordings have provided useful information about the origins of the various waves of the ERG.

Glial currents

The ERG waveform is also affected by glial cell and RPE cell currents. Retinal glial cells whose currents affect the ERG include Müller cells and radial astrocytes in the optic nerve head. One crucial function of

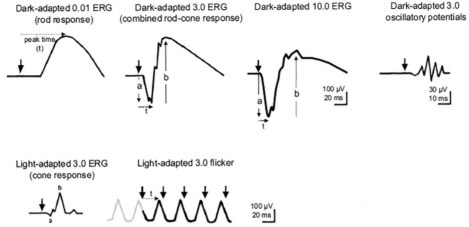

Fig. 24.1 Standard tests for full-field clinical electrophysiology. The Society for the Clinical Electrophysiology of Vision (ISCEV) has recommended five standard electroretinogram (*ERG*) tests with full-field stimulation for use worldwide in clinical electrodiagnostic facilities. This figure, from the 2015 update of *ISCEV Standard for Full-Field Clinical Electroretinography*[1] shows examples, but not norms, of ERGs elicited using the recommended tests in normal humans. Light calibrations in candela seconds per meter squared (cd.s.m^{-2}) for each test appear above the ERGs. *Large arrowheads* indicate the time at which the stimulus flash occurred. *Dashed arrows* show common ways to measure time-to-peak ("t," implicit time), and a- and b-wave amplitudes. For some purposes, for example, quantitative analyses to separate various ERG components, amplitude measurements at a fixed time after stimulus onset are more appropriate (see Fig. 24.12). (From McCulloch DL, Marmor MF, Brigell MG, et al. ISCEV Standard for full-field clinical electroretinography (2015 update). *Doc Ophthalmol.* 2015;130:1–12, used with permission.)

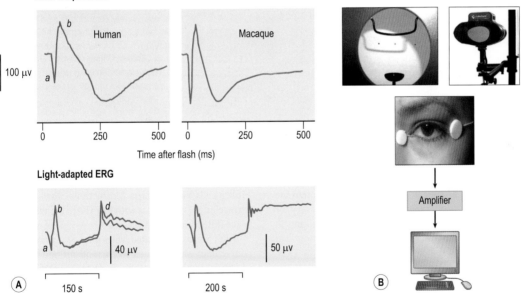

Fig. 24.2 Full-field flash electroretinograms (*ERGs*) of human subjects and macaque monkeys. (**A**) *Top*: Dark-adapted ERG responses to brief high energy flashes of ~400 scotopic troland seconds (sc td.s) from darkness that occurred at time zero for a normal alert human subject *(left)* and an anesthetized macaque *(right)*. For macaque ERGs, and ERGs from all animals in subsequent figures, subjects were anesthetized. *Bottom*: Light-adapted ERGs in response to longer duration flashes (150 or 200 ms). For both subjects, white Ganzfeld flashes of 4.0 log photopic (ph) td were presented on a steady rod-saturating background of 3.3 log sc td. (*Top* modified from Robson JG, Frishman LJ. Dissecting the dark-adapted electroretinogram. *Doc Ophthalmol.* 1998; 95(3–4):187–215 used with permission; *bottom* modified from Sieving PA, Murayama K, Naarendorp F. Push-pull model of the primate photopic electroretinogram: a role for hyperpolarizing neurons in shaping the b-wave. *Vis Neurosci.* 1994;11(3):519–532, used with permission.) (**B**) ERG recording setup: recordings made using a traditional Ganzfeld bowl *(left)* or more modern LED-based full-field stimulator. Use of DTL fiber electrodes[7] is illustrated. ERG recordings are amplified and sent to a computer for averaging, display, and analysis.

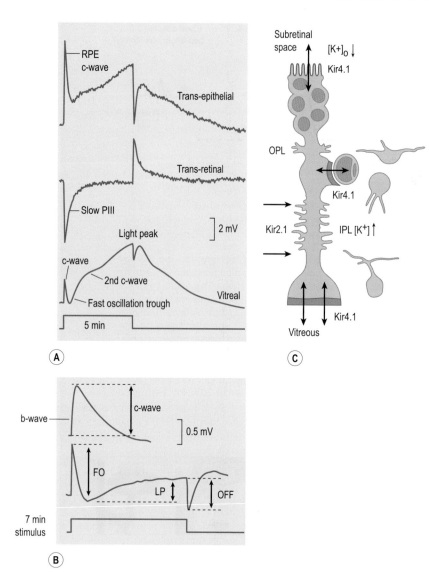

Fig. 24.3 Distal retinal components of the direct-current electroretinogram (dc-ERG), and distribution of inward-rectifying potassium channels, Kir2.1 and Kir4.1, in Müller cells. **(A)** Simultaneous intraretinal (local) and vitreal (global) ERG recordings from the intact eye of the cat. *Top:* Transretinal potentials and transepithelial potentials (TEP) were recorded in response to a 5-minute period of illumination. The a- and b-waves cannot be seen due to the compressed time scale. The intraretinal recordings show the two (sub)components of the c-wave: (1) the retinal pigment epithelium (RPE) c-wave, which is the TEP recorded between a microelectrode in the subretinal space and a retrobulbar reference, and (2) slow PIII, the cornea-negative transretinal component generated by Müller cell currents (see text), recorded between the same microelectrode and the vitreal electrode. The vitreal ERG *(bottom)*, recorded between the vitreal electrode and retrobulbar reference, is the sum of the RPE c-wave and slow PIII. The c-wave is followed by the fast oscillation (FO) trough and then the light peak (LP), both of which are exclusively RPE responses. (From Steinberg RH, Linsenmeier RA, Griff ER. Retinal pigment epithelial cell contributions to the electroretinogram and electrooculogram. *Prog Retin Res.* 1985;4:33–66, used with permission.) **(B)** Direct-current electroretinogram (dc-ERG) recorded from a C57BL/6 mouse in response to a 7-minute period of illumination. FO, LP, and OFF-response amplitudes are marked by *arrows. Upper* record shows the early portion of the response on an expanded (×5) time scale. Amplitude calibration: 0.5mV. (From Kofuji P, Biedermann B, Siddharthan V, et al. Kir potassium channel subunit expression in retinal glial cells: implications for spatial potassium buffering. *Glia.* 2002;39(3):292–303, used with permission.) **(C)** Strongly rectifying Kir2.1 channels are widely distributed in the Müller cell membrane. K+ in synaptic regions enters Müller cells through strongly rectifying Kir2.1 channels and exits through weakly rectifying (bidirectional) Kir4.1 channels concentrated in the ILM, inner limiting membrane OLL, outer limiting lamina and Müller cell processes around blood vessels. *IPL,* Inner plexiform layer; *OPL,* outer plexiform layer. (Modified from Kofuji P, Biedermann B, Siddharthan V, et al. Kir potassium channel subunit expression in retinal glial cells: implications for spatial potassium buffering. *Glia.* 2002;39(3):292–303, used with permission.)

glia is to regulate extracellular K+ concentration, $[K^+]_o$, to maintain the electrochemical gradients across cell membranes that are necessary for normal neuronal function. Membrane depolarization and spiking in retinal neurons that occur in response to changes in illumination lead to leak of K+ from the neurons and to K+ accumulation in the ECS. Membrane hyperpolarization, in contrast, leads to lower $[K^+]_o$ as the membrane leak conductance is reduced, but the Na+ K+-ATPase in the membrane continues to transport K+ into the cell.

K+ currents in Müller cells move excess K+ from areas of high $[K^+]_o$ to areas of lower $[K^+]_o$ by a process called spatial buffering.[15,16] Return currents in the retina are formed by Na+ and Cl-. The regional distribution and electrical properties of inward-rectifying K+ (Kir) channels in Müller cells (see Fig. 24.3C) are critical for the spatial buffering capacity of the cells. Studies by Kofuji and coworkers have shown that strongly rectifying Kir2.1 channels in Müller cells are located in "source" areas, particularly in synaptic regions where $[K^+]_o$ is elevated due to local neuronal activity.[19,20] In contrast, Kir4.1 channels (weakly rectifying) are densest in Müller cell endfeet, in inner and outer limiting membranes, and in processes around blood vessels. K+ enters Müller cells through Kir2.1 channels that minimize K+ outflow and K+ exits the

Müller cells via the more bidirectional Kir4.1 channels to enter the extracellular "sink" areas with low $[K^+]_o$: the vitreous humor, subretinal space (SRS), and blood vessels.[19]

ERG waves associated with glial K+ currents have a slower time course than waves related to currents around the neurons, the activity of which causes the changes in $[K^+]_o$. As $[K^+]_o$ increases or decreases with neuronal activity, the resulting glial K+ currents will be related to the integral of the K+ flow rate.[5] Other waves generated by glial K+ currents in Müller cells, or other retina cells that move K+ such as the RPE cells, include the c-wave and slow PIII (Fig. 24.3A,B), both related to the reduction in $[K^+]_o$ in the SRS that occurs when photoreceptors hyperpolarize in response to a strong flash of light.[17,20–25] The negative scotopic threshold response (nSTR) and photopic negative response (PhNR), both originating from inner retinal activity, are also thought to be mediated by glial K+ currents resulting from that activity, in the retina or optic nerve head.[26–33]

Stimulus conditions

Aside from structural and functional aspects of the retina, stimulus conditions are of great importance in determining the extent to which particular retinal cells and circuits contribute to the ERG. Signals will be generated in rod pathways, in cone pathways, or in both, depending upon the stimulus energy, wavelength, and temporal characteristics, as well as upon the extent of background illumination, with rods responding to, and being desensitized by, lower light levels than cones. Fully dark-adapted ERGs driven by rods only (i.e., scotopic ERGs) are thus useful for assessing rod pathway function (dark-adapted ERGs in Figs. 24.1 and 24.2, *top*), and light-adapted ERGs driven only by cones (i.e., photopic ERGs), for assessing cone pathway function (Figs. 24.1 and 24.2, *bottom*). Fig. 24.1, *bottom right*, also shows responses to 30 Hz flicker, which isolates cone-driven responses because rod circuits do not resolve high frequencies well. Bright light flashes elicit small wavelets superimposed on the b-wave called oscillatory potentials (OPs) that are generated by circuits proximal to bipolar cells.[34,35] OPs can be isolated by bandpass filtering: 75 to 300 Hz in Fig. 24.1, *top right*.

The spatial extent of the stimulus is an important factor in ERG testing. For standard clinical tests, as illustrated in Fig. 24.1, and listed in Box 24.1A, as well as for most testing of animal models, a full-field (Ganzfeld) flash of light is used (Fig. 24.2B). A full-field stimulus generally elicits the largest responses because more retinal cells are activated and the extracellular current is larger than for focal stimuli. Full-field stimulation also has the advantage that all regions of retina are evenly illuminated and, with respect to background illumination, evenly adapted. Pupils are generally dilated for full-field stimulation. More spatially localized (focal) stimuli are useful for analysis of function of particular retinal regions, for example, foveal versus peripheral regions in primates. Multifocal stimulation allows assessment of many small regions simultaneously.

ERG responses for a minimum set of stimuli were selected by the International Society for the Clinical Electrophysiology of Vision (ISCEV) to efficiently acquire standard, comparable data on rod and cone pathway function from clinics and laboratories around the world (illustrated in Fig. 24.1).[1] Names of the standard tests are listed in Box 24.1A. Tests using stimuli presented over a fuller range of stimulus conditions to allow more complete or specific evaluation of retinal function, are listed in Box 24.1B, and a few of these tests will be described later in this chapter.

NONINVASIVE RECORDING OF THE ELECTRORETINOGRAM

ERGs can be recorded from the corneal surface using various types of electrodes. A commonly used electrode, with good signal-to-noise characteristics, is a contact lens with a conductive metal electrode set into it (Burian Allen electrode). It has a lid speculum to reduce effects of blinking and eye closure. In the bipolar form of the electrode, the outer surface of the lid speculum is coated with conductive material that serves as the reference. This type of electrode is best tolerated (in alert subjects) when a topical anesthetic is used. Other types of contact lens electrodes have also been used, for example, the jet electrode, which is disposable. Some clinicians and researchers use thin mylar fibers impregnated with silver particles, called DTL electrodes,[7] as illustrated in Fig. 24.2B, or gold foil, or wire loop electrodes (H-K loop) that hook over the lower eyelid. For rodents, metal wires in loops or other configurations, placed in contact with the corneal surface, are often used. Some labs use cotton wick electrodes and some use DTL fibers under contact lenses or another form of contact lens electrode.[30,41] Corneas are kept hydrated with a lubricating conductive solution in all cases. The reference electrode can be placed under the eyelid, for example, the speculum of a contact lens electrode as described previously, or remotely, for example, on the temple, the forehead, or the cornea of the fellow eye. ERG signals ranging from microvolts to a millivolt or

more, peak to peak, for responses to strong stimuli, are amplified and digitized for computer averaging and analysis. Filtering is carried out to remove signals outside the frequency range of retinal responses to stimulation (<1 and >300 Hz), and to remove line frequency noise (e.g., 50 or 60 Hz).

CLASSICAL DEFINITION OF COMPONENTS OF THE ELECTRORETINOGRAM

The origins of the various waves of the ERG have been of long-standing interest to clinicians and researchers. Our current understanding of the cellular origins of the ERG profits from extensive knowledge, as described in previous chapters, of the functional microcircuitry of the retina, and particularly of the physiology and cell biology of the retinal cell types, and the identity and action of retinal neurotransmitters, their receptors, transporters, and release mechanisms. However, a classical study using ether anesthesia provided the first pharmacologic separation of ERG components.

Granit's[42] classical pharmacologic dissection of the ERG (illustrated in Fig. 24.4) provided valuable insights on origins of ERG waves, as well as a nomenclature for waves based on their distinct retinal origins. Component "processes" were found to disappear from the ERG during the induction of ether anesthesia in the following order: process (P)I—the slow c-wave response that follows the b-wave, generated predominantly by the RPE; PII—the b-wave, generated by bipolar cells; and eventually PIII—the photoreceptor-related responses that remained the longest during ether anesthesia. PII and PIII are still commonly used terms for ERG components generated by ON bipolar cells and photoreceptors, respectively.

SLOW PIII, THE C-WAVE, AND OTHER SLOW COMPONENTS OF THE DIRECT-CURRENT (DC)- ELECTRORETINOGRAM

PIII of the ERG can be separated into a fast and a slow portion: fast PIII is the a-wave, which reflects photoreceptor current (see further), and slow PIII results from Müller cell currents induced by photoreceptor-dependent reduction in $[K^+]_o$ in the SRS (Fig. 24.3C). Negative-going slow PIII and the positive-going pigment epithelial response to the same reduction in subretinal $[K^+]_o$ add together to form the c-wave,[20–23,43] which is positive-going in the dark-adapted ERG of the cat (Figs. 24.3 and 24.4). This is because the positive-going RPE contribution is larger than the negative-going Müller cell contribution (illustrated by the intraretinal recordings from intact cat eye in Fig. 24.3A). In mice, the c-wave is also positive-going.[18] (Fig. 24.3B). In humans and monkeys, slow PIII and the RPE c-wave are more equal in amplitude, and the corneal c-wave is less positive. Two slower potentials that arise from the RPE, the fast oscillation potential (FO) and light peak (LP), are also present in cat and mouse dc-ERG recordings (Fig. 24.3). The mouse LP is much smaller in amplitude than that in the cat. The cellular mechanisms that generate these slow waves were reviewed in more detail in previous reviews of ERG origins.[44,45]

In alert human subjects it is not possible to obtain stable dc-ERG recordings necessary for recording slow events, for example, those arising from the RPE, that occur over seconds or minutes, because the eyes move too frequently. Therefore, to measure slow potentials, the electro-oculogram (EOG), an eye movement–dependent voltage, is recorded. The EOG is a corneo-fundal potential that originates largely from the RPE; its amplitude changes with illumination, being maximal at the peak of the LP. Use of EOGs to evaluate retinal/RPE function is described in an ISCEV standard publication on clinical EOG.[38]

FULL-FIELD DARK-ADAPTED (GANZFELD) FLASH ELECTRORETINOGRAM

In Fig. 24.5, full-field dark-adapted ERG responses to a range of stimulus strengths for a human subject *(left)*, a macaque monkey, whose retina and ERG are similar to that of human *(middle)*, and a C57BL/6 mouse *(right)*. The mouse ERG is similar to the primate ERG but larger in amplitude (see calibrations). For higher stimulus strengths than shown in the figure, the mouse ERG develops larger OPs than those generally seen in the primate ERGs (e.g., Fig. 24.6). The ERGs in Fig. 24.5 were generated almost entirely, except for responses to the strongest stimuli, by the primary rod circuit, which is the most sensitive retinal circuit.

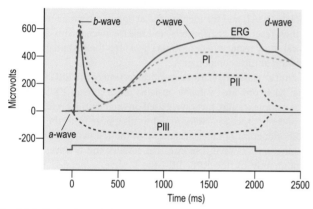

Fig. 24.4 Dark-adapted electroretinogram (*ERG*) of the cat and its three component processes revealed by induction of ether anesthesia. The *solid red line* indicates the ERG of the intact cat eye in response to a 2 s flash (14 Lamberts) from darkness. *Dashed lines* indicate three processes (*PI, PII,* and *PIII*), numbered in the order in which they disappeared from the ERG during induction of ether anesthesia. (Modified from Granit R. The components of the retinal action potential in mammals and their relation to the discharge in the optic nerve. *J Physiol.* 1933; 77(3):207–239, used with permission.)

For all three species, the strongest stimuli evoked an a-wave, followed by a b-wave. For stimuli more than two log units weaker than the strongest one, b-waves were still present, but a-waves were no longer visible. B-waves can be seen in responses to weaker stimuli than a-waves partly because of the convergence of many rods (20–40) onto each rod bipolar cell, which increases their sensitivity,[47–49] and partly because of the large radial extent of ON bipolar cells in the retina. The slow negative wave in the ERGs of the three subjects in response to the weakest stimuli, called the (negative) scotopic threshold response (nSTR), and the equally sensitive positive (p)STR are related to amacrine and/or ganglion cell activity.[26,29–31,50] The high sensitivity of the STRs relative to b-waves (and a-waves) reflects the additional convergence of rod signals in the primary rod circuit in the inner retina proximal to the rod bipolar cells.[47,51,52]

Dark-adapted a-wave

It has long been appreciated that the dark-adapted a-wave primarily reflects the rod receptor photocurrent. The a-wave generator was localized to photoreceptors in classical intraretinal recording studies in mammalian retinas, some of which included current source density (CSD), or source-sink, analyses.[13,14,53–55] The most direct demonstration of the a-wave's cellular origin was provided in such experiments by Penn and Hagins[54,55] in isolated rat retina. These experiments produced evidence that light suppressed the circulating (i.e., dark) current of the photoreceptors, and the investigators proposed that this suppression is seen in the ERG as the a-wave.

Negative electroretinograms

The receptoral origin of the a-wave was also demonstrated in early studies in amphibians using compounds that blocked synaptic transmission, Mg^{2+}, Co^{2+}, and Na^+-aspartate, and isolated photoreceptor signals in the ERG while abolishing responses of postreceptoral neurons.[56,57] These manipulations also caused the b-wave to disappear, indicating its postreceptoral origin. As our understanding of synaptic pharmacology has improved, it has become more common to use glutamate agonists and antagonists to block transfer of signals from

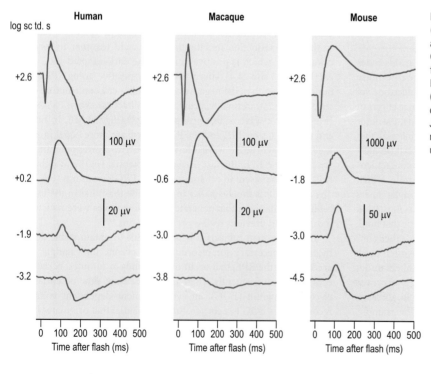

Fig. 24.5 Dark-adapted full-field electroretinogram (ERGs) of a human subject, a macaque monkey, and a mouse. The ERGs are of a human, macaque, and C57BL/6 mouse in response to brief (<5 ms) flashes from darkness generated by computer-controlled LEDs. Responses to the weakest stimuli were rod-driven (scotopic), whereas for the strongest stimuli they were driven by both rods and cones. (Modified from Robson JG, Frishman LJ. Dissecting the dark-adapted electroretinogram. *Doc Ophthalmol.* 1998; 95(3–4):187–215, used with permission.)

photoreceptors to specific second-order neurons. For example, blocking metabotropic transmission to depolarizing (ON) bipolar cells with L-2-amino-4-phosphonobutyric acid (APB or AP4), an mGluR6 receptor agonist,[58] eliminates the b-wave and produces a negative ERG.[59,60] Much of the remaining ERG is the rod photoreceptor response, although late negative signals also arise from OFF pathway neurons.[39,61]

An essentially identical negative ERG to that after APB administration occurs in mice in which the mGluR6 receptor is genetically deleted,[62] or when there are mutations in the mGluR6 receptor or other proteins whose function is necessary for normal signal transduction in ON bipolar cells.[63] For example, Fig. 24.6 shows the typical negative ERG of the dark-adapted *Nob1*, that is, no b-wave, mouse.[46,64] The *Nob1* mouse has a mutation in the *Nyx* gene that encodes nyctalopin, a protein found in ON bipolar cell dendrites.[65,66] Mutation of this protein produces a negative ERG in human patients who are diagnosed with X-linked complete congenital stationary night blindness (CSNB-1).[67,68] Negative ERGs also occur for other forms of CSNB caused by mutations in mGlur6 receptors, and in *Nob3* and *Nob4* mice with such mutations,[63,69] as well as in *Nob2* mice in which glutamatergic transmission from photoreceptors is compromised.[70] Although the ERG of the *Nob1* and other mice lacking b-waves is almost entirely negative-going, it rises from its trough at the time course of the c-wave. Photoreceptor-dependent slow responses such as c-wave and slow PIII are not affected by blockade of postreceptoral responses in neural retina.

Retinal ischemia owing to compromised inner retina circulation also isolates the a-wave and eliminates postreceptoral ERG components. This was demonstrated in early experiments in monkeys by occlusion of the central retinal artery.[71,72] A "negative ERG" in which b-waves are reduced or missing is a common clinical readout of central retinal artery and vein occlusions, as well as other disorders affecting postreceptoral retina such as melanoma-associated retinopathy, X-linked retinoschisis, complete CSNB, or toxic conditions.[10,12]

Modeling

The utility of the a-wave in studies of normal and abnormal photoreceptor function was advanced by the development of quantitative models based on single-cell physiology that could predict the behavior both of the isolated photoreceptor cell outer segment currents and

ERG a-wave in the same or similar species. Hood and Birch[73,74] demonstrated that the behavior of the leading edge of the dark-adapted a-wave in the human ERG can be predicted by a model of photoreceptor function derived to describe in vitro suction electrode recordings of currents around the outer segments of single primate rod photoreceptors.[75] Lamb and Pugh[76,77] followed a simplified kinetic model of the leading edge of the photoreceptor response (in vitro current recordings initially in amphibians) that took account of the stages of the biochemical phototransduction cascade in the outer segments of vertebrate rods. This model was subsequently shown to predict the leading edge of the human dark-adapted a-wave generated by strong stimuli[78] and has been used extensively in clinical studies of retinal disease, and in analyses of photoreceptor function in animal models. A simplified formulation presented by Hood and Birch[79–81] is often used (see legend of Fig. 24.7) and can also be adjusted to application to cone signals. Fig. 24.7 shows fits of Hood and Birch's model to the dark-adapted a-wave of a normal human subject and a patient with retinitis pigmentosa (RP).

Photoreceptor models of Hood and Birch,[79–81] Lamb and Pugh,[77] and recent ones with improved fits[39] provide parameters to represent the maximum amplitude of the a-wave, R_{max} in equations of Hood and Birch, and the sensitivity (S) of the response. R_{max} and S vary depending upon the pathology and stimulus conditions (e.g., adaptation level), and both parameters may be affected by RP. For example, S is thought to be more affected than R_{max} in eyes in which the photoreceptors are hypoxic and more generally for abnormalities in the transduction cascade or increases in retinal illumination, whereas R_{max} is more affected by photoreceptor loss (as illustrated in Fig. 24.7).[82]

Although models of the leading edge of the a-wave yield useful parameters for describing the health of the photoreceptor outer segments, simpler approaches using stronger flashes than those advised by the ISCEV standard (Fig. 24.1 and Box 24.1)[1] are helpful. Hood and Birch[82,83] and other investigators[84] have noted that a pair of strong flashes, or even a single flash that nearly or just saturates the rod response, can be analyzed without fitting a model to make a rough estimate of R_{max} and to measure a peak time that is related to S. Such measurements for a single flash[82] are illustrated in the *bottom row* of Fig. 24.7. The flash strength used was 4.0 log sc td.s, which is 63 times (1.8 log units) higher than the current ISCEV standard flash[1] for mixed rod-cone ERG (assuming an 8-mm pupil).

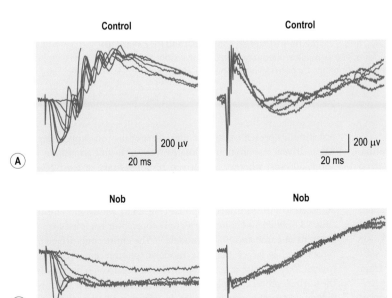

Fig. 24.6 Negative electroretinogram (ERG) of mouse lacking a b-wave. Single-flash responses on short *(left)* and long *(right)* time scales from a control C57BL/6 mouse (**A**) and a *Nob1* mouse (**B**). ERGs on the *left* are responses to flashes of 0.11, 0.98, 2.57, 4.37, 17.4, 27.5, and 348 sc cd.s.m⁻², and on the *right* to flashes of 40.0, 68.4, 102, 170, and 348 sc cd.s.m⁻². (From Kang Derwent JJ, Saszik SM, Maeda H, et al. Test of the paired-flash electroretinographic method in mice lacking b-waves. *Vis Neurosci.* 2007; 24(2):141–149, used with permission.)

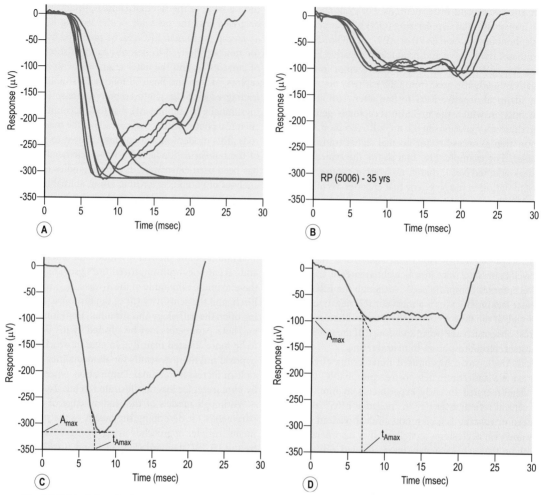

Fig. 24.7 Modeling the leading edge of the dark-adapted a-wave. (**A**) and (**B**) Rod-isolated electroretinogram (ERG) of a normal human subject (**A**), and a retinitis pigmentosa (RP) patient (**B**) in response to flashes of increasing strengths near a-wave saturation. Responses are fit with the Hood and Birch[80] adaptation of the Lamb and Pugh[77] model, expressed in the following equation:

$$R(I,t) = (1 - \exp[-I * S * (t - td)^2 \ ]) * R_{max} \text{For } t > t_d \qquad \textbf{(Eq. 24.1)}$$

where response amplitude, R, is a function of flash strength, I, and the time, t, after the occurrence of brief (impulse) flash of light. S is the sensitivity that scales the stimulus strength, R_{max} is the maximum amplitude, and t_d, a brief delay commonly between 2.4 to 4 ms. (**C**) and (**D**) A simple approach is shown for estimating A_{max}, and t_{max}, indicators for model parameters, R_{max} and S for the normal human subject (**C**) and RP patient (**D**). (Heckenlively JR, Arden GB, eds. *Principles and Practice of Clinical Electrophysiology of Vision.* 2nd ed. Fig. 35.13 (p. 498), © 2006 Massachusetts Institute of Technology, by permission of The MIT Press.)

Mixed rod-cone a-wave

For weak to moderate stimulus flashes to the dark-adapted retina, a-waves are dominated by rod signals, but stronger flashes elicit mixed rod-cone ERGs (*top row* of Fig. 24.5). To investigate relative contributions of rod- and cone-driven responses to the ERG, it is necessary to separate them. Fig. 24.8 shows ERG (*red circles*) of a dark-adapted macaque in response to two different flash strengths and individual rod- and cone-driven contributions.

Rod-driven responses (*blue circles* in Fig. 24.8) are extracted by subtracting the isolated cone-driven response to the same stimulus from the full mixed rod-cone response. Isolated cone-driven responses (*triangles*) are obtained by briefly (1 s) suppressing rod-driven responses with an adapting flash and then measuring the response to the original test stimulus presented 300 ms after offset of the rod-suppressing flash. Cone-driven responses in primates recover to full amplitude within about 300 ms, whereas rod-driven responses take at least 1 second, making it possible to isolate the cone-driven responses. The cone photoreceptor–driven portion of the leading edge of the a-wave represents about 20% of the saturated response (Fig. 24.8). Model lines for the rod (Fig. 24.8, *blue*) and cone (*purple*) photoreceptor responses are modifications of Lamb and Pugh's model.[39,77] The entire cone-driven a-wave (*green line*) is larger than the modeled photoreceptor contribution (*purple line*) because it includes additional negative-going signals from the postreceptoral OFF pathway that can be eliminated with ionotropic glutamate receptor antagonists, as described in a later section on light-adapted ERG.

Time course of the rod photoreceptor response recorded as the a-wave

The leading edge of the a-wave is the only portion of the photoreceptor response that normally is visible in the brief flash ERG. As seen in the *Nob1* mouse that has no b-wave (Fig. 24.6), elimination of the major postreceptoral contributions (i.e., the b-wave) to the dark-adapted ERG leaves the c-wave present at late times. For high energy stimuli, the mouse ERG a-wave recovers toward baseline, forming a "nose" in response to strong stimuli (Fig. 24.6B). The a-wave nose is a common feature of the mammalian ERG. It also can be seen in the macaque (Fig. 24.9) when post receptor responses are eliminated by pharmacologic blockade, and in humans in whom complete CSNB has eliminated the ON bipolar cell–dependent b-wave. This indicates that the b-wave does not have a role in truncating the negative-going a-wave response, although this has been commonly assumed to be the case. The presence of a nose generated by the photoreceptors also is in conflict with the models of a-wave generation described previously in the chapter and illustrated in Fig. 24.7A. These models assume that the a-wave reflects only the outer segment photocurrent response and not currents generated by more proximal portions of the photoreceptor cells.[80] Note that the model line in Fig. 24.7A, based only on outer segment photocurrents, does not recover toward baseline despite the presence of the a-wave nose. In a study investigating the origin of the "nose" of the a-wave Robson and Frishman[84] provided evidence that recovery of the a-wave toward baseline is shaped by currents around more proximal portions of the rod photoreceptor cell than the outer segments. They used SPICE (Simulation Program and Integrated Circuit Emphasis) to generate a-waves that took account of the electrical properties (resistance and capacitance) and spatial dimensions of the rat rod (outer segments, axons, nucleus, spherule) from classical studies of Hagins et al.[86] and Penn and Hagins.[55] The simulations demonstrated that the recovery from the a-wave trough (shaping the a-wave nose) can be attributed to the rod photoreceptor itself, as is suggested by the presence of a nose in ERGs of subjects lacking b-waves (Fig. 24.9).[85] They proposed that the initial recovery of the a-wave nose reflects the large capacitive currents observed by Hagins et al.[86] to occur in the outer nuclear layer in rat

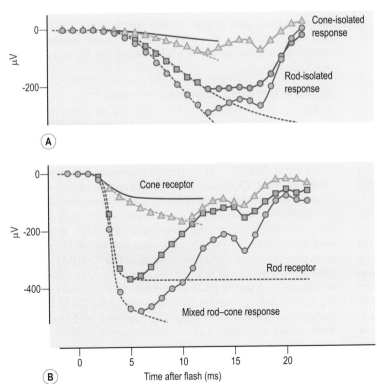

Fig. 24.8 Mixed rod-cone dark-adapted electroretinogram (ERG) of macaque monkey showing separate components. (**A**) ERG responses of a macaque to a brief blue LED flash of 188 sc td.s (57 ph td.s) and (**B**) to a xenon-white flash of 59,000 sc td.s (34,000 ph td.s). In both plots, the largest response *(red circles)* is the mixed rod-cone a-wave; the *red dashed line* shows the modeled mixed rod/cone response. The second largest response is the (isolated) rod-driven response *(filled blue squares and circles)*, and the *dashed blue line* is the modeled rod photoreceptor contribution. The second to smallest response *(filled triangles)* is the isolated cone-driven response, and the *dashed green line* shows the modeled response (including postreceptoral portion). The smallest response *(purple line)* is the modeled cone photoreceptor contribution, based on findings after intravitreal injection of PDA (5 mM intravitreal concentration, assuming a vitreal volume of 2.1 mL in macaque eye in this and subsequent figures). The stimulus for part A (for 8.5 mm pupil) was 1 ph cd.s.m[−2], that is, about three times weaker (for cones) than the ISCEV standard flash of 3 cd.s.m[−2], whereas for part B it was 200 times stronger than the standard flash. (From Robson JG, Saszik SM, Ahmed J, Frishman LJ. Rod and cone contributions to the a-wave of the electroretinogram of the macaque. *J Physiol.* 2003;547(Pt 2):509–530, used with permission.)

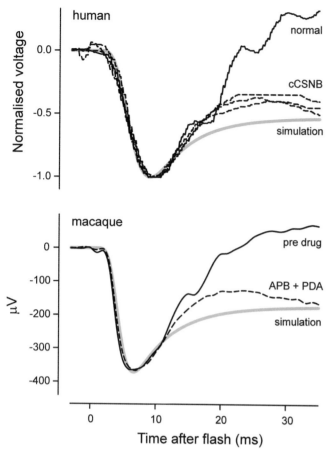

Fig. 24.9 Electroretinograms (ERGs) lacking ON bipolar cell components. Normalized ERGs from three patients with complete congenital stationary night blindness (cCSNB) and a normal control (upper records redrawn from Nakamura M, Sanuki R, Yasuma TR, et al. TRPM1 mutations are associated with the complete form of congenital stationary night blindness. *Mol Vis.* 2010:16;425–437) and the ERG from a macaque (lower records from Robson JG, Frishman LJ. The rod-driven a-wave of the dark-adapted mammalian electroretinogram. *Prog Retin Eye Res.* 2014;39:1–22.) before and after pharmacologic suppression of both ON and OFF bipolar cell responses with a mixture of APB and PDA.

retina. The capacitive currents are largest around the stout nuclear region of the photoreceptor cell, when strong stimulus flashes are used.

Dark-adapted b-wave (PII)

It is well accepted that the dark-adapted b-wave arises primarily from ON bipolar cells. Results of intraretinal recording and CSD analyses were consistent with the b-wave originating primarily from bipolar cells with contributions from Müller cell currents.[13,14,71] Also, pharmacologic blockade of postreceptoral responses and specifically those of ON bipolar cells or mutations that prevent signaling by ON bipolar cells can eliminate the b-wave[60] (e.g., Fig. 24.6).[63,64]

There is also good evidence that for most of its dynamic range, the dark-adapted b-wave is generated by rod bipolar cells in the primary rod circuit. Only for very strong stimuli will rod signals pass via gap junctions to cones and then to cone bipolar cells, which will also then contribute to the dark-adapted flash response.[48,51,87,88] For the dark-adapted, scotopic ERGs it has been possible to isolate Granit's PII from other ERG components and to compare its characteristics with those of rod bipolar cells recorded in retinal slices. One approach is to pharmacologically isolate PII.

Intravitreal injection of the inhibitory neurotransmitter γ-aminobutyric acid (GABA) has been used to suppress inner retinal activity in order to isolate PII in the dark-adapted retina of the C57BL/6 mouse (Fig. 24.10A). GABA receptors are present on bipolar cell terminals, as well as on amacrine and ganglion cells of inner retina. Following GABA inhibition,[30,89] inner retinal responses involved in generating the very sensitive pSTR and nSTR are blocked, leaving a pharmacologically isolated PII, likely generated by rod bipolar cells. Loss of the sensitive STRs was not due to a general loss of retinal sensitivity; a-wave amplitude and kinetics, reflecting photoreceptor function, did not change after GABA injection (Fig. 24.10C).

PII isolated by intravitreal GABA from ERG responses of C57BL/6 mice to very weak stimuli are similar to PII isolated in humans using a weak adapting light to suppress the very sensitive STRs.[90] Moreover, isolated PII has a remarkably similar time course of patch electrode current recordings from rod bipolar cells in a mouse retinal slice preparation in response to similarly weak stimuli.[91] This supports the view that isolated PII reflects rod bipolar cell activity. A primary role for an alternative generator for PII, the Müller cells, is unlikely in mice because mice with genetically inactivated Kir4.1 channels in their retinas still produce b-waves.[20]

After GABA injection, with the pSTR removed, the PII response rises in proportion to stimulus energy and then saturates in a manner that is adequately described by a simple hyperbolic function (see Fig. 24.10 legend). These findings are consistent with a single mechanism, that is, one retinal cell type, the rod bipolar cell, producing the isolated PII component of the ERG.[89,92]

Although bipolar cells play a major role in generating b-waves, Müller cells also contribute to the b-wave. The PII component, pharmacologically isolated from macaque ERG (Fig. 24.11B), is similar in its rising phase to PII of the other species (illustrated in Fig. 24.11A). However, PII in macaque (and cat) recovers more slowly to baseline. Macaque PII can be analyzed into a fast component and a slow component that is a low-pass filtered version of the fast component (Fig. 24.11B). In cat, intravitreal injection of Ba^{2+} to block inward-rectifying K$^+$ channels in Müller cells did not eliminate the b-wave[29,93] but did remove a slow portion of isolated PII that is similar in time course to a low-pass filtered version of the response.[45] With longer-duration stimuli such as those used in early studies in amphibians,[94] glial contributions to the b-wave become more significant, and contributions of neuronal and glial generators of the b-wave could be equal.

Scotopic threshold response

As illustrated in Figs. 24.5 and 24.10, for very weak flashes from darkness, near psychophysical threshold in humans,[31,95] the nSTR and pSTR dominate the ERG of most mammals studied. The nSTR has been shown in intraretinal analyses in cat to be generated more proximally in the retina than PII.[31] As described just previously, in noninvasive recordings the pSTR and nSTR can be suppressed and thus separated from PII using a weak adapting background or by injection of inhibitory neurotransmitters (GABA, as illustrated in Figs. 24.10 and 24.11, or by another inhibitory neurotransmitter, glycine).[96] Blockade by ionotropic glutamate receptor antagonists (see legend to Fig. 24.11) or use of an agonist for N-methyl-D-aspartate (NMDA) receptors present on inner retinal neurons will also remove the STRs.[37,92] The effects of GABA on the pSTR in mouse and the nSTR are shown in Fig. 24.10B and D, respectively. In both cases, after GABA injection, as described previously, the remaining responses can be modeled as the PII component alone.

Based on the pharmacologic isolation studies, a linear model of the dark-adapted ERG can be proposed that takes into account contributions

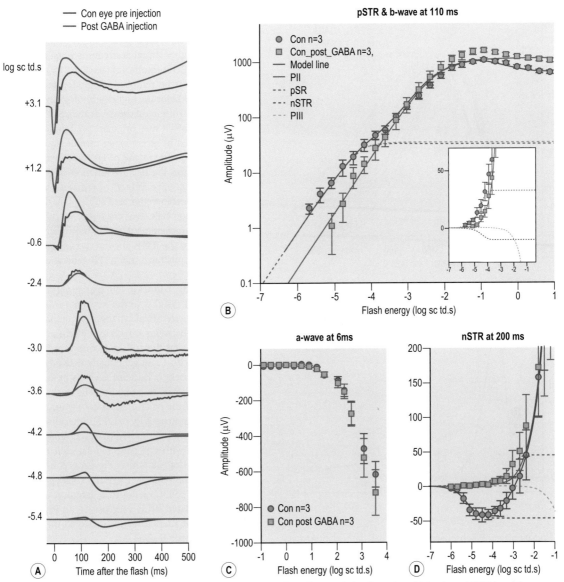

Fig. 24.10 Dark-adapted mouse electroretinogram (ERG) before and after intravitreal injection of GABA: analysis of ERG components. (**A**) ERG of a C57BL/6 mouse in response to brief flashes of increasing stimulus strength recorded before and after intravitreal injection of GABA (30 mM intravitreal concentration assuming for this and subsequent panels, a 20 μL vitreal volume in mouse). (**B**) ERGs of three mice measured at 110 ms (mean ± standard error of mean) after a brief flash, at the peak of the positive scotopic threshold response (*pSTR*) and b-wave. The modeled full ERG *(blue line)* includes four components: PII, pSTR, negative STR (*nSTR*), and PIII. All components are assumed to increase in proportion to stimulus strength before saturating. Explicitly, the exponential saturation of the pSTR, nSTR and PIII is defined by:

$$V = V_{max}(1 - \exp(-I/I_0) \qquad \textbf{(Eq. 24.2)}$$

where V_{max} is the maximum saturated amplitude, and I_0 the stimulus strength for an amplitude of $(1 - 1/e)V_{max}$. The hyperbolic relation used for PII is described by the function:

$$V = V_{max}I/(I + I_0) \qquad \textbf{(Eq. 24.3)}$$

where V_{max} has the same meaning as for the exponential function but I_0 is the stimulus strength at which the amplitude is $V_{max}/2.30$ (**C**) ERGs measured at 6 ms after a brief flash, to measure a-wave amplitude on its leading edge. (**D**) ERGs measured at 200 ms to measure nSTR amplitude. Model lines for the full response and for component parts are as described for panel B.

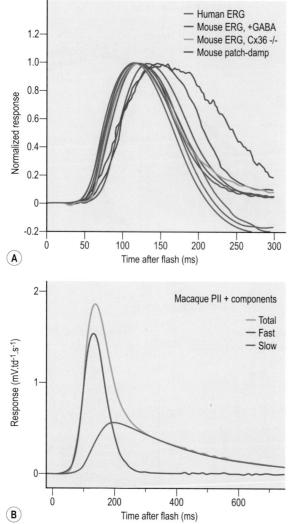

(A)

(B)

Fig. 24.11 Rod bipolar cell component, PII, of the dark-adapted electroretinogram (*ERG*) of a human subject, macaque monkey, and mouse. (**A**) Comparison of rod bipolar cell current from patch recordings in mouse retinal slice (Field GD, Rieke F. Non-linear signal transfer from mouse rods to bipolar cells and implications for visual sensitivity. Neuron. 2002;34(5):773-785) with isolated PII (by weak light adaptation) from humans, isolated PII from ERGs of six C57BL/6 mice by intravitreal injection of GABA (32–46 mM) and from a Cx36(−/−) mouse lacking ganglion cells. (From Cameron AM, Mahroo OA, Lamb TD. Dark adaptation of human rod bipolar cells measured from the b-wave of the scotopic electroretinogram. *J Physiol.* 2006;575(Pt 2):507–526, which was modified from Robson JG, Maeda H, Saszik SM, Frishman LJ. In vivo studies of signaling in rod pathways of the mouse using the electroretinogram. *Vision Res.* 2004; 44(28):3253–3268, used with permission.) (**B**) PII of macaque, isolated by pharmacologic blockade (6,7-dinitroquinoxaline-2,3-dione [DNQX], 0.1 mM; N-methyl-D-aspartic acid [NMDA], 3 mM) of inner retinal responses. PII has been analyzed into a fast component, proposed to be a direct reflection of the postsynaptic current, and a slow component that is a low-pass filtered version of the faster component, believed to be the Müller-cell contribution. (From Robson JG, Frishman LJ. Dissecting the dark-adapted electroretinogram. *Doc Ophthalmol.* 1998;95(3–4):187–215, and unpublished observations.)

not only from PII but also from the pSTR and nSTR (and PIII) components of the mouse ERG (see Fig. 24.10B–D). These components add together to form the ERG response (*blue solid line* in Fig. 24.10B) at a particular time after the stimulus flash. The model assumes that each ERG component (*dashed and red lines*) initially rises in proportion to

stimulus strength and then saturates in a characteristic manner. This behavior was demonstrated in single-cell recordings in mammalian retinas,[75,97] as well as for a- and b-waves in numerous other studies. To isolate PII at higher stimulus strengths when the photoreceptor contribution to the ERG is significant (see Fig. 24.9), the PIII (photoreceptor) component must be removed. A model line for PIII is included in Fig. 24.10B and D for the higher stimulus strengths.[30]

The neuronal origins of the nSTR and pSTR are species dependent. In macaques, the nSTR may originate predominantly from ganglion cells; it was eliminated in severe experimental glaucoma with selective ganglion cell death, whereas the pSTR remained.[50] In contrast, in rodents the pSTR requires the healthy function of ganglion cells.[26] The pSTR was eliminated in mice and rats by removing ganglion cells (optic nerve crush [ONC] or transection and subsequent degeneration) and in mice in which ganglion cells were deleted genetically, whereas the nSTR was only partially removed in rat, and of normal amplitude in mice.[26,98–100] In cat (and human) the nSTR also survives ganglion cell loss,[101] and in cat it has been demonstrated that nSTR generation involves K^+ currents in Müller cells.[28]

Mice lacking connexin 36 gap junction proteins (Cx36) provide additional insights to the neuronal origins of the STR. Cx36 is expressed in the electrical synapses (gap junctions) between AII amacrine cells and between AII amacrine cells and ON cone bipolar cells, as well as between the rod and cone terminals.[88,102] In the scotopic ERG of mice with Cx36 genetically deleted, pSTR remains, whereas the nSTR is absent.[51] Because Cx36 is essential for transmission of ON pathway signals to ganglion cells in the primary rod pathway,[88] preservation of the pSTR in Cx36(−/−) mice suggests that the pSTR must depend upon activity of OFF rather than ON ganglion cells. The nSTR depends on the syncytium of AII amacrine cells and their electrical synapses with ON cone bipolar cells and was no longer functional in Cx36-deficient mice. Fig. 24.11A includes an example of PII isolated from the scotopic ERG of a Cx36(−/−) mouse that lacks the nSTR and the pSTR, owing to a ganglion cell lesion subsequent to ONC. This isolated PII is very similar to PII isolated pharmacologically or by light adaptation, as well as to the rod bipolar cell recordings from the retinal slice.

Because of their specific inner retinal origins, the nSTRs and pSTRs are of particular interest in animal models of diseases that affect the inner retina, such as glaucoma. They provide noninvasive readouts of pathologic changes in function and can be used to document effects of neuroprotective agents.[26,50,103]

LIGHT-ADAPTED, CONE-DRIVEN ELECTRORETINOGRAMS

Isolating cone-driven responses

To study the cone-driven (photopic) flash ERG, rods must be suppressed, or unable to respond because of characteristics of stimuli selected to test the cones. Typically for recording photopic ERGs, rods are rendered unresponsive by imposing a steady background light sufficient to saturate their responses (i.e., >25 cd.m⁻²). Another approach is to briefly saturate rod responses and to wait for cones to recover. Cones recover more quickly than rods: in primates, in about 300 ms as described previously for results in Fig. 24.8.[39] In mice and rats, the recovery time of cone signals is longer, about 1 second.[98,104]

Rod and cone signals can also be separated by selection of appropriate stimulus wavelength. In trichromatic primates, L-cones can be isolated using red light at wavelengths greater than 630 nm and excluding wavelengths much shorter. However, mice and rats do not have L-cones, and the spectral sensitivity of their medium wavelength M-cones peaks near 515 and 510 nm, respectively,[104,105] and overlaps with that of rods, which peaks around 500 nm. Scotopic stimulus calibrations are thus adequate for the rodent M-cone responses, and more appropriate than photopic calibrations, which are based on human spectral sensitivity. However, for any subject, spectral separation of responses of individual cone types is possible using ERG flicker photometry.[106] In mice and rats such studies have isolated short-wavelength UV (S-) cones that peak around 358 or 359 nm.[105,107]

Separation of rod and cone signals in mice can also be achieved using genetically manipulated models in which either rods or cones have been inactivated. Examples of such models include Rho(−/−) (rod opsin knockout) mice that have cone function only, but also eventual cone degeneration,[108] Tra(−/−) (transducin α knockout) with cone function only,[109] Cnga3(−/−) (cone cyclic nucleotide channel deficient) mice,[4] or *GNAT 2*[cpfl3] (G_T protein) mutant mice with rod function only.[110] Mice with inactivated or degenerated rods and cones, i.e., rodless, coneless mice,[111] can be used to study function of a more recently identified photoreceptor pigment, melanopsin, found in a small population of retinal ganglion cells. Contributions to ERGs from melanopsin-driven responses are thought to be minimal.[112]

Similar to the dark-adapted ERG, the photopic ERG responses to brief stimulus flashes on a rod-saturating background are similar in man and macaque (Fig. 24.12). In mice, however, the b-wave rises more slowly to its peak, does not return to baseline as early, and OPs are more prominent. Very strong stimuli produce more prolongation of responses in mice and produce larger OPs (*inset on the right* of Fig. 24.12) than in primates. For macaques, a second peak after the b-wave emerges and is believed to be an OFF pathway response (i-wave).[113] In some cases, (not shown) more of the i-wave response is below the baseline level.

Light-adapted a-wave

The a-waves in the photopic ERG are smaller than those in the scotopic ERG, reflecting the large difference in retinal densities of cones versus rods. In human and macaque, about 5% of the photoreceptors are cones. Cones comprise up to 3% of photoreceptors in mice, and fewer in rats. In addition, use of glutamate analogs has shown that much of cone-driven a-wave is postreceptoral in origin. In macaques, the a-wave is reduced in amplitude by the ionotropic glutamate receptor antagonists *cis*-2,3-piperidine-dicarboxylic acid (PDA) (and kynurenic acid [KYN], not shown) that block kainate and AMPA receptors of OFF bipolar and horizontal cells, as well as cells of inner retina (Fig. 24.13).[109,110] In contrast, L-2-amino-4-phosphonobutyric acid (APB) eliminates the b-wave, but does not reduce the amplitude of the leading edge of the a-wave. PDA has a similar effect for signal transmission to postreceptoral neurons as aspartate, which blocks all glutamatergic transmission, and cobalt (Co^{2+}), which blocks voltage-gated Ca^{2+} channels that are essential for vesicular release of the neurotransmitter glutamate (Fig. 24.13).

PDA-sensitive postreceptoral neurons, rather than cones, were found to generate the leading edge of the a-wave for the first 1.5 log units of increasing flash strength that elicited a cone-driven a-wave in macaque (Fig. 24.13).[114] Postreceptoral cells contribute 25% to 50% of the leading edge of the a-wave for higher stimulus strengths when cone photoreceptor contributions are also present. The relative sizes of the postreceptor and receptor-driven portions of the photopic a-wave for cone-isolated responses in the macaque dark-adapted ERG are modeled in Fig. 24.8B. Responses up to approximately 5 ms after the flash are cone photoreceptor responses.[39]

Experiments in mouse to investigate the origins of the photopic a-wave yielded similar results to those in macaque. PDA-sensitive

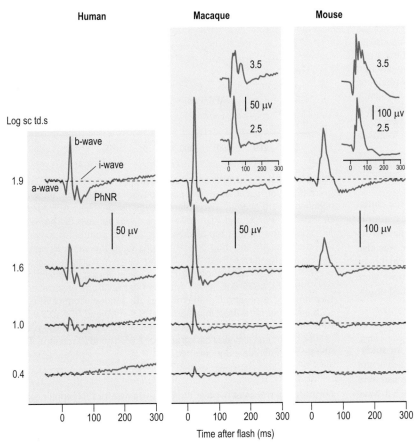

Fig. 24.12 Light-adapted full-field electroretinogram (ERG) of a human subject, macaque monkey, and mouse. ERGs measured in response to brief (<5 ms) white LED flashes for the human and monkey, green flashes for mouse, except for insets at the *top* for the macaque and mouse showing responses from different subjects to intense white xenon flashes. Steady background was 100 sc cd.m⁻² for primates, 63 sc cd.m⁻² for mice. *PhNR*, Photopic negative response. (Unpublished observations.)

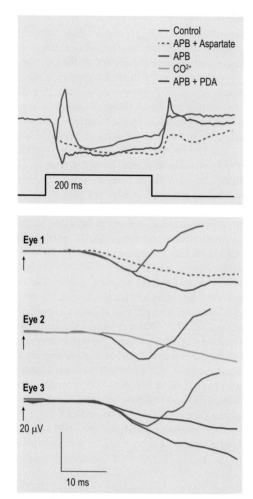

Fig. 24.13 Postreceptoral contributions to the a-wave of the macaque monkey electroretinogram (ERG). Comparison of effects of intravitreally injected APB (1 mM) and APB + PDA (5 mM) with effects of aspartate (0.05 M) and cobalt (Co^{2+}, 1 mM); on photopic a-waves of three different eyes of two macaques. The inset at the *top* shows the control response of eye #1 to the 200 ms stimulus of 3.76 log td (100 cd.m^{-2}) on a steady background of 3.3 log td (35.5 cd.m^{-2}). The a-waves are shown *below* on an expanded time scale. For the stimulus used, the a-wave leading edge (10 µV) was mostly postreceptoral in origin. *APB*, L-2-amino-4-phosphonobutyric acid.

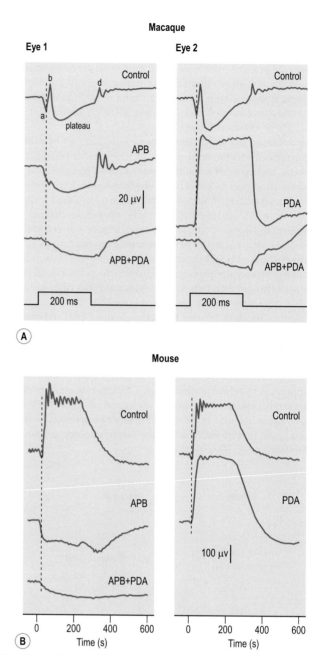

Fig. 24.14 Effects of APB and PDA on the light-adapted electroretinogram (ERG) of macaque monkey and mouse. (**A**) Macaque: Intravitreal injections were given in two different eyes sequentially: APB followed by PDA for eye 1, and PDA followed by APB for eye 2. The *vertical line* shows the time of the a-wave trough in the control response. The 200 ms stimulus and drug concentrations were the same as reported for Fig. 24.15. (From Bush RA, Sieving PA. A proximal retinal component in the primate photopic ERG a-wave. *Invest Ophthalmol Vis Sci.* 1994;35(2):635–645, used with permission from Association for Research in Vision and Ophthalmology.) (**B**) Mouse: Control ERG and response after intravitreal injection of APB (1 mM) and PDA (0.5 mM) + APB in a C57BL/6 mouse. The 200 ms stimulus was 4.6 log sc td (3.9 log cd.m^{-2}) on a steady background of 2.6 log sc td (63 cd.m^{-2}). (From Shirato and Frishman, unpublished.)

responses dominated the leading edge of the a-wave for the initial 1.5 log units, and at least half of the response to stronger stimuli. Photoreceptor signals were present in response to strong flashes up to 8 ms after the flash. A significant portion of the a-wave was also removed by NMDA, which suppresses responses of inner retinal neurons, indicating contributions to the leading edge of the a-wave were from more proximal neurons in the OFF pathway (unpublished observations, Maeda, Kaneko, and Frishman).

Light-adapted b-wave

Intraretinal CSD studies such as those described previously for studying origins of the dark-adapted ERG indicated an ON bipolar cell origin for light-adapted b-waves.[53,115] Origins of the photopic b-wave also were studied in the same series of experiments in macaques in which a-wave origins were studied (illustrated in Fig. 24.13). Macaque photopic ERG responses to long-duration flashes have been studied before and after intravitreal injection of APB (Fig. 24.14A, *top right*, eye 1, *left*).[6] APB

removed the transient b-wave, supporting a role for ON bipolar cells in generating the response (although the possibility of glial mediation was not eliminated in these studies). In contrast, when PDA was injected first (eye 2, *right*) to remove OFF pathway and inner retinal influences, including horizontal cell inhibitory feedback, the b-wave was larger in amplitude and the maximum amplitude was sustained for the duration of the stimulus. These findings indicate that cone-driven b-waves in primates are normally transient because they are truncated by PDA-sensitive horizontal cell inhibition[118] or OFF pathway contribution of opposite polarity to the ON bipolar cell contribution. This observation has been called a push-pull effect.[6,114,] Only an isolated photoreceptor response of slow onset in response to the light flash remained after all postreceptoral activity was eliminated either by APB followed by PDA or PDA followed by APB.

The outcome in a parallel mouse experiment to that in macaque (Fig. 24.14A) helped determine origins of the photopic b-wave in mice. The control response to a 200 ms stimulus in a C57BL/6 mouse differed from that in primates. The b-wave looked similar to the response in macaque after PDA. APB removed the b-wave in the mouse but did not reveal a d-wave; only a tiny positive intrusion was present (Fig. 24.16).[117,119] Similar results have been observed in rat.[120] PDA injection in mouse produced only a small increase in b-wave amplitude but removed OPs and the small positive intrusion. APB combined with PDA produced a negative ERG of slower onset than in the control ERG, owing to removal of the leading edge of the a-wave. The slow recovery of the isolated photoreceptor-related response, compared with that of the macaque, was due to the presence of slow PIII in the ERG in the mouse.[121]

Recent studies in mice and rats found that tetrodotoxin (TTX) significantly reduced the amplitude of the light-adapted b-wave.[98,121] This finding is consistent with presence of TTX-sensitive voltage-gated sodium channels in cone bipolar cells in rats.[122] In contrast, the light-adapted b-wave amplitude increased in macaques, believed to be due to removal of the PhNR that originates from spiking neurons in inner retina.[32,113,118]

Light-adapted d-wave

The d-wave is a positive-going wave at light offset that is a characteristic of the photopic ERG. The d-wave is prominent in all-cone retinas but also can be seen in the photopic ERG of the mixed rod-cone retina of human and macaque monkey for stimulus durations of 150 or 200 ms (Figs. 24.2A and 24.14A). The mouse and rat photopic ERG does not include a d-wave in response to offset of light flashes of only a few hundred ms in duration.[119-121]

Intraretinal analysis in macaque retina initially indicated that d-waves represent a combination of a rapid positive-going offset of cone receptors followed by the negative-going offset of the b-wave.[71,72,123] However, at light offset, intravitreal injection of glutamate analogs in macaques revealed a prominent role for OFF cone bipolar cells, as well in generating d-waves (see Fig. 24.14).[6,124] The relatively slower offset of cone photoreceptor responses in rodents may explain, in part, the lack of d-waves for stimuli that elicit them in primates. The lack of d-waves in rodents is not due to differences in relative numbers of ON and OFF cone bipolar cells compared with primates, because the proportions of each cell type are similar.[125]

Flicker electroretinogram

The fast flicker ERG (nominally 30 Hz flicker) is used to assess the health of cone-driven responses in humans because rod-driven responses do not respond to such fast flicker and only resolve stimuli up to about 20 Hz. Flicker ERG is a particularly valuable test to monitor residual cone function in degenerative diseases such as RP. Studies using APB and PDA in macaques have shown that most of the fast flicker response (e.g., Fig. 24.1) is generated by postreceptoral cells in ON and OFF pathways.[126,127] Intravitreal injection of APB to block the b-wave left a delayed peak in the flicker waveform

that was practically eliminated by addition of PDA to block OFF pathway responses.

The interactions of ON and OFF pathways in flicker ERGs have been examined in macaque over a wide range of temporal frequencies.[126] The typical temporal frequency response function of the photopic ERG of the macaque (Fig. 24.15A) is similar to that seen in humans.[116,128] Response amplitude dips at frequencies around 8 to 12 Hz before rising to a maximum amplitude around 50 Hz. Injections of APB and PDA revealed that the dip is due to cancellation of contributions to the response at different phases from ON and OFF pathways. Other experiments in macaques demonstrated small, more proximal retinal contributions to the flicker responses, at the fundamental frequency of stimulation, and prominent TTX-sensitive contributions to the second harmonic component of the response that peaked around 8 to 10 Hz.[127]

The second harmonic component appears to be larger in macaque recordings than in humans.[116]

Flicker ERGs in mice differ from those in primates in several ways. The frequency response for the primary rod pathway in mice extends up to 30 Hz and secondary rod pathway responses up to 50 Hz.[87] These ranges overlap substantially with the range for cone pathway responses for a control C57BL/6 mouse (Fig. 24.15B).[87,117,128] The overlap of rod- and cone-driven frequency responses means that flicker cannot easily be used in rodents to selectively stimulate cone-driven responses. The lower photopic frequency response of mice relative to primates is due at least in part to the slower recovery of cone photoreceptors in mice.[117] The low amplitude of responses in *Nob1* mice, which lack ON pathway responses, indicates that OFF pathway contributions to the light-adapted frequency response are smaller in mice than in primates (Fig. 24.17B). The ON and OFF pathway responses do not interact to cancel responses at midrange frequencies in mice. Similar to macaques, however, the photoreceptors, whose contribution was isolated by injection of PDA, contributed only a small signal.[117] Second harmonic responses in C57BL/6 mice that peak around 17 Hz were found to be greatly reduced either by loss of ON pathway responses[117] or injection of TTX.

Oscillatory potentials

OPs in flash ERG responses to strong stimuli consist of a series of high-frequency, low-amplitude wavelets superimposed on the b-wave. OPs are present under dark- and light-adapted conditions. The mixed rod-cone flash ERG of a human (Fig. 24.2, *top*) includes at least four OPs that can be extracted by filtering the response to remove signals of frequencies lower than around 75 Hz. The number of wavelets varies between 4 and 10 depending upon stimulus conditions. The temporal characteristics of OPs also vary. As an example, a recent study described dark-adapted OPs in humans as ranging in frequency from 100 Hz or less to more than 200 Hz. The peak occurred around 150 Hz for moderate stimulus strengths but was closer to 100 Hz for the strongest stimuli.[129] Light-adapted OPs also include a high-frequency band peaking around 150 Hz with a lower-frequency band peaking around 75 Hz and extending to frequencies of about 50 Hz, which is below the low-frequency cutoff (75 Hz) for isolating OPs recommended by ISCEV.

OPs are numbered in order from the first to occur in the ERG. There is consensus from experiments in amphibians and mammals that OPs are generated by inner retinal neurons,[34] making them useful for evaluating inner retinal function. However, the discrete origins of different OPs and mechanisms of their generation are not well understood. Intraretinal studies using stimuli that elicited responses from both rod and cone systems in macaques localized OPs, as a group, to inner retina.[35] For a brief light flash, the major OPs in the photopic

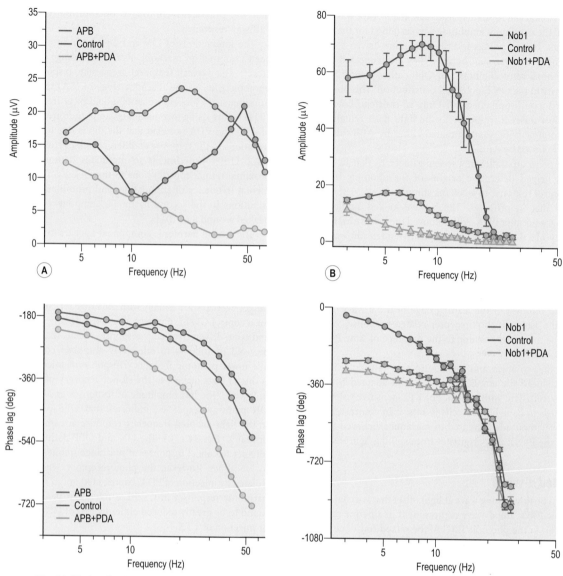

Fig. 24.15 Amplitude and phase of the temporal frequency response of the light-adapted electroretinogram (ERG) in macaque monkey and mouse. (**A**) Flicker ERG response of three macaques (mean ± standard error of mean [SEM]) to sinusoidal stimulation before and after pharmacologic separation of ON and OFF pathway components of the fundamental response. Flicker mean luminance was 457 cd.m^{-2}; 80% contrast, on a 40 cd.m^{-2} white background. *Blue circles:* control; *red circles:* after APB (1 mM); *green circles:* after APB + PDA, 5 mM). (From Kondo M, Sieving PA. Primate photopic sine-wave flicker ERG: vector modeling analysis of component origins using glutamate analogs. *Invest Ophthalmol Vis Sci.* 2001;42(1):305–312, used with permission.) (**B**) Flicker ERG responses of three C57BL/6 mice (mean ± SEM) and three *Nob1* mice to sinusoidal stimulation. Mean luminance was 63 cd.m^{-2}, 100% contrast. *Blue circles:* fundamental response of control; *red circles: Nob1* mice; *triangles: Nob1* mice after intravitreal injection of PDA (5.2–6.2 mM). (From Shirato S, Maeda H, Miura G, Frishman LJ. Postreceptoral contributions to the light-adapted ERG of mice lacking b-waves. *Exp Eye Res.* 2008;86(6):914–928. https://doi.org/10.1016/j.exer.2008.03.008, used with permission from Association for Research in Vision and Ophthalmology.)

ERG were found to be APB-sensitive, indicating an origin in the ON pathway. However, later OPs in the brief flash response and at light off-set for longer-duration stimuli were found to originate from OFF pathway.[130,131] TTX reduced amplitudes of later OPs more than early ones in rabbits, but this finding has not been consistent across species.[131,132] Inhibitory neurotransmitters glycine and GABA suppress OPs in monkeys and other mammals, as do iontotropic glutamate receptor antagonists that block transmission of signals from bipolar cells to amacrine and ganglion cells. Consistent with this, PDA removed OPs from the mouse light-adapted ERG (illustrated in Fig. 24.16B). GABAergic involvement is limited to specific receptor types. Genetic deletion of GABAC receptors in mice enhanced amplitudes of the OPs,[133] whereas blockade of GABAA receptors removed OPs in C57BL/6 mice (unpublished observations).

Although the observations described previously indicate involvement of amacrine or retinal ganglion cells in generating OPs, the role of

Macaque PhNR - Experimental glaucoma

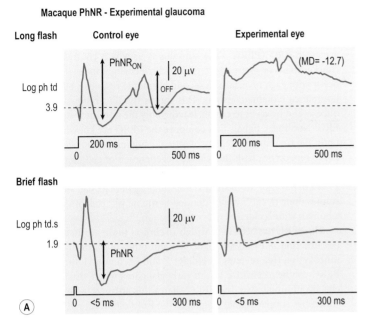

Human PhNR - Primary open angle glaucoma

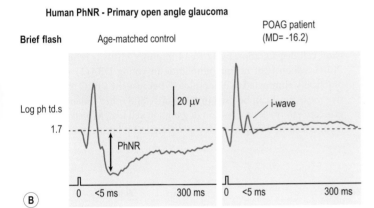

Fig. 24.16 Photopic negative response (*PhNR*) in macaque monkey and human in normal and glaucomatous eyes. (**A**) Full-field flash electroretinogram (ERG) showing the PhNR of a macaque in response to long (*top*) and brief (*middle*) red LED flashes on a rod-saturating blue background (3.7 log sc td) from the control (*left*) and "experimental" (*right*) fellow eye with laser-induced glaucoma. *Arrows* mark the amplitude of the PhNR. *MD*, Mean deviation. (Modified from Viswanathan S, Frishman LJ, Robson JG, Harwerth RS, Smith III EL. The photopic negative response of the macaque electroretinogram: reduction by experimental glaucoma. *Invest Ophthalmol Vis Sci.* 1999;40(6): 1124–1136, used with permission from Association for Research in Vision and Ophthalmology.) (**B**) Full-field flash ERGs of an age-matched 63-year-old normal human subject and a patient with primary open angle glaucoma (*POAG*) under similar stimulus conditions to those used in (**A**) for monkeys. (Modified from Viswanathan S, Frishman LJ, Robson JG, Walters JW. The photopic negative response of the flash electroretinogram in primary open angle glaucoma. *Invest Ophthalmol Vis Sci.* 2001;42(2):514–522, used with permission from Association for Research in Vision and Ophthalmology.)

ganglion cells has been controversial. Loss of OPs after ganglion cell death has not been observed consistently across species, making amacrine cells more likely to be the generators. Reductions in OPs have been reported in conditions such as diabetic retinopathy that compromise inner retinal circulation, but not in conditions that selectively reduce ganglion cell function. However, in Ogden's studies in macaques, optic nerve section and subsequent ganglion cell degeneration led to disappearance of the OPs.[134] Further, in the macaque photopic "flash" ERG studies in macular regions using a multifocal stimulus, both severe experimental glaucoma and TTX removed a high-frequency band of OPs (centered at 143 Hz), while a lower-frequency band (at 77 Hz) remained intact.[132,135] In contrast, OPs were still present in full-field dark-adapted ERGs.[50]

The mechanisms for generating OPs are likely to involve both intrinsic membrane properties of cells and neuronal interactions/feedback circuits. Oscillatory activity has been observed most frequently in amacrine cells. For example, GABAergic wide-field amacrine cells (WFAC) isolated from white bass retina generated high-frequency (>100 Hz) oscillatory membrane potentials (OMPs) in response to extrinsic depolarization.[136] These OMPs were shown to arise from "a complex interplay between voltage-dependent Ca^{2+} currents and voltage- and Ca^{2+}-dependent K^{+} currents."[136]

A feedback mechanism is consistent with effects on OPs of GABA and glycine, both of which participate widely in feedback circuits in inner retina, for example, between amacrine cells and bipolar cells or other amacrine cells. A feedback model has been proposed to account for high-frequency oscillatory (or "rhythmic") activity seen in some mammalian ganglion cell recordings from whole retina that involves electrical synapses, indicated by tracer coupling patterns, as well as inhibitory feedback circuits between amacrine and ganglion cells.[137]

OPs are more prominent in mice than in primates or rats. Similar to humans, peak temporal frequencies of OPs in dark-adapted C57BL/6J mice range from 100 to 120 Hz or higher, whereas they are about 70 to 85 Hz in light-adapted mice.[138] In rats, in which OPs are much smaller overall, two frequency bands of OPs have been reported for dark-adapted ERG, one peaking around 70 Hz and the other, more like other species, around 120 to 130 Hz. In the light-adapted ERG, only the lower-frequency band is present, similar to the findings in mice.[139] In mice and rats, OPs under dark- and light-adapted conditions are present at frequencies lower than common in primates, i.e., down to 50 Hz, and in mice small OPs can occur at frequencies as low as 30 to 40 Hz.[138]

Photopic negative response

A slow negative wave after the b-wave, called the photopic negative response (PhNR), can be seen in the light-adapted ERG and is more prominent in primates than in mice and rats. In humans and monkeys, the PhNR is thought to reflect spiking activity of retinal ganglion cells.[32,33,127] The PhNR is reduced in macaque eyes with experimental glaucoma or after TTX injection (Fig. 24.16)[32] and in humans with primary open angle glaucoma (POAG).[33] The PhNR also is reduced in several other disorders affecting the optic nerve head and inner retina. The slow time course of the PhNR suggests glial involvement, perhaps via K^+ currents in astrocytes in the optic nerve head set up by increased $[K^+]_o$ from spiking of ganglion cells. PhNRs can be evoked using white flashes on a white background if the flash is very bright. However, a red LED flash on a blue background elicits PhNRs over a wider range of stimulus strengths (Fig. 24.16). The red flash may minimize spectral opponency that would reduce ganglion cell responses, and the use of a blue background suppresses rods while minimizing light adaptation of L-cone signals.[118] The PhNR can be exaggerated relative to other major ERG components using slowed focal stimuli confined to the macula.[140]

In rodents, with relatively few ganglion cells compared to primates, the PhNR is small and probably originates mainly from amacrine cells. It is reduced in amplitude by TTX, PDA blockade of transmission to the inner retina, or NMDA suppression of inner retinal activity,[141] but not by loss of ganglion cells in mice (Fig. 24.17)[121] or rat.[98] In rodents, glia are believed to be involved in the generation of the PhNR. In Royal College of Surgeons rats, a large photopic ERG-negative response develops in the degenerating retina,[141] owing at least in part to increased density of Kir4.1 channels in Müller cell endfeet. These channels are critical for producing glial currents that contribute to the ERG.[19,20]

Pattern electroretinogram

A commonly used technique to assess ganglion cell function is to record a pattern ERG (PERG). The stimulus is usually a contrast-reversing checkerboard or grating pattern for which changes in local luminance occur with each reversal as a second harmonic response, but the mean luminance remains constant. This causes the linear signals that produce a- and b-waves to cancel, leaving only the nonlinear signals in the ERG. Nonlinear signals that compose the PERG are known to depend upon the functional integrity of retinal ganglion cells. Following optic nerve section or crush that causes degeneration of ganglion cell axons and cell bodies in several mammals, PERGs are eliminated, while a- and b-waves of the flash ERG are still present (e.g., Fig. 24.17). Initial studies done in cat[142] were extended to monkey,[143] rodents,[121,144–147] and a human with accidental nerve transection.[148]

The PERG has been used widely in clinical studies to assess ganglion cell function in eyes with glaucoma and other diseases that affect the inner retina (see reviews by Holder[149] and Bach and Hoffman[150]). The PERG can be a sensitive test in early glaucoma when visual field deficits are minimal.[150,151] The PERG shares this attribute with the PhNR, which has similar retinal origins to the PERG in macaque.[127,152] In the macaque, and likely in humans, PhNRs induced by each local change in local retinal luminance contribute to the PERG.

The PERG is also useful in the study of rodent models of glaucoma. The DBA/2J mouse model of inherited glaucoma has normal ganglion cell numbers at 2 months of age and progresses to massive retinal ganglion cell degeneration by 12 to 14 months.[153] This is reflected in the PERG, which is of normal amplitude in young DBA/2J mice but is practically eliminated in older mice.[147] Because the PERG is a noninvasive measure, it can be used in these mice and other rodent models of glaucoma to track progression of ganglion cell loss, as well as to document effects of therapies to slow progression and protect neurons.

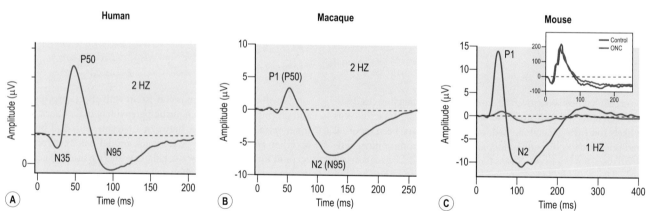

Fig. 24.17 Transient pattern electroretinogram (PERG) of human, macaque monkey, and mouse. (**A**) Representative transient PERG of a normal human subject, elicited with a contrast-reversing checkerboard pattern (0.8-degree checks), mean luminance greater than 80 cd.m⁻², modulated at 2 Hz, 100% contrast. Amplitude for normal humans ranges from 2 to 8 μV, according to the *ISCEV Standard for Clinical Pattern Electroretinography (PERG): 2012 Update* from which the figure was adapted. (From Bach M, Brigell MG, Hawlina M, Holder GE, Johnson MA, McCulloch, DL, Meigen T, Viswanathan S. ISCEV standard for clinical pattern electroretinography (PERG)—2012 update. *Doc Ophthalmol.* 2013;126:1–7, used with permission.) (**B**) Transient PERG of a macaque, elicited with a checkerboard (0.5-degree checks), mean luminance of 55 cd.m⁻² modulated at 2 Hz, 84% contrast. (Unpublished, Luo and Frishman). (**C**) PERG of a C57BL/6 mouse before (*blue line*) and 40 days after (*red line*) unilateral optic nerve crush (ONC) when ganglion cells had degenerated. The pattern was a 0.05 c/degree horizontal bar grating, mean luminance 45 sc cd.m⁻², contrast-reversed at 1 Hz, 90% contrast. *Inset* shows brief flash ERGs for the same eye: 57 cd.s.m⁻² flash on a 63 sc cd.m⁻² background before (*blue line*) and 40 days after (*red line*) ONC. (From Miura G, Wang MH, Ivers KM, Frishman LJ. Retinal pathway origins of the pattern ERG of the mouse. *Exp Eye Res.* 2009;89(1):49–62, used with permission.)

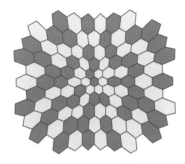

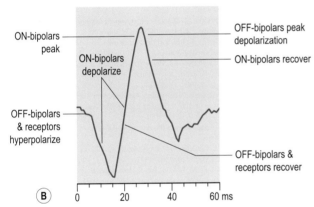

(A) 500 nv ⌐ 0 100 ms

(B)

ON-bipolars peak

ON-bipolars depolarize

OFF-bipolars & receptors hyperpolarize

OFF-bipolars peak depolarization

ON-bipolars recover

OFF-bipolars & receptors recover

0   20   40   60 ms

Fig. 24.18 Multifocal electroretinogram (mfERG) and its major components. (**A**) mfERG trace array (field view) using 103 hexagons scaled with eccentricity and covering about 35 degrees of visual angle, as illustrated *above* the traces. (From Hoffmann MB, Bach M, Kondo M, Li S, Walker S, Holopigian K et al. ISCEV standard for clinical multifocal electroretinography (mfERG) (2021 update). *Doc Ophthalmol.* 2021;142:5–16, used with permission.) (**B**) Model for the retinal contributions to the human mfERG based on results from the macular region of a macaque after pharmacologic separation of components. (From Hood DC, Frishman LJ, Saszik S, Viswanathan S. Retinal origins of the primate multifocal ERG: implications for the human response. *Invest Ophthalmol Vis Sci.* 2002;43(5):1673–1685, used with permission from Association for Research in Vision and Ophthalmology.)

PERGs can be recorded as transient responses to low reversal frequencies (1–2 Hz) or as steady state responses to higher frequencies (e.g., 8 Hz). The transient PERG has prominent early positive and later negative waves named, respectively, P50 and N95 (see Fig. 24.17) in humans, denoting the timing of the peak and trough following each pattern reversal.[37] Both P50 and N95 waves reflect ganglion cell activity, although P50 may include some nonspiking input.[154] The early positive (P1) and later negative (N2) component (Fig. 24.17) in the mouse transient PERG differ in exact timing but have similar general appearance to P50 and N95 in primates.[121,147]

MULTIFOCAL ELECTRORETINOGRAM

The multifocal ERG (mfERG) provides a technique to simultaneously record local ERG responses from many small retinal regions, typically 60 or 103, over 35 to 40 degrees of the visual field. Focal ERGs from individual regions are recorded in some clinics and labs,[155] but sampling more than a couple of regions is time consuming. The stimulus and mfERG records from a normal human subject are illustrated (Fig. 24.18A). The individual hexagons of the stimulus are reversed in contrast following a long pseudorandom (m-) sequence, which is shifted in time uniquely for each hexagon to enable extraction of responses to individual hexagons using cross-correlation of stimulus timing and the recorded response.[157,158] The reversal rate is locked to the frame rate of the visual stimulator, 75 Hz for CRTs, 60 Hz for LCD. Each hexagon had a 50% chance of reversing contrast on each frame change. The test is usually performed under light-adapted conditions, for which the foveal response is large, and allows changes in function to be detected in Stargardt's disease or other macular dystrophies. The scotopic mfERG was found to be more susceptible to effects of scattered light than light-adapted recordings and is rarely attempted.[159] Dark-adapted recordings in rodents require use of large focal regions.[160] Although difficult, some light-adapted recordings in rodents have been possible.[161]

Studies using glutamate analogs have shown that despite different methods of generation and response timing of the mfERG, the cellular origins of the major positive and negative waves are essentially the same as the light-adapted flash ERG (Fig. 24.18B).[156] This was the case for the standard fast mfERG, as well as when the stimulus presentation was slowed by interleaving blank frames between m-steps to allow the full ERG to form.[162]

A small optic nerve head component from axons of retinal ganglion cells may also be observed in the mfERG, especially when stimuli are arranged to optimize the response.[163,164] The optic nerve head component is the likely involved in the generation of high-frequency OPs in the slow sequence mfERG that are reduced in experimental glaucoma in macaques.[132,135]

BOX 24.3   Retinal cells contributing to the electroretinogram in specialized testing

Scotopic threshold response	Inner retinal neurons
Positive scotopic threshold response (pSTR)	Amacrine cells (monkey)
Negative scotopic threshold response (nSTR)	Retinal ganglion cells (rodents)
	Retinal ganglion cells (monkey)
	Partially retinal ganglion cells (rats, human?)
	Amacrine cells (AII) (mice)
	Partially amacrine cells (rats, human)
	Glial currents
Photopic negative response (PhNR)	Retinal ganglion cells (human, monkey)
	Amacrine cells (rodents)
	Glial currents
Pattern electroretinogram (PERG)	Retinal ganglion cells (human, monkey, rodent)
	Glial currents (transient PERG: N95, N2?)
Multifocal ERG	Initial negative and positive waves have similar origins to a- and b-waves in photopic ERG (monkey, and presumably human)

CLOSING COMMENTS

The ERG provides a means for noninvasive evaluation of normal and abnormal retinal function in humans and in animal models. Its value as a test of retinal function has increased as we have gained a better understanding of the retinal circuits involved and mechanisms of generation for each wave. Our current understanding of the origins of the ERGs recording in standard testing, and in more specialized testing, as reviewed in this chapter, are summarized in Boxes 24.2 and 24.3, respectively.

Looking to the future, promising early reports of the application of machine learning approaches to classification of ERGs in inherited retinal disease[165] may improve the value of the ERG in retinal testing.

REFERENCES

1. McCulloch DL, Marmor MF, Brigell MG, et al. ISCEV Standard for full-field clinical electroretinography (2015 update). *Doc Ophthalmol.* 2015;130:1–12.
2. Perlman I. Testing retinal toxicity of drugs in animal models using electrophysiological and morphological techniques. *Doc Ophthalmol.* 2009;118(1):3–28.
3. Tanimoto N, Muehlfriedel RL, Fischer MD, et al. Vision tests in the mouse: Functional phenotyping with electroretinography. *Frontiers Biosci.* 2009;14:2730–2737.
4. Vijayasarathy C, Sardar Pasha SPB, Sieving PA. Of men and mice: Human X-linked retinoschisis and fidelity in mouse modeling. *Prog Retin Eye Res.* 2021:100999.
5. Robson JG, Frishman LJ. Dissecting the dark-adapted electroretinogram. *Doc Ophthalmol.* 1998;95(3–4):187–215.
6. Sieving PA, Murayama K, Naarendorp F. Push-pull model of the primate photopic electroretinogram: a role for hyperpolarizing neurons in shaping the b-wave. *Vis Neurosci.* 1994;11(3):519–532.
7. Dawson WW, Trick GL, Litzkow CA. Improved electrode for electroretinography. *Invest Ophthalmol Vis Sci.* 1979;18(9):988–991.
8. Dowling JE. *The retina: an approachable part of the brain.* Cambridge, MA: The Belknap Press; 1987.
9. Li L, Jiao X, D'Atri I, et al. Mutation in the intracellular chloride channel CLCC1 associated with autosomal recessive retinitis pigmentosa. *PLoS Genet.* 2018;14:e1007504.
10. Robson AG, Nilsson J, Li S, et al. ISCEV guide to visual electrodiagnostic procedures. *Doc Ophthalmol.* 2018;136:1–26.
11. Heckenlively J, Arden GB. *Principles and practice of clinical electrophysiology of vision.* 2nd edn. Cambridge, MA: MIT Press; 2006.
12. Lam BL. *Electrophysiology of vision; Clinical testing and applications.* Boca Raton, FL: Taylor and Francis; 2005.
13. Brown KT, Wiesel TN. Localization of origins of electroretinogram components by intraretinal recording in the intact cat eye. *J Physiol.* 1961;158:257–280.
14. Brown KT, Wiesel TN. Analysis of the intraretinal electroretinogram in the intact cat eye. *J Physiol.* 1961;158:229–256.
15. Newman E, Reichenbach A. The Muller cell: a functional element of the retina. *Trends Neurosci.* 1996;19(8):307–312.
16. Newman EA, Frambach DA, Odette LL. Control of extracellular potassium levels by retinal glial cell K₊ siphoning. *Science.* 1984;225(4667):1174–1175.
17. Steinberg RH, Linsenmeier RA, Griff ER. Retinal pigment epithelial cell contributions to the electroretinogram and electrooculogram. *Prog Retin Res.* 1985;4:33–66.
18. Wu J, Peachey NS, Marmorstein AD. Light-evoked responses of the mouse retinal pigment epithelium. *J Neurophysiol.* 2004;91(3):1134–1142.
19. Kofuji P, Biedermann B, Siddharthan V, et al. Kir potassium channel subunit expression in retinal glial cells: implications for spatial potassium buffering. *Glia.* 2002;39(3):292–303.
20. Kofuji P, Ceelen P, Zahs KR, Surbeck LW, Lester HA, Newman EA. Genetic inactivation of an inwardly rectifying potassium channel (Kir4.1 subunit) in mice: phenotypic impact in retina. *J Neurosci.* 2000;20(15):5733–5740.
21. Steinberg RH, Linsenmeier RA, Griff ER. Three light-evoked responses of the retinal pigment epithelium. *Vision Res.* 1983;23(11):1315–1323.
22. Steinberg RH, Oakley 2nd B, Niemeyer G. Light-evoked changes in [K+]0 in retina of intact cat eye. *J Neurophysiol.* 1980;44(5):897–921.
23. Witkovsky P, Dudek FE, Ripps H. Slow PIII component of the carp electroretinogram. *J Gen Physiol.* 1975;65(2):119–134.
24. Oakley 2nd B. Potassium and the photoreceptor-dependent pigment epithelial hyperpolarization. *J Gen Physiol.* 1977;70(4):405–425.
25. Oakley 2nd B, Green DG. Correlation of light-induced changes in retinal extracellular potassium concentration with c-wave of the electroretinogram. *J Neurophysiol.* 1976;39(5):1117–1133.
26. Bui BV, Fortune B. Ganglion cell contributions to the rat full-field electroretinogram. *J Physiol.* 2004;555(Pt 1):153–173.
27. Frishman LJ, Sieving PA, Steinberg RH. Contributions to the electroretinogram of currents originating in proximal retina. *Vis Neurosci.* 1988;1(3):307–315.
28. Frishman LJ, Steinberg RH. Light-evoked increases in [K+]o in proximal portion of the dark-adapted cat retina. *J Neurophysiol.* 1989;61(6):1233–1243.
29. Frishman LJ, Steinberg RH. Intraretinal analysis of the threshold dark-adapted ERG of cat retina. *J Neurophysiol.* 1989;61(6):1221–1232.
30. Saszik SM, Robson JG, Frishman LJ. The scotopic threshold response of the dark-adapted electroretinogram of the mouse. *J Physiol.* 2002;543(Pt 3):899–916.
31. Sieving PA, Frishman LJ, Steinberg RH. Scotopic threshold response of proximal retina in cat. *J Neurophysiol.* 1986;56(4):1049–1061.
32. Viswanathan S, Frishman LJ, Robson JG, Harwerth RS, Smith 3rd EL. The photopic negative response of the macaque electroretinogram: reduction by experimental glaucoma. *Invest Ophthalmol Vis Sci.* 1999;40(6):1124–1136.
33. Viswanathan S, Frishman LJ, Robson JG, Walters JW. The photopic negative response of the flash electroretinogram in primary open angle glaucoma. *Invest Ophthalmol Vis Sci.* 2001;42(2):514–522.
34. Wachtmeister L. Oscillatory potentials in the retina: what do they reveal? *Progr Retin Eye Res.* 1998;17(4):485–521.
35. Heynen H, Wachtmeister L, van Norren D. Origin of the oscillatory potentials in the primate retina. *Vision Res.* 1985;25(10):1365–1373.
36. Hoffmann MB, Bach M, Kondo M, Li S, Walker S, Holopigian K, et al. ISCEV standard for clinical multifocal electroretinography (mfERG) (2021 update). *Doc Ophthalmol.* 2021;142:5–16.
37. Bach M, Brigell MG, Hawlina M, Holder GE, Johnson MA, McCulloch DL, et al. ISCEV standard for clinical pattern electroretinography (PERG)—2012 update. *Doc Ophthalmol.* 2013;126:1–7.
38. Constable PA, Bach M, Frishman L, Jeffrey BG, Robson AG. ISCEV Standard for Clinical Electro-oculography (2017 Update). *Doc Ophthalmol.* 2017;131(1):1–9.
39. Robson JG, Saszik SM, Ahmed J, Frishman LJ. Rod and cone contributions to the a-wave of the electroretinogram of the macaque. *J Physiol.* 2003;547(Pt 2):509–530.
40. Fulton AB, Brecelj J, Lorenz B, Moskowitz A, Thompson D, Westall CA. Pediatric clinical visual electrophysiology: a survey of actual practice. *Doc Ophthalmol.* 2006;113(3):193–204.
41. Kinoshita J, Peachey NS. Noninvasive electroretinographic procedures for the study of the mouse retina. *Curr Protoc Mouse. Biol.* 2018;8:1–16.
42. Granit R. The components of the retinal action potential in mammals and their relation to the discharge in the optic nerve. *J Physiol.* 1933;77(3):207–239.
43. Linsenmeier RA, Steinberg RH. Origin and sensitivity of the light peak in the intact cat eye. *J Physiol.* 1982;331:653–673.
44. Frishman LJ. Electrogenesis of the ERG. In: Schachat Andrew P, ed. *Ryan's Retina.* 6th edition. Elsevier; 2017:224–248.
45. Frishman LJ. Origins of the ERG. In: Heckenlively J, Arden GB, eds. *Principles and practice of clinical electrophysiology of vision.* Cambridge, Mass: MIT Press; 2006:139–183.
46. Kang Derwent JJ, Saszik SM, Maeda H, et al. Test of the paired-flash electroretinographic method in mice lacking b-waves. *Vis Neurosci.* 2007;24(2):141–149.
47. Freed MA, Smith RG, Sterling P. Rod bipolar array in the cat retina: pattern of input from rods and GABA-accumulating amacrine cells. *J Comp Neurol.* 1987;266(3):445–455.
48. Smith RG, Freed MA, Sterling P. Microcircuitry of the dark-adapted cat retina: functional architecture of the rod-cone network. *J Neurosci.* 1986;6(12):3505–3517.
49. Tsukamoto Y, Morigiwa K, Ueda M, Sterling P. Microcircuits for night vision in mouse retina. *J Neurosci.* 2001;21(21):8616–8623.
50. Frishman LJ, Shen FF, Du L, et al. The scotopic electroretinogram of macaque after retinal ganglion cell loss from experimental glaucoma. *Invest Ophthalmol Vis Sci.* 1996;37(1):125–141.
51. Abd-El-Barr MM, Pennesi ME, Saszik SM, et al. Genetic dissection of rod and cone pathways in the dark-adapted mouse retina. *J Neurophysiol.* 2009;102:1945–1955.
52. Sterling P, Freed MA, Smith RG. Architecture of rod and cone circuits to the on-beta ganglion cell. *J Neurosci.* 1988;8(2):623–642.

53. Heynen H, van Norren D. Origin of the electroretinogram in the intact macaque eye – II. Current source-density analysis. *Vision Res.* 1985;25(5):709–715.
54. Penn RD, Hagins WA. Signal transmission along retinal rods and the origin of the electroretinographic a-wave. *Nature.* 1969;223(5202):201–204.
55. Penn RD, Hagins WA. Kinetics of the photocurrent of retinal rods. *Biophys J.* 1972;12(8): 1073–1094.
56. Furukawa T, Hanawa I. Effects of some common cations on electroretinogram of the toad. *Japn J Physiol.* 1955;5(4):289–300.
57. Sillman AJ, Ito H, Tomita T. Studies on the mass receptor potential of the isolated frog retina. II. On the basis of the ionic mechanism. *Vision Res.* 1969;9(12):1443–1451.
58. Slaughter MM, Miller RF. 2-amino-4-phosphonobutyric acid: a new pharmacological tool for retina research. *Science.* 1981;211(4478):182–185.
59. Knapp AG, Schiller PH. The contribution of on-bipolar cells to the electroretinogram of rabbits and monkeys. A study using 2-amino-4-phosphonobutyrate (APB). *Vision Res.* 1984;24(12):1841–1846.
60. Stockton RA, Slaughter MM. B-wave of the electroretinogram. A reflection of ON bipolar cell activity. *J Gen Physiol.* 1989;93(1):101–122.
61. Robson JG, Frishman LJ. Photoreceptor and bipolar cell contributions to the cat electroretinogram: a kinetic model for the early part of the flash response. *J Optical Soc Am A Optics Image Sci Vis.* 1996;13(3):613–622.
62. Masu M, Iwakabe H, Tagawa Y, et al. Specific deficit of the ON response in visual transmission by targeted disruption of the mGluR6 gene. *Cell.* 1995;80(5):757–765.
63. McCall MA, Gregg RG. Comparisons of structural and functional abnormalities in mouse b-wave mutants. *J Physiol.* 2008;586(Pt 18):4385–4392.
64. Pardue MT, McCall MA, LaVail MM, Gregg RG, Peachey NS. A naturally occurring mouse model of X-linked congenital stationary night blindness. *Invest Ophthalmol Vis Sci.* 1998;39(12):2443–2449.
65. Gregg RG, Mukhopadhyay S, Candille SI, et al. Identification of the gene and the mutation responsible for the mouse nob phenotype. *Invest Ophthalmol Vis Sci.* 2003;44(1): 378–384.
66. Pesch K, Zeitz C, Fries JE, et al. Isolation of the mouse nyctalopin gene nyx and expression studies in mouse and rat retina. *Invest Ophthalmol Vis Sci.* 2003;44(5):2260–2266.
67. Bech-Hansen NT, Naylor MJ, Maybaum TA, et al. Mutations in NYX, encoding the leucine-rich proteoglycan nyctalopin, cause X-linked complete congenital stationary night blindness. *Nature Genet.* 2000;26(3):319–323.
68. Boycott KM, Pearce WG, Musarella MA, et al. Evidence for genetic heterogeneity in X-linked congenital stationary night blindness. *Am J Hum Genet.* 1998;62(4):865–875.
69. Dryja TP, McGee TL, Berson EL, et al. Night blindness and abnormal cone electroretinogram ON responses in patients with mutations in the GRM6 gene encoding mGluR6. *Proc Natl Acad Sci USA.* 2005;102(13):4884–4889.
70. Chang B, Heckenlively JR, Bayley PR, et al. The nob2 mouse, a null mutation in Cacna1f: anatomical and functional abnormalities in the outer retina and their consequences on ganglion cell visual responses. *Vis Neurosci.* 2006;23(1):11–24.
71. Brown KT. The electroretinogram: its components and their origins. *Vision Res.* 1968;8(6): 633–677.
72. Brown KT, Watanabe K, Murakami M. The early and late receptor potentials of monkey cones and rods. *Cold Spring Harbor Symp Quant Biol.* 1965;30:457–482.
73. Hood DC, Birch DG. A quantitative measure of the electrical activity of human rod photoreceptors using electroretinography. *Vis Neurosci.* 1990;5(4):379–387.
74. Hood DC, Birch DG. The A-wave of the human electroretinogram and rod receptor function. *Invest Ophthalmol Vis Sci.* 1990;31(10):2070–2081.
75. Baylor DA, Nunn BJ, Schnapf JL. The photocurrent, noise and spectral sensitivity of rods of the monkey Macaca fascicularis. *J Physiol.* 1984;357:575–607.
76. Lamb TD, Pugh Jr. EN. G-protein cascades: gain and kinetics. *Trends Neurosci.* 1992;15(8):291–298.
77. Lamb TD, Pugh Jr. EN. A quantitative account of the activation steps involved in phototransduction in amphibian photoreceptors. *J Physiol.* 1992;449:719–758.
78. Breton ME, Schueller AW, Lamb TD, Pugh Jr. EN. Analysis of ERG a-wave amplification and kinetics in terms of the G-protein cascade of phototransduction. *Invest Ophthalmol Vis Sci.* 1994;35(1):295–309.
79. Hood DC, Birch DG. Human cone receptor activity: the leading edge of the a-wave and models of receptor activity. *Vis Neurosci.* 1993;10(5):857–871.
80. Hood DC, Birch DG. Light adaptation of human rod receptors: the leading edge of the human a-wave and models of rod receptor activity. *Vision Res.* 1993;33(12):1605–1618.
81. Hood DC, Birch DG. Phototransduction in human cones measured using the alpha-wave of the ERG. *Vision Res.* 1995;35(20):2801–2810.
82. Hood DC, Birch DG. Measuring the health of the human photoreceptors with the leading edge of the a-wave. In: Heckenlively J, Arden GB, eds. *Principles and practice of clinical electrophysiology of vision.* Chicago: CV Mosby; 2006:487–502.
83. Cideciyan AV, Jacobson SG. An alternative phototransduction model for human rod and cone ERG a-waves: normal parameters and variation with age. *Vision Res.* 1996;36(16): 2609–2621.
84. Robson JG, Frishman LJ. The rod-driven a-wave of the dark-adapted mammalian electroretinogram. *Prog Retin Eye Res.* 2014;39:1–22.
85. Nakamura M, Sanuki R, Yasuma TR, et al. TRPM1 mutations are associated with the complete form of congenital stationary night blindness. *Mol Vis.* 2010;16:425–437.
86. Hagins WA, Penn RD, Yoshikami S. Dark current and photocurrent in retinal rods. *Biophys J.* 1970;10:380–412.
87. Nusinowitz S, Ridder 3rd WH, Ramirez J. Temporal response properties of the primary and secondary rod-signaling pathways in normal and Gnat2 mutant mice. *Exp Eye Res.* 2007;84(6):1104–1114.
88. Deans MR, Volgyi B, Goodenough DA, Bloomfield SA, Paul DL. Connexin36 is essential for transmission of rod-mediated visual signals in the mammalian retina. *Neuron.* 2002; 36(4):703–712.
89. Robson JG, Maeda H, Saszik SM, Frishman LJ. In vivo studies of signaling in rod pathways of the mouse using the electroretinogram. *Vision Res.* 2004;44(28):3253–3268.
90. Cameron AM, Mahroo OA, Lamb TD. Dark adaptation of human rod bipolar cells measured from the b-wave of the scotopic electroretinogram. *J Physiol.* 2006;575(Pt 2): 507–526.
91. Field GD, Rieke F. Non-linear signal transfer from mouse rods to bipolar cells and implications for visual sensitivity. *Neuron.* 2002;34(5):773–785.
92. Robson JG, Frishman LJ. Response linearity and kinetics of the cat retina: the bipolar cell component of the dark-adapted electroretinogram. *Vis Neurosci.* 1995;12(5):837–850.
93. Frishman LJ, Yamamoto F, Bogucka J, Steinberg RH. Light-evoked changes in $[K^+]o$ in proximal portion of light-adapted cat retina. *J Neurophysiol.* 1992;67(5):1201–1212.
94. Miller RF, Dowling JE. Intracellular responses of the Muller (glial) cells of mudpuppy retina: their relation to b-wave of the electroretinogram. *J Neurophysiol.* 1970;33(3): 323–341.
95. Frishman LJ, Reddy MG, Robson JG. Effects of background light on the human dark-adapted electroretinogram and psychophysical threshold. *J Optical Soc Am A Optics Image Sci Vis.* 1996;13(3):601–612.
96. Naarendorp F, Sieving PA. The scotopic threshold response of the cat ERG is suppressed selectively by GABA and glycine. *Vision Res.* 1991;31(1):1–15.
97. Barlow HB, Levick WR, Yoon M. Responses to single quanta of light in retinal ganglion cells of the cat. *Vision Res.* 1971;Suppl 3:87–101.
98. Mojumder DK, Sherry DM, Frishman LJ. Contribution of voltage-gated sodium channels to the b-wave of the mammalian flash electroretinogram. *J Physiol.* 2008;586(10): 2551–2580.
99. Moshiri A, Gonzalez E, Tagawa K, et al. Near complete loss of retinal ganglion cells in the math5/brn3b double knockout elicits severe reductions of other cell types during retinal development. *Dev Biol.* 2008;316(2):214–227.
100. Saszik SM. *The dark-adapted electroretinogram (ERG) of the mouse: inner retinal contributions and the effects of light adaptation.* College of Optometry. Houston: University of Houston; 2003.
101. Sieving P.A. Retinal ganglion cell loss does not abolish the scotopic threshold response (STR) of the cat and human ERG Clin Vis Sci 1991; 2:149–158.
102. Guldenagel M, Ammermuller J, Feigenspan A, et al. Visual transmission deficits in mice with targeted disruption of the gap junction gene connexin36. *J Neurosci.* 2001;21(16): 6036–6044.
103. Bui BV, Edmunds B, Cioffi GA, Fortune B. The gradient of retinal functional changes during acute intraocular pressure elevation. *Invest Ophthalmol Vis Sci.* 2005;46(1):202–213.
104. Lyubarsky AL, Falsini B, Pennesi ME, Valentini P, Pugh Jr. EN. UV- and midwave-sensitive cone-driven retinal responses of the mouse: a possible phenotype for coexpression of cone photopigments. *J Neurosci.* 1999;19(1):442–455.
105. Jacobs GH, Fenwick JA, Williams GA. Cone-based vision of rats for ultraviolet and visible lights. *J Exp Biol.* 2001;204(Pt 14):2439–2446.
106. Jacobs GH, Neitz J, Krogh K. Electroretinogram flicker photometry and its applications. *J Optical Soc Am A Optics Image Sci Vis.* 1996;13(3):641–648.
107. Jacobs GH, Neitz J, Deegan 2nd JF. Retinal receptors in rodents maximally sensitive to ultraviolet light. *Nature.* 1991;353(6345):655–656.
108. Toda K, Bush RA, Humphries P, Sieving PA. The electroretinogram of the rhodopsin knockout mouse. *Vis Neurosci.* 1999;16(2):391–398.
109. Calvert PD, Krasnoperova NV, Lyubarsky AL, et al. Phototransduction in transgenic mice after targeted deletion of the rod transducin alpha-subunit. *Proc Natl Acad Sci USA.* 2000;97(25):13913–13918.
110. Chang B, Dacey MS, Hawes NL, et al. Cone photoreceptor function loss-3, a novel mouse model of achromatopsia due to a mutation in Gnat2. *Invest Ophthalmol Vis Sci.* 2006;47(11):5017–5021.
111. Lucas RJ, Freedman MS, Lupi D, Munoz M, David-Gray ZK, Foster RG. Identifying the photoreceptive inputs to the mammalian circadian system using transgenic and retinally degenerate mice. *Behav Brain Res.* 2001;125(1–2):97–102.
112. Fu Y, Zhong H, Wang MH, et al. Intrinsically photosensitive retinal ganglion cells detect light with a vitamin A-based photopigment, melanopsin. *Proc Natl Acad Sci USA.* 2005;102(29):10339–10344.
113. Rangaswamy NV, Frishman LJ, Dorotheo EU, Schiffman JS, Bahrani HM, Tang RA. Photopic ERGs in patients with optic neuropathies: comparison with primate ERGs after pharmacologic blockade of inner retina. *Invest Ophthalmol Vis Sci.* 2004;45(10):3827–3837.
114. Bush RA, Sieving PA. A proximal retinal component in the primate photopic ERG a-wave. *Invest Ophthalmol Vis Sci.* 1994;35(2):635–645.
115. Heynen H, van Norren D. Origin of the electroretinogram in the intact macaque eye I. Principal component analysis. *Vision Res.* 1985;25(5):697–707.
116. Kremers J, Aher A, Parry N, Patel NB, Frishman LJ. Comparisons of macaque and human L- and M-cone driven ERGs. *Exp Eye Res.* 2021 May;206:108556.
117. Shirato S, Maeda H, Miura G, Frishman LJ. Postreceptoral contributions to the light-adapted ERG of mice lacking b-waves. *Exp Eye Res.* 2008;86(6):914–928.
118. Rangaswamy NV, Shirato S, Kaneko M, Digby BI, Robson JG, Frishman LJ. Effects of spectral characteristics of Ganzfeld stimuli on the photopic negative response (PhNR) of the ERG. *Invest Ophthalmol Vis Sci.* 2007;48(10):4818–4828.
119. Sharma S, Ball SL, Peachey NS. Pharmacological studies of the mouse cone electroretinogram. *Vis Neurosci.* 2005;22(5):631–636.
120. Xu L, Ball SL, Alexander KR, Peachey NS. Pharmacological analysis of the rat cone electroretinogram. *Vis Neurosci.* 2003;20(3):297–306.
121. Miura G, Wang MH, Ivers KM, Frishman LJ. Retinal pathway origins of the pattern ERG of the mouse. *Exp Eye Res.* 2009;89(1):49–62.
122. Cui J, Pan ZH. Two types of cone bipolar cells express voltage-gated Na^+ channels in the rat retina. *Vis Neurosci.* 2008;25(5–6):635–645.
123. Whitten DN, Brown KT. The time courses of late receptor potentials from monkey cones and rods. *Vision Res.* 1973;13(1):107–135.

124. Ueno S, Kondo M, Ueno M, Miyata K, Terasaki H, Miyake Y. Contribution of retinal neurons to d-wave of primate photopic electroretinograms. *Vision Res.* 2006;46(5):658–664.

125. Strettoi E, Volpini M. Retinal organization in the bcl-2-overexpressing transgenic mouse. *J Comp Neurol.* 2002;446(1):1–10.

126. Kondo M, Sieving PA. Primate photopic sine-wave flicker ERG: vector modeling analysis of component origins using glutamate analogs. *Invest Ophthalmol Vis Sci.* 2001;42(1):305–312.

127. Viswanathan S, Frishman LJ, Robson JG. Inner-retinal contributions to the photopic sinusoidal flicker electroretinogram of macaques. Macaque photopic sinusoidal flicker ERG. *Doc Ophthalmol.* 2002;105(2):223–242.

128. Krishna VR, Alexander KR, Peachey NS. Temporal properties of the mouse cone electroretinogram. *J Neurophysiol.* 2002;87(1):42–48.

129. Hancock HA, Kraft TW. Human oscillatory potentials: intensity-dependence of timing and amplitude. *Doc Ophthalmol.* 2008;117(3):215–222.

130. Rangaswamy NV, Hood DC, Frishman LJ. Regional variations in local contributions to the primate photopic flash ERG: revealed using the slow-sequence mfERG. *Invest Ophthalmol Vis Sci.* 2003;44(7):3233–3247.

131. Dong CJ, Agey P, Hare WA. Origins of the electroretinogram oscillatory potentials in the rabbit retina. *Vis Neurosci.* 2004;21(4):533–543.

132. Zhou W, Rangaswamy N, Ktonas P, Frishman LJ. Oscillatory potentials of the slow-sequence multifocal ERG in primates extracted using the Matching Pursuit method. *Vision Res.* 2007;47(15):2021–2036.

133. McCall MA, Lukasiewicz PD, Gregg RG, Peachey NS. Elimination of the rho1 subunit abolishes GABA(C) receptor expression and alters visual processing in the mouse retina. *J Neurosci.* 2002;22(10):4163–4174.

134. Ogden TE. The oscillatory waves of the primate electroretinogram. *Vision Res.* 1973;13(6):1059–1074.

135. Rangaswamy NV, Zhou W, Harwerth RS, Frishman LJ. Effect of experimental glaucoma in primates on oscillatory potentials of the slow-sequence mfERG. *Invest Ophthalmol Vis Sci.* 2006;47(2):753–767.

136. Vigh J, Solessio E, Morgans CW, Lasater EM. Ionic mechanisms mediating oscillatory membrane potentials in wide-field retinal amacrine cells. *J Neurophysiol.* 2003;90(1):431–443.

137. Kenyon GT, Moore B, Jeffs J, et al. A model of high-frequency oscillatory potentials in retinal ganglion cells. *Vis Neurosci.* 2003;20(5):465–480.

138. Lei B, Yao G, Zhang K, Hofeldt KJ, Chang B. Study of rod- and cone-driven oscillatory potentials in mice. *Invest Ophthalmol Vis Sci.* 2006;47(6):2732–2738.

139. Forte JD, Bui BV, Vingrys AJ. Wavelet analysis reveals dynamics of rat oscillatory potentials. *J Neurosci Methods.* 2008;169(1):191–200.

140. Kondo M, Kurimoto Y, Sakai T, et al. Recording focal macular photopic negative response (PhNR) from monkeys. *Invest Ophthalmol Vis Sci.* 2008;49(8):3544–3550.

141. Machida S, Raz-Prag D, Fariss RN, Sieving PA, Bush RA. Photopic ERG negative response from amacrine cell signaling in RCS rat retinal degeneration. *Invest Ophthalmol Vis Sci.* 2008;49(1):442–452.

142. Maffei L, Fiorentini A. Electroretinographic responses to alternating gratings in the cat. *Exp Brain Res.* 1982;48(3):327–334.

143. Maffei L, Fiorentini A, Bisti S, Hollander H. Pattern ERG in the monkey after section of the optic nerve. *Exp Brain Res.* 1985;59(2):423–425.

144. Berardi N, Domenici L, Gravina A, Maffei L. Pattern ERG in rats following section of the optic nerve. *Exp Brain Res.* 1990;79(3):539–546.

145. Porciatti V. The mouse pattern electroretinogram. *Doc Ophthalmol.* 2007;115(3):145–153.

146. Porciatti V, Pizzorusso T, Cenni MC, Maffei L. The visual response of retinal ganglion cells is not altered by optic nerve transection in transgenic mice overexpressing Bcl-2. *Proc Natl Acad Sci USA.* 1996;93(25):14955–14959.

147. Porciatti V, Saleh M, Nagaraju M. The pattern electroretinogram as a tool to monitor progressive retinal ganglion cell dysfunction in the DBA/2J mouse model of glaucoma. *Invest Ophthalmol Vis Sci.* 2007;48(2):745–751.

148. Harrison JM, O'Connor PS, Young RS, Kincaid M, Bentley R. The pattern ERG in man following surgical resection of the optic nerve. *Invest Ophthalmol Vis Sci.* 1987;28(3):492–499.

149. Holder GE. Pattern electroretinography (PERG) and an integrated approach to visual pathway diagnosis. *Progr Retin Eye Res.* 2001;20(4):531–561.

150. Bach M, Hoffmann MB. Update on the pattern electroretinogram in glaucoma. *Optom Vis Sci.* 2008;85(6):386–395.

151. Ventura LM, Porciatti V, Ishida K, Feuer WJ, Parrish 2nd RK. Pattern electroretinogram abnormality and glaucoma. *Ophthalmology.* 2005;112(1):10–19.

152. Luo X, Frishman LJ. Retinal pathway origins of the pattern electroretinogram (PERG). *Invest Ophthalmol Vis Sci.* 2011;52(12):8571–8584.

153. John SW, Smith RS, Savinova OV, et al. Essential iris atrophy, pigment dispersion, and glaucoma in DBA/2J mice. *Invest Ophthalmol Vis Sci.* 1998;39(6):951–962.

154. Viswanathan S, Frishman LJ, Robson JG. The uniform field and pattern ERG in macaques with experimental glaucoma: removal of spiking activity. *Invest Ophthalmol Vis Sci.* 2000;41(9):2797–2810.

155. Miyake Y. Focal macular electroretinography. *Nagoya J Med Sci.* 1998;61(3–4):79–84.

156. Hood DC, Frishman LJ, Saszik S, Viswanathan S. Retinal origins of the primate multifocal ERG: implications for the human response. *Invest Ophthalmol Vis Sci.* 2002;43(5):1673–1685.

157. Sutter EE. The fast m-transform: a fast computation of cross-correlations with binary m-sequences. *SIAM J Computing.* 1991;20(4):686–694.

158. Sutter EE, Tran D. The field topography of ERG components in man—I. The photopic luminance response. *Vision Res.* 1992;32(3):433–446.

159. Hood DC, Wladis EJ, Shady S, Holopigian K, Li J, Seiple W. Multifocal rod electroretinograms. *Invest Ophthalmol Vis Sci.* 1998;39(7):1152–1162.

160. Nusinowitz S, Ridder 3rd WH, Heckenlively JR. Rod multifocal electroretinograms in mice. *Invest Ophthalmol Vis Sci.* 1999;40(12):2848–2858.

161. Paskowitz DM, Nune G, Yasumura D, et al. BDNF reduces the retinal toxicity of verteporfin photodynamic therapy. *Invest Ophthalmol Vis Sci.* 2004;45(11):4190–4196.

162. Hood DC, Seiple W, Holopigian K, Greenstein V. A comparison of the components of the multifocal and full-field ERGs. *Vis Neurosci.* 1997;14(3):533–544.

163. Sutter EE, Shimada Y, Li Y, Bearse MA. Mapping inner retinal function through enhancement of adaptive components in the m-ERG. *Vision Sci Appl OSA Tech Dg Ser.* 1999;1:52–55.

164. Sutter EE, Bearse Jr. MA. The optic nerve head component of the human ERG. *Vision Res.* 1999;39(3):419–436.

165. Müller PL, Treis T, Odainic A, Pfau M, Herrmann P, Tufail A, et al. Prediction of function in ABCA4-related retinopathy using ensemble machine learning. *J Clin. Med.* 2020 Aug;9(8):2428.

Regulation of Light Through the Pupil

Randy H. Kardon and Edward Linton

The pupil is a dynamic aperture that regulates the entry of light destined for the retina. Its usefulness is illustrated by the fact that it is a relatively conserved structure among essentially all vertebrates, and it is present through a completely separate evolutionary process in cephalopods.[1] The major functions of the pupil are outlined in Fig. 25.1 and are summarized below.

The human visual system is able to adapt to large changes in illumination, in part through constriction and dilation of the pupil. The retina has a dynamic range of around 12 log units that allows both excellent vision in daylight and some useful vision under starlight, which is between 1 million and 100 million times dimmer (6–8 log units). Pupil movement in response to changing light intensity aids in optimizing retinal illumination to maximize visual perception, and can account for 1.5 log units or an approximately 30-fold change in retinal illumination in half a second. This provides an important immediate mechanism for light and dark adaptation, supplementing slower retinal processes.[2] However, the ability of the pupil to regulate retinal illumination also depends on iris pigmentation; a blue, lightly pigmented iris allows light to pass through to the retina with very little influence of pupil size.[3] Patients with a fixed immobile pupil are usually symptomatic during an abrupt change in illumination; they may be photophobic when they are subjected to sudden increases in light, and they may not be able to discern objects in their environment when they first enter dim lighting conditions. These symptoms are described by patients with an immobile pupil because compensatory retinal photoreceptor adaptation is not fast enough. This emphasizes the important role of the pupil in optimizing visual perception in a timely fashion over a wide range of lighting conditions of the environment.

In addition to regulating retinal illumination, the pupil can also contribute to improving (up to a point) the image quality at the retina. A small pupil reduces the degree of chromatic and spherical aberration.[4,5] Part of the reason for this is that a smaller aperture size limits the light rays entering the optical system to the central cornea and lens, avoiding more peripheral portions of the cornea and lens, where refractive power and aberrations are greater (Box 25.1). Image quality can also be affected by depth of focus.

A small pupil aperture increases the depth of focus of the eye's optics by filtering out fewer parallel light rays from a given object. This is the principle used to create a sharp image with a pinhole camera.[7] When attempting near gaze, the accommodative power of the eye moves the focal plane from distance to near, and pupil miosis aids accommodation by bringing objects into better focus by increasing the depth of focus afforded by the smaller aperture size.

Besides the physiologic functions of the pupil explained earlier and outlined in Fig. 25.1, the pupil diameter and its movement under different conditions also provide important indicators used for clinical assessment of a patient. The clinical aspects of pupil function (Fig. 25.2; Box 25.2) consist of (1) pupil movement as an objective indicator of afferent input, (2) pupil inequality as a reflection of asymmetric autonomic nerve output to each iris, (3) the influence of pupil diameter and morphology on the optical properties of the eye, (4) pupil behavior as an indicator of various central nervous system (CNS) states and conditions, and (5) the pupil response to topical and systemic drugs for diagnostic, therapeutic, and investigational purposes.

The pupil response to light is routinely used clinically to compare the magnitude of the afferent signal that is generated by each eye and transmitted along the afferent pupil pathway in response to a bright light presented sequentially to one eye and then the other. Under normal conditions, there should be minimal difference in the magnitude of reflex pupil constriction to the same stimulus presented to each eye; however various injuries and disease states can cause a noticeable asymmetry in this signal, termed a *relative afferent pupil defect*, or RAPD. This is an important sign because the afferent pupil pathway travels along the anterior portion of the visual pathway and an RAPD can be a critically important clinical sign in evaluating afferent visual dysfunction.

Inequality of the pupils, termed *anisocoria*, is another important clinical state of the pupils because it may represent autonomic nerve interruption to the iris from the sympathetic or parasympathetic nervous system, direct damage to the iris sphincter or dilator muscle, or pharmacologic exposure of the iris to mydriatic or miotic drugs. The clinical significance of anisocoria, its causes, and an approach to pharmacologic evaluation are covered in more detail later in this chapter. Generalized changes in autonomic function can cause symmetric changes in pupil size, which can also be a useful clinical sign for diagnosis or pharmacologic monitoring.

Given that the round, (nearly) centered, dynamic pupil serves to modulate light entry and image quality, it follows that large and/or irregular pupils may produce clinically significant visual symptoms in the form of photophobia and optical aberrations, particularly at night or after dilating drops, when pupil diameter is largest. A large immobile pupil resulting from scarring, dilating drops, or damage to the iris sphincter muscle or its nerve supply may produce extreme sensitivity to light and glare in dim light. This is because the normal function of the pupil in controlling retinal illumination is impaired.

Pupillary responses to light, psychosensory stimuli, and resting pupillomotor tone have also been precisely quantified by computerized

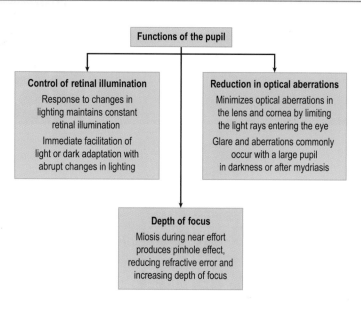

Fig. 25.1 Functions of the pupil include control of retinal illumination, reduction in optical aberrations, and improved depth of focus.

---

pupillometry in laboratory settings to aid in diagnosis and the monitoring of treatment in many eye and CNS disorders, including retinal disorders, optic neuropathies, neurologic diseases such as multiple sclerosis and Parkinson disease, psychiatric disorders such as depression and schizophrenia, and as an objective indicator of cognitive function.

The pupil response to cholinergic or adrenergic drops has long been used to clinically differentiate causes of anisocoria. Emerging evidence shows the pupil may also be used as a pharmacologic indicator of peripheral or central drug effects. The pupil response to topical inhibitors of narcotics (naloxone) has also been used to study the effect of narcotic tolerance in addicted individuals.

In this chapter the physiology of the normal pupil is discussed, and examples of abnormalities of pupil function are also shown. Knowledge of normal pupil physiology is key to understanding various pathologic states. The reader who is interested in pursuing these subjects in much greater detail is advised to consult the excellent book by Loewenfeld.[8]

THE NEURONAL PATHWAY OF THE PUPIL LIGHT REFLEX AND NEAR PUPIL RESPONSE

To understand the major factors that can affect the diameter and movement of the pupil to various stimuli, it is important to know the basic neuronal pathway for the pupil light reflex and near response. This is

schematically depicted in Fig. 25.3. The pupil light reflex consists of three major divisions of neurons that integrate the light stimulus to produce a pupil contraction: (1) an afferent division, (2) an interneuron division, and (3) an efferent division.

The afferent division consists of retinal input from photoreceptors, bipolar neurons, and ganglion cells. Axons of retinal ganglion cells from each eye provide light input information that is conveyed by synapses to interneurons located in the pretectal olivary nucleus of the midbrain. In turn, these interneurons distribute pupil light input to neurons in the right and left Edinger–Westphal nuclei through crossed (decussating) and uncrossed (nondecussating) connections. From here, the neurons of the Edinger–Westphal nucleus send their preganglionic parasympathetic axons along the oculomotor nerve to synapse at the ciliary ganglion in each orbit. The neurons in the ciliary ganglion give rise to postganglionic parasympathetic axons that travel in the short ciliary nerves to the globe (passing through the suprachoroidal space), where they synapse with the iris sphincter muscle.

The pupil constriction to a near stimulus involves activation of neurons in the rostral brainstem that relay their signal to the same Edinger–Westphal neurons that are activated in the light reflex. Therefore, the efferent pathway for the near pupil constriction is the same as for the light reflex, but the input pathway to the Edinger–Westphal nucleus differs.

The integration of the pupil light reflex and pupil near response, including the anatomy of the involved neurons, their receptive field properties, and their response to various attributes of light stimuli, has been reviewed.[9] In the following sections, these neuronal pathways are summarized.

Afferent arm of the pupil light reflex

The neural integration of the pupil light reflex begins with the afferent pathway in the retina, consisting of the photoreceptors, bipolar cells, and ganglion cells. For many years, it was disputed whether it was the rods or cones that contribute to the pupil light reflex and whether these were the same photoreceptors as those contributing to visual perception. Extensive experimental and psychophysical work has shown that the neuronal pathways mediating the pupil light reflex and visual perception share the same photoreceptors. Until recently, it was thought that all photoreceptor input was shared by both conscious perception of light and the pupil light reflex. In previous studies, almost all changes in light input producing a change in visual perception also produced a comparable change in pupil size. In fact, in almost every way measured, the pupil responses to light parallel those of visual perception. For example, the wavelength-sensitivity profile of pupil threshold for a

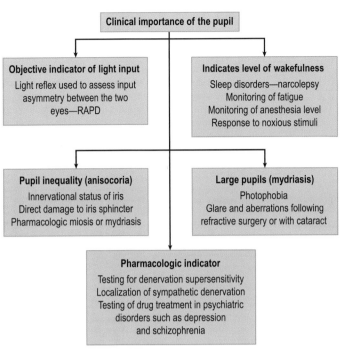

BOX 25.2 Diagnosis and the relative afferent pupillary defect

The amount of transient pupil contraction to a light stimulus or the steady-state diameter of the pupil under constant illumination can reflect the health of the retina and optic nerve and may be used to detect disease.

The most common clinical test for assessing input asymmetry between the two eyes is the alternating light test, commonly referred to as the swinging flashlight test. As a light is alternated back and forth between the right and left eyes, the clinician observes the pupil movements in response to the light.

If the two eyes are matched with respect to retinal and optic nerve input, the pupil movements appear similar when either eye is stimulated. However, if one eye's input has been diminished because of disease affecting the retina or optic nerve, the pupil responses to light shown in that eye become noticeably less during the alternating light test.

When this input asymmetry is observed during the alternating light test, it is called a relative afferent pupillary defect (RAPD): RAPDs are discussed in greater length in a subsequent portion of this chapter.

Pupil diameter can also be used to determine the extent of midbrain supranuclear inhibition, which is also related to an individual's state of wakefulness.

An excited, aroused person will have larger-diameter pupils because of the increase in central inhibition of the parasympathetic nerves innervating the iris sphincter, which originate in the midbrain, and the increase in sympathetic tone to the dilator muscle.

Conversely, a sleepy individual, a fatigued individual, or one under the influence of general anesthesia or narcotics will have smaller pupils as a result of central disinhibition at the level of the midbrain. Careful monitoring of the diameter of the pupil in this setting may be clinically useful for ascertaining the presence of sleep disorders such as narcolepsy, the level of anesthesia, or the presence of narcotics.

The extent of pupil dilation to sensory stimuli such as pain or sound may also serve as an objective indicator of how intact the sensory input is.

---

small transient contraction as the color of light is changed from blue to red exactly parallels the same wavelength-sensitivity profile of visual perception. The shift in sensitivity is also the same as the eye is changed from a condition of light adaptation to dark adaptation (Purkinje shift), providing further evidence that the same photoreceptors are used for both pupil and vision. Patients with various abnormalities of rods and cones can be shown to have the same deficits in color vision or lack of appropriate sensitivity change during dark adaptation when the results of visual threshold are compared with pupil threshold for small contractions to light stimuli.[10] Both rods and cones contribute to the pupil light reflex, but to a different extent depending on the lighting conditions.

Under conditions of dark adaptation and in response to low-intensity lights, the pupil light reflex becomes a sensitive light meter and is mediated primarily by rods, giving rise to low-amplitude pupil contractions. However, with brighter light stimuli and under conditions of greater light adaptation, the cones dominate most of the transient

pupil light contractions. Therefore, the rods are primarily responsible for the pupil's ability to give rise to small contractions in response to low-intensity lights under conditions of dark adaptation—they provide a high sensitivity to the pupil light reflex at low light levels, just as they do for visual perception. The cones provide the input responsible for the larger transient pupil contractions that are easily observed under direct clinical observation, occurring at suprathreshold levels of light, mainly under photopic conditions. Loewenfeld[11] has summarized the extensive literature on this subject and her text should be consulted by the reader desiring a more complete discussion of this topic. It is also believed that the bipolar cells, which receive input from the photoreceptors, are the same neurons providing input to the pupil light reflex as those mediating visual perception.

Although it appears that the pupil and visual systems share rod and cone photoreceptor input, a number of interesting observations in recent years has revealed a previously unrecognized and important aspect of light transduction through the pupil pathway.

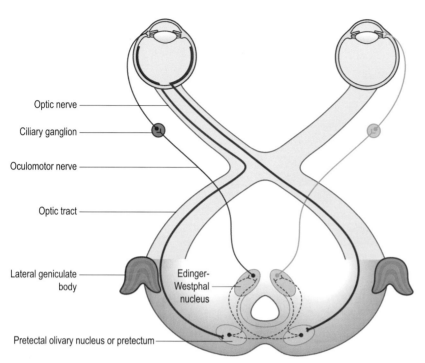

Fig. 25.3 Diagram of the nerve pathways involved in the pupil light reflex. Afferent input from the nasal retina crosses to the contralateral side, and the pupil input from retinal ganglion cell axons exits the optic tract in the brachium of the superior colliculus to synapse at the pretectal olivary nucleus. The temporal retinal input from the same eye follows a similar course on the ipsilateral side. The neurons in the pretectal olivary nucleus send crossed and uncrossed fibers by way of the posterior commissure to the Edinger–Westphal nucleus on each side. From here, the preganglionic parasympathetic fibers travel with the oculomotor nerve and then synapse at the ciliary ganglion. The postganglionic parasympathetic neurons pass from the ciliary ganglion by way of the short ciliary nerves to the iris sphincter muscle.

Evidence in the last 20 years has shown that the rod and cone input to the pupil light reflex is mediated by a special class of retinal ganglion cells containing the primitive visual pigment melanopsin found in the retina of lower animals.[12–23] Besides being activated by rod and cone input causing a transient pupil response, the intrinsically photosensitive retinal ganglion cell (ipRGC) is also directly sensitive to light, providing a sustained steady-state pupil constriction to light. This intrinsic, direct activation pathway of the melanopsin-containing RGCs causes the cell to discharge in a sustained way and is directly proportional to steady-state light input, similar to a direct current (DC) light meter, which does not show classical light adaptation properties. In genetically altered mice that completely lack functional rods and cones, it was discovered that a rather robust pupil light reflex was still present. This unexpected finding was followed by a series of studies to identify what retinal element could be contributing to the pupil light reflex in the absence of rod and cone input. Through clever labeling experiments, a specific ganglion cell was identified containing melanopsin, which was itself photosensitive, with a broad spectral peak centering on about 480 nm, which is blue light. These melanopsin ganglion cells have been found to project to a number of locations, with a large projection to the suprachiasmatic nucleus in the hypothalamus and also to the pretectal nucleus, the site of the first midbrain interneuron synapse for the pupil light reflex pathway (Box 25.3). Additional details about ipRGCs can be found in Chapter 26.

Elegant electrophysiologic recordings coupled with the study of response properties of these ganglion cells have revealed that the melanopsin-containing RGCs provide the midbrain pathway for the pupil light reflex and also provide light sensing information for the diurnal regulating areas of the hypothalamus that modulate the circadian rhythm. These melanopsin ganglion cells also receive rod and cone input to the pupil light reflex, but are also capable of transduction of light directly (under photopic conditions), without photoreceptor input, and may be responsible for providing more of steady-state light input to the brain.

Chromatic pupillary light responses, those measured using stimuli with blue wavelengths targeting the spectral sensitivity of ipRGCs, have been shown to be sensitive to changes in ipRGC function. The postillumination

> ## BOX 25.3 Melanopsin-containing retinal ganglion cells and the pupil
>
> Activation properties of the melanopsin retinal ganglion cells via input from rods, cones, or intrinsic light stimulus can be assessed in humans by recording pupil light reflexes at different wavelengths of light under scotopic and photopic states of retinal adaptation.
>
> Application of the newly discovered physiology of the pupil light reflex may provide an objective clinical means of differentiating retinal from optic nerve disease and determining which class of photoreceptive neurons is being affected by disease (see Chapter 26).[24]

pupil response (PIPR), which is the sustained pupillary contraction after light offset, is now an established marker of direct, intrinsic melanopsin–mediated activation of ipRGCs, and protocols for its measurement have been developed in recent years, although inconsistency between methods has led to variable results among different studies.[25] Nevertheless, the PIPR has been shown to be reduced in moderate- and severe-stage glaucoma, correlated to RGC thickness, and correlated to visual field loss on automated perimetry. It has also been shown to be abnormal in milder stages of glaucoma with more specifically defined testing paradigms. Similar work is being done in other optic neuropathies including Leber's hereditary optic neuropathy (LHON), anterior ischemic optic neuropathy (AION), idiopathic intracranial hypertension (IIH), and demyelinating diseases such as multiple sclerosis.

Interestingly, these ipRGCs have also been shown in recent years to be dysfunctional in various neurologic disorders, including Parkinson disease, which supports evidence that there is a significant prevalence of circadian disorders in patients with Parkinson disease. Other neurodegenerative diseases, including Alzheimer disease and Huntington disease, which have prominent circadian disturbances, are also being investigated.

There is also recent evidence of input from melanopsin-sensitive RGCs to brain structures important for mood, and the PIPR has been shown to be diminished in patients with seasonal affective disorder.

This helps to explain why some patients blind from photoreceptor loss still exhibit a pupil light reaction to bright blue light[26] and also maintain a circadian rhythm, while patients blind from optic nerve lesions (loss of melanopsin ganglion cell input) often lack a normal circadian rhythm.

The interneuron arm of the pupil light reflex

The ganglion cell axons conveying light input to the classic, main pupil light reflex pathway segregate from the rest of the visual ganglion cell axons at the distal portion of the optic tract before the lateral geniculate nucleus. As in the visual input pathway, the pupil ganglion cell axons from the nasal retina (temporal field) decussate at the chiasm to the opposite side, and the axons from the temporal retina (nasal field) stay on the same side. Therefore, pupil ganglion cell axons from homonymous areas of the visual field (temporal field from the contralateral eye and nasal field from the ipsilateral eye) distribute within the optic tract. From there, they travel in the brachium of the superior colliculus and synapse in the midbrain with the next neurons in the light reflex located at the olivary pretectal nucleus. These neurons represent interneurons because they serve to integrate the afferent input coming from the retina with the efferent output of the pupil light reflex exiting the midbrain from the Edinger–Westphal nucleus.

The receptive field properties of the pretectal neurons have been elucidated in the awake primate.[27,28] These interneurons are the way-station for the converging receptive field impulses of the RGCs from the retina and are fewer in number, summating the ganglion cell input at this location. The receptive field of each pretectal neuron has been found to receive input from ganglion cells over a large area of retina (up to 20 degrees). Some of these neurons exhibit a "flat" response, firing equally well from input over its entire receptive field. However, another subset exhibits a "foveal-weighted" response, discharging at a higher frequency when a stimulus is placed near the center of the visual field (and receptive field of the neuron). This may partly explain why the pupil light reflex appears to be more sensitive to light coming from the center of the visual field.

Patients with a relatively small area of damage to their central visual field have also been found to show an obvious decrease in the pupil light reflex in the affected eye compared with the fellow eye (an RAPD), which may relate to the receptive field properties of the pretectal interneurons. The pretectal neurons discharge at a frequency that is linear to the log of intensity of the light stimulus given. However, not all of these neurons respond in the same range; it appears that some are more sensitive in different ranges of intensities, so together there is an interneuron response covering at least a 4 log unit range of input. Neurons in the pretectum send crossed and uncrossed fibers, through the posterior commissure, to the small population of neurons comprising the paired Edinger–Westphal nuclei. This allows afferent input from the pretectal nucleus on each side to be distributed almost equally to the pupil efferent pathway originating in the Edinger–Westphal nucleus (Box 25.4).

The uncrossed pathway appears to have evolved during development of binocularity and stereovision. Animals with eyes located more to the side of the head (e.g., birds, rabbits) have almost completely crossed pathways, with no significant uncrossed component. That is why shining a light in one eye of these animals produces an almost totally crossed input to the pretectum, which then sends an almost completely crossed output to the Edinger–Westphal nucleus. The result is that only the pupil of the eye being stimulated will contract. Cats are between birds and primates in this evolutionary respect, with approximately 70% of their pupil pathway crossed. Placing a pet cat so that one of its eyes points more toward a light produces a greater reaction of the pupil in the eye facing the light, causing an anisocoria. In humans, in whom the crossed and uncrossed pathways are almost equal, the direct and consensual pupil light reflex is equal. This is why illuminating one eye normally does not result in pupil inequality (anisocoria). Similarly, input deficits to one eye caused by damage to the retina or optic nerve should not normally produce an anisocoria in humans.

In some individuals the crossed pathway slightly exceeds the uncrossed pathway in both the retina and midbrain, leading to a slightly greater pupil response in the eye stimulated compared with the pupil contraction of the fellow eye, similar to cats, but not to the same extent. This consensual deficit, termed *contraction anisocoria*, is small and can usually be recognized only with the aid of pupillographic recordings.

As stated earlier, the melanopsin-containing RGCs appear to mediate the classic midbrain pathway of the pupil light reflex. However, there is also evidence that ganglion cells conveying visual information to the occipital cortex may also play a role in modulation of pupil movement in response to different types of visual stimuli, which is likely mediated through cortical projection onto supranuclear interneurons.

For example, patients with isolated occipital infarcts have homonymous visual field defects that show corresponding pupil defects to small (2 degrees in diameter) focal lights presented to the same cortically blind visual field area. This phenomenon has been reported previously, but only in subsequent studies utilizing pupil perimetry has the correspondence between the shape characteristic of the homonymous pupil and visual field defect been fully appreciated.[29–40] This correspondence provides compelling evidence for a role of cortical mediation of the pupil light reflex when small, focal light stimuli are used. In addition, the pupil has been shown to respond to changes in complex stimuli such as spatial frequency, motion, and contrast, providing additional evidence for a higher-level cortical process that is capable of mediating pupil contractions to visual stimuli.[41–47]

There is also evidence that visual attention can modulate the pupil light response, an idea that fits with the above observations and dates back to the 1940s, when the pupil light reflex was found to be influenced by ocular dominance in retinal rivalry.[48] Evidence followed that the pupil light reflex was suppressed while planning a saccade, and can be influenced by task demands.[49]

Recently, an elegant set of primate experiments showed that the pupil light reflex gain can be modulated by cortical stimulation of the frontal eye fields below the threshold required for a saccade, which recruits visual attention to a specific location. The pupil response to a light stimulus is potentiated when the stimulus is presented in the attended area, and dampened when it is presented elsewhere.[50] It is theorized that this spatial influence of the frontal eye field is mediated through its substantial projection to the olivary pretectal nucleus. Similar findings have recently been reported in humans. Covert attention (without eye movement) significantly potentiates the pupil light reflex to stimuli presented in the region of attention. These experiments supported growing evidence that the olivary pretectal nucleus not only

> ## BOX 25.4 Dorsal midbrain lesions and the pupil
>
> Damage to the posterior commissure from tumors compressing the dorsal midbrain from above (e.g., pinealomas) or from encephalitis (e.g., tertiary syphilis) may block the impulse pathway from the pretectal neurons to the Edinger–Westphal nucleus.
>
> This situation can result in a loss of the pupil light reflex but spares the near pupil response (which originates from a more rostral location in the midbrain, before synapsing with the Edinger–Westphal nucleus), causing a light-near dissociation of the pupil.

receives ascending inputs from melanopsin RGCs, but may be modulated in a spatially specific manner from descending cortical inputs.

In addition to modulation of the pupil light reflex, there is experimental evidence of pupil contraction with orienting visual attention to a bright area, purportedly to prepare pupil size for the next saccadic goal. This effect was abolished by lidocaine injection to the superior colliculus,[51] which is known to be involved in spatial attention. These experiments are part of a growing body of evidence that intermediate layers of the superior colliculus, which receive inputs primarily from cortical areas, are responsible for mediating the pupil response to reorienting attention. These reorienting pupil responses are dependent on an intact visual cortex.

Recent studies show direct evidence that the activity of the locus coeruleus, an area responsible for broad adrenergic innervation to many brain areas, is associated with changes in pupil size. Electrical microstimulation in mice, rats, and monkeys can cause pupil dilation, and functional imaging studies also show that pupil size changes during some visual tasks localize to the locus coeruleus. Baseline pupil size is influenced by tonic locus coeruleus activity, which may be an indicator of vigilance, arousal, and other activation states. Transient phasic activity in the locus coeruleus has been associated with surprise, which is a well-known behavioral cause of pupil dilation.[52] As evidence grows for cortical influences on pupil size, there has been a surge of interest in using pupil measurement as an indicator of neural processes, which appears at least possible in well-controlled activities mediated by the pretectal olivary nucleus, intermediate layers of the superior colliculus, and locus coeruleus. There is hope that precise measurements of pupil responses to various changes in cognitive function can bring new insights into the physiology and pathophysiology of these fundamental neural systems in health and disease.

The efferent arm of the pupil light reflex

The efferent arm of the pupil light reflex is diagrammatically summarized in Fig. 25.4, which also shows the site of common lesions along this pathway that may be encountered in clinical practice. The neurons in the Edinger–Westphal nucleus send preganglionic axons into the right and left fascicle of the oculomotor nerve (third nerve) to join the motor axons destined for the eye muscles, as well as the preganglionic accommodative fibers that originate in nearby nuclei. The right and left fascicles of the third nerve exit the midbrain through the subarachnoid space, where each continues as the third nerve toward the orbital apex (Box 25.5).

After passing through the cavernous sinus to the orbital apex, the preganglionic pupillary fibers and accommodative fibers synapse in the ciliary ganglion (parasympathetic ganglion). A lesion at this site may produce an Adie's pupil. From here, the last neurons in the chain, the postganglionic neurons, pass into the eye by way of the short ciliary nerves, located in the suprachoroidal space, where they distribute to the anterior segment of the eye to innervate the iris sphincter muscle. The postganglionic accommodative fibers, which outnumber the pupil fibers 30:1, supply the ciliary muscle within the ciliary body of the eye. The postganglionic pupillary neurons appear to innervate the iris sphincter muscle in a segmental distribution over approximately 20 clock-hour sections. This is why lesions of the ciliary ganglion, such as in Adie syndrome, usually cause a number of sectors of the iris sphincter to become acutely denervated, with loss of the pupil contraction only in these segments (Box 25.6).

The pupil near reflex and accommodation

When fixation of the eye is shifted from a far to a near object of interest, the eyes converge, the intraocular lenses accommodate, and both pupils constrict. This triad of ocular vergence, accommodation, and

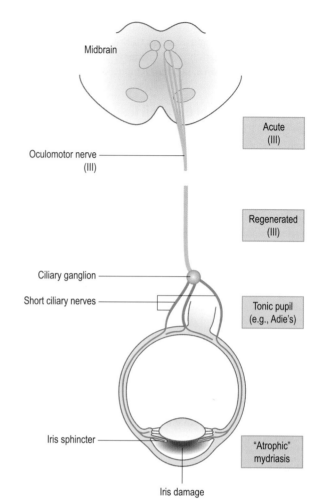

Fig. 25.4 Innervation of the iris sphincter, from the Edinger–Westphal nucleus by way of the oculomotor nerve, ciliary ganglion, and short ciliary nerves, with some of the causes of a fixed dilated pupil.

BOX 25.5   **Pupil-involving third nerve palsy**

The pupillary preganglionic fibers are located on the superior aspect of the oculomotor nerve as it exits the midbrain, but soon come to lie on the medial aspect.[53]

This is the reason aneurysms of the circle of Willis that lie in this area, such as aneurysms of the posterior communicating artery, often cause pupillary efferent deficits early on, because of the medial location of the artery with respect to the oculomotor nerve.

---

pupil contraction is called the *near response*. Despite many contentions in the literature claiming that this pupil constriction is exclusively dependent on either convergence or accommodation, clinical and experimental data indicate that any one of the three functions can be selectively abolished or elicited without affecting the others. These experimental and clinical observations have resulted in general agreement that the impulses that cause accommodation, convergence, and pupil constriction must arise from different cell groups within the oculomotor nucleus and travel by way of separate fibers to their effector muscles. Accommodation, convergence, and pupillary constriction are associated movements and are not tied to one another in the manner usually referred to by the term *reflex*. They are controlled, synchronized, and associated by supranuclear connections, but they are not

BOX 25.6 Light-near dissociation

The postganglionic parasympathetic accommodative axons, which innervate the smooth muscle of the ciliary body, outnumber the postganglionic light reflex axons, which innervate the iris sphincter muscle in a ratio of 30 to 1.

Damage to the postganglionic parasympathetic axons can occur as a result of an Adie's pupil or trauma or after orbital surgery. After acute injury, the surviving nerve cell bodies within the ciliary ganglion sprout axons and grow toward the ciliary body muscle and the iris sphincter after about 8 to 12 weeks.

Because the accommodative cell bodies outnumber the pupil light reflex cell bodies, almost all of the axonal sprouts reaching the iris sphincter muscle originate from the accommodative cell bodies. This reinnervation of the iris sphincter is therefore aberrant because the pupil sectors that were denervated still do not respond to light, but they now contract in response to activation of the accommodative neurons, hence producing a light-near dissociation of the pupil reflex.

caused by one another. The components of the near pupil reflex were recently summarized.[9,53]

The miosis of the near response and the pupillary constriction to light have a single final common efferent pathway from the Edinger–Westphal nucleus to the iris sphincter by way of the ciliary ganglion. They primarily differ in the origin of the supranuclear pathways that are elicited by light and near that both converge on the Edinger–Westphal nucleus. With a near stimulus such as accommodation, the pupil normally constricts, even with no change in retinal luminance. It is important to realize that this near reflex of the pupil is mediated by the same efferent nerve pathway originating from the same neurons in the Edinger–Westphal nucleus that mediate the pupil light reflex. There does not appear to be a separate neuronal efferent pathway that mediates the near pupil constriction.

However, the supranuclear control over this response is different from the one mediating the light reflex. In the case of the light reflex, the supranuclear input comes from the pretectal nucleus, as described in the previous section. In the case of the near reflex involving accommodation, convergence, and miosis, the supranuclear input is thought to originate from cortical areas surrounding visual cortex and from cortical areas within the frontal eye fields. The cortical neurons providing input for the near reflex are thought to synapse at least once, before passing ventral toward the visceral neurons overlying the oculomotor complex in the midbrain. This is because a cortical lesion in this area does not produce atrophy within the oculomotor nuclear complex (it is at least one synapse removed). It is also important to realize that the near reflex consists of convergence of the eyes, accommodation, and pupil contraction, all of which should be thought of as comovements and, as stated earlier, are not strictly dependent on one another. Any one of the three comovements may occur in the absence of the others, as discussed by Loewenfeld.[11] Because the supranuclear pathway for the near reflex passes ventral in the midbrain and the supranuclear pathway for the light reflex passes dorsal in the midbrain, the two systems may be differentially affected by disease processes (Box 25.4).

The supranuclear neuronal input from a near visual task stimulates the pupil constrictor neurons located in the visceral part of the Edinger–Westphal nuclei. The same supranuclear neuronal input also stimulates the more numerous accommodative neurons, located nearby in the remaining visceral portion of the Edinger–Westphal nucleus. These preganglionic neurons give rise to accommodative axons that travel together with the pupil preganglionic light reflex neurons within the oculomotor nerve to synapse at the ciliary ganglion in the orbit (see previous section).

In summary, with a near stimulus, both the accommodative neurons (which mediate ciliary muscle contraction) and light reflex neurons (which mediate iris sphincter contraction) in the Edinger–Westphal visceral motor nuclei are stimulated from a supranuclear level. This gives rise to a separate neuronal output of accommodative and light reflex preganglionic neurons by way of the oculomotor nerve to the ciliary ganglion, which in turn gives off separate postganglionic innervation to the ciliary body and iris sphincter muscles. The preganglionic and postganglionic light reflex pathways make use of the same neurons to mediate pupil contraction to either near or light stimuli.[37]

Pupil reflex dilation: central and peripheral nervous system integration

Normally, when the pupil dilates, two integrated processes take place: the iris sphincter relaxes and the iris dilator contracts, actively helping pull the pupil open.[54,55] Because the iris sphincter is stronger than the dilator muscle, pupil dilation does not readily occur until the sphincter muscle relaxes. Relaxation of the iris sphincter is accomplished by supranuclear inhibition of the Edinger–Westphal nucleus at a CNS level, most notably from the reticular activating formation in the brainstem. It appears from animal studies that this neuronal inhibitory pathway involves the CNS's sympathetic class of neurons. These sympathetic neurons pass through the periaqueductal gray area and innervate the pupil efferent neurons at the Edinger–Westphal nucleus, and at the synapse there is α2-adrenergic receptor activation.[56] When this central inhibition is active, the preganglionic parasympathetic output from the Edinger–Westphal nucleus is suppressed, resulting in a relative relaxation of the iris sphincter and pupil dilation. When this inhibition is inactive, such as during sleep, with anesthesia, or with narcotics, the preganglionic neurons fire at a high rate, causing miosis. The neurons of the Edinger–Westphal nucleus are unique in this respect because their baseline discharge frequency, without any input, is high. If all input to these neurons is disconnected, they fire at a high rate, which results in a sustained pupil contraction and miosis. This is why deep sleep or anesthesia, which reduces almost all inhibitory supranuclear input to the Edinger–Westphal nucleus, results in small pupils.

Alternatively, during a state of wakefulness, the supranuclear inhibition is active and the neurons of the Edinger–Westphal nucleus are suppressed, causing the pupils to become larger again. If a light stimulus is given at this point, a train of neuronal impulses from the retina and then the pretectal interneuron will arrive at the Edinger–Westphal nucleus, which momentarily overcomes this inhibition, causing the pupil to constrict. If the light is turned off or the retina begins to become light adapted, the supranuclear inhibition again dominates, causing a reflex dilation of the pupil.

Almost all of the conditions mentioned previously cause changes in pupil diameter resulting from the modulation of the neuronal output from the Edinger–Westphal nucleus. In addition, the same factors causing a reflex dilation of the pupil also result in an increase in output to the peripheral sympathetic nervous system innervating the iris dilator muscle. The sympathetic nerve activity can be thought of as a "turbo-charge" for pupil dilation. Peripheral sympathetic nerve activation is not a requirement for pupil dilation to occur (parasympathetic inhibition alone can accomplish that to some extent), but it greatly enhances the dynamics of pupil dilation in terms of speed and maximal pupil diameter attained.

The sympathetic outflow to the iris dilator muscle can be thought of as a paired three-neuron chain (Fig. 25.5) on both the right and left side of the central and peripheral nervous system without decussations. The first neuron originates in the hypothalamus and descends through the brainstem on each side into the lateral column of the spinal cord, where it synapses at the cervicothoracic level of C7–T2. The second

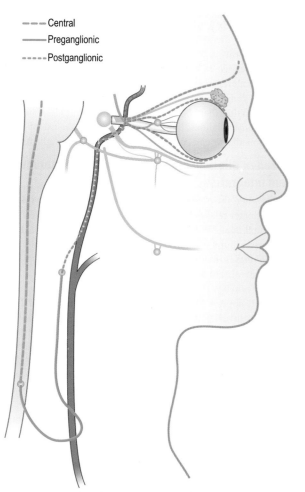

Central
Preganglionic
Postganglionic

Fig. 25.5 Sympathetic innervation to the eye, showing the three-neuron chain of central, preganglionic, and postganglionic fibers. (Modified from Maloney WF, Younge BR, Moyer NJ. Evaluation of the causes and accuracy of pharmacologic localization in Horner's syndrome. *Am J Ophthalmol.* 1980;90(3):394–402. https://doi.org/10.1016/S0002-9394(14)74924-4.)

preganglionic neuron leaves this level of the spinal cord and travels over the apical pleura of the lung and into the spinal rami to synapse at the superior cervical ganglion at the level of the carotid artery bifurcation on the right and left side of the neck. The third neuron, the postganglionic neuron, follows a long course along the internal carotid artery into the head and orbit. As these neurons pass through the cavernous sinus, they are associated with the abducens and then the trigeminal nerve before entering the orbit and distributing to the iris dilator muscle via the long ciliary nerves.[57]

In addition to the neuronal mechanisms involved in pupil dilation, humoral mechanisms may contribute to pupil diameter. Circulating catecholamines in the blood (e.g., a bolus released from the adrenal glands) may act directly on the iris dilator muscle either through the bloodstream or, potentially, indirectly through the tears, resulting in mydriasis. Clinical conditions that influence the integration of the parasympathetic inhibition, sympathetic stimulation, and humoral release of neurotransmitters may take various forms and may affect the dynamics of reflex dilation in a characteristic manner that may be diagnostic of clinical conditions. This is revisited later in this chapter when pupil inequality and conditions that impede pupil dilation are discussed.

Other neuronal input to the iris

In addition to the autonomic nerves supplying the iris, sensory innervation to the iris is provided by the ophthalmic division of the trigeminal nerve.[58,59] However, these sensory nerves may play an additional role in modulating pupil diameter. It is well known to cataract surgeons that mechanical and chemical irritation of the eye can cause a strong miotic response that is noncholinergic and fails to reverse with autonomically acting drugs. In rabbits and cats the response seems to be caused by the release of substance P or closely related peptides from the sensory nerve endings, but in monkeys and humans substance P has little or no miotic effect. Cholecystokinin (in nanomolar amounts) caused contraction of isolated iris sphincter from monkeys and humans.[60] Intracameral injections in monkeys caused miosis that was not prevented by tetrodotoxin or indomethacin, indicating that the miosis was not caused by either stimulation of nerve endings or release of prostaglandins but by direct action on sphincter receptors. The cholecystokinin antagonist lorglumide caused competitive inhibition of the response.

STRUCTURE OF THE IRIS

Iris sphincter, iris dilator, and iris color

It is important to understand the structure of the iris and its histology to understand how the iris tissue accommodates changes in pupil diameter during contraction and dilation and how disorders of the iris tissue affect pupil movement. The iris can be divided into two main layers: the posterior leaf and the anterior leaf (Fig. 25.6). The posterior iris leaf contains the dilator muscle, the sphincter muscle, and the posterior pigmented epithelium. From a front view of the iris, the dilator muscle is located circumferentially, in the midperiphery of the iris.

The sphincter muscle is located just inside the pupillary border; its circumference is made up of approximately 20 motor segments connected together but innervated individually by postganglionic branches of the ciliary nerve. In the normal iris these segments receive nerve excitation in a roughly simultaneous fashion, and the entire circumference contracts in concert. Both the dilator and sphincter muscles are derived embryologically from the anterior layer of the two layers of posterior pigmented epithelium.

The more superficial, anterior iris leaf consists of connective tissue stroma with cells, blood vessels, and nerves supplying the sphincter and dilator, but there is no epithelial layer in primate species. The different components of the posterior and anterior iris undergo structural alterations to accommodate changes in pupil diameter during contraction and dilation.[61] These alterations in structure confer mechanical nonlinearities influencing how much the pupil can constrict or dilate in response to changes in light or pharmacologic stimulus and was extensively studied by Loewenfeld.[62]

The mechanical nonlinearities are important because they impose limitations on the range of pupil diameter over which the extent of pupil movement can be used for assessing neuronal reflexes to light stimuli or near stimuli or for pharmacologic testing of the pupil. For example, a person with small, 3-mm diameter pupils in dim light would obviously not show as large a pupil contraction to a standard light stimulus as a person with 5-mm diameter pupils, but the retina and optic nerves of both persons may be completely normal. A similar situation would occur if one attempted to quantify the response to a topical miotic or mydriatic agent. Therefore, the structure of the iris can pose physical constraints on pupil movement in response to sensory stimuli or pharmacologic agents, and this should be considered carefully when comparing the response in different eyes. It has been shown that calculating the percent change in pupil contraction (e.g., change in diameter from baseline to peak contraction divided by the baseline pupil diameter) helps to normalize the pupil light reflex across a range of pupil sizes.[63]

The color of the iris is determined by its mesodermal and ectodermal components. In Caucasians, the stroma is relatively free of pigment at birth. The stroma absorbs the long wavelengths of light, allowing the shorter (blue) wavelengths to pass through to the pigmented epithelium where they are reflected back, causing the iris to appear blue. If pigmentation does not develop in the anterior stromal layers, the iris remains blue throughout life. If the stroma becomes denser and contains significant numbers of melanosomes, the blue color gives way to gray. The accumulation of pigment in the iris melanocytes of individuals destined to have nonblue irides occurs during the first year of life and is dependent on sympathetic innervation of the melanocytes (derived from neural crest cells). Interruption of the oculosympathetic nerve supply to one eye during this time period usually results in heterochromia, with the denervated iris remaining blue. In a heavily pigmented iris, the fine pattern of iris vessels is hidden by pigment and the surface of the iris looks brown and velvety.

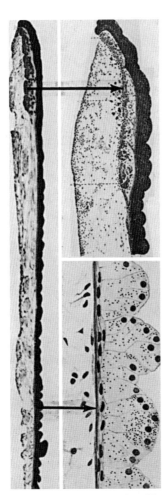

Fig. 25.6 Histology of the iris in cross section. *Upper arrow* points to sphincter muscle drawn in higher magnification; *lower arrow* points to dilator muscle of bleached preparation drawn in higher magnification. (From Saltzmann M. *Anatomy and Histology of the Human Eye-ball.* Chicago, IL: University of Chicago Press; 1912.)

PROPERTIES OF LIGHT AND THEIR EFFECT ON PUPIL MOVEMENT

Properties of light stimulating the retina that affect the pupil response include intensity, duration, temporal frequency, area, perimetric location, state of retinal adaptation, wavelength, and spatial frequency. There is a wealth of information on how these properties of light stimuli affect the pupillary response with regard to latency and amplitude of movement. Loewenfeld[8,64] has presented the most complete review of this topic in her book on the pupil, which should be consulted for a detailed literature review and for examples illustrating these different light effects. In general, the amplitude of pupil movement increases in proportion to the log light intensity of the stimulus, whereas the latency time of the pupil light reflex (time from stimulus onset to beginning of pupil contraction) becomes shorter (Fig. 25.7). With increasing duration of light stimulus, the contraction amplitudes become greater and more prolonged. With long-duration light stimuli, after an initial contraction the pupil may undergo oscillations (hippus) and undergo slow dilation, or "pupil escape," because of light adaptation (Fig. 25.7). Table 25.1 summarizes the different light effects.

Most investigations of the pupillary light reflex have focused on the response of the pupil to changes in light level because the neuronal pathway for this reflex was thought to respond only to stepwise changes in light intensity. With the advent of computer graphics and sophisticated software programs, more complex stimuli can be presented to allow properties of spatial frequency, color, motion, and luminance to be controlled more carefully. A number of investigators have taken advantage of this technology to investigate whether the pupil is capable of responding to visual stimuli that change in color or spatial frequency when the average luminance does not change.[9,34–36,57,58,65]

The results of these studies provide evidence that the pupil contracts to either an onset or offset of spatial frequency or color exchanges. From a practical standpoint, these responses allow the pupil response to be used as an objective indicator of visual acuity and color discrimination. From a theoretical standpoint, the pupil response to isoluminant

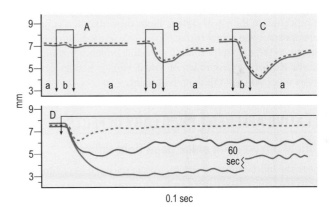

Fig. 25.7 (A), (B), and **(C)** Dark-adapted normal subject. Light flashes, interval b, of increasing intensity were given to the right eye to produce increasing pupillary constriction. Latent period decreases with intensity of flash. Both pupils were recorded simultaneously using an infrared pupillography device. The right pupil tracing *(solid line)* and the left pupil tracing *(broken line)* move in synchrony. **(D)** Reactions of the pupil to prolonged light of different intensities. At the dimmest intensity there was a short pupil light constriction and the pupil dilated (escaped) during the light stimulus. At the brighter intensities, the contractions were larger and more sustained, also exhibiting oscillations (hippus). (From Lowenstein O, Loewenfeld IE. In: Davso H, ed. *The Eye.* Vol. 3. New York: Academic Press; 1962.)

TABLE 25.1	Effect of properties of light stimuli on the pupillary light reflex
Stimulus property	**Effect on pupillary light reflex**
Light intensity	Amplitude of contraction increases linearly over at least a 3 log unit range of stimulus intensity (stimulus under photopic conditions). The entire stimulus-response function resembles an "S"-shaped curve. Latency time, the time from stimulus onset to the start of pupil contraction (200–450 ms), becomes more prolonged with dimmer light stimuli (in the range of 20–40 ms further delay/log unit decrement of light intensity).
State of light adaptation	In the dark-adapted state, the threshold light intensity needed to produce a pupil contraction becomes less as rods are brought into play. However, rods in the dark-adapted state do not produce as much increase in pupil contraction in response to increases in stimulus intensity, compared with cones in the mesopic and photopic states.
Duration	When stimulus duration is shorter than 70 ms, there is a reciprocal relationship between the duration and intensity, which is required to produce a given pupil contraction amplitude. With longer-duration stimuli, the pupil contracts more, there is a shorter latency time (up to a point), and the pupillary contraction is more sustained; however, pupil escape (relative dilation) may occur as a result of light adaptation.
Area	The pupillary light reflex shows much greater area summation properties than visual perception (for visual threshold of perception, summation is minimal with stimuli greater than 1 degree). With full-field Ganzfeld stimuli, the pupil threshold can be equal to visual threshold (or even smaller); with stimuli smaller than 1–2 degrees, visual threshold is usually more sensitive (by 0.5–1.0 log units).
Perimetric location	Under dark adaptation, the fovea shows a decreased sensitivity compared with surrounding retinal areas because of the lack of rods here. In mesopic and photopic adaptation, the pupil responds greatest in the central field; the temporal field response is usually greater than the nasal field response.
Spectral sensitivity	The wavelength sensitivity of the pupillary light reflex follows that of visual perception with a blue shift under dark adaptation and a peak sensitivity at green under photopic conditions.
Temporal frequency	The normal pupil cannot move much faster than 4 Hz because of the relatively slow contraction of smooth muscle. Animals with striated iris muscle (pigeons) can easily follow a 10-Hz stimulus. At frequencies of 9–25 Hz, the steady-state pupil diameter increases, indicating loss of sensitivity in neuronal integration of light within this frequency range.
Spatial frequency	When the change in average luminance across a stimulus patch is kept constant, the pupil undergoes small contractions when a sinusoidal grating is presented or when the grating bars are alternated between dark and light. The mechanism is thought to be independent of a luminance response. The greater the spatial frequency, the less the pupil contracts to the stimulus and this has been correlated with visual acuity.
Motion	Recent evidence suggests that the pupil may respond to a motion stimulus even under isoluminant conditions.

stimuli provides a means to explore how and where different signals are processed in the visual system. From these studies it is becoming more apparent that visual cortex plays a role in modulating the pupil response to these complex stimuli, providing evidence that small pupil reflexes elicited by properties of visual stimuli besides luminance involve more than just midbrain processing.

RELATIVE AFFERENT PUPILLARY DEFECTS

Clinical observation of the pupil light reflex

One of the most important clinical uses of the pupil has to do with its role in assessing afferent input from the retina, optic nerve, and anterior visual pathways (chiasm, optic tract, and midbrain pathways). The pupil light reflex sums the entire neuronal input from the photoreceptors, bipolar cells, ganglion cells, and axons of ganglion cells. Therefore, damage at any one of these sites along the visual pathway will reduce the amplitude of pupil movement in response to a light stimulus.[8,66] The pupil light reflex can show considerable variation, even among normal individuals as a result of supranuclear influences on the midbrain pupillomotor center that are not related to afferent input of the retina and optic nerve. However, the pupil light reflex is symmetric between the two eyes of a normal individual. The normal symmetry of input between the two eyes allows the clinician to pick up any asymmetric damage between the two eyes by simply comparing how well the pupil contracts to a standard light shined into

one eye compared with alternating the light over to the other eye.[67] Observation of the pupil movement in response to alternating the light back and forth between the two eyes (Figs. 25.8 and 25.9) is the basis for the alternating light test or swinging flashlight test for assessing the RAPD.[68,69] The RAPD, or input asymmetry, can be quantified in log units using neutral density filters of increasing strength placed in front of the better responding eye. A log density filter that neutralizes or balances the asymmetry of pupil movement between the two eyes, until they are matched, is chosen and is taken as the log unit RAPD.

Another important property of the pupil light reflex is that when a diffuse light stimulus enters the eye, the entire area of the visual field is summated into the pupil response, with some increased weight given to the central 10 degrees.[8] The area summating properties of the pupil light reflex make the amplitude of its movement roughly proportional to the amount of working visual field. Therefore, damage to peripheral portions of the retina and visual field defects outside of the central field can also reduce the amplitude of the pupil light reflex. This is in contrast to other objective tests of visual function such as the Ganzfeld electroretinogram (which measures diffuse damage to the retina and not local damage) and visual evoked potentials (which are center weighted and therefore affected mainly by central field loss). The pupil light reflex is one of the few objective reflexes that can be used as a clinical test for detecting and quantifying abnormalities in the retina, optic nerve, optic chiasm, or optic tract, and is also able to detect regional visual field damage in the center or periphery.

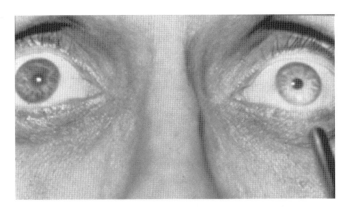

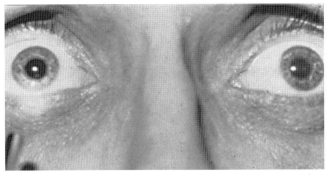

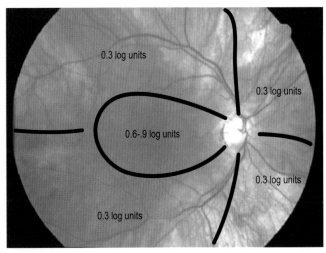

Fig. 25.10 Approximate distribution of the amount of log unit relative afferent pupil defect expected for corresponding loss of input in the regions of the retina shown, assuming the other eye is normal.

Fig. 25.8 A patient is shown with a large relative afferent pupil defect of the right eye. In the *top* photograph a light is shined in the normal left eye and both pupils constrict to a small diameter. When the light is alternated to stimulate the right eye (*bottom* photograph), the pupils hardly constrict at all.

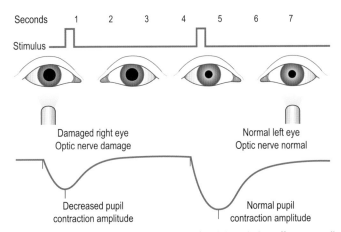

Fig. 25.9 Pupillographic demonstration of a right relative afferent pupil defect. With short light pulses the pupil light reflex (*bottom* tracings) are of lesser amplitude when the stimulus was given to the right eye compared with stimulus to the left eye.

Estimating the amount of the RAPD in log units is important to confirm and validate how much visual field damage (asymmetry between the two eyes) is present and whether it is consistent with the results of the visual field test. For example, a patient with a small amount of macular degeneration in one eye and not the other might be expected to have only a 0.3 log unit RAPD. However, if that patient had a 1.0 log unit RAPD, some other cause of visual loss, such as a previous branch retinal artery occlusion or optic neuropathy, would have to be considered. In addition, the area and extent of visual field loss

would be expected to be more than that caused by a small amount of macular degeneration. The importance of quantifying the RAPD cannot be overemphasized. In general, in the case of unilateral visual damage, loss of the central 5 degrees of the visual field results in an RAPD of approximately 0.3 log units. Loss of the entire central area of field (10 degrees) causes about a 0.6 to 0.9 log unit RAPD. Each visual field quadrant outside of the macula is worth about 0.3 log units (Fig. 25.10), but the temporal field loss seems to result in more loss of pupil input compared with the nasal field quadrants. Examples of the log unit magnitude of the RAPD expected for common clinical disorders are given in Table 25.2. The correlation between the relative afferent defect and the area and extent of visual field loss, however, is only approximate. Differences between the two may be important clues as to the cause and extent of damage to the anterior visual system (Box 25.7).

Recent studies using computerized pupillography to quantify the log unit RAPD more precisely have also revealed that some normal subjects with normal visual fields and examination can have a small 0.3 log unit RAPD.[57,72,73] Therefore small RAPDs discovered incidentally in a patient without ocular complaints and a normal examination can probably be dismissed.

Estimating the amount of the pupillomotor input asymmetry (the RAPD) can also be done more subjectively, without using neutral density filters, by grading the asymmetry of pupil response as +1, +2, +3, or +4. This subjective grading can also be classified according to the amount of pupil escape or dilation of the pupils as the light is alternated to the other eye.[74] However, most subjective grading of the RAPD has serious limitations; it is subject to some large errors resulting from age variations in pupil diameter and pupil mobility. For example, a patient with small pupils and small pupil contractions to light may have a large RAPD that may appear deceptively small on the basis of the small differences in pupil excursion observed as the light is alternated between the two eyes. However, the amount of neutral density filter needed to dim the better eye until the small contractions are equal could easily approach 0.9 to 1.2 log units, representing substantial input damage. Estimating the size of an RAPD without using filters is much like estimating an ocular deviation "by Hirschberg" without doing a prism cover test. More accurate quantification of the RAPD is accomplished by determining the log unit difference needed to balance the pupil reaction between the two eyes using photographic neutral density filters, as described previously. If one pupil does not move well because

TABLE 25.2   Common diseases producing relative afferent pupillary defects and expected magnitude of defect

Condition	Site	Log unit relative afferent pupillary defects	Influencing factors
Intraocular hemorrhage	Anterior chamber or vitreous (dense)	0.6–1.2	Density of hemorrhage
Intraocular hemorrhage	Anterior chamber (diffuse)	0.0–0.3	Density of hemorrhage
Intraocular hemorrhage	Preretinal (central vein occlusion or diabetic)	0.0	Preretinal location does not significantly reduce light
Diffusing media opacity	Cataract or corneal scar	0.0–0.3 (in opposite eye)	Dispersion of light producing increase in light input
Unilateral functional visual field loss	None	0	
Central serous retinopathy (CSR) or cystoid macular edema (CME)	Retina (fovea)	0.3	Area of retina involved
Central or branch retinal vein occlusion (CRVO, BRVO)	Inner retina	0.3–0.6 (nonischemic) 0.9 (ischemic)	Area of visual field defect and degree of ischemia
Central or branch retinal artery occlusion (CRAO, BRAO)	Inner retina	0.3–3.0	Area and location of retina involved
Retinal detachment	Outer retina	0.3–2.1	Area and location of detached retina (e.g., 0.6 log units for macula + 0.3 log units for each quadrant)
Anterior ischemic optic neuropathy	Optic nerve head	0.6–2.7	Extent and location of visual field defect
Optic neuritis (acute)	Optic nerve	0.6–3.0	Extent and location of visual field defect
Optic neuritis (recovered)	Optic nerve	0.0–0.6	No visual field defect, residual RAPD
Glaucoma	Optic nerve	Usually none if symmetric damage to both eyes	Degree of visual field asymmetry between the two eyes correlates with the log unit RAPD
Compressive optic neuropathy	Optic nerve	0.3–3.0	Extent and location of visual field defect
Chiasmal compression	Optic chiasm	0.0–1.2	Asymmetry of visual field loss, unilateral central field involvement
Optic tract lesion	Optic tract	0.3–1.2 (in the eye with temporal field loss)	Incongruity of homonymous field defect, hemifield pupillomotor input asymmetry
Postgeniculate damage	Visual radiations Visual cortex	0.0	Stimulus light area (no RAPD but definite pupil perimetry defects)
Midbrain tectal damage	Olivary pretectal area of pupil light input region of midbrain	0.3–1.0	Similar to optic tract lesions, but no visual field defect

BOX 25.7   Relative afferent pupillary defect and management

The amount of the relative afferent papillary defect (RAPD) is correlated largely with the amount of asymmetry of visual field deficit between the two eyes, and helps substantiate abnormal results of visual field testing.[57,65,70,71] This can often help the clinician determine whether a patient's visual field defects are reliable and reflect the true pathologic state.

The correlation between the visual field asymmetry and the RAPD is also useful in following the course of disease to determine whether there is a worsening or improvement in function over time.

The RAPD is a relative measure of the input of one eye compared with the other. Bilateral symmetric damage should not produce an RAPD.

A patient who exhibited a definite RAPD in one eye on the first visit may show no RAPD at all on the follow-up visit. This may represent improvement in the previously damaged eye. However, it may also indicate that there is now damage in what was previously the better eye, matching the damage to the other eye, so that there are now symmetric visual field defects and no RAPD.

of weakness of the sphincter or pharmacologic immobility, one can still check for a RAPD by observing the pupil that still works—and comparing its direct reaction with its consensual reaction.

Computerized pupillometry

Various computerized, infrared-sensitive pupillometers are commercially available. Most of these elegant instruments can precisely record the dynamics of pupillary movement in the light or in the dark (Fig. 25.11). Once recorded, the pupillary information can be analyzed by sophisticated software (see pupil tracings in the alternating light test, shown in Fig. 25.9). This allows quantitative information about the pupillary light reflex to be assessed.[65,72,75–78] Such instrumentation is also useful for detecting and diagnosing causes of anisocoria (unequal pupils) when both pupils are recorded simultaneously (refer to the section on oculosympathetic defects). There has been increasing interest in using computerized pupillography to help nonophthalmologists quantify pupil responses to evaluate a wide array of neurologic conditions from movement disorders, neurodegenerative conditions, and autism spectrum to neurologic status in the intensive care unit.[79–83]

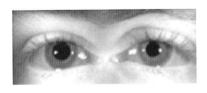
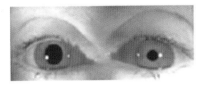
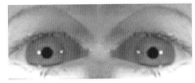

Fig. 25.11 The cause of anisocoria in room light *(top panel)* is determined by first adding bright light to determine whether the anisocoria increases *(middle panel)* or decreases *(bottom panel)*.

Pupil perimetry

The pupil light reflex may also be used to obtain objective information about the sensitivity of local areas of the visual field by recording small pupil contractions in response to focal light stimuli placed in different perimetric locations. An automated perimeter can be modified to record pupil responses to each focal light stimulus to produce a form of objective pupil perimetry.[37,38] Multifocal pupillographic objective perimetry is accomplished by measuring pupil constriction in response to various stimuli presented to different areas of the visual field in each eye. This technology is actively being developed for detection of visual pathway diseases, including glaucoma and macular degeneration among others. Recent experiments have also shown that pupil responses to peripheral stimuli are changed when attention is cued to the location, which is in keeping with the previously mentioned work in cortical modulation of the pupillary light reflex. This paradigm has the advantage of being objective, as it does not rely on the patient to respond and is faster than automated perimetry.[84–88] Pupil perimetry may be helpful as an objective form of perimetry and as a way to localize lesions along the visual pathways. Pupil perimetry can also be useful in cases of nonorganic, functional visual loss to show objectively that visual input is indeed going normally into the brain from parts of the visual field in which the patient claims to see nothing.

EFFERENT PUPILLARY DEFECTS

Anisocoria

When a pupil inequality is seen, it can mean that damage has occurred to either the iris sphincter or dilator muscle, their innervation has been interrupted, or there are external pharmacologic factors influencing pupil movement. To sort out which muscle is not working normally, it helps to know how the anisocoria is influenced by light (Fig. 25.11). It is worth noting that an anisocoria always increases in the direction of action of the paretic iris muscle, just as an esotropia increases when gaze is in the direction of action of a weak lateral rectus muscle. If the iris sphincter is paretic, the lighting condition that normally brings into action that muscle accentuates the weakness; adding bright light tends to increase the anisocoria. Alternatively, if the iris dilator is paretic, the anisocoria is expected to increase as light is taken away

because reflex dilation to darkness is impaired. Table 25.3 provides a summary of the common causes of anisocoria that are discussed in the following section.

Pupil inequality that increases in the dark

In patients who have pupil inequality that increases in the dark, the problem is distinguishing Horner syndrome (Fig. 25.12) from a simple anisocoria (also termed physiologic anisocoria). In both of these conditions, the pupil inequality becomes greater in dim light; however, the dynamics of pupil dilation are impaired in oculosympathetic defects but not in simple anisocoria. Other features also characterize simple anisocoria from Horner syndrome.

A simple anisocoria may vary from day to day, or even from hour to hour, and it is visible in about one-fifth of the normal population. In some people it may be present most of the time, and the larger pupil may always be in the same eye. In other people it may come and go, and the larger pupil may often switch to the other eye. Physiologic anisocoria is not related to refractive error. The cause of physiologic anisocoria is not known with certainty, but current evidence favors a transient, asymmetric, supranuclear inhibition of the Edinger–Westphal nucleus. This would cause the pupil on the more inhibited side to be larger. If this mechanism is correct, it would also explain why any stimulus that transiently overcomes supranuclear inhibition, such as bright light, near stimulus, sleep, or anesthesia, causes the physiologic anisocoria to decrease. Simple anisocoria is considered benign.

The characteristic dilation lag of the Horner's pupil can easily be seen in the office with a hand light shining from below. At the time the room lights are switched off, the reflex dilation of the two pupils should be simultaneously observed and the smaller pupil assessed to see whether it dilates more slowly than the other pupil (Box 25.8). Pupil dilation is normally a combination of sphincter relaxation and dilator contraction. This combination produces a prompt dilation in a normal pupil when the illumination is abruptly decreased. The patient with unilateral Horner syndrome has a weak dilator muscle in the iris ipsilateral to the oculosympathetic defect and as a result that pupil dilates more slowly than the normal pupil (Fig. 25.13). If the sympathetic lesion is complete, the affected pupil will dilate only by sphincter relaxation; this process takes longer than with an intact sympathetic innervation to the dilator muscle. This asymmetry of pupil dilation produces an anisocoria that becomes largest 4 to 5 seconds after the lights are turned out. Dilation of the eye with the oculosympathetic defect is a much slower process than most people imagine. After the lights have been out for 10 to 20 seconds, the anisocoria lessens as the sympathectomized pupil gradually catches up because of continual relaxation of the iris sphincter owing to central inhibition of the parasympathetic pathway at the Edinger–Westphal nucleus. The delayed dilation of the involved eye owing to a deficit of sympathetic innervation to the dilator muscle is a process referred to as *dilation lag* (Fig. 25.13).

Often, the initial increase in anisocoria during the first few seconds of darkness can be accentuated by adding an auditory stimulus or even an auxiliary electrical transcutaneous stimulation ("buzzing the sympathetic nerves")[89] just after the lights are turned out. This causes the normal pupil to dilate forcefully in response to the extra sympathetic stimulation evoked by a loud noise or other external stimuli, but in the eye with the oculosympathetic defect, this maneuver has little effect. Comparison of the dynamics of dilation of the two pupils is a quick and simple way of distinguishing Horner syndrome from simple anisocoria, and it is a test that does not require pupillary drug testing. It works well most of the time, especially in young people with mobile pupils, but if the dilation lag is inconclusive, apraclonidine or cocaine eye drops should be used to confirm the diagnosis of Horner syndrome (see further).

TABLE 25.3   Common causes of anisocoria and associated features

Condition	Cause	Anisocoria	Light response	Near response	Slit lamp	Pharmacologic testing
Acute Adie's pupil	Denervation of parasympathetic postganglionic nerves to pupillary sphincter (segmental)	Anisocoria increases in bright light	Segmental loss of light reaction in some sphincter areas around the circumference	Same areas where light response is lost also show loss of near constriction	Remaining innervated sphincter areas pucker with light and pull denervated segments	Supersensitivity to 0.1% pilocarpine; check response of both pupils in darkness after 30 minutes
Chronic Adie's pupil (more than 8 weeks after event)	Reinnervation of denervated sphincter segments by postganglionic accommodative nerves	May be no anisocoria in room light or affected pupil may be the smaller pupil	Poor response to light; poor dilation in darkness as a result of tonically contracted segments that have reinnervation	Light-near dissociation is present with good near effort from the patient	Similar appearance as in the acute state, reinnervated segments show diffuse contraction to near	As segments become reinnervated, cholinergic supersensitivity is lost; small, tonic pupil dilates normally to anticholinergics
Pharmacologic mydriasis (anticholinergic)	Scopolamine patch, eyedrops, plants (jimson weed)	Anisocoria increases in bright light	Loss of response to light; residual small reaction may occur with submaximal exposure or after sufficient time has elapsed	Same degree of loss of near response as loss of light response; near point of accommodation is more remote	Any residual light response of the sphincter is diffuse and not segmental	Subsensitivity to pilocarpine of all concentrations compared with the opposite unaffected eye (observed in dim light or darkness)
Pharmacologic mydriasis (adrenergic)	Low concentration of adrenergics found in over-the-counter eyedrops for red eyes, cocaine, Neo-Synephrine	Anisocoria increases in bright light, but not as much as in anticholinergic mydriasis	Diminished response to light, but dilator muscle can be overcome by strong sphincter constriction to bright light	Same diminished response as light reaction; near point of accommodation is unaffected and is normal	Besides diminished reaction, the pupil movement looks normal and is not segmental	Reversal of anisocoria with adrenergic blockade (dipyridamole or thymoxamine); may be overcome with pilocarpine
Damage to iris sphincter	Ischemia, angle-closure glaucoma, herpes zoster iritis, trauma, after anterior segment surgery, moxifloxacin toxicity	Anisocoria increases in bright light	Loss of response to light, some sphincter segments may be more affected than others	Usually affected to the same degree as the light reflex; may have normal accommodative amplitude	Transillumination defects may be present	Lack of response to 1% pilocarpine in damaged areas of the iris sphincter
Iron or copper mydriasis	Intraocular foreign body	Anisocoria increases in bright light	Loss of response to light, not usually segmental	Usually affected to the same degree as the light reflex	Usually heterochromia is present, with the iris being darker	May show cholinergic supersensitivity
Third nerve palsy	Trauma, compression, rarely ischemia	Anisocoria increases in bright light	Loss of response to light, not usually segmental unless aberrant regeneration is present	Usually affected to the same degree as the light reflex; accommodative amplitude is decreased	Usually symmetric weakness along the circumference of the sphincter to light reaction	May show cholinergic supersensitivity
Mechanically scarred iris	Trauma, iritis	Anisocoria increases in bright light	Loss of response to light when viewed without slit lamp	Usually affected to the same degree as the light reflex; accommodative amplitude is normal	Small movement of the scarred down iris can usually be observed; synechiae can often be seen after dilation	Lack of response to 1% pilocarpine
Physiologic anisocoria	Asymmetric inhibition at the Edinger–Westphal nucleus	Anisocoria increases in bright light	Normal; normal dilation in response to darkness and auditory stimulation	Normal; anisocoria lessens with a good near response	Normal	Normal response to topical agents; cocaine lessens the anisocoria
Oculosympathetic defect (Horner syndrome)	Sympathetic nerve palsy; ptosis is usually present of the upper and lower lid; anhidrosis may be present	Anisocoria increases in bright light	Normal; slow dilation in response to darkness and auditory stimulation	Normal; anisocoria lessens with a good near response	Normal; heterochromia is common if palsy occurred early in life	Cocaine increases the anisocoria; supersensitivity is usually demonstrated to adrenergic agents
Congenital pseudo-Horner syndrome	Unknown; anisocoria is often present in old photographs from infancy	Anisocoria increases in bright light	Appears normal, but the smaller pupil does not dilate well to darkness or auditory stimulation	Normal; anisocoria lessens with a good near response	Normal	May give a false-positive cocaine test; when direct-acting agents or anticholinergic drops are used, the pupil still fails to dilate as well as the fellow eye

BOX 25.8   Horner syndrome

Clinically, Horner syndrome is recognized by looking for the associated signs, such as ptosis, "upside-down ptosis" of the lower lid, and in a fresh case, conjunctival injection, decreased sweating on the involved side, and in some cases, lowered intraocular pressure on the affected side.

Pain on the side of the face with the smaller pupil (jaw, ear, and cheek pain) is often an important sign pointing to a carotid artery dissection as a cause of the Horner syndrome (Fig. 25.14).

Pharmacologic diagnosis of Horner syndrome with cocaine or apraclonidine

Cocaine's action is to block the reuptake of the norepinephrine that is normally released from the nerve endings so that norepinephrine accumulates at the synapse. If, because of an interruption in the sympathetic pathway, norepinephrine is not being released, cocaine has little to no adrenergic effect. A Horner's pupil will dilate less to cocaine than the normal pupil, regardless of the location of the lesion. Forty-five

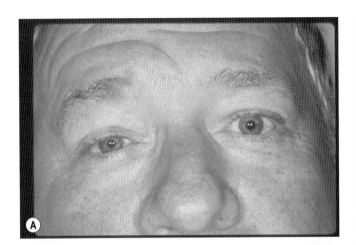
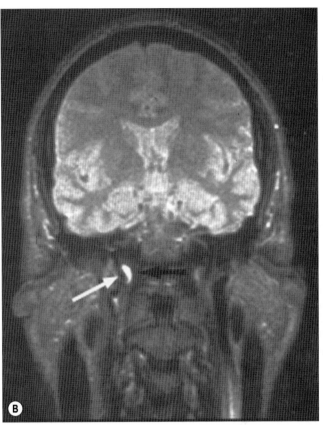
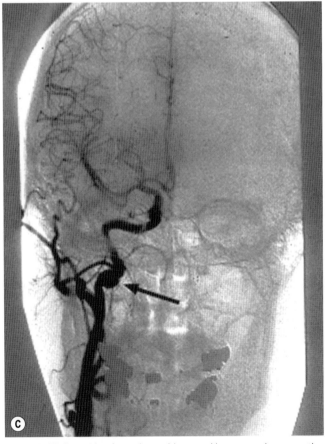

Fig. 25.12 (A) Example of a patient with acute Horner syndrome on the right with accompanying facial pain. Note the miosis and ptosis on the right eye. This patient had a dissection of the internal carotid artery demonstrated by the magnetic resonance imaging scan **(B)** showing a bright signal in the wall of the carotid artery resulting from blood (*white* "comma" adjacent to carotid lumen in lower left; *arrow*). The dissection created a false lumen that appears as a focal enlargement of the lumen of the carotid artery demonstrated in the carotid angiogram on the right *(arrow)* **(C)**.

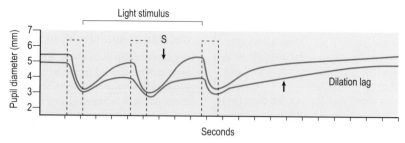

Fig. 25.13 Example of a pupillographic demonstration of dilation lag of the pupil in the eye with Horner syndrome. The smaller pupil is slow to dilate, causing an increase in anisocoria during the early phase of dilation and accentuated by a loud sound (S). In the last part of the tracing, no further stimulus was given to allow the dilation lag to be observed in the tracing. The dilation lag is a delayed dilation of the smaller pupil; after 5 seconds in darkness, the smaller pupil slowly dilates as a result of inhibition of the sphincter muscle, despite loss of sympathetic nerve contribution to pupil dilation.

minutes after cocaine drops have been placed in both eyes, the anisocoria should have clearly increased because the normal pupil has dilated more than the Horner's pupil.

A solution of 4% or 10% cocaine HCl drops in both eyes can be used (never more than two drops) to be sure that the iris gets a full mydriatic dose; this amount of cocaine does not normally produce a corneal epithelial defect. The pH of the solution usually causes significant burning after topical application. Preapplication of topical anesthetic helps counteract the discomfort. After 40 to 60 minutes have elapsed, the anisocoria is measured in room light. The patient should stay active during that time so that adequate sympathetic discharge is occurring (sleeping during this time might result in neither pupil dilating to cocaine). If there is little dilation of the eye with a suspected oculosympathetic defect and this pupil never dilated well in darkness before the drop was given, even after 30 seconds of darkness, a false-positive cocaine test also must be considered. This can occur if the iris is in some way held in a miotic state by either scarring or aberrant reinnervation of the iris sphincter. In such cases, adding a direct-acting sympathomimetic agent to both eyes (i.e., 2.5% phenylephrine) at the conclusion of a positive cocaine test should easily dilate the iris of the suspected eye if there really is an oculosympathetic defect, and the cocaine-induced anisocoria should almost be eliminated. In some cases, the 2.5% phenylephrine may even cause the eye with the oculosympathetic defect to have the larger pupil as a result of supersensitivity. Pseudo-Horner syndrome, caused by the reasons stated earlier, results in inadequate dilation to direct-acting sympathetic agents.

The likelihood of a diagnosis of Horner syndrome with cocaine testing increases in proportion to the amount of anisocoria (measured 50 to 60 minutes after the instillation of cocaine). Unlike the hydroxyamphetamine test (used for localizing the lesion to either the preganglionic or postganglionic neuron), calculation of the change in the anisocoria from before to after cocaine application is unnecessary. It has been found that if there is at least 0.8 mm of pupillary inequality after cocaine, the presence of Horner syndrome is highly likely.[90]

In recent years, it has been proposed that a new pharmacologic test using 0.5% apraclonidine be used for the diagnosis of Horner's syndrome in place of cocaine.[91-95] Apraclonidine has strong α2-adrenergic agonist properties (blocking the release of norepinephrine from the synaptic terminal) and weak α1-agonist properties. Typically, 30 minutes following topical apraclonidine administered to both eyes, the miotic eye with the oculosympathetic defect dilates and, if anything, the normal pupil becomes smaller (in dim light), causing the anisocoria to reverse, or at least lessen. In patients with anisocoria of other causes such as physiologic anisocoria, no mydriasis occurs. Apraclonidine has

an advantage over cocaine in that in most cases it will actively dilate the affected eye and induce miosis in the normal eye, making its action a positive (mydriatic) one in the affected eye and a negative one in the unaffected eye, opposite to the cocaine test. Unlike phenylephrine, the corneal penetration of which varies widely among individuals, apraclonidine readily penetrates the cornea and gains access to the iris, so the limiting factor to its mydriatic effect is whether α1 supersensitivity is present in the iris dilator muscle. Adrenergic supersensitivity is usually present about 48 hours after a decrease in sympathetic nerve activity. Apraclonidine has potential advantages over phenylephrine, not only in its ease of corneal penetration, but also because it does not need to be diluted.

Pharmacologic localization of the denervation in Horner syndrome

The site of the oculosympathetic lesion in Horner syndrome is a question of considerable clinical importance because many postganglionic defects are caused by benign vascular headache syndromes or more serious carotid dissections, and a preganglionic lesion is sometimes the result of the spread of a malignant neoplasm or brainstem stroke.

Hydroxyamphetamine eye drops help localize the site of the lesion in Horner syndrome. The clinician would like to know where the lesion is because that knowledge directs the radiographic workup (e.g., to the internal carotid artery rather than to the pulmonary apex). Horner syndrome sometimes presents itself in such a characteristic setting that further efforts at localizing the lesion are not needed. This is true of patients with cluster headaches or after surgical procedures that interrupt the oculosympathetic chain in a known location.

Hydroxyamphetamine acts by releasing norepinephrine from storage in the sympathetic nerve endings. When the lesion is postganglionic, most, if not all, of the nerves are dead, and no norepinephrine stores are available for release. When the lesion is complete, a pupil like this will not dilate at all in response to hydroxyamphetamine. However, a period of almost 1 week from the onset of damage may be needed before the dying neurons and their stores of norepinephrine are gone. Postganglionic lesions (along the carotid artery) can be separated from the nonpostganglionic lesions (in the brainstem, spinal cord, upper lung, and lower neck) with a degree of certainty that varies with the amount of change in anisocoria induced when the drops are put in both eyes.[96] An increase in the anisocoria of greater than 0.5 mm (change in anisocoria from prehydroxyamphetamine to posthydroxyamphetamine) makes a postganglionic lesion highly likely. Unfortunately, pharmacies are currently not allowed by the Drug Enforcement Administration to formulate hydroxyamphetamine, owing to the widespread abuse of amphetamines.

Congenital and childhood Horner syndrome

When a child has a unilateral ptosis and miosis, the first question is whether it is really Horner syndrome. The ptosis of Horner syndrome is moderate, and never complete. Sometimes, the elevation of the lower lid (upside-down ptosis) helps to make the diagnosis, as the sympathetically innervated Mueller's smooth muscle is present in both the upper and lower eyelids. A child with congenital Horner syndrome and naturally curly hair has hair that will seem limp and lank on the affected side of the head. The shape of the hair follicles appears to depend on intact sympathetic innervation, as does the iris pigment. In children, iris color is usually acquired after the first 9 to 12 months of life because of accumulation of melanosomes in iris melanocytes that are innervated by the sympathetic nerves. Therefore, if the iris in the eye with Horner syndrome does not develop pigmentation during this period, heterochromia is present, indicating that an oculosympathetic defect was present early in life. However, the presence of heterochromia does not indicate the cause or whether it was congenital versus acquired during the first year of life.

Cocaine eye drops may be of some help in diagnosing Horner syndrome in children. If there is no significant dilation of the smaller pupil, a drop of 2.5% phenylephrine should then be administered to each eye to substantiate that the pupil can dilate to a direct-acting sympathomimetic agent and that this is not pseudo-Horner syndrome (see previous section on the cocaine test). Topical apraclonidine testing in children under age 2 years should be done only with close monitoring of respiration for the subsequent hours, since there have been reports of central respiratory depression after topical testing. Other signs may also be helpful for diagnosing Horner syndrome in children. The most telling sign is a hemifacial flush that can occur on the normally innervated side in contrast to the blanch that occurs on the side with the oculosympathetic defect when the infant is nursing or crying. In an air-conditioned office it may be hard to decide whether there is an asymmetry of sweating. A cycloplegic refraction can sometimes produce an atropinic flush everywhere except on the affected face and forehead and thus can unexpectedly solve the diagnostic problem. Horner syndrome that clearly has been acquired in infancy should be evaluated for neuroblastoma, a treatable tumor, using a combination of imaging and testing the urine for metabolites of adrenergic compounds secreted from the tumor.

Pupil inequality that is increased in bright light

When the anisocoria increases with bright light, this implies that the larger pupil is abnormal and may not contract well to light because of direct damage to the iris sphincter muscle from trauma or surgery or because of ischemic atrophy, scarring (synechia) of the iris to the lens from previous inflammation, pharmacologic mydriasis, or denervation of the parasympathetic nerve supply to the iris sphincter (see Fig. 25.4). The following sections outline the most important clinical observations and tests that may be needed to sort out the cause of the efferent pupil defect (see Table 25.3).

Examination of the iris with high magnification using the slit-lamp biomicroscope

Trauma to the globe usually results in a torn sphincter or an iris that shows transillumination defects at the slit lamp. The pupil is often not round, and there may be other evidence of ocular injury. Naturally, such a pupil does not constrict well to light. The residual reaction is often associated with the remaining normal sectors of the iris sphincter because the traumatic tears are usually segmental. An atrophic sphincter resulting from previous herpes zoster iritis may also reveal large geographic areas of transillumination defects seen with the slit lamp

from previous ischemic vasculitic insults to the iris during the uveitis. Similar findings may be observed in essential iris atrophy, which is usually unilateral.

However, if the iris tissue looks normal, the examination is focused on whether any part of the iris sphincter is contracting with light. If some contraction occurs, it should be determined whether the residual contraction is diffuse over the whole circumference or segmental. If there is no segmental movement of the iris, the possibility of atropinic mydriasis should be considered.[97] However, a completely blocked light reaction can sometimes be seen when the sphincter is totally denervated by a preganglionic lesion (third nerve palsy) or a postganglionic lesion (fresh tonic pupil), in acute angle closure (iris ischemia), or in the presence of an intraocular iron foreign body that has been present for some time (iron mydriasis). If the dilated pupil still has some response to light, the dilation could be caused by partial denervation of the sphincter or by incomplete atropinization or adrenergic mydriasis. When the light reaction is poor because the dilator muscle is in spasm (because of adrenergic mydriatics such as phenylephrine), the pupil is large, the conjunctiva blanched, and the lid retracted. In such a case, the near point of accommodation is usually normal but may be slightly decreased as a result of spherical aberration and a shallow depth of field caused by the dilated pupil. However, in the case of adrenergic mydriasis, there usually is some light reaction to very bright lights because the stronger iris sphincter can usually overcome pulling by the adrenergic effects on the dilator muscle.

If there is some residual light reaction, the next step is to look with the slit lamp for sector palsy of the iris sphincter. When the dilator is in a drug-induced adrenergic spasm or when the cholinergic receptors in the iris sphincter are blocked by an atropine-like drug, the entire 360 degrees of the sphincter muscle is affected. This is not the case when the postganglionic nerve fibers have been interrupted: Adie's pupils with a residual light reaction (about 90% of them) have segmental contractions of the remaining normal segments of the sphincter. Some preganglionic partial third-nerve palsies also have regional sphincter palsies, but these can usually be attributed to an associated preexisting diabetic autonomic neuropathy or aberrant regeneration. This means that when the examiner sees a pupil with a weak light reaction but no segmental palsy, he or she should consider a drug-induced mydriasis or a preganglionic lesion, in which case one should look again for lid and motility signs of a third nerve paresis.

Pharmacologic response of the iris sphincter to cholinergic drugs
Cholinergic supersensitivity

If weak pilocarpine (0.0625%, 0.1%, or 0.125%) is applied to both eyes and the affected (dilated) pupil constricts more than the normal pupil (actually becoming the smaller pupil in darkness), the iris sphincter has probably lost some of its innervation and has become supersensitive (Fig. 25.14). Cholinergic supersensitivity can occur within 5 to 7 days. The conclusion that cholinergic supersensitivity exists assumes that corneal penetration of the drug is the same in each eye (i.e., both corneas are healthy and untouched, tear function is normal, and the eyelids are working properly in both eyes). It would seem likely that with postganglionic denervation (damage at the ciliary ganglion or distal to it) the sphincter will show more supersensitivity than in the preganglionic case (third nerve palsy). However, it appears that the differences are not great. For all of these reasons, cholinergic supersensitivity of the iris sphincter is now considered only a confirmatory sign of Adie syndrome. In fact, the results of supersensitivity testing may be ambiguous in Adie syndrome, depending on the chronicity of the condition. As reinnervation takes place over time in Adie syndrome (with accommodative cholinergic nerves growing into the iris sphincter), the

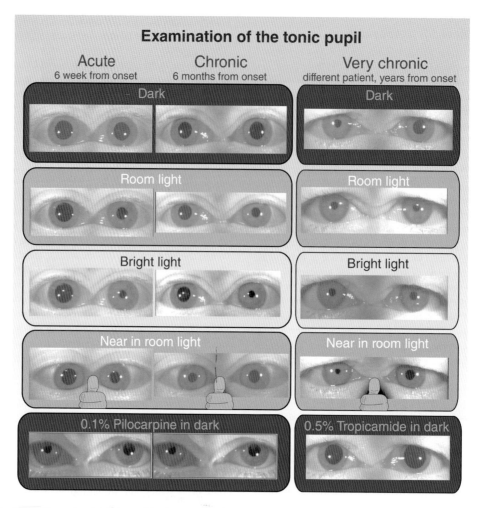

Fig. 25.14 Example of Adie's pupil in the same patient at presentation *(left column)* and 6 months later *(middle column)*, as well as a separate patient with a tonic right pupil that has become miotic, the "little old Adie's pupil" *(right column)*. The *left* two panels demonstrate the typical signs of a tonic pupil, showing little anisocoria in darkness and an increasing anisocoria in room light. In the acute setting, fixation to a near target fails to induce miosis, in the tonic right pupil, however after 3 months a light-near dissociation develops after the iris sphincter is reinnervated by accommodative neurons. In the middle "chronic" column we see the pupil fails to constrict to a room or bright light stimulus but constricts tonically when fixating at near. Acutely and at 6 months, the patient still exhibited signs of cholinergic supersensitivity *(bottom middle)*, with the involved pupil contracting more to 0.1% pilocarpine than the fellow pupil. After several years, some tonic pupils become miotic at baseline *(right column)*, with little response to light, but intact constriction with an accommodative target. Pharmacologic dilation can overcome the pupil sphincter tone in these cases.

reinnervated sphincter segments may lose their cholinergic supersensitivity.[47] If a patient shows the presence of cholinergic supersensitivity in one eye without any segmental palsies, other causes besides Adie's pupil should be reconsidered. Subtle signs of ptosis or diplopia should be looked for once more to leave no doubt that the oculomotor nerve is not affected. It is rare for an ambulatory patient to have an isolated sphincter palsy without other signs of oculomotor nerve palsy as a result of compressive damage to the intracranial third nerve caused by a tumor or aneurysm.

Testing of iris cholinergic sensitivity is best performed when comparing an affected eye with its fellow, normal eye. Testing for whether cholinergic supersensitivity is present in both eyes, without comparing the response with the normal fellow eye in the same subject, is problematic because there is considerable variation in the cholinergic response among different individuals. Even some normal eyes can respond to 0.05% pilocarpine, so for supersensitivity testing to be the most meaningful, the test is best used in the setting of unilateral causes.

Undersensitivity of the iris sphincter to cholinergic testing

If the normal pupil constricts only a small amount to dilute cholinergic agents and the dilated pupil not at all, the mydriasis may be caused by the presence of an anticholinergic drug such as atropine, which inhibits the receptors on the iris sphincter muscle. A stronger concentration of pilocarpine is then needed to settle this point. If, on application of 1% pilocarpine in each eye, the affected pupil does little or nothing and the unaffected pupil constricts normally, the pupil is not larger because of nerve denervation but rather because of a problem in the sphincter muscle itself. The following are different non-neuronal causes of mydriasis:

- Anticholinergic mydriasis (e.g., scopolamine, cyclopentolate, atropine)
- Moxifloxacin-induced iris sphincter damage with transillumination defects (e.g., occurring after cataract surgery)
- Traumatic iridoplegia (look for sphincter tears, appearing as divots at the pupil border; pigment dispersion on the corneal endothelium of lens; and angle recession)

- Angle-closure glaucoma (ischemia of the iris sphincter that occurs during the time when the intraocular pressure is high)
- Previous herpes zoster iritis causing direct damage to the iris sphincter
- Synechiae causing a bound-down iris that is mechanically immobile
- Fixed pupil following anterior segment surgery
- Ocular ischemia to the anterior segment, damaging the iris sphincter.

The cause for a loss of function of the iris muscle following anterior segment surgery is unknown. In some cases, with a postoperative rise in intraocular pressure, the cause may be an ischemic insult to the iris sphincter. An autoimmune process may be responsible, but it has not been proven. It may be related to the same process as Urrets-Zavalia syndrome, in which a dilated, fixed pupil may occur following penetrating keratoplasty. Another cause may be moxifloxacin-induced iris toxicity after topical or intracameral injection.

Adie's tonic pupil: postganglionic parasympathetic denervation

Young adults (more commonly women than men) may suddenly find that one pupil is large or that they cannot focus as well with one eye at near. Slit-lamp examination usually shows segmental denervation of the iris sphincter, with some remaining normal segments still reacting to light. Within the first week, supersensitivity of the iris and ciliary muscle to cholinergic substances can be demonstrated. After about 2 months, nerve regrowth is active and fibers originally bound for the ciliary muscle (they outnumber the iris sphincter fibers by 30 to 1) start arriving (aberrantly) at the iris sphincter and the ciliary muscle. The light reaction of the denervated segments does not return, but the reinnervated segments now show contraction to a near stimulus. This produces the characteristic "light-near dissociation" of Adie syndrome (Fig. 25.14), as well as a return of some accommodative amplitude. Therefore, the presence of light-near dissociation in this setting is a sign of a chronic Adie's pupil with reinnervation and is not a sign of an acute Adie's pupil. The pupil contraction to a near stimulus is often tonic, being slow to dilate when gaze is shifted to a distant target. Although there is also some return of accommodative amplitude, the dynamics of focusing in the affected eye are also slowed and not normal. Patients often complain of difficulties when trying to refocus from near to far because the relaxation of accommodation is slower in the affected eye. Eventually, the affected pupil becomes the smaller of the two pupils, especially in dim light, as a result of the amount of reinnervation by cholinergic accommodative neurons, which keep the sphincter in a contracted state. It turns out that the segmental palsy of the iris sphincter in Adie syndrome and the individual sphincter segment responses to light, near, and pilocarpine can be seen especially well by infrared video recording of transillumination of the iris (Fig. 25.15).

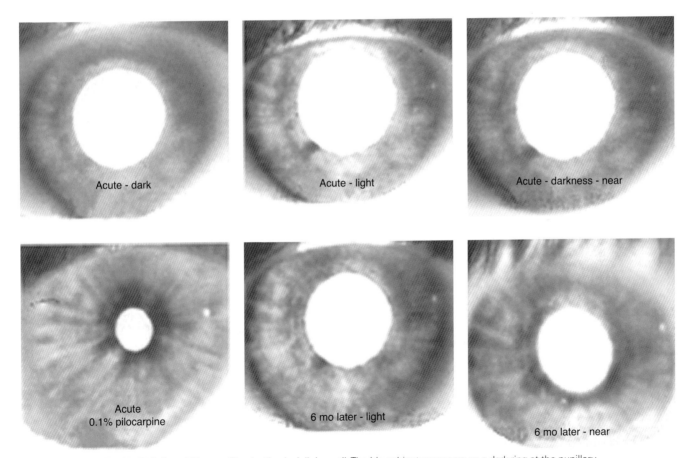

Fig. 25.15 Infrared iris transillumination in Adie's pupil. The iris sphincter appears as a dark ring at the pupillary border when it contracts, as observed with infrared iris transillumination. In the patient shown, almost all of the iris sphincter was denervated, except for the segment at the 7 o'clock meridian, which darkened when made to contract with light or near *(top row, center and right panels)*. With low-dose pilocarpine, the rest of the sphincter muscle that was denervated is the area where supersensitivity was present *(bottom row, left panel)*. Every area darkened after the pilocarpine, except the normal segment at the 7 o'clock position, which remains lighter (not contracted), as shown in the *upper right panel*. After 6 months, the pupil started to become smaller and contracted to near *(bottom right panel)*, but it remained unresponsive to light, except for the 7 o'clock segment *(center right panel)*.

Many of these patients also lack normal motor jerk reflexes and may also have decreased vibratory sensation, indicating a similar process occurring in the spinal cord neurons. However, Adie syndrome is not associated with any major neurologic disorder or significant dysfunction. The cause of Adie's pupil is not well understood, but it has been hypothesized that an immune reaction may mediate the damage to ciliary ganglion and spinal neurons. Younger children may get an Adie's pupil after having chickenpox. After about 10 years, almost 50% of patients with Adie's pupil show evidence of a similar process occurring in the other eye. There are some reports of a positive test for syphilis in patients with bilateral Adie's pupil, so in some cases this diagnosis should be considered.[98,99]

Pupil involvement in third nerve palsy

There is an old clinical rule of thumb stating that if the pupillary light reaction is spared in the setting of a complete third nerve palsy, the palsy is probably not caused by compression or injury but is more likely caused by small vessel disease, such as might be seen in diabetes. It is still a fairly good rule (but there are rare exceptions), provided one bears in mind that a small but definite number of pupil-sparing third nerve palsies are caused by midbrain infarcts and should have neuroimaging studies. Because the preganglionic parasympathetic nerves for the pupil light reflex are located on the medial side of the intracranial portion of the third nerve as it exits the midbrain, compression of the third nerve in this location results in some element of iris sphincter palsy (Box 25.5). The most common cause of this would be an aneurysm (i.e., of the posterior communicating artery) or pituitary apoplexy (sudden lateral expansion of a pituitary adenoma pressing on the medial aspect of the third nerve). However, other causes of pupil-involving third nerve palsies also occur, such as from giant cell arteritis, Tolosa-Hunt syndrome, ophthalmoplegic migraine, and posterior draining–dural cavernous fistulae ("white eye shunt"). Rarely, ischemic third nerve palsies can involve the pupil. Pupil involvement is often incomplete in cases of pupil involvement from various causes, so it is important to look for iris sphincter weakness by observing for anisocoria in bright light, which may help to decide if urgent neuroimaging is needed. In the absence of aberrant regeneration (from chronic compression), we have yet to observe a case of a pupil-involving third nerve palsy from an aneurysm or compression that showed segmental palsies; all of the cases so far have shown symmetric involvement of the iris sphincter over its circumference. Some patients with ischemic third nerve palsy and diabetes have shown mild pupil involvement with elements of segmental palsies. It appears that these patients may have had preexisting pupil involvement from diabetic autonomic neuropathy. Nearly all cases of pupil-involving third nerve palsies will involve some other sign of oculomotor dysfunction including ptosis or an ocular motility abnormality; however, this involvement may be subtle. Pupil involvement from a third nerve palsy distinguishes itself from pharmacologic mydriasis by constricting to 1% pilocarpine.

Aberrant regeneration in the third nerve

The third cranial nerve carries bundles of nerves supplying different extraocular muscles (medial rectus, inferior rectus, inferior oblique, superior rectus, and levator palpebrae muscles), as well as preganglionic parasympathetic nerves to the iris sphincter and ciliary body. Injury to the third nerve and glial scaffolding, through which individual nerve bundles pass, causes the nerve fibers to regrow, and they often end up in the wrong place. For example, the eye may inappropriately turn in when the patient is trying to look down, or the pupil may inappropriately constrict with depression, adduction, or supraduction of the globe (Fig. 25.16). With eyelid involvement, the lid fissure may widen with infraduction, adduction, or supraduction of the

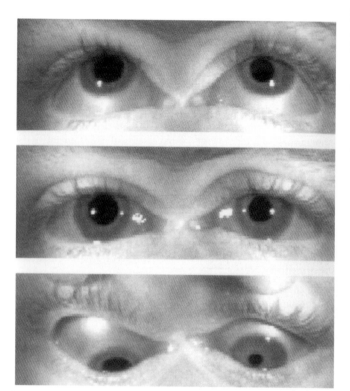

Fig. 25.16 Primary aberrant regeneration of the left third nerve following chronic compression of the oculomotor nerve by a meningioma. In darkness (*top and center panels*) the left pupil is the smaller of the two pupils as a result of innervation by motor nerves. Nerves that normally would have supplied the inferior rectus muscle now are innervating the iris sphincter muscle, causing pupil contraction on down-gaze (*lower panel*).

eye. Aberrant regeneration of the oculomotor nerve may be primary or secondary. In secondary aberrant regeneration, a third nerve palsy precedes the aberrant regeneration by at least 8 weeks. In primary aberrant regeneration, there is no preceding nerve palsy; the damage to the nerve slowly progresses simultaneous with the process of aberrant regeneration. Primary aberrant regeneration is clinically important to recognize because it is almost always caused by a slow compression of the intracranial third nerve by a tumor or aneurysm.

Light-near dissociation: evaluation of the near response

The pupil response to a near effort should be observed as a standard part of the pupil evaluation. Any time the pupil light reaction seems weak, it is important to check to see whether the pupils constrict better to near than they do to light. If they do, this is called a *light-near dissociation*. Causes of light-near dissociation are summarized in Table 25.4. These are categorized by three major mechanisms:

1. Loss of light input resulting from severe damage to the afferent visual system (retina or optic nerve pathways)
2. Interruption of the light input pathways to the Edinger–Westphal nucleus from the pretectum (Argyll Robertson pupils, dorsal midbrain syndrome)
3. Aberrant regeneration of the pupillary sphincter from accommodative fibers (Adie syndrome) or extraocular muscle neurons from the oculomotor nerve (medial rectus fibers or accommodative fibers from third nerve aberrant regeneration).

When the pupil fails to dilate

When one or both pupils stay small and miotic, even in darkness, a number of reasons may be responsible. To better understand the

TABLE 25.4 Causes of light-near dissociation of the pupil

Cause	Location	Mechanism
Severe loss of afferent light input to both eyes	Anterior visual pathway (retina, optic nerves, chiasm)	Damage to the retina or optic nerve pathways
Loss of pretectal light input to Edinger–Westphal nucleus	Tectum of the midbrain	Infectious (Argyll Robertson pupils) or compression (pinealoma) or ischemia (stroke)
Adie syndrome	Iris sphincter	Aberrant reinnervation of sphincter by accommodative neurons
Third nerve aberrant reinnervation	Iris sphincter	Aberrant reinnervation of sphincter by accommodative neurons or medial rectus neurons

TABLE 25.5 Causes of poor pupil dilation in darkness

Cause	Location	Mechanism
Past inflammation or surgical trauma	Posterior iris surface or sphincter	Scarring or synechiae of the iris resulting from past iritis
Acute trauma	Sphincter	Prostaglandin release causing sphincter spasm
Adie tonic pupil Third nerve aberrant reinnervation	Sphincter	Aberrant reinnervation of iris sphincter by accommodative or extraocular motor neurons that are not inhibited in darkness
Pharmacologic miosis	Iris sphincter	Cholinergic influence
Unilateral episodic spasm of miosis	Postganglionic parasympathetic neuron	Uninhibited episodic activation of postganglionic neurons
Congenital miosis (bilateral)	Sphincter	Developmental abnormality
Fatigue, sleepiness	Edinger–Westphal nucleus	Loss of inhibition at midbrain from reticular activating formation
Lymphoma, inflammation, infection	Periaqueductal gray matter	Interruption of inhibitory fibers to the Edinger–Westphal nucleus
Central acting drugs	Reticular activating formation, midbrain	Narcotics, general anesthetics
Old age (bilateral miosis)	Reticular activating formation, midbrain	Loss of inhibition at midbrain from reticular activating formation
Oculosympathetic defect	Sympathetic neuron interruption	Horner syndrome

different possible mechanisms, it is important to understand what normally happens in darkness to allow the pupil to dilate. When a light stimulus is terminated, two mechanisms cause the pupil to dilate. The majority of pupil dilation comes about from inhibition to the Edinger–Westphal nucleus in the midbrain. This reduces the firing of the preganglionic parasympathetic neurons in the Edinger–Westphal nucleus, causing relaxation of the iris sphincter. Within a few seconds, sympathetic nerve firing increases, serving to augment the pupil dilation by active contraction of the dilator muscle. The combined inhibition of the iris sphincter and stimulation of the iris dilator is a carefully integrated neuronal reflex. The inability of the pupil to dilate in darkness may result from the following causes (Table 25.5):

1. Mechanical limitations of the pupil (scarring)
2. Pharmacologic miosis
3. Aberrant reinnervation of cholinergic neurons to the iris sphincter that are not normally inhibited in darkness (accommodative or extraocular motor neurons)
4. Lack of inhibitory input signal getting to the Edinger–Westphal nucleus
5. Lack of sympathetic input to the dilator muscle.

REFERENCES

1. Douglas RH. The pupillary light responses of animals; a review of their distribution, dynamics, mechanisms and functions. *Prog Retin Eye Res.* 2018;66:17–48.
2. Rushton WAW. Visual adaptation: the Ferrier lecture. *Proc R Soc Biol Lond.* 1965;162:20.
3. Kardon RH, Hong S, Kawasaki A. Entrance pupil size predicts retinal illumination in darkly pigmented eyes, but not lightly pigmented eyes. *Invest Ophthalmol Vis Sci.* 2013 Aug 15;54(8):5559–5567.
4. Campbell FW, Green DG. Optical and retinal factors affecting visual resolution. *J Physiol.* 1965;181:576.
5. Westheimer G. Pupil diameter and visual resolution. *Vis Res.* 1964;4:39.
6. Charman WN, Jenning JAM, Whitefoot H. The refraction of the eye in relation to spherical aberration and pupil diameter. *Vis Res.* 1978;17:737.
7. Campbell FW. The depth of field of the human eye. *Optica Acta.* 1957;4:157.
8. Loewenfeld IE, Newsome DA. Iris mechanics: I. Influence of pupil diameter on dynamics of pupillary movements. *Am J Ophthalmol.* 1971;71:347.
9. Kardon RH, Corbett JJ, Thompson HS. Segmental denervation and reinnervation of the iris sphincter as shown by infrared videographic transillumination. *Ophthalmology.* 1998;105:313.
10. Ten Doesschate J, Alpern M. Response of the pupil to steady state retinal illumination: contribution by cones. *Science.* 1965;149:989.
11. Loewenfeld IE and Lowenstein O. The light reflex *The pupil: anatomy, physiology and clinical applications.* vol 1. Ames, IO & Detroit, MI: Iowa State University Press and Wayne State University Press; 1993.
12. Hannibal J, Hindersson P, Knudson SM, Georg B, Fahrenkrug J. The photopigment melanopsin is exclusively present in pituitary adenylate cyclase-activating polypeptide-containing retinal ganglion cells of the retinohypothalamic tract. *J Neurosci.* 2002:22.
13. Hattar S, Liao HW, Takao M, Berson DM, Yau KW. Melanopsin containing retinal ganglion cells: architecture, projections, and intrinsic photosensitivity. *Science.* 2002;295:1065–1070.
14. Fu Y, Liao HW, Do MTH, Yau KW. Non-image-forming ocular photoreception in vertebrates. *Curr Opin Neurobiol.* 2005;15:415–422.
15. Berson DM. Strange vision: ganglion cells as circadian photoreceptors. *Trends Neurosci.* 2003;26:314–320.
16. Lucas RJ, Freedman MS, Lupi D, et al. Identifying the photoreceptive inputs to the mammalian circadian system using transgenic and retinally degenerate mice. *Behav Brain Res.* 2001;125:97–102.
17. Gamlin PDR, McDougal DH, Pokorny J, et al. Human and macaque pupil responses driven by melanopsin-containing retinal ganglion cells. *Vision Res.* 2007;47:946–954.
18. Dacey DM, Liao HW, Peterson BB, et al. Melanopsin-expressing ganglion cells in primate retina signal colour and irradiance and project to the LGN. *Nature.* 2005;433:749–754.
19. Van Gelder RN. Non-visual ocular photoreception. *Ophthalm Genet.* 2001:195–205.
20. Peirson S, Foster RG. Melanopsin: another way of signaling light. *Neuron.* 2006; 49:331–339.
21. Gooley JJ, Lu J, Fischer D, Saper CB. A broad role for melanopsin in non-visual photoreception. *J Neurosci.* 2003;23:7093–7106.
22. Provencio I, Rollag MD, Castrucci AM. Photoreceptive net in the mammalian retina. *Nature.* 2002;415:493.
23. Hattar S, Lucas RJ, Mrosovsky N, et al. Melanopsin and rod–cone photoreceptor systems account for all major accessory visual functions in mice. *Nature.* 2003;424:76–81.

24. Kardon R, Anderson SC, Damarjian TG, Grace EM, Stone E, Kawasaki A. Chromatic pupil responses: preferential activation of the melanopsin-mediated versus outer photoreceptor-mediated pupil light reflex. *Ophthalmology.* 2009;116(8):1564–1573.

25. Adhikari P, Zele AJ, Feigl B. The post-illumination pupil response (PIPR). *Invest Ophthalmol Vis Sci.* 2015 Jun;56(6):3838–3849.

26. Kawasaki A, Kardon RH. Intrinsically photosensitive retinal ganglion cells. *J Neuro-ophthalmol.* 2007;27(3):195–204.

27. Gamlin PDR, Clarke RJ. The pupillary light reflex pathway of the primate. *J Am Optom Assoc.* 1995;66:415.

28. Gamlin PDR, Zhang H, Clarke RJ. Luminance neurons in the pretectal olivary nucleus mediate the pupillary light reflex in the rhesus monkey. *Exp Brain Res.* 1995;106:177.

29. Alexandridis E, Krastel H, Reuther R. Disturbances of the pupil reflex associated with lesions of the upper visual pathway. *Albrecht von Graefes Arch Klin Exp Ophthalmol.* 1979;209:199.

30. Barbur JL, Forsyth PM. Can the pupil response be used as a measure of visual input associated with the geniculo-striate pathway? *Clin Vis Sci.* 1986;1:107.

31. Barbur JL, Harlow AJ, Sahraie A. Pupillary responses to stimulus structure, colour, and movement. *Ophthal Physiol Opt.* 1992;12:137.

32. Cibis G, Campos E, Aulhorn E. Pupillary hemiakinesia in suprageniculate lesions. *Arch Ophthalmol.* 1975;93:1252.

33. Hamann K, Hellner KA, Müller-Jensen A, Zschocke S. Videopupillographic and VER investigations in patients with congenital and acquired lesions of the optic radiation. *Ophthalmologica.* 1979;178:348.

34. Grundlagen Harms H. Methodik und Bedeutung der Pupillenperimetrie fur die Physiologie und Pathologie des Schorgans. *Albrecht von Graefes Arch Klin Exp Ophthalmol.* 1949;149:1.

35. Hellner KA, Jensen W, Muller A. Video processing pupillographic perimetry in hemianopsia. *Klin Mbl Augenheik.* 1978;172:731.

36. Hellner K, Jensen W, Muller-Jensen A. Video-processing pupillography as a method for objective perimetry in pupillary hemiakinesia. In: Greve EL, editor. *The proceedings of the second international visual field symposium, Tubingen, 1976. Doc Ophthalmol Proc Series.* vol 14. The Hague: Dr W Junk Publishers; 1977.

37. Kardon RH. Pupil perimetry. *Curr Opin Ophthalmol.* 1992 Oct;3(5):565-70.

38. Kardon RH, Kirkali PA, Thompson HS. Automated pupil perimetry. *Ophthalmology.* 1991;98:485.

39. Narasaki S, Kawai K, Kubota S, Noguchi J. Videopupillographic perimetry and its clinical application. *Jpn J Ophthalmol.* 1974;18:253.

40. Reuther R, Alexandridis E, Krastel H. Disturbances of the pupil reflex associated with cerebral infraction in the posterior cerebral artery territory. *Arch Psychiatr Nervenkr.* 1981;229:249.

41. Barbur JL, Keenleyside MS, Thomson WD. Investigation of central visual processing by means of pupillometry. In: Kulikowski JJ, Dickinson CM, Murray IJ, eds. *Seeing colour and contour.* Oxford: Pergamon Press; 1989.

42. Barbur JL, Thomson WD. Pupil response as an objective measure of visual acuity. *Ophthal Physiol Opt.* 1987;7:425.

43. Cocker KD, Moseley MJ. Visual acuity and the pupil grating response. *Clin Vis Sci.* 1992;7:143.

44. Slooter JH, van Noren D. Visual acuity measured with pupil responses to checkerboard stimuli. *Invest Ophthalmol Vis Sci.* 1980;19:105.

45. Ukai K. Spatial pattern as a stimulus to the pupillary system. *J Opt Soc Am.* 1985:1094.

46. Young RSL, Han B, Wu P. Transient and sustained components of the pupillary responses evoked by luminance and color. *Vis Res.* 1993;33:437.

47. Young RSL, Kennish J. Transient and sustained components of the pupil response evoked by achromatic spatial patterns. *Vis Res.* 1993;33:2239.

48. Barany EH, Hallden U. Phasic inhibition of the light reflex of the pupil during retinal rivalry. *J Neurophysiol.* 1948 Jan;11(1):25–30.

49. Benedetto A, Binda P. Dissociable saccadic suppression of pupillary and perceptual responses to light. *J Neurophysiol.* 2016 Mar;115(3):1243–1251.

50. Ebitz RB, Moore T. Selective modulation of the pupil light reflex by microstimulation of prefrontal cortex. *J Neurosci.* 2017 May 10;37(19):5008–5018.

51. Wang CA, Munoz DP. Neural basis of location-specific pupil luminance modulation. *Proc Natl Acad Sci U S A.* 2018 Oct 9;115(41):10446–10451.

52. Joshi S, Gold JI. Pupil size as a window on neural substrates of cognition. *Trends Cogn Sci.* 2020 Jun;24(6):466–480.

53. Kerr FWL, Hollowell OW. Location of pupillomotor and accommodation fibres in the oculomotor nerve: experimental observations on paralytic mydriasis. *J Neurol Neurosurg Psychiatr.* 1964;27:473.

54. Loewenfeld IE and Lowenstein O. Methods of pupil testing *The pupil: anatomy, physiology and clinical applications.* vol 1. Ames, IO & Detroit, MI: Iowa State University Press and Wayne State University Press; 1993.

55. Loewenfeld IE and Lowenstein O. Reactions to darkness *The pupil: anatomy, physiology and clinical applications.* vol 1. Ames, IO & Detroit, MI: Iowa State University Press and Wayne State University Press; 1993.

56. Koss MC. Pupillary dilation as an index of central nervous system alpha2-adrenoceptor activation. *J Pharmacol Methods.* 1986;15:1.

57. Johnson LN, Hill RA, Bartholomew MJ. Correlation of afferent pupillary defect with visual field loss on automated perimetry. *Ophthalmology.* 1988;95:1649.

58. Huhtala A. Origin of myelinated nerves in the rat iris. *Exp Eye Res.* 1976;22:259.

59. Saari M, Kiviniemi P, Johansson G, Huhtala A. Wallerian degeneration of the myelinated nerves of cat iris after denervation of the ophthalmic division of the trigeminal nerve: an electron microscopic study. *Exp Eye Res.* 1973;17:281.

60. Almegrad B, Stjernschantz J, Bill A. Cholecystokinin contracts isolated human and monkey iris sphincters: a study with CCK receptor antagonists. *Eur J Pharmacol.* 1992;211:183.

61. Newsome DA, Loewenfeld IE. Iris mechanics: II. Influence of pupil diameter on details of iris structure. *Am J Ophthal.* 1971;71:553.

62. Loewenfeld IE and Lowenstein O. The reaction to near vision *The pupil: anatomy, physiology and clinical applications.* vol 1. Ames, IO & Detroit, MI: Iowa State University Press and Wayne State University Press; 1993.

63. Chen Y, Kardon RH. Studying the effect of iris mechanics on the pupillary light reflex using brimonidine-induced anisocoria. *Invest Ophthalmol Vis Sci.* 2013 Apr 26;54(4):2951–2958.

64. Loewenfeld IE and Lowenstein O. Reflex dilation *The pupil: anatomy, physiology and clinical applications.* vol 1. Ames, IO & Detroit, MI: Iowa State University Press and Wayne State University Press; 1993.

65. Kardon RH, Denison CE, Brown CK, Thompson HS. Critical evaluation of the cocaine test in the diagnosis of Horner's syndrome. *Arch Ophthalmol.* 1990;108:384.

66. Lowenstein O, Kawabata H, Loewenfeld I. The pupil as indicator of retinal activity. *Am J Ophthalmol.* 1964;57:569.

67. Levatin P. Pupillary escape in disease of the retina or optic nerve. *Arch Ophthalmol.* 1959;62:768.

68. Thompson HS, Corbett JJ. Asymmetry of pupillomotor input. *Eye.* 1991;5:36.

69. Thompson HS, Corbett JJ, Cox TA. How to measure the relative afferent pupillary defect. *Surv Ophthalmol.* 1981;26:39.

70. Brown RH, Zilis JD, Lynch MG, Sanborn GE. The afferent pupillary defect in asymmetric glaucoma. *Arch Ophthalmol.* 1987;105:1540.

71. Thompson HS, Montague P, Cox TA, Corbett JJ. The relationship between visual acuity, pupillary defect, and visual field loss. *Am J Ophthalmol.* 1982;93:681.

72. Kawasaki A, Moore P, Kardon RH. Long-term fluctuation of relative afferent pupillary defect in subjects with normal visual function. *Am J Ophthalmol.* 1996;122:875.

73. Volpe NJ, Plotkin ES, Maguire MG, Hariprasad R, Galetta SL. Portable pupillography of the swinging flashlight test to detect afferent pupillary defects. *Ophthalmology.* 2000;107:1913.

74. Bell RA, Waggoner PM, Boyd WM, Akers RE, Yee CE. Clinical grading of relative afferent pupillary defects. *Arch Ophthalmol.* 1993;111:938.

75. Cox TA. Pupillography of a relative afferent pupillary defect. *Am J Ophthalmol.* 1986;101:250.

76. Cox TA. Pupillographic characteristics of simulated relative afferent pupillary defects. *Invest Ophthalmol Vis Sci.* 1989;30:1127.

77. Fison PN, Garlick DJ, Smith SE. Assessment of unilateral afferent pupillary defects by pupillography. *Br J Ophthalmol.* 1979;63:195.

78. Kawasaki A, Moore P, Kardon RH. Variability of the relative afferent pupillary defect. *Am J Ophthalmol.* 1995;120:622.

79. De Vries L, Fouquaet I, Boets B, Naulaers G, Steyaert J. Autism spectrum disorder and pupillometry: A systematic review and meta-analysis. *Neurosci Biobehav Rev.* 2021

80. Wang CH, Wu CY, Liu CC, et al. Neuroprognostic accuracy of quantitative versus standard pupillary light reflex for adult postcardiac arrest patients: A systematic review and meta-analysis. *Crit Care Med.* 2021 Oct 1;49(10):1790–1799.

81. Pinheiro HM, da Costa RM. Pupillary light reflex as a diagnostic aid from computational viewpoint: A systematic literature review. *J Biomed Inform.* 2021 May;117:103757.

82. Zafar SF, Suarez JI. Automated pupillometer for monitoring the critically ill patient: a critical appraisal. *J Crit Care.* 2014 Aug;29(4):599–603.

83. Olson DM, Fishel M. The use of automated pupillometry in critical care. *Crit Care Nurs Clin North Am.* 2016 Mar;28(1):101–107.

84. Sabeti F, Maddess T, Essex RW, James AC. Multifocal pupillographic assessment of age-related macular degeneration. *Optom Vis Sci.* 2011 Dec;88(12):1477–1485.

85. Maddess T, Bedford SM, Goh XL, James AC. Multifocal pupillographic visual field testing in glaucoma. *Clin Exp Ophthalmol.* 2009 Sep;37(7):678–686.

86. Maddess T, Essex RW, Kolic M, Carle CF, James AC. High- versus low-density multifocal pupillographic objective perimetry in glaucoma. *Clin Exp Ophthalmol.* 2013 Mar;41(2):140–147.

87. Sabeti F, James AC, Essex RW, Maddess T. Multifocal pupillography identifies retinal dysfunction in early age-related macular degeneration. *Graefes Arch Clin Exp Ophthalmol.* 2013 Jul;251(7):1707–1716.

88. Rosli Y, Carle CF, Ho Y, et al. Retinotopic effects of visual attention revealed by dichoptic multifocal pupillography. *Sci Rep.* 2018 Feb 14;8(1):2991.

89. Omary R, Bockisch CJ, Landau K, Kardon RH, Weber KP. Buzzing sympathetic nerves: A new test to enhance anisocoria in Horner's syndrome. *Front Neurol.* 2019 Feb 21;10:107.

90. Kardon RH, Haupert C, Thompson HS. The relationship between static perimetry and the relative afferent pupillary defect. *Am J Ophthalmol.* 1993;115:351.

91. Kardon RH. Are we ready to replace cocaine with apraclonidine in the pharmacologic diagnosis of Horner syndrome? *J Neuro-ophthalmol.* 2005;25:69–70.

92. Morales J, Brown S, Abdul-Rahim AS, Crosson C. Ocular effects of apraclonidine in Horner's syndrome. *Arch Ophthalmol.* 2000;118:951–954.

93. Brown SM, Aouchiche R, Freedman KA. The utility of 0.5 percent apraclonidine in the diagnosis of Horner syndrome. *Arch Ophthalmol.* 2003;121:1201–1203.

94. Chen PL, Chen JT, Lu DW, Chen YC, Hsiao CH. Comparing efficacies of 0.5 percent apraclonidine with 4 percent cocaine in the diagnosis of Horner syndrome in pediatric patients. *J Ocul Pharmacol Ther.* 2006;22:182–187.

95. Koc F, Kavuncu S, Kansu T, Acaroglu G, Firat E. The sensitivity and specificity of 0.5 percent apraclonidine in the diagnosis of oculosympathetic paresis. *Br J Ophthalmol.* 2005;89:1442–1444.

96. Cremer SA, Thompson HS, Digre KB, Kardon RH. Hydroxyamphetamine mydriasis in Horner's syndrome. *Am J Ophthalmol.* 1990;110:71.

97. Kardon RH. Anatomy and physiology of the pupil. Section III. The autonomic nervous system: pupillary function, accommodation, and lacrimation. 5th edn. In: Miller NM, Newman NJ, eds. *Walsh and Hoyt's clinical neuro-ophthalmology.* vol 1 Baltimore: Williams & Wilkins; 1998.

98. Thompson HS, Kardon RH. The Argyll Robertson pupil. *J Neuroophthalmol.* 2006;26(2):134–138.

99. Weinstein JM, Zweifel TJ, Thompson HS. Congenital Horner's syndrome. *Arch Ophthalmol.* 1980;98:1074.

26

Ganglion-Cell Photoreceptors

Kwoon Y. Wong, David M. Berson, and Ignacio Provencio

Overview

Since the turn of this century, compelling evidence has emerged for a novel class of photoreceptors in the mammalian retina. These neurons are ganglion cells that express the photopigment melanopsin and respond autonomously to relatively bright light with a sustained depolarization and increase in spike frequency. Named intrinsically photosensitive retinal ganglion cells (ipRGCs), they differ radically in form and function from the classical rod and cone photoreceptors. In this chapter, we discuss the origins of this discovery, the idiosyncratic physiology of these cells, and the roles they play in retinal processing and visual behavior in health and disease.

HISTORICAL ROOTS

The discovery of photoreceptors in the inner retina may have come as a shock initially to many retinal scientists, but the roots of the idea are actually traceable to the very beginnings of retinal science (reviewed in[1-3]). Beginning with Descartes and through the first half of the 19th century, it was assumed that the photoreceptive elements of the retina lined its inner surface, nearest the incoming light.[3] For example, Treviranus,[4] the first to conduct systematic microscopic studies of the retina, suggested that optic fibers passed through all retinal layers to end as photosensitive papillae at the vitreal surface. Bidder[5] accurately described the outer retinal location of the rods, but hypothesized that they served a reflective function, like a tapetum, and continued to view optic fibers in the inner retina as the locus of phototransduction. The lack of photosensitivity of the fibers of the optic disc, as indicated by the blind spot, eventually undermined this view, and prompted Bowman[6] and Helmholtz[7] to propose ganglion cells as the true photoreceptors. It was not until the latter half of the 19th century that photoreception was convincingly localized to the outer retina. The key insights were made by Heinrich Müller, who inferred the retinal depth of the photoreceptors by a clever geometric analysis of the parallactic displacement of shadows of retinal vasculature (the "Purkinje tree"). He also detected "visual purple" or rhodopsin in the rods, which Franz Boll soon thereafter demonstrated was a photosensitive pigment.[8]

Fifty years would pass before interest in the possibility of inner retinal photoreception would reemerge. The catalyst was the groundbreaking work of Clyde Keeler, who identified the first animal model of inherited retinal degeneration. This strain of mice, which Keeler termed "rodless," is allelic with the *rd1* strain (formerly *rd*); both carry the *Pde6b^rd1* mutation and phenotypically resemble human autosomal recessive retinitis pigmentosa (OMIM database number 180072).[9,10] Keeler eventually achieved wide acclaim for this seminal contribution to the genetics of retinal disease, but a key observation he made in these mice received little notice at the time. Although his *rodless* mice were apparently blind when tested behaviorally or electroretinographically,

they unexpectedly retained robust pupillary responses to light.[11] This led him to suggest that "in mammals the iris may function independent of vision" either through intrinsic photosensitivity of the smooth muscle itself or by "direct stimulation of the internal nuclear or ganglionic cells" by light.[11,12]

Over the next 70 years, a series of studies in retinally degenerate mammals confirmed the persistence of the pupillary response but suggested that the functional blindness might not be as complete as Keeler had believed. Various photic effects on behavior or physiology were noted, despite the absence of an outer retina in histologic material or a detectable electroretinogram (reviewed in[13,14]). These included avoidance of a visual cliff, photic suppression of activity in open field test, visually guided avoidance of shock in a shuttlebox, chromatic discrimination, entrainment of circadian rhythms, suppression of pineal melatonin synthesis, and suppression of spontaneous firing in the superior colliculus.[13,15-20] A number of these studies demonstrated that eye removal abolished these residual photoresponses and overtly echoed Keeler's speculation about the possible existence of inner retinal photoreceptors, including ganglion cells.[16,18,19] These suggestions gained only limited currency, probably because improved anatomical studies had begun to cast doubt on the completeness of the loss of outer retinal photoreceptors, especially in the peripheral retina. These studies showed that the mouse retina, once believed to possess only rod photoreceptors, in fact also had a modest population of cones, and that these degenerated far more slowly than rods in the *rd1* model. Perhaps 20% survived beyond 80 days of age, albeit without intact outer segments, and a few lasted at least a year.[21] This clouded the interpretation of the behavioral studies, virtually all of which had been conducted in mice young enough to have had many surviving cones. With the benefit of hindsight, however, it seems plausible that at least some of the residual light-driven effects reported in these early studies were indeed mediated by inner retinal photoreceptors. Even in *rd1* animals as young as 6 to 10 weeks old, surviving rods or cones seem unable to support visual function: silencing ganglion-cell phototransduction in such animals abolishes the photic influences on circadian rhythms, the pupil, locomotor activity, and melatonin synthesis that these mice would otherwise exhibit[22] (see "Central projections" further in the chapter).

In the 1990s, Russell Foster and colleagues took up the work on retinally degenerate mice, applying more rigorous methods to provide compelling evidence for inner retinal photoreception.[14,23-29] Their innovations included appropriate controls for genetic background and the use of very old *rd1* animals and several genetically modified mice strains in which they confirmed nearly complete loss of cones, as well as rods. They also showed that there was little loss of sensitivity of circadian photoreception as rod and cone degeneration progressed and that the residual visually evoked behaviors extended beyond circadian regulation to other outputs of what they called the nonimage-forming (NIF) visual centers of the brain. These included pupillary constriction, acute suppression of locomotor activity, and acute suppression of pineal melatonin release by light. The case for novel inner photoreceptors was bolstered by parallel observations in human patients with advanced outer retinal disease[30] (see also[31,32]) and by assessment of the spectral tuning of residual photoresponses in retinally degenerate animals. Yoshimura and Ebihara[33] (see also[34]) showed that the photic influence on circadian rhythms in retinally degenerate mice was most effective at 480 nm, clearly distinct from the optimal wavelengths for activating the known rod and cone photopigments. Remarkably similar spectral data were obtained for residual pupillary responses.[27]

DISCOVERY OF MELANOPSIN AND GANGLION-CELL PHOTORECEPTORS

The identities of the mysterious inner retinal photoreceptors and their photopigment were established in a flurry of studies in the period 2000 to 2005. These developments have been thoroughly reviewed elsewhere,[29,35–38] so we provide only an abbreviated summary here. A pivotal contribution was the discovery of melanopsin.[4,39] This novel opsin (coded by the *Opn4* gene) derives its name from the dermal melanophores of frogs, the photosensitive cells of the skin in which the gene was first identified.[39] It was shown subsequently that in mice and primates, including humans, the protein was expressed solely in a small minority of cells in the inner retina, mainly in the ganglion-cell layer (GCL).[40] It was speculated that melanopsin could be the photopigment of the postulated inner retinal photoreceptors and that the neurons expressing it might be the cells of origin of the retinohypothalamic tract. These ideas were at odds with an alternative suggestion, introduced a few years earlier, that the relevant photopigment might not be an opsin but, rather, a cryptochrome, a blue light–absorbing flavoprotein (reviewed in[36,41]). However, overwhelming evidence for melanopsin's central role soon emerged from studies in rodents and in heterologous expression systems.

Two key studies in this cohort focused on rat retinal ganglion cells shown by retrograde axonal tracing to innervate the suprachiasmatic nucleus (SCN) of the hypothalamus, the brain's circadian pacemaker.[42–45] The first showed that these ganglion cells expressed melanopsin[46] (see also[47,48]), while the second demonstrated that they generated robust electrical responses to light even when pharmacologically or mechanically isolated from other retinal neurons[49] (see also[50]). Because this capacity for autonomous phototransduction distinguishes these cells from all other RGCs, they are termed intrinsically photosensitive retinal ganglion cells (ipRGCs), or photoreceptive ganglion cells, or ganglion-cell photoreceptors. Soon, both mice and primates were shown also to possess ipRGCs with structural and functional properties much like those in the rat.[47,51–54] See Box 26.1 for an example of the impact of this discovery on ophthalmic practice.

The presence of melanopsin within physiologically identified ipRGCs was first demonstrated directly by Hattar *et al.*[47] (see also[51,54]). The opsin was found not only in the cell body, but also in their dendrites[47,55] which, like the soma, are directly photosensitive.[49] Further support for the view that melanopsin was the sensory photopigment in these cells came from the opsin-like action spectrum of the light response in ipRGCs[49,52,54] and from the observation that the intrinsic photosensitivity of these cells was abolished in melanopsin knockout mice.[52,56] The capacity of melanopsin to function as a sensory photopigment was first demonstrated biochemically,[57] and subsequently confirmed by electrophysiology and calcium imaging in heterologous expression systems.[58–60] There is remarkably good concordance in the spectral sensitivity in this system, as assessed from absorbance of

heterologously expressed or purified melanopsin, from the action spectrum of ipRGCs, and from behaviors mediated by inner retinal photoreceptors; all closely adhere to a retinaldehyde template function with a best wavelength at approximately 480 nm[27,33,34,49,52,54,59–65] (but see[57,58]).

DISTINCTIVE FUNCTIONAL PROPERTIES OF ipRGCS

Ganglion-cell photoreceptors have physiologic properties that are optimized for their roles in NIF vision and contrast markedly with those of the rod and cone photoreceptors that feed the cortical circuits mediating the perception of form, color, and motion. The photoresponse kinetics of ipRGCs also differs drastically from those of conventional, nonphotoreceptive ganglion cells.

Melanopsin chromophore and pigment bistability

In both vertebrate and invertebrate photopigments, the opsin apoprotein is covalently linked to a retinaldehyde molecule derived from vitamin A that serves as the light-absorbing moiety, or chromophore. In darkness, the retinaldehyde is in the 11-*cis* form. Absorption of a photon converts it into all-*trans* retinaldehyde. This triggers a conformational change in the opsin which in turn activates a G protein, initiating the transduction cascade. Before the photopigment can undergo another cycle of photoexcitation, the all-*trans* retinaldehyde must be reisomerized to 11-*cis*. For rod and cone photoreceptors, such reisomerization is carried out through multiple enzymatic steps after bleaching, that is, the dissociation of all-*trans* retinaldehyde from the opsin apoprotein. Several of these enzymatic steps occur in cells of the retinal pigment epithelium (RPE), which are essential for the visual cycle in rods and important, if not obligatory, for cones (see Chapter 13 for more information). The visual cycle in invertebrate photoreceptors appears to be radically different, in part because their photopigments are bistable: after photoexcitation, all-*trans* retinaldehyde remains covalently bound to the opsin and is reisomerized to 11-*cis* by subsequent absorption of light in a process known as photoreversal.[66]

The chromophore of melanopsin in situ is 11-*cis* retinaldehyde.[57-60,62,64,67,68] Sequence homology indicates that melanopsin resembles invertebrate opsins more than it does vertebrate ones,[39,40] implying that it might be bistable. There is growing evidence in support of this view[58,62,67-72] (but see[73]). If melanopsin is indeed bistable, it would be expected to be less reliant than rods or cones on the enzymatic machinery of the RPE for the regeneration of its chromophore, and might be utterly independent. Indeed, ipRGC photoresponses appear highly resistant to lighting conditions that fully bleach rod and cone photopigments, suggesting that all-*trans* retinaldehyde remains covalently bound to melanopsin following photoexcitation.[74] Furthermore, neither acute pharmacologic disruption of the retinoid cycle nor genetic deletion of the essential isomerohydrolase of the RPE (RPE65) abolishes the melanopsin-based photoresponse of ipRGCs or their ability to photoentrain circadian rhythms[69,75] (but see[67]). The evidence implies that to a remarkable degree, the melanopsin in ipRGCs can be loaded with its chromophore and can recover from photoactivation independent of retinoid processing by RPE. Melanopsin might acquire its retinoid mainly in the form of all-*trans* retinal which it then photoisomerizes to a *cis* isomer to form a photoexcitable pigment. This autonomy is important for the intrinsic photosensitivity of ipRGCs because these cells are located far (>100 μm) from the RPE (see Box 26.2). Nevertheless, during prolonged exposure to bright light, melanopsin regeneration in ipRGCs depends partly on 11-*cis* retinaldehyde supplied by the RPE,[76] analogous to the partial dependence of *Drosophila* rhodopsin regeneration on the enzymatic visual cycle in RPE-like retinal pigment cells.[77] During prolonged stimulation by bright light, 11-*cis* retinaldehyde appears to be transported from the RPE to ipRGCs by cellular retinaldehyde-binding protein (CRALBP) in Müller glial cells, which span the thickness of the retina.[76,78]

Spectral tuning

As noted previously, melanopsin has peak sensitivity in the blue region at around 480 nm, different from the spectral sensitivities of the rod and cone visual pigments (Fig. 26.1). This wavelength roughly coincides with the peak of solar emission, perhaps the result of

evolutionary pressures to optimize the sensitivity of this system to daylight. Although melanopsin is often described as a blue light–sensitive pigment, it is important to recognize that, like other opsin-based photopigments, its spectral tuning is rather broad. Throughout the spectral range from 340 to 580 nm, sensitivity is within 2 log units of that seen with the optimal wavelength (Fig. 26.1). Although there is evidence that ipRGCs project to the lateral geniculate nucleus and could thus contribute to cortical function[54,79-81] (see "Central projections" further in the chapter), we are unaware of any evidence that the unique spectral tuning of melanopsin is exploited in the conscious appreciation of color, which is well accounted for by the three cone photopigments and trichromatic theory (but see[82-84]). Melanopsin's spectral tuning, however, should be considered in the design of intraocular lenses (see Box 26.3).

The spectral behavior of the ipRGC output signal is much more complex than predicted simply from the action spectrum of the intrinsic light response as measured in dark-adapted ipRGCs. This is in part because melanopsin appears to be a bistable photopigment (see the previous section). The absorption spectrum of the activated form of the pigment, and thus of photoreversal, is shifted to longer wavelengths with respect to that of melanopsin in the dark state (e.g.,[62,70,72]), and this suggests the possibility of a form of spectral opponency under some conditions. A second source of complexity is the functional input to the ipRGCs from rod and cone photoreceptors, discussed in detail in "Synaptic input" further in the chapter. Because the intensity threshold for melanopsin activation is above that for rods and cones, the spectral tuning of ipRGCs can be expected to be intensity dependent. Furthermore, there is evidence in primates that the cone input to ipRGCs is itself spectrally opponent, with activation of short-wavelength cones driving OFF responses in ipRGCs, and activation of mid- and long-wavelength cones driving ON responses.[54]

Invertebrate-like phototransduction cascade

In a photoreceptor cell, the light-absorbing pigment signals through an intracellular biochemical pathway to transduce light into electrical activity across the cell membrane.[85] Despite its discovery in vertebrate tissues, melanopsin shares greater sequence homology to that of the rhabdomeric opsins (R-opsins) of invertebrates rather than the ciliary opsins (C-opsins) typically found among vertebrate species.[39,62,86] This similarity to R-opsins suggested that melanopsin might activate a phototransduction cascade similar to that found in *Drosophila* photoreceptors rather than that in vertebrate rods and cones (see Chapter 18). In rhabdomeric phototransduction, R-opsins couple to Gq proteins, which activate phospholipase Cβ4 (PLCβ4), an enzyme that hydrolyzes the membrane phospholipid phosphatidylinositol (4,5)-bisphosphate (PIP2) into two second messengers: membrane-delimited diacylglycerol, and cytosolic inositol 1,4,5 trisphosphate (IP3).[87] Canonical transient receptor potential (TRPC) channels are the terminal effectors of this cascade, mediating an influx of cations that results in depolarization across the plasma membrane.[88]

Early melanopsin phototransduction experiments were conducted in heterologous expression systems, and melanopsin expression was found to render nonphotosensitive cells light-responsive, a necessary characteristic of a putative photopigment. With melanopsin introduced into cultured HEK-293 cells and *Xenopus* oocytes, illumination could activate Gq proteins and the downstream target, PLCβ4.[59,60] Additionally, these HEK-293 cells, which were engineered to express TRPC channels, exhibited membrane depolarization in response to light, a quantitative experimental end point. This response, however, could be blocked by pharmacologic inhibition of Gq proteins or PLC.[60] Similarly, in an oocyte expression system, light-induced inward currents were diminished by blockers of Gq and PLC.[59] In cultured dermal

---

BOX 26.2 Sparing of intrinsically photosensitive retinal ganglion cell function in conditions involving retinal detachment and Leber's congenital amaurosis

There are at least two clinical conditions in which disruption of normal interactions between retinal pigment epithelium (RPE) and neural retina compromise rod and cone function but may permit continued phototransduction by intrinsically photosensitive retinal ganglion cells (ipRGCs). Retinal detachment disrupts the close contact between rod/cone outer segments and the RPE. This compromises the bidirectional exchange of retinoids across the subretinal space and thus the photosensitivity of rods and cones. Leber's congenital amaurosis (LCA), an autosomal recessive, early onset form of retinitis pigmentosa, is caused in some cases by mutations in the *Rpe65* gene. This disrupts the function of RPE65, a retinoid isomerase essential for the regeneration of 11-*cis* chromophore for rod and cone photopigments. Both retinal detachment and LCA have devastating consequences for photosensitivity of rods and cones. Evidence from animal studies (see main text) predicts that photosensitivity of ipRGCs should be substantially preserved under these conditions and should thus provide some useful photic information to the brain.

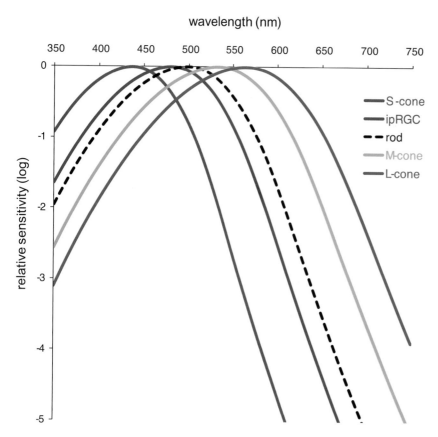

Fig. 26.1 Spectral tuning of human retinal photoreceptors. The spectral sensitivity of melanopsin-based phototransduction in intrinsically photosensitive retinal ganglion cells (ipRGCs) differs from that of the other four types of human retinal photoreceptors. The best wavelength for stimulating melanopsin in ipRGCs is at about 480 nm, compared with 437 nm for the short-wavelength cone ("S-cone"), 498 nm for the rod, 533 nm for the midwavelength cone ("M-cone"), and 564 nm for the long-wavelength cone ("L-cone").

BOX 26.3   Spectral issues in the design of intraocular lens implants

Designers of intraocular lens implants must grapple with the fact that there are both harmful and salutary effects of short-wavelength visible light. The goal must be to strike the appropriate balance between photoprotection and photoreception. High-pass filters that block blue, as well as ultraviolet, wavelengths offer better retinal photoprotection than those that block only ultraviolet light, while leaving rod and cone photoresponses (which peak near 500 nm and 555 nm respectively) relatively unaffected. However, because melanopsin is most sensitive to blue light with peak sensitivity at 480 nm, lenses that block blue wavelengths could compromise nonimage-forming (NIF) photoreception.[297,298] On the other hand, reducing NIF photoreception in this manner might have the benefit of reducing the harmful effects of light exposure at night on the NIF visual system, as discussed in the main text. These factors need to be considered in the design and selection of lens implants. It has been shown that for the typical person, long-pass filtering with a sharp filter cutoff near 445 nm may provide the best compromise between photoprotection and light reception.[299]

---

melanophores, a native expression system in which melanopsin was originally identified, light increased IP3 levels and inhibition of PLC blocked light-induced dispersion of melanosomes, again implicating a rhabdomeric phototransduction pathway.[89]

Electrophysiological studies in rodent ipRGCs have similarly shown the involvement of Gq and PLCβ4.[90–94] The light-gated channel mediating membrane depolarization has remained elusive although a heterotetramer of TRPC6 and TRPC7 seems likely.[92,94] These TRPC subunits have been identified in ipRGCs, and mice null for TRPC6 and TRPC7 show no photoresponses in M1-type ipRGCs[94] (Fig. 26.2 top).

The subsequent discovery and characterization of multiple types of physiologically diverse ipRGCs, named M1–M6 (see "Morphological types" further in the chapter), raised the possibility that melanopsin-initiated signaling might also be more diverse than previous believed. Indeed, two isoforms of melanopsin have been identified.[95] Moreover, while both M1 and M2 cells activate a typical rhabdomeric phototransduction cascade, as described previously, that terminates in the opening of heteromeric TRPC6/7 channels,[90,93,94,96–98] M2 cells simultaneously activate a yet-to-be-characterized pathway that opens hyperpolarization-activated cyclic nucleotide–gated (HCN) cation channels[97] (Fig. 26.2 bottom). The fast and slow components of photocurrents observed in cells have been attributed to the TRPC and HCN channels, respectively.[97] As mentioned, the intermediate G proteins, effectors, and second messengers leading to the gating of HCN channels remain to be identified.

The melanopsin signaling pathways in M4 cells are less clear.[96] Two hypotheses have been proposed. The first posits that the rhabdomeric cascade observed in M1 and M2 cells is conserved in M4 cells with the additional feature that a class of potassium leak channel closes in response to light.[98] The second hypothesis suggests that the M2 cell pathway leading to HCN channel opening is also at play in M4 cells.[97] These competing hypotheses are difficult to reconcile and require further investigation. Further study will also be necessary to characterize the phototransduction cascades of M3, M5, and M6 cells, which are yet to be elucidated.

Depolarizing photoresponse with action potentials

As mentioned in the previous section, an end point of the melanopsin phototransduction cascade is the opening of cation-selective channels in the plasma membrane. As for all other RGCs, the interior of an ipRGC is negatively charged relative to the extracellular space; thus, the

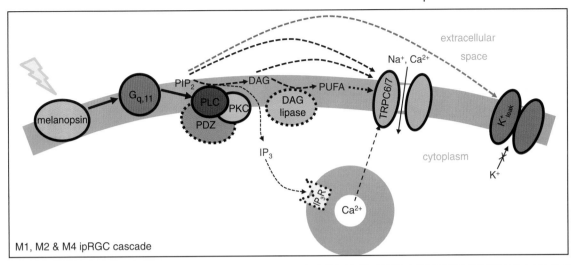

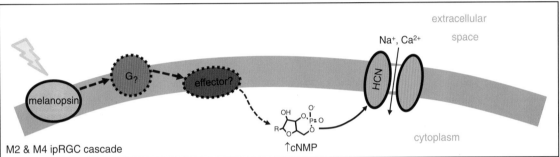

Fig. 26.2 Phototransduction cascades in ganglion-cell photoreceptors. *Solid lines* indicate established components and pathways; *dotted lines* indicate those that are possible but not proven. *Top:* Phototransduction cascade in M1, M2, and M4 intrinsically photosensitive retinal ganglion cells (ipRGCs). When melanopsin is excited by light, it signals through a G protein of the $G_{q/11}$ family to activate phospholipase C (*PLC*). This ultimately opens heteromeric TRPC6/7 cation channels, but the gating mechanism remains unknown. The signaling pathway is closely linked to the membrane and may involve depletion of the PLC substrate phosphatidyl 4,5-bisphosphate (PIP2), its metabolite diacylglycerol (*DAG*), or polyunsaturated fatty acids (*PUFA*) generated from DAG by DAG lipase. An isoform of protein kinase C (*PKC*) also appears to play an important role and, by analogy with *Drosophila* phototransduction, may be linked to PLC by an inactivation-no-afterpotential D (INAD)-like scaffolding protein that contains PDZ domains. The cytosolic product of PIP2 hydrolyisis, inositol 1,4,5-trisphosphate (IP3), acts at its cognate receptor (IP3-R) to liberate calcium from intracellular stores. Though such calcium mobilization is not necessary for phototransduction, it appears to play a significant modulatory role. In M4 ipRGCs, a potassium leak channel closes in response to this pathway (*blue dotted line*) resulting in a positive shift in membrane potential, making the cells more excitable to subsequent stimulation. *Bottom:* Phototransduction cascade in M2 and M4 ipRGCs. In addition to the phosphoinositide pathways described in the top panel, M2 and M4 cells show evidence of an alternate, cyclic nucleotide monophosphate (*cNMP*)–mediated cascade targeting a hyperpolarization-activated cyclic nucleotide–gated (*HCN*) cation channel. The identities of the cyclic nucleotide that opens the HCN channel and of the G protein and effector(s) that regulate its intracellular concentration remain to be determined.

opening of light-gated cation channels results in net influx of cations and membrane depolarization. In this, ipRGCs once again resemble invertebrate rhabdomeric receptors, which likewise depolarize when illuminated, but differ from the vertebrate rods and cones, which are hyperpolarized by light (see Chapter 19). If the depolarizing ipRGC light response is large enough, it brings the membrane potential above the threshold for activating voltage-gated sodium channels, triggering action potentials (Fig. 26.3). This represents yet another divergence from the rod/cone photoreceptors, which do not spike. Action potentials are necessary for ipRGCs, as for other RGCs, to propagate electrical information faithfully along the optic nerve and tract to relatively distant central visual centers. By contrast, rod and cone axons are very short, and passive spread of the electrical signals generated in the outer

segment is sufficient for appropriate voltage modulation of the axon terminal.

Sensitivity

A salient feature of ipRGCs is the relative insensitivity of their melanopsin-mediated responses to light. The threshold intensity for the ipRGC intrinsic photoresponse is 1 to 2 orders of magnitude (i.e., 10–100 times) higher than that for cones, and up to 5 log units higher than that for rods.[49,54,99,100] Such insensitivity is apparently due mainly to the low abundance of melanopsin molecules in ipRGCs, and the resulting low probability of photon absorption.[101] This in turn is related to the fact that ipRGCs lack any structural specialization for increasing the packing of pigment-laden membrane in the cell, such as the discs in

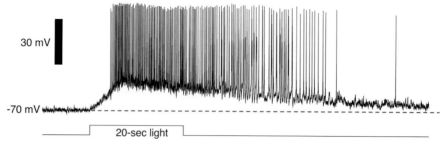

30 mV

-70 mV

20-sec light

Fig. 26.3 Melanopsin-driven light response of an intrinsically photosensitive retinal ganglion cell (ipRGC). Ganglion-cell photoreceptors can respond to light through not only their melanopsin phototransduction but also rod/cone-driven synaptic input. Here, the light-evoked response of a rat ipRGC was recorded intracellularly in the presence of pharmacologic agents that blocked synaptic input, thus isolating the intrinsic photosensitivity of this cell. The *dotted red line* marks the prestimulus level of the membrane potential. Notice that the light-evoked action potentials begin long after stimulus onset and that they persist throughout and even long after the stimulus. (From KY Wong, unpublished).

the outer segments of rods and cones or the rhabdomeric microvilli of invertebrate photoreceptors. The insensitivity of intrinsic, melanopsin-based responses in ipRGCs means that such responses are triggered mainly by relatively bright light. Because the dynamic range of these responses complements those of the rod and cone photoreceptors, and because all three of these signals converge on ipRGCs (see "Synaptic input" further in the chapter), these retinal output neurons and at least some of the NIF visual responses they drive are able to function over the entire intensity range of naturally encountered light stimuli.[54,56]

Kinetics

The temporal characteristics of the melanopsin-based ipRGC photoresponse are different from those of the outer retinal photoreceptors, with remarkably slower onset and termination than both rod and cone photoresponses, and greater stability in the face of sustained illumination than for the cone response. Rod and cone photoresponses begin within several milliseconds of light onset and peak within tens of milliseconds. Even the fastest ipRGC intrinsic responses, evoked by very high light intensities ($>10^{14}$ photons/cm^2 per second at 480 nm; for reference, direct sunlight is approximately 10^{17} photons/cm^2 per second), are much slower, with the first action potential appearing no earlier than a few hundred milliseconds after light onset and peak firing rate achieved only after several seconds. Latencies rise dramatically for less intense flashes, and for near-threshold light stimuli ($\sim10^{11}$ photons/cm^2 per second at 480 nm) can be as long as tens of seconds to the first spike and several minutes before the peak discharge is reached.[49,102] The basis for such sluggish onset arises in part from the phosphorylation of melanopsin: when melanopsin was engineered to contain reduced numbers of phosphorylable sites, photoresponse latency was reduced by as much as approximately threefold.[103] However, this relatively modest effect of phosphorylation cannot account for the very long latencies near threshold, which seem more likely to result from the temporal integration of many low-amplitude, long-lasting, single-photon events.[101]

In response to a prolonged light step, the melanopsin-driven response gradually decays from an early peak to a lower steady-state level. This reflects light adaptation, which prevents saturation of the phototransduction cascade, and it is partly calcium dependent as in the outer retinal photoreceptors[104,105] (see also Chapter 20). After light adaptation is complete (which typically requires several minutes), membrane potential and thus spike frequency remain elevated above baseline levels for as long as the light stimulus persists. Electrophysiological recordings from ipRGCs have shown melanopsin-based photoresponses lasting at least 10 hours,[102] while analysis of activity-dependent induction of the immediate early

gene *cFos* in putative ipRGCs implies that these photoreceptors can respond continuously to light for at least 19 hours.[106] Thus, the ipRGC intrinsic photoresponse is far more sustained (Fig. 26.3) than the cone response, which adapts much faster and more completely, making the response very transient. The ability of ipRGCs to continuously signal the presence of bright light for many hours is a key characteristic of the NIF visual system, which features tonic responses to steady diffuse illumination and the ability to integrate photon flux over periods of more than an hour, as explained in more detail in "Central projections" further in the chapter.

The termination of the melanopsin light response is extraordinarily slow. After the cessation of light stimulation, cone and rod responses terminate within hundreds of milliseconds and several seconds, respectively. But termination of the intrinsic photoresponse of ipRGCs takes up to several minutes, especially for very high light intensities.[49,52,54] The reason for this slow recovery is not established, but the similarity of melanopsin to invertebrate rhabdomeric opsins suggests that it results in part from the thermal stability of the light-activated (metarhodopsin) form of the photopigment.[62,71] If so, the slowly decaying poststimulus voltage response is directly analogous to the persistent depolarizing afterpotential of invertebrate photoreceptors.[66] This is supported by the observation that the poststimulus depolarization can be suppressed by exposure to long-wavelength light, presumably by triggering photoreversal of the pigment.[71,72] However, light is not required for response termination, because this can occur in complete darkness. As expected for all G protein–coupled receptors, the light-independent mechanisms for response termination involve phosphorylation of melanopsin followed by arrestin binding.[107]

The very sustained nature of ipRGC photoresponses is unique among ganglion cells. In response to a light step, nearly all other ganglion cells respond to the stimulus in a far more transient manner, with spike rate changes that last for no more than several seconds,[99,102] indicating that whereas ipRGCs stably encode absolute light intensity, most conventional ganglion cells detect mainly changes in light intensity. This sustained versus transient dichotomy reflects differences in synaptic inputs and in biophysical properties intrinsic to the ganglion cells.[108]

Morphologic types

In all mammals studied to date, melanopsin-expressing ganglion cells represent a small minority of all RGCs. These are now recognized as comprising multiple cell types, which have been studied most extensively in the mouse, in which six types of melanopsin-expressing RGCs have been identified. They can be distinguished by their differing morphologies, melanopsin expression levels, and central targets. As form tracks function, the distinct configurations and projections of the ipRGC types also suggest different physiologic properties and behavioral roles,[109] as is explained in subsequent sections.

Schematics of the six mouse ipRGC types, named M1–M6, are shown in Fig. 26.4. M1 and M2 were the first two types to be identified due to their robust melanopsin immunoreactivity.[49,55] Mouse M1 cells have relatively small soma diameters of around 15 μm on average, and sparsely branched, broad dendritic arbors (~350 μm average field diameter) that stratify in the OFF sublayer of the inner plexiform layer (IPL), abutting the inner nuclear layer (INL).[109–113] As explained in "Synaptic input" further on, despite such stratification, M1 cells and the other ipRGC types that contain OFF-stratifying dendrites do not exhibit OFF responses under normal conditions. M1d is a displaced subset of the M1 type, differing only in having somas within the innermost aspect of the INL.[47,110] Additionally, two subsets of M1 cells differentially express the POU-domain transcription factor Brn3b, which correlates to the central targets and potential functions of those cells[114,115] (see "Central projections" further in this chapter), suggesting that the M1 type consists of two subtypes. On the whole, M1 cells exhibit the highest intrinsic photosensitivity among the known types

of mouse ipRGCs,[116–118] although substantial heterogeneity in intensity dynamic range has been noted among M1 cells, which has been proposed to allow the M1 population to collectively encode a wide range of absolute light intensities.[119]

Compared with M1 cells, mouse M2 cells have slightly larger somas averaging around 18 μm in diameter and broad, sparse arbors (~380 μm field diameter) that ramify in the ON sublayer of the IPL.[109–113,118] They are also less melanopsin immunoreactive than M1 cells, suggesting a lower level of melanopsin expression. Accordingly, in terms of autonomous phototransduction, M2 ipRGCs are an order of magnitude less sensitive to light.[116,120]

M3 somas can be visualized using antimelanopsin antisera but the neurites are difficult to resolve with standard immunohistochemical techniques, suggesting relatively low melanopsin expression, and indeed M3 cells generate weaker intrinsic photoresponses than both M1 and M2.[116,121] M3 somas are intermediate in size to M1 and M2 somas, and their sparse dendrites bistratify in both ON and OFF sublaminae of the IPL, with an average dendritic field diameter of ~460 μm, the largest among mouse ipRGCs.[109,110,113,121,122]

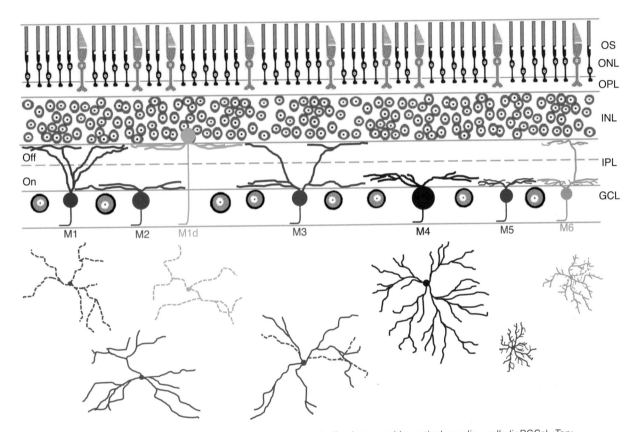

Fig. 26.4 The six morphologic types of mouse intrinsically photosensitive retinal ganglion cells (ipRGCs). *Top:* Dendritic stratification of the six known types of ipRGCs as seen in a schematic cross-section of the retina. M1 cells have sparse dendrites that terminate in the OFF sublamina of the inner plexiform layer (*IPL*) and their cell bodies are located either in the ganglion-cell layer (*GCL; dark green cell*) or displaced to the inner nuclear layer (*INL; light green cell*). The other types of ipRGCs have somas exclusively in the GCL. Like M1, the M2 type (*red cell*) has sparse dendrites, but these are restricted to the ON sublamina of the IPL. M3 cells (*magenta*) similarly have sparse dendrites, although they stratify in both ON and OFF sublaminas. The M4 type (*brown*), also called the ON alpha cell, has denser, radiate dendrites that stratify slightly more distally than the dendrites of M2 cells. M5 cells (*blue*) have compact, bushy ON-stratifying dendrites. M6 cells (*orange*) have M5-like dendrites in the ON sublamina, and additional dendrites that terminate in the OFF sublamina. The dendrite fields have been shrunk relative to the somas owing to space constraints. *OS,* Outer segments; *ONL,* outer nuclear layer; *OPL,* outer plexiform layer. *Bottom:* Schematic drawings of the dendritic fields of the ipRGC types, illustrating their diverse morphologies and field sizes. Dendrites terminating in the OFF sublamina of the IPL are depicted as *dashed lines.*

It is now understood that M4 cells correspond to what have been previously characterized as ON alpha RGCs.[112,123] ON alpha RGCs were originally not believed to be intrinsically photoreceptive, but now are known to express a very low level of melanopsin and possess autonomous photosensitivity.[112,118] The M4 type has the largest soma (~24 μm) of any class of mouse RGC, with dendritic field diameter ranging from approximately 270 μm to approximately 370 μm, depending on retinal location.[109,112,118,123–126] The entire extent of the cells can be labeled using antibodies against SMI-32, which stain both ON alpha and OFF alpha RGCs.[123,127,128] Owing to the low melanopsin content of M4 cells, their intrinsic photoresponse has an even higher threshold than that of M2 cells.[112,116]

Because M5 and M6 cells express the lowest melanopsin levels among mouse ipRGC types, they have been identified using Cre recombinase–based melanopsin-specific reporter mice, or tyramide-enhanced melanopsin immunoreactivity.[129,130] M5 cells have small somas of around 14 μm in diameter and compact, bushy dendritic arbors (~220 μm diameter) that terminate in the ON sublamina of the IPL.[118,127,130,131] M6 cell morphology resembles that of M5 cells with small somas (~12 μm diameter) and small dendritic arbors (~220 μm diameter), except that M6 cells show slightly more exuberant branching than M5 cells and are bistratified, with additional dendrites terminating in the OFF sublamina of the IPL.[129] As expected from the very low melanopsin expression in M5 cells, the peak amplitude of their intrinsic photoresponse appears even smaller than that for M3 cells.[116] The intrinsic response of M6 cells is likewise relatively small, although it has not been systematically compared with those of the other ipRGCs types.[129,131a]

In addition to having diverse intrinsic photoresponse sensitivities reflecting different melanopsin expression levels (see previously) and differential expression of melanopsin isoforms,[95] the various mouse ipRGC types have been shown to differ in terms of additional physiologic measures such as resting membrane potential, membrane resistance, spontaneous spike rate, spike waveform, and voltage-gated currents.[111,116,121,131,132] These ipRGC types also exhibit diverse extrinsic photoresponses reflecting differences in synaptic input from rod/cone-driven circuits, as explained in "Synaptic input" further in the chapter.

The morphology and distribution of human ipRGCs have been described in detail.[53,54,133–135] Of the approximately 1.5 million RGCs in a human, only about 7300, or 0.5%, express melanopsin.[133] They comprise five morphologic types, four of which appear homologous to mouse ipRGCs: a strongly melanopsin-immunoreactive M1-like type with OFF-stratifying dendrites; an M2-like ON-stratifying type with somewhat weaker melanopsin immunoreactivity; a relatively rare M3-like ON/OFF–bistratifying type; and an M4-like ON-stratifying type with very weak melanopsin immunoreactivity. The fifth type of human ipRGC, named "gigantic M1" or "GM1," has OFF-stratifying dendrites and very large somas averaging about 33 μm. For both M1-like and GM1 types, a subset of cells have somas displaced to the INL.[133] The dendritic fields of human ipRGCs are the largest of any ganglion cell type, ranging from 300 μm in the central retina to 1200 μm in the periphery (Fig. 26.5). The dendrites of neighboring cells overlap extensively so that the entire retina, except for the fovea, is covered by a network of melanopsin-containing processes (Fig. 26.6). Because both the cell bodies and the dendrites of these cells are intrinsically photosensitive,[49,54] each ipRGC integrates photons over a region comparable to its dendritic field size. These large receptive fields and low spatial densities make ipRGCs ill-suited for fine spatial discriminations, but ideal for the pronounced spatial integration that characterizes NIF functions. They contrast sharply with the very small receptive fields of rods and cones (<10 μm in diameter), the foundation for the fine-grained retinal representations at the cortical level that permit high acuity spatial vision (see Chapter 33). The melanopsin-mediated photoresponses of human ipRGCs have been investigated using extracellular spike recording and were found to comprise three physiologic varieties with different intensity thresholds and response kinetics.[136]

Multiple ipRGC types have also been identified in many other species. The rat retina contains M1–M5, the morphologic properties and physiologic diversity of which are remarkably similar to their mouse counterparts.[49,50,137–139] M1-like OFF-stratifying ipRGCs and M2-like ON-stratifying ipRGCs are present in nonhuman primates, including macaque and marmoset.[54,134,140,141] Both rabbit and tree shrew possess three morphologic types of melanopsin-immunopositive RGCs that somewhat resemble M1–M3,[142,143] whereas only M1-like and M3-like ipRGCs have been detected in the Mongolian gerbil retina.[144] Extracellular spike recording has revealed three physiologic types of ipRGCs in the Sudanian grass rat, a diurnal rodent.[145]

Resistance to pathologic states

Compared to other types of ganglion cell, ipRGCs appear more resistant to a variety of acute insults including *N*-methyl-D-aspartic acid–induced excitotoxicity,[146–150] optic nerve transection,[149,151,152] and optic nerve crush.[153–155] Two weeks following optic nerve crush, M1 ipRGCs are reduced by 30%, whereas "few if any" M2 cells survive.[153] In experimental models of glaucoma, ipRGCs also exhibit some resilience relative to other (i.e., conventional) RGCs. After 6 to 8 months of experimentally

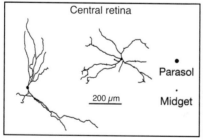 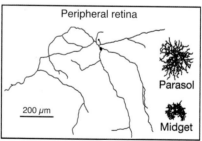

Fig. 26.5 Morphology of primate intrinsically photosensitive retinal ganglion cells (ipRGCs) as seen in whole-mounted retina. The dendritic arbors of these cells cover much less area in the central retina (*left*) than they do in the periphery (*right*), but at all eccentricities they have among the largest fields of any primate ganglion cells. For comparison, the much smaller and more densely branching dendritic fields of midget and parasol cells (two ganglion cell types mediating image-forming vision) are also shown. (Reproduced with permission from Dacey DM, Liao HW, Peterson BB et al. Melanopsin-expressing ganglion cells in primate retina signal color and irradiance and project to the LGN. *Nature.* 2005;433(7027):749–754.)

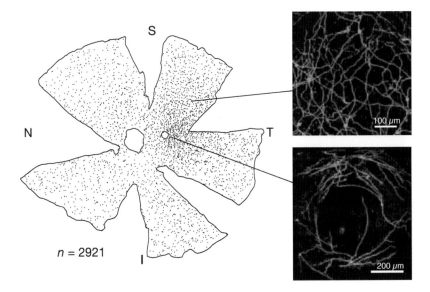

Fig. 26.6 Distribution of melanopsin-expressing ganglion cells in the primate retina. In this experiment, intrinsically photosensitive retinal ganglion cells (ipRGCs) in a macaque retina were revealed by antimelanopsin immunofluorescence. *Left:* Plot of a flattened whole retina, with each dot representing the cell body of a melanopsin-immunopositive cell. In this retina, a total of 2921 melanopsin-expressing ganglion cells were found. *S*, Superior; *I*, inferior; *N*, nasal; *T*, temporal. *Right:* The network of melanopsin-immunoreactive dendrites in the peripheral retina *(top)* and around the fovea *(bottom)*. Notice the absence of melanopsin staining in the fovea. (Reproduced with permission from Dacey DM, Liao HW, Peterson BB et al. Melanopsin-expressing ganglion cells in primate retina signal color and irradiance and project to the LGN. *Nature.* 2005;433(7027):749–754.)

BOX 26.4   Promise of melanopsin-based gene therapy for blindness

Transient transfection with the melanopsin gene is sufficient to induce photosensitivity in a variety of cell types in culture[58–60,65,95] (Fig. 26.7 *top*). Introduction of melanopsin into inner retinal cells thus holds promise as a candidate gene therapy for restoring sight in retinitis pigmentosa and other forms of outer retinal blindness. The practicality of this approach is enhanced by the fact that intrinsically photosensitive retinal ganglion cells (ipRGCs) do not absolutely require the retinal pigment epithelium for chromophore regeneration. Another advantage is that all of the critical elements of melanopsin-driven phototransduction appear to be associated with the plasma membrane, thus reducing the requirements for specialized cytosolic machinery. Indeed, three studies using a mouse model of retinitis pigmentosa report that transfecting conventional RGCs with the melanopsin gene renders most of them photosensitive and can rescue some light-driven behavioral responses[172,179a,300] (Fig. 26.7 *bottom*).

However, several disadvantages of this approach need to be considered. First, in both ipRGCs and the various heterologous expression systems, the melanopsin-based photoresponse is far more sluggish than those of the rods and cones. Thus, even if image-forming vision is restored, the patient's perception of stimulus motion and of the timing of transient visual events would

presumably be highly distorted. Second, ipRGCs are even less sensitive to light than cones, so visual threshold would be even higher than for people suffering from night blindness. Still, melanopsin is more light sensitive than the most promising alternative candidate for gene therapeutic induction of inner retinal photosensitivity, namely the microbial light-gated ionophore channelrhodopsin-2.[301–303] Third, if melanopsin is targeted to RGCs, all of which have dendritic fields vastly larger than the profile of rod and cone outer segments, then spatial resolution would be quite poor. The average receptive field diameter of melanopsin-transfected mouse RGCs in one study was about $100\,\mu m$.[179a] To improve spatial resolution, it might be better to selectively target bipolar cells for melanopsin transfection (see for example[302]). It is unknown if these cells express critical components of the melanopsin phototransduction cascade, and so Van Wyk and colleagues developed a chimeric protein containing the light-sensitive domains of melanopsin and the intracellular domains of the ON bipolar cell–specific metabotropic glutamate receptor type 6, to ensure that photostimulation of this protein can activate the G protein transduction cascade in ON bipolar cells. Introducing this chimeric protein into the ON bipolar cells of *rd1* mice improved visual function.[304]

---

elevated intraocular pressure (IOP) by laser coagulation, the general population of RGCs is reduced by 25% to 33%, while ipRGCs are reduced by only about 17%.[128] Like optic nerve crush, ipRGC types are differentially affected by IOP elevation. At least 6 months after elevated IOP, M1 ipRGCs show no significant decline in number. Yet, M4 cells are reduced by 25%, in line with the reduction observed in the general RGC population. Additionally, chronically elevated IOP has no impact on circadian entrainment, a primarily M1-mediated NIF visual function. Contrast sensitivity, however, is diminished in these animals, consistent with the loss of image-forming RGCs including M4 ipRGCs.[128]

The participation of several ipRGC types in image-forming vision will be described in "Central projections" further in the chapter.

The molecular basis for these kinds of injury resistance is largely unknown, although the PI3K/Akt signaling pathway appears to be involved.[149] Moreover, melanopsin expression levels seem to correlate with resilience to insult. Overexpression of melanopsin in RGCs promotes axonal regeneration by activating the mammalian target of rapamycin (mTOR) pathway.[156] Further investigation into the molecular basis of ipRGC survival after retinal injuries may lead to novel strategies for preventing and/or treating various retinal diseases (see also Box 26.4).

SYNAPTIC INPUT

Unlike conventional RGCs, ipRGCs do not require synaptic input to respond to light because they are directly photosensitive. Nonetheless, both primate and rodent ipRGCs receive synaptic inputs from bipolar and amacrine cells and thereby generate rod/cone-driven, as well as melanopsin-based, light responses. Receiving these inputs has consequences for the timing, spectral behavior, and sensitivity of the light-evoked discharges of these cells. A schematic diagram summarizing the intraretinal synaptic inputs to M1 and M2 ipRGCs appears in Fig. 26.8.

Bipolar cell input

There is strong structural and physiologic evidence for synaptic contacts from bipolar cell axons onto ipRGC dendrites. The earliest anatomical evidence came from electron-microscopic immunohistochemical data in mice showing ribbon synaptic (bipolar) contacts onto melanopsin-expressing dendrites[157] and this has been supported by subsequent structural observations.[122,134,140,143,158–161] Bipolar cell input to ipRGCs has also been confirmed electrophysiologically. Rodent ipRGCs are excited by applied glutamate, the transmitter released by bipolar cell terminals. Spontaneous glutamate-mediated excitatory postsynaptic currents are detectable in ipRGCs, and these almost certainly derive from bipolar cell synapses.[99,162] Under appropriate recording conditions, broad-spectrum (white) light elicits two excitatory ON response components in ipRGCs. One has a high threshold, is sluggish in its onset and termination, and is insensitive to synaptic blockers; these properties testify to its origin in intrinsic melanopsin-based phototransduction. The other component occurs much more rapidly after light onset, can be abolished by pharmacologic blockade of synaptic transmission, and is attributable to excitatory synaptic input from ON bipolar cells.[54,99,116,120,162] Both rods and cones contribute to these extrinsic light responses, making them as many as five orders of magnitude more sensitive to light than the melanopsin photoresponse[54,99,100,120,137] (Fig. 26.9).

It is surprising that the ON channel provides the dominant bipolar input to all ipRGCs. For decades, ON bipolar cell axons were thought to contact ganglion cell dendrites only in the inner half of the IPL, that is, in the ON sublamina[163,164] ("IPL: On" in Fig. 26.8). Whereas this arrangement is congruent with the ON input to M2–M6 ipRGCs, which

possess ON-stratifying dendrites, it seems at odds with the observation that the ON channel also dominates the synaptic inputs to the OFF-stratifying M1 and M1-like ipRGCs, which arborize largely or exclusively within the OFF sublamina.[49,54,55,118,122,137,140,165] Because most of the OFF-stratifying cells have somas in the GCL, their dendrites must traverse the ON sublayer en route to the OFF sublayer, so some of the ON channel input could conceivably occur in the ON sublayer on proximal dendrites (Fig. 26.4 top). Indeed, Belenky et al.[157] reported that virtually all bipolar cell contacts onto melanopsin dendrites were found in the inner half of the IPL, although they did not indicate whether these dendrites derived from the outer- or inner-stratifying types of melanopsin RGCs. Two studies[133,158] have also suggested that rod bipolar cells (a type of ON bipolar cell) make direct contact onto the GCL somas and proximal dendrites of melanopsin-expressing RGCs, including M1 cells (but see[160]). However, contacts solely on the soma or proximal dendrites would severely restrict the size of the synaptically driven receptive fields of these ipRGCs, when in fact they are large and coextensive with the dendritic arbor.[54,99,116] This suggests that there must be additional ON bipolar input to the distal dendrites of M1 cells in the OFF sublayer. This inference is further supported by the observation that displaced M1 ipRGCs, which have somas in the INL and dendrites restricted to the OFF sublamina, nonetheless exhibit synaptically mediated ON responses.[54,159] There is compelling evidence that these paradoxical ON bipolar inputs are made by ectopic ON bipolar cell axon terminals and synaptic release sites in the OFF sublamina, belonging primarily to type-6 ON cone bipolar cells[134,143,159–161] (Fig. 26.8 top).

Anatomical studies have not detected any direct synaptic contact between OFF bipolar cells and ipRGCs. However, pharmacologic blockade of ON bipolar cells and amacrine cells reveals in some rat M1 ipRGCs a very small depolarizing ipRGC response at light offset, consistent with a weak input from OFF bipolar cells.[99] It is plausible that these M1 cells receive OFF bipolar input polysynaptically, via gap junctional electrical synapses with OFF bipolar–driven amacrine cells, as has been documented for certain conventional ON ganglion cells.[166]

Amacrine cell input and neuromodulation

Ganglion-cell photoreceptors also receive substantial synaptic input from amacrine cells. Initial evidence came from an electron-microscopic study in mouse documenting amacrine cell synaptic release

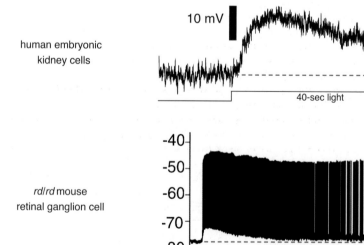

human embryonic kidney cells

10 mV

40-sec light

rd/rd mouse retinal ganglion cell

-40
-50
-60
-70
-80

1-sec light

10 sec

Fig. 26.7 Induction of photosensitivity by ectopic melanopsin expression. Artificially expressing the gene for melanopsin in cells that normally lack photosensitivity can render them light-responsive. *Top:* Intracellular recording of the light-evoked depolarization in a human embryonic kidney cell transiently transfected with the mouse melanopsin gene. *Bottom:* An intracellular recording of light response in a ganglion cell in a retinally degenerate mouse retina virally transfected with the melanopsin gene. This light sensitivity was induced by the genetic manipulation because this morphologic type of ganglion cell is not intrinsically photosensitive in control retinas. In both cases, the artificially induced light responses resemble the intrinsic light response of intrinsically photosensitive retinal ganglion cells (compare with Fig. 26.3). (*Top.* from KY Wong, unpublished; *bottom,* reproduced with permission from Lin B, Koizumi A, Tanaka N, Panda S, Masland RH. Restoration of visual function in retinal degeneration mice by ectopic expression of melanopsin. *Proc Natl Acad Sci U S A.* 2008;105(41):16009–16014.)

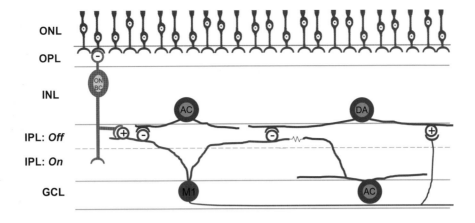

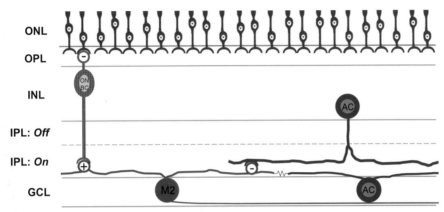

Fig. 26.8 Synaptic circuits involving M1 and M2 intrinsically photosensitive retinal ganglion cells (ipRGCs). *Top:* Mouse M1 cells are known to receive direct synaptic inputs from ON bipolar cells (*ON BC*) and amacrine cells (*AC*). ON BCs normally innervate ganglion cells in the proximal, ON sublamina of the inner plexiform layer (*IPL*), but because the dendrites of M1 ipRGCs are mainly in the distal, OFF sublamina, ON BC use ectopic glutamatergic synapses in the OFF sublamina to signal to M1 cells. ACs provide a strong inhibitory input to these ipRGCs via GABAergic and glycinergic synapses. Additionally, M1 cells signal in the retrograde direction to some dopaminergic AC (*DAs*) via glutamate release from axon collaterals, and to some ON-OFF–bistratifying displaced ACs via gap junctional electrical synapses. *Bottom:* Mouse M2 cells receive glutamatergic input from the axon terminals of ON BCs in the ON sublamina. These ipRGCs also receive inhibitory input from ACs and signal through gap junctions to some ON-stratifying displaced ACs. *GCL,* ganglion-cell layer; *ONL,* outer nuclear layer; *INL,* inner nuclear layer; *OPL,* outer plexiform layer.

A rat ipRGC generating rod/cone-driven and melanopsin-based light responses.

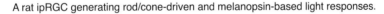
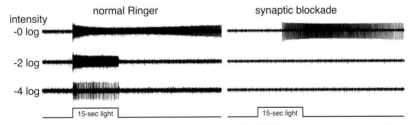

Fig. 26.9 A rat intrinsically photosensitive retinal ganglion cell (ipRGC) generating rod/cone-driven and melanopsin-based light responses. Extracellular recordings of spiking in a rat ipRGC evoked by light stimuli at three intensities (dimmest at *bottom,* brightest at *top*); the *vertical lines* in the traces are action potentials. *Left:* Under normal physiologic conditions, this cell is capable of generating both rod/cone-driven and melanopsin-based light responses. At the two dimmest light intensities, only rod/cone-mediated responses are induced, and they have fast onset and termination. At the highest intensity, the melanopsin response is also activated, resulting in prolonged poststimulus spiking. *Right:* In the presence of drugs that block synaptic transmission, only the intrinsic melanopsin light response is induced. Notice the slow response onset and prolonged poststimulus persistence, which are similar to those in the intracellular recording shown in Fig. 26.3. (From KY Wong, unpublished.)

sites in close apposition to melanopsin-containing dendrites in the IPL.[157] The dominant effect of these inputs is almost certainly inhibitory because the vast majority of amacrine cells contain one of two major inhibitory transmitters: γ-aminobutyric acid (GABA) or glycine. Studies in rodent retina have demonstrated that exogenously applied or endogenously released GABA and/or glycine trigger inhibitory chloride currents in ipRGCs and that such currents can be activated by light, primarily at light onset.[99,116,122,162,167] In primate ipRGCs, amacrine inputs have not been investigated electrophysiologically but there is extensive anatomical evidence for them in marmoset and macaque, where they contact both outer- and inner-stratifying melanopsin-expressing dendrites.[133,134,140,141,168]

There are at least 50 types of amacrine cells in mammalian retinas, differing in dendritic stratification and field size, as well as in their neurochemical signature.[169–176] Several amacrine cell types have been found to form chemical synapses with ipRGCs,[122,133,167,177] and the best understood is the dopaminergic amacrine cell,[122,133,134,158,178] which has processes stratifying almost exclusively in the most distal sublayer of the IPL,[179] the same stratum in which dendrites of outer-stratifying ipRGCs arborize.[47,49,54,55] Dopamine is a key retinal neuromodulator, and its primary role is to help retinal cells and circuits adapt to different background lighting conditions.[169,180] Thus, ipRGCs can potentially adapt to light not only through intrinsic mechanisms ("photoreceptor adaptation"[104,105]), but also through synaptic inputs ("network adaptation"). Supporting this possibility, dopamine has been shown to regulate the transcription of melanopsin in rat over a time course of several hours,[181] and electrophysiological studies have demonstrated additional, more acute effects of dopamine on the intrinsic photoresponse of ipRGCs.[182,183] There is emerging evidence that ipRGC electrophysiology can also be influenced by several additional neuromodulators. Some of these substances exert inhibitory effects on ipRGCs, such as opioids,[184,185] somatostatin,[186] and adenosine,[187] whereas orexin-A has been found to potentiate spontaneous spiking and light-evoked responses in M2 ipRGCs.[188]

In addition to being regulated by amacrine cell neuromodulators, ipRGCs express receptors for melatonin,[183,189] a hormone secreted at night by outer retinal photoreceptors,[190,191] and melatonin has been shown to alter synaptic inputs to M4 ipRGCs.[183] Moreover, various aspects of ipRGC electrophysiology are under circadian control, causing these neurons to exhibit different photoresponses, resting membrane potentials, and spontaneous spike rates at different times of day.[183,192] Such time-dependent variations could contribute to a circadian rhythm in the ipRGC-mediated pupillary light reflex (PLR).[193]

Extrinsic versus intrinsic photoresponses

In primate M1- and M2-like ipRGCs, the intrinsic melanopsin-based responses are invariably depolarizing, but the polarity of the extrinsic, synaptically mediated light response is wavelength-dependent[54]: blue light elicits hyperpolarizing extrinsic responses, whereas longer wavelengths evoke depolarizing ones (Fig. 26.10). Whereas the depolarizing responses are driven by ON bipolar cells, the hyperpolarizing response to short-wavelength light is mediated by an amacrine cell type that receives input exclusively from blue cone–selective ON bipolar cells.[168] In mice, M5 ipRGCs also exhibit color opponency, with green cone input in the surround region of the receptive field driving amacrine-mediated inhibitory responses.[130] The overall spectral behavior of these color-opponent ipRGCs is unusually complex, because it is shaped not only by their synaptic inputs but also by the two spectrally distinct states of their melanopsin photopigment, which exert opposing photic effects on the phototransduction cascade (see "Spectral tuning" previously in the chapter).

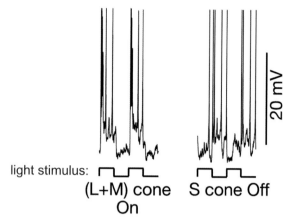

Fig. 26.10 Color-opponent light responses in macaque intrinsically photosensitive retinal ganglion cells (ipRGCs). Light stimuli selectively modulating L-cone and M-cone influences on ipRGCs drive depolarizing or "ON" responses to light (*left*), whereas S-cone–isolating stimuli trigger hyperpolarizing or "OFF" responses (*right*). (Reproduced with permission from Dacey DM, Liao HW, Peterson BB et al. Melanopsin-expressing ganglion cells in primate retina signal color and irradiance and project to the LGN. *Nature.* 2005;433(7027):749–754.)

In addition to altering spectral sensitivity, synaptic input to ipRGCs expands their intensity dynamic range, temporal bandpass, and sensitivity to spatial contrast. The rod input evokes a depolarizing photoresponse that is as sustained as the melanopsin-based response, lasting for the duration of illumination, but it is about 5 log units more light sensitive and has a much faster onset.[54,100,102] Although the cone input likewise evokes ipRGC responses with very short latencies, these responses decay within a few seconds, and for primate ipRGCs are only about 1 log unit more sensitive than the intrinsic light response.[54] Accordingly, ipRGCs rely on the rod input to measure absolute light intensities in the low to moderate range, but use intrinsic, as well as extrinsic, responses to measure higher light intensities. Further, because the sluggish intrinsic response can only track slow fluctuations in light intensity,[99,139] ipRGCs require rod/cone input to track intensity changes above approximately 0.5 Hz.[194] Because the cone input adapts especially rapidly, it is activated mainly at the beginning of prolonged illumination,[54,99,120,195] or during repeated, intermittent photostimulation.[196,197] Finally, synaptic input to M2–M6 cells creates a receptive field that consists of antagonistic center versus surround regions, conferring these ipRGCs with an ability to detect spatial contrast within the receptive field.[112,116,129] The receptive field of M1 cells lacks center/surround antagonism,[116] consistent with this cell type's primary role in NIF visual functions.

SYNAPTIC OUTPUT AND PHYSIOLOGIC FUNCTIONS

Ganglion-cell photoreceptors send axons to various brain regions involved in NIF visual functions, such as the PLR, circadian photoentrainment, and acute induction of sleep. Melanopsin phototransduction enables ipRGCs to drive these visual behaviors in the absence of functional rods and cones. Conversely, when the melanopsin gene is genetically knocked out in mice, abolishing the intrinsic photosensitivity of ipRGCs, these behaviors are largely, although not completely, preserved (see "Central projections" further in chapter), indicating that rod/cone photoreceptors can also drive these visual functions.[22,34,56,198–200] However, when the ganglion-cell photoreceptors are selectively killed either genetically or pharmacologically, leaving the rest of the retina, including the rods and cones, intact, these NIF behavioral responses to light are largely abolished.[201–204] Thus, ipRGCs are essential for channeling rod/cone-driven light signals to the various NIF visual brain centers, presumably by relaying their synaptic inputs from bipolar and amacrine cells, as described earlier. ipRGCs also make synaptic outputs within the retina and to some brain regions involved in image-forming vision. This section surveys both the intraretinal and extraretinal outputs of these ganglion cells and their functional roles.

Intraretinal output

The first suggestion of a possible intraretinal output of ganglion-cell photoreceptors emerged almost simultaneously with the definitive proof of their existence. Hankins and Lucas [205] reported that light alters the latency of the human cone electroretinogram (ERG) (see Chapter 24) through an intraretinal mechanism driven by a nonclassical opsin (Fig. 26.11 *bottom*). Although their study did not identify that opsin, subsequent work leaves little doubt that it is melanopsin. The spectral tuning, high threshold, and extensive temporal integration of the ERG modulation they reported closely parallel those of the melanopsin-dependent responses of ipRGCs and the behavioral responses they mediate. Related findings in the mouse support a role for melanopsin in the regulation of the ERG, although the nature of that regulation appears somewhat different than in the human eye.[206,207] Chemogenetic stimulation of ipRGCs has been reported to potentiate the photoresponses of conventional RGCs, suggesting that intraretinal signaling by ipRGCs modulates the retinal output.[208]

Another early indication of possible intraretinal outputs of ipRGCs came from the imaging study of Sekaran et al.[51] In retinas of retinally degenerate mice, they detected light-evoked calcium signals in many more cells of the GCL than were melanopsin immunoreactive. Similar findings were reported in a study using photic induction of the immediate early gene *cFos* to identify retinal neurons activated directly or indirectly by ipRGCs in a functionally rodless/coneless mouse.[209] The interpretation of these results has been complicated somewhat by the subsequent evidence that immunohistochemical staining underestimates the number and diversity of ganglion cells expressing melanopsin.[118] However, the prevalence of Fos immunopositive cells in the INL[209] seems greater than can be accounted for by the rare displaced ipRGCs and seems to suggest that some amacrine and/or bipolar cells might receive excitatory input from ipRGCs.

Evidence strongly indicating just such an input has emerged from studies of dopaminergic amacrine (DA) cells. As mentioned previously, ipRGC dendrites costratify with those of DA cells and receive synaptic inputs from them. Studies of the light responses of the dopamine cells suggest that this synaptic input is reciprocated.[210–212] Most DA cells have brisk, relatively transient ON responses to light. These are abolished by the ON bipolar cell blocker L-(+)-2-amino-4-phosphonobutyric acid (L-AP4),[213] indicating that they are driven exclusively by ON bipolar cell input. However, about 20% to 40% of DA cells continue to be excited by light in the presence of L-AP4. These residual responses have all the hallmarks of mediation by melanopsin-expressing ipRGCs: they are sluggish, very sustained

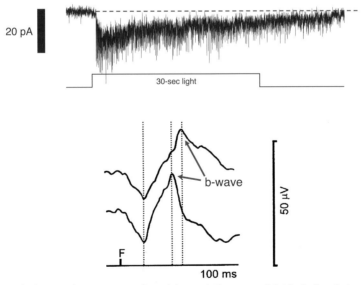

Fig. 26.11 Intraretinal synaptic outputs and modulatory influences of intrinsically photosensitive retinal ganglion cells (ipRGCs). *Top:* Intracellular recording of a dopaminergic amacrine cell made under conditions blocking rod/cone-driven inputs and revealing excitation from ipRGCs. The signatures of melanopsin photo-responses—sustained excitation, slow onset, and poststimulus persistence—are evident. Unlike the intracellular recordings shown in the previous figures, this is a "voltage clamp" recording, which monitors the ionic currents across the cell membrane. Downward deflection indicates that light induces an inward flow of cations into the dopaminergic amacrine cell. The *red dotted line* marks the prestimulus baseline level. *Bottom:* ipRGC signaling to dopaminergic amacrine cells and/or electrically coupled amacrine cells might modulate the image-forming visual system in human. These electroretinograms were recorded from a human subject at night under dark-adapted conditions. The top recording was obtained at 9:00 p.m., showing a b-wave (which arises from ON bipolar cell light responses) with a relatively long latency to peak. A 15-min bright light pulse delivered at 11:00 p.m. accelerated the b-wave recorded at 3:00 a.m. (*bottom*). A plausible explanation for this phenomenon is that the bright light stimulated ipRGCs and consequently ipRGC-driven amacrine cells, elevating the release of dopamine and/or other neuromodulators which then modulated the kinetics of the ON bipolar cell photoresponse. F, Flash. (*Top*, from KY Wong, unpublished; *bottom*, reproduced with permission from Hankins MW, Lucas RJ. The primary visual pathway in humans is regulated according to long-term light exposure through the action of a nonclassical photopigment. *Curr Biol.* 2002;12(3):191–198.)

(Fig. 26.11 *top*), and exhibit the action spectrum of melanopsin-based phototransduction, peaking in sensitivity near 480 nm. The inference that ipRGCs mediate this excitatory influence is further supported by the finding that it can be recorded from about 25% of the DA cells in *rd/rd* mice,[210,211] and light-dependent Fos expression suggests that this percentage increases over the course of aging.[214] This centrifugal transmission of ipRGC signals can potentially regulate the intraretinal release of dopamine. In fact, two studies have shown significant light-evoked retinal dopamine release in retinally degenerate rats lacking virtually all rod and cone photoreceptors,[215,216] and melanopsin deficiency prevents light-evoked dopamine release in mice[217] (but see[218–221]). Because retinal dopamine plays a key role in modulation of retinal physiology by light adaptation and circadian phase, the influence of ipRGCs on DA cells may mediate the centrifugal influences of melanopsin on the ERG discussed earlier. Additionally, in mice lacking melanopsin, clock gene rhythms normally present in the rod/cone layer are absent.[217] These centrifugal influences are mediated at least in part by the intraretinal axon collaterals of M1 ipRGCs, which are branches of the axon that project back to the IPL to terminate on DA cells,[222,223] releasing glutamate in an action potential–dependent manner onto ionotropic glutamate receptors on DA cells[210,222,224–226] (Fig. 26.8 *top*). This is the first known instance in the mammalian retina of a ganglion cell's neurites as the presynaptic element at a chemical synapse, although there is a precedent in catfish.[227]

Gap junctional contacts constitute an additional route by which ipRGCs can influence other retinal neurons. Sekaran et al.[51] argued for just such communication based on their observation that the gap junctional blocker carbenoxylone abolished the light-evoked calcium increase in some neurons in *rd* mice. However, a later paper reported that carbenoxolone blocks the light-evoked calcium rise even in mechanically isolated ipRGCs, suggesting that at least some of the carbenoxolone-sensitive cells in the study of Sekaran et al.

could have been ipRGCs.[228] Nonetheless, at around the same time, gap junction–permeable tracers injected into individual M1–M3 mouse ipRGCs were found to label nearby amacrine cells in the GCL (i.e., displaced amacrine cells), raising the possibility of gap junctional transmission from ipRGCs to some amacrine cells.[113] This possibility was subsequently confirmed in the rat retina, where all spiking, sustained ON displaced amacrine cells were found to remain photosensitive even when rod/cone signaling was pharmacologically blocked. These rod/cone-independent photoresponses had melanopsin-like spectral tuning and kinetics, and could be blocked by the gap junction blocker meclofenamic acid but not by antagonists for chemical synapses.[229] Gap junctional signaling from ipRGCs to displaced amacrine cells has likewise been demonstrated in mouse retinas,[229–231] and could potentially also occur in primate retinas where ipRGC-amacrine tracer coupling has been reported.[134] All six mouse ipRGC types form gap junctions with displaced amacrine cells and with a few conventionally placed amacrine cells.[231,232] M1 and M3 ipRGCs couple mainly with ON/OFF–bistratifying amacrine cells, whereas the other four ipRGC types couple mostly with ON-stratifying ones[231] (Fig. 26.8). Most if not all ipRGC-coupled amacrine cells contain GABA,[113] and some have been found to also accumulate serotonin, or contain nitric oxide synthase, neuropeptide Y,[232] or corticotropin-releasing hormone,[233] although ipRGC-coupled amacrine cells do not contain dopamine[229] or vasoactive intestinal peptide.[232] Thus, gap junctional signaling from ipRGCs to coupled amacrine cells should cause the release of a variety of chemicals, which are likely to exert diverse modulatory effects on retinal function.

Central projections

The axonal projections of melanopsin RGCs have been characterized in greatest detail in rodents[46,47,79,114,118,129,234–238] (Fig. 26.12), although some data are available in primates.[239] Ganglion-cell photoreceptors

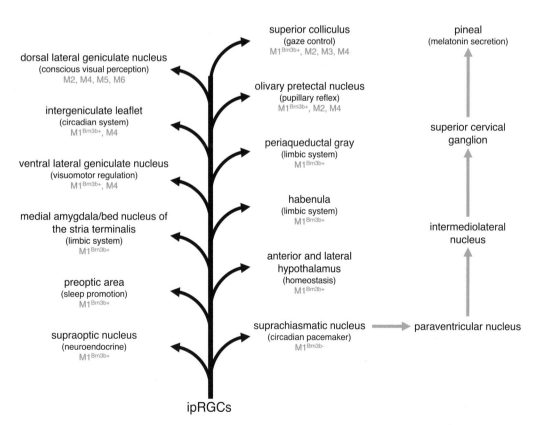

Fig. 26.12 Central projections and possible functional roles of intrinsically photosensitive retinal ganglion cells (*ipRGCs*). The major brain nuclei receiving axonal innervations from melanopsin RGCs are listed in this diagram, with the monosynaptic projections in *black* and the indirect pathway leading to the pineal in *gray*. ipRGC types known to project to a given site are indicated in *blue*.

are believed to influence their postsynaptic targets by releasing L-glutamate, pituitary adenylate cyclase–activating polypeptide (PACAP), or GABA.[48,53,240–242] With the exception of the SCN, almost all central sites that receive ipRGC afferents also receive, to varying degrees, axons from conventional, nonphotosensitive RGCs.[243] The roles of these conventional RGC projections to sites not involved in pattern vision remain to be determined.

The pupillary light reflex

Brn3b-positive M1 ipRGCs project to the shell of the olivary pretectal nucleus (OPN),[47,79,114,115,244] while M2 and M4 ipRGCs project to the core.[114,118,129,234,238] The OPN, a small component of the pretectal region that lies just rostral to the superior colliculus, is an essential link in the polysynaptic circuit driving the PLR. The direct input from ganglion-cell photoreceptors to the OPN is thought to account for the persistence of the PLR when rod and cone contributions are lost either through inherited degeneration, or by genetic or pharmacologic manipulation.[11,12,27,56,245] The properties of this persistent PLR are strikingly concordant with those of the direct light responses of ipRGCs, including a very high intensity threshold, an action spectrum peaking near 480 nm, and a complete loss of the response when the melanopsin gene is deleted.[27,32,56,245] Rods and cones also clearly drive the PLR. Thus, in melanopsin knockout mice with intact rods and cones, the PLR is normal at low or moderate light intensities that are subthreshold for melanopsin activation; it is only at higher intensities ($>10^{11}$ photons/cm^2 per second) that the PLR is incomplete.[56] The outer and inner retinal photoreceptor contributions to the PLR differ in terms of kinetics, as revealed by experiments involving humans and macaques. The time course of the PLR closely mirrors that of the light response in ipRGCs, with rod/cone photoreceptors mediating the fast component and the endogenous phototransduction generating most of the slower component, which outlasts the light stimulus[195,245,246] (Fig. 26.13; see also Box 26.5). When pharmacologic agents were injected into the eye of a macaque to block rod/cone signaling to the inner retina but leaving melanopsin phototransduction intact, only the sluggish component, of the ipRGC light response and of the PLR remained.[245] Thus, the classical photoreceptors mediate brisk pupillary responses to dim and moderate intensities, whereas melanopsin-based phototransduction by ipRGCs drives sluggish pupillary responses to bright light. As noted earlier, ipRGCs receive substantial synaptic inputs from rod and cone circuits and are thus a likely conduit for the influence of classical photoreceptors on the PLR. Indeed, when most ipRGCs are killed by genetic modification, the rod/cone component of the PLR is effectively abolished.[201] Available evidence leaves no doubt that the outer-stratifying type of ipRGCs contributes to the pupillomotor circuit, but leaves open the possibility that inner-stratifying types such as M2 may also contribute.[188,234] See also Chapter 25 for more information on the PLR.

Circadian photoentrainment and photic modulation of the pineal gland

The SCN and the intergeniculate leaflet (IGL), which is a part of the lateral geniculate nucleus of the thalamus, receive the densest projections from ipRGCs.[47] Both of these are components of the circadian visual system. Brn3b-negative M1 ipRGCs constitute around 80% of the retinal innervation to the SCN, with the balance being M2 cell projections.[114,234] In all living organisms, many physiologic processes (e.g., sleep-wake cycles, body temperature, food intake) display daily rhythms that help the organisms cope with predictable environmental change. In mammals, the central pacemaker for these rhythms is the SCN. Clock cells in the SCN have neuronal activities that exhibit intrinsic rhythms with a period of about 24 hours. These rhythms

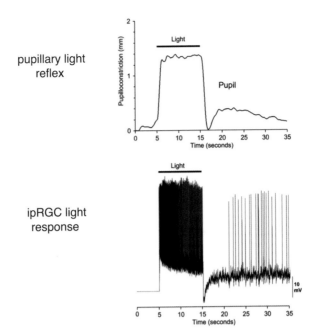

Fig. 26.13 Similarity between the intrinsically photosensitive retinal ganglion cell (*ipRGC*) photoresponse and the pupillary light reflex in macaque. The time course of the macaque pupillary light reflex closely follows that of the ipRGC light response. In both cases, a fast component that is mediated mainly by rods and cones is detected during the light stimulus, whereas a more sluggish, melanopsin-based component is evident after the light is off. This temporal separation of rod/cone- and melanopsin-driven components may allow the pupillary light reflex to serve as a diagnostic test to reveal rod/cone versus ganglion cell defects in patients (see Box 26.5). (Reproduced with permission from Gamlin PD, McDougal DH, Pokorny J, Smith VC, Yau KW, Dacey DM. Human and macaque pupil responses driven by melanopsin-containing retinal ganglion cells. *Vision Res.* 2007;47(7):946–954.)

BOX 26.5 The pupillary light reflex as a diagnostic test

The pupillary light reflex (PLR) has potential utility as a diagnostic tool to differentiate between outer retinal disorders affecting rod or cone circuits and inner retinal diseases affecting ganglion cells.[296] As illustrated in Fig. 26.13, components of the PLR mediated by the rod and cone photoreceptors are temporally separable from those mediated by melanopsin. The earliest component of the light-driven constriction is mediated almost exclusively by rods and/or cones. By contrast, the slowly decaying poststimulus constriction is driven mainly by melanopsin; this presumably reflects the persistent depolarizing afterpotential in intrinsically photosensitive retinal ganglion cells (ipRGCs) that, in turn, is thought to be supported by a slowly depleting pool of photoactivated (meta) melanopsin (see "Melanopsin chromophore and pigment bistability" in the main text). It should also be possible to tease out specific photoreceptor contributions by exploiting differences among them in threshold and saturating intensities and in spectral sensitivity. Red light may be presented under rod-saturating photopic conditions to selectively evoke a cone-driven PLR, whereas bright blue light is most effective for inducing a melanopsin-mediated response that persists beyond stimulus termination. To elicit a response driven mainly by the rods, a dim green light presented under a dark-adapted condition is ideal.[305]

---

are known as circadian rhythms (*circa* = approximately; *dies* = day). During the "subjective night," the SCN coordinates hormonal, physiologic, and behavioral adaptations to the nocturnal environment, and

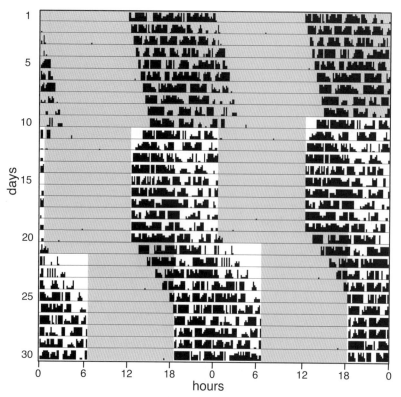

Fig. 26.14 Photoentrainment of a diurnal animal. In this simulated actogram, the locomotor activity of a diurnal animal is plotted as *vertical black bars* for about a month. This diagram is double-plotted, with each row displaying two consecutive 24-hour periods and each 24-hour period plotted twice. During the first 10 days, the animal is kept in constant darkness, allowing its circadian pacemaker to "free run." Because this animal's circadian clock has a period that is slightly longer than 24 hours, its locomotor activity starts slightly later each day, as reflected in the gradual rightward shift of the period of activity. On days 11 through 20, however, a 12-hour light:12-hour dark lighting schedule is presented, and the animal's active period becomes synchronized or "entrained" to the light-dark cycle. On day 21, the light-dark cycle is abruptly delayed by 6 hours, mimicking the consequences of a westward flight that crosses six time zones. It takes the circadian clock several days to re-entrain the animal to this new cycle.

during the "subjective day," it adapts the brain and body to the daytime world. The internal clockworks of the SCN consist of transcription/translation feedback loops of clock genes and their attendant gene products.[247] The period of one molecular cycle is around 24 hours. Because the period is not exactly 24 hours, these rhythms must be reset periodically so that the internal clock remains in phase with the external light/dark cycles. In other words, subjective day (or night) needs to be synchronized, or "entrained," with the environmental light cycle (Fig. 26.14). Such entrainment is accomplished mainly by the phase-shifting effects of light on the SCN and its transcriptional machinery, mediated by its direct input from the retina. If the SCN clock is too fast, subjective night starts too early, so the organism is exposed to environmental light during early subjective night, which delays the clock. On the other hand, if the clock is too slow, subjective night starts and ends too late, so the SCN gets photic input during late subjective night, which advances the clock.[42,44,45,248] The same mechanism is responsible for the recovery from jet let when traveling across time zones. While both classical and ganglion-cell photoreceptors can mediate photoentrainment, all light signals are channeled through ipRGCs.[201–203] These reach the circadian pacemaker through a monosynaptic pathway called the retinohypothalamic tract, and also through an indirect pathway involving the IGL.[249] Because a diurnal organism is typically exposed to daylight for 8 to 16 hours per day but light can phase-shift a misaligned clock only at the transitions between the light and dark phases, it is crucial that the retinal signal to SCN is sustained throughout those 8 to 16 hours so that it is still active near the end of the light phase. Therefore, the persistence of the ipRGC photoresponse is important for entraining diurnal animals like humans. Indeed, ipRGCs can continuously signal light for at least 10 hours,[102] and light responses recorded from the SCN retain the sustained nature of the ipRGC photoresponse.[99,242,250–252] Melanopsin is sufficient for photoentrainment, not only in rodents but also in primates, including humans.[31,32,253] Whereas rods likewise drive

prolonged light responses in ipRGCs[54,102] and can effectively mediate photoentrainment,[200] cones generate transient light responses[54,195] and are therefore less suited for entrainment,[22,196] although they are required for normal circadian phase-shift responses to short light pulses.[254]

The SCN sends several output signals to drive circadian rhythms throughout the organism. One of the primary outputs is a polysynaptic circuit that leads to the pineal gland, which releases the hormone melatonin (Fig. 26.12). Under the influence of the SCN clock, melatonin release is lowest at subjective day and highest at subjective night. This hormone induces a range of physiologic responses throughout the body that are suitable to the nighttime, such as sleepiness for diurnal animals.[255] In addition to entraining the circadian rhythm of melatonin secretion, light can acutely suppress secretion of this molecule during the subjective night. When illuminated at night, melanopsin-deficient *rd1* mice fail to downregulate the transcription of pineal arylalkylamine-*N*-acetyltransferase, the rate-limiting enzyme in the melatonin biosynthetic pathway, indicating the crucial role of ipRGCs.[22] This NIF response to light may be associated with significant adverse health consequences. For example, there is a high correlation between the amount of light exposure at night and the incidence of breast cancer.[256–258] This may be attributable in part to the photic suppression of nocturnal melatonin, which has been shown to exert various oncostatic and antitoxic effects.[259,260] Melatonin suppression by light at night may therefore be one risk factor responsible for the higher incidence of breast cancer in industrialized countries. Thus, it is important to minimize light exposure at subjective night, especially for night shift workers whose subjective night is during the daylight hours. It has been shown that in humans, melatonin release is most effectively suppressed by blue light close to the best wavelength for melanopsin phototransduction.[61,261] Therefore, if exposure to light at subjective night is unavoidable, red light would presumably be less harmful than broad-spectrum light (see also Box 26.6).

BOX 26.6 Inner retinal photoreception, seasonal affective disorder, and sleep in the blind

In seasonal affective disorder (SAD), patients suffer recurring bouts of depression, fatigue, and lethargy in fall and winter, when days are short.[306] Although the etiology of the disease is unknown, several observations, including the effectiveness of phototherapy[307–309] point to a possible defect in nonimage-forming (NIF) photoreception and prolonged periods of nocturnal melatonin release in winter.[310] While bright, white light phototherapy can ameliorate SAD in some patients, low-intensity, narrow-band (~470-nm) blue light treatment centered near melanopsin's peak spectral sensitivity is just as efficacious.[311] A specific missense variant of the melanopsin gene occurs at higher frequency in SAD patients than in healthy control subjects.[312] The functional consequences of this variation for melanopsin-based signaling or the intrinsic photosensitivity of ipRGCs are unknown. Additionally, SAD patients demonstrate a reduced melanopsin-driven pupillary response in the winter compared with healthy controls.[313] Together these data suggest that a melanopsin subsensitivity to low wintertime environmental light conditions may trigger SAD in some patients.

Some blind people retain inner retinal photosensitivity and hence NIF visual functions despite the total loss of functional rods and cones[30–32]; others suffer more serious retinal degenerations and do not have any capacity to support NIF vision. One of the major problems experienced by this latter group is their complete lack of photoentrainment, causing their sleep-wake cycle to be uncoupled from the solar cycle. An often-effective treatment is the daily administration of melatonin, to mimic the suprachiasmatic nucleus output signal that normally occurs once every 24 hours in properly entrained sighted individuals.[295,314] Tasimelteon, a melatonin receptor agonist, has also been shown to help blind individuals entrain their circadian rhythms to the prevailing day:night cycle, although continued treatment is necessary to maintain these improvements in quality of life.[315,316]

Acute regulation of sleep and activity

The daily sleep-wake cycle is controlled by the interaction of a homeostatic drive—the accrual of sleep debt after prolonged wakefulness—and the circadian clock.[262] Sleep is also acutely impacted by light. In humans, light disrupts sleep and is alerting,[263] but in nocturnal rodents, light induces sleep.[264,265] These effects of light are independent of the SCN and, accordingly, are mediated by Brn3b-positive M1 ipRGCs that project to the preoptic area (POA), a brain region containing nuclei implicated in the regulation of sleep.[79,235,266,267] It has been proposed that these target cells in the POA send inhibitory projections to the tuberomammillary nucleus, lateral hypothalamus, ventral tegmental area, and raphe nucleus, which are known wakefulness-promoting sites.[267] It should be noted that the phenomenon of "negative masking," that is, the acute photic suppression of wheel-running activity in nocturnal rodents, is now known to be a photic induction of sleep and an attendant drop in body temperature rather than a direct inhibition of the circuitry driving activity in animals that remain awake[264,268] (reviewed in[269]).

Lateral habenula and modulation of mood

Light has been shown to modulate mood, and ipRGCs are now known to mediate this effect. For example, mice maintained in an ultradian (i.e., very short) light:dark cycle show an increased level of corticosterone, impaired learning, and depression-like behaviors.[270,271] However, animals whose ipRGCs have been ablated are resistant to these experimentally induced deficits in cognition and mood. Additionally, housing mice in constant light[272] or interrupting their night with a 2-hour block of light[273] also can induce depression-like behavior. However, this light-induced disruption of euthymic mood appears independent of light-driven induction of sleep.[271] These profound effects of light on mood are routed through a projection from Brn3b-positive M1 ipRGCs to neurons in the perihabenular nucleus,[271,273] which in turn project to the nucleus accumbens,[273] a region implicated in mood control and depression.[274] An alternate, indirect M1 ipRGC projection relays in the ventral lateral geniculate and intergeniculate leaflet prior to extending to the perihabenula.[275]

Besides depressive symptoms, light can enhance fear and lead to anxiety-like behaviors.[276,277] Chemogenetic activation of ipRGCs is sufficient to mimic such behaviors in mice.[277] In addition to the habenula, several other mood-related central structures receive direct input from ipRGCs, including the amygdala, lateral hypothalamus, bed nucleus of the stria terminalis, and periaqueductal gray[79] (reviewed in[278]). The roles of these sites in the photic regulation of mood and the types of ipRGCs that innervate them remain to be established.

Lateral geniculate nucleus, superior colliculus, and conscious light perception

ipRGCs have been implicated increasingly in playing a role in pattern vision (reviewed in[279]). In primates and rodents, melanopsin RGCs make substantial projections to the dorsal lateral geniculate nucleus (dLGN), the thalamic relay of retinal signals in the image-forming visual pathway[54,118] (see Chapter 29). A blind woman evidently lacking functional rods and cones reported conscious perception of light, with peak sensitivity near 480 nm, as expected for a melanopsin-based mechanism.[32] Thus, whereas the sluggish light responses and large dendritic fields of ipRGCs make them ill-suited for the analysis of fine details or motion in the retinal image, they may nevertheless contribute to conscious appreciation of ambient illumination, presumably through their projection to the dLGN.

In mice, non-M1 ipRGCs appear critical for normal contrast sensitivity as genetic ablation of these cells results in a deficit in contrast sensitivity, a phenotype consistent with the projection of several non-M1 ipRGC types to the dLGN.[112,123] In fact, contrast sensitivity is substantially reduced even when only melanopsin is eliminated, with rod/cone input to ipRGCs left intact.[123,194] The unique phototransduction pathway of M4 cells allows their relatively weak intrinsic photoresponse to close potassium leak channels (Fig. 26.2 *top*), thereby increasing their excitability and, consequently, the contrast sensitivity of these cells.[98]

The contribution of ipRGCs to color vision remains an area of debate. Some effects of color vision attributed to melanopsin may, in fact, be mediated by cones.[83] Nevertheless, synaptic input to ipRGCs in primates is color-opponent.[54] Thus, it is conceivable that ipRGCs contribute in some way to conscious discrimination of color. In mice, M5 cells also demonstrate color opponency[130] and murine color-opponent processes have been mapped to the dLGN,[280] a target of M5 cells.[130] Interestingly, the potential involvement of ipRGCs in color vision may provide an algorithm for encoding time-of-day as the different chromatic characteristics of twilight versus midday vary in a reliably predictable diurnal manner.[168]

There are also weak projections from ipRGCs to the superior colliculus (SC),[79] a midbrain center involved in redirecting gaze to visual targets and, in rodents, predatory hunting and defensive responses.[281] M1–M4 cells are tuned to different speeds of stimuli traversing the visual field, and these four ipRGC types project to the SC, suggesting a role for these cells in the tracking of moving objects.[116]

DEVELOPMENT

Studies in rodents clearly demonstrate that ipRGCs are the first photoreceptors to become fully functional in the developing retina.[52,282,283] This is likely to be true also in the human eye, as melanopsin is expressed in human fetuses by 9 weeks postconception,[284] many weeks before the appearance of rod and cone opsins.[285,286] There is evidence that sufficient environmental light can reach the fetal mouse eye to stimulate melanopsin phototransduction, activating an intraretinal signaling pathway that reduces the number of retinal neurons, suppresses hypoxia, and consequently restricts the growth of the retinal vasculature.[287] In neonatal mice, spontaneous spiking events called retinal waves propagate through the retina to help refine RGC projections to central targets.[288] Between postnatal days 4 and 7, when rods and cones are not yet light sensitive in mice,[289] photostimulation of melanopsin in ipRGCs prolongs spiking in the retinal waves and enhances the segregation of left-eye and right-eye RGC inputs in the dLGN.[290] Melanopsin-based photoreception in the neonatal mouse retina also regulates retinal development. Specifically, ablation of ipRGCs or dark rearing has been found to cause the mislocalization of cone photoreceptors, and this effect appears to be mediated by ipRGC signaling to DA cells[291] (see also "Intraretinal output" previously).

REFERENCES

1. Polyak SL. In: Klüver H, ed. *The Vertebrate Visual System; Its Origin, Structure, and Function and its Manifestations in Disease with an Analysis of its Role in the Life of Animals and in the Origin of Man, Preceded by a Historical Review of Investigations of the Eye, and of the Visual Pathways and Centers of the Brain*. Chicago, IL: University of Chicago Press; 1957.
2. Finger S. *Origins of Neuroscience: A History of Explorations Into Brain Function*. New York, NY: Oxford University Press; 2001.
3. Wade NJ. Visual neuroscience before the neuron. *Perception*. 2004;33(7):869–889.
4. Treviranus GR. *Beiträge zur Aufklärung der Erscheinungen und Gesetze des organischen Lebens. Volume 1, issue 1. Ueber die blättige Textur der Crystalllinse des Auges als Grund des Vermögens, einerlei Gegenstand in verschiedener Entfernung deutlich zu sehen, und über den innern Bau der Retina*. Bremen: Heyse; 1835.
5. Bidder F. Zur Anatomie der Retina, insbesondere zur Würdigung der stabförmigen Körper in derselben. *Archiv für Anatomie, Physiologie und wissenschaftliche Medicin*. 1839:371–384.
6. Bowman W. *Lectures on the Parts Concerned in the Operations on the Eye, and on the Structure of the Retina, Delivered at the Royal London Ophthalmic Hospital, Moorfields, June 1847. To Which Are Added, a Paper on the Vitreous Humor; and also a Few Cases of Ophthalmic Disease*. London, United Kingdom: Longman, Brown, Green and Longmans; 1849.
7. Helmholtz H. Beschreibung eines Augenspiegels zur Untersuchung der Netz haut im lebenden Auge. *Arch Physiol Heilk*. 1851;11:827–830.
8. Boll F. On the anatomy and physiology of the retina. *Vision Res*. 1977;17(11–12):1249–1265.
9. Pittler SJ, Keeler CE, Sidman RL, Baehr W. PCR analysis of DNA from 70-year-old sections of rodless retina demonstrates identity with the mouse rd defect. *Proc Natl Acad Sci U S A*. 1993;90(20):9616–9619.
10. Chang B, Hawes NL, Hurd RE, Davisson MT, Nusinowitz S, Heckenlively JR. Retinal degeneration mutants in the mouse. *Vision Res*. 2002;42(4):517–525.
11. Keeler CE. Iris movements in blind mice. *Am J Physiol*. 1927;81:107–112.
12. Keeler CE. Blind mice. *J Exp Zool*. 1928;51(4):495–508.
13. Dräger UC, Hubel DH. Studies of visual function and its decay in mice with hereditary retinal degeneration. *J Comp Neurol*. 1978;180(1):85–114.
14. Foster RG, Provencio I, Hudson D, Fiske S, De Grip W, Menaker M. Circadian photoreception in the retinally degenerate mouse (rd/rd). *J Comp Physiol*. 1991;169(1):39–50.
15. Hopkins AE. Vision and retinal structure in mice. *Proc Natl Acad Sci U S A*. 1927;13(7):488–492.
16. Karli P. Étude de la valeur fonctionnelle d'une rétine dépourvue de cellules visuelles photo-réceptrices. *Arch Sci Physiol (Paris)*. 1954;8:305–327.
17. Bovet D, Bovet-Nitti F, Oliverio A. Genetic aspects of learning and memory in mice. *Science*. 1969;163(863):139–149.
18. Dunn J, Dryer R, Bennett M. Diurnal variation in plasma corticosterone following long term exposure to continuous illumination. *Endocrinology*. 1972;90(6):1660–1663.
19. Ebihara S, Tsuji K. Entrainment of the circadian activity rhythm to the light cycle: effective light intensity for a Zeitgeber in the retinal degenerate C3H mouse and the normal C57BL mouse. *Physiol Behav*. 1980;24(3):523–527.
20. Goto M, Ebihara S. The influence of different light intensities on pineal melatonin content in the retinal degenerate C3H mouse and the normal CBA mouse. *Neurosci Lett*. 1990;108(3):267–272.
21. Carter-Dawson LD, LaVail MM, Sidman RL. Differential effect of the rd mutation on rods and cones in the mouse retina. *Invest Ophthalmol Vis Sci*. 1978;17(6):489–498.
22. Panda S, Provencio I, Tu DC, et al. Melanopsin is required for non-image-forming photic responses in blind mice. *Science*. 2003;301(5632):525–527.
23. Colwell CS, Foster RG. Photic regulation of Fos-like immunoreactivity in the suprachiasmatic nucleus of the mouse. *J Comp Neurol*. 1992;324(2):135–142.
24. Provencio I, Wong S, Lederman AB, Argamaso SM, Foster RG. Visual and circadian responses to light in aged retinally degenerate mice. *Vision Res*. 1994;34(14):1799–1806.
25. Freedman MS, Lucas RJ, Soni B, et al. Regulation of mammalian circadian behavior by non-rod, non-cone, ocular photoreceptors. *Science*. 1999;284(5413):502–504.
26. Lucas RJ, Freedman MS, Munoz M, Garcia-Fernandez JM, Foster RG. Regulation of the mammalian pineal by non-rod, non-cone, ocular photoreceptors. *Science*. 1999;284(5413):505–507.
27. Lucas RJ, Douglas RH, Foster RG. Characterization of an ocular photopigment capable of driving pupillary constriction in mice. *Nat Neurosci*. 2001;4(6):621–626.
28. Mrosovsky N, Lucas RJ, Foster RG. Persistence of masking responses to light in mice lacking rods and cones. *J Biol Rhythms*. 2001;16(6):585–588.
29. Foster RG. Keeping an eye on the time: the Cogan Lecture. *Invest Ophthalmol Vis Sci*. 2002;43(5):1286–1298.
30. Czeisler CA, Shanahan TL, Klerman EB, et al. Suppression of melatonin secretion in some blind patients by exposure to bright light. *N Engl J Med*. 1995;332(1):6–11.
31. Klerman EB, Shanahan TL, Brotman DJ, et al. Photic resetting of the human circadian pacemaker in the absence of conscious vision. *J Biol Rhythms*. 2002;17(6):548–555.
32. Zaidi FH, Hull JT, Peirson SN, et al. Short-wavelength light sensitivity of circadian, pupillary, and visual awareness in humans lacking an outer retina. *Curr Biol*. 2007;17(24):2122–2128.
33. Yoshimura T, Ebihara S. Spectral sensitivity of photoreceptors mediating phase-shifts of circadian rhythms in retinally degenerate CBA/J (rd/rd) and normal CBA/N (+/+)mice. *J Comp Physiol*. 1996;178(6):797–802.
34. Hattar S, Lucas RJ, Mrosovsky N, et al. Melanopsin and rod-cone photoreceptive systems account for all major accessory visual functions in mice. *Nature*. 2003;424(6944):76–81.
35. Berson DM. Strange vision: ganglion cells as circadian photoreceptors. *Trends Neurosci*. 2003;26(6):314–320.
36. Van Gelder RN. Making (a) sense of non-visual ocular photoreception. *Trends Neurosci*. 2003;26(9):458–461.
37. Fu Y, Liao HW, Do MT, Yau KW. Non-image-forming ocular photoreception in vertebrates. *Curr Opin Neurobiol*. 2005;15(4):415–422.
38. Provencio I. Melanopsin cells. In: Masland RH, Albright TD, editors. The Senses: A Comprehensive Reference, Vol 1, Vision I. San Diego, CA: Academic Press; 2008.
39. Provencio I, Jiang G, De Grip WJ, Hayes WP, Rollag MD. Melanopsin: An opsin in melanophores, brain, and eye. *Proc Natl Acad Sci U S A*. 1998;95(1):340–345.
40. Provencio I, Rodriguez IR, Jiang G, Hayes WP, Moreira EF, Rollag MD. A novel human opsin in the inner retina. *J Neurosci*. 2000;20(2):600–605.
41. Sancar A. Regulation of the mammalian circadian clock by cryptochrome. *J Biol Chem*. 2004;279(33):34079–34082.
42. Klein DC, Moore RY, Reppert SM. *Suprachiasmatic Nucleus: The Mind's Clock*. New York, NY: Oxford University Press; 1991:230.
43. van Esseveldt KE, Lehman MN, Boer GJ. The suprachiasmatic nucleus and the circadian time-keeping system revisited. Brain Res. *Brain Res Rev*. 2000;33(1):34–77.
44. DeCoursey PJ. Functional organization of circadian systems in multicellular animals. In: Dunlap JC, Loros JL, DeCoursey PJ, eds. *Chronobiology*. Sunderland, MA: Sinauer Assoc., Inc; 2004:145–178.
45. Hastings MH, Herzog ED. Clock genes, oscillators, and cellular networks in the suprachiasmatic nuclei. *J Biol Rhythms*. 2004;19(5):400–413.
46. Gooley JJ, Lu J, Chou TC, Scammell TE, Saper CB. Melanopsin in cells of origin of the retinohypothalamic tract. *Nat Neurosci*. 2001;4(12):1165.
47. Hattar S, Liao HW, Takao M, Berson DM, Yau KW. Melanopsin-containing retinal ganglion cells: architecture, projections, and intrinsic photosensitivity. *Science*. 2002;295(5557):1065–1070.
48. Hannibal J, Hindersson P, Knudsen SM, Georg B, Fahrenkrug J. The photopigment melanopsin is exclusively present in pituitary adenylate cyclase-activating polypeptide-containing retinal ganglion cells of the retinohypothalamic tract. *J Neurosci*. 2002;22(1):RC191.
49. Berson DM, Dunn FA, Takao M. Phototransduction by retinal ganglion cells that set the circadian clock. *Science*. 2002;295(5557):1070–1073.
50. Warren EJ, Allen CN, Brown RL, Robinson DW. Intrinsic light responses of retinal ganglion cells projecting to the circadian system. *Eur J Neurosci*. 2003;17(9):1727–1735.
51. Sekaran S, Foster RG, Lucas RJ, Hankins MW. Calcium imaging reveals a network of intrinsically light-sensitive inner-retinal neurons. *Curr Biol*. 2003;13(15):1290–1298.
52. Tu DC, Zhang D, Demas J, et al. Physiologic diversity and development of intrinsically photosensitive retinal ganglion cells. *Neuron*. 2005;48(6):987–999.
53. Hannibal J, Hindersson P, Ostergaard J, et al. Melanopsin is expressed in PACAP-containing retinal ganglion cells of the human retinohypothalamic tract. *Invest Ophthalmol Vis Sci*. 2004;45(11):4202–4209.
54. Dacey DM, Liao HW, Peterson BB, et al. Melanopsin-expressing ganglion cells in primate retina signal colour and irradiance and project to the LGN. *Nature*. 2005;433(7027):749–754.
55. Provencio I, Rollag MD, Castrucci AM. Photoreceptive net in the mammalian retina. This mesh of cells may explain how some blind mice can still tell day from night. *Nature*. 2002;415(6871):493.
56. Lucas RJ, Hattar S, Takao M, Berson DM, Foster RG, Yau KW. Diminished pupillary light reflex at high irradiances in melanopsin-knockout mice. *Science*. 2003;299(5604):245–247.
57. Newman LA, Walker MT, Brown RL, Cronin TW, Robinson PR. Melanopsin forms a functional short-wavelength photopigment. *Biochemistry*. 2003;42(44):12734–12738.
58. Melyan Z, Tarttelin EE, Bellingham J, Lucas RJ, Hankins MW. Addition of human melanopsin renders mammalian cells photoresponsive. *Nature*. 2005;433(7027):741–745.
59. Panda S, Nayak SK, Campo B, Walker JR, Hogenesch JB, Jegla T. Illumination of the melanopsin signaling pathway. *Science*. 2005;307(5709):600–604.

60. Qiu X, Kumbalasiri T, Carlson SM, et al. Induction of photosensitivity by heterologous expression of melanopsin. *Nature.* 2005;433(7027):745–749.
61. Brainard GC, Hanifin JP, Greeson JM, et al. Action spectrum for melatonin regulation in humans: evidence for a novel circadian photoreceptor. *J Neurosci.* 2001;21(16):6405–6412.
62. Koyanagi M, Kubokawa K, Tsukamoto H, Shichida Y, Terakita A. Cephalochordate melanopsin: evolutionary linkage between invertebrate visual cells and vertebrate photosensitive retinal ganglion cells. *Curr Biol.* 2005;15(11):1065–1069.
63. Torii M, Kojima D, Okano T, et al. Two isoforms of chicken melanopsins show blue light sensitivity. *FEBS Lett.* 2007;581(27):5327–5331.
64. Walker MT, Brown RL, Cronin TW, Robinson PR. Photochemistry of retinal chromophore in mouse melanopsin. *Proc Natl Acad Sci U S A.* 2008;105(26):8861–8865.
65. Bailes HJ, Lucas RJ. Human melanopsin forms a pigment maximally sensitive to blue light (lambdamax approximately 479 nm) supporting activation of G(q/11) and G(i/o) signalling cascades. *Proc Biol Sci.* 2013;280(1759):20122987.
66. Hillman P, Hochstein S, Minke B. Transduction in invertebrate photoreceptors: role of pigment bistability. *Physiol Rev.* 1983;63(2):668–772.
67. Fu Y, Zhong H, Wang MH, et al. Intrinsically photosensitive retinal ganglion cells detect light with a vitamin A-based photopigment, melanopsin. *Proc Natl Acad Sci U S A.* 2005;102(29):10339–10344.
68. Matsuyama T, Yamashita T, Imamoto Y, Shichida Y. Photochemical properties of mammalian melanopsin. *Biochemistry.* 2012;51(27):5454–5462.
69. Tu DC, Owens LA, Anderson L, et al. Inner retinal photoreception independent of the visual retinoid cycle. *Proc Natl Acad Sci U S A.* 2006;103(27):10426–10431.
70. Mure LS, Rieux C, Hattar S, Cooper HM. Melanopsin-dependent nonvisual responses: evidence for photopigment bistability in vivo. *J Biol Rhythms.* 2007;22(5):411–424.
71. Qiu X, Berson DM. Melanopsin bistability in ganglion-cell photoreceptors. *Invest Ophthalmol Vis Sci.* 2007;48:612 E-Abstract.
72. Emanuel AJ, Do MT. Melanopsin tristability for sustained and broadband phototransduction. *Neuron.* 2015;85(5):1043–1055.
73. Mawad K, Van Gelder RN. Absence of long-wavelength photic potentiation of murine intrinsically photosensitive retinal ganglion cell firing in vitro. *J Biol Rhythms.* 2008;23(5):387–391.
74. Sexton TJ, Golczak M, Palczewski K, Van Gelder RN. Melanopsin is highly resistant to light and chemical bleaching in vivo. *J Biol Chem.* 2012;287(25):20888–20897.
75. Doyle SE, Castrucci AM, McCall M, Provencio I, Menaker M. Nonvisual light responses in the Rpe65 knockout mouse: rod loss restores sensitivity to the melanopsin system. *Proc Natl Acad Sci U S A.* 2006;103(27):10432–10437.
76. Zhao X, Pack W, Khan NW, Wong KY. Prolonged inner retinal photoreception depends on the visual retinoid cycle. *J Neurosci.* 2016;36(15):4209–4217.
77. Wang X, Wang T, Jiao Y, von Lintig J, Montell C. Requirement for an enzymatic visual cycle in Drosophila. *Curr Biol.* 2010;20(2):93–102.
78. Harrison KR, Reifler AN, Chervenak AP, Wong KY. Prolonged melanopsin-based photoresponses depend in part on RPE65 and cellular retinaldehyde-binding protein (CRALBP). *Curr Eye Res.* 2021;46(4):515–523.
79. Hattar S, Kumar M, Park A, et al. Central projections of melanopsin-expressing retinal ganglion cells in the mouse. *J Comp Neurol.* 2006;497(3):326–349.
80. Brown TM, Gias C, Hatori M, et al. Melanopsin contributions to irradiance coding in the thalamo-cortical visual system. *PLoS Biol.* 2010;8(12):e1000558.
81. Procyk CA, Eleftheriou CG, Storchi R, et al. Spatial receptive fields in the retina and dorsal lateral geniculate nucleus of mice lacking rods and cones. *J Neurophysiol.* 2015;114(2):1321–1330.
82. Horiguchi H, Winawer J, Dougherty RF, Wandell BA. Human trichromacy revisited. *Proc Natl Acad Sci U S A.* 2013;110(3):E260–E269.
83. Spitschan M, Aguirre GK, Brainard DH. Selective stimulation of penumbral cones reveals perception in the shadow of retinal blood vessels. *PLoS One.* 2015;10(4):e0124328.
84. Zele AJ, Feigl B, Adhikari P, Maynard ML, Cao D. Melanopsin photoreception contributes to human visual detection, temporal and colour processing. *Sci Rep.* 2018;8(1):3842.
85. Yau KW, Hardie RC. Phototransduction motifs and variations. *Cell.* 2009;139(2):246–264.
86. Koyanagi M, Terakita A. Gq-coupled rhodopsin subfamily composed of invertebrate visual pigment and melanopsin. Photochem Photobiol. 2008;84(4):1024–1030.
87. Hardie RC, Raghu P. Visual transduction in Drosophila. *Nature.* 2001;413(6852):186–193.
88. Hardie RC. A brief history of trp: commentary and personal perspective. *Pflugers Arch.* 2011;461(5):493–498.
89. Isoldi MC, Rollag MD, Castrucci AM, Provencio I. Rhabdomeric phototransduction initiated by the vertebrate photopigment melanopsin. *Proc Natl Acad Sci U S A.* 2005;102(4):1217–1221.
90. Graham DM, Wong KY, Shapiro P, Frederick C, Pattabiraman K, Berson DM. Melanopsin ganglion cells use a membrane-associated rhabdomeric phototransduction cascade. *J Neurophysiol.* 2008;99(5):2522–2532.
91. Hartwick AT, Bramley JR, Yu J, et al. Light-evoked calcium responses of isolated melanopsin-expressing retinal ganglion cells. *J Neurosci.* 2007;27(49):13468–13480.
92. Perez-Leighton CE, Schmidt TM, Abramowitz J, Birnbaumer L, Kofuji P. Intrinsic phototransduction persists in melanopsin-expressing ganglion cells lacking diacylglycerol-sensitive TRPC subunits. *Eur J Neurosci.* 2011;33(5):856–867.
93. Warren EJ, Allen CN, Brown RL, Robinson DW. The light-activated signaling pathway in SCN-projecting rat retinal ganglion cells. *Eur J Neurosci.* 2006;23(9):2477–2487.
94. Xue T, Do MT, Riccio A, et al. Melanopsin signalling in mammalian iris and retina. *Nature.* 2011;479(7371):67–73.
95. Pires SS, Hughes S, Turton M, et al. Differential expression of two distinct functional isoforms of melanopsin (Opn4) in the mammalian retina. J *Neurosci.* 2009;29(39):12332–12342.
96. Contreras E, Nobleman AP, Robinson PR, Schmidt TM. Melanopsin phototransduction: beyond canonical cascades. *J Exp Biol.* 2021;224(23).
97. Jiang Z, Yue WWS, Chen L, Sheng Y, Yau KW. Cyclic-nucleotide- and HCN-channel-Mediated phototransduction in intrinsically photosensitive retinal ganglion cells. *Cell.* 2018;175(3):652–664. e12.
98. Sonoda T, Lee SK, Birnbaumer L, Schmidt TM. Melanopsin phototransduction is repurposed by ipRGC subtypes to shape the function of distinct visual circuits. *Neuron.* 2018;99(4):754–767. e4.
99. Wong KY, Dunn FA, Graham DM, Berson DM. Synaptic influences on rat ganglion-cell photoreceptors. *J Physiol.* 2007;582(Pt 1):279–296.
100. Weng S, Estevez ME, Berson DM. Mouse ganglion-cell photoreceptors are driven by the most sensitive rod pathway and by both types of cones. *PLoS One.* 2013;8(6):e66480.
101. Do MT, Kang SH, Xue T, et al. Photon capture and signalling by melanopsin retinal ganglion cells. *Nature.* 2008
102. Wong KY. A retinal ganglion cell that can signal irradiance continuously for 10 hours. *J Neurosci.* 2012;32(33):11478–11485.
103. Mure LS, Hatori M, Zhu Q, et al. Melanopsin-encoded response properties of intrinsically photosensitive retinal ganglion cells. *Neuron.* 2016;90(5):1016–1027.
104. Wong KY, Dunn FA, Berson DM. Photoreceptor adaptation in intrinsically photosensitive retinal ganglion cells. *Neuron.* 2005;48(6):1001–1010.
105. Do MT, Yau KW. Adaptation to steady light by intrinsically photosensitive retinal ganglion cells. *Proc Natl Acad Sci U S A.* 2013;110(18):7470–7475.
106. Hannibal J, Vrang N, Card JP, Fahrenkrug J. Light-dependent induction of cFos during subjective day and night in PACAP-containing ganglion cells of the retinohypothalamic tract. *J Biol Rhythms.* 2001;16(5):457–470.
107. Cameron EG, Robinson PR. beta-Arrestin-dependent deactivation of mouse melanopsin. *PLoS One.* 2014;9(11):e113138.
108. Zhao X, Reifler AN, Schroeder MM, Jaeckel ER, Chervenak AP, Wong KY. Mechanisms creating transient and sustained photoresponses in mammalian retinal ganglion cells. *J Gen Physiol.* 2017;149(3):335–353.
109. Sondereker KB, Stabio ME, Renna JM. Crosstalk: The diversity of melanopsin ganglion cell types has begun to challenge the canonical divide between image-forming and non-image-forming vision. *J Comp Neurol.* 2020;528(12):2044–2067.
110. Berson DM, Castrucci AM, Provencio I. Morphology and mosaics of melanopsin-expressing retinal ganglion cell types in mice. *J Comp Neurol.* 2010;518(13):2405–2422.
111. Schmidt TM, Kofuji P. Functional and morphological differences among intrinsically photosensitive retinal ganglion cells. *J Neurosci.* 2009;29(2):476–482.
112. Estevez ME, Fogerson PM, Ilardi MC, et al. Form and function of the M4 cell, an intrinsically photosensitive retinal ganglion cell type contributing to geniculocortical vision. *J Neurosci.* 2012;32(39):13608–13620.
113. Muller LP, Do MT, Yau KW, He S, Baldridge WH. Tracer coupling of intrinsically photosensitive retinal ganglion cells to amacrine cells in the mouse retina. *J Comp Neurol.* 2010;518(23):4813–4824.
114. Chen SK, Badea TC, Hattar S. Photoentrainment and pupillary light reflex are mediated by distinct populations of ipRGCs. *Nature.* 2011;476(7358):92–95.
115. Jain V, Ravindran E, Dhingra NK. Differential expression of Brn3 transcription factors in intrinsically photosensitive retinal ganglion cells in mouse. *J Comp Neurol.* 2012;520(4): 742–755.
116. Zhao X, Stafford BK, Godin AL, King WM, Wong KY. Photoresponse diversity among the five types of intrinsically photosensitive retinal ganglion cells. *J Physiol.* 2014;592(7): 1619–1636.
117. Lee SK, Sonoda T, Schmidt TM. M1 Intrinsically photosensitive retinal ganglion cells integrate rod and melanopsin inputs to signal in low light. *Cell Rep.* 2019;29(11):3349–3355. e2.
118. Ecker JL, Dumitrescu ON, Wong KY, et al. Melanopsin-expressing retinal ganglion-cell photoreceptors: cellular diversity and role in pattern vision. *Neuron.* 2010;67(1):49–60.
119. Milner ES, Do MTH. A population representation of absolute light intensity in the mammalian retina. *Cell.* 2017;171(4):865–876. e16.
120. Schmidt TM, Kofuji P. Differential cone pathway influence on intrinsically photosensitive retinal ganglion cell subtypes. *J Neurosci.* 2010;30(48):16262–16271.
121. Schmidt TM, Kofuji P. Structure and function of bistratified intrinsically photosensitive retinal ganglion cells in the mouse. *J Comp Neurol.* 2011;519(8):1492–1504.
122. Viney TJ, Balint K, Hillier D, et al. Local retinal circuits of melanopsin-containing ganglion cells identified by transsynaptic viral tracing. *Curr Biol.* 2007;17(11):981–988.
123. Schmidt TM, Alam NM, Chen S, et al. A role for melanopsin in alpha retinal ganglion cells and contrast detection. *Neuron.* 2014;82(4):781–788.
124. Sun W, Li N, He S. Large-scale morphological survey of mouse retinal ganglion cells. *J Comp Neurol.* 2002;451(2):115–126.
125. Kong JH, Fish DR, Rockhill RL, Masland RH. Diversity of ganglion cells in the mouse retina: unsupervised morphological classification and its limits. *J Comp Neurol.* 2005; 489(3):293–310.
126. Coombs J, van der List D, Wang GY, Chalupa LM. Morphological properties of mouse retinal ganglion cells. *Neuroscience.* 2006;140(1):123–136.
127. Sonoda T, Okabe Y, Schmidt TM. Overlapping morphological and functional properties between M4 and M5 intrinsically photosensitive retinal ganglion cells. *J Comp Neurol.* 2020;528(6):1028–1040.
128. Gao J, Griner EM, Liu M, Moy J, Provencio I, Liu X. Differential effects of experimental glaucoma on intrinsically photosensitive retinal ganglion cells in mice. *J Comp Neurol.* 2022;530(9):1494-1506.
129. Quattrochi LE, Stabio ME, Kim I, et al. The M6 cell: A small-field bistratified photosensitive retinal ganglion cell. *J Comp Neurol.* 2019;527(1):297–311.
130. Stabio ME, Sabbah S, Quattrochi LE, et al. The M5 cell: A color-opponent intrinsically photosensitive retinal ganglion cell. *Neuron.* 2018;97(1):150–163. e4.
131. Hu C, Hill DD, Wong KY. Intrinsic physiological properties of the five types of mouse ganglion-cell photoreceptors. *J Neurophysiol.* 2013;109(7):1876–1889.
131a. Reifler AN, Wong KY. Adeno-associated virus (AAV)-mediated Cre recombinase expression in melanopsin ganglion cells without leaky expression in rod/cone photoreceptors. *J Neurosci Methods.* 2023;384:109762.
132. Stinchcombe AR, Hu C, Walch OJ, Faught SD, Wong KY, Forger DB. M1-type, but not M4-type, melanopsin ganglion cells are physiologically tuned to the central circadian clock. *Front Neurosci.* 2021;15:652996.

133. Hannibal J, Christiansen AT, Heegaard S, Fahrenkrug J, Kiilgaard JF. Melanopsin expressing human retinal ganglion cells: Subtypes, distribution, and intraretinal connectivity. *J Comp Neurol.* 2017;525(8):1934–1961.

134. Liao HW, Ren X, Peterson BB, et al. Melanopsin-expressing ganglion cells on macaque and human retinas form two morphologically distinct populations. *J Comp Neurol.* 2016;524(14):2845–2872.

135. Nasir-Ahmad S, Lee SCS, Martin PR, Grunert U. Melanopsin-expressing ganglion cells in human retina: Morphology, distribution, and synaptic connections. *J Comp Neurol.* 2019;527(1):312–327.

136. Mure LS, Vinberg F, Hanneken A, Panda S. Functional diversity of human intrinsically photosensitive retinal ganglion cells. *Science.* 2019;366(6470):1251–1255.

137. Reifler AN, Chervenak AP, Dolikian ME, et al. The rat retina has five types of ganglion-cell photoreceptors. *Exp Eye Res.* 2015;130:17–28.

138. Esquiva G, Lax P, Cuenca N. Impairment of intrinsically photosensitive retinal ganglion cells associated with late stages of retinal degeneration. *Invest Ophthalmol Vis Sci.* 2013; 54(7):4605–4618.

139. Walch OJ, Zhang LS, Reifler AN, Dolikian ME, Forger DB, Wong KY. Characterizing and modeling the intrinsic light response of rat ganglion-cell photoreceptors. *J Neurophysiol.* 2015;114(5):2955–2966.

140. Jusuf PR, Lee SC, Hannibal J, Grunert U. Characterization and synaptic connectivity of melanopsin-containing ganglion cells in the primate retina. *Eur J Neurosci.* 2007;26(10): 2906–2921.

141. Neumann S, Haverkamp S, Auferkorte ON. Intrinsically photosensitive ganglion cells of the primate retina express distinct combinations of inhibitory neurotransmitter receptors. *Neuroscience.* 2011;199:24–31.

142. Johnson EN, Westbrook T, Shayesteh R, et al. Distribution and diversity of intrinsically photosensitive retinal ganglion cells in tree shrew. *J Comp Neurol.* 2019;527(1):328–344.

143. Hoshi H, Liu WL, Massey SC, Mills SL. ON inputs to the OFF layer: bipolar cells that break the stratification rules of the retina. *J Neurosci.* 2009;29(28):8875–8883.

144. Jeong MJ, Jeon CJ. Localization of melanopsin-immunoreactive cells in the Mongolian gerbil retina. *Neurosci Res.* 2015;100:6–16.

145. Karnas D, Hicks D, Mordel J, Pevet P, Meissl H. Intrinsic photosensitive retinal ganglion cells in the diurnal rodent, Arvicanthis ansorgei. *PLoS One.* 2013;8(8):e73343.

146. DeParis S, Caprara C, Grimm C. Intrinsically photosensitive retinal ganglion cells are resistant to N-methyl-D-aspartic acid excitotoxicity. *Mol Vis.* 2012;18:2814–2827.

147. Fogo GM, Shuboni-Mulligan DD, Gall AJ. Melanopsin-containing ipRGCs are resistant to excitotoxic injury and maintain functional non-image forming behaviors after insult in a diurnal rodent model. *Neuroscience.* 2019;412:105–115.

148. Honda S, Namekata K, Kimura A, et al. Survival of alpha and intrinsically photosensitive retinal ganglion cells in NMDA-induced neurotoxicity and a mouse model of normal tension glaucoma. *Invest Ophthalmol Vis Sci.* 2019;60(12):3696–3707.

149. Li SY, Yau SY, Chen BY, et al. Enhanced survival of melanopsin-expressing retinal ganglion cells after injury is associated with the PI3 K/Akt pathway. *Cell Mol Neurobiol.* 2008

150. Wang S, Gu D, Zhang P, et al. Melanopsin-expressing retinal ganglion cells are relatively resistant to excitotoxicity induced by N-methyl-d-aspartate. *Neurosci Lett.* 2018;662: 368–373.

151. Perez de Sevilla Muller L, Sargoy A, Rodriguez AR, Brecha NC. Melanopsin ganglion cells are the most resistant retinal ganglion cell type to axonal injury in the rat retina. *PLoS One.* 2014;9(3):e93274.

152. Robinson GA, Madison RD. Axotomized mouse retinal ganglion cells containing melanopsin show enhanced survival, but not enhanced axon regrowth into a peripheral nerve graft. *Vision Res.* 2004;44(23):2667–2674.

153. Duan X, Qiao M, Bei F, Kim IJ, He Z, Sanes JR. Subtype-specific regeneration of retinal ganglion cells following axotomy: effects of osteopontin and mTOR signaling. *Neuron.* 2015;85(6):1244–1256.

154. Tran NM, Shekhar K, Whitney IE, et al. Single-cell profiles of retinal ganglion cells differing in resilience to injury reveal neuroprotective genes. *Neuron.* 2019;104(6):1039–1055. e12.

155. VanderWall KB, Lu B, Alfaro JS, et al. Differential susceptibility of retinal ganglion cell subtypes in acute and chronic models of injury and disease. *Sci Rep.* 2020;10(1):17359.

156. Li S, Yang C, Zhang L, et al. Promoting axon regeneration in the adult CNS by modulation of the melanopsin/GPCR signaling. *Proc Natl Acad Sci U S A.* 2016;113(7):1937–1942.

157. Belenky MA, Smeraski CA, Provencio I, Sollars PJ, Pickard GE. Melanopsin retinal ganglion cells receive bipolar and amacrine cell synapses. *J Comp Neurol.* 2003;460(3):380–393.

158. Østergaard J, Hannibal J, Fahrenkrug J. Synaptic contact between melanopsin-containing retinal ganglion cells and rod bipolar cells. *Invest Ophthalmol Vis Sci.* 2007;48(8):3812–3820.

159. Dumitrescu ON, Pucci FG, Wong KY, Berson DM. Ectopic retinal ON bipolar cell synapses in the OFF inner plexiform layer: contacts with dopaminergic amacrine cells and melanopsin ganglion cells. *J Comp Neurol.* 2009;517(2):226–244.

160. Grunert U, Jusuf PR, Lee SC, Nguyen DT. Bipolar input to melanopsin containing ganglion cells in primate retina. *Vis Neurosci.* 2011;28(1):39–50.

161. Sabbah S, Papendorp C, Koplas E, et al. Synaptic circuits for irradiance coding by intrinsically photosensitive retinal ganglion cells. *bioRxiv.* 2018:442954.

162. Perez-Leon JA, Warren EJ, Allen CN, Robinson DW, Lane Brown R. Synaptic inputs to retinal ganglion cells that set the circadian clock. *Eur J Neurosci.* 2006;24(4):1117–1123.

163. Famiglietti Jr. EV, Kolb H. Structural basis for ON-and OFF-center responses in retinal ganglion cells. *Science.* 1976;194(4261):193–195.

164. Nelson R, Famiglietti Jr. EV, Kolb H. Intracellular staining reveals different levels of stratification for on- and off-center ganglion cells in cat retina. *J Neurophysiol.* 1978;41(2):472–483.

165. Schmidt TM, Taniguchi K, Kofuji P. Intrinsic and extrinsic light responses in melanopsin-expressing ganglion cells during mouse development. *J Neurophysiol.* 2008;100(1):371–384.

166. Ackert JM, Farajian R, Volgyi B, Bloomfield SA. GABA blockade unmasks an OFF response in ON direction selective ganglion cells in the mammalian retina. *J Physiol.* 2009;587(Pt 18):4481–4495.

167. Lee S, Chen M, Shi Y, Zhou ZJ. Selective glycinergic input from vGluT3 amacrine cells confers a suppressed-by-contrast trigger feature in a subtype of M1 ipRGCs in the mouse retina. *J Physiol.* 2021;599(22):5047–5060.

168. Patterson SS, Kuchenbecker JA, Anderson JR, Neitz M, Neitz J. A color vision circuit for non-image-forming vision in the primate retina. *Curr Biol.* 2020;30(7):1269–1274. e2.

169. Dowling JE. *The Retina: An Approachable Part of the Brain. Revised ed.* Cambridge, MA: The Belknap Press of. Harvard University Press; 2012.

170. Mariani AP. Amacrine cells of the rhesus monkey retina. *J Comp Neurol.* 1990;301(3): 382–400.

171. Kolb H, Linberg KA, Fisher SK. Neurons of the human retina: a Golgi study. *J Comp Neurol.* 1992;318(2):147–187.

172. Lin B, Masland RH. Populations of wide-field amacrine cells in the mouse retina. *J Comp Neurol.* 2006;499(5):797–809.

173. MacNeil MA, Masland RH. Extreme diversity among amacrine cells: implications for function. *Neuron.* 1998;20(5):971–982.

174. Helmstaedter M, Briggman KL, Turaga SC, Jain V, Seung HS, Denk W. Connectomic reconstruction of the inner plexiform layer in the mouse retina. *Nature.* 2013;500(7461): 168–174.

175. Peng YR, Shekhar K, Yan W, et al. Molecular classification and comparative taxonomics of foveal and peripheral cells in primate retina. *Cell.* 2019;176(5):1222–1237. e22.

176. Yan W, Laboulaye MA, Tran NM, Whitney IE, Benhar I, Sanes JR. Mouse retinal cell atlas: molecular identification of over sixty amacrine cell types. *J Neurosci.* 2020;40(27): 5177–5195.

177. Christiansen AT, Kiilgaard JF, Klemp K, Woldbye DPD, Hannibal J. Localization, distribution, and connectivity of neuropeptide Y in the human and porcine retinas-A comparative study. *J Comp Neurol.* 2018;526(12):1877–1895.

178. Vugler AA, Redgrave P, Semo M, Lawrence J, Greenwood J, Coffey PJ. Dopamine neurones form a discrete plexus with melanopsin cells in normal and degenerating retina. *Exp Neurol.* 2007;205(1):26–35.

179. Zhang DQ, Stone JF, Zhou T, Ohta H, McMahon DG. Characterization of genetically labeled catecholamine neurons in the mouse retina. *Neuroreport.* 2004;15(11):1761–1765.

179a. Zhang Y, Meister M, Pawlyk BS, Bulgakov OV, Li T, Sandberg MA. Responses of intrinsically-photosensitive retinal ganglion cells after melanopsin-gene transfection. *Invest Ophthalmol Vis Sci.* 2007;48:E-Abstract 4604.

180. Witkovsky P. Dopamine and retinal function. *Doc Ophthalmol.* 2004;108(1):17–40.

181. Sakamoto K, Liu C, Kasamatsu M, Pozdeyev NV, Iuvone PM, Tosini G. Dopamine regulates melanopsin mRNA expression in intrinsically photosensitive retinal ganglion cells. *Eur J Neurosci.* 2005;22(12):3129–3136.

182. Van Hook MJ, Wong KY, Berson DM. Dopaminergic modulation of ganglion-cell photoreceptors in rat. *Eur J Neurosci.* 2012;35(4):507–518.

183. Pack W, Hill DD, Wong KY. Melatonin modulates M4-type ganglion-cell photoreceptors. *Neuroscience.* 2015;303:178–188.

184. Cleymaet AM, Berezin CT, Vigh J. Endogenous opioid signaling in the mouse retina modulates pupillary light reflex. *Int J Mol Sci.* 2021;22(2).

185. Cleymaet AM, Gallagher SK, Tooker RE, et al. mu-Opioid receptor activation directly modulates intrinsically photosensitive retinal ganglion cells. *Neuroscience.* 2019;408:400–417.

186. Vuong HE, Hardi CN, Barnes S, Brecha NC. Parallel inhibition of dopamine amacrine cells and intrinsically photosensitive retinal ganglion cells in a non-image-forming visual circuit of the mouse retina. *J Neurosci.* 2015;35(48):15955–15970.

187. Sodhi P, Hartwick AT. Adenosine modulates light responses of rat retinal ganglion cell photoreceptors througha cAMP-mediated pathway. *J Physiol.* 2014;592(19):4201–4220.

188. Zhou W, Wang LQ, Shao YQ, et al. Orexin-A intensifies mouse pupillary light response by modulating intrinsically photosensitive retinal ganglion cells. *J Neurosci.* 2021;41(12):2566–2580.

189. Sheng WL, Chen WY, Yang XL, Zhong YM, Weng SJ. Co-expression of two subtypes of melatonin receptor on rat M1-type intrinsically photosensitive retinal ganglion cells. *PLoS One.* 2015;10(2):e0117967.

190. Wiechmann AF, Sherry DM. Role of melatonin and its receptors in the vertebrate retina. *Int Rev Cell Mol Biol.* 2013;300:211–242.

191. Huang H, Wang Z, Weng SJ, Sun XH, Yang XL. Neuromodulatory role of melatonin in retinal information processing. *Prog Retin Eye Res.* 2013;32:64–87.

192. Weng S, Wong KY, Berson DM. Circadian modulation of melanopsin-driven light response in rat ganglion-cell photoreceptors. *J Biol Rhythms.* 2009;24(5):391–402.

193. Zele AJ, Feigl B, Smith SS, Markwell EL. The circadian response of intrinsically photosensitive retinal ganglion cells. *PLoS One.* 2011;6(3):e17860.

194. Schroeder MM, Harrison KR, Jaeckel ER, et al. The roles of rods, cones, and melanopsin in photoresponses of m4 intrinsically photosensitive retinal ganglion cells (ipRGCs) and optokinetic visual behavior. *Front Cell Neurosci.* 2018;12:203.

195. McDougal DH, Gamlin PD. The influence of intrinsically-photosensitive retinal ganglion cells on the spectral sensitivity and response dynamics of the human pupillary light reflex. *Vision Res.* 2010;50(1):72–87.

196. Lall GS, Revell VL, Momiji H, et al. Distinct contributions of rod, cone, and melanopsin photoreceptors to encoding irradiance. *Neuron.* 2010;66(3):417–428.

197. Gooley JJ, Ho Mien I, St Hilaire MA, et al. Melanopsin and rod-cone photoreceptors play different roles in mediating pupillary light responses during exposure to continuous light in humans. *J Neurosci.* 2012;32(41):14242–14253.

198. Ruby NF, Brennan TJ, Xie X, et al. Role of melanopsin in circadian responses to light. *Science.* 2002;298(5601):2211–2213.

199. Panda S, Sato TK, Castrucci AM, et al. Melanopsin (Opn4) requirement for normal light-induced circadian phase shifting. *Science.* 2002;298(5601):2213–2216.

200. Altimus CM, Guler AD, Alam NM, et al. Rod photoreceptors drive circadian photoentrainment across a wide range of light intensities. *Nat Neurosci.* 2010;13(9): 1107–1112.

201. Güler AD, Ecker JL, Lall GS, et al. Melanopsin cells are the principal conduits for rod-cone input to non-image-forming vision. *Nature*. 2008;453(7191):102–105.
202. Hatori M, Le H, Vollmers C, et al. Inducible ablation of melanopsin-expressing retinal ganglion cells reveals their central role in non-image forming visual responses. *PLoS ONE*. 2008;3(6):e2451.
203. Göz D, Studholme K, Lappi DA, Rollag MD, Provencio I, Morin LP. Targeted destruction of photosensitive retinal ganglion cells with a saporin conjugate alters the effects of light on mouse circadian rhythms. *PLoS ONE*. 2008;3(9):e3153.
204. Ostrin LA, Strang CE, Chang K, et al. Immunotoxin-induced ablation of the intrinsically photosensitive retinal ganglion cells in rhesus monkeys. *Front Neurol*. 2018;9:1000.
205. Hankins MW, Lucas RJ. The primary visual pathway in humans is regulated according to long-term light exposure through the action of a nonclassical photopigment. *Curr Biol*. 2002;12(3):191–198.
206. Barnard AR, Hattar S, Hankins MW, Lucas RJ. Melanopsin regulates visual processing in the mouse retina. *Curr Biol*. 2006;16(4):389–395.
207. Milosavljevic N, Allen AE, Cehajic-Kapetanovic J, Lucas RJ. Chemogenetic activation of ipRGCs drives changes in dark-adapted (scotopic) electroretinogram. *Invest Ophthalmol Vis Sci*. 2016;57(14):6305–6312.
208. Milosavljevic N, Storchi R, Eleftheriou CG, Colins A, Petersen RS, Lucas RJ. Photoreceptive retinal ganglion cells control the information rate of the optic nerve. *Proc Natl Acad Sci U S A*. 2018;115(50):E11817–E11826.
209. Barnard AR, Appleford JM, Sekaran S, et al. Residual photosensitivity in mice lacking both rod opsin and cone photoreceptor cyclic nucleotide gated channel 3 alpha subunit. *Vis Neurosci*. 2004;21(5):675–683.
210. Zhang DQ, Wong KY, Sollars PJ, Berson DM, Pickard GE, McMahon DG. Intraretinal signaling by ganglion cell photoreceptors to dopaminergic amacrine neurons. *Proc Natl Acad Sci U S A*. 2008
211. Zhang DQ, Belenky MA, Sollars PJ, Pickard GE, McMahon DG. Melanopsin mediates retrograde visual signaling in the retina. *PLoS One*. 2012;7(8):e42647.
212. Zhao X, Wong KY, Zhang DQ. Mapping physiological inputs from multiple photoreceptor systems to dopaminergic amacrine cells in the mouse retina. *Sci Rep*. 2017;7(1):7920.
213. Slaughter MM, Miller RF. 2-amino-4-phosphonobutyric acid: a new pharmacological tool for retina research. *Science*. 1981;211(4478):182–185.
214. Semo M, Coffey P, Gias C, Vugler A. Retrograde melanopsin signaling increases with age in retinal degenerate mice lacking rods and the majority of cones. *Invest Ophthalmol Vis Sci*. 2016;57(1):115–125.
215. Morgan WW, Kamp CW. Dopaminergic amacrine neurons of rat retinas with photoreceptor degeneration continue to respond to light. *Life Sci*. 1980;26(19):1619–1626.
216. Vugler AA, Redgrave P, Hewson-Stoate NJ, Greenwood J, Coffey PJ. Constant illumination causes spatially discrete dopamine depletion in the normal and degenerate retina. *J Chem Neuroanat*. 2007;33(1):9–22.
217. Dkhissi-Benyahya O, Coutanson C, Knoblauch K, et al. The absence of melanopsin alters retinal clock function and dopamine regulation by light. *Cell Mol Life Sci*. 2013;70(18):3435–3447.
218. Boelen MK, Boelen MG, Marshak DW. Light-stimulated release of dopamine from the primate retina is blocked by 1-2-amino-4-phosphonobutyric acid (APB). *Vis Neurosci*. 1998;15(1):97–103.
219. Munteanu T, Noronha KJ, Leung AC, Pan S, Lucas JA, Schmidt TM. Light-dependent pathways for dopaminergic amacrine cell development and function. *Elife*. 2018;7
220. Perez-Fernandez V, Milosavljevic N, Allen AE, Vessey KA, Jobling AI, Fletcher EL, et al. Rod photoreceptor activation alone defines the release of dopamine in the retina. *Curr Biol*. 2019;29(5):763–774. e5.
221. Cameron MA, Pozdeyev N, Vugler AA, Cooper H, Iuvone PM, Lucas RJ. Light regulation of retinal dopamine that is independent of melanopsin phototransduction. *Eur J Neurosci*. 2009;29(4):761–767.
222. Prigge CL, Yeh PT, Liou NF, Lee CC, You SF, Liu LL, et al. M1 ipRGCs Influence visual function through retrograde signaling in the retina. *J Neurosci*. 2016;36(27):7184–7197.
223. Joo HR, Peterson BB, Dacey DM, Hattar S, Chen SK. Recurrent axon collaterals of intrinsically photosensitive retinal ganglion cells. *Vis Neurosci*. 2013;30(4):175–182.
224. Liu LL, Alessio EJ, Spix NJ, Zhang DQ. Expression of GluA2-containing calcium-impermeable AMPA receptors on dopaminergic amacrine cells in the mouse retina. *Mol Vis*. 2019;25:780–790.
225. Liu LL, Spix NJ, Zhang DQ. NMDA receptors contribute to retrograde synaptic transmission from ganglion cell photoreceptors to dopaminergic amacrine cells. *Front Cell Neurosci*. 2017;11:279.
226. Zhang DQ, Zhou TR, McMahon DG. Functional heterogeneity of retinal dopaminergic neurons underlying their multiple roles in vision. *J Neurosci*. 2007;27(3):692–699.
227. Sakai HM, Naka K, Dowling JE. Ganglion cell dendrites are presynaptic in catfish retina. *Nature*. 1986;319(6053):495–497.
228. Bramley JR, Wiles EM, Sollars PJ, Pickard GE. Carbenoxolone blocks the light-evoked rise in intracellular calcium in isolated melanopsin ganglion cell photoreceptors. *PLoS One*. 2011;6(7):e22721.
229. Reifler AN, Chervenak AP, Dolikian ME, et al. All spiking, sustained ON displaced amacrine cells receive gap-junction input from melanopsin ganglion cells. *Curr Biol*. 2015;25(21):2763–2773.
230. Sabbah S, Berg D, Papendorp C, Briggman KL, Berson DM. A Cre mouse line for probing irradiance- and direction-encoding retinal networks. *eNeuro*. 2017;4(2).
231. Zhao X, Wong KY. Structure and function of the gap junctional network of photoreceptive ganglion cells. *Vis Neurosci*. 2021;38:E014.
232. Harrison KR, Chervenak AP, Resnick SM, Reifler AN, Wong KY. Amacrine cells forming gap junctions with intrinsically photosensitive retinal ganglion cells: ipRGC types, neuromodulator contents, and connexin isoform. *Invest Ophthalmol Vis Sci*. 2021;62(1):10.
233. Pottackal J, Walsh HL, Rahmani P, Zhang K, Justice NJ, Demb JB. Photoreceptive ganglion cells drive circuits for local inhibition in the mouse retina. *J Neurosci*. 2021;41(7):1489–1504.
234. Baver SB, Pickard GE, Sollars PJ. Two types of melanopsin retinal ganglion cell differentially innervate the hypothalamic suprachiasmatic nucleus and the olivary pretectal nucleus. *Eur J Neurosci*. 2008;27(7):1763–1770.
235. Gooley JJ, Lu J, Fischer D, Saper CB. A broad role for melanopsin in nonvisual photoreception. *J Neurosci*. 2003;23(18):7093–7106.
236. Hannibal J, Fahrenkrug J. Target areas innervated by PACAP-immunoreactive retinal ganglion cells. *Cell Tissue Res*. 2004;316(1):99–113.
237. Morin LP, Blanchard JH, Provencio I. Retinal ganglion cell projections to the hamster suprachiasmatic nucleus, intergeniculate leaflet, and visual midbrain: bifurcation and melanopsin immunoreactivity. *J Comp Neurol*. 2003;465(3):401–416.
238. Delwig A, Larsen DD, Yasumura D, Yang CF, Shah NM, Copenhagen DR. Retinofugal projections from melanopsin-expressing retinal ganglion cells revealed by intraocular injections of Cre-dependent virus. *PLoS One*. 2016;11(2):e0149501.
239. Hannibal J, Kankipati L, Strang CE, Peterson BB, Dacey D, Gamlin PD. Central projections of intrinsically photosensitive retinal ganglion cells in the macaque monkey. *J Comp Neurol*. 2014;522(10):2231–2248.
240. Hannibal J, Moller M, Ottersen OP, Fahrenkrug J. PACAP and glutamate are co-stored in the retinohypothalamic tract. *J Comp Neurol*. 2000;418(2):147–155.
241. Sonoda T, Li JY, Hayes NW, et al. A noncanonical inhibitory circuit dampens behavioral sensitivity to light. *Science*. 2020;368(6490):527–531.
242. Wong KY, Graham DM, Berson DM. The retina-attached SCN slice preparation: an in vitro mammalian circadian visual system. *J Biol Rhythms*. 2007;22(5):400–410.
243. Beier C, Zhang Z, Yurgel M, Hattar S. Projections of ipRGCs and conventional RGCs to retinorecipient brain nuclei. *J Comp Neurol*. 2021;529(8):1863–1875.
244. Li JY, Schmidt TM. Divergent projection patterns of M1 ipRGC subtypes. *J Comp Neurol*. 2018;526(13):2010–2018.
245. Gamlin PD, McDougal DH, Pokorny J, Smith VC, Yau KW, Dacey DM. Human and macaque pupil responses driven by melanopsin-containing retinal ganglion cells. *Vision Res*. 2007;47(7):946–954.
246. Zhu Y, Tu DC, Denner D, Shane T, Fitzgerald CM, Van Gelder RN. Melanopsin-dependent persistence and photopotentiation of murine pupillary light responses. *Invest Ophthalmol Vis Sci*. 2007;48(3):1268–1275.
247. Takahashi JS. Transcriptional architecture of the mammalian circadian clock. *Nat Rev Genet*. 2017;18(3):164–179.
248. Hastings MH, Maywood ES, Brancaccio M. The mammalian circadian timing system and the suprachiasmatic nucleus as its pacemaker. *Biology (Basel)*. 2019;8(1).
249. Morin LP, Allen CN. The circadian visual system, 2005. *Brain Res Rev*. 2006;51(1):1–60.
250. Drouyer E, Rieux C, Hut RA, Cooper HM. Responses of suprachiasmatic nucleus neurons to light and dark adaptation: relative contributions of melanopsin and rod-cone inputs. *J Neurosci*. 2007;27(36):9623–9631.
251. Van Diepen HC, Ramkisoensing A, Peirson SN, Foster RG, Meijer JH. Irradiance encoding in the suprachiasmatic nuclei by rod and cone photoreceptors. *FASEB J*. 2013;27(10):4204–4212.
252. van Diepen HC, Schoonderwoerd RA, Ramkisoensing A, Janse JAM, Hattar S, Meijer JH. Distinct contribution of cone photoreceptor subtypes to the mammalian biological clock. *Proc Natl Acad Sci U S A*. 2021;118(22).
253. Silva MM, Albuquerque AM, Araujo JF. Light-dark cycle synchronization of circadian rhythm in blind primates. *J Circadian Rhythms*. 2005;3:10.
254. Dollet A, Albrecht U, Cooper HM, Dkhissi-Benyahya O. Cones are required for normal temporal responses to light of phase shifts and clock gene expression. *Chronobiol Int*. 2010;27(4):768–781.
255. Pandi-Perumal SR, Srinivasan V, Spence DW, Cardinali DP. Role of the melatonin system in the control of sleep: therapeutic implications. *CNS Drugs*. 2007;21(12):995–1018.
256. Jasser SA, Blask DE, Brainard GC. Light during darkness and cancer: relationships in circadian photoreception and tumor biology. *Cancer Causes Control*. 2006;17(4):515–523.
257. Stevens RG, Brainard GC, Blask DE, Lockley SW, Motta ME. Breast cancer and circadian disruption from electric lighting in the modern world. *CA Cancer J Clin*. 2014;64(3):207–218.
258. Mao L, Summers W, Xiang S, et al. Melatonin represses metastasis in Her2-postive human breast cancer cells by suppressing RSK2 expression. *Mol Cancer Res*. 2016;14(11):1159–1169.
259. Hoang BX, Shaw DG, Pham PT, Levine SA. Neurobiological effects of melatonin as related to cancer. *Eur J Cancer Prev*. 2007;16(6):511–516.
260. Kong X, Gao R, Wang Z, et al. Melatonin: A potential therapeutic option for breast cancer. *Trends Endocrinol Metab*. 2020;31(11):859–871.
261. Thapan K, Arendt J, Skene DJ. An action spectrum for melatonin suppression: evidence for a novel non-rod, non-cone photoreceptor system in humans. *J Physiol*. 2001;535 (Pt 1):261–267.
262. Borbely AA. A two process model of sleep regulation. *Hum Neurobiol*. 1982;1(3):195–204.
263. Lockley SW, Evans EE, Scheer FA, Brainard GC, Czeisler CA, Aeschbach D. Short-wavelength sensitivity for the direct effects of light on alertness, vigilance, and the waking electroencephalogram in humans. *Sleep*. 2006;29(2):161–168.
264. Altimus CM, Guler AD, Villa KL, McNeill DS, Legates TA, Hattar S. Rods-cones and melanopsin detect light and dark to modulate sleep independent of image formation. *Proc Natl Acad Sci U S A*. 2008;105(50):19998–20003.
265. Morin LP, Studholme KM. Separation of function for classical and ganglion cell photoreceptors with respect to circadian rhythm entrainment and induction of photosomnolence. *Neuroscience*. 2011;199:213–224.
266. Rupp AC, Ren M, Altimus CM, et al. Distinct ipRGC subpopulations mediate light's acute and circadian effects on body temperature and sleep. *Elife*. 2019;8
267. Zhang Z, Beier C, Weil T, Hattar S. The retinal ipRGC-preoptic circuit mediates the acute effect of light on sleep. *Nat Commun*. 2021;12(1):5115.
268. Studholme KM, Gompf HS, Morin LP. Brief light stimulation during the mouse nocturnal activity phase simultaneously induces a decline in core temperature and locomotor

activity followed by EEG-determined sleep. *Am J Physiol Regul Integr Comp Physiol.* 2013;304(6):R459–R471.

269. Morin LP. A path to sleep is through the eye. *eNeuro.* 2015;2(2).

270. LeGates TA, Altimus CM, Wang H, et al. Aberrant light directly impairs mood and learning through melanopsin-expressing neurons. *Nature.* 2012;491(7425):594–598.

271. Fernandez DC, Fogerson PM, et al.Lazzerini Ospri L, Light Affects mood and learning through distinct retina-brain pathways. *Cell.* 2018;175(1):71–84. e18.

272. Fonken LK, Finy MS, Walton JC, et al. Influence of light at night on murine anxiety- and depressive-like responses. *Behav Brain Res.* 2009;205(2):349–354.

273. An K, Zhao H, Miao Y, et al. A circadian rhythm-gated subcortical pathway for nighttime-light-induced depressive-like behaviors in mice. *Nat Neurosci.* 2020;23(7):869–880.

274. Francis TC, Lobo MK. Emerging role for nucleus accumbens medium spiny neuron subtypes in depression. *Biol Psychiatry.* 2017;81(8):645–653.

275. Huang L, Xi Y, Peng Y, et al. A visual circuit related to habenula underlies the antidepressive effects of light therapy. *Neuron.* 2019;102(1):128–142. e8.

276. Warthen DM, Wiltgen BJ, Provencio I. Light enhances learned fear. *Proc Natl Acad Sci U S A.* 2011;108(33):13788–13793.

277. Milosavljevic N, Cehajic-Kapetanovic J, Procyk CA, Lucas RJ. Chemogenetic activation of melanopsin retinal ganglion cells induces signatures of arousal and/or anxiety in mice. *Curr Biol.* 2016;26(17):2358–2363.

278. Aranda ML, Schmidt TM. Diversity of intrinsically photosensitive retinal ganglion cells: circuits and functions. *Cell Mol Life Sci.* 2021;78(3):889–907.

279. Lucas RJ, Allen AE, Milosavljevic N, Storchi R, Woelders T. Can we see with melanopsin? *Annu Rev Vis Sci.* 2020;6:453–468.

280. Denman DJ, Siegle JH, Koch C, Reid RC, Blanche TJ. Spatial organization of chromatic pathways in the mouse dorsal lateral geniculate nucleus. *J Neurosci.* 2017;37(5):1102–1116.

281. Cang J, Savier E, Barchini J, Liu X. Visual function, organization, and development of the mouse superior colliculus. *Annu Rev Vis Sci.* 2018;4:239–262.

282. Hannibal J, Fahrenkrug J. Melanopsin containing retinal ganglion cells are light responsive from birth. *Neuroreport.* 2004;15(15):2317–2320.

283. Sekaran S, Lupi D, Jones SL, et al. Melanopsin-dependent photoreception provides earliest light detection in the mammalian retina. *Curr Biol.* 2005;15(12):1099–1107.

284. Tarttelin EE, Bellingham J, Bibb LC, et al. Expression of opsin genes early in ocular development of humans and mice. *Exp Eye Res.* 2003;76(3):393–396.

285. Bibb LC, Holt JK, Tarttelin EE, et al. Temporal and spatial expression patterns of the CRX transcription factor and its downstream targets. Critical differences during human and mouse eye development. *Hum Mol Genet.* 2001;10(15):1571–1579.

286. Hendrickson A, Bumsted-O'Brien K, Natoli R, Ramamurthy V, Possin D, Provis J. Rod photoreceptor differentiation in fetal and infant human retina. *Exp Eye Res.* 2008;87(5):415–426.

287. Rao S, Chun C, Fan J, et al. A direct and melanopsin-dependent fetal light response regulates mouse eye development. *Nature.* 2013;494(7436):243–246.

288. Arroyo DA, Feller MB. Spatiotemporal features of retinal waves instruct the wiring of the visual circuitry. *Front Neural Circuits.* 2016;10:54.

289. Bonezzi PJ, Stabio ME, Renna JM. The development of mid-wavelength photoresponsivity in the mouse retina. *Curr Eye Res.* 2018;43(5):666–673.

290. Renna JM, Weng S, Berson DM. Light acts through melanopsin to alter retinal waves and segregation of retinogeniculate afferents. *Nat Neurosci.* 2011;14(7):827–829.

291. Tufford AR, Onyak JR, Sondereker KB, et al. Melanopsin retinal ganglion cells regulate cone photoreceptor lamination in the mouse retina. *Cell Rep.* 2018;23(8):2416–2428.

292. Shah-Desai SD, Tyers AG, Manners RM. Painful blind eye: efficacy of enucleation and evisceration in resolving ocular pain. *Br J Ophthalmol.* 2000;84(4):437–438.

293. Merbs SL. Management of a blind painful eye. *Ophthalmol Clin North Am.* 2006;19(2):287–292.

294. Wilhelm H. The pupil. *Curr Opin Neurol.* 2008;21(1):36–42.

295. Skene DJ, Arendt J. Circadian rhythm sleep disorders in the blind and their treatment with melatonin. *Sleep Med.* 2007;8(6):651–655.

296. Kawasaki A, Kardon RH. Intrinsically photosensitive retinal ganglion cells. *J Neuroophthalmol.* 2007 Sep;27(3):195–204.

297. Mainster MA. Violet and blue light blocking intraocular lenses: photoprotection versus photoreception. *Br J Ophthalmol.* 2006;90(6):784–792.

298. Mainster MA, Turner PL. Blue-blocking IOLs decrease photoreception without providing significant photoprotection. *Surv Ophthalmol.* 2010;55(3):272–289.

299. Van de Kraats J, Van Norren D. Sharp cutoff filters in intraocular lenses optimize the balance between light reception and light protection. *J Cataract Refract Surg.* 2007;33(5):879–887.

300. Liu M-M, Dai J-M, Liu W-Y, Zhao C-J, Lin B, Yin Z-Q. Human melanopsin-AAV2/8 transfection to retina transiently restores visual function in rd1 mice. *Int J Ophthalmol.* 2016;9:655–661.

301. Bi A, Cui J, Ma YP, et al. Ectopic expression of a microbial-type rhodopsin restores visual responses in mice with photoreceptor degeneration. *Neuron.* 2006;50(1):23–33.

302. Lagali PS, Balya D, Awatramani GB, et al. Light-activated channels targeted to ON bipolar cells restore visual function in retinal degeneration. *Nat Neurosci.* 2008;11(6):667–675.

303. Lu Q, Pan Z-H. Optogenetic strategies for vision restoration. *Adv Exp Med Biol.* 2021;1293:545–555.

304. Van Wyk M, Pielecka-Fortuna J, Löwel S, Kleinlogel S. Restoring the ON switch in blind retinas: Opto-mGluR6, a next-generation, cell-tailored optogenetic tool. *PLoS Biol.* 2015;13(5):e1002143.

305. Park JC, Moura AL, Raza AS, Rhee DW, Kardon RH, Hood DC. Toward a clinical protocol for assessing rod, cone, and melanopsin contributions to the human pupil response. *Invest Ophthalmol Vis Sci.* 2011;52(9):6624–6635.

306. Rosenthal NE, Sack DA, Gillin JC, et al. Seasonal affective disorder. A description of the syndrome and preliminary findings with light therapy. *Arch Gen Psychiatry.* 1984;41(1):72–80.

307. Macchi MM, Bruce JN. Human pineal physiology and functional significance of melatonin. *Front Neuroendocrinol.* 2004;25(3–4):177–195.

308. Golden RN, Gaynes BN, Ekstrom RD, et al. The efficacy of light therapy in the treatment of mood disorders: a review and meta-analysis of the evidence. *Am J Psychiatry.* 2005;162(4):656–662.

309. Pjrek E, Friedrich ME, Cambioli L, et al. The efficacy of light therapy in the treatment of seasonal affective disorder: a meta-analysis of randomized controlled trials. *Psychother Psychosom.* 2020;89(1):17–24.

310. Wehr TA, Duncan Jr. WC, Sher L, et al. A circadian signal of change of season in patients with seasonal affective disorder. *Arch Gen Psychiatry.* 2001;58(12):1108–1114.

311. Meesters Y, Duijzer WB, Hommes V. The effects of low-intensity narrow-band blue-light treatment compared to bright white-light treatment in seasonal affective disorder. *J Affect Disord.* 2018;232:48–51.

312. Roecklein KA, Rohan KJ, Duncan WC, et al. A missense variant (P10L) of the melanopsin (OPN4) gene in seasonal affective disorder. *J Affect Disord.* 2008;Sep 17.

313. Roecklein KA, Franzen PL, Wescott DL, et al. Melanopsin-driven pupil response in summer and winter in unipolar seasonal affective disorder. *J Affect Disord.* 2021;291:93–101.

314. Sack RL, Brandes RW, Kendall AR, Lewy AJ. Entrainment of free-running circadian rhythms by melatonin in blind people. *N Engl J Med.* 2000;343(15):1070–1077.

315. Lockley SW, Dressman MA, Licamele L, et al. Tasimelteon for non-24-hour sleep-wake disorder in totally blind people (SET and RESET): two multicentre, randomised, double-masked, placebo-controlled phase 3 trials. *Lancet.* 2015;386(10005):1754–1764.

316. Quera Salva MA, Hartley S, Leger D, Dauvilliers YA. Non-24-hour sleep-wake rhythm disorder in the totally blind: Diagnosis and management. *Front Neurol.* 2017;8:686.

27

Overview of the Central Visual Pathways

Janine D. Mendola

The eye is a complex organ responsible for collecting, focusing, and processing light. Modern genetic analysis indicates that there are many different classes of ganglion cells in the retina that act to initially select and segregate visual information. However, it is the central visual pathways that continue to segregate, combine, and ultimately interpret this information. Distinct pathways are responsible for a range of functions including conscious visual perception, sensory-motor integration, eye movements, and circadian rhythms. The central visual pathways refer broadly to all the regions of the brain conveying or receiving either direct or indirect retinal input. The system begins via the projection targets of the retina, comprised of several midbrain structures with diverse functions. However, certain targets such as the thalamic lateral geniculate nucleus (LGN) participate in a far more expansive and complex elaboration than others. This is the critical system for conscious perception and cognition that is so highly developed in primates and humans. In this overview, we will first introduce the central visual pathways with a brief review of the targets of the retinal projections (Figs. 27.1 and 27.2). Second, by reviewing the types of conscious vision loss that occur after damage along the major visual pathways we provide a concise summary of their basic organization (Fig. 27.3). We conclude the chapter with a brief mention of the relatively new neuroimaging techniques that have greatly expanded our ability to study the human visual system directly (Fig. 27.4). Whereas Chapter 26 outlined predominantly subconscious, nonimage-forming visual pathways in the brain that receive input from melanopsin-expressing intrinsically photosensitive retinal ganglion cells, the subsequent chapters consider the conscious visual system in more detail. Also, in Chapter 28, the optic nerve that carries retinal ganglion cell axons toward their targets is fully discussed in terms of development, structure, and potential injury. The LGN, described in detail in Chapter 29, is an important relay in the visual pathway involved with form vision. The precision and specificity of the retinogeniculate connections are crucial to subsequent stages. From the LGN, the visual pathway proceeds to the primary visual cortex, V1. It is at the level of V1 that visual signals undergo more complex processing, which is detailed in Chapter 30. Visual processing of a combination of stimulus features such as shape, color, contrast, motion, texture, and depth is further enhanced by over 30 extrastriate cortical areas, some of which are described in Chapter 31.

TARGETS OF THE RETINAL PROJECTIONS

We begin with a brief review of the intricate but well described functional anatomy of the retinal projections (Fig. 27.1). Although there are systematic variations in the size of optic nerves, the LGN,

and primary visual cortex in humans,[1] the basic pattern is the same. Axons from the output cells of the retina (ganglion cells) are specifically directed to the area of the blind spot and exit to form the optic nerve. Ganglion cells representing both the nasal and temporal sides of the retina all exit at this juncture but axons retain their spatial positions with respect to axons from neighboring regions. This precise preservation of the neighborhood relations (or "map") of the retina is the basis for the retinotopic organization that defines these projections. This organization is of profound importance for understanding the visual system and is elaborated upon repeatedly in the chapters that follow. When optic nerve axons reach the optic chiasm (located above the pituitary gland), only those representing the temporal visual field (those located in the *nasal* side of the retina) cross contralaterally. These crossing fibers from nasal retina are known to slightly outnumber those that do not cross (53%–47%).[2] Incidentally, some fibers from the nasal side representing the far edge of peripheral vision (in the temporal visual field) are known to deviate slightly anterior and form a structure referred to as Wilbrand's knee (see Fig. 27.3 for the clinical relevance). The remaining axons from the *temporal* retina remain segregated to comprise the ipsilateral optic tract (along with fibers from the nasal retinal from the other side). Hence the optic tract and all subsequent connections receive information from the contralateral visual field. In other words, both sides of the brain receive input from both the left and right eye (although this information may not be truly integrated by single neurons until later stages, such as primary visual cortex).

The major targets of the retinal ganglion cell axons are (1) the LGN, (2) the superior colliculus (SC), (3) the pretectum, and (4) the pulvinar. There is a weaker projection to several small hypothalamic nuclei including (5) the suprachiasmatic, supraoptic, paraventricular nuclei, and to (6) the accessory optic system (AOS), including the nucleus of the optic tract (NOT) and the dorsal, medial, and terminal nuclei (Fig. 27.1; Box 27.1; and see Fig. 9.8).

The most significant projection, in terms of the number of optic nerve fibers, is to the lateral LGN in the thalamus. The LGN is the major termination site of the retinal ganglion cells and plays an important role in the visual pathway leading to the primary visual cortex. Approximately 90% of all retinal ganglion cells project to the LGN, which is laminated. An important function of the LGN is to organize its retinal inputs by their receptive field properties. Although only a small fraction of the inputs to the LGN are from the retina, they create a strong excitatory drive, and are precisely retinotopic. Other LGN synapses reflect either local interneurons, inputs from other midbrain

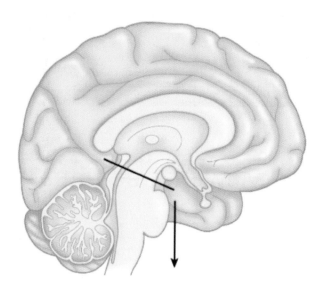

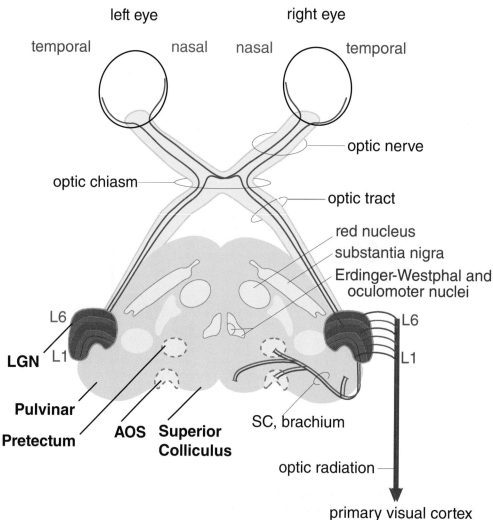

Fig. 27.1 Schematic illustration of five major retinal midbrain targets, labeled in bold. Blue color represents the temporal visual field (corresponding to the nasal retina), and Wilbrand's knee is depicted near the level of the optic chiasm. *Red* represents nasal visual field (corresponding to the temporal retina). Axons from nasal retina (from the contralateral eye) and temporal retina (from the ipsilateral eye) remain segregated in the lateral geniculate nucleus (*LGN*) layers. From layer 1 (L1) to layer 6 (L6) input is ordered as follows: contra, ipsi, ipsi, contra, ipsi, contra. *AOS*, accessory optic system; *SC*, superior colliculus.

(e.g., SC) or brain stem sources, or feedback from visual cortex, all generally thought to provide modulatory input. Each LGN layer receives input from a specific eye and class of ganglion cell. Whereas electrophysiological studies suggest that the neuronal signals coming into and leaving the LGN are quite similar, the LGN appears to be involved in regulating information flow between the retina and primary visual cortex, the major projection target of the LGN (see Chapter 29). The left and right eye segregation of axons in the six major LGN layers synapse in layer 4 of V1, and form the basis for monocular dominance columns, which form the substrate for binocularity, as discussed in detail in Chapter 30. Also noteworthy is that the magnification of the central visual field that originates in the retina, owing to a greater density of ganglion cells, is maintained in the LGN, and is exaggerated even further at the level of V1 (see Fig. 27.3).

The SC is a midbrain structure that, in conjunction with the cortical frontal eye fields and the brainstem reticular formation, is involved in the generation of visually guided saccadic eye movements[3,4] (see Chapter 9). The SC is a laminated, retinotopically organized nucleus, and, as seen in the LGN, the retinal projection retains eye segregation with alternating columns of left and right eye terminals forming a banded pattern throughout the superficial layers. Approximately 10% of all retinal ganglion cells project to the SC. The majority of retinal axons that terminate in the SC are small caliber, originate from ganglion cells with small dendritic fields, and do not project to other retinal targets.[5] The SC is an evolutionarily conserved sensorimotor structure that integrates visual and other sensory information to drive reflexive behaviors. Nevertheless, more modern studies also emphasize a role in complex behaviors such as attention and decision-making, even contributing to object selectivity in certain extrastriate cortical regions to which it projects.[6,7] An interesting feature of the SC is a lack of input from S-cones, and clever experiments have thus simulated "SC lesions" by studying the effects of stimuli carried only by S-cone input.[8]

The pretectal complex, a group of small midbrain nuclei, is just rostral to the SC. It receives signals from a group of small-diameter retinal ganglion cells with large receptive fields and is involved with the control of the pupillary light reflex (see Chapter 25) by means of a projection to the Edinger-Westphal nucleus of the oculomotor complex. The pupillary light reflex demonstrates a consensual response primarily resulting from crossed and uncrossed optic nerve fibers that enter each pretectal complex, which in turn sends a bilateral projection to the Edinger-Westphal nucleus (see Chapter 9).

Retinal ganglion cells also project to three of four major subdivisions of the pulvinar nucleus of the thalamus.[9,10] The pulvinar is the largest nuclear mass in the primate thalamus and receives a projection from the small-caliber fibers from the optic nerve and the SC. It projects to several visual cortical areas, including V1, extrastriate, and parietal areas. Thus, the pulvinar represents a pathway that can bypass the LGN to get to V1 and may play a role in processing form vision. More recent studies point to a role for the pulvinar in the coding of the "importance" of visual stimuli (i.e., visual salience or "attention").[11] In some case studies, damage to the pulvinar has been reported to cause a visual neglect of the contralateral visual field (e.g.,[12]). It has been shown that the pulvinar integrates neural signals associated with eye and hand and arm movements and may receive signals associated with saccadic eye movements, which suggests its role is also one of formulating reference frames for hand-eye coordination.[13–15]

The AOS consists of several small nuclei, the lateral terminal nucleus (LTN), the medial terminal nucleus (MTN), and the dorsal terminal nucleus (DTN), as well as the NOT in the midbrain.[16] The AOS plays an important role in optokinetic nystagmus (OKN) in which slow

compensatory and pursuit-type eye movements alternate with fast saccadic-type eye movements in response to viewing prolonged large field motion (see Chapter 9). In primates, lesions of the NOT and the DTN have been shown to modify the OKN and reduce or abolish optokinetic after nystagmus (OKAN).[17]

Finally, we consider that several small hypothalamic nuclei receive a direct retinal projection (Fig. 27.2). The suprachiasmatic nucleus receives a sparse projection from fibers that leave the dorsal surface of the optic chiasm and has been implicated in the synchronization of circadian rhythms.[18] The paraventricular and supraoptic nuclei are likely also involved with the regulation of the light-dark cycle for neuroendocrine functions. It is worth noting that the superchiasmatic nucleus is one of the recipients of intrinsically light sensitive ganglion cells that contain a unique opsin (melanopsin) unlike the four opsins found in rods or cones. These ganglion cells are few in number but have very large dendritic trees. This is the basis for the photoentrainment of the circadian rhythm (see Chapter 26).

RETINOTOPIC PATHWAYS AND VISUAL FIELD LESIONS

Much of our early knowledge of the retinotopic organization of the human central visual system derived from the visual field defects associated with lesions along the major pathway leading to form vision, the retinogeniculocortical pathway. Fig. 27.3 illustrates several known anatomical lesions, from the retina to the occipital lobes, and their subsequent effect on the visual fields. In the first example shown, complete interruption of one optic nerve, which may occur with severe degenerative disease or injury, results in permanent blindness in the affected eye. Partial interruption of the nerve fibers results in a partial loss of the visual field and can occur with glaucoma, optic disc drusen, pits, infarcts, or optic neuritis. Regions of local blindness are often referred to as scotomata (derived from Greek meaning darkness).

It is of clinical relevance to note that interruption of the optic nerve closer to the junction of the optic chiasm (#2 in Fig. 27.3) can also include loss of vision in the far temporal periphery, owing to Wilbrand's knee, an abnormality resulting from chronic optic neuropathy on that side.[19] In humans, a sheet of inferonasal fibers of the optic nerve deviate slightly toward the contralateral optic nerve before crossing over to the opposite optic tract.[19]

Slightly further along the visual pathway, interruption of the decussating optic nerve fibers in the optic chiasm (#3 in Fig. 27.3) results in loss of vision in the temporal visual hemifields of both eyes called bitemporal hemianopia. Damage of this type commonly occurs with pituitary tumors as they grow and compress the overlying optic chiasm. Rarely, if pressure is exerted on the lateral edge of the optic chiasm (#4 in Fig. 27.3) damage arises primarily in the uncrossed fibers, resulting in loss of vision in the nasal hemifield, or nasal hemianopia, ipsilateral to the compression.

Lesions that occur after the chiasm are characterized by visual field defects that involve the temporal hemifield of the contralateral eye and the nasal hemifield of the ipsilateral eye; this is because of the partial decussation of optic nerve fibers at the optic chiasm. In this type of lesion, visual field loss occurs on the side contralateral to the lesion. Complete interruption at the level of the optic tract (#5 in Fig. 27.3) or beyond results in this type of vision loss. Homonymous hemianopia is the clinical term used to describe such loss of the contralateral visual field. It is usually difficult to determine whether the site of the lesion is at the level of the optic tract, LGN, or visual cortex for most homonymous hemianopias. In cases in which the lesion is in the optic tract, the homonymous hemianopia may be accompanied by an afferent pupillary defect in the contralateral eye (Box 27.2). The likely reason for

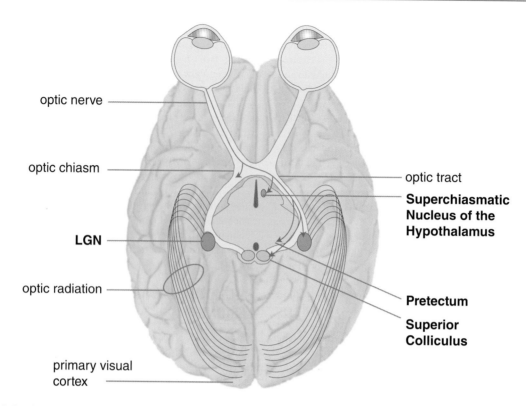

optic nerve

optic chiasm

LGN

optic radiation

primary visual
cortex

optic tract

**Superchiasmatic
Nucleus of the
Hypothalamus**

Pretectum

**Superior
Colliculus**

Fig. 27.2 Central visual pathways highlighting retinal projections to the superchiasmatic nucleus of the hypothalamus, as well as the pretectum and superior colliculus (SC). *LGN,* Lateral geniculate nucleus.

this is because ganglion cells in the nasal retina outnumber those in the temporal retina (53%–47%), thus causing a greater loss of fibers for the pupillary response of the contralateral eye[20] (however, also see[3]). Lesions at the level of the brachium of the SC (#7 in Fig. 27.1) may result in an afferent pupillary defect in the contralateral eye, but with intact, normal visual fields because lesions at this level spare the retinogeniculate fibers. Lesions involving the LGN (#6 in Fig. 27.1) are often difficult to distinguish from other optic tract lesions, but usually present with a visual field defect and an intact contralateral afferent pupillary reflex because lesions at this level normally spare the retinal fibers terminating in the pretectum responsible for the afferent pupillary reflex.

Cortical projections from both LGN form a prominent set of white matter bundles called the optic radiations. It is worth noting that the ventral bundle makes an anterior loop (called Meyer's loop) to travel around the lateral ventricle before reaching V1 in the calcarine occipital cortex. This explains why more anterior lesions can produce visual field loss in the upper contralateral sector (#8 in Fig. 27.3). Further along, lesions involving the posterior optic radiation (#9–#11 in Fig. 27.3) or the visual cortex also result in homonymous hemianopia, but often with sparing of the central, macular field. Several hypotheses have been put forward to explain macular sparing, but in many patients macular sparing is likely more apparent than real because it is likely an artifact of visual field testing caused by poor foveal fixation or eye movements. In other patients in whom macular sparing is not artifactual, the most likely explanation is the immense areal dimension (magnification) of the cortical representation of the retinal fovea in the far posterior of primary visual cortex above and below the calcarine sulcus. The posterior cerebral artery supplies the occipital poles, but in some individuals they are supplied by both the posterior and middle cerebral arteries. Thus infarcts of the posterior cerebral artery would

affect only part of the occipital poles, sparing portions of the foveal representation and sparing macular vision. Finally, also of clinical relevance, certain lesions of the anterior calcarine cortex that represents the far peripheral contralateral visual field can lead to the "monocular occipital temporal crescent syndrome" (#12 in Fig. 27.3). This is because this region of the visual field is represented by one eye only, as a consequence of the greater extent of the temporal visual field and slight bias in weight of nasal retinal projections.

Before concluding this chapter it is appropriate to mention that direct knowledge of the human central visual pathways has improved dramatically in the past 30 years as a result of major advances in noninvasive neuroimaging, such as structural and functional MRI. For example, diffusion tensor imaging (DTI) of white matter tracts is allowing unprecedented visualization of the optic radiations in single subjects (Fig. 27.4, with permission from Hofer et al., see also Box 27.3 on DTI). Work still needs to be done to refine and validate these techniques, but the ultimate impact will be substantial. Similarly, functional MRI (fMRI) makes possible retinotopic localization of many visual areas beyond primary visual cortex with only a few hours of testing. We need only consider that prior to this era of human neuroimaging, the state-of-the-art method for localizing such boundaries was to complete weeks of laborious postmortem histologic analysis of very rare patient samples (e.g.,[21]). Now, human neuroimaging data can be compared with and sometimes directly validated by experiments in animal models. It should become evident in the next chapters considering the LGN, primary visual cortex, and extrastriate cortex that this fruitful exchange of ideas between clinical and experimental work is ongoing.

In summary, and in anticipation of the following chapters, we recap as follows. Starting with the many different types of ganglion cells that are suggested by genetic analysis, the central visual pathways continue to segregate many important parallel features, such as

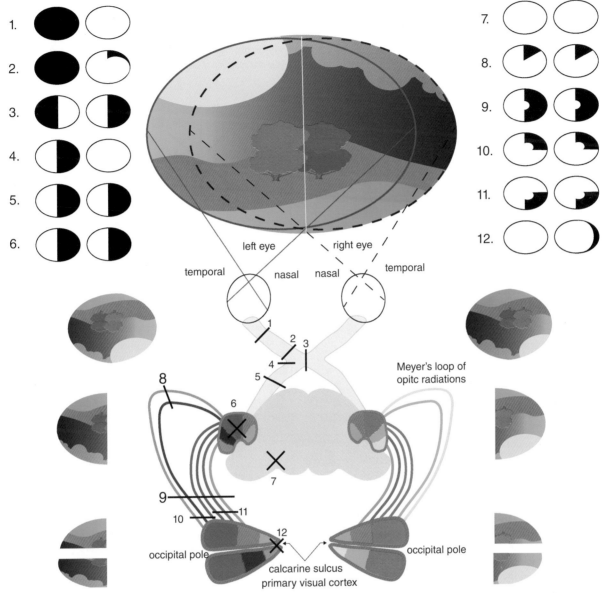

Fig. 27.3 Schematic description of retinotopic pathways and visual field lesions.

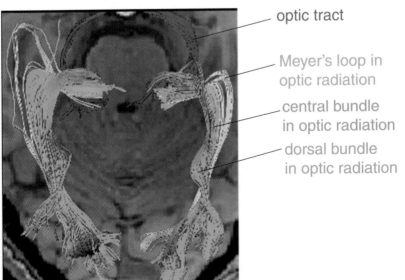

Fig. 27.4 Diffusion tensor imaging of optic tract and optic radiations in a single subject, with permission from Hoffer et al., 2010.

BOX 27.1 Central targets of the optic nerves

- Lateral geniculate nucleus
- Superior colliculus
- Pretectum
- Pulvinar
- Hypothalamic nuclei
- Accessory optic system

BOX 27.2 Blindsight

Blindsight is a phenomenon in which people with lesions of primary visual cortex and hemifield defects are unconsciously aware of visual stimuli presented in their blind hemifield. Methodology used to obtain these results may be responsible for the apparent visual awareness and thus the concept of blindsight is surrounded heavily by controversy. However, when methodology can be ruled out, blindsight has been explained by the existence of retinal inputs to central targets other than the LGN, specifically the superior colliculus and pulvinar, and their projections to extrastriate cortical areas,[22] or by direct connections from the LGN to motion-sensitive extrastriate cortical regions.[23] Blindsight is discussed in more detail in Chapters 29 and 31.

BOX 27.3 Diffusion tensor imaging

Diffusion tensor imaging (DTI) is an important brain imaging modality that is already playing a clinical role in ophthalmology in terms of diagnosis, prognosis, and selection of biomarkers.

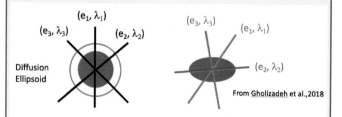

From Gholizadeh et al.,2018

FA = the ratio of anisotropic to isotropic diffusion
MD = $(\lambda 1 + \lambda 2 + \lambda 3)/3$
RD = $(\lambda 2 + \lambda 3)/2$
AD = $\lambda 1$ (largest eigenvalue)

DTI allows for advanced visualization of white matter tracts across the brain by measuring the diffusion of water along axon clusters; this is sensitive to both cellular and microstructural changes.[24] Each voxel measured from a DTI volume can be represented by an ellipsoid with three principal axes and eigenvectors (see figure). The longest axis, which runs parallel to the measured axon, is referred to as axial diffusivity (AD), while the mean of the two perpendicular axes is referred to as the radial diffusivity (RD). AD and RD measures have already shown value in diagnosing axonal damage and myelin damage, respectively.[25,26] Aside from these principal eigenvector-based measures, two additional global measures are derived from the three principal axes, specifically fractional anisotropy (FA) and mean diffusivity (MD—identical to the apparent diffusion coefficient). FA is a scale of the relative anisotropic to isotropic nature of the diffusion, with perfectly isotropic diffusion having a value of 0 and perfectly anisotropic diffusion having a value of 1. FA is argued to be quite sensitive in detecting white matter integrity as it is decreased when the axonal architecture is disrupted and when there is a loss of myelin,[24] and thus represents a loss of organized structure and coherent diffusion.[27,28] This is because many factors, including cell death, changes in myelination, and intra/extracellular water, may affect FA. MD, however, has been proposed to be the simplest and potentially the most useful DTI derived scalar,[29] representing the average of all principal eigenvalues. An increased MD is common with damaged tissue because of the resulting increase of free diffusion,[27] and a relatively high MD can characterize a high level of disorganization, while a low MD represents a highly organized structure. Finally, it is possible to use DTI-based tractography methods to reconstruct complete fiber tracts in three dimensions, like that shown in Fig. 27.4. The method is impressive, but still faces challenges in resolving crossing fibers in complex structures (like Meyer's loop). Nevertheless, methodology continues to advance, and significant clinical impact will only increase in the future.[30–34]

eye of origin, visual field location, and several distinct LGN neuron types (Chapter 29). The central visual pathways are also generally recurrent, and often maintain feedforward, lateral, and feedback connections between sites at different hierarchical levels. At the level of primary visual cortex, new segregations emerge such as selectively for the orientation of contrast edges (Chapter 30). Beyond V1, additional retinotopic cortical areas are often categorized into two functional networks (dorsal or ventral) with at least partially different functional specializations (visually driven action or pattern recognition, respectively) but, again, there is significant cross-talk, and substantial feedback connections (Chapter 31). A final important theme is the gradual increase in the amount of visual information necessary to maximally activate neurons at progressively higher tiers of the visual system. From LGN to higher-tier extrastriate areas, we will see that neurons integrate larger portions of the visual field, and achieve sensitivity to increasingly complex features. This is the crowning achievement of the global perception that enables navigation and object classification of our complex world.

ACKNOWLEDGMENTS

A previous version of this chapter was written by Joanne A. Matsubara and Jamie D. Boyd. Portions of the current text were adapted from the previous version. Austin C. Cooper assisted with Box 28.3.

REFERENCES

1. Andrews TJ, Halpern SD, Purves D. Correlated size variations in human visual cortex, lateral geniculate nucleus, and optic tract. *J Neurosci*. 1997;17(8):2859–2868.

2. Kupfer C, Chumbley L, De J, Downer C. Quantitative histology of optic nerve, optic tract and lateral geniculate nucleus of man. *J. Anat*. 1967;101(Pt 3):393–401.

3. Munoz DP, Dorris MC, Paré M, Everling S. On your mark, get set: brainstem circuitry underlying saccadic initiation. *Can J Physiol Pharmacol*. 2000;78:934 2000 11100942.

4. Schall JD. Neural basis of saccade target selection. *Rev Neurosci*. 1995;6(63):7633641:63–85.

5. Rodieck RW, Watanabe M. Survey of the morphology of macaque retinal ganglion cells that project to the pretectum, superior colliculus, and parvicellular laminae of the lateral geniculate nucleus. *J Comp Neurol*. 1993;338:289–303 8308173.

6. Basso MA, Bickford ME, Cang J. Unraveling circuits of visual perception and cognition through the superior colliculus. *Neuron*. 2021;109(6):918–937.

7. Bogadhi AR, Katz LN, Bollimunta A, Leopold DA, Krauzlis RJ. Midbrain activity shapes high-level visual properties in the primate temporal cortex. *Neuron*. 2021;109(4):690–699.

8. Smithson HE. S-cone psychophysics. *Vis Neurosci*. 2014;31(2):211–225.

9. Grieve KL, Acuna C, Cudeiro J. The primate pulvinar nuclei: vision and action. *Trends Neurosci*. 2000;23:35–9 10631787.

10. O'Brien BJ, Abel PL, Olabvarria JF. The retinal input to calbindin-D28k-defined subdivisions in macaque inferior pulvinar. *Neurosci Lett*. 312:145–148 200111602331

11. Robinson DL, Petersen SE. The pulvinar and visual salience. *Trends Neurosci*. 1992;15:127–32 1374970.

12. Lucas N, Bourgeois A, Carrera E, Landis T, Vuilleumier P. Impaired visual search with paradoxically increased facilitation by emotional features after unilateral pulvinar damage. *Cortex*. 2019;120:223–239.

13. Acuna C, Gonzalez F, Dominguez R. Sensorimotor unit activity related to intention in the pulvinar of behaving Cebus apella monkeys. *Exp Brain Res*. 1983;52:411–22 6653702.

14. Cudeiro J, González F, Pérez R, Alonso JM, Acuña C. Does the pulvinar-LP complex contribute to motor programming? *Brain Res*. 1989;484:367–70 2713694.

15. Robinson DL, McClurkin JW, Kertzman C. Orbital position and eye movement influences on visual responses in the pulvinar nuclei of the behaving macaque. *Exp Brain Res*. 1990;82:235–46 2286229.

16. Fredericks CA, Giolli RA, Blanks RH, Sadun AA. The human accessory optic system. *Brain Res*. 1988;454:116–22 3408998.

17. Schiff D, Cohen B, Buttner-Ennever J, Matsuo V. Effects of lesions of the nucleus of the optic tract on optokinetic nystagmus and after-nystagmus in the monkey. *Exp Brain Res*. 1990;79(2):225–39 2323371.

18. Moore RY. Organization of the primate circadian system. *J Biol Rhythms*. 1993;8(S3-9): 8274760.

19. Horton JC. Wilbrand's Knee: To Be or Not to Be a Knee? *J Neuroophthalmol*. 2020 Sep;40 Suppl 1(Suppl 1):S7-S14.

20. Schmid R, Wilhelm B, Wilhelm H. Naso-temporal asymmetry and contraction anisocoria in the pupillomotor system. *Grafes arch Clin Exp Ophthalmol*. 2000;238(2):123–8.

21. Clarke S, Miklossy J. Occipital cortex in man: organization of callosal connections, related myelo- and cytoarchitecture, and putative boundaries of functional visual areas. *J Comp Neurol*. 1990;298(2):188–214.

22. Stoerig P. Blindsight, conscious vision, and the role of primary visual cortex. In: Martinex-Conde S, Macknik S, Martinez L, Alonso J-M, Tse PU, eds. *Fundamentals of Awareness, Multi-Sensory Integration and High-Order Perception. Visual Perception Part 2. Progress in Brain Research*. Vol. 155. Amsterdam: Elsevier; 2006:217–234.

23. Ajina S, Bridge H. Blindsight relies on a functional connection between hMT+ and the lateral geniculate nucleus, not the pulvinar. *PLoS Biol*. 2018;16(7):e2005769.

24. Alexander AL, Lee JE, Lazar M, Field AS. Diffusion tensor imaging of the brain. *Neurotherapeutics*. 2007;4(3):316–29. 11.

25. Sbardella E, Tona F, Petsas N, Pantano P. DTI measurements in multiple sclerosis: Evaluation of brain damage and clinical implications. *Multe Scler Int*. 2013:671730.

26. Aung WY, Mar S, Benzinger TL. Diffusion tensor MRI as a biomarker in axonal and myelin damage. *Imaging in Medicine*. 2013;5(5):427–440.

27. Soares JM, Marques P, Alves V, Sousa N. A hitchhiker's guide to diffusion tensor imaging. *Frontiers in Neuroscience*. 2013:7:31.

28. Stebbins G, T. Diffusion tensor imaging in Parkinson's disease. *Encyclopedia of Movement Disorders*. Elsevier. 2010;Volume 1:308–310.

29. O'Donnell LJ, Westin C-F. An introduction to diffusion tensor image analysis. *Neurosurgery Clinics of North America*. 2011;22(2):185–196.

30. Calabrese E. Diffusion tractography in deep brain stimulation surgery: A review. *Front Neuroanat*. 2016;10:45.

31. Setsompop K, Fan Q, Stockmann J, et al. High-resolution in vivo diffusion imaging of the human brain with generalized slice dithered enhanced resolution: Simultaneous multislice (gSlider-SMS). *Magn Reson Med*. 2018;79(1):141–151.

32. Curcio CA, Allen KA. Topography of ganglion cells in human retina. *J Comp Neurol*. 1990;300(1):5–25 2229487.

33. Gholizadeh N, Greer PB, Simpson J, et al. Characterization of prostate cancer using diffusion tensor imaging: A new perspective. *Eur J Radiol*. 2019;110:112–120.

34. Markwell EL, Feigl B, Zele AJ. Intrinsically photosensitive melanopsin retinal ganglion cell contributions to the pupillary light reflex and circadian rhythm. *Clin Exp Optom*. 2010;93(3):137–149.

28

Optic Nerve

Jeffrey L. Goldberg

Introduction

The optic nerves carry the axons of retinal ganglion cells (RGCs), and these axons transmit all the visual information from the inner retina to the brain. The retina and optic nerve are developmentally an outgrowth of the forebrain, and, like other white matter tracts of the central nervous system (CNS), the optic nerve does not repair itself after most types of injury. Thus, diseases that affect the optic nerve commonly cause vision loss, and blindness from optic nerve injury or degenerative disease is typically irreversible. This chapter reviews the principal aspects of optic nerve anatomy, development, and physiology, and discusses the pathologic changes at the molecular and cellular levels in the context of clinical disease.

OPTIC NERVE ANATOMY

Retinal ganglion cell axons within the nerve fiber layer

RGC axons begin at the RGC cell bodies in the innermost layer of the retina. Although most neurons in this layer are RGCs and the layer is commonly referred to as the *ganglion cell layer*, in humans approximately 3% of cells in the central retina and up to 80% in the peripheral retina may be other cell types, primarily "displaced" amacrine cells.[1] In addition, studies in mammals have demonstrated the presence of "displaced" RGCs located in the inner nuclear layer.[2] As discussed in Chapter 21, each RGC receives input from bipolar cells and amacrine cells, and projects its axon toward the vitreous, whereupon the axon turns approximately 90 degrees and projects toward the optic nerve head in the nerve fiber layer. The nerve fiber layer is not quite radially arranged around the optic nerve head (optic disc), as axons temporal to the foveal center of the retina course away from the fovea, and then toward the optic disc, entering in the superior and inferior portions of the disc (Fig. 28.1). This interesting anatomy prevents axons from crossing the high-sensitivity fovea, where they might otherwise scatter light and degrade visual acuity. The axons from more peripheral RGCs are more superficial (vitread) to those arising from less peripheral ganglion cells[3] (Fig. 28.2). In addition, there is strict segregation of those fibers arising from RGCs located superior to the temporal horizontal meridian (raphe) and those fibers arising from RGCs located inferior to the horizontal raphe. Because of this anatomical segregation of nerve fiber bundles, visual field defects corresponding to RGC axon injury typically have stereotyped patterns, for example, superior or inferior nasal steps, temporal wedges, or arcuate scotomas, that do not cross the horizontal meridian (Box 28.1).

Intrascleral optic nerve

The optic nerve itself is considered to begin at the optic nerve head which, when viewed through the front of the eye, is observed as the optic disc. There is an approximately 1 mm component of optic nerve within the intrascleral part of the globe, which includes the lamina cribrosa (Fig. 28.3). Once at the optic disc, ganglion cell axons turn away from the vitreous and dive into the optic disc toward the brain. Axons arising from more peripheral RGCs are peripheral within the optic nerve head.[4] The optic disc contains the nerve fibers around its edge, the neuroretinal rim, and the central cup, which does not contain RGC axons. The cup-to-disc ratio may range from 0 to 1.0, depending on natural variation in the size of the disc, and whether there is less than a full complement of axon fibers, for example, as a result of damage from glaucomatous optic neuropathy (see further in chapter). More updated estimates of the complement of axon-containing tissue entering the intrascleral optic nerve include the *Bruch's membrane opening minimum rim width*, typically measured from ocular coherence tomography (OCT) imaging.[5,6]

Intraorbital optic nerve

The optic nerve extends approximately 30 mm from the globe to the optic canal.[7] The straight-line distance from the back of the globe to the optic canal is much less (the exact amount depending on individual orbital depth), with the excess optic nerve laxity allowing for free movement of the globe during eye movements. In some cases excessive proptosis of the globe stretches the optic nerve tautly, resulting in direct injury to or even avulsion of the nerve itself. Beginning behind the globe, the nerve is ensheathed by the layered meninges extending from the brain, bathing the optic nerve in cerebrospinal fluid and providing vascular support along the length of the nerve (see further).

The initially retinotopic correspondence of optic nerve fibers to retinal location, including the segregation between axons arising from the superior and inferior retina, is gradually lost as the axons course through the nerve (Fig. 28.2). There is only moderate retinotopy in the initial segment of the optic nerve.[8] The retinotopy decreases distally,[9,10] and then becomes ordered vertically for eventual nasal decussation near the chiasm.[11] The loss of retinotopy is not absolute, because the fibers from the nasal (but not temporal) macula continue to be located centrally within the nerve over a considerable distance.[12] Fibers from large RGCs are less retinotopically organized than those from smaller RGCs.[12] Although studies in humans are difficult to do antemortem, postmortem studies of nerves with specific visual field defects demonstrate similar findings, and postmortem studies of developing fetuses and adult eyes also show loss of retinotopy within the transition from the optic nerve head to the more distal nerve.[8,13] Within the orbit, the optic nerve travels within the muscle cone formed by the superior rectus, lateral rectus, inferior rectus, and medial rectus muscles. Tumors within the cone are common sources of compression of the optic nerve, or compressive optic neuropathy. Examples of these tumors include cavernous hemangioma, hemangiopericytoma, fibrous histiocytoma, lymphoma, and schwannoma. In addition, enlargement of the muscles themselves, particularly the inferior rectus and/or the medial rectus in Grave's ophthalmopathy, may also compress the optic nerve.

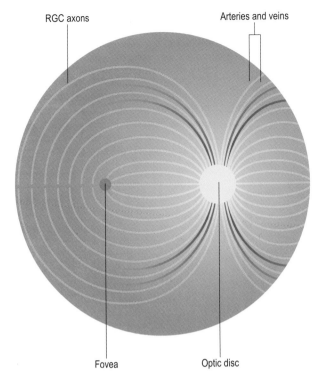

Fig. 28.1 Axons of retinal ganglion cells (*RGCs*) take a specific course through the retina, such that fibers more temporal to the fovea skirt around the edge of the macula and enter the optic nerve head closer to the superior or inferior poles. Neither the axons nor the blood vessels typically cross the horizontal meridian of the retina.

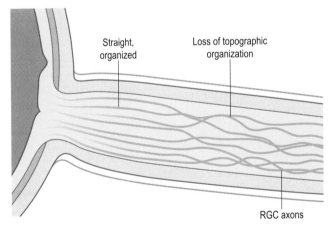

Fig. 28.2 Retinal ganglion cell (*RGC*) axons enter the optic nerve head with specific retinotopic organization (as in Fig. 28.1). With increasing distance from the optic nerve head, however, the axons become increasingly jumbled, losing their topographic organization. Thus focal damage to nerve at the nerve head will produce specific retinotopic defects, while focal damage to axons further posterior to the eye will produce scotomas that lack retinotopic organization.

The optic canal

The optic nerve enters the cranium via the optic canal, a 5- to 12-mm passage that lies immediately superonasal to the superior orbital fissure.[14] The optic canal contains some axons of sympathetic neurons destined for the orbit, as well as the ophthalmic artery. The latter lies

immediately inferolateral to the optic nerve itself, covered in dura. At the distal end of the canal, there is a half-moon–shaped segment of dura which overhangs the optic nerve superiorly, and thereby lengthens the canal by a few millimeters. As in the intraorbital portion of the optic nerve, within and immediately posterior to the optic canal, meningeal tissue ensheathes the optic nerve. Benign tumors of the meninges, or meningiomas, are frequent causes of compressive optic neuropathies in these locations. Small tumors within the canal itself, where there is very little free space, may lead to compressive optic neuropathy without a radiographically visible tumor.

Intracranial optic nerve and the optic chiasm

Once the nerve has entered the cranium, there is a highly variable length of nerve (8–19 mm, mean of 12 mm) until the optic chiasm is reached.[15] The length of the chiasm itself is approximately 8 mm. The intracranial optic nerve and chiasm are immediately above the planum sphenoidale and sella turcica, the latter of which contains the pituitary gland. There is approximately 10 mm between the inferior part of the nerve and the superior part of the pituitary. Tumors of the pituitary that increase its size enough to impinge upon the chiasm cause compressive optic neuropathy.

At the optic chiasm, RGC axons from the temporal retina remain ipsilateral, and those from the nasal retina cross the chiasm and course toward the contralateral brain; in humans this ratio has been estimated at 47% ipsilateral anatomically[16] and 48% ipsilateral functionally.[17] This small difference between the number of crossing and noncrossing fibers is commonly reported to be responsible for the relative afferent pupillary defect seen in disorders of the optic tract, in which an afferent pupillary defect is seen contralateral to the injured tract, but may reflect the fact that some fibers from specialized cells within the retina responsible for the pupillary reflex may cross from the temporal retina into the contralateral optic tract.[17]

The optic tract and lateral geniculate nucleus

Although the optic nerve ends anatomically at the chiasm, the RGC axons continue within the optic tract to the lateral geniculate nucleus (LGN), superior colliculus, pretectal nuclei, or hypothalamus (see further). Circuitry and processing by some of these targets are discussed in Chapters 27 and 29.

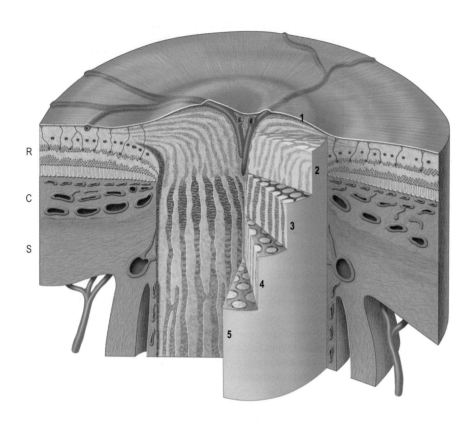

Fig. 28.3 The optic nerve head is at various points adjacent to retina (*R*), choroid (*C*), and sclera (*S*), and demonstrates a varied cellular morphology along this distance. (*1*) Superficial nerve fiber layer; (*2*) anterior prelaminar region; (*3*) posterior prelaminar region; (*4*) laminar region; (*5*) retrolaminar region. (Scheme 1 in Trivino A, Ramírez JM, Salazar JJ, Ramírez AI, Garcia-Sánchez J. Immunohistochemical study of human optic nerve head astroglia. *Vision Res.* 1996;36(14):2015–2028.)

OPTIC NERVE AXON COUNTS AND DIMENSIONS

In the normal adult human optic nerve, manual techniques have demonstrated an estimated 1,200,000 RGC axons per nerve.[18–20] There is a strong correlation between the size of the neuroretinal rim and the number of axons,[20,21] and between the number of axons and the size of the scleral canal in primates,[22] although the degree of correlation is controversial.[20,23]

Many factors affect the number of axons within the optic nerve, from inherited differences to damage from diseases, i.e., optic neuropathies (see further in chapter). In addition, there is a gradual loss of RGCs during normal human aging, with approximately 5000 to 7000 axons lost per year of life.[18,19,24,25] For unclear reasons, there is a smaller degree of loss of macular RGCs with age compared with peripheral RGCs, and this may reflect contraction of the macula with time.[26]

Although the number of RGC axons entering the optic nerve is fairly constant, the diameter of the optic nerve varies widely. At the disc itself, where the fibers are completely unmyelinated, the mean vertical diameter of the disc is 1.9 mm (range 1.0–3.0 mm) and the mean horizontal diameter is 1.7–1.8 mm (range 0.9–2.6 mm).[21,27] The mean area of the disc is 2.7 mm² (range 0.8–5.5 mm²). The mean area of the neuroretinal rim (not including the cup) is 2.0 mm² (range 0.8–4.7 mm²). Because the axonal tissue entering the optic disc varies much less than the size of the optic disc itself, the optic cup in the center of the disc can vary greatly without necessarily reflecting any underlying deficit in the number of RGC axons. The diameter of the optic nerve approximately doubles posterior to the globe as a result of myelination of the axons.

MICROSCOPIC ANATOMY AND CYTOLOGY

Axons

There are no other neuronal cell bodies within the optic nerve, making it a pure white matter tract of the CNS. Although the optic nerve itself may contain other small nerves, particularly tiny peripheral nerves (branches of the trigeminal system) which carry pain sensation or control vascular tone, the vast majority of the optic nerve is composed of the approximately 1,200,000 axons of the RGCs. Optic nerve axons are collected in fascicles, which are separated by pia-derived septa. The number of fascicles ranges from approximately 50 to 300, maximal immediately retrobulbar and at the optic canal.[28] The mean axon diameter is slightly less than 1 μm, with a unimodal skewed distribution. Compared with the optic tract, there is relatively little segregation of axons by size within the optic nerve, except for a tendency for thinner axons to be located inferocentrotemporally.[9,29]

There is variability of axonal diameter and myelin thickness from the retina to the brain. Studies in other mammals show that the diameters of the largest axons increase as the distance from the retina increases.[30] The diameter of individual axons is regulated by multiple factors including oligodendrocytes[31] and electrical activity,[32] increases during development, and decreases during aging, either through loss of large-diameter axons[33] or from a general, aging-induced atrophy.

Oligodendrocytes and myelin

Conduction of nerve impulses down the axons in the optic nerve depends on the presence of myelin, a fatty, multilaminated structure which insulates each axon and greatly increases the speed and efficiency of conduction (discussed further). The RGC axons in the retrolaminar optic nerve are completely myelinated under nonpathologic circumstances (Fig. 28.4). The occasional axons of the peripheral nervous system running within the adventitia of the central retinal artery and in the outer dura may be nonmyelinated or myelinated by peripheral nerve Schwann cells.[34,35] Each axon is myelinated with several lamellae of myelin bilayers, the number of which vary from axon to axon but in proportion to the diameter of the axon.[36] Individual oligodendrocytes elaborate an average of 20 to 30 processes per oligodendrocyte, and each process myelinates 150 to 200 microns of axon length.[37]

Oligodendrocytes and axons regulate each other during development and throughout adulthood. Oligodendrocytes depend on the presence of axons for their survival[38] and production of myelin proteins.[39] Axons regulate oligodendrocyte survival and proliferation, and thus their number, through expression of specific signaling proteins[40] and through axonal electrical activity,[41] thus controlling oligodendrocyte numbers to match the number of axons.[42] Conversely, axons are signaled by oligodendrocytes to regulate axon diameter, and to prevent axons sprouting or branching within the optic nerve.[31,43] Later, in the adult, oligodendrocytes and myelin are partially responsible for inhibition of axon regeneration after optic nerve damage or degeneration (see further).[44,45]

Astrocytes

Astrocytes, named for their stellate appearance, are ubiquitous glial components of the CNS and function in white matter tracts such as the optic nerve to regulate ionic and energy homeostasis. Astrocytes are highly efficient at transporting potassium, and increases in the level of extracellular potassium as a result of axon repolarization are buffered by astrocytes. Their ability to accumulate glycogen may allow them to serve as an energy source for the optic nerve in the absence of glucose (e.g., ischemia), by shuttling lactate to adjacent axons,[46] a mechanism that may play a role in injury response.[47] Astrocytes form the glial-limiting membrane,[48] and their processes are concentrated at the nodes of Ranvier and in contact with nearby capillaries. This positions the astrocyte to play a role in transportation of substances between the local circulation and the axons; in inducing endothelial cells to form the blood-brain barrier[49]; and perhaps in signaling blood vessels to dilate or constrict according to local metabolic needs. Astrocytes also mediate connectivity between optic nerve axons and the adjacent connective tissues, such as the pial septa, the adventitia of the central retinal artery and vein, and the pia in a layer named the glial mantle of Fuchs.[34] Recent data in rodents suggest that optic nerve head astrocytes also play a role in phagocytosing discarded material from axons, including extruded degenerating mitochondria.[50]

Interestingly, the most common intrinsic tumor of the optic nerve is astrocytoma, or optic nerve glioma. This is usually a low-grade tumor of well-differentiated astrocytic cells that appear hair-like, or "pilocytic." Pilocytic astrocytomas are usually seen in childhood and have a favorable prognosis. They are also commonly seen in association with neurofibromatosis. Rarely, more malignant neoplasms of astrocytic origin develop in adults. These resemble the higher-grade astrocytic neoplasms found elsewhere in the CNS, and are usually fatal.

Microglia

Microglia, a type of resident macrophage, are an important cellular component of the optic nerve. Although their origin was debated for decades, they have been shown experimentally to be of peripheral, bone marrow origin, and are not derived from the neuroectoderm that yields neurons, astrocytes, and oligodendrocytes.[51,52] Microglia share several markers with macrophages, with both having Fc receptors (for immunoglobulin), C3 receptors (for complement), binding of Griffonia isolectin B4, and antigenicity for F4/80 and ED1 monoclonal antibodies.[53] In the human optic nerve, microglia can be seen at 8 weeks after conception, when they are relatively undifferentiated. Microglia become more differentiated during fetal development, going from tuberous to amoeboid to a ramified morphology.[54] They are associated with axon bundles, but not necessarily with blood vessels, and are found in both the nerve parenchyma and its meninges. Nerve and meningeal microglia are similar ultrastructurally except for vacuoles and endoplasmic reticulum in the former. This may be due to their phagocytosis of dying axons during development.[55] Microglia

share several characteristics of immune capacities of macrophages. By phagocytosing extracellular material, degradation within intracellular compartments can occur. This may be followed by antigen presentation on the cell surface. In combination with certain histocompatibility antigens, this presented antigen can cause stimulation of T lymphocytes and subsequent immune system activation (see further).

Meninges and meningothelial cells

The optic nerve is covered with three layers of meninges: dura, arachnoid, and pia. The meninges can also be divided up into *pachymeninges* (dura) and *leptomeninges* (arachnoid and pia). The outermost dura is a thick fibrovascular tissue, which is in immediate contiguity with the sclera, the periorbita, and the dural layer of the lining of the cranial contents. The middle arachnoid layer is a loose, thin, fibrovascular tissue. The innermost pia is a thin, tightly adherent layer with extensions into the nerve itself forming the pial septae, through which the fascicles of ganglion cell axons course.[28] In the optic canal, there are numerous trabeculae connecting the dura through the arachnoid to the pia, which reduce the free space of the nerve sheath in this area.[56]

The space between the dura and arachnoid is the subdural space, while the space between the arachnoid and pia is the subarachnoid space. The subdural space around the optic nerve is small, and is not in communication with the intracranial subdural space. Meningothelial cells may have several functions[57] including that of wound repair and scarring, phagocytosis, and collagen production. The subarachnoid space, on the other hand, is in communication with the intracranial subarachnoid space. The optic nerve subarachnoid space ends anteriorly within a blind pouch just before the optic disc. There is an appreciable pressure within the subarachnoid space, measuring from 4 to 14 mmHg.[58] This extension of the subarachnoid space from the brain into the orbit explains why elevated intracranial pressure may cause compression of the optic nerve by elevating the hydraulic pressure, and differences between intracranial pressure and intraocular pressure (IOP), measured across the thin tissue of the optic nerve head, are now linked to the pathophysiology of glaucoma.[59–61]

BLOOD SUPPLY

Optic nerve head

Studies of histologic sections and of corrosion casting of the vessels themselves have added greatly to our understanding of the optic nerve blood supply[62] (Fig. 28.5). The ophthalmic artery provides the major vascular supply to the inner retina and optic nerve. The central retinal artery branches off from the intraorbital ophthalmic artery and enters the optic nerve approximately 12 mm behind the globe. In the retina, RGC bodies and the nerve fiber layer are supplied by capillary branches derived primarily from the central retinal artery arising out of the optic nerve head. As it branches on the optic disc into the retinal arterioles, the central retinal artery provides partial perfusion of the superficial optic disc via small capillaries. Along the optic nerve itself, however, the central retinal artery provides minimal perfusion of the nerve.[63]

In contrast, branches of the medial and lateral short posterior ciliary arteries, originating from the ophthalmic artery, as well as the choroid, provide the major blood supply to the optic nerve head. Their branches perfuse the optic nerve, both anteriorly via direct branches and posteriorly via a retrograde arteriolar investiture of the optic nerve (see further). Anastomoses of posterior ciliary artery branches form the circle of Zinn-Haller,[64,65] which contributes significant perfusion to the optic nerve head. In addition, there are contributions from recurrent choroidal arterioles to the prelaminar and laminar optic nerve head, and contributions from recurrent pial arterioles to the laminar and retrolaminar optic nerve head. A clinical implication of

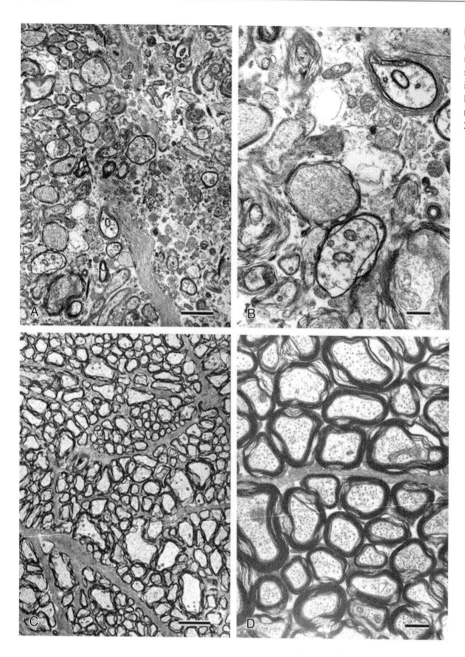

Fig. 28.4 Transverse sections through the adult rat optic nerve demonstrate typical profiles of myelinated axons and the fibrous glial septae that separate bundles of axons. Scale bars are 4 μm in panels A and C, and 500 nm in panels B and D. (From Figure 3 in Gong H, Amemiya T. Optic nerve changes in zinc-deficient rats. *Exp Eye Res.* 2001;72:363–369.)

the common posterior ciliary arterial source of the choroid and deep optic nerve head is that they will fluoresce simultaneously during the earliest phase of fluorescein angiography, before the retinal arterioles transit dye.

Unlike the choroidal vessels, which have fenestrated endothelial cells, optic nerve vessels have nonfenestrated endothelial cells with tight junctions, surrounded by pericytes. Optic nerve vessels therefore share the same blood-nerve barrier characteristics as the blood-brain barrier. Only a restricted number of molecules can cross the blood-nerve barrier. For example, gadolinium enhancement on magnetic resonance imaging is not seen unless there is some pathologic process within the optic nerve that would disrupt the blood-nerve barrier, for example, inflammation.[66,67] Another major difference between choroidal and optic nerve head vessels is that only the latter can autoregulate, i.e., maintain approximately constant blood flow despite most changes in intravascular or extravascular (intraocular) pressure.[68–70] Thus there is compensation of perfusion for a wide range of IOPs in normal individuals. A dysregulation in optic nerve head autoregulation, and any

ischemia that would follow, may contribute to the pathophysiology of glaucoma (see further).

Intraorbital optic nerve and optic canal

The intraorbital optic nerve is perfused primarily by the pial circulation, which branches from the ophthalmic artery either directly or indirectly via recurrent branches of the short posterior ciliary arteries. The pia sends penetrating vessels into the intraorbital optic nerve along the fibrovascular pial septae, from which a capillary network extends into neural tissue (axons and glia). Similarly, the intracanalicular optic nerve is perfused by up to three branches of the ophthalmic artery, namely a medial collateral, lateral collateral, and ventral branch,[71,72] which perfuse the pial surface and then penetrate the nerve. An important clinical implication of the pial supply relates to optic nerve sheath meningiomas. If a surgeon strips the meningioma away from the nerve, then the pia will also be removed, resulting in loss of the blood supply to the nerve and possible infarction and blindness. Another clinical correlation is related to the small amount of free space within the canal,

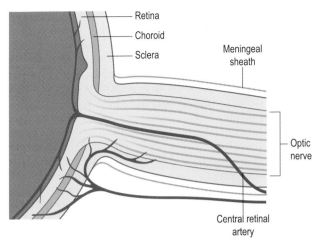

Fig. 28.5 Vascular anatomy of the optic nerve head. The optic nerve is supplied by branches from the central retinal artery, from penetrating meningeal arterioles, from recurrent arterioles off of the inner retinal vasculature, and from diffusion from the fenestrated blood supply of the choroid.

which when occupied by hematoma from shearing of the delicate vessels there may result in a sight-threatening compressive hematoma[72] (and see further).

Intracranial optic nerve, chiasm, and optic tract

The intracranial optic nerve and chiasm are perfused by the internal carotid artery and its branches, primarily the anterior cerebral, the anterior communicating, and the superior hypophyseal artery. The posterior chiasm may also be perfused by branches of the posterior communicating artery. The optic tract is predominantly perfused by branches of the posterior communicating and anterior choroidal arteries. Similar to the intraorbital and intracanalicular optic nerve, the blood supply occurs via small pial penetrating vessels. However, there is no dura or arachnoid surrounding the optic nerve posterior to the optic canal, and thus the risk of infarction is not from stripping a tumor off the nerve, but from inadvertent detachment of the fine vessels during surgical manipulation.

Vascular biology

Vessels of the human optic nerve contain endothelial cells separated from pericytes by a basement membrane, with endfeet of astrocytes surrounding the two.[73] The tight junctions between endothelial cells contribute to the blood-nerve barrier, which is present in the normal optic nerve throughout its length. The anterior part of the optic nerve, however, shares a distinctive feature with the area postrema, choroid plexus, and median eminence, in that there is local disturbance of the blood-brain barrier. Although the optic nerve capillary endothelial cells in the anterior optic nerve have tight junctions, leakage can occur from adjacent choriocapillaris through the border tissue of Elschnig at the level of the lamina choroidalis.[74,75] Further leakage from this area into the subretinal space may be prevented by tight junctions between the glia making up the intermediary tissue of Kuhnt.[74,76] The blood-nerve barrier may be incompetent in focal inflammatory disorders such as optic neuritis.[77]

The optic nerve differs from almost all other areas of the CNS in that there is connective tissue around vessels.[34] The vessels are closely surrounded by morphologically specialized collagen[78] and pial fibroblasts, beyond which are astrocytic foot processes.[34,73,79] These pial septa are not a constant factor of mammalian optic nerves; rats, for example, do not have septa.

The vessels within the nerve have their own innervation. These nervi vasorum contain multiple neurotransmitters[80] including adrenergic, cholinergic, and calcitonin gene–related peptide; neuropeptide Y; substance P; and vasoactive intestinal peptide.[81] Human posterior ciliary arteries respond to the potent vasoconstrictor angiotensin II.[82]

OPTIC NERVE DEVELOPMENT

Generation of optic nerve oligodendrocytes and myelination

Oligodendrocytes develop from oligodendrocyte precursor cells (OPCs). OPCs migrate from the brain into the optic nerve, perhaps from the base of the preoptic recess, and this migration may continue during adult life.[83] The OPC has a complex regulatory mechanism, with in vitro and animal studies implicating platelet-derived growth factor (PDGF) and ciliary neurotrophic factor (CNTF). Other factors in the differential control of differentiation, division, and renewal of the stem cell population, such as basic fibroblast growth factor, are likewise involved.[84,85] An intrinsic developmental clock controls the differentiation of OPCs into oligodendrocytes,[86] after which the cell is mitotically unresponsive to PDGF.[87–91] In normal development, some OPCs persist into the adult and may participate in remyelination.[92]

After oligodendrocyte differentiation from OPCs, there is typically a short delay before myelination starts, which may be regulated by inhibitory signals from axons activating the notch signaling pathway.[93] The developmental regulation of myelination of the optic nerve and tract occurs earliest at the brain end of the optic nerve, then travels distally toward the eye, (i.e., proximally with respect to the ganglion cell axon). This is in contradistinction to myelination elsewhere in the CNS, which usually occurs from the neuron cell body outward along the axon. The brain-to-eye direction of myelination correlates with animal studies demonstrating OPC migration and then differentiation outward along the optic nerve.[94,95] In humans, oligodendrocytes are not seen in the optic nerve before 18 weeks of gestation.[94] Later, optic tract and intracranial nerve axons begin myelination at 32 weeks of gestation, with the process virtually complete at birth. The axons adjacent to the globe begin myelination only at birth; all are myelinated by about 7 months of age.[96] Further myelination continues, however, and thickening of axonal myelin may continue past 2 years or longer.

In longitudinal studies of rat optic nerve development,[97] axons that become myelinated increase in diameter. The signal for change in caliber is generated by the oligodendrocyte.[31,98] Although unmyelinated and not yet myelinated axons can conduct electrical impulses in the developing optic nerve, there is a surprising increase in conduction velocity during development, independent of diameter or myelination status, the reasons for which are unclear.[99]

Interestingly, intraretinal RGC axons are not normally myelinated in most species; indeed, there are normally no oligodendrocytes in the retina. Studies of rat optic nerve head and anterior optic nerve demonstrate an abnormal transition zone from unmyelinated axons to myelinated axons, with varying lengths and thicknesses of myelin, unusual nodal region morphology, and few normal oligodendrocytes.[100] Studies of rat optic nerve suggest that a signal found at the lamina cribrosa blocks the migration of OPCs into the retina.[101] This barrier is possibly due to the presence of specialized optic nerve head astrocytes,[83] serum factors from a focally deficient blood-nerve barrier[102,103] or the adhesion substrate tenascin.[104] In rabbits, which have no lamina cribrosa, there are axons myelinated by oligodendrocytes in the retina, and intraretinal OPCs can be identified.[101] Further, the retinal portion of the ganglion cell axon has no constitutive barrier to myelination because ganglion cell axons of retina transplanted into rat midbrain can be myelinated,[103] and OPCs injected intraretinally can differentiate and myelinate RGC axons.[105] Myelination may also be artifactually induced by injuring the retina from the scleral side. This trauma leads to migration of Schwann cells and subsequent intraretinal myelination.[106] In human eyes, myelination of part of the nerve fiber layer is occasionally seen; it is assumed that this is secondary to ectopic oligodendrocytes, although there are reports of Schwann cells myelinating intraretinal axons in the cat[107] and rat.[108] Although oligodendrogliomas within other parts of the CNS are sometimes seen, neoplasms of oligodendrocytes within the optic nerve are very rare.

Generation of optic nerve astrocytes

Astrocyte precursor cells have been considerably less well studied. Like oligodendrocytes, developmental regulation of astrocyte number is determined by RGCs.[109] Astrocyte precursor cells may depend on CNTF or leukemia inhibitory factor (LIF) for differentiation into astrocytes,[110] at which point they upregulate the expression of glial fibrillary acidic protein (GFAP), an intermediate filament protein. GFAP itself is important to optic nerve development, as transgenic mice lacking GFAP demonstrate abnormal myelination and blood-brain barriers.[111] Astrocytes may also be critical for optic nerve development in that they may serve as the substrate over which extending ganglion cell axons grow.[112]

Development of optic nerve meninges

The anatomy and development of the optic nerve meninges have been well described.[35,57] All three meningeal layers are formed from fibroblast-like cells, which vary in ultrastructural appearance from typical process-bearing fibroblasts to mesothelial cells lining the subdural and subarachnoid space. The meningeal layers are particularly rich in collagen and elastin. Trabeculae between the arachnoid and pia are formed from collagen and are lined with the same mesothelial cells that line the subarachnoid space. The most rapid proliferation of human meningeal cells during development occurs within 8 to 18 weeks of conception, with centrally located fibroblasts and peripherally located cells containing glycogen that increase during this time.[35,113] By 14 weeks, the three layers of the meninges can be distinguished. These glycogen-rich cells go on to produce large amounts of collagen, which is deposited in the dura after 14 or 15 weeks.

Axon number

Studies in animals suggest that approximately 50% to 100% excess RGCs are produced in the retina. During early development, the number of RGCs decreases by programmed cell death called apoptosis (discussed in the context of axon injury, further), in many cases because not all of the axons properly connect to their target regions within the brain.[114,115] This form of programmed cell death may be adaptive if it does not release toxic intracellular components into the extracellular environment and thereby does not affect neighboring cells that are already integrated to survive. Likewise, in humans, up to two-thirds of developing RGCs die, predominantly during the second trimester.[116]

Axon growth

Considerable progress has been made in recent years in our understanding of the development of the optic nerve, particularly at the level of molecular and cellular regulation. Axon growth requires specific extracellular signals—merely inhibiting cell death is not sufficient for inducing axon growth in developing RGCs.[117,118] The most potent signals for axon growth are the same peptide trophic factors that most strongly promote RGC survival, and multiple trophic factors can often combine to induce even greater axon growth.[118-121] The best studied peptide trophic factors for RGC axon growth are brain-derived

neurotrophic factor (BDNF), CNTF, insulin-like growth factor (IGF), basic fibroblast growth factor (bFGF), and glial cell line–derived neurotrophic factor (GDNF), although it is not clear how critical any of these are singly for axon growth during normal development.[117,122,123] Other than peptide trophic factors, extracellular matrix molecules such as laminin and heparin sulfate proteoglycans, and cell adhesion molecules such as L1 and N-cadherin are expressed in the visual pathway[124,125] and provide a critical substrate along which axons extend.[126]

Electrical activity (discussed further in the chapter) is not required for axon growth, but likely plays a role in sculpting axonal morphology. After injecting tetrodotoxin into the eye to block action potentials,[127] or in experimental mice in which synaptic release of neurotransmitters is essentially eliminated,[128] RGCs and other CNS neurons successfully elongate their axons to their targets in the absence of electrical activity. RGC activity may increase the rate of axon arborization in their target fields by stabilizing growing branches,[129-131] and may influence the specificity of local connectivity and targeting of axons.[132-134] Considerable progress has been made in understanding these molecular mechanisms for axon growth, and these have been reviewed elsewhere.[135]

Axon guidance

Optic nerve axon guidance is heavily influenced by the earliest pathfinding axons,[136] which serve as a substrate and guidance cue for the growth of the axons that follow. During development, RGC axons are guided by neuronal and glial molecules that attract and repel axonal growth cones.[137,138] For example, embryonic RGC axons are repelled by Müller glia away from deeper retinal layers into the nerve fiber layer.[139,140] Within the retina, the interesting course of retinal axons in the macular nerve fiber layer is likely due to a foveal repellant combined with an optic disc attractant.[141] RGC axons are directed centrally in the retina away from chondroitin sulfate proteoglycans (CSPGs)[142] and are attracted into the optic nerve head by netrins.[143,144] A semaphorin, sema5A, may contribute to keeping the developing axons within the substance of the developing optic nerve.[145] Ipsilateral-projecting axons are repelled at the optic chiasm by Slit1 and Slit2,[146] ephrin-B,[147,148] and CSPGs.[149] The developmental ordering of the axons as they pass through the chiasm and go on to innervate the LGN primarily reflects their time of arrival.[150,151]

RGC axons reach four main targets: (1) the LGN of the thalamus; (2) the superior colliculus; (3) the pretectal nucleus; and (4) the suprachiasmatic nucleus, although several other targets exist.[152] Most axons course unbranched to the LGN, but studies in many animals,[153] including primates,[154] have demonstrated the existence of axon collaterals to the other targets, suggesting that the same may be true for human optic nerves.

The LGN is the primary synaptic target for visual information processing on the way to the visual cortex (discussed at length in Chapter 29). The primate LGN has six layers: layers 1 and 2 consist of large (magnocellular) cells, and layers 3, 4, 5, and 6 consist of small (parvocellular) cells. The magnocellular layers receive input from the midget RGCs, while the parvocellular layers receive input from the parasol RGCs. Layers 2, 3, and 5 receive input from the ipsilateral retina, while layers 1, 4, and 6 receive input from the contralateral retina. In addition, there are interlaminar cells forming the koniocellular layers. These cells are smaller than those of the parvocellular layers, and receive synaptic input in part from blue-yellow RGCs.[155]

A second set of optic nerve axons project to the superior colliculus, a paired structure of the dorsal midbrain. In lower animals, for example, rodents, the majority of fibers of the optic nerve project to the superior colliculus. In primates, including humans, only a minority does so, with the majority of axons destined instead for the LGN.[156] The superior colliculus has a laminar organization and is retinotopically mapped.[157] Most studies of superior colliculus architecture have been done in animals, although the human superior colliculus appears to have similar anatomy.[158] The function of the superior colliculus is to coordinate retinal and cortical control of saccades and fixation.[157] Fibers branching to midbrain terminal nuclei stabilize the retinal image during movement of the eye, head, or body.[159]

The pretectal nucleus in the midbrain receives RGC fibers important for the pupillary response.[160,161] The pretectal projection is bilateral, and in addition, fibers from each pretectal nucleus project both ipsilaterally and contralaterally to the Edinger-Westphal subnuclei of the third nerve nucleus. The latter then projects parasympathetic axons along the course of the third nerve to the ciliary ganglion within the orbit, where a synapse is made. Postsynaptic parasympathetic fibers continue to the pupilloconstrictor muscle, constriction of which is visible as the pupillary light reflex. The combined ipsilateral and contralateral projections from the retina to the pretectal nuclei, and from the pretectal nuclei to the Edinger-Westphal subnuclei necessitate that a light stimulus causing impulses along either optic nerve will cause equal constriction of both pupils. This is the physiologic basis for detecting an afferent pupillary defect (also called the swinging flashlight test or Marcus Gunn pupil). If there is a functional difference in the number of optic nerve axons carrying impulses from each retina, then light shined into the eye with fewer axons will cause a lesser amount of (bilaterally symmetric) pupillary constriction than light shined into the other eye. By alternating the light between the two eyes and observing the difference in pupil size dependent on which eye the light is shined into, one can detect which optic nerve is functionally conducting less than the other. This measure is highly correlated with differences in the number of surviving RGCs.[162] It has been proposed that there are differences between the myelin surrounding axons destined for the LGN and those responsible for the pupillomotor reflex because of the existence, albeit rare, of patients with demyelinative optic neuropathies and monocular blindness with preserved pupillary reflexes.[163] More details about the pupil light reflex can be found in Chapter 25.

A fourth projection of optic nerve axons is via the retinohypothalamic tract to the suprachiasmatic nucleus and the paraventricular nucleus[164–166] within the hypothalamus. These fibers are responsible for circadian control of the sleep-wake cycle (mediated by a population of intrinsically photosensitive RGCs [ipRGCs][167] that express the photopigment melanopsin[168–170]), temperature, and other systemic functions. Roles for ipRGCs are described in detail in Chapter 26.

OPTIC NERVE PHYSIOLOGY

Retinal ganglion cell electrophysiology and synaptic transmission

In the retina, RGCs receive synaptic input from bipolar and amacrine cells, which primarily use glutamate as the major excitatory neurotransmitter. RGCs have both NMDA and non-NMDA ionotropic glutamate receptors, as well as metabotropic receptors.[171–176] Other neurotransmitters modulating RGCs include GABA,[175] acetylcholine,[177,178] and aspartate (acting on NMDA receptors).[179] Within the retina itself the levels of glutamate are controlled by Müller cells, which have glutamate transporters, and which contain the enzyme glutamine synthetase, converting glutamate to the amino acid glutamine. Glutamate reuptake within the retina is necessary for maintaining appropriate RGC function.[180–183] The electrophysiology of RGCs is complex,[184–189] and is discussed at length in Chapter 23 and elsewhere.[190] RGCs themselves are glutamatergic, but they also use other neurotransmitters, including substance P and serotonin.[191–195] Furthermore, RGCs are extensively interconnected with other RGCs and amacrine cells via gap junctions, which enables sharing of electrical signals but also affects susceptibility to trauma.[196]

Axonal conduction
Action potentials

RGC axons transmit information via action potentials, which are all-or-nothing spikes of electrical activity. This is in contrast with intercellular communication within the retina, where graded potentials are predominantly used to transmit information. With action potentials, the actual amount of voltage change, (i.e., depolarization), is the same, while the number of impulses per second and the distribution of impulses within various axons is the mechanism by which visual information is carried down the optic nerve. Conduction down individual axons occurs via the same biophysical mechanisms which occur in any myelinated axon (see section on myelin further in the chapter). Variations in conduction velocity of individual axons may help coordinate conduction time between RGCs located at differing distances between their retinal location and the optic nerve.[197]

The mechanism of axonal conduction is straightforward. At rest, the inside of an axon is at a negative voltage with respect to the outside of the axon. This resting potential is negative, and primarily results from the fact that the concentration of potassium is much higher within the axon compared with its extracellular concentration. As a small number of potassium ions flow down their concentration gradient from the inside of the axon to the outside, this movement of positive charge out of the axon results in a negative potential within the axon. Outward flux of potassium continues until the charge separation becomes too great and can no longer be driven by the concentration difference between the inside and outside of the axon. The point at which the gradient for potassium concentration is balanced by the gradient for separation of charge results in an equilibrium potential for potassium. While the resting potential is primarily determined by potassium, there is also a smaller contribution from sodium flowing down its concentration gradient. In the case of sodium, the concentration in the extracellular space is high, compared with a low concentration within the axon. This concentration gradient would induce sodium to enter the axon, and movement of a small number of sodium ions results in a positive sodium equilibrium potential. However, in a resting (nondepolarizing) axon the conductance for sodium is much smaller than that for potassium, and therefore the final resting potential is weighted much more by the equilibrium potential for potassium than for sodium.

The situation changes during axonal conduction. Partial axon depolarization (resulting from an upstream section of membrane that is already depolarized—with the initial trigger starting at the axon hillock near the cell body) induces opening of voltage-sensitive sodium channels located within the membrane. These allow much greater amounts of sodium to enter the axon, and the positive sodium ions cause the axon to become more positive, (i.e., depolarized). In this case, the potential across the membrane is now weighted far more by the sodium equilibrium potential than by the potassium equilibrium potential. Increased potential within the axon rapidly affects adjacent sections of the axon and causes sodium channels in downstream areas of the axonal membrane to likewise become partially depolarized, in turn initiating the process of activating voltage-gated sodium channels. This chain of events continues down the axon, resulting in long-range transmission of an action potential.

Repolarization is the return of the axonal membrane potential to the original (negative resting potential) state and is necessary for more than a single action potential to be transmitted down the axon (while also ensuring action potentials do not propagate in the incorrect direction). Repolarization is due to the closure of the voltage-sensitive sodium channels and a transient opening of voltage-sensitive potassium channels. Once the latter occurs, the membrane resting potential is weighted more by the potassium equilibrium potential than by the sodium equilibrium potential. This results in a restoration of membrane potential to the resting state.

In the process of transmission of an action potential there is movement of sodium and potassium ions along their concentration gradients. If action potentials continued indefinitely, the sodium and potassium concentrations would reach equilibrium across the axonal membrane, resulting in loss of their concentration gradients and blocking conduction. Therefore, in order to re-establish their concentration gradients, there is a relatively slow redistribution process of these ions via the Na^+K^+-ATPase that takes place. This is a highly energy-dependent process and will fail to happen if axonal metabolism is significantly disturbed.

Role of oligodendrocytes and myelin

Myelin confers two electrophysiological functions. First, it decreases capacitance, meaning less sodium ion positive charge needs to enter the axon to depolarize the membrane. Second, it increases resistance, meaning that there is less leakage of charge across the membrane. Together, these properties decrease the amount of ionic flux needed to achieve changes in voltage across the membrane, saving on Na^+K^+-ATPase activity and thus energy needed to maintain ionic homeostasis after conduction.

Oligodendrocytes and myelin confer other critical properties for axonal conduction. Neonatal unmyelinated axons have a low density of sodium channels spread along the length of the axon, which allows a measure of axon conduction. In adults, however, ion channels are not distributed uniformly along a myelinated axon. Instead, the channels are segregated into patches located within the small areas where the axon is unmyelinated, called nodes of Ranvier.[198] Conduction in a myelinated axon, called *saltatory* conduction, becomes much faster, as depolarization "jumps" from one node to the next. The clustering of sodium channels into nodes, as well as an important developmental switch in sodium channel isoforms, are also induced by oligodendrocytes.[199-201]

Role of astrocytes

Although neurons are classically considered the only electrically active cell population in the CNS, astrocytes also have ion channels. For example, multiple voltage-sensitive sodium channels have been demonstrated in rat optic nerve astrocytes.[198,202,203] Both sodium and potassium channels have been studied electrophysiologically in cultured astrocytes.[204,205] Within the intact optic nerve, nonvesicularly released glutamate from the axon may induce glial cell spiking[206] and possibly other effects.[207] Whether ion channels or neurotransmitter receptors on optic nerve glia are physiologically important in vivo has yet to be demonstrated, but their presence suggests that optic nerve astrocytes may be more functionally specialized than previously recognized.

Axonal transport

The entire length of the RGC axon must be maintained by transporting proteins, mRNA, mitochondria, and other subcellular constituents many centimeters from the cell body, where the nucleus and most of the protein synthetic machinery resides. Axonal transport occurs in two directions, orthograde (away from the cell body and toward the brain), and retrograde (toward the cell body and away from the brain). By injecting radioactive, fluorescent, or enzymatically active macromolecular tracers into either the eye or the terminal fields of the axons, the course and timing of orthograde and retrograde transport can be determined. The rates of transport of specific moieties may vary as a function of stage of optic nerve development, suggesting a developmental

regulation of axonal transport.[208] Different rates of axonal transport may be related to differences in the motor proteins interacting with microtubules, for example, kinesin[209] for fast transport and dynein[210] for slow transport.

Fast axonal transport, at 90 to 350 mm/day,[211,212] carries several subcellular organelles, such as the vesicles of neurotransmitter used in synaptic transmission, toward the axon terminal.[213] This class of transport continues despite transection of the axon distal to the cell body, suggesting that intra-axonal components are sufficient for the process to occur. Slow axonal transport is divided into two classes, a slower class at 0.2 to 1 mm/day that carries cytoskeletal proteins, such as neurofilament proteins and the tubulins that make up microtubules,[214] and a more rapid class at 2 to 8 mm/day, which carries proteins such as actin and myosin, metabolic enzymes, and mitochondria.[215-217]

Retrograde transport occurs at about half the velocity of fast orthograde transport. Retrograde transport of neurotrophic molecules during development may signal the cell body that the axon is reaching its targets in the brain. How do growth signals at the axon get passed along to the distant cell body, where gene transcription and translation are induced to support survival and axon growth? Neurotrophin-mediated activation of Trk receptors leads to endocytosis of activated, ligand-bound receptors into clathrin-coated vesicles. These signaling endosomes carry with them the machinery of the ras-raf-MAP kinase signaling cascades, and can continue to activate these pathways once inside the cell.[218] Neurotrophin signaling endosomes may then be retrogradely transported back to the cell body along microtubules, where they can activate transcriptional regulators and induce new gene expression.[219-221]

Recent studies in rodent optic nerve have greatly expanded the characterization and understanding of the mRNAs and proteins transported down axons.[222-224] With advances in mass spectrometry and RNA sequencing, the cohort of transported proteins has been named the *axon transportome*. Differential transport of mitochondria, proteins of various classes, and mRNAs during axon development, in response to visual/electrical activity, and after injury explain changing physiology of the axon and likely the axon terminals and synapses in various brain regions.

OPTIC NERVE INJURY

Clinical implications

The optic nerve is commonly involved in disease, resulting in optic neuropathy and vision loss. Glaucoma is the most common optic neuropathy; others include inflammatory optic neuropathies such as optic neuritis associated with the demyelinating disease multiple sclerosis; ischemic optic neuropathy usually affecting older adults; and compressive optic neuropathy, commonly associated with a tumor or aneurysm. Most optic neuropathies are due to damage to the optic nerve, or pathophysiology occurring at least partially in the optic nerve.

Types of optic nerve injury
Traumatic optic neuropathy

Although traumatic optic neuropathy, particularly optic nerve transection, is one of the least common human scenarios in which RGC axons are injured, it has been the best studied animal model by far. In humans, concussive injury can indirectly traumatize the optic nerve and injure axons, as might happen after a car accident or other blunt injury. Direct transection, although rarer, might result from a foreign body such as a bullet or a fragment of broken orbital bone, or in optic nerve avulsion. In animal models, typically the optic nerve is surgically cut or crushed within the orbit behind the eye,[225] although approaches crushing the nerve intracranially[226] or traumatizing the optic nerve using concussive injury have also been studied.[227] Regenerative response is assayed by labeling RGC axons and determining whether any extend past the lesion site.[225] Interestingly, although injuring the optic nerve at increasing distances from the eye delays the onset of RGC death,[228] there may be less regenerative response with more distal injury.[229]

Ischemic optic neuropathy

Because the vascular supply to the optic nerve is complex and varies qualitatively along its course, a variety of clinical syndromes may result from ischemia or infarction at each location. Arteritic and nonarteritic anterior ischemic optic neuropathies are associated with histopathologically verifiable occlusion of posterior ciliary arteries. An infarction of the central retinal artery or one of its branches will result in RGC axon loss, with a pale disc and loss of axons within the optic nerve itself. Ischemia may also result from hypotension or severe blood loss, although the resulting pathophysiology may vary.[230,231] Finally, there is controversy as to the degree to which the effects of IOP causing axonal damage in glaucomatous optic neuropathy are an ischemic or compressive process.

The pathophysiology of myelinated axonal ischemia is complex.[232,233] The presence of myelination affects the metabolism of the axon. Because less current is necessary for depolarization to occur, less ATP is needed for transmission of action potentials. At the same time, the myelinated axon is more sensitive to anoxic damage. Although neonatal optic nerve, which is not myelinated, does not easily suffer irreversible damage from anoxia, more mature nerves from animals that have just undergone myelination are highly sensitive to anoxia. Similarly, optic nerves from *md* rats, a myelin-deficient rat strain, are sensitive to anoxia.[234] Nonetheless, even myelinated axons (white matter) are relatively less sensitive to ischemia than neuronal cell bodies (gray matter).[235]

Ischemic optic nerve injury can be modeled in experimental animals via a variety of approaches. A powerful method is to occlude the posterior ciliary arteries, best done in primate animals, but which has the disadvantage of also affecting the choroidal circulation.[236,237] Infusion of the vasoconstrictor endothelin-1 into the perineural space is a good model of subacute to chronic ischemia, and can be performed in a variety of species.[238–244] The best models involve direct vascular damage, tissue edema, and vascular compromise at the optic disc[245,246] and at the retrobulbar optic nerve.[247]

Optic neuritis and inflammation

Inflammation of the optic nerve, or optic neuritis, is the most common form of acute optic neuropathy in young and middle-aged adults, and is a frequent harbinger of multiple sclerosis.[248,249] Demyelination is the most common pathologic accompaniment of optic nerve inflammation, and conduction block owing to this or other effects of inflammation[250] is responsible for the usually temporary loss of visual function seen in patients with optic neuritis. Demyelination itself would not necessarily cause loss of RGCs, and, as in multiple sclerosis, multiple rounds of demyelination and associated inflammation may be required for axonal loss.[251–253] Axonal loss in optic neuritis has been long appreciated clinically as optic atrophy and loss of the nerve fiber layer,[254] and experimental models of optic nerve inflammation can be used to elucidate how this axonal damage occurs.[255–257] It is likely that one major effect of inflammation is on the axonal cytoskeleton, as witnessed by changes in microtubule and neurofilament organization,[257] and by changes in axonal transport.[258–260]

In cases of acquired loss of myelin, for example, in idiopathic optic neuritis, there is abnormal conduction because of the changes in resistive and capacitive properties of the membrane brought about by demyelination. This can happen via loss of the compact morphology of the myelin alone, i.e., without frank demyelination.[261] A low density of internodal sodium channels in adult optic nerve may allow some conduction after demyelination, as in optic neuritis.[262] Axonal conduction becomes slowed, however, and in some cases may be blocked ("conduction block"), both resulting in decreased visual function. Even in a completely demyelinated axon, a low density of internodal sodium channels in demyelinated optic nerve may still allow conduction.[262] Another phenomenon peculiar to demyelination is worsening of vision with heat or exercise, or *Uhthoff's phenomenon*. Increased temperature and exercise are thought to decrease the sodium channel open-time during depolarization, resulting in less charge entering the axon, and a decreased likelihood that an adjacent section of demyelinated axon will be able to depolarize enough to cause opening of its own voltage-sensitive sodium channels. This leads to temperature-sensitive conduction block.

Optic neuritis has been modeled in rat and mouse models of experimental autoimmune encephalomyelitis, in which the immune systems of rodents are stimulated to react against myelin-associated proteins. Immunization against myelin-oligodendrocyte glycoprotein (MOG) induces multiple sclerosis–like demyelination throughout the brain including in the optic nerve.[263] However, creating transgenic mice with T-cells directed against MOG or passively transferring anti-MOG T-cells in rats creates demyelinating disease largely confined to the optic nerve, mimicking optic neuritis.[264,265] In such models, RGC axons are incidentally severed and fail to regenerate and, as after optic nerve trauma, RGCs die with a 1- to 2-week delay.[266]

Compressive optic neuropathy

Compression of the optic nerve is a common clinical correlate of a large number of optic neuropathies. Besides the obvious causes such as neoplasms and aneurysms, the optic nerve can also be compressed by enlarged extraocular muscles (as in Grave's ophthalmopathy), edema (as seen with indirect traumatic optic neuropathy, in which the nerve is contused within the optic canal), or optic disc drusen. Compression intrinsic to the nerve itself may occur in some forms of glaucomatous optic neuropathy in which increased IOP may cause bowing out and shifting of the lamina cribrosa, constricting the bundles of optic nerve axons within the lamina cribrosa pores.[267] Although all three layers of meninges are present in the intraorbital and intracanalicular optic nerve, only the pia continues along the intracranial optic nerve. The clinical relevance of this is that a tumor arising from the optic nerve meninges themselves, (i.e., an optic nerve sheath meningioma), will normally continue through the optic canal but then extend along the sphenoid bone, and not along the course of the intracranial optic nerve or optic chiasm. This means that it is extremely rare for an optic nerve sheath tumor to extend toward the chiasm and thereby affect the other side. The more common way for optic nerve sheath meningiomas to become bilateral is by directly extending along the sphenoid bone meninges.

The effects of chronic experimental compression of the intraorbital optic nerve were delineated at the microscopic and ultrastructural level in a classic series of experiments by Clifford-Jones and colleagues.[268,269] They found demyelination initially, followed by remyelination, even while the axons were still compressed. There were relatively minor findings of direct axonal loss. Demyelinated axons or the direct effects of pressure might be expected to lead to conduction block, which would be reversible. This could therefore explain the remarkable return of visual function after removal of tumors compressing the optic nerve.[270]

Glaucoma

The most common optic neuropathy is glaucomatous optic neuropathy, distinguished by a distinct morphology of progressive excavation of the nerve head without significant pallor of the remaining neuroretinal rim. Within the retina, there are decreased numbers of RGC bodies in glaucoma,[271–273] and this likely reflects death by apoptosis.[274–277] The number of RGCs lost correlates with the visual field deficit.[278] In addition to the RGC body loss, there is loss of the ganglion cell axons, manifested by segmental loss of the nerve fiber layer,[279–283] increased cup-to-disc ratio, thinning of the optic nerve[284] and chiasm,[285] and changes in postsynaptic cell counts within the LGN[286–289] (the main target of RGC axons in higher animals) and even the cerebral cortex.[290,291]

A wide variety of pathologic evidence suggests that the optic disc is the primary site of injury.[292] The focal areas of optic nerve axonal injury correlate with the focal areas of cell body loss in the retina and visual field defects.[24,25] Thus the most typical glaucomatous visual field defects spread in an arcuate pattern but stop at the horizontal meridian in the nasal field. This site corresponds to the temporal raphe of the nerve fibers within the retina. The reason for this is that while there is a small distance between adjacent RGCs across the temporal raphe, the axons that correspond to these RGCs are separated by a large distance at the optic disc. In those cases when defects are seen on both sides of the horizontal meridian, it can be seen that spread has occurred in both the superior and inferior visual fields, but not directly across the meridian.

What mechanisms induce RGC death in glaucoma? Glaucoma has been extensively modeled in animals (reviewed in[293,294]). Studies of tissue from human patients with glaucoma and nonhuman primates and other mammals with experimental glaucoma confirm changes at the optic nerve head, such as with respect to bowing out of the lamina cribrosa, intra-axonal accumulation of organelles (consistent with blocked axonal transport; see Fig. 28.6), and Wallerian degeneration distal to the lamina cribrosa.[267,295,296] Whether owing to mechanical trauma of axons,[228,297–299] ischemia, generation of nitric oxide, or other causes, axonal injury causes changes in RGCs, eventually resulting in death.[292] Increased IOP perturbs rapid anterograde and retrograde axonal transport at the lamina cribrosa.[300–303] This may cause RGCs to be deprived of neurotrophic factors or other survival signals produced by brain targets.

Papilledema

Papilledema is defined as optic disc edema secondary to elevated intracranial pressure, and should not be used nonspecifically to denote disc edema. Pathologic examination of optic nerve heads with papilledema reveals intra-axonal edema, consistent with abnormalities of axonal transport. It is unclear whether the visual loss associated with chronic papilledema results from disturbances of axonal transport, or from ischemia owing to congestion of the optic nerve head, but the premise that an imbalance between the intracranial pressure and eye pressure contributes to glaucomatous injury has gained support from both animal and human data.[59–61]

Retinal ganglion cell death after optic nerve injury

Death of RGCs is the final common pathway underlying virtually all diseases of the optic nerve, including glaucomatous optic neuropathy, anterior ischemic optic neuropathy, optic neuritis, and compressive optic neuropathy. In many diseases affecting the RGC axons (e.g., glaucoma or arteritic ischemia), the visual loss is permanent, reflecting the fact that RGC loss is irreversible. In some cases (e.g., chronic compressive optic neuropathy, acute optic neuritis, or papilledema) the visual loss can be reversed when the axonal damage is relieved, presumably because RGC death has not yet occurred. Even in glaucoma, there is now evidence that there is some period of RGC electrophysiological dysfunction and visual field defects that precedes frank cell death.[304–306] However, if allowed to continue, these disorders can result eventually in permanent RGC death.

Apoptosis

A variety of techniques have been used to show that the death of RGCs after axotomy occurs by apoptosis.[228,274,307–310] Pathologic studies show condensation of the nucleus and cytoplasm, budding of the cytoplasmic membrane, cleavage of DNA into 180 to 200 bp fragments, fragmentation of the cell into membrane-bound bodies, and heterophagy of these bodies.[311,312] The apoptosis program is an intricate and sequential activation of multiple intracellular enzymes, including cysteine-dependent aspartate-directed proteases (caspases) and endonucleases regulated from the mitochondrial membrane by the Bcl-2 family of proteins. Proapoptotic family members such as Bax, Bak, and Bok are held in check by antiapoptotic members such as Bcl-2 and Bcl-xL. A third group in this family, including Bim and Bad, cannot activate apoptosis by themselves but can facilitate apoptosis by interfering with Bcl-2 or Bcl-xL's ability to regulate Bax, for example. If antiapoptotic proteins are unable to balance the proapoptotic family members, either because they are sequestered by Bim-like proteins or are in short supply due to inadequate production, the anti-apoptotic proteins will increase mitochondrial membrane permeability and enhance release of cytochrome C into the cytoplasm. Cytochrome C binds to an adaptor

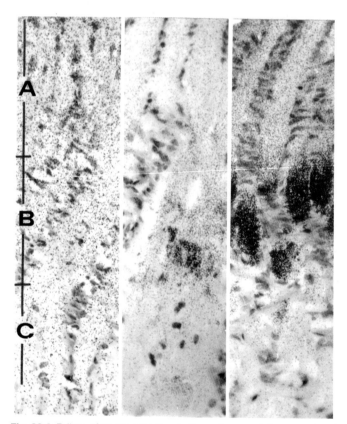

Fig. 28.6 Failure of axoplasmic flow in the optic nerve injury associated with elevated intraocular pressure (IOP). The radiographs capture the optic nerve through the prelaminar region (A), the lamina cribrosa (B), and the postlaminar orbital optic nerve (C). Optic nerves were harvested after tritiated leucine was injected into the eyes of normal monkeys *(left)*, or eyes of monkeys with moderately *(center)* or more severely *(right)* experimentally elevated IOP. With increasing IOP, increasing accumulation of radioactive label is appreciated at the lamina cribrosa, with an associated decrease in grains transported posterior to this point. (From Figures 2–4 of Anderson DR, Hendrickson A. Effect of intraocular pressure on rapid axoplasmic transport in monkey optic nerve. *Invest Ophthalmol.* 1974;13(10):771. Reproduced with permission from Association of Research in Vision and Ophthalmology.)

protein Apaf-1, forming a complex that can initiate a cascade of enzymatic degradation of cellular components by a family of enzymes called caspases, beginning with the activation of procaspase-9. Also released from the mitochondria, a protein called Smac/Diablo binds to and inactivates an antiapoptotic protein called Inhibitor of Apoptosis (IAP), which normally represses activation of procaspases. Thus by at least two mechanisms, mitochondrial permeabilization by Bax inclines the balance toward apoptosis. Once the apoptosome is formed from the factors released from the mitochondria, the activation of caspases takes place. These in turn activate other caspases, and this cascade of events results in the activation of other enzymes within the cell that results in the breakdown of DNA and other macromolecules, membrane-bound compartmentalization of cell components, and then phagocytosis by adjacent cells.

Besides axonal injury, several other modes of cell death may induce apoptosis. For example, the binding of tumor necrosis factor to tumor necrosis factor receptors may induce apoptosis via death domain signaling and subsequent activation of caspase-8, initially bypassing the caspase-9 activation by the mitochondria. Glutamate excitotoxicity may also induce apoptosis,[313] and RGCs are particularly susceptible to high levels of glutamate in the extracellular space.[176,314-316] It has been proposed that excitotoxic RGC death may explain pathologic conditions such as glaucoma.[317] The evidence supporting this is that antagonists of glutamate excitotoxicity mediated by NMDA receptors generally decrease RGC death after optic nerve injury,[318,319] and that there may be elevations of glutamate levels within the eye after optic nerve injury,[320] or experimental or human glaucoma.[321] Changes in NMDA receptor subunit expression follow axonal injury[322] and may underlie changes in susceptibility to excitotoxicity. Variability in the sensitivity of RGCs to excitotoxicity in animal models,[323] and the failure of clinical efficacy of NMDA receptor inhibition for prevention of progression in glaucoma, however, raises significant questions about this mechanism.[324]

Time course

The rate and timing of RGC death after optic nerve injury depends on the species, age, RGC body size, and subtype of RGC, and the distance from the site of injury to the RGC. For example, after optic nerve injury in goldfish and frogs, ganglion cells do not die, but hypertrophy and regenerate axons within 1 to 2 months.[325-327] Conversely, in adult rodents, optic nerve injury leads to initiation of cell death within 5 to 7 days, and 50% to 90% cell death occurring within weeks to months.[297-299,328-331] Similarly, ganglion cells from squirrel and owl monkeys die approximately 4 to 6 weeks after axotomy.[332,333] In humans with chiasmal compression for at least 6 months, there is extensive loss of ganglion cells from the nasal hemiretinas; yet even 35 days after transection of the ipsilateral optic tract there is sparing of some temporal ganglion cells.[334] In contrast, neonatal RGCs are far more sensitive to axotomy than adults,[297,335,336] perhaps because naturally occurring developmental cell death is taking place at the same time. As an example, in postnatal rodents, 90% of RGCs die within 48 hours of optic nerve crush.

There are many subtypes of RGCs, which can be defined by differences in dendrite morphology, target field innervation, electrophysiology, visual stimulus response properties, and gene expression. Different subtypes of RGCs show varying susceptibility to death after optic nerve injury in animal models of trauma or glaucoma. Originally this was discovered in animal models using measures of cell size, with data suggesting that large RGCs with alpha-type physiology die sooner after optic nerve insult.[337] These data were called into question as it was not technologically easy at the time to assess whether cells changed morphology or physiology after injury, for example, to distinguish whether

large RGCs died or atrophied to appear smaller, or similarly whether RGCs changed their physiology or response patterns after axon injury. More recent use of in vivo imaging and tracking of individual RGCs, as well as single cell RNA sequencing of RGCs over a time course after injury, have improved on these formative observations. Together these data suggest that RGCs do indeed change in size, response physiology, and gene expression after injury, confirming some of confounding results of the older data, but also suggesting that different subtypes of RGCs are indeed differentially susceptible to axon injury and death.[338] Furthermore, limited data from human electrophysiology measurements in patients with glaucoma, for example, confirm that some of the same observations from animal models are seen similarly in human disease, such as preferential loss of OFF-pathway compared with ON-pathway RGCs.[339,340]

It is controversial whether the response of ganglion cells to axotomy depends on the distance between the lesion and the cell body. Some studies have shown that the shorter that distance, the more rapid the degeneration[328,329] and the more severe the effect.[341-344] This could be due to lack of a trophic signaling along a length of residual axon or more rapid transmission of a signal mediating cell death, with either mechanism possibly mediated through retrograde axonal transport.[299,333,345] Others have suggested that the timing of ganglion cell degeneration is not correlated with the distance to the lesion.[332,333] Axotomized fibers from the macula degenerate later than those more peripheral, suggesting that the distance from the site of axotomy to the retina does not affect timing of RGC death.[333] Differences in ganglion cell survival also depend on the site of optic nerve transection in relation to the vascular supply of the retina. If the ophthalmic or central retinal arteries are transected, then the inner retina, including the ganglion cell layer, will be infarcted,[346] confusing interpretation of RGC survival.

Signaling of axonal injury

How does axonal injury result in induction of apoptosis? RGC death after optic nerve injury or target removal appears to take place through several mechanisms, including lack of neurotrophic factors from the target tissue, excitotoxicity from physiologic or pathologic levels of glutamate, free radical formation, leakage of cellular constituents from the end of the axon, proliferation of macroglia, activation of microglia, buildup of excess retrogradely transported macromolecules, and breakdown of the blood-brain barrier.[122,319,328,341,343,347-349] Even the contralateral retina may be affected by a unilateral optic nerve injury, suggesting the involvement of intrachiasmal signaling or retinopetal fibers.[350]

RGCs are highly dependent on neurotrophic factors during development and in the adult for their survival.[117] Responsiveness to neurotrophic factors also appears to require physiologic levels of electrical activity.[118] If the optic nerve is injured and CNTF or other neurotrophic factors are introduced into the vitreous or retina, there is increased survival of RGCs compared with control eyes.[31,122,123,351-353] It is possible that the increased survival seen after neurotrophin administration is not a *specific* rescue effect from neurotrophin deprivation, but rather a generalized prosurvival effect. Neurotrophic factor restoration and electrical activation have moved into clinical trials in recent years with some suggestion of positive effect,[292,354] but much work remains to be done to identify dosing and delivery regimens with consistent and meaningful effects.

Phagocytosis and immune activation

Optic nerve injury also leads to activation of local glial cells and recruitment of immune cells. For example, during Wallerian degeneration, resident microglia, as well as circulating monocytes, phagocytose myelin debris,[76] although there may be a contribution from oligodendrocytes and astrocytes.[81,108,355–357] Probably most phagocytes in the degenerating optic nerve are derived from the circulation, although not all studies are in agreement.[358,359] Deficiencies in the activation of microglia may lead to decreased clearance of myelin debris, and subsequent inhibition of axonal regeneration[360]; conversely, increasing macrophage-mediated clearance of debris can increase regeneration.[361] Broadly speaking, interfering with microglial and macrophage recruitment and activation is very effective in preventing RGC death in animal models of optic neuropathies.[362]

More recent data has strongly implicated innate immune regulation of RGC death in glaucoma models. Innate immunity is driven by many components of genetics and environment, including exposure to pathogens and formation of the gut commensal microflora (called the microbiome). Microbiome effect on neurodegeneration by way of regulation of innate immunity is now gathering support from both human research subjects and animal models. For example, in mice raised in clean environments where the relative lack of diversity in the microbiome does not stimulate innate immune recognition of certain epitopes, elevating IOP does not lead to ganglion cell death, whereas elevating IOP in mice raised in normal environments does. The link to innate immunity is demonstrated by the observation that transfer of CD4+ T-cells from the latter to the former mice leads to IOP-induced ganglion cell degeneration.[363]

Astrogliosis

The role of optic nerve astrocytes in the pathologic processes of gliosis is complex.[364,365] As a reaction either to local injury or to remote death of adjacent axons, astrocytes are observed to hypertrophy and extend processes, partly as a type of scar formation, but likely also as part of the process of recruiting or modulating other cell types. Recent data suggest that some astrocytic responses lead to neuronal death[366] whereas other astrocytic responses lead to adaptive or even neuroprotective effects.[367,368] Such so-called neurotoxic and neuroprotective astrocytes, broadly referred to as A1 and A2 astrocytes, likely represent a useful if oversimplified construct. Astrocyte activation after injury may also explain in part the failure of ganglion cell axons to regenerate after injury[45] (see further).

Failure of axon regeneration

In adult mammals, there is essentially no axon regenerative response after optic nerve injury. This contrasts with lower vertebrates—for example, not only do goldfish RGCs survive after their axons are transected,[369] but they are also able to extend neurites and ultimately establish correct connections with their targets.[370] Research in the early 20th century showed that mammalian RGCs, like other centrally projecting neurons, make only abortive attempts to regenerate their axons. Even when conditions permit axonal extension, only a small minority of RGCs eventually extend their axons. For example, severed rodent RGC axons approach the optic nerve head but then reverse and meander in another direction.[371] Analysis of the proximal stump of the transected optic nerve just posterior to the optic nerve head shows early regenerating axons, which then die off.[372]

Thus in most cases, optic nerve injury and axon loss leads to permanent vision loss. Our understanding of the mechanisms preventing axon regeneration in adult mammals continues to advance, particularly with respect to the role of inflammation, discussed previously, and of glial-associated inhibitory signals, and neuron-intrinsic limitations to axon repair, discussed further.

Glial inhibition of neurite extension

Since the early experiments of Aguayo and colleagues, it has long been known that RGCs and other CNS neurons regenerate axons into peripheral nervous system (PNS) grafts (e.g., sciatic nerve), but not into CNS tissue.[373,374] Because RGCs do not extend axons in the absence of specific extracellular signals (discussed previously), regenerative failure might be explained in part by a relative inability of mature CNS astrocytes and oligodendrocytes to secrete trophic signals after injury. Evidence has supported this hypothesis, but it turns out that astrocytes and oligodendrocytes also actively inhibit axons from regenerating. The nonpermissive nature of the CNS (but not PNS) substrate for axonal elongation is therefore of great interest and has resulted in a large number of candidate molecules. The most studied inhibitory molecules are components of oligodendrocyte myelin and proteoglycans expressed by astrocytes, and these molecules and their signaling mechanisms have been reviewed recently in detail.[375]

Resident microglia and/or macrophages recruited to the site of injury may also inhibit or fail to support axon growth. Although macrophages/microglia do increase in number at the site of injury,[376,377] they may not be appropriately activated for support of axonal extension,[361,378] and may differ from other macrophages in fundamental ways.[379] If activated macrophages/microglia are poorly able to phagocytose degraded myelin, the inhibitory signals found in myelin may prevent axonal regeneration.[360]

Neuron-intrinsic limitations to axon regeneration

Interest has also focused on the possibility that failure of regeneration reflects a specific inability of an adult RGC to extend its axon because embryonic axons are able to do so when transplanted into adult tissue. Recent research has focused on determining whether the rate and extent of axon growth depends purely on extracellular signals and substrates, as discussed previously in regard to optic nerve development, or also on the intrinsic state of the neuron. Elsewhere in the CNS, embryonic neurons can regenerate their axons quite readily, but they lose their capacity to regenerate with age.[380–382] This developmental loss of regenerative ability has generally been attributed to the maturation of astrocytes and oligodendrocytes, and to the production of myelin, all of which strongly inhibit axon growth after injury. In experiments in which the inhibitory environment is removed or molecularly blocked, however, only a few percent of axons regenerate, and functional recovery typically proceeds remarkably slowly (discussed further). For example, RGCs take 2 months to regenerate through a peripheral nerve graft.[383,384]

These experiments indicate that the neurons themselves are partly responsible. For example, axons from postnatal day 2 or older hamster retinas lose the ability to reinnervate even embryonic tectal explants.[385] When cultured in the complete absence of CNS glia, embryonic RGCs extend their axons 10 times faster than postnatal or adult RGCs.[386] Interestingly, the decrease in the axon growth ability of RGCs occurs sharply at birth during the period of target innervation, but target contact may not be responsible for this change. Rather, retinal maturation, and possibly a membrane-associated signal from retinal amacrine cells, may be sufficient to induce the developmental decrease in RGC axon growth ability.[386] Once this signal is sent, the loss is permanent—removal of the amacrine cells does not allow the RGCs to speed up again. This may explain the failure of RGC regeneration, at least in part—even in a perfect environment, RGCs may lack the intrinsic capacity to rapidly grow their axons again, after they have done it once during development.

What molecular changes underlie the developmental loss in rapid axon growth ability? RGCs could gradually increase expression of genes that limit axon growth or decrease expression of genes necessary for faster axonal elongation, or both. For example, recent data has pointed to a family of transcription factors that may regulate axon regenerative ability in RGCs.[387,388] Cytoplasmic kinases or phosphatases such as Ca^{2+}-dependent signaling kinases and calmodulin kinases (CaMKs) may also provide a downstream mechanism for axon growth control.[389,390] Second messengers such as cAMP and cGMP have also been implicated in the intrinsic axon regenerative control of the RGC, perhaps by modulating responsiveness to positive neurotrophic factors[118] or to myelin-associated axon growth inhibitors.[391] Finding the molecules that, when modified, truly enhance functional regenerative repair remains a major ongoing goal in optic nerve research today.

OPTIC NERVE REPAIR

The major goal of any optic nerve repair strategy must be to protect or regenerate the connections of RGC axons to their targets in the brain, as these connections are ultimately what serve vision.

Neuroprotection and retinal ganglion cell survival

A first step to protecting optic nerve axons from a degenerative process is preventing RGC death. Neuroprotection, first proposed for other CNS diseases, has been considered in recent years as a possible treatment for optic neuropathies.[392] There is a variety of laboratory evidence using cell culture or animal models of optic nerve disease to suggest that one or more neuroprotective methodologies eventually may be successful in clinical disease, but thus far no strategy has been successfully proven in large, randomized controlled clinical trials in human patients with glaucoma. A number of clinical trials are now in progress and it is likely that small molecule or gene therapy approaches will prove neuroprotective in the coming years.

Regeneration of retinal ganglion cell axons

The same factors that strongly promote RGC survival also tend to strongly promote RGC axon regeneration, with few exceptions. Furthermore, our understanding of the mechanisms of axon growth has generated much progress in understanding regenerative failure. As mentioned previously, reversing the developmental decrease in intrinsic axon growth ability could also be leveraged to promote axon regeneration. Targeting the immune system, retinal or optic nerve cell metabolism, or astrogliosis could also prove effective strategies. A combinatorial approach may be required—both the intrinsic neuronal growth state and the extrinsic environment may have to be optimized for successful regeneration after injury. A major challenge to translating axon regenerative therapies to the clinic, however, will be the length of time it takes for axons to grow down the lengthy optic pathways to their targets in the brain and create and refine new connections to their postsynaptic partners. This longer period will imply that long clinical trials may be required—a barrier to translation in chronic disease.

Optic nerve remyelination

In the case of optic neuritis, where the primary defect in RGC function is attributable to oligodendrocyte demyelination, strategies to enhance remyelination are paramount. Currently, the major approach involves treating patients with steroids, which presumably interferes with the ongoing inflammatory insult and allows a faster rewrapping of optic nerve axons and return to baseline vision. In the presence of demyelination, oligodendrocytes may reconstitute themselves and remyelinate axons,[393] although the nature of the inducing chemical signals has not been well characterized.[394] Similarly, chronic treatment with immune modulators decreases the risk of subsequent demyelinating events. Cell transplant therapy with oligodendrocytes or progenitor cells may prove fruitful in such disease, as has been explored for multiple sclerosis.[395]

"Neuroenhancement" of retinal ganglion cell function

Before RGCs have died, and even before their axons are fully damaged in the optic nerve and would require a proregenerative therapy, RGCs may be partially inhibited in the optic nerve from their full functional capacity. For example, glaucoma causes dysfunction and then death of RGCs, but the window between dysfunction and death in humans is not currently known. Acute studies of IOP raising and lowering in humans and chronic studies of IOP raising and lowering in animal models both suggest that a window between dysfunction and death exist in this degenerative disease.[304-306] Thus, factors known to enhance RGC health and, ultimately, survival could be applied to intervene before death and potentially reverse dysfunction, here termed "neuroenhancement." These remain major goals for the biomedical community for patients with glaucoma.

Neuroenhancement has been used in the literature either generically to refer to improvement of axon regeneration, or more specifically to improvement of cognitive function in degenerative brain disease.[396-398] Compared to the many years it would take a glaucoma trial to demonstrate neuroprotection (e.g., one would ideally demonstrate that progression of visual field losses is slowed or halted), it may be possible to measure an enhancement of RGC structure or function acutely. A potential "neuroenhancement" therapy would target RGCs that are dysfunctional and/or atrophic. With the same neurotrophic factors that stimulate neuroprotection in the long term, such dysfunctional RGCs could hypertrophy to their normal size, or resume normal electrical responsiveness or optic nerve transmission of visual information, or both. Novel approaches to measuring RGC structure and function, referred to as optic neuropathy *biomarkers*, will likely prove critical to advancing such therapeutic candidates through early phase clinical trials.[339,399]

CONCLUSIONS

The optic nerve is the critical conduit for visual information to pass from the eye to the brain. The past decade has seen dramatic increases in our fundamental understanding of optic nerve physiology and pathophysiology, particularly at the cellular and molecular levels, but much remains to address the many optic neuropathies that lead to vision loss and blindness. The next decade will likely prove even more exciting, as advances in regenerative medicine begin to transition from the bench to the clinic.

ACKNOWLEDGEMENTS

Supported by the National Eye Institute (P30-EY026877) and an unrestricted grant from Research to Prevent Blindness, Inc. The author is indebted to Leonard Levin for the foundations of this chapter carried from prior editions.

REFERENCES

1. Curcio CA, Allen KA. Topography of ganglion cells in human retina. *J Comp Neurol.* 1990;300(1):5–25.
2. Linden R. Displaced ganglion cells in the retina of the rat. *J Comp Neurol.* 1987;258(1):138–143.
3. Ogden TE. Nerve fiber layer of the macaque retina: retinotopic organization. *Invest Ophthalmol Vis Sci.* 1983;24(1):85–98.
4. Minckler DS. The organization of nerve fiber bundles in the primate optic nerve head. *Arch Ophthalmol.* 1980;98(9):1630–1636.
5. Chauhan BC, O'Leary N, AlMobarak FA, et al. Enhanced detection of open-angle glaucoma with an anatomically accurate optical coherence tomography-derived neuroretinal rim parameter. *Ophthalmology.* 2013;120(3):535–543.
6. Gardiner SK, Boey PY, Yang H, Fortune B, Burgoyne CF, Demirel S. Structural Measurements for Monitoring Change in Glaucoma: Comparing Retinal Nerve Fiber Layer Thickness With Minimum Rim Width and Area. *Invest Ophthalmol Vis Sci.* 2015;56(11):6886–6891.
7. Wolff E. *The Anatomy of the Eye and Orbit.* Philadelphia: Blakiston; 1948:263.
8. Fitzgibbon T, Taylor SF. Retinotopy of the human retinal nerve fibre layer and optic nerve head. *J Comp Neurol.* 1996;375(2):238–251.
9. Reese BE, Ho KY. Axon diameter distributions across the monkey's optic nerve. *Neuroscience.* 1988;27:205.
10. Jeffery G. Distribution and trajectory of uncrossed axons in the optic nerves of pigmented and albino rats. *J Comp Neurol.* 1989;289:462.
11. Chan SO, Guillery RW. Changes in fiber order in the optic nerve and tract of rat embryos. *J Comp Neurol.* 1994;344(1):20–32.
12. Naito J. Retinogeniculate projection fibers in the monkey optic nerve: a demonstration of the fiber pathways by retrograde axonal transport of WGA-HRP. *J Comp Neurol.* 1989;284(2):174–186.
13. FitzGibbon T. The human fetal retinal nerve fiber layer and optic nerve head: a DiI and DiA tracing study. *Vis Neurosci.* 1997;14(3):433–447.
14. Maniscalco JE, Habal MB. Microanatomy of the optic canal. *J Neurosurg.* 1978;48(3):402–406.
15. Renn WH, Rhoton Jr. AL. Microsurgical anatomy of the sellar region. *J Neurosurg.* 1975;43(3):288–298.
16. Kupfer C, Chumbley L, Downer JC. Quantitative histology of optic nerve, optic tract and lateral geniculate nucleus of man. *J Anat.* 1967;101(3):393–401.
17. Schmid R, Wilhelm B, Wilhelm H. Naso-temporal asymmetry and contraction anisocoria in the pupillomotor system. *Graefes Arch Clin Exp Ophthalmol.* 2000;238(2):123–128.
18. Balazsi AG, Rootman J, Drance SM, et al. The effect of age on the nerve fiber population of the human optic nerve. *Am J Ophthalmol.* 1984;97:760.
19. Mikelberg FS, Drance SM, Schulzer M, et al. The normal human optic nerve: Axon count and axon diameter distribution. *Ophthalmology.* 1989;96:1325.
20. Mikelberg FS, Yidegiligne HM, White VA, Schulzer M. Relation between optic nerve axon number and axon diameter to scleral canal area. *Ophthalmology.* 1991;98(1):60–63.
21. Quigley HA, Brown AE, Morrison JD, Drance SM. The size and shape of the optic disc in normal human eyes. *Arch Ophthalmol.* 1990;108(1):51–57.
22. Quigley HA, Coleman AL, Dorman-Pease ME. Larger optic nerve heads have more nerve fibers in normal monkey eyes. *Arch Ophthalmol.* 1991;109(10):1441–1443.
23. Falck FY, Klein TB, Higginbotham EJ. Larger optic nerve heads have more nerve fibers in normal monkey eyes. *Arch Ophthalmol.* 1992;110(8):1042–1043.
24. Harwerth RS, Quigley HA. Visual field defects and retinal ganglion cell losses in patients with glaucoma. *Arch Ophthalmol.* 2006;124(6):853–859.
25. Kerrigan-Baumrind LA, Quigley HA, Pease ME, Kerrigan DF, Mitchell RS. Number of ganglion cells in glaucoma eyes compared with threshold visual field tests in the same persons. *Invest Ophthalmol Vis Sci.* 2000;41(3):741–748.
26. Harman A, Abrahams B, Moore S, Hoskins R. Neuronal density in the human retinal ganglion cell layer from 16-77 years. *Anat Rec.* 2000;260(2):124–131.
27. Jonas JB, Gusek GC, Naumann GO. Optic disc, cup and neuroretinal rim size, configuration and correlations in normal eyes. *Invest Ophthalmol Vis Sci.* 1988;29(7):1151–1158.
28. Jeffery G, Evans A, Albon J, Duance V, Neal J, Dawidek G. The human optic nerve: fascicular organisation and connective tissue types along the extra-fascicular matrix. *Anat Embryol.* 1995;191(6):491–502.
29. Sanchez RM, Dunkelberger GR, Quigley HA. The number and diameter distribution of axons in the monkey optic nerve. *Invest Ophthalmol Vis Sci.* 1986;27:1342.
30. Baker GE, Stryker MP. Retinofugal fibres change conduction velocity and diameter between the optic nerve and tract in ferrets. *Nature.* 1990;344:342.
31. Colello RJ, Pott U, Schwab ME. The role of oligodendrocytes and myelin on axon maturation in the developing rat retinofugal pathway. *J Neurosci.* 1994
32. Fernandez E, Cuenca N, Cerezo JR, De J. Juan, *Visual experience during postnatal development determines the size of optic nerve axons.* Neuroreport. 1993;5(3):365–367.
33. Repka MX, Quigley HA. The effect of age on normal human optic nerve fiber number and diameter. *Ophthalmology.* 1989;96:26.
34. Anderson DR, Hoyt WF. Ultrastructure of intraorbital portion of human and monkey optic nerve. *Arch Ophthalmol.* 1969;82:506.
35. Sturrock RR. Development of the meninges of the human embryonic optic nerve. *J Hirnforsch.* 1987;28:603.
36. Friedrich VL, Mugnaini E. Myelin sheath thickness in the CNS is regulated near the axon. *Brain Res.* 1983;274:329.
37. McLoon SC, McLoon LK, Palm SL, et al. Transient expression of laminin in the optic nerve of the developing rat. *J Neurosci.* 1988 1981;8
38. Ludwin SK. Oligodendrocyte survival in Wallerian degeneration. *Acta Neuropathol (Berl).* 1990;80:184.
39. Kidd GJ, Hauer PE, Trapp BD. Axons modulate myelin protein messenger RNA levels during central nervous system myelination in vivo. *J Neurosci Res.* 1990;26:409.
40. Barres BA, Jacobson MD, Schmid R, Sendtner M, Raff MC. Does oligodendrocyte survival depend on axons? *Curr Biol.* 1993;3(8):489–497.
41. Barres BA, Raff MC. Proliferation of oligodendrocyte precursor cells depends on electrical activity in axons. *Nature.* 1993;361(6409):258–260.
42. Burne JF, Staple JK, Raff MC. Glial cells are increased proportionally in transgenic optic nerves with increased numbers of axons. *J Neurosci.* 1996;16(6):2064–2073.
43. Colello RJ, Schwab ME. A role for oligodendrocytes in the stabilization of optic axon numbers. *J Neurosci.* 1994;14(11 Pt 1):6446–6452.
44. Savio T, Schwab ME. Rat CNS white matter, but not gray matter, is nonpermissive for neuronal cell adhesion and fiber outgrowth. *J Neurosci.* 1989;9:1126.
45. Schwab ME. Myelin-associated inhibitors of neurite growth. *Exp Neurol.* 1990;109:2.
46. Wender R, Brown AM, Fern R, Swanson RA, Farrell K, Ransom BR. Astrocytic glycogen influences axon function and survival during glucose deprivation in central white matter. *J Neurosci.* 2000;20(18):6804–6810.
47. Cooper ML, Pasini S, Lambert WS, et al. Redistribution of metabolic resources through astrocyte networks mitigates neurodegenerative stress. *Proc Natl Acad Sci U S A.* 2020;117(31):18810–18821.
48. ffrench-Constant C, Raff MC. The oligodendrocyte-type-2 astrocyte cell lineage is specialized for myelination. *Nature.* 1986;323:335.
49. Janzer RC, Raff MC. Astrocytes induce blood-brain barrier properties in endothelial cells. *Nature.* 1987;325:253.
50. Davis CH, Kim KY, Bushong EA, et al. Transcellular degradation of axonal mitochondria. *Proc Natl Acad Sci U S A.* 2014;111(26):9633–9638.
51. Chan WY, Kohsaka S, Rezaie P. The origin and cell lineage of microglia: new concepts. *Brain Res Rev.* 2007;53(2):344–354.
52. Hickey WF, Kimura H. Perivascular microglial cells of the CNS are bone marrow-derived and present antigen in vivo. *Science.* 1988;239:290.
53. Stoll G, Trapp BD, Griffin JW. Macrophage function during Wallerian degeneration of rat optic nerve: Clearance of degenerating myelin and Ia expression. *J Neurosci.* 1989;9:2327.
54. Sturrock RR. Microglia in the human embryonic optic nerve. *J Anat.* 1984;139:81.
55. Sturrock RR. An electron microscopic study of macrophages in the meninges of the human embryonic optic nerve. *J Anat.* 1988;157:145.
56. Hayreh SS. The sheath of the optic nerve. *Ophthalmologica.* 1984;189:54.
57. Anderson DR. Ultrastructure of meningeal sheaths: Normal human and monkey optic nerves. *Arch Ophthalmol.* 1969;82:659.
58. Liu D, Michon J. Measurement of the subarachnoid pressure of the optic nerve in human subjects. *Am J Ophthalmol.* 1995;119(1):81–85.
59. Ford RL, Frankfort BJ, Fleischman D. Cerebrospinal fluid and ophthalmic disease. *Curr Opin Ophthalmol.* 2022;33(2):73–79.
60. Jonas JB, Wang N, Yang D, Ritch R, Panda-Jonas S. Facts and myths of cerebrospinal fluid pressure for the physiology of the eye. *Prog Retin Eye Res.* 2015;46:67–83.
61. Shalaby WS, Ahmed OM, Waisbourd M, Katz LJ. A review of potential novel glaucoma therapeutic options independent of intraocular pressure. *Surv Ophthalmol.* 2021
62. Anderson DR, Braverman S. Reevaluation of the optic disk vasculature. *Am J Ophthalmol.* 1976;82(2):165–174.
63. Lieberman MF, Maumenee AE, Green WR. Histologic studies of the vasculature of the anterior optic nerve. *Am J Ophthalmol.* 1976;82(3):405–423.
64. Olver JM, Spalton DJ, McCartney AC. Microvascular study of the retrolaminar optic nerve in man: the possible significance in anterior ischaemic optic neuropathy. *Eye.* 1990;4 (Pt 1):7–24.
65. Olver JM. Functional anatomy of the choroidal circulation: methyl methacrylate casting of human choroid. *Eye.* 1990;4(Pt 2):262–272.
66. Guy J, McGorray S, Fitzsimmons J, Beck B, Rao NA. Disruption of the blood-brain barrier in experimental optic neuritis: immunocytochemical co-localization of H2O2 and extravasated serum albumin. *Invest Ophthalmol Vis Sci.* 1994;35(3):1114–1123.
67. Guy J, Fitzsimmons J, Ellis EA, Beck B, Mancuso A. Intraorbital optic nerve and experimental optic neuritis. Correlation of fat suppression magnetic resonance imaging and electron microscopy. *Ophthalmology.* 1992;99(5):720–725.
68. Geijer C, Bill A. Effects of raised intraocular pressure on retinal, prelaminar, laminar, and retrolaminar optic nerve blood flow in monkeys. *Invest Ophthalmol Vis Sci.* 1979;18(10):1030–1042.
69. Weinstein JM, Duckrow RB, Beard D, Brennan RW. Regional optic nerve blood flow and its autoregulation. *Invest Ophthalmol Vis Sci.* 1983;24(12):1559–1565.
70. Riva CE, Grunwald JE, Petrig BL. Autoregulation of human retinal blood flow. An investigation with laser Doppler velocimetry. *Invest Ophthalmol Vis Sci.* 1986;27(12):1706–1712.
71. Francois J, Fryczkowski A. The blood supply of the optic nerve. *Adv Ophthalmol.* 1978;36:164–173.
72. Chou PI, Sadun AA, Lee H. Vasculature and morphometry of the optic canal and intracanalicular optic nerve. *J Neuroophthalmol.* 1995;15(3):186–190.
73. Sturrock RR. Vascularization of the human embryonic optic nerve. *J Hirnforsch.* 1987;28:615.
74. Rao K, Lund RD. Degeneration of optic axons induces the expression of major histocompatibility antigens. *Brain Res.* 1989;488:332.
75. Flage T. Permeability properties of the tissues in the optic nerve head region in the rabbit and the monkey: An ultrastructural study. *Acta Ophthalmol.* 1977;55:652.
76. Tsukahara I, Yamashita H. An electron microscopic study on the blood-optic nerve and fluid-optic nerve barrier. *Graefes Arch Clin Exp Ophthalmol.* 1975;196:239.
77. Guy J, Rao NA. Acute and chronic experimental optic neuritis: Alteration in the blood-optic nerve barrier. *Arch Ophthalmol.* 1984;102:450.
78. Sawaguchi S, Yue BY, Abe H, Iwata K, Fukuchi T, Kaiya T. The collagen fibrillar network in the human pial septa. *Curr Eye Res.* 1994;13(11):819–824.
79. Cohen AI. Ultrastructural aspects of the human optic nerve. *Invest Ophthalmol.* 1967;6:294.

80. Lincoln J, Milner P, Appenzeller O, Burnstock G, Qualls C. Innervation of normal human sural and optic nerves by noradrenaline- and peptide-containing nervi vasorum and nervorum: effect of diabetes and alcoholism. *Brain Res.* 1993;632(1-2):48–56.

81. Ye XD, Laties AM, Stone RA. Peptidergic innervation of the retinal vasculature and optic nerve head. *Invest Ophthalmol Vis Sci.* 1990;31:1731.

82. Nyborg NC, Nielsen PJ. Angiotensin-II contracts isolated human posterior ciliary arteries. *Invest Ophthalmol Vis Sci.* 1990;31:2471.

83. Ling TL, Mitrofanis J, Stone J. Origin of retinal astrocytes in the rat: evidence of migration from the optic nerve. *J Comp Neurol.* 1989;286:345.

84. David S. Neurite outgrowth from mammalian CNS neurons on astrocytes in vitro may not be mediated primarily by laminin. *J Neurocytol.* 1988;17:131.

85. Dreyer EB, Leifer D, Heng JE, et al. An astrocytic binding site for neuronal Thy-1 and its effect on neurite outgrowth. *Proc Natl Acad Sci USA.* 1995;92(24):11195–11199.

86. Tang DG, Tokumoto YM, Raff MC. Long-term culture of purified postnatal oligodendrocyte precursor cells. Evidence for an intrinsic maturation program that plays out over months. *J Cell Biol.* 2000;148(5):971–984.

87. Leifer D, Lipton SA, Barnstable CJ, et al. Monoclonal antibody to Thy-1 enhances regeneration of processes by rat retinal ganglion cells in culture. *Science.* 1984;224:303–306.

88. Bartsch U, Kirchhoff F, Schachner M. Immunohistological localization of the adhesion molecules L1, N-CAM, and MAG in the developing and adult optic nerve of mice. *J Comp Neurol.* 1989;284:451.

89. Skoff RP. The fine structure of pulse labeled (3H-thymidine cells) in degenerating rat optic nerve. *J Comp Neurol.* 1975;161:595.

90. Bogler O, Noble M. Measurement of time in oligodendrocyte-type-2 astrocyte (O-2A) progenitors is a cellular process distinct from differentiation or division. *Dev Biol.* 1994;162(2):525–538.

91. Gao FB, Durand B, Raff M. Oligodendrocyte precursor cells count time but not cell divisions before differentiation. *Curr Biol.* 1997;7(2):152–155.

92. Shi J, Marinovich A, Barres BA. Purification and characterization of adult oligodendrocyte precursor cells from the rat optic nerve. *J Neurosci.* 1998;18(12):4627–4636.

93. Givogri MI, Costa RM, Schonmann V, Silva AJ, Campagnoni AT, Bongarzone ER. Central nervous system myelination in mice with deficient expression of Notch1 receptor. *J Neurosci Res.* 2002;67(3):309–320.

94. Politis MJ. Exogenous laminin induces regenerative changes in traumatized sciatic and optic nerve. *Plast Reconstr Surg.* 1989;83:228.

95. Colello RJ, Devey LR, Imperato E, Pott U. The chronology of oligodendrocyte differentiation in the rat optic nerve: evidence for a signaling step initiating myelination in the CNS. *J Neurosci.* 1995;15(11):7665–7672.

96. Magoon EH, Robb RM. Development of myelin in human optic nerve and tract: A light and electron microscopic study. *Arch Ophthalmol.* 1981;99:655.

97. Lev-Ram V, Grinvald A. Ca2+- and K+-dependent communication between central nervous system myelinated axons and oligodendrocytes revealed by voltage-sensitive dyes. *Proc Natl Acad Sci USA.* 1986;83:6651.

98. Sanchez I, Hassinger L, Paskevich PA, Shine HD, Nixon RA. Oligodendroglia regulate the regional expansion of axon caliber and local accumulation of neurofilaments during development independently of myelin formation. *J Neuroscience.* 1996;16(16):5095–5105.

99. Foster RE, Connors BW, Waxman SG. Rat optic nerve: electrophysiological, pharmacological and anatomical studies during development. *Brain Res.* 1982;255:371.

100. Hildebrand C, Remahl S, Waxman SG. Axo-glial relations in the retina-optic nerve junction of the adult rat: electron-microscopic observations. *J Neurocytol.* 1985;14:597.

101. ffrench-Constant C, Miller RH, Burne JF, et al. Evidence that migratory oligodendrocyte-type-2 astrocyte (O-2A) progenitor cells are kept out of the rat retina by a barrier at the eye-end of the optic nerve. *J Neurocytol.* 1988;17:13.

102. Tso MO, Shih CV, McLean IW. Is there a blood brain barrier at the optic nerve head? *Arch Ophthalmol.* 1975;93:815.

103. Perry VH, Lund RD. Evidence that the lamina cribrosa prevents intraretinal myelination of retinal ganglion cell axons. *J Neurocytol.* 1990;19:265.

104. Bartsch U, Faissner A, Trotter J, et al. Tenascin demarcates the boundary between the myelinated and nonmyelinated part of retinal ganglion cell axons in the developing and adult mouse. *J Neurosci.* 1994;14(8):4756–4768.

105. Laeng P, Molthagen M, Yu EG, Bartsch U. Transplantation of oligodendrocyte progenitor cells into the rat retina: extensive myelination of retinal ganglion cell axons. *Glia.* 1996;18(3):200–210.

106. Perry VH, Hayes L. Lesion-induced myelin formation in the retina. *J Neurocytol.* 1985;14:297.

107. Bussow H. Schwann cell myelin ensheathing CNS axons in the nerve fibre layer of the cat retina. *J Neurocytol.* 1978;7:207.

108. Jung HJ, Raine CS, Suzuki K. Schwann cells and peripheral nervous system myelin in the rat retina. *Acta Neuropathol (Berl).* 1978;44:245.

109. Burne JF, Raff MC. Retinal ganglion cell axons drive the proliferation of astrocytes in the developing rodent optic nerve. *Neuron.* 1997;18(2):223–230.

110. Mi H, Barres BA. Purification and characterization of astrocyte precursor cells in the developing rat optic nerve. *J Neurosci.* 1999;19(3):1049–1061.

111. Liedtke W, Edelmann W, Bieri PL, et al. GFAP is necessary for the integrity of CNS white matter architecture and long-term maintenance of myelination. *Neuron.* 1996;17(4):607–615.

112. Lucius R, Young HP, Tidow S, Sievers J. Growth stimulation and chemotropic attraction of rat retinal ganglion cell axons in vitro by co-cultured optic nerves, astrocytes and astrocyte conditioned medium. *Int J Develop Neurosci.* 1996;14(4):387–398.

113. Sturrock RR. A quantitative histological study of cell division and changes in cell number in the meningeal sheath of the embryonic human optic nerve. *J Anat.* 1987;155:133.

114. Penfold PL, Provis JM. Cell death in the development of the human retina: phagocytosis of pyknotic and apoptotic bodies by retinal cells. *Graefes Arch Clin Exp Ophthalmol.* 1986;224(6):549–553.

115. Ilschner SU, Waring P. Fragmentation of DNA in the retina of chicken embryos coincides with retinal ganglion cell death. *Biochem Biophys Res Comm.* 1992;183(3):1056–1061.

116. Provis JM, van DD, Billson FA, et al. Human fetal optic nerve: overproduction and elimination of retinal axons during development. *J Comp Neurol.* 1985;238:92.

117. Goldberg JL, Barres BA. The relationship between neuronal survival and regeneration. *Annu Rev Neurosci.* 2000;23:579–612.

118. Goldberg JL, Espinosa JS, Xu Y, Davidson N, Kovacs GT, Barres BA. Retinal ganglion cells do not extend axons by default: promotion by neurotrophic signaling and electrical activity. *Neuron.* 2002;33(5):689–702.

119. Jo SA, Wang E, Benowitz LI. Ciliary neurotrophic factor is and axogenesis factor for retinal ganglion cells. *Neuroscience.* 1999;89(2):579–591.

120. Logan A, Ahmed Z, Baird A, Gonzalez AM, Berry M. Neurotrophic factor synergy is required for neuronal survival and disinhibited axon regeneration after CNS injury. *Brain.* 2006;129(Pt 2):490–502.

121. Loh NK, Woerly S, Bunt SM, Wilton SD, Harvey AR. The regrowth of axons within tissue defects in the CNS is promoted by implanted hydrogel matrices that contain BDNF and CNTF producing fibroblasts. *Exp Neurol.* 2001;170(1):72–84.

122. Mansour-Robaey S, Clarke DB, Wang YC, Bray GM, Aguayo AJ. Effects of ocular injury and administration of brain-derived neurotrophic factor on survival and regrowth of axotomized retinal ganglion cells. *Proc Natl Acad Sci USA.* 1994;91(5):1632–1636.

123. Mey J, Thanos S. Intravitreal injections of neurotrophic factors support the survival of axotomized retinal ganglion cells in adult rats in vivo. *Brain Res.* 1993;602(2):304–317.

124. Lafont F, Rouget M, Triller A, Prochiantz A, Rousselet A. In vitro control of neuronal polarity by glycosaminoglycans. *Development.* 1992;114(1):17–29.

125. Reichardt LF, Tomaselli KJ. Extracellular matrix molecules and their receptors: functions in neural development. *Annu Rev Neurosci.* 1991;14:531–570.

126. Riehl R, Johnson K, Bradley R, et al. Cadherin function is required for axon outgrowth in retinal ganglion cells in vivo. *Neuron.* 1996;17(5):837–848.

127. Shatz CJ, Stryker MP. Prenatal tetrodotoxin infusion blocks segregation of retinogeniculate afferents. *Science.* 1988;242(4875):87–89.

128. Verhage M, Maia AS, Plomp JJ, et al. Synaptic assembly of the brain in the absence of neurotransmitter secretion. *Science.* 2000;287(5454):864–869.

129. Cantallops I, Haas K, Cline HT. Postsynaptic CPG15 promotes synaptic maturation and presynaptic axon arbor elaboration in vivo. *Nat Neurosci.* 2000;3(10):1004–1011.

130. Cohen-Cory S. BDNF modulates, but does not mediate, activity-dependent branching and remodeling of optic axon arbors in vivo. *J Neurosci.* 1999;19(22):9996–10003.

131. Rashid NA, Cambray-Deakin MA. N-methyl-D-aspartate effects on the growth, morphology and cytoskeleton of individual neurons in vitro. *Brain Res Dev Brain Res.* 1992;67(2):301–308.

132. Catalano SM, Shatz CJ. Activity-dependent cortical target selection by thalamic axons. *Science.* 1998;281(5376):559–562.

133. Kalil RE, Dubin MW, Scott G, Stark LA. Elimination of action potentials blocks the structural development of retinogeniculate synapses. *Nature.* 1986;323(6084):156–158.

134. Katz LC, Shatz CJ. Synaptic activity and the construction of cortical circuits. *Science.* 1996;274(5290):1133–1138.

135. Goldberg JL. How does an axon grow? *Genes Dev.* 2003;17(8):941–958.

136. Sretavan DW, Pure E, Siegel MW, Reichardt LF. Disruption of retinal axon ingrowth by ablation of embryonic mouse optic chiasm neurons. *Science.* 1995;269(5220):98–101.

137. Goodman CS. Mechanisms and molecules that control growth cone guidance. *Annu Rev Neurosci.* 1996;19:341–377.

138. Haupt C, Huber AB. How axons see their way--axonal guidance in the visual system. *Front Biosci.* 2008;13:3136–3149.

139. Bauch H, Stier H, Schlosshauer B. Axonal versus dendritic outgrowth is differentially affected by radial glia in discrete layers of the retina. *J Neurosci.* 1998;18(5):1774–1785.

140. Stier H, Schlosshauer B. Axonal guidance in the chicken retina. *Development.* 1995;121(5):1443–1454.

141. Airaksinen PJ, Doro S, Veijola J. Conformal geometry of the retinal nerve fiber layer. *Proc Natl Acad Sci U S A.* 2008;105(50):19690–19695.

142. Brittis PA, Silver J. Multiple factors govern intraretinal axon guidance: a time-lapse study. *Mol Cell Neurosci.* 1995;6(5):413–432.

143. de la Torre JR, Hopker VH, Ming GL, et al. Turning of retinal growth cones in a netrin-1 gradient mediated by the netrin receptor DCC. *Neuron.* 1997;19(6):1211–1224.

144. Deiner MS, Kennedy TE, Fazeli A, Serafini T, Tessier-Lavigne M, Sretavan DW. Netrin-1 and DCC mediate axon guidance locally at the optic disc: loss of function leads to optic nerve hypoplasia. *Neuron.* 1997;19(3):575–589.

145. Oster SF, Bodeker MO, He F, Sretavan DW. Invariant Sema5A inhibition serves an ensheathing function during optic nerve development. *Development.* 2003;130(4):775–784.

146. Plump AS, Erskine L, Sabatier C, et al. Slit1 and Slit2 cooperate to prevent premature midline crossing of retinal axons in the mouse visual system. *Neuron.* 2002;33(2):219–232.

147. Nakagawa S, Brennan C, Johnson KG, Shewan D, Harris WA, Holt CE. Ephrin-B regulates the Ipsilateral routing of retinal axons at the optic chiasm. *Neuron.* 2000;25(3):599–610.

148. Williams SE, Mann F, Erskine L, et al. Ephrin-B2 and EphB1 mediate retinal axon divergence at the optic chiasm. *Neuron.* 2003;39(6):919–935.

149. Chung KY, Taylor JS, Shum DK, Chan SO. Axon routing at the optic chiasm after enzymatic removal of chondroitin sulfate in mouse embryos. *Development.* 2000;127(12):2673–2683.

150. Reese BE. The chronotopic reordering of optic axons. *Perspect Dev Biol.* 1996;3(3):233–242.

151. Chalupa LM, Meissirel C, Lia B. Specificity of retinal ganglion cell projections in the embryonic rhesus monkey. *Perspect Dev Biol.* 1996;3(3):223–231.

152. Martersteck EM, Hirokawa KE, Evarts M, et al. Diverse Central Projection Patterns of Retinal Ganglion Cells. *Cell Rep.* 2017;18(8):2058–2072.

153. Bowling DB, Michael CR. Projection patterns of single physiologically characterized optic tract fibres in cat. *Nature.* 1980;286(5776):899–902.

154. Kondo Y, Takada M, Kayahara T, Yasui Y, Nakano K, Mizuno N. Single retinal ganglion cells sending axon collaterals to the bilateral superior colliculi: a fluorescent

retrograde double-labeling study in the Japanese monkey (Macaca fuscata). *Brain Res.* 1992;597(1):155–161.
155. Hendry SH, Reid RC. The koniocellular pathway in primate vision. *Annu Rev Neurosci.* 2000;23:127–153.
156. Bunt AH, Hendrickson AE, Lund JS, Lund RD, Fuchs AF. Monkey retinal ganglion cells: morphometric analysis and tracing of axonal projections, with a consideration of the peroxidase technique. *J Comp Neurol.* 1975;164(3):265–285.
157. Wurtz RH. Vision for the control of movement. The Friedenwald Lecture. *Invest Ophthalmol Vis Sci.* 1996;37(11):2130–2145.
158. Hilbig H, Bidmon HJ, Zilles K, Busecke K. Neuronal and glial structures of the superficial layers of the human superior colliculus. *Anat Embryol (Berl).* 1999;200(1):103–115.
159. Fredericks CA, Giolli RA, Blanks RHI, et al. The human accessory optic system. *Brain Res.* 1988;454:116.
160. Itoh K, Takada M, Yasui Y, et al. A pretectofacial projection in the cat: a possible link in the visually-triggered blink reflex pathways. *Brain Res.* 1983;275:332.
161. Baleydier C, Magnin M, Cooper HM. Macaque accessory optic system: II: Connections with the pretectum. *J Comp Neurol.* 1990;302:405.
162. Lagreze WA, Kardon RH. Correlation of relative afferent pupillary defect and estimated retinal ganglion cell loss. *Graefes Arch Clin Exp Ophthalmol.* 1998;236(6):401–404.
163. Lhermitte F, Guillaumat L, Lyon CO. Monocular blindness with preserved direct and consensual pupillary reflex in multiple sclerosis. *Arch Neurol.* 1984;41:993.
164. Sadun AA, Schaechter JD, Smith LE. A retinohypothalamic pathway in man: light mediation of circadian rhythms. *Brain Res.* 1984;302:371.
165. Schaecter JD, Sadun AA. A second hypothalamic nucleus receiving retinal input in man: the paraventricular nucleus. *Brain Res.* 1985;340:243.
166. Johnson RF, Morin LP, Moore RY. Retinohypothalamic projections in the hamster and rat demonstrated using cholera toxin. *Brain Res.* 1988;462:301.
167. Berson DM, Dunn FA, Takao M. Phototransduction by retinal ganglion cells that set the circadian clock. *Science.* 2002;295(5557):1070–1073.
168. Gooley JJ, Lu J, Chou TC, Scammell TE, Saper CB. Melanopsin in cells of origin of the retinohypothalamic tract. *Nat Neurosci, 2001.* **4***(12).* :1165.
169. Provencio I, Rodriguez IR, Jiang G, Hayes WP, Moreira EF, Rollag MD. A novel human opsin in the inner retina. *J Neurosci.* 2000;20(2):600–605.
170. Provencio I, Rollag MD, Castrucci AM. Photoreceptive net in the mammalian retina. This mesh of cells may explain how some blind mice can still tell day from night. *Nature.* 2002;415(6871):493.
171. Ohishi H, Shigemoto R, Nakanishi S, Mizuno N. Distribution of the messenger RNA for a metabotropic glutamate receptor, mGluR2, in the central nervous system of the rat. *Neuroscience.* 1993;53(4):1009–1018.
172. Rothe T, Bigl V, Grantyn R. Potentiating and depressant effects of metabotropic glutamate receptor agonists on high-voltage-activated calcium currents in cultured retinal ganglion neurons from postnatal mice. *Pflugers Arch.* 1994;426(1-2):161–170.
173. Li X, Hallqvist A, Jacobson I, Orwar O, Sandberg M. Studies on the identity of the rat optic nerve transmitter. *Brain Res.* 1996;706(1):89–96.
174. Matsui K, Hosoi N, Tachibana M. Excitatory synaptic transmission in the inner retina: paired recordings of bipolar cells and neurons of the ganglion cell layer. *J Neurosci.* 1998;18(12):4500–4510.
175. Rorig B, Grantyn R. Rat retinal ganglion cells express Ca(2+)-permeable non-NMDA glutamate receptors during the period of histogenetic cell death. *Neurosci Lett.* 1993;153(1):32–36.
176. Siliprandi R, Canella R, Carmignoto G, et al. N-methyl-D-aspartate-induced neurotoxicity in the adult rat retina. *Vis Neurosci.* 1992;8(6):567–573.
177. Feller MB, Wellis DP, Stellwagen D, Werblin FS, Shatz CJ. Requirement for cholinergic synaptic transmission in the propagation of spontaneous retinal waves. *Science.* 1996;272(5265):1182–1187.
178. Keyser KT, MacNeil MA, Dmitrieva N, Wang F, Masland RH, Lindstrom JM. Amacrine, ganglion, and displaced amacrine cells in the rabbit retina express nicotinic acetylcholine receptors. *Vis Neurosci.* 2000;17(5):743–752.
179. Kubrusly RC, de Mello MC, de Mello FG. Aspartate as a selective NMDA receptor agonist in cultured cells from the avian retina. *Neurochem Int.* 1998;32(1):47–52.
180. Matsui K, Hosoi N, Tachibana M. Active role of glutamate uptake in the synaptic transmission from retinal nonspiking neurons. *J Neurosci.* 1999;19(16):6755–6766.
181. Higgs MH, Lukasiewicz PD. Glutamate uptake limits synaptic excitation of retinal ganglion cells. *J Neurosci.* 1999;19(10):3691–3700.
182. Pow DV, Barnett NL, Penfold P. Are neuronal transporters relevant in retinal glutamate homeostasis? *Neurochem Int.* 2000;37(2-3):191–198.
183. Barnett NL, Pow DV. Antisense knockdown of GLAST, a glial glutamate transporter, compromises retinal function. *Invest Ophthalmol Vis Sci.* 2000;41(2):585–591.
184. Taschenberger H, Grantyn R. Several types of Ca2+ channels mediate glutamatergic synaptic responses to activation of single Thy-1-immunolabeled rat retinal ganglion neurons. *J Neurosci.* 1995;15(3 Pt 2):2240–2254.
185. Schmid S, Guenther E. Developmental regulation of voltage-activated Na+ and Ca2+ currents in rat retinal ganglion cells. *Neuroreport.* 1996;7(2):677–681.
186. Schmid S, Guenther E. Alterations in channel density and kinetic properties of the sodium current in retinal ganglion cells of the rat during in vivo differentiation. *Neuroscience.* 1998;85(1):249–258.
187. Guenther E, Schmid S, Reiff D, Zrenner E. Maturation of intrinsic membrane properties in rat retinal ganglion cells. *Vision Res.* 1999;39(15):2477–2484.
188. Schmid S, Guenther E. Voltage-activated calcium currents in rat retinal ganglion cells in situ: changes during prenatal and postnatal development. *J Neurosci.* 1999;19(9):3486–3494.
189. Taschenberger H, Juttner R, Grantyn R. Ca2+-permeable P2X receptor channels in cultured rat retinal ganglion cells. *J Neurosci.* 1999;19(9):3353–3366.
190. Velte TJ, Masland RH. Action potentials in the dendrites of retinal ganglion cells. *J Neurophysiol.* 1999;81(3):1412–1417.
191. Caruso DM, Owczarzak MT, Pourcho RG. Colocalization of substance P and GABA in retinal ganglion cells: a computer-assisted visualization. *Vis Neurosci.* 1990;5(4):389–394.
192. Caruso DM, Owczarzak MT, Goebel DJ, Hazlett JC, Pourcho RG. GABA-immunoreactivity in ganglion cells of the rat retina. *Brain Res.* 1989;476(1):129–134.
193. Ehrlich D, Keyser K, Manthorpe M, Varon S, Karten HJ. Differential effects of axotomy on substance P-containing and nicotinic acetylcholine receptor-containing retinal ganglion cells: time course of degeneration and effects of nerve growth factor. *Neuroscience.* 1990;36(3):699–723.
194. Ehrlich D, Keyser KT, Karten HJ. Distribution of substance P-like immunoreactive retinal ganglion cells and their pattern of termination in the optic tectum of chick (Gallus gallus). *J Comp Neurol.* 1987;266(2):220–233.
195. Pickard GE, Rea MA. Serotonergic innervation of the hypothalamic suprachiasmatic nucleus and photic regulation of circadian rhythms. *Biol Cell.* 1997;89(8):513–523.
196. Akopian A, Kumar S, Ramakrishnan H, Roy K, Viswanathan S, Bloomfield SA. Targeting neuronal gap junctions in mouse retina offers neuroprotection in glaucoma. *J Clin Invest.* 2017;127(7):2647–2661.
197. Stanford LR. Conduction velocity variations minimize conduction time differences among retinal ganglion cell axons. *Science.* 1987;238(4825):358–360.
198. Black JA, Friedman B, Waxman SG, et al. Immuno-ultrastructural localization of sodium channels at nodes of Ranvier and perinodal astrocytes in rat optic nerve. *Proc R Soc Lond [Biol].* 1989;238:39.
199. Kaplan MR, Cho MH, Ullian EM, Isom LL, Levinson SR, Barres BA. Differential control of clustering of the sodium channels Na(v)1.2 and Na(v)1.6 at developing CNS nodes of Ranvier. *Neuron.* 2001;30(1):105–119.
200. Kaplan MR, Meyer-Franke A, Lambert S, et al. Induction of sodium channel clustering by oligodendrocytes. *Nature.* 1997;386(6626):724–728.
201. Van Wart A, Matthews G. Impaired firing and cell-specific compensation in neurons lacking nav1.6 sodium channels. *J Neurosci.* 2006;26(27):7172–7180.
202. Black JA, Waxman SG, Friedman B, et al. Sodium channels in astrocytes of rat optic nerve in situ: immuno-electron microscopic studies. *Glia.* 1989;2:353.
203. Oh Y, Black JA, Waxman SG. *The expression of rat brain voltage-sensitive Na+ channel mRNAs in astrocytes.* Molec. *Brain Res.* 1994;23(1-2):57–65.
204. Bevan S, Lindsay RM, Perkins MN, et al. Voltage gated ionic channels in rat cultured astrocytes, reactive astrocytes and an astrocyte-oligodendrocyte progenitor cell. *J Physiol (Paris).* 1987;82:327.
205. Barres BA, Chun LLY, Corey DP. Ion channels in vertebrate glia. *Annu Rev Neurosci.* 1990;13:441.
206. Kriegler S, Chiu SY. Calcium signaling of glial cells along mammalian axons. *J Neurosci.* 1993;13(10):4229–4245.
207. Jeffery G, Sharp C, Malitschek B, Salt TE, Kuhn R, Knopfel T. Cellular localisation of metabotropic glutamate receptors in the mammalian optic nerve: a mechanism for axon-glia communication. *Brain Res.* 1996;741(1-2):75–81.
208. Willard M, Simon C. Modulations of neurofilament axonal transport during the development of rabbit retinal ganglion cells. *Cell.* 1983;35:551.
209. Amaratunga A, Morin PJ, Kosik KS, Fine RE. Inhibition of kinesin synthesis and rapid anterograde axonal transport in vivo by an antisense oligonucleotide. *J Biol Chem.* 1993;268(23):17427–17430.
210. Dillman JFI, Dabney LP, Pfister KK. Cytoplasmic dynein is associated with slow axonal transport. *Proc Natl Acad Sci USA.* 1996;93(1):141–144.
211. Aschner M, Rodier PM, Finkelstein JN. Increased axonal transport in the rat optic system after systemic exposure to methylmercury: differential effects in local vs systemic exposure conditions. *Brain Res.* 1987;401(1):132–141.
212. Crossland WJ. Fast axonal transport in the visual pathway of the chick and rat. *Brain Res.* 1985;340:373.
213. Morin PJ, Liu NG, Johnson RJ, et al. Isolation and characterization of rapid transport vesicle subtypes from rabbit optic nerve. *J Neurochem.* 1991;56:415.
214. Mercken M, Fischer I, Kosik KS, Nixon RA. Three distinct axonal transport rates for tau, tubulin, and other microtubule-associated proteins: evidence for dynamic interactions of tau with microtubules in vivo. *J Neuroscience.* 1995;15(12):8259–8267.
215. Black MM, Lasek RJ. Axonal transport of actin: Slow component b is the principal source of actin for the axon. *Brain Res.* 1979;171:401.
216. Willard M, Wiseman M, Levine J, et al. Axonal transport of actin in rabbit retinal ganglion cells. *J Cell Biol.* 1979;81:581.
217. Giorgi PP, DuBois H. Labelling by axonal transport of myelin-associated proteins in the rabbit visual pathway. *Biochem J.* 1981;196:537.
218. Howe CL, Valletta JS, Rusnak AS, Mobley WC. NGF signaling from clathrin-coated vesicles: evidence that signaling endosomes serve as a platform for the Ras-MAPK pathway. *Neuron.* 2001;32(5):801–814.
219. MacInnis BL, Campenot RB. Retrograde support of neuronal survival without retrograde transport of nerve growth factor. *Science.* 2002;295(5559):1536–1539.
220. Riccio A, Pierchala BA, Ciarallo CL, Ginty DD. An NGF-TrkA-mediated retrograde signal to transcription factor CREB in sympathetic neurons. *Science.* 1997;277(5329): 1097–1100.
221. Watson FL, Heerssen HM, Moheban DB, et al. Rapid nuclear responses to target-derived neurotrophins require retrograde transport of ligand-receptor complex. *J Neurosci.* 1999;19(18):7889–7900.
222. Schiapparelli LM, Shah SH, Ma Y, et al. The Retinal Ganglion Cell Transportome Identifies Proteins Transported to Axons and Presynaptic Compartments in the Visual System In Vivo. *Cell Rep.* 2019;28(7):1935–1947.:e5.
223. Schiapparelli LM, Sharma P, He HY, et al. Proteomic screen reveals diverse protein transport between connected neurons in the visual system. *Cell Rep.* 2022;38(4):110287.
224. Shah SH, Goldberg JL. The Role of Axon Transport in Neuroprotection and Regeneration. *Dev Neurobiol.* 2018;78(10):998–1010.
225. Cameron EG, Xia X, Galvao J, Ashouri M, Kapiloff MS, Goldberg JL. Optic Nerve Crush in Mice to Study Retinal Ganglion Cell Survival and Regeneration. *Bio Protoc.* 2020;10(6).

226. Bei F, Lee HHC, Liu X, et al. Restoration of Visual Function by Enhancing Conduction in Regenerated Axons. *Cell*. 2016;164(1-2):219–232.

227. Bricker-Anthony C, Hines-Beard J, Rex TS. Molecular changes and vision loss in a mouse model of closed-globe blast trauma. *Invest Ophthalmol Vis Sci*. 2014;55(8):4853–4862.

228. Berkelaar M, Clarke DB, Wang YC, Bray GM, Aguayo AJ. Axotomy results in delayed death and apoptosis of retinal ganglion cells in adult rats. *J Neurosci*. 1994;14(7):4368–4374.

229. You SW, So KF, Yip HK. Axonal regeneration of retinal ganglion cells depending on the distance of axotomy in adult hamsters. *Invest Ophthalmol Vis Sci*. 2000;41(10):3165–3170.

230. Johnson MW, Kincaid MC, Trobe JD. Bilateral retrobulbar optic nerve infarctions after blood loss and hypotension. A clinicopathologic case study. *Ophthalmology*. 1987;94(12):1577–1584.

231. Connolly SE, Gordon KB, Horton JC. Salvage of vision after hypotension-induced ischemic optic neuropathy. *Am J Ophthalmol*. 1994;117(2):235–242.

232. Stys PK. Anoxic and ischemic injury of myelinated axons in CNS white matter: from mechanistic concepts to therapeutics. *J Cereb Blood Flow Metab*. 1998;18(1):2–25.

233. Petty MA, Wettstein JG. White matter ischaemia. *Brain Res Brain Res Rev*. 1999;31(1):58–64.

234. Waxman SG, Davis PK, Black JA, et al. Anoxic injury of mammalian central white matter: decreased susceptibility in myelin-deficient optic nerve. *Ann Neurol*. 1990;28:335.

235. Marcoux FW, Morawetz RB, Crowell RM, DeGirolami U, Halsey Jr. JH. Differential regional vulnerability in transient focal cerebral ischemia. *Stroke*. 1982;13(3):339–346.

236. Hayreh SS, Baines JA. Occlusion of the posterior ciliary artery. 3. Effects on the optic nerve head. *Br J Ophthalmol*. 1972;56(10):754–764.

237. Hayreh SS, Baines JA. Occlusion of the posterior ciliary artery. I. Effects on choroidal circulation. *Br J Ophthalmol*. 1972;56(10):719–735.

238. Cioffi GA, Van EM. Buskirk, *Microvasculature of the anterior optic nerve. Surv Ophthalmol*. 1994;38(Suppl):S107–S116.

239. Cioffi GA, Orgul S, Onda E, Bacon DR, Van EM. Buskirk, *An in vivo model of chronic optic nerve ischemia: the dose-dependent effects of endothelin-1 on the optic nerve microvasculature. Curr Eye Res*. 1995;14(12):1147–1153.

240. Orgul S, Cioffi GA, Bacon DR, Van EM. Buskirk, *An endothelin-1-induced model of chronic optic nerve ischemia in rhesus monkeys. J Glaucoma*. 1996;5(2):135–138.

241. Nishimura K, Riva CE, Harino S, Reinach P, Cranstoun SD, Mita S. Effects of endothelin-1 on optic nerve head blood flow in cats. *J Ocul Pharmacol Ther*. 1996;12(1):75–83.

242. Orgul S, Cioffi GA, Wilson DJ, Bacon DR, Van EM. Buskirk, *An endothelin-1 induced model of optic nerve ischemia in the rabbit. Invest Ophthalmol Vis Sci*. 1996;37(9):1860–1869.

243. Cioffi GA, Sullivan P. The effect of chronic ischemia on the primate optic nerve. *Eur J Ophthalmol*. 1999;9(Suppl 1):S34–S36.

244. Oku H, Sugiyama T, Kojima S, Watanabe T, Azuma I. Experimental optic cup enlargement caused by endothelin-1-induced chronic optic nerve head ischemia. *Surv Ophthalmol*. 1999;44(Suppl 1):S74–S84.

245. Bernstein SL, Guo Y, Kelman SE, Flower RW, Johnson MA. Functional and cellular responses in a novel rodent model of anterior ischemic optic neuropathy. *Invest Ophthalmol Vis Sci*. 2003;44(10):4153–4162.

246. Chen CS, Johnson MA, Flower RA, Slater BJ, Miller NR, Bernstein SL. A primate model of nonarteritic anterior ischemic optic neuropathy. *Invest Ophthalmol Vis Sci*. 2008;49(7):2985–2992.

247. Duan Y, Kong W, Watson BD, Goldberg JL. *Retinal Ganglion Cell Survival and Optic Nerve Glial Response after Rat Optic Nerve Ischemic Injury*. New Orleans, LA: American Heart Association Investigators' Meeting; 2008.

248. Rizzo JFd, Lessell S. Risk of developing multiple sclerosis after uncomplicated optic neuritis: a long-term prospective study. *Neurology*. 1988;38(2):185–190.

249. Optic Neuritis Study Group The 5-year risk of MS after optic neuritis. Experience of the optic neuritis treatment trial. *Neurology*. 1997;49(5):1404–1413.

250. Yarom Y, Naparstek Y, Lev-Ram V, Holoshitz J, Ben-Nun A, Cohen IR. Immunospecific inhibition of nerve conduction by T lymphocytes reactive to basic protein of myelin. *Nature*. 1983;303(5914):246–247.

251. Trapp BD, Peterson J, Ransohoff RM, Rudick R, Mork S, Bo L. Axonal transection in the lesions of multiple sclerosis. *N Engl J Med*. 1998;338(5):278–285.

252. Perry VH, Anthony DC. Axon damage and repair in multiple sclerosis. *Philos Trans R Soc Lond B Biol Sci*. 1999;354(1390):1641–1647.

253. Evangelou N, Esiri MM, Smith S, Palace J, Matthews PM. Quantitative pathological evidence for axonal loss in normal appearing white matter in multiple sclerosis. *Ann Neurol*. 2000;47(3):391–395.

254. MacFadyen DJ, Drance SM, Douglas GR, Airaksinen PJ, Mawson DK, Paty DW. The retinal nerve fiber layer, neuroretinal rim area, and visual evoked potentials in MS. *Neurology*. 1988;38(9):1353–1358.

255. Hayreh SS, Massanari RM, Yamada T, Hayreh SM. Experimental allergic encephalomyelitis. I. Optic nerve and central nervous system manifestations. *Invest Ophthalmol Vis Sci*. 1981;21(2):256–269.

256. Sergott RC, Brown MJ, Silberberg DH, Lisak RP. Antigalactocerebroside serum demyelinates optic nerve in vivo. *J Neurol Sci*. 1984;64(3):297–303.

257. Zhu B, Moore GR, Zwimpfer TJ, et al. Axonal cytoskeleton changes in experimental optic neuritis. *Brain Res*. 1999;824(2):204–217.

258. Guy J, Ellis EA, Tark EFd, Hope GM, Rao NA. Axonal transport reductions in acute experimental allergic encephalomyelitis: qualitative analysis of the optic nerve. *Curr Eye Res*. 1989;8(3):261–269.

259. Guy J, Ellis EA, Kelley K, Hope GM, Rao NA. Quantitative analysis of labelled inner retinal proteins in experimental optic neuritis. *Curr Eye Res*. 1989;8(3):253–260.

260. Rao NA, Guy J, Sheffield PS. Effects of chronic demyelination on axonal transport in experimental allergic optic neuritis. *Invest Ophthalmol Vis Sci*. 1981;21(4):606–611.

261. Gutierrez R, Boison D, Heinemann U, Stoffel W. Decompaction of CNS myelin leads to a reduction of the conduction velocity of action potentials in optic nerve. *Neurosci Lett*. 1995;195(2):93–96.

262. Waxman SG, Black JA, Kocsis JD, et al. Low density of sodium channels supports action potential conduction in axons of neonatal rat optic nerve. *Proc Natl Acad Sci USA*. 1989;86:1406.

263. Storch MK, Stefferl A, Brehm U, et al. Autoimmunity to myelin oligodendrocyte glycoprotein in rats mimics the spectrum of multiple sclerosis pathology. *Brain Pathol*. 1998;8(4):681–694.

264. Bettelli E, Pagany M, Weiner HL, Linington C, Sobel RA, Kuchroo VK. Myelin oligodendrocyte glycoprotein-specific T cell receptor transgenic mice develop spontaneous autoimmune optic neuritis. *J Exp Med*. 2003;197(9):1073–1081.

265. Shao H, Huang Z, Sun SL, Kaplan HJ, Sun D. Myelin/oligodendrocyte glycoprotein-specific T-cells induce severe optic neuritis in the C57BL/6 mouse. *Invest Ophthalmol Vis Sci*. 2004;45(11):4060–4065.

266. Guan Y, Shindler KS, Tabuena P, Rostami AM. Retinal ganglion cell damage induced by spontaneous autoimmune optic neuritis in MOG-specific TCR transgenic mice. *J Neuroimmunol*. 2006;178(1-2):40–48.

267. Fontana L, Bhandari A, Fitzke FW, Hitchings RA. In vivo morphometry of the lamina cribrosa and its relation to visual field loss in glaucoma. *Curr Eye Res*. 1998;17(4):363–369.

268. Clifford-Jones RE, McDonald WI, Landon DN. Chronic optic nerve compression. An experimental study. *Brain*. 1985;108(Pt 1):241–262.

269. Clifford-Jones RE, Landon DN, McDonald WI. Remyelination during optic nerve compression. *J Neurol Sci*. 1980;46(2):239–243.

270. Guyer DR, Miller NR, Long DM, Allen GS. Visual function following optic canal decompression via craniotomy. *J Neurosurg*. 1985;62(5):631–638.

271. Giles CL, Soble AR. Intracranial hypertension and tetracycline therapy. *Am J Ophthalmol*. 1971;72(5):981–982.

272. Minckler DS. Histology of optic nerve damage in ocular hypertension and early glaucoma. *Surv Ophthalmol*. 1989;33(Suppl):401–411.

273. Quigley HA. Ganglion cell death in glaucoma: pathology recapitulates ontogeny. *Aust N Z J Ophthalmol*. 1995;23(2):85–91.

274. Quigley HA, Nickells RW, Kerrigan LA, Pease ME, Thibault DJ, Zack DJ. Retinal ganglion cell death in experimental glaucoma and after axotomy occurs by apoptosis. *Invest Ophthalmol Vis Sci*. 1995;36(5):774–786.

275. Kerrigan LA, Zack DJ, Quigley HA, Smith SD, Pease ME. TUNEL-positive ganglion cells in human primary open-angle glaucoma. *Arch Ophthalmol*. 1997;115(8):1031–1035.

276. Okisaka S, Murakami A, Mizukawa A, Ito J. Apoptosis in retinal ganglion cell decrease in human glaucomatous eyes. *Jpn J Ophthalmol*. 1997;41(2):84–88.

277. Dkhissi O, Chanut E, Wasowicz M, et al. Retinal TUNEL-positive cells and high glutamate levels in vitreous humor of mutant quail with a glaucoma-like disorder. *Invest Ophthalmol Vis Sci*. 1999;40(5):990–995.

278. Quigley HA, Dunkelberger GR, Green WR. Retinal ganglion cell atrophy correlated with automated perimetry in human eyes with glaucoma. *Am J Ophthalmol*. 1989;107(5):453–464.

279. Hoyt WF, Frisen L, Newman NM. Fundoscopy of nerve fiber layer defects in glaucoma. *Invest Ophthalmol*. 1973;12(11):814–829.

280. Quigley HA, Miller NR, George T. Clinical evaluation of nerve fiber layer atrophy as an indicator of glaucomatous optic nerve damage. *Arch Ophthalmol*. 1980;98(9):1564–1571.

281. Airaksinen PJ, Drance SM, Douglas GR, Mawson DK, Nieminen H. Diffuse and localized nerve fiber loss in glaucoma. *Am J Ophthalmol*. 1984;98(5):566–571.

282. Iwata K, Kurosawa A, Sawaguchi S. Wedge-shaped retinal nerve fiber layer defects in experimental glaucoma preliminary report. *Graefes Arch Clin Exp Ophthalmol*. 1985;223(4):184–189.

283. Drance SM. The early structural and functional disturbances of chronic open-angle glaucoma. Robert N. Shaffer lecture. *Ophthalmology*. 1985;92(7):853–857.

284. Stroman GA, Stewart WC, Golnik KC, Cure JK, Olinger RE. Magnetic resonance imaging in patients with low-tension glaucoma. *Arch Ophthalmol*. 1995;113(2):168–172.

285. Iwata F, Patronas NJ, Caruso RC, et al. Association of visual field, cup-disc ratio, and magnetic resonance imaging of optic chiasm. *Arch Ophthalmol*. 1997;115(6):729–732.

286. Weber AJ, Chen H, Hubbard WC, Kaufman PL. Experimental glaucoma and cell size, density, and number in the primate lateral geniculate nucleus. *Invest Ophthalmol Vis Sci*. 2000;41(6):1370–1379.

287. Yücel YH, Zhang Q, Gupta N, Kaufman PL, Weinreb RN. Loss of neurons in magnocellular and parvocellular layers of the lateral geniculate nucleus in glaucoma. *Arch Ophthalmol*. 2000;118(3):378–384.

288. Vickers JC, Hof PR, Schumer RA, Wang RF, Podos SM, Morrison JH. Magnocellular and parvocellular visual pathways are both affected in a macaque monkey model of glaucoma. *Aust N Z J Ophthalmol*. 1997;25(3):239–243.

289. Chaturvedi N, Hedley-Whyte ET, Dreyer EB. Lateral geniculate nucleus in glaucoma. *Am J Ophthalmol*. 1993;116(2):182–188.

290. Crawford ML, Harwerth RS, Smith 3rd EL, Mills S, Ewing B. Experimental glaucoma in primates: changes in cytochrome oxidase blobs in V1 cortex. *Invest Ophthalmol Vis Sci*. 2001;42(2):358–364.

291. Crawford ML, Harwerth RS, Smith 3rd EL, Shen F, Carter-Dawson L. Glaucoma in primates: cytochrome oxidase reactivity in parvo- and magnocellular pathways. *Invest Ophthalmol Vis Sci*. 2000;41(7):1791–1802.

292. Chang EE, Goldberg JL. Glaucoma 2.0: neuroprotection, neuroregeneration, neuroenhancement. *Ophthalmology*. 2012;119(5):979–986.

293. Morrison JC, Johnson EC, Cepurna W, Jia L. Understanding mechanisms of pressure-induced optic nerve damage. *Prog Retin Eye Res*. 2005;24(2):217–240.

294. Whitmore AV, Libby RT, John SW. Glaucoma: thinking in new ways-a role for autonomous axonal self-destruction and other compartmentalised processes? *Prog Retin Eye Res*. 2005;24(6):639–662.

295. Quigley HA, Addicks EM. Chronic experimental glaucoma in primates. II. Effect of extended intraocular pressure elevation on optic nerve head and axonal transport. *Invest Ophthalmol Vis Sci*. 1980;19(2):137–152.

296. Quigley HA, Addicks EM, Green WR, Maumenee AE. Optic nerve damage in human glaucoma. II. The site of injury and susceptibility to damage. *Arch Ophthalmol.* 1981;99(4):635–649.

297. Allcutt D, Berry M, Sievers J. A qualitative comparison of the reactions of retinal ganglion cell axons to optic nerve crush in neonatal and adult mice. *Brain Res.* 1984;318(2):231–240.

298. Allcutt D, Berry M, Sievers J. A quantitative comparison of the reactions of retinal ganglion cells to optic nerve crush in neonatal and adult mice. *Brain Res.* 1984;318(2):219–230.

299. Barron KD, Dentinger MP, Krohel G, Easton SK, Mankes R. Qualitative and quantitative ultrastructural observations on retinal ganglion cell layer of rat after intraorbital optic nerve crush. *J Neurocytol.* 1986;15(3):345–362.

300. Anderson DR, Hendrickson A. Effect of intraocular pressure on rapid axoplasmic transport in monkey optic nerve. *Invest Ophthalmol.* 1974;13:771.

301. Quigley HA, Guy J, Anderson DR. Blockade of rapid axonal transport. Effect of intraocular pressure elevation in primate optic nerve. *Arch Ophthalmol.* 1979;97(3):525–531.

302. Radius RL. Pressure-induced fast axonal transport abnormalities and the anatomy at the lamina cribrosa in primate eyes. *Invest Ophthalmol Vis Sci.* 1983;24:343.

303. Minckler DS, Bunt AH, Johanson GW. Orthograde and retrograde axoplasmic transport during acute ocular hypertension in the monkey. *Invest Ophthalmol Vis Sci.* 1977;16(5):426–441.

304. Ventura LM, Porciatti V. Restoration of retinal ganglion cell function in early glaucoma after intraocular pressure reduction: a pilot study. *Ophthalmology.* 2005;112(1):20–27.

305. Ventura LM, Sorokac N, De Los Santos R, Feuer WJ, Porciatti V. The relationship between retinal ganglion cell function and retinal nerve fiber thickness in early glaucoma. *Invest Ophthalmol Vis Sci.* 2006;47(9):3904–3911.

306. Ventura LM, Venzara 3rd FX, Porciatti V. Reversible dysfunction of retinal ganglion cells in non-secreting pituitary tumors. *Doc Ophthalmol.* 2008

307. Garcia-Valenzuela E, Gorczyca W, Darzynkiewicz Z, Sharma SC. Apoptosis in adult retinal ganglion cells after axotomy. *J Neurobiol.* 1994;25(4):431–438.

308. Rehen SK, Linden R. Apoptosis in the developing retina: paradoxical effects of protein synthesis inhibition. *Braz J Med Biol Res.* 1994;27(7):1647–1651.

309. Levin LA, Louhab A. Apoptosis of retinal ganglion cells in anterior ischemic optic neuropathy. *Arch Ophthalmol.* 1996;114(4):488–491.

310. Cellerino A, Galli-Resta L, Colombaioni L. The Dynamics of Neuronal Death: A Time-Lapse Study in the Retina. *J Neurosci.* 2000;20(16):RC92.

311. Kerr JF, Wyllie AH, Currie AR. Apoptosis: a basic biological phenomenon with wide-ranging implications in tissue kinetics. *Br J Cancer.* 1972;26(4):239–257.

312. Gavrieli Y, Sherman Y, Ben-Sasson SA. Identification of programmed cell death in situ via specific labeling of nuclear DNA fragmentation. *J Cell Biol.* 1992;119(3):493–501.

313. Ankarcrona M, Dypbukt JM, Bonfoco E, et al. Glutamate-induced neuronal death: a succession of necrosis or apoptosis depending on mitochondrial function. *Neuron.* 1995;15(4):961–973.

314. Lucas M, Solano F, Sanz A. Induction of programmed cell death (apoptosis) in mature lymphocytes. *FEBS Letters.* 1991;279(1):19–20.

315. Olney JW. The toxic effects of glutamate and related compounds in the retina and the brain. *Retina.* 1982;2(4):341–359.

316. Sisk DR, Kuwabara T. Histologic changes in the inner retina of albino rats following intravitreal injection of monosodium L-glutamate. *Graefes Arch Clin Exp Ophthalmol.* 1985;223(5):250–258.

317. Schumer RA, Podos SM. The nerve of glaucoma! *Arch Ophthalmol.* 1994;112(1):37–44.

318. Russelakis-Carneiro M, Silveira LC, Perry VH. Factors affecting the survival of cat retinal ganglion cells after optic nerve injury. *J Neurocytol.* 1996;25(6):393–402.

319. Yoles E, Muller S, Schwartz M. NMDA-receptor antagonist protects neurons from secondary degeneration after partial optic nerve crush. *J Neurotrauma.* 1997;14:665–675.

320. Yoles E, Schwartz M. Elevation of intraocular glutamate levels in rats with partial lesion of the optic nerve. *Arch Ophthalmol.* 1998;116(7):906–910.

321. Dreyer EB, Zurakowski D, Schumer RA, Podos SM, Lipton SA. Elevated glutamate levels in the vitreous body of humans and monkeys with glaucoma. *Arch Ophthalmol.* 1996;114(3):299–305.

322. Kreutz MR, Bockers TM, Bockmann J, et al. Axonal injury alters alternative splicing of the retinal NR1 receptor: the preferential expression of the NR1b isoforms is crucial for retinal ganglion cell survival. *J Neurosci.* 1998;18(20):8278–8291.

323. Ullian EM, Barkis WB, Chen S, Diamond JS, Barres BA. Invulnerability of retinal ganglion cells to NMDA excitotoxicity. *Mol Cell Neurosci.* 2004;26(4):544–557.

324. Levin LA, Peeples P. History of neuroprotection and rationale as a therapy for glaucoma. *Am J Manag Care.* 2008;14(1 Suppl):S11–S14.

325. Murray M, Grafstein B. Changes in the morphology and amino acid incorporation of regenerating goldfish optic neurons. *Exp Neurol.* 1969;23:544–560.

326. Humphrey MF, Beazley LD. Retinal ganglion cell death during optic nerve regeneration in the frog Hyla moorei. *J Comp Neurol.* 1985;263:382–402.

327. Humphrey MF. A morphometric study of the retinal ganglion cell response to optic nerve severance in the frog Rana pipiens. *J Neurocytol.* 1988;17:293–304.

328. Grafstein B, Ingoglia NA. Intracranial transection of the optic nerve in adult mice: Preliminary observations. *Exp Neurol.* 1982;76:318–330.

329. Misantone LJ, Gershenbaum M, Murray M. Viability of retinal ganglion cells after optic nerve crush in adult rats. *J Neurocytol.* 1984;13(3):449–465.

330. Villegas-Perez MP, Vidal-Sanz M, Rasminsky M, Bray GM, Aguayo AJ. Rapid and protracted phases of retinal ganglion cell loss follow axotomy in the optic nerve of adult rats. *J Neurobiol.* 1993;24(1):23–36.

331. Peinado-Ramon P, Salvador M, Villegas-Perez MP, Vidal-Sanz M. Effects of axotomy and intraocular administration of NT-4, NT-3, and brain-derived neurotrophic factor on the survival of adult rat retinal ganglion cells. A quantitative in vivo study. *Invest Ophthalmol Vis Sci.* 1996;37(4):489–500.

332. Radius RL, Anderson DR. Retinal ganglion cell degeneration in experimental optic atrophy. *Am J Ophthalmol.* 1978;86(5):673–679.

333. Quigley HA, Anderson DR. Descending optic nerve degeneration in primates. *Invest Ophthalmol Vis Sci.* 1977;16:841–849.

334. Kupfer C. Retinal ganglion cell degeneration following chiasmal lesions in man. *Arch Ophthalmol.* 1963;70:256–260.

335. Goldberg S, Frank B. Do young axons regenerate better than old axons? *Exp Neurol.* 1981;74:245–259.

336. Stone J. The naso-temporal division of the cat's retina. *J Comp Neurol.* 1966;126:585–600.

337. Watanabe M, Fukuda Y. Survival and axonal regeneration of retinal ganglion cells in adult cats. *Prog Retin Eye Res.* 2002;21(6):529–553.

338. Tran NM, Shekhar K, Whitney IE, et al. Single-Cell Profiles of Retinal Ganglion Cells Differing in Resilience to Injury Reveal Neuroprotective Genes. *Neuron.* 2019;104(6):1039–1055.:e12.

339. Beykin G, Norcia AM, Srinivasan VJ, Dubra A, Goldberg JL. Discovery and clinical translation of novel glaucoma biomarkers. *Prog Retin Eye Res.* 2021;80:100875.

340. Norcia AM, Yakovleva A, Hung B, Goldberg JL. Dynamics of Contrast Decrement and Increment Responses in Human Visual Cortex. *Transl Vis Sci Technol.* 2020;9(10):6.

341. Thanos S, Pavlidis C, Mey J, Thiel HJ. Specific transcellular staining of microglia in the adult rat after traumatic degeneration of carbocyanine-filled retinal ganglion cells. *Exp Eye Res.* 1992;55(1):101–117.

342. Leinfelder PJ. Retrograde degeneration in the optic nerves and tracts. *Am J Ophthalmol.* 1940;23:796–802.

343. Watson WE. Cellular responses to axotomy and to related procedures. *Br Med Bull.* 1974;30:112–115.

344. Lieberman AR. A review of the principal features of perikaryal responses to axon injury. *Int Rev Neurobiol.* 1971;14:49–124.

345. Anderson DR. Ascending and descending optic atrophy produced experimentally in squirrel monkeys. *Am J Ophthalmol.* 1973;76:693–711.

346. Madison R, Moore MR, Sidman RL. Retinal ganglion cells and axons survive optic nerve transection. *Int J Neurosci.* 1984;23(1):15–32.

347. Cragg BG. What is the signal for chromatolysis? *Brain Res.* 1970;23:1–21.

348. Schnitzer J, Scherer J. Microglial cell responses in the rabbit retina following transection of the optic nerve. *J Comp Neurol.* 1990;302:779–791.

349. Cui Q, Harvey AR. At least two mechanisms are involved in the death of retinal ganglion cells following target ablation in neonatal rats. *J Neurosci.* 1995;15:8143–8155.

350. Bodeutsch N, Siebert H, Dermon C, Thanos S. Unilateral injury to the adult rat optic nerve causes multiple cellular responses in the contralateral site. *J Neurobiol.* 1999;38(1):116–128.

351. Maffei L, Carmignoto G, Perry VH, Candeo P, Ferrari G. Schwann cells promote the survival of rat retinal ganglion cells after optic nerve section. *Proc Natl Acad Sci USA.* 1990;87(5):1855–1859.

352. Castillo BJ, del CM, Breakefield XO, et al. Retinal ganglion cell survival is promoted by genetically modified astrocytes designed to secrete brain-derived neurotrophic factor (BDNF). *Brain Res.* 1994;647(1):30–36.

353. Weibel D, Kreutzberg GW, Schwab ME. Brain-derived neurotrophic factor (BDNF) prevents lesion-induced axonal die-back in young rat optic nerve. *Brain Res.* 1995;679(2):249–254.

354. Beykin G, Stell L, Halim MS, et al. Phase 1b Randomized Controlled Study of Short Course Topical Recombinant Human Nerve Growth Factor (rhNGF) for Neuroenhancement in Glaucoma: Safety, Tolerability, and Efficacy Measure Outcomes. *Am J Ophthalmol.* 2022;234:223–234.

355. Cook RD, Wisniewski HM. The role of oligodendroglia and astroglia in Wallerian degeneration of the optic nerve. *Brain Res.* 1973;61:191.

356. Ludwin SK. Phagocytosis in the rat optic nerve following Wallerian degeneration. *Acta Neuropathol (Berl).* 1990;80:266.

357. Stoll G, Mueller HW. Lesion-induced changes of astrocyte morphology and protein expression in rat optic nerve. *Ann NY Acad Sci.* 1988;540:461.

358. Ling EA. Electron microscopic studies of macrophages in Wallerian degeneration of rat optic nerve after intravenous injection of colloidal carbon. *J Anat.* 1978;126:111.

359. Stevens A, Bahr M. Origin of macrophages in central nervous tissue. A study using intraperitoneal transplants contained in Millipore diffusion chambers. *J Neurol Sci.* 1993;118(2):117–122.

360. Reichert F, Rotshenker S. Deficient activation of microglia during optic nerve degeneration. *J Neuroimmunol.* 1996;70(2):153–161.

361. Lazarov-Spiegler O, Solomon AS, Zeev-Brann AB, Hirschberg DL, Lavie V, Schwartz M. Transplantation of activated macrophages overcomes central nervous system regrowth failure. *FASEB Journal.* 1996;10(11):1296–1302.

362. Baris M, Tezel G. Immunomodulation as a Neuroprotective Strategy for Glaucoma Treatment. *Curr Ophthalmol Rep.* 2019;7(2):160–169.

363. Chen H, Cho KS, Vu THK, et al. Commensal microflora-induced T cell responses mediate progressive neurodegeneration in glaucoma. *Nat Commun.* 2018;9(1):3209.

364. Butt AM, Colquhoun K. Glial cells in transected optic nerves of immature rats. I. An analysis of individual cells by intracellular dye-injection. *J Neurocytol.* 1996;25(6):365–380.

365. Butt AM, Kirvell S. Glial cells in transected optic nerves of immature rats. II. An immunohistochemical study. *J Neurocytol.* 1996;25(6):381–392.

366. Liddelow SA, Guttenplan KA, Clarke LE, et al. Neurotoxic reactive astrocytes are induced by activated microglia. *Nature.* 2017;541(7638):481–487.

367. Anderson MA, Burda JE, Ren Y, et al. Astrocyte scar formation aids central nervous system axon regeneration. *Nature.* 2016;532(7598):195–200.

368. Sofroniew MV. Astrocyte barriers to neurotoxic inflammation. *Nat Rev Neurosci.* 2015;16(5):249–263.

369. Wanner M, Lang DM, Bandtlow CE, Schwab ME, Bastmeyer M, Stuermer CA. Reevaluation of the growth-permissive substrate properties of goldfish optic nerve myelin and myelin proteins. *J Neurosci.* 1995;15(11):7500–7508.

370. Matsumoto N, Kometani M, Nagano K. Regenerating retinal fibers of the goldfish make temporary and unspecific but functional synapses before forming the final retinotopic projection. *Neuroscience.* 1987;22(3):1103–1110.

371. Sawai H, Clarke DB, Kittlerova P, Bray GM, Aguayo AJ. Brain-derived neurotrophic factor and neurotrophin-4/5 stimulate growth of axonal branches from regenerating retinal ganglion cells. *J Neurosci*. 1996;16(12):3887–3894.

372. Zeng BY, Anderson PN, Campbell G, Lieberman AR. Regenerative and other responses to injury in the retinal stump of the optic nerve in adult albino rats: transection of the intraorbital optic nerve. *J Anat*. 1994;185(Pt 3):643–661.

373. So KF, Aguayo AJ. Lengthy regrowth of cut axons from ganglion cells after peripheral nerve transplantation into the retina of adult rats. *Brain Res*. 1985;328(2):349–354.

374. Aguayo AJ, David S, Bray GM. Influences of the glial environment on the elongation of axons after injury: transplantation studies in adult rodents. *J Exp Biol*. 1981;95:231–240.

375. Yiu G, He Z. Glial inhibition of CNS axon regeneration. *Nat Rev Neurosci*. 2006;7(8):617–627.

376. Frank M, Wolburg H. Cellular reactions at the lesion site after crushing of the rat optic nerve. *Glia*. 1996;16(3):227–240.

377. Podhajsky RJ, Bidanset DJ, Caterson B, Blight AR. A quantitative immunohistochemical study of the cellular response to crush injury in optic nerve. *Exp Neurol*. 1997;143(1):153–161.

378. Zeev-Brann AB, Lazarov-Spiegler O, Brenner T, Schwartz M. Differential effects of central and peripheral nerves on macrophages and microglia. *Glia*. 1998;23(3):181–190.

379. Castano A, Bell MD, Perry VH. Unusual aspects of inflammation in the nervous system: Wallerian degeneration. *Neurobiol Aging*. 1996;17(5):745–751.

380. Kalil K, Reh T. A light and electron microscopic study of regrowing pyramidal tract fibers. *J Comp Neurol*. 1982;211(3):265–275.

381. Reh T, Kalil K. Functional role of regrowing pyramidal tract fibers. *J Comp Neurol*. 1982;211(3):276–283.

382. Saunders NR, Balkwill P, Knott G, et al. Growth of axons through a lesion in the intact CNS of fetal rat maintained in long-term culture. *Proc R Soc Lond B Biol Sci*. 1992;250(1329):171–180.

383. Aguayo AJ, Vidal-Sanz M, Villegas-Perez MP, Bray GM. Growth and connectivity of axotomized retinal neurons in adult rats with optic nerves substituted by PNS grafts linking the eye and the midbrain. *Ann N Y Acad Sci*. 1987;495:1–9.

384. Bray GM, Villegas-Perez MP, Vidal-Sanz M, Aguayo AJ. The use of peripheral nerve grafts to enhance neuronal survival, promote growth and permit terminal reconnections in the central nervous system of adult rats. *J Exp Biol*. 1987;132:5–19.

385. Chen DF, Jhaveri S, Schneider GE. Intrinsic changes in developing retinal neurons result in regenerative failure of their axons. *Proc Natl Acad Sci U S A*. 1995;92(16):7287–7291.

386. Goldberg JL, Klassen MP, Hua Y, Barres BA. Amacrine-signaled loss of intrinsic axon growth ability by retinal ganglion cells. *Science*. 2002;296(5574):1860–1864.

387. Blackmore MG, Moore DL, Goldberg JL, Bixby JL, Lemmon VP. *A developmentally regulated family of transcription factors controls axon growth in CNS neurons*, in *Society for Neuroscience. Washington, D.C.* 2008:725.23.

388. Moore, D.L., M.G. Blackmore, and J.L. Goldberg, *Transcriptional control of intrinsic axon growth ability in retinal ganglion cells, in Society for Neuroscience*. 2008: Washington, D. C. p. 725.24.

389. Wayman GA, Kaech S, Grant WF, et al. Regulation of axonal extension and growth cone motility by calmodulin-dependent protein kinase I. *J Neurosci*. 2004;24(15):3786–3794.

390. Guo X, Zhou J, Starr C, et al. Preservation of vision after CaMKII-mediated protection of retinal ganglion cells. *Cell*. 2021;184(16):4299–4314. e12.

391. Cai D, Qiu J, Cao Z, McAtee M, Bregman BS, Filbin MT. Neuronal cyclic AMP controls the developmental loss in ability of axons to regenerate. *J Neurosci*. 2001;21(13):4731–4739.

392. Williams PR, Benowitz LI, Goldberg JL, He Z. Axon Regeneration in the Mammalian Optic Nerve. *Annu Rev Vis Sci*. 2020;6:195–213.

393. Carroll WM, Jennings AR, Mastaglia FL. The origin of remyelinating oligodendrocytes in antiserum-mediated demyelinative optic neuropathy. *Brain*. 1990;113:953.

394. Stanhope GB, Billings-Gagliardi S, Wolf MK. Myelination requirements of central nervous system glia in vitro: statistical validation of differences between glia from adult and immature mice. *Glia*. 1990;3:125.

395. Goldman SA, Mariani JN, Madsen PM. Glial progenitor cell-based repair of the dysmyelinated brain: Progression to the clinic. *Semin Cell Dev Biol*. 2021;116:62–70.

396. Brenner MJ, Fox IK, Kawamura DH, et al. Delayed nerve repair is associated with diminished neuroenhancement by FK506. *Laryngoscope*. 2004;114(3):570–576.

397. Normann C, Berger M. Neuroenhancement: status quo and perspectives. *Eur Arch Psychiatry Clin Neurosci*. 2008;258(Suppl 5):110–114.

398. Schloesser RJ, Chen G, Manji HK. Neurogenesis and neuroenhancement in the pathophysiology and treatment of bipolar disorder. *Int Rev Neurobiol*. 2007;77:143–178.

399. Beykin G, Goldberg JL. Molecular Biomarkers for Glaucoma. *Curr Ophthalmol Rep*. 2019;7(3):171–176.

29

Processing in the Lateral Geniculate Nucleus

José Manuel Alonso and Arjun Krishnaswamy

THE LATERAL GENICULATE NUCLEUS: THE GATEWAY TO CONSCIOUS VISUAL PERCEPTION

Located one synapse from the retina, the lateral geniculate nucleus (LGN) of the thalamus is the main link between eye and cortex. Although the retina connects with other subcortical structures, the route through the LGN is required for conscious visual perception. Connections between retinal ganglion cells (RGCs) and LGN neurons are highly specific and establish channels of visual information that preserve the encoding of visual stimuli within the retina. Rather than transform visual information originating in its RGC inputs, the LGN modulates the transfer of retinal information to cortex based on visual demands, changes in brain state (sleep, arousal), and attention. The LGN modulation by sleep-arousal is thought to be mediated by inputs from the brain stem and the modulation by attention by inputs from the visual cortex. In addition, inputs from the superior colliculus (SC) to the koniocellular layers of the LGN may also contribute to a form of subconscious vision known as blindsight. The purpose of this chapter is to illuminate the structure and function of the LGN by first reviewing LGN anatomy and physiology, incorporating new genetic insights into the LGN's cellular taxonomy, following the flow of information into LGN and out to the cortex, and, finally, reviewing the functional impact of attention. The final section summarizes the key points.

LATERAL GENICULATE NUCLEUS ANATOMY

The human LGN is an elongated, layered structure with the shape of a small bean (Fig. 29.1A) and a volume that can range from 77 to 152 cubic millimeters across individual subjects.[1] All human LGNs have six main layers in the posterior half of the nucleus representing central vision and two layers in the smaller segment representing monocular peripheral vision (Fig. 29.1B). The six main layers of the LGN are classified by cell size as parvocellular (parvo: small in Latin) or magnocellular (magno: big in Latin), and they are separated by thin koniocellular layers with sparse small cells (konio: dust in Greek). The layers are numbered, from ventral to dorsal, as M1 to M2 for the magnocellular layers, P3 to P6 for the parvocellular layers, and K1 to K6 for the koniocellular layers (Fig. 29.1C).

Every LGN layer represents half of the contralateral visual field. The LGN layers of the left hemisphere represent the right visual hemifield and the layers of the right hemisphere the left visual hemifield. Because each visual hemifield is seen with the nasal retina from one eye and temporal retina from the other, the two eyes need to be represented in the same LGN. The representations of each eye are segregated into different LGN layers. The nasal retina from the contralateral eye is represented in layers M1, P4, P6, K1, ventral K2, K4, and K6, whereas the temporal retina from the ipsilateral eye is represented in layers M2, P3, P5, dorsal K2, K3, and K5 (Fig. 29.1C).[2] The layers

receiving contralateral input are the only ones representing the monocular peripheral region; therefore, those representing the ipsilateral eye are always shorter because they represent a smaller visual field.

The repeated representations of the visual hemifield in the different LGN layers are precisely aligned such that one point in visual space is represented along a line crossing all layers roughly perpendicularly. This retinotopic alignment is so precise that the blind spot caused by the optic nerve is represented by a gap of LGN tissue free of cells, which maintains the retinotopic alignment of the contralateral and ipsilateral layers (see Fig. 29.6). The laminar organization of the LGN is similar in humans and other primates such as macaques[2,3] but differs across mammalian species.[4] In spite of these variations, several organizing principles are evolutionarily preserved in the LGN, including the segregation of eye inputs and the basic neuronal circuitry.

LATERAL GENICULATE NUCLEUS DEVELOPMENT AND CELLULAR TAXONOMY

Work in mice shows that the LGN is generated alongside approximately 50 other thalamic nuclei from a small patch of neuroepithelium located in the embryonic diencephalon. Under the control of developmental programs, a small group of neural precursors bud off this patch to create the nascent LGN, differentiating in the womb to create excitatory neurons and glia.[5,6] LGN is among the only dorsal thalamic nuclei possessing inhibitory interneurons, which in rodents are born in the ventral LGN and forebrain, and migrate into the LGN after the excitatory neurons are generated.[7,8] Primate LGN development is likely to follow a similar plan, as recent comparative genetic analyses reveal that rodent, macaque, and human LGN neurons can be divided into transcriptomically similar subclasses.[9]

Droplet sequencing methods allow investigators to acquire millions of individual neural transcriptomes from human, macaque, and mouse LGN, and then group neurons according to their gene expression (Box 29.1).[9] Comparing such transcriptomic cellular atlases across species reveals that primate magnocellular and parvocellular LGN cells selectively express the calcium buffer parvalbumin-1 (Pvalb1), whereas koniocellular LGN cells express the calcium buffer calbindin-1 (Calb1). Interestingly, this pair of genes labels largely exclusive subpopulations of excitatory neurons that reside in the core (Pvalb1) or shell (Calb1) regions of rodent LGN. Atlas comparisons also show a diversity of interneurons for each species and predict three or four different inhibitory types for primates occurring at an abundance of about one-quarter that of their excitatory counterparts. These new data confirm older evidence showing that magnocellular LGN cells selectively express genes such as neurofilament heavy chain and Robo2,[10] whereas parvocellular LGN cells express the transcription factor Foxp2.[10,11]

A notable omission from this effort is a lack of genetic analyses in cats, in which morphologic and functional characterization of LGN

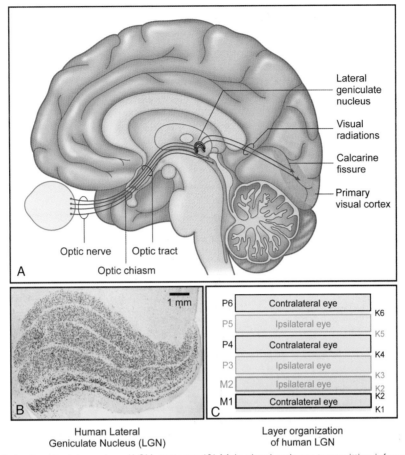

Fig. 29.1 Lateral geniculate nucleus (*LGN*) anatomy. (**A**) Main visual pathway transmitting information from retina to primary visual cortex through the LGN in the human brain. (**B**) Coronal section of human LGN (Reproduced with permission from Andrews TJ, Halpern SD, Purves D. Correlated size variations in human visual cortex, lateral geniculate nucleus, and optic tract. *J Neurosci* 1997:17;2859–2868.). (**C**) Cartoon illustrating the laminar organization of human LGN in the parvocellular (P3–P6), magnocellular (M1–M2), and koniocellular layers (K1–K6) representing the contralateral and ipsilateral eyes.

neural types is most complete. In this species, relay neurons are categorized into X-, Y-, and W-cells, which each possess a characteristic dendritic structure, laminar organization, and visual response.[12] W-cells are believed to be analogous to koniocellular cells in primates and shell neurons in mouse.[12] A well-accepted correspondence between the remaining LGN types in cats, primates, and mice does not exist currently. However, several functional studies suggest that magnocellular and parvocellular cells are composed of several subtypes, consistent with recent work in rodents showing 20 functionally distinct LGN neuron classes.[13] A clearer picture of the cell-type diversity in the LGN is important to our understanding of how this structure combines inputs originating from retina, cortex, midbrain, and brainstem. We consider major sources of input in the next section.

LATERAL GENICULATE NUCLEUS INPUTS

The LGN is the main link between eye and cortex. Its excitatory neurons, called relay cells, integrate excitatory input from RGC axons and transfer this information to the cortex for further analysis. Only a relatively small percentage of the LGN synapses are made by RGC axons,[14] whereas many others arise from axons originating in the visual cortex and brain stem. Thus, the LGN has been proposed to act as a "smart" filter that titers visual input reaching the V1 according to internal feedback. Next we briefly overview the main LGN inputs (Fig. 29.2D).

Retinal inputs

A family of RGC types decompose incoming visual stimuli. Some RGCs compare stimuli falling in their receptive field center with stimuli in their surround. ON RGCs fire when the stimulus luminance is higher at the center than surround, whereas OFF RGCs fire when the stimulus luminance is higher at the surround than the center. In humans, midget RGCs receive center input from a single cone.[15] Parasol RGCs boast larger dendritic arbors that integrate from several cones, making their view of the world larger but devoid of color information.[16] Yet other RGCs have been described in the peripheral parts of the primate retina that encode other features such as stimulus motion. These three RGC classes project to specific layers within the LGN, with midget RGCs providing input to the parvocellular layers, parasol RGCs to the magnocellular layers, and all other RGC types innervating the koniocellular layers (Fig. 29.2A–C). New genetic methods (see Box 29.1) have provided a nearly complete cellular atlas of primate RGCs and predict a total of 22 primate RGC types.[17] As expected from previous work, midget and parasol types are the most abundant (~90% of all peripheral and foveal RGCs), but a sizable fraction of primate RGCs with unknown function remain. Such non-midget, non-parasol RGC types likely drive the koniocellular pathway[2] and express genes that are also expressed by the approximately 50 feature-detecting RGCs types found in mice.[18] Whether this transcriptomic similarity also reflects a functional similarity across species is not known, but the type-specific

---

BOX 29.1   Droplet sequencing

Neural circuits are viewed through the lens of their man-made electrical counterparts—the brain's many individual circuits are thought to wire unique subsets of neural types together so they can perform computations. Thus, defining a full list of the brain's neural types (parts list) has become a central goal in the neurosciences. A marriage of combinatorics, microfluidics, and deep sequencing has yielded a new technology to fuel this effort. This approach, called droplet sequencing,[95] works as follows. (1) A brain or brain region is dissociated into a suspension of individual cells. (2) Each cell is then encapsulated in a droplet of oil using a microfluidic device that collides such cell-containing droplets with another droplet containing lysis buffer, an inert bead decorated with DNA primers, and reverse transcriptase. (3) Upon collision, cells release mRNAs that bind the bead-anchored primers and permit reverse transcriptase to

copy their code into a DNA compliment (cDNA). Thus, each bead contains cDNA strands bearing a unique barcode, a communal bead barcode. (4) After all cells have been processed, the droplets are combined and broken open for a final round of amplification, and the entire library is subjected to deep sequencing. Comparing mRNA species bearing one bead barcode to another permits individual cells to be grouped into transcriptomic atlases that describe cell types. Each single-cell transcriptome costs fractions of a cent, making large-scale analysis of neural genomes relatively cheap—atlases now exist for every principal type in the retina,[17,95–99] the lateral geniculate nucleus,[9] and visual cortex[100] of several species providing a tangible route to translate insights from experimental models, such as mouse, to man.

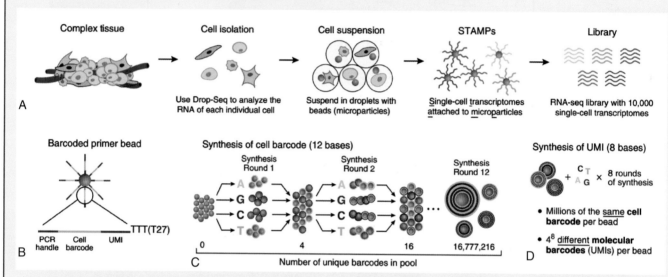

Molecular barcoding of cellular transcriptomes in droplets. (**A**) Complex tissue is dissociated into individual cells, which are then encapsulated in droplets together with microparticles *(gray circles)* that deliver barcoded primers. Each cell is lysed within a droplet; its mRNAs bind to the primers on its companion microparticle. The mRNAs are reverse-transcribed into cDNAs, generating a set of beads called "single-cell transcriptomes attached to microparticles" (STAMPs). The barcoded STAMPs can then be amplified in pools for high-throughput mRNA-seq to analyze any desired number of individual cells. (**B**) The primers on all beads contain a common sequence ("Polymerase chain reaction (PCR) handle") to enable PCR amplification after STAMP formation. Each microparticle contains more than [108] individual primers that share the same "cell barcode" (panel **C**) but have different unique molecular identifiers (UMIs), enabling mRNA transcripts to be digitally counted (panel **D**). A 30 bp oligo dT sequence is present at the end of all primer sequences for capture of mRNAs. (**C**) To generate the cell barcode, the pool of microparticles is repeatedly split into four equally sized oligonucleotide synthesis reactions, to which one of the four DNA bases is added, and then pooled together after each cycle, in a total of 12 split-pool cycles. The barcode synthesized on any individual bead reflects that bead's unique path through the series of synthesis reactions. (**D**) Following the completion of the "split-and-pool" synthesis cycles, all microparticles are together subjected to eight rounds of degenerate synthesis with all four DNA bases available during each cycle, such that each individual primer receives one of[48] (65,536) possible sequences, called a unique molecular identifier (UMI). (Figure and legend modified from Macosko EZ, Basu A, Satija R, et al. Highly parallel genome-wide expression profiling of individual cells using nanoliter droplets. *Cell.* 2015;161:1202–1214. https://doi:10.1016/j.cell.2015.05.002.)

---

marker genes provide a clear way to address this idea. Indeed, early comparative studies appear to have found a direction-selective primate RGC type with morphology and function matching that seen in mice.[19]

Cortical inputs

Nearly 30% of the LGN excitatory synapses form between relay cells and the axons of layer 6 (L6) pyramidal cells projecting from cortex.[20,21] Such feedback connections are stream specific. For example, the magnocellular LGN layers receive input from a population of L6 cortical neurons that are anatomically and functionally distinct from those providing input to the parvocellular layers.[22–24] Unlike their RGC counterparts, these cortical feedback axons connect only with relay cells and not with resident interneurons.[21] L6 neurons form small boutons

located on the distal dendrites of relay cells that cannot drive LGN spiking on their own. Instead, these inputs are thought to modulate ongoing relay neuron activity.

Inputs from the thalamic reticular nucleus

The antero-latero-dorsal surface of the entire thalamus is wrapped in a thin nucleus that exhibits a strong suppressive effect on every thalamic nucleus including the LGN. This shell, called the thalamic reticular nucleus (TRN), contains inhibitory neurons and has a loose topographic organization that matches the inputs it receives from sensory cortices, motor regions, and brainstem structures.[25] Remarkably little is known about these neurons, but several recent genetic studies have identified a host of disease-relevant mutations that affect genes strongly

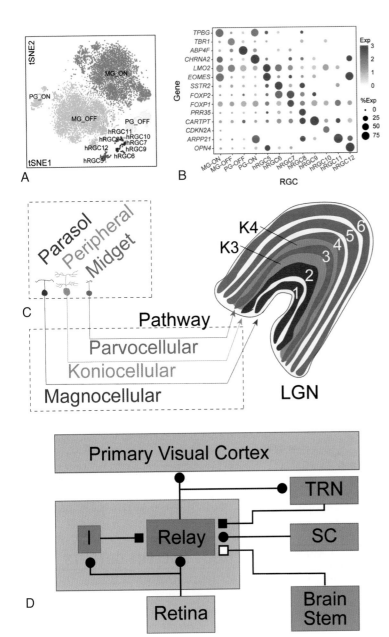

Fig. 29.2 (A, B) Gene expression–defined human retinal ganglion cell (*RGC*) clusters visualized using t-Stochastic Neighbourhood Embedding (tSNE) (**A**), and the same clusters ranked according to expression of key genes. (Reproduced from Yan W, Peng Y-R, van Zyl T, et al. Cell atlas of the human fovea and peripheral retina. *Sci Rep.* 2020;10(1):9802. https://doi.org/10.1038/s41598-020-66092-9). (**C**) Cartoon shows the type-specific RGC input to specific layers of primate lateral geniculate nucleus (*LGN*). (Modified from Monavarfeshani A, Sabbagh U, Fox MA. Not a one-trick pony: Diverse connectivity and functions of the rodent lateral geniculate complex. *Vis Neurosci.* 2017;34: E012. https://doi:10.1017/S0952523817000098.) (**D**) Diagram of feedforward, feedback, and modulatory inputs to the LGN. *Filled circles* are excitatory connections, *filled squares* are inhibitory, and *open squares* are modulatory. *SC,* Superior colliculus; *TRN,* thalamic reticular nucleus.

expressed by the TRN.[26] Visual TRN integrates descending input from L6 V1 neurons with ascending input from LGN relay cells to deliver feedback inhibition to LGN neurons.

Inputs from the brain stem

The LGN is a major target of neuromodulatory inputs emanating from diverse brain regions that include histaminergic inputs from the hypothalamus, serotonergic inputs from the dorsal raphe, cholinergic inputs from pontine nuclei, and noradrenergic inputs from the locus coeruleus. These inputs are believed to diffusely release their neuromodulators onto LGN neurons and activate G-protein–coupled receptors that hyperpolarize or depolarize the membrane potential of LGN relay neurons, LGN inhibitory neurons, and retinal inputs.[27]

Inputs from the superior colliculus

Visual input from the eye is forked—RGC axons branch to innervate both the LGN and a midbrain sensorimotor area called the superior

colliculus (SC). Inputs in this latter structure are organized retinotopically in the superficial-most layers of SC, which are registered to a trio of lower layers containing maps of auditory, somatosensory, and motor space.[28] LGN is a major target of the SC. In primates, SC inputs target the koniocellular layers of the LGN and recent work in cats and mice suggest that such inputs can "drive" LGN neurons to fire action potentials.[29] Thus, some LGN spikes sent to cortex appear to take a scenic route through the SC. This strong SC input remains poorly studied; however, the SC→LGN projection has been found in over 15 different mammalian species,[30] suggesting a conserved evolutionary function. This function is likely related to motion processing, as most of the SC inputs target thalamic structures (koniocellular LGN layers, pulvinar) that project to the middle-temporal area (area MT).

Inputs from local interneurons

Local interneurons comprise approximately 25% to 30% of LGN neurons in macaques,[31] approximately 20% to 25% in cats,[32–35] and 10%

to 20% in rats and mice.[32,36,37] These neurons extend large dendritic arbors with short axons that ramify within the extent of their dendritic arbor.[38,39] They integrate feedforward input from RGCs and from other LGN interneurons and use this output to inhibit relay neurons. Interneurons in the LGN are atypical—both axons and dendrites are capable of releasing neurotransmitter. Modeling studies indicate that dendritic release sites are electrically insulated from each other, and the axonal compartment isolated from the dendrites.[40] In cats, dendritic synapses participate in triads that inhibit X-cells, whereas axonal synapses form preferentially on Y-cells.[41] It is also worth noting that dendritic synapses are considerably more common than axonal synapses in cats.[41] Whether these arrangements are present in other species is not clear.

LATERAL GENICULATE NUCLEUS CIRCUITRY

The remarkable diversity of inputs to the LGN runs at odds with the synapses they form in this structure—most connections can be easily categorized into three classes based on their ultrastructure. One class bears large terminals housing hundreds of round vesicles docked at multiple release sites (called RL), another has small terminals with round vesicles (RS), and the last has a flat nerve terminal with pleomorphic vesicles (F).[42] Retinal axons form all RL terminals (~5–10% of LGN synapses), internal inputs from cortex and elsewhere form all RS terminals (~80% of LGN synapses), and inhibitory inputs form all F synapses (~15% of LGN synapses). Local interneuron dendrites form F1 synapses with high synaptic vesicle density and interneuron or reticular axons form F2 synapses with lower synaptic vesicle density.[21,42] Next we highlight three commonly observed microcircuit arrangements and discuss their potential roles in LGN function.

Retinal ganglion cell synapses localize to the soma and proximal dendrites of LGN neurons

Synapses from RGCs account for only a small fraction of the total number of synapses with the LGN. However, these connections are by far the strongest.[21] Their outsized influence on relay neuron firing arises in part from the unique, multivesicular RL morphology and their subcellular location on the proximal dendrites and somata of LGN neurons (Fig. 29.3). This places their excitatory potentials close to the axon hillock where LGN neurons initiate action potentials. Convergence estimates in slice recordings from cat and rodent LGN suggest that an adult LGN neuron receives input from between one and four different retinal axons, with one RGC input providing most of the excitatory drive.[43,44] The weaker RGC inputs are thought to synapse on the distal

dendrites of an LGN neuron's arbor and often show a more RS-like appearance. Thus, an LGN neuron's view of the world is shaped predominantly by a small number of RGCs.

Retinal and local interneuron synapses are arranged as triads

The RL terminals of retinal axons often synapse with the dendrites of the LGN relay cell dendrites and those of the relay cell's presynaptic interneuron. This unit, termed a *triad*, positions feedforward excitatory and inhibitory synapses within a few microns of one another and often encapsulates these two structures within a glial sheath. Triads impose an exacting form of feedforward inhibition upon RL terminal activation because inhibition from adjacent F terminals would shunt excitatory drive within milliseconds. This arrangement is thought to favor retinal inputs that fire in tight synchrony, as lagging or leading inputs are likely to be silenced by local inhibition. Whether such synchrony is used to encode different features of a stimulus is currently unknown.

Drivers and modulators

Although the exact significance of the RL, RS, and F stereotypy is not clear, the consistency of these morphologic definitions across the LGN of rodents, cats, primates, and humans indicates a conserved computational role in the LGN.[21] A prominent view of LGN function posits that inputs bearing RL versus RS terminals can be defined as being drivers or modulators, respectively. In this scheme, only RL inputs can evoke spikes from LGN relay cells; RS inputs modulate resting potential and therefore the burst versus tonic firing status of the relay cell. There is significant morphologic and ex vivo functional data in support of this hypotheses, but in vivo evidence is lacking. Although a large body of in vivo work is consistent with the notion that feedback inputs (bearing RS terminals) cannot evoke action potentials in LGN neurons, many of these studies were performed under anesthesia, which is now known to exert a powerful suppression of geniculate circuitry. Repeating these studies, perhaps with new optogenetic tools, would offer a way to resolve this issue.

LATERAL GENICULATE NUCLEUS OUTPUTS

The main output of the LGN goes to the primary visual cortex and is essential for the emergence of conscious visual perception. In macaques, the axons from magnocellular, parvocellular, and koniocellular LGN neurons are vertically segregated in different cortical layers (Fig. 29.4A). The LGN axons are densest in layer 4Cα for magnocellular neurons, 4Cβ for parvocellular neurons, and layers 4A and

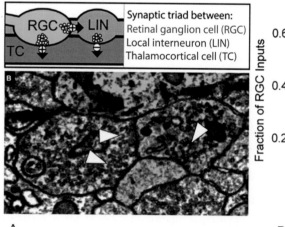
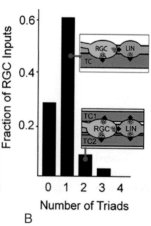

Fig. 29.3 Lateral geniculate nucleus (LGN) circuitry. (**A**) *Top:* Diagram of synaptic RGC→LIN→TC synaptic triad showing excitatory RGC synapses with a TC and an LIN. *Bottom:* electron micrograph showing RGC→LIN→TC triad pseudocolored to indicated RGC terminals, TC dendrites, and LIN dendrites. (**B**) Distribution of the number of triadic relationships (RGC→TC + LIN1→TC pairs) within 5 μm of each of 135 analyzed RGC→LIN1 synapses. *LIN,* Local interneuron; *RGC,* retinal ganglion cell; *TC,* thalamocortical cell. (Modified from Morgan JL, Lichtman JW. An individual interneuron participates in many kinds of inhibition and innervates much of the mouse visual thalamus. *Neuron.* 2020:106(3):468–481. e462. https://doi:10.1016/j.neuron.2020.02.001)

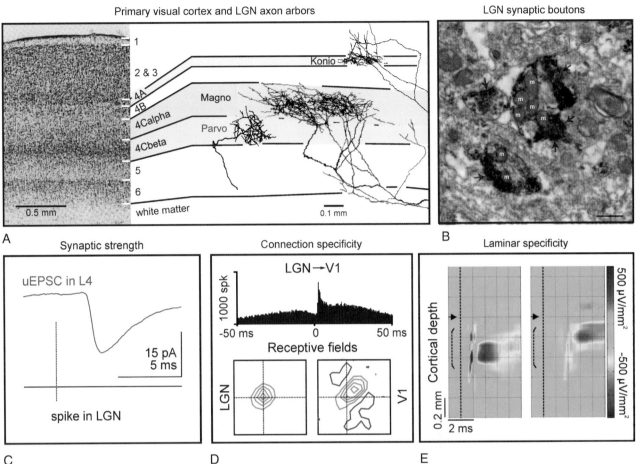

Fig. 29.4 Lateral geniculate nucleus (LGN) main output: the primary visual cortex. (**A**) Coronal section of macaque primary visual cortex (*left*) with main layer limits (*white lines*) and LGN axons targeting different cortical layers (*right*). The parvocellular LGN cells (parvo) have the smallest axon arbors and target layer 4Cβ (*in red*). The magnocellular LGN cells (magno) have the largest axon arbors and target layer 4Cα (*in gray*). The koniocellular LGN cells (konio) have axon arbors of diverse sizes and target layer 4 A (*in blue*). (Reproduced from Blasdel GG, Lund JS. Termination of afferent axons in macaque striate cortex. *J Neurosci.* 1983;3:1389–1413. Copyright 1983 Society for Neuroscience.) (**B**) Synaptic boutons (*green*) of LGN axon arbors in macaque primary visual cortex are large, have many mitochondria (m) and make multiple synapses (*arrows*). (Image provided by Dr. Virginia Garcia-Marin et al. from Garcia-Marin V, Kelly JG, Hawken MJ. Major feedforward thalamic input into layer 4 C of primary visual cortex in primate. *Cereb Cortex.* 2019;29:134–149. https://doi:10.1093/cercor/bhx311.) (**C**) Unitary excitatory postsynaptic current (uEPSC in *red*) from a neuron in layer 4 (L4) of the mouse primary visual cortex (V1) triggered by a single LGN afferent (*dotted line* marks time of LGN spike). (Data from Lien AD, Scanziani M. Cortical direction selectivity emerges at convergence of thalamic synapses. *Nature.* 2018;558;80–86.) (**D**) Crosscorrelogram between the spikes from a neuron in cat primary visual cortex (V1) and a neuron in LGN (*top*) and receptive fields (LGN: OFF-center in *blue*, cortex: OFF-center in *blue* with two ON flanks in *red*). (Data from Alonso JM, Usrey WM, Reid RC. Rules of connectivity between geniculate cells and simple cells in cat primary visual cortex. *J Neurosci.* 2001;21:4002–4015.) (**E**) Current source density triggered by two LGN afferents projecting at the *top* (afferent on the *right*) and *bottom* (afferent on the *left*) of layer 4 in the rabbit primary visual cortex. *Dotted lines* mark time of LGN spikes and *arrows* mark top of layer 4. (Reproduced from Stoelzel CR, Bereshpolova Y, Gusev AG, Swadlow HA. The impact of an LGNd impulse on the awake visual cortex: synaptic dynamics and the sustained/transient distinction. *J Neurosci.* 2008;28:5018–5028. https://doi:10.1523/JNEUROSCI.4726-07.2008. Copyright 2008 Society for Neuroscience.)

3 for koniocellular neurons.[45,46] The LGN axons are also horizontally segregated. The axons from the contralateral and ipsilateral eyes segregate horizontally in different ocular dominance columns[47] and the LGN axons from koniocellular neurons also segregate horizontally in patches of cells with high cytochrome oxidase activity known as blobs.[46] Such blobs correlate with dense thalamic innervation and are believed to reflect the energy demands of high firing rates in geniculocortical transmission.

The synaptic boutons made by LGN axons are large, are located proximally in the dendrites of cortical neurons, make multiple synaptic contacts with each cortical target, and have multiple mitochondria to maintain high metabolic activity[48] (Fig. 29.4B). Consistent with the large size of the synaptic boutons, the excitatory postsynaptic currents generated by single geniculocortical axons are strong (Fig. 29.4C) and show robust synaptic depression.[49–51] Moreover, the arrival of a spike

through a single geniculocortical axon is strongly correlated with a rapid increase in the spiking activity of the cortical targets (Fig. 29.4D), which are tightly restricted to the cortical layer targeted by the axon[51,52] (Fig. 29.4E). As expected from a strong monosynaptic connection, the receptive field properties of each geniculate neuron and its cortical targets are precisely matched in spatial position, ocular dominance, and ON-OFF receptive field polarity[49,52–56] (Fig. 29.4D). The number of LGN neurons varies greatly across species and individuals of the same species, but is strongly correlated with the volume of primary visual cortex[4,57] and the cortical resources available to process visual information.

In addition to the primary visual cortex, the LGN also projects to the visual sector of the TRN, a nucleus with inhibitory neurons that regulate the LGN output through feedforward inhibition. The LGN also projects to several extrastriate visual cortical areas such as area V2

BOX 29.2   Blindsight

The bilateral removal of primary visual cortex causes limited deficits in the visual acuity of cats[101] and tree shrews.[102] However, similar lesions in macaques and humans cause severe cortical blindness[62,103–105] while leaving intact a form of subconscious vision known as blindsight.[106] Human patients with blindsight are not aware that a stimulus is present but, when asked to guess, their percentage of correct trials is above chance, particularly when the stimulus is large, has high contrast, and is moving. Inactivation studies indicate that several subcortical structures are likely to play a role in blindsight, including the lateral geniculate nucleus (LGN),[107] the superior colicullus, and the pulvinar.[108] In addition, direct connections from thalamus to extrastriate cortex[58] and spared tissue in area V1 are likely to play a role.[109] Across the animal kingdom, there are two major types of pathways that transmit information from thalamus to visual cortex—retino-geniculate pathways and tectogeniculate pathways. The retinogeniculate pathways reach the primary visual cortex through the parvocellular, magnocellular, and koniocellular layers of the LGN (Box 29.2A). The tectogeniculate pathways reach both the primary visual cortex and extrastriate visual cortex through a network of subcortical structures that connect the tectum (superior colliculus) with the koniocellular layers of LGN and the pulvinar. The relative dominance of retinogeniculate and tectogeniculate pathways varies greatly across species and could explain why lesions in primary visual cortex can cause severe blindness in primates but have less of an effect on the visual acuity of carnivores.

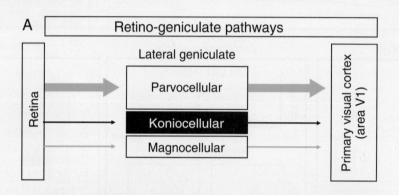

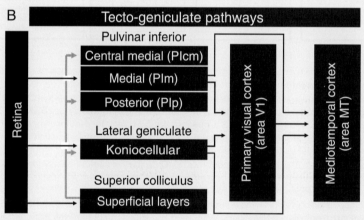

Blindsight. (**A**) The lateral geniculate nucleus (LGN) transmits information from the retina to the primary visual cortex through retinogeniculate pathways that make connection in the parvocellular, magnocellular, and koniocellular layers. (**B**) The LGN also transmits information from the retina to the extrastriate cortex through a network of subcortical structures that include the superior colliculus, the pulvinar, and the koniocellular layers of LGN.

and the area MT.[58–60] Specifically, the LGN projection to area MT originates in a small number of koniocellular LGN cells that do not project to primary visual cortex[61] and may mediate the residual vision referred to as "blindsight" in patients with large lesions in primary visual cortex[62] (Box 29.2).

LATERAL GENICULATE NUCLEUS RECEPTIVE FIELDS

In macaques and cats, every LGN neuron is strongly dominated by just one retinal input[63–65] that makes LGN receptive fields very similar to the retinal afferents.[66] Like its retinal afferents, most macaque LGN receptive fields have a circular concentric organization with spatial antagonism between center and surround. The optimal stimulation of the receptive field center drives an increment in the activity of the LGN cell. Conversely, the optimal stimulation of the receptive field surround can completely suppress the activity.

As a group, parvocellular LGN neurons have the highest spatial resolution, respond well to low temporal frequencies, and generate sustained responses that can last for several seconds to effectively signal the stimulus duration. By comparison, magnocellular LGN neurons have lower spatial resolution, respond better to higher temporal frequencies, have higher contrast sensitivity, and generate more transient responses that can rapidly signal the onset of a stimulus. Koniocellular LGN neurons fall in between the parvocellular and magnocellular types in terms of spatial and temporal resolution. Both the parvocellular and koniocellular pathways are likely to contribute to color vision, with parvocellular LGN cells transmitting information about red/green opponency and koniocellular LGN neurons about blue/yellow opponency. The strength and specificity of retinogeniculate connections make most LGN response properties to be inherited from the retina rather than being computed de novo.[63–65]

Parvocellular layers

In the parvocellular layers of the macaque LGN, the optimal colors stimulating receptive field center and surround can be different, a property termed *color opponency*. The most common receptive field type in the macaque parvocellular LGN layers is the red ON-center.[67] This cell type fires when a stimulus containing long-wavelength light (red, L+) is presented in the receptive field center and is suppressed when a stimulus containing middle-wavelength light (blue-green, M–) is presented in the receptive field surround.[67] Thus, this neuron responds best to red stimuli of any size but is inhibited by large green-blue stimuli (Fig. 29.5A). Other receptive field types in the parvocellular layers of the macaque LGN are green ON-center, red OFF-center, and green OFF-center receptive fields with no center-surround organization, and receptive fields with no color opponency.

Magnocellular layers

Neurons in the magnocellular LGN layers do not show color opponency and respond only to monochromatic luminance contrast (as if they were "seeing" the images in black and white). ON-center LGN neurons are best driven by small light stimuli on a dark background, like stars in the night sky. Conversely, OFF-center LGN neurons are best driven by small dark stimuli on a bright background, like the punctuation on this page. Both types of neurons are suppressed when the stimulus covers both the receptive field center and surround (Fig. 29.5B). The receptive field structure of ON- and OFF-center LGN neurons is highly conserved across mammals and has been directly measured in different species of primates, carnivores, rodents, and lagomorphs. In all species with form vision, including invertebrates and fish, ON and OFF receptive fields are constructed at the first synapse of the visual pathway, between photoreceptors and bipolar cells in the retina, and are important to measure light and dark contrast in the visual world. In mammals, ON and OFF visual pathways differ not only in their stimulus preferences for light or dark contrast but also in their contrast sensitivity, temporal resolution, spatial resolution, and cortical representations.[68]

Koniocellular layers

The koniocellular layers are likely to be an evolutionarily conserved feature of LGN.[30] Yet, their receptive field properties remain poorly studied.[2,69] In the macaque LGN, the dorsal koniocellular layers appear to relay information about short-wavelength light and low visual acuity to the superficial layers of the cortex, whereas the ventral koniocellular layers seem more related to visual motion and receive input from the SC.[30] In marmosets, some neurons in the koniocellular ventral layers of LGN (K1 and K2) respond to all stimuli falling within their receptive field center that have different luminance than the receptive field surround. That is, they respond equally well to stimuli darker or lighter than the background but are suppressed by any stimuli fully covering the receptive field surround.[70] Because these ON-OFF koniocellular cells are driven by both light and dark stimuli, their responses

to patterns, such as sinusoidal drifting gratings, resemble a step more than a sinusoidal function (Fig. 29.5C). Like magnocellular LGN cells, koniocellular ON-OFF cells have high contrast sensitivity, generate transient responses, and can rapidly signal the appearance of small low-contrast stimuli or motion within the visual field. The location of these ON-OFF cells in the ventral koniocellular layers allows them to receive input from the SC and project to cortical area MT. Therefore, they could play an important role in the tectogeniculate-MT pathway and the residual vision (blindsight) of patients with damaged primary visual cortex[70] (Box 29.3).

LATERAL GENICULATE NUCLEUS MAP OF VISUAL SPACE

An important function of the LGN is to organize its retinal inputs by receptive field properties, which include spatial position in the retina (retinotopy), eye input (contralateral or ipsilateral to each LGN), contrast polarity (light or dark), and response time course (sustained or transient). This functional organization varies greatly across species and increases in complexity as the LGN becomes larger during evolution. In spite of large species variations in LGN volume, shape and laminar segregation, all mammals with form vision organize their LGN retinal inputs in a map of visual/retinal space known as visuotopic/retinotopic map (Fig. 29.6).

In both humans and macaques, the LGN map of visual space magnifies central vision. This magnification is a direct consequence of the higher cell density sampling foveal than peripheral vision in the retina. The density of RGCs sampling the human fovea is greater than 30,000 per mm^2 but can fall to 5000 per mm^2 within just 3 mm of visual eccentricity.[71] The LGN map of visual space (Fig. 29.6A)[72] is accurately replicated across all the LGN layers, making each isoretinotopic line form paths that are nearly straight that cross both the coronal (Fig. 29.6B) and sagittal LGN axes (Fig. 29.6C). Within each isoretinotopic line, LGN neurons in different layers respond to the same stimulus position but have different eye inputs, light-dark contrast polarities, color opponency, and response time course. LGN neurons receiving input from the contralateral eye respond with an activity increment to the contralateral eye only, and those receiving input from the ipsilateral eye respond to the ipsilateral eye only. Neurons in the magnocellular LGN layers generate fast response transients that signal the appearance of the stimulus, whereas neurons in the parvocellular LGN layers generate sustained responses that signal the stimulus duration. The LGN map of visual space is closely replicated in the primary visual cortex, including the magnification of central vision. However, the contribution of the magnocellular pathway is greatly amplified in the primary visual cortex through a dramatic expansion of the axon arbor size, which is several times larger in magnocellular than parvocellular LGN neurons, as expected from the larger receptive field size (Fig. 29.4A).

RETINOGENICULATE TRANSMISSION

The retinogeniculate connection is one of the strongest connections within the visual pathway. In the cat, a single RGC can make more than 170 synapses with the same LGN neuron and provide its sole retinal input[64] (Fig. 29.7A). Retinogeniculate synapses are large and are located proximally in the LGN dendrites; the excitatory postsynaptic potential generated by a single retinal input is so large that it can be recorded from outside the LGN neuron with an extracellular electrode, an extracellular LGN signal frequently referred as s-potential[65,73] (Fig. 29.7B,C). In primates and carnivores, many LGN neurons receive more than one retinal input; however, one input is much stronger than the rest.[63,66] A retinal dominant input is strong enough to make its main

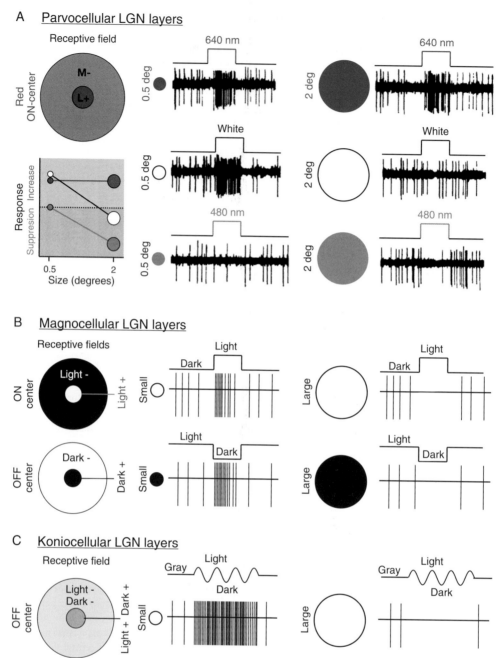

Fig. 29.5 Lateral geniculate nucleus (*LGN*) receptive fields. (**A**) Receptive field from a red ON-center cell in the parvocellular layers of the macaque LGN. *Left:* The receptive field (*top*) is stimulated by long-wavelength red light (L+) at the center and suppressed by middle-wavelength light (M−) at the surround. *Middle and right:* Small stimuli with long-wavelength light (e.g., red or white) drive spiking activity whereas large stimuli with middle-wavelength light (e.g., blue or white) suppress it. (Reproduced from Wiesel TN, Hubel DH. Spatial and chromatic interactions in the lateral geniculate body of the rhesus monkey. *J Neurophysiol.* 1966;29:1115–1156. https://doi:10.1152/jn.1966.29.6.1115.) (**B**) Cartoon illustrating receptive fields (*left*) and visual responses (*middle and right*) of ON- and OFF-center cells in macaque LGN. Small white stimuli drive spiking activity in ON-center cells and large white stimuli suppress it (the reverse for OFF-center cells). (**C**) Cartoon illustrating receptive field (*left*) and responses (*middle, right*) of a cell in the koniocellular layers intercalated with magnocellular layers of the marmoset LGN. Small stimuli that are lighter (*light*) or darker (*dark*) than the surround drive spiking activity and large stimuli suppress activity. (Based on data from Eiber CD, Rahman AS, Pietersen ANJ et al. Receptive field properties of koniocellular on/off neurons in the lateral geniculate nucleus of marmoset monkeys. *J Neurosci.* 2018;38:10384–10398.)

BOX 29.3 Linking physiology to behavior

The contributions of parvocellular and magnocellular lateral geniculate nucleus (LGN) pathways to visual behavior have been studied by making restricted lesions within either the parvocellular or magnocellular layers of the macaque LGN (and their adjacent koniocellular layers). Macaques were trained to discriminate stimuli in the part of the visual field corresponding to the damaged portion of the LGN.[110] Macaques with LGN lesions could discriminate form and motion with either pathway, as long as the stimuli had high contrast and were presented at the optimal spatial and temporal frequency for each pathway. Macaques with lesions in the magnocellular LGN layers lost the ability to discriminate high temporal frequencies and fast movements. Conversely, macaques with lesions in the parvocellular LGN layers lost the ability to discriminate high spatial frequencies and color and had a major deficit in contrast sensitivity. These studies demonstrate that lesions in different LGN layers can cause different deficits in visual perception and provide a classical example linking neuronal physiology with visual behavior.

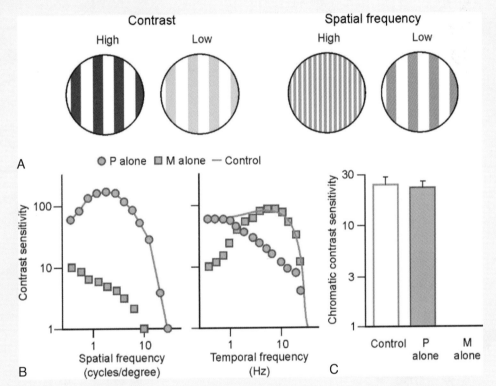

Visual loss after selective ablation of lateral geniculate nucleus (LGN) layers. (**A**) Stimuli used to test visual loss. (**B**) Lesions in the parvocellular layers (M alone) reduce contrast sensitivity for all spatial frequencies (*left*) and low temporal frequencies (*right*). Lesions in the magnocellular layers (M alone) reduce contrast sensitivity at high temporal frequencies (*right*). (**C**) Lesions in the parvocellular layers (M alone) cause a major loss in color contrast sensitivity. (Reproduced from Kandel ER, Schwartz JH, Jessell TM. *Principles of Neural Science*. McGraw Hill; 2000.)

LGN targets fire many spikes in precise 1 millisecond synchrony and replicate the input receptive field. Moreover, LGN neurons precisely synchronized by common retinal inputs converge at the same cortical targets.[74] Therefore, because synchronous spikes are more effective at driving cortical cells to threshold, the divergence from a strong retinal input into two LGN cells can play an important role in transmitting visual information from retina to visual cortex.[75]

In primates and carnivores, retinogeniculate connections are also highly specific (Fig. 29.7). Because the connections are dominated by a single retinal afferent, they relay very efficiently the receptive field properties of the retinal inputs. ON LGN neurons responding to stimulation of the contralateral eye are driven by an ON RGC from the contralateral eye, and LGN neurons generating sustained responses are driven by RGCs that also generate sustained responses.[76] The exquisite retinogeniculate specificity demonstrated in carnivores and primates[63,64,66,73,74,76] may be reduced in animals with low spatial resolution.

For example, in mice, LGN neurons processing the binocular field can receive retinal inputs from both eyes.[77] However, even in mice, the inputs from one eye dominate spiking activity while the inputs from the nondominant eye appear to remain functionally silent.[78]

Retinogeniculate connections are also highly reliable. A single spike from a single retinal ganglion can generate synaptic currents strong enough to drive a spike in an LGN neuron without the help from additional retinal inputs.[63,65,66,79] In fact, under certain stimulation conditions, nearly all spikes from a single RGC can generate LGN spikes, effectively bypassing the LGN connection on its way to the cortex.[79] This high reliability in retinogeniculate transmission is continuously fluctuating with changes in alertness and visual stimulation. Low alertness, drowsiness, sleep, and general anesthesia all cause a pronounced reduction in retinogeniculate transmission and LGN activity. Even under general anesthesia, many retinal spikes generate LGN spikes, but only when separated by short interspike intervals.[66]

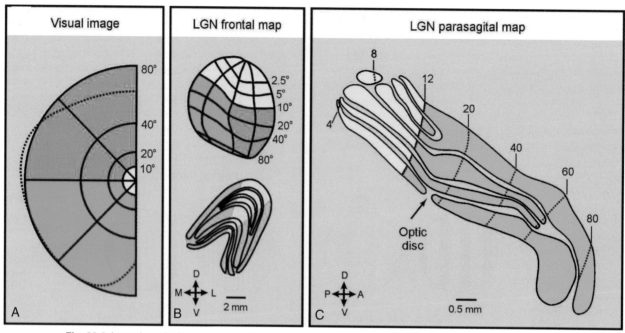

Fig. 29.6 Lateral geniculate nucleus (*LGN*) map of visual space. (**A**) Half of the human visual field (hemifield) illustrated as a *dotted line* superimposed on semicircular sectors shown as *yellow* (central 10 degrees), *blue* (upper visual field), and *green* (lower visual field). (**B**) Cartoon illustrating frontal view of macaque LGN (*top*) and coronal slice (*bottom*). (**C**) Cartoon illustrating a sagittal slice of macaque LGN. *D*, Dorsal; *L*, lateral; *V*, ventral; *M*, medial; *A*, anterior; *P*, posterior.

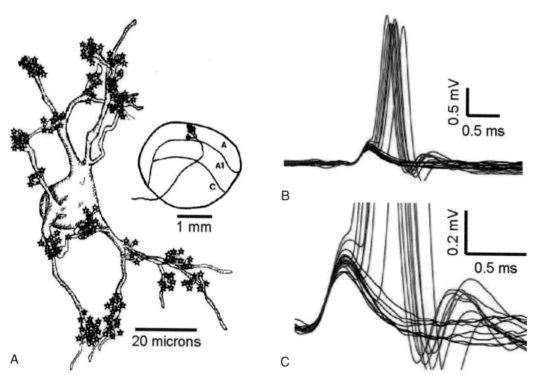

Fig. 29.7 Retinogeniculate transmission. (**A**) Synapses made by a single retinal afferent (*stars*) in a single lateral geniculate nucleus (LGN) cell (*left*) and axon arbor of the retinal afferent in layer A of cat LGN (*right*). (Reproduced from Hamos JE, Van Horn SC, Raczkowski D, Sherman SM. Synaptic circuits involving an individual retinogeniculate axon in the cat. *J Comp Neurol.* 1987;259:165–192. https://doi:10.1002/cne.902590202.) (**B**) Extracellularly recorded synaptic potentials *(black)* generated by a single retinal afferent driving spikes *(red)* in a single LGN cell in the awake cat. (Reproduced from Weyand TG. Retinogeniculate transmission in wakefulness. *J Neurophysiol.* 2007;98:769–785.) (**C**) Same as (**B**), expanded to show the synaptic potentials in more detail.

MODULATION OF LATERAL GENICULATE NUCLEUS ACTIVITY

LGN activity is modulated by global changes in brain state (Fig. 29.8A) and selective spatial attention (Fig. 29.8B). Current models suggest that the changes in state arise from cortical and brainstem inputs to LGN neurons, which hyperpolarize or depolarize the resting potential on these neurons to regulate their firing properties. LGN activity can be also modulated by eye movements such as saccades but the mechanisms remain poorly understood[80] (Fig. 29.8C).

Cortical and reticular modulation

The projection from the visual cortex targets distal LGN cell dendrites and mediates modulations of LGN activity by selective spatial attention. Paying selective attention to a stimulus increases the activity of LGN neurons from both the magnocellular and parvocellular layers while decreasing the activity of inhibitory neurons from the TRN[81] (Fig. 29.8B). The attentional modulation of LGN are subtle but strong enough to be measured with functional magnetic resonance imaging in humans.[82]

Current models suggest that cortical layer 6 (L6) neurons play a key role in this process. In these models, L6 neurons amplify responses from retinotopically aligned LGN neurons and suppress responses from misaligned ones via neurons in the TRN. The inhibition from the TRN can be very powerful. During sleep, rhythmic firing patterns from the TRN hyperpolarize the majority of LGN neurons, making them burst en masse when excited by their L6 cortical inputs.[83] Such synchronous bursting disconnects the LGN from its retinal inputs and disrupts the flow of visual information to cortex.[83,84] Whether this switch in firing mode is regulated during awake states is not well understood. However, TRN feedback inputs to LGN are retinotopically ordered, and a handful of studies in primates show that TRN inhibition hyperpolarizes LGN neurons viewing unattended locations in visual space.[81] LGN neurons viewing attended locations in visual space are spared, making their signals to V1 more salient.

Brainstem modulation

In awake rabbits, alertness can increase the number of LGN spikes by two times or more,[85,86] dramatically reducing bursting activity (Fig. 29.8A). In the alert state, LGN visual responses reliably reproduce temporal fluctuations in stimulus luminance; however, general anesthesia, sleep, or drowsiness reduce the LGN tonic activity, increase bursting, and reduce the ability of the LGN to reliably signal the spatiotemporal properties of visual stimuli.[85,87] The pronounced fluctuations

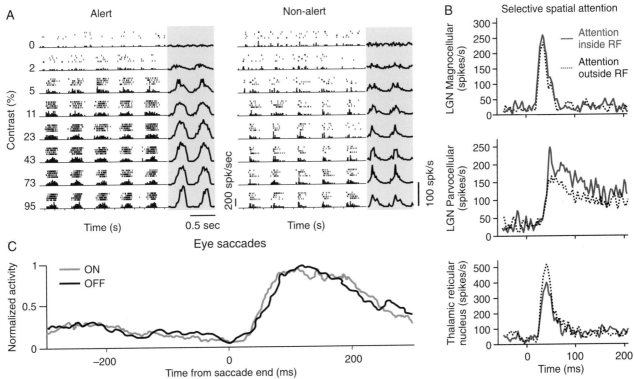

Fig 29.8 Modulation of retinogeniculate transmission at the lateral geniculate nucleus (LGN). **(A)** Responses from a single LGN neuron in the awake rabbit measured during two brain states, alert (*left*) and nonalert/drowsy (*right*). Responses driven by drifting sinusoidal gratings with different contrasts (numbers on the *left*) are shown as rasters on top of peristimulus time histograms for each grating cycle (*left*) and the average of two grating cycles (*right*). (Reproduced from Cano M, Bezdudnaya T, Swadlow HA, Alonso JM. Brain state and contrast sensitivity in the awake visual thalamus. *Nat Neurosci.* 2006;9:1240–1242. https://doi:10.1038/nn1760.) **(B)** Responses from single thalamic neurons in the awake macaque to a light spot presented inside the receptive field for 500–1000 ms. The responses are from single neurons recorded in the LGN magnocellular layers (*top*), LGN parvocellular layers (*middle*), and thalamic reticular nucleus (*bottom*). They were measured when the macaque was paying attention to the stimulus inside the receptive field (*red*) and when it was paying attention to another stimulus outside the receptive field (*black*). (Reproduced from McAlonan K, Cavanaugh J, Wurtz RH. Guarding the gateway to cortex with attention in visual thalamus. *Nature.* 2008;456:391–394. https://doi:10.1038/nature0738.) **(C)** Normalized average of spike density functions from 10 ON-center and 15 OFF-center LGN cells in the macaque (5 magnocellular, 19 parvocellular, 1 koniocellular) that demonstrated significant saccadic suppression and postsaccadic facilitation during spontaneous saccades. Trials are aligned on the saccade end (0 ms) to demonstrate the time course of the postsaccadic facilitation. (Reproduced from Royal DW, Sary G, Schall JD, Casagrande VA. Correlates of motor planning and postsaccadic fixation in the macaque monkey lateral geniculate nucleus. *Exp Brain Res.* 2006;168:62–75. https://doi:10.1007/s00221-005-0093-z.)

in LGN activity with global changes in brain state are mediated by the dense projections from the brain stem (see previously) that innervate the proximal dendrites of LGN neurons.

The model of action for these inputs remains unknown but could resemble their cortical and reticular cousins—altering the resting potential of LGN neurons to switch them between burst and tonic modes.[84,88,89] However, there is little direct circuit-level evidence to support this scheme. On the other hand, recent work in rodents suggests that noradrenergic and cholinergic inputs are important for the locomotion-related enhancement of LGN visual responses that occur in this species.[90] The increased cholinergic LGN tone during locomotion is consistent with the loss of acetylcholine-muscarinic LGN transmission that precedes burst firing in sleep and drowsiness.[84,88,89]

The firing mode of lateral geniculate nucleus neurons is controlled by changes in V_m

The cellular mechanisms underlying LGN modulations by brain state, attention, and eye movements are likely to involve changes in the cell resting potential, which controls the firing rate behavior.[21] Resting potential is a major determinant of thalamic neuron firing. All LGN relay neurons possess T-type calcium channels that recover from inactivation when the membrane potential is sufficiently negative (approximately −85 mV). Once recovered, these channels lead thalamic neurons to burst when depolarized rather than firing tonically.[91–94] In burst mode, these neurons encode both strong and weak retinal stimulation similarly; in tonic mode, differences in incoming retinal activity can be read out linearly in LGN neuron firing rate.[86] Evidence for this form of regulation exists for cholinergic brain stem inputs that depolarize LGN neurons and switch them from burst to tonic mode, but whether other brain stem inputs and cortical inputs act similarly is unknown. One important caveat is that the hyperpolarization needed to enter burst mode is significant and it is unclear whether it can be generated during alert states as demonstrated for nonalert awake states.[85] If it cannot, then cortical and noncholinergic brainstem inputs will likely modulate LGN activity during alert states through alternate mechanisms.

CONCLUSIONS

The LGN provides the main entrance of visual information to the cerebral cortex. In primates and carnivores, retinogeniculate connections are among the strongest and most specific connections within the visual pathway. The transfer of visual information through the LGN is continuously regulated by modulatory inputs originating in the brain stem and visual cortex, which adjust information transfer based on behavioral demand, alertness, and attention. The basic circuitry of the LGN is well preserved across species and can be studied in different animal models from rodents to primates. However, other features of LGN function vary greatly across species as is the case for visual acuity, binocular vision, and vision without primary visual cortex (blindsight in humans). In the years to come, the development of specific markers for cell types will provide a more detailed understanding of the basic cell taxonomy and LGN connectivity as cell atlases for different species become available. The challenge of future work will be to use all these tools to finally understand how the inputs from retina, cortex, brain stem, and SC interact in the LGN to generate vision.

REFERENCES

1. Andrews TJ, Halpern SD, Purves D. Correlated size variations in human visual cortex, lateral geniculate nucleus, and optic tract. *J Neurosci.* 1997;17:2859–2868.
2. Hendry SH, Reid RC. The koniocellular pathway in primate vision. *Annu Rev Neurosci.* 2000;23:127–153.
3. Malpeli JG, Baker FH. The representation of the visual field in the lateral geniculate nucleus of Macaca mulatta. *J Comp Neurol.* 1975;161:569–594.
4. Mazade R, Alonso JM. Thalamocortical processing in vision. *Vis Neurosci.* 2017;34:E007.
5. Scholpp S, Lumsden A. Building a bridal chamber: development of the thalamus. *Trends Neurosci.* 2010;33:373–380.
6. Nakagawa Y, Shimogori T. Diversity of thalamic progenitor cells and postmitotic neurons. *Eur J Neurosci.* 2012;35:1554–1562.
7. Golding B, et al. Retinal input directs the recruitment of inhibitory interneurons into thalamic visual circuits. *Neuron.* 2014;81:1057–1069.
8. Jager P, Ye Z, Yu X, et al. Tectal-derived interneurons contribute to phasic and tonic inhibition in the visual thalamus. *Nat Commun.* 2016;7:13579. Epub 2016/12/09. https://doi.org/10.1038/ncomms13579. PubMed PMID: 27929058; PMCID: PMC5155147.
9. Bakken TE, van Velthoven CT, Menon V, et al. Single-cell and single-nucleus RNA-seq uncovers shared and distinct axes of variation in dorsal LGN neurons in mice, non-human primates, and humans. *Elife.* 2021;10. Epub 2021/09/03. https://doi.org/10.7554/eLife.64875. PubMed PMID: 34473054; PMCID: PMC8412930.
10. Murray KD, Rubin CM, Jones EG, Chalupa LM. Molecular correlates of laminar differences in the macaque dorsal lateral geniculate nucleus. *J Neurosci.* 2008;28:12010–12022.
11. Iwai L, Ohashi Y, van der List D, Usrey WM, Miyashita Y, Kawasaki H. FoxP2 is a parvocellular-specific transcription factor in the visual thalamus of monkeys and ferrets. *Cereb Cortex.* 2013;23(9):2204–2212. Epub 2012/07/14. https://doi.org/10.1093/cercor/bhs207. PubMed PMID: 22791804; PMCID: PMC3729200.
12. Usrey WM, Alitto HJ. Visual functions of the thalamus. *Annu Rev Vis Sci.* 2015;1:351–371.
13. Roman Roson M, Bauer Y, Kotkat AH, Berens P, Euler T, Busse L. Mouse dLGN receives functional input from a diverse population of retinal ganglion cells with limited convergence. *Neuron.* 2019;102(2):462–476. e8. Epub 2019/02/26. https://doi.org/10.1016/j.neuron.2019.01.040. PubMed PMID: 30799020.
14. Bickford ME. Synaptic organization of the dorsal lateral geniculate nucleus. *Eur J Neurosci.* 2019;49:938–947.
15. Masri RA, Grunert U, Martin PR. Analysis of parvocellular and magnocellular visual pathways in human retina. *J Neurosci.* 2020;40:8132–8148.
16. Dacey DM. Parallel pathways for spectral coding in primate retina. *Annu Rev Neurosci.* 2000;23:743–775.
17. Yan W, Peng YR, van Zyl T, et al. Cell atlas of the human fovea and peripheral retina. *Sci Rep.* 2020;10(1):9802. Epub 2020/06/20. https://doi.org/10.1038/s41598-020-66092-9. PubMed PMID: 32555229; PMCID: PMC7299956.
18. Sanes JR, Masland RH. The types of retinal ganglion cells: current status and implications for neuronal classification. *Annu Rev Neurosci.* 2015;38:221–246.
19. Detwiler PB, Crook DK, Packer O, Robinson F, Dacey DM. The recursive bistratified ganglion cell type of the macaque monkey retina is ON-OFF direction selective. *Invest. Ophthalmol. Vis. Sci.* 2019;60:3884.
20. Erisir A, Van Horn SC, Sherman SM. Relative numbers of cortical and brainstem inputs to the lateral geniculate nucleus. *Proc Natl Acad Sci U S A.* 1997;94:1517–1520.
21. Sherman, S.M. & Guillery, R.W. *Thalamus.* 5th ed. (2004).
22. Conley M, Raczkowski D. Sublaminar organization within layer VI of the striate cortex in Galago. *J Comp Neurol.* 1990;302:425–436.
23. Fitzpatrick D, Usrey WM, Schofield BR, Einstein G. The sublaminar organization of corticogeniculate neurons in layer 6 of macaque striate cortex. *Vis Neurosci.* 1994;11:307–315.
24. Briggs F, Usrey WM. Parallel processing in the corticogeniculate pathway of the macaque monkey. *Neuron.* 2009;62:135–146.
25. Pinault D. The thalamic reticular nucleus: structure, function and concept. *Brain Res Brain Res Rev.* 2004;46:1–31.
26. Krol A, Wimmer RD, Halassa MM, Feng G. Thalamic reticular dysfunction as a circuit endophenotype in neurodevelopmental disorders. *Neuron.* 2018;98:282–295.
27. Varela C. Thalamic neuromodulation and its implications for executive networks. *Front Neural Circuits.* 2014;8:69.
28. Allen KM, Lawlor J, Salles A, Moss CF. Orienting our view of the superior colliculus: specializations and general functions. *Curr Opin Neurobiol.* 2021;71:119–126.
29. Bickford ME, Zhou N, Krahe TE, Govindaiah G, Guido W. Retinal and tectal "driver-like" inputs converge in the shell of the mouse dorsal lateral geniculate nucleus. *J Neurosci.* 2015;35:10523–10534.
30. Harting JK, Huerta MF, Hashikawa T, van Lieshout DP. Projection of the mammalian superior colliculus upon the dorsal lateral geniculate nucleus: organization of tectogeniculate pathways in nineteen species. *J Comp Neurol.* 1991;304:275–306.
31. Montero VM, Zempel J. The proportion and size of GABA-immunoreactive neurons in the magnocellular and parvocellular layers of the lateral geniculate nucleus of the rhesus monkey. *Exp Brain Res.* 1986;62:215–223.
32. Arcelli P, Frassoni C, Regondi MC, De Biasi S, Spreafico R. GABAergic neurons in mammalian thalamus: a marker of thalamic complexity? *Brain Res Bull.* 1997;42:27–37.
33. Arcelli P, Frassoni C, Regondi MC, De Biasi S, Spreafico R. GABAergic neurons in mammalian thalamus: a marker of thalamic complexity? *Brain Res Bull.* 1997;42(1):27–37. Epub 1997/01/01. https://doi.org/10.1016/s0361-9230(96)00107-4. PubMed PMID: 8978932.
34. Fitzpatrick D, Penny GR, Schmechel DE. Glutamic acid decarboxylase-immunoreactive neurons and terminals in the lateral geniculate nucleus of the cat. *J Neurosci.* 1984;4:1809–1829.
35. Madarasz M, Somogyi G, Somogyi J, Hamori J. Numerical estimation of gamma-aminobutyric acid (GABA)-containing neurons in three thalamic nuclei of the cat: direct GABA immunocytochemistry. *Neurosci Lett.* 1985;61:73–78.
36. Gabbott PL, Somogyi J, Stewart MG, Hamori J. A quantitative investigation of the neuronal composition of the rat dorsal lateral geniculate nucleus using GABA-immunocytochemistry. *Neuroscience.* 1986;19:101–111.
37. Gabbott PL, Somogyi J, Stewart MG, Hamori J. A quantitative investigation of the neuronal composition of the rat dorsal lateral geniculate nucleus using GABA-

immunocytochemistry. *Neuroscience*.. 1986;19(1):101–111. Epub 1986/09/01. https://doi.org/10.1016/0306-4522(86)90008-4. PubMed PMID: 3537838.
38. Montero VM. Ultrastructural identification of synaptic terminals from the axon of type 3 interneurons in the cat lateral geniculate nucleus. *J Comp Neurol*. 1987;264:268–283.
39. Hamos JE, Van Horn SC, Raczkowski D, Uhlrich DJ, Sherman SM. Synaptic connectivity of a local circuit neurone in lateral geniculate nucleus of the cat. *Nature*. 1985;317:618–621.
40. Bloomfield SA, Sherman SM. Dendritic current flow in relay cells and interneurons of the cat's lateral geniculate nucleus. *Proc Natl Acad Sci U S A*. 1989;86:3911–3914.
41. Sherman SM, Friedlander MJ. Identification of X versus Y properties for interneurons in the A-laminae of the cat's lateral geniculate nucleus. *Exp Brain Res*. 1988;73:384–392.
42. Van Horn SC, Erisir A, Sherman SM. Relative distribution of synapses in the A-laminae of the lateral geniculate nucleus of the cat. *J Comp Neurol*. 2000;416:509–520.
43. Morgan JL, Berger DR, Wetzel AW, Lichtman JW. The fuzzy logic of network connectivity in mouse visual thalamus. *Cell*. 2016;165:192–206.
44. Sherman SM. Interneurons and triadic circuitry of the thalamus. *Trends Neurosci*. 2004;27: 670–675.
45. Blasdel GG, Lund JS. Termination of afferent axons in macaque striate cortex. *J Neurosci*. 1983;3:1389–1413.
46. Hendry SH, Yoshioka T. A neurochemically distinct third channel in the macaque dorsal lateral geniculate nucleus. *Science*. 1994;264:575–577.
47. Hubel DH, Wiesel TN, LeVay S. Plasticity of ocular dominance columns in monkey striate cortex. *Philos Trans R Soc Lond B Biol Sci*. 1977;278:377–409.
48. Garcia-Marin V, Kelly JG, Hawken MJ. Major feedforward thalamic input into layer 4c of primary visual cortex in primate. *Cereb Cortex*. 2019;29:134–149.
49. Lien AD, Scanziani M. Cortical direction selectivity emerges at convergence of thalamic synapses. *Nature*. 2018;558:80–86.
50. Boudreau CE, Ferster D. Short-term depression in thalamocortical synapses of cat primary visual cortex. *J Neurosci*. 2005;25:7179–7190.
51. Stoelzel CR, Bereshpolova Y, Gusev AG, Swadlow HA. The impact of an LGNd impulse on the awake visual cortex: synaptic dynamics and the sustained/transient distinction. *J Neurosci*. 2008;28:5018–5028.
52. Reid RC, Alonso JM. Specificity of monosynaptic connections from thalamus to visual cortex. *Nature*. 1995;378:281–284.
53. Alonso JM, Usrey WM, Reid RC. Rules of connectivity between geniculate cells and simple cells in cat primary visual cortex. *J Neurosci*. 2001;21:4002–4015.
54. Tanaka K. Cross-correlation analysis of geniculostriate neuronal relationships in cats. *J Neurophysiol*. 1983;49:1303–1318.
55. Tanaka K. Cross-correlation analysis of geniculostriate neuronal relationships in cats. *J Neurophysiol*. 1983;49(6):1303–1318. Epub 1983/06/01. https://doi.org/10.1152/jn.1983.49.6.1303. PubMed PMID: 6875624.
56. Bereshpolova Y, Hei X, Alonso JM, Swadlow HA. Three rules govern thalamocortical connectivity of fast-spike inhibitory interneurons in the visual cortex. *Elife*. 2020;9
57. Stevens CF. An evolutionary scaling law for the primate visual system and its basis in cortical function. *Nature*. 2001;411:193–195.
58. Sincich LC, Park KF, Wohlgemuth MJ, Horton JC. Bypassing V1: a direct geniculate input to area MT. *Nat Neurosci*. 2004;7:1123–1128.
59. Yukie M, Iwai E. Direct projection from the dorsal lateral geniculate nucleus to the prestriate cortex in macaque monkeys. *J Comp Neurol*. 1981;201:81–97.
60. Bullier J, Kennedy H. Projection of the lateral geniculate nucleus onto cortical area V2 in the macaque monkey. *Exp Brain Res*. 1983;53:168–172.
61. Nassi JJ, Callaway EM. Multiple circuits relaying primate parallel visual pathways to the middle temporal area. *J Neurosci*. 2006;26:12789–12798.
62. Stoerig P, Cowey A. Blindsight in man and monkey. *Brain*. 1997;120(Pt 3):535–559.
63. Cleland BG, Dubin MW, Levick WR. Simultaneous recording of input and output of lateral geniculate neurones. *Nat New Biol*. 1971;231:191–192.
64. Hamos JE, Van Horn SC, Raczkowski D, Sherman SM. Synaptic circuits involving an individual retinogeniculate axon in the cat. *J Comp Neurol*. 1987;259:165–192.
65. Sincich LC, Adams DL, Economides JR, Horton JC. Transmission of spike trains at the retinogeniculate synapse. *J Neurosci*. 2007;27:2683–2692.
66. Usrey WM, Reppas JB, Reid RC. Specificity and strength of retinogeniculate connections. *J Neurophysiol*. 1999;82:3527–3540.
67. Wiesel TN, Hubel DH. Spatial and chromatic interactions in the lateral geniculate body of the rhesus monkey. *J Neurophysiol*. 1966;29:1115–1156.
68. Kremkow J, Alonso JM. Thalamocortical circuits and functional architecture. *Annu Rev Vis Sci*. 2018;4:263–285.
69. Martin PR, White AJ, Goodchild AK, Wilder HD, Sefton AE. Evidence that blue-on cells are part of the third geniculocortical pathway in primates. *Eur J Neurosci*. 1997;9:1536–1541.
70. Martin PR, White AJ, Goodchild AK, Wilder HD, Sefton AE. Evidence that blue-on cells are part of the third geniculocortical pathway in primates. *Eur J Neurosci*. 1997;9(7):1536–1541. Epub 1997/07/01. https://doi.org/10.1111/j.1460-9568.1997.tb01509.x. PubMed PMID: 9240412.
71. Curcio CA, Allen KA. Topography of ganglion cells in human retina. *J Comp Neurol*. 1990;300:5–25.
72. Traquair HM. *An Introduction to Clinical Perimetry*. London: Kimpton H; 1938:4–5.
73. Bishop PO, Burke W, Davis R. The interpretation of the extracellular response of single lateral geniculate cells. *J Physiol*. 1962;162:451–472.
74. Alonso JM, Usrey WM, Reid RC. Precisely correlated firing in cells of the lateral geniculate nucleus. *Nature*. 1996;383:815–819.
75. Dan Y, Alonso JM, Usrey WM, Reid RC. Coding of visual information by precisely correlated spikes in the lateral geniculate nucleus. *Nat Neurosci*. 1998;1:501–507.
76. Cleland BG, Dubin MW, Levick WR. Sustained and transient neurones in the cat's retina and lateral geniculate nucleus. *J Physiol*. 1971;217:473–496.
77. Cleland BG, Dubin MW, Levick WR. Sustained and transient neurones in the cat's retina and lateral geniculate nucleus. *J Physiol*. 1971;217(2):473–496. Epub 1971/09/01. https://doi.org/10.1113/jphysiol.1971.sp009581. PubMed PMID: 5097609; PMCID: PMC1331787.
78. Rompani SB, Mullner FE, Wanner A, et al. Different modes of visual integration in the lateral geniculate nucleus revealed by single-cell-initiated transsynaptic tracing. *Neuron*. 2017;93(4):767–776. e6. Epub 2017/02/24. https://doi.org/10.1016/j.neuron.2017.01.028. PubMed PMID: 28231464; PMCID: PMC5330803.
79. Weyand TG. Retinogeniculate transmission in wakefulness. *J Neurophysiol*. 2007;98:769–785.
80. Royal DW, Sary G, Schall JD, Casagrande VA. Correlates of motor planning and postsaccadic fixation in the macaque monkey lateral geniculate nucleus. *Exp Brain Res*. 2006;168:62–75.
81. McAlonan K, Cavanaugh J, Wurtz RH. Guarding the gateway to cortex with attention in visual thalamus. *Nature*. 2008;456:391–394.
82. O'Connor DH, Fukui MM, Pinsk MA, Kastner S. Attention modulates responses in the human lateral geniculate nucleus. *Nat Neurosci*. 2002;5:1203–1209.
83. McCormick DA, McGinley MJ, Salkoff DB. Brain state dependent activity in the cortex and thalamus. *Curr Opin Neurobiol*. 2015;31:133–140.
84. Brown RE, Basheer R, McKenna JT, Strecker RE, McCarley RW. Control of sleep and wakefulness. *Physiol Rev*. 2012;92:1087–1187.
85. Bezdudnaya T, et al. Thalamic burst mode and inattention in the awake LGNd. *Neuron*. 2006;49:421–432.
86. Cano M, Bezdudnaya T, Swadlow HA, Alonso JM. Brain state and contrast sensitivity in the awake visual thalamus. *Nat Neurosci*. 2006;9:1240–1242.
87. Livingstone MS, Hubel DH. Effects of sleep and arousal on the processing of visual information in the cat. *Nature*. 1981;291:554–561.
88. Steriade M. Acetylcholine systems and rhythmic activities during the waking--sleep cycle. *Prog Brain Res*. 2004;145:179–196.
89. Jones BE. Activity, modulation and role of basal forebrain cholinergic neurons innervating the cerebral cortex. *Prog Brain Res*. 2004;145:157–169.
90. Aydin C, Couto J, Giugliano M, Farrow K, Bonin V. Locomotion modulates specific functional cell types in the mouse visual thalamus. *Nat Commun*. 2018;9:4882.
91. Jahnsen H, Llinas R. Electrophysiological properties of guinea-pig thalamic neurones: an in vitro study. *J Physiol*. 1984;349:205–226.
92. Jahnsen H, Llinas R. Ionic basis for the electro-responsiveness and oscillatory properties of guinea-pig thalamic neurones in vitro. *J Physiol*. 1984;349:227–247.
93. Guido W, Lu SM, Sherman SM. Relative contributions of burst and tonic responses to the receptive field properties of lateral geniculate neurons in the cat. *J Neurophysiol*. 1992;68:2199–2211.
94. Lu SM, Guido W, Sherman SM. Effects of membrane voltage on receptive field properties of lateral geniculate neurons in the cat: contributions of the low-threshold Ca2+ conductance. *J Neurophysiol*. 1992;68:2185–2198.
95. Macosko EZ, Basu A, Satija R, et al. Highly parallel genome-wide expression profiling of individual cells using nanoliter droplets. *Cell*. 2015;161:1202–1214.
96. Macosko EZ, Basu A, Satija R, et al. Highly parallel genome-wide expression profiling of individual cells using nanoliter droplets. *Cell*. 2015;161(5):1202–1214. Epub 2015/05/23. https://doi.org/10.1016/j.cell.2015.05.002. PubMed PMID: 26000488; PMCID: PMC4481139.
97. Shekhar K, Lapan SW, Whitney IE, et al. Comprehensive classification of retinal bipolar neurons by single-cell transcriptomics. *Cell*. 2016;166(5):1308–1323. e30. Epub 2016/08/28. https://doi.org/10.1016/j.cell.2016.07.054. PubMed PMID: 27565351; PMCID: PMC5003425.
98. Tran NM, Shekhar K, Whitney IE, et al. Single-cell profiles of retinal ganglion cells differing in resilience to injury reveal neuroprotective genes. *Neuron*. 2019;104(6):1039–1055. e12. Epub 2019/12/01. https://doi.org/10.1016/j.neuron.2019.11.006. PubMed PMID: 31784286; PMCID: PMC6923571.
99. Yan W, Laboulaye MA, Tran NM, Whitney IE, Benhar I, Sanes JR. Mouse retinal cell atlas: molecular identification of over sixty amacrine cell types. *J Neurosci*. 2020;40(27):5177–5195. Epub 2020/05/28. https://doi.org/10.1523/JNEUROSCI.0471-20.2020. PubMed PMID: 32457074; PMCID: PMC7329304.
100. Peng YR, Shekhar K, Yan W, et al. Molecular classification and comparative taxonomics of foveal and peripheral cells in primate retina. *Cell*. 2019;176(5):1222–1237. e22. Epub 2019/02/05. https://doi.org/10.1016/j.cell.2019.01.004. PubMed PMID: 30712875; PMCID: PMC6424338.
101. Berkley MA, Sprague JM. Striate cortex and visual acuity functions in the cat. *J Comp Neurol*. 1979;187:679–702.
102. Ware CB, Casagrande VA, Diamond IT. Does the acuity of the tree shrew suffer from removal of striate cortex? A commentary on the paper by ward and Masterton. *Brain Behav Evol*. 1972;5:18–29.
103. Pasik T, Pasik P. The visual world of monkeys deprived of striate cortex: effective stimulus parameters and the importance of the accessory optic system. *Vision Res* Suppl. 1971; 3:419–435.
104. Weiskrantz L, Warrington EK, Sanders MD, Marshall J. Visual capacity in the hemianopic field following a restricted occipital ablation. *Brain*. 1974;97:709–728.
105. Poppel E, Held R, Frost D. Leter: Residual visual function after brain wounds involving the central visual pathways in man. *Nature*. 1973;243:295–296.
106. Sanders MD, Warrington EK, Marshall J, Wieskrantz L. "Blindsight": Vision in a field defect. *Lancet*. 1974;1:707–708.
107. Schmid MC, et al. Blindsight depends on the lateral geniculate nucleus. *Nature*. 2010;466: 373–377.
108. Schmid MC, Mrowka SW, Turchi J, et al. Blindsight depends on the lateral geniculate nucleus. *Nature*. 2010;466(7304):373–377. Epub 2010/06/25. https://doi.org/10.1038/nature09179. PubMed PMID: 20574422; PMCID: PMC2904843.
109. Kinoshita M, Kato R, Isa K, et al. Dissecting the circuit for blindsight to reveal the critical role of pulvinar and superior colliculus. *Nat Commun*. 2019;10(1):135. Epub 2019/01/13. https://doi.org/10.1038/s41467-018-08058-0. PubMed PMID: 30635570; PMCID: PMC6329824.
110. Merigan WH, Maunsell JH. How parallel are the primate visual pathways? *Annu Rev Neurosci*. 1993;16:369–402.

30

Primary Visual Cortex

Alessandra Angelucci and Stuart Trenholm

OVERVIEW

In many ways, primary visual cortex can be thought of as our mind's eye. It sits at a pivotal location in our visual system, such that losing primary visual cortex results in total loss of conscious visual perception. It is the site where visual information first enters cortex from the eyes, via the thalamus. As nearly all visual information passing to extrastriate visual areas first passes through primary visual cortex, the processing that it undertakes serves a critical and holistic role in our visual system.

Until the Renaissance, it was generally thought that the optic nerves terminated in the ventricles, which were supposed to house the animal spirits that drove our nervous system. In the 17th century, Thomas Willis was able to trace the optic nerves to the thalamus,[1] establishing it for a time as the highest level of vision. However, evidence of an even higher visual center in cortex would soon begin to emerge. One early such example can be found in an anecdote given by the Dutch physician Herman Boerhaave during one of his popular medical lectures, in which he described the tale of a Parisian pauper with an exposed brain who would supposedly solicit alms while holding his own calvarium:

> "He would frequently permit experiments to be made for a small trifle of money. Upon gently pressing the dura mater with one's finger, he suddenly perceived as it were, a thousand sparks before his eyes, and upon pressing a little more forcibly, and then his eyes lost all their sight..."[2]

More substantial evidence of a cortical seat for vision would soon be found. In the 19th century, Albrecht von Graefe developed an early form of perimetry to study visual fields in humans, and by examining medical cases of homonymous hemianopia and relating these to hemiplegias he was able to posit a role for cortex in visual perception.[3,4] Around the same time, cortical lesion studies in animal models by researchers including David Ferrier and Hermann Munk would further suggest a cortical seat of vision, with Munk placing visual cortex in the occipital lobe.[5]

In humans, primary visual cortex takes up a significant portion of our occipital lobe, extending from the posterior pole along the medial wall of the hemisphere (Fig. 30.1). It is made up of six principal layers and is roughly 2 mm thick.[6] Primary visual cortex goes by many other names, including "V1," "striate cortex," named as such because the 18th century Italian anatomist Francesco Gennari noted a white stripe running through the middle of the occipital lobe when he sliced through the brain,[7] and "Area 17," based on a numerical map of cortical areas generated by Korbidian Brodmann at the turn of the 20th century.[8]

Within a given hemisphere, V1 receives information from both eyes, but only regarding the contralateral hemifield. In V1, the visual world is mapped onto cortical space in a retinotopic manner, meaning that neighboring portions of V1 encode neighboring portions of the visual field. The fovea—which takes up a much larger share of V1 per visual degree than more peripheral parts of the visual field—is represented in the occipital pole, while the far periphery is represented in the anterior margin of the calcarine fissure.[9] The upper and lower visual fields are mapped onto the lower (lingual gyrus) and upper (cuneus gyrus) banks, respectively.[9] Evidence for such arrangement of V1 in humans comes from experimental evidence using methods such as positron emission tomography (PET)[10] or, more commonly, functional magnetic resonance imaging (fMRI).[11] Perturbations to the brain in humans using either electrical stimulation or transcranial magnetic stimulation (TMS) have validated these maps,[12] as have years of clinical work mapping scotomas related to damage in specific portions of V1. Our modern view of V1 starts with the work of Nobel laureates David Hubel and Torsten Wiesel, whose work studying light-evoked responses of individual neurons in V1 is described below in further detail.

VISUAL INPUTS TO V1 AND LOCAL CORTICAL CIRCUITS

The six layers of V1 comprise several different cell types, with approximately 80% of cells being excitatory and approximately 20% being inhibitory.[13] As is seen further, these six layers are further broken down based on the specific cell types in each layer and the specific types of connections the cells make. In broad strokes, thalamic input to V1 is focused in layer 4 (except for the koniocellular geniculocortical pathway), inhibitory neurons tend to modify local cortical processing, and excitatory neurons in both superficial (above layer 4) and deep (below layer 4) layers undertake tasks related to local, long-range cortical, and long-range subcortical signaling.

Bottom-up visual inputs to V1 from the lateral geniculate nucleus

V1 receives its predominant, driving visual input from the lateral geniculate nucleus (LGN). Work in nonhuman primates has shown that LGN axons carry signals from both left and right eyes, and from the parvocellular, magnocellular, and koniocellular (P, M, and K, respectively) layers, and that all these inputs remain segregated as they first synapse in V1 (Fig. 30.2). The left and right eye segregation of axons from the M and P LGN layers into layer 4C of V1 forms the anatomical basis for ocular dominance columns, which represent the substrate for binocularity, as discussed in detail further on. In V1, K, M, and P LGN axons terminate in separate layers and sublayers (see Fig. 30.2 for details). K LGN axons are likely made up of several classes, as those that end in different V1 layers appear to come from different populations of LGN cells.[14]

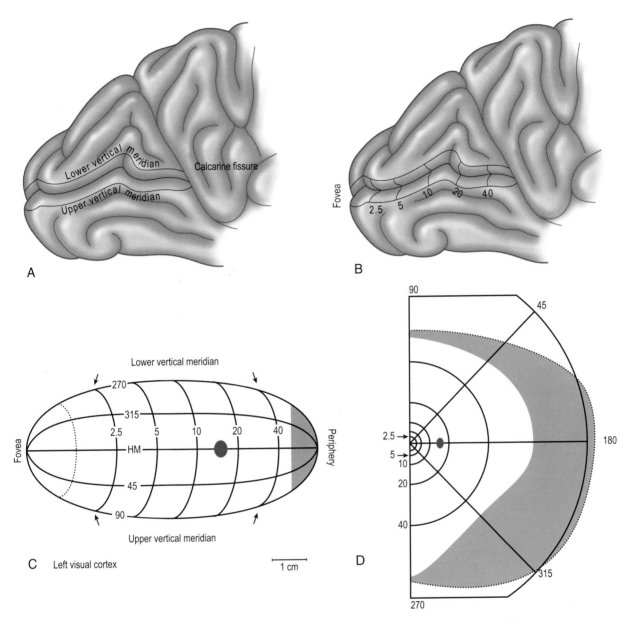

Fig. 30.1 Representation of the visual field in V1. (A) Left occipital lobe showing the location of V1 within the calcarine fissure. (B) View of calcarine fissure of V1. The *lines* indicate the coordinates of the visual field map. The representation of the horizontal meridian runs approximately along the base of the calcarine fissure. The *vertical lines* mark the isoeccentricity contours from 2.5 degrees to 40 degrees. V1 wraps around the occipital pole to extend about 1 cm onto the lateral convexity where the fovea is represented. (C) Schematic map showing the projection of the right visual hemifield upon the left visual cortex by transposing the map illustrated in (B) onto a flat surface. The *row of dots* indicates approximately where V1 folds around the occipital tip. The *blue oval* marks the region of V1 corresponding to the contralateral eye's blind spot. It is important to note that considerable variation occurs among individuals in the exact dimensions and location of V1. *HM*, Horizontal meridian. (D) Right visual hemifield plotted with a Goldmann perimeter. The *purple* region corresponds to the monocular temporal crescent which is mapped within the most anterior 8% to 10% of V1. (Reproduced from Horton JC, Hoyt WF. Quadrantic visual field defects: A hallmark of lesions in extrastriate (V2/V3) cortex. *Brain.* 1991;114:1703–1718.)

Other inputs to V1

Besides the LGN, V1 receives a variety of other modulatory inputs both from subcortical and cortical areas. These inputs include serotonergic, noradrenergic, and cholinergic inputs from the brainstem and basal forebrain nuclei, respectively.[17] The latter inputs show differences in density in V1 layers, but a much less specific pattern of innervation than do LGN inputs. Other input sources include the intralaminar nuclei of the thalamus and the pulvinar, both of which send broad projections most heavily to layers 1 and 2 of V1. Additionally, there are retinotopically more specific sources of input to V1, including from the claustrum and visual (V) areas 2, 3, 4, and 5 (V3, V4, and V5 are also referred to as the dorsomedial [DM], dorsolateral [DL] and

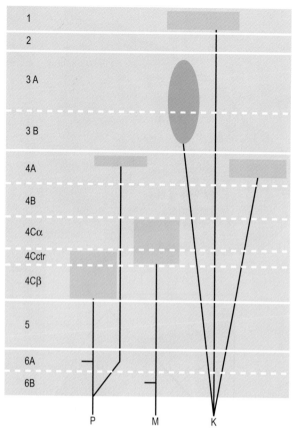

Fig. 30.2 A schematic of the main lateral geniculate nucleus (LGN) projection patterns to visual cortex in macaque monkeys. M LGN afferents project to sublayer 4Cα, P afferents to sublayer 4Cβ and layer 4A; M and P afferents additionally send collaterals to layers 6B and 6A, respectively, while K LGN afferents project to 4A, the cytochrome oxidase blobs in layer 3, and layer 1. LGN projections to 4A have been shown in macaques but appear to be absent in humans and apes.[15] Numbers refer to V1 layers; *P*, parvocellular; *M*, magnocellular; *K*, koniocellular. (Reproduced from Casagrande VA, Kaas JH. The afferent, intrinsic, and efferent connections of primary visual cortex in primates. In: Peters A, Rockland KS, eds. *Primary Visual Cortex in Primate*. New York: Springer; 1994:201–259. https://doi.org.10.1007/978-1-4757-9628-5_5.)

middle-temporal [MT] visual areas, respectively[16,18]). As a rule, any area to which V1 projects also sends feedback to V1. However, some higher-order visual areas in the temporal and parietal lobes that do not receive direct projections from V1 send axons to V1.[19] With the exception of the claustrum, the axons of which overlap with M and P axons in layer 4C, the other extrastriate visual inputs to V1 terminate outside of layer 4C. Some specific roles of such "top-down" inputs to V1 are described in more detail in the feedback section further.

Interlaminar circuitry and cell types
Feedforward pathways
The main thalamic inputs to V1 terminate in layer 4C (except for K visual channels). Signals next propagate to layers 2/3, where they are sent intracortically to higher visual areas, as well as locally to layer 5. Layer 5 provides input to layer 6. Layers 5 and 6 send signals primarily to subcortical nuclei. These are by no means the only interlaminar feedforward pathways in V1, but they are the most well described across species and likely the most robust (Fig. 30.3).

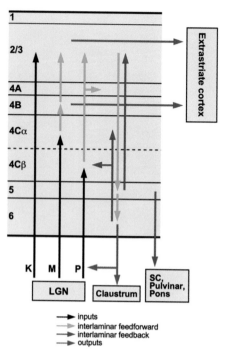

Fig. 30.3 A schematic of intracortical connectivity and signal flow in monkey V1. Magnocellular (M) and parvocellular (P) lateral geniculate nucleus (*LGN*) inputs terminate predominantly in layer 4Cα and 4Cβ, respectively. Signals from layer 4Cα propagate to layer 3 via an intermediate synapse in layer 4B; signals from layer 4Cβ propagate to layers 4A and 3B. There are also weaker projections from 4C directly to 3B (not shown). Layer 3B projects upward. Signals then pass from layer 2/3 onto higher cortical areas, as well as locally onto layer 5. Layer 5 relays visual signals subcortically (for instance to the superior colliculus) and projects locally to layer 6, where collaterals from M and P LGN axons also terminate. Layers 5 and 6 relay feedback signals to layers 2/3 and 4, respectively, and layer 6 also sends significant feedback signals to the LGN.[16,20–22] *SC*, Superior colliculus.

Intralaminar and feedback pathways
There is dense connectivity within each cortical layer enabling significant intralaminar processing. Additionally, there is significant feedback connectivity between connected cortical layers (Fig. 30.3), meaning that upon receiving input from a given layer, the recipient layer processes the information and then relays a signal back to the input layer, thus resulting in highly recurrent processing. Such extensive recurrent processing has made it particularly complicated for researchers to gain a holistic view of how exactly information is processed locally in cortex and what kind of signal transformations are taking place.

Parallel streams within V1
In primate V1, beyond the thalamic input layers, where geniculate M, P, and K axons remain segregated, the three streams significantly intermingle. Whereas layer 4B receives inputs from M-dominated layer 4Cα, and layer 4A mainly from P-dominated layer 4Cβ (in addition to direct geniculate K and P inputs to 4A; Fig. 30.3), outputs from all subdivisions of 4C converge onto the same regions in layer 3B, where inputs from K LGN axons also terminate.[23] Layer 3A, the major output layer to the secondary visual cortical area (V2), in turn, receives inputs from layer 3B, thus relaying a mixture of M, P, and K information to V2. Layer 4B sends mixed M and P signals to V2. Layer 4B also directly projects to area MT, a dorsal stream area specialized in motion processing, but only conveys M signals to MT, an area in the dorsal stream specialized in motion processing.[24]

Thus, except for the V1 output pathway to MT, there is not strict segregation of geniculate streams beyond layer 4 of V1.

Cell types making up the cortical circuit

Recent RNA sequencing work in the visual cortex of mice has found that V1 is comprised of approximately 20 different types of excitatory neurons and 20 different types of inhibitory neurons, with many of these cell types being specific to distinct cortical layers.[25] Subsequent single cell RNA sequencing data from human cortex (the middle-temporal gyrus—obtained from surgical resections in epileptic patients) revealed that human cortex comprises roughly 75 transcriptionally unique cell types, with some of the cell types exhibiting strong transcriptional similarity to cell types found in mouse V1.[26] Within cortex, excitatory neurons release the neurotransmitter glutamate from their axon terminals, and can be grossly separated based on morphology into pyramidal cells, which exhibit a long primary dendrite that streams out of the cell body up toward the cortical surface, and stellate cells, which comprise layer 4 excitatory neurons. Inhibitory cells (interneurons) release the neurotransmitter GABA from their axon terminals. Whereas many different morphologic, electrophysiological, and genetic types of inhibitory neurons have been described, recent work—largely in mice—has identified three major nonoverlapping classes of inhibitory neurons expressing unique molecular markers. Studies on the connectivity and functional properties of these inhibitory neuron types have further indicated that each type plays a unique role in cortical computations.[27] Parvalbumin-expressing (PV) interneurons synapse onto the cell body/axon hillock region of nearby excitatory neurons, which provides them with a strong ability to veto the spiking of excitatory cells. In contrast, somatostatin-expressing (SST) interneurons synapse onto the dendrites of excitatory neurons, thus modulating the input-output transformation occurring in excitatory cells. Both PV and SST cells can also inhibit other interneurons. Another well-studied group of interneurons are vasoactive intestinal peptide–expressing (VIP) cells, which receive significant long-range cortical inputs and in turn provide inhibitory inputs to nearby SST interneurons. Thus, VIP cells can telegraph long-range information via local disinhibition: excitation of VIP cells can inhibit local SST neurons, which leads to disinhibition (i.e., removal of inhibition) of the dendrites of excitatory neurons. It remains unknown whether these three major classes of interneurons correspond to nonoverlapping populations in primate

V1. However, the seminal studies of Lund and colleagues,[28–31] which have identified a variety of morphologic interneuron types and their connections, indicate that primate V1 includes most morphologic types identified in rodents.

PROCESSING IN V1: CLASSICAL AND EXTRACLASSICAL RECEPTIVE FIELDS, FUNCTIONAL ARCHITECTURE, AND LONG-RANGE CONNECTIONS

The early visual pathway performs a local analysis of the visual scene. This analysis begins in the retina and LGN, where circular receptive fields with a center-antagonistic surround organization process contrast, brightness, and color. This analysis continues in V1, where major changes in receptive field structure endow V1 cells with new response properties, including binocularity, sensitivity to stimulus orientation, spatial frequency, motion direction, and binocular disparity. Like LGN, V1 retains an orderly retinotopic organization, but V1 neurons have larger receptive field sizes than LGN cells.

The classical receptive field

The seminal studies of Hubel and Wiesel in cat and monkey V1[32,33] led to the discovery of *orientation selectivity*, the property of V1 cells to respond to a narrow range of edge orientations. Thus, the analysis of object contour, which represents the first step in the processing of object form, begins in V1. Hubel and Wiesel identified three types of orientation-selective receptive fields arranged in serial order of complexity: simple, complex, and hypercomplex. *Simple cells* have receptive fields with spatially segregated ON and OFF subregions, and dominate in the thalamic input layers of V1[34] (Fig. 30.4). The response of these cells depends on the spatial arrangement of their inhibitory and excitatory subregions; when presented with an oriented moving bar of light, they respond optimally when the bar leaves the OFF region and enters the ON region. Hubel and Wiesel proposed a model in which orientation selectivity in simple cells results from the convergence of inputs from LGN cells with spatially aligned circular symmetric receptive fields (Fig. 30.4). Although the mechanisms for the generation of orientation selectivity have been debated for decades,[35,36] there is now good evidence that feedforward LGN inputs generate an orientation bias or preference in V1 neurons, according to a feedforward

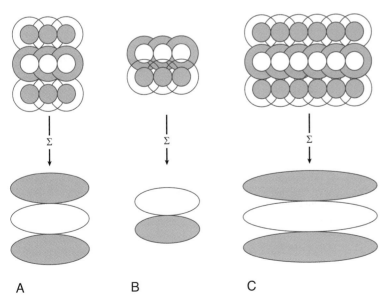

A   B   C

Fig. 30.4 Simple cells. Orientation-selective receptive fields of simple cells can be created by summing the responses of LGN neurons with nonoriented, circularly symmetric receptive fields. The receptive fields of three hypothetical simple cells are shown. Each hypothetical receptive field has adjacent excitatory and inhibitory regions. A comparison of (**A**) and (**C**) illustrates that the degree of orientation selectivity can vary depending on the number of neurons combined along the main axis. (Reproduced from Wandell BA. *Foundations of Vision: Behavior, Neuroscience and Computation.* (Sinauer Associates Inc, 1995).)

mechanism similar to that proposed by Hubel and Wiesel; however, intra-V1 recurrent excitatory and inhibitory connections amplify such bias and sharpen orientation tuning, respectively.[37]

Complex cells have overlapping ON and OFF subregions and dominate outside the geniculate input layers. Unlike simple cells, complex cells show positional invariance, that is, they respond to an oriented bar presented at any location inside their receptive field and respond continuously to a moving bar of light in their receptive field. *Hypercomplex* or *end-stopped cells* respond to oriented bars of restricted length and are suppressed by long bars extending beyond their receptive field, suggesting they may signal more complex contours such as curves or corners. Hubel and Wiesel originally proposed that the receptive fields of each cell class (simple, complex, and hypercomplex) resulted from the convergence of inputs from the lower-order class in a hierarchical fashion. However, it appears that this is not the case, as many complex cells can receive direct inputs from the LGN, both simple and complex cells are found in all V1 layers,[38] and length-tuning (or more generally size-tuning) is a general property of V1 cells, both simple and complex, now termed *surround modulation* or *surround suppression*.[39]

The processing of object form requires more than just information about the orientation of contours. One can reconstruct any visual pattern when, in addition to edge orientation, information about the spatial frequency, contrast, and phase content is also available. To probe how the visual system analyzes spatial patterns, visual psychophysicists and neurophysiologists use *grating stimuli*. Fig. 30.5A shows an example of sinusoidal gratings in which the intensity of the light and dark bars changes gradually around the mean as a sinusoidal function of space. Gratings possess the four image properties listed above, and each can be varied systematically while keeping the others constant. The spatial frequency of the grating is the number of pairs of bars (or cycles) per degree of visual angle. The contrast is the difference in light intensity between the light and dark bars of the grating: when this difference is large the grating is said to have high contrast (Fig. 30.5A, left and middle), when it is low the grating has low contrast (Fig. 30.5A, right). The spatial phase refers to the position of the bars relative to some landmark. Using these grating stimuli, it has been shown that, in addition to orientation selectivity, V1 neurons show selectivity for *spatial frequency* (Fig. 30.5B–K). Broad tuning for spatial frequency is first established in the retina by the center-surround organization of its receptive fields.[40] In V1, spatial frequency tuning becomes narrower than in retina and LGN. Furthermore, whereas in LGN cells spatial frequency tuning has low-pass characteristics, in V1 the majority of cells exhibit bandpass spatial frequency tuning[41,42] (Fig. 30.5B–K). Early models of form vision suggested that the visual system's spatial frequency selectivity is the basis for coding visual images by Fourier analysis,[43] an idea that was not supported by experimental evidence. However, a number of subsequent models have used local spatial frequency filters with properties similar to the receptive fields of cells in the primate visual system to successfully describe the visual system's ability to detect and discriminate visual objects, suggesting that even if the Fourier model is not fully accurate, some form of spatial frequency analysis does occur in the cortex.

It is also in V1 that the initial analysis of object motion is performed. *Direction selectivity*, the preferential response of a neuron to an object moving in a particular direction, is another receptive field property that, in primates, emerges predominantly in V1 (in rabbits and mice, direction-selective cells are commonly found in the retina, whereas only a sparse population of cells in the primate retina and LGN shows direction selectivity). Many models of direction selectivity[45] require a time delay in the inputs to distinct parts of a cell's receptive field, such that an object moving in the optimal direction first encounters a long-response latency region and subsequently a short latency region, so

that signals from both regions arrive simultaneously at the cell body where they summate, leading the cell to firing; in contrast, when the object is moving in the nonoptimal direction, signals from the different regions do not temporally summate and the cell does not reach its firing threshold.

Another receptive field property that emerges outside the geniculate input layers of V1 is *binocularity*, the integration of inputs from the two eyes. Most binocular cells in V1 are dominated by signals from one or the other eye, a property called *ocular dominance*[32] (see Fig. 30.9). Many binocular neurons are also selective for *retinal disparity*,[46] a cue for stereoscopic depth perception. Retinal disparity results because objects located in front or behind the observer's plane of fixation hit slightly different locations on the two retinas. Individual V1 cells are tuned to a narrow range of retinal disparities.

Functional architecture
Columns and maps

As described in Fig. 30.1, V1 contains a systematic map of the visual field. This retinotopic organization imposes constraints on how object features and attributes are represented in cortex, requiring them to be encoded at each visual field location to avoid gaps in the overall representation. Using single microelectrode recordings, Hubel and Wiesel[34] discovered that neurons recorded in a vertical electrode penetration shared similar orientation preference, ocular dominance and retinotopic location, but when the electrode was inserted at an oblique angle relative to the cortical surface, orientation preference, ocularity, and retinotopic position shifted in an orderly fashion. Near the fovea representation of V1, visuotopic location shifted approximately every 2 mm, while a full cycle of orientations and ocular dominance columns were represented approximately every 800 and 1000 μm, respectively; thus, both eyes and a full set of orientations are represented at each spatial location. Based on these findings, Hubel and Wiesel proposed the concept of the *hypercolumn* as the processing unit or module of V1. However, it was not until the advent of intrinsic signal optical imaging that we gained an understanding of how different feature maps are represented in V1 (Fig. 30.6). This technique is based on differences in reflectance of red light (when the latter is shone on the cortical surface while presenting visual stimuli to the animal's eyes), between oxygenated and deoxygenated blood that occurs as a result of changes in neural activity.[47-49] Using this approach, it was discovered that in cat and primates, orientation-preference maps have a *pinwheel-like* organization: domains/columns representing all orientations around the clock are represented in an orderly manner as the spokes of a pinwheel around a pinwheel center or singularity; abrupt changes in orientation preference occur at singularities and regions of the map called *fractures* (Fig. 30.6A). Eye preference is also organized into a map consisting of alternating bands of eye preference, the *ocular dominance bands*, repeating along the tangential domain of V1 (Fig. 30.6B). Orientation singularities align preferentially with the center of ocular dominance bands (Fig. 30.6D). Superimposed to these maps is also a *direction-preference* map, whereby each orientation domain is split into two subdomains preferring opposite directions for that given orientation.[50]

Single microelectrode recording studies demonstrated that, similar to orientation, cells with similar spatial frequency tuning are also clustered together in V1. Studies using C-2-deoxyglucose uptake showed that presentation of gratings of high or low spatial frequency results in patchy activation patterns, with low spatial frequency responses coinciding with the cytochrome oxidase blobs in V1 (discussed further in chapter).[52] However, because the clustering of spatial frequency tuning is looser than that for orientation tuning, it has long been difficult to demonstrate whether spatial frequency is mapped continuously in V1. Using two-photon calcium imaging, which allows recording from large

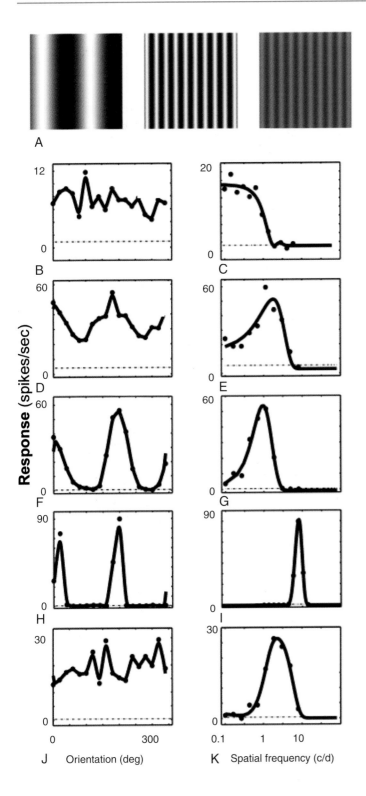

A

B
C

D
E

F
G

H
I

J   Orientation (deg)
K   Spatial frequency (c/d)

Response (spikes/sec)

Fig. 30.5 Orientation and spatial frequency tuning in V1. (**A**) Three example sinusoidal grating stimuli: a low spatial frequency and high contrast grating (*left*), a high spatial frequency and high contrast grating (*middle*), and a high spatial frequency and low contrast grating (*right*). (**B–K**) Example tuning functions from five cells showing the range of orientation (*left column*) and spatial frequency (*right column*) tuning found in macaque V1. The cell in (**H–I**) is sharply tuned for both orientation and spatial frequency. The cell in (**J–K**) is sharply tuned for spatial frequency but poorly tuned for orientation. (Modified from Xing D, Ringach DL, Shapley R, Hawken MJ. Correlation of local and global orientation and spatial frequency tuning in macaque V1. *J Physiol.* 2004;557:923–933.[44])

neuronal populations at single cell resolution, it has been recently demonstrated that spatial frequency in layer 2/3 of macaque V1 is indeed organized into a highly structured and continuous map, the contours of which run orthogonally to the contours of the orientation map.[53]

Cytochrome oxidase blobs

Embedded into the computational module of V1 (the hypercolumn) are the cytochrome oxidase (CO) blobs and interblobs (Fig. 30.6C).

The CO blobs are clusters of cells, about 400 μm in diameter, prominent in the superficial layers of V1, which receive direct inputs from the K layers of the LGN, and stain darkly for CO; the latter is a metabolic enzyme of the Krebs cycle, which is particularly rich within the more metabolically active regions of V1, (i.e., those receiving direct inputs from the LGN). Blobs lie preferentially at the center of ocular dominance columns and align with the centers of orientation pinwheels (Fig. 30.6D; however, pinwheels are more numerous than blobs, thus

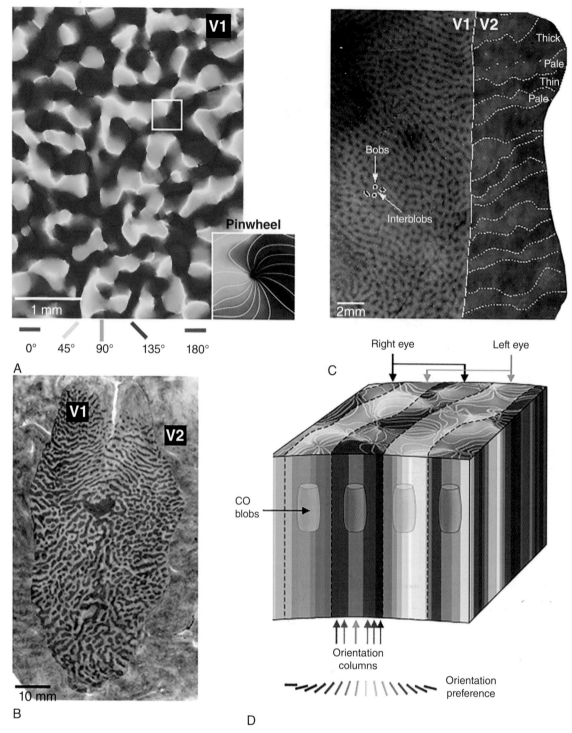

Fig. 30.6 Functional architecture of V1 in macaque and humans. (**A**) The orientation map in macaque V1. The *white square* points to an orientation pinwheel in the map shown at higher magnification in the inset (Unpublished data from M. Hassanpour and A. Angelucci). (**B**) The complete pattern of ocular dominance columns in human V1. (Modified from Adams DL, Sinich LC, Horton JC. Complete pattern of ocular dominance columns in human primary visual cortex. *J Neurosci.* 2007;27:10391–10403. Copyright 2007 Society for Neuroscience.) (**C**) The cytochrome oxidase (CO) map in macaque V1 and V2. CO histochemistry reveals a pattern of *dark patches* (the *blobs*) amidst *pale regions* (the *interblobs*) in V1, while in V2 it reveals a repeating pattern of *dark thick and thin stripes* with interleaved two *pale stripes* (Modified from Federer F, Williams D, Ichida JM, Merlin, S, Angelucci A. Two projection streams from macaque V1 to the pale cytochrome oxidase stripes of V2. *J Neurosci.* 2013;33:11530–11539.) (**D**) The computational module of V1 consists of at least one orientation *hypercolumn* (a full cycle of orientation columns/domains), one cycle of ocular dominance columns, and blobs and interblobs.(Modified from Kandel ER, Schwartz JH, Jessell TM, Siegelbaum SA, and Hudspeth AJ. In Principles of Neural Science (2013). McGraw Hill.)

while most blobs align with pinwheel centers, not all pinwheel centers align with blobs). Physiologically, neurons in the CO blobs have been reported to have receptive fields that are tuned for low spatial frequency, exhibit broader tuning for orientation, and are color selective. In contrast, neurons in the interleaving CO-pale interblobs prefer medium and high spatial frequencies, and are more sharply tuned for orientation.[54,55] However, it has long been debated whether CO blobs uniquely contain color-selective cells and are, thus, devoted to color processing, and whether color and orientation are processed by distinct channels. A recent two-photon imaging study in macaque V1 has shown that a significant proportion of color-selective cells, which prefer isoluminant color over achromatic gratings, are also orientation selective, suggesting that color and orientation in V1 can be processed by similar circuits.[56] However, unoriented, color-preferring neurons are predominantly located in the blobs, whereas oriented and color-selective cells dominate in the interblobs.[56,57] Altogether, physiologic and imaging studies point to the blobs as regions specialized in the processing of surface properties, such as brightness and color, and the interblobs as regions specialized in the processing of contours.

The extraclassical receptive field: surround modulation in V1

Hubel and Wiesel, and many visual neurophysiologists after them, characterized the receptive field properties of single V1 cells to isolated grating or bar stimuli. This led to the concept of the classical receptive field as the visual field region where presentation of stimuli of optimal parameters for the neuron evokes a spiking response.[58] However, it was later discovered that a visual stimulus extending beyond a neuron's receptive field, or presentation of stimuli outside the receptive field, modulate the neuron's response to stimuli inside its receptive field, a property that was termed *surround modulation* (reviewed in[39]). Surround modulation is an integral part of visual information processing because natural visual stimuli do not activate neurons in isolation, but within the context of other stimuli. Indeed, it has been described at all levels of the visual system, from the retina to extrastriate cortex,

across many species and sensory modalities. A fundamental property of surround modulation is its orientation-dependence, that is gratings of different orientations presented inside and outside a neuron's receptive field typically evoke a higher response from the neuron compared with stimuli of the same orientation. Thus, orientation discontinuities in a visual stimulus (as well as motion or texture discontinuities) enhance a neuron's response. Because of this property, it was proposed that surround modulation serves to compute visual saliency, pop-out, object boundary detection, or figure-ground segregation.[59,60] However, using iso-oriented and collinearly aligned small bar stimuli presented inside and outside the receptive field of a neuron, other researchers found response enhancement, leading these investigators to suggest that surround modulation serves *contour integration*,[61-63] i.e., to group together collinear elements into elongated contours. Theoretical[64] and experimental[65] work has additionally suggested that the function of surround modulation may be to reduce redundancies in the responses of neurons to natural images/movies (which contain strong spatiotemporal correlations) and to increase response sparseness, which could lead to more efficient coding of natural stimuli.

Circuits for surround modulation

Surround modulation requires integration of visual signals across distant visual field locations. Because feedforward afferents from the LGN are spatially restricted to the receptive field size of their target V1 cells[66] and LGN cells are not orientation tuned (in monkey), feedforward mechanisms are insufficient to account for orientation-tuned surround modulation in V1. Intra-areal *long-range horizontal connections* within V1 and interareal *feedback connections* from extrastriate cortex to V1 are two sets of connections thought to provide the spatial integration of signals and tuning required for surround modulation (reviewed in[67]) (Fig. 30.7).

Horizontal connections in V1 are millimeters-long intralaminar connections made by excitatory neurons predominantly in layers 2/3 and 5.[68] They encompass visual field regions extending two to three times the size of their receptive field,[69] contact both excitatory and

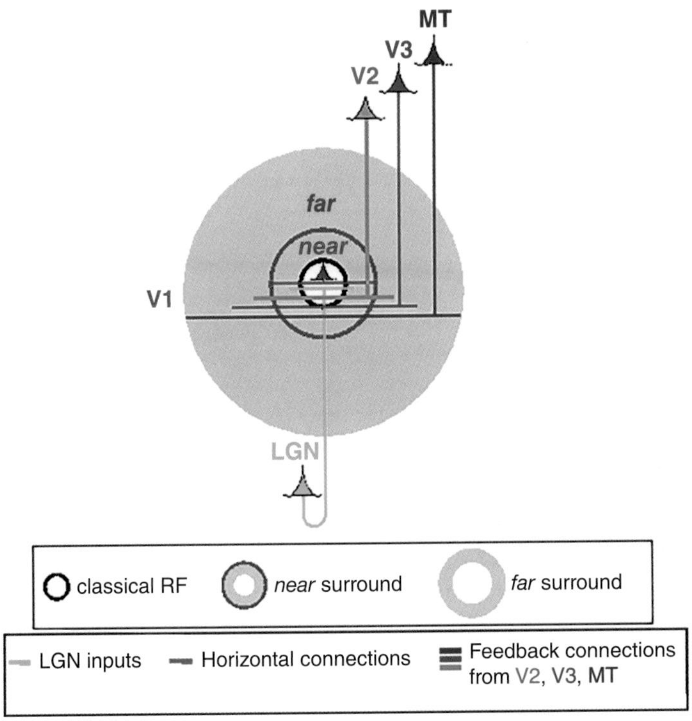

Fig. 30.7 Circuits for surround modulation in macaque V1. Lateral geniculate nucleus (*LGN*) inputs contribute primarily to generating the size and tuning properties of the classical receptive field (RF). Horizontal and feedback connections all contribute to the RF and the near RF surround, but only feedback connections contribute to surround modulation arising from the far surround, with feedback arising from areas V2, V3, and middle-temporal (*MT*) contributing to progressively more extensive surround regions, respectively. (Reproduced with permission from the Annual Review of Neuroscience, Volume 40 © 2017 by Annual Reviews, http://www.annualreviews.org.)

inhibitory neurons and, at least in layers 2/3, link preferentially neurons with similar and collinear orientation preference.[70]

Corticocortical feedback connections, in macaque V1, arise from excitatory neurons in the superficial and deep layers of extrastriate cortical areas (predominantly V2, V3/DM, MT) and terminate densely in layers 1/upper 2 and 5/6, and sparsely in layers 3 and 4B.[71,72] In V1, they contact both excitatory and inhibitory neurons,[73] also making direct contacts with the V1 neurons sending feedforward inputs to their home area.[74] Feedback projections encompass visual field regions extending 5–25 times the receptive field diameter of their targeted V1 cells, with feedback from progressively higher extrastriate areas providing progressively larger terminal fields in V1.[69] Moreover, feedback connections conduct signals 10 times faster (2–6 m/s) than horizontal connections (0.1–0.3 m/s).[75]

Because of these properties both horizontal and feedback connections are well suited to generate orientation-tuned surround modulation at different spatial scales, with horizontal connections subserving surround modulation and contour integration from just outside the receptive field of V1 neurons (the *near* surround) and feedback from progressively higher areas providing modulation from progressively more distant surround regions (the *far* surround) (Fig. 30.7). Recent optogenetic studies have provided direct causal evidence for a role of both horizontal and feedback connections in surround modulation.[76,77] Finally, both theoretical and experimental evidence suggests that horizontal and feedback connections generate surround modulation through a common mechanism involving both increased inhibition and reduced recurrent excitation, via interactions with local inhibitory (SST) neurons and local recurrent networks[78-83] (reviewed in[67]).

OUTPUT STREAMS FROM V1

Pyramidal neurons in all layers, and the spiny stellate cells of layer 4B, send outputs outside of V1.

Subcortical outputs

Layer 6 sends direct excitatory feedback to the LGN and indirect inhibitory feedback to the LGN via axon collaterals to the thalamic reticular nucleus. The direct corticogeniculate feedback is organized into parallel streams, each targeting distinct streams of the feedforward geniculocortical inputs. Anatomically, separate populations of neurons having distinct morphologies and arising from distinct sublayers of layer 6 innervate the M, P, and K layers of the LGN.[84-86] Physiologically, three classes of corticogeniculate cells with properties closely resembling those of neurons in the LGN M, P, and K layers have been identified[87]; these connections serve to modulate the activity of LGN cells, filtering or gating the incoming feedforward information in a stream-specific fashion.

In primates, cells in layer 5 send a major driving output to the inferior subdivision of the pulvinar nucleus of the thalamus, which, in turn, sends driving feedforward-like inputs to layers 3 and/or 4 of extrastriate cortex (sometimes with collaterals to layer 5), as well as modulatory feedback inputs to layer 1 of V1. Moreover, layer 5 projects to the superficial layers of the superior colliculus and other midbrain nuclei such as the pretectum and the pons nuclei, centers that are concerned with eye movements (Fig. 30.3).

Corticocortical outputs
Parallel streams from V1 to V2

The superficial layers of V1 provide the major output to other cortical areas in the visual hierarchy. The latter also receive sparser projections from V1 layers 5/6. These output projections emerge from different layers and CO compartments of V1, suggesting they carry distinct

information. In primates, the largest output connection from V1 is to area V2. CO staining in primate V2 reveals a repeating pattern of alternating dark-thick/pale/dark-thin/pale stripes (Fig. 30.5C). These CO patterns, together with those in V1, have been shown to form the scaffold around which connections between V1 and V2 are organized. Livingstone and Hubel[54,88] first proposed a tripartite division of V1-to-V2 connections, according to which the CO blobs in layers 2/3 of V1 project to the V2 thin stripes, the interblobs in V1 layers 2/3 to the pale stripes, and V1 layer 4B to the thick V2 stripes. It was then shown that the thick stripes project to MT (an area specialized in processing motion and stereopsis), and the thin and pale stripes to V4 (an area specialized in processing color and form),[89,90] and that there is segregation of receptive field properties in the different V2 stripes.[89,91] Based on this evidence, Livingstone and Hubel[92] proposed that these V1-to-V2 pathways subserve a tripartite division of color (blob-to-thin stripes), form (interblobs-to-pale stripes), and motion/depth (4B-to-thick stripes) information processing.

Recent anatomical studies in macaque monkeys have led to a revision of this model. In contrast to the classic tripartite model, Sincich and Horton[93] found that V1 projections to all stripe types arise from layers 2/3, 4A, 4B, and 5/6, but in proportions that depend on the target V2 stripe type. Thus, whereas thin and pale stripes receive a predominant projection from V1 layers 2/3, the thick stripes receive an almost equal contribution from layers 2/3 and 4B. Moreover, these authors showed that interblobs project to both thick and pale stripes, but these two stripe types receive inputs from largely distinct neuronal populations in the interblobs. Federer et al.[94] additionally demonstrated that in the New World primate marmoset, like in macaque, the projections to the thick and pale stripes arise from distinct populations of interblob neurons, but in the marmoset these two populations are additionally spatially segregated, with projections to the thick stripes arising from the blob border region, and those to pales tripes from the middle of the interblobs (Fig. 30.8). These authors also found that in both marmoset and macaque the two pale stripes receive distinct inputs from V1 interblobs: only the pale stripes located laterally to thick stripes (pale-lateral) receive projections from layer 4B, whereas the pale-medial stripes receive little (macaque) or no (marmoset) projections from 4B.[51] Moreover 97%–99% of V1 inputs to the two pale stripe types arise from distinct neuronal populations, i.e., individual cells project to one or the other pale stripe type and only rarely to both. Optical imaging studies have additionally demonstrated functional differences between the two pale stripes, suggesting they represent distinct compartments.[5,95] Overall results from these more recent studies suggest the existence of four parallel streams of information processing between V1 and V2 (Fig. 30.8).

V1 outputs to other cortical areas

In addition to V2, V1 sends direct feedforward connections to visual areas V3/DM, V4/DL, and V5/MT. V1 layer 4B is the major source of V1 inputs to V3/DM, and V5/MT (Fig. 30.8). The V1 projection to V4 is sparse at best and originates mainly from the superficial layers of V1 from the region representing the central few degrees of the visual field. There are also extremely sparse direct projections from V1 to inferior temporal cortex.

How do parallel input streams relate to parallel output streams?

It was originally proposed that there is a direct link between the parallel M and P geniculate pathways to V1 and the output pathways from V1 to extrastriate cortex. Specifically, it was thought that M signals feed directly into the dorsal stream to parietal cortex, via the thick CO stripes of V2 and area MT (the *where* pathway specialized in

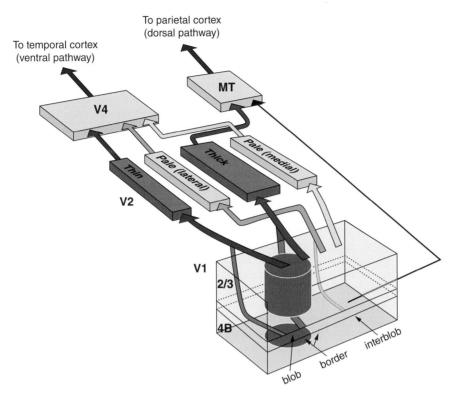

Fig. 30.8 Parallel pathways from V1. Four parallel output pathways from V1 to V2. Each pathway is represented by *arrows* of different colors. *Lighter colors* indicate the inputs from V1 layer 4B to V2. Sparser inputs from V1 layer 4A and 5/6 to V2 are not shown. *Arrow thickness* indicates the relative density of projections from V1 to V2. One pathway (*red*) projects from the cytochrome oxidase (CO) blob columns (predominantly cells in layers 2/3 and less so in layers 4A–B and 5/6) to the thin stripes. A second pathway (*blue*) projects from the blob-border columns (predominantly and equally from layers 2/3 and 4B, and less so from 4A and 5/6) to the thick stripes. Two additional pathways project from the interblobs to either the pale-lateral or the pale-medial stripes, with inputs to the pale-lateral stripes arising predominantly from layers 2/3 and less so from layer 4A–B and 5/6, while those to the pale-medial stripes arising exclusively (marmoset) or overwhelmingly (macaque) from layer 4B. Thin and pale stripes project to area V4 and the ventral stream, while thick stripes project to area middle-temporal (MT) in the dorsal stream. There is also a direct projection from layer 4B of V1 to area MT in the dorsal pathway. (Federer F, Williams D, Ichida JM, Merlin,S, Angelucci A. Two projection streams from macaque V1 to the pale cytochrome oxidase stripes of V2. *J Neurosci.* 2013;33:11530–11539 and Federer F, Ichida JM, Jeffs J, Schiessl I, McLoughlin N, Angelucci A. Four projection streams from primate V1 to the cytochrome oxidase stripes of V2. *J Neurosci.* 2009;29(49):15455–15471.)

spatial vision), while P signals feed into the ventral stream to temporal cortex, via the thin and pale V2 stripes and area V4 (the *what* pathway specialized in object vision). However, the subsequent discovery of the K pathways did not fit this simple two-pathway scheme. Moreover, additional experimental evidence demonstrated that M, P, and K signals are not strictly segregated beyond the input layers of V1. Anatomically, as discussed in the earlier chapter section "Visual inputs to V1 and local cortical circuits", the output pathways from both sublayers of 4C converge onto the same regions in layer 3, leading to intermingling of M and P information in the superficial layers of V1 (where K inputs also terminate), which provide the strongest projection to V2. Moreover, V1 layer 3 cells respond well with either the M or P LGN layers blocked, while responses in area V4 are affected by silencing either the M or P pathway,[96] suggesting V1 layer 3 and area V4 receive inputs from both pathways. However, silencing the M pathway eliminates responses in the majority of MT cells[97] (MT receives a direct visual input from K LGN cells, as well as visual inputs via the superior colliculus-to-pulvinar pathway[98,99]), and there is anatomical evidence for a predominant M input to MT from layer 4B of V1.[24] Thus, unlike other areas such as V2 and V4, where both M

and P signals contribute to neuronal responses, MT cell responses are dominated by M inputs. However, cells in layer 4B of V1 and in MT do not simply show the same receptive field properties as M LGN cells. For example, layer 4B cells, but not their M LGN afferents, have direction-selective receptive fields, and cells in MT, unlike M cells and most V1 cells, are selective for the direction of complex moving patterns, such as plaids, independent of the direction of motion of their components.[100] The latter are constructed through complex local and interareal circuitry.

Parallel feedback streams from V2 to V1

A recent study has demonstrated that the parallel feedforward pathways from V1 to V2 described previously are reciprocated by similar parallel feedback pathways from V2 to V1: thin stripes feedback to CO blobs, and thick and pale stripes to interblobs.[72] Feedback connections are thought to mediate the modulatory influences of visual context (or surround modulation) as outlined previously, as well as the modulatory influences of attention and predictions, as outlined further. The finding of stream-specific feedback channels suggests that feedback-mediated modulations are functionally specialized, meaning that each channel modulates responses related to a specific stimulus attribute (e.g., color, or motion).

PLASTICITY, LEARNING AND CONTEXT-DEPENDENT PROCESSING IN V1

Although initial recordings in V1 suggested a system of stable visual filters (i.e., fixed orientation filters), subsequent work has shown that responses of individual V1 neurons can be highly plastic, and that response properties can be modulated by things such as learning, attention, and context. Many of these plastic changes in V1 response properties are likely modulated by top-down inputs from higher cortical areas (as discussed previously).

Ocular dominance plasticity and a critical period for "learning to see"

Soon after their breakthrough work characterizing the response properties of individual neurons in V1, Hubel and Wiesel made another ground-breaking discovery: obstructing vision to one eye during early postnatal development drastically reduced the extent to which that eye could subsequently drive activity in V1 (Fig. 30.9). They showed this first in cats, and subsequently in monkeys.[101,102] What they showed amounted to a *critical period* during development: restoring vision to the deprived eye after the critical period was insufficient for it to regain its ability to activate visual cortex; performing monocular deprivation in adult animals showed no comparable deficit in the deprived eye's ability to activate V1. Clinically, this finding has proven important as a guideline for correcting amblyopia in childhood before the end of the critical period, in order to ensure that both eyes can effectively drive V1 later in life.[103]

Attention affects V1 responses

Attention can enhance our ability to perceive certain things, while also enabling us to filter out and ignore other things. Spatial attention (i.e., attending to a particular part of the visual field) has been shown to modify neuronal responses throughout much of the visual system. Although much work on attention has been focused on higher visual areas, such as V4, there is ample evidence that responses in V1 are also affected. In V1, attention appears capable of modulating firing rates, enhancing the efficacy of thalamocortical synapses and modulating trial-by-trial response variability.[104]

Learning affects V1 responses

Aside from ocular dominance plasticity during development, neurons in V1 can modulate their response properties following visual perceptual learning. One recent study in mice has provided insights into how this can happen at a cellular and circuit level[105] (Fig. 30.10). Mice were placed in a virtual reality environment that allowed them to walk down a virtual corridor. They were trained to distinguish between black and white bars of different orientations that were projected onto the virtual corridor walls. By recording from many V1 neurons in layers 2/3 of V1 and being able to distinguish which cells were excitatory and which were inhibitory (either PV-, SST-, or VIP-expressing), it was found that learning increased the tuning selectivity of excitatory, PV, and SST neurons, with some cells becoming more tuned to the reward stimulus and some becoming more tuned to the distractor stimulus. Furthermore, the correlations between specific neurons changed following learning in distinct ways. Thus, to learn a given visual stimulus, the feature selectivity of neurons can change at the microcircuit level, within only a subset of the overall V1 population changing for a particular type of learning. A follow-up study examined in further detail how learning versus attention differentially modify neuronal activity patterns in V1 in cell type–specific ways.[106] Whether learning occurs in a similar manner in primate V1 remains to be examined.

Behavioral context affects V1 responses

In the previous section on surround modulation, it was discussed how the stimulus content in the receptive field surround can modify the responses of V1 neurons. In addition to this, situational or behavioral contexts that are independent of changes in the visual stimulus can also affect our visual perception, a phenomenon that is likely controlled via similar top-down influences. A nice demonstration of this phenomenon comes from a study recording from individual V1 neurons in macaque monkeys.[107] In this experiment, animals were trained on a task involving five short line segments, each roughly corresponding to the receptive field of a single V1 neuron. Three of the line segments were horizontally aligned along their long axis, and the middle line had lines both above and below it (all together, the five line segments were arranged like a "plus" sign). The monkeys were trained on two specific contexts: for one context, they needed to judge whether the center line was horizontally aligned closer to the left or right flanking lines; for the second context, the monkeys needed to assess if the center

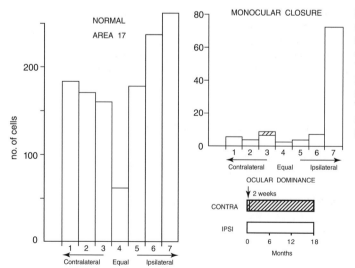

Fig. 30.9 Ocular dominance plasticity. *Left:* A histogram showing the distribution of cells recorded in V1 of macaque monkeys, plotted in accordance with their ocular dominance preference (1 being exclusively driven by the contralateral eye, 4 being equally driven by both eyes, 7 being exclusively driven by the ipsilateral eye). *Right:* The same plot but following 16 weeks of monocular deprivation (to the contralateral eye), from 2 weeks of age to 18 weeks of age. (From Hubel DH, Wiesel TN, LeVay S, Barlow HB, Gaze RM. Plasticity of ocular dominance columns in monkey striate cortex. *Philos Trans R Soc Lon B Biol Sci.* 2017;278:377–409.)

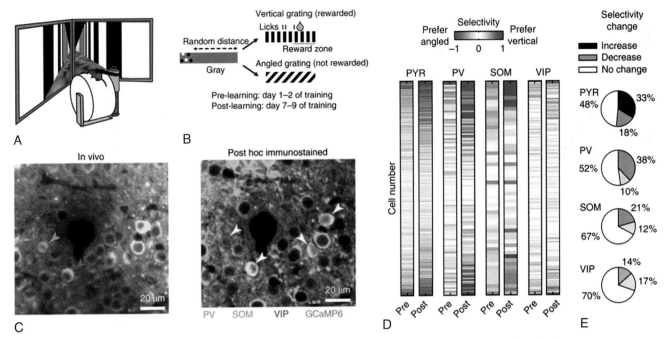

Fig 30.10 (**A**) A head-fixed mouse is placed on a running wheel, and the movement of the running wheel controls a virtual environment on computer monitors, allowing the mouse to virtually navigate through a corridor. (**B**) The experimental paradigm. Animals saw vertical and angled gratings while walking down the virtual corridor and were only rewarded with water during a zone of vertical gratings. (**C**) *Left:* In vivo two-photon calcium imaging of neurons in layer 2/3 of mouse V1 (*white circles* are cell bodies labeled with a calcium indicator dye that can be used to monitor neuronal activity). *Right:* Posthoc immunohistochemistry of the same cells imaged in vivo, enabling categorization of the cells as either excitatory (GCaMP6 only), or different inhibitory cell types (parvalbumin-expressing [*PV*], somatostatin-expressing [SOM], and vasoactive intestinal peptide-expressing [VIP]). (**D**) For different types of cortical neurons (excitatory = pyramidal = PYR), the number of cells showing a tuning preference for angled versus vertical gratings is shown before and after a week-long training. (**E**) A subset of each neuronal class changes its tuning preferences following learning. (From Khan AG, Poort J, Chadwick J, et al. Distinct learning-induced changes in stimulus selectivity and interactions of GABAergic interneuron classes in visual cortex. *Nat Neurosci.* 2018;21:851–859.

line was closer to the line directly above or below it. Once animals were trained, the researchers recorded from a V1 neuron whose receptive field matched the location of the center line. What they found was that the responses of individual V1 neurons were strongly modulated by the specific context, even though what was presented within their receptive field center was constant across both contexts.

Expectation affects V1 responses

When you walk into a familiar room and a piece of furniture has been moved or an object has been removed, this can quickly draw your attention. It turns out that neuronal responses in V1 are modulated by deviations from expectation, and these modulations of V1 responses appear to also arise from top-down influences. For example, brain recordings in humans have shown that omitting a visual stimulus among a series of regularly repeated stimuli appears to result in distinct "visual" related activity even during omitted stimulus trials.[108] Related, in mice trained to run on a treadmill that controls a virtual reality environment through which they are navigating, it has been shown that instantaneously decoupling the link between the treadmill and the virtual reality display (i.e., decoupling expected optic flow from experienced optic flow) can result in distinct neuronal activity in V1.[109] This could arise from "predictive coding," whereby visual cortex compares incoming sensory inputs (in the case of V1, this would be signals coming from the retina via LGN) to expected signals (for instance, prediction signals sent to V1 via feedback connections from higher visual

areas about what is expected to be seen given then current environment/context and the current motor plan).[110,111]

WHEN THINGS GO WRONG

As outlined in Chapter 27, lesions to different parts of the visual system reliably cause scotomas in distinct parts of the visual field. Whereas damage to higher visual areas can often cause deficits in specific aspects of visual processing (as discussed in Chapter 31), lesions to V1 tend to result in a complete loss of vision in the part of the visual field that was damaged. As such, damage to V1 results in complete loss of conscious visual perception previously supported by the damaged area. When this damage is extensive and covers significant portions of visual space, it can lead to the interesting phenomenon of blindsight, in which although the person with V1 damage has no conscious awareness of visual events happening within their scotoma, they maintain "subconscious" access to vision in this visual field region via other preserved visual pathways. Blindsight appears to rely on remnant processing between thalamus and/or superior colliculus and higher visual areas, and it is discussed in more detail in Chapters 29 and 31. Cortical (or cerebral) visual impairment (CVI) is relatively common in both children and adults. In children, it is thought that CVI most commonly arises from injuries to the brain occurring before, during, or shortly after birth. In adults, some of the most common causes of CVI are stroke and traumatic brain damage.

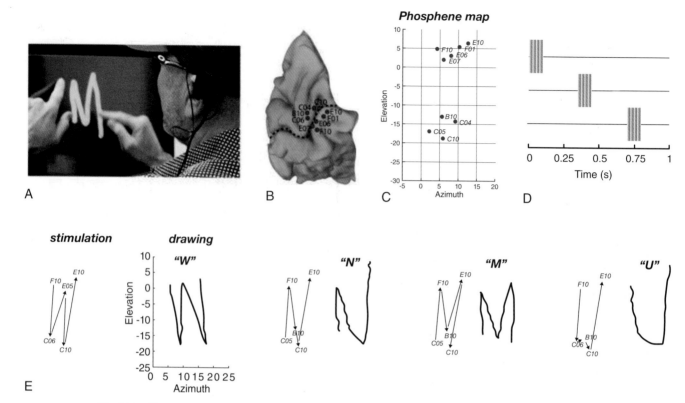

Phosphene map

Fig. 30.11 Electrical stimulation of visual cortex drives visual percepts. (**A**) Photo of a participant tracing out an evoked percept that was seen following electrical stimulation of visual cortex. (**B**) Location of the stimulating electrodes in visual cortex. (**C**) Phosphene maps, corresponding to where the participant 'viewed' phosphenes following stimulation of each individual electrode. (**D**) Example of a dynamic stimulation protocol, where electrical pulses are delivered sequentially from one electrode (*top*), to an adjacent electrode (*middle*), to a third adjacent electrode (*bottom*). (**E**) "Drawing" activity patterns with electrical stimulation in cortex evoked percepts of shapes that the participants could trace out. (From Beauchamp MS, Oswalt D, Sun P, et al. Dynamic stimulation of visual cortex produces form vision in sighted and blind humans. *Cell.* 2020;181:774–783.e5.)

Possible rehabilitation strategies

One emerging strategy for treating CVI, as discussed in more detail in Chapter 31, is to train patients to view images on the edge of their scotoma, and this has shown limited success in partially shrinking the size of the scotoma. Another strategy that has shown some promise involves directly electrically stimulating the cortical tissue to directly evoke visual perceptions. Electrical stimulation in visual cortex of a visually impaired patient was first performed in the 1960s.[112] More recently, researchers used temporally offset stimulation patterns with multiple stimulation probes located in different retinotopic regions of visual cortex, which enabled blind participants to successfully report "seeing" different letters[113] (Fig. 30.11; similar results have also been recently reported in monkey experiments[114]). However, such stimulation does not drive "natural" vision, but instead generates visual phosphenes, and perception arises via the patient making sense of the phosphenes.

CONCLUSIONS

V1 sits at a critical place in our visual system, receiving bottom-up visual information from the retina via the thalamus, and processing these signals in a variety of ways before passing them onto higher visual areas, while also incorporating top-down feedback and contextual signals from many other areas. As such, not only is V1 the central hub for conscious visual perception, it is also a key brain region where visual stimulus context and various other forms of context (expectations, goals, attention, etc.) modify responses. As a result, the signals V1 sends to higher visual areas (Chapter 31) reflect both the visual stimuli in the outside world and the internal state of the organism.

ACKNOWLEDGMENTS

We acknowledge funding from the Canada Research Chairs program to ST, the National Institute of Health and the National Science Foundation to AA, and Research to Prevent Blindness to the Department of Ophthalmology at the University of Utah. A previous version of this chapter was written by Vivien Casagrande and Roan Marion. Portions of the current text were adapted from the previous version, and some of the figures were reprinted from the previous chapter. We thank Christopher Pack for commenting on the manuscript.

REFERENCES

1. Molnár Z. Thomas Willis (1621–1675), the founder of clinical neuroscience. *Nat. Rev. Neurosci.* 2004;5:329–335.
2. Fishman RS. Boerhaave's Tale. *Surv. Ophthalmol.* 2005;50:226–228.
3. Simpson DA, Crompton JL. The visual fields: An interdisciplinary history I. The evolution of knowledge. *J. Clin. Neurosci.* 2008;15:101–110.
4. Ivanišević M, Stanić R, Ivanišević P, Vuković A. Albrecht von Graefe (1828–1870) and his contributions to the development of ophthalmology. *Int. Ophthalmol.* 2020;40:1029–1033.
5. Fishman RS. Brain wars: Passion and conflict in the localization of vision in the brain. In: Albert DM, Zrenner C, eds. *History of Ophthalmology: Sub auspiciis Academiae Ophthalmologicae Internationalis.* Netherlands: Springer; 1995:173–184.
6. Andrews TJ, Halpern SD, Purves D. Correlated size variations in human visual cortex, lateral geniculate nucleus, and optic tract. *J. Neurosci.* 1997;17:2859–2868.
7. Glickstein M, Rizzolatti G. Francesco Gennari and the structure of the cerebral cortex. *Trends Neurosci.* 1984;7:464–467.
8. Brodmann K. *Vergleichende Lokalisationslehre der Grosshirnrinde in ihren Prinzipien dargestellt auf Grund des Zellenbaues.* Leipzig: Barth; 1909.
9. Horton JC, Hoyt WF. Quadrantic visual field defects: A hallmark of lesions in extrastriate (V2/V3) cortex. *Brain.* 1991;114:1703–1718.
10. Fox PT, Miezin FM, Allman JM, Essen DV, Raichle ME. Retinotopic organization of human visual cortex mapped with positron- emission tomography. *J. Neurosci.* 1987;7:913–922.
11. Engel SA, Rumelhart DE, Wandell BA, et al. fMRI of human visual cortex. *Nature.* 1994 Jun 16;369(6481):525.
12. Meyer BU, Diehl R, Steinmetz H, Britton TC, Benecke R. Magnetic stimuli applied over motor and visual cortex: influence of coil position and field polarity on motor responses, phosphenes, and eye movements. *Electroencephalogr. Clin. Neurophysiol. Suppl.* 1991;43:121–134.
13. Harris KD, Shepherd GMG. The neocortical circuit: themes and variations. *Nat. Neurosci.* 2015;18:170–181.
14. Casagrande V, Yazar F, Jones K, Ding Y. The morphology of the koniocellular axon pathway in the macaque monkey. *Cereb. Cortex.* 2007;17:2334–2345.
15. Casagrande VA, Khaytin I, Boyd J. Evolution of the visual system in mammals—color vision and the function of parallel visual pathways in primates. In: Binder MD, Hirokawa N, Windhorst U, eds. *Encyclopedia of Neuroscience.* Berlin: Springer; 2009:1472–1475.
16. Casagrande VA, Kaas JH. The afferent, intrinsic, and efferent connections of primary visual cortex in primates. In: Peters A, Rockland KS, eds. *Primary Visual Cortex in Primates.* New York: Springer; 1994:201–259.
17. Jones EG. Chapter I. The thalamus of primates. In: Bloom FE, Björklund A, Hökfelt T, eds. *Handbook of Chemical Neuroanatomy.* vol. 14. Amsterdam: Elsevier; 1998.
18. Lyon DC, Kaas JH. Connectional and architectonic evidence for dorsal and ventral v3, and dorsomedial area in marmoset monkeys. *J. Neurosci.* 2001;21:249–261.
19. Rockland KS, Ojima H. Multisensory convergence in calcarine visual areas in macaque monkey. *Int. J. Psychophysiol.* 2003;50:19–26.
20. Lund JS, Yoshioka T, Levitt JB. Substrates for interlaminar connections in area V1 of macaque monkey cerebral cortex. In: Peters A, Rockland KS, eds. *Primary Visual Cortex in Primates.* New York: Springer; 1994:37–60.
21. Callaway EM. Cell types and local circuits in primary visual cortex of the macaque monkey. In: Chalupa LM, Werner JS, eds. *The Visual Neurosciences 680–694.* Cambridge, MA: The MIT Press; 2004.
22. Douglas RJ, Martin KAC. Neuronal circuits of the neocortex. *Annu. Rev. Neurosci.* 2004;27:419–451.
23. Yabuta NH, Callaway EM. Functional streams and local connections of layer 4C neurons in primary visual cortex of the macaque monkey. *J. Neurosci.* 1998;18:9489–9499.
24. Nassi JJ, Callaway EM. Specialized circuits from primary visual cortex to V2 and area MT. *Neuron.* 2007;55:799–808.
25. Tasic Bosiljka, Menon Vilas, Nghi Nguyen Thuc, et al. Adult mouse cortical cell taxonomy revealed by single cell transcriptomics. *Nat Neurosci.* 2016 Feb;19(2):335–346. https://doi.org/10.1038/nn.4216. Epub 2016 Jan 4.
26. Hodge Rebecca D, Bakken Trygve E, Miller Jeremy A, et al. Conserved cell types with divergent features in human versus mouse cortex. *Nature.* 2019 Sep;573(7772):61–68. https://doi.org/10.1038/s41586-019-1506-7. Epub 2019 Aug 21.
27. Tremblay R, Lee S, Rudy B. GABAergic Interneurons in the Neocortex: From Cellular Properties to Circuits. *Neuron.* 2016;91:260–292.
28. Lund JS. Local circuit neurons of macaque monkey striate cortex: I. Neurons of laminae 4C and 5A. *J. Comp. Neurol.* 1987;257:60–92.
29. Lund JS. Anatomical organization of macaque monkey striate visual cortex. *Annu. Rev. Neurosci.* 1988;11:253–288.
30. Lund JS, Yoshioka T. Local circuit neurons of macaque monkey striate cortex: III. Neurons of laminae 4B, 4A, and 3B. *J. Comp. Neurol.* 1991;311:234–258.
31. Lund JS, Wu CQ. Local circuit neurons of macaque monkey striate cortex: IV. neurons of laminae 1–3A. *J. Comp. Neurol.* 1997;384:109–126.
32. Hubel DH, Wiesel TN. Receptive fields, binocular interaction and functional architecture in the cat's visual cortex. *J. Physiol.* 1962;160:106–154.
33. Hubel DH, Wiesel TN. Receptive fields and functional architecture of monkey striate cortex. *J. Physiol.* 1968;195:215–243.
34. Hubel DH, Wiesel TN. Ferrier lecture. Functional architecture of macaque monkey visual cortex. *Proc. R. Soc. Lond. B Biol. Sci.* 1977;198:1–59.
35. Sompolinsky H, Shapley R. New perspectives on the mechanisms for orientation selectivity. *Curr. Opin. Neurobiol.* 1997;7:514–522.
36. Ferster D, Miller KD. Neural mechanisms of orientation selectivity in the visual cortex. *Annu. Rev. Neurosci.* 2000;23:441–471.
37. Shapley R, Hawken M, Ringach DL. Dynamics of orientation selectivity in the primary visual cortex and the importance of cortical inhibition. *Neuron.* 2003;38:689–699.
38. Ringach DL, Shapley RM, Hawken MJ. Orientation selectivity in macaque V1: Diversity and laminar dependence. *J. Neurosci.* 2002;22:5639–5651.
39. Angelucci, A. & Shushruth, S. Chapter 30. Beyond the classical receptive field: Surround modulation in primary visual cortex. in The New Visual Neurosciences (2013). https://mitpress.mit.edu/9780262019163/the-new-visual-neurosciences/
40. Kuffler SW. Discharge patterns and functional organization of mammalian retina. *J. Neurophysiol.* 1953;16:37–68.
41. Campbell FW, Cooper GF, Enroth-Cugell C. The spatial selectivity of the visual cells of the cat. *J. Physiol.* 1969;203:223–235.
42. De Valois RL, Albrecht DG, Thorell LG. Spatial frequency selectivity of cells in macaque visual cortex. *Vision Res.* 1982;22:545–559.
43. Westheimer G. The Fourier theory of vision. *Perception.* 2001;30:531–541.
44. Xing D, Ringach DL, Shapley R, Hawken MJ. Correlation of local and global orientation and spatial frequency tuning in macaque V1. *J. Physiol.* 2004;557:923–933.
45. Mauss AS, Vlasits A, Borst A, Feller M. Visual circuits for direction selectivity. *Annu. Rev. Neurosci.* 2017;40:211–230.
46. Poggio GF, Fischer B. Binocular interaction and depth sensitivity in striate and prestriate cortex of behaving rhesus monkey. *J. Neurophysiol.* 1977;40:1392–1405.
47. Blasdel GG, Salama G. Voltage-sensitive dyes reveal a modular organization in monkey striate cortex. *Nature.* 1986;321:579–585.
48. Grinvald A, Lieke E, Frostig RD, Gilbert CD, Wiesel TN. Functional architecture of cortex revealed by optical imaging of intrinsic signals. *Nature.* 1986;324:361–364.
49. Blasdel GG. Orientation selectivity, preference, and continuity in monkey striate cortex. *J. Neurosci.* 1992;12:3139–3161.
50. Shmuel A, Grinvald A. Functional organization for direction of motion and its relationship to orientation maps in cat area 18. *J. Neurosci.* 1996;16:6945–6964.
51. Federer F, Williams D, Ichida JM, Merlin,S, Angelucci A. Two projection streams from macaque V1 to the pale cytochrome oxidase stripes of. *J Neurosci.* 2013;33:11530–11539.
52. Tootell RB, Silverman MS, Hamilton SL, Switkes E, Valois RD. Functional anatomy of macaque striate cortex. V. Spatial frequency. *J. Neurosci.* 1988;8:1610–1624.
53. Nauhaus I, Nielsen KJ, Disney AA, Callaway EM. Orthogonal micro-organization of orientation and spatial frequency in primate primary visual cortex. *Nat. Neurosci.* 2012;15:1683–1690.
54. Livingstone MS, Hubel DH. Anatomy and physiology of a color system in the primate visual cortex. *J. Neurosci.* 1984;4:309–356.
55. Economides JR, Sincich LC, Adams DL, Horton JC. Orientation tuning of cytochrome oxidase patches in macaque primary visual cortex. *Nat. Neurosci.* 2011;14:1574–1580.
56. Garg AK, Li P, Rashid MS, Callaway EM. Color and orientation are jointly coded and spatially organized in primate primary visual cortex. *Science.* 2019;364:1275–1279.
57. Lu HD, Roe AW. Functional organization of color domains in V1 and V2 of macaque monkey revealed by optical imaging. *Cereb. Cortex.* 2008;18:516–533.
58. Hubel DH, Wiesel TN. Receptive fields of single neurones in the cat's striate cortex. *J. Physiol.* 1959;148:574–591.
59. Knierim JJ, van Essen DC. Neuronal responses to static texture patterns in area V1 of the alert macaque monkey. *J. Neurophysiol.* 1992;67:961–980.
60. Lamme VA. The neurophysiology of figure-ground segregation in primary visual cortex. *J. Neurosci.* 1995;15:1605–1615.
61. Kapadia MK, Ito M, Gilbert CD, Westheimer G. Improvement in visual sensitivity by changes in local context: Parallel studies in human observers and in V1 of alert monkeys. *Neuron.* 1995;15:843–856.
62. Polat U, Mizobe K, Pettet MW, Kasamatsu T, Norcia AM. Collinear stimuli regulate visual responses depending on cell's contrast threshold. *Nature.* 1998;391:580–584.
63. Field, D.J., Golden, J. & Hayes, A. Chapter 44. The New Visual Neurosciences 627–638 (2013). https://mitpress.mit.edu/9780262019163/the-new-visual-neurosciences/
64. Simoncelli EP, Olshausen BA. Natural image statistics and neural representation. *Annu. Rev. Neurosci.* 2001;24:1193–1216.
65. Vinje WE, Gallant JL. Natural stimulation of the nonclassical receptive field increases information transmission efficiency in V1. *J. Neurosci.* 2002;22:2904–2915.
66. Angelucci A, Sainsbury K. Contribution of feedforward thalamic afferents and corticogeniculate feedback to the spatial summation area of macaque V1 and LGN. *J. Comp. Neurol.* 2006;498:330–351.
67. Angelucci A, Bijanzadeh M, Nurminen L, Federer F, Merlin S, Bressloff PC. Circuits and mechanisms for surround modulation in visual cortex. *Annu Rev Neurosci.* 2017;40:425–451.
68. Rockland KS, Lund JS. Intrinsic laminar lattice connections in primate visual cortex. *J. Comp. Neurol.* 1983;216:303–318.
69. Angelucci Alessandra, Levitt Jonathan B, Walton Emma JS, Hupe Jean-Michel, Bullier Jean, Lund. Jennifer S. Circuits for local and global signal integration in primary visual cortex. *J Neurosci.* 2002 Oct 1;22(19):8633–8646. https://doi.org/10.1523/JNEUROSCI.22-19-08633.2002.
70. Bosking WH, Zhang Y, Schofield B, Fitzpatrick D. Orientation selectivity and the arrangement of horizontal connections in tree shrew striate cortex. *J. Neurosci.* 1997;17:2112–2127.
71. Rockland KS, Pandya DN. Laminar origins and terminations of cortical connections of the occipital lobe in the rhesus monkey. *Brain Res.* 1979;179:3–20.
72. Federer F, Ta'afua S, Merlin S, Hassanpour MS, Angelucci A. Stream-specific feedback inputs to the primate primary visual cortex. *Nat. Commun.* 2021;12:228.
73. Anderson JC, Martin KAC. The synaptic connections between cortical areas V1 and V2 in macaque monkey. *J. Neurosci.* 2009;29:11283–11293.
74. Siu C, Balsor J, Merlin S, Federer F, Angelucci A. A direct interareal feedback-to-feedforward circuit in primate visual cortex. *Nat. Commun.* 2021;12:4911.
75. Girard P, Hupé JM, Bullier J. Feedforward and feedback connections between areas V1 and V2 of the monkey have similar rapid conduction velocities. *J. Neurophysiol.* 2001;85:1328–1331.
76. Adesnik H, Bruns W, Taniguchi H, Huang ZJ, Scanziani M. A neural circuit for spatial summation in visual cortex. *Nature.* 2012;490:226–231.

77. Nurminen L, Merlin S, Bijanzadeh M, Federer F, Angelucci A. Top-down feedback controls spatial summation and response amplitude in primate visual cortex. *Nat. Commun.* 2018;9:2281.

78. Schwabe L, Obermayer K, Angelucci A, Bressloff PC. The role of feedback in shaping the extra-classical receptive field of cortical neurons: A recurrent network model. *J. Neurosci.* 2006;26:9117–9129.

79. Ozeki H, Finn IM, Schaffer ES, Miller KD, Ferster D. Inhibitory stabilization of the cortical network underlies visual surround suppression. *Neuron.* 2009;62:578–592.

80. Haider Bilal, Krause Matthew R, Duque Alvaro, Yu Yuguo, Touryan Jonathan, Mazer James A, McCormick. David A. Synaptic and network mechanisms of sparse and reliable visual cortical activity during nonclassical receptive field stimulation. *Neuron.* 2010;65(1):107–121. https://doi.org/10.1016/j.neuron.2009.12.005.

81. Shushruth S, Mangapathy Pradeep, Ichida Jennifer M, Bressloff Paul C, Schwabe Lars, Angelucci. Alessandra. Strong recurrent networks compute the orientation tuning of surround modulation in the primate primary visual cortex. *J Neurosci.* 2012 Jan 4;32(1):308–321. https://doi.org/10.1523/JNEUROSCI.3789-11.2012.

82. Rubin DB, Van Hooser SD, Miller KD. The stabilized supralinear network: A unifying circuit motif underlying multi-input integration in sensory cortex. *Neuron.* 2015;85:402–417.

83. Sato TK, Haider B, Häusser M, Carandini M. An excitatory basis for divisive normalization in visual cortex. *Nat. Neurosci.* 2016;19:568–570.

84. Fitzpatrick D, Usrey WM, Schofield BR, Einstein G. The sublaminar organization of corticogeniculate neurons in layer 6 of macaque striate cortex. *Vis. Neurosci.* 1994;11:307–315.

85. Ichida JM, Casagrande VA. Organization of the feedback pathway from striate cortex (V1) to the lateral geniculate nucleus (LGN) in the owl monkey (Aotus trivirgatus). *J. Comp. Neurol.* 2002;454:272–283.

86. Briggs F, Kiley CW, Callaway EM, Usrey WM. Morphological substrates for parallel streams of corticogeniculate feedback originating in both V1 and V2 of the macaque monkey. *Neuron.* 2016;90:388–399.

87. Briggs F, Usrey WM. Parallel processing in the corticogeniculate pathway of the macaque monkey. *Neuron.* 2009;62:135–146.

88. Livingstone MS, Hubel DH. Connections between layer 4B of area 17 and the thick cytochrome oxidase stripes of area 18 in the squirrel monkey. *J. Neurosci.* 1987;7:3371–3377.

89. DeYoe EA, Van Essen DC. Segregation of efferent connections and receptive field properties in visual area V2 of the macaque. *Nature.* 1985;317:58–61.

90. Shipp S, Zeki S. Segregation of pathways leading from area V2 to areas V4 and V5 of macaque monkey visual cortex. *Nature.* 1985;315:322–324.

91. Hubel DH, Livingstone MS. Segregation of form, color, and stereopsis in primate area 18. *J. Neurosci.* 1987;7:3378–3415.

92. Livingstone M, Hubel D. Segregation of form, color, movement, and depth: anatomy, physiology, and perception. *Science.* 1988;240:740–749.

93. Sincich LC, Horton JC. Divided by cytochrome oxidase: A map of the projections from V1 to V2 in macaques. *Science.* 2002;295:1734–1737.

94. Federer F, Ichida JM, Jeffs J, Schiessl I, McLoughlin N, Angelucci A. Four projection streams from primate V1 to the cytochrome oxidase stripes of V2. *J Neurosci.* 2009;29(49):15455–15471.

95. Felleman Daniel J, Lim Heejin, Xiao Youping, Wang Yi, Eriksson Anastasia, Parajuli. Arun. The Representation of Orientation in Macaque V2: Four Stripes Not Three. *Cereb Cortex.* 2015 Sep;25(9):2354–2369. https://doi.org/10.1093/cercor/bhu033. Epub 2014 Mar 9.

96. Ferrera VP, Nealey TA, Maunsell JH. Responses in macaque visual area V4 following inactivation of the parvocellular and magnocellular LGN pathways. *J. Neurosci.* 1994;14:2080–2088.

97. Nealey TA, Maunsell JH. Magnocellular and parvocellular contributions to the responses of neurons in macaque striate cortex. *J. Neurosci.* 1994;14:2069–2079.

98. Rodman HR, Gross CG, Albright TD. Afferent basis of visual response properties in area MT of the macaque. II. Effects of superior colliculus removal. *J. Neurosci.* 1990;10:1154–1164.

99. Kinoshita Masaharu, Kato Rikako, Isa Kaoru, Kobayashi Kenta, Kobayashi Kazuto, Onoe Hirotaka, Isa. Tadashi. Dissecting the circuit for blindsight to reveal the critical role of pulvinar and superior colliculus. *Nat Commun.* 2019 Jan 11;10(1):135. https://doi.org/10.1038/s41467-018-08058-0.

100. Movshon JA, Adelson EH, Gizzi MS, Newsome WT. The analysis of moving visual patterns. In: Chagas C, Gattass R, Gross C, eds. *Pattern recognition mechanisms.* Rome: Vatican Press; 1985.

101. Wiesel TN, Hubel DH. Single-cell responses in striate cortex of kittens deprived of vision in one eye. *J. Neurophysiol.* 1963;26:1003–1017.

102. Hubel DH, Wiesel TN, LeVay S, Barlow HB, Gaze RM. Plasticity of ocular dominance columns in monkey striate cortex. *Philos Trans R Soc Lon. B Biol Sci.* 2017;278:377–409.

103. Hensch TK, Quinlan EM. Critical periods in amblyopia. *Vis. Neurosci.* 2018;35:E014.

104. Maunsell JHR. Neuronal mechanisms of visual attention. *Annu. Rev. Vis. Sci.* 2015;1:373–391.

105. Khan AG, Poort J, Chadwick J, et al. Distinct learning-induced changes in stimulus selectivity and interactions of GABAergic interneuron classes in visual cortex. *Nat Neurosci.* 2018;21:851–859.

106. Poort Jasper, Wilmes Katharina A, Blot Antonin, et al. Learning and attention increase visual response selectivity through distinct mechanisms. *Neuron.* 2022 Feb 16;110(4):686–697.e6. https://doi.org/10.1016/j.neuron.2021.11.016. Epub 2021 Dec 13.

107. Li W, Piëch V, Gilbert CD. Perceptual learning and top-down influences in primary visual cortex. *Nat. Neurosci.* 2004;7:651–657.

108. Simson R, Vaughan HG, Walter R. The scalp topography of potentials associated with missing visual or auditory stimuli. *Electroencephalogr. Clin. Neurophysiol.* 1976;40:33–42.

109. Keller GB, Bonhoeffer T, Hübener M. Sensorimotor mismatch signals in primary visual cortex of the behaving mouse. *Neuron.* 2012;74:809–815.

110. Rao RPN, Ballard DH. Predictive coding in the visual cortex: a functional interpretation of some extra-classical receptive-field effects. *Nat. Neurosci.* 1999;2:79–87.

111. Keller GB, Mrsic-Flogel TD. Predictive processing: A canonical cortical computation. *Neuron.* 2018;100:424–435.

112. Brindley GS, Lewin WS. The sensations produced by electrical stimulation of the visual cortex. *J. Physiol.* 1968;196:479–493.

113. Beauchamp MS, Oswalt D, Sun P, et al. Dynamic stimulation of visual cortex produces form vision in sighted and blind humans. *Cell.* 2020;181:774–783. e5.

114. Chen X, Wang F, Fernandez E, Roelfsema PR. Shape perception via a high-channel-count neuroprosthesis in monkey visual cortex. *Science.* 2020;370:1191–1196.

31

Extrastriate Visual Cortex

Carlos R. Ponce and Christopher C. Pack

INTRODUCTION TO THE EXTRASTRIATE CORTEX

The goal in this chapter is to develop a basic understanding of the function of extrastriate cortex. This is a collection of brain regions concerned with visual processing and that receive strong driving input from the primary visual cortex (V1). The function of these areas has historically been inferred from studies of patients with punctate lesions. In these patients, the visual deficits are highly specific, causing impairments in functions such as face recognition (prosopagnosia) or color perception (achromatopsia). These impairments are quite different from those caused by V1 lesions, which typically result in phenomenological blindness in affected portions of the contralateral visual field.

Extrastriate cortex regions are found proximally anterior to the primary visual cortex (Fig. 31.1). They can be identified anatomically in some cases, or more frequently by the presence of a distinct retinotopic map. As noted in Chapter 30, this is a point-by-point mapping of retinal space onto the cortical sheet, and it is important to appreciate that the cortex contains dozens of these maps. In extrastriate cortex, the purpose is to analyze specific aspects of the visual scene, and this localization of function explains the highly specific nature of the corresponding deficits following extrastriate lesions.

Although there are many different extrastriate areas, it was pointed out nearly 40 years ago that they can be categorized into two functional networks (Fig. 31.2). This "two-stream" hypothesis was developed based on anatomical studies,[1] as well as behavioral studies that showed a dissociation between perception and action.[2] The behavioral studies yielded a particularly intriguing set of observations suggesting that people experience visual stimuli quite differently depending on whether they are physically interacting with them or simply recognizing them passively.[2]

The first network is located ventrally, neighboring the hippocampus, and it is concerned with visual analyses that might be considered as the "passive" formation of visual memories. The second network is located dorsally, neighboring parietal and premotor cortex, and it is concerned with visual analyses necessary for actions such as navigating and grasping. Both are involved in visual perception, with the ventral network being most concerned with static images, and the dorsal network with moving ones. Each network comprises dozens of cortical regions arranged into a hierarchy, with each region processing visual signals and relaying them to the next. Along these "feedforward" pathways, regions proximal to V1 are often described as "early" stages in visual processing, and distal regions as "late" or "deep" stages. This picture is complicated somewhat by the existence of numerous "feedback" pathways that send signals in the opposite direction (from "late" to "early" stages), and whose function is poorly understood. There are also "lateral" connections within areas and across the two networks. In the following sections, we will briefly examine evidence from lesion studies that illustrate the differences between these networks, and then we will consider how each network performs particular visual functions, with an emphasis on the feedforward processing of signals along each pathway.

THE VENTRAL VISUAL NETWORK

Here we describe the primary functions of a major portion of extrastriate cortex called the ventral network, which encompasses large regions of the occipital and temporal lobes. Ventral network dysfunction can result in agnosias related to form and color.[1] This is well illustrated by the example of subject J, a 30-year-old woman who contacted research investigators at Bielefeld University in Germany circa 2018, presenting with a chief complaint of an inability to recognize faces, including those of her family, her husband, or even her own face in the mirror. J suffers from developmental prosopagnosia, a lifelong debilitating condition with serious social and socioeconomic consequences: "If you have a job where you sit in your office and people come to you at previously appointed times, it is easy. But if you have to actively approach people... you can't do it if you don't know who is who." J suffered several job losses because of her condition.[3] Although the first case was only formally recognized as recently as 1976,[3] developmental prosopagnosia is now known to occur at an estimated prevalence of 2.5% across the population.[4] Although the pathophysiology behind developmental prosopagnosia is poorly understood, cases of *acquired* prosopagnosia can be directly related to damage to inferior occipital and temporal cortex,[5] a region that functional imaging has confirmed responds most strongly to pictures of faces.[6,7]

The best-known cases of prosopagnosia show little to no recognition impairment of other object categories (e.g., cars, tools), but this is relatively rare; most cases of face recognition impairments are associated with general recognition deficits.[8] This reflects the underlying architecture of the ventral network: it comprises a set of cortical areas, each with relative functional specializations, yet still highly interconnected. In the macaque monkey brain, ventral network areas include seven main regions: primary visual cortex (V1), V2, V3, V4, posterior inferotemporal cortex (PIT, sometimes labeled as TEO in the early anatomy literature, this latter term's origins are uncertain but often interpreted as temporo-occipital), and central/anterior inferotemporal cortex (C/AIT, or temporal area E), with parts of the ventral temporal pole (PG).[9] Human ventral network regions also include areas V1–V3, a V4/V8 complex, followed by the lateral occipital complex (LOC) and ventral occipitotemporal cortex (VOT).[10] In the monkey, these ventral network areas have been defined using anatomical tracing, single-cell electrophysiology, targeted lesions, and imaging, whereas in humans most of these areas have only been identified using functional imaging. For this reason, this section will focus mostly on the monkey ventral network.

Areas of the ventral network are interconnected with other brain regions involved in memory (hippocampus and parahippocampal regions), action association (striatum), and flexible planning (prefrontal cortex); these different outputs suggest that the larger ventral

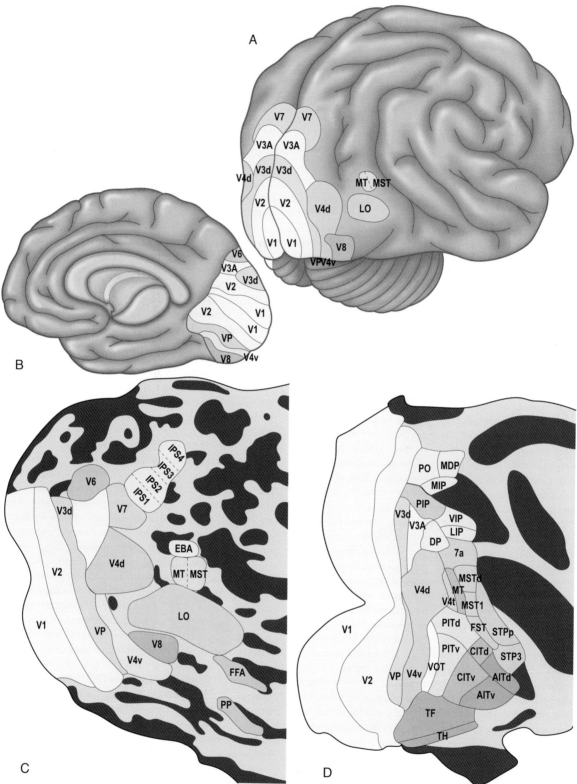

Fig. 31.1 Human (A–C) and monkey (D) visual cortical areas. Visual cortical areas are shown on a schematic diagram of the human brain from the posterior aspect (**A**) and midsagittal plane (**B**). Many of the areas cannot be appreciated on the surface view of the brain, and a flat map of the human (**C**) visual cortical areas is also shown. Areas involved in vision are colored and labeled. The depths of the sulci are shown in *black* and gyri in *white* to give a perspective to location relative to the sulcal patterns. For comparison, a flat map of visual areas in the macaque monkey is shown in (**D**). Homologous areas, insofar as they can be identified, are given the same color and nomenclature, but many more areas have been studied in monkey brain than in human one. In the occipital cortex of humans are the second visual area (V2); the third visual area, broken into a dorsal (V3d) and a posterior half (VP); V3 anterior (V3A); the ventral (V4v) and dorsal (V4d) subdivisions of V4; and the sixth, seventh, and eighth visual areas (V6, V7, and V8). Visual responsive areas in the parietal lobes include the middle-temporal area (MT); the medial superior temporal area (MST); the lateral occipital area (LO), and the extrastriate body area (ERA). Several visual areas in the intraparietal sulcus have been recently studied and named (IPS1, IPS2, IPS3,

IPS4). In the occipitotemporal cortex are found the fusiform face area (FFA) and the parahippocampal place area (PPA). Monkey extrastriate areas shown in (**D**) include, in the temporal lobe, the posterior inferotemporal area, with dorsal (PITd) and ventral (PITv) subdivisions; the central infero-temporal area, with dorsal (CITd) and ventral (CITv) subdivisions; the anterior inferotemporal area, with dorsal (AITd) and ventral (AITv) subdivisions; the superior temporal polysensory area, with anterior (STPa) and posterior (STPp) subdivisions; the floor of the superior temporal sulcus (FST); and temporal areas F (TF) and H (TH). In the parietal lobe are found the medial and superior temporal area, with dorsal (MSTd) and lateral (MSTl) subdivisions; the parietooccipital area (PO); the posterior intraparietal area (PIP); the lateral intraparietal area (LIP); the ventral intraparietal area (VIP); the medial intraparietal area (MIP); the medial dorsal parietal area (MDP); the dorsal prelunate area (DP); and Brodmann's area 7a (7a). (Extrastriate areas have been variously named by the order in which they were studied, by their position relative to sulci and gyri, and by the classical histologic areas to which they most closely correspond. A single area can be named by all three methods, as for the middle-temporal area (MT), known also as V5 and as Brodmann's area 37, and similar sounding names can refer to unrelated areas, as for V7, named in order of its discovery, and 7a, a completely unrelated visual area located in Brodmann's cytoarchitectonic area 7). (Modified from Swisher JD, Halko MA, Merabet LB, McMains SA, Somers DC. Visual topography of human intraparietal sulcus. *J Neurosci.* 2007;27:5326–5337; Larsson J, Heeger DJ. Two retinotopic visual areas in human lateral occipi-tal cortex. *J Neurosci.* 2006;26:13128–13142; Sereno MI, Tootell RB. From monkeys to humans: what do we now know about brain homologies? *Curr Opin Neurobiol.* 2005;15:135–144; and Tootell RB, Tsao D, Vanduffel W. Neuroimaging weighs in: humans meet macaques in "primate" visual cortex. *J Neurosci.* 2003;23:3981–3989.)

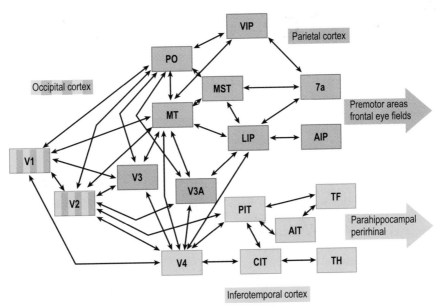

Fig. 31.2 Summary diagram depicting the hierarchy of visual areas associated with the ventral and dorsal pro-cessing streams in monkey and the major interconnections between them. All connections are shown with bidirectional arrows to emphasize that each projection to a higher-level visual area is matched by a feedback projection. Areas V1 and V2 are colored both *red* and *green* to depict their contributions to processing both "what" and "where" information for further, more segregated processing in extrastriate cortex. The dorsal stream areas, colored in *red*, process information about object location (where stream) and project to premo-tor and frontal eye fields. The ventral stream areas, colored in *green*, process details of the form, color, and shape of objects (what stream) and project to the inferotemporal cortical zones and parahippocampal and perirhinal areas.

network comprises multiple subspecialized pathways.[9] However, the overall functions of these subnetworks are all constrained by three major principles: (1) they are bounded by topographical maps present at birth[11]; (2) neurons in anterior cortical regions (e.g., anterior inferotemporal cortex [IT], temporal area G or TG) show larger receptive field (RF) sizes than those in more posterior regions (e.g., V1–posterior IT [PIT]); and (3) neurons with larger RFs tend to respond to more complex images, such as faces or places, in ways that are reminiscent of perception. We review these principles next.

Topographical features of the ventral network

From birth, the ventral network is defined by topography.[12] The ventral network comprises retinotopic maps like the one defining area V1—maps of neighboring neurons in cortex also respond to neighboring regions of the visual field. These retinotopic maps are arranged back-to-back along the anterior-posterior axis, aligned such that their corresponding foveal representations merge along *confluences*, where, for example, V1 neurons with foveal RFs are located close to V2 neurons with foveal RFs (both sets being along the lateral occipitotemporal lobes).[13-15] As in V1, the rest of the ventral network devotes more neurons to processing information at the fovea, both because V2, V4, and IT inherit architectural con-straints from V1 and likely because shape- and texture-based rec-ognition tasks require high-acuity vision for fine discrimination. Subsequently, both at the higher spatial scale detectable by func-tional magnetic resonance imaging (fMRI) and at the level of sin-gle-electrode electrophysiology,[16] the entire ventral network shows stronger responses when objects are presented at or near the fovea versus the periphery.

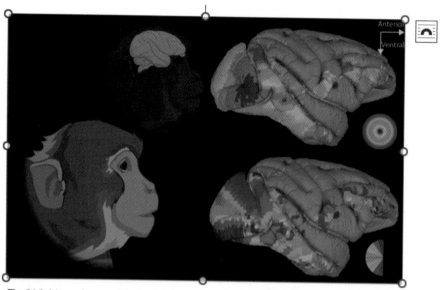

Fig. 31.3 Maps of eccentricity (*top*) and polar angle (*bottom*) in visual space in macaque visual cortex. Foveal confluences are indicated by *red* on the top brain schematic. (Brain maps courtesy of Michael Arcaro and macaque images from BioRender.com.)

There are at least three major foveal confluences within the occipitotemporal lobes (see Fig. 31.4, top right)[13,15]: one confluence is shared by the retinotopic maps of areas V1, V2, and V3, another confluence by the maps of V4 and the PIT, and the last one is contained within the central and anterior IT.[11]

Besides being organized around these three supra-areal confluence maps, ventral network neurons also share other features as a whole, including a bias for responding to objects presented in the contralateral visual field. Posterior ventral network neurons have RFs fully contained within the contralateral visual field, and although anterior network neurons can also respond to stimuli in the ipsilateral hemifield, extending their RFs past the vertical midline of the visual field, they remain heavily biased in responding largely to contralateral stimulation. In fact, this bias is present throughout all visually responsive regions of the brain, including associative regions like prefrontal cortex. One final common topographical feature across the visual recognition network is that neurons responding to the upper visual field are situated in more ventral cortex, whereas neurons responding to the lower field are located more dorsolaterally on the occipital and temporal cortex (Fig. 31.3); this anatomical segregation may provide a substrate for functional differences among neurons, even within the same area[17]—such as some neuronal RFs becoming more selective for face-like patterns and others becoming more selective for body-like patterns, or some RFs becoming more sensitive for some colors over others.[18,19]

Receptive fields and visual selectivity

Primary visual cortex contains neurons that respond to stimulation in locations as eccentric as ±80 degrees along the horizontal axis, and 40 to 60 degrees along the vertical axis.[20] Although this rather large visual field appears perceptually continuous, neurons in every visual area sample this space discretely—for any given neuron, this visual field region is defined as its RF. Neurons in anterior IT can have RFs that capture large regions of the visual field (with RF sizes between 10 and 40 degrees of visual field, with *size* defined as the square root of the RF area), compared with 5 degrees in PIT and V4, and 2 degrees in V2.[21] Although it is unclear whether every cortical area captures the same retinotopic coverage as V1 does (this partially depends on how one defines a cortical area), it is clear that every retinotopic location is covered along different stages of the ventral network.[12,22]

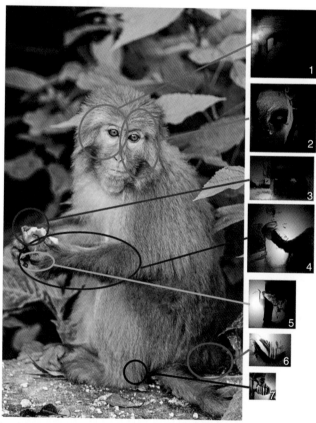

Fig. 31.4 Hierarchical processing in the ventral network. When presented with natural scenes, observers are able to recognize features at different spatial scales, from the overall gist and shape of whole objects to focused details such as texture or line orientations. This fine-level examination of the visual scene is processed locally by neurons in V1, with small receptive fields (RFs) shaped to respond maximally to oriented lines (see inset image **1**, showing a computer-generated image of an actual V1 receptive field). These neurons project to V2 and V4, where neurons have larger RFs (insets **2–3**, and these latter regions project to inferotemporal cortex, where neurons are capable of integrating larger object features such as parts of foods, faces, and bodies (**4–7**).

Neurons with large RFs are also activated by more complex visual images. This was well characterized by a series of experiments by Tanaka and others, in which they stimulated neurons along the ventral network using simple images such as bars, discs, and other simple geometric patterns, and with physical objects and images of animals, foodstuffs, and other multifeature stimuli. They showed a gradual, continuous increase in the amount of visual information necessary to maximally activate neurons, starting from the posterior (caudal) to anterior (rostral) direction of the ventral network.[21] This suggests a generalization of the fundamental principle postulated by Hubel and Wiesel about V1 (see previous chapter), where primary visual cortex neurons derive their selectivity as an elaboration of simpler inputs from neurons in earlier visual regions—a selectivity to oriented contours derived through spatially aligned inputs from the lateral geniculate nucleus.[23] This recombination of inputs from neurons encoding simpler motifs gives rise to RFs that respond to more elaborate visual stimuli, and this algorithm appears to occur repeatedly over the ventral network. The result is neurons that combine simple oriented contours to derive sensitivity to curvature and broader spatiotemporal frequencies (present in V1, V2,[24] and V4[25,26]), followed by neurons that combine curvature, colors, and textures (in V4[27] and PIT[28,29]), and finally followed by neurons that respond maximally to photographs of real-world objects such as faces, body parts, and places (in central and anterior IT).[30–32] This clear, unidirectional increase in both RF size and in stimulus complexity has led many investigators to refer to the ventral network as the *ventral stream* or *ventral pathway*,[1,2] viewing it as a feedforward hierarchy of regions culminating in cortical stages of neurons with functional properties that approximate abstract perceptual judgments. Neurons at the end of this pathway then serve as inputs for more flexible, multisensory neurons in associative regions that truly encode abstract concepts, such as those in the medial temporal lobe that respond not only to images of a given individual but also to images of the individual's written name (as exemplified by neurons tuned to information as specific as those related to the actor Jennifer Aniston[33]).

When it comes to the ventral stream, the leading edge of knowledge stops at the question of what visual attributes are meant to be encoded by IT neurons. What are the real-world features that best trigger responses from IT neurons? We have described these neurons as being attuned for the presence of "faces," "body parts," and "places," and related their common absence or dysfunction to category-specific visual impairments such as prosopagnosia. Yet much like the idea of describing a highly interconnected recurrent network as a "stream," this is only a correct *first* approximation that eventually runs into trouble.

Just as disorders of face perception are frequently associated with other kinds of object recognition issues, studies of neurons at the individual level reveal that neurons do not respond exclusively to images defined by semantic, categorical labels. For example, neurons that are strongly activated by photographs of faces will also respond to photographs of objects that are round and containing curved and straight contours, such as clocks or cut oranges.[34,35] Most commonly, neurons will respond to randomly selected natural images belonging to no semantic category. Whereas there are strong arguments that the organization of the human ventral stream can be understood semantically (at least partially, by mapping neuronal function to word-based atlases[36]), it is not clear how this organization arises in nonhuman primates and other taxonomic groups lacking language. It is possible that language has developed around the preexisting organization of visually selective neurons in the ventral stream; this makes elucidating the fundamental principles behind this organization one of the most exciting current lines of work in this field.

These lines of work spring from several overlapping questions. One issue, raised previously in the chapter, relates to whether the functional organization is based on semantic, conceptual objects of social and ecological significance ("faces,"[37] "animate"[38]), or if it is based on lower-level visual attributes correlated to but not identical to objects.[39,40] Another question is whether these visual attributes are linked by a simple yet-undiscovered parametric relationship, as simple as the orientation-dependent topography of V1,[41] the curvature-dependent topography of V4,[42] or the direction-dependent topography of MT neurons[43] (see next section). It is possible that instead, IT neurons are organized around a set of learned attributes defined by low-level visual similarity, much like current deep-learning models (i.e., convolutional neural networks) abstract the visual world.[44]

How distributed is coding?

One well-established way to think about functional organization in the ventral stream is to ask whether a given visual percept is encoded by a small group of neurons in a sea of many otherwise silent neurons, or whether it is encoded in the distributed, concurrent activity of a much larger population of neurons. We previously described the existence of individual neurons in the human medial temporal lobe that responded when a subject was shown images or written references to the actor Jennifer Aniston.[45] This finding is reminiscent of a philosophical concept made famous by Jerzy Konorski—the *gnostic* or *"grandmother" cell*,[46] a theoretical neuron whose activity would reflect a subject's perception of a given concept, such as their grandmother. In this scenario, an independent observer would only need to monitor the activity of that single cell to predict a subject's responses. In the opposite scenario—that of a fully distributed code—the observer would never be able to ascertain the subject's perceptual responses without monitoring the full population of neurons in a given region. Neither (extreme) scenario finds many defenders in the field of visual neuroscience—both scenarios are rendered implausible by the problem of efficiency: if the visual brain operated with gnostic cells, there would not be enough neurons to represent the astronomical number of concepts and patterns forming our perception.[47] Similarly, if the visual brain required all of its neurons to represent every concept, energy costs would likely set up a lethal disadvantage to the organism. However, there remains abundant disagreement about intermediate scenarios. The idea that a given neuron represents particular values within a population-wide code (e.g., an axis-based, parametric space such as orientation) is prevalent in many research programs[48]; this idea is reminiscent of classic distributed coding views. In contrast, there is the idea that a given neuron's activity represents the presence of a learned visual pattern; this idea is reminiscent of the grandmother cell hypothesis, only substituting a very complex abstract concept (grandmother) with a local combination of visual attributes (a given oriented contour). Convolutional neural networks have shown how difficult it is to defend either intermediate scenario as mutually exclusive of the other. Like mild versions of theoretical grandmother cells, hidden units in a neural network learn specific combinations of visual attributes from their training image sets, yet when presented with random photographs, nearly all of these hidden units can "respond" (i.e., emit nonzero outputs), providing information useful for downstream units. So do CNN hidden units implement distributed coding or more localist operations? The answer is that as convolutional filters, hidden units are capable of responding to any input but still show stronger responses to particular patterns. This is a combination of distributed and localist operations (see Box 31.1), and one that appears to be a good first-order description of neurons in the ventral stream.

BOX 31.1   Artificial neural networks and the brain

Computational models are becoming integral to more and more biological vision research programs. Specifically, deep-learning models such as convolutional neural networks (CNNs), autoencoders, and vision transformers can serve as testing grounds for new hypotheses of neuronal function in the brain. As image-computable models, they can be used (1) to identify unexpected patterns or biases in preselected stimulus sets, (2) to streamline code for real-time closed-loop experiments,[88] or (3) to perform companion *in silico* simulations complementing more expensive and time-consuming neuronal experiments.[27,28] Although computational models are common in many other branches of neuroscience, CNNs have been particularly natural additions to vision studies because in fact they are algorithmic relatives of the mammalian visual system itself. One of the first image-computable models of vision was Kunihiko Fukushima's *Neocognitron*,[90] a deep-layer network directly inspired by Hubel and Wiesel's findings in primary visual cortex (one of many of Fukushima's neuroscience-inspired models[91,92]). Like V1, the Neocognitron comprised (1) units that worked like simple cells, combining geometrically simpler inputs to derive filters with elaborated selectivity, and (2) units that worked like complex cells, pooling the outputs of simple cells to attain invariance to position changes. The simple cell-like units also relied on a nonlinearity operation that limited their responses to positive values, like neurons show in their all-or-none, action potential–based responses. These three biologically inspired operations—filtering, pooling, and rectification, with the later addition of normalization—have been staples of CNNs from their earliest incarnations,[93,94] and these operations have been generally accepted as mechanisms of neuronal function in the visual system.[95-98] In addition to this overlap in local mechanisms, CNNs also share major architectural motifs characteristic of the visual system, including a hierarchical arrangement of layers ("areas"), and receptive fields that increase both in size[99] and in shape complexity.[100] However, one major difference between the biological visual system and CNNs is how they learn. CNNs are trained via supervised learning, specifically with backpropagation,[101] an algorithm that adjusts each connection weight in the network based on errors between the CNN output and the label of the training example, and which naturally requires access to every weight in the model. Cortical areas do not show the type of precise, neuron-to-neuron symmetric projections that would make this algorithm biologically plausible—cortical feedback connections are diffuse,[102] often linking nonvisuotopically corresponding regions.[103,104] Although biologically plausible alternatives for CNN training are being explored, it does not seem as if any of them work as well as backpropagation.[105] This raises two possibilities: either current theories lack the actual unsupervised learning mechanisms used by the brain, or current theories do have them (e.g., Hebbian plasticity–like algorithms,[106] using rate of change of firing responses, feedback alignment[107]), which would mean that CNNs lack an important architectural feature that makes those learning mechanisms effective. This is one of many exciting questions at the intersection of neuroscience and machine learning.

How does the ventral stream acquire its anatomical organization?

A third important question about the ventral network's functional organization is whether it is present at birth, formed by yet-undiscovered mechanisms engrained genetically by natural selection, or whether it develops through experience, based on the individual animal's exposure to the statistics and content of the visual world. This is an active debate in studies of the ventral stream. Definitive data are lacking to settle this question, but there are tantalizing discoveries on either side of this innateness (or *nativist*) versus *bottom-up* (or *experience*) debate. Evidence for the nativist camp include the

following observations: (1) V1 neurons appear to be arranged based on their preferences for orientation even before eye-opening[49] (so it follows that selectivity-map-shaping mechanisms could also exist in deeper stages of the ventral stream); (2) a functional imaging study has shown that some temporal cortical regions will respond preferentially to photographs of faces in sighted subjects, and these same cortical regions will respond preferentially to touching of faces in subjects with full loss of sight[50]; and, finally, (3) clusters of neurons that share preferential responses to photographs of faces, body parts, and places—these clusters are frequently described as "patches" or "domains"[6,51]—tend to occur in relatively similar locations across all primates, something that would be unlikely if experience was the only way to seed the locations of these patches. One explanation for the systematic location of face and place patches ties back to the (less controversially innate) retinotopic maps that define the ventral stream. Face patches appear near the foveal confluences of the temporal lobe,[52] whereas place patches appear along more peripheral representations of visual space[9]; this correlation is illuminated by the fact that in baby monkeys, the foveal bias precedes the development of face patches.[12] One explanation for this relationship is that neurons that respond preferentially near the fovea also tend to have smaller RFs, better suited for processing high curvature, whereas neurons that respond preferentially at the periphery of vision tend to have larger RFs, better suited for extended contours.[53] Thus neurons may not be innately tuned for faces, but rather will be more likely to develop face tuning because they have smaller RFs situated near the fovea.[11] A second observation emphasizing the importance of experience is that animals that grow without early experience to faces will not develop face patches and instead develop other kinds of patches, such as some focusing on hands.[52] Equally relevant is that given intensive experience, humans and monkeys can develop cortical patches for letters and numbers,[54,55] a finding that cannot be explained by innate or genetic mechanisms.

Although these categorical patches are useful measures in the nativism versus experience discussion, they also raise the question of their functional purpose. Why does the ventral stream develop patches at all? It is a general principle of cortical organization that neurons with similar visual tuning properties tend to cluster into groups as small as tens of micrometers and up to several millimeters.[56,57] Clusters could be the result of neurons receiving similar inputs, grouping owing to activity-dependent interactions.[11] However, some theories suggest that clusters serve as functional subsystems, where neurons with similar but nonidentical response properties can work together to overcome noise and variability in the visual input, variability brought about, for example, by incidental changes in viewing distance or angle.[58]

Invariance

Solving the problem of selectivity in the ventral stream is a primary concern in the field; another is the question of invariance. A given object in the real world can project to the retina in a practically infinite number of ways, depending on its position relative to the viewer, current light conditions, and partial occlusion. These *nuisance* variables can be overcome by perception—we can recognize and keep track of the same object as it moves through a scene, passing through shadows, for example. This raises the question of how the ventral stream achieves this so-called *invariance* at the level of neurons. Most tests of invariance have involved a given set of images that are then presented at various positions, sizes, or even viewpoints. A given neuron responds differently to each image, allowing for these images to be sorted by the neuron's "preference." The most common way to define invariance is by measuring if the neuron demonstrates the same preference ranking across different nuisance transformations. This has revealed that neurons of the ventral stream show limited invariance to position,[59] size,[60] texture,[61,62] and rotation.[59] However, no neuron shows as much robustness to nuisance changes as the full perceptual system does, suggesting that this is a distributed property across subnetworks of the ventral stream.[63] Invariance to face rotation, for example, is achieved by a subnetwork of *face patches* spanning all of IT cortex.[64]

Applications

Beyond basic knowledge, what is to be gained by defining the mechanisms and representational content of the ventral stream? The second decade of the 21st century has seen an acceleration in the performance of neural networks and other machine intelligence (MI) models, many of which are trained to perform object classification,[65–67] object detection and segmentation,[68,69] and other visual recognition tasks. These computational models include a variety of architectures (such as convolutional neural networks, variational autoencoders, and vision transformers), and they have enormous potential to transform many industries, such as health care (assisting physicians in screening radiology[70] and pathology[71,72] imaging data), transportation[73] (assisting drivers in monitoring hazardous situations), and security.[74] If they worked as intended, an immediate concern would be their colossal potential for misuse, for example, by minimizing privacy. However, most current CNNs pose little threat because they do not work that well. Current models are not as robust as the visual system when presented with noisy or distorted images,[75] and they can fail in unexpected ways when presented with images having different low-level statistical properties than those involved in their training image sets (for example, evaluating cartoon-like images if the networks were trained only with photographs). The visual system does not exhibit these issues. Further, these models can be vulnerable to so-called *adversarial attacks*, where photographs can be altered with nearly imperceptible noise patterns in order to change the classification offered by the models[76,77]—a potentially disastrous vulnerability that could be exploited by bad actors in the context of self-driving cars, for example, causing models to ignore stop signs or misclassify pedestrians. Finding solutions to these problems is complicated by the fact that these multistage models have many degrees of freedom, learning features from data on their own—optimizing their internal weights according to relatively simple *cost functions* imposed at their output layer.[78] Computer scientists and engineers are working to improve these systems using many approaches, and many believe that more improvements will arise from a better understanding of the brain's ventral stream.[79]

Fortunately, it is becoming easier and more commonplace to perform investigations of the ventral stream in the context of theories of MI. An increasing number of visual neuroscience laboratories are regularly using CNNs as part of their investigations of the brain, largely because both ventral stream and CNNs appear to converge to similar solutions. Investigators at the Massachusetts Institute of Technology showed that the more accurate a CNN is at classification, the more useful it is at fitting IT neuronal responses to photographs,[80] presumably because accurate CNNs learn to represent similar visual features about photographs as the ventral stream does about the natural world. But this has not been easy to show, because as long sequences of functions, CNNs filter, recombine, and threshold pixel information, making it difficult to keep track of which visual features (which combinations of colors, shapes, textures) are ultimately emphasized or eliminated on their way to the output classification layer. This opaqueness has motivated engineers to develop methods for so-called *explainable artificial intelligence* (XAI),[81,82] meant to provide rationales for the solutions found by deep networks. One popular XAI algorithm relevant to the ventral stream is DeepDream,[83] which generates images that maximally activate units within a given CNN. This algorithm allows a reversal of the functionality of CNNs, where instead of propagating an image into the network to consequently measure a hidden unit's response, one can perturb images at the pixel, input level using a function that optimizes the activation of that same hidden unit. This results in artificially reconstructed images containing the unique visual attributes that for a CNN make a dog a "dog," for example, at least based on training data.[84] In many ways, the goal of explaining artificial intelligence (AI) mirrors the goal of understanding neurons deep in the ventral stream, such as those in IT, and subsequently these XAI algorithms have been modified to be helpful in visual neuroscience studies. For example, one can fit pretrained CNNs to replicate the responses of given ventral stream neurons and then apply the DeepDream algorithm to the proxy CNN model, to visualize the visual features putatively learned by the neuron[85,86] (Fig. 31.4). Alternatively and more directly, one can bypass the CNN model and functionally link image-generating, deep-learning models[87] with ventral stream neurons, even as deep in the hierarchy as IT. When applied to neurons in nonhuman primate IT cortex, this latter approach results in highly activating images that often resemble visual attributes commonly present in animals such as monkeys or dogs.[88,89] However, more often, these neuron-guided synthetic images contain visual attributes that are not constrained to any given semantic category, and thus provide exciting new clues in the exploration about the types of visual information are encoded by IT neurons.

THE DORSAL VISUAL NETWORK

The functional specialization of the dorsal visual network is most apparent in patients with *akinetopsia*. This is a rare condition in which visual deficits are largely limited to the perception of moving stimuli. Perception of static stimuli, colors, and depths are for the most part intact.[108] In akinetopsia, patients have difficulty with navigation, particularly for complex tasks like walking in crowds or driving a car. Even simple tasks, such as pouring tea into a cup, can be difficult, as patients do not perceive the fluid motion of the liquid into the cup, but rather a sequence of snapshots, often at a delay.

Akinetopsia had been reported sporadically in the early 20th century, but without detailed psychophysical examinations of the patients. Thus, it was difficult to distinguish it from a more generalized disorder of vision or awareness.[108] However, in 1983, an unambiguous case of akinetopsia was reported by Zihl et al.,[109] who described a 42-year-old female patient (LM), who had lost the ability to perceive motion following a bilateral vascular cortical lesion. Interestingly, the lesions spared the primary visual cortex, and so her presentation was not typical of a cortical deficit such as hemianopsia.

Receptive fields and visual selectivity

Brain imaging revealed that patient LM's lesion included the posterior portion of the middle-temporal gyrus and the nearby white matter. Around the same time, experiments in monkeys revealed that the brain regions homologous to the lesion sites in LM were highly specialized for processing visual motion. The most well studied of these areas is V5, and it was first identified anatomically in owl monkeys by Allman and Kass.[110] In the same year, Dubner and Zeki performed the first electrophysiological recordings in this area, which revealed that nearly all neurons were selective for the direction of stimulus motion.[111] The same neurons had almost no selectivity for color and weak selectivity for orientation, suggesting a highly specialized representation of motion. Starting from the 1980s and continuing to the present day, area MT/V5 has been the target of intense study, as a model of the link between neural activity and conscious perception.[112]

Link to perception and action

Importantly, this link is *causal*. Chemical inactivation of MT neurons can produce a transient akinetopsia in monkeys: during inactivation, the animals lose the ability to perceive the motion of most stimulus patterns, while most other visual capabilities remain intact.[113,114] Permanent lesions of MT lead to profound deficits in motion perception, some of which never recover.[115] At the same time, direct electrical stimulation of clusters of MT neurons causes a percept of moving stimuli, with the perceived motion direction matching the direction that elicits the strongest neural response in the electrically stimulated neurons during normal vision.[116] These results indicate that neural activity in MT is both necessary and sufficient for the perception of visual motion, at least under the experimental conditions used in these studies (we revisit this later). A more direct role for MT in controlling action has been revealed through studies of smooth pursuit eye movements.[117,118] These are tracking movements that are made to keep a moving object's image stationary on the retina; they are significantly impaired following MT lesions[118] and modulated by electrical stimulation of MT.[119]

The essential role of area MT in motion processing suggests a localization of function similar to that discussed in the context of prosopagnosia: in both cases, small clusters of neurons are critical for the integrity of certain kinds of visual-feature processing. For motion perception, this kind of localization might seem surprising, given that many other parts of the visual cortex contain neurons with clear selectivity for stimulus direction. Indeed, the main source of input to MT is layer 4B of the primary visual cortex, where neurons are themselves highly selective for motion direction. These neurons are spared in patients like LM,[108] so why do the perceptual deficits persist?

The answer to this question reflects the hierarchical nature of visual processing, which is quite similar in the dorsal and ventral networks.[120] In this sense, the dorsal network is also a feedforward *pathway*. We have seen that in the ventral pathway, selectivity for complex objects and faces is constructed from successive transformations of signals representing simple features. The dorsal pathway is no different: V1 neurons are selective for what might be called *simple* motion patterns, wherein the motion is confined to a small range of spatial and temporal patterns at a particular point in space. As in the ventral pathway, the neurons that receive input from V1 are tasked with integrating these inputs to gather information across different stimulus features.[121,122] Thus in both dorsal and ventral streams, signals in V1 are necessary but not sufficient to support normal visual perception. They are necessary because they provide the main link between the retina and higher-order cortex, but they are insufficient because individual V1 neurons convey very limited information about the global properties of a stimulus.

A large body of computational and experimental work has examined the mechanisms that characterize the integration of motion signals in MT.[123,124] The consensus is that the hierarchical processing of information serves to establish both selectivity for complex stimuli and invariance to irrelevant properties. This was discussed previously for the ventral pathway, but for the dorsal pathway it means that MT neurons integrate output from lower-level neurons with different preferences for features such as orientation or spatial position, to obtain a measure of object motion that is both specific for a particular motion direction and independent of the structure of the stimulus. In other words, the responses of these neurons are related mostly to the stimulus motion direction and little else. More recent theoretical investigations have shown that deep neural networks trained to estimate self-motion (i.e., the direction in which the observer is moving) can recapitulate many of the detailed properties of neural responses in the dorsal visual pathway[125] (Box 31.1).

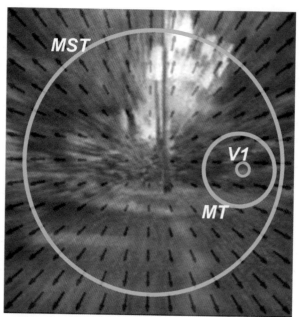

Fig. 31.5 Hierarchical processing in the dorsal network. During navigation, observers most often experience motion that expands outwards from a point in visual space. This motion is processed locally by neurons in V1, with small receptive fields. These neurons project to the middle-temporal area (MT), where neurons have larger receptive fields, and to the medial superior temporal area (MST), where neurons are capable of integrating the entire complex motion stimulus, to evaluate the direction of self-motion.

This emphasis on the computation of self-motion fits with the neural selectivity observed in other regions of the dorsal visual pathway. For example, area V3A contains a preponderance of direction-selective neurons, many of which respond to complex motion patterns of the kind seen during self-motion.[126] This selectivity becomes clearest in area MST, which receives its strongest input from MT. As such, it appears to be the next hierarchical stage along the dorsal pathway. Neurons in MST are selective for the kind of motion stimuli that are represented in MT, but also for complex motion, such as expanding and rotating patterns.[127–129]

Complex motion selectivity suggests a clear behavioral function in guiding navigation. In the simplest case, when the observer is moving toward a fixed, stationary object, retinal stimulation involves motion expanding outward from a point that corresponds to the direction of self-motion (Fig. 31.5). MST neurons are highly sensitive to these patterns[130] and, as in MT, this sensitivity is causally related to behavior. Transient inactivation of MST leads to impaired navigation through simulated environments[131] and electrical stimulation of MST alters the subject's perceived direction of self-motion.[132] MST is considered the terminal node of the dorsal pathway, with efferent projections going to parietal lobe structures that are concerned with spatial orientation[133] and brainstem structures that are concerned with eye movements.[134]

Subcortical inputs and subconscious vision

A final aspect of the dorsal visual pathway is that it receives direct input from subcortical structures, including the lateral geniculate nucleus[135] and the pulvinar.[136] These inputs bypass the primary visual cortex, and as a result they are capable of supporting visual function following lesions to the occipital lobe. As mentioned in the Introduction, such lesions are a common consequence of stroke and traumatic brain injury, and they result in homonymous visual field deficits on the contralateral side, known as *cortical blindness* (or cortical visual impairment).

Cortically blind patients lack phenomenological awareness of stimuli in their blind visual fields, but often exhibit a kind of subconscious vision known as *blindsight*.[137] In some forms of blindsight, patients are able to make judgments about visual stimuli with above-chance performance, despite not being aware that a stimulus was even presented. In other cases, there is a vague awareness of a stimulus. Importantly, the stimuli that are most effective at eliciting blindsight are those that best activate the dorsal visual pathway, namely moving stimuli that are large and high in contrast. This suggests a role for subcortical inputs in supporting dorsal pathway functions like navigation in cortically blind patients, and indeed some patients are capable of navigating on foot or even on a bicycle, based on motion information processed through the lesioned visual field. Such functionality might also be supported in part by spared V1 tissue.[138] In any case, the residual pathways reaching the dorsal pathway after V1 damage, as well as potentially similar inputs to the ventral pathway,[139] suggest a potential avenue for vision rehabilitation in these patients.[140] Blindsight is discussed further in Chapter 29.

PLASTICITY AND REHABILITATION

Cortical blindness

Rehabilitation protocols in cortical blindness typically involve having patients perform simple tasks, such as discriminating the direction of motion of a small stimulus. When the stimulus is placed in the blind visual field, the hope is that training can strengthen the connections from spared visual structures to the recipient dorsal pathway neurons, thereby restoring function. This kind of rehabilitation is still an active area of research,[140] and no specific therapy has yet found widespread clinical acceptance.

The prospects for vision rehabilitation

From the perspective of fundamental science, there is good evidence that the cortical circuitry for motion perception is quite plastic, even in adults. Generally speaking, the close connection between visual motion perception and neural activity in areas such as MT/V5 can be strengthened or diminished through training. Although the rules that govern this kind of plasticity are still unclear, it does seem that the stimulus used during training powerfully modulates the connection between neural activity and perception.[141] In one study,[114] monkeys trained with a simple motion stimulus (a drifting grating) showed accurate motion perception when area MT was chemically inactivated. The same animals, when subsequently trained on a more complex motion stimulus (random dots), were sharply impaired on the initial motion perception task following MT inactivation. Interestingly, the properties of the MT neurons themselves did not change with training, indicating that what changes is the connection with perception, rather than the stimulus representation itself. These findings mirror those observed with permanent lesions of MT[115]: perception of simple moving stimuli eventually recovers, but perception of complex ones does not.

These kinds of observations have motivated a search for training paradigms that can restore function in the cortically blind. Early attempts at vision restoration relied on training with very simple stimuli, and the results were equivocal at best. However, more recent studies have used complex motion stimuli of the kind that were found specifically to engage area MT. When cortically blind patients were trained to report the motion of these stimuli, they showed clear improvement in visual function, with some perceptual capabilities in the blind visual field returning to normal levels.[142] Consistent with the monkey studies, training with more complex stimuli was shown to yield better improvements and better generalization than training with simpler motion stimuli.[142] However, overall visual acuity in the blind field remained far below normal, and the training was quite laborious, requiring several months of daily engagement. Thus, the prospects for vision restoration remain limited, particularly in the chronic phase (>6 months) after a stroke. It remains to be seen whether particular stimuli or tasks improve the effectiveness of vision restoration, and whether the gains seen with motion stimuli can be extended to other stimuli such as shapes. However, there is hope that MI models (such as CNNs currently being used for driver assistance in modern automobiles) will soon become accurate enough to be used in portable devices and complement the limits of plasticity in therapy.

REFERENCES

1. Mishkin M, Ungerleider LG, Macko KA. Object vision and spatial vision: two cortical pathways. *Trends in Neurosciences.* 1983;6:414–417.
2. Goodale MA, Milner AD. Separate visual pathways for perception and action. *Trends in Neurosciences.* 1992;15:20–25.
3. McConachie HR. Developmental prosopagnosia. A single case report. *Cortex.* 1976;12:76–82.
4. Corrow SL, Dalrymple KA, Barton JJS. Prosopagnosia: current perspectives. *Eye and Brain.* 2016;8:165–175.
5. Damasio AR, Tranel D, Damasio H. Face agnosia and the neural substrates of memory. *Annual Review of Neuroscience.* 1990;13:89–109.
6. Kanwisher N, McDermott J, Chun MM. The fusiform face area: a module in human extrastriate cortex specialized for face perception. *The Journal of neuroscience.* 1997;17:4302–4311.
7. Sergent J, Signoret J-L, Bruce V, Rolls ET. Functional and anatomical decomposition of face processing: Evidence from prosopagnosia and pet study of normal subjects [and discussion]. *Philosophical Transactions: Biological Sciences.* 1992;335:55–62.
8. Geskin, J. & Behrmann, M. Congenital prosopagnosia without object agnosia? A literature review. 35, 4–54, (2017).
9. Kravitz DJ, Saleem KS, Baker CI, Ungerleider LG, Mishkin M. The ventral visual pathway: An expanded neural framework for the processing of object quality. *Trends in Cognitive Sciences.* 2013;17:26–49.
10. Grill-Spector K, Malach R. The human visual cortex. *Annual Review of Neuroscience.* 2004;27:649–677.
11. Arcaro MJ, Livingstone MS. On the relationship between maps and domains in inferotemporal cortex. *Nature Reviews Neuroscience.* 2021;22:573–583.
12. Arcaro MJ, Livingstone MS. A hierarchical, retinotopic proto-organization of the primate visual system at birth. *eLife.* 2017;6
13. Rosa MGP. Visual maps in the adult primate cerebral cortex: some implications for brain development and evolution. *Braz J Med Biol Res.* 2002;35:1485–1498.
14. Rosa MGP, Tweedale R. Brain maps, great and small: lessons from comparative studies of primate visual cortical organization. *Society.* 2005:665–691.
15. Wandell BA, Dumoulin SO, Brewer AA. Visual field maps in human cortex. *Neuron.* 2007;56:366–383.
16. Gattass R, Gross CG. Visual topography of striate projection zone (MT) in posterior superior temporal sulcus of the macaque. *J Neurophysiol.* 1981;46:621–638.
17. Hafed Ziad M, Chen C-Y. Sharper, stronger, faster upper visual field representation in primate superior colliculus. *Current Biology.* 2016;26:1647–1658.
18. Denman DJ, et al. Mouse color and wavelength-specific luminance contrast sensitivity are non- uniform across visual space. *eLife.* 2018;7
19. Rhim I, Coello-Reyes G, Ko HK, Nauhaus I. Maps of cone opsin input to mouse V1 and higher visual areas. *Journal of Neurophysiology.* 2017;117:1674–1682.
20. Van Essen DC, Newsome WT, Maunsell JH. The visual field representation in striate cortex of the macaque monkey: asymmetries, anisotropies, and individual variability. *Vision Res.* 1984;24:429–448.
21. Kobatake E, Tanaka K. Neuronal selectivities to complex object features in the ventral visual pathway of the macaque cerebral cortex. *Journal of neurophysiology.* 1994;71:856–867.
22. Boussaoud D, Desimone R, Ungerleider LG. Visual topography of area TEO in the macaque. *J Comp Neurol.* 1991;306:554–575.
23. Hubel DH, Wiesel TN. Receptive fields, binocular interaction and functional architecture in the cat's visual cortex. *The Journal of Physiology.* 1962;160:106–154.
24. Hubel DH, Wiesel TN. Receptive fields and functional architecture of monkey striate cortex. *J Physiol.* 1968;195:215–243.
25. Carlson ET, Rasquinha RJ, Zhang K, Connor CE. A sparse object coding scheme in area. *Current biology.* 2011;21:288–293.
26. David SV, Hayden BY, Gallant JL. Spectral receptive field properties explain shape selectivity in area V4. *J Neurophysiol.* 2006;96:3492–3505.
27. Srinath R, et al. Early emergence of solid shape coding in natural and deep network vision. *Current Biology.* 2021;31:51–65. e55.
28. Rose OO, Johnson JK, Wang B, Ponce CRR. Visual prototypes in the ventral stream are attuned to complexity and gaze behavior. *Nature Commun.* 2021;12:1–16.
29. Rust NC, DiCarlo JJ. Selectivity and tolerance ("invariance") both increase as visual information propagates from cortical area V4 to IT. *The Journal of Neuroscience.* 2010;30:12978–12995.

30. Desimone R, Albright TD, Gross CG, Bruce C. Stimulus-selective properties of inferior temporal neurons in the macaque. *Journal of Neuroscience*. 1984;4:2051–2062.

31. Popivanov ID, Schyns PG, Vogels R. Stimulus features coded by single neurons of a macaque body category selective patch. *Proceedings of the National Academy of Sciences of the United States of America*. 2016;113:E2450–E2459.

32. Tsao DY, Livingstone MS. Mechanisms of face perception. *Annual Review of Neuroscience*. 2008;31:411–437.

33. Quiroga RQ, Reddy L, Kreiman G, Koch C, Fried I. Invariant visual representation by single neurons in the human brain. *Nature*. 2005;435:1102–1107.

34. Meyers EM, Borzello M, Freiwald WA, Tsao D. Intelligent information loss: the coding of facial identity, head pose, and non-face information in the macaque face patch system. *Journal of Neuroscience*. 2015;35:7069–7081.

35. Tsao DY, Freiwald WA, Tootell RB, Livingstone MS. A cortical region consisting entirely of face-selective cells. *Science*. 2006;311:670–674.

36. Huth AG, de Heer WA, Griffiths TL, Theunissen FE, Gallant JL. Natural speech reveals the semantic maps that tile human cerebral cortex. *Nature*. 2016;532:453–458.

37. Kanwisher N, Dilks D. In: Chalupa L, Werner J, eds. *The New Visual Neurosciences*. Cambridge, MA: MIT Press; 2013.

38. Kriegeskorte N, *et al.* Matching categorical object representations in inferior temporal cortex of man and monkey. *Neuron*. 2008;60:1126–1141.

39. Coggan DD, Liu W, Baker DH, Andrews TJ. Category-selective patterns of neural response in the ventral visual pathway in the absence of categorical information. *NeuroImage*. 2016;135:107–114.

40. Long B, Yu C-P, Konkle T. Mid-level visual features underlie the high-level categorical organization of the ventral stream. *Proceedings of the National Academy of Sciences*. 2018;115:E9015 LP–E9024.

41. Hubel DH, Wiesel TN. Shape and arrangement of columns in cat's striate cortex. *J Physiol*. 1963;165:559–568.

42. Hu JM, Song XM, Wang Q, Roe AW. Curvature domains in v4 of macaque monkey. *eLife*. 2020;9:1–21.

43. Albright TD, Desimone R, Gross CG. Columnar organization of directionally selective cells in visual area MT of the macaque. *J Neurophysiol*. 1984;51:16–31.

44. Bao P, She L, McGill M, Tsao DY. A map of object space in primate inferotemporal cortex. *Nature*. 2020;583:103–108.

45. Quiroga RQ, Reddy L, Kreiman G, Koch C, Fried I. Invariant visual representation by single neurons in the human brain. *Nature*. 2005;435:1102–1107.

46. Konorski J. Some new ideas concerning the physiological mechanisms of perception. *Acta Biol Exp (Warsz)*. 1967;27:147–161.

47. Mineault PJ, Pack CC. The cerebral emporium of benevolent knowledge. *Neuron*. 2013;79:833–835.

48. Ma WJ, Beck JM, Latham PE, Pouget A. Bayesian inference with probabilistic population codes. *Nat Neurosci*. 2006;9:1432–1438.

49. Hubel DH, Wiesel TN. Receptive fields of cells in striate cortex of very young, visually inexperienced kittens. *J Neurophysiol*. 1963;26:994–1002.

50. Murty NAR, *et al.* Visual experience is not necessary for the development of face-selectivity in the lateral fusiform gyrus. *Proceedings of the National Academy of Sciences*. 2020;117:23011–23020.

51. Downing PE, Chan AWY, Peelen VM, Dodds CM, Kanwisher N. Domain specificity in visual cortex. *Cerebral cortex 1991*. 2006;16:1453–1461. d.

52. Arcaro MJ, Schade PF, Vincent JL, Ponce CR, Livingstone MS. Seeing faces is necessary for face-domain formation. *Nature Neuroscience*. 2017;20

53. Ponce CR, Hartmann TS, Livingstone MS. End-stopping predicts curvature tuning along the ventral stream. *Journal of Neuroscience*. 2017;37

54. Ben-Shachar M, Dougherty RF, Deutsch GK, Wandell BA. The development of cortical sensitivity to visual word forms. *Journal of Cognitive Neuroscience*. 2011;23:2387–2399.

55. Srihasam K, Vincent JL, Livingstone MS. Novel domain formation reveals proto-architecture in inferotemporal cortex. *Nature Neuroscience*. 2014;17:1776–1783.

56. Tsao DY, Freiwald WA, Tootell RBH, Livingstone MS. A cortical region consisting entirely of face-selective cells. *Science*. 2006;311:670–674.

57. Tsunoda K, Yamane Y, Nishizaki M, Tanifuji M. Complex objects are represented in macaque inferotemporal cortex by the combination of feature columns. *Nat Neurosci*. 2001;4:832–838. d.

58. Leibo JZ, Liao Q, Anselmi F, Poggio T. The invariance hypothesis implies domain-specific regions in visual cortex. *PLoS Comput Biol*. 2015;11:e1004390.

59. Logothetis NK, Pauls J, Poggio T. Shape representation in the inferior temporal cortex of monkeys. *Current Biology*. 1995;5:552–563.

60. Ito M, Tamura H, Fujita I, Tanaka K. Size and position invariance of neuronal responses in monkey inferotemporal cortex. *Journal of Neurophysiology*. 1995;73:218–226.

61. Sáry G, Vogels R, Orban GA. Cue-invariant shape selectivity of macaque inferior temporal neurons. *Science*. 1993;260:995–997.

62. Vogels, R. & Orban, G.A. in *Extrageniculostriate Mechanisms Underlying Visually-Guided Orientation Behavior* Vol. 112 (eds Masao Norita *et al.*) 195–211 (1996).

63. Clarke A, Poggio TA, Anselmi F, Poggio TA, Anselmi F, eds. Visual cortex and deep networks—learning invariant representations. *Perception*. 2017;47:355–356.

64. Hesse JK, Tsao DY. The macaque face patch system: a turtle's underbelly for the brain. *Nat Rev Neurosci*. 2020;21:695–716.

65. Huang G, Liu Z, van der Maaten L, Weinberger KQ. Densely connected convolutional networks. *Proceedings—30th IEEE Conference on Computer Vision and Pattern Recognition, CVPR*. 2017;2016:2261–2269.

66. Krizhevsky A, Sutskever I, Hinton GE. ImageNet classification with deep convolutional neural networks. *Advances in Neural Information Processing Systems*. 2012:1097–1105.

67. Simonyan, K. & Zisserman, A. Very deep convolutional networks for large-scale image recognition. (2014).

68. Girshick, R. in *Proceedings of the IEEE International Conference on Computer Vision*. 1440–1448 (2015).

69. Girshick R, Donahue J, Darrell T, Malik J. Rich feature hierarchies for accurate object detection and semantic segmentation. *Proceedings of the IEEE Computer Society Conference on Computer Vision and Pattern Recognition*. 2013:580–587.

70. Hosny A, Parmar C, Quackenbush J, Schwartz LH, Aerts HJWL. Artificial intelligence in radiology. *Nature Reviews Cancer*. 2018;18:500–510.

71. Bera K, Schalper KA, Rimm DL, Velcheti V, Madabhushi A. Artificial intelligence in digital pathology—new tools for diagnosis and precision oncology. *Nature Reviews Clinical Oncology*. 2019;16:703–715.

72. Moxley-Wyles B, Colling R, Verrill C. Artificial intelligence in pathology: an overview. *Diagnostic Histopathology*. 2020;26:513–520.

73. Grigorescu S, Trasnea B, Cocias T, Macesanu G. A survey of deep learning techniques for autonomous driving. *Journal of Field Robotics*. 2019;37:362–386.

74. Cameron JAD, Savoie P, Kaye ME, Scheme EJ. Design considerations for the processing system of a CNN-based automated surveillance system. *Expert Systems with Applications*. 2019;136:105–114.

75. Geirhos, R. *et al.* Comparing deep neural networks against humans: object recognition when the signal gets weaker. (2017).

76. Nguyen, A., Yosinski, J. & Clune, J. Deep neural networks are easily fooled: high confidence predictions for unrecognizable images. (2014).

77. Szegedy, C. *et al.* Intriguing properties of neural networks. (2013).

78. Goodfellow, I. & Bengio, Y. *Deep Learning*. (2016).

79. Simonite, T. (2018).

80. Yamins DLK, *et al.* Performance-optimized hierarchical models predict neural responses in higher visual cortex. *Proceedings of the National Academy of Sciences of the United States of America*. 2014;111:8619–8624.

81. Gunning D, *et al.* XAI-Explainable artificial intelligence. *Science Robotics*. 2019;4

82. Samek, W. & Müller, K.-R. Towards explainable artificial intelligence. (2019).

83. Mordvintsev, A., Olah, C. & Tyka, M. in *Google AI Blog* (2015).

84. Nguyen A, Dosovitskiy A, Yosinski J, Brox T, Clune J. Synthesizing the preferred inputs for neurons in neural networks via deep generator networks. *Proceedings of the 30th International Conference on Neural Information Processing Systems*. 2016

85. Bashivan P, Kar K, DiCarlo JJ. Neural population control via deep image synthesis. *Science*. 2019;364

86. Walker EY, *et al.* Inception loops discover what excites neurons most using deep predictive models. *Nature Neuroscience*. 2019;22:2060–2065.

87. Goodfellow I, *et al.* Generative adversarial networks. *Communications of the ACM*. 2020;63: 139–144.

88. Ponce CR, *et al.* Evolving images for visual neurons using a deep generative network reveals coding principles and neuronal preferences. *Cell*. 2019

89. Xiao W, Kreiman G. XDream: Finding preferred stimuli for visual neurons using generative networks and gradient-free optimization. *PLOS Computational Biology*. 2020;16:e1007973.

90. Fukushima K. Neocognitron: a self organizing neural network model for a mechanism of pattern recognition unaffected by shift in position. *Biological cybernetics*. 1980;36: 193–202.

91. Fukushima K. A feature extractor for curvilinear patterns: a design suggested by the mammalian visual system. *Kybernetik*. 1970;7:153–160.

92. Fukushima K. Cognitron: a self-organizing multilayered neural network. *Biological cybernetics*. 1975;20:121–136.

93. LeCun Y, *et al.* Backpropagation applied to handwritten zip code recognition. *Neural Computation*. 1989;1:541–551.

94. Lindsay G. *Models of the Mind: How Physics, Engineering and Mathematics Have Shaped Our Understanding of the Brain*. New York: Bloomsbury; 2021.

95. Carandini M, Heeger DJ. Normalization as a canonical neural computation. *Nature Reviews Neuroscience*. 2012;13:51–62.

96. Hubel DH. Single unit activity in striate cortex of unrestrained cats. *J Physiol*. 1959;147:226–238.

97. Riesenhuber M, Poggio T. Hierarchical models of object recognition in cortex. *Nature Neuroscience*. 1999;2:1019–1025.

98. Van Essen DC, Anderson CH, Felleman DJ. Information processing in the primate visual system: an integrated systems perspective. *Science*. 1992;255:419–423.

99. Araujo A, Norris W, Sim J. Computing receptive fields of convolutional neural networks. *Distill*. 2019;4:e21. https://distill.pub/2019/computing-receptive-fields/.

100. OpenAi. (2020).

101. Rumelhart DE, Hinton GE, Williams RJ. Learning representations by back-propagating errors. *Nature*. 1986;323:533–536.

102. Rockland KS. Morphology of individual axons projecting from area V2 to MT in the macaque. *J. Comp. Neurol*. 1995;355:15–26.

103. Salin PA, Bullier J, Kennedy H. Convergence and divergence in the afferent projections to cat area 17. *Journal of Comparative Neurology*. 1989;283:486–512.

104. Salin PA, Girard P, Kennedy H, Bullier J. Visuotopic organization of corticocortical connections in the visual system of the cat. *J. Comp. Neurol*. 1992;320:415–434.

105. Bartunov, S. *et al.* Assessing the Scalability of Biologically-Motivated Deep Learning Algorithms and Architectures. (2018).

106. Whittington JCR, Bogacz R. Theories of error back-propagation in the brain. *Trends in Cognitive Sciences*. 2019;23:235–250.

107. Lillicrap TP, Cownden D, Tweed DB, Akerman CJ. Random synaptic feedback weights support error backpropagation for deep learning. *Nature Communications*. 2016;7:13276. https://doi.org/10.1038/ncomms13276.

108. Zeki S. Cerebral akinetopsia (visual motion blindness): a review. *Brain*. 1991;114(Pt 2):811–824.

109. Zihl J, von Cramon D, Mai N. Selective disturbance of movement vision after bilateral brain damage. *Brain*. 1983;106(Pt 2):313–340.

110. Allman JM, Kaas JH. A representation of the visual field in the caudal third of the middle temporal gyrus of the owl monkey (*Aotus Trivirgatus*). *Brain Res*. 1971;31:85–105.

111. Dubner R, Zeki SM. Response properties and receptive fields of cells in an anatomically defined region of the superior temporal sulcus in the monkey. *Brain Res*. 1971;35:528–532.

112. Born RT, Bradley DC. Structure and function of visual area MT. *Annu Rev Neurosci*. 2005; 28:157–189.

113. Chowdhury SA, DeAngelis GC. Fine discrimination training alters the causal contribution of macaque area MT to depth perception. *Neuron*. 2008;60:367–377.

114. Liu LD, Pack CC. The contribution of area MT to visual motion perception depends on training. *Neuron*. 2017;95:436–446. e433.

115. Rudolph K, Pasternak T. Transient and permanent deficits in motion perception after lesions of cortical areas MT and MST in the macaque monkey. *Cereb Cortex*. 1999;9:90–100.

116. Salzman CD, Britten KH, Newsome WT. Cortical microstimulation influences perceptual judgements of motion direction. *Nature*. 1990;346:174–177.

117. Lisberger SG, Movshon JA. Visual motion analysis for pursuit eye movements in area MT of macaque monkeys. *J Neurosci*. 1999;19:2224–2246.

118. Newsome WT, Wurtz RH, Dursteler MR, Mikami A. Deficits in visual motion processing following ibotenic acid lesions of the middle temporal visual area of the macaque monkey. *J Neurosci*. 1985;5:825–840.

119. Groh JM, Born RT, Newsome WT. How is a sensory map read out? Effects of microstimulation in visual area MT on saccades and smooth pursuit eye movements. *J Neurosci*. 1997;17:4312–4330.

120. Krause MR, Pack CC. Contextual modulation and stimulus selectivity in extrastriate cortex. *Vision Res*. 2014;104:36–46.

121. Movshon JA, Adelson EH, Gizzi MS, Newsome WT. In: Chagas C, Gattass R, Gross C, eds. *Pattern Recognition Mechanisms*. Vatican City: Vatican Press; 1985:117–151.

122. Tsui JM, Hunter JN, Born RT, Pack CC. The role of V1 surround suppression in MT motion integration. *J Neurophysiol*. 2010;103:3123–3138.

123. Pack CC, Born RT. Temporal dynamics of a neural solution to the aperture problem in visual area MT of macaque brain. *Nature*. 2001;409:1040–1042.

124. Simoncelli EP, Heeger DJ. A model of neuronal responses in visual area MT. *Vision Res*. 1998;38:743–761.

125. Mineault PJ, Bakhtiari S, Richards B, Pack CC. Your head is there to move you around: Goal-driven models of the primate dorsal pathway. *Advances in Neural Information Processing Systems 35 pre-proceedings (NeurIPS 2021)*. 2021.

126. Nakhla N, Korkian Y, Krause MR, Pack CC. Neural Selectivity for Visual Motion in Macaque Area V3A. *eNeuro*. 2021;8.

127. Duffy CJ, Wurtz RH. Sensitivity of MST neurons to optic flow stimuli. II. Mechanisms of response selectivity revealed by small-field stimuli. *J Neurophysiol*. 1991;65:1346–1359.

128. Mineault PJ, Khawaja FA, Butts DA, Pack CC. Hierarchical processing of complex motion along the primate dorsal visual pathway. *Proc Natl Acad Sci U S A*. 2012;109: E972–980.

129. Tanaka K, Saito H. Analysis of motion of the visual field by direction, expansion/contraction, and rotation cells clustered in the dorsal part of the medial superior temporal area of the macaque monkey. *J Neurophysiol*. 1989;62:626–641.

130. Graziano MS, Andersen RA, Snowden RJ. Tuning of MST neurons to spiral motions. *J Neurosci*. 1994;14:54–67.

131. Gu Y, Deangelis GC, Angelaki DE. Causal links between dorsal medial superior temporal area neurons and multisensory heading perception. *J Neurosci*. 2012;32:2299–2313.

132. Britten KH, van Wezel RJ. Electrical microstimulation of cortical area MST biases heading perception in monkeys. *Nat Neurosci*. 1998;1:59–63.

133. Boussaoud D, Ungerleider LG, Desimone R. Pathways for motion analysis: cortical connections of the medial superior temporal and fundus of the superior temporal visual areas in the macaque. *J Comp Neurol*. 1990;296:462–495.

134. Boussaoud D, Desimone R, Ungerleider LG. Subcortical connections of visual areas MST and FST in macaques. *Vis Neurosci*. 1992;9:291–302.

135. Sincich LC, Park KF, Wohlgemuth MJ, Horton JC. Bypassing V1: a direct geniculate input to area MT. *Nat Neurosci*. 2004;7:1123–1128.

136. Berman RA, Wurtz RH. Exploring the pulvinar path to visual cortex. *Prog Brain Res*. 2008;171:467–473.

137. Stoerig P, Cowey A. Blindsight in man and monkey. *Brain*. 1997;120(Pt 3):535–559. https://doi.org/10.1093/brain/120.3.535.

138. Barbot A, *et al*. Spared perilesional V1 activity underlies training-induced recovery of luminance detection sensitivity in cortically-blind patients. *Nat Commun*. 2021;12:6102.

139. Schmid MC, *et al*. Blindsight depends on the lateral geniculate nucleus. *Nature*. 2010;466:373–377.

140. Melnick MD, Tadin D, Huxlin KR. Relearning to See in Cortical Blindness. *Neuroscientist*. 2016;22:199–212. https://doi.org/10.1177/1073858415621035.

141. Bakhtiari S, Awada A, Pack CC. Influence of stimulus complexity on the specificity of visual perceptual learning. *Journal of Vision*. 2020;20:13.

142. Das A, Tadin D, Huxlin KR. Beyond blindsight: properties of visual relearning in cortically blind fields. *J Neurosci*. 2014;34:11652–11664.

32

Visual Processing of Spatial Form

Daniel H. Baker

Introduction

The preceding chapters have described how visual signals pass from the retina to the visual regions of the brain. In this chapter we discuss how processing of these signals results in our ability to perceive spatial form, such as the outlines of objects, textures, and other patterns. This ability is crucial for mobile species (including humans) to interact with the world around them, and our understanding of the underlying mechanisms has increased rapidly over the past century.

The chapter begins by considering how the tuning of visual cortical neurons performs a local analysis of the content of an image, and how the combined responses of many such neurons determines the limits of our visual abilities. A key method supporting our understanding of low-level vision is the adaptation paradigm, in which neurons temporarily change their tuning following repeated stimulation. Experiments using this technique indicate that many visual features, including orientation, size, shape, and motion, are represented by populations of neurons tuned along these dimensions.

Next we consider how object boundaries are identified, and introduce the concept of second-order vision, which detects changes in contrast and texture information. We discuss how our sensitivity varies across the visual field, becoming poorer away from the fovea. Computational analyses of functional magnetic resonance imaging (fMRI) data allow us to quantify how receptive field sizes change across the visual field, and also increase along the visual hierarchy. These changes have implications both for our ability to detect faint patterns and our perception of higher contrast textures. This *contrast constancy* effect differentially interacts with visual disorders such as amblyopia and optic neuritis.

Finally, we discuss how information from low-level units is combined to represent important image features such as edges and extended textures, and ultimately more specific categories of object such as faces. Recent fMRI work has demonstrated how a spatially local representation of basic image features at early stages transitions to more spatially invariant object representations in higher visual areas. Overall, this chapter aims to give the reader an understanding of how the early stages of vision contribute to our perceptual experience of the world and allow us to localize and recognize the objects we interact with and the environment we navigate.

EARLY VISUAL MECHANISMS AS FEATURE DETECTORS

Neurons in primary visual cortex (area V1, at the very back of the brain) have receptive fields that are orientation selective and also tuned to particular spatial frequencies (spatial frequency describes the coarseness of a texture, or the width of the grating bars in a receptive field). For example, a neuron with a vertically oriented receptive field will respond strongly to vertical stripes but remain silent when shown horizontal stripes. Fig. 32.1 shows example receptive field profiles for some simulated neurons (*middle column*), as well as an image (*left*) filtered by each receptive field (*right*). These filtered images simulate what the world looks like to a population of neurons that tile the image (technically, the image has been *convolved* with each filter). One way to think about the function these cells perform is to think of them as feature detectors—they respond only when the part of an image they are centered on contains orientation and spatial frequency information close to the neuron's preferred values. In the example images, you can see how sections of the border of the banana are picked out by neurons with different orientation preferences.

Why do neurons have such specific characteristics? One very likely explanation is that their tuning allows them to efficiently represent the information they encounter in the natural world. For example, Field[1] showed that the statistics of natural images were well captured by banks of filters with similar properties to early visual neurons, in a way that reduces redundancy in the signal. Furthermore, Olshausen and Field[2] showed that an algorithm trained on sets of natural images spontaneously develops receptive field properties similar to those found in biological visual systems. This general approach of applying a bank of orientation- and spatial frequency-selective filters to an image is also a critical first step for contemporary computer vision models. In particular, a class of machine learning methods called *deep convolutional neural networks* uses this method, and they have been very successful at performing useful categorization tasks, such as object identification and image labeling.[3,4] So, V1 neurons behave in this way because filtering allows the visual cortex to simplify the incoming information from the eyes in an efficient and principled way.

The combined response of populations of tuned neurons determines the limits of our perceptual abilities. These limits can be summarized by the *contrast sensitivity function* (CSF), which describes how sensitive an individual is to stimuli of different spatial frequencies.[5] In Fig. 32.2A, an example CSF (*thick line*) is shown to be the envelope of many mechanisms with narrower tuning (e.g., populations of neurons, given by the *thinner lines*). For any given spatial frequency, our sensitivity will be governed by the most responsive neurons, assuming some appropriate read-out rule.[6] The individual mechanisms typically have bandwidths of just over an octave,[7] whereas the CSF covers several octaves of spatial frequency (an octave is a factor of two difference).

Filters   Output

Image

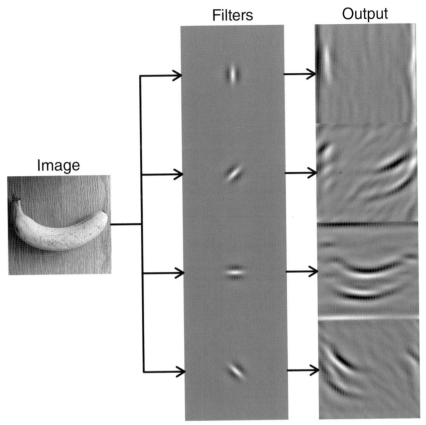

Fig. 32.1 Illustration of image filtering by a bank of oriented filters. The banana image (*left*) is convolved with a series of linear filters with oriented receptive fields (*middle*), resembling the properties of early visual neurons. The *right* column shows the filtered image "seen" through each filter (i.e., the energy passed by the filter). Notice the *left*, *right*, and *middle* of the banana are represented by filters with different orientation preferences.

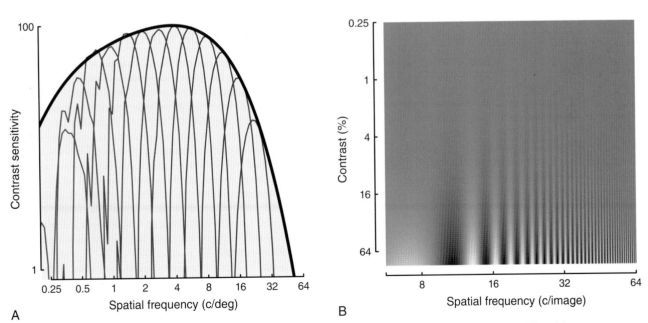

Fig. 32.2 Figure illustrating the contrast sensitivity function (CSF) and individual mechanism tuning (**A**) and the window of visibility (**B**). In (**A**), individual mechanisms (*thin curves*) have a bandwidth of 1.4 octaves, consistent with neurophysiological recordings, and the black curve shows the overall sensitivity of the (*model*) system. In (**B**), spatial frequency and contrast are modulated on the x- and y-axes respectively (after Campbell and Robson). Although the modulations change smoothly (in logarithmic units), most viewers perceive an inverted U-shaped region determined by their own CSF (observe the similarity with the curve in **A**). Note that for (**B**) the spatial frequency in cycles per degree depends on viewing distance.

The CSF is normally measured in psychophysical experiments, in which participants are asked to detect faint grating patterns of different spatial frequencies. Typical CSFs, such as the one shown in Fig. 32.2A, have a characteristic peak at frequencies around 2–4 c/deg, and a fall-off to either side.[5] Any visual signals falling outside of the envelope of the CSF (i.e., outside of the *gray shaded region*) will be invisible. This means that by knowing an individual's contrast sensitivity, we can predict what they will be able to see. Notice that the point at which the rightmost limb of the function reaches 1 determines the highest spatial frequency (e.g., the finest detail) that the observer can resolve, which sets the limits of visual acuity (discussed further in Chapter 33). However, the CSF provides much more detailed information on visual health and function, which can be useful for understanding and diagnosing visual disorders, as we discuss later in the chapter.

It is possible to visualize one's own CSF by looking at the image in Fig. 32.2B. In this pattern, spatial frequency increases smoothly along the (logarithmic) x-axis, and contrast decreases smoothly along the (logarithmic) y-axis. At each frequency, the perceived height of the bars is governed by the viewer's contrast sensitivity, and a "hump" peaking at midrange spatial frequencies is apparent (although note that the placement of the hump will depend on viewing distance). Of course different people have different contrast sensitivities. If you wear glasses, you might notice that removing them shifts the peak of the hump to the left, as the high spatial frequencies are blurred by the eye's optics.

Interestingly, different animal species have different contrast sensitivities to humans (for examples of experimental paradigms see[8]). Birds of prey like eagles have a CSF tuned to quite high spatial frequencies,[9] presumably so they can spot small prey animals far away on the ground. Ground-dwelling animals like mice are better adapted to low spatial frequencies[10] for seeing close up food and large predators! But in all known cases, animals share the inverted U-shaped function found in humans, albeit shifted to higher or lower frequencies.

ADAPTATION AS A TOOL FOR UNDERSTANDING VISION

How do we know that the CSF is the envelope of many mechanisms with narrower tuning? Early evidence for this idea came from studies using adaptation paradigms.[11] In an adaptation experiment, a high intensity stimulus is shown repeatedly for a long time (usually several minutes). This has the effect of desensitizing the neurons that represent that stimulus, but having little or no effect on neurons with different tuning (see Fig. 32.3). For example, adapting to a vertical stimulus of 4 c/deg will produce a "notch" of lower sensitivity in the CSF centered at the adapting frequency. But it will not affect sensitivity to spatial frequencies that are much higher or lower, or to stimuli with horizontal orientations. This specificity indicates that an apparently continuous function such as the CSF is really the envelope of several more narrowly tuned mechanisms. If instead our sensitivity were determined by a single broadband mechanism, then adaptation would affect sensitivity at all frequencies equally.

Adaptation has other effects on our perception besides reducing sensitivity. Stimuli adjacent to the adaptor (e.g., with slightly higher or lower spatial frequencies) appear increased or decreased in spatial frequency, as though they were "repelled" away from the adaptor.[12] This happens because adaptation differentially alters the tuning of nearby mechanisms, shifting their peaks away from the adapting frequency. Such after-effects occur not just for spatial frequency,[12] but also for orientation,[13] motion,[14] and higher-order stimulus properties

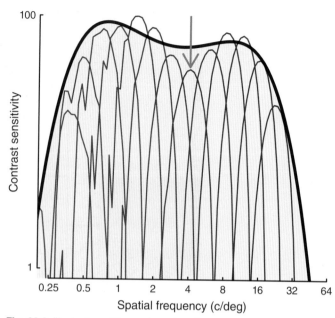

Fig. 32.3 Illustration of how adaptation changes the shape of the contrast sensitivity function (CSF). The model described in Fig. 32.2 is adapted at 4 c/deg *(see arrow)*. This reduces the sensitivity of mechanisms that peak close to the adapting stimulus and creates a notch in the CSF *(black curve)*.

including object size,[15] depth,[16] aspect ratio,[17] numerosity,[18] and even facial expression.[19] The prevalence of repulsive after-effects suggests that many sensory dimensions are represented by an underlying population code comprising multiple narrowly tuned units, and that this is a general organizing principle for sensory systems.

OBJECTS ARE DEFINED BY SPATIAL CHANGES IN LUMINANCE, COLOR, CONTRAST, AND TEXTURE

Visual mechanisms that can detect changes in luminance are critical for perceiving the form and location of objects in the environment. This is primarily because most objects have different surface and reflectance properties from their backgrounds, and in natural light will appear brighter or darker. An object like the circle shown in Fig. 32.4A is brighter than its surround, and will therefore produce strong responses in mechanisms matched to the object's approximate spatial frequency. For example, a filter such as those shown in Fig. 32.1, in which the excitatory central region (shown in *white*) is approximately the same width as the circle in Fig. 32.4A, would be expected to respond strongly, signaling the presence of an object. Additionally, mechanisms tuned to higher spatial frequencies will respond strongly to the edges of the object, indicating the location of the border between it and the surround.

Changes in luminance across space are referred to as *first-order* information, and neurons that can detect them are *first-order mechanisms* (see Fig. 32.1 for an illustration of how first-order edges are detected). These are the most critical aspect of our spatial visual abilities, and demonstrate why the concept of contrast sensitivity is so important—luminance modulations outside of the envelope of the CSF (Fig. 32.2) are literally invisible to us. In evolutionary terms, the ability to detect luminance variation has obvious survival benefit for identifying predators, food, and other beneficial or harmful aspects of the environment.

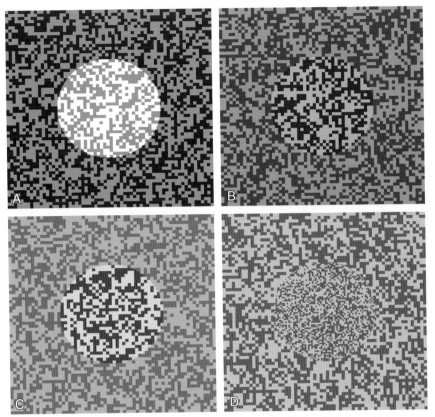

Fig. 32.4 Examples of shape segmentation from different cues. In (**A**) the circle has a higher average luminance than its surround. In (**B**) the circle is defined by chromatic information. In (**C**) the contrast (differences between light and dark regions) is higher inside the circle than outside of it. In (**D**) the grain of the carrier texture is finer inside the circle than outside it (e.g., the spatial frequency content is different).

Sometimes objects do not differ much in luminance from their background. However, there are other cues that might reveal them, such as differences in color (Fig. 32.4B), contrast (Fig. 32.4C), or texture (Fig. 32.4D). Color vision processes are explained further in Chapter 34, so are not discussed in detail here other than to mention that the contrast sensitivity of color channels is much coarser than for the achromatic (luminance) system. This means that we are less able to resolve fine spatial details when they are defined by color than by luminance, and the CSF is shifted downwards and to the left (Fig. 32.5A), but plateaus at low spatial frequencies (based on data from[20]).

Cues such as contrast and texture are referred to as *second-order* information. These are invisible to first-order mechanisms, which respond only to changes in luminance. Instead, second-order mechanisms are constructed from the outputs of multiple first-order mechanisms. The classic circuit for second-order vision is the filter-rectify-filter (FRF) arrangement, whereby the outputs of first-order filters are rectified, and then form the input into second-order mechanisms.[22,23] This places a fundamental limit on second-order vision, in that the carrier texture must be detectable by first-order mechanisms. Because of these limitations, and the additional processing stages required, sensitivity to second-order modulations is much lower than for achromatic first-order vision (see Fig. 32.5B, based on data from Schofield and Georgeson[21]). In ecological terms, sensitivity to second-order information allows us to break camouflage, for example, to detect animals such as moths and cuttlefish[24] that have evolved to blend in with their backgrounds, and also to distinguish differences in lighting conditions from changes in material properties.[25]

SENSITIVITY AND RECEPTIVE FIELD SIZE VERSUS ECCENTRICITY

A key limit on our visual abilities is the fall-off in sensitivity across the visual field. Foveal vision is generally more sensitive than vision in the periphery, yet this decline is not constant across spatial frequency, or different types of cue. Pointer and Hess[26] found that contrast sensitivity declined most rapidly at high spatial frequencies, when data were plotted as a function of eccentricity in degrees. However, replotting the data as a function of the number of cycles of the grating makes these differences much less marked. Baldwin, Meese, and Baker[27] found that the decline in sensitivity was steepest over about the first eight cycles of the stimulus, and somewhat shallower at greater eccentricities. Sensitivity across the visual field can therefore be characterized by an approximately bilinear function of eccentricity expressed in stimulus cycles, as shown in Fig. 32.6. Notice, however, that there are asymmetries, particularly about the horizontal meridian, with sensitivity declining more gradually in the lower visual field than the upper visual field.

Sensitivity also declines differentially for different cues. For example, Hess et al.[28] compared sensitivity as a function of eccentricity for first- and second-order stimuli. The decline was much more rapid for second-order (contrast modulated) stimuli than for first-order stimuli, although this appeared to be mostly governed by the fall-off in carrier sensitivity (i.e., the sensitivity to the texture, which has been contrast modulated). In other words, when high frequency carriers become harder to see, this limits the detectability of second-order modulations. Sensitivity to chromatic information is also poor away from the

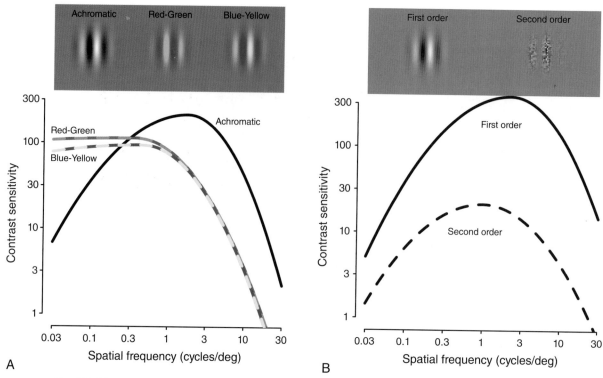

Fig. 32.5 Example contrast sensitivity functions for chromatic (**A**) and second-order vision (**B**). The *black curve* in both panels shows an achromatic first-order contrast sensitivity function for reference. Icons above each panel illustrate each type of stimulus, although note that these images are not identical to those used in the original experiments and are not calibrated for luminance. (Curves are based on model fits to the data from Figs. 8 and 9 of Mullen KT. The contrast sensitivity of human colour vision to red-green and blue-yellow chromatic gratings. *J Physiol.* 1985;359:381–400, and Fig. 1a of Schofield AJ, Georgeson MA. Sensitivity to modulations of luminance and contrast in visual white noise: Separate mechanisms with similar behaviour. *Vision Res.* 1999;39[16]:2697–2716.)

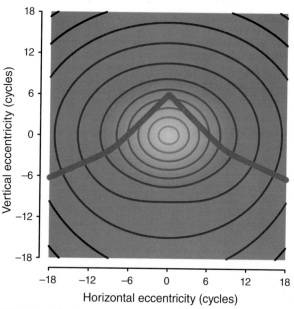

Fig. 32.6 The fall-off in contrast sensitivity as a function of eccentricity. (Based on the work of Baldwin AS, Meese TS, Baker DH. The attenuation surface for contrast sensitivity has the form of a witch's hat within the central visual field. *J Vis.* 2012;12(11):23.). Contour lines are spaced every 1.5 dB of sensitivity loss. The *red curve* shows a cross-section through the horizontal meridian to illustrate the bilinear fall-off.

fovea, and declines more rapidly than sensitivity to luminance modulations,[29–31] largely because of the low density of color-sensitive cones (see Chapter 34) in the peripheral regions of the retina.

Part of the reason that sensitivity declines away from the fovea may also be that receptive field sizes grow larger with eccentricity. This finding is well established neurophysiologically (e.g.,[32]), and can also be demonstrated in humans using fMRI. The population receptive field (pRF) technique[33] typically involves presenting observers with drifting bar textures moving across the visual field at different angles. The time course of fMRI activity is then fitted using a computational model to determine, for each voxel in the cortex, the region of the visual field to which it is most responsive. Many studies have used this technique to show that receptive field sizes (i.e., the area over which a voxel is responsive) increase with distance from the foveal representation. Figs 32.7A and B show example pRF data for one participant from a study by Lygo et al.[34] Note that the regions of cortex representing more peripheral locations in Fig. 32.7A (*dark red*) also correspond to larger pRF diameters in Fig. 32.7B (*yellow and green*). The figure also illustrates that a far greater proportion of visual cortex is responsive to stimuli in the central few degrees around the fovea than to stimuli in the periphery. It is likely that this reduced cortical representation of peripheral locations also contributes to our poorer sensitivity away from the fovea.

As well as varying across the visual field, pRFs become larger as we ascend the visual hierarchy beyond primary visual cortex (V1). Whereas V1 neurons typically have pRF sizes below 1 degree of visual

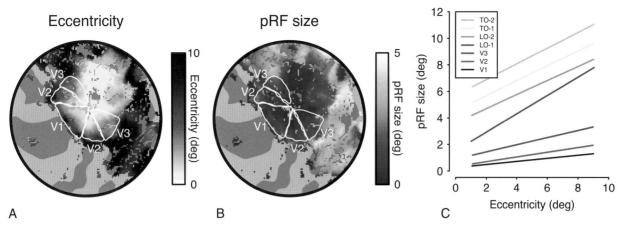

Fig. 32.7 Example population receptive field (*pRF*) maps using data from the study of Lygo FA, Richard B, Wade RA, Morland AB, Baker DH. Neural markers of suppression in impaired binocular vision. *Neuroimage*. 2021;230:117780. (**A**) and (**B**) show flattened regions of cortex from the occipital lobe of the right hemisphere for a single participant. In (**A**) colors indicate the eccentricity of the mid-point of each pRF. In (**B**) colors indicate the standard deviation of the fitted Gaussian receptive field. (**C**) illustrates how pRF width increases with eccentricity and across visual areas (based on Fig. 6A of Amano K, Wandell BA, Dumoulin SO. Visual field maps, population receptive field sizes, and visual field coverage in the human MT+ complex. *J Neurophysiol*. 2009;102(5):2704–2718). *LO*, Lateral occipital; *TO*, temporal-occipital; *V*, visual area.

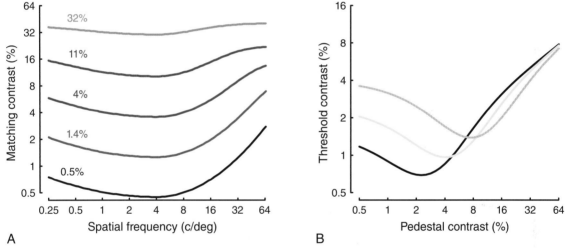

Fig. 32.8 Illustration of contrast matching (**A**) and contrast discrimination (**B**). In (**A**), matches at low contrast (*black, red*) follow the bandpass shape of the contrast sensitivity function (inverted here because the y-axis plots contrast rather than sensitivity), but matches at high contrasts (*green*) are flatter. In (**B**), differences in discrimination near detection threshold (low pedestal contrasts at the *left of the plot*) disappear at high pedestal contrasts where the functions converge (*right of plot*).

angle, this increases to around 3 degrees in V3. Voxels in lateral and temporal occipital cortex can have receptive fields spanning as much as 10 degrees. Fig. 32.7C summarizes this relationship (based on data from Amano, Wandell, and Dumoulin[35]). The increase in receptive field size across the visual hierarchy might be due to increased spatial pooling in higher visual areas, or the transition to a spatially invariant representation of specific categories of object, as we discuss later in this chapter.

SUPRATHRESHOLD VISION AND CONTRAST CONSTANCY

Although experiments at detection threshold have revealed much about the limitations of visual perception, it is also reasonable to ask what happens at the higher contrast levels we might encounter outside

of the laboratory. To study suprathreshold (i.e., above-threshold) perception, two key paradigms have been developed: contrast matching and contrast discrimination. In both types of experiment, participants are typically asked to judge which of two stimuli appear higher in contrast. In the matching paradigm, the two stimuli will also differ along some other dimension, such as spatial frequency, spatial position, or adaptation status. The participant's task is to indicate which stimulus appears higher in contrast, or to adjust the contrast of one stimulus so that it appears the same as the other. In the discrimination paradigm, the two stimuli are usually spatially identical and differ only in contrast. One stimulus, known as the pedestal, has a fixed contrast. The other stimulus contains the pedestal with a contrast increment added (i.e., it is slightly higher in contrast than the pedestal on its own). The participant's task is to identify which stimulus contains the increment.

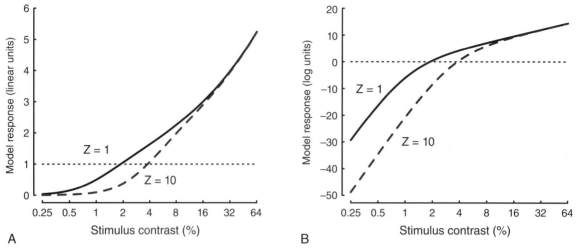

Fig. 32.9 Example contrast-response functions generated by equation 1, plotted in linear units (**A**), and logarithmic (dB) units (**B**). Each plot shows two functions, with different values of the saturation constant (Z = 1, *black*; Z = 10, *blue*). Note that the x (contrast) axis is scaled logarithmically in both cases.

Contrast-matching experiments typically find that differences in perceived contrast near threshold disappear at higher contrasts. This is the case across spatial frequency, where the CSF flattens at high contrasts—an effect known as contrast constancy[36]—as illustrated in Fig. 32.8A. Notice that the differences between perceived contrast at middling spatial frequencies and the extreme ends of the curve start to disappear as contrast is increased. This means that although two stimuli might vary greatly in their detectability, at high contrast they will appear equivalent in their perceived contrast. The same is true across the visual field. As we see in Fig. 32.6, sensitivity is much lower in the periphery. However, high-contrast stimuli do not appear reduced in contrast when they are presented away from where we are fixating[37]—the contrast constancy effect ensures that, when they are visible, images appear at their true contrast.

Similar findings are apparent for the contrast discrimination paradigm. Thresholds from discrimination experiments have a characteristic "dipper" shape, whereby low-contrast pedestals make increment detection easier, and high-contrast pedestals make it harder.[38] This is illustrated in Fig. 32.8B, which plots thresholds as a function of pedestal contrast (thresholds are defined as the minimum detectable increment contrast required for some criterion level of performance, such as 75% correct). Much as for the matching paradigm, differences at detection threshold between two conditions (e.g., two spatial frequencies, eccentricities, or stimulus sizes) disappear at high pedestal contrasts, where the dipper "handle" regions converge.[39] Again, this means that our perception of high-contrast images is invariant with sensitivity limits at detection threshold.

How can we understand why vision above threshold is relatively independent of limitations at threshold? The effects for both matching and discrimination paradigms can be considered in a common framework in which we model the underlying contrast-response function (the function that maps physical stimulus intensity to the resulting neural activity). This response is well described by the following canonical equation[40,41]:

$$resp = \frac{C^{2.4}}{Z + C^2},$$

in which C is the stimulus contrast, and Z is the "saturation constant"—a parameter that governs the lateral placement of the response curve.

Fig. 32.9 shows example contrast-response functions for two different values of Z. At low contrasts, the curves are very different—the smaller value of Z produces a larger response, which will translate to better detection performance (lower thresholds). The *horizontal dotted line* in each panel of Fig. 32.9 shows a threshold criteria (of 1 unit of response), which is reached at much lower contrasts (around 2%) by the model with $Z = 1$, than by the model with $Z = 10$ (around 4%). However, at high contrasts, the curves superimpose, and perceived contrast (determined by the height of the curve) does not depend on sensitivity at threshold. This happens because at high contrasts the denominator of the equation is dominated by the contrast term (C^2), and the value of Z does not substantially influence the response.

We can therefore understand and model differences in sensitivity across spatial frequency, retinal location, and adaptation history within a common framework in which the saturation constant varies. This is referred to as *contrast gain*, which is a fundamental concept in our understanding of early spatial vision. The idea is that the saturation constant is like the volume control on a hi-fi—it turns the responsiveness of our neurons up and down in different situations. Adaptation is a good example of this: our sensitivity adjusts to take the recent history of stimulation into account. If contrasts have been high, we reduce the gain so that the system is less responsive and more energy efficient. If contrasts have been low, we increase the gain and become more sensitive to weak signals. But, critically, none of these changes affect our stable, veridical percept of contrast at high intensities, meaning that our everyday perception is robust to differences in the underlying neural code.

THE EFFECT OF DISEASE ON SPATIAL VISION

Many visual disorders affect the perception of contrast and spatial form. In this section we discuss the effects of two conditions: strabismic amblyopia and optic neuritis. Strabismic amblyopia is a condition in which one eye is misaligned with the other, usually due to problems with the muscles that control eye position. During development, the brain learns to ignore (or suppress) the inputs from this "amblyopic" eye, and so its neural representation is reduced. Note that this occurs even though the eyeball itself is healthy—it is a neural adjustment that has traditionally been thought to be irreversible after a critical period in childhood (up to around the age of 7).

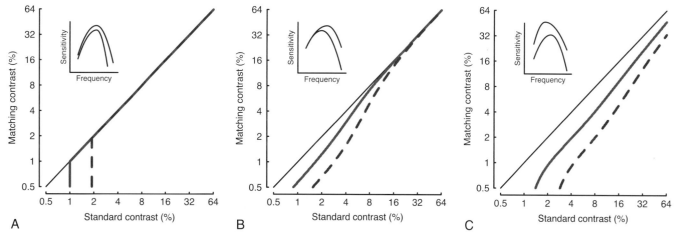

Fig. 32.10 Illustration of contrast-matching data for different visual disorders. (**A**) shows matching functions based on data from a strabismic amblyope reported by Hess RF, Howell ER. The threshold contrast sensitivity function in strabismic amblyopia: Evidence for a two type classification. *Vision Res.* 1977;17(9):1049–1055. The *blue* and *red* functions represent different spatial frequencies with increasing amounts of threshold elevation relative to the nonamblyopic eye. For contrasts above threshold, perception is veridical, and matching data fall on the oblique line of unity. (**B**) shows data consistent with anisometropic amblyopia, where perceived contrast shows a more gradual return to veridical perception. (**C**) shows the pattern observed in optic neuritis, where perceived contrast is reduced across the whole range (based on data from Hess RF. Contrast vision and optic neuritis: Neural blurring. *J Neurol Neurosurg Psychiatry.* 1983;46[11]:1023–1030.) *Insets* in each panel show example contrast sensitivity functions for the affected and fellow eyes.

Many individuals with strabismic amblyopia have contrast sensitivity deficits in their affected eye across the full range of spatial frequencies.[37,42,43] The inset to Fig. 32.10A illustrates this by showing the CSF for the amblyopic and fellow (i.e., unaffected) eyes. This means the window of visibility is smaller in the amblyopic eye, and many low-contrast images may be invisible to that eye, but visible to the fellow eye. On the other hand, above detection threshold, perceived contrast is relatively unaffected. The main panel of Fig. 32.10A shows how stimuli above detection threshold are perceived veridically at the same contrast as in the fellow eye. Interestingly, although contrast perception may be veridical, strabismic amblyopes often report substantial spatial distortions through their amblyopic eye, such that a regular pattern such as a grating can appear scrambled.[44] This is thought to be due to a "miswiring" of neurons representing signals from the affected eye.[45]

Individuals with anisometropic amblyopia, caused by a difference in optical power between the eyes, typically show a different pattern. In these patients (and in some individuals with strabismus), the loss of contrast sensitivity is restricted to high spatial frequencies (see inset to Fig. 32.10B), meaning that they lose the ability to see fine detail with their affected eye.[42,47] Above threshold, there may also be a more gradual restoration of perceived contrast, such that contrasts are attenuated over a wide range (main panel of Fig. 32.10B). Furthermore, whereas strabismus affects central vision more than vision in the periphery, the deficits for anisometropic amblyopes are consistent across the visual field.

Contrast sensitivity loss, and reduction of perceived contrast, is also observed in patients with optic neuritis. This is the visual form of multiple sclerosis, where degeneration of the myelin sheath that insulates nerve fibers causes a loss of function in one eye. Many optic neuritis patients experience pain on eye movements, temporary vision loss, and reduced color perception. In addition, there is a sensitivity loss,[48] similar to that seen in strabismic amblyopia (see inset to Fig. 32.10C). However, in optic neuritis, perceived contrast is uniformly reduced across the entire contrast range.[46] This means that even at high contrasts stimuli appear reduced in contrast through the affected eye (see Fig. 32.10C).

We can consider these quite different forms of visual loss in the context of the nonlinear transducer equation introduced in the previous chapter section. The visual loss in amblyopia might be explained by changes in the saturation constant, as this affects detection thresholds but leaves contrast perception above threshold untouched. Contemporary models of vision in amblyopia are generally consistent with such an attenuation at an early stage of processing.[49] However, the losses in optic neuritis cannot be explained in this way, and might instead point to an increase in neural noise, or generally slower signal transmission, caused by the demyelination. This can be modeled as a subtractive effect, where the output of the nonlinearity is reduced by a fixed amount.

SUMMATION AND SUPPRESSION OF SIGNALS ACROSS SPACE AND FEATURE

The early stages of visual cortex process changes in luminance over small, local regions of the visual field. But we also need to perceive the extended surfaces and textures that make up objects and our environment. Beyond primary visual cortex, there must therefore be some form of spatial pooling that combines information across larger regions. Classical psychophysical work measured detection thresholds for stimuli of different sizes to plot an area summation curve.[50] Fig. 32.11A shows an example area summation curve showing threshold as a function of stimulus diameter (expressed in grating cycles). For very small stimuli at the *left* of the plot there is a rapid decrease in threshold that is attributable to pooling within the receptive field of early-stage neurons. In the *middle* of the plot the threshold improvement is more modest, with a slope consistent with pooling after a squaring nonlinearity and the increased levels of noise that result from attending over a wider area.[51] This *fourth root summation* regime is attributable to signal aggregation across many early-stage units (such as V1 simple cells) by

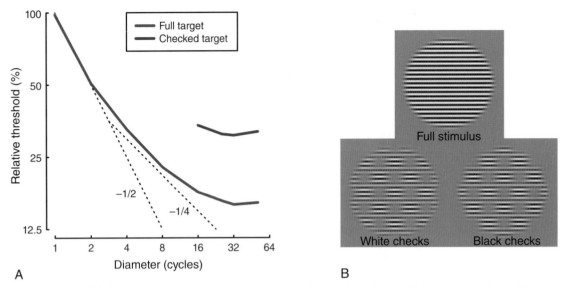

Fig. 32.11 (**A**) shows an example area summation curve, showing how thresholds (the inverse of sensitivity) decrease for stimuli of increasing size, based on data from Meese TS, Summers RJ. Area summation in human vision at and above detection threshold. *Proc Biol Sci.* 2007;274(1627):2891–2900. The *dotted lines* show square root and fourth root predictions for area. (**B**) shows "Swiss cheese" stimuli used to study area summation by keeping the window of attention constant but manipulating the total contrast energy. The *white and black check* stimuli sum to produce the *full stimulus*.

some higher-level mechanism with a larger receptive field (note that the fourth root terminology refers to the slope of the function when the x-axis plots stimulus area). Finally, for very large stimuli (>32 cycles wide) there is no further improvement, likely because the improved sensitivity from increasing area is offset by the reduced sensitivity away from the fovea (see Fig. 32.6).

The flattening of the area summation curve makes it difficult to estimate the range over which contrast information is pooled. Baldwin and Meese[52] compensated for the peripheral loss of sensitivity by scaling contrasts according to detailed threshold measurements across the visual field (see Fig. 32.6). They found that fourth root improvements continued even out to 32 grating cycles when measured in this way. Other attempts to estimate the extent of spatial pooling have used specially constructed stimuli (see Fig. 32.11B) in which sections are missing (i.e., regularly spaced holes in an extended texture) to fix the window of attention (and the pooling of noise over space) while manipulating the total amount of contrast energy.[51] This approach indicates that within-mechanism signal summation extends over at least 12 grating cycles.[53]

Spatial pooling is also evident in fMRI data. For example, the increasing pRF size in higher visual areas (see Fig. 32.7C) is well explained by a corticocortical circuit that pools activity from lower visual areas nonlinearly over an increasing spatial extent.[54] In some visual areas, this pooling eventually results in a relatively size- and position-invariant representation of high-level object classes, such as faces,[55,56] allowing us to recognize objects wherever they appear in our field of view.

Of course our visual environment is not usually filled with narrowband sine-wave gratings! Instead, most real-world objects contain energy at a range of spatial frequencies and orientations, and so the visual system must also pool over stimulus feature to bind this information together. This pooling is particularly apparent in our perception of edges. A sharp-edged luminance transition from black to white contains energy across multiple spatial frequencies—formally, these are the odd-numbered harmonic frequencies of the lowest frequency (known as the fundamental; see Fig. 32.12 for an illustration). Accurate

perception of edge location involves combining these signals together, taking their relative phases into account, and the results may be used to generate a "sketch" of object boundaries.[57] The phase component is critical here, as if this is lost then precise information about edge location is destroyed (see Fig. 32.12F).

To balance the pooling of information across space and feature, early visual processing also involves a complementary process of suppression. This is known as *contrast gain control*,[41] and it is the process by which neurons with different tuning properties can reduce each other's firing. Gain control suppression is most evident when the contrast-response function of a neuron being shown its preferred stimulus is altered by the presence of another stimulus, to which it would not usually respond (such as a grating with orthogonal orientation). The contrast-response function is shifted to the right, which changes the range over which it is activated (similar to the two curves shown in Fig. 32.9). In terms of perception, contrast gain control can affect contrast detection and discrimination performance in a similar way to adaptation—reducing sensitivity and shifting dipper functions diagonally (as in Fig. 32.8B).[40] There are many accounts of why contrast gain control is necessary,[58] including to reduce redundancy in the neural code, maximize sensitivity, and optimize metabolic activity. More recently it has been demonstrated that the strength of suppression can itself adapt based on recent stimulation history,[59] which may be consistent with a process of optimal signal combination.[60] Studying this canonical cortical circuit in the visual system may also reveal more generally how neural populations interact throughout the brain.

A DISTRIBUTED REPRESENTATION ALONG THE VENTRAL STREAM

Visual brain regions along the ventral surface of the occipital and temporal lobes show specialization for different stimulus features. For example, an area of lateral occipital cortex called LO2 appears to be responsive to different object outlines, and may therefore represent global shape.[61] An adjacent area of cortex called LO1 is instead sensitive to object orientation.[62] Temporarily disrupting one of these areas

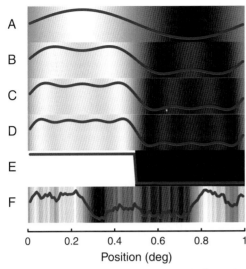
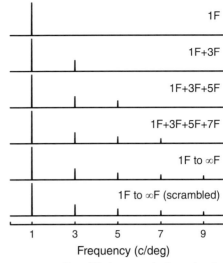

Fig. 32.12 Illustration of edge synthesis from sine-wave components. Row (**A**) shows a single cycle of a sine wave at the fundamental (lowest) frequency, which here is 1 c/deg. The *right panel* shows the frequency spectrum, with energy only at the fundamental frequency (1 F). Rows (**B–D**) show how the waveform changes as more odd harmonics are added, until eventually the edge is sharp (row **E**). However, scrambling the phase relationship between the different frequency components (row **F**) destroys the edge and makes its location uncertain, even though the component amplitudes are unchanged.

using powerful magnetic fields (a technique called transcranial magnetic stimulation [TMS]) has a selective effect only on the information it represents[63]: TMS to LO1 impairs orientation perception, and TMS to LO2 impairs shape perception. Both of these regions also contain retinotopic representations of the visual field,[61] though with much larger receptive field sizes than earlier visual areas (see Fig. 32.7C). In addition to representing orientation and shape, the lateral occipital complex (which includes LO1 and LO2) signals other global properties of an object or scene, such as symmetry,[64,65] that require integration across large portions of the visual field.

Other visually responsive parts of ventral-temporal cortex appear to show selectivity for different categories of input, such as faces,[66] bodies,[67] and scenes or locations.[68] These brain regions are less sensitive to an object's position in the visual field than the earlier retinotopic visual areas. However, despite the intuitive appeal of a modular account, where specific brain regions represent different classes of object, the true story may be rather different. Haxby and colleagues[69] showed that many arbitrary categories of object produce unique and complex patterns of response across a broad swathe of cortex. This was even the case when regions that are maximally selective to each category were excluded. This more distributed representation has since been shown to be partly driven by the low-level image statistics common to a class of objects,[70] such as their typical combinations of orientation and spatial frequency. So it may be that the apparent selectivity of some brain regions is driven by more global changes in preference for different low-level image statistics that are naturally confounded with object category.[71] This idea that the cortex represents continuous gradients along several low-level feature dimensions is quite different from the classical modular view. In either case, the precise transformations that are required to move from the sparse, retinotopic code in early visual cortex to a positionally invariant categorical representation are still being determined.

CONCLUSION

In this chapter we have seen how local processing of fundamental image properties is the first stage of building high-level representations of real-world objects and textures. Populations of orientation- and spatial frequency-selective neurons in V1 determine our window of visibility onto the external world and are augmented by subsequent mechanisms that code second-order information that can disambiguate objects from shadows and break camouflage. Our sensitivity is highest where we are looking (in the fovea) and declines lawfully and predictably with eccentricity. But these absolute limits at threshold are invisible to us at high contrasts, where the contrast constancy effect means that images are perceived at their true contrasts. We can understand these effects through computational modeling, which is also helpful for explaining deficits in visual disorders such as amblyopia. Finally, we have seen how information is pooled over space and feature to represent extended textures and key image features such as edges. These allow our visual systems to build positionally invariant representations of object form and also identify global properties of regularity, such as symmetry. Overall, our ability to perceive spatial form is fundamental to our interactions with the environment. The past century has provided ample new knowledge about how form is processed in the brain, and begun to reveal the details of neural visual representation.

REFERENCES

1. Field DJ. Relations between the statistics of natural images and the response properties of cortical cells. *J Opt Soc Am A*. 1987;4(12):2379–2394.
2. Olshausen BA, Field DJ. Emergence of simple-cell receptive field properties by learning a sparse code for natural images. *Nature*. 1996;381(6583):607–609.
3. Girshick R, Donahue J, Darrell T, Malik J. Rich feature hierarchies for accurate object detection and semantic segmentation. *IEEE Conference on Computer Vision and Pattern Recognition*. Columbus, Ohio, USA: 2014:580–587.
4. Redmon J, Farhadi A. YOLO9000: Better, faster, stronger. 2017 IEEE Conference on Computer Vision and Pattern Recognition (CVPR). Los Alamitos, CA, USA: *IEEE Computer Society*, 2017:6517–6525.
5. Campbell FW, Robson JG. Application of Fourier analysis to the visibility of gratings. *J Physiol*. 1968;197(3):551–566.
6. Jazayeri M, Movshon JA. Optimal representation of sensory information by neural populations. *Nat Neurosci*. 2006;9(5):690–696.
7. De Valois RL, Albrecht DG, Thorell LG. Spatial frequency selectivity of cells in macaque visual cortex. *Vision Res*. 1982;22(5):545–549.
8. Harmening WM. Contrast sensitivity and visual acuity in animals. *Ophthalmologe*. 2017; 114(11):986–996.
9. Reymond L, Wolfe J. Behavioural determination of the contrast sensitivity function of the eagle *Aquila audax*. *Vision Res*. 1981;21(2):263–271.

10. Histed MH, Carvalho LA, Maunsell JHR. Psychophysical measurement of contrast sensitivity in the behaving mouse. *J Neurophysiol.* 2012;107(3):758–765.

11. Blakemore C, Campbell FW. On the existence of neurones in the human visual system selectively sensitive to the orientation and size of retinal images. *J Physiol.* 1969;203(1):237–260.

12. Blakemore C, Sutton P. Size adaptation: A new aftereffect. *Science.* 1969;166(3902):245–247.

13. Gibson JJ, Radner M. Adaptation, after-effect and contrast in the perception of tilted lines. I. Quantitative studies. *Journal of Experimental Psychology.* 1937;20(5):453–467.

14. Mather G, Pavan A, Campana G, Casco C. The motion aftereffect reloaded. *Trends Cogn Sci.* 2008;12(12):481–487.

15. Meese TS, Baker DH. Object image size is a fundamental coding dimension in human vision: new insights and model. *Neuroscience.* 2023;514:79-91.

16. Blakemore C, Julesz B. Stereoscopic depth aftereffect produced without monocular cues. *Science.* 1971;171(3968):286–288.

17. Storrs KR, Arnold DH. Shape adaptation exaggerates shape differences. *J Exp Psychol Hum Percept Perform.* 2017;43(1):181–191.

18. Burr David, Ross John. A visual sense of number. *Curr Biol.* 2008;18(6):425–428.

19. Russell JA, Fehr B. Relativity in the perception of emotion in facial expressions. *J Exp Psychol Gen.* 1987;116:223–237.

20. Mullen KT. The contrast sensitivity of human colour vision to red-green and blue-yellow chromatic gratings. *J Physiol.* 1985;359:381–400.

21. Schofield AJ, Georgeson MA. Sensitivity to modulations of luminance and contrast in visual white noise: Separate mechanisms with similar behaviour. *Vision Res.* 1999;39(16):2697–2716.

22. Chubb C, Sperling G. Drift-balanced random stimuli: A general basis for studying non-fourier motion perception. *J Opt Soc Am A.* 1988;5(11):1986–2007.

23. Malik J, Perona P. Preattentive texture discrimination with early vision mechanisms. *J Opt Soc Am A.* 1990;7(5):923–932.

24. Zylinski S, Osorio D, Shohet AJ. Perception of edges and visual texture in the camouflage of the common cuttlefish, *Sepia officinalis. Philos Trans R Soc Lond B Biol Sci.* 2009;364(1516):439–448.

25. Schofield AJ, Rock PB, Sun P, Jiang X, Georgeson MA. What is second-order vision for? Discriminating illumination versus material changes. *J Vis.* 2010;10(9):2.

26. Pointer JS, Hess RF. The contrast sensitivity gradient across the human visual field: With emphasis on the low spatial frequency range. *Vision Res.* 1989;29(9):1133–1151.

27. Baldwin AS, Meese TS, Baker DH. The attenuation surface for contrast sensitivity has the form of a witch's hat within the central visual field. *J Vis.* 2012;12(11).

28. Hess RF, Baker DH, May KA, Wang J. On the decline of 1st and 2nd order sensitivity with eccentricity. *Journal of Vision.* 2008;8(1):19.

29. Hansen T, Pracejus L, Gegenfurtner KR. Color perception in the intermediate periphery of the visual field. *J Vis.* 2009;9(4):26 1–12.

30. Mullen KT, Kingdom FAA. Differential distributions of red-green and blue-yellow cone opponency across the visual field. *Vis Neurosci.* 2002;19(1):109–118.

31. Mullen KT, Sakurai M, Chu W. Does L/M cone opponency disappear in human periphery? *Perception.* 2005;34(8):951–959.

32. Van Essen DC, Newsome WT, Maunsell JH. The visual field representation in striate cortex of the macaque monkey: Asymmetries, anisotropies, and individual variability. *Vision Res.* 1984;24(5):429–448.

33. Dumoulin SO, Wandell BA. Population receptive field estimates in human visual cortex. *Neuroimage.* 2008;39(2):647–660.

34. Lygo FA, Richard B, Wade AR, Morland AB, Baker DH. Neural markers of suppression in impaired binocular vision. *Neuroimage.* 2021;230:117780.

35. Amano K, Wandell BA, Dumoulin SO. Visual field maps, population receptive field sizes, and visual field coverage in the human MT+ complex. *J Neurophysiol.* 2009;102(5):2704–2718.

36. Georgeson MA, Sullivan GD. Contrast constancy: Deblurring in human vision by spatial frequency channels. *J Physiol.* 1975;252(3):627–656.

37. Hess RF, Bradley A. Contrast perception above threshold is only minimally impaired in human amblyopia. *Nature.* 1980;287(5781):463–464.

38. Nachmias J, Sansbury RV. Letter: Grating contrast: Discrimination may be better than detection. *Vision Res.* 1974;14(10):1039–1042.

39. Legge GE, Foley JM. Contrast masking in human vision. *J Opt Soc Am.* 1980;70(12):1458–1471.

40. Foley JM. Human luminance pattern-vision mechanisms: Masking experiments require a new model. *J Opt Soc Am A Opt Image Sci Vis.* 1994;11(6):1710–1719.

41. Heeger DJ. Normalization of cell responses in cat striate cortex. *Vis Neurosci.* 1992;9(2):181–197.

42. Hess RF, Howell ER. The threshold contrast sensitivity function in strabismic amblyopia: Evidence for a two type classification. *Vision Res.* 1977;17(9):1049–1055.

43. Levi DM, Harwerth RS. Spatio-temporal interactions in anisometropic and strabismic amblyopia. *Invest Ophthalmol Vis Sci.* 1977;16(1):90–95.

44. Hess RF, Campbell FW, Greenhalgh T. On the nature of the neural abnormality in human amblyopia; neural aberrations and neural sensitivity loss. *Pflugers Arch.* 1978;377(3):201–207.

45. Hess RF, Field DJ. Is the spatial deficit in strabismic amblyopia due to loss of cells or an uncalibrated disarray of cells? *Vision Res.* 1994;34(24):3397–3406.

46. Hess RF. Contrast vision and optic neuritis: Neural blurring. *J Neurol Neurosurg Psychiatry.* 1983;46(11):1023–1030.

47. Gstalder RJ, Green DG. Laser interferometric acuity in amblyopia. *Journal of Pediatric Ophthalmology & Strabismus.* 1971;8(4):251–256.

48. Kersten D, Hess RF, Plant GT. Assessing contrast sensitivity behind cloudy media. *Clinical Vision Science.* 1988;2:143–158.

49. Baker DH, Meese TS, Hess RF. Contrast masking in strabismic amblyopia: Attenuation, noise, interocular suppression and binocular summation. *Vision Res.* 2008;48(15):1625–1640.

50. Robson JG, Graham N. Probability summation and regional variation in contrast sensitivity across the visual field. *Vision Res.* 1981;21(3):409–418.

51. Meese TS, Summers RJ. Area summation in human vision at and above detection threshold. *Proc Biol Sci.* 2007;274(1627):2891–2900.

52. Baldwin AS, Meese TS. Fourth-root summation of contrast over area: No end in sight when spatially inhomogeneous sensitivity is compensated by a witch's hat. *J Vis.* 2015;15(15):4.

53. Baker DH, Meese TS. Contrast integration over area is extensive: A three-stage model of spatial summation. *J Vision.* 2011;11(14):14.

54. Kay KN, Winawer J, Mezer A, Wandell BA. Compressive spatial summation in human visual cortex. *J Neurophysiol.* 2013;110(2):481–494.

55. Desimone R, Albright TD, Gross CG, Bruce C. Stimulus-selective properties of inferior temporal neurons in the macaque. *J Neurosci.* 1984;4(8):2051–2062.

56. Perrett DI, Rolls ET, Caan W. Visual neurones responsive to faces in the monkey temporal cortex. *Exp Brain Res.* 1982;47(3):329–342.

57. Marr D, Hildreth. E. Theory of edge detection. *Proc R Soc Lond B Biol Sci.* 1980;207(1167):187–217.

58. Carandini M, Heeger DJ. Normalization as a canonical neural computation. *Nat Rev Neurosci.* 2012;13:51–62.

59. Aschner Amir, Solomon Samuel G, Landy Michael S, Heeger DJ, Kohn A. Temporal contingencies determine whether adaptation strengthens or weakens normalization. *J Neurosci.* 2018;38(47):10129–10142.

60. Baker DH, Wade AR. Evidence for an optimal algorithm underlying signal combination in human visual cortex. *Cereb Cortex.* 2017;27(1):254–264.

61. Larsson J, Heeger DJ. Two retinotopic visual areas in human lateral occipital cortex. *J Neurosci.* 2006;26(51):13128–13142.

62. Larsson J, Landy MS, Heeger DJ. Orientation-selective adaptation to first- and second-order patterns in human visual cortex. *J Neurophysiol.* 2006;95(2):862–881.

63. Silson EH, McKeefry DJ, Rodgers J, Gouws AD, Hymers M, Morland AB. Specialized and independent processing of orientation and shape in visual field maps LO1 and LO2. *Nat Neurosci.* 2013;16(2):267–269.

64. Tyler CW, Baseler HA, Kontsevich LL, Likova LT, Wade AR, Wandell BA. Predominantly extra-retinotopic cortical response to pattern symmetry. *Neuroimage.* 2005;24(2):306–314.

65. Bertamini M, Makin ADJ. Brain activity in response to visual symmetry. *Symmetry.* 2014;6(4):975–996.

66. Kanwisher N, McDermott J, Chun MM. The fusiform face area: A module in human extrastriate cortex specialized for face perception. *J Neurosci.* 1997;17(11):4302–4311.

67. Downing PE, Jiang Y, Shuman M, Kanwisher N. A cortical area selective for visual processing of the human body. *Science.* 2001;293(5539):2470–2473.

68. Epstein R, Kanwisher N. A cortical representation of the local visual environment. *Nature.* 1998;392(6676):598–601.

69. Haxby JV, Gobbini MI, Furey ML, Ishai A, Schouten JL, Pietrini P. Distributed and overlapping representations of faces and objects in ventral temporal cortex. *Science.* 2001;293(5539):2425–2430.

70. Rice GE, Watson DM, Hartley T, Andrews TJ. Low-level image properties of visual objects predict patterns of neural response across category-selective regions of the ventral visual pathway. *J Neurosci.* 2014;34(26):8837–8844.

71. Coggan DD, Giannakopoulou A, Ali S, Goz B, Watson DM, Hartley T, Baker DH, Andrews TJ. A data-driven approach to stimulus selection reveals an image-based representation of objects in high-level visual areas. *Hum Brain Mapp.* 2019;40(16):4716–4731.

33

Visual Acuity

Dennis M. Levi

Visual acuity is a measure of the keenness of sight. The Egyptians used the ability to distinguish double stars as a measure of visual acuity more than 5000 years ago.[1] Over the centuries visual acuity has been studied, measured, and analyzed because it represents a fundamental limit in our ability to see. Consequently, visual acuity has been used as a criterion for military service and various other occupations, driving, and for receiving social security benefits.

Visual acuity is limited primarily by the optics of the eye and by the anatomy and physiology of the visual system. As such, visual acuity is perhaps the key clinical measure of the integrity of the optical and physiologic state of the eye and visual pathways (Box 33.1).

DEFINING AND SPECIFYING VISUAL ACUITY

How do we define the keenness of sight? Visual acuity is used to specify a spatial limit (i.e., a threshold in the spatial dimension).[2] Over the centuries there have been a large number of different ideas about how to define, measure, and specify visual acuity, and these can be distilled down to four widely accepted criteria:

- Minimum visible acuity—detection of a feature
- Minimum resolvable acuity—resolution of two features
- Minimum recognizable acuity—identification of a feature
- Minimum discriminable acuity—discrimination of a change in a feature (e.g., a change in size, position, or orientation).

These different criteria actually represent different limits and may be determined by different aspects of the visual pathway (Table 33.1).

Minimum visible acuity

- Minimum visible acuity refers to the smallest object that one can detect.

As early as the 17th century, de Valdez measured the distance at which a row of mustard seeds could no longer be counted, and early astronomers such as Robert Hooke were interested in the size of stars that could be detected and their relation to retinal anatomy.[1] In this context, the minimum visible acuity refers to the smallest target that can be detected. Under ideal conditions, humans can detect a long, dark wire (like the cables of the Golden Gate bridge) against a very bright background (like the sky on a bright sunny day) when they subtend an angle of just 0.5 arc seconds (~0.00014 degrees). It is widely accepted that the minimum visible acuity is so small because the optics of the eye (described further in the chapter) spread the image of the thin line, so that on the retina it is much wider, and the fuzzy retinal image of the wire casts a shadow which reduces the light on a row of cones to a level which is just detectably less than the light on the row of cones on either side. In other words, although we specify the minimum visible acuity in terms of the angular size of the target at the retina, it is actually limited by our ability to discriminate the intensity of the target relative to its background.

Increasing the target size, up to a point, is equivalent to increasing its relative intensity. Hecht and Mintz[3] measured the visual resolution of a black line against a background over a large range of background brightness. They found that the minimum visible acuity varied from about 10 minutes at the lowest background levels, to about 0.5 arc seconds at the highest. The limiting factor in the case of minimum visible acuity is the observers' sensitivity to small variations in the stimulus intensity ($\Delta I/I$), i.e., their contrast sensitivity (discussed further in the chapter). Indeed, Hecht and Mintz[3] state that the retinal image produced by the 0.5 arc second line represents a "fine fuzz of a shadow extending over several cones," and they calculated that at the highest intensity levels tested, the foveal cones occupying the center of the shadow suffer a drop in intensity (relative to the neighboring cones) of approximately 1%—just at the limit of intensity discrimination.

Although the minimum visible acuity represents one limit to spatial vision, it is in fact a limit in the ability to discern small changes in contrast, rather than a spatial limit per se, and minimum visible acuity is not used clinically.

Minimum resolvable acuity

- Minimum resolvable acuity refers to the smallest angular separation between neighboring objects that one can resolve.

Resolving double stars is an example of what is now known as minimal resolvable acuity, which is limited by the eyes' imperfect optics. There is currently still debate about how best to define and measure resolution. However, today, the minimum resolvable acuity is much more likely to be assessed by determining the finest black and white stripes that can be resolved. Under ideal conditions (e.g., high contrast and luminance), humans with very good vision can resolve black and white stripes when one cycle subtends an angle of approximately 1 minute of arc (0.017 degrees). This minimum resolvable acuity represents one of the fundamental limits of spatial vision: it is the finest high-contrast detail that can be resolved. In foveal vision the limit is determined primarily by the spacing of photoreceptors in the retina. The visual system "samples" the stripes discretely, through the array of receptors at the back of the retina (Fig. 33.1). If the receptors are spaced such that the whitest and blackest parts of the grating fall on separate cones (Fig. 33.1B), we should be able to make out the grating. But if the entire cycle falls on a single cone (Fig. 33.1C), we will see nothing but a gray field (or we may experience a phenomenon called **aliasing**, in which we misperceive the width or orientation of the stripes). Cones in the fovea have a center-to-center separation of about 0.5 minutes of arc (0.008 degrees), which fits nicely with the observed acuity limit of 1 minute of arc (0.017 degrees—as we need two cones per cycle to be able to perceive it accurately), and each foveal cone has a "private" line to a ganglion cell. Rods and cones in the retinal periphery are less tightly packed together, and many receptors converge on each ganglion cell. As a result, visual acuity is much poorer in the periphery than in the fovea.

Minimum recognizable acuity

- Minimum recognizable acuity refers to the angular size of the smallest feature that one can recognize or identify.

Although this method has been used since the 17th century, the approach still used by eye doctors today was introduced more than a century ago by Herman Snellen and his colleagues. Snellen

---

BOX 33.1   Visual acuity

Visual acuity is a measure of the keenness of sight. Visual acuity is limited primarily by the optics of the eye and by the anatomy and physiology of this visual system. As such, visual acuity is perhaps the key clinical measure of the integrity of the optical and physiologic state of the eye and visual pathways.

TABLE 33.1   Summary of the different forms of acuity and their limits

Type of acuity	Measured	Acuity (degrees)
Minimum visible	Detection of a feature	0.00014
Minimum resolvable	Resolution of two features	0.017
Minimum recognizable	Identification of a feature	0.017
Minimum discriminable	Discrimination of a change in a feature	0.00024

---

constructed a set of block letters for which the letter as a whole was five times as large as the strokes that formed the letter (Fig. 33.2). The distance of the patient was varied until they could no longer accurately read the letters. In later adaptations of the Snellen test, the viewer was positioned at a constant distance (typically 20 feet [6 meters]), and the size of the letters, rather than the position of the viewer, was altered. Visual acuity, measured in this way was defined as:

The distance at which the patient can just identify the letters / The distance at which a person with "normal" vision can just identify the letters

Thus, "normal" vision came to be defined as 20/20 (6/6 in metric units). To relate this back to visual angle, a 20/20 letter is designed to subtend an angle of 5 arc minutes (0.083 degrees) at the eye, and each stroke of a 20/20 letter subtends an angle of 0.017 degrees (1 arc minute). Thus, if one can read a 20/20 letter, one can discern detail that subtends 1 minute of arc. If one has to be at 20 feet to read a letter that someone with normal vision can read at 40 feet, one has 20/40 vision (worse than normal). Although 20/20 is often considered the gold standard, most healthy young adults have an acuity level considerably better than 20/20.[4] Illiterate E and Landolt C charts are based on the same principles as the Snellen chart.

Although Snellen's notation for visual acuity is commonly used, there are other schemes for specifying acuity (Table 33.2). For example, the minimum angle of resolution (MAR) is the angular size of detail of the visual acuity letter in minutes of arc—it is the Snellen denominator (the number below the line, e.g., 40) over the Snellen numerator (the number above the line, e.g., 20). Thus, for example, a Snellen acuity of 20/20 is equivalent to an MAR of 1′; 20/40 to an MAR of 2′,

Spatial frequency lower than sampling limit

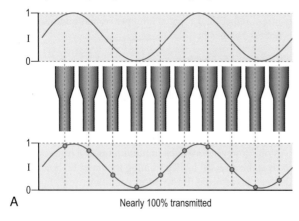

A   Nearly 100% transmitted

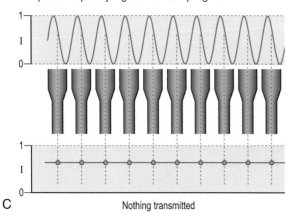

Spatial frequency higher than sampling limit

C   Nothing transmitted

Spatial frequency equal to sampling limit

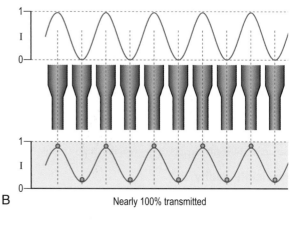

B   Nearly 100% transmitted

Fig. 33.1 Spatial sampling of a sinusoid whose spatial frequency is (**A**) lower than the sampling limit set by the spacing of the cones, (**B**) equal to the sampling limit set by the spacing of the cones, (**C**) higher than the sampling limit set by the spacing of the cones.

and 20/100 an MAR of 5′. Another method for specifying acuity is the Snellen fraction (the Snellen numerator divided by the denominator or 1/MAR). Acuity is sometimes specified as log MAR (the logarithm of the minimum angle of resolution) and sometimes as log visual acuity (the logarithm of the Snellen fraction). Snell and Sterling[5] developed a metric for quantifying visual loss due to injury or disease. The Snell-Sterling efficiency scale sets 20/20 (MAR = 1′) as 100% efficiency and reduces the efficiency by a fixed percentage (~84%) for every 1-minute loss of acuity.

There are many stimulus and subject variables that influence the minimum recognizable visual acuity (discussed further).

Minimum discriminable acuity

- Minimum discriminable acuity refers to the angular size of the smallest *change* in a feature (e.g., a change in size, position, or orientation) that one can discriminate.

Perhaps the most studied example of minimum discriminable acuity is our ability to discern a difference in the relative positions of two features. Our visual systems are very good at telling where things are. Consider two abutting horizontal lines, one slightly higher than the other (Fig. 33.3A). It is very easy to discern that, for example, the right line is higher than the left (i.e., discriminate the relative positions of the two lines) even from a long way away. This is an example of a class of visual tasks that have been given the label "hyperacuity" by Gerald Westheimer.[6] These tasks all have in common that they involve judging the relative position of objects, and Westheimer coined the term hyperacuity because, under ideal conditions, humans can make these judgments with a precision that is finer than the size or spacing of foveal cones.

The smallest misalignment that we can reliably discern is known as Vernier acuity—named after the Frenchman, Pierre Vernier, whose scale, developed in the 17th century, was widely used to aid ship's navigators. The success of the Vernier scale was based on the fact that humans are very adept at judging whether nearby lines are lined up or not. Thus, Vernier alignment is still widely used in precision machines, and even in the dial switches in modern ovens. Under ideal conditions, Vernier acuity may be just three arc seconds (~0.0008 degrees)! This performance is even more remarkable when you consider that it is about 10 times smaller than even the smallest foveal cones. Note that the optics of the eye spread the image of a thin line over a number of retinal cones, and that the eyes are in constant motion, and this performance appears even more remarkable.

Vernier acuity is not the most remarkable form of hyperacuity. Guinness World Records 2005 describes the "highest hyperacuity" as follows: In April 1984, Dr. Dennis M. Levi (the author of this chapter) "...repeatedly identified the relative position of a thin, bright green line within 0.8 seconds of arc (0.00024 deg). This is equivalent to a displacement of some 0.25 inches (6 mm) at a distance of 1 mile (1.6 km)." This "remarkable" position acuity was accomplished with a bisection task (Fig. 33.3B), but can actually be understood based on the ability to discern small changes in local contrast (i.e., minimum detectable acuity).[7]

As remarkable as the other hyperacuities (sometimes also called "position" acuities) might seem, they do not defy the laws of physics. Geisler[8] calculated that if one placed a machine (known as an ideal discriminator) at the retina, and this machine knew precisely the pattern of photons absorbed by the retinal photoreceptors when the stripes were aligned and the pattern of photons absorbed when they were misaligned, this machine could actually perform an order of magnitude better than even the best humans. So, the information about the Vernier offset is present in the pattern of photons absorbed by the photoreceptors; however, humans must be able to

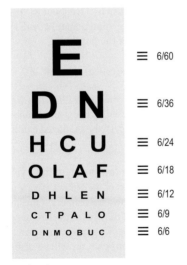

Fig. 33.2 Snellen acuity chart.

E	≡ 6/60
D N	≡ 6/36
H C U	≡ 6/24
O L A F	≡ 6/18
D H L E N	≡ 6/12
C T P A L O	≡ 6/9
D N M O B U C	≡ 6/6

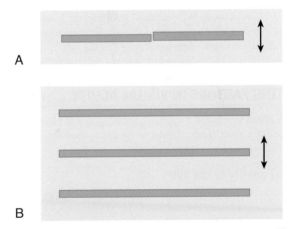

Fig. 33.3 Two "hyperacuity" configurations: Vernier acuity (**A**) and bisection acuity (**B**). In both cases, the subject's task is to judge the relative position of the features.

TABLE 33.2 Different acuity notations

Snellen (imperial)	Notation (metric)	Minimum angle of resolution (MAR)	log MAR	Decimal	Spatial Frequency (SF) (c/deg)
20/200	6/60	10	1	0.1	3
20/20	6/6	1	0.0	1.00	30
20/10	6/3	0.5	−0.3	2	60

interpret the information despite the constant motion of the eyes. Thus, hyperacuity must ultimately be limited by neurons in the visual cortex that are able to interpolate positional information with high resolution.

There is a good deal of evidence that different mechanisms limit position judgments for closely spaced (or abutting) targets, and for widely separated targets. In the nearby case, both contrast and contrast polarity are important. For example, in a two-line Vernier target, Vernier acuity is better when the lines are both either bright or dark than if one line is bright and the other dark. For longer-range position judgments where the targets are well separated, neither contrast nor contrast polarity nor the local stimulus details matter very much. For long-range position judgments the visual system must localize each of the features, and then compare the position labels of separate cortical mechanisms. The idea that cortical receptive fields have position labels (in addition to labels for other stimulus dimensions) is consistent with the topographical mapping of visual space in the brain (i.e., each point in space is systematically mapped onto the visual cortex). More than a century ago, Hermann Lotze[9] wrote:

"So long as the opinion is maintained that the space relations of impressions pass as such into the soul, it must of course, in the interest of the soul, be further held that each impression is conveyed to it by a distinct fibre, and that the fibres reach the seat of the soul with their relative situation wholly undisturbed."

Although we now know much more about the anatomy and physiology of the visual system than was known in the 1880s, Lotze clearly recognized that there must be a topographical representation of the world in the visual nervous system (if not the soul!), and that each "fiber" must carry a label about the position of the "impression" that it carried. For this reason, position labels were called "Lotze's local signs." Lotze also concluded that local signs played an important role in directing eye movements toward stimuli in the peripheral field of vision. So how accurate is "local sign" information? It turns out that humans can localize the position of a single peripheral feature to within about 1% to 2% of the eccentricity of the target, a little more precisely than our saccadic eye movements to peripheral targets.[10]

LIMITING FACTORS IN VISUAL ACUITY

In this section we explore the optical, anatomical, and physiologic factors that limit visual acuity. In the fovea, optics, anatomy, and neural mechanisms conspire to limit our visual acuity.

Optical quality of the eye

The optics of the eye spread the retinal image. Consider the retinal image of a distant star. Because stars are very far away, they are considered to be a "point source," that is, if they were in perfect focus and the eye's optics were perfect, they would subtend an infinitely small angle at the eye. Point sources are useful if one wants to learn about the quality of the eye's optics. As it turns out, the eye's optics are far from perfect; in fact, a camera might have better optical quality. The eye's optics spread the image, so that a point in space forms a distribution (e.g., a Gaussian) on the retina, as illustrated in Fig. 33.4A. This distribution, not to be confused with the office football pool, is known as the *point spread* function (if the source is a line, it is called the line spread function). Fig. 33.4B–D shows the retinal light distribution for a pair of nearby stars. As the stars become closer and closer together, their images overlap to a greater and greater degree, so that when they are very close, they look like a single distribution. When the separation between the stars on the retina is less than half the spread of each

image, they will appear as a single star. This is known as the Rayleigh limit (Fig. 33.4D). The Rayleigh limit is determined mainly by the wavelength of the light and the size of the pupil (we soon discuss why). As noted earlier, the ability to distinguish double stars was one of the earliest measures of visual acuity.[1] In a similar vein, an important ritual of certain wedding ceremonies involves the groom showing the bride the double star pair Mizar and Alcor in the handle of the big dipper. Successful sighting of the nearly invisible Alcor portends a successful marriage, so good optics may be the key to a happy marriage!

Another way to determine the quality of an optical system is to measure its modulation transfer function. This is typically done by passing test patterns of sinusoidal gratings (Fig. 33.5) of known contrast through the optical system and measuring the contrast in the image. Sine waves are characterized by their spatial frequency (i.e., the number of stripes in a given distance, usually specified in cycles per degree), their contrast (i.e., the difference in the luminance of the peaks and troughs divided by the sum of the luminance of the peaks and troughs), and their phase (the position of the peaks). Sine waves are especially useful because even after they are degraded by an optical system, they maintain their characteristic shape (i.e., once a sine wave, always a sine wave) and just become smaller in amplitude (and may shift in phase). The ratio of image contrast to object contrast is a measure of image quality. By measuring the ratio of image contrast to object contrast for a range of object spatial frequencies, one can measure the modulation transfer of any optical system. The *red line* in Fig. 33.6A shows the average modulation transfer functions of a large group of observers with 3-mm pupils (about the average size of the pupil in a well-lighted room). As the object spatial frequency increases, the modulation transfer declines, falling to near zero at a spatial frequency of around 80 cycles per degree. The spatial frequency at which the modulation transfer function falls to zero is called the cutoff spatial frequency. At this spatial frequency the optics do not transmit the sinusoidal variations in the luminance of the object. The theoretical cutoff spatial frequency (SF; in cycles/degree), like the Rayleigh limit, is determined mainly by the wavelength of the light (λ), and the diameter of the pupil (d):

$$\text{Cutoff SF}(c/\text{deg}) = \pi/180^\circ \ d/\lambda$$

where d and λ are both specified in millimeters (mm). For red light (630 nm or 0.000630 mm as used by Liang and Williams[11]) and a 3-mm pupil (about as small as they get), the predicted cutoff spatial frequency is 83 c/deg.

What limits optical image formation of the eye?

As noted previously, the optics of the human eye are imperfect. Why do the eye's optics not match up to a fine camera? One limitation is diffraction produced by the pupil of the eye (or the lens aperture of a camera). For example, when light passes through the aperture, instead of staying in a straight line, the light from each ray will be scattered into different directions. This scatter is known as diffraction, and its consequence is to spread or defocus the image and to reduce the transfer of high spatial frequencies in the modulation transfer function. The *blue lines* in Fig. 33.6 show the diffraction limit (i.e., the modulation transfer of an aberration-free optical system). As noted, the cutoff spatial frequency in the modulation transfer function depends on the pupil diameter. The *red line* in Fig. 33.6B shows the modulation transfer function of a large group of human eyes for a large (7-mm) pupil size. Note that for the large pupil diameter the modulation transfer function is much poorer than predicted by the theoretical limit set by diffraction.

In both panels of Fig. 33.6, the eye's optics are always worse than the theoretical limit, especially when the pupil is large. One important

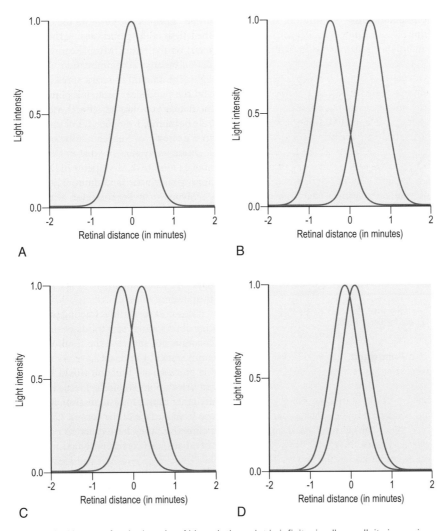

Fig. 33.4 (**A**) Retinal image of a single point. Although the point is infinitesimally small, its image is spread on the retina. (**B–D**) Retinal image of a pair of nearby points, separated by distances equal to two (**B**), one (**C**), and half (**D**) the spread of each image. The latter case is known as the Rayleigh limit.

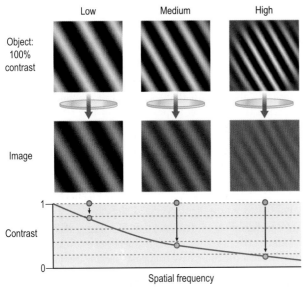

Fig. 33.5 The modulation transfer function.

reason is that the eye exhibits aberrations. One form of aberration in the eye is known as spherical aberration, in which light rays passing through different parts of the eye's optics are focused at slightly different points in the image plane. Larger pupils will result in more aberrations because more peripheral rays of light will enter the eye. There is also chromatic aberration. If the light source (like starlight) is a mixture of light of different wavelengths, then not all of the wavelengths will be in focus on the retina (at any given time), so the eye will have different point spreads for different wavelengths.

Refractive error and defocus results in a marked loss of image quality

The refractive error of the eye is determined by the refractive power of the optical components of the eye (i.e., the power of the cornea and lens) and the length of the eyeball. To focus a distant point source on the retina, the refractive power of the optical components of the eye must be perfectly matched to the length of the eyeball. This perfect match is known as emmetropia. If there is an uncorrected refractive error or the optics of the eye are defocused, the image of a distant object on the retina will be spread out (i.e., the point spread function will widen) and the modulation transfer function will be low (*green line* in Fig. 33.6A).

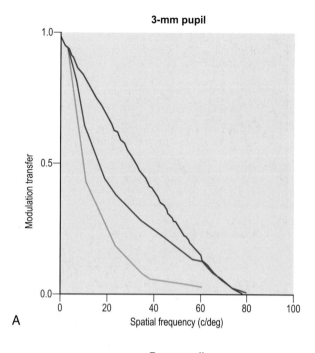

3-mm pupil

A

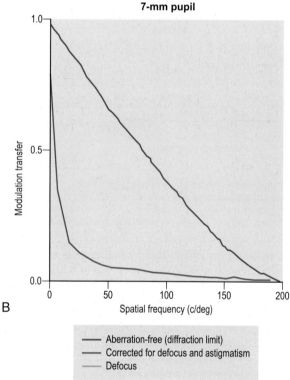

7-mm pupil

B

— Aberration-free (diffraction limit)
— Corrected for defocus and astigmatism
— Defocus

Fig. 33.6 The modulation transfer function (MTF) of the human eye. (**A**) The *red line* is the mean MTF of 12 eyes with a 3-mm pupil with refractive error corrected. The *blue line* is the MTF of an aberration-free eye (i.e., limited by diffraction only). The *green line* shows schematically the effect of uncorrected refractive error. (Reprinted with permission from Liang J, Williams DR. Aberrations and retinal image quality of the normal human eye. *J Opt Soc Am A Opt Image Sci Vis.* 1997;14:2873–2883.) (**B**) The *red line* is the mean MTF of 14 eyes with a 7.3-mm pupil with refractive error corrected. The *blue line* is the MTF of an aberration-free eye (i.e., limited by diffraction only). (Modified from Campbell FW, Green DG. Optical and retinal factors affecting visual resolution. *J Physiol.* 1965;181:576–593.)

For myopes, the power of the optical components is too strong for the length of the globe, causing the light rays to converge too much to focus on the retina. Myopia cannot be remedied through accommodation because accommodation will increase the convergence of the light. The amount of image spread depends on the amount of defocus and the pupil size. Reducing pupil size increases the depth of focus, so that defocus has less effect with small than with large pupils. As a rule of thumb, 1 diopter (D) of uncorrected simple myopia will result in a decrease of Snellen acuity, on average, to approximately 20/60. A recent study suggests that in children visual acuity was reduced by about 1 minute of MAR per 0.70 D of spherical refractive error and by approximately the same amount per 1.5 D of astigmatism.[12]

Myopia can be corrected with negative (minus) lenses, which diverge the rays. On the other hand, hyperopia (far-sightedness) occurs when the power of the optical components is too weak for the length of the eyeball, causing the light rays to not converge enough to focus on the retina (the image plane lies behind the retina in an unaccommodated hyperopic eye). If the hyperopia is not too severe, a young hyperope can compensate by accommodating, and thereby increasing the power of the eye.

The most powerful refracting surface in the eye is the cornea, which contributes about two-thirds of the eye's refracting power. When the cornea is not spherical the result is astigmatism. With astigmatism, a point source would not have a single point focus on the retina (i.e., the point spread function would be asymmetric), and lines of different orientations would be focused in different planes. Although there are other causes for astigmatism, it is usually caused by asymmetry of the front surface of the cornea. Cylindrical lenses that have two focal points (e.g., they have different power in the horizontal and vertical meridians) can correct astigmatism.

Photoreceptor size and spacing; aperture size; the "Nyquist" limit; aliasing

Retinal anatomy plays a very important role in setting the limits for foveal resolution acuity. Foveal cones are arranged in a regular arrangement (sometimes called a triangular array) and are densely packed (see Fig. 33.7). This dense packing is critical to fine resolution. The reason is simple. The visual world is represented by continuous variations in light intensity. However, our visual system "samples" the world discretely, (i.e., by looking at the light distribution through many small individual photoreceptors). The more closely packed the photoreceptors, the better the light distribution can be represented to the visual nervous system. As illustrated in Fig. 33.1, there is a sampling limit. To properly represent the peaks and troughs in the intensity profile of a sine wave, there must be at least two cones for each cycle of the grating. This is known as the Nyquist limit and is represented in Fig. 33.1B. More formally, the Nyquist limit occurs when the sine wave has a spatial period (i.e., the peak-to-peak distance) that is two times the cone spacing. When the spatial period is smaller than twice the cone spacing (i.e., when the sine wave spatial frequency is higher than the Nyquist frequency), the phenomenon known as "aliasing" may occur, i.e., rather than the cones signaling a perfect replica of the sine wave on the retina, the signal is distorted—it appears to be a sine wave with a lower spatial frequency than the original (Fig. 33.8). Because cones in the fovea have a center-to-center separation of around 0.5 arc minutes, the cone sampling (or Nyquist) limit is a grating spatial period of about 1 minute (i.e., a grating spatial frequency of 60 cycles per degree. Note that because the cones have triangular packing, geometry dictates that the Nyquist frequency will actually be about 15% higher or ~69 c/deg). This represents a fundamental limitation set by the spacing of the

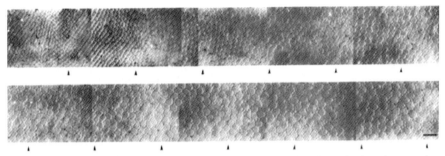

Fig. 33.7 Inner segments of a human cone mosaic in a strip extending from the foveal center (*upper left arrow*) along the temporal horizontal meridian. The large cells are cones, and the small cells are rods. The horizontal scale bar indicates 10 μm. (From Hirsch J, Curcio C. The spatial resolution capacity of human foveal retina. *Vision Res.* 1989;29:1095–1101.)

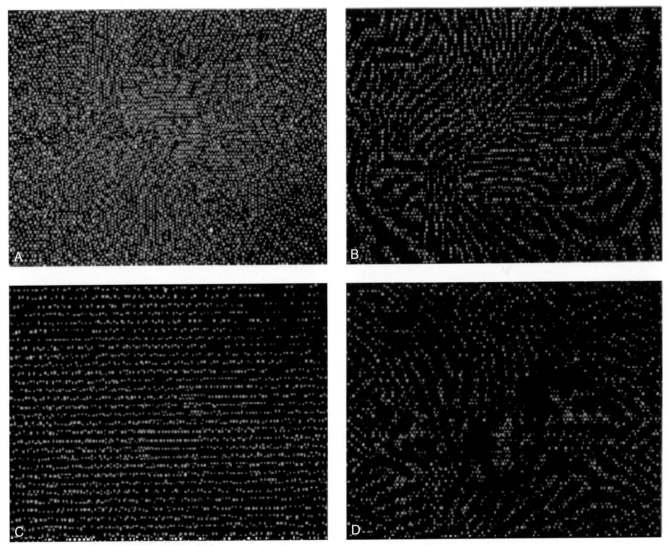

Fig. 33.8 (**A**) The foveal cone mosaic is represented as sample points (*bright dots*). In the other panels it has been sandwiched with gratings of 40 cpd (**C**), 80 cpd (**B**), and 110 cpd (**D**). (From Williams DR. Topography of the foveal cone mosaic in the living human eye. *Vision Res.* 1988;28:433–454. Copyright Elsevier 1988.)

foveal cones, and it is not far off the limitations set by the eye's optics. Thus, in the fovea, the cone spacing is nicely matched to the eye's optics. As seen later in this chapter, cone spacing in peripheral vision changes dramatically, whereas the optics change only a little.

The notion that there is a "highest" spatial frequency that can be accurately represented by the visual system (the Nyquist frequency)

raises the interesting question of whether aliasing actually occurs in human vision. Fortunately for us, our optics "protect" us from the effects of aliasing in the fovea by reducing the contrast of high spatial frequencies. Interestingly, it is possible to create a very high spatial frequency pattern on the retina bypassing the optics of the eye (this can be accomplished using lasers to create interference patterns). Under these conditions, humans report the appearance of aliasing—fine gratings appear coarse (and often appear to change their orientation). Fig. 33.8 illustrates how viewing a grating through too coarse a grid produces the kind of wavy, coarse appearance produced by aliasing.

Cone to ganglion cell convergence

If many cones converged on a single ganglion cell, the advantage of having closely spaced cones would be lost. Recall, however, that in the fovea each cone effectively has a "private line" to the brain via the midget bipolar and ganglion cells. So, the receptive field centers of midget ganglion cells are effectively one cone wide. In peripheral vision resolution is limited by the retinal ganglion cells that are widely spaced (sparsely sampled) and that pool information from many cones.

Eccentricity

In contrast to the tightly packed cones in the fovea, cone density decreases dramatically with retinal eccentricity, and there is substantial convergence of cones to ganglion cells (Chapter 26). Humans have many more rods (~90 million) than cones (about 4–5 million), and they have very different geographical distributions on the retina (Fig. 33.9). The cones are most concentrated in the center of the fovea, and their density drops off dramatically with retinal eccentricity. Rods are missing from the center of the fovea, and their density increases to a peak at about 20 degrees, and then declines again. As can be seen in Fig. 33.7, the cones in the fovea are much more densely packed than in the peripheral retina, and there are no rods in the section from the foveal center. This "rod-free" area (~300 micrometers on the retina) subtends a visual angle of about 1 degree. Moreover, unlike the fovea, in the retinal periphery there is considerable convergence of cones onto ganglion cells.

Almost 140 years ago, Aubert and Forster[13] demonstrated that visual acuity declines in an orderly fashion with eccentricity—an important observation that has been often repeated and extended to a multiplicity of tasks over the years. About 100 years later, Weymouth[14] showed that many visual functions degrade approximately linearly with eccentricity, and we can characterize the rate of fall-off of many visual functions (as well as the anatomical structures that limit performance) by the gradient, which can be represented by a single number called E_2. E_2 represents the eccentricity at which the foveal value has doubled.[15]

Daniel and Whitteridge[16] coined the term "cortical magnification factor" or CMF, to describe the cortical distance (usually specified in mm) devoted to 1 degree in the visual field. Although there are still uncertainties about the precise CMF of the fovea in humans, the best estimates (based on functional imaging) suggest that it is about 20 mm/deg (i.e., 1 degree in visual space is represented over a distance of ~20 mm in the cortical representation of the fovea). In contrast, at an eccentricity of 10 degrees, 1 degree in visual space is represented over a distance of only about 1.5 mm in the cortex.

The CMF is generally specified in mm/deg. A convenient simplification is that the inverse CMF (i.e., the number of degrees per millimeter) varies approximately linearly with eccentricity (Fig. 33.10A). Thus, in the human fovea, approximately 0.05 degrees of visual space (3′) is represented in 1 mm of striate cortex, while at 10 degrees eccentricity,

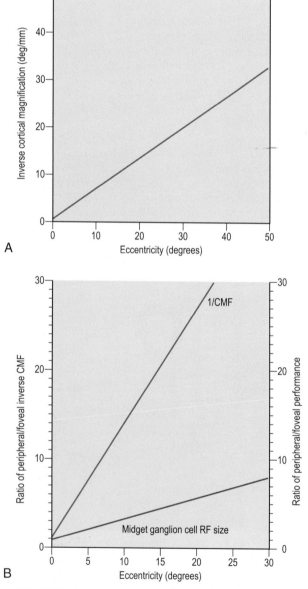

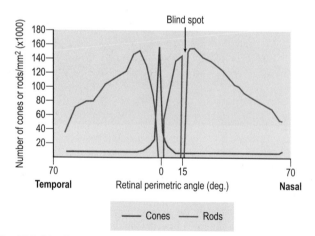

Fig. 33.9 Distribution of cones (*blue*) and rods (*red*) across the retina. (Modified from Osterberg G. Topography of the layer of rods and cones in the human retina. *Acta Ophthal.* 1935;Suppl 6:1–102.)

Fig. 33.10 (**A**) The inverse cortical magnification factor (*CMF*; in degrees per millimeter) versus eccentricity. (**B**) The *red line* shows the gradient (i.e., the rate of variation) of inverse magnification with eccentricity, by plotting the ratio of peripheral to foveal inverse magnification at each eccentricity. For inverse cortical magnification the gradient is steep. In contrast, the gradient for midget retinal ganglion cell size (*the blue line*) is shallow. *RF*, Receptive Field.

about 0.67 degrees is represented in 1 mm. The *red line* in Fig. 33.10B shows the gradient (i.e., the rate of variation of inverse magnification with eccentricity), by plotting the ratio of peripheral to foveal inverse magnification at each eccentricity. Essentially, this normalizes inverse magnification at each eccentricity by the foveal value. An advantage of using the gradient is that it makes it simple to compare changes in anatomy or performance with eccentricity for different structures and functions.

For inverse cortical magnification (the *red line* in Fig. 33.10B), the gradient is steep and E_2 is approximately 0.77 degrees.[15] In contrast, the gradient for midget retinal ganglion cell size (the *blue line* in Fig. 33.10B—from[17]) is shallow, and E_2 is about 3.7 degrees. The importance of the gradients of performance is that they may provide clues as to the structures, at various levels of the visual pathway, that limit performance. Indeed, one of the reasons Polyak[18] gave for undertaking his classical study of the retina was to obtain a better understanding of the "striking difference between central and peripheral acuity." Different psychophysical tasks also have different gradients. For example, Vernier acuity has a steep gradient, whereas contrast sensitivity (discussed further in the chapter) has a shallow gradient.

Fig. 33.11 shows a visual acuity chart in which the letters are "scaled" in size, so that each letter covers an approximately equal cortical distance, and interestingly, the letters should be approximately equally visible!

Why is the foveal representation in the cortex so highly magnified? The visual system must make a trade off. High resolution (like our foveas) requires a great deal of resources—a dense array of photoreceptors, a one-to-one line from photoreceptors to retinal ganglion cells, and a large chunk of cortex. If we could see the entire visual field with such high resolution, we might need to have eyes and brains too large to fit in our heads! Thus, we have evolved a visual system that provides high resolution in the center, and lower resolution in the periphery. In large part, the high foveal magnification in the cortex reflects the topography of the retina[19] (see Fig. 33.7); however, there appears to be

additional magnification of the foveal representation in the cortex,[20] and the striate cortex contains more than 100 times more cells than the lateral geniculate nucleus (LGN).

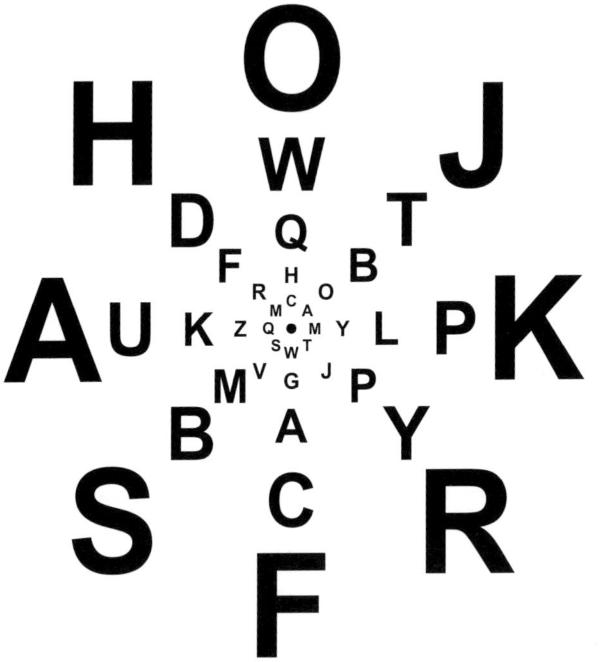

Crowding in peripheral vision

In peripheral vision, the identification of a letter is severely impaired by neighboring letters (Box 33.2). This "crowding" phenomenon has been discussed scientifically for some 60 years but is only beginning to be understood (for reviews see[21,22]). The reader can experience this phenomenon by viewing Fig. 33.12. When looking at the fixation point, the letter R is clearly legible in the top panel, where it is presented in isolation. However, it is much more difficult to read in the lower panel, when flanked by other letters.

Inspection of Fig. 33.12 makes it obvious that crowding does not result in reduced apparent contrast—rather, crowded letters are high contrast but indistinct or jumbled together. Tyler and Likova[23] also note their strong subjective impression of a "gray, or inchoate, smudge between the two outer letters, including the inner parts of those letters."

In peripheral vision, the spatial extent of crowding depends on eccentricity, and can be as large as approximately 0.5 times the target eccentricity. Several recent studies have varied both target size and eccentricity and show that the extent of peripheral crowding is more or less invariant to target size.[24–27]

The strength and extent of peripheral crowding are much greater than the strength and extent of masking,[24,28] so that in peripheral vision, the suppressive spatial interactions due to nearby flanks are not likely to be a consequence of simple contrast masking.

A number of studies, using very different stimuli and tasks, have shown convincingly that crowding is indifferent to whether the target and flanks are presented to the same eye or to different eyes (target to one eye, flanks to the other[29–31]). The fact that crowding occurs when target and flanks are presented to separate eyes immediately places the site of the interaction at or beyond the site of combination of information of the two eyes. Remarkably, this dichoptic interaction even occurs when the flankers are presented around the blind spot of one eye and the target in the "monocular" region corresponding to the blind spot of the other eye.[32] This is both surprising and interesting because there is a complete absence of direct retinal afferents from one eye to this region of cortex.

Note that it is easy to resolve the letters in Fig. 33.12 when viewing them directly (with the fovea). Except near the limit of resolution[33] in the normal fovea, the extent of "crowding" is proportional to stimulus size and cannot easily be distinguished from ordinary masking.[34,35] At the limit, foveal crowding extends over a tiny distance just 4 to 5 minutes of arc.[33,36,37] Interestingly, recent work using adaptive optics to bypass the optical limitations imposed by the human eye suggests that foveal and peripheral crowding differ in several ways.[38] The critical spacings for foveal targets of different size were nicely captured by edge-to-edge spacing, rather than center-to-center spacing, and the robust recovery for flankers closer than the critical distance, while common in foveal contour interaction studies, is generally absent in peripheral experiments. With adaptive optics maximal edge-to-edge

Fig. 33.11 A visual acuity chart in which the letter size has been "scaled" according to the cortical magnification factor. (From Anstis SM. A chart demonstrating variations in acuity with retinal position. *Vision Res.* 1974;14:589–592. Copyright Elsevier 1974.)

BOX 33.2 Crowding

In peripheral vision and in the central field in strabismic amblyopia, the identification of a letter, which can be easily identified in isolation, is severely impaired by neighboring letters. This "crowding" phenomenon has been discussed scientifically for some 60 years but is only beginning to be understood. Crowding represents an essential bottleneck for object recognition and reading.

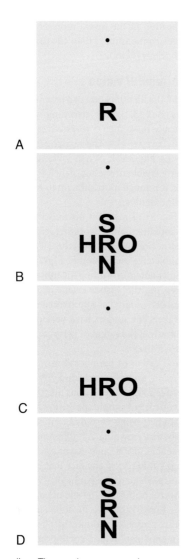

A

B

C

D

Fig. 33.12 Crowding. The reader can experience crowding by fixating the dot and trying to identify one letter: in isolation (**A**), surrounded by four random flanking letters (**B**), surrounded by two horizontally placed random flanking letters (**C**), surrounded by two vertically placed random flanking letters (**D**). (From Levi DM. Crowding—An essential bottleneck for object recognition: A mini-review. *Vision Res.* 2008;48:635–654. Copyright Elsevier 2008.)

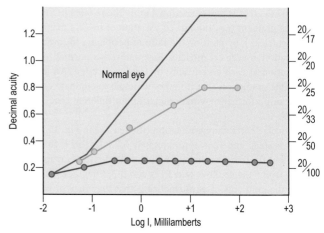

Fig. 33.13 Acuity versus log luminance for normal fovea (*red*) and for patients with retinal lesions owing to a disease of Bruch's membrane (*green*) and macular toxoplasmosis (*blue*). (Modified from Sloan LL. Variation of acuity with luminance in ocular diseases and anomalies. *Doc Ophthalmol.* 1969;26:384–393.)

Similarly, Vernier acuity for abutting lines is markedly reduced at low luminance levels.[41] Reducing luminance alters the visibility of a stimulus. For example, the contrast ($\Delta I/I$) necessary to detect a thin line increases as retinal illumination is reduced. Specifically, both line detection thresholds and (abutting) Vernier thresholds decrease with the square root of retinal illuminance, suggesting that photon statistics may be the main source of information loss.[8,41,42] Interestingly, when the effect of luminance on target visibility is taken into account (by making the target contrast a fixed multiple of the detection threshold at each luminance level), Vernier acuity becomes independent of target luminance.[42]

Contrast

Visual acuity is generally tested with high-contrast (~100% contrast) optotypes, and reducing the contrast results in a systematic reduction of acuity.[43–46] Fig. 33.14 (from[47]) shows that visual acuity for Sloan letters varies linearly on log-log coordinates, with a log-log slope of approximately −0.5. In other words, visual acuity improves in proportion to the square root of the target contrast. Similarly, other types of acuity (e.g., abutting Vernier acuity) depend strongly on target contrast. Interestingly, relative position judgments with widely separated targets show little dependence on contrast, luminance, or polarity, as might be expected if these judgments are limited by a local sign mechanism (discussed earlier).

Time

For many visual tasks including visual acuity and abutting Vernier acuity, performance is degraded when the stimulus presentation is brief.[48,49] This effect can largely be understood on the basis of stimulus energy or visibility (i.e., reducing the duration below a "critical" duration) reduces the number of quanta and the visibility of the stimulus. This effect of duration can be canceled by increasing the illumination or contrast of the stimulus to maintain a constant visibility (or a constant number of absorbed quanta[2,49,50]).

Motion

Even when you try to hold your eyes completely stationary, they continue to execute small but important movements. These involuntary eye drifts and small jerks keep the retinal image "fresh"; if the eye muscles are temporarily paralyzed—say, as a result of taking curare[51]—the

interference was found to occur with flankers approximately 0.75 to 1.3 minutes from the target.[38]

The issue of crowding is discussed further in the section on amblyopia.

Luminance

Visual acuity is usually measured under moderate photopic luminance conditions (80–320 cd/m²), and under those conditions (and indeed luminance levels ranging from full moonlight to a bright sunny sky) visual acuity remains fairly constant.[2,39,40] At very low luminance levels, visual acuity is markedly reduced. Under very low (scotopic) luminance conditions visual acuity is mediated by rods, and rod acuity asymptotes at an acuity level between 20/100 and 20/200. Fig. 33.13 shows the acuity versus log luminance function for normal fovea (*red*) and for patients with retinal lesions owing to a disease of Bruch's membrane (*green*) and macular toxoplasmosis (*blue*). Retinal disease lowers both the upper asymptote and the slope of the acuity versus luminance function.

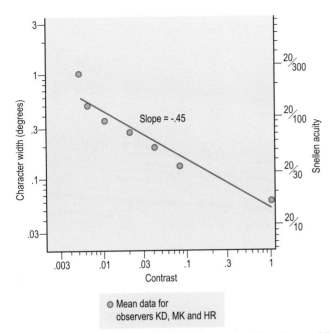

Fig. 33.14 The effect of contrast on Snellen acuity. (From Legge GE, Rubin GS, Luebker A, et al. Psychophysics of reading—V. The role of contrast in normal vision. *Vision Res.* 1987;27:1165–1177. Copyright Elsevier 1987.)

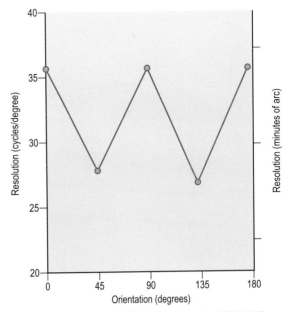

Fig. 33.15 Oblique effect. (Modified from Campbell FW, Kulikowski JJ, Levinson J. The effect of orientation on the visual resolution of gratings. *J Physiol.* 1966;187:427–436.)

entire visual world gradually fades from view. Using retinal image stabilization, Keesey[52] showed that these small involuntary eye movements have little or no effect on visual acuity. Indeed, visual acuity measured with Landolt Cs and Vernier acuity are unaffected by retinal image motion of up to approximately 2.5 degrees/second.[53] Beyond that, Vernier acuity for targets consisting of closely spaced dots or lines is strongly degraded by fast motion. For very large, blurred stimuli (low spatial frequency sinusoids), Vernier acuity is quite robust to even very high velocities.[54]

Anisotropies

There are anisotropies in visual acuity. For example, in the fovea visual acuity and contrast sensitivity at high spatial frequencies are better for horizontal and vertical gratings than for oblique (Fig. 33.15). The W-shaped function shown in Fig. 33.15 is known as the oblique effect.[55] It is not an optical effect because it occurs when interference fringes are imaged directly on the retina, thus bypassing the optics of the eye.[56] In peripheral vision the oblique effect gives way to a radial organization, with acuity being better for gratings oriented along a line connecting the fovea to the peripheral location (radial orientation) and worse for the orthogonal orientation. The most profound anisotropy is found under conditions of crowding. Crowding in peripheral vision is much more extensive when the flankers are radially arranged than when they are tangentially arranged (Fig. 33.16).[27,38] The reader can see this effect for themselves in the lower two panels of Fig. 33.12. In panel (D), the flanks are arranged radially, in panel (C), tangentially.

Visual acuity and reading

The ability to read quickly and accurately is crucial in our society, and difficulty in reading is one of the most frequent reasons that patients visit their eye doctor. Clearly, if acuity is substantially reduced, reading will be impaired. However, recent work shows that it is text spacing and not text size that limits reading speed. When the text spacing is closer than a critical spacing, reading is slowed. The critical spacing for

reading is equal to the critical spacing for crowding[22,27,57] (Fig. 33.17). The notion that crowding limits reading is surprising and perhaps controversial, because reading rate has generally been thought to be linked to letter size rather than spacing. Changing the viewing distance for normal reading material changes both size and spacing; however, experiments measuring reading performance versus letter size with normal and doubled letter spacing (i.e., 1.1 and 2.2 times the letter size) reveal that it is spacing that matters.[57] Thus crowding appears to represent a limit for reading in normal and amblyopic central vision.[57] This is consistent with the conclusions of Legge and his coworkers that the "visual span" (i.e., the number of letters in a line of text that can be recognized reliably without moving the eyes) represents a sensory bottleneck for reading.[58–60]

Whereas the critical spacing for crowding and reading are also identical in peripheral vision (suggesting that crowding represents one limit to fast reading in the periphery), reading slows with increasing eccentricity even when crowding is controlled for (by scaling with eccentricity), for reasons that remain mysterious.

SPATIAL VISION WITH LOW CONTRAST

Until now the focus has been the smallest high-contrast details that can be resolved; however, most of the objects in our world are larger than the resolution limit and have lower contrast.

How can we measure and quantify how well we see objects that are larger than the resolution limit? Recall how the performance of an optical system was measured earlier in this chapter. Test patterns consisting of sinusoidal gratings (see Fig. 33.5) of known contrast and a range of sizes (spatial frequencies) were passed through the optical system, and the ratio of image contrast to object contrast was used as a measure of modulation transfer of the optical system. Sinusoidal gratings have some important advantages for testing optical systems, and therefore should be useful in characterizing human pattern vision. There is, however, a problem. In an optical system, it is relatively easy to measure the contrast of the image; however, that is not so easily done in human vision, because the image is on the retina. More

Subject AT

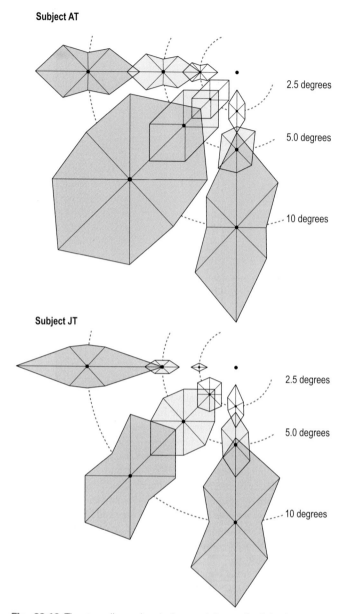

Subject JT

Fig. 33.16 The two-dimensional shape of "crowding" in foveal (*the small dot in the center*) and peripheral vision (at 2.5, 5, and 10 degrees). (From Toet A, Levi DM. The two-dimensional shape of spatial interaction zones in the parafovea. *Vision Res.* 1992;32:1349–1357. Copyright Elsevier 1992.)

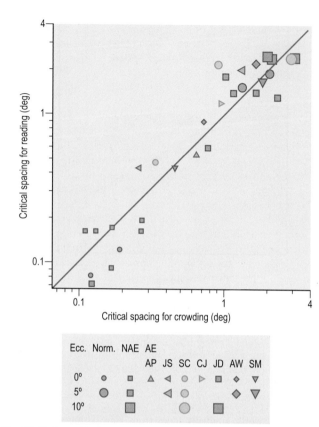

Ecc.	Norm.	NAE	AE						
			AP	JS	SC	CJ	JD	AW	SM
0°	○	■	△	◁	○	▷	■	◆	▽
5°	◯	■		◁	◯			◆	▽
10°	◯	■			◯		■		

Fig. 33.17 The critical spacing for reading is equal to the critical spacing for crowding for normal foveal, peripheral, and amblyopic vision. *AE*, Amblyopic Eye; *ECC*, Eccentricity; *Norm*, Normal; *NAE*, Non-amblyopic eye; *AP, JS,* etc. are subjects initials. (Levi DM, Song S, Pelli DG. Amblyopic reading is crowded. *J Vision.* 2007;7[2]:1–17, reproduced with permission from Association for Research in Vision and Ophthalmology.)

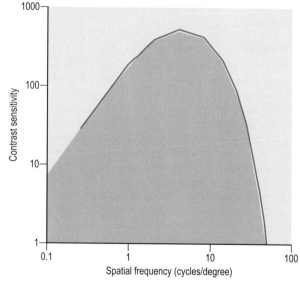

Fig. 33.18 The contrast sensitivity function: our window of visibility.

The contrast sensitivity function represents our window of visibility

The *red line* in Fig. 33.18 shows a CSF. The vertical axis shows the observer's contrast sensitivity plotted as a function of the spatial frequency of the sinusoidal gratings (with low spatial frequencies, or broad stripes represented on the *left*, and high spatial frequencies or

importantly, how well we see sinusoidal gratings will be determined by both the optical components of the eye and by any neural processing in the visual pathway. Thus, what we really want to know is about the quality of the image that reaches the brain and gives rise to perception. Schade[61] first addressed this by showing people sinusoidal gratings and asking them to adjust the contrast of the gratings until they could just be detected. By repeating these measurements for a wide range of different spatial frequencies (stripe widths), Schade was able to describe the "contrast sensitivity function", i.e., contrast sensitivity for gratings of different spatial frequencies. Almost 10 years later, Campbell and Green[55] published what is widely regarded as a classical paper, describing a relatively simple method for measuring the contrast sensitivity function, and showed that both optical and neural processes influence the function.

fine stripes, on the *right*). Surprisingly, the function is shaped like an upside-down U. The modulation transfer of the eye (or any other optical system) reduces the contrast of high spatial frequencies, so the fall-off of sensitivity at high spatial frequencies is to be expected based on the optics of the eye. However, the fall-off of sensitivity at low spatial frequencies is unexpected. Poor optics will not reduce sensitivity at low spatial frequencies, so this low spatial frequency fall-off must be due to neural factors (we discuss these later).

Contrast sensitivity is obtained by measuring the smallest amount of contrast needed to detect the target (the contrast threshold), and sensitivity is defined as the reciprocal of the threshold contrast. Thus, if the contrast at threshold is 0.01, contrast sensitivity will be 100, and a contrast threshold of 0.1 will give a contrast sensitivity of 10. Thus, the *red line* in Fig. 33.18 corresponds to the lowest contrast one can see, and the *pink region* under the curve represents the window of visibility. Any pattern whose spatial frequency and contrast fall within the *pink region* will be visible, while any combination of spatial frequency and contrast in the region above the curve will be invisible. For example, a spatial frequency of 1 c/degree will be invisible if its contrast is less than 0.01 and will be visible with any contrast greater than 0.01. For this spatial frequency, the contrast sensitivity is 100. Note that contrast sensitivity equal to 1 corresponds to a contrast of 100%. This is the rightmost point on the CSF (at around 50 c/degree) and corresponds to the observer's resolution limit. It is the finest grating the observer can detect with 100% contrast.

Fig. 33.19 allows you to visualize your own CSF. This figure shows a sinusoidal grating whose contrast increases continuously from the top of the figure to the bottom, and whose spatial frequency increases continuously from the left side of the graph to the right side. If you hold the figure at a distance of about 50 cm, you will notice the inverted U shape where the grating fades from visibility to invisibility. This is your own CSF—because it tells us how your sensitivity varies over a wide range of target sizes, it is more informative than visual acuity.

Fig. 33.18 illustrates a typical CSF, obtained with foveal viewing of stationary gratings at high levels of illumination (i.e., using cone vision). The CSF changes its shape at low luminance (Fig. 33.20). For example, at very low (scotopic) luminance levels, sensitivity is markedly reduced at all spatial frequencies, and the low spatial frequency fall-off is less pronounced. At intermediate (mesopic) luminance levels, CSF is reduced mainly at high spatial frequencies. The CSF also changes its shape when the gratings are moved, flickered on and off or temporally modulated in other ways (Fig. 33.21). These changes in the shape of the CSF reflect neural changes.

The contrast sensitivity function in peripheral vision

Visual resolution declines with eccentricity. How the CSF changes with eccentricity depends in large part on how it is measured. In early studies, peripheral CSFs were measured with a patch of gratings that was fixed in size (e.g., 1 degree). As illustrated in Fig. 33.22A, when a fixed-size patch is viewed in the periphery, contrast sensitivity decreases

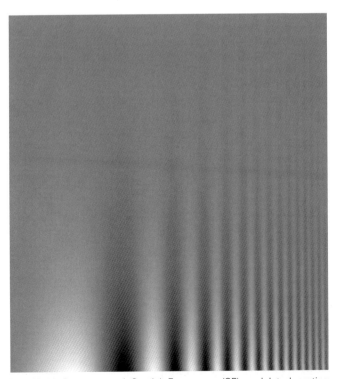

Fig. 33.19 Contrast- and Spatial Frequency (SF)-modulated grating. (From Robson J, Campbell F. A quick demonstration of your own contrast sensitivity function. In: Pelli DG, Torres AM. *Thresholds: Limits of Perception*. New York: NY Arts Magazine; 1977.)

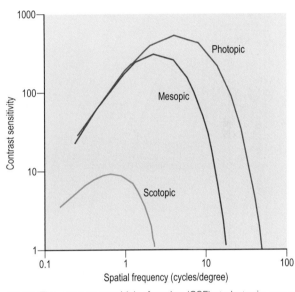

Fig. 33.20 The contrast sensitivity function (CSF) at photopic, mesopic, and scotopic luminance levels.

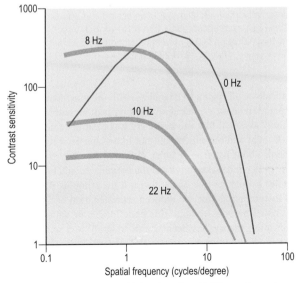

Fig. 33.21 The contrast sensitivity function (CSF) at three temporal frequencies. Note that it changes its shape at higher temporal frequencies.

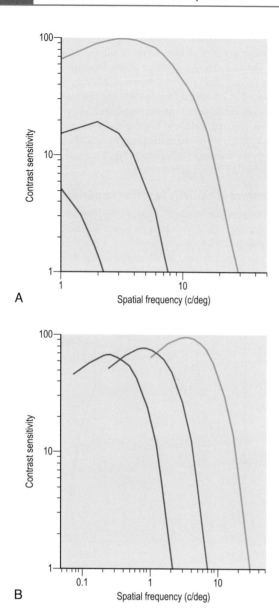

A

B

Fig. 33.22 Contrast sensitivity functions at three eccentricities: fovea (*green*), 7.5 degrees (*red*), and 30 degrees (*blue*). (**A**) With fixed field size (2-degree half circle). (**B**) With field size scaled in proportion to ganglion cell density at each eccentricity. (From Rovamo J, Virsu V, Näsänen R. Cortical magnification factor predicts the photopic contrast sensitivity of peripheral vision. *Nature.* 1978;271:54–56.)

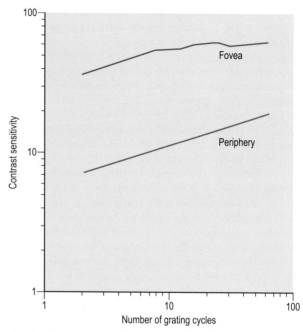

Fig. 33.23 Contrast sensitivity versus number of cycles for fovea (*blue*) and periphery (*red*). (Modified from Robson JG, Graham N. Probability summation and regional variation in contrast sensitivity across the visual field. *Vision Res.* 1981;21:409–418. Copyright Elsevier 1981.)

dramatically at all spatial frequencies—with the most marked effect at high spatial frequencies. Based on these types of measurements, it was commonly assumed that the periphery was basically able to function to detect light and movement, but not to be capable of making useful judgments about patterns or form. However, Rovamo et al.[62] showed that the peak contrast sensitivity of the periphery could be almost (but not quite) as high as that of the fovea, if the stimulus size was magnified to compensate for the reduced representation of the periphery in the visual nervous system. This basic idea, now widely known as magnification theory, has been shown to apply to a wide variety of visual stimuli and tasks. Rovamo et al.[62] magnified the stimulus size by a scale factor that was actually based on retinal ganglion cell density at each eccentricity, so in essence they equated the number of ganglion cells that were stimulated by the patch of grating at each eccentricity. (This "scaling" was accomplished by viewing the same patch on the screen from successively closer viewing distances as the eccentricity

increased, thus increasing the angular size of the stimulus patch.) The result is that peak contrast sensitivity is almost the same at each eccentricity (Fig. 33.22B). Note, however, that even with the larger field size, both the peak of the CSF and the cutoff spatial frequency shift toward lower spatial frequencies as eccentricity increases.

How is it that peripheral contrast sensitivity improves so much at low spatial frequencies when the patch size is increased? Robson and Graham[63] showed that the improvement could largely be explained by a process known as probability summation. They measured contrast sensitivity for patches with different numbers of grating cycles. They found that contrast sensitivity improved as they added cycles, and the improvement followed a power function (i.e., a straight line on log-log axes). In the fovea, the function saturated when there were around 8 cycles, so that adding yet more cycles did not improve sensitivity much (Fig. 33.23, *blue line*). However, in peripheral vision sensitivity improved up to 64 cycles (the maximum number they tested; see Fig. 33.23, *red line*). Recall that the scaling method of Rovamo et al. increased the field size when testing the periphery. Thus, the periphery would get the benefit of having more cycles of the grating than the fovea, and as Robson and Graham showed, the periphery uses every cycle it gets! Robson and Graham argued that the improvement in sensitivity as more cycles are presented accrues from having more opportunities to detect the pattern. Their notion of probability summation across space was that the grating would be detected if it landed on a mechanism (receptive field) that was sensitive to the target, and signaled its presence, and they further assumed that each receptive field acted independently. Based on these simple assumptions, they were able to predict the effect of the number of cycles by simply pooling the responses of independent mechanisms sensitive to the target.

Clinical testing of visual acuity
Visual acuity chart design considerations

The original Snellen chart consisted of seven letter sizes, with a single (20/200) letter at the top, two (20/100) letters on the next line, the number of characters (letters and numbers) increasing on each subsequent line, and the interletter spacing varying from line to line (Fig. 33.2). Moreover, the change in letter size between the 20/200 and 20/100 lines is very coarse (50%), whereas the change from 20/50 to 20/40 is much finer (20%), so that testing accuracy varies depending on the acuity level.

Most contemporary charts incorporate some or all of the design principles (Box 33.3) proposed by Bailey and Lovie[64]; the same number of letters on each line; a constant ratio from one letter size to the next (i.e., each line is a fixed percentage smaller than the previous line); spacing between letters and lines proportional to letter size; and nearly equal legibility to the optotypes (or nearly equal average legibility at each letter size). A distinguishing feature of charts that incorporate these principles is the V-shaped appearance, as each line is proportionally smaller than the preceding line. Fig. 33.24 shows two such charts, the Bailey-Lovie chart and the Early Treatment of Diabetic Retinopathy Study (ETDRS) charts. The constant ratio (logarithmic) size scaling is based on the psychophysical principle that just-noticeable differences and their variability scale logarithmically.[65]

BOX 33.3 Chart design

Most contemporary charts incorporate some or all of the following design principles: the same number of letters on each line; a constant ratio from one letter size to the next (i.e., each line is a fixed percentage smaller than the previous line); spacing between letters and lines proportional to letter size, and nearly equal legibility the optotypes (or nearly equal average legibility at each letter size). Clinically, acuity can be measured with a variety of optotypes and charts. These include illiterate Es, Landolt Cs, and letters. Operationally, visual acuity charts come in several formats: printed, projected, and computer generated.

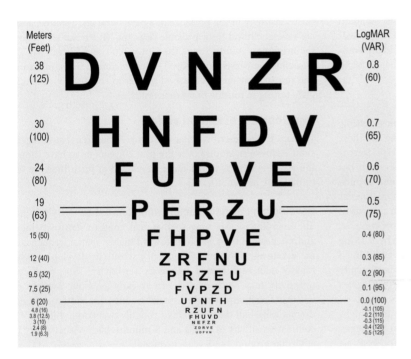

A

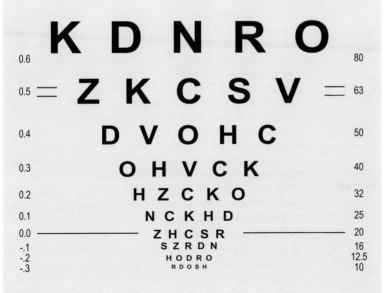

B

Fig. 33.24 The Bailey-Lovie chart (**A**) and the Early Treatment of Diabetic Retinopathy Study (ETDRS) charts (**B**). *MAR*, Minimum Angle of Resolution; *VAR*, xxx. (Courtesy of Dr. Ian Bailey.)

One impetus for using proportional spacing is the idea that letter spacing should be proportional to letter size to keep the effect of contour interaction consistent across acuity levels.[36] However, in peripheral vision[24] and in the central field of strabismic amblyopes, crowding[66] is a fixed spatial distance, not a fixed multiple of the target size.

Clinically, acuity can be measured with a variety of optotypes and charts. These include illiterate Es, Landolt Cs, and letters. One of the great advantages of using letters for measuring acuity is that the likelihood of randomly guessing the correct letter is low (~4% or 1 out of 26 if all the letters are used). Many charts used a reduced letter set, and for these the guess rate will be higher. For example, the ETDRS chart uses the Sloan letter set (C, D, H, K, N, O, R, S, V, Z), while the Bailey-Lovie chart uses the British letter set (D, E, F, H, N, P, R, U, V, Z). For both of these, the guess rate is 10% (1 out of 10). Operationally, visual acuity charts come in several formats: printed, projected, and computer generated.

There is a wide range of special methods for testing infants, toddlers, and others who have limited capacity to respond to standard acuity charts. These run the gamut from objective tests such as visual-evoked potentials (VEP), optokinetic nystagmus (OKN), and preferential looking (PL), often used for infants and discussed in Chapter 38, to symbol and picture charts.

Clinical tests for contrast sensitivity function

Contrast sensitivity is not routinely measured in the clinical setting; however, there are now several methods available for doing so. These include the Functional Acuity Contrast Test (FACT CS Test—Stereo-Optical Co) that replaced the original Vistech chart.[67] This chart has five different sinusoidal grating frequencies, each presented at nine contrast levels, allowing determination of the full CSF. A more popular approach is the Pelli-Robson CS chart[68] (Fig. 33.25), which consists of 16 "triplets" of letters. The letters in each triplet have the same contrast, with the contrast between successive triplets decreasing by 0.15 log units. Because the patient's task is to simply read the letters as far down the chart as they can, it is essentially identical to other visual acuity measures. What is different is that letter size is constant (0.5 degrees at 3 meters or 20/120) and contrast varies. There are also several conventional charts (varying letter size) that are available in both high- and low-contrast versions (e.g., the Bailey-Lovie chart and the Regan low-contrast chart). It should be noted that different clinical contrast sensitivity tests measure different aspects of vision. For example, the

Pelli-Robson test (fixed large letter size) provides information about the sensitivity near the peak of the CSF, whereas the low-contrast variable letter size tests (e.g., Bailey-Lovie and Regan charts) provide information about sensitivity along the high-frequency limb of the CSF (i.e., the smallest letter size that can be resolved at a fixed low contrast). Although contrast sensitivity testing provides useful information for clinical trials, assessing treatment outcomes, and so on, it is not clear how widely used it is in clinical practice. For example, fewer than 20% of eyecare practitioners who responded in a survey frequently or always measured contrast sensitivity in preoperative cataract patients.[69]

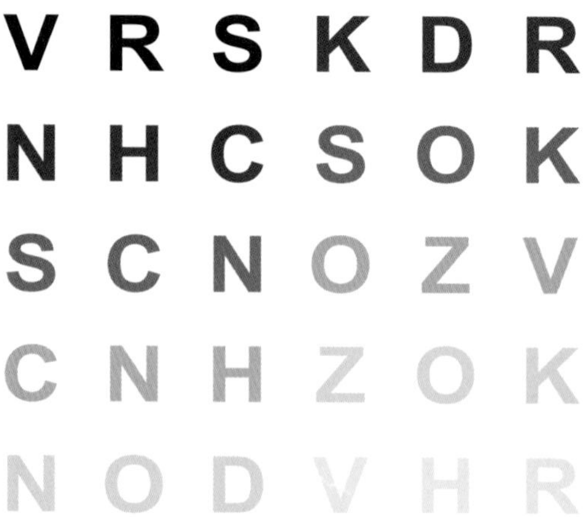

Glare

Glare—the effect of a bright or dazzling light source—can be uncomfortable and can lead to a loss of visual function (known as disability glare). Disability glare is a consequence of excessive light scatter that reduces the contrast of the retinal image. Clinically, disability glare can be estimated by measuring the reduction in visual acuity or contrast sensitivity in the presence of a peripheral glare source, and there are several clinical tests available (e.g., the Miller-Nadler Glare tester, the Brightness Acuity Tester, the Optec 3000, and Vistech MCT8000). Disability glare tests have proved useful in clinical trials (for example[70]) and research on aging (discussed further in chapter), but the utility of glare testing in routine practice is not clear.

Development of spatial vision

William James described infant vision as "a buzzing, blooming, confusion."[71] However, studies over the past 20 years or so have shown that the visual system is much more developed at birth than we used to think (see Chapter 38).

Development of visual acuity and contrast sensitivity function

The emerging picture suggests that peak contrast sensitivity increases, and the peak of the CSF shifts toward higher spatial frequencies with increasing age. Low spatial frequency sensitivity develops much more rapidly than high spatial frequency sensitivity. Thus, peak contrast sensitivity may reach adult levels as early as about 9 weeks of age, whereas sensitivity at higher spatial frequencies continues to develop dramatically, and there remains a roughly twentyfold difference in the contrast sensitivity of adults and 8-month-olds.[72] Visual acuity is only adult-like around 3 to 5 years postnatal.[73]

Development of hyperacuity

The early development of Vernier actually appears to be somewhat delayed, compared to resolution. Shimojo and coworkers[74,75] suggested that Vernier acuity is initially worse than grating acuity, and then shows a dramatic improvement (relative to grating acuity) between about 2 and 8 months. At 8 months, Vernier acuity was about twice as good as grating acuity. The Vernier acuity of very young infants remains controversial. However, the important point is that Vernier acuity and grating acuity reach adult levels of performance at different ages. The attainment of adult levels of hyperacuity—which is 6 to 10 times better than grating acuity—is delayed compared with resolution.

It is interesting to speculate why Vernier acuity has a slow, late development, reaching adult levels considerably later than resolution. If we consider that Vernier acuity is limited by the precision with which the brain "knows" the position of each afferent, then it is perhaps not so surprising that intrinsic positional uncertainty can only reach adult levels after retinal development is fully complete. The primary postnatal changes in the retina concern differentiation of the macular region.[73] After birth, foveal receptor density and cone outer segment length both increase as foveal cones become thinner and more elongated. There is a dramatic migration of ganglion cells and inner nuclear layers from

Fig. 33.25 The Pelli-Robson chart for measuring contrast sensitivity. (From Pelli DG, Robson JG, Wilkins AJ. The design of a new letter chart for measuring contrast sensitivity. *Clin Vision Sci.* 1988;2:187–199. Copyright Elsevier 1988.)

the foveal region, as the foveal pit develops during the first 4 months of life, and it is not until about 4 years of age that the fovea is fully adult-like.[76] From birth to beyond 4 years of age, cone density increases in the central region, owing both to migration of receptors and decreases in their dimensions. Both of these factors result in finer cone sampling (by decreasing the distance between neighboring cones). It is likely that alterations in cone spacing and the light-gathering properties of the cones during early development contribute a great deal toward the improvements in acuity and contrast sensitivity during the first months of life. The massive migration of retinal cells, and the alterations in the size of retina and eyeball (along with changes in interpupillary distance), may necessitate the plasticity of cortical connections early in life. It seems reasonable to speculate that the brain cannot "know" the positions of foveal cones with high levels of precision, until after these changes in the retina are complete. Interestingly, the peripheral retina appears to develop much more rapidly than the fovea.[76]

Visual acuity through the lifespan

Visual acuity reaches adult levels around 3 to 5 years of age, and remains rather constant until around 55 to 60 years of age, after which it begins to decline.[77] The decline is important because of the graying of the population of the United States. According to US Census 2000, 35 million Americans are 65 years and over (12.4% of the population). Those over 85 years are growing at roughly three times the rate of the general population—50,000 Americans are over 100 years old.

There are a number of reasons why one might expect visual function to decline with age. These include:

- Decreased pupil size, particularly in dim light
- Decreased lens transmission particularly, for short-wavelength (blue) light
- Increased intraocular light scattering.

All of these result in reduced retinal image contrast (particularly for small targets) and reduced retinal illumination. Thus, one might expect that visual performance is impaired most under low-contrast and low-light conditions, NOT the high-luminance and high-contrast conditions normally used to test visual acuity.

Until around 10 years ago, only high-contrast acuity was known in elders. However, the Smith-Kettlewell Institute (SKI) study, which has followed some 900 elderly persons from Marin County, California, over a period of about 7 years, suggests that high-contrast acuity greatly underestimates the loss of visual function in the elderly.[78] Fig. 33.26 shows this graphically by presenting the letter **m**, sized in proportion to the median acuity for four measures of visual acuity in 60- to 65-year-olds and in 85- to 90-year-olds.

For high-contrast, high-illumination targets, acuity is reduced by about a factor of 1.8 in the older group (i.e., the "m" must be about 1.8 times larger). Low-contrast acuity with glare is reduced by about a factor of three in the younger (60–65 years) group, but by almost a factor of seven in the older group. Although the SKI study population is probably not representative of the population at large (it is primarily white and well-educated with high socioeconomic status), it has important implications for understanding the visual problems of the elderly. Specifically, it shows that high-contrast visual acuity greatly underestimates the true age-related decline in vision, and that older persons with good standard visual acuity may be visually impaired under conditions of reduced contrast, reduced lighting, changing light level, or reduced contrast in the presence of glare.

Amblyopia

Amblyopia is a developmental disorder of spatial vision usually associated with the presence of strabismus, anisometropia, or form deprivation early in life (Box 33.4).[79] Amblyopia is clinically important because, aside from refractive error, it is the most frequent cause of vision loss in infants and young children,[80] and it is of basic interest because it reflects the neural impairment that can occur when normal visual development is disrupted. The damage produced by amblyopia is generally expressed in the clinical setting as a loss of visual acuity in an apparently healthy eye, despite appropriate optical correction; however, there is a great deal of evidence showing that amblyopia results in a broad range of neural, perceptual, and clinical abnormalities.[81–84] Currently there is no positive diagnostic test for amblyopia. Instead, amblyopia is diagnosed by exclusion: in patients with conditions such as strabismus and anisometropia, a diagnosis of amblyopia is made through exclusion of uncorrected refractive error and underlying ocular pathology.

In humans, amblyopia occurs naturally in about 2% to 4% of the population[79] and the presence of amblyopia is almost always associated with an early history of abnormal visual experience: binocular misregistration (strabismus), image degradation (high refractive error and astigmatism, anisometropia), or form deprivation (congenital cataract, ptosis). The severity of the amblyopia appears to be associated with the degree of imbalance between the two eyes (e.g., dense unilateral cataract results in severe loss), and to the age at which the amblyogenic factor occurred. Precisely how these factors interact is as yet unknown, but it is evident that different early visual experiences result in different functional losses in acuity and contrast sensitivity amblyopia[85] (Fig. 33.27), and a significant factor that distinguishes performance among amblyopes is the presence or absence of binocular function. Amblyopes who lack binocularity (primarily strabismic amblyopes) show much greater losses in Vernier and Snellen acuity than in grating resolution.[86,87]

Crowding and amblyopia

Extensive crowding occurs in the central field of strabismic amblyopes. As first reported by Irvine:[88] "single letters or direction of ... an E could be identified by the amblyopic eye, if viewed one letter at a

	Bright light high contrast	Bright light low contrast	Dim light low contrast	Glaring light low contrast
Age group (years)				
60–65	m	m	m	m
85–90	m	m	m	m

Fig. 33.26 The letter m sized in proportion to the median acuity for four measures of visual acuity in 60- to 65-year-olds and in 85- to 90-year-olds. (Haegerstrom-Portnoy G. The Glenn A Fry Award Lecture 2003: Vision in elders—summary of findings of the SKI study. *Optom Vis Sci.* 2005;82:87–93.)

BOX 33.4 Amblyopia

Amblyopia is a developmental disorder of spatial vision usually associated with the presence of strabismus, anisometropia, or form deprivation early in life.[79] Reduced visual acuity in an apparently healthy eye despite appropriate optical correction is the sine qua non of amblyopia. However, there is a great deal of evidence showing that amblyopia results in a broad range of neural, perceptual, and clinical abnormalities.

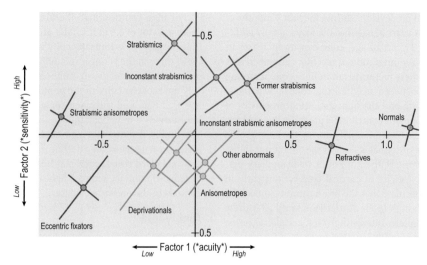

Fig. 33.27 Mean locations of the 11 clinically defined categories in the two-factor space. The diagonal bars show 1 standard error of the mean (SEM) measured along the principal axes of the elliptical distributions, which we use only as descriptive indicators of dispersion. (Mckee SP, Levi DM, Movshon JA. The pattern of visual deficits in amblyopia. *J Vis.* 2003;3:380–405.)

time, but when placed in conjunction with other letters in a line, confusion affected the interpretation." The ophthalmologist Hermann Burian noted that his orthoptist recorded better visual acuities in amblyopic patients than he did. The orthoptist used isolated letters to measure acuity, whereas he used letters arranged in a row.[89] The phenomenon of crowding in strabismic amblyopia has been repeatedly confirmed.[20,35,36,66,86,87,90–93]

Although the extent of crowding in the central field of amblyopic observers was originally thought to be proportional to the amblyope's uncrowded acuity, and similar to normal observers when the resolution deficit was taken into account,[36] the story seems to be a bit more complicated. Recent studies suggest that crowding is qualitatively different in strabismic and anisometropic amblyopes.[88,89] In anisometropic amblyopes, crowded acuity is proportional to the amblyope's uncrowded acuity, similar to normal vision with blur, whereas in strabismic amblyopes it is worse, often very much so, similar to normal peripheral vision.

REFERENCES

1. Wade NJ. Image, eye and retina (invited review). *J Opt Soc Am.* 2007;24:1229–1249.
2. Westheimer G. Visual acuity. In: Kaufman PL, Alm A, Adler FH, eds. *Adler's physiology of the eye: clinical application.* St. Louis, MO: CV Mosby; 2003:453–469.
3. Hecht S, Mintz EU. The visibility of single lines at various illuminations and the retinal basis of visual resolution. *J Gen Physiol.* 1939;22:593–612.
4. Frisén L, Frisén M. How good is normal visual acuity? A study of letter acuity thresholds as a function of age. *Albrecht Von Graefes Arch Klin Exp Ophthalmol.* 1981;215(3):149–157.
5. Snell AC, Sterling S. The percentage evaluation of macular vision. *Trans Am Ophthalmol Soc.* 1925;23:204–227.
6. Westheimer G. Visual hyperacuity. *Progress in Sensory Physiology.* Vol. 1. New York: Springer; 1981:1–30.
7. Klein SA, Levi DM. Hyperacuity thresholds of 1 second: Theoretical predictions and empirical validation. *J Opt Soc Am A.* 1985;2:1170–1190.
8. Geisler WS. Physical limits of acuity and hyperacuity. *J Opt Soc Am A.* 1984;1:775–782.
9. Lotze H. *Microcosmus: An essay concerning man and his relation to the world.* Edinburgh, Scotland: TT Clark,; 1885.
10. Levi DM, Tripathy SP. Localization of a peripheral patch: The role of blur and spatial frequency. *Vision Res.* 1996;36:3785–3803.
11. Liang J, Williams DR. Aberrations and retinal image quality of the normal human eye. *J Opt Soc Am A Opt Image Sci Vis.* 1997;14:2873–2883.
12. Kleinstein RN, et al. Uncorrected refractive error and distance visual acuity in children aged 6 to 14 years. *Optom Vis. Sci.* 2021;98(1):3–12.
13. Aubert H, Foerster K. Beitraege zur Kenntnisse der indirecten Sehens. *Graefes Archiv fur Ophthalmologie.* 1857;3:1–37.
14. Weymouth FW. Visual sensory units and the minimal angle of resolution. *Am J Ophthalmol.* 1958;46:102.
15. Levi DM, Klein SA, Aitsebaomo AP. Vernier acuity, crowding and cortical magnification. *Vision Res.* 1985;25:963–977.
16. Daniel PM, Whitteridge D. The representation of the visual field on the cerebral cortex in monkeys. *J Physiol.* 1961;159:203–221.
17. Peterson BB, Dacey DM. Morphology of human retinal ganglion cells with intraretinal axon collaterals. *Vis Neurosci.* 1998;15:377–387.
18. Polyak S. *The vertebrate visual system.* Chicago: University of Chicago Press; 1957.
19. Wässle H, Grünert U, Röhrenbeck J, Boycott BB. Cortical magnification factor and the ganglion cell density of the primate retina. *Nature.* 1989;341:643–646.
20. Azzopardi P, Cowey A. The overrepresentation of the fovea and adjacent retina in the striate cortex and dorsal lateral geniculate nucleus of the macaque monkey. *Neuroscience.* 1996;72:627–639.
21. Whitney D, Levi DM. Visual crowding: A fundamental limit on conscious perception and object recognition. *Trends In Cognitive Sciences.* 2011;15:160–168.
22. Strasburger H. Seven myths on crowding and peripheral vision. *Iperception.* 2020;11(3):1–46.
23. Tyler CW, Likova LT. Crowding: A neuroanalytic approach. *J Vision.* 2007;7:1–9.
24. Levi DM, Hariharan S, Klein SA. Suppressive and facilitatory spatial interactions in peripheral vision: Peripheral crowding is neither size invariant nor simple contrast masking. *J Vision.* 2002;2:167–177.
25. Tripathy SP, Cavanagh P. The extent of crowding in peripheral vision does not scale with target size. *Vision Res.* 2002;42:2357–2369.
26. Pelli DG, Palomares M, Majaj NJ. Crowding is unlike ordinary masking: Distinguishing feature integration from detection. *J Vision.* 2004;4:1136–1169.
27. Pelli DG, Tillman KA, Freeman J, Su M, Berger T, Majaj NJ. Crowding and eccentricity determine reading rate. *J Vision.* 2007;7(2):1–36.
28. Andriessen JJ, Bouma H. Eccentric vision: Adverse interactions between line segments. *Vision Res.* 1976;16:71–78.
29. Flom MC, Heath GG, Takahashi E. Contour interaction and visual resolution: Contralateral effect. *Science.* 1963;142:979–980.
30. Westheimer G, Hauske G. Temporal and spatial interference with Vernier acuity. *Vision Res.* 1975;15:1137–1141.
31. Kooi FL, Toet A, Tripathy SP, Levi DM. The effect of similarity and duration on spatial interaction in peripheral vision. *Spatial Vision.* 1994;8:255–279.
32. Tripathy SP, Levi DM. Long-range dichoptic interactions in the human visual cortex in the region corresponding to the blind spot. *Vision Res.* 1994;34:1127–1138.
33. Danilova MV, Bondarko VM. Foveal contour interactions and crowding effects at the resolution limit of the visual system. *J Vision.* 2007;7(2):25. 1–18.
34. Levi DM, Klein SA, Hariharan S. Suppressive and facilitatory spatial interactions in foveal vision: Foveal crowding is simple contrast masking. *J Vision.* 2002;2:140–166.
35. Hariharan S, Levi DM, Klein SA. "Crowding" in normal and amblyopic vision assessed with Gaussian and Gabor C's. *Vision Res.* 2005;45:617–633.

36. Flom MC, Weymouth FW, Kahneman D. Visual resolution and contour interaction. *J Opt Soc Am*. 1963;53:1026–1032.
37. Toet A, Levi DM. The two-dimensional shape of spatial interaction zones in the parafovea. *Vision Res*. 1992;32:1349–1357.
38. Coates DR, Levi DM, Touch P, Sabesan R. Foveal crowding resolved. *Scientific Reports*. 2018;8(1):9177. https://doi.org/10.1038/s41598-018-27480-4.
39. Shlaer S. The relation between visual acuity and illumination. *J Gen Physiol*. 1937;21:165–188.
40. Sloan LL. Variation of acuity with luminance in ocular diseases and anomalies. *Doc Ophthalmol*. 1969;26:384–393.
41. Geisler WS, Davila KD. Ideal discriminators in spatial vision: Two-point stimuli. *J Opt Soc of Am A*. 1985;2:1483–1497.
42. Waugh SJ, Levi DM. Visibility, luminance and Vernier acuity. *Vision Res*. 1993;33:527–538.
43. Ludvigh EJ. Effect of reduced contrast on visual acuity as measured with Snellen test letters. *Arch Ophthalmol*. 1941;25:469–474.
44. Herse PR, Bedell HE. Contrast sensitivity for letter and grating targets under various stimulus conditions. *Optom Vis Sci*. 1989;66:774–781.
45. Rabin J, Wicks J. Measuring resolution in the contrast domain: The small letter contrast test. *Optom Vis Sci*. 1996;73:398–403.
46. Johnson CA, Casson EJ. Effects of luminance, contrast, and blur on visual acuity. *Optom Vis Sci*. 1995;72:864–869.
47. Legge GE, Rubin GS, Luebker A. Psychophysics of reading—V. The role of contrast in normal vision. *Vision Res*. 1987;27:1165–1177.
48. Baron WS, Westheimer G. Visual acuity as a function of exposure duration. *J Opt Soc Am*. 1973;63:212–219.
49. Waugh SJ, Levi DM. Visibility, timing and Vernier acuity. *Vision Res*. 1993;33:505–526.
50. Hadani I, Meiri AZ, Guri M. The effects of exposure duration and luminance on the 3-dot hyperacuity task. *Vision Res*. 1984;24:871–874.
51. Matin L, Picoult E, Stevens JK, Edwards MW Jr, Young D, MacArthur R. Oculoparalytic illusion: Visual-field dependent spatial mislocalizations by humans partially paralyzed with curare. *Science*. 1982;216:198–201.
52. Keesey UT. Effects of involuntary eye movements on visual acuity. *J Opt Soc Am*. 1960;50:769–774.
53. Westheimer G, McKee SP. Visual acuity in the presence of retinal-image motion. *J Opt Soc Am*. 1975;65:847–850.
54. Levi DM. Pattern perception at high velocities. *Current Biol*. 1996;6:1020–1024.
55. Campbell FW, Green DG. Optical and retinal factors affecting visual resolution. *J Physiol*. 1965;181:576–593.
56. Mitchell DE, Freeman RD, Westheimer G. Effect of orientation on the modulation sensitivity for interference fringes on the retina. *J Opt Soc Am*. 1967;57:246–249.
57. Levi DM, Song S, Pelli DG. Amblyopic reading is crowded. *J Vision*. 2007;7(2):1–17.
58. Legge GE, Mansfield JS, Chung STL. Psychophysics of reading. XX. Linking letter recognition to reading speed in central and peripheral vision. *Vision Res*. 2001;41(6):725–743.
59. Yu D, Cheung S-H, Legge GE, Chung STL. Effect of letter spacing on visual span and reading speed. *J Vision*. 2007;7(2):1–10.
60. Legge GE, Cheung S-H, Yu D, Chung STL, Lee H-W, Owens DP. The case for the visual span as a sensory bottleneck in reading. *J Vision*. 2007;7(2):1–15.
61. Schade OH Sr. Optical and photoelectric analog of the eye. *J Opt Soc Am*. 1956;46:721–739.
62. Rovamo J, Virsu V, Näsänen R. Cortical magnification factor predicts the photopic contrast sensitivity of peripheral vision. *Nature*. 1978;271:54–56.
63. Robson JG, Graham N. Probability summation and regional variation in contrast sensitivity across the visual field. *Vision Res*. 1981;21:409–418.
64. Bailey IL, Lovie JE. New design principles for visual acuity letter charts. *Am J Optom Physiol Opt*. 1976;53:740–745.
65. Westheimer G. Scaling of visual acuity measurements. *Arch Ophthalmol*. 1979;97:327–330.
66. Levi DM, Hariharan S, Klein SA. Suppressive and facilitatory interactions in amblyopic vision. *Vision Res*. 2002;42:1379–1394.
67. Ginsburg AP. A new contrast sensitivity vision test chart. *Am J Optom Physiol Opt*. 1984;61:403–407.
68. Pelli DG, Robson JG, Wilkins AJ. The design of a new letter chart for measuring contrast sensitivity. *Clin Vis Sci*. 1988;2:187–199.
69. Bass EB, Steinberg EP, Luthra R, et al. Variation in ophthalmic testing prior to cataract surgery. Results of a national survey of optometrists. Cataract Patient Outcome Research Team. *Arch Ophthalmol*. 1995;113:27–31.
70. Chylack LT Jr, Wolfe JK, Friend J, et al. Validation of methods for the assessment of cataract progression in the Roche European-American Anticataract Trial (REACT). *Ophthalmic Epidemiol*. 1995;2:59–75.
71. James W. *Principles of psychology*. Henry Holt & Co. 1890. Republished. Cambridge, MA: Harvard University Press; 1981.
72. Norcia AM, Tyler CW, Hamer RD. Development of contrast sensitivity in the human infant. *Vision Res*. 1990;30:1475–1486.
73. Boothe RG, Dobson V, Teller DY. Postnatal development of vision in human and non-human primates. *Ann Rev Neurosci*. 1985;8:495–545.
74. Shimojo S, Birch EE, Gwiazda J, Held R. Development of Vernier acuity in infants. *Vision Res*. 1984;24:721–728.
75. Shimojo S, Held R. Vernier acuity is less than grating acuity in 2- and 3-month-olds. *Vision Res*. 1987;27:77–86.
76. Yuodelis C, Hendrickson A. A qualitative and quantitative analysis of the human fovea during development. *Vision Res*. 1986;26:847–855.
77. Hirsch MJ, Wick RE, eds. *Vision of the aging patient: An optometric symposium*. Philadelphia: Chilton Co; 1960.
78. Haegerstrom-Portnoy G. The Glenn A Fry Award Lecture 2003: Vision in elders—summary of findings of the SKI study. *Optom Vis Sci*. 2005;82:87–93.
79. Ciuffreda KJ, Levi DM, Selenow A. *Amblyopia: Basic and clinical aspects*. Boston: Butterworth-Heinemann; 1991.
80. Sachsenweger R. Problems of organic lesions in functional amblyopia. In: Arruga H, ed. International Strabismus Symposium. Basel: Karger, 1968.
81. Kiorpes L. Visual processing in amblyopia: Animal studies. *Strabismus*. 2006;14:3–10.
82. Levi DM. Visual processing in amblyopia: Human studies. *Strabismus*. 2006;14:11–19.
83. Barrett BT, Bradley A, McGraw PV. Understanding the neural basis of amblyopia. *Neuroscientist*. 2004;10:106–117.
84. Hess RF. Amblyopia: Site unseen. *Clin Exp Optom*. 2001;84:321–336.
85. Mckee SP, Levi DM, Movshon JA. The pattern of visual deficits in amblyopia. *J Vis*. 2003;3:380–405.
86. Levi DM, Klein SA. Hyperacuity and amblyopia. *Nature*. 1982;298:268–270.
87. Levi DM, Klein SA. Vernier acuity, crowding and amblyopia. *Vision Res*. 1985;25:979–991.
88. Irvine RS. Amblyopia Ex Anopsia. Observations on retinal inhibition, scotoma, projection, light difference discrimination and visual acuity. *Trans Am Ophthalmol Soc*. 1948;46:527–575.
89. Burian HM, von Noorden GK. *Binocular vision and ocular motility. Theory and management of strabismus*. St. Louis, Missouri: CV Mosby; 1974.
90. Bonneh YS, Sagi D, Polat U. Local and non-local deficits in amblyopia: Acuity and spatial interactions. *Vision Res*. 2004;44:3099–3110.
91. Song S., Pelli D.G., Levi D.M. *Three limits on letter identification by normal and amblyopic observers*. In preparation.
92. Hess RF, Jacobs RJ. A preliminary report of acuity and contour interactions across the amblyope's visual field. *Vision Res*. 1979;19:1403–1408.
93. Hess RF, Dakin SC, Tewfik M, Brown B. Contour interaction in amblyopia: Scale selection. *Vision Res*. 2001;41:2285–2296.

34

Color Vision

Jay Neitz, Katherine Mancuso, James A. Kuchenbecker, and Maureen Neitz

The ability to perceive color is a highly valued sensory capacity, and it has been a subject of experimental inquiry for over 200 years. Before the development of modern biological techniques, breakthroughs in color vision research stemmed from careful consideration of perceptual experiences. From color mixing and matching experiments, it was deduced that three different receptors in the eye, each maximally sensitive to a different region of the visible spectrum, were required to explain normal color vision. Thus, the three-component theory of Young and Helmholtz, as well as Hering's conflicting hypothesis of three paired, opponent color processes, were developed in the 1800s, long before the three types of retinal cone photopigment were isolated and characterized. It is now understood that normal, or trichromatic, color vision is mediated by three types of cone photoreceptor—designated short- (S), middle- (M), and long- (L) wavelength sensitive—the activities of which are, indeed, combined in later opponent organization to provide color perception. The first direct measurements of the absorption properties of primate cone photopigments occurred in the 1960s using a technique called microspectrophotometry. Since then, additional techniques, including electrophysiological recordings from individual cones and molecular genetics, have allowed the refinement of the spectral sensitivity curves for the S, M, and L pigments, shown in Fig. 34.1.

The fact that most humans have trichromatic color vision explains why computer monitors and televisions mix just three primary colors, red, green, and blue, to produce colors that match almost all those seen in the real world. Likewise, if humans were tetrachromatic, having four cone photopigments, televisions with four primaries would be required. The presence of three classes of cone photoreceptor also explains color blindness. That is, loss of function of each individual cone class is associated with an inherited form of color vision deficiency: protan defects involve loss of L-cone function, deutan defects with loss of M-cone function, and tritan defects with loss of S-cone function (Box 34.1). Each type of color vision defect results from rearrangements, deletions, or mutations in the genes encoding the corresponding L, M, or S photopigment. Color vision tests have been developed to detect changes in the cone complement. Observations that cannot be fully explained just by the presence of three types of cone photoreceptor, however, involve the appearance of color. The neural circuitry for color vision extracts signals from only three cone types and yet gives rise to six color percepts arranged in opponent pairs: blue-yellow, red-green, and black-white. These topics, including the molecular genetics of color vision deficiencies, tests of color vision, and the neural circuitry of color perception, are discussed in detail in the following sections.

MOLECULAR GENETICS OF COLOR VISION AND COLOR DEFICIENCIES

Although the tendency for color vision defects to run in families and to be more prevalent among men had long been recognized, a major advancement in understanding the biological basis of color vision and its defects came in 1986 when Jeremy Nathans and colleagues cloned and sequenced the genes encoding the S-, M-, and L-cone opsins and determined that the L- and M-opsin genes are in adjacent positions on the X-chromosome.[1,2] Further breakthroughs in understanding differences in the quality of color vision among individuals with anomalous trichromacy followed with identification of the amino acids involved in spectral tuning, which are responsible for the approximately 30 nm difference in peak sensitivity of the L and M pigments underlying normal color vision.[3,4]

Most inherited red-green color vision defects are caused by rearrangement and deletions of the L- and M-opsin genes on the X-chromosome that come about by meiotic recombination during oogenesis in females.[5,6] A dichromatic phenotype results in males who inherit an X-chromosome in which all but one of the opsin genes have been deleted. A protanopic type defect is characterized by the absence of L-opsin gene expression or function. A deuteranopic type defect is characterized by the lack of M-opsin gene expression or function (Box 34.2). Although humans often have more than just two opsin genes on the X-chromosome, only two are typically expressed, and these determine color vision phenotype. If meioic recombination creates an array in which the first two genes encode pigments with identical spectral properties, a male who inherits the array will be dichromatic, either protanopic or deuteranopic. However, a male with an array in which the first two genes encode opsins of the same class (M or L), but differ slightly in spectral sensitivities, will be an anomalous trichromat. He will be protanomalous if the genes encode two M-opsins or deuteranomalous if they encode two L-opsins. The extent of color vision loss in anomalous trichromats is determined by the degree of similarity in the spectral peaks of the two pigments.[7,8]

It has been assumed that the 30-nm spectral separation between the L and M pigments was optimized during evolution and that there is also an optimal ratio of L and M-cones. However, recent studies have shown that much smaller spectral separations between, and skewed proportions of, L and M-cones still provide robust red-green color vision. For example, observers do not show a reduction in color discrimination that can be reliably classified as just outside the normal range until the L/M separation is reduced to about 12 nm or less[6] and anomalous trichromats with spectral separations between pigments on the order of only 3 nm still have 10 times better red-green color vision

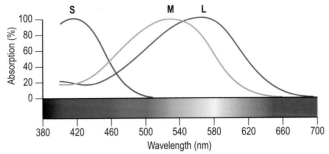

Fig. 34.1 Absorption spectra of the three types of cone photopigment, short- (S), middle- (M), and long- (L) wavelength sensitive. The S photopigment is maximally sensitive to wavelengths near 419 nm, the M pigment to wavelengths near 530 nm, and the L pigment to wavelengths near 560 nm. Neural comparison of the rates of quantal absorption by the three cone types gives rise to four unique hue percepts—blue, yellow, red, and green—and hundreds of intermediate colors in the visible spectrum. Outputs of the L- and M-cones are used together by our visual system to mediate black and white percepts.

BOX 34.1 Nomenclature for inherited color vision deficiencies

Protan defects are the least common form of red-green color vision defects affecting about 2% of males in the US. There are two categories: dichromatic (protanopia) and anomalous trichromatic (protanomaly), each affecting about 1% of males. The severity of protan defects varies over a relatively narrow range. Protan comes from the Greek root for "the first." S-cones and M-cones mediate protan color vision.

Deutan defects are the most common form of red-green color vision defects, affecting about 6% of males in the United States. There are two categories: dichromatic (deuteranopia) and anomalous trichromatic (deuteranomaly). Deuteranomaly and deuteranopia affect about 5% and about 1% of males, respectively. The severity of deutan defects varies over a relatively broad range, from nearly normal to moderately red-green deficient. Deutan comes from the Greek root for "the second." S-cones and L-cones mediate deutan color vision.

Tritan defects are relatively rare and are characterized by impaired blue-yellow color vision. Tritan defects are autosomal dominant, and they display "incomplete penetrance," meaning there is variability in the degree to which color vision is impaired among individuals with the same underlying gene defect, even within a family. Tritan defects are also "acquired," meaning they are not usually present from birth. Both of these observations are explained by the degenerative nature of tritan defects. Inheriting one mutant copy of the S-opsin gene causes the S-cones to degenerate. However, the cones function early in life because they express normal S-opsin from a normal copy of the gene.

BOX 34.2 Visual pigments, cone opsins, and official gene designations

Visual pigments, also known as photopigments, are composed of an apoprotein and an 11-*cis* retinal chromophore. The genes OPN1LW, OPN1MW, and OPN1SW each encode an apoprotein (termed opsin). The chromophore is a vitamin A derivative that absorbs ultraviolet light; when covalently bound to an opsin, the chromophore absorption spectrum is shifted to longer wavelengths. Amino acid differences among the opsins are responsible for the differences in the absorption spectra of the three cone classes (Fig. 34.1). Within the L and M classes, variations or polymorphisms in the amino acid sequences produce relatively small spectral shifts, giving rise to L and M photopigment variants.

- OPN1MW: middle wavelength-sensitive cone opsin, expressed in M-cones, commonly referred to as "green" cones. OPN1MW is on the X-chromosome at location Xq28. Deutan defects are most commonly associated with the absence or lack of expression of the OPN1MW gene(s).
- OPN1LW: long wavelength-sensitive cone opsin, expressed in L-cones, commonly referred to as "red" cones. OPN1LW is on the X-chromosome at location Xq28 adjacent to OPN1MW. Protan defects are most commonly associated with the absence or lack of expression of the OPN1LW gene(s).
- OPN1SW: short wavelength-sensitive cone opsin, expressed in S-cones, commonly referred to as "blue" cones. OPN1SW is on chromosome 7 at 7q32.1. Tritan defects are caused by a missense mutation in one copy of the OPN1SW gene. A missense mutation is a change in a gene's amino acid coding sequence that substitutes one amino acid for another in the encoded protein.

Inherited blue-yellow color vision, or tritan, defects are considerably more rare than red-green defects. They are caused by mutations in the S-opsin gene,[13–16] and are inherited in an autosomal-dominant fashion, meaning that an individual who is heterozygous for an S-opsin gene mutation will often exhibit the phenotype. Evidence from adaptive optics imaging of tritan subjects indicates that the defect is an S-cone dystrophy, similar to the rod dystrophy caused by heterozygous mutations in the rod pigment rhodopsin in retinitis pigmentosa.[16] Tritan defects are said to be incompletely penetrant, meaning that not everyone with an S-opsin gene defect exhibits the phenotype, but this is due to a progressive loss of S-cones, which must reach a critical threshold before the phenotype is manifested.

TESTS OF COLOR VISION

As described in the previous section, color vision defects result from genetic changes responsible for either the alteration or loss of cone photopigments. Because color vision is based on neural comparisons between different classes of cone photoreceptor, both the loss of a photopigment type and changes in the peak sensitivity of a photopigment such that there is a reduction in the differential responses of the two cone classes will result in a reduced ability to distinguish colors.

Pseudoisochromatic plate tests are perhaps the most familiar tool for diagnosing color vision deficiencies. Popular examples include Ishihara's test of color vision and the Hardy, Rand, and Rittler (HRR) pseudoisochromatic plates. The plates consist of printed pages with dots of various colors and shades of gray, each containing a colored symbol(s) that is visible to individuals with normal color vision but invisible to those with certain color vision defects. Subjects are asked to identify the symbols. The specific pattern of errors in a test allows for diagnosis of the likely presence or absence of a color vision defect and an indication of the type and severity for some tests.

A fundamentally different testing strategy is used with arrangement tests, in which subjects are asked to arrange a series of colored

than the corresponding dichromat. Such anomalous trichromats can discern primary colors in their environment and perform basic color vision tasks.[9] Another surprising finding occurred with the development of adaptive optics, a technique that allows visualization of the cone photoreceptor mosaic in living humans. Selective bleaching combined with adaptive optics imaging allowed identification of the different cone types and revealed that individuals with normal color vision have roughly the same number and arrangement of S-cones, but there is tremendous variation in the ratios of L- and M-cones.[10,11] This was startling in light of the widely held belief that the quality of red-green color vision would be affected by extreme cone ratios. Instead, because normal color vision has low spatial resolution, it can be adequately served by a sparse mosaic of one of the cone types.[12]

discs "in order" so that each disc is placed adjacent to the discs that are most similar in color appearance. Misordering of the discs allows a diagnosis of the presence or absence of a color vision defect. Examples of arrangement tests are the Farnsworth-Munsell 100 Hue Test which involves arranging 85 discs (not 100 as the name suggests), and the much more practical Farnsworth-Munsell Dichotomous D-15 Test, which was designed to use the arrangement of 12 discs to separate strongly color deficient individuals from those with milder color vision deficiencies or normal color vision.

The Rayleigh color match is often referred to as the "gold standard" for color vision testing. It is performed on the anomaloscope, an instrument that contains an optical system that produces two side-by-side lighted fields. One field, the "test light," is a monochromatic amber color, and the other is a mixture of red and green light. The person being tested adjusts the ratio of red-to-green light in the mixture until it exactly matches the amber test light. Setting a match with a higher or lower ratio of red-to-green light compared with the match made by a person with normal color vision is diagnostic of an inherited color vision abnormality caused by a shift in the spectral peak of either the L or M pigment. This test is extraordinarily sensitive and can detect genetically specified alterations in the spectral sensitivities of the photopigments, even in subjects in whom the alteration in the photopigment has little or no effect on the person's ability to discriminate between different colors. Its extreme sensitivity in detecting the presence of anomalous photopigments is why the anomaloscope has been widely adopted as the "gold standard." However, it must be emphasized that mild photopigment abnormalities may be associated with little loss in color discrimination ability. Even with shifted visual pigments, the quality of color vision may still be quite good.[9]

Each of the widely used color vision tests has its distinct advantages and is considered to be best under different circumstances. Because of this, for general diagnosis of color vision defects, the results from a battery of tests can provide the most complete picture from which to make a differential diagnosis. Ideally, for diagnosis of color vision defects one should obtain information on the "type" of problem. Is it a red-green or blue-yellow deficiency or mixed? If it is red-green, is it a "protan" or "deutan" defect? Is it a genetic disorder, or is it caused by damage to the visual system by disease or injury? The test should also provide information about severity. Does the person have dichromatic color vision or a milder "anomalous" form of deficiency? If

it is an anomalous form, is it very mild, mild, or moderate? Under some conditions, it is impractical to administer a battery of tests. Cole et al.[17] recommended the fourth edition of the Richmond HRR Pseudoisochromatic test as the "one of choice for clinicians who wish to use a single test for color vision." It has plates for detecting protan, deutan, and tritan defects, and its classification of mild, medium, and strong categories for deutan and protan defects is useful. Still, the HRR is not perfect at distinguishing dichromats from anomalous trichromats. The anomaloscope in the hands of a skilled practitioner is better at separating dichromats from anomalous trichromats, but it is not widely available. Administering the D-15 in conjunction with a pseudoisochromatic plate test can be helpful in discriminating dichromats from anomalous trichromats.

Genetic testing is the most reliable means of distinguishing acquired color vision defects from inherited color vision defects. Presently, genetic tests are not commercially available; however, the technology exists to perform such tests because the molecular genetics of inherited color vision defects is well understood, as described in the previous section.

COLOR APPEARANCE

The neural circuitry for color vision receives input from only three cone types (Fig. 34.2) and yet gives rise to six hue percepts arranged in opponent pairs: blue-yellow, red-green, and black-white. The orthodox view has been that for blue-yellow opponency, signals from S-cones are combined antagonistically with an additive signal from M- and L-cones, abbreviated as S-(M+L); and for red-green opponency, signals from L-cones are combined antagonistically with those from M-cones (abbreviated as L-M). However, color vision testing in humans has established that the spectral signatures of hue perception actually involve neurons that receive contributions from all three cone types combined in the following manner: blue = (S+M)-L; yellow = L-(S+M); red = (S+L)-M; and green = M-(S+L). Therefore, although much progress has been made in identifying neurons in the visual system with color opponent responses, those matching the spectral signatures of human perception remain to be found. Results from molecular biology have shed new light on the evolution of primate color vision, imposing constraints on the possibilities for the underlying circuitry. Evolutionary constraints coupled with recent observations from

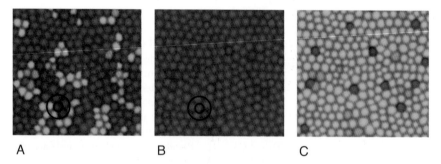

A   B   C

Fig. 34.2 **(A)** Illustration of the arrangement of the three cone classes in a trichromat. S-cones (*colored blue*) represent a minority, approximately 6% of the total, and are roughly evenly spaced across the retinal mosaic. The arrangement of L-cones (*colored red*) and M-cones (*colored green*) is very close to random for trichromats. Midget ganglion cells have center-surround receptive fields with the center derived from a single cone (for example, within the inner ring of the two concentric circles). The six adjacent cones are the most important contributors to the surround (enclosed by the outer ring). Midget ganglion cells with single cone centers usually have mixed L- and M-cone surrounds. **(B)** Arrangement of cones in a deuteranope, a dichromat with only two different cone classes, L and S. In a dichromat, all the cones in the surround are of the same class as the center input to a midget ganglion cell. **(C)** Arrangement of cones in a protanope, a dichromat with only M- and S-cones.

human subjects with a retinal circuitry deficit are leading toward a new understanding of the color vision circuits.

Blue-yellow circuitry

To understand the neural operations responsible for transforming the cone signals into perception, it is helpful to consider reduced color vision systems with fewer cone types and fewer fundamental sensations. S-cones are an evolutionarily ancient photoreceptor type, and blue-yellow color vision appears to be the ancestor from which all other color vision evolved. Our dichromatic primate ancestors had two types of cone: short- and long-wavelength sensitive. Presumably, they also had similar circuits underlying their vision as modern-day dichromats, including a high-acuity spatial vision circuit served by the midget ganglion cell system (introduced in Chapter 21), in addition to the blue-yellow color vision circuit.

It is not completely clear which ganglion cell subtypes are specialized for carrying information corresponding to blue-yellow color vision. In primates, the S-cones have only two significant output pathways described thus far (Fig. 34.3, left). One pathway is the straight-through output to bipolar cells. S-cone ON bipolar cells, in turn, output to the *small bistratified ganglion cells*, which transmit a "blue-on" signal to the brain.[18] The second pathway from S-cones occurs through H2 horizontal cells,[19–21] which then output to *midget ganglion cells* via midget bipolar cells; however, the physiologic role of this anatomical connection has remained unclear. Historically, the small bistratified ganglion cells have been viewed as the primary candidate to serve as a neural substrate for blue-yellow color vision. However, a recent assessment of human subjects with a genetic mutation that renders the ON bipolar pathways inactive casts doubt on the role of small bistratified cells in blue perception. Specifically, the mutation occurs in the metabotropic glutamate receptor expressed on the ON bipolar cells, and clinically, these subjects present with congenital stationary night blindness (CSNB)[22] (Box 34.3). If small bistratified cells were the physiologic substrate for blue perception, with no input from the S-cone ON-bipolars, CSNB patients would be expected to have a tritan color vision defect. However, standard tests indicate that they have normal, trichromatic color vision. Although the visual mechanisms associated with this ON-pathway deficit require further inquiry, these results suggest that blue perceptions are mediated by a separate pathway, leading us to consider the possible role of the second anatomical S-cone output, via H2 horizontal cells, to the midget ganglion cell pathway.

In the region of the primate retina that serves the highest visual acuity, the fovea, 80% to 90% of ganglion cells are of the "midget" variety, so-called because of their small dendritic arbors, which in the central 7 to 10 degrees connect to a single cone via a "midget" bipolar cell. There are two types of midget ganglion cells, ON and OFF center, which receive input through a corresponding pair of ON and OFF midget bipolar cells, which have opposite responses to the neurotransmitter, glutamate, released by cones (Chapters 22 and 23). In a dichromatic ancestor to humans that had only S- and L-cones, about 94% of the cones were L. Thus, the midget ganglion cell system's primary function was to compare absorptions of S- vs. L-cones to provide achromatic luminance signals (Fig. 34.2B), presumably giving rise to white percepts through the ON pathway and black percepts through the OFF pathway (Fig. 34.3, top right). Because S-cones are sparse and roughly evenly spaced across the retina, and the signal strength to neighboring cones falls off exponentially with distance, only a small number of midget ganglion cells would receive significant input from S-cones from H2 horizontal cells, providing a possible substrate for L- vs. S-cone comparisons required for blue-yellow opponency (Fig. 34.3, top left).

Red-green circuitry

The idea that midget ganglion cells with S-cone input from H2 horizontal cells may serve as a substrate for blue-yellow perception seems plausible when considering the effects produced when the third type of cone was added during evolution.[23] Results from molecular genetics indicate that trichromatic color vision arose recently from a gene duplication event that added M-cones. For this low-probability genetic event to get passed on and eventually confer routine trichromacy to Old World primates, including humans, it must have produced an immediate advantage for the primate ancestor by adapting a pre-existing visual circuit for a new dimension of red-green color vision. In ancestral primates with only S- and L-cones, the small bistratified ganglion cell circuitry would have been little affected in its spectral response characteristics by the addition of M-cones (Fig. 34.3, bottom left). The center would remain unaltered owing to the S-cone-specific connections made by small bistratified cells, and the surround would be transformed from "L'" to "L+M." Thus, the simple addition of a third cone type would not "split" this ganglion cell class into two spectral types, one for blue-yellow and one for red-green color vision, as required by the evolutionary constraint that an immediate advantage was produced.

In contrast, when M-cones were randomly added to the pre-existing midget system, the small subset of spectrally opponent midget ganglion cells would have automatically become segregated into two different classes. The center of the receptive field would have become either "L" or "M," making an M-center, L-surround opponent type and an L-center, M-surround opponent type. A subset of midget bipolar cells would receive S-cone opponent input, making M-ON-center midget ganglion cells (M-S)-L-cone opponent and L-ON-center midget ganglion cells (L-S)-M-cone opponent. The S-cone opponent input to the corresponding OFF midget ganglion cells makes them (S-M)+L and (S-L)+M. Thus, midget ganglion cells with S-cone input and M-cone centers would exist as an OFF-ON pair for red-green color vision. Midget ganglion cells with S-cone input and L-cone centers would exist as an OFF-ON pair for blue-yellow color vision (Fig. 34.3, inset).

In summary, it is plausible that midget ganglion cells receiving S-cone opponent input via H2 horizontal cells may provide the physiologic substrate giving rise to hue circuits. The cone forming the receptive field center can be either L or M and the ganglion cells can be either ON or OFF center. The resulting four possible combinations would correspond to the known spectral signatures of the four main hue percepts of trichromats. M-ON-center midget ganglion cells with S-cone input and L-cones in the surround would be M-(S+L) for green percepts; this same receptive field through an OFF-center ganglion cell produces (S+L)-M for red percepts. An L-cone center with S-cone input and an M-cone surround would result in L-(S+M) for yellow percepts; this same receptive field through an OFF-center ganglion cell produces (S+M)-L for blue percepts.

Black-white circuitry

A remaining unresolved mystery in color vision is that the addition of a randomly distributed long-to-middle wavelength-sensitive cone type during primate evolution causes almost every midget ganglion cell in the retina to respond to spatially uniform red or green lights in addition to dark-light edges. The midgets are the only ganglion cells in the retina with high enough spatial density and small enough receptive fields to explain human high-acuity black-and-white spatial vision. They are also the only ganglion cells in the retina with L vs. M spectral opponency required to explain color vision. Thus, midget ganglion cells must do "double duty," serving both high-acuity

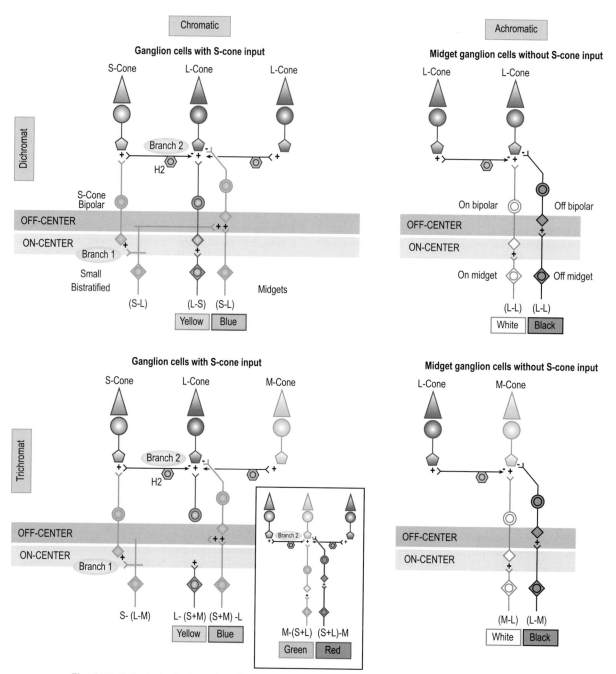

Fig. 34.3 Retinal circuits based on known anatomical connections that would give rise to signals matching the spectral signatures of human perception following the addition of a third cone type. The top two figures represent the circuitry for a dichromatic primate ancestor to modern humans with only two cone types, S and L. "Branch 1" indicates the straight-through S-cone output via an S-cone bipolar cell to the *small bistratified ganglion cell pathway*; "branch 2" is a second known anatomical connection that may provide S-cone opponent signals to the *midget ganglion cell center* via H2 horizontal cells (see text). Most midget ganglion cells in the dichromat with S- and L-cones (but no M-cones) compare L-cone centers to L-cone surrounds, mediating achromatic, black-and-white vision (*top right*). The bottom two panels show how the cone inputs to retinal circuits were changed with the addition of a third cone type (M-cones) when trichromatic color vision evolved. The addition of M-cones to a dichromat only changes the "surrounds" of small bistratified ganglion cell receptive fields. They would continue to have similar spectral response properties, making them an unlikely substrate for red, green, blue, and yellow hue sensations. In contrast, the addition of M-cones split the pre-existing blue-yellow midget circuit into two organizations with distinct spectral response properties, one with L-cone centers for blue-yellow and one with M-cone centers for red-green color vision (*inset*). Midget ganglion cells in trichromats without S-cone inputs (*bottom right*) respond to diffuse red or green lights and dark-light edges. L-ON and M-ON midget ganglion cells both respond to white, making their responses highly correlated, and thus their signals would be combined in the cortex. L-OFF and M-OFF signals would be similarly combined, providing the substrate for black and white perception.

BOX 34.3 Congenital stationary night blindness

The two types of photoreceptor in the human eye, rods and cones serve different functions. Rods provide vision only under very low light levels, such as when little light is available at night. In contrast, cones serve color and black-and-white vision at relatively higher light levels, such as daylight and standard indoor lighting.

Whereas cones synapse with both ON and OFF bipolar cells, the rods synapse with only ON-type bipolar cells. The dendrites of ON bipolar cells express a metabotropic glutamate receptor, mGluR6, and mutations in this receptor result in ON-pathway deficit. Curiously, while rod-mediated vision is severely compromised in congenital stationary night blindness (CSNB) patients, producing loss of nocturnal vision, cone-mediated vision appears to be unaffected even though direct signaling between cones and ON bipolar cells is disrupted.

black-and-white vision and color vision. L- and M-cones are about 94% of the cone population, while just about 6% of cones are S-cones. However, red-green and blue-yellow color vision have similar acuities indicating that only a subset of L/M spectrally opponent ganglion cells contribute to hue perception, whereas the preponderance of L/M opponent midget ganglion cells are used for high-acuity dark-light detection. This idea is plausible considering recordings from neurons in the primary visual cortex (V1) which receive direct input from the axons in the lateral geniculate nucleus (LGN) that relay signals from midget ganglion cells in the retina. Most V1 neurons respond well to achromatic (dark-light) modulation but not chromatic (color) modulation. In contrast, about 5% to 10% of neurons in V1 respond robustly to purely chromatic modulation and little, if at all, to achromatic modulation[24] (Fig. 34.3, bottom right). Thus, the outputs of the midget ganglion cells are somehow split to form a large population of cortical cells that respond well to black-white edges responsible for high-acuity achromatic vision and a second smaller population of color cells that do not respond to black-and-white. S-cone input (described previously) that produces midget ganglion cells corresponding to the known spectral signatures of trichromats' four main hue percepts may explain how this happens.

For the small population of midget ganglion cells that receive S-cone input from H2 horizontal cells, the S-cone input is always opposite in sign to L- or M-cone center. An S- vs. L- or S- vs. M-cone center will not respond to white light because white contains short, middle, and long wavelengths that stimulate S-, M-, and L-cones equally. Equal stimulation of S- and L-cones or S- and M-cones by white light will cancel the response of S- vs. M- and S- vs. L-center midget ganglion cells. The four versions of such cell centers, S-M, S-L, M-S, and L-S, will all have L+M surrounds. The centers and surrounds are balanced so that when there is an M-cone in the center, M-cone input in the surround cancels a fraction of that in the center, and a fraction of the L-cone center cancels the L-cone input in the surround. Thus, as introduced in the previous section, according to this hypothesis, midget ganglion cells with S-cone inputs are of four types (S-M)+L, (S-L)+M, (M-S)-L, and (L-S)-M. They are tuned to respond to distinct but overlapping regions of the spectrum and mediate the hues of red, blue, green, and yellow, respectively, but they do not respond to black or white. A theory of cortical wiring, originated by Donald Hebb,[25] is often summarized as "Cells that fire together wire together." M vs. L midget ganglion cells without S-cone input respond strongly to black-white edges. M-ON and L-ON midget ganglion cells are excited by white and inhibited by black; being highly correlated in their responses, neurons carrying their signals are likely to be wired together in the cortex, as will neurons carrying midget cell M-OFF and L-OFF signals. So wired, these

could correspond to the achromatic neurons in V1. Because they do not respond to black or white, neurons with S-cone inputs carrying hue signals to the cortex would not be correlated to each other or the achromatic neurons. Thus, they would not "wire together" but instead form separate classes of cortical neurons responsible for color vision. Accordingly, only the small subset of midget ganglion cells receiving input from all three cone types would pass hue signals to higher cortical levels (Fig. 34.3, bottom left), and M versus L midget ganglion cells that respond to black and white edges are responsible for high-acuity vision and percepts of black and white.

FUTURE DIRECTIONS

Much has been learned about the neural types and their interconnections in the retina responsible for luminance and color. There is a growing body of information about the higher visual centers; yet, how these ultimately operate to provide vision remains a fascinating puzzle. Many clues have come from information about the evolution of the visual system[23] and about its anatomy and physiology, and continued progress will undoubtedly arise from rapidly emerging technologies. One such example has resulted from the development of viral vector-mediated gene therapy to address human visual disorders. Using recombinant adenoassociated virus containing cone-specific promoter elements, it is possible to target transgene expression to subclasses of mammalian cone, including in primates.[26] Introducing new cone photopigments into animal models with reduced color vision provides an experimental tool for probing the neural circuitry for color vision and understanding the evolutionary requirements for developing a new dimension of red-green color vision.

There is currently no cure for red-green color vision deficiency. However, in most cases, the cone photoreceptors are healthy and viable, and viral-mediated gene therapy is feasible for delivering the missing cone-opsin gene to photoreceptors to rescue the deficit. The successful gene therapy for color blindness in primates[26] indicates that the neural circuitry required for taking advantage of a third cone type is present in dichromatic individuals, as was the case in dichromatic primate ancestors. Thus, gene therapy holds promise for providing red-green color-blind adults with full trichromatic color vision.

REFERENCES

1. Nathans J, Thomas D, Hogness DS. Molecular genetics of human color vision: The genes encoding blue, green, and red pigments. *Science*. 1986;232:193–202.
2. Nathans J, Piantanida TP, Eddy RL, Shows TB, Hogness DS. Molecular genetics of inherited variation in human color vision. *Science*. 1986;232:203–210.
3. Neitz M, Neitz J, Jacobs GH. Spectral tuning of pigments underlying red-green color vision. *Science*. 1991;252:971–974.
4. Asenjo AB, Rim J, Oprian DD. Molecular determinants of human red/green color discrimination. *Neuron*. 1994;12:1131–1138.
5. Neitz J, Neitz M. The genetics of normal and defective color vision. *Vision Research*. 2011;51(7):633–651.
6. Davidoff C, Neitz M, Neitz J. Genetic testing as a new standard for clinical diagnosis of color vision deficiencies. *Translational vision science & technology*. 2016;5(5):2.
7. Neitz J, Neitz M, Kainz PM. Visual pigment gene structure and the severity of human color vision defects. *Science*. 1996;274:801–804.
8. Sharpe LT, Stockman A, Jägle H, et al. Red, green, and red-green hybrid pigments in the human retina: Correlations between deduced protein sequences and psychophysically measured spectral sensitivities. *Journal of Neuroscience*. 1998;18:10053–10069.
9. Rezeanu D, Barborek R, Neitz M, Neitz J. Potential value of color vision aids for varying degrees of color vision deficiency. *Opt Express*. 2022;30(6):8857–8875.
10. Roorda A, Williams DR. The arrangement of the three cone classes in the living human eye. *Nature*. 1999;397:520–522.
11. Hofer H, Carroll J, Neitz J, Neitz M, Williams DR. Organization of the human trichromatic cone mosaic. *Journal of Neuroscience*. 2005;25(42):9669–9679.
12. Neitz A, Jiang X, Kuchenbecker JA, et al. Effect of cone spectral topography on chromatic detection sensitivity. *J Opt Soc Am A Opt Image Sci Vis*. 2020;37(4):A244–A254.
13. Weitz CJ, Miyake Y, Shinzato K, et al. Human tritanopia associated with two amino acid substitutions in the blue sensitive opsin. *American Journal of Human Genetics*. 1992;50:498–507.

14. Weitz CJ, Went LN, Nathans J. Human tritanopia associated with a third amino acid substitution in the blue sensitive visual pigment. *American Journal of Human Genetics*. 1992;51:444–446.

15. Gunther KL, Neitz J, Neitz M. A novel mutation in the short-wavelength sensitive cone pigment gene associated with a tritan color vision defect. *Visual Neuroscience*. 2006;23: 403–409.

16. Baraas RC, Carroll J, Gunther KL, et al. Adaptive optics retinal imaging reveals S-cone dystrophy in tritan color-vision deficiency. *Journal of the Optical Society of America A*. 2007;24:1438–1447.

17. Cole BL, Lian K-Y, Lakkis C. The new Richmond HRR pseudoisochromatic test of colour vision is better than the Ishihara test. *Clinical and Experimental Optometry*. 2006;89:73–80.

18. Dacey DM, Lee BB. The blue-ON opponent pathway in primate retina originates from a distinct bistratified ganglion cell type. *Nature*. 1994;367:731–735.

19. Dacey DM, Lee BB, Stafford DK, Pokorny J, Smith VC. Horizontal cells of the primate retina: Cone specificity without spectral opponency. *Science*. 1996;271:656–659.

20. Puller C, Haverkamp S, Neitz M, Neitz J. Synaptic elements for GABAergic feed-forward signaling between HII horizontal cells and blue cone bipolar cells are enriched beneath primate S-cones. *PloS One*. 2014;9(2):e88963.

21. Puller C, Manookin MB, Neitz M, Neitz J. Specialized synaptic pathway for chromatic signals beneath S-cone photoreceptors is common to human, Old and New World primates. *Journal of the Optical Society of America*. 2014;31(4):A189–A194.

22. Dryja TP, McGee TL, Berson EL, et al. Night blindness and abnormal cone electroretinogram ON responses in patients with mutations in the GRM6 gene encoding mGluR6. *Proceedings of the National Academy of Sciences of the United States of America*. 2005;102(13):4884-4889.

23. Neitz J, Neitz M. Evolution of the circuitry for conscious color vision in primates. *Eye*. 2017; 31(2):286–300.

24. Solomon SG, Lennie P. The machinery of colour vision. *Nature Reviews Neuroscience*. 2007; 8(4):276–286.

25. Hebb D. Organization of behavior. New York: Wiley. *J Clin Psychol*. 1949;6(3):335–307.

26. Mancuso K, Hauswirth WW, Li Q, et al. Gene therapy for red-green colour blindness in adult primates. *Nature*. 2009;461:784–787.

35

The Visual Field

Chris A. Johnson and Michael Wall

INTRODUCTION AND HISTORICAL BACKGROUND

Perimetry and visual field testing have been used as diagnostic procedures for evaluation of visual function for approximately 200 years. A historical review of these techniques may be found in several publications,[1–5] with the onset of visual field testing occurring more than 2000 years ago.[6] Particularly within recent times, a variety of new techniques for performing tests and interpreting results have been developed, but the primary method of assessing the visual field has been the detection of a small white stimulus superimposed on a uniform white background. Perimetry is used clinically to detect functional losses produced by pathology to the visual pathways, to provide differential diagnostic information concerning the location of a visual deficit, to monitor the status of the visual field over time to determine the efficacy of treatment and the stability of vision impairment, and to evaluate the condition of visual mechanisms subserving the peripheral visual fields. Recent enhancements of the test and analysis procedures have made it possible to automate the techniques, standardize the methodology, perform sophisticated statistical and mathematical evaluation of results, and allow rapid exchange of information among clinical sites.

In this chapter the psychophysical basis for visual field testing is discussed and an overview of the various forms of visual field testing that are available is provided. In addition, guidelines for interpretation of visual field results are presented, and determinations of the pattern, shape, and location of visual field losses are reported. A presentation of artifactual test results and how to avoid them is offered and methods of assessing progression and improvement of visual fields over time are evaluated. The chapter also provides a set of recommendations for clinical visual field testing, and introduces new methods of performing portable, accurate visual field testing in a variety of settings using tablets and virtual reality headsets. It is hoped that the reader will find this information helpful and be able to incorporate these techniques into their daily clinical regimen.

THE PSYCHOPHYSICAL BASIS FOR PERIMETRY AND VISUAL FIELD TESTING

The most common form of perimetric testing is performed monocularly with the fellow eye occluded. The patient's task is to detect a small white target stimulus briefly superimposed on a uniform background luminance at different visual field locations to determine the minimum increment of light needed to detect the stimulus (the differential light threshold or increment threshold), often referred to as Weber's law ($L/L = C$, where L is the background luminance, ΔL is the increment of light, and C is a constant).[7] Light sensitivity, the reciprocal of threshold, is presented either as the size and intensity of the stimulus that could be just noticeably detected at a particular visual field location for manual testing, or as a decibel (dB) value in automated perimetry, where 0 dB represents the maximum intensity that can be achieved by the device, and higher dB values indicating lower intensities on a log scale times 10 (inverse log scale). The dynamic range of an automated perimeter is typically from 0 to greater than 40 dB to cover the range of possible sensitivity thresholds for various stimulus sizes and eccentricities. There are a number of factors that affect the ability to detect a stimulus (visual field location, size, duration, color, flicker, motion, adaptation level, etc.) that will only partially be discussed in this chapter but have been reported elsewhere.[8]

A standard background luminance of 31.5 apostilbs (10 candelas per meter squared [cd/m^2]) is typically employed to provide a photopic level of adaptation, maintain the consistency of Weber's law, and provide the most stable testing conditions. Additionally, it is important to have a pupil diameter that is greater than 2 mm, an optimal refractive correction for the testing distance, and appropriate testing conditions (stimulus size and duration, interval between presentations, steady fixation, etc.). Under these conditions, the fovea is the most sensitive visual field location, thereby able to detect the smallest and dimmest stimulus. Sensitivity decreases systematically as one moves from the fovea toward greater visual field eccentricities, as indicated in Fig. 35.1 for a right eye, for which sensitivity is plotted three-dimensionally (x and y position coordinates and a z intensity coordinate) for the visual field. In view of this shape, this representation has often been called the "hill of vision" or the "island of vision in a sea of blindness."[9] The shape of the visual field will vary slightly when different stimulus sizes and durations are used. The dark hole in the hill of vision is the blind spot, where the optic nerve exits the eye to connect with the brain. It is a region of nonseeing because there are no photoreceptors or other retinal sensors present there. The location of the blind spot is approximately 15 degrees from the fovea on the temporal side of the visual field with about one-third of the blind spot above the horizontal meridian (2 degrees) and roughly two-thirds below the horizontal meridian (4 degrees). The overall size of the visual field is greater than 90 degrees temporally (away from the nose), 60 degrees nasally (toward the nose), 60 to 70 degrees superiorly, and 80 degrees inferiorly for a young, normal healthy eye.[4]

In addition to testing conditions that can affect visual field sensitivity, properties of the visual pathways also influence differential light sensitivity. The ability to detect an increment of light is not all or nothing, but is probabilistic, which can result in variability of 2 to 3 dB in normal visual field areas and up to 10 or more dB in damaged visual field regions.[10–18] This probabilistic aspect of detection sensitivity can be described by a frequency of seeing curve.[11–16] Very dim stimuli are rarely or never seen, whereas high-intensity stimuli are nearly always detected. As a consequence, the frequency of seeing curve is S-shaped and spans a range of approximately 3 dB for locations near the center of the visual field and 4 to 5 dB for stimuli at more eccentric locations for a normal eye, and 10 dB or more in damaged visual field areas. The variability is usually different for individuals, depending on age, attentiveness, cognitive abilities, and related factors.

Another factor that can affect visual field sensitivity is damage produced by disease or other impairments to the visual pathways, which is its most important attribute as a clinical diagnostic test procedure. As indicated in later portions of this chapter, the pattern, shape, and location of visual field sensitivity losses can be helpful in identifying the location of visual pathway dysfunction and the potential disorders that may have produced this loss. In addition to overall sensitivity loss in damaged visual field areas, these compromised regions typically have much higher variability, making it more difficult to determine the amount of sensitivity loss. One of the objectives of clinical visual field testing is to utilize methods that minimize the amount of variability in perimetric results.

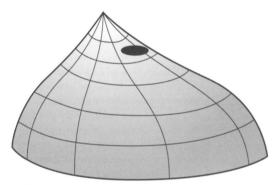

Fig. 35.1 Three-dimensional representation of sensitivity of the eye to light throughout the visual field. An illustration for a right eye is presented.(OD)

THE PHYSIOLOGIC BASIS FOR PERIMETRY

One of the advantages of perimetry and visual field testing is that the pattern, shape, and location of sensitivity losses reflect the anatomical arrangement of the visual pathways Fig. 35.2 presents a basic cross-sectional view of the visual pathways from the eye to the visual centers of the brain. It is important to note that the temporal visual field projects to the nasal portion of the retina, the nasal visual field is represented in the temporal retina, and the superior visual field projects to inferior retina and inferior visual field is imaged on the superior retina. All designations in this chapter are with reference to the visual field location rather than the retinal area. The optics of the eye form an image on the retina, where light intensities are converted into electrical impulses by approximately 100 million photoreceptors (rods and cones), which transmit the electrical signals to neural mechanisms in the inner retina (bipolar, horizontal, amacrine, inter-plexiform, and retinal ganglion cells). The optic nerve consists of retinal ganglion cell axons that then leave the eye and travel back to the brain. The ganglion cell fibers from the temporal retina (representing the nasal visual field) are shown in *red* in Fig. 35.2 and remain on the same side, while the retinal ganglion cell fibers from the nasal retina (representing the temporal visual field) are shown in *blue* and cross over to the opposite side at the optic chiasm. At this point, the information from both eyes is combined so that the right half of the visual field processing is sent to the left hemisphere and the left half of the visual field information goes to the right hemisphere. The fibers terminate in the lateral geniculate body in the thalamus, and from there fibers from the lateral geniculate are sent to primary visual cortex. Between the optic chiasm and primary visual cortex, the fibers are still arranging themselves to be able to produce a point-by-point mapping of the visual field for both eyes. This anatomical arrangement provides clinically useful information in determining the locus of damage to the visual pathways. A highly detailed description of the anatomy and physiology of the visual system may be found elsewhere in this volume, as well as in *Webvision: The Organization of the Retina and Visual System*.[19]

Fig. 35.2 Schematic illustration of the human visual pathways.

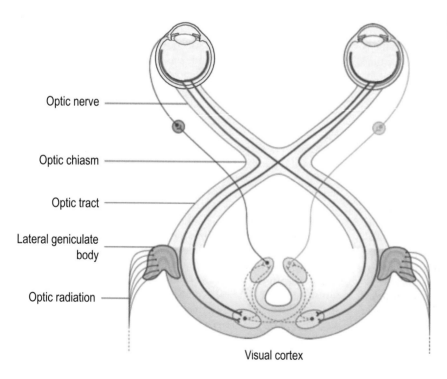

Optic nerve

Optic chiasm

Optic tract

Lateral geniculate body

Optic radiation

Visual cortex

COMMON FORMS OF PERIMETRIC TESTING

Usually, three primary methods of visual field testing are performed clinically: (1) static perimetry, (2) kinetic perimetry, and (3) suprathreshold static perimetry. These procedures have specific advantages and disadvantages, and each can be useful for clinical evaluation. In this view, these procedures should be regarded as complementary and fulfilling particular requirements for diagnostic purposes. Selection of which procedure to use depends on the capabilities, attention and cooperation of the patient, and the relative importance of perimetry as part of the eye examination.

Static perimetry

The most common form of visual field testing conducted by automated perimeters is static perimetry, consisting of detection of a small white stimulus superimposed on a uniform white background at various locations in the field of view. At each location, the minimum amount of light needed to detect the stimulus is determined and is referred to as the differential or increment sensitivity threshold. The pattern of stimulus locations corresponds to either a polar coordinate system (radius and meridian) or a Cartesian coordinate arrangement (a grid bracketing the horizontal and vertical meridians). A number of test procedures have been developed for measuring threshold sensitivities (method of limits, staircase, Swedish Interactive Threshold Algorithm [SITA], ZEST, TOP, GATE).[20–28] In addition to the sensitivity threshold measurements, procedures for estimating test reliability (false positives, false negatives, fixation losses, alignment [eye and head tracking]) and variability are also included.[29]

Visual field results are typically presented in a composite framework that includes demographic information and testing conditions, a graphical representation of visual field sensitivity (grayscale or color map), general or widespread sensitivity in comparison to an average normal person of the same age, an assessment of localized sensitivity loss, alignment during the test (eye and head tracking), and summary statistics that provide the amount of diffuse loss, localized damage, consistency, reliability, compatibility with glaucomatous deficits, and stage of visual field normality. Each device has its own terminology and analysis methods for providing this information. Fig. 35.3 presents a representative print out of visual field results obtained using a Humphrey field analyzer, and Fig. 35.4 demonstrates a similar arrangement for the Octopus perimeter. An example of grayscale representations in Fig. 35.5 is presented for a normal visual field (A), a visual field with widespread or diffuse sensitivity loss (B), and localized sensitivity reductions (C). Note that the grayscale or color map representation provides a useful method for evaluating the pattern and shape of visual field sensitivity characteristics.

Among the advantages of automated static perimetry are the use of a standardized test procedure, the ability to easily exchange information from one device and office to another, comparisons to age-corrected normal population characteristics for a single visit or for changes over time, methods for monitoring response reliability, eye and head tracking, and assessments of variability within and between tests. Also, database programs such as FORUM for the Humphrey field analyzer allow visual field information to be stored concurrently with retinal photographs, optical coherence tomography results, intraocular pressure, and other relevant information obtained during a clinic visit. Disadvantages of current automated static perimetry tests include limitations in the ability to efficiently evaluate the entire field of view, less flexible test procedures that are not adaptive, a significant burden on the patient's continual attention and performance throughout the test, higher variability in damaged visual field regions, and limited interactive capabilities between the patient and the examiner.

Kinetic perimetry

Kinetic perimetry consists of moving a stimulus of predetermined size and intensity on a uniform background luminance to determine the locations at which the stimulus can first be detected. Although this form of visual field testing was the preferred method approximately 40 years ago by presenting small stimuli on either a dark 1- or 2-meter tangent screen or a lit bowl perimeter, it is not used as frequently today. Only a limited number of older practitioners are able to perform this test manually, and only partial forms of kinetic perimetry are available on a few automated perimeters. To become proficient in conducting kinetic perimetry requires a considerable amount of time (6–12 months), practice, and experience, with most of the training mentored and hands-on. An excellent description of how to perform kinetic perimetry is found in the book authored by Anderson.[4]

Most kinetic perimetry is conducted using either a black tangent screen (1 or 2 meters) or a Goldmann or Goldmann-like perimeter with the examiner performing the test manually. A few automated devices have a limited kinetic perimetry test, and the Octopus 900 perimeter has the most advanced semiautomatic kinetic perimetry test.[30–33] The visual field (hill of vision) is mapped by moving a stimulus of specified size and luminance from the periphery toward the central fixation point along radial meridians until the patient responds when they can first detect the stimulus. The rate of motion should be constant and is typically 4 to 5 degrees per second for locations in the far periphery, and 1 to 2 degrees per second for more-central visual field locations. Once these kinetic scans have been made for meridians around the visual field, the detection points are connected by lines that denote an isopter (region of equal sensitivity). In a normal eye, isopters are elliptical, with the long axis in the inferior temporal quadrant and the short axis in the superior nasal quadrant. Departures from the egg-shaped normal isopter require additional scans to properly characterize the contour of the isopter. Multiple isopters can be derived by using different stimulus size and luminance combinations. Areas of nonseeing (scotomas) are mapped by placing a stimulus near the center of the deficit and moving outward from the center in all directions to define the outer contour of the scotoma. To evaluate visual field locations between isopters to search for possibly scotomas, static spot checks are performed by briefly flashing a stimulus at various locations. When the visual field has been completely evaluated, a two-dimensional map of sensitivity to light is produced. A representative example of a kinetic perimetry test result for a normal healthy right eye is presented in Fig. 35.6.

Kinetic perimetry used to be the predominant method of visual field testing about 40 years ago, but with the advent of automated perimetry, static testing is now the primary method. However, kinetic perimetry is still a valuable technique for assessing visual field status in patients with retinal or neuro-ophthalmologic conditions, and for patients with limited attention spans or cognitive impairment. There are distinct advantages and disadvantages associated with kinetic perimetry. The test is highly interactive between the examiner and the patient, so flexible test procedures can readily be implemented and adjusted throughout the test procedure. Kinetic perimetry testing permits accurate mapping of the location, pattern, and shape of visual field losses to assist in differential diagnostic evaluation. The far peripheral visual field can be assessed in a much more efficient manner when compared with static perimetry. The disadvantages of kinetic perimetry include a greater amount of variability when compared with static perimetry, large individual differences among examiners in their technique, lack of standardized procedures, limited normal population characteristics, and difficulty in properly representing widespread or diffuse visual field sensitivity loss. Whereas static perimetry has a well-defined procedure and may be likened to the types of strategies used in the game of

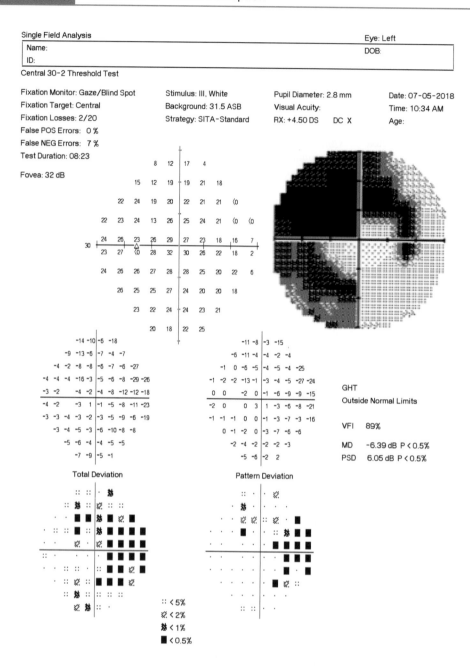

Single Field Analysis

Eye: Left

Name:
ID:

DOB:

Central 30-2 Threshold Test

Fixation Monitor: Gaze/Blind Spot
Fixation Target: Central
Fixation Losses: 2/20
False POS Errors: 0%
False NEG Errors: 7%
Test Duration: 08:23

Fovea: 32 dB

Stimulus: III, White
Background: 31.5 ASB
Strategy: SITA-Standard

Pupil Diameter: 2.8 mm
Visual Acuity:
RX: +4.50 DS   DC X

Date: 07-05-2018
Time: 10:34 AM
Age:

Total Deviation

Pattern Deviation

GHT
Outside Normal Limits

VFI   89%

MD   −6.39 dB P < 0.5%
PSD   6.05 dB P < 0.5%

:: < 5%
⌀ < 2%
⌘ < 1%
■ < 0.5%

Fig. 35.3 An example of a printed visual field report from the Humphrey field analyzer for the left eye of a glaucoma patient who was tested with the 30-2 SITA Standard test procedure.

checkers, kinetic perimetry is a heuristic, interactive series of strategies that may be more representative of chess. It is probably for this reason that there has been limited implementation of kinetic test strategies for automated perimetry.

Suprathreshold static perimetry

Although there have been significant advances in deriving more efficient test strategies for static and kinetic perimetry, they still require more time to achieve quantitative perimetry results compared with a rapid screening to determine whether the visual field is within or outside normal limits. For a general eye examination or for population-based screening, it is desirable to have a very efficient test procedure that also has good performance. The basic strategy behind suprathreshold static perimetry is to present stimuli at key locations in the visual field using stimuli that should be easily seen by individuals with normal visual function (normal versus abnormal visual field) or to further characterize areas of loss as being mild, moderate, or advanced.[34-41] Unfortunately, there have been some drawbacks to determining optimal suprathreshold static test procedures: (1) the vast majority of test procedures that have undergone rigorous evaluations have been quantitative static and kinetic visual field test procedures rather than visual field screening tests, with a few exceptions[34-41]; (2) the information concerning performance characteristics of suprathreshold static perimetry is quite limited; (3) whereas there are many potential suprathreshold static test procedures, it is not known which provides better performance, and there are few comparisons of various methods; (4) quantitative static perimetry test procedures have become more efficient, reducing the advantage of condensed testing time with suprathreshold

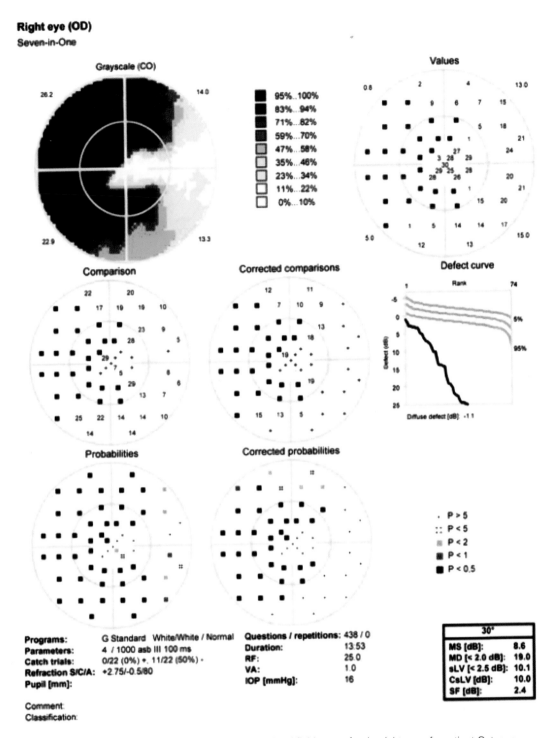

Fig. 35.4 An example of the seven-in-one printed visual field report for the right eye of a patient Octopus 900 perimeter.

static perimetry;[42–47] and (5) properties of the test procedures (underlying assumptions, number of locations tested, stimulus properties, test strategy, guidelines for interpretation of results, etc.) vary widely from one test to another. Therefore, it is of interest to note that frequency doubling technology (FDT) has two screening tests (one with higher specificity and one with higher sensitivity) that have good performance

and can provide a screening of a normal eye in less than 30 seconds and an eye with visual field loss in 1 to 1.5 minutes.[41]

Suprathreshold static perimetry provides a standardized test procedure that is efficient and is quite suitable for screening purposes, either within a clinical office environment or for large-scale population-based screening. It can also be used to provide an assessment of the entire

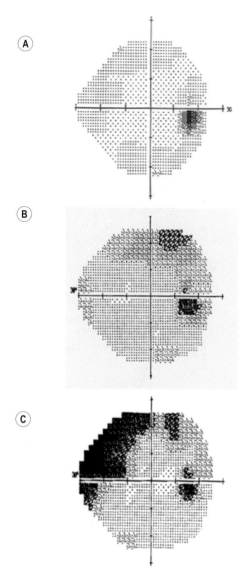

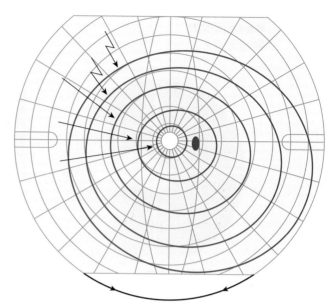

Fig. 35.6 Illustration of a normal visual field for kinetic perimetry of the right eye that was tested with a Goldmann-type manual perimeter.

Fig. 35.5 Humphrey field analyzer 24-2 grayscale presentations for (**A**) a normal visual field, (**B**) widespread or diffuse visual field loss, and (**C**) localized visual field deficits.

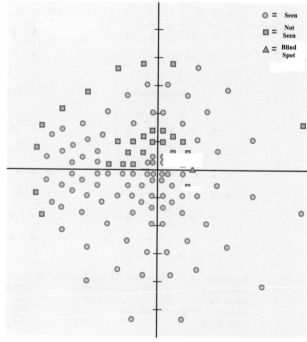

Fig. 35.7 An example of a two-zone, threshold-related 120-point visual field screening test on the Humphrey field analyzer for the right eye of a glaucoma patient with a superior arcuate visual field defect.

visual field. However, it provides only limited quantitative information. An example of a suprathreshold static perimetry result for the right eye obtained using the two-zone 120 location test on the Humphrey field analyzer is presented in Fig. 35.7.

DETECTION OF SENSITIVITY LOSS AND INTERPRETATION OF RESULTS

Information for evaluating and interpreting the results of a single visual field test can be found on the printed output of the test results. Fig. 35.8 presents the results of a visual field test performed on the Humphrey field analyzer using the 30-2 SITA Standard test procedure to assess the left eye of a patient with superior and inferior partial arcuate glaucomatous visual field defects.

On the top portion of the visual field printout is the patient's name, eye that was tested, the patient ID code, and date of birth. Below this are listed the test conditions that were used (background luminance, stimulus size, fixation target, fixation monitoring method, etc.), the test strategy, reliability characteristics (false-positive responses,

false-negative responses, fixation losses), and the patient's age and ocular conditions (distance refraction, pupil size and best-corrected visual acuity). This listing makes it possible to immediately determine whether proper testing conditions were employed, whether the test was reliable, and whether other information (distance refraction, visual acuity, date of birth, etc.) is correct.

If there are excessive false-positive responses (pressing the response button when no stimulus was presented), this indicates that the patient was pressing the button too frequently ("trigger happy"), and it is likely that there will also be excessive fixation losses and extremely high (nonphysiologic) threshold sensitivity values. If the patient becomes

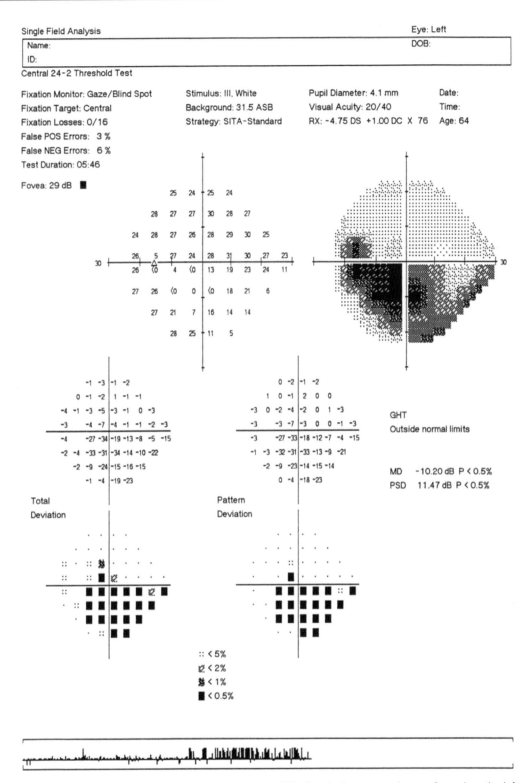

Fig. 35.8 Humphrey field analyzer results for the 24-2 SITA Standard test procedure performed on the left eye of a glaucoma patient with a superior paracentral deficit and inferior arcuate sensitivity loss. As indicated at the *bottom* of the printed output, gaze tracking and eye-head alignment was very good at first and then become quite variable during later portions of the test.

drowsy or inattentive, a high number of false negatives (not pressing the response button when a stimulus 9 to 10 times greater than a previously determined threshold value) can occur. However, it should also be noted that if the patient has more advanced visual field loss, the damaged areas will have higher variability, which can also result in high false negatives. [48-52]

Below this information is the visual field data. The foveal threshold sensitivity value is presented, along with a probability level if it is below the lower 5%, 2%, 1%, or 0.5% of values for a normal individual of the same age. This is followed by an X/Y plot of threshold sensitivity values in decibels (dB) at each of the visual field locations on the left, and a grayscale representation of visual field sensitivity on the right.

The decibel scale is a relative logarithmic scale (log threshold sensitivity ×10). A value of 0 dB is defined as the maximum luminance intensity that the Humphrey field analyzer can produce (10,000 apostilbs, or 3175 cd/m²). The gray scale provides an interpolated two-dimensional graphic of the pattern and shape of visual field deficits for differential diagnostic purposes. (It should be noted that this scale is coarse, and subtle defect patterns are often not visualized, for example, subtle defects that are shown on the total and pattern deviation plots, discussed further on.) The lower left graphs present the numerical deviation of threshold sensitivity values from the average normal observer of the same age at each visual field location (top graph) and the probability that it is lower than the 5%, 2%, 1%, or 0.5% probability of the normal population (bottom graph). On the top graph, positive numbers reflect threshold sensitivity values that are above the average normal of the same age, and negative numbers indicate threshold sensitivity values that are below the average normal. The lower graph with probability levels demonstrates the locations with reduced sensitivity and the magnitude of this deficit. This data representation is referred to as the Total Deviation plot.

Visual field sensitivity loss can be widespread (diffuse or generalized) or it can be localized to a specific region. To partially disconnect the widespread and localized visual field loss components, the Humphrey field analyzer adjusts the individual threshold sensitivity values by the general height value. The general height is determined by ranking all the threshold sensitivity values from highest to lowest and selecting the value corresponding to the 85th percentile (for the 24-2 pattern, this is the seventh-highest threshold sensitivity value). All the threshold sensitivity values are adjusted by this value, which diminishes all or most of the widespread sensitivity loss to reveal the localized deficits. The deviation values and probability levels are similar to those of the Total Deviation plots, and this representation is referred to as pattern deviation. Fig. 35.9 presents examples of the clinical benefit of comparing the total deviation *(left)* and pattern deviation *(right)* plots to illustrate: (A) a right eye of a trigger-happy patient where total deviation values are normal and pattern deviation is outside of normal, (B) a right eye of a patient with widespread or diffuse loss where total deviation is outside of normal and pattern deviation is mostly within normal limits, (C) a superior arcuate deficit for a right eye that depicts localized loss, and (D) a left eye that has a combination of both localized and widespread or diffuse loss.

This point-by-point characterization contains a substantial amount of information, so general summary statistics are also available. Mean deviation (MD) is the average deviation of threshold sensitivity values from the average normal individual of the same age. However, not all locations have the same effect, as more-central visual field locations are given more weight than ones that are peripheral. Pattern standard deviation is the amount of irregularity or perturbation of the normal slope of the visual field that is calculated as the root mean square deviation. Areas of visual field sensitivity loss are the primary sources responsible for producing deviations from the normal slope. Most visual fields are performed on glaucoma patients, so there is also an analysis that is designed for identifying visual field sensitivity loss patterns that are characteristic of glaucoma. The glaucoma hemifield test (GHT) contains five superior and five mirror image inferior clusters of visual field locations that mimic the pattern of losses that typically occur with glaucoma. It then compares the asymmetry between the average sensitivity for each cluster for mirror image regions in the superior and inferior visual field. There are only minor differences in the average values for superior and inferior clusters for normal healthy visual fields. However, visual field losses produced by glaucoma will result in values that are often outside of the normal asymmetry values. There are five designations that are presented as a result of this analysis: (1) within

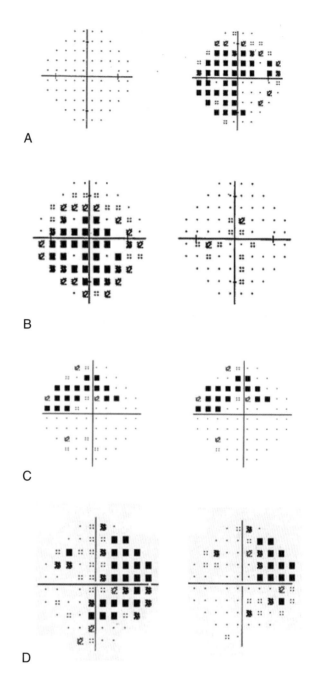

Fig. 35.9 Examples of the results for total and pattern deviation probability plots for (**A**) a "trigger-happy" patient with abnormally high sensitivity, produced by pressing the response button too often, (**B**) generalized or widespread visual field loss, (**C**) localized visual field loss, and (**D**) a combination of widespread and localized visual field sensitivity deficits. Examination of the relationship between Total and Pattern Deviation patterns can be very useful clinically.

normal limits, if all cluster asymmetries correspond to normal values; (2) outside normal limits, if one or more of the cluster comparisons is outside of the 1% probability level for normal; (3) borderline, if one or more of the cluster comparisons are outside of the 3% probability level; (4) depressed sensitivity, if the overall threshold sensitivity values are below the lower 0.5% probability level; and (5) abnormally high sensitivity, if the overall threshold sensitivity values are above the upper 0.5% probability level. Fig. 35.10 presents the five superior and five inferior clusters represented in a 30-2 test presentation pattern.

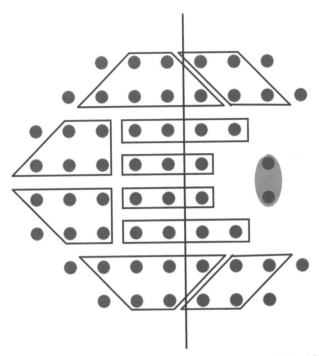

Fig. 35.10 The 10 clusters (five superior and five inferior) of visual field locations used to assess superior and inferior hemifield asymmetry for the glaucoma hemifield test. The 10 clusters are designed to correspond to the pattern of arcuate nerve fiber bundles entering the optic nerve head.

The visual field index (VFI) is the final summary statistic, which determines the percentage of the visual field that is within normal limits by comparing the visual field to a population of normal healthy eyes.[53–56] A normal visual field has a VFI value of 100% and a perimetrically blind visual field has a VFI score of 0%. This can then provide a simple value that can be used to track the rate of change over time. To minimize the influence of cataract on the VFI that would result in widespread or diffuse loss, only points that are represented as beyond normal limits for the Pattern Deviation plot are considered. Additionally, greater weight is provided to more-central points than peripheral points in accordance with cortical magnification factors. Although this is a simple representation of overall visual field status, it should be kept in mind that it has both ceiling and floor effects.[54–56] Not only do normal visual fields have a VFI of 100%, but small deficits where the MD is better than –5 or –6 dB will also elicit a VFI of 100%, which results in a ceiling effect. When there is advanced glaucomatous visual field loss, the raw dB sensitivity values are beyond the range of pattern deviation values, so the algorithm switches to total deviation probabilities. This produces a discontinuity in the VFI values that represents a floor effect and makes it difficult to determine a rate of progression.

Finally, at the bottom of the visual field printout is a graph of gaze tracking that monitors the patient's alignment with the perimeter and fixation accuracy. Gaze tracking is a most valuable component because it provides the examiner with valuable information about the patient's performance during the test.[4,29,57–61] Gaze tracking uses infrared light that will not interfere with the test procedure and uses a video camera to capture the location of the first Purkinje image (corneal reflex) in relation to the edges of the pupil (retinal red reflex). The gaze tracking graph presents the status of alignment throughout the test procedure. By examining this graph, it is possible not only to determine the quality

of alignment and fixation throughout the procedure but also to provide an indication of droopy upper eyelids, inattention and fatigue, excessive blinking and dry eye, and consistency of alignment. Upper bar deflections indicate departures from fixation, using three bar sizes of small (approximately 2–4 degrees of fixation loss), medium (about 4–6 degrees of fixation loss), and large (>6 degrees of fixation loss). Lower bar deflections indicate interruptions of the infrared beam reflections (e.g., blinks) or dry eye (tear film breakup). Fig. 35.11 presents several examples of gaze tracking: (A) good gaze tracking and accurate fixation; (B) excessive blinking or dry eye; (C) droopy eyelid or fatigue; (D) inattention and fatigue near the end of the test; and (E) generally poor alignment throughout the test.

Overall, the single visual field analysis that is produced on the printed output contains a wealth of information concerning visual field status, interpretation of results and comparison with a healthy normal population, reliability, alignment, and other properties that can be most helpful for clinical assessment. It is important to keep in mind that everything that is provided on the visual field printout is important—it is not useful to only concentrate on selected portions of the output. It is also helpful to remember that visual field testing is only one of many items that are part of the eye examination.

VISUAL FIELD LOSS PATTERNS CREATED BY VARIOUS PATHOLOGIES

Careful clinical assessment of the pattern and shape of visual field deficits is probably the most critical component of visual field interpretation. Although printed output of the visual field is two-dimensional, it is important to keep in mind the three-dimensional properties of the visual field (length, width, and depth). There are many features that can provide clinical insights into the disease process and locus of involvement of the visual pathways, including the pattern and shape of areas of sensitivity loss, whether the transition from normal to impaired areas has steep or gradual boundaries, and whether the deficit "respects" (terminates abruptly) at specific locations that correspond to anatomical properties of the visual pathways. Fig. 35.12 presents a general representation of damage to fibers at different location in the visual pathways (*blue lines*) and the resulting patterns of visual field loss that are associated with this impairment. More detailed examples of visual field losses resulting from injuries to specific portions of the visual system may be found in other literature sources.[4,29,30,62–65]

It is critical to have a systematic approach to use for interpreting the visual field. In this view, the next segment of this chapter provides a listing of key pattern and shape characteristics of visual field losses, followed by a set of sequential guidelines for performing the assessment of a single visual field.

PATTERNS OF VISUAL FIELD LOSS

- *Generalized or widespread visual field sensitivity loss.* This is a nonspecific type of visual field loss because it can be produced by a variety of sources (ocular media, small pupil, visual pathology to many regions of the visual pathways, cognitive and attentional lapses).
- *Visual field constriction.* This is a narrowing of the field of vision that is often referred to as tunnel vision, due to its characteristic shape. A variety of insults to the visual pathways can create a constricted visual field.
- *Ring scotomas.* These losses tend to occur in the midperipheral visual field as a total or partial ring of sensitivity loss surrounded by regions of higher sensitivity. They are typically produced by retinitis pigmentosa or another type of retinal degeneration.

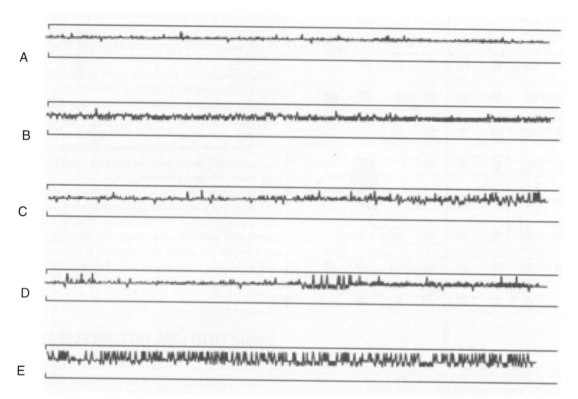

Fig. 35.11 Examples of gaze tracking results for the Humphrey field analyzer. Upward deflections indicate alignment difficulties (eye and head movements), and downward deflections indicate blinking, droopy upper eyelids, or tear film breakup. (**A**) Good gaze tracking, (**B**) excessive blinking, (**C**) droopy upper eyelid, (**D**) fatigue and misalignment in the latter part of the test, and (**E**) major alignment problems and poor initialization.

- *Central scotomas.* In general, these deficits are produced by damage to mechanisms in the macular region or by certain types of optic neuropathies.
- *Arcuate scotomas.* These defects are produced by damage to the arcuate nerve fiber bundles that are produced by glaucoma, other optic neuropathies, or vascular insults (branch artery occlusion), as the vascular supply of the eye travels in an arcuate fashion.
- *Nasal steps.* This can be regarded as a part of the arcuate defect that has a distinct sharp transition from seeing to nonseeing at the horizontal meridian. It most commonly occurs in glaucoma.
- *Defects that "respect" the horizontal meridian.* This is a sharp boundary between seeing and nonseeing at the horizontal meridian on the nasal side of the visual field, and is usually associated with glaucoma, other optic neuropathies, or branch artery occlusions.
- *Centrocecal scotomas.* This pattern denotes visual damage that includes the blind spot (ceco) and fixation. This deficit has a candle flame shape and is associated with damage to fibers in the papillomacular bundle that subserve the macula and the region between fixation and the optic disc. Most optic nerve fibers are contained in the papillomacular bundle. Some optic neuropathies and macular damage can produce this deficit.
- *Defects that "respect" the vertical meridian.* The fibers conveying information from the left and right sides of vision for both eyes separate at the central vertical meridian or midline when the information from both eyes is combined at the chiasm and after the chiasm. Damage to nerve fibers at the chiasm and beyond results in a steep, abrupt transition in sensitivity at the vertical meridian.
- *Bitemporal visual field deficits.* A bitemporal visual field deficit that respects the vertical meridian is characteristic of damage to the optic chiasm.

- *Visual field losses that resemble a horizontal wedge.* This is a very uncommon visual field deficit in which the area of visual field loss resembles a horizontal wedge or tongue along the horizontal meridian or a tongue of remaining visual field sensitivity along the horizontal meridian. When homonymous, this pattern corresponds to damage of neural fibers at the level of the lateral geniculate body. Bitemporal horizontal wedge defects along the horizontal are usually congenital in origin.
- *Homonymous visual field loss.* Visual field losses that occur on the same side of vision (left or right) for both eyes are homonymous (the nasal visual field of one eye combined with the temporal visual field of the other eye). The vertical meridian is respected, and the visual pathway damage is in the optic radiations posterior to the optic chiasm. A total homonymous hemianopsia (complete homonymous loss of vision for the left or right visual field) indicates that all of the fibers in the optic radiations have been damaged at some location after the optic chiasm.
- *Congruous and incongruous visual field loss.* As a rule, the greater the amount of incongruity of loss between the two eyes (i.e., one eye has more a more extensive deficit than the other eye), the closer the damage is to the optic chiasm. Deficits to the optic radiations in the optic tract produce incongruous visual field deficits between the two eyes, whereas damage to the optic radiations in the temporal and parietal lobe are semicongruous. Primary visual cortex lesions produce visual field deficits that are highly congruous.
- *Pie in the sky visual field deficits.* A homonymous semicongruous visual field deficit the appears as if a piece of a pie is missing from the superior visual field that respects the vertical meridian is typically associated with temporal lobe lesions, in accordance with the arrangement of the optic radiations traveling through the temporal lobe.

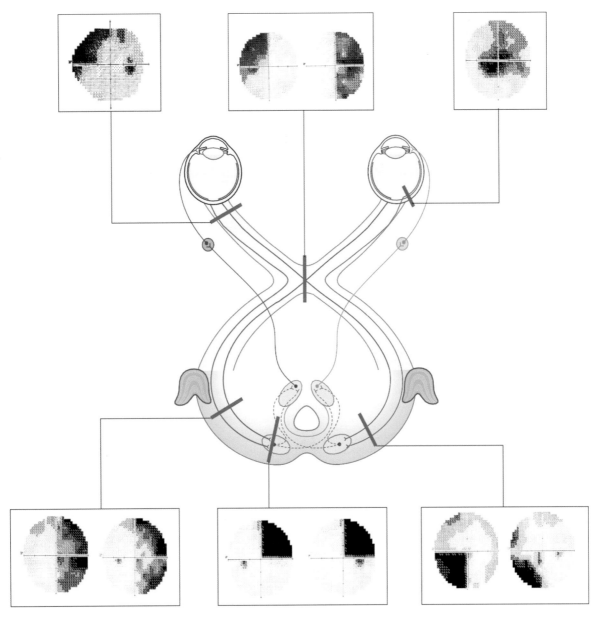

Fig. 35.12 Examples of visual field loss produced by damage to the visual pathways at various locations from the retina to primary visual cortex.

- *Pie on the floor visual field loss.* Conversely, a semicongruous homonymous visual field deficit that respects the vertical meridian that resembles a missing piece of pie that has fallen to the floor is usually associated with parietal lobe damage to the optic radiations traveling through the parietal lobe.
- *Cookie cutter punched-out deficits.* Visual field losses that appear to be nearly identical between the two eyes, as if a hole punch or cookie cutter had removed a portion of the visual field is indicative of an occipital lobe (primary visual cortex) deficit.

Although there will sometimes be exceptions to these general principles, these guidelines will be helpful in properly interpreting visual field information and determining the most likely locus of damage to the visual pathways. There are many excellent sources that provide examples of visual field deficits associated with damage to specific regions of the visual pathways.[4,29,30,62–65]

VISUAL FIELD INTERPRETATION GUIDELINES

1. Place the visual field printout of the left eye on the left and the right eye on the right.
2. Determine whether the appropriate test was performed, the date of birth is correct, pupil size is 3 mm or greater, visual acuity is listed, the near refractive correction is appropriate, the tests were reliable, and the results are consistent with the status of the visual pathways are not artifactual (droopy lid, small pupil, lens rim, etc.).
3. For each eye, evaluate whether the visual field is within normal limits or has sensitivity loss.
   a. If the visual field is reliable and within normal limits for both eyes, the assessment is complete.
   b. If one or both visual fields are unreliable or there are eye and head tracking problems, determine whether the tests should be repeated.

4. If there is evidence of sensitivity loss, determine whether it is just one eye or both eyes that have evidence of impairment.
   a. If the loss is in just one eye, then the damage occurred prior to the location where the information from both eyes is combined (optic chiasm), indicating that the deficit is produced by damage to the retina or the optic nerve, or by ocular media problems.
   b. If the visual field loss is in both eyes, then the damage may be present at the chiasm or postchiasmal, but it can also be due to retinal or optic nerve damage in both eyes.
5. What is the general location of the loss (superior, inferior, nasal, temporal)? If the loss is extensive, where is the most prominent region of visual field loss?
6. What is the shape and location of the visual field deficit (central, centrocecal, arcuate, nasal step, bitemporal, quadrant, hemifield, constricted, respect the horizontal meridian, respect the vertical meridian)?
7. How do deficits from the two eyes compare to each other?
   a. Is the deficit binasal (probably glaucoma, optic neuropathy, or retinal disease)?
   b. Is the deficit bitemporal (chiasmal lesion)?
   c. Is the deficit homonymous (same side of vision)?
      i. Is it a total homonymous hemianopia (all visual pathway fibers are damaged past the chiasm)?
      ii. If it is not a total homonymous hemianopia, is it a quadrant deficit?
      iii. How congruous is the deficit between the two eyes? (The more congruous, the farther back the damage is present in the visual pathways.)
      iv. What is the shape of the area of loss? Pie in the sky (deficit in the superior visual field) is most common for temporal lobe deficits, while pie on the floor (deficit in the inferior visual field) occurs more often with parietal lobe lesions.
8. Once this has been completed, the visual field interpretation should be combined with other clinical findings to determine a final lesion localization and differential diagnosis.

Box 35.1 provides a brief summary of the visual field interpretation guidelines.

ASSESSING VISUAL FIELD PROGRESSION

Analysis of a single visual field is a critical component of a clinical eye examination, keeping in mind that it is useful to have the first visual field as an educational experience for the patient to minimize practice and learning effects. In conjunction with other information obtained during the eye examination, visual field information can be helpful in identifying the source and potential site of visual damage. However, it is also important to determine the status of the visual field during follow-up appointments to determine whether visual function is improving, remaining stable, or deteriorating, as well as to assess its impact on quality of life and activities of daily living. Many approaches for evaluating visual field properties over time have been reported, but only a few have achieved consensus among practitioners. Some are too complicated for routine use in a busy clinic, some are restricted to a small subgroup of patients, and some are not available for general clinical use. This chapter presents the main techniques being used for longitudinal evaluation of perimetric test results, along with their advantages and disadvantages. A more thorough review of methods to determine visual field change over time has recently been published for those who wish to receive more detailed information.[66] However, note that several publications from independent groups have reported

---

> ### BOX 35.1 Visual field interpretation guidelines[67–70]
>
> - **Detection**
>   - Is the visual field of each eye within normal limits or are there abnormalities?
> - **Identification**
>   - What is the pattern of visual field loss?
>   - Is the visual field loss in one eye or both eyes?
> - **Differential diagnosis**
>   - What location or locations in the visual pathways could account for this loss?
>   - What is the general location of the defect? (superior, inferior, nasal, temporal)
>   - What is the shape and specific location of the visual field defect?
>   - Does the defect correlate with anatomical features of the visual pathways and boundaries?
> - **Staging of visual field loss**
>   - What is the severity of visual field loss?
>   - Is the loss abrupt and steep or gradually sloping?
> - **Artifactual visual field loss**
>   - Does the deficit reflect a lens rim obstruction, a droopy upper eyelid, or some other nonpathologic or physiologic result?
> - **Functional visual field loss**
>   - Does the pattern and severity of visual field loss exceed that expected on the basis of other clinical findings?
> - **Longitudinal follow-up of visual field loss**
>   - Is the visual field loss improving, getting worse, or remaining stable over time?
>   - What is the rate of change?
>   - Do visual field results suggest a change in clinical management?
> - **Practical visual field issues**
>   - Does visual field impairment affect quality of life and activities of daily living?
>   - Do visual field results impair navigation (driving, use of stairs, etc.) or object identification, or result in employment restrictions?

---

that the various methods that are used for assessing visual field change only agree with each other about 50% to 60% of the time.[67–70] The most common methods of determining visual field changes over time include clinical judgment, classification systems, event analysis, trend analysis, and a hybrid event-trend–based evaluation.

Clinical judgment

Clinical judgment of visual field properties over extended time periods is probably the most common method of assessment, particularly within the context of a typical eye examination in a busy clinic. The eye care specialist uses his/her knowledge, training, and experience to determine whether the visual field has undergone any positive (improvement) or negative (progression) changes during the management of their ocular or neurologic condition. The primary advantages of clinical judgment of perimetric findings are that it is an efficient means of assessing visual field status, as well as being an important indicator of the effectiveness of the treatment regimen. Shortcomings of clinical judgment include the high variability of determinations among different eye care specialists,[71] the higher level of agreement and consistency of statistical analysis procedures in comparison with highly skilled clinical practitioners,[71] and the tendency for highly experienced clinicians to overcall visual field progression.[72]

Classification systems

Classification systems are designed to produce a staging of the amount of visual field loss into a series of separate categories. A historical review of visual field staging and classification systems has been published that indicates that many different classification systems utilize five to seven different levels of visual field loss to cover the spectrum from normal visual field properties to perimetric blindness.[73] However, the Advanced Glaucoma Intervention Study (AGIS) and the Collaborative Initial Glaucoma Treatment Study (CIGTS) multicenter clinical trials used classification systems that consisted of 20 stages.[74,75] The methods used by AGIS and CIGTS to determine the 20 stages was different, resulting in AGIS having higher specificity and CIGTS having higher sensitivity.[74,75] Advantages of the classification systems included a consistent systematic method of performing the analysis that could be performed by different centers and practitioners, and a system that could be adopted by any clinician wishing to utilize this method of evaluating visual field change over time. Disadvantages were use of a discrete rather than a continuous outcome, decisions based on opinion rather than evidence-based findings, and uncertainty regarding the measurement scale (linear, nonlinear, etc.). It was not clear that a difference between 4 and 7 was equivalent to a difference between 13 and 16. However, these classification systems did provide a consistent scoring procedure for all participating clinical centers in these two multicenter clinical trials (AGIS and CIGTS).

Event analysis

Typically, event analysis consists of comparing the current visual field to those that were obtained at baseline. The evaluation can be either on a point-by-point basis (or groups of points) or by visual field summary statistics.[76–79] Changes between the current visual field and baseline values are then compared with the test-retest variability of multiple examinations performed over a short time period to determine whether the deviations are within or outside of expected variability limits. The early manifest glaucoma treatment (EMGT) multicenter study utilized event analysis as a means of assessing visual field changes over time.[76,77] There are several advantages of event analysis: (1) it is a consistent methodology that is evidence based; (2) it is able to detect changes rapidly to produce a higher sensitivity; and (3) it applies a rigorous statistical model for quantitative analysis. There are also several disadvantages: (1) if the current visual field or the baseline is in error or is atypical, erroneous results will occur; (2) interim visual fields are not considered, making it difficult to determine a rate of change over time; and (3) the procedure yields a higher number of false-positive results that reduce its specificity.

Trend analysis

Another common method of determining visual field change over time is trend analysis, a technique that has also been used in several multicenter trials.[80–84] This procedure analyzes all the visual field data to determine the best fitting equation to describe the data. In most cases this is an ordinary least squares linear regression, but for long time periods or during changes in therapeutic management, a bilinear or "hockey stick" approach may also be used.[85–88] Advantages of this procedure include the inclusion of all visual field data, the generation of the goodness of the linear fit and an assessment of test-to-test variability, and the ability to derive a slope of visual field change over time that can be evaluated statistically.[79–87] The limitations of this approach include the requirement that between six and eight visual fields are needed to have the best performance (high sensitivity and specificity) and the requirement that the slope be statistically significantly different from zero to have confidence in the evaluated change.[80–88] There have been many attempts to refine trend analysis, but most of these approaches have achieved only modest improvements in performance. There remain many possibilities for using techniques such as machine learning, artificial intelligence, and related sophisticated approaches to create further improvement. However, it should be kept in mind that new procedures must be simple for the clinician to utilize without requiring extensive additional training to properly incorporate the approach into routine clinical examinations.

Hybrid combined event and trend analysis

Event analysis tends to be able to detect visual field changes before trend analysis (higher sensitivity), but event analysis has poorer specificity than trend analysis. Given the advantages and disadvantages of event analysis and trend analysis, recent attempts have been directed toward combining the best qualities of each method. For example, a procedure such as the guided progression analysis (GPA) will utilize an event analysis approach but will require confirmation of the change on the next visual field (two confirmed changes in a row) or persistent changes (three similar changes in a row) as a means of maintaining high sensitivity while preserving specificity.[77–79,89–91] Additional modifications that alter the weighting of various visual field results have also been attempted. Currently, it appears that event analysis and trend analysis are the most common simple methods of evaluating visual field progression, although there is certainly an incentive for new investigators to generate more effective predictive models for determining perimetric changes over time.

ALTERNATIVE AND NEW VISUAL FIELD TEST PROCEDURES

There are a number of new visual field test procedures that have been introduced within the last 20 to 30 years (see Box 35.2 for a brief summary). Some tests have been found to be useful clinical diagnostic instruments for general clinical use, whereas others are primarily suited for clinical research studies requiring more advanced procedures. In this chapter, we discuss only those methods that are beneficial for routine clinical diagnostic testing. Additional information regarding other test procedures is available in other publications.[92–96]

SITA Faster and 24-2 C visual field tests

The SITA is a Bayesian test strategy that is available on the Humphrey field analyzer. The primary method is referred to as SITA Standard, although there is a version called SITA Fast that has reduced testing time but produces slightly greater variability for determinations in damaged visual field areas. Because visual field testing is demanding and can produce fatigue, there is an incentive to develop more rapid visual field test procedures. Recently a third SITA program known as SITA Faster has been introduced.[97] It produces significantly shorter test times by implementing seven modifications to SITA Fast: (1) the starting stimulus intensities are presented at the age-adjusted average normal sensitivity values rather than their previous starting value in SITA Fast; (2) there is only one reversal of the staircase strategy instead of two; (3) SITA Faster uses the distribution of SITA Fast normal values rather than the previous distribution; (4) perimetrically blind areas are not retested; (5) false-negative trials are not performed; (6) there are no blind spot catch trials because gaze tracking monitors eye and head alignment; and (7) the extra time delay between presentations has been eliminated.

Preliminary studies indicate that SITA Faster reduced testing time by more than 50% compared with SITA Standard. All but a few of the test results for SITA Faster are highly similar to SITA Standard and SITA

BOX 35.2   Other visual field test procedures

- **Contrast sensitivity and incremental light detection**
  - Standard automated perimetry—Detection of a small light projected onto a uniform background at various visual field locations.
  - Contrast sensitivity perimetry—Determination of minimum contrast needed to detect an alternating light and dark grating at different visual field locations.
- **Spatial visual field tests**
  - High pass resolution perimetry—Determination of the minimum size of a low contrast optotype stimulus that can be detected at various visual field locations.
  - Rarebit perimetry—Fine detail mapping of the visual field by determining detectability of small light dots (pixels).
- **Temporal visual field tests**
  - Flicker perimetry—The ability to detect a flickering stimulus on a uniform background at various visual field locations. There are three forms:
    (1) Determining the highest flicker rate that can be detected (critical flicker fusion or CFF).
    (2) Determining the minimum flicker amplitude that can be detected (temporal modulation perimetry).
    (3) Determining the minimum light increment of a superimposed flickering stimulus on a uniform background to detect flicker (luminance pedestal flicker perimetry).
  - **Motion perimetry—Measurement of motion sensitivity at various visual field locations. There are three methods:**
    (1) Determination of the minimum displacement of a stimulus necessary to detect motion.
    (2) Determination of the amount of coherence of a series of dots, some of which are moving in the same direction while others are moving in random directions.
    (3) Determination of the size of a visual field region needed to detect the motion of a series of dots.
- **Spatiotemporal visual field tests**
  - Frequency doubling technology (FDT) perimetry—The minimum amount of contrast needed to detect a low spatial frequency sinusoidal grating undergoing high temporal frequency counterphase flicker.
  - Pulsar perimetry—Similar to FDT perimetry except that it uses a two-dimensional bull's eye pattern of light and dark sectors.
- **Color visual field tests**
  - Opponent process perimetry—Isolation and measurement of color vision mechanisms at various visual field locations, using a large color target superimposed on a chromatic background.
- **Electrophysiology perimetry**
  - Multifocal electroretinography (MERG)—Recording of local electroretinography signals from various visual field locations using a modified binary M sequence while viewing an alternating checkerboard pattern.
  - Multifocal visual evoked potentials (MVEP)—Recording of primary visual cortex signals similar to MERG while viewing an alternating checkerboard pattern.

Fast, except that MD is slightly higher and Pattern Standard Deviation (PSD) is slightly lower for SITA Faster.[98–102] It has also been reported that there are a higher number of false-positive responses with SITA Faster, and it has anecdotally been observed that if the initial primary points (one oblique location in each quadrant) have determinations that are in error, it can result in an entire quadrant of the visual field having slightly incorrect threshold sensitivities. Because SITA Faster dramatically reduces test time, it has been reported that it is possible to perform two tests during a single visit with minimal changes in the overall time to conduct perimetry.[101,102]

To provide a more thorough assessment of the macular region, particularly for glaucoma, 10 stimuli have been introduced into the central region of the 24-2 pattern to produce the 24-2 C procedure.[103–107] The 10 stimulus locations were selected by evaluating a number of program 10-2 test results to identify the locations that were most likely to detect glaucomatous visual field losses in the macular region. The 24-2 C test does not add much additional time to the 24-2 test. Overall, with the advent of the 24-2 C pattern, faster test times, and greater preferences by both the patient and the examiner, the SITA Faster has many advantages over the previous SITA procedures. However, additional research investigations by practitioners that are independent of the manufacturer will help establish its role in clinical diagnostic testing. Fig. 35.13 presents an example of SITA Faster that incorporates the 24-2 C test procedure.

Short Wavelength Automated Perimetry

Short wavelength automated perimetry (SWAP) is a visual field test procedure that determines the threshold sensitivity for large (Goldmann Size V) short wavelength (blue) stimuli that are projected onto a bright (100 cd/m²) broadband yellow background.[108–112] The yellow background decreases the sensitivity of the middle (green) and long (red) wavelength mechanisms to allow the short wavelength mechanisms to be isolated and measured. The procedure was first introduced by Stiles and his associates[113] and was later adapted for clinical use in perimetry by Kitahara[114] and King-Smith.[115] Sample and colleagues[116,117] and Johnson and associates[118–124] were able to modify existing Humphrey field analyzers to be able to perform SWAP, conducting extensive longitudinal studies, as well as determining optimal clinical testing conditions.[111] Fig. 35.14 presents an example of SITA SWAP in the right eye of a patient with glaucomatous visual field loss.

Although it was reported that SITA SWAP was a more sensitive test than SITA Standard,[118–125] two recent independent studies have now reported that there was essentially no meaningful difference in the ability of SWAP to detect glaucomatous visual field loss when compared with standard automated perimetry.[126,127] Essentially for all of the cases where SWAP detected a glaucomatous visual field deficit earlier than standard automated perimetry, there were an equivalent number of cases where standard automated perimetry identified a deficit that was not identified by SWAP. Moreover, it is clear that SWAP is affected by yellowing of the lens and early cataract development, is a more difficult task, and requires additional instruction. A more efficient SWAP test procedure has also been developed,[128,129] and it should also be noted that SWAP has been found to be useful in performing testing of neuro-ophthalmologic conditions, diabetic retinopathy, and other retinal conditions.[130–135]

Frequency doubling technology perimetry

When a low spatial frequency sinusoidal grating (≤1 cycle per degree of visual angle) undergoes high temporal frequency counterphase square wave flicker (≥15 hertz), there appears to be approximately twice as many light and dark bars than are physically present, and this phenomenon has been referred to as frequency doubling. Kelly[136,137] originally described frequency doubling and evaluated its properties, while Maddess and colleagues[138] applied frequency doubling for clinical ophthalmic detection and evaluation of diseases affecting the visual pathways. Subsequently, this was refined by Johnson and associates[139–141] to develop a commercial device referred to as frequency doubling technology (FDT) and a more elaborate second generation instrument called the Humphrey matrix.

The FDT device presents a 0.25 cycle per degree vertical sinusoidal grating that undergoes 25 hertz counterphase flicker at 19 locations (10 degrees by 10 degrees) in the visual field, superimposed on a 50-cd/m²

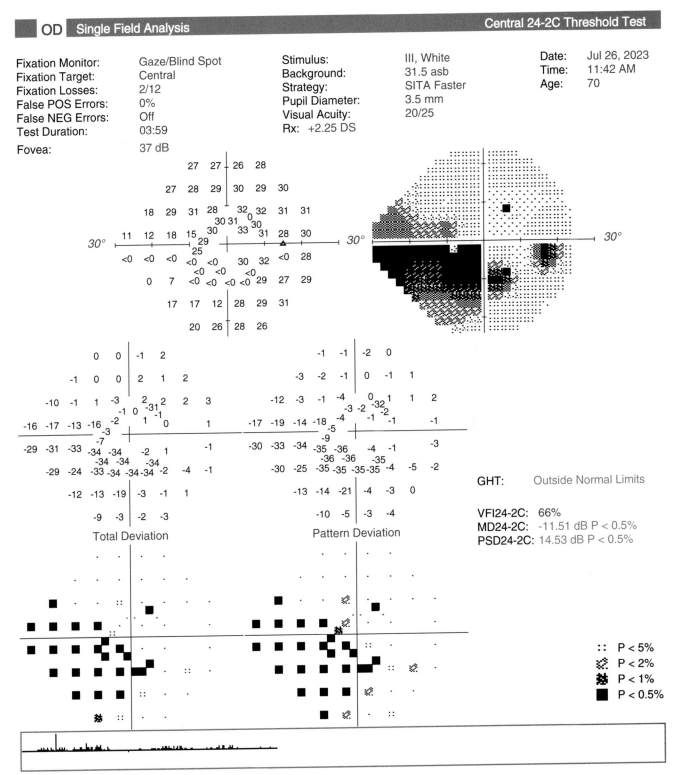

OD | Single Field Analysis   Central 24-2C Threshold Test

Fixation Monitor: Gaze/Blind Spot
Fixation Target: Central
Fixation Losses: 2/12
False POS Errors: 0%
False NEG Errors: Off
Test Duration: 03:59
Fovea: 37 dB

Stimulus: III, White
Background: 31.5 asb
Strategy: SITA Faster
Pupil Diameter: 3.5 mm
Visual Acuity: 20/25
Rx: +2.25 DS

Date: Jul 26, 2023
Time: 11:42 AM
Age: 70

GHT: Outside Normal Limits

VFI24-2C: 66%
MD24-2C: -11.51 dB P < 0.5%
PSD24-2C: 14.53 dB P < 0.5%

Total Deviation

Pattern Deviation

:: P < 5%
▨ P < 2%
▩ P < 1%
■ P < 0.5%

Fig. 35.13 A printed output of a 24-2C SITA Faster test procedure performed on the right eye of a patient with superior arcuate and inferior nasal step visual field deficits. Ten stimuli have been added to the macular region to detect central glaucomatous deficits and changes have been made to the SITA algorithm to reduce testing time.

uniform white background. Each stimulus is presented for 720 milliseconds. To avoid temporal transients at the onset and offset of the stimulus, the contrast is ramped up to the designated contrast for 160 milliseconds, remains at the designated contrast for 400 milliseconds, and then is ramped down to zero contrast for 160 milliseconds. The observer's task is to detect the presence of the frequency doubling stimulus, and contrast is varied according to a modified binary search (MOBS) procedure. Fig. 35.15 presents an example of a frequency doubling test result for the left eye of a patient with a superior arcuate visual field deficit. Many investigations have reported that this procedure is

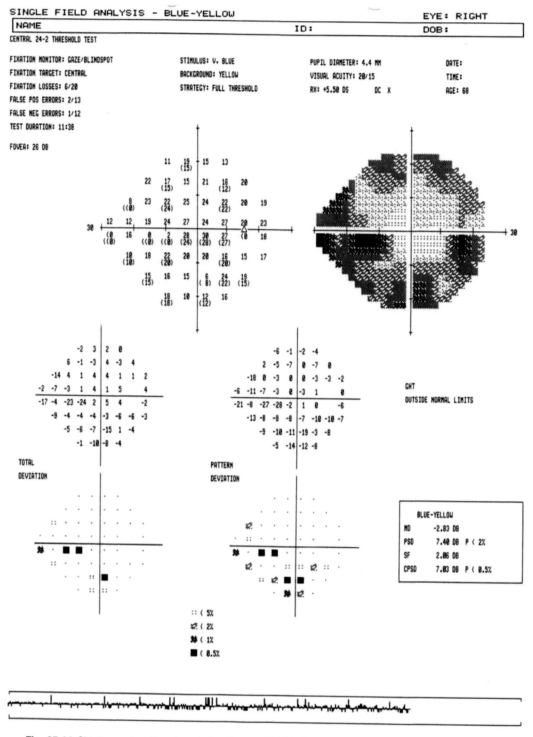

Fig. 35.14 Short wavelength automated perimetry (SWAP) findings for the right eye of a patient with an inferior partial arcuate visual field loss.

effective in detecting and characterizing visual field loss from glaucoma and other diseases affecting the visual pathways, with more limited changes in variability in damaged visual field areas.[142–148]

The second-generation Humphrey matrix perimeter expanded the capabilities of FDT by increasing the spatial frequency of the sinusoidal grating to 0.5 cycles per degree, reducing the stimulus size to 5-degree by 5-degree stimuli, and reducing the temporal frequency to 18 hertz. In this manner, it was possible to construct 24-2 and 30-2 stimulus test patterns that had a 6-degree center-to-center spacing for stimulus locations horizontally and vertically. Additionally, to test the macular region, the stimulus size was further reduced to 2-degree by 2-degree stimuli with a center-to-center spacing of 2 degrees to produce 10-2

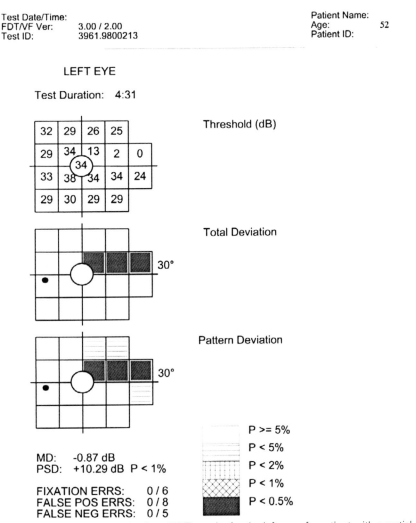

FULL THRESHOLD N-30

Test Date/Time:
FDT/VF Ver: 3.00 / 2.00
Test ID: 3961.9800213

Patient Name:
Age: 52
Patient ID:

LEFT EYE

Test Duration: 4:31

Threshold (dB)

Total Deviation

30°

Pattern Deviation

30°

P >= 5%
P < 5%
P < 2%
P < 1%
P < 0.5%

MD: -0.87 dB
PSD: +10.29 dB P < 1%

FIXATION ERRS: 0 / 6
FALSE POS ERRS: 0 / 8
FALSE NEG ERRS: 0 / 5

Fig. 35.15 Frequency doubling technology (FDT) results for the left eye of a patient with a partial superior arcuate deficit as obtained on the original FDT device evaluating 19 visual field regions.

and macula tests. The stimulus consisted of a 0.5 cycles per degree sinusoidal grating undergoing counterphase flicker at 12 hertz. The higher spatial frequency in combination with the lower temporal flicker rate did not produce a frequency doubling effect, so the test results reflected flicker sensitivity. Decreasing the flicker frequency to 12 hertz increased the dynamic range of the test procedure. A number of studies have indicated that the Humphrey matrix is able to detect and follow visual field loss related to macular degeneration, glaucoma, neuro-ophthalmologic conditions and other diseases affecting the afferent visual pathways[149–156] It has a robust screening test that is a highly effective visual field screener. Fig. 35.16 presents the results of a Humphrey matrix 24-2 test procedures for the left eye of a patient with a superior partial arcuate deficit produced by glaucoma.

TABLETS AND VIRTUAL REALITY HEADSETS

New advances in procedures and technology have made it possible to perform visual field testing on tablets, virtual reality headsets, and secure internet web sites for screening and quantitative evaluations. Many of these devices are currently available for visual field examinations and other visual function tests, and results have been generally positive.[157–179] However, any new methodology typically includes advantages and limitations. Beneficial aspects of this form of testing include (1) portability, (2) results highly comparable to automated bowl perimetry, (3) capabilities for home testing, (4) minimal effect from ambient room illumination, (5) fewer restrictions on testing location (e.g., waiting room, home, population screening), (6) rapid sanitization between uses, (7) rapid, accurate eye tracking, and (8) ability to incorporate state of the art test procedures. Limitations of this form of testing are (1) a limited field of view for tablets and some internet display systems, (2) a smaller intensity range in comparison to automated bowl perimeters, (3) variation of stimulus size with eccentricity to increase the dynamic response range, (4) lack of familiarity with the display system, especially for older patients, and (5) difficulty translating prior test results obtained from a bowl perimeter. This new form of testing represents a paradigm shift that will require additional familiarity and experience, similar to the transition from manual visual field testing to automated procedures. It is anticipated that these limitations will be minimized in the future.

Fig. 35.17 presents a printout of a visual field obtained with a tablet, and Fig. 35.18 illustrates results obtained with a similar test procedure on a virtual reality headset.

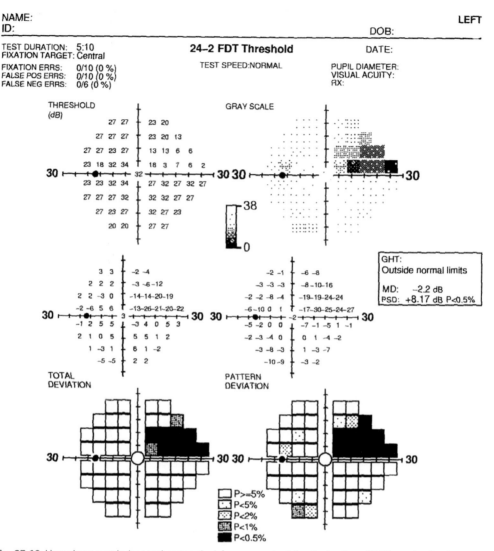

Fig. 35.16 Humphrey matrix (second-generation) frequency doubling technology (FDT) results for the same left eye shown in Fig. 35.15 revealing a superior partial arcuate glaucomatous visual field deficit for the 24-2 stimulus presentation pattern.

ARTIFACTUAL VISUAL FIELD RESULTS

Visual field testing will usually produce results that are useful in detecting, diagnosing, and monitoring disorders affecting the visual pathways, assuming that the patient is cooperative and the findings are reliable. However, there are also testing conditions that can produce visual field deficits that occur because of improper methods or patient-related issues that are not the result of pathologic causes.[180-183] This section of the chapter presents some of the more common examples of artifactual visual field test results.

To maintain the adaptation state of the eye at a level that is photopic and produces the most stable and reliable findings, it is important that the eye being tested has a pupil diameter of more than 2 millimeters in diameter. Fig. 35.19 presents a visual field that was obtained when the eye had a 1-millimeter diameter pupil (*left*) and the same test performed with a 3-millimeter diameter pupil (*right*). When the pupil diameter is small, less light enters the eye, and the adaptation state is no longer photopic or stable.

The upper eyelid will sometimes sag down (ptosis), resulting in obstruction of a portion of the superior visual field that produces an area of superior visual field loss. This can occur quite often in older

patients and can sometimes be confused with a superior arcuate deficit that is associated with glaucoma. To minimize the occurrence of visual field loss related to a droopy upper eyelid, one can elevate the upper eyelid by using surgical tape to keep the eyelid out of the field of view. Although surgical tape will keep the upper eyelid elevated, it is still possible for the patient to blink. A hallmark of this type of artifact is an abrupt change from 0 dB to normal or near normal sensitivities. Fig. 35.20 presents a visual field obtained with a droopy upper eyelid (*left*) and a similar visual field when the eyelid was taped (*right*).

The surface of the perimeter bowl is located at a near distance of one-third of a meter (33 centimeters). Because of this, a patient's distance correction may not provide a sharply focused image of the fixation point and stimulus targets, particularly if the patient is older and presbyopic. A blurred image of the perimeter bowl and fixation prompts will result in lower sensitivity values. It is therefore important to provide a near addition correction over the distance refraction of up to 3 diopters. A graduated scale of near addition lens corrections, based on the patient's age, is available for most commercial visual field devices. Fig. 35.21 presents the visual field of a patient with no near lens correction in place during testing (*left*) and a subsequent visual field when the appropriate near lens correction was added (*right*).

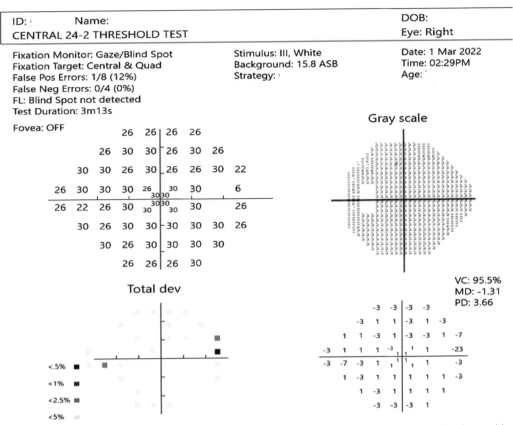

ID: Name:
CENTRAL 24-2 THRESHOLD TEST

DOB:
Eye: Right

Fixation Monitor: Gaze/Blind Spot
Fixation Target: Central & Quad
False Pos Errors: 1/8 (12%)
False Neg Errors: 0/4 (0%)
FL: Blind Spot not detected
Test Duration: 3m13s

Stimulus: III, White
Background: 15.8 ASB
Strategy:

Date: 1 Mar 2022
Time: 02:29PM
Age:

Fovea: OFF

```
            26  26 | 26  26
        26  30  30 ⌐26  30  26
    30  30  26  30 ⌊26  26  30  22
26  30  30  30  26 |  30  30       6
              30 30
26  22  26  30  30 30  30  30      26
              30   30
    30  26  30  30 ⊢30  30  30  26
        30  26  30 | 30  30  30
            26  26 | 26  30
```

Gray scale

VC: 95.5%
MD: -1.31
PD: 3.66

Total dev

```
              -3  -3 | -3  -3
          -3   1   1 | -3   1  -3
       1   1  -3   1 | -3  -3   1  -7
      -3   1   1   1 | -3   1   1  -23
                       1 1
      -3  -7  -3   1 | 1 1  1   1   -3
       1  -3   1   1 | 1   1   1  -3
       1  -3   1 |  1   1   1
          -3  -3 | -3   1
```

<.5% ■
<1%   ■
<2.5% ■
<5%

Fig. 35.17 The printed output of test results obtained using the 24-2 stimulus pattern obtained using a tablet display system.

To position the near correction lens there is a lens holder that can be adjusted and centered close to the eye for the test procedure. When the lens holder and lens are placed close to the eye and outside of the excursion of eyelashes, it does not obstruct any portion of the visual field. However, patients do not like to sit near a featureless white hemispherical bowl and sometimes have a tendency to back away or become misaligned during the test. This can produce a trial lens rim artifactual visual field loss. Fig. 35.22 left presents an example of a trial lens rim visual field deficit that produces an outer ring of sensitivity loss (*left*) adjacent to normal sensitivity that was created by the patient backing away from the perimeter bowl. Sometimes the patient may move on the chin rest and become misaligned, resulting in a partial lens rim artifactual visual field loss over part of the field of view, as shown in the right panel of Fig. 35.22.

An automated visual field test may initially evaluate sensitivity of the fovea by presenting a small stimulus in the center of a diamond of red fixation spots that are projected below the center of the perimeter bowl. After this, the patient is instructed to look at the center of the perimeter bowl to evaluate the remainder of the visual field. If the examiner does not instruct the patient to move fixation to the center of the perimeter bowl or the patient neglects to do so, the test will be misaligned because of the patient's incorrect fixation. Fig. 35.23 presents an example of incorrect fixation below the center of the perimeter bowl (*left*) and the subsequent visual field when fixation was performed properly (*right*).

Older patients have lower sensitivity than younger patients, so the automated perimeter adjusts the test procedure and subsequent analysis of results to account for this. Because of this, it is important to enter the proper date of birth for the patient. Fig. 35.24 presents the visual field results for the right eye of a 47-year-old patient for whom

the date of birth was entered incorrectly, resulting in an age that was 40 years older at 87 (*left*), and the *right* panel demonstrates the visual field obtained when the correct date of birth was entered. Note that the grayscale representation is highly similar for both tests, but the analysis of results for total and pattern deviation is different.

Patients often want to do well performing visual field testing and are eager to produce results that are normal or minimally reduced. As a consequence, they may be motivated to press the response button often, even when they are unsure that they saw the stimulus, (i.e., they are "trigger happy.") This can result in sensitivity values that are higher than is physiologically possible, and can lead to unreliable results (high fixation losses and false positives). Fig. 35.25 presents an example of a trigger-happy individual that has very high sensitivity values (note that the grayscale representation has large regions that are white), and also high fixation losses and high false-positive responses.

Finally, it is clear that a visual field test is not the most exciting procedure for patients, and they are sometimes tested after many other examinations and procedures in the clinic. As a result, it is sometimes difficult for the patient to maintain attention and alertness to the test procedure for extended minutes. Fig. 35.26 presents an example of a patient that had a good attention span of about 1 minute and then faded. Fig. 35.26 presents an example of this type of visual field result. The four lighter regions that are located obliquely in each of the visual field quadrants are the first locations that are tested (the seed points that inform the adjacent locations). In this example, the patient was alert for those presentations. However, after these are performed the test undergoes a growth pattern where neighbors of these primary locations are tested. It can be seen that the patient lost attention and concentration on the test and produced low sensitivities. This has often been called a cloverleaf pattern or resembling Mickey Mouse ears. If

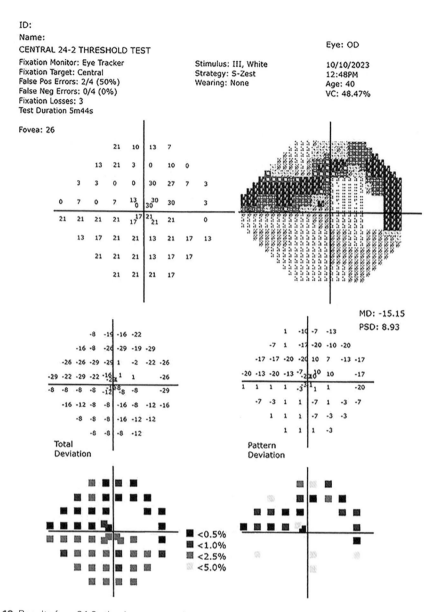

ID:
Name:
CENTRAL 24-2 THRESHOLD TEST
Fixation Monitor: Eye Tracker
Fixation Target: Central
False Pos Errors: 2/4 (50%)
False Neg Errors: 0/4 (0%)
Fixation Losses: 3
Test Duration 5m44s

Eye: OD

Stimulus: III, White
Strategy: S-Zest
Wearing: None

10/10/2023
12:48PM
Age: 40
VC: 48.47%

Fovea: 26

MD: -15.15
PSD: 8.93

Total Deviation

Pattern Deviation

■ <0.5%
▦ <1.0%
▨ <2.5%
▧ <5.0%

Fig. 35.18 Results for a 24-2 stimulus presentation pattern performed using a virtual reality headset with rapid (60 hertz) and accurate (<0.2 degree) resolution.

1-mm diameter pupil   **3-mm diameter pupil**

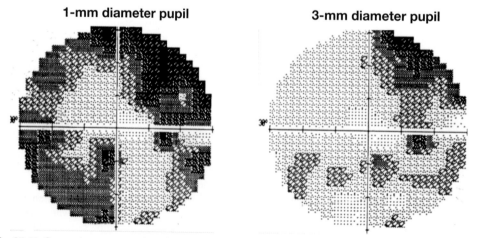

Fig. 35.19 Grayscale representation of visual field results for the right eye of a glaucoma patient with a 1-mm (*left*) and a 3-mm (*right*) pupil diameter. It is recommended that the pupil diameter is 2 mm or greater for visual field testing to avoid artifactual results.

Droopy eyelid (ptosis) | **Upper eyelid taped**

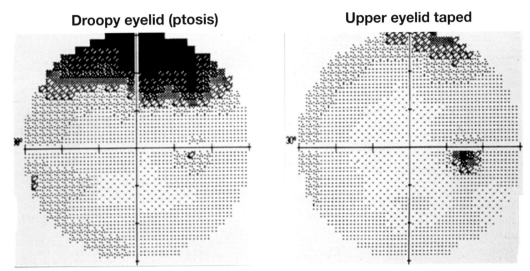

Fig. 35.20 A grayscale representation of visual field results obtained for the right eye of a patient with a droopy upper eyelid (*left*) and with the upper eyelid taped (*right*). Note that droopy eyelid results can mimic the appearance of a superior arcuate visual field loss.

Incorrect lens | **Correct lens**

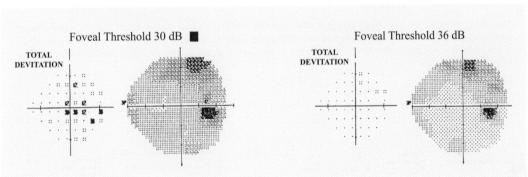

Fig. 35.21 Visual field results for the right eye of a patient when an incorrect near lens correction was employed (*left*) and when the appropriate lens correction was provided (*right*).

Lens rim artifact | **Partial lens rim artifact**

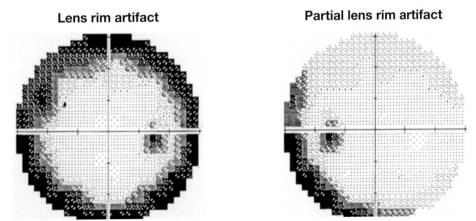

Fig. 35.22 Examples of a trial lens rim artifact (*left*) and a partial trial lens rim artifact (*right*). A complete trial lens rim artifact typically occurs when the patient's eye is back too far from the lens, so its rim obscures a portion of the visual field. A partial lens rim artifact can be produced by misalignment of the eye and the lens.

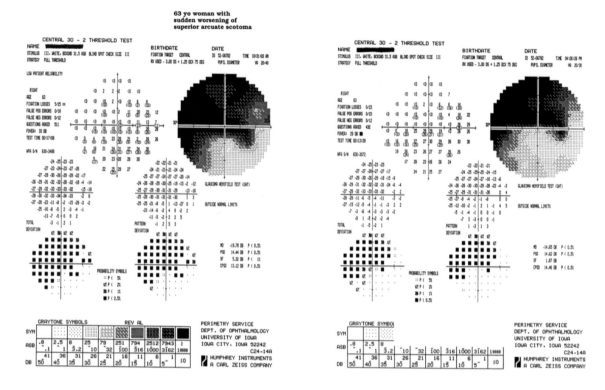

Fig. 35.23 An example of a displaced horizontal meridian (*left*) and correct placement of fixation (*right*). Foveal testing is performed with fixation directed toward a diamond pattern below the center of the perimeter bowl. If the patient is not instructed to change fixation to the center of the perimeter bowl, the visual field will be displaced inferiorly.

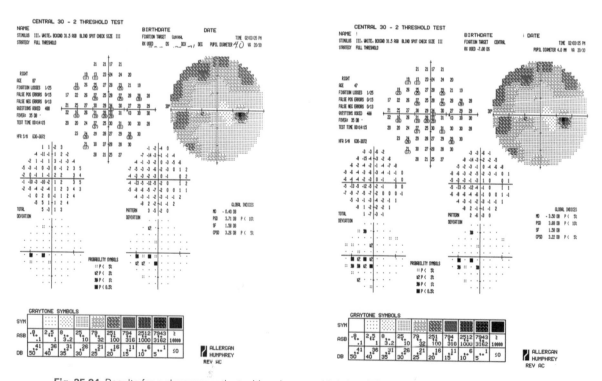

Fig. 35.24 Results for a glaucoma patient with an incorrect birthdate (40 years too old) that was entered (*left*) and the same visual field with the appropriate birthdate (*right*).

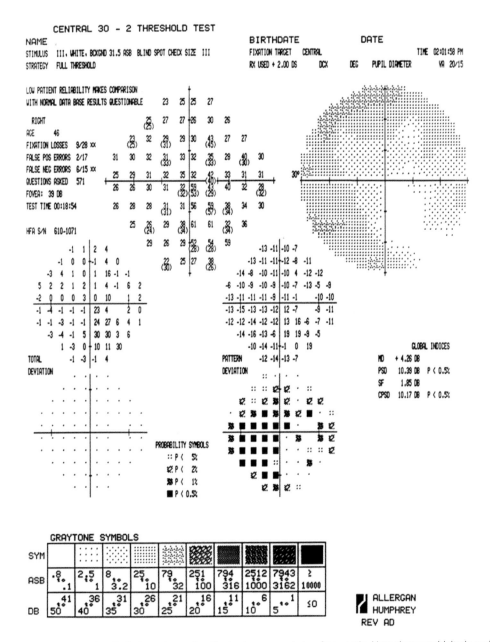

Fig. 35.25 An example of a "trigger-happy" patient who responds too frequently. Note that sensitivity is well above normal limits for portions of the visual field (*white areas* on the grayscale representation) and that there are high fixation losses and false positives present due to excessive response button pressing.

this occurs, it is important to provide the patient with brief rest periods to minimize attention losses and reinstruct them about the test.

We have presented the most common artifactual results that can occur, but it should also be kept in mind that other inappropriate findings can occur. It is important for the person administering to test to be aware of these situations and to provide continuous monitoring of the patient during the test procedure to minimize the likelihood that poor results will occur. Establishing good test procedures and keeping high-quality control assessments will produce a larger number of high-quality clinical visual field results.

CONCLUSIONS

Perimetry and visual field testing are important diagnostic procedures that can provide a wealth of useful clinical information about a person's functional vision status, their ability to detect and identify objects in

the periphery and navigate through the environment, and the influence on their quality of life and activities of daily living. They also provide useful guides concerning the location of damage to the visual pathways and the disease entity that is producing visual field loss. The pattern and shape of visual field loss in conjunction with the degree of correspondence of affected areas between the two eyes can provide specific valuable insights in terms of the location of involvement for pathology that is impairing the visual pathways. Visual acuity, on the other hand, is quite nonspecific because a reduced visual acuity of 20/200 can be produced by optical aberrations, uncorrected refractive error, macular dysfunction, optic nerve disease, or anomalies of the visual cortex and central visual pathways. Visual field information can be critical for determining the most likely location of damage to the visual pathways and, subsequently, where to focus any imaging procedure such as MRI.

It is important to remember that no single diagnostic test procedure or clinical assessment provides complete information about the

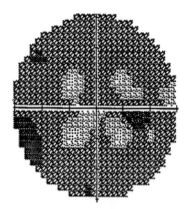

TOTAL DEVIATION 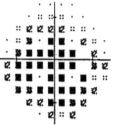 **PATTERN DEVIATION**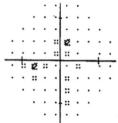

Rx Used: +3.00 DS
Pupil Diameter: 4.0 mm

GHT: General Reduction
CPSD: *normal*

Fig. 35.26 An example of a cloverleaf visual field display produced by a patient that was attentive for the initial portion of the test (light oblique areas that were tested first) but had limited attention span and vigilance for the remainder of the test.

status of the visual system, including visual fields. Perimetry test results should be regarded as providing complementary information within the context of the complete clinical examination, the patient's prior history and visual complaints, and the relationship between structural and functional deficits relating to various insults to the visual pathways.

It is hoped that this chapter has provided the reader with a background and guidelines for performing and interpreting visual fields, for distinguishing artifactual visual field results, assessing the capabilities and limitations of alternate forms of visual field procedures, and its role in the clinical evaluation of the patient. It is recommended to personally undergo visual field testing to gain an appreciation of the demands and involvement that patients undergo when performing a visual field test. Experience can always be a most important learning tool, as well as feedback from patients about their capabilities and limitations when completing visual field testing.

REFERENCES

1. Duke-Elder S, Scott GI. *System of Ophthalmology Vol VII – The Foundations of Ophthalmology, Visual Fields.* London: Henry Plimpton; 1971:393–425.
2. Aulhorn E, Harms H. Visual Perimetry. In: Jameson D, Hurvich L, eds. *Visual Psychophysics: Handbook of Sensory Physiology.* Vol VII/4. New York: Springer-Verlag; 1972.
3. Harrington DO, Drake MV. *The Visual Fields: Text and Atlas of Visual Perimetry.* St Louis, MO: CV Mosby; 1990.
4. Anderson DR. *Perimetry With and Without Automation.* St Louis: CV Mosby; 1987.
5. Greve EL. *Single and Multiple Stimulus Static Perimetry: The Two Phases of Perimetry.* The Hague: Dr. W Junk Publishers; 1971.
6. Johnson CA, Wall M, Thompson HS. A history of perimetry and visual field testing. *Optom Vis Sci.* 2011;88:8–15.
7. Boring EG. *A History of Experimental Psychology.* New York: Appleton-Century-Crofts; 1950.
8. Jameson D, Hurvich L. *Visual Psychophysics: Handbook of Sensory Physiology.* Vol VII/4. New York: Springer Verlag; 1972.
9. Traquair HM. *An Introduction to Clinical Perimetry.* St Louis, MO: CV Mosby; 1927.
10. Weber J, Rau S. The properties of perimetric thresholds in normal and glaucomatous eyes. *Ger J Ophthalmol.* 1992;1:79085.
11. Chauhan BC, Tompkins JD, LeBlanc RP, McCormick TA. Characteristics of frequency-of-seeing curves in normal subjects, patients with suspected glaucoma and patients with glaucoma. *Investig Ophthalmol Vis Sci.* 1993;34:3534–3540.
12. Spenceley SE, Henson DB. Visual field test simulation and error in threshold estimation. *British J Ophthalmol.* 1996;80:304–308.
13. Wall M, Maw RJ, Stanek KE, Chauhan BC. The psychometric function and reaction times of automated perimetry in normal and abnormal areas of the visual field in patients with glaucoma. *Investig Ophthalmol Vis Sci.* 1996;37:878–885.
14. Wall M, Kutzko KE, Chauhan BC. Variability in patients with glaucomatous visual field damage is reduced using size V stimuli. *Investig Ophthalmol Vis Sci.* 1997;38:426–435.
15. Henson DB, Chaudry S, Artes PH, Faragher EB, Ansons A. Response variability in the visual field: comparison of optic neuritis, glaucoma, ocular hypertension and normal eyes. *Investig Ophthalmol Vis Sci.* 2000;41:417–421.
16. Spry PGD, Johnson CA, McKendrick AM, Turpin A. Variability components of standard automated perimetry and frequency doubling technology perimetry. *Investig Ophthalmol Vis Sci.* 2001;42:1404–1410.
17. Chauhan BC, Garway-Heath DE, Goni FJ, et al. Practical recommendations for measuring rates of visual field change in glaucoma. *British J Ophthalmol.* 2008;92:569–573.
18. Chauhan BC, Johnson CA. Test-retest variability characteristics of frequency doubling perimetry and conventional perimetry in glaucoma patients and normal controls. *Investig Ophthalmol Vis Sci.* 1999;40:648–656.
19. Kolb H., Nelson R., Fernandez E., Jones B. Webvision: The Organization of the Retina and Visual System (located on the internet at webvision.med.utah.edu)
20. Bengtsson B, Olsson J, Heijl A, Rootzen H. A new generation of algorithms for computerized threshold perimetry, SITA. *Acta Ophthalmol.* 1997;75:368–375.
21. Bengtsson B, Heijl A, Olsson J. Evaluation of a new threshold visual field strategy SITA, in normal subjects, Swedish Interactive Thresholding Algorithm. *Acta Ophthalmol.* 1998;76:165–169.
22. Bengtsson B, Heijl A. Evaluation of a new perimetric threshold strategy, SITA, in patients with manifest and suspect glaucoma. *Acta Ophthalmol.* 1998;76:268–272.
23. McKendrick AM. Recent developments in perimetry: test stimuli and procedures. *Clin Exp Optom.* 2005;88:73–80.
24. Johnson CA. Recent developments in automated perimetry in glaucoma diagnosis and management. *Curr Opin Ophthalmol.* 2002;13:77–84.
25. Anderson AJ. Spatial resolution of the tendency-oriented perimetry algorithm. *Investig Ophthalmol Vis Sci.* 2003;44:1962–1968.
26. Turpin A, McKendrick AM, Johnson CA, Vingrys AJ. Properties of perimetric threshold estimates from full threshold, ZEST, and SITA-like strategies, as determined by computer simulation. *Investig Ophthalmol Vis Sci.* 2003;44:4787–4795.
27. Luithardt AF, Meisner C, Monhart M, Krapp E, Mast A, Schiefer U. Validation of a new static perimetric thresholding strategy (GATE). *British J Ophthalmol.* 2015;99:11–15.
28. Schiefer U, Pascual JP, Edmunds B, et al. Comparison of the new perimetric GATE strategy with conventional full-threshold and SITA standard strategies. *Investig Ophthalmol Vis Sci.* 2009;50:488–494.
29. Anderson DR, Patella VM. *Automated Static Perimetry.* St Louis: CV Mosby; 1999.
30. Racette L, Fischer M, Bebie H, Hollo G, Johnson CA, Matsumoto C. *Visual Field Digest.* Koniz, Switzerland: Haag-Streit,; 2016.
31. Dolderer J, Vonthein R, Johnson CA, Schiefer U, Hart W. Scotoma mapping by semi-automated kinetic perimetry: the effects of stimulus properties and the speed of subjects' responses. *Acta Ophthalmol.* 2006;84:338–344.
32. Schiefer U, Nowomiejska K, Krapp E, Patzold J, Johnson CA. K-TRAIN—A computer-based interactive training program for practicing kinetic perimetry: evaluation of acceptance and success rate. *Graefes Arch. Clin. Exp. Ophthalmol.* 2006;244:1300–1309.
33. Nevalainen J, Paetzold J, Krapp E, Vonthein R, Johnson CA, Schiefer U. The use of semiautomated kinetic perimetry (SKP) to monitor advanced glaucomatous visual field loss. *Graefes Arch. Clin. Exp. Ophthalmol.* 2008;246:1331–1339.
34. Johnson CA, Keltner JL, Balestrery FG. Suprathreshold static perimetry in glaucoma and other optic nerve disease. *Ophthalmology.* 1979;86:1278–1286.
35. Johnson CA, Keltner JL. Automated suprathreshold static perimetry. *Am J Ophthalmol.* 1980;89:731–741.
36. Henson DB. Visual field screening and development of a new screening program. *J Am Optom Assoc.* 1989;60:893–898.
37. Langerhorst CT, Bakker D, Raakman MA. Usefulness of the Henson Central Field Screener for the detection of visual field defects, especially in glaucoma. *Doc Ophthalmol.* 1989;72:279–285.
38. Siakowski RM, Lam BL, Anderson DR, Feuer WJ, Halikman AM. Automated suprathreshold static perimetry screening for detecting neuro-ophthalmologic disease. *Ophthalmology.* 1996;103:907–917.
39. Artes PH, Henson DB, Harper R, McLeod D. Multisampling suprathreshold perimetry: A comparison with conventional suprathreshold and full-threshold strategies by computer simulation. *Investig Ophthalmol Vis Sci.* 2003;44:2582–2587.

40. Artes PH, McLeod D, Henson DB. Response time as a discriminator between true- and false-positive responses in suprathreshold perimetry. *Investig Ophthalmol Vis Sci.* 2002;43:129–132.
41. Johnson CA, Cioffi GA, Van Buskirk EM. *Evaluation of two screening tests for frequency doubling technology perimetry. Perimetry Update 1998/1999.* Amsterdam: Kugler Publications; 1999:103–109.
42. Heijl A, Patella VM, Chong LX, et al. A new SITA perimetric threshold testing algorithm: construction and a multicenter clinical trial. *Am J Ophthalmol.* 2019;198:154–165.
43. Thulasidas M, Patyal S. Comparison of 24-2 Faster, Fast and Standard programs of Swedish Interactive Threshold Algorithm of Humphrey Field Analyzer for perimetry in patients with manifest and suspect glaucoma. *J Glaucoma.* 2020;29:1070–1076.
44. Phu J, Kalloniatis M. Viability of performing multiple 24-2 visual field examinations at the same clinical visit: The Frontloading Fields Study (FFS). *Am J Ophthalmol.* 2021;230: 48–59.
45. Phu J, Kalloniatis M. The Frontloading Fields Study (FFS): Detecting changes in mean deviation in glaucoma using multiple visual field tests per clinical visit. *Transl Vis Sci Technol.* 2021;10(13):21.
46. Qian CX, Chen Q, Cun Q, et al. Comparison of the SITA Faster: a new visual field strategy with SITA Fast strategy. *Int J Ophthalmol.* 2021;14:1185–1191.
47. Pham AT, Ramulu PY, Boland MV, Yohannan J. The effect of transitioning from SITA Standard to SITA Faster on visual field performance. *Ophthalmology.* 2021;128:1417–1425.
48. Vingrys AJ, Demirel S. False-response monitoring during automated perimetry. Optometry and Visual. *Sciences.* 1998;75:513–517.
49. Nelson-Quigg JM, Twelker JD, Johnson CA. Response properties of normal observers and patients during automated perimetry. *Arch Ophthal.* 1989;107:1612–1615.
50. Johnson CA, Nelson-Quigg JM. A prospective three-year study of response properties of normals and patients during automated perimetry. *Ophthalmology.* 1993;100:269–274.
51. Bengtsson B, Heijl A. indicators of patient performance or test reliability? *Investig Ophthalmol Vis Sci.* 2000;41:2201–2204.
52. Johnson CA, Sherman K, Doyle C, Wall M. A Comparison of false negative responses for full threshold and SITA standard perimetry in glaucoma patients and normal observers. *J Glaucoma.* 2014;23:288–292.
53. Bengtsson B, Heijl A. A visual field index for calculation of glaucoma rate of progression. *Am J Ophthalmol.* 2009;145:343–353.
54. Artes PH, O'Leary N, Hutchison DM, et al. Properties of the Statpac visual field index. *Investig Ophthalmol Vis Sci.* 2011;52:4030–4038.
55. Rao HL, Senthil S, Choudhari NS, Mandal AK, Garudadri CS. Behavior of visual field index in advanced glaucoma. *Investig Ophthalmol Vis Sci.* 2013;54:307–312.
56. Talbot R, Goldberg I, Kelly P. Evaluating the accuracy of the visual field index for the Humphrey Visual Field Analyzer in patients with mild to moderate glaucoma. *Am J Ophthalmol.* 2013;156:1272–1276.
57. Ishiyama Y, Murata H, Mayama C, Asaoka R. An objective evaluation of gaze tracking in Humphrey perimetry and the relation with the reproducibility of visual fields: a pilot study in glaucoma. *Investig Ophthalmolo Vis Sci.* 2014;55:8149–8152.
58. Ishiyama Y, Murata H, Asaoka R. The usefulness of gaze tracking as an index of visual field reliability in glaucoma patients. *Investig Ophthalmol Vis Sci.* 2015;56:6233–6236.
59. Ishiyama Y, Murata H, Hirasawa H, Asaoka R. Estimating the usefulness of Humphrey perimetry gaze tracking for evaluating structure-function relationships in glaucoma. *Investig Ophthalmol Vis Sci.* 2015;56:7801–7805.
60. Arai T, Murata H, Matsuura M, Usui T, Asaoka R. The association between ocular surface measurements with visual field reliability indices and gaze tracking results in preperimetric glaucoma. *British J Ophthalmol.* 2018;102:525–530.
61. Asaoka R, Fujino Y, Aoki S, Matsuura M, Murata H. Estimating the reliability of glaucomatous visual field for the accurate assessment of progression using the gaze tracking and reliability indices. *Ophthalmol Glaucoma.* 2019;2:111–119.
62. Johnson CA, Keltner JL. Principles and techniques of examination of the visual sensory system. In: Miller NR, Newman NJ, eds. *Walsk and Hoyt's Textbook of NeuropOphthalmology*, 5th ed. Vol. 1. Philadelphia: Lippincott, Williams and Wilkins, 1998:153–235 [Chapter 7]
63. Wall M, Johnson CA. Principles and Techniques of the examination of the visual sensory system. In: Miller NR, Newman NJ, eds. *Walsh and Hoyt's Clinical Ophthalmology.*, Vol.1. Philadelphia: Lippincott, Williams and Wilkens; 2005:83–149 [Chapter 2].
64. Rowe F. *Visual Fields Via the Visual Pathway.* 2nd edition. London: CRC Press; 2016.
65. Choplin N, Edwards R. *Visual Fields.* West Depford, NJ: Slack Publishing; 1998.
66. Hu R, Racette L, Chen KS, Johnson CA. Functional assessment of glaucoma: Uncovering progression. *Surv Ophthalmol.* 2020;65:639–661.
67. Vesti E, Johnson CA, Chauhan BC. Comparison of different methods for detecting glaucomatous visual field progression. *Investig Ophthalmol Vis Sci.* 2003;44:3873–3879.
68. Vesti, E, Chauhan BC, Johnson CA. Comparison of different methods for detecting glaucomatous visual field progression. In: Henson D, Wall M, eds. *Perimetry Update 2002/2003.* the Hague: Kugler Publications, 2004:39–40.
69. Katz J. Scoring systems for measuring progression of visual field loss in clinical trials of glaucoma treatment. *Ophthalmology.* 1999;106:391–395.
70. Heijl A, Bengtsson B, Chauhan BC, et al. A comparison of visual field progression criteria of 3 major glaucoma trials in early manifest glaucoma trial patients. *Ophthalmology.* 2008;115:1557–1565.
71. Viswanathan AC, Crabb DP, McNaught AI, et al. Interobserver agreement on visual field progression in glaucoma: a comparison of methods. *British J Ophthalmol.* 2003;87: 726–730.
72. Schulzer M, Anderson DR, Drance SM. Sensitivity and specificity of a diagnostic test determined by repeated observations in the absence of an external standard. *J Clin Epidemiol.* 1991;44:1167–1179.
73. Brusini P, Johnson CA. Staging functional damage in glaucoma: review of different classification methods. *Surv Ophthalmol.* 2007;52:156–179.
74. Advanced Glaucoma Intervention Study. 2 Visual field scoring and reliability. *Ophthalmology.* 1994;101:1445–1455.
75. Musch DC, Lichter PR, Guire KE, Standardi CL. The Collaborative Initial Glaucoma Treatment Study: study design, methods and baseline characteristics of enrolled patients. *Ophthalmology.* 1999;106:653–662.
76. Leske MC, Heijl A, Hyman L, Bengtsson B. Early Manifest Glaucoma Trial: Design and baseline data. *Ophthalmology.* 1999;106:2144–2153.
77. Heijl A, Leske MC, Bengtsson B, Bengtsson B, Hussein M. Early Manifest Glaucoma Trial Group. Measuring visual field progression in the Early Manifest Glaucoma Trial. *Acta Ophthalmol.* 2003;81:286–293.
78. Artes PH, O'Leary N, Nicolela MT, Chauhan BC, Crabb DP. Visual field progression in glaucoma: what is the specificity of the Guided Progression Analysis? *Ophthalmology.* 2014;121:2023–2027.
79. Nguyen AT, Greenfield DS, Bhakta AS, Lee J, Feuer WJ. Detecting glaucoma progression using Guided Progression Analysis with OCT and visual field assessment in eyes classified by international classification of disease severity codes. *Ophthalmol Glaucoma.* 2019;2:36–46.
80. Hitchings RA, Migdal CS, Wormald R, Poinooswamy D, Fitze F. The primary treatment trial: changes in the visual field analysis by computer assisted perimetry. *Eye.* 1994;8:117–120.
81. Kummet CM, Zamba KD, Doyle CK, Johnson CA, Wall M. Refinement of pointwise linear regression criteria for determining glaucoma progression. *Investig Ophthalmol Vis Sci.* 2013;54:6234–6241.
82. Naghizadeh F, Hollo G. Detection of glaucomatous progression with Octopus cluster trend analysis. *J Glaucoma.* 2014;23:269–275.
83. Gardiner SK, Mansberger SL. Detection of functional deterioration in glaucoma analysis by trend analysis using overlapping clusters of locations. *Transl Vis Sci Technol.* 2020;9:12.
84. Wu Z, Medeiros FA. Comparison of visual field point-wise event-based and global trend-based analysis for detecting glaucomatous progression. *Transl Vis Sci Technol.* 2018;7:20.
85. Gardiner SK, Demirel S, DeMoraes CG, et al. Ocular Hypertension Treatment Study Group. Series length used during trend analysis affects sensitivity to changes in progression rate in the ocular hypertension treatment study. *Investig Ophthalmol Vis Sci.* 2013;54:1252–1259.
86. Pathak M, Demirel S, Gardiner SK. Nonlinear, multilevel mixed-effects approach for modeling longitudinal standard automated perimetry data in glaucoma. *Investig Ophthalmol Vis Sci.* 2013;54:5505–5513.
87. Alasil T, Wang K, Yu F, et al. Correlation of retinal nerve fiber layer thickness and visual fields in glaucoma: a broken stick model. *Am J Ophthalmol.* 2014;157:953–959.
88. Wollstein G, Kagemann L, Bilonick RA, et al. Retinal nerve fibre layer and visual function loss in glaucoma: the tipping point. *British J Ophthalmol.* 2012;95:47–52.
89. Rao HL, Kumbar T, Kumar AU, Babu JG, Senthil S, Garudadri CS. Agreement between event-based and trend-based glaucoma progression analysis. *Eye.* 2013;27:803–808.
90. Aref AA, Budenz DL. Detecting visual field progression. *Ophthalmology.* 2017;124:S51–S56.
91. Medeiros FA, Weinreb RN, Moore G, Liebmann JM, Girkin CA, Zangwill LM. Integrating event- and trend-based analyses to improve detection of glaucomatous visual field progression. *Ophthalmology.* 2012;119:458–467.
92. McKendrick AM. Recent developments in perimetry: test stimuli and procedures. *Clin Exp Optom.* 2005;88:73–80.
93. Johnson C.A. Chapter 8: Psychophysical and electrophysiological testing in glaucoma: visual fields and other functional tests. in Choplin N. and Traverso C eds, *Atlas of Glaucoma*, Third Edition, 2014, pp 87-112.
94. Johnson CA. Advanced psychophysical tests for glaucoma. In: Yanoff M, Duker J, eds. *Ophthalmology.* 3rd edition. New York: Elsevier; 2009:1137–1140.
95. Johnson CA. Detecting functional changes in the patient's vision—Visual field analysis. In: Schecknow P, Samples J, eds. *Schacknow and Samples: The Glaucoma Book (Paul Schecknow and John Samples, eds)*, Wilmington, PA: Springer, 2010:239–264 [CHapter 23].
96. Rodriguez-Una I, Azuara-Blanco A. New technologies for glaucoma detection. *Asia Pac, J Ophthalmol.* 2018;7:394–404.
97. Heijl A, Patella VM, Chong LX, et al. A new SITA perimetric threshold testing algorithm: Construction and a multicenter clinical study. *Am J Ophthalmol.* 2019;198:154–165.
98. Qian CX, Chen Q, Cun Q, et al. Comparison of the SITA Faster: a new visual field strategy with SITA Fast strategy. *Int J Ophthalmol.* 2021;14:1185–1191.
99. Pham AT, Ramulu PY, Boland MV, Yohannan J. The effect of transitioning from SITA Standard to SITA Faster on visual field performance. *Ophthalmology.* 2021;128:1417–1425.
100. Lavanya R, Riyazuddin M, Dasari S, et al. A comparison of the visual field parameters of SITA Faster and SITA Standard strategies in glaucoma. *J Glaucoma.* 2020;29:783–788.
101. Phu J, Kalloniatis M. Viability of performing multiple 24-2 visual field examinations at the same clinical visit: The Frontloading Fields Study. *Am J Ophthalmol.* 2021;230:48–59.
102. Phu J, Kalloniatis M. The Frontloading Fields Study (FFS): detecting changes in mean deviation in glaucoma using multiple visual field tests per clinical visit. *Transl Vis Sci Technol.* 2021;10(13):21.
103. Chakravarti T, Moghadam M, Proudfoot JA, Weinreb RN, Bowd C, Zangwill LM. Agreement between 10-2 and 24-2C visual field test protocols for detecting glaucomatous central visual field defects. *J Glaucoma.* 2021;30:e285–e291.
104. Phu J, Kalloniatis M. Comparison of 10-2 and 24-2C test grids for identifying central visual field defects in glaucoma and suspect patients. *Ophthalmology.* 2021;128:1405–1416.
105. Phu J, Kalloniatis M. Ability of 24-2C and 24-2 grids to identify central visual field defects and structure-function concordance in glaucoma and suspects. *Am J Ophthalmol.* 2020;219:317–331.
106. Hong JW, Baek MS, Lee JY, Song MK, Shin JW, Kook MS. Comparison of the 24-2 and 24-2C visual field grids in determining the macular structure-function relationship in glaucoma. *J Glaucoma.* 2021;30:887–894.
107. Yamane MLM, Odel JG. Introducing the 24-2C visual field test in neuro-ophthalmology. *Journal of Neuroophthalmology.* 2021;41:e606–e611.
108. Johnson CA, Adams AJ, Twelker JD, QUigg JM. Age-related changes in the central visual field for short wavelength sensitive pathways. *J Opt Soc Am A.* 1988;5:2131–2139.
109. Johnson CA. Diagnostic value of short wavelength automated perimetry. *Curr Opin Ophthalmol.* 1996;7:54–58.
110. Sample PA. Short wavelength automated perimetry: its role in the clinic and for understanding ganglion cell function. *Prog Retin Eye Res.* 2000;19:369–383.
111. Sample PA, Johnson CA, Haegerstrom-Portnoy G, Adams AJ. Optimum parameters for short wavelength automated perimetry. *J Glaucoma.* 1996;5:375–383.

112. Racette L, Sample PA. Short wavelength automated perimetry. *Ophthalmol Clin North Am.* 2003;16:227–236.
113. Stiles WS. Increment thresholds and the mechanisms of color vision. *Doc Ophthalmol.* 1949;3:138–165.
114. Kitahara K, Tamaki R, Noji J, Kandatsu A, Matsuzaki H. Extrafoveal Stiles'π mechanisms. In: Greve EL, Heijl A, eds. *Fifth International Visual Field Symposium. Documenta Ophthalmologica Proceedings Series.* vol 35. Dordrecht: Springer; 1983.
115. Kranda K, King-Smith PE. What can color thresholds tell us about the nature of underlying detection mechanisms? *Ophthal Physiol Opt.* 1984;4:83–87.
116. Sample PA, Weinreb RN. Progressive color visual field loss in glaucoma. *Investig Ophthalmol Vis Sci.* 1992;33:2068–2071.
117. Sample PA, Martinez GA, Weinreb RN. Color visual fields: a five-year prospective study in eyes with primary open angle glaucoma. In: Mills RP, ed. *Perimetry Update 1992/93.* New York: Kugler Publications; 1993:473–476.
118. Johnson CA, Sample PA, Cioffi GA, Liebmann JR, Weinreb RN. Structure and Function Evaluation (SAFE): I. Criteria for glaucomatous visual field loss. *Am J Ophthalmol.* 2002;134:177–185.
119. Johnson CA, Sample PA, Zangwill LM, et al. Structure and Function Evaluation (SAFE): II. Comparison of optic disc and visual field characteristics. *Am J Ophthalmol.* 2003;135:148–154.
120. Johnson CA, Adams AJ, Casson EJ, Brandt JD. Blue-on-yellow perimetry can predict the development of glaucomatous visual field loss. *Arch Ophthal.* 1993;111:645–650.
121. Johnson CA, Adams AJ, Casson EJ, Brandt JD. Progression of early glaucomatous visual field loss for blue-on-yellow and standard white-on-white automated perimetry. *Arch Ophthal.* 1993;111:651–656.
122. Johnson CA, Brandt JD, Khong AM, Adams AJ. Short wavelength automated perimetry (SWAP) in low-, medium- and high-risk ocular hypertensives: Initial baseline findings. *Arch Ophthal.* 1995;113:70–76.
123. Johnson CA, Adams AJ, Casson EJ. Blue-on-yellow perimetry: a five-year overview. In: Mills RP, ed. *Perimetry Update 1992/93.* New York: Kugler Publications; 1993:459–466.
124. Demirel S, Johnson CA. Isolation of short wavelength sensitive mechanisms in normal and glaucomatous visual field regions. *J Glaucoma.* 2000;9:63–73.
125. Sit AJ, Medieros FA, Weinreb RN. Short wavelength automated perimetry can predict glaucomatous visual field loss by ten years. *Semin Ophthalmol.* 2004;19:122–124.
126. Van der Schoot J, Reus NJ, Colen TP, Lemij HG. The ability of short wavelength automated perimetry to predict conversion to glaucoma. *Ophthalmology.* 2010;117:30–34.
127. Bengtsson B, Heijl A. Diagnostic sensitivity of fast blue-yellow standard automated perimetry in early glaucoma: a comparison between different test programs. *Ophthalmology.* 2006;113:1092–1097.
128. Turpin A, Johnson CA, Spry PGD. Development of a maximum likelihood procedure for short wavelength automated perimetry (SWAP). In: Wall M, Mills RP, eds. *Perimetry Update 2000/2001.* The Hague: Kugler Publications; 2001:139–147.
129. Bengtsson B. A new rapid threshold algorithm for short wavelength automated perimetry *Investig Ophthalmol and Vis Sci.* 4420031388–1394.
130. McKendrick AM, Cioffi GA, Johnson CA. Short wavelength sensitivity deficits in patients with migraine. *Arch Ophthal.* 2002;120:154–161.
131. Keltner JL, Johnson CA. Short wavelength automated perimetry in neuro-ophthalmologic disorders. *Arch Ophthal.* 1995;113:475–481.
132. Zhou HP, Asaoka R, Inoue T, et al. Short wavelength automated perimetry and standard automated perimetry in central serous chorioretinopathy. *Sci Rep.* 2020;10(1):16451.
133. Walters JW, Gaume A, Pate L. Short wavelength automated perimetry compared with achromatic perimetry in autosomal dominant optic atrophy. *British J Ophthalmol.* 2006;90:1267–1270.
134. Abrishami M, Daneshvar R, Yaghubi Z. Short wavelength automated perimetry in type I diabetic patients without retinal involvement: a test modification to decrease test duration. *Eur J Ophthalmol.* 2012;22:203–209.
135. Remky A, Weber A, Hendricks S, Lichtenberg K, Arend O. Short wavelength automated perimetry in patients with diabetes mellitus without macular edema. *Graefes Arch Clin Exp Ophthalmol.* 2003;241:468–471.
136. Kelly DH. Frequency doubling in visual responses. *J Opt Soc Am A.* 1966;56:1628–1633.
137. Kelly DH. Non-linear visual responses to flickering sinusoidal gratings. *J Opt Soc Am.* 1981;71:1051–1055.
138. Maddess T, Henry H. Performance of non-linear visual units in ocular hypertension and glaucoma. *Clin Vis Sci.* 1992;7:371–383.
139. Johnson CA, Samuels SJ. Screening for glaucomatous visual field using the frequency doubling contrast test. *Investigative Ophthalmology and Visual Sciences.* 1997;38:413–425.
140. Johnson CA, Wall M, Fingeret M, Lalle P. *A Primer for Frequency Doubling Technology Perimetry.* Skaneateles, New York: Welch Allyn; 1998.
141. Spry PGD, Johnson CA, Anderson AJ, et al. *A Primer for frequency Doubling Technology Perimetry Using The Humphrey Matrix.* Dublin, CA: Carl Zeiss Meditec; 2008.
142. Chauhan BC, Johnson CA. Test-retest variability characteristics of Frequency Doubling Perimetry and conventional perimetry in glaucoma patients and normal controls. *Investig Ophthalmol Vis Sci.* 1999;40:648–656.
143. Cello KE, Nelson-Quigg JM, Johnson CA. Frequency doubling technology (FDT) perimetry for detection of glaucomatous visual field loss. *Am J Ophthalmol.* 2000;129:314–322.
144. Anderson A.J. and Johnson C.A.: Frequency-doubling technology perimetry. In Sample PA and Girkin CA, ed., *Ophthalmology Clinics of North America*, Philadelphia: W.B. Saunders, 2003, vol 16, number 2, 213-225.
145. Johnson CA, Fingeret M, Iwase I. Frequency doubling technology perimetry. In: Weinreb RN, Greve EL, eds. *Glaucoma Diagnosis, Structure and Function.* The Hague: Kugler Publications; 2004:109–117.
146. Johnson CA. Frequency doubling technology perimetry for neuro-ophthalmological diseases. (Editorial). *British J Ophthalmol.* 2004;88:1232–1233.
147. Takahashi G, Demirel S, Johnson CA. Predicting conversion to glaucoma using standard automated perimetry and frequency doubling perimetry. *Graefes Arch. Clin. Exp. Ophthalmol.* 2017;255(4):797–803.
148. Quinn LM, Wheeler DT, Gardiner SK, Newkirk M, Johnson CA. Frequency doubling technology (FDT) perimetry in normal children. *Am J Ophthalmol.* 2006;142:983–989.
149. Huang C, Carolan J, Redline D, et al. Humphrey matrix frequency doubling perimetry for neuro-ophthalmic disorders of the optic nerve and chiasm: comparison with Humphrey SITA Standard 24-2. *Investig Ophthalmol Vis Sci.* 2008;49:917–923.
150. Tavarati P, Woodward K, Keltner J, et al. Sensitivity and specificity of the Humphrey matrix to detect homonymous hemianopsias. *Investig Ophthalmol Vis Sci.* 2008;49:924–928.
151. Anderson AJ, Johnson CA, Werner JS. Measuring central visual function in age-related maculopathy with frequency-doubling (Matrix) perimetry. *Optom Vis Sci.* 2011;88:806–815.
152. Anderson AJ, Johnson CA, Fingeret M, et al. Characteristics of the normative database for the Humphrey matrix perimeter. *Investig Ophthalmol Vis Sci.* 2005;46:1540–1548.
153. Hu R, Wang C, Racette L. Comparison of matrix frequency-doubling technology perimetry and standard automated perimetry in monitoring the development of visual field defects for glaucoma suspect eyes. *PLoS One.* 2017;12(5):e0178079.
154. Racette L, Medeiros FA, Zangwill LM, Ng D, Weinreb RN, Sample PA. Diagnostic accuracy of the Matrix 24-2 and original N-30 frequency-doubling technology tests compared with standard automated perimetry. *Investig Ophthalmol Vis Sci.* 2008;49:954–960.
155. Yoon MK, Hwang TN, Day S, Hong J, Porce T, McCulley TJ. Comparison of Humphrey matrix frequency doubling technology to standard automated perimetry in neuro-ophthalmic disease. *Middle East Afr J Ophthalmol.* 2012;19:211–215.
156. Sakai T, Matsushima M, Shikishima K, Kitahara K. Comparison of standard automated perimetry with matrix frequency doubling technology in patients with resolved optic neuritis. *Ophthalmology.* 2007;114:949–956.
157. Prager AJ, Kang JM, Tanna AP. Advances in perimetry for glaucoma. *Curr Opin Ophthalmol.* 2021;32:92–97.
158. Johnson CA, Thapa S, Kong YXG, Robin AL. Performance of an iPad application to detect moderate and advanced visual field loss in Nepal. *Am J Ophthalmol.* 2017;182:147–154.
159. Livingstone I, Butler A, Masanjo E, et al. Testing pediatric acuity with an iPad: Validation of "Peekaboo Vision" in Malawi and the UK. *Transl Vis Sci Technol.* 2018;8(1):8.
160. Aslam TM, Perry NRA, Murray IJ, et al. Development and testing of an automated computer tablet-based method for self-testing of high and low contrast near visual acuity in ophthalmic patients. *Graefes Arch Clin Exp Ophthalmol.* 2016;254:591–599.
161. Prea SM, Kong GYX, Guymer RH, Sivarajah P, Baglin EK, Vingrys AJ. The short-term compliance and concordance to in clinic testing for tablet-based home monitoring in age-related macular degeneration. *Am J Ophthalmol.* 2021;235:280–290.
162. Varadaraj V, Assi L, Gajwani P, et al. Evaluation of tablet-based tests of visual acuity and contrast sensitivity in older adults. *Ophthalmic Epidemiol.* 2021;28:293–300.
163. Chacon A, Rabin J, Yu D, Johnston S, Bradshaw T. Quantification of color vision using a tablet display. *Aerosp Med Hum Perf.* 2015;86:56–58.
164. Vingrys AJ, Healey JK, Liew S, et al. Validation of a tablet as a tangent perimeter. *Transl Vis Sci Technol.* 2016, 14;5(4):3.
165. Jones PR, Lindfield D, Crabb DP. Using an open-source perimeter (Eyecatcher) as a rapid triage measure for glaucoma clinic waiting areas. *British J Ophthalmol.* 2021;105:681–686.
166. Dorr M, Lesmes LA, Elze T, Wang H, Lu ZL, Bex PJ. Evaluation of the precision of contrast sensitivity function assessment on a tablet device. *Sci Rep.* 2017;7:46706.
167. Dorr M, Lesmes LA, Lu ZL, Bex PJ. Rapid and reliable assessment of the contrast sensitivity function on an iPad. *Investig Ophthalmol Vis Sci.* 2013;54:7266–7273.
168. Jones PR, Campbell P, Callagan T, et al. Glaucoma home monitoring using a tablet-based visual field test (Eyecatcher): an assessment of accuracy and adherence over 6 months. *Am J Ophthalmol.* 2021;223:42–52.
169. Wu Z, Guymer RH, Jung CJ, et al. Measurement of retinal sensitivity on tablet devices in age-related macular degeneration. *Transl Vis Sci Technol.* 2015;4(3):13.
170. Nesaratnam N, Thomas PBM, Kirollos R, Vingrys AJ, Kong GYX, Martin KR. Tablets at the bedside: iPad-based visual field test used in the diagnosis of intrasellar haemangiopericytoma: A case report. *BMC Ophthalmol.* 2017;17(1):53.
171. Harris P, Johnson CA, Chen Y, et al. Evaluation of the Melbourne Rapid Fields (MRF) test procedure. *Optom Vis Sci.* 2022;99:372–382.
172. Vivas-Mateos G., Boswell S., Livingstone I.A.T., Delafield -Butt J., Giardini M.E. Screen and virtual reality-based testing of contrast sensitivity. Annual International Conference of IEEE Engineering Medicine and Biology Society, 2020, 2054–6067.
173. Lynn MH, Luo G, Tomasi M, Pundlik S, Houston KE. Measuring virtual reality headset resolution and field of view: implications for vision care applications. *Optom Vis Sci.* 2020;97:573–582.
174. Montelongo M, Gonzalez A, Morganstern F, Donahue SP, Groth SL. A virtual reality-based automated perimeter, device and pilot study. *Transl Vis Sci and Technol.* 2021;10(3):20.
175. Jones T, Troscianko T. Mobility performance of low-vision adults using an electronic mobility aid. *Clin Exp Optom.* 2006;89:20–27.
176. Hollander DA, Volpe NJ, Moster ML, Balcer LJ, Judy KD, Galetta SL. Use of a portable head mounted perimetry system to assess bedside visual fields. *British J Ophthalmol.* 2000;84:1185–1190.
177. Stapefeidt J, Kucur SS, Huber N, Hohn R, Sznitman R. Virtual reality-based and conventional visual field examination comparison in healthy and glaucoma patients. *Transl Vis Sci Technol.* 2021;10(12):10.
178. Sayad AM, Abdel-Mottaleb M, Kashem R, et al. Expansion of peripheral visual field with novel virtual reality digital spectacles. *Am J Ophthalmol.* 2020;210:125–135.
179. Mees L, Upadhayaya S, Kumar P, et al. Validation of a head-mounted virtual reality visual field screening device. *J Glaucoma.* 2020;29:86–91.
180. Herse PR. Factors influencing normal perimetric thresholds obtained using the Humphrey field analyzer. *Investig Ophthalmol Vis Sci.* 1992;33:611–617.
181. Keltner JL, Johnson CA, Spurr JO, Kass MA, Gordon MO, the Ocular Hypertension Study Group Confirmation of visual field abnormalities in the Ocular Hypertension Treatment Study (OHTS). *Arch Ophthal.* 2000;118:1187–1194.
182. Keltner JL, Johnson CA, Cello KE, et al. Classification of visual field abnormalities in the ocular hypertension treatment study. *Arch Ophthal.* 2003;121:643–650.
183. Keltner JL, Johnson CA, Spurr JO, Beck RW, the Optic Neuritis Study Group Baseline visual field profile of optic neuritis: the experience of the Optic Neuritis Treatment Trial. *Arch Ophthal.* 1993;111:231–234.

36

Binocular Vision

Dennis M. Levi and Clifton M. Schor

INTRODUCTION

"No question relating to vision has been so much debated as the cause of the single appearance of objects seen by both eyes" (Charles Wheatstone, 1838[1])

The question has been discussed at least since Aristotle (384–322 BC) and subject to empirical investigation since Ptolemy (ca. 100–170). For a scholarly discussion of the origin of the many of the terms encountered in this chapter on binocular vision, see Wade (2021).[2]

Humans and many other animals with frontally located eyes achieve binocular vision from the two retinal images through a series of sensory and motor processes that result in our rich percept of single objects and stereoscopic (three-dimensional [3D]) depth. Achieving "normal" single binocular vision and keen stereoscopic depth perception requires:

1. Accurate central monocular fixation with each eye.
2. Accurate simultaneous binocular fixation.
3. Integrated neuromuscular activity of both the intra- and extraocular muscles.
4. A sensory correspondence system organized about the two foveas.
5. Similarity of the final ocular images from each eye (i.e., similar size, acuity, and contrast sensitivity).
6. A neural mechanism to combine the images from the two eyes to compute binocular disparity and estimate stereoscopic depth intervals by scaling disparity with distance cues.

"Normal" binocular vision represents a highly coordinated organization of sensory and motor processes. Failure of any component may result in compromised binocular vision and stereopsis. Indeed, the evaluation of binocular vision is clinically very important because it tells us about the integrity of the underlying visual processes. Aside from refractive error, binocular vision anomalies are among the most common problems encountered in optometry and ophthalmology. About 7% of the population is stereoblind[3]; as much as 30% of the population may have poor stereopsis[4]; approximately 3% to 5% has strabismus; approximately 3% has amblyopia; and many more have high phorias, convergence insufficiency, etc. The topics that follow are intended to provide the foundation for the clinical science of binocular vision.

WHY TWO EYES?

Perhaps most fundamentally, having two eyes confers the same evolutionary advantage as having two lungs or two ears: redundancy—it is good to have spare parts in case of loss. And having two eyes, like having two ears, provides for facial symmetry. A second functional advantage is that two eyes enable you to see more of the world. Each stationary eye alone can see about 150 degrees from side to side, but the binocular field of view is about 190 degrees, with a central 120 degrees of overlap of the monocular visual fields. Moreover, image distortions or scotomas in one eye, such as the blind spot, can be masked by a normal image in the other eye. Third, in normal vision, visual sensitivity for near-threshold stimuli is greater with two eyes than with one (by about a factor of 1.5),[5] through the process of binocular summation. Indeed, it has been suggested that binocular summation may have provided the evolutionary pressure that first moved eyes toward the front of the faces of some birds and mammals.[6] This advantage is reduced at suprathreshold levels by gain control mechanisms.[7,8] Finally, two frontal eyes enable stereopsis, the vivid impression of three-dimensionality—of objects "popping out in depth"—that most humans get when viewing real-world objects with both eyes. This is based on binocular disparity—the differences between the two retinal images of the same world that are not available with purely monocular vision. At its most elementary level, acute stereopsis benefits both the predator, at the point of attack, and the prey, by unmasking the camouflage of predators.[9]

MAPPING THE TWO EYE'S IMAGES INTO A SINGLE PERCEPT

Given that we see a single, unified world, intuitively it makes sense that information from the two eyes should be brought together at some point. However, until Hubel and Wiesel's Nobel prize–winning discovery that this convergence is first evident in the primary visual cortex, where most neurons can be influenced by input from both the left and right eyes (that is, they are binocular),[10,11] there were strong arguments about whether the information converged at all, and if so, whether it was in a specialized "fusion center" in the brain—a notion that dates back to Descartes (1664; see ref 12).

A full description of the neural basis of binocular vision is beyond the scope of this chapter. In brief, the story begins with the semidecussation of the optic fibers at the optic chiasm. Axons from the retinal ganglion cells (RGCs) form the optic nerves of each eye. When they reach the chiasm, fibers from the nasal half of each retina cross to the opposite side of the brain; axons from the temporal half do not cross. Axons from the left half of each retina end up in the left lateral geniculate nucleus (LGN), while the axons from the right end up in the right LGN. Thus, the right LGN receives projections from the left visual field, and vice versa. Each LGN layer contains a highly ordered "map" of half of the visual field. This "topographic" mapping provides us with a neural basis for knowing where things are in space. Excitatory inputs from the two eyes do not converge onto a binocular map in the LGN (because each eye's map is in a different layer), and there is limited functional binocular convergence of the eye-specific inputs in the retinogeniculate pathway.[13] However, information from the same part of the visual field is mapped to corresponding regions in adjacent layers. This binocular convergence does not happen until the primary visual cortex, where most neurons can be influenced by input from both the left and right eyes—that is, they are binocular.[11] A binocular neuron has two receptive fields, one in each eye. In binocular primary visual cortex neurons, the receptive fields in the two eyes are generally quite similar, sharing nearly identical orientation and spatial-frequency tuning, as well as the same preferred speed and direction of motion.[14] Thus, these cells are well suited to the task of matching images in the two eyes. This is a remarkable transformation, because up to this point information from the two eyes is separated. However, this changes dramatically in striate cortex, where a majority of cells can be influenced through <u>both</u> the left eye and the right eye.

Many binocular neurons respond best when the retinal images are on corresponding points in the two retinas, that is, the two eyes' images appear in identical visual directions (i.e., they appear in the same spatial location), thereby providing a neural basis for the horopter, which is normally located close to the plane of fixation and where objects appear single. However, many other binocular neurons respond best when similar images occupy slightly *different* or disparate positions[15–17] on the retinas of the two eyes or when images fall on receptive fields with different spatial phases.[18–20] In other words, these neurons are tuned to a particular binocular disparity. Binocular neurons in V1 may provide a neural substrate for detecting absolute disparity,[21] i.e., the depth-distance from the horopter. Other cortical areas (e.g., V2, V4) may be the substrate for computing relative disparity,[22,23] that is, depth discrimination (discussed later).

VISUAL DIRECTION

Locating objects in 3D space requires knowing the relationship between the locations of objects in physical space and their perceived (subjective) spatial locations,[24] as illustrated in Fig. 36.1. This simple figure illustrates several important concepts. The perceived visual directions of objects depends on the retinal locations of their images. Each retinal image location is associated with a specific visual direction, called its local sign or oculocentric direction.[24,25] The primary visual direction is the oculocentric direction of an object that is fixated along the primary line of sight and is imaged on the center of the fovea (represented by the *diamond* in Fig. 36.1). Secondary lines of sight are the oculocentric directions of other retinal image locations relative to the primary visual direction. As illustrated in Fig. 36.1, the perceived visual directions of nonfixated objects (represented by the *circle* and *square*) are relative to the visual direction of a fixated object (represented by the *diamond*). In the example, an image located to the left side of the fovea is perceived to the right of the fixated object, (e.g., the visual direction of the square). The normal ability to distinguish differences in oculocentric directions is extremely accurate, as demonstrated by Vernier alignment thresholds, which are in the order of 6 arc seconds for foveal viewing (see Chapter 33).

However, retinal image location alone is not sufficient to define the relationship between the physical and perceived locations of objects in space. The perceived direction of an object in space relative to the body, the egocentric direction, is derived from the combination of its oculocentric visual direction with information about version eye orientation in the head (i.e., direction of gaze) and head position relative to the trunk of the body. Egocentric localization is referenced to an egocenter, which is generally located at a point midway between the two eyes where a cyclopean eye represents binocular visual directions. The retina of the cyclopean eye is a metaphorical representation of a binocular map of oculocentric directions computed in the visual cortex. The gaze direction of the cyclopean eye equals the version gaze position of the two eyes. Projected visual directions from the cyclopean retina are egocentric (i.e., they are the combination of oculocentric direction and version eye position). The combined information of

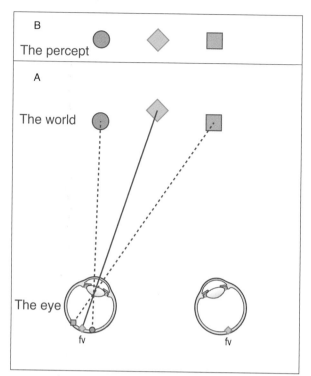

Fig. 36.1 Perceived visual direction as a function of retinal image location. (**A**) The relationships between objects in physical space and their retinal images. The *square* represents a fixated object (primary line of sight) and the nonfixated objects (*circle and square*) are secondary lines of sight. (**B**) The relationships between retinal image locations and their visual directions (oculocentric directions). The perceived visual directions of the nonfixated objects (secondary visual directions of the circle and square) are relative to the primary visual direction of the fixated diamond. *fv,*

retinal position and versional eye position is critical to distinguishing between retinal image motion caused by eye movements and movement of the object.[26]

Fig. 36.2 illustrates the concept of egocentric direction: The retinal oculocentric directions from the two retinal images of a single object at (Fig. 36.2A) or close to (Fig. 36.2B, circle) the plane of fixation are combined to produce a single direction (haplopia) relative to the observer's egocenter. Note that in this example, the binocular egocentric direction deviates slightly from either of the monocularly perceived directions by one-half of the angular disparity. If the retinal images have unequal contrast or luminance, the perceived direction will be biased or weighted toward the direction of the higher-contrast image.[27–29]

In contrast, for objects that are outside the range of single vision, either nearer or farther than the plane of fixation, a single object has two separate egocentric directions that correspond to two separate positions (i.e., oculocentric directions) on the cyclopean retina. Different directions are stimulated when the two eye's retinal images are formed on noncorresponding retinal locations. When combined with version eye position information, they are perceived in separate egocentric directions (i.e., diplopia, Fig. 36.2C). The egocentric directions of the diplopic images are perceived as though both monocular components had paired images on corresponding points in the contralateral eye (Fig. 36.2C). The relative egocentric direction of each of the diplopic images depends on whether the object is nearer or farther than the plane of fixation. For an object closer than the plane of fixation, the egocentric direction associated with the retinal image of the right eye is to the left of the egocentric direction produced by the image of the left

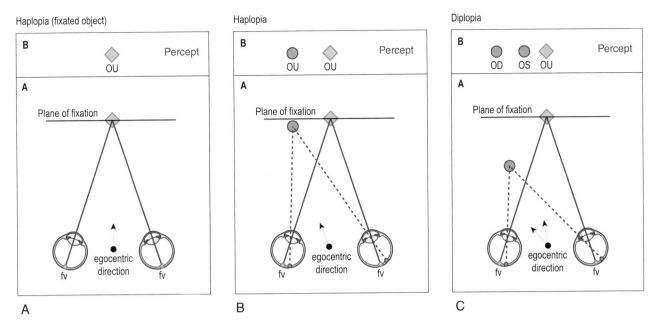

Fig. 36.2 Egocentric directions for haplopia and diplopia. (**A**) The oculocentric directions of a fixated object are combined to produce a single egocentric direction. (**B**) The retinal images of nonfixated objects that are near the plane of fixation also will be combined to produce a single egocentric direction. (**C**) When the disparity of retinal images is larger than the normal fusion range (Panum's fusional area), the oculocentric directions are not combined and the object has two egocentric directions (physiologic diplopia). *fv,* Fovea; *OD,* right eye; *OS,* left eye; *OU,* both eyes.

eye. This form of diplopia, produced by near objects, is called "crossed" diplopia due to the right-left/left-right relationship between the eyes and perceived locations of the object. Conversely, objects farther than the plane of fixation will be perceived with "uncrossed" diplopia, where the right eye sees an object located on the right side and the left eye sees an object located on the left side.

In normal binocular vision, diplopia of nonfixated objects lying nearer or farther than the plane of fixation, called physiologic diplopia, occurs as a natural consequence of the lateral separation of frontally located eyes and the topographical organization of binocularly corresponding visual directions across the retina. In contrast, patients with a late-onset strabismus may experience pathologic diplopia, wherein objects in the plane of fixation are perceived as doubled. In pathologic diplopia, the retinal image location caused by misalignment of the visual axis of the deviating eye causes a fixated target to be seen in different egocentric directions by the two eyes during binocular viewing. In addition to diplopia, an object imaged on the fovea of the deviating eye may have the same egocentric direction as another object imaged on the fovea of the fixating eye, resulting in visual confusion. Because diplopia and visual confusion may create an existential threat, most strabismic patients adapt by suppressing input from the deviating eye, and/or by developing anomalous retinal correspondence (discussed further in the chapter).

BINOCULAR EYE MOVEMENTS

Our eyes are in constant motion, making versions (conjugate changes in the visual axes of the two eyes in the same direction and magnitude) and vergences (rotations of the visual axes in opposite directions) as we look at and track objects in the world (see Chapter 9). However, in normal binocular vision, only versions influence the perception of egocentric direction, which is sensed as the average position of the two eyes. If vergence movements also influenced perception of egocentric directions, then vergence would produce disparities between visual directions of foveal images and would be in conflict with bifoveal retinal correspondence. Because vergence movements of the two eyes are in opposite directions, they do not change the computation of the average position of the two eyes. Thus, when the two eyes fixate objects to the left or right of the midline in asymmetric convergence, only the version, or conjugate, component of eye position contributes to perceived direction.[30]

NORMAL RETINAL CORRESPONDENCE AND THE HOROPTER

Fig. 36.2 illustrates the relationship between retinal image locations and perceived visual directions. The two foveal images of a fixated object (Fig. 36.2A diamond) share a common visual direction and are fused to produce the percept of a single haplopic object in subjective space (Fig. 36.2B). Points in the two retinae, that when stimulated result in the perception of the same visual direction, are defined as corresponding points. The foveas represent an important pair of corresponding retinal points, but there are many other pairs associated with secondary lines of sight and visual directions. For example, in Fig. 36.3 the *square* represents the location of an object in the right visual field that falls on paired retinal areas with a common visual direction for the two eyes, thus defining another set of corresponding retinal areas. Similarly, the *circle* in the left visual field represents a location of an object in the left visual field that is imaged on corresponding retinal points. Identical visual directions associated with corresponding points depend primarily on retinal image locations and their associated oculocentric directions. For a given fixation distance, the location of objects (in space) whose images lie on corresponding points in the two eyes define a surface called the horopter. In effect, the horopter is a map in space where binocularly viewed objects appear single.

The longitudinal (horizontal) horopter is illustrated by the *black curved line* in Fig. 36.3A. The shape of the horopter depends on the viewing distance (Fig. 36.4), as well as physiologic and optical factors that affect the retinal images and their cortical representations. The abathic distance is the distance at which the empirical horopter is a straight line (matching the apparent frontoparallel plane or AFPP). If the locations of corresponding points were simply determined by equal angular distances from the primary line of sight, then the horopter would be a circle passing through the fixation point and the entrance

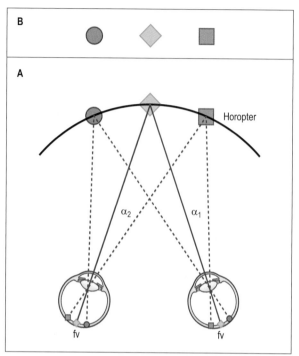

Fig. 36.3 Corresponding retinal points. Retinal areas in the two eyes with identical oculocentric directions (**B**) are corresponding retinal points. The locations of objects along the horizontal meridian that are imaged on corresponding points (**A**) define the longitudinal horopter. The physical location of an object that is on the horopter is quantified by the longitudinal visual angles (α_1 and α_2). *fv*, fovea.

pupil of each eye[24,31] (geometric or theoretical horopter or Vieth-Muller [V-M] circle—Fig. 36.4, *black circles*). Curvature changes in the horopter with viewing distance result from increases in the radius of the horopter circle (V-M circle) as viewing distance increases. Note, however, the measured (empirical) longitudinal horopter rarely coincides with the V-M circle. The horopter only equals the V-M circle when corresponding points are equidistant from their respective foveas. The deviation of the empirical horopter from the geometric horopter (the Hering-Hillebrand deviation) has been taken as evidence of an asymmetry between the locations of corresponding points on the nasal and temporal retinas. Compression of points on the nasal retinae compared with the temporal cause the horopter to be more curved, and compression on the temporal retinae cause it to be less curved than the V-M circle.

Pairs of retinal points with identical visual directions in the two eyes also define a vertical horopter (i.e., locations of object points in the midsagittal plane that are imaged on corresponding points along the vertical meridian; Fig. 36.5).[32–34.] The empirical vertical horopter is pitched top-back, with the degree of pitch increasing with viewing distance.[35,37] Fig. 36.6 shows both the horizontal and vertical empirical horopters (Fig. 36.6A) measured at different viewing distances. While fixating points at different distances along the ground plane, the declination or backward pitch of the vertical horopter expands the range of single vision by making objects along the ground plane appear fused during any single fixation distance.[36]

Disparities in the natural environment

The heatmap (Fig. 36.6B) shows the distribution of binocular disparities across the central visual field for a fixed viewing distance (100 cm), with darker colors representing greater uncrossed disparity (Fig. 8 from[38]). It is interesting to note that the upper visual field tends to have uncrossed (far) disparities, whereas the lower field has more crossed (near) disparities, closely matching the distribution of retinal disparities encountered in the natural environment[36,37] (Fig. 36.6C) (G & B 19 fig. 9B); indeed, the binocular sensory and motor systems are nicely adapted to the statistics of the natural environment.

Fig. 36.4 The empirical horopter (*thick solid line*) in relation to the Vieth-Muller circle (VMO; *circles*), defined by the locations of objects with equal longitudinal visual angles (α_1 and α_2), and the objective frontoparallel plane (OFPP; *dot-dot-dash line*), defined by a plane at the fixation distance that is parallel to a line passing through the entrance pupils of the two eyes.

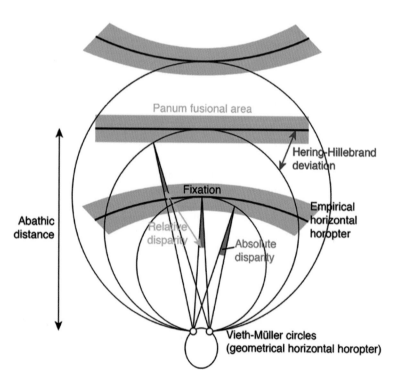

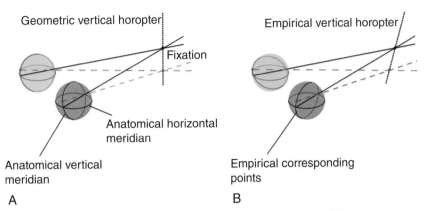

Fig. 36.5 (**A**) The geometric vertical horopter. The anatomical vertical meridians of the eyes are geometric corresponding points. When these points are projected into the world, they intersect at a vertical line in the head's midsagittal plane–the geometric vertical horopter. (**B**) The empirical vertical horopter has crossed disparity below fixation and uncrossed disparity above fixation, causing a top-back pitch. (From Cooper EA, Burge J, Banks MS. The vertical horopter is not adaptable, but it may be adaptive. *J Vis.* 2011;11(3).)

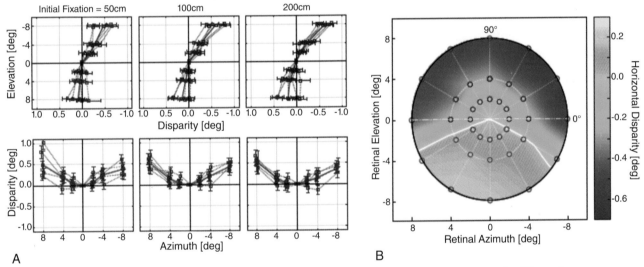

Fig. 36.6 Binocular horopter. (**A**) Binocular horopter along the vertical and horizontal meridians for different fixation distances (50, 100, and 200 cm) along the vertical (*top*) and horizontal (*bottom*) meridians. (**B**) Binocular horopter across the central visual field. Fixation distance was 100 cm. The abscissa and ordinate indicate azimuth and elevation, respectively. Median horizontal disparity for corresponding points is indicated by color: darker colors represent greater uncrossed disparity. *White curve* indicates where disparity changes sign from crossed to uncrossed. *Red dots* represent the tested field positions. (From Gibaldi A, Banks MS. Binocular eye movements are adapted to the natural environment. *J Neurosci* 2019;39(15):2877–2888.)

PANUM'S FUSIONAL AREA

The retinal images of objects in the world need not fall on precisely corresponding points in the two retinae to be perceived as single. The horopter represents the specific locations of objects the world that have zero retinal image disparity. For individuals with normal binocular vision there is a small range of distances (both behind and in front of the horopter), where objects are seen single. This range, illustrated by the shaded areas in Fig. 36.4, is Panum's fusional area.[38] Objects within Panum's area have some finite amount of binocular (retinal) disparity. However, the size and shape of Panum's area depends both on the eccentricity of the objects (the larger the eccentricity, the larger Panum's

area) and the spatial and temporal properties of the targets—smallest for small, rapidly varying (high spatial and temporal frequency) targets and larger for large, slowly varying (low spatial and temporal frequency) targets.[39] Panum's area allows for some useful vergence errors that assist vergence stability in binocular fixation without the penalty of diplopia.[40] Indeed, persons with normal binocular vision often manifest a fixation disparity, a small error in convergence under conditions of fusion—that is, while maintaining single binocular vision.[40–42] Fixation disparity is generally not measured in the clinic; however, the amount of prism required to eliminate the fixation disparity (known as the associated phoria) is used to prescribe prism to relieve the asthenopia that can occur in patients with large heterophorias[40] (see Box 36.1).

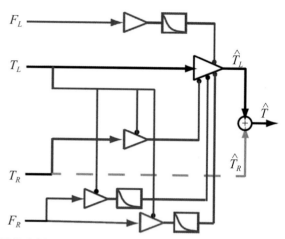

Fig. 36.7 A binocular gain control model with target-flanker interactions. (From Lev M, Ding J, Polat U, Levi DM. Nearby contours abolish the binocular advantage. *Sci Rep* 2021;11(1):16920. https://doi.org/10.1038/s41598-021-96053-9.)

BINOCULAR COMBINATION AND BINOCULAR SUPPRESSION IN NORMAL VISION

The superiority of binocular over monocular viewing for detecting near-threshold isolated targets, about a factor of 1.5, has been documented and quantified in hundreds of studies (reviewed in ref 44). We still do not have a full understanding of how the inputs to the two eyes are combined; however, to account for the complexity of binocular interactions under a broad range of different stimuli and tasks (including contrast detection, discrimination, and matching, as well as phase discrimination), almost all recent models of binocular combination incorporate dynamic gain control.[28,29,43,44] Dynamic gain control in the visual system is somewhat akin to automatic gain control (AGC) of image contrast in cameras. Separate AGCs for each eye serve to equalize the perceived contrast of the two eye images. Importantly, this class of models can predict the effects of having different stimulus contrast in the two eyes. When the stimuli in the two eyes differ substantially in contrast, the "winner takes all" (i.e., the eye with the higher contrast dominates). Indeed, a complex gain control model with flank-to-target and target-to-flank interactions (Fig. 36.7 shows the structure of this model) also predicts the effects of nearby flanking contours on monocular and binocular contrast detection, discrimination, and matching, and the complete failure of binocular summation when the separation of the flanking contours is too small.[45]

When the retinal images have significant differences in defocus or contrast interocular blur, suppression may occur. A wide range of conditions can produce unequal contrast of the two ocular images, including anisometropia, unequal amplitudes of accommodation, and asymmetric convergence on targets that are closer to one eye than to the other. Interocular blur suppression is requisite for adaptation to a monovision correction of presbyopia (in which one eye is corrected for distance viewing and the other for near). Monovision suppression allows clear, nonblurred, binocular percepts and retention of stereopsis, albeit with the stereo-threshold elevated by approximately twofold.[46–51]

However, when the stimuli to the two eyes differ substantially, a form of suppression known as binocular rivalry takes place.[52] The classic example of binocular rivalry occurs when nonfusible images such as orthogonally oriented gratings, for example horizontal in one eye and vertical in the other, are presented to corresponding retinal areas in the two eyes. Under these conditions, only one set of gratings (say horizontal) will be seen and, after several seconds, the image of the other set of gratings (say vertical) will appear to wash over the first (wholesale suppression). At other times, the two monocular images become fragmented, and small interwoven retinal patches from each eye alternate independently of one another. In this case, piecemeal suppression is regional, localized to the vicinity of the contour intersections.

The rivalrous patches appear to alternate between the two images approximately once every 4 seconds, but the rate of oscillation and its duty cycle vary with the degree of difference between the two ocular images and with the stimulus strength. The rate of rivalry increases as the orientation difference between the targets increases beyond 22 degrees,[52,53] indicating that rivalry is not likely to occur within the tuned range for cortical orientation columns. Levelt[54] formulated a series of rules describing how the dominance and suppression phases of binocular rivalry vary with the strength of stimulus variables such as brightness, contrast, and motion. He concluded that the duration of the suppression phase of one of the retinal images decreases when its stimulus visibility or strength is increased relative to the retinal image of the fellow eye. If the strengths of the stimuli for both eyes are increased, then the suppression phase for each eye decreases, and the oscillation rate of rivalry increases. Reducing the stimulus contrast of both eyes also reduces the oscillation rate until, at a very low level of contrast, rivalry is replaced with a binocular summation of nonfusible targets.[55,56]

The perception of rivalry has a latency of approximately 200 ms so that briefly presented nonfusible patterns appear superimposed.[57] However, rivalry occurs between dichoptic patterns that are alternated rapidly at 7 Hz or faster, indicating an integration time of at least 150 ms.[58] When rivalrous and fusible stimuli are presented simultaneously, fusion takes precedence over rivalry,[59] and the onset of a fusible target can terminate suppression, although the fusion mechanism takes time (150–200 ms) to become fully operational.[58,60] Suppression and stereo-fusion appear to be mutually exclusive outcomes of binocular rivalry stimuli presented at a given retinal location,[61,62] but stereoscopic depth and rivalry can be observed simultaneously when fusible contours are superimposed on rivalrous backgrounds.

The classic demonstrations of rivalry pit a stimulus in one eye against a stimulus in the other eye. However, rivalry can also occur between fragments of images in the same eye, and it is now clear that rivalry is part of a larger effort by the visual system to deal with ambiguity and come up with the most likely version of the world, given the current retinal images.[63,64]

Binocular rivalry is not the only form of suppression that takes place in normal binocular vision. Indeed, we rarely experience double vision in our everyday lives; however, as we view the world, much of the information lands on noncorresponding areas in the two eyes. Objects that are at some distance in front of or behind the plane of fixation (with binocular disparities that are well outside the limits of Panum's fusional areas) are rarely diplopic under normal casual viewing conditions because of the suppression of one image. The suppression of physiologic diplopia is called suspension because, unlike the binocular rivalry discussed previously, this form of suppression does not alternate between the two images. Instead, only one image is continually suppressed, favoring visibility of the target imaged on the nasal hemiretina.[53,65] However, calling attention to the disparate target can evoke physiologic diplopia.

More profound forms of suppression known as permanent suppression and continuous flash suppression (CFS) can also occur in normal vision.[66–68] Permanent suppression occurs when one eye views a contoured stimulus while the other eye views a spatially homogeneous field.[66] Under these conditions, the image of the eye viewing the contoured field dominates, while the image of the eye viewing the homogeneous field is almost continually suppressed. Permanent suppression occurs for the normal blind spot, which appears filled in, even under monocular viewing conditions. Because of the stability of the dominance/suppression percept under these viewing conditions, the term *permanent suppression* is used to distinguish this type of suppression from binocular rivalry suppression. You can experience a powerful demonstration of permanent suppression by holding a cylindrical tube in front of your right eye and placing the palm of your left hand in front of the left eye near the far end of the tube. The combined stable percept is that of a hole in the left hand. The hand is seen as the region surrounding the aperture through which the background is viewed. This ecologically valid example of occlusion gives priority to the background seen through the aperture.

A similar profound suppression of one eye takes place when a rapidly changing sequence of high-contrast, contour-rich patterns is presented to one eye and a static stimulus is presented to the other eye. Under these conditions, the static stimulus is suppressed from awareness.[67,68] CFS appears to selectively suppress low spatial frequency and cardinally oriented features in the image.[68]

BINOCULAR (RETINAL) DISPARITY AND DEPTH PERCEPTION

Objects that are not on the horopter will have some amount of binocular retinal disparity. Objects with horizontal retinal disparity are imaged on laterally separated noncorresponding retinal areas and, as in the case of the empirical horopter, the longitudinal visual angles (α_1 and α_2, the angles subtended by the primary and secondary lines of sight—Fig. 36.3) are unequal. Horizontal binocular disparity is a unique binocular stimulus for stereoscopic depth perception, horizontal disparity vergence eye movements, and horizontal diplopia, either physiologic or pathologic. In each case, the perceptual or motor response is a consequence of the relationship between the object's disparate images and the horopter. Crossed disparities give rise to a perception of "near" stereoscopic depth or crossed diplopia, and elicit convergence eye movements, while uncrossed disparities give rise to

a sense of relative "far" stereoscopic depth or uncrossed diplopia and divergence eye movements.

Absolute and relative disparity

The absolute disparity of an object is the difference between the angle subtended by the target at the two entrance pupils of the eyes and the angle of convergence. Absolute disparity is the optimal cue or stimulus for vergence eye movements. The *square* in Fig. 36.8 is farther away than the *diamond* (where the observer is fixating), the secondary lines of sight for the square intersect behind the horopter, which coincides with the angle of convergence. The absolute disparity produced by the square is uncrossed (it can be quantified by the difference between the longitudinal visual angles α_1 and α_2), and uncrossed disparities (outside of Panum's fusional area) evoke divergence eye movements. Uncrossed disparities may also give rise to the percept of relative "far" stereoscopic depth or, if the disparity is large, to uncrossed diplopia (i.e., double vision with the right eye's image seen to the right of the left eye's image). Crossed disparities give rise to the percept of relative "near" stereoscopic depth or, if the disparity is large, to crossed diplopia (i.e., double vision with the right eye's image seen to the left of the left eye's image), and uncrossed disparities (outside of Panum's fusional area) evoke convergence eye movements.

The judgment of relative depth (for instance, the distance of square relative to the diamond in Fig. 36.8) is based on relative disparity (i.e., the difference between the absolute disparities of two objects). Horizontal relative disparity provides the cue for high-resolution stereopsis or stereo-depth discrimination. Humans are an order-of-magnitude more sensitive to relative than to absolute disparity.[69]

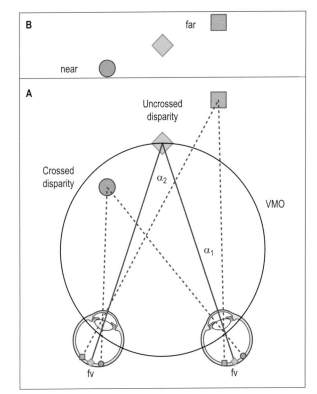

Fig. 36.8 Binocular disparity and the perception of stereoscopic depth. Objects that are not located on the longitudinal horopter have binocular disparity, which may be crossed disparity (*circle* in panel **A**) and be perceived as nearer than the fixated object (the relative depth of the *circle* with respect to the *diamond* in panel **B**) or uncrossed disparity (*square* in **A**) and be perceived as farther than the fixated reference object (**B**). *fv*, fovea; *VMO*, Vieth Muller Circle.

Stereoacuity

In normal foveal vision under optimal conditions, stereoacuity (the smallest detectable depth difference, that is, the difference in the longitudinal visual angles (α_1 and α_2 in Fig. 36.8) is a "hyperacuity" (Westheimer), with thresholds as low as 3 arc seconds! These hyperacuity thresholds are smaller than the width of a single photo receptor. Of course, normal stereoacuity depends on a number of stimulus conditions, including contrast,[70-72] spatial frequency,[73-75] and viewing duration,[76,77] as well as the degree of the similarity between the stimuli to each eye.[78] For example, optical defocus of the retinal images due to uncorrected refractive errors degrades stereoacuity in proportion to the magnitude of defocus.[79,80] The effect of blurring the retinal images is greater for stereoacuity than for other resolution tasks, such as Vernier acuity,[81] visual acuity, and instantaneous displacement thresholds.[82]

Surprisingly, unilateral optical defocus produces a greater reduction of stereoacuity than does symmetrical bilateral defocus,[83,84] consistent with other paradoxical effects on stereoacuity caused by interocular differences in stimulus parameters.[71-73,85] For example, improving the focus in one eye will, paradoxically, degrade stereopsis more than equal defocus in both eyes (stereo-contrast paradox). With unilateral defocus, stereoacuity decreases as the amount of defocus increases until stereopsis is suspended by interocular differences greater than about two diopters.[83,84] The filtering of high spatial frequencies that occurs in defocused images cannot fully explain the resulting reduction in stereoacuity, and foveal suppression may also play a role.[86]

Because of the effect of optical defocus on stereoacuity, usually a clinician's primary goal is to provide an accurate refractive correction for each eye to optimize binocular vision and stereoacuity. However, for one group of patients—presbyopes—interocular refractive error corrections are often purposely unbalanced to correct one eye for distance vision and the other eye for near vision.[52] The scheme of providing an ocular correction for distance vision with one eye and a near vision correction for the other eye, either with single vision contact lenses,[49-51] refractive surgery,[87-89] or intraocular lens implants,[90-92] is called monovision.[92,93] The monovision procedure appears to be well tolerated by many (but by no means all) patients with normal binocular vision, and patients seem to experience less disorientation during perceptual adaptation when the dominant eye is corrected for distance vision.[50,94] Following a period of adaptation, most patients do not experience symptoms of asthenopia, nor are they aware of blurred vision at far or near viewing distances.[93-95] Although their binocular field of view and motor fusion ranges are generally normal, many monovision patients will experience diplopia at night or in dim illumination (when their pupils are dilated), or when they view bright targets of high contrast.[92,93] Some visual functions do not adapt to unilateral optical defocus, resulting in a loss of binocular summation for high spatial frequencies, reduced binocular visual acuity, and degraded stereoacuity with foveal suppression.[48,50,94,95]

However, a recently discovered unwanted effect of monovision correction is the misperception of the distance of moving objects, which may pose a potential public safety hazard.[96] What Burge and colleagues discovered[96,97] is that the effect of having one retinal image blurred and the other clear can introduce a motion illusion because the two images are processed at different speeds. The blurred image is actually processed faster than the clear image (because blur removes the high spatial frequency information, which is processed more slowly than the remaining low spatial frequency information). The difference in processing speeds results in a dramatic illusion in the perceived depth of moving targets, analogous to the well-known Pulfrich effect[98] (described next), but in reverse. Indeed, they calculate that a monovision correction that induces a +1.5 D difference in

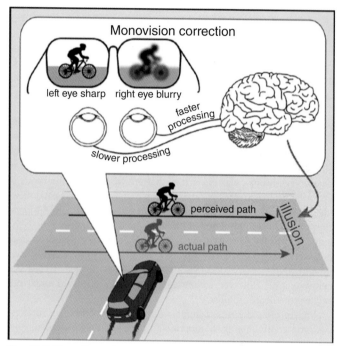

Fig. 36.9 The effect of a monovision lens on perceived distance. The interocular blur differences caused by a monovision correction can cause dramatic misperceptions of motion. (From Burge J, Rodriguez-Lopez V, & Dorronsoro C. Monovision and the misperception of motion. *Curr Biol* 2019;29(15):2586–2592, e2584. https://doi.org/10.1016/j.cub.2019.06.070.)

the two retinal images will result in an overestimation of the distance a target moving at 15 miles per hour by more than 9 feet (2.8 m, illustrated in Fig. 36.9).

It has been known for about a century that interocular differences in the retinal illuminance or contrast result in a misperception of the depth of moving objects, known as the Pulfrich effect,[98] because reduced illuminance or contrast in one eye slows the processing of motion, causing a delay relative to the other eye and introducing a neural disparity. Depth distortion with the Pulfrich effect increases with target velocity.

Stereoacuity also provides a very important clinical assay for the integrity of binocular vision. Normal stereoscopic vision is experience dependent and requires normal binocular visual experience over a period of early childhood (see Chapter 38). Moreover, stereopsis may also be impacted by in older patients by disease (e.g., age-related macular degeneration), so clinical testing of stereopsis is important to detect binocular abnormalities in children or adults, and most of the clinical tests are designed as screening tools for distinguishing between normal and abnormal binocular vision. It is important to note that there are a wide range of clinical stereoacuity tests; however, clinicians should be aware that many of these contain either monocular cues or nonstereoscopic binocular cues that can enable patients to "pass" the test despite being stereo blind or stereo deficient[99] (see Box 36.2).

Fig. 36.10 shows examples of two classes of stereograms used for testing stereopsis. The top stereogram is an example of a contour stereogram that tests "local" stereopsis: it consists of high-contrast test figures having unambiguous features, and relative disparities that can be detected by all patients with normal binocular vision. However, these stereograms contain monocular (i.e., local) cues that are discernable in targets with large disparities. When properly fused, the contours in this stereogram provide clear stereoscopic depth perception from binocular disparity, but the relative differences in the positions of the stimuli may be apparent without fusion or stereopsis.

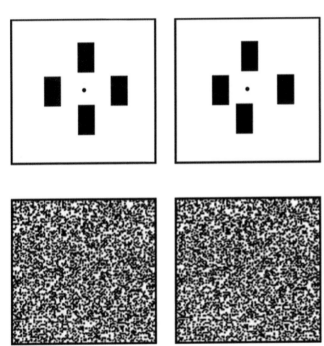

Fig. 36.10 Examples of stereograms with contour-defined objects (local stereopsis) or disparity-defined objects (global stereopsis or cyclopean perception). The disparity patterns in the contour and random-dot stereograms are identical in size and disparity magnitude. Most individuals with normal binocular vision can learn to free-fuse the stereograms by either overconvergence or underconvergence and observe the stereoscopic depth in each example. However, it should be noted that the two viewing strategies produce opposite directions of relative depth.

The lower panels in Fig. 36.10 shows an example of a random-dot stereogram (RDS) that tests "global" stereopsis. While the locations, directions, and disparity magnitudes of the stimuli of the RDS and contour stereograms are identical, the pattern is more difficult to see in the RDS.[100] Because the form information in RDSs is not available with one eye, that is, global (fusion and stereopsis are necessary to see the form), this form of stereopsis has also been called "cyclopean." The correct identification of a disparity-defined form embedded into the RDS is definitive evidence that the patient has stereopsis. The global image is defined by its binocular disparity, and cyclopean stereoscopic

depth reveals the global image. However, global stereopsis tests generally consist of small, dense, low-contrast elements, which make them especially challenging for patients with binocular anomalies (e.g., amblyopia), even though they may actually have the neural mechanisms necessary for global stereopsis.

Stereopsis and the "matching problem"

Each half of the RDS illustrated in Fig. 36.8 (*top*) contains 1000 by 1000 dots! This leads to the matching or correspondence problem in binocular vision (i.e., the problem of figuring out which bit of the image in the left eye should be matched with which bit in the right eye). The problem is particularly vexing in images like RDSs. Matching thousands of left-eye dots to thousands of right-eye dots in Fig. 36.8 would require a lot of work for any computational system. However, the visual system adopts a number of strategies to simplify the problem. These include blurring, which reduces the high spatial frequency information, and adopting certain heuristicws or constraints.[101] The uniqueness constraint asserts that a wfeature in the world is represented exactly once in each retinal image (i.e., each monocular image feature should be paired with exactly one feature in the other monocular image). The continuity or smoothness constraint holds that, except at the edges of objects, neighboring points in the world lie at similar distances from the viewer. Accordingly, disparity should change smoothly at most places in the image. These (and possibly additional) constraints make the matching problem much more tractable by reducing the number of possible solutions. However, recent work suggests that identifying correct matches may not be the optimal strategy.[102] Rather, they suggest that the brain uses "what not detectors" that sense dissimilar features in the two eyes, and suppress unlikely interpretations of the scene, thus facilitating stereopsis by providing evidence against interpretations that are incompatible with the true structure of the scene. Note that this scheme would mean that a large (perhaps infinite) number of matches are considered and rejected.

Retinal disparity, perceptual constancy, and perceived depth

The retinal disparity associated with the physical depth of an object can be determined by the relationship:

$$\eta = [(a * \Delta b/d^2)] * c \qquad \text{(Eq. 36.1)}$$

where a is the interpupillary distance (IPD), d is the viewing distance, Δb is the depth interval that is equal to the distance between the disparate object and the viewing distance, and c is a constant to convert the stereo-angle to arc minutes ($c = 3438$) or arc seconds ($c = 206{,}264$). The function shows that, for any given fixation distance, the relationship between depth interval and retinal disparity is linear, but the relationship varies across fixation distances by the square of the distance (Fig. 36.9). This means that an individual with a 60-mm IPD whose stereoacuity is 10 arc seconds, will be able to discriminate a depth difference of 0.12 mm at a 40-cm viewing distance. However, they would require a 3-cm depth difference at 6 m, or an 800-m depth difference at a 1000 m viewing distance.

The properties of objects in the world (such as their size, color, etc.) are stable, while the retinal information may vary substantially from moment to moment. To maintain perceptual constancy between perceived depth and disparity requires an observer to scale the horizontal disparity with viewing distance. There are several potential sources of perceptual information about viewing distance. These include the vertical disparity gradients that occur naturally in tertiary directions of gaze, in which a nearby target subtends a larger visual angle vertically in one eye than in the other.[103–108] For example,

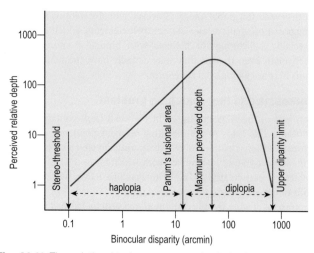

Fig. 36.11 The relationship between perceived depth and binocular disparity for disparities from the lower to the upper limits of stereoscopic depth perception. (Modified from Tyler CW. Sensory processing of binocular disparity. In Schor CM, Ciuffreda KJ, eds. Vergence Eye Movements. Basic and Clinical Aspects. Boston: Butterworths, 1983:199–295.)

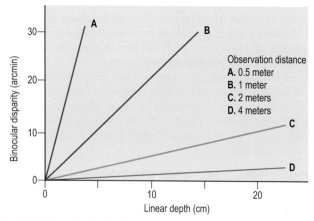

Fig. 36.12 The relationship between binocular disparity and linear depth for four fixation distances. The disparity-depth relationship is linear for any constant fixation distance, but nonlinear across fixation distances.

if a target is elevated above the visual plane, it has a vertical disparity that increases with horizontal eccentricity and inversely with viewing distance. Other sources of perceptual information about viewing distance and azimuth include the convergence and version angles,[109,110] retinal cues, such as oblique disparities,[111] and nonstereoscopic or perspective cues.[6.] For example, perception of depth in slanted surfaces (slant depth) can be derived from horizontal disparity using azimuth, elevation, and distance (obtained from vertical disparity gradients, convergence, and version).

How does perceived depth (at a fixed viewing distance) depend on disparity? Fig. 36.11 shows that for disparities below the smallest detectable depth (Dmin), no depth is perceived. Beyond that limit, perceived depth increases proportionally with increasing disparity (this has been referred to as quantitative or fine stereopsis; Fig. 36.12), even when the disparity exceeds the limit of fusion (Panum's area), and the maximum perceived stereoscopic depth occurs when the stimulus is clearly diplopic. With larger binocular disparities (referred to as qualitative or coarse stereopsis), the perception of depth decreases as the upper disparity limit of stereopsis (Dmax) is approached where the relative depth of diplopic objects can no longer be resolved. In this regime, depth has a direction (near or far), but the depth magnitude is uncertain.[112]

TABLE 36.1   Coarse versus fine stereopsis

Fine stereopsis	Coarse stereopsis
Small disparities	Large disparities
Within Panum's area	Beyond Panum's area (diplopic images)
High resolution (threading needle)	
Strict matching (first order)	Low resolution
Slow development	Relaxed matching (second order)
Requires good acuity and alignment	Rapid development
	Robust to acuity and misalignment

Quantitative (fine) and qualitative (coarse) stereopsis differ in important ways (Table 36.1): quantitative depth perception improves with exposure duration,[77] whereas qualitative depth perception is optimal with briefly presented stimuli and fades with long exposures.[112] Additionally, quantitative stereopsis requires similar stimuli in the two eyes.[111] However, qualitative stereopsis arises for briefly presented stimuli even when the two eyes' retinal images differ in size, shape, and/or contrast polarity.[113–116] Qualitative stereopsis is a useful alerting percept for the approximate location in depth of objects that appear suddenly, and may also be a stimulus to initiate vergence alignment of the eyes to transient changes in both small and large retinal disparities.[114–116] Quantitative stereopsis, on the other hand, is useful for precise judgment of the 3D shape, depth, and orientation of continuously viewed features near the plane of fixation.

Coarse and fine stereopsis also differ in their developmental time course. Coarse stereo may be used by the typically developing visual system to achieve binocular fusion, which, in turn, can be used to align the two eyes, permitting the eventual development of the high-resolution, fine stereoscopic system.[117] Moreover, coarse and fine stereopsis are differently impacted by binocular abnormalities such as amblyopia[118] (discussed further in the chapter).

Nonstereoscopic cues to depth and distance

Stereopsis is based on triangulation, that is, on seeing the world from two different vantage points (i.e., two laterally separated eyes). However, there are other triangulation cues to depth or distance: motion cues based on seeing the world from multiple points by moving the head from side to side,[119] and focus cues based on seeing the world from various points across the pupil.[120] In principle, one computes absolute distance based on these cues. However, the reliability of these cues is determined by the triangulation baseline (i.e., IPD) relative to the scene distance, so they are most effective for relatively close viewing distances.

There are also a number of cues to depth and distance, based on perspective projection. These include relative (i.e., the size of the retinal image is inversely proportional to distance) and familiar size, linear perspective (owing to projection of parallel and perpendicular structure in world), texture gradient (density, size, and foreshortening owing to projection of textures), and height relative to the horizon (closer objects are lower). With the exception of familiar size, these cues can only be used to estimate distance ratios.

A third set of cues is based on light transport (i.e., on how light is transmitted through materials and air and reflects off surfaces). These cues include occlusion (which can provide depth order) and aerial perspective because light traveling through air results in a reduction in contrast, saturation, and change in hue toward blue owing to scattering and absorption. Light transport cues can provide highly uncertain information about absolute distance, but generally only over long distances.

Combining depth cues

Our rich perceptual experience of the 3D world is more than the stimuli on our retinae. Perception is a construct or estimate of our environment, based upon current stimulus cues and our past experience or knowledge of the world. The Bayesian approach is a useful statistical modeling tool in probability theory for estimating perceptual outcomes based upon a combination of current stimulus cues and our knowledge about the conditions of the world—what is and is not likely to occur. As noted, there are a host of different cues to depth and distance. How does the visual system combine these cues? A number of studies[121–124] suggest that the brain estimates the reliability of each cue, and weights them accordingly. Thus, disparity cues may be most reliable at relatively close distances, while other cues may be more reliable at larger distances.

ANOMALIES OF BINOCULAR VISION

Anisometropia, astigmatism, and aniseikonia

Normal binocular vision requires the retinal images in the two eyes to be similar in size, shape and clarity. Anisometropia (i.e., unequal refractive error in the two eyes) can have profound effects on binocular vision resulting in image blur, reduced resolution, and reduced image contrast, and may also result in reduced stereopsis, aniseikonia (i.e., unequal retinal image size), and amblyopia.

Amblyopia is a common neurodevelopmental abnormality that results in physiologic alterations in the visual pathways and impaired vision in one eye, less commonly in both. It reflects a broad range of neural, perceptual, oculomotor, and clinical abnormalities that can occur when normal visual development is disrupted early in life. Fig. 36.13 shows the likelihood that pure anisometropia (*red symbols*) and the combination of anisometropia and strabismus (*blue symbols*) will result in amblyopia (A) or a reduction of stereoacuity (B) as a function of the degree of anisometropia. With four diopters of aniso-hyperopia there is an approximately 38% probability of amblyopia, and a greater than 60% probability of reduced stereoacuity.

Anisometropia may be a consequence of the two eyes having different axial lengths (axial anisometropia) or because the optical components of the two eyes differ in power (refractive anisometropia). Spherical optical differences produce a relative overall size discrepancy in the two retinal images, and astigmatic optical differences produce a relative meridional size difference in the two retinal images. Whereas anisometropia (and the associated aniseikonia) often results from the natural development of refractive errors, aniseikonia is often associated with anisometropia as a result of intraocular lens implantation (Box 36.3), refractive surgery, or penetrating keratoplasty.[125–129]

There are large individual differences in both the symptoms and tolerance of aniseikonia. Aniseikonia is usually considered clinically significant when the image size difference is greater than 4%, but many patients experience distortions in spatial perception and/or uncomfortable binocular vision, headaches, and eyestrain with differences as small as 2%.[19,130,131] The symptoms of eyestrain (asthenopia) are not specific[129] and the diagnosis of aniseikonia in a patient with fusion and stereopsis must be made from measurements of retinal image

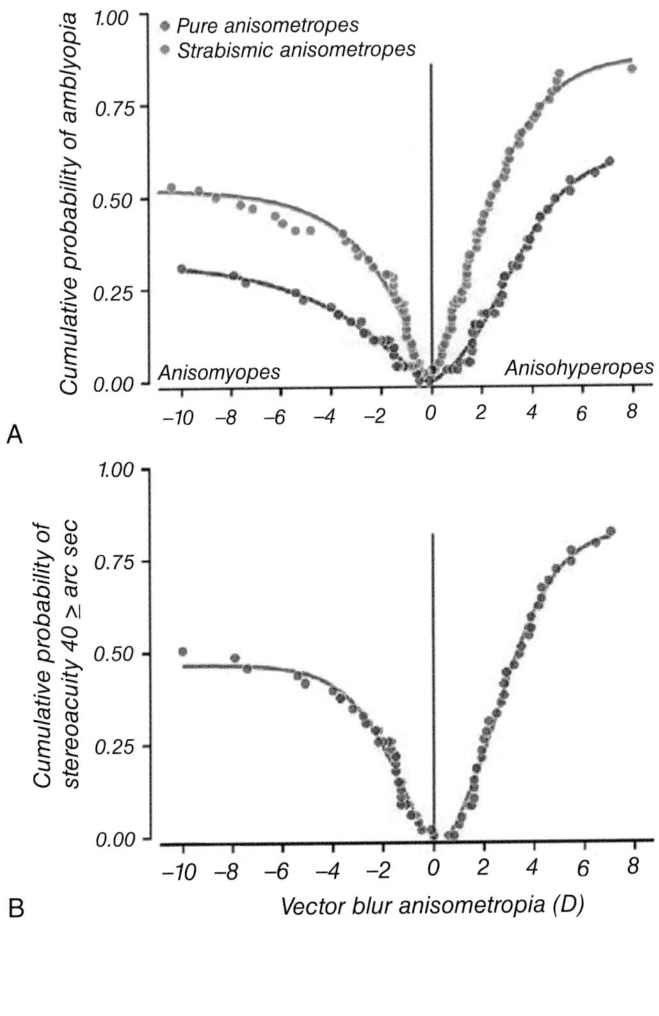

Fig. 36.13 The effect of anisometropia on visual acuity (**A**) and stereoacuity (**B**). Specifically, the cumulative probability of being amblyopic (defined as a two-line difference between the two eyes **A**) or having reduced stereoacuity (≥40 arc sec **B**) as a function of the amount of anisometropia. (From Levi DM, Mckee SP, & Movshon JA. Visual deficits in anisometropia. *Vis Res* 2011;51:48–57. https://doi:10.1016/j.visres.2010.09.029.)

BOX 36.3   Spatial distortions caused by aniseikonia

- Electronics technician, 58 years old
- Cataract surgery for left eye with an intraocular lens (IOL) implant
- Refractive errors before surgery
  OD: +3.25 −1.25 × 010
  OS: +2.25 −0.50 × 180
- Refractive errors after surgery
  OD: +3.25 −1.25 × 010
  OS: +0.50 −2.75 × 005
- Symptoms after IOL surgery: Clear vision with each eye, but while reading a newspaper binocularly, the pages looked farther away on the left side and they appeared trapezoidal. He also complained of problems with depth perception, such as reaching and pressing the floor button in the elevator or soldering on a circuit board.

  Comment: Using the rough rule-of-thumb of 1% magnification per diopter of anisometropia, the patient has an overall magnification of 2.75% with the right-eye image larger, plus an additional 1.5% magnification in the vertical meridian of the right-eye image. Thus, the anisometropia following the cataract surgery has both an overall and meridional component, but the meridional component is the more likely cause of spatial distortions. The patient's complaints are consistent with an induced effect from the aniseikonia, and although a 1.5% image size difference may not cause symptoms in all patients, this electronics technician was quite disturbed by his altered perception.

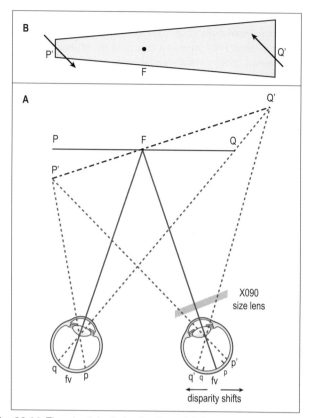

Fig. 36.14 The physiologic basis of spatial distortions caused by the aniseikonia from meridional magnification in the horizontal meridian of the right eye. The frontoparallel plane PFQ appears to be rotated to a plane P'FQ' as a result of the binocular disparity produced by meridional magnification. See the text for details. (Adapted from Ogle KN. *Researches in Binocular Vision.* New York: Hafner Publishing Co, 1964.)

size differences[129–133] or from assessment of the aniseikonic spatial distortions[24,130,131].

The retinal image size difference poses problems both for stereopsis and for control of eye alignment. The size discrepancy generated by an anisometropic spectacle correction produces disparities that vary with eye position, causing a noncomitant variation of heterophoria (anisophoria).[134,135] The oculomotor system can adapt tonic vergence to compensate for anisophoria. However, when a person is unable to adapt to the correction, the symptoms of eyestrain occur with attempts to adjust binocular eye alignment as gaze shifts from one direction to another. These motor symptoms can be confused with sensory disorders normally assumed to result from aniseikonia.[135] Anisometropic contact lens corrections do not produce anisophoria because the optical center of the lens remains fixed with respect to the pupil center during eye movements.

The types of spatial distortions perceived from the relative magnification of one retinal image can be understood by the altered perception of the orientation of the frontoparallel plane that is associated with aniseikonia.[24] The AFPP is the orientation of a flat plane when it appears parallel to the facial plane. Its orientation is influenced by the orientation of the identical visual direction horopter, by optical distortions that influence horizontal and vertical retinal image disparity and by adaptations of stereoscopic depth that compensate for optical distortions. Prior to adaptation, unequal retinal image sizes cause the AFPP to be slanted around a vertical axis at the fixation point by an amount and direction determined by two components of aniseikonia: the geometric effect, the induced effect, and a third component, declination errors, slanted about a horizontal axis.

The geometric effect occurs with retinal image size differences in the horizontal meridian and is a consequence of the horizontal disparity caused by lateral magnification. The frontoparallel plane appears slanted toward, (i.e., facing, the eye with the larger horizontal magnification). The physiologic basis for the apparent slant in

the geometric effect is illustrated in Fig. 36.14. The geometric effect can be simulated by viewing an objectively flat frontoparallel plane (plane PFQ) through a ×090 horizontal size lens or afocal magnifier. A size lens is a small Galilean telescope without refractive power for objects at infinity. In this example, it produces magnification in the horizontal meridian of the right eye (×090). When viewed through the size lens, the plane does not appear parallel to the face, but rotated about the fixation point to the plane P'FQ'; that is, such that point P is perceived as nearer and point Q as farther. The amount of perceived rotation is proportional to the magnification difference between the two retinal images produced by the size lens. The direction and magnitude of rotation result from the change in the horizontal disparity gradient produced by the uniocular horizontal magnification. The disparities across the gradient are in opposing directions in the left and right visual fields. In this example the gradient produces crossed disparities for objects in the left visual field and uncrossed disparities for objects in the right visual field. The perceptually slanted plane illustrated in Fig. 36.14B shows both a perceptual surface rotation and an apparent change in perceived size. Objects in the left visual field appear smaller than in the right. The size distortion is consistent with learned relationships between size and distance, for example, if one object appears farther than another but without a correlated difference in retinal image sizes, the cue conflict causes the farther object to be perceived as larger.

The induced effect is caused by a relative magnification difference in the vertical meridians of the two eyes and can be simulated by a ×180 or vertical meridional magnifier. The induced effect is interesting because vertical binocular disparities, by themselves, do not result in the perception of stereoscopic depth, but vertical meridional aniseikonia in a real-world visual environment causes a perceived rotation of the AFPP. The induced effect is similar to the geometric effect in that it is perceived as a rotation of the frontoparallel plane about a vertical axis, but the induced effect is in the opposite direction. The objective frontoparallel plane (OFPP) appears tilted away from the eye viewing through the vertical magnifier. Because the phenomenon is similar in form, but opposite in direction to the geometric effect, it is called the *induced effect* to convey the notion that the distortion is the same, as if it was "induced" by a horizontal meridional magnifier over the fellow eye.

The induced effect results from the magnification of the vertical disparities, which are inherently present in tertiary gaze at relatively near viewing distances due to differences in ocular perspective of the target. Naturally occurring vertical disparities increase as the horizontal eccentricity (azimuth) of the target from straight ahead increases and as the viewing distance decreases.[136] Normally, the viewing distance is sensed from convergence, and target azimuth can be derived from the rate of increase of vertical disparity with horizontal eccentricity with respect to the head, from the vertical disparity gradient and/or extraretinal signals for horizontal version eye position. Without estimates of distance and eccentricity, horizontal disparity alone is an ambiguous stimulus for slant perception. Identical horizontal disparity patterns can correspond to different slant patterns for surfaces seen in symmetrical and asymmetrical convergence. For example, while a zero-disparity pattern describes the V-M circle, this constant disparity pattern also describes a surface slant that increases with horizontal gaze eccentricity.[137] To interpret slant from horizontal disparity correctly, knowledge of target distance and gaze eccentricity are needed. The combination of vertical disparity gradients, horizontal version eye position, and convergence provides this information.[138,139] When vertical magnifiers distort vertical disparity gradients, the surface slant is changed to conform to the erroneous estimates of distance and eccentricity produced by the vertical meridional magnifier.[12] This induced effect is weak, or absent, for targets located at an infinite viewing distance because retinal images of remote targets lack a difference in perspective with eccentricity that is significant enough to produce a vertical disparity gradient. For most observers, induced and geometric effects are about equal in magnitude and opposite in direction.[24] Thus, overall magnification differences, as opposed to meridional magnification differences, have little effect on the perception of space.

The third component of aniseikonia is a declination error (perceived tilt about a horizontal axis) that arises from retinal image shear, or magnifications in oblique meridians. The direction of rotation (inclination or declination) of the oblique magnifier is predicted from the combined vertical and horizontal disparity components of the magnified retinal images. Oblique magnification can also cause horizontal tilt about a vertical axis if the horizontal and vertical components are unequal. Magnifiers at ×45 and ×135 degrees have equal horizontal and vertical magnification components, so that the resulting geometric and induced effects tend to cancel one another. However, oblique magnification along other meridians produces unequal amounts of geometric and induced distortion, and the stronger distortion usually dominates the horizontal tilt percept.

In the final analysis, the perceptual distortions from aniseikonia are a combination of the three components, geometric effect, induced effect, and declination error, with individual variability in the degree of tolerance and ability to adapt to stereoscopic misrepresentation of relative depth. These principles are illustrated by the case described in Box 36.3, where a relatively small induced effect caused disturbing spatial distortions for an electronics technician.

Strabismus

Strabismus, or heterotropia (the British refer to it as "squint"), is a commonly occurring binocular anomaly (prevalence of approximately 2–4%), in which one eye fixates, and the other eye is directed at some point other than fixation.[140] The term *squint* refers to a strabismic patient closing one eye to avoid diplopia. A discussion of the causes, diagnosis, classification, and treatment of strabismus is beyond the scope of this chapter; however, strabismus can have profound effects on visual processing and visual perception. An adult with a sudden onset of strabismus due to injury or disease is likely to experience pathologic diplopia because images of the same object fall on noncorresponding areas in the two eyes, causing the fixated target to be seen in different egocentric directions (diplopia) during binocular viewing. They may also experience visual confusion because an object imaged on the fovea of the deviating eye has the same egocentric direction as a different object imaged on the fovea of the fixating eye, even though their physical locations are much different (Fig. 36.15). However, most patients experience strabismus early in life, and adapt by developing strabismic suppression[141,142] and/or anomalous retinal correspondence (i.e., an alteration of the normal topography of oculocentric directions).[143–145]

Strabismic suppression

Suppression causes the perception of objects normally visible to the deviating eye to be eliminated during simultaneous binocular viewing to provide single vision.[146] Patients with exotropia may suppress an entire hemifield,[147] but for esotropes the suppression is limited to a specific area (sometimes called a "suppression scotoma"), bounded by the fovea of the deviating eye and the area stimulated by the object that is fixated by the nondeviating eye[142] (the diplopia point; X (i.e., the area on which the image is formed in the left (deviated) eye, sometimes referred to as point X.) in Fig. 36.15). This pattern of suppression results from stimulation of the fixating eye's fovea. However, when targets are imaged eccentrically away from the fovea of the fixating eye,

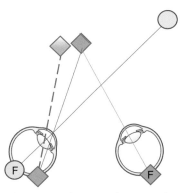

Fig. 36.15 Retinal correspondence and suppression in strabismus. A strabismic patient with normal retinal correspondence and without suppression would have diplopia, two egocentric directions of single objects (represented by *solid and dashed images*) and visual confusion, a common visual direction for two separate objects (represented by the superimposition of the images of the fixated *diamond* and the *circle*, which is imaged on the fovea of the deviating eye).

the suppression moves to a corresponding retinal region of the deviating eye.[148]

Anomalous binocular correspondence

Anomalous binocular correspondence (ABC) (Fig. 36.5C) is an adapted shift in the visual directions of the deviated eye relative to the normal visual directions of the fixating eye. The result is that during binocular viewing a peripheral retinal area of the deviating eye acquires a common visual direction to that of the fovea of the fixating eye.[143,149,150] This apparent shift in retinal correspondence produces a difference in the visual directions between the two eyes for foveally imaged objects, which can be demonstrated clinically with the Hering-Bielschowsky afterimage test for anomalous correspondence.[145] For this test, afterimages are formed on the foveas of both eyes. Even with an interocular deviation from strabismus, a patient with normal correspondence will perceive the afterimages in a common direction, but a patient with deep anomalous binocular correspondence will perceive the afterimages in different visual directions. The subjective separation of the monocular foveal afterimages is referred to as the angle of anomaly, which represents the magnitude of the perceptual shift from the normal corresponding relationship between the two foveas. When the magnitude of the angle of anomaly is equal to the magnitude of the oculomotor misalignment (harmonious anomalous retinal correspondence), then objects in space can appear single even though one of the eyes is deviated. On the other hand, when the angle of anomaly is less than the objective angle of strabismus (unharmonious anomalous retinal correspondence), the residual disparity will cause diplopia unless suppression is also present. The angular separation of the diplopic images of the fixation point is referred to as the subjective angle and in unharmonious anomalous retinal correspondence, the subjective angle is usually smaller than the angle of strabismus (objective angle). The relationship between the objective angle of strabismus (H), the subjective angle (S), and the angle of anomaly (A) is $H = S + A$. This formula is used clinically to compute the angle of anomaly from measures of the objective and subjective angles of strabismus.

Tests for the sensory adaptations of a strabismic patient are variable,[151–157] and generally the diagnosis of anomalous binocular correspondence for a given strabismic patient is test dependent.[155] Tests for anomalous correspondence either locate the extrafoveal point in the deviating eye that has the same visual direction as fovea in the fixating eye (i.e., subjective angle), or quantify the angular separation of the visual directions of the foveas of the two eyes (i.e., angle of anomaly).[145] Tests in the former category (e.g., Bagolini striated lenses or the Worth four-dot test) have a higher probability of being positive for anomalous correspondence than tests in the latter category, such as the Hering-Bielschowsky afterimage procedure.[155] The dependence of the state of a patient's binocular correspondence on the clinical procedure may be the result of variation in the angle of anomaly across the retina[148] or some other property of the mechanisms underlying anomalous retinal correspondence.[148,154–156] Thus, a patient may demonstrate harmonious anomalous correspondence with the Bagolini striated lens test and normal correspondence with the major amblyoscope and afterimage tests.

Three main theories on anomalous correspondence have been proposed.[148] The first (anomalous retinal correspondence [ARC]) proposes that there is a shift in retinal correspondence[143,145] so that retinal points that are normally disparate are shifted to acquire an anomalous coupling in the striate cortex,[157,158] for example, the fovea of the fixating eye is anomalously coupled with a peripheral area of the deviating eye. It is unclear how this could be accomplished by the visual nervous system, particularly when the deviation is large and variable. The second theory (expanded fusion range) proposes

that strabismics who have no suppression[159] are able to perceive space singly owing to enlarged Panum's fusional areas.[160–162] This type of adaptation might apply to those with a small angle of deviation. The third, and most likely, theory (anomalous binocular correspondence) is that the two eyes perceive space independently, much like the two hands explore space. Each eye computes egocentric visual direction from its own sense of eye position and oculocentric retinal image location. In ABC, the angle of anomaly can change from moment to moment, either during vergence movements or while the eyes are stationary. In effect, there is a lack of binocular retinal correspondence.[163,164] All three models achieve binocular sensory fusion by moving the horopter to the distance of the fusion stimulus. The main difference between the models is how the distance of the horopter is changed to achieve binocular sensory fusion. NRC (normal retinal correspondence) and ARC use vergence to move the horopter to different distances, whereas ABC uses perceived distance to move the horopter and achieves sensory fusion without changing vergence.

Over two centuries ago, Wells (1818)[165] described binocular vision in strabismus as organized without binocular retinal correspondence. In essence, strabismics with ABC derived binocular disparity from differences between separate egocentric directions of the two eyes rather than from a binocular retinal correspondence system that compares oculocentric directions. A century later, three related versions of a head-centric anomalous motor fusion mechanism were described by Verhoeff[164] (1938), Brock[163,166] (1939), and Morgan[167] (1961). A computational model published by Schor describes how diplopia, binocular fusion, and stereopsis can be derived in strabismus with a lack of binocular retinal correspondence.[168]

Patients with ABC have binocular fusion while manifesting a large variable amplitude of strabismus,[169] and some demonstrate crude stereopsis while squinting.[170,171] ABC is distinguished from ARC (Von Graefe 1854, discussed in ref 172) if there is a developmental absence of binocular retinal correspondence that can result from suppression of one eye in congenital and early-onset strabismus, if suppression deprives development of binocular cortical neurons.[173–175] The two forms of anomalous correspondence (ABC and ARC) interact differently with vergence eye movements. Vergence is not predicted to influence the amplitude of perceived disparity between two foveal afterimages (i.e., angle of anomaly) either in normal retinal correspondence NRC or in ARC, whereas vergence is predicted to influence the amplitude of disparity between foveal afterimages in ABC (i.e., covariation).[172,176] How is it possible to have binocular disparity, fusion, diplopia, and stereopsis without retinal correspondence?

VISUAL DIRECTIONS AND THE HOROPTER IN ANOMALOUS BINOCULAR CORRESPONDENCE

NRC, ARC, and ABC all derive absolute disparity from a reference binocular parallax angle (β_R) that serves as a zero-disparity reference or horopter. Binocular parallax is the angle subtended by a point in space at the entrance pupils of the two eyes. Historically it has been referred to as a longitudinal angle that lies in the visual plane.[24] In NRC and ARC, the classical definition of the horopter is the locus of points in space that are imaged on fixed pairs of binocular corresponding retinal points. Said in another way, it is the locus of points in space where identical visual directions (IVDs) of pairs of corresponding retinal points intersect. The intersections are quantified by their longitudinal angles or binocular parallax angles. When corresponding points are equidistant from their respective foveas, β_R is constant with retinal eccentricity and the horopter equals the V-M circle. The horopter in ABC is also defined as the locus of points in space where IVDs intersect; however, these IVDs are not linked to fixed pairs of binocular corresponding retinal points. IVDs in ABC correspond to egocentric directions of two independent eyes that intersect at points on the horopter. In ABC, the distance that IVDs intersection in space (d') is quantified from β_R and the interpupillary distance, where d' = IPD / tanβ_R. In ABC, β_R is independent of the vergence angle and is determined by the perceived distance of the intended fixation target (d').

The horopter was first measured in strabismus with anomalous correspondence by Flom, who demonstrated binocular disparity in anomalous correspondence with both a singleness criterion (i.e., IVDs horopter) and diplopia criterion for targets located farther and nearer than the horopter surface.[177] The horizontal (i.e., longitudinal) horopter in NRC and ARC moves in depth with horizontal vergence eye movements, and corresponding retinal points, whose visual directions intersect at the horopter, are unaffected by vergence. Consequently, the separation of foveal afterimages in NRC remains unchanged during vergence because in NRC, vergence signals do not influence egocentric direction. Unlike the horopter in NRC and ARC, the distance of the horizontal horopter in ABC (d') does not change with horizontal vergence eye movements, and empirically measured pairs of binocular corresponding points (i.e., points with IVDs) continually change their retinal locations with the changing vergence angle to maintain a single fused percept of a stationary fixation target (i.e., covariation). Stationary objects in space positioned on the horopter do not become disparate or diplopic with registered vergence movements. However, the separation

of foveal afterimages in ABC does change during vergence eye movements because vergence signals combine with the fixed retinal image locations of afterimages (oculocentric directions) to change their egocentric directions. The horopter in ABC changes distance with changes in the perceived zero-disparity reference-fixation distance (d'), independent of vergence eye movements, just as size-distance constancy scales the perceived size of the retinal image with perceived distance,[178] and stereo-depth scales binocular disparity with perceived distance. Perceived distance changes that stimulate vergence (i.e., proximal vergence) in ABC can also change the zero-disparity reference distance (d') and its binocular parallax angle (β_R) that quantifies the horopter.

COMPUTATION OF BINOCULAR DISPARITY IN ANOMALOUS BINOCULAR CORRESPONDENCE

In NRC, ARC, and ABC, absolute binocular disparity (δ) is calculated as the difference in the binocular parallax angle subtended by a target (β_T) and the binocular parallax angle subtended by the horopter (β_P): $\delta = \beta_{T-\theta}\,\beta_P$. Fig. 36.16 and its caption illustrates a block diagram of retinocentric ($_{RET}$; i.e., oculocentric) and head-centric ($_{H-C}$; i.e., egocentric) models for deriving binocular disparity in NRC and ABC, respectively. β_T in NRC and ARC equals the physical binocular parallax

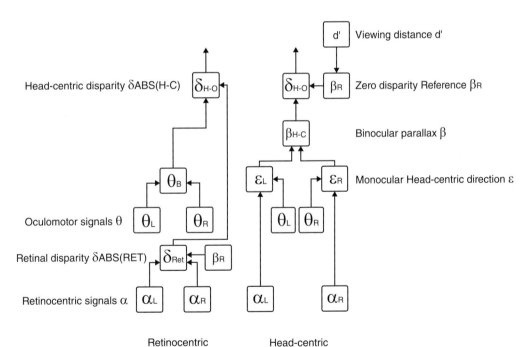

Fig. 36.16 Block diagram of retino-centric ($_{RET}$), that is, oculocentric, and head-centric ($_{H-C}$), that is, egocentric, disparity models. Retinocentric and head-centric disparity models differ by where disparity is computed in the sequence of operations that transform oculocentric to egocentric direction (either before or after the transformation to head-centric coordinates). In NRC, the transformation combines version eye position signals (θ) with oculocentric direction (α) to yield egocentric direction (ϵ). In anomalous binocular correspondence (ABC), the transformation combines a combination of version and vergence signals (θ) with oculocentric directions to yield egocentric direction (ϵ). Absolute binocular retinal disparity in oculocentric coordinates (δ_{RET}) is computed before the transformation to head-centric coordinates from the difference between right eye and left eye oculocentric directions ($\delta_{RET} = \alpha_L - \alpha_R$) of matched features of the two retinal images, and then the binocular retinal disparity is combined with averaged eye position (i.e., version) signals (θ_B) to form a head-centric, egocentric representation (δ_{H-C}). Absolute binocular egocentric disparity in head-centric coordinates (δ_{H-C}) is computed from the difference in monocular egocentric directions ($\beta_{H-C} = \epsilon_L\,\epsilon_R$) and a reference binocular parallax angle for zero disparity β_R), where absolute egocentric disparity δ_{H-C} equals $\beta_{H-C} - \beta_R$.

angle subtended by a target at the two eyes' entrance pupils. β_T in ABC equals the difference between the egocentric directions of a target viewed by the two eyes. In ABC, when sensed eye position and retinal image position are accurate, then the physical and perceptual estimates of binocular parallax (β_T) are equal.

In NRC, β_R at the fovea equals the angle of vergence. In ARC, β_R equals the angle of vergence minus the angle of anomaly. In ABC, β_R is computed from an estimate of a zero-disparity reference distance (d') and the IPD, where $\tan\beta_R$ = IPD/d'. Binocular fusion in NRC, ARC, and ABC is achieved by changing β_R (i.e., changing the horopter distance) to equal β_T. In NRC and ARC, β_R is changed with vergence eye movements. In ABC, β_R is changed by selecting a new perceived zero-disparity reference distance (d') independent of vergence.

In ABC, interactions between a target's binocular parallax angle (β_T) and variations of d', that is, the binocular parallax reference distance for zero disparity (β_R), result in variations of the sign and magnitude of absolute binocular disparity. This is illustrated in Fig. 36.17, using a cyclopean eye reference for visual directions. The figure shows the influence of the perceived reference distance for zero disparity (d') on absolute disparity. The absolute disparity of foveal images (T) is shown for NRC (*left panel*) and ABC (*right panel*) with variations of the perceived reference distance (d'). In NRC (*left panel*), binocular disparity is computed between oculocentric directions of foveal images in the left and right eyes that have been mapped (*curved black lines*) onto a common cyclopean retina (C). Here, binocular retinal disparity equals the angle between the two eyes' oculocentric directions represented by the cyclopean eye. Disparity in this example equals zero (*vertical green line*) at the nodal point of the cyclopean eye. The oculocentric directions of the two eyes images (α) and the absolute binocular retinal disparity (δ_{RET}) between foveal images are independent of both extra-retinal signals for vergence and estimated viewing distance (d'). For a fixation target in space (T), they only rely upon the distance of the horopter (i.e., β_R), as determined by vergence, and the binocular parallax angle subtended by the fixation target (β_T).

In the ABC (Fig. 36.17, right panel), absolute binocular disparity ($\delta_{H\text{-}C}$) of foveal images of the fixation target T equals the angle subtended at a cyclopean reference point for egocentric directions (*green dashed lines*), by the points where the left- and right-eye foveal

egocentric directions of T (*black lines*) intersect the perceived fronto-parallel zero-disparity reference distance (d'). The sign of perceived direction (crossed vs. uncrossed) and magnitude (azimuth) or horizontal eccentricity (E) of each of the intersection points in the horopter plane depends on both their egocentric directions (ϵ) and the perceived distance (d') of the intended fixation target (T), where E = d'tan ϵ. In ABC, intended fixation distance (d') refers to distance of attention rather than distance of convergence. Technically, the zero-disparity reference should be the V-M circle to maintain a constant β_R with horizontal eccentricity. When the estimated reference distance d' is accurate and equals the physical distance of the fixation target (T), the egocentric directions of the two eyes' foveal images (T) intersect at a single point in the zero-disparity reference plane. Then β_T = β_R and absolute egocentric disparity ($\delta_{H\text{-}C}$) is zero. When the estimated zero-disparity reference distance (d') of the intended fixation target and its corresponding binocular parallax reference (β_R) are in error, then d' differs from the physical distance of the fixation target. Then the two foveal egocentric directions of the fixation target (*black lines*) intersect two points in the reference plane (i.e., diplopia), and absolute egocentric disparity subtended at the cyclopean reference point is nonzero. For example, when the reference distance d' is perceived farther away than the physical distance of the fixation target, the sign of absolute binocular disparity of the bifoveal fixation target is crossed ($\beta_T > \beta_R$), and when d' is perceived nearer than the physical distance of the fixation target, the sign of the absolute binocular disparity of the bifoveal fixation target is uncrossed ($\beta_T < \beta_R$). The sign or direction of disparity is unambiguous in NRC because of the fixed nature of binocular retinal correspondence and the intersection of the bifoveal point of convergence with the horopter. Note that in NRC the magnitude of the perceived horizontal separation of disparate images (i.e., diplopia) is scaled with perceived distance, just as the linear stereoscopic depth interval scales disparity with perceived distance. However, because the zero-disparity reference distance in strabismus with ABC depends upon an estimated reference viewing distance for zero disparity (d') that is independent of vergence, errors or variation in estimates of d' can influence both the sign and magnitude of disparity computed under different viewing conditions, such as in a dark room or with Bagolini striated glasses.

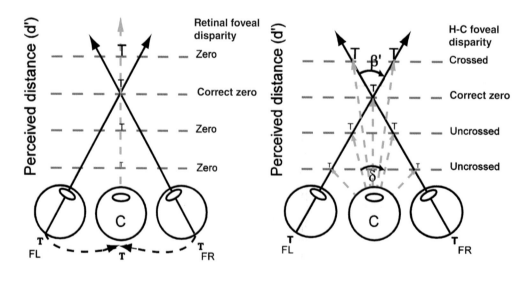

Retinocentric correspondence   **Head-centric correspondence**

Fig. 36.17 The influence of differences between perceived distance of the intended fixation target (d') and its physical distance on the sign and magnitude of binocular disparity for retinocentric, that is, NRC (*left panel*) and head-centric, that is, anomalous binocular correspondence (ABC; *right panel*) coordinate systems. C, FL, FR, T.

SUBCLASSES OF ANOMALOUS CORRESPONDENCE AND ERRORS OF PERCEIVED DISTANCE

When associated with the same vergence angle, the angle of anomaly equals the difference between the bifoveal zero-disparity reference horopter in NRC and the zero-disparity reference horopter in strabismus (β_R). When the estimated zero-disparity reference distance d' (i.e., β_R) of the intended fixation target is accurate, the angle of anomaly equals the angle of strabismus and is classified as harmonious anomalous correspondence. When the estimated reference distance (β_R) is inaccurate and the estimated reference distance is nearer or farther than the physical distance of the intended fixation target (β_T), the angle of anomaly is classified as unharmonious (less than the angle of strabismus) or paradoxical (greater than the angle of strabismus or opposite in sign).

BINOCULAR FUSION IN ANOMALOUS BINOCULAR CORRESPONDENCE

Two components of binocular fusion in ABC were demonstrated by Alpern and Hofstetter[176] who showed that when a base-out prism was presented to an esotrope diagnosed with harmonious anomalous binocular correspondence, the prism disparity of the fixation target was perceived as fused (i.e., single) without suppression and without changing vergence, both before and after the prism was present. Then, over the course of the next few hours, the eyes made a gradual slow-vergence response to the prism disparity, while single vision persisted throughout the motor response. Hallden[175] refers to these two responses in anomalous correspondence as sensory and motor fusion mechanisms, respectively.

ANOMALOUS SENSORY FUSION MECHANISMS IN ANOMALOUS BINOCULAR CORRESPONDENCE

When a base-out prism places the fixation target on the fovea of the deviating eye in esotropia with harmonious ABC, initially there is a crossed disparity in which β_T is greater than β_R. The sensory fusion mechanism quickly reduces the crossed disparity to zero without changing vergence by adjusting β_R until it equals β_T. Prism disparity is reduced by shifting the perceived zero-disparity reference distance d' inward, that is, moving the zero-disparity reference (β_R) closer to β_T. This sensory fusion response is followed by slow-vergence movements that increase vergence by an amount equal to the added prism (i.e., prism adaptation), without changing perceived binocular disparity.[179]

ANOMALOUS MOTOR FUSION MECHANISMS IN ANOMALOUS BINOCULAR CORRESPONDENCE

After obtaining binocular sensory fusion with ABC, vergence slowly moves retinal images out of a foveal suppression scotoma[143] (i.e., onto the nasal retina in esotropia). Jampolsky showed that the suppression scotoma in esotropia extends from the fovea to the retinal point that the fixation target is normally imaged in the turned (strabismic) eye.[142] In ABC, the target remains fused during the slow-vergence response because neither β_T nor β_R change during vergence, such that there is no change in their absolute disparity ($\delta = \beta_T - \beta_R$). The objective angle of strabismus and the angle of anomaly increase together (i.e., covariation),[175] while the subjective angle remains constant. Although this slow vergence has been described as a motor fusion response, its purpose is not to move β_R to match β_T, but rather to move the retinal images out of the foveal suppression scotoma to allow disparity to be sensed for stereoscopic depth perception.

If the suppression scotoma could be eliminated, then the slow vergence would be unnecessary and ABC would fuse the bifoveal retinal images stimulated by the prism. This is the rationale for a clinical treatment of ABC that focuses on eliminating foveal suppression scotomas by rapid alternate flashing of targets onto the two foveas with an amblyoscope until bifoveal fusion is obtained without interference by slow-vergence movements, that is, Walraven technique.[180] When successful, antisuppression treatment can result in single binocular vision in ABC with stereopsis and bifoveal fixation, and for all intents and purposes, patients behave just like a person with NRC. However they still do not have binocular retinal correspondence; they are "differently abled."

Nonstrabismic binocular anomalies

There are a broad range of nonstrabismic binocular anomalies. These include large heterophorias, reduced fusional reserves, and abnormal accommodative-vergence relationships. Although these often go undiagnosed, they may influence visual performance and quality of life.[181] These nonstrabismic binocular anomalies are quite common in the young, and increase with age.[182,183] Importantly, whereas many of these patients may be asymptomatic under normal viewing, they may suffer from visual stress when using 3D viewing devices (e.g., virtual reality displays).[184-186] In natural viewing conditions, accommodation and convergence are tightly linked—we converge and focus on the same plane. However, this tight linkage is often violated in 3D displays where accommodation is determined by the (virtual) screen distance in order to see clearly, but vergence is either closer or farther than the screen in order to see single. This vergence-accommodation conflict places stress on the visual system and leads to asthenopia and other symptoms of discomfort,[186] and reduced performance.[187-189] Clinical measures of the zone of clear single binocular vision (ZCSBV)[190] test binocular motor fusion and accommodation under a variety of stimulus conflicts between accommodation and vergence that can be used to predict performance on virtual reality displays,[187] as well as with any prescribed optical aid. For these reasons it is important to test a broad range of visual functions in clinical patients, including heterophorias, stereopsis, vergence ranges, and accommodative functions.

SUMMARY

Binocular vision represents the exquisite integration of biological and psychological components to provide clear single binocular vision and a precise, veridical subjective representation of the depth and distance of objects in the environment. This chapter has presented some of the basic principles of the normal and abnormal sensory processes, but they represent just one component of the system. Equally important are the oculomotor components (Chapter 9), which in normal binocular vision interact with sensory mechanisms to place the ocular images on appropriate retinal areas to support fusion and stereopsis, or to engage adaptive sensory mechanisms such as suppression and ARC in patients with strabismus. Further, whether an individual has normal or abnormal binocular vision is a product of environmental influences in infancy (Chapters 38 and 40). During an early sensitive period, normal visual experience is required to develop the full capacity of the visual system, otherwise abnormal visual experience will produce abnormal monocular and/or binocular visual processes. Clinical application of the science of binocular vision involves all of these components with the goal of alleviating any interference with clear, single binocular vision.

ACKNOWLEDGMENTS

The authors and editors would like to acknowledge the contributions of Dr. Ronald Harwerth for his coauthorship of this chapter in a previous edition.

REFERENCES

1. Wheatstone C. Contributions to the physiology of vision. I. On some remarkable, and hitherto unobserved, phenomena of binocular vision. *Phil Trans R Soc Lond.* 1938;128: 371–394.
2. Wade NJ. On the origin of terms in binocular vision. *I-Perception.* 2021;12:1–19.
3. Chopin A, Bavelier D, Levi DM. The prevalence and diagnosis of 'stereoblindness' in adults less than 60 years of age: a best evidence synthesis. *Ophthalmic Physiol Opt.* 2019, Mar;39(2):66–85.
4. Hess RF, To L, Zhou J, Wang G, Cooperstock JR. Stereo vision: The haves and have-nots. *Iperception.* 2015;6(3):2041669515593028.
5. Baker DH, Lygo FA, Meese TS, Georgeson MA. Binocular summation revisited: Beyond √2. *Psychol Bull.* 2018, Nov;144(11):1186–1199.
6. Wolfe JM, Kluender KR, Levi DM, Bartoshuk LM, Hertz RS, Klatzky RL, Lederman SJ, Merfield DM. *Sensation & Perception.* Sixth Edition. Oxford, UK: Oxford University Press; 2021.
7. Ding J, Sperling G. A gain-control theory of binocular combination. *Proc Natl Acad Sci U S A.* 2006;103(4):1141–1146.
8. Ding J, Levi DM. Binocular combination of luminance profiles. *J Vis.* 2017;17(13):4.
9. Bishop PO. Binocular vision. In: Moses RA, Hart WM, eds. *Adler's Physiology of the Eye.* 8th edn. St Louis: CV Mosby; 1987:619–689.
10. Hubel DH, Wiesel TN. Receptive fields, binocular interaction and functional architecture in the cat's visual cortex. *J Physiol.* 1962, Jan;160:106–154.
11. Hubel DH, Wiesel TN. Ferrier lecture. Functional architecture of macaque monkey visual cortex. *Proc R Soc Lond B Biol Sci.* 1977;198:1–59.
12. Howard IP, Rogers BJ. *Seeing in Depth Depth Perception.* Vol 2. Ontario, Canada: Porteous Thornhill, 2002.
13. Bauer J, Weiler S, Fernholz MHP, Laubender D, Scheuss V, Hübener M, Bonhoeffer T, Rose T. Limited functional convergence of eye-specific inputs in the retinogeniculate pathway of the mouse. *Neuron.* 2021;109(15):2457–2468.e12.
14. Hubel DH, Wiesel TN. A re-examination of stereoscopic mechanisms in area 17 of the cat. *J Physiol.* 1973, Jul;232(1):29P–30P.
15. Barlow HB, Blakemore C, Pettigrew JD. The neural mechanism of binocular depth discrimination. *J Physiol.* 1967;193(2):327–342.
16. Pettigrew JD, Nikara T, Bishop PO. Binocular interaction on single units in cat striate cortex: simultaneous stimulation by single moving slit with receptive fields in correspondence. *Exp Brain Res.* 1968;6(4):391–410.
17. Poggio G, Fischer B. Binocular interaction and depth sensitivity in striate and prestriate cortex of behaving rhesus monkey. *J Neurophysiol.* 1977;40(6):1392–1405.
18. DeAngelis GC, Ohzawa I, DeAngelis, GC, Ohzawa, I and Freeman, RD. Depth is encoded in the visual cortex by a specialized receptive field structure. *Nature.* 1991;352(6331):156.
19. Ohzawa I, DeAngelis GC, et al. Stereoscopic depth discrimination in the visual cortex: neurons ideally suited as disparity detectors. *Science.* 1990;249(4972):1037–1041.
20. Read JC, Cumming BG. Sensors for impossible stimuli may solve the stereo correspondence problem. *Nat Neurosci.* 2007;10(10):1322–1328.
21. Cumming BG, Parker AJ. Binocular neurons in V1 of awake monkeys are selective for absolute, not relative, disparity. *J Neurosci.* 1999;19(13):5602–5618.
22. Thomas OM, Cumming BG, Parker AJ. A specialization for relative disparity in V2. *Nat Neurosci.* 2002, May;5(5):472–478.
23. Pasupathy A, Popovkina DV, Kim T. Visual functions of primate area V4. *Annu Rev Vis Sci.* 2020;6:363–385.
24. Ogle KN. *Researches in Binocular Vision.* New York: Hafner Publishing Co, 1964.
25. Klein S.A. and Levi D.M. The position sense of the peripheral retina. *Journal of the Optical Society of America* A 4, 1543–1553, 1987.
26. Harwerth RS, Smith EL, Crawford MLJ. Motor and sensory fusion in monkeys: psychophysical measurements. *Eye.* 1996;10:209–216.
27. Banks MS, van Ee R, Backus BT. The computation of binocular visual direction. A re-examination of Manfield and Legge (1996). *Vision Res.* 1997;37:1605–1613.
28. Ding J, Sperling G. A gain-control theory of binocular combination. *Proc Natl Acad Sci U S A.* 2006;103(4):1141–1146.
29. Ding J, Klein SA, et al. Binocular combination of phase and contrast explained by a gain-control and gain-enhancement model. *J Vis.* 2013;13(2):13 11–37.
30. Howard IP. *Human Visual Orientation.* Chichester: Wiley; 1982.
31. The problem of visual orientation, Part I. The history to 1900. WALLS GL. *Am J Optom Arch Am Acad Optom.* 1951 Feb;28(2):55–83.
32. Schreiber KM, Hillis JM, Filippini HR, Schor CM, Banks MS. The surface of the empirical horopter. *J Vis.* 2008;8(3):7:1–20.
33. Shipley T, Rawlings SC. The nonius horopter—I. History and theory. *Vision Res.* 1970;10: 1255–1262.
34. Von Helmholtz H. *Treatise on Physiological Optics,* vol III (Translated from the 3rd German edition and edited by JPC Southhall). New York: Dover; 1962.
35. Cooper EA, Burge J, Banks MS. The vertical horopter is not adaptable, but it may be adaptive. *J Vis.* 2011;11(3).
36. Gibaldi A, Banks MS. Binocular eye movements are adapted to the natural environment. *J Neurosci.* 2019;39(15):2877–2888.
37. Sprague WW, Cooper EA, Tosic I, Banks MS. Stereopsis is adaptive for the natural environment. *Sci Adv.* 2015;1(4).
38. Mitchell DE. A review of the concept of "Panum's fusional areas." *Am J Optom Physiol Optics.* 1966;43:387–401.
39. Schor CM, Tyler CW. Spatio-temporal properties of Panum's fusional area. *Vision Res.* 1981;21:683–692.
40. Schor CM. The relationship between fusional vergence eye. Movements and fixation disparity. *Vision Res.* 1979;19:1359–1367.
41. Ogle KN, Martens TG, Dyer JA. *Oculomotor Imbalance in Binocular Vision and Fixation Disparity.* Philadelphia: Lea & Febiger; 1967.
42. Ogle KN, Mussey F, Prangen AD. Fixation disparity and fusional processes in binocular single vision. *Am J Ophthalmol.* 1949;32:1069–1087.
43. Campbell FW and Green DG. Monocular versus binocular visual acuity. Nature, 1965 Oct 9;208(5006):191–2. http://doi.org/10.1038/208191.
44. Yehezkel O, Ding J, Sterkin A, Polat U, Levi DM. Binocular combination of stimulus orientation. *R Soc Open Sci.* 2016;3(11):160534.
45. Lev M, Ding J, Polat U, Levi DM. Nearby contours abolish the binocular advantage. *Sci Rep.* 2021;11(1):16920.
46. Shortess GK, Krauskopf J. Role of involuntary eye movements in stereoscopic acuity. *J Opt Soc Am.* 1961;51:555–559.
47. Du Toit R, Ferreira JT, Nel ZJ. Visual and non-visual variables implicated in monovision wear. *Optom Vis Sci.* 1998;75:119–125.
48. Schor CM, Landsman L, Erickson P. Ocular dominance and interocular suppression of blur in monovision. *Am J Optom Physiol Optics.* 1987;64:723–730.
49. Erickson P, McGill EC. Role of visual acuity, stereoacuity, and ocular dominance in monovision patient success. *Optom Vis Sci.* 1992;69:761–764.
50. Erickson P, Schor CM. Visual function with presbyopic contact lens correction. *Optom Vis Sci.* 1990;67:22–28.
51. Evans BJW. Monovision: A review. *Ophthal Physiol Opt.* 2007;27:417–439.
52. Fahle M. Binocular rivalry. Suppression depends on orientation and spatial frequency. *Vision Res.* 1982;22:787–800.
53. Schor CM. Visual stimuli for strabismic suppression. *Perception.* 1977;6:583–593.
54. Levelt W. *Psychological Studies On Binocular Rivalry.* The Hague: Mouton. 1968
55. Liu L, Tyler CW, Schor CM. Failure of rivalry at low contrast: evidence of a suprathreshold binocular summation process. *Vision Res.* 1992;32:1471–1479.
56. Hering E. *Beitrage zur Physiologie.* Vol 5. Leipzig: Engelmann, 1861.
57. Wolfe JM. Stereopsis and binocular rivalry. *Psychol Rev.* 1986;93:269–282.
58. Blake R, Logothetis NK. Visual competition. *Nat Rev Neurosci.* 2002;3:13–21.
59. Harrad RA, McKee SP, Blake R, Yang Y. Binocular rivalry disrupts stereopsis. *Perception.* 1994;23:15–28.
60. Blake R, O'Shea RP. "Abnormal fusion" of stereopsis and binocular rivalry. *Psychol Rev.* 1988;95:151–154.
61. Timney B, Wilcox St LM, John R. On the evidence for a 'true' binocular process in human vision. *Spatial Vis.* 1989;4:1–15.
62. Clifford CW. Binocular rivalry. *Curr Biol.* 2009, Dec 1;19(22):R1022–R1023.
63. Blake R, Wilson H. Binocular vision. *Vision Res.* 2011;51(7):754–770.
64. Crovitz HF, Lipscomb DB. Dominance of the temporal visual fields at a short duration of stimulation. *Am J Psychol.* 1963;76:631–637.
65. Kollner H. Das funktionelle Uberwiegen der nasalen Netzhauthalften im gemeinschaftlichen Sehfeld. *Archiv Augenheilkunde.* 1914;76:153–164.
66. Mauk D, Francis EL, Fox R. The selectivity of permanent suppression. *Invest Ophthalmol Vis Sci.* 1984;25s:294.
67. Tsuchiya N, Koch C. Continuous flash suppression reduces negative afterimages. *Nat Neurosci.* 2005;8(8):1096–1101.
68. Yang E, Blake R. Deconstructing continuous flash suppression. *J Vis.* 2012;12(3):8.
69. Chopin A, Levi D, Knill D, Bavelier D. The absolute disparity anomaly and the mechanism of relative disparities. *J Vis.* 2016;16(8):2.
70. Halpern DL, Blake R. How contrast affects stereoacuity. *Perception.* 1988;17:3–13.
71. Legge GE, Gu Y. Stereopsis and contrast. *Vision Res.* 1989;29:989–1004.
72. Schor CM, Heckman T. Interocular differences in contrast and spatial frequency. Effects on stereopsis and fusion. *Vision Res.* 1989;29:837–847.
73. Hess RF, Wilcox LM. Linear and non-linear filtering in stereopsis. *Vision Res.* 1994;34: 2431–2438.
74. Schor CM, Wood I. Disparity range for local stereopsis as a function of luminance spatial frequency. *Vision Res.* 1983;23:1649–1654.
75. Schor CM, Wood IC, Ogawa J. Spatial tuning of static and dynamic local stereopsis. *Vision Res.* 1984;24:573–578.
76. Harwerth RS, Rawlings SC. Viewing time and stereoscopic threshold with random-dot stereograms. *Am J Optom Physiol Optics.* 1977;54:452–457.
77. Ogle KN, Weil MP. Stereoscopic vision and the duration of the stimulus. *Arch Ophthalmol.* 1958;59:4–17.
78. Ding J, Levi DM. A unified model for binocular fusion and depth perception. *Vision Res.* 2021;180:11–36.
79. Lovasik J, Szymkiw M. Effects of aniseikonia, retinal illuminance and pupil size on stereopsis. *Invest Ophthalmol Vis Sci.* 1985;26:741–750.

80. Schmidt PP. Sensitivity of random-dot stereoacuity and Snellen acuity to optical blur. *Optom Vis Sci.* 1994;71:466–471.

81. Westheimer G. The spatial sense of the eye. *Invest Ophthalmol Vis Sci.* 1979;18:893–912.

82. Enoch JM, Lakshminarayanan V. Vernier acuity and aging. *International Ophthalmology.* 1995;19(2):109–115.

83. Ong J, Burley WS. Effect of induced anisometropia on depth perception. *Am J Optom Arch Am Acad Optom.* 1972;49:333–335.

84. Westheimer G, Pettet MW. Detection and processing of vertical disparity by the human observer. *Proc R Soc Lond B Biol Sci.* 1992;250:243–247.

85. Cormack LK, Stevenson SB, Landers DD. Interactions of spatial frequency and unequal monocular contrasts in stereopsis. *Perception.* 1997;26:1121–1136.

86. Stevenson SB, Cormack LK. A contrast paradox in stereopsis, motion detection, and vernier acuity. *Vision Res.* 2000;40:2881–2884.

87. Braun EHP, Lee J, Steinert RF. Monovision in LASIK. *Ophthalmology.* 2008;115:1196–1202.

88. Jain S, Ou R, Azar DT. Monovision outcomes in presbyopic individuals after refractive surgery. *Ophthalmology.* 2001;108:1430–1433.

89. Gobin L, Rozema JJ, Tassignon MJ. Predicting refractive aniseikonia after cataract surgery in anisometropia. *J Cataract Refract Surg.* 2008;34:1353–1361.

90. Greenbaum S. Monovision pseudophakia. *J Cataract Refract Surg.* 2002;28:1439–1443.

91. Handa T, Mukuno K, Uozato N, et al. Ocular dominance and patient satisfaction after monovision by intraocular lens implantation. *J Cataract Refract Surg.* 2004;30:769–774.

92. Snyder C. Monovision: A clinical review. *Spectrum.* 1989;4:30–36.

93. McGill EC, Erickson P. Sighting dominance and monovision distance binocular fusional ranges. *J Am Optom Assoc.* 1991;62:738–742.

94. Schor CM, McCandless JW. An adaptable association between vertical and horizontal vergence. *Vision Res.* 1995;35:3519–3527.

95. Fawcett SL, Herman WK, Alferi CD, Castleberry KA, Parks MM, Birch EE. Stereoacuity and foveal fusion in adults with long-standing surgical monovision. *J Pediatr Ophthalmol Strabismus.* 2001;5:342–347.

96. Burge J, Rodriguez-Lopez V, Dorronsoro C. Monovision and the misperception of motion. *Curr Biol.* 2019;29(15):2586–2592. e2584.

97. Rodriguez-Lopez V, Dorronsoro C, Burge J. Contact lenses, the reverse Pulfrich effect, and anti-Pulfrich monovision corrections. *Sci Rep.* 2020;10(1):16086.

98. Pulfrich C. Die Stereoskopie im Dienste der isochromen und heterochromen Photometrie. *Naturwissenschaften.* 1922;10:553–564.

99. Chopin A, Bavelier D, Levi DM. The prevalence and diagnosis of 'stereoblindness' in adults less than 60 years of age: a best evidence synthesis. *Ophthalmic Physiol Opt.* 2019;39(2):66–85.

100. Bradshaw MF, Rogers BJ, De Bruyn B. Perceptual latency and complex random-dot stereograms. *Perception.* 1995;24:749–759.

101. Marr D, Poggio T. A computational theory of human stereo vision. *Proc R Soc Lond B Biol Sci.* 1979;204(1156):301–328.

102. Goncalves NR, Welchman AE. "What not" detectors help the brain see in depth. *Curr Biol.* 2017, May 22;27(10):1403–1412. e1408.

103. Garding J, Porrill J, Mayhew JEW, Frisby JP. Stereopsis, vertical disparity and relief transformations. *Vision Res.* 1995;35:703–722.

104. Gillam B, Lawergren B. The induced effect, vertical disparity, and stereoscopic theory. *Percept Psychol.* 1983;34:121–130.

105. Liu L, Stevenson SB, Schor CM. A polar coordinate system for describing binocular disparity. *Vision Res.* 1994;34:1205–1222.

106. Rogers BJ, Bradshaw MF. Vertical disparities, differential perspective and binocular stereopsis. *Nature.* 1993;361:253–255.

107. Schreiber KM, Hillis JM, Filippini HR, Schor CM, Banks MS. The surface of the empirical horopter. *J Vis.* 2008;8(3):7:1–20.

108. Westheimer G, McKee SP. Stereoscopic acuity with defocused and spatially filtered images. *J Opt Soc Am.* 1980;70:772–778.

109. Brown JP, Ogle KN, Reiher L. Stereoscopic acuity and observation distance. *Invest Ophthalmol.* 1965;4:894–900.

110. Foley JM. Binocular distance perception. *Psychol Rev.* 1980;87:411–434.

111. Beverly KI, Regan D. Evidence for the existence of neural mechanisms selectively sensitive to the direction of movement in space. *J Physiol Lond.* 1973;235:17–29.

112. Westheimer G, Pettet MW. Detection and processing of vertical disparity by the human observer. *Proc R Soc Lond B Biol Sci.* 1992;250:243–247.

113. Pope DR, Edwards M, Schor CM. Extraction of depth from opposite-contrast stimuli. Transient system can, sustained system can't. *Vision Res.* 1999;39:4010–4017.

114. Edwards M, Pope DR, Schor CM. Luminance contrast and spatial-frequency tuning of the transient-vergence system. *Vision Res.* 1998;38:705–717.

115. Hess RF, Baker CL, Wilcox LM. Comparison of motion and stereopsis: linear and non-linear performance. *J Opt Soc Am A Opt Image Sci Vis.* 1999;16:987–994.

116. Schor CM, Edwards M, Pope D. Spatial-frequency tuning of the transient-stereopsis system. *Vision Res.* 1998;38:3057–3068.

117. Giaschi D, Narasimhan S, Solski A, Harrison E, Wilcox LM. On the typical development of stereopsis: fine and coarse processing. *Vision Res.* 2013;89:65–71.

118. Giaschi D, Lo R, Narasimhan S, Lyons C, Wilcox LM. Sparing of coarse stereopsis in stereodeficient children with a history of amblyopia. *J Vis.* 2013;13(10):17.

119. Rogers B, Graham M. Motion parallax as an independent cue for depth perception. *Perception.* 1979;8(2):125–134.

120. Watt SJ, Akeley K, Ernst MO, Banks MS. Focus cues affect perceived depth. *J Vis.* 2005; 5(10):834–862.

121. Gepshtein S, Burge J, Ernst MO, Banks MS. The combination of vision and touch depends on spatial proximity. *J Vis.* 2005;5(11):1013–1023.

122. Hillis JM, Ernst MO, Banks MS, Landy MS. Combining sensory information: mandatory fusion within, but not between, senses. *Science.* 2002;298(5598):1627–1630.

123. Ernst MO, Banks MS. Humans integrate visual and haptic information in a statistically optimal fashion. *Nature.* 2002;415(6870):429–433.

124. Ernst MO, Banks MS, Bulthoff HH. Touch can change visual slant perception. *Nat Neurosci.* 2000;3(1):69–73.

125. Binder PS. The effect of suture removal on keratoplasty astigmatism. *Am J Ophthalmol.* 1988;105:637–645.

126. Genvert GI, Cohen EJ, Arentsen JJ, Laibson PR. Fitting gas-permeable contact lenses after penetrating keratoplasty. *Am J Ophthalmol.* 1985;99:511–514.

127. Gobin L, Rozema JJ, Tassignon MJ. Predicting refractive aniseikonia after cataract surgery in anisometropia. *J Cataract Refract Surg.* 2008;34:1353–1361.

128. Holladay JT, Prager TC, Ruiz RS, Lewis JW, Rosenthal H. Improving the predictability of intraocular lens power calculations. *Arch Ophthalmol.* 1986;104:539–541.

129. Borish IM. *Anisometropia and aniseikonia. Clinical Refraction.* 3rd edn. Chicago, Professional Press; 1975:257–306.

130. Kramer P, Shippman S, Bennett G, Meininger D, Lubkin V. A study of aniseikonia and Knapp's law using a projection space eikenometer. *Binocul Vis Strabismus Q.* 1999;14: 197–201.

131. Lubkin LV, Shippman S, Bennett G, Meininger D, Kramer P, Poppinga P. Aniseikonia quantification: Error rate of rule of thumb estimation. *Binocul Vis Strabismus Q.* 1999; 14:191–196.

132. Stephens GL, Polasky M. New options for aniseikonia correction: The use of high index materials. *Optom Vis Sci.* 1991;68:899–906.

133. Musch DC, Farjo AA, Meyer RF, Waldo MN, Janz NK. Assessment of health-related quality of life after corneal transplantation. *Am J Ophthalmol.* 1997;124:1–8.

134. Schor CM, Gleason G, Lunn R. Interactions between short-term vertical phoria adaptation and non-conjugate adaptation of vertical pursuits. *Vision Res.* 1993;33:55–63.

135. Schor CM, McCandless JW. An adaptable association between vertical and horizontal vergence. *Vision Res.* 1995;35:3519–3527.

136. van Ee R, Schor CM. Unconstrained stereoscopic matching of lines. *Vision Res.* 2000;40: 151–162.

137. Backus BT, Banks MS, van Ee R, Crowell JA. Horizontal and vertical disparity, eye position, and stereoscopic slant perception. *Vision Res.* 1999;39:1143–1170.

138. Ogle KN. The optical space sense. In: Davson H, editor. *The Eye.* vol 4. New York: Academic Press; 1962.

139. Banks MS, Backus BT. Extra-retinal and perspective cues cause the small range of the induced effect. *Vision Res.* 1998;38(2):187–194.

140. Morgan Jr. MW. Methods used in the treatment of squint. *Am J Optom Arch Am Acad Optom.* 1948;25(2):57–74.

141. Schor CM. Zero retinal image disparity: a stimulus for suppression in small angle strabismus. *Doc Ophthalmol.* 1978;46:149–160.

142. Jampolsky A. Characteristics of suppression in strabismus. *Arch Ophthalmol.* 1955;54: 683–696.

143. Boeder P. The response shift. *Doc Ophthalmol.* 1967;23:88–100.

144. Von Noorden GK. Amblyopia: A multidisciplinary approach. Proctor lecture. *Invest Ophthalmol Vis Sci.* 1985;26:1704–1716.

145. Von Noorden GK. *Binocular Vision and Ocular Motility.* St Louis: CV Mosby; 1990.

146. Wensveen JM, Harwerth RS, Smith EL. Clinical suppression in monkeys reared with abnormal visual experience. *Vision Res.* 2001;41:1593–1609.

147. Gobin MH. The limitation of suppression to one half of the visual field in the pathogenesis of strabismus. *Br Orthop J.* 1968;25:42–49.

148. Schor CM. Binocular sensory disorders. In: Regan D, editor. *Vision and Visual Dysfunction.* vol 9. Boca Raton: CRC Press; 1991:179–223.

149. Bagolini B. Anomalous correspondence: Definition and diagnostic methods. *Doc Ophthalmol.* 1967;23:346–398.

150. Burian HM. Anomalous retinal correspondence: its essence and its significance in diagnosis and treatment. *Am J Ophthalmol.* 1951;34:237–253.

151. Harwerth RS, Fredenberg PM. Binocular vision with primary microstrabismus. *Invest Ophthalmol Vis Sci.* 2003;44:4293–4306.

152. Jampolsky A. Esotropia and convergent fixation disparity of small degree: differential diagnosis and management. *Am J Ophthalmol.* 1956;41:825–833.

153. Parks MM. Monofixation syndrome. *Trans Am Ophthalmol Soc.* 1969;67:609–657.

154. von Noorden GK. Infantile esotropia. A continuing riddle. *Am Orthop J.* 1984;34:52–62.

155. Flom MC, Kerr KE. Determination of retinal correspondence. Multiple-testing results and the depth of anomaly concept. *Arch Ophthalmol.* 1967;77:200–213.

156. Kerr KE. Anomalous correspondence—the cause or consequence of strabismus? *Optom Vis Sci.* 1998;75:17–22.

157. Tychsen L. Causing and curing infantile esotropia in primates: The role of decorrelated binocular input. *Trans Am Ophthalmol Soc.* 2007;105:564–593.

158. Wong AM, Lueder GT, Burkhalter A, Tychsen L. Anomalous retinal correspondence: neuroanatomic mechanism in strabismic monkeys and clinical findings in strabismic children. *J AAPOS.* 2000;4:168–174.

159. Crone RA. *Diplopia.* Amsterdam: Excerpta Medica, 1973.

160. Awaya S, von Noorden GK, Romano PE. Sensory adaptations in strabismus. Anomalous retinal correspondence in different positions of gaze. *Am Orthopt J.* 1970;20:28–35.

161. Bagolini B, Capobianco NM. Subjective space in comitant squint. *Am J Ophthalmol.* 1965;59:430–442.

162. Helveston EM, von Noorden GK, Williams F. Sensory adaptations in strabismus. Retinal correspondence in the "A" or "V" pattern. *Am Orthopt J.* 1970;20:22–27.

163. Brock FW. Projection habits in alternate squints. *Am J Optom.* 1940;17:193–207.

164. Verhoeff FH. Anomalous projection and other visual phenomena associated with strabismus. *Arch Ophthalmol.* 1938;19:663–699.

165. Wells WC. *Two Essays: One Upon Single Vision With Two Eyes; the Other on Dew.* Part III. Of some consequences from the foregoing theory of objects being seen single with two eyes, together with the explanation of several other phenomena of vision. London: A. Constable; 1818.

166. Brock FW. Anomalous projection in squint. Its cause and effect. New methods of correction. *Am J Optom.* 1939;16:201–221.

167. Morgan MW. Anomalous correspondence interpreted as a motor phenomenon. *Am J Optom.* 1961;38:131–148.
168. Schor CM. Perceptual-motor computational model of anomalous binocular correspondence. *Optometry and Vision Science.* 2015;92(5):544–550.
169. Serrano-Pedraza I, Clarke MP, Read JC. Single vision during ocular deviation in intermittent exotropia. *Ophthalmic and Physiological Optics.* 2011;31:45–55.
170. Sireteanu R. Binocular vision in strabismic humans with alternating fixation. *Vision Research.* 1982;22:889–896.
171. Dengler B, Kommerell G. Stereoscopic cooperation between the fovea of one eye and the periphery of the other eye at large disparities. Implications for anomalous retinal correspondence in strabismus. *Graefes Arch Clin Exp Ophthalmol.* 1993;231:199–206.
172. Alpern M, Hofstetter H. The effect of prism on esotropia—A case report. *Am J Optom Arch Am Acad Optom.* 1948;25:80–91.
173. Hubel DH, Wiesel TN. Binocular interaction in striate cortex of kittens reared with artificial squint. *J Neurophysiol.* 1965;28:1041–1059.
174. Kumagami T, Zhang B, Smith EL, Chino YM. Effect of onset age of strabismus on the binocular responses of neurons in the monkey visual cortex. *Invest Ophthalmol Vis Sci.* 2000;41:948–954.
175. Tychsen L, Wong AM, Burkhalter A. Paucity of horizontal connections for binocular vision in V1 of naturally strabismic macaques: cytochrome oxidase compartment specificity. *J Comp Neurol.* 2004;474:261–275.
176. Hallden U. Fusional phenomena in anomalous correspondence. *Acta Ophthalmol Suppl.* 1952;37:1–93.
177. Flom MC. Corresponding and disparate retinal points in normal and anomalous correspondence. *Am J Optom Physiol Opt.* 1980;57(9):656–665.
178. Kaufman L, Kaufman JH, Noble R, Edlund S, Bai S, King T. Perceptual distance and the constancy of size and stereoscopic depth. *Spat Vis.* 2006;19(5):439–457.
179. Bagolini B. Sensorial anomalies in strabismus, (suppression, anomalous correspondence, amblyopia). *Doc. Ophthalmol.* 1976;41(1):1–22.
180. Walraven FC. A discussion of anomalous retinal correspondence. *Am Orthopt J.* 1957;7:162–175.
181. Cacho-Martínez P, García- Muñoz Á, Ruiz- Cantero MT. Do we really know the prevalence of accommodative and nonstrabismic binocular dysfunctions? *Journal of Optometry.* 2010;3(4):185–197.
182. Paniccia SM, Ayala A. Prevalence of accommodative and non-strabismic binocular anomalies in a Puerto Rican pediatric population. *Optometry & Visual Performance.* 2015;3(3):158–164.
183. Pladere T, Luguzis A, Zabels R, et al. When virtual and real worlds coexist: Visualization and visual system affect spatial performance in augmented reality. *J Vis.* 2021;21(8):17.
184. Mon-Williams M, Wann JP, Rushton S. Binocular vision in a virtual world: visual deficits following the wearing of a head-mounted display. *Ophthalmic Physiol Opt.* 1993;13(4):387–391.
185. Yoon HJ, Kim J, Park SW, Heo H. Influence of virtual reality on visual parameters: immersive versus non-immersive mode. *BMC Ophthalmol.* 2020;20(1):200.
186. Shibata T, Kim J, Hoffman DM, Banks MS. Visual discomfort with stereo displays: Effects of viewing distance and direction of vergence-accommodation conflict. *Proc SPIE Int Soc Opt Eng.* 2011;7863:78630P78631–78630P78639.
187. Shibata T, Kim J, Hoffman DM, Banks MS. The zone of comfort: Predicting visual discomfort with stereo displays. *J Vis.* 2011;11(8):11.
188. Wee SW, Moon NJ, Lee WK, Jeon S. Ophthalmological factors influencing visual asthenopia as a result of viewing 3D displays. *Br J Ophthalmol.* 2012;96(11):1391–1394.
189. Hoffman DM, Girshick AR, Akeley K, Banks MS. 2008 Vergence-accommodation conflicts hinder visual performance and cause visual fatigue. *J Vis.* 2008;8(3):33. 1–30.
190. Hofstetter HW. Zone of clear single binocular vision. *Am J Optom Arch Am Acad Optom.* 1945;22(301–333):361–384.

37

Temporal Properties of Vision

Allison M. McKendrick and Andrew J. Anderson

Our visual perception arises from the interpretation of light information, which varies in space, wavelength, and time. It is the latter of these attributes that is explored in this chapter. The amount of light falling on a particular retinal location may alter over time because a target changes luminance (e.g., a light is abruptly turned on [an *aperiodic* stimulus], or a light is repeatedly flashing [a *periodic* stimulus]) or because of image motion (e.g., a steadily illuminated light sweeps over the retinal location). Retinal image motion is extremely common—even for nominally stationary objects—because people's eyes and heads are commonly moving relative to their surroundings. How does the visual system respond to and interpret light variations that occur as a function of time?

This chapter summarizes several basic phenomena that describe the sensitivity of our visual system to temporal information, including how some of these are influenced by spatial properties, chromaticity, background features, and surround characteristics. The application of these phenomena to the clinical study of abnormalities of visual processing, such as in disease, is also discussed.

TEMPORAL SUMMATION AND THE CRITICAL DURATION FOR SINGLE PULSES OF LIGHT (APERIODIC STIMULI)

To detect the presence of something in the visual world, it must be present for a finite period. Although a single quantum of light may be sufficient to generate a neural response, multiple quanta are generally required within a particular period before the light is reliably seen, a property known as *temporal summation*. In the human visual system, temporal summation occurs for durations of approximately 40 to 100 milliseconds, depending on the spatial and temporal properties of the object and its background, the adaptation level, and the eccentricity of the stimulus.[1-5] The maximum time over which temporal summation occurs is the *critical duration*.

Let's say we wish to determine how long a light needs to be presented on a dark background to be visible. In general terms, a more intense light does not need to be presented for as long as a less intense one to reach threshold visibility. Provided that the light pulse is shorter than the critical duration, it will be at threshold when the product of its duration and its intensity equals a constant. The formula that describes this time-intensity reciprocity is *Bloch's law*[6]:

$$Bt = K \qquad \textbf{(Eq. 37.1)}$$

where B = luminance of the light, t = duration, and K = a constant value.

Bloch's law is shown schematically in Fig. 37.1A. When stimulus intensity and duration are plotted on log-log coordinates, as in Fig. 37.1A, Bloch's law describes a line with a slope of −1. When the critical duration is exceeded, the threshold intensity versus duration function is described by a horizontal line; that is, a constant intensity is now required to reach threshold, irrespective of the stimulus duration. Bloch's law has been shown to be generally valid for a wide range of stimulus and background conditions, including both foveal and peripheral viewing.

The preceding discussion assumes that whenever the observer's threshold is exceeded, they will respond accurately to the stimulus. This predicts an abrupt and idealized transition between the two curves, as depicted in Fig. 37.1A. In reality, both visual stimuli and the physiologic mechanisms that we use to detect them are subject to random fluctuations. We may consider the length of the stimulus presentation to be divided into a number of discrete time intervals. The signal is detected when the response exceeds threshold in at least one interval and the probability of detection in each interval is considered independent. This description of the probabilistic nature of visual detection is known as *probability summation over time*.[7] The concept of probability summation is included in many models of temporal visual processing and is thought to be at least partly responsible for the less-than-abrupt transition between the region of temporal summation and constant intensity that occurs under some experimental conditions.[3] This can be seen in Fig. 37.1B. Here we see the amount of contrast required to detect a grating as initially decreasing with increased stimulus duration, as we would expect from Bloch's law. However, there is not an abrupt transition to where threshold contrast is independent of stimulus duration, particularly for higher spatial frequency gratings (lower curves). However, Gorea and Tyler[3] concluded that critical duration is minimally affected by spatial frequency once the effects of probability summation were factored in.

Factors affecting the critical duration

The critical duration depends on properties of both the stimulus and the background. At least in part, differences in critical duration reflect differences in neural response latencies for the relevant neural pathways. The latency of a neural response likely sets a limit to critical duration as it is this duration over which temporal summation for a single neuronal response occurs. The critical duration varies with light adaptation level; that is, with brighter backgrounds, the critical duration decreases.[8-12] Conversely, with dark adaptation, the critical duration increases.[13,14] Unless dark adapted, the size of the stimulus also affects the critical duration, with larger stimuli having a decreased critical duration.[9,12,15] Retinal eccentricity also influences the critical duration, as does the visual task.[16,17] Temporal summation is also affected by the spectral composition (wavelength or color) of the light stimuli, with purely chromatic stimuli having longer temporal integration than achromatic (luminance) stimuli.[18-20] For colored lights, the critical duration decreases with increased chromatic saturation of the background, similar to the decrease in critical duration with increased luminance for achromatic stimuli.[21] Fig. 37.2 demonstrates how increased retinal

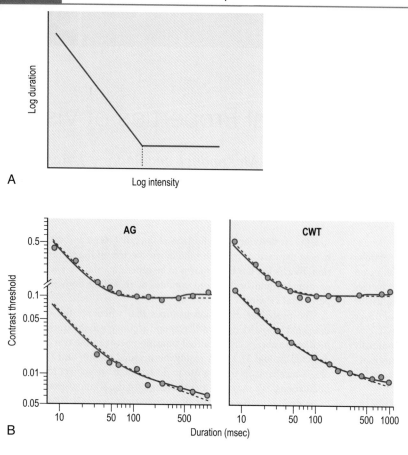

Fig. 37.1 (**A**) Schematic of the idealized relationship between threshold light intensity and the duration for it to reach visibility. For durations less than the critical duration, the threshold intensity is linearly related to duration, as described by Bloch's law. (**B**) The relationship between threshold light intensity and duration for flickering grating stimuli for two observers (AG, CWT) as measured by Gorea and Tyler. *Upper curves* represent data from 0.8 cycle per degree gratings, whereas *lower curves* show data for an 8 degree per cycle grating stimulus. Note that for the higher spatial frequency (lower curve), there is a more gradual transition between the two curves depicted schematically in (**A**). (B, from Gorea A, Tyler CW. New look at Bloch's law for contrast. *J Opt Soc Am A.* 1986;3(1): 52–61.)

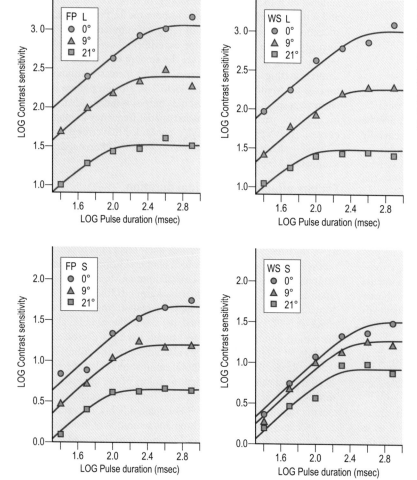

Fig. 37.2 Log contrast sensitivity versus pulse duration for equiluminant chromatic pulses. Data are shown for two observers (FP, WS). The upper panels show performance for "red-green" modulation (long wavelength sensitive (L) and medium wavelength sensitive cone modulation) whereas the lower panels show data for short-wavelength modulation (S). (From Swanson WH, Pan F, Lee BB. Chromatic temporal integration and retinal eccentricity: Psychophysics, neurometric analysis and cortical pooling. *Vision Res.* 2008;48:2657–2662.).

eccentricity markedly reduces the critical duration, although by similar amounts for both the "red-green" and S-cone chromatic pathways.[20] Note Fig. 37.2 plots the inverse of the threshold (i.e., sensitivity).

TEMPORAL SENSITIVITY TO PERIODIC STIMULI

In contrast to the aperiodic stimuli considered in the previous section (e.g., single pulses of light), periodic stimuli have luminance changes over time that repeat at a given frequency. Most research examining periodic stimuli has been directed to explore the following questions: (1) What is the fastest flicker rate that can be detected by the human visual system (the critical flicker fusion frequency [CFF]); and (2) What factors influence sensitivity to flicker slower than this critical rate?

Critical flicker fusion frequency

When a light is turned on and off repeatedly in rapid succession, the light appears to flicker, provided the on and off intervals are greater than some finite time interval. If the lights are flickered fast enough, we perceive the flashes as a single fused light rather than a series of flashes. In simple terms, when the perception of fusion occurs, we have reached the limit of the temporal-resolving ability of our visual system. The transition from the perception of flicker to that of fusion occurs at the *critical flicker fusion (CFF) frequency*. The value of the CFF varies, depending on characteristics of the stimulus and the observer. Some of the important factors that influence the CFF are discussed in the following sections.

Effect of stimulus luminance on critical flicker fusion

In general, the CFF increases as the luminance of the flashing stimulus increases. This relationship is known as the *Ferry-Porter law*, which states that CFF increases as a linear function of log luminance.[22,23] The Ferry-Porter law is valid for a wide range of stimulus conditions and is illustrated in Fig. 37.3.[24] The lower curves (*solid lines* and *symbols*) show data collected in the fovea, and the upper curves show data collected at 35 degrees eccentricity. For both locations the upper curves are for smaller targets (0.05 degrees foveally and 0.5 degree eccentrically), and the lower curves are for larger targets (0.5 degrees foveally and 5.7 degrees eccentrically). Fig. 37.3 demonstrates several interesting observations about the relationship between CFF and luminance. First, the Ferry-Porter law holds despite changes in stimulus size. Second, the linear relationship between log luminance and CFF predicted by the Ferry-Porter law is present for both central and peripheral viewing, although the slope of this relationship increases in the periphery, implying faster processing.[24] The Ferry-Porter law holds not only for spot targets but also for grating stimuli.[24] For scotopic luminance levels, at which rods mediate detection, CFF decreases substantially to approximately 20 Hz and no longer obeys the Ferry-Porter law.[23,25,26]

Effect of stimulus chromaticity on critical flicker fusion

The linear relationship between CFF and log luminance (the Ferry-Porter law) is also valid for purely chromatic stimuli.[27-30] However, the slope of the relationship has been shown to vary with stimulus wavelength.[28] This relationship is demonstrated in Fig. 37.4, which shows foveal CFF versus illuminance functions from four separate studies.[27-30] In all four studies the CFF illuminance functions were well fit by Ferry-Porter lines, and in all cases the functions for green (middle-wavelength) lights were found to be steeper than those for red (long-wavelength) lights. The steeper slope for green stimuli has been interpreted as evidence supporting the green cone pathways being inherently faster than the red cone pathways for the transmission of information near the CFF.[28] The CFF is lowest for blue stimuli detected by the short-wavelength pathways.[31,32]

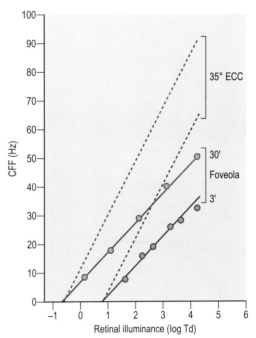

Fig. 37.3 Photopic critical flicker fusion (CFF) versus intensity functions measured in the fovea (*solid symbols and lines*) and at 35 degrees (*dashed lines*) from Tyler and Hamer.[24] The test stimulus was 660 nm presented on a equiluminant white surround. Foveal test stimuli were 0.5 degree (*red filled circles*) and 0.05 degree (*blue filled circles*). Eccentric stimuli were 5.7 degrees (*red dashed line*) and 0.5 degrees (*blue dashed line*). Results for the eccentric stimuli are represented here by a line fitted to the data, as an adherence to the Ferry-Porter law was found for all test conditions. *ECC*, Eccentricity. (Reprinted with permission from Tyler CW and Hamer RD. Analysis of visual modulation sensitivity. IV. Validity of the Ferry-Porter law. *J Opt Soc Am A*. 1990;7:743–758. © The Optical Society.

Effect of eccentricity on critical flicker fusion

The CFF varies as a function of eccentricity in the visual field. If the stimulus size and luminance are kept constant, the CFF increases with eccentricity over the central 50 degrees or so of the visual field and then decreases with further increases in eccentricity.[33,34] This is illustrated in Fig. 37.5, which plots the CFF as a function of eccentricity in the temporal visual field.

Effect of stimulus size on critical flicker fusion: the Granit-Harper law

As shown in Fig. 37.3, the CFF increases with stimulus size. For a wide range of luminances, CFF increases linearly with the logarithm of the stimulus area. This relationship is known as the *Granit-Harper law*, named after the investigators who first reported it.[35] The Granit-Harper law holds for a wide range of luminances, retinal eccentricities out to 10 degrees, and stimuli as large as almost 50 degrees diameter. However, subsequent investigators have determined that it is not the overall area of the stimulus that is critical, but rather the local retinal area with the best temporal resolution. This was demonstrated by Roehrig,[36,37] who measured the same value for the CFF for a complete 49.6-degree field in comparison to an annulus of the same diameter, with its central 66% not illuminated. Because the midperiphery has better temporal resolution than central vision, an eccentric annulus produced the same CFF as the full 49.6-degree stimulus. The Granit-Harper law does not hold under dim light conditions in which rods mediate performance.[35]

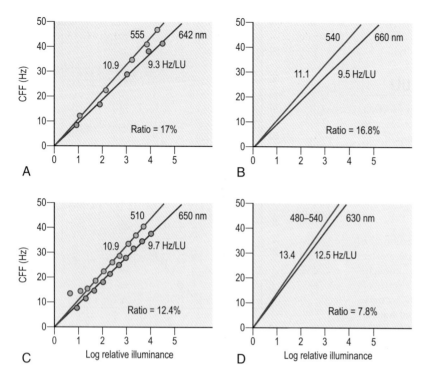

Fig. 37.4 Critical flicker fusion (*CFF*) versus illuminance functions for red and green flicker measured by Hamer and Tyler. Note that all data are well fit by the Ferry-Porter law, with green lights having a steeper slope than red. (**A**) Data for one subject from Hamer and Tyler. The green light function is steeper by 17%. (**B**) CFF data for red (660 nm) and green (540 nm) flickering stimuli for a single observer tested by Pokorny and Smith The green light function is steeper by 16.8%. (**C**) CFF data from Ives for red (650 nm) and green (510 nm) flicker stimuli viewed foveally. The green light function is steeper by 12.4%. (**D**) CFF data for green light (mean of 480 and 540 nm data) and red light (630 nm) flicker from Giorgi. The green light function is steeper than the red by 7.8%. *LU*, (A, from Hamer RD, Tyler CW. Analysis of visual modulation sensitivity. V. Faster visual response for G- than R-cone pathway. *J Opt Soc Am A.* 1992;9(11):1889–1904; B, from Pokorny J, Smith VC. Luminosity and CFF in deuteranopes and protanopes. *J Opt Soc Am.* 197;62:111–117; C, from Ives HE. Studies in the photometry of lights of different colours. II. Spectral luminosity curves by the method of critical frequency. *Philos Mag.* 1912;24:352–370; D, from Giorgi A. Effect of wavelength on the relationship between critical flicker frequency and intensity in foveal vision. *J Opt Soc Am.* 1963;53:480–486.)

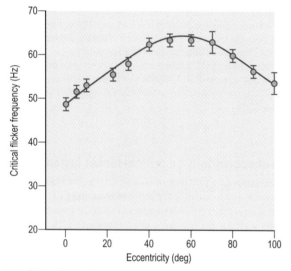

Fig. 37.5 Critical flicker frequency (mean ± standard deviation) as a function of eccentricity in the temporal visual field of the right eye of one observer. Stimulus area was 88.4 degrees², pupil diameter was 8 mm, and retinal illuminance was 2510 photopic trolands. (From Rovamo J, Raninen A. Critical flicker frequency and M-scaling of stimulus size and retinal illuminance. *Vision Res.* 1984;24:1127–1131.)

Outside 10 degrees eccentricity, a revised form of the Granit-Harper law is required to fit the changes in CFF with stimulus area. Rovamo and Raninen[38] have shown that the Granit-Harper law can be generalized across the visual field by replacing the retinal stimulus area with the number of ganglion cells stimulated. In this more general case, the CFF increases linearly with the logarithm of the number of ganglion cells stimulated. This is illustrated in Fig. 37.6. Fig. 37.6A plots CFF against eccentricity for three different stimulus areas. The CFF decreases with increasing eccentricity irrespective of the stimulus area. Fig. 37.6B plots the same CFF data as a function of the number

of retinal ganglion cells stimulated at each eccentricity and results in a linear relationship between these two parameters.

Temporal contrast sensitivity

The CFF defines an upper limit for temporal sensitivity, beyond which we can no longer detect that a light is flickering. How sensitive are we to flicker below the CFF, and how does the visual system respond to more complex temporal variations of light than simple flashes or trains of flashes? Classical work on human temporal contrast sensitivity was performed by De Lange in the 1950s, who mathematically analyzed temporal waveforms and employed linear filter theory.[39–41]

Fig. 37.7 shows the results from flicker-sensitivity experiments by Kelly, who continued the analytical approach pioneered by De Lange.[42] The stimulus was a very wide (68 degree diameter), uniform field, with indistinct edges. The vertical axis of the *left panel* indicates the "threshold modulation ratio," which is the extent that the sinusoidally modulated light deviates from its average (the direct current [DC] component). A modulation ratio of one means the stimulus modulates over time between zero luminance and two times the average, which is the maximum modulation possible. The axis is reversed so that higher points on the axis indicate higher sensitivity to flicker (i.e., only a very small modulation ratio is required for the flicker to be detected).

A series of curves are shown, each obtained at a different average retinal illumination or adaptation level. The curves define the flicker detection boundary for the particular level of adaptation, with the flicker rate specified by its temporal frequency in cycles per second (cps), or hertz (Hz). For a given level of adaptation, any combination of frequency and modulation amplitude below the curve is seen as flickering, whereas any combination above the curve is perceived as a steady light. The point at which the curve intersects the abscissa (x-axis) corresponds to the CFF. Note that at low adaptation levels, the shape of the curve is low pass, meaning that modulation sensitivity is similar for low temporal frequencies and then falls off systematically for higher temporal frequencies. At high adaptation levels, the shape of the curve is bandpass, meaning that modulation sensitivity is greatest for a band of

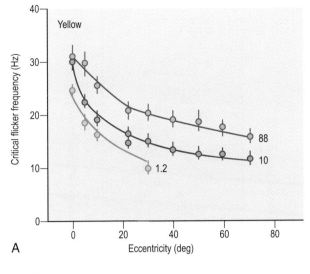

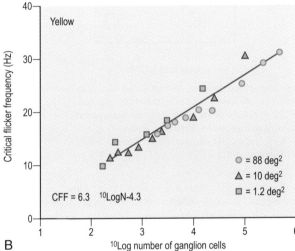

Fig. 37.6 (**A**) Critical flicker frequency (*CFF*; mean ± standard deviation) for targets viewed eccentrically for one observer reported by Rovamo and Raninen. Similar target sizes were used at all eccentricities, but retinal illuminance was F scaled by reducing the average stimulus luminance in inverse proportion to photopic Ricco's area. The numbers on the right of the curves refer to the stimulus area in degrees². When eccentricity increased from 0 to 70 degrees, the stimulus luminance nominally decreased from 50 to 0.80 photopic cd/m². Note that CFF decreases with increasing eccentricity irrespective of stimulus area when this luminance scaling is applied (in contrast to the results from a fixed luminance stimulus seen in Fig. 37.5). (**B**) CFF data from (**A**) plotted as a function of the number of retinal ganglion cells stimulated. (From Rovamo J, Raninen A. Critical flicker frequency as a function of stimulus area and luminance at various eccentricities in human cone vision: a revision of Granit-Harper and Ferry-Porter laws. *Vision Res.* 1988;28(7):785–790; Livingstone MS, Hubel DH. Connections between layer 4B of area 17 and the thick cytochrome oxidase stripes of area 18 in the squirrel monkey. *J Neurosci.* 1987;7:3371–3377.)

intermediate temporal frequencies and systematically falls off for lower and higher temporal frequencies.

With increasing retinal illuminance, more conditions are seen as flickering, consistent with the simpler Ferry-Porter law. At low frequencies the curves are similar, indicating that low-frequency flicker reaches threshold at a similar value of modulation ratio for all levels of photopic adaptation. This is not the case for high frequencies, at which the threshold is determined by both adaptation

level and frequency. At higher luminance levels the sensitivity for flicker detection peaks at frequencies of approximately 15 to 20 Hz. This is similar to the Brücke brightness enhancement effect, which is discussed later.

The right panel of Fig. 37.7 replots the data of Fig. 37.7A as a function of the absolute amplitude of the high-frequency flicker (rather than this amplitude expressed as a fraction of the average luminance, as given on the *left*). This has the effect of reversing the curves so that the amplitude sensitivity is greatest at the lowest adaptation level. The curves of Fig. 37.7B approach a common asymptote at high frequencies. This implies that, at high temporal frequencies, sensitivity is predicted by the absolute amplitude of the signal, independent of adaptation level. This behavior is not apparent at the low temporal frequency range.

Chromatic temporal sensitivity

Chromatic temporal contrast sensitivity measured with sinusoidally modulating stimuli also varies with retinal illuminance,[43] but there are two key differences when compared with performance measured with achromatic stimuli. First, chromatic functions are generally low pass, that is, sensitivity is similar for a range of low temporal frequencies before falling off at higher temporal frequencies. Second, the high-frequency cutoff is at lower temporal frequencies, that is, a lower CFF is found for chromatic in comparison to achromatic stimuli for a given retinal illuminance.[43]

Spatial effects on temporal sensitivity

The work of De Lange[40] and Kelly[42] describes our sensitivity to temporal sinusoidal variations in stimulus contrast but does not consider the effect that the spatial characteristics of the light source have on sensitivity. This can be investigated by using grating stimuli—rather than spatially uniform spots—the contrast of which can be modulated over time. When this is done, contrast sensitivity is found to depend on both the spatial and temporal properties of the stimulus.[44,45] Fig. 37.8 shows a surface plot of the human *spatiotemporal contrast sensitivity* function, as derived by Kelly, from a large number of psychophysical measurements.[44,46,47] One axis of the graph shows the temporal frequency of the stimulus; the other shows the spatial frequency. The height represents the observer's contrast sensitivity for the particular spatial and temporal conditions.[44,47,48] Paths running through the curve parallel to the temporal frequency axis represent the temporal contrast sensitivity functions for gratings of a particular spatial frequency, and those running parallel to the spatial frequency axis represent the spatial contrast sensitivity functions for gratings of a particular temporal frequency. The temporal contrast sensitivity function is bandpass at low spatial frequencies, becoming low pass at high spatial frequencies.

Mechanisms underlying temporal sensitivity

The shape of the human spatial contrast sensitivity function has been explained in terms of a multiple-channel model in which the overall function actually represents the summed sensitivity of a number of separate channels, each sensitive to a comparatively narrower range of temporal frequencies and tuned to a different peak spatial frequency.[49–51] The possible physiologic basis for these channels is considered at the end of this section. Similar to spatial processing, there is experimental evidence for a discrete number of channels for temporal processing, each tuned to a different peak temporal frequency.[52–55] However, there appear to be fewer independent temporal frequency filters than there are filters conveying spatial frequency information. The number of temporal mechanisms identified has been shown to be dependent on the spatial frequency of the stimulus, in addition to the retinal location.

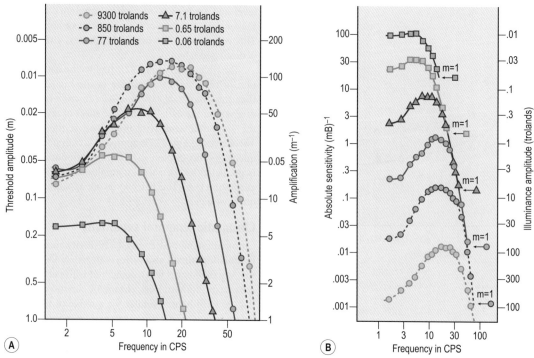

Fig. 37.7 Temporal sensitivity data collected by Kell Visual attenuation characteristics, as measured with sinu- soidal variation about different levels of retinal illuminance, are shown. (**A**) Threshold modulation ratios for just- detectable flicker plotted as a function of temporal frequency. (**B**) Absolute amplitudes of retinal illuminance variation for just-noticeable flicker plotted as a function of temporal frequency. Absolute sensitivity is the reciprocal of threshold absolute amplitude at each frequency. *CPS*, cycles per second. (From Kelly D. Visual responses to time-dependent stimuli. I. Amplitude sensitivity measurements. *J Opt Soc Am.* 1961;51:422.)

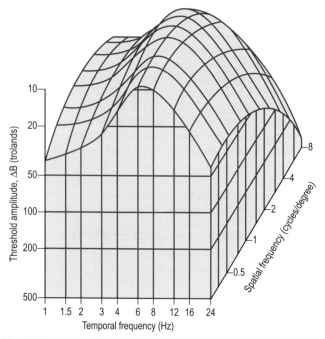

Fig. 37.8 Human spatiotemporal amplitude threshold surface obtained with circular gratings of 16 degrees viewed binocularly with natural pupils. (From Kelly D. Adaptation effects on spatio-temporal sine-wave thresholds. *Vision Res.* 1972;12:89–101.)

How can we determine whether different mechanisms are gov- erning performance? One method relies on the assumption that dif- ferent mechanisms result in distinct subjective representations of the stimulus; that is, when different mechanisms are responding to the stimulus, the stimulus looks different. Kelly[44] and Kulikowski[56] report that flickering gratings at threshold produce one of three percepts depending on the spatiotemporal parameters of the grating: slow flicker, apparent motion, or frequency doubling (i.e., the perceived spatial frequency is twice the actual spatial frequency). This is consis- tent with three mechanisms underlying temporal processing. Further support for multiple mechanisms comes from studies of *temporal dis- crimination*, or the ability to determine that stimuli are flickering at different rates. For grating patches of 0.25 cycles per degree, Watson and Robson[54] found there were three temporal frequencies that were uniquely discriminable, which they interpreted as evidence for three unique filters mediating temporal processing. Mandler and Makous[53] modeled temporal discrimination performance and also found evi- dence for three mechanisms underlying temporal processing.

An alternative method for identifying mechanisms underlying visual processing is that of *selective adaptation*. Adaptation is where sensitivity is depressed when a mechanism is exposed to a stimulus for a protracted period, with *selective adaptation* highlighting that mecha- nisms will have their sensitivities reduced in proportion to their indi- vidual sensitivities to the adapting—also called the *masking*—stimulus. Selective adaptation has been widely used to isolate the mechanisms underlying color vision processing.[57] Hess and Snowden[52] used a selec- tive adaptation approach to examine temporal processing with tempo- ral stimuli to uncover temporal mechanisms; an example of their data is displayed in Fig. 37.9. The first stage of these experiments (not shown in the figure) involved measuring foveal contrast detection thresholds for a wide range of spatial and temporal conditions. These measures were used to set the contrast of the *probe* stimulus, which was set to be just detectable (4 dB above threshold). The detectability of this probe

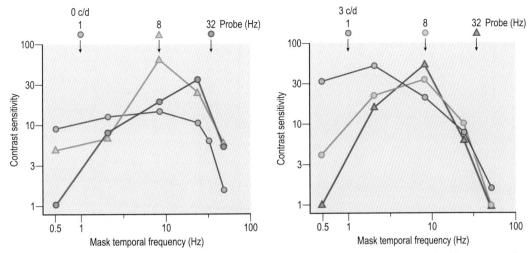

Fig. 37.9 Properties of temporal mechanisms identified using a selective adaptation method by Hess and Snowden. Mask contrast sensitivity is plotted against mask temporal frequency for detection of a just-suprathreshold probe. Data are for probes of 1, 8, and 32 Hz. The *left panel* shows data for a probe of 0 cycles per degree, for which three mechanisms are revealed: one low-pass and two bandpass. The *right panel* shows data for a 3 cycle per degree probe, and only two mechanisms are revealed. (From Hess RF, Snowden RJ. Temporal properties of human visual filters: Number, shapes and spatial covariation. *Vision Res.* 1992;32:47–59.)

stimulus was then measured in the presence of masking stimuli of the same spatial frequency but different temporal frequency. The contrast of the masking stimulus was varied until the probe was just visible.

Fig. 37.9A shows the contrast sensitivity (the reciprocal of contrast) of the mask plotted against the mask temporal frequency, for foveally presented stimuli of no spatial content (i.e., 0 cycles per degree). Three mechanisms are revealed by the probe stimuli: one low pass (*solid circles*) and two bandpass (*open circles, solid triangles*). Fig. 37.9B shows data for a probe of 3 cycles per degree, and only two mechanisms are revealed. The bandpass mechanism, centered on higher temporal frequencies in Fig. 37.9A, disappears when the spatial frequency content of the stimulus increases. Using a similar method, Snowden and Hess[58] have shown that for retinal eccentricities of 10 degrees, only two mechanisms are found, reducing to a single mechanism at eccentricities of greater than 30 degrees.

More recent evidence suggests that these channels are not as independent as initially thought. Using a masking paradigm, Cass and Alais[59] demonstrated two channels underlying human temporal vision. High-frequency masks were able to suppress low-frequency targets, suggesting an interaction between temporal channels. The high-frequency channel was orientation invariant which suggests a precortical origin, given that significant orientation selectively of visual neurons is not apparent until area V1 in the brain. In contrast, the low-frequency filter demonstrated orientation dependence, suggesting a cortical origin.

So, what is the neural basis of these psychophysically measured temporal channels? Visual information from the retina is carried to the visual cortex, via the lateral geniculate nucleus, by several major neural pathways (magnocellular, parvocellular, and koniocellular). These pathways have been shown to carry largely independent, but sometimes overlapping, visual information to the cortex, although significant convergence arises at the cortical level.[60] Magnocellular neurons are capable of processing achromatic fast flicker,[61,62] with neuronal temporal contrast sensitivity data resembling the form of that of human observers.[63] Parvocellular retinal ganglion cells are well established to be the physiologic substrate for red-green chromatic modulation.[62] It is important to note, however, that retinal ganglion cell responses persist at considerably higher temporal frequencies than the human

psychophysical CFF.[63] This is particularly the case for chromatic modulation in which the human psychophysical function limit is approximately 10 to 15 Hz, yet parvocellular retinal ganglion cells will respond up to 30 to 40 Hz.[64] These differences are explained by models in which responses from multiple single retinal cells converge on cortical detection mechanisms. The exact manner in which this convergence occurs and how the site of convergence is represented in the visual cortex is an ongoing area of debate.[20,64–67]

Surround effects on temporal sensitivity

Our sensitivity to temporal variations depends not only on the properties of the flickering light but also on those of the background surrounding the light. In the dark (scotopic conditions), detection of light increments is mediated by rods, and in the light (photopic conditions), detection is mediated by cones. For flicker sensitivity, it has been shown that when photopic flickering lights are presented on dark backgrounds, the dark-adapted rods surrounding the stimulus act to decrease cone-mediated flicker sensitivity via suppressive rod-cone interactions.[68–73] These suppressive rod-cone interactions are most significant at high temporal frequencies (see Fig. 37.10) and in the retinal periphery. Suppressive effects between cone mechanisms of flicker thresholds (e.g., long wavelength–sensitive cones and medium wavelength–sensitive cones) have also been demonstrated.[74,75]

Within the photopic range, luminance differences between a flickering target and its surround are particularly important in determining temporal contrast sensitivity for low temporal frequencies.[76–79] This is illustrated in Fig. 37.11. The *triangles* represent the temporal contrast sensitivity for a surround equal to the average luminance of the flickering light (25 cd/m²), and sensitivity at low temporal frequencies is constant under this condition. For either a dark surround (0 cd/m², *squares*) or a light surround (50 cd/m², *circles*), the sensitivity drops off at low temporal frequencies.

The presence of a surround differing in luminance from that of the flickering target creates a contrast border at the edge of the target. Spehar and Zaidi[79] have demonstrated that such a border decreases temporal contrast sensitivity. Whether the background is brighter or dimmer is not important; rather the decrease in temporal contrast sensitivity depends on the magnitude of the border contrast, with larger

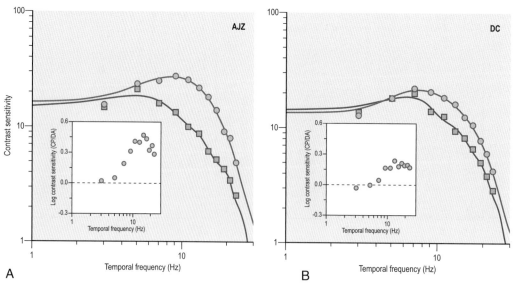

Fig. 37.10 The effect of rod-cone interactions on temporal contrast sensitivity. Temporal contrast sensitivity to an 80-photopic troland sinusoidal stimulus measured after (A) 30 minutes of dark adaptation (closed blue squares) where the rods are fully sensitive; and (B) during the first 5 minutes following the termination of a 2-minute exposure to a 10,000 troland broad band light (partial rod bleach: filled red circles). After dark adaptation, temporal contrast sensitivity is attenuated for temporal frequencies above 6–8 Hz. *Panel insets* show the difference in log contrast sensitivity between the two conditions for each observer (AJZ, DC). (Reproduced with permission from Zele AJ, Cao D, Porkorny D. Rod-cone interactions and the temporal impulse response of the cone pathway. *Vision Res.* 2008;48:2593–2598.)

contrasts resulting in larger decreases in temporal contrast sensitivity at low temporal frequencies. In short, we are most sensitive to temporal changes when the luminance of the background is matched to the average of the flickering target. One experimental paradigm in which such surround effects become important is the case of luminance-pedestal flicker, which is discussed in the following section.

Influence of local changes in luminance: the luminance pedestal

Historically, studies of temporal sensitivity have generated flicker using one of two methodologies, which are illustrated schematically in Fig. 37.12.[80] The upper panel of Fig. 37.12 illustrates where the flicker produces no change in average luminance over time; examples of studies using such stimuli include those by De Lange[40] and Roufs.[78] The lower panel of Fig. 37.12 illustrates flicker generated by modulating a light increment over time. This results in both a flickering component and an increase in time-averaged luminance—here called the *luminance pedestal*—above the background level (examples of studies using such stimuli include those of Alexander and Fishman[72]; Eisner[81]; Eisner, Shapiro, and Middleton[82]; and Anderson and Vingrys[80]). Because both methods have been used to assess temporal sensitivity, it is important to understand whether they yield equivalent or differing results.

The two stimulus types can only yield equivalent results if the luminance pedestal has no effect on thresholds, which seems unlikely. In the previous section, we discussed how flicker sensitivity changes with light adaptation (see Fig. 37.10); as such, it may be expected that the local increase in luminance created by the luminance pedestal may act to increase thresholds. This is the case and has been reported by Anderson and Vingrys.[80]

Furthermore, the presence of the pedestal causes a difference between the surround and the flickering target. Specifically, it allows the surround to remain more dark adapted (allowing suppressive rod-cone interactions to decrease high-frequency flicker sensitivity) and

creates a border contrast (decreasing sensitivity at low flicker rates).[83] Overall, it has been shown that both local adaptation mechanisms and surround interactions are important to explaining the differences in thresholds measured with these two types of stimuli.[83,84]

The effects of flicker on perception

The presence of flicker can alter both the apparent color and brightness of a light.[85–91] When a light is flickered, its apparent brightness varies depending on the frequency of the flicker, with maximum apparent brightness occurring between 5 and 20 Hz. This phenomenon is known as the *Brücke brightness enhancement effect*.[92] Such brightness enhancement can be demonstrated experimentally by matching the brightness of a flickering light to that of a nonflickering standard.[88] When the light is flickered at rates faster than those that result in brightness enhancement, the apparent brightness of the flickering light decreases. Eventually, the apparent brightness plateaus, and at rates beyond the CFF, the apparent brightness is the same as the apparent brightness of a steady light equal to the time-averaged luminance of the flickering light. This observation was made by Talbot[93] and Plateau[94] and is known as the *Talbot-Plateau law*. Lights flickering above the CFF, at which point flicker is invisible, appear identical to steady lights of the same chromaticity and time-averaged luminance. Under most conditions of adaptation, the Talbot-Plateau law appears to hold. One exception is the case of blue targets presented on bright yellow backgrounds, in which case the target appears more yellow than a steady light, even when it is not visibly flickering.[91]

Temporal phase segmentation

An important task of the visual system is to distinguish objects from their background, a task known as *image segmentation* (see Chapter 32). Useful information for the process of image segmentation includes differences in luminance and color between the image and its background. Differences in temporal phase are also sufficient for image

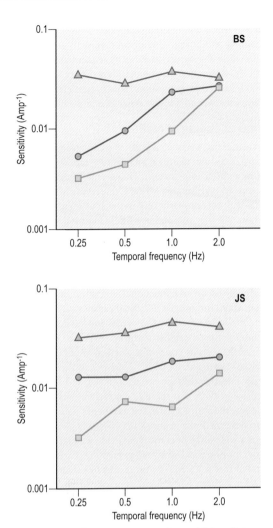

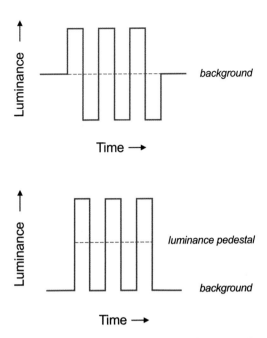

Fig. 37.12 Schematic of flickering stimuli that do (lower panel) or do not (lower panel) also produce a change in average luminance. The time-averaged luminance during the presentation of flicker is represented by the *dashed lines*. Note that for stimuli produced by interrupting a light increment, the time-averaged luminance is greater than the background by an amount that is the luminance pedestal. (Modified from Anderson AJ, Vingrys AJ. Interactions between flicker thresholds and luminance pedestals. *Vision Res.* 2000;40:2579-2588.)

Fig. 37.11 Surround effects on temporal sensitivity. Data are from Spehar and Zaidi for two observers (BS, JS). Amplitude sensitivity is plotted as a function of temporal frequency for different surround conditions: green squares, 0 cd/m² (dark surround); red triangles, 25.0 cd/m² (equiluminant surround); and blue circles, 50 cd/m² (light surround). (From Spehar B, Zaidi Q. Surround effects on the shape of the temporal contrast-sensitivity function. *J Opt Soc Am A.* 1997;14(9):2517-2525.)

segmentation.[95–98] For example, if a field of identical dot elements is rapidly flickered from black to white in phase (i.e., all dots appear white simultaneously, then black simultaneously), the field appears to be uniformly flickering. If, however, elements in a subregion flicker in counterphase to the rest (i.e., within the subregion the dots are white when those outside are black), a contour between the subregion and the rest of the display is observed. At high temporal frequencies (greater than approximately 10 Hz), the difference in phase of individual elements cannot be detected; however, the contour between regions is easily visualized provided the gap between regions is less than about 0.4 degrees.[96,98] Temporal image segmentation is possible for chromatic stimuli, although only at low temporal frequencies.[98]

Clinical applications of temporal sensitivity measurements

Measurements of temporal processing have been used extensively for clinical testing. Both measures of CFF and temporal contrast sensitivity have been used to explore visual function in disease (for example, see 99, 100). Spatiotemporal contrast sensitivity (see Fig. 37.8) has also

been explored in clinical disorder, with a notable example being the study of amblyopia,[101] where sensitivity to stimuli of high temporal but low spatial frequency is largely preserved.

Often, clinical measures of temporal sensitivity are performed across the visual field, with use of perimetric strategies (see Chapter 35). There are several perimetric techniques for exploring temporal sensitivity across the visual field: CFF perimetry (which measures the CFF for small spot targets at various field locations), temporal modulation perimetry (which measures temporal contrast sensitivity for small spot targets either about a mean luminance or displayed on a luminance pedestal), and frequency-doubling perimetry. Frequency-doubling perimetry measures contrast sensitivity for patches of sinusoidal grating of low spatial and high temporal frequency, parameters that result in the grating appearing to have twice its actual spatial frequency. The CFF has also been used as a measure of task-induced visual fatigue.[102,103]

The development of perimetric methods for measuring temporal sensitivity has been largely directed to the detection of glaucoma or identification of glaucomatous visual field progression.[104–112] Abnormalities in temporal processing have also been identified in a range of other diseases, using perimetric and other strategies, including Parkinson disease, dyslexia, age-related macular degeneration, multiple sclerosis, optic neuritis, high-risk drusen, central serous chorioretinopathy, and migraine.[113–124]

Temporal segmentation stimuli have also been used in a clinical setting to assess the patency of the magnocellular system. Letters created from small rapidly flickering dots are presented, and the subject must then identify the letters. The dots within the letters flicker in opposite phase to the dots external to the letter. Temporal segmentation stimuli have been used to identify abnormalities in temporal sensitivity in dyslexia and glaucoma.[125–128]

MOTION PROCESSING

The detection of motion is an extension of temporal processing that forms a far-reaching separate area of study. *Motion* is a change in spatial position over time. Indeed, practically everything of visual interest in the world is moving, if not as a result of movement of the object itself, then by movement of the observer's head or eyes, causing the image on the retina to move. As we have already discussed, the ability of the visual system to detect temporal changes in luminance at a given location is exquisite. Such exquisite temporal sensitivity is important for processing motion, as the ability to follow local variations in luminance over time—and to compare these variations to those occurring in neighboring locations—is critical for determining if an image is moving across the retina. Indeed, some of the earliest models for motion detection involved mechanisms that sought correlations between temporal variations in luminance in one area, and those in an adjacent area following a short delay.[129] However, human motion perception mechanisms are more complex than a simple model that compares separate measures of an object's location with excellent temporal sensitivity. The visual system needs to detect such local motion cues, but also to globally integrate complex motion cues that may occur across the visual field (for example, owing to movement of the observer in addition to the movement of objects in the environment), and then to interpret the meaning of these cues. This section briefly describes some perceptual and psychophysical data on human motion perception. A brief description of the neurophysiologic substrates underlying motion perception is included because this provides a basis for understanding the applications of motion tasks to the study of functional visual loss in disease. There are several detailed reviews of motion processing elsewhere.[130,131]

Psychophysical and perceptual evidence for unique motion processing

Several perceptual phenomena provide evidence for the existence of mechanisms designed specifically to process motion information. One of these is known as the *motion aftereffect*, which occurs after prolonged viewing of a moving stimulus (this is also known as *motion adaptation*).[132–135] After prolonged staring at a moving stimulus, stationary objects appear to move in the opposite direction and the apparent speed of moving objects is distorted. Importantly, the apparent position of such stationary objects does not change, suggesting that motion and position are encoded separately.

Another example demonstrating that the perception of motion is not merely a simple representation of physical motion is that of *apparent motion*. Apparent motion occurs when spatially separate lights are

flashed in sequence, giving the perception of movement despite each light remaining stationary. This phenomenon is sometimes used in shop fronts, where the motion induced by sequential flashing of lights is designed to draw attention. Apparent motion can be induced by a single pair of lights flashed in succession. This movement is also known as the *phi phenomenon*, and was first described in detail by Wertheimer.[136]

The neural encoding of motion

Further evidence for motion as a primary sensory dimension arises from the existence of distinct neuronal architecture capable of supporting the encoding of motion information. Hubel and Wiesel[137] observed that some neurons in cortical area V1 have directionally selective receptive fields. Cells with this property respond well when a stimulus moves in one direction, but they respond in a limited fashion, or not at all, when the stimulus moves in the opposite direction. Direction-selective neurons are not evenly distributed throughout area V1; they are predominantly located in layers 4A, 4B, 4Cα, and 6.[138] Layer 4Cα receives its main input from magnocellular pathways,[139] suggesting that the magnocellular pathway is part of a functional specialization designed to carry information about motion. As discussed earlier, magnocellular neurons are preferentially involved in the visual processing of flicker.[61,140–142] Signals from the magnocellular pathway are passed from 4Cα to layer 4B, from which neurons connect to cortical area MT (medial temporal, otherwise known as area V5).[143–146] In area MT a high proportion of directionally selective cells are present (~80%), and these neurons have large receptive fields.[147,148] It should be noted that not all magnocellular neurons follow the path to V5/MT; a number of neurons converge with the parvocellular neurons in area V1.[149,150]

There is a wide body of convergent evidence that links area V5/MT to aspects of motion processing and perception. Early work in primates demonstrated that a V5/MT lesion results in performance deficits for motion tasks, without corresponding losses to visual acuity or color perception.[151,152] Newsome and Paré[151] investigated motion perception in the presence of MT lesions in rhesus monkeys, with monkeys required to identify the direction of motion of a subset of dots moving in a common direction within a field of randomly moving dots (Fig. 37.12). The proportion of dots moving in a common direction (coherence ratio) was varied to determine the direction identification threshold. Key to this task is that the moving dots be selected randomly for each frame of presentation so that the direction of motion cannot be determined by tracking the location of a single dot. Rather, the local motion signals must be combined over a large area of the visual field to determine the global motion percept (Fig. 37.13).[153] This type of stochastic random dot motion stimulus has been widely used to explore mechanisms that pool motion information across space because it

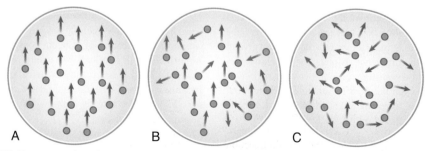

Fig. 37.13 Representation of a global-dot motion stimulus. The subject is required to identify the overall direction of motion of the dots (up/down). The signal strength is varied by changing the number of signal dots moving in that direction in successive frames. The remaining dots, the noise dots, moved in random directions. The dots that comprise the signal dots are chosen at the start of each frame. (**A**) A 100% signal strength condition. (**B**) A 50% signal strength condition. (**C**) A 0% signal strength condition; there is no global motion of the dots, only random local motion. (From Edwards M, Badcock DR. Global motion perception: Interaction of on and off pathways. *Vision Res.* 1994;34:2849–2858.)

allows variation of the predominant motion cue without varying the magnitude of local motion information. Newsome and Paré[151] found striking elevations in such motion thresholds when they made selective lesions to area MT. Newsome, Britten, and Movshon[154] further demonstrated that the activity in a single MT cell correlated directly with the monkey's trial by trial performance in a motion discrimination task. They also demonstrated that microstimulation of tiny regions of MT can bias a monkey's motion perception in a manner predictable from the response characteristics of cells adjacent to the stimulating electrode.

Zihl, Von Cramon, and Mai[155]; Hess, Baker, and Zihl[156]; and Baker, Hess, and Zihl[157] provide a series of reports investigating the motion perception of a human patient with a bilateral loss of the superior temporal cortical region. This patient was found to have a specific deficit to motion processing while other measured forms of visual processing were normal or relatively intact. In particular, the patient performed poorly on a random-dot motion task similar to that used by Newsome and Paré[151] This pattern of deficit is consistent with that found when area V5/MT is lesioned in primates, providing evidence for a similar specialized area for motion processing in humans. Seeded by this earlier work, numerous studies have demonstrated the importance of area V5/MT to human motion perception, using techniques such as functional magnetic resonance imaging[158,159] and transcranial magnetic stimulation.[160,161]

There is general consensus that the detection of moving stimuli and the integration of motion cues across space relies on the visual neural pathway leading from the magnocellular layers of the lateral geniculate nucleus through area V1 to area MT. However, it is also recognized that some aspects of how humans integrate and segregate motion signals across space, including for large fields of motion such as optic flow, are better explained by models of broader networks of neurons (for review see[131]). Furthermore, the pathway from V1 does not represent the only input to V5/MT; area MT also receives input from the superior colliculus via the pulvinar.[162] The pathway via the pulvinar contributes to the phenomenon of "blindsight," where patients with clinical lesions to V1 can still have some residual conscious or unconscious sensitivity to moving stimuli.[163,164] In addition, Nawrot and Rizzo[165] have demonstrated that the cerebellum may also play an important role in human motion processing. In their study, motion direction discrimination deficits were found in a group of patients with acute midline cerebellar lesions. These patients were unable to discern the direction of motion in a global motion task, similar to the deficit reported following MT lesions in primates.[151,152] Area V3 is also important to human motion perception, particularly for the interpretation of self-motion in the environment[166] and the encoding of three-dimensional structure from motion cues.[167] More complex neural networks are required to explain aspects of motion interpretation in the human brain; for example, the understanding that an object is animate. These are reviewed elsewhere.[131]

Applications of motion processing to the clinic and other contexts

Motion perception has been explored extensively in a range of clinical conditions because motion is a unique sensory dimension, processed by a relatively well-understood neural pathway, at least for the earlier stages of motion perception such as motion detection and the integration of motion cues across space. As discussed in the preceding section, the detection of stimulus motion occurs early in the motion pathway (retina to V1), the ability to discriminate the direction of motion is present in cortical neurons within V1, and the ability to extract global motion information occurs in the extrastriate visual areas (V5/MT or higher). The clinical study of motion processing often selects

stimuli designed to inform about the stage of motion processing that is impacted. For example, if the ability to detect stimulus motion and discriminate its direction is intact yet the ability to integrate or segregate motion cues across space is impaired, this suggests damage within extrastriate areas.

The ability to both detect motion and discriminate its direction declines with age,[168,169] although the effects of aging can differ depending upon the type of motion task, as well as the location of the motion (central versus peripheral vision).[170] Motion processing abnormalities have been documented as a consequence of a variety of neurological conditions, including Parkinson disease,[171,172] Alzheimer disease,[173] and in people who experience migraine.[174]

Visual motion processing has also been extensively studied in individuals with glaucoma, sometimes with perimetric approaches to testing motion perception across the visual field (see Chapter 35). For example, random-dot motion perimetry assesses the ability to globally integrate local motion cues across space at discrete locations across the visual field. Several studies have found random-dot motion perimetric deficits in glaucoma.[175–182] The magnitude of such motion deficits in glaucoma is correlated with the extent of loss for contrast discrimination tasks designed to assess magnocellular processing, consistent with the source of the motion perception loss arising prior to cortical processing.[178] Peripheral motion displacement thresholds (the minimum distance a line or random-dot pattern must jump in order to appear to move) are also elevated in glaucoma.[180,183–185]

CONCLUSION

The human visual system's ability to encode and interpret temporal cues in the visual world is critical to human visual perception. The basic attributes of human temporal visual perception, such as the ability to detect and distinguish pulses of light, have been understood for decades. Human motion perception is one of the best studied and most completely understood areas of human perceptual function. Nevertheless, the ability to interpret complex motion cues in the visual world is an active research field and is far from completely understood. Motion perception is considered critical to our interaction with the world, including navigation, driving, and interpretation of the motion of ourselves and others. Improved understanding of the ways in which humans extract and interpret complex motion cues will be important to understand integrative brain function and to predict and interpret the effects of brain disorders and will also have applications in improving machine vision and robotics.

REFERENCES

1. Breitmeyer BG, Ganz L. Temporal studies with flashed gratings: inferences about human transient and sustained channels. *Vision Res.* 1977;17:861–865.
2. Burr DC. Temporal summation of moving images by the human visual system. *Proc R Soc Lond B Biol Sci.* 1981;211(1184):321–339.
3. Gorea A, Tyler CW. New look at Bloch's law for contrast. *J Opt Soc Am A.* 1986;3(1):52–61.
4. Legge GE. Sustained and transient mechanisms in human vision: temporal and spatial properties. *Vision Res.* 1978;18:69–81.
5. Snowden RJ, Braddick OJ. The temporal integration and resolution of velocity signals. *Vision Res.* 1991;31(5):907–914.
6. Bloch A. Experience sur la vision. *C R Soc Biol.* 1885;37:493–495.
7. Watson AB. Probability summation over time. *Vision Res.* 1979;19:515–522.
8. Sperling HG, Jolliffe CL. Intensity-time relationship at threshold for spectral stimuli in human vision. *J Opt Soc Am.* 1965;55:191–199.
9. Saunders RM. The critical duration of temporal summation in the human central fovea. *Vision Res.* 1975;15:699–703.
10. Mitsuboshi M, Kawabata Y, Aiba TS. Color-opponent characteristics revealed in temporal integration time. *Vision Res.* 1987;27:1197–1206.
11. Krauskopf J, Mollon JD. The independence of the temporal integration properties of the individual chromatic mechanisms. *J Physiol, Lond.* 1971;219:611–623.
12. Barlow HB. Temporal and spatial summation in human vision at different background intensities. *J Physiol Lond.* 1958;141:337–350.
13. Stewart BR. Temporal summation during dark adaptation. *J Opt Soc Am.* 1972;62:449–457.

14. Montellese S, Sharpe LT, Brown JL. Changes in critical duration during dark-adaptation. *Vision Res.* 1979;19:1147–1153.
15. Graham CH, Margaria R. Area and intensity-time relation in the peripheral retina. *Am J Physiol.* 1935;113:299–305.
16. Baumgardt E, Hillman B. Duration and size as determinants of peripheral retinal response. *J Opt Soc Am.* 1961;51:340–344.
17. Connors MM. Luminance requirements for hue perception and identification, for a range of exposure durations. *J Opt Soc Am.* 1970;60:958–965.
18. Dain SJ, King-Smith PE. Visual thresholds in dichromats and normals: The importance of post-receptoral processes. *Vision Res.* 1981;21:573–580.
19. Smith VC, Bowen RW, Pokorny J. Threshold temporal integration of chromatic stimuli. *Vision Res.* 1984;24(7):653–660.
20. Swanson WH, Pan F, Lee BB. Chromatic temporal integration and retinal eccentricity: Psychophysics, neurometric analysis and cortical pooling. *Vision Res.* 2008;48:2657–2662.
21. Kawabata Y. Temporal integration at equiluminance and chromatic adaptation. *Vision Res.* 1994;34(8):1007–1018.
22. Ferry E. Persistence of vision. *Am J Sci.* 1892;44:192–207.
23. Porter T. Contributions to the study of flicker. *Proc R Soc A.* 1902;62:313–329.
24. Tyler CW, Hamer RD. Analysis of visual modulation sensitivity. IV. Validity of the Ferry-Porter law. *J Opt Soc Am A.* 1990;7:743–758.
25. Hecht S, Verrijp C. Intermittent stimulation by light. III. The relation between intensity and critical flicker fusion frequency for different retinal locations. *J Gen Physiol.* 1933;17:251–265.
26. Ives HE. A theory of intermittent vision. *J Opt Soc Am Rev Sci Instrum.* 1922;6:343–361.
27. Giorgi A. Effect of wavelength on the relationship between critical flicker frequency and intensity in foveal vision. *J Opt Soc Am.* 1963;53:480–486.
28. Hamer RD, Tyler CW. Analysis of visual modulation sensitivity. V. Faster visual response for G- than R-cone pathway. *J Opt Soc Am A.* 1992;9(11):1889–1904.
29. Ives HE. Studies in the photometry of lights of different colours. II. Spectral luminosity curves by the method of critical frequency. *Philos Mag.* 1912;24:352–370.
30. Pokorny J., Smith V.C. Luminosity and CFF in deuteranopes and protanopes. *J Opt Soc Am.* 197;62:111–117.
31. Brindley GS, JJ, Du Croz Rushton WAH. The flicker fusion frequency of the blue-sensitive mechanism of colour vision. *J. Physiol (Lond).* 1966;183:497–500.
32. Hess RF, Mullen KT, Zrenner E. Human photopic vision with only short wavelength cones: post-receptoral properties. *J Physiol.* 1989;417:151–172.
33. Hartmann E, Lachenmayr B, Brettel H. The peripheral critical flicker frequency. *Vision Res.* 1979;19:1019–1023.
34. Rovamo J, Raninen A. Critical flicker frequency and M-scaling of stimulus size and retinal illuminance. *Vision Res.* 1984;24:1127–1131.
35. Granit R, Harper P. Comparitive studies on the peripheral and central retina. II Synaptic reactions in the eye. *Am J Physiol.* 1930;95:211–227.
36. Roehrig W. The influence of area on the critical flicker fusion threshold. *J Psychol.* 1959;47:317–330.
37. Roehrig W. The influence of the portion of the retina stimulated on the critical flicker-fusion threshold. *J Psychol.* 1959;48:57–63.
38. Rovamo J, Raninen A. Critical flicker frequency as a function of stimulus area and luminance at various eccentricities in human cone vision: a revision of Granit-Harper and Ferry-Porter laws. *Vision Res.* 1988;28(7):785–790.
39. De Lange H. Relationship between critical flicker frequency and a set of low-frequency characteristics of the eye. *J Opt Soc Am.* 1954;44:380.
40. De Lange H. Research into the dynamic nature of the human fovea-cortex systems with intermittent and modulated light. I. Attenuation characteristics with white and colored light. *J Opt Soc Am.* 1958;48:777.
41. De Lange H. Research into the dynamic nature of the human fovea-cortex systems with intermittent and modulated light. II. Phase shift in brightness and delay in color perception. *J Opt Soc Am.* 1958;48:784.
42. Kelly D. Visual responses to time-dependent stimuli. I. Amplitude sensitivity measurements. *J Opt Soc Am.* 1961;51:422.
43. Swanson WH, Ueno T, Smith VC. Pokorny J. Temporal modulation sensitivity and pulse-detection thresholds for chromatic and luminance perturbations. *J Opt Soc Am A.* 1987;4(10):1992–2005.
44. Kelly DH. Frequency doubling in visual responses. *J Opt Soc Am.* 1966;56:1628–1633.
45. Robson JG. Spatial and temporal contrast-sensitivity functions of the visual system. *J Opt Soc Am.* 1966;56:1141–1142.
46. Kelly D. Adaptation effects on spatio-temporal sine-wave thresholds. *Vision Res.* 1972;12:89–101.
47. Kelly DH. Motion and vision. II. Stabilized spatio-temporal threshold surface. *J Opt Soc Am.* 1979;69(10):1340–1349.
48. Kelly DH. Motion and vision. I. Stabilized images of stationary gratings. *J Opt Soc Am.* 1979;69:1266–1274.
49. Blakemore C, Campbell FW. On the existence of neurones in the human visual system selectively sensitive to the orientation and size of retinal images. 1969;203:237–261.
50. Campbell, F.W. and J.G. Robson, Applications of Fourier Analysis to the visibility of gratings. 1968;197:551–566.
51. Graham N, Nachmias J. Detection of grating patterns containing two spatial frequencies: a comparison of single channel and multiple -channels models. *Vision Res.* 1971;11(3):251–259.
52. Hess RF, Snowden RJ. Temporal properties of human visual filters: Number, shapes and spatial covariation. *Vision Res.* 1992;32:47–59.
53. Mandler MB, Makous W. A three channel model of temporal frequency perception. *Vision Res.* 1984;24:1881–1887.
54. Watson AB, Robson JA. Discrimination at threshsolds: Labelled detectors in human vision. *Vision Res.* 1981;21:1115–1122.
55. Yo C, Wilson HR. Peripheral temporal frequency channels code frequency and speed inaccurately but allow accurate discrimination. *Vision Res.* 1993;33:33–45.
56. Kulikowski JJ. Effect of eye movements on the contrast sensitivity of spatio-temporal patterns. *Vision Res.* 1971;11:261–273.
57. Stiles WS. Separation of the "blue" and "green" mechanisms of foveal vision by measurements of increment thresholds. In: Stiles WS, ed. *Mechanisms of colour vision.* London: Academic Press; 1978:418–434.
58. Snowden RJ, Hess RF. Temporal frequency filters in the human peripheral visual field. *Vision Res.* 1992;32(1):61–72.
59. Cass J, Alais D. Evidence for two interacting temporal channels in human visual processing. *Vision Res.* 2006;46:2859–2868.
60. Sawatari A, Callaway EM. Convergence of magno- and parvocellular pathways in layer 4B of macaque primary visual cortex. *Nature.* 1996;380(6573):442–446.
61. Kaplan E, Shapley R. The primate retina contains two types of ganglion cells, with high and low contrast sensitivity. *Proc Nat Acad Sci USA.* 1986;83:2755–2757.
62. Lee BB. Receptive field structure in the primate retina. *Vision Res.* 1996;36:631–644.
63. Lee BB, Pokorny J, Smith VC, Martin PR, Valberg A, Luminance and chromatic modulation sensitivity of macaque ganglion cells and human observers. *J Opt Soc Am A.* 1990;7:2223–2236.
64. Lee BB, Sun H, Zucchini W. The temporal properties of the response of macaque ganglion cells and central mechanisms of flicker detection. *J Vis.* 2007;7(14):(1):1–6.
65. Smith VC, Pokorny J, Lee BB, Dacey DM, Sequential processing in vision: The interaction of sensitivity regulation and temporal dynamics. *Vision Res.* 2008;48:2649–2656.
66. D'Souza DV, Auer T, Strasburger H, Frahm J, Lee BB. Temporal frequency and chromatic processing in humans: An fMRI study of the cortical visual areas. *J Vis.* 2011;11(8).
67. Lee BB. Sensitivity to chromatic and luminance contrast and its neuronal substrates. *Curr Opin Behav Sci.* 2019;30:156–162.
68. Zele AJ, Cao D, Pokorn D. Rod-cone interactions and the temporal impulse response of the cone pathway. *Vision Res.* 2008;48:2593–2598.
69. Lange G, Denny N, Frumkes TE. Suppressive rod-cone interactions: Evidence for separate retinal (temporal) and extraretinal (spatial) mechanisms in achromatic vision. *J Opt Soc Am A.* 1997;14:2487–2498.
70. Goldberg SH, Frumkes TE, Nygaard RW. Inhibitory influence of unstimulated rods in the human retina: Evidence provided by examining cone flicker. *Science.* 1983;221:180–182.
71. Coletta NJ, Adams AJ. Rod-cone interaction in flicker detection. *Vision Res.* 1984;24:1333–1340.
72. Alexander KR, Fishman GA. Rod-cone interaction in flicker perimetry. *Br J Ophthalmol.* 1984;68:303–309.
73. Arden GB, Hogg CR. Rod-cone interactions and analysis of retinal disease. *Br J Ophthalmol.* 1985;69:404–415.
74. Coletta NJ, Adams AJ. Spatial extent of rod-cone and cone-cone interaction for flicker detection. *Vision Res.* 1986;26:917–925.
75. Eisner A. Non-monotonic effect of test illuminance on flicker detection: A study of foveal light adaptation with annular surrounds. *J Opt Soc Am A.* 1994;11:33–47.
76. Harvey LO. Flicker sensitivity and apparent brightness as a function of surround luminance. *J Opt Soc Am.* 1970;60:860–864.
77. Keesey UT. Variables determining flicker sensitivity in small fields. *J Opt Soc Am.* 1970;60:390–398.
78. Roufs JAJ. Dynamic properties of vision. I. Experimental relationships between flicker and flash thresholds. *Vision Res.* 1972;12:261–278.
79. Spehar B, Zaidi Q. Surround effects on the shape of the temporal contrast-sensitivity function. *J Opt Soc Am A.* 1997;14(9):2517–2525.
80. Anderson AJ, Vingrys AJ. Interactions between flicker thresholds and luminance pedestals. *Vision Res.* 2000;40:2579–2588.
81. Eisner A. Suppression of flicker response with increasing test illuminance: roles of temporal waveform, modulation depth and frequency. *J Opt Soc Am A.* 1995;12:214–224.
82. Eisner A, Shapiro AG, Middleton J. Equivalence between temporal frequency and modulation depth for flicker response suppression: analysis of a three-process model of visual adaptation. *J Opt Soc Am A.* 1998;15:1987–2002.
83. Anderson AJ, Vingrys AJ. Multiple processes mediate flicker sensitivity. *Vision Res.* 2001;41:2449.
84. Zele AJ, Vingrys AJ. Defining the detection mechanisms for symmetric and rectified flicker stimuli. *Vision Res.* 2007;47(21):2700–2713.
85. Ball RJ. An investigation of chromatic brightness enhancement tendencies. *Am J Optom Physiol Opt.* 1964;41:333–361.
86. Ball RJ, Bartley SH. Changes in brightness index, saturation, and hue produced by luminance-wavelength-temporal interactions. *J Opt Soc Am.* 1966;66:695–699.
87. Bartley SH. Some effects of intermittent photic stimulation. *J Exp Psychol.* 1939;25:462–480.
88. Bartley SH. Brightness comparisons when one eye is stimulated intermittently and the other steadily. *J Psychol.* 1951;34:165–167.
89. Bartley SH. Brightness enhancement in relation to target intensity. *J Psychol.* 1951;32:57–62.
90. Bartley SH, Nelson TM. Certain chromatic and brightness changes associated with rate of intermittency of photic stimulation. *J Psychol.* 1960;50:323–332.
91. Stockman A, Plummer DJ. Color from invisible flicker: A failure of the Talbot-Plateau law caused by an early 'hard' saturating nonlinearity used to partition the human short-wave cone pathway. *Vision Res.* 1998;38:3703–3728.
92. Brucke E. Uber die Nutzeffect intermitterender Netzhautreizungen. Sitzungsberichte der Mathematisch-Naturwissenschaftlichen. *Classe der Kaiserlichen Akademie der Wissenschaften.* 1848;49:128–153.
93. Talbot HF. Experiments on light. *Philos Mag Ser.* 1834;3(5):321–334.
94. Plateau J. Sur un principe de photometrie. *Bulletins de L'Academie Royale des Sciences et Belles-lettres de Bruxelles.* 1835;2:52–59.
95. Fahle M. Figure-ground discrimination from temporal information. *Proc Royal Soc Lond B Biol Sci.* 1993;254:199–203.

96. Forte J, Hogben JH, Ross J. Spatial limitations of temporal segmentation. *Vision Res.* 1999;39:4052–4061.

97. Leonards U, Singer W, Fahle M. The influence of temporal phase differences on texture segmentation. *Vision Res.* 1996;36:2689–2697.

98. Rogers-Ramachandran DC, Ramachandran VS. Psychophysical evidence for boundary and surface systems in human vision. *Vision Res.* 1998;38:71–77.

99. Bierings R, de Boer MH, Jansonius NM. Visual performance as a function of luminance in glaucoma: The De Vries-Rose, Weber's, and Ferry-Porter's Law. *Invest Ophthalmol Vis Sci.* 2018;59(8):3416–3423.

100. João CAR, Scanferla L, Jansonius NM. Retinal contrast gain control and temporal modulation sensitivity across the visual field in glaucoma at photopic and mesopic light conditions. *Invest Ophthalmol Vis Sci.* 2019;60(13):4270–4276.

101. Manny RE, Levi DM. Psychophysical investigations of the temporal modulation sensitivity function in amblyopia: spatiotemporal interactions. *Invest Ophthalmol Vis Sci.* 1982;22(4):525–534.

102. Maeda E, Yoshikawa T, Hayashi N. Radiology reading-caused fatigue and measurement of eye strain with critical flicker fusion frequency. *Jpn J Radiol.* 2011;29(7):483.

103. Singh S, Downie LE, Anderson AJ. Do blue-blocking lenses reduce eye strain from extended screen time? A double-masked randomized controlled trial. *Am J Ophthalmol.* 2021;226:243–251.

104. Lachenmayr BJ, Drance SM, Douglas GR. Light-sense, flicker and resolution perimetry in glaucoma: A comparative study. *Graefe's Arch Clin Exp Ophthalmol.* 1991;229:246–251.

105. Cello KE, Nelson-Quigg JM, Johnson CA. Frequency doubling technology perimetry for detection of glaucomatous visual field loss. *Am J Ophthalmol.* 2000;129:314–322.

106. Johnson CA, Samuels SJ. Screening for glaucomatous visual field loss with frequency-doubling perimetry. *Invest Ophthalmol Vis Sci.* 1997;38:413.

107. Maddess T, Henry GH. Performance of nonlinear visual units in ocular hypertension and glaucoma. *Clin Vis Sci.* 1992;7(5):371–383.

108. Yoshiyama KK, Johnson CA. Which method of flicker perimetry is most effective for detection of glaucomatous visual field loss? *Invest Ophthalmol Vis Sci.* 1997;38:2270–2277.

109. Casson EJ, Johnson CA, Shapiro LR. A longitudinal comparison of temporal modulation perimetry to white-on-white and blue-on-yellow perimetry in ocular hypertension and early glaucoma. *J Opt Soc Am.* 1993;10:1792–1806.

110. Casson EJ, Johnson CA. Temporal modulation perimetry in glaucoma and ocular hypertension. In: Mills RP, ed. *Perimetry Update 1992/3.* Amsterdam: Kugler Publications; 1993.

111. Casson EJ, Johnson CA, Nelson-Quigg JM. Temporal modulation perimetry: the effects of aging and eccentricity on sensitivity in normals. *Invest Ophthalmol Vis Sci.* 1993;34:3096–3102.

112. Fidalgo BR, Jindal A, Tyler CW, Ctori I, Lawrenson JG. Development and validation of a new glaucoma screening test using temporally modulated flicker. *Ophthalmic Physiol Opt.* 2018;38(6):617–628.

113. Bodis-Wollner I. Visual deficits related to dopamine deficiency in experimental animals and Parkinson's disease patients. *Trends Neurosci.* 1990;13(7):296–302.

114. Coleston DM, Chronicle E, Ruddock KH, Kennard C. Precortical dysfunction of spatial and temporal visual processing in migraine. *J Neurol Neurosurg Psychiatry.* 1994;57:1208–1211.

115. Coleston DM, Kennard C. Responses to temporal visual stimuli in migraine, the critical flicker fusion test. *Cephalalgia.* 1995;15:396–398.

116. Evans BJ, Drasdo N, Richards IL. An investigation of some sensory and refractive visual factors in dyslexia. *Vision Res.* 1994;34(14):1913–1926.

117. Fujimoto N, Adachi-Usami E. Frequency doubling perimetry in resolved optic neuritis. *Invest Ophthalmol Vis Sci.* 2000;41:2558–2560.

118. Grigsby SS, Vingrys AJ, Benes SC, King-Smith PE. Correlation of chromatic, spatial, and temporal sensitivity in optic nerve disease. *Invest Ophthalmol Vis Sci.* 1991;32:3252–3262.

119. Mason RJ, Snelgar RS, Foster DH, Heron JR, Jones RE. Abnormalities of chromatic and luminance critical flicker frequency in multiple sclerosis. *Invest Ophthalmol Vis Sci.* 1982;23:246–252.

120. Mayer MJ, Spiegler SJ, Ward B, Glucs A, Kim CB. Foveal flicker sensitivty discriminates ARM-risk from healthy eyes. *Invest Ophthalmol Vis Sci.* 1992;33(11):3143–3149.

121. McKendrick AM, Vingrys AJ, Badcock DR, Heywood JT. Visual field losses in subjects with migraine headaches. *Invest Ophthalmol Vis Sci.* 2000;41(5):1239–1247.

122. McKendrick AM, Vingrys AJ, Badcock DR, Heywood JT. Visual dysfunction between migraine events. *Invest Ophthalmol Vis Sci.* 2001;42:626.

123. Phipps JA, Guymer RH, Vingrys AJ. Temporal sensitivity deficits in patients with high-risk drusen. *Aust NZ J Ophthalmol.* 1999;27:265–267.

124. Vingrys AJ, Pesudovs K. Localised scotomata detected with temporal modulation perimetry in central serous chorioretinopathy. *Aust NZ J Ophthalmol.* 1999;27(2):109–116.

125. Barnard N, Crewther SG, Crewther DP. Development of a magnocellular function in good and poor primary school-age readers. *Optom Vis Sci.* 1998;75(1):62–68.

126. Flanagan JG, Williams-Lyn D, Trope GE. The phantom contour illusion letter test: A new psychophysical test for glaucoma?. In: Mills RP, Wall M, eds. *Perimetry Update 1994/1995.* Amsterdam/New York: Kugler Publications; 1995.

127. Quaid PT, Flanagan JG. Defining the limits of flicker defined form: effect of stimulus size, eccentricity and number of random dots. *Vision Res.* 2005;45:1075–1084.

128. Goren D, Flanagan JG. Is flicker-defined form (FDF) dependent on the contour? *J Vis.* 2008;8(4):(15):1–11.

129. Reichardt W. Autocorrelation, a principle for the evaluation of sensory information by the central nervous system. In: Rosenblith WA, ed. *Sensory Communication.* New York: Wiley; 1961:303–317.

130. Nishida S. Advancement of motion psychophysics: Review 2001–2010. *J Vis.* 2011;11(11):1–10.

131. Nishida S, Kawabe T, Sawayama M, Fukiage T. Motion perception: From detection to interpretation. *Annu Rev Vis Sci.* 2018;4:501–523.

132. Hiris E, Blake R. A new perspective on the visual motion aftereffect. *Proc Nat Acad Sci USA.* 1992;89:9025–9028.

133. Nishida S, Sato T. Positive motion after-effect induced by bandpass-filtered random-dot kinematograms. *Vision Res.* 1992;32(9):1635–1646.

134. Sekuler RW, Ganz L. Aftereffect of seen motion with a stabilized retinal image. *Science.* 1963;139:419–420.

135. Mather G, Pavan A, Campana G, Casco C. The motion aftereffect reloaded. *Trends Cogn Sci.* 2008;12:481–487.

136. Wertheimer M. Experimentelle Studien uber das Sehen von Bewegung. *Zietschrift fur Psychologie.* 1912;61:161–265.

137. Hubel D, Weisel T. Receptive fields and functional architecture of monkey striate cortex. 1968;**195**:215–243.

138. Hawken, M.J., A.J. Parker, and J.S. Lund, Laminar organisation and contrast sensitivity of direction-selective cells in the striate cortex of the Old World monkey. 1988;10:3541–3548.

139. Hendrickson AE, Wilson JR, Ogren MP. The neuroanatomical organisation of pathways between the dorsal lateral geniculate nucleus and visual cortex in Old World and New World primates. *J Comp Neurol.* 1978;182:123–136.

140. Merigan W, Maunsell J. Macaque vision after magnocellular lateral geniculate lesions. 1990;5:347–352.

141. Schiller P, Malpeli J. Functional specificity of lateral geniculate nucleus laminae of the rhesus monkey. 1978;41:788–797.

142. Callaway EM. Structure and function of parallel pathways in the primate early visual system. *J Physiol.* 2005;566:13–19.

143. DeYoe EA, Van DC, Essen, Segregation of efferent connections and receptive field properties in visual area V2 of the macaque. *Nature.* 1985;317:58–61.

144. Livingstone MS, Hubel DH. Connections between layer 4B of area 17 and the thick cytochrome oxidase stripes of area 18 in the squirrel monkey. *J Neurosci.* 1987;7:3371–3377.

145. Shipp S, Zeki S. The organisation of connections between areas V5 and V1 in macaque monkey visual cortex. *Eur J Neurosci.* 1989;1:309–332.

146. Shipp S, Zeki S. The organisation of connections between areas V5 and V2 in macaque monkey visual cortex. *Eur J Neurosci.* 1989;1:333–354.

147. Albright TD. Direction and orientation selectivity of neurons in visual area MT of the macaque. *J Neurophysiol.* 1984;52(6):1106–1130.

148. Maunsell JH, Van DC, Essen, Functional properties of neurons in middle temporal visual area of the macaque monkey. I. Selectivity for stimulus direction, speed, and orientation. *J Neurophysiol.* 1983;49:1127–1147.

149. Malpeli JG, Schiller PH, Colby CL. Response properties of single cells in monkey striate cortex during reversible inactivation of indiviual lateral geniculate laminae. *J Neurophysiol.* 1981;46:1102–1119.

150. Nealey TA, Maunsell JHR. Magnocellular and parvocellular contributions to the responses of neurons in macaque striate cortex. *J Neurosci.* 1994;14:2069–2079.

151. Newsome WT, Pare EB. A selective impairment of motion perception following lesions of the middle temporal visual area (MT). *J Neurosci.* 1988;8:2201–2211.

152. Schiller PH. The effects of V4 and middle temporal (MT) area lesions on visual performance in the rhesus monkey. *J Neurosci.* 1993;10:717–746.

153. Edwards M, Badcock DR. Global motion perception: Interaction of on and off pathways. *Vision Res.* 1994;34:2849–2858.

154. Newsome WT, Britten KH, Movshon JA. Neuronal correlates of a perceptual decision. *Nature.* 1989;341:52–54.

155. Zihl J, von Cramon D, Mai N. Selective disturbance of movement vision after bilateral brain damage. *Brain.* 1983;106(Pt 2):313–340.

156. Hess RH, Baker CL, Zihl J. The "motion-blind" patient: Low-level spatial and temporal filters. *J Neurosci.* 1989;9:1628–1640.

157. Baker CL, Hess RF, Zihl J. Residual motion perception in a "motion-blind" patient, assessed with limited-lifetime random dot stimuli. *J Neurosci.* 1991;11:454–461.

158. Seiffert AE, Somers DC, Dale AM, Tootell RB. Functional MRI studies of human visual motion perception: Texture, luminance, attention and after-effects. *Cereb Cortex.* 2003;13(4):340–349.

159. Smith AT, et al. Sensitivity to optic flow in human cortical areas MT and MST. *Eur J Neurosci.* 2006;23(2):561–569.

160. Matsuyoshi D, Hirose N, Mima T, Fukuyama H, Osaka N. Repetitive transcranial magnetic stimulation of human MT+ reduces apparent motion perception. *Neurosci Lett.* 2007;429(2–3):131–135.

161. McKeefry D, Burton MP, Vakrou C, Barrett BT, Morland AB, Induced deficits in speed perception by transcranial magnetic stimulation of human cortical areas V5/MT+ and V3A. *J Neurosci.* 2008;28(27):6848–6857.

162. Berman RA, Wurtz RH. Exploring the pulvinar path to visual cortex. *Prog Brain Res.* 2008;171:467–473.

163. Barleben M, Stoppel CM, Kaufmann J. Neural correlates of visual motion processing without awareness in patients with striate cortex and pulvinar lesions. *Hum Brain Mapp.* 2015;36(4):1585–1594.

164. Fox DM, Goodale MA, Bourne JA. The age-dependent neural substrates of blindsight. *Trends Neurosci.* 2020;43(4):242–252.

165. Nawrot M, Rizzo M. Motion perception deficits from midline cerebellar lesions in human. *Vision Res.* 1995;35(5):723–731.

166. Kuai SG, Shan ZK, Chen J, Integration of motion and form cues for the perception of self-motion in the human brain. *J Neurosci.* 2020;40(5):1120–1132.

167. Paradis AL, Cornilleau-Pérès V, Droulez J. Visual perception of motion and 3-D structure from motion: An fMRI study. *Cereb Cortex.* 2000;10(8):772–783.

168. Bennett PJ, Sekuler R, Sekuler AB. The effects of aging on motion detection and direction identification. *Vision Res.* 2007;47(6):799–809.

169. Willis A, Anderson SJ. Effects of glaucoma and aging on photopic and scotopic motion perception. *Invest Ophthalmol Vis Sci.* 2000;41(1):325–335.

170. Sepulveda JA, Anderson AJ, Wood JM, McKendrick AM. Differential aging effects in motion perception tasks for central and peripheral vision. *J Vis.* 2020;20(5):8.

171. Castelo-Branco M, Mendes M, Silva F, Massano J, Januário G, Januário C, et al. Motion integration deficits are independent of magnocellular impairment in Parkinson's disease. *Neuropsychologia.* 2009;47:314–320.

172. Trick GL, Kaskie B, Steinman SB. Visual impairment in Parkinson's disease: deficits in orientation and motion discrimination. *Optom Vis Sci.* 1994;71(4):242–245.

173. Rizzo M, Nawrot M. Perception of movement and shape in Alzheimer's disease. *Brain.* 1998;121:2259–2270.

174. McKendrick AM, Badcock DR. Motion processing deficits in migraine. *Cephalalgia.* 2004;24(5):363–372.

175. Bosworth CF, Sample PA, Gupta N, Bathija R, Weinreb RN. Motion automated perimetry identifies early glaucomatous field defects. *Arch Ophthalmol.* 1998;116(9):1153–1158.

176. Joffe KM, Raymond JE, Chrichton A. Motion coherence perimetry in glaucoma and suspected glaucoma. *Vision Res.* 1997;37(7):955–964.

177. Wall M, Ketoff KM. Random dot motion perimetry in patients with glaucoma and in normal subjects. *Am J Ophthalmol.* 1995;120(5):587–596.

178. McKendrick AM, Badcock DR, Morgan WH. The detection of both global motion and global form is disrupted in glaucoma. *Invest Ophthalmol Vis Sci.* 2005;46(10):3693–3701.

179. Wall M, Jennisch CS, Munden PM. Motion perimetry identifies nerve fiber bundlelike defects in ocular hypertension. *Arch Ophthalmol.* 1997;115:26–33.

180. Bosworth CF. P.A. Sample, and Weinreb.R.N., *Perimetric motion thresholds are elevated in glaucoma suspects and glaucoma patients. Vision Res.* 1997;37:1989–1997.

181. Karwatsky P, Bertone A, Overbury O, Faubert J. Defining the nature of motion perception deficits in glaucoma using simple and complex motion stimuli. *Optom Vis Sci.* 2006;83:466–472.

182. Wall M, Woodward KR, Doyle CK, Artes PH. Repeatability of automated perimetry: a comparison between standard automated perimetry with stimulus size II and V, Matrix and motion perimetry. *Invest Ophthalmol Vis Sci.* 2009;50:974–979.

183. Bullimore MA, Wood JM, Swenson K. Motion perception in glaucoma. *Invest Ophthalmol Vis Sci.* 1993;34:3526–3533.

184. Westcott MC, Fitzke FW, Hitchings RA. Abnormal motion displacement thresholds are associated with fine scale luminance sensitivity loss in glaucoma. *Vision Res.* 1998;38:3171–3180.

185. Verdon-Roe GM, Westcot MC, Viswanathan AC, Fitzke FW, Garway-Heath DF. Exploration of the psychophysics of a motion displacement hyperacuity stimulus. *Invest Ophthalmol Vis Sci.* 2006;47:4847–4855.

38

Development of Vision in Infancy

Anthony M. Norcia

The limited behavioral repertoire of the infant and the impossibility of instructing the test participant have made it necessary for vision scientists interested in human visual development to adapt the classical methods of psychophysics and electrophysiology for use with infants and preverbal children. These methodological adaptations and their interpretation are considered in the context of a hierarchical model of visual processing that organizes the discussion of empirical studies of development at different levels of processing.

METHODOLOGIES FOR ASSESSING INFANT VISION AND THEIR INTERPRETATION

Preferential looking

Infants' spontaneous visual fixation is attracted to certain stimuli more readily than to others.[1,2] In particular, infants prefer to look at patterned stimuli rather than regions of uniform brightness. This spontaneous behavior has served as the basis for a quantitative measure of stimulus visibility known as *forced-choice preferential looking* (FPL).[3] In the FPL task, the infant is confronted with a randomized series of patterns of varying visibility, presented either on the left or the right of a test screen. An observer judges whether the infant's fixation behavior is biased to the left or the right on a trial-by-trial basis. If the observer's judgments agree (or disagree) systematically with the actual position of the stimulus, it can be said that the infant's behavior is under the control of the stimulus. Distributions of the observer's judgments for a series of stimulus values are used to plot a psychometric function that relates the observer's percent correct to the stimulus values presented to the infant. Thresholds are estimated by curve fitting and interpolation to a criterion value of percent correct.

Visual evoked potentials

Visual evoked potentials (VEPs) are electrical brain responses that are triggered by the presentation of a visual stimulus. VEPs are distinguished from the spontaneous electroencephalogram (EEG) due to their consistent time of occurrence after the presentation of the stimulus (time-locking). For example, the abrupt contrast reversal of a checkerboard pattern consistently produces a positive potential on the scalp at a latency of approximately 100 ms in adults.[4] Time-locked responses to abrupt presentations are referred to as *transient VEPs*. A second method of recording VEPs, the steady-state method, uses temporally periodic stimuli.[5] For commonly used pattern reversal stimuli, the frequency of the repetition is often specified as the pattern reversal rate

in reversals per second. This rate is twice the stimulus fundamental frequency (in Hz), which is more commonly used to describe the temporal frequency of pattern onset-offset stimuli. As the stimulus repetition rate increases, the responses to successive stimuli begin to overlap. At high stimulation rates, the response comprises only a small number of components that occur at exact integer multiples of the stimulus frequency. Activity at each of the frequency components of the steady-state response is characterized by its amplitude and phase, where phase represents the temporal delay between the stimulus and the evoked response.

The surface-recorded VEP reflects the activity of cortical visual areas, with contributions from subcortical generators being apparent only under highly specialized recording conditions.[6–8] The primary adaptations of adult VEP recording techniques for infants involve the control of fixation with fixation toys or superimposed video images and the rejection of trials when the infant's fixation was not centered on the stimulus.

Ocular following movements

Both infants and adults make reflexive eye movements following the presentation of a moving target. Optokinetic nystagmus (OKN) is characterized by a repetitive saw-tooth waveform. Rapid displacement of large fields also elicits short-latency ocular following movements.[9] Ocular following can also take the form of slower, pursuit-like movements.[10] Reflexive eye movements are controlled by a combination of cortical and subcortical mechanisms.[11] Infrared tracking, electrooculography, and naked-eye observation of the preponderant direction of eye motion (DEM) are the primary assays of ocular following used in infants and preverbal children.[10,12,13]

HIERARCHY OF VISUAL PROCESSING

Fig. 38.1 presents the schematic framework of visual processing that will be used to focus the discussion of empirical studies of visual function in infants and young children. The visual processing hierarchy is divided into three stages: early, middle, and late. The progression from early to late correlates roughly with an ascent from the retina to the cortex and with a functional hierarchy corresponding to the complexity of the information extracted at each level. In this view, early vision begins in the retina and continues through the lateral geniculate and on into primary visual cortex. By the level of primary visual cortex, stimulus attributes such as orientation, direction of motion, and disparity have been extracted from the retinal images.[14–16] Middle

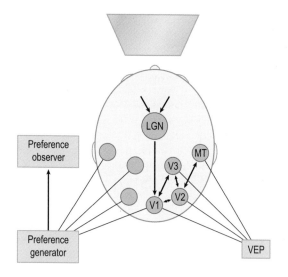

Visual hierarchies

	Early	**Middle**	**Late**
Attributes	Contrast Color Disparity Direction Speed Orientation	Collinearity Symmetry Figure/ground Occlusion Texture Depth Shape	Object categories recognition
Where	Retina, LGN, and V1	V1-Vn	Face area, Place area Temporal lobe
When	Up to 100 msec Sensation	100 to 200 msec Perception	After 200 msec Cognition

Fig. 38.1 Visual processing hierarchy. *Top panel:* schematic diagram of early visual pathways. The visual evoked potential (*VEP*) method records activity directly from several early visual areas. Preference-based behavioral measures require an additional "stage" at which preference and spontaneous fixation behavior is generated, as well as a behavioral observation stage. *LGN*, lateral geniculate nucleus; *MT*, middle-temporal (area).

vision—the processes by which local measurements of image features such as line orientation are integrated across space—begins no sooner than primary visual cortex and no doubt extends through a number of first- and second-tier extrastriate visual areas. The content of the representation at the level of middle vision includes information regarding the shape of extended contours, figure/ground relationships, the symmetry of objects, and surface depths, but not the identity of the objects in the scene. The identification of objects (object recognition), which involves not only visual perception but also memory, is conceptualized as occurring in higher-order visual and visual association areas functionally associated with "late vision."

Each of the different methods for assessing visual function in the preverbal child has a different relationship to the visual processing hierarchy. The FPL technique depends on the integrity of the early visual system, as well as additional mechanisms responsible for the spontaneous preference for pattern (labeled "preference generator" in Fig. 38.1).Whether or not middle or late mechanisms are invoked may depend on the discrimination the infant is called on to perform. Orienting behaviors could be driven from many levels of the cortical

hierarchy or from subcortical structures. In any case, the output of the preference generator must produce robust fixation behavior that can be detected reliably by the FPL observer. Information regarding the location of the stimulus can be lost at the level of early vision, or at the level of the preference generator or by the observer of the infant's behavior. Given the additional sites for potential information loss after early vision, FPL is a conservative estimator of the function of the early part of the visual pathway.

Like FPL, the VEP depends on the integrity of the retina and an unknown amount of cortical processing. Fixation, in the sense that the stimulus must fall on central retina, is required, but spontaneous orientation to a preferred stimulus is not. Electrical activity in the visual pathway is obscured by non-stimulus-related electrical activity associated with the EEG and muscle activity, as well as electrode-motion artifacts. The obscuring experimental noise can be reduced effectively, either through time-locked averaging or spectral analysis. At this point, relatively little is known about the contribution of extrastriate cortical areas to the VEP. Given this, the VEP is quite likely to reflect the capabilities of early vision, but caution must be used in inferring the integrity of later stages of processing—especially if simple stimuli are used.

Ocular following movements require the integrity of the retina, certainly, but given the substantial role of subcortical mechanisms in the control of eye movements,[11] it is difficult to specifically relate eye movement data to the hierarchy of cortical mechanisms shown in Fig. 38.1.

This review emphasizes developmental studies that have used the VEP. The rationale for this choice is several-fold. First, there is now sufficient evidence to indicate that the infant VEP is generated after the site of orientation selectivity,[17,18] direction selectivity,[19–21] Vernier offset detection,[22] and binocular correlation detection.[23,24] All these features are considered to be the outputs of early vision. In adults, it has been found that the VEP reflects both rivalry and suppression,[25–29] as well as several aspects of middle vision, including figure-ground segmentation based on either texture or motion.[30] Second, the VEP does not require visual preference or transfer of information through the observation of spontaneous behavior and is thus less likely to underestimate the capabilities of early vision. Third, the VEP provides a rich source of information regarding the temporal dynamics of the visual response and, through the use of high-density recording arrays, source localization.[31] Finally, there are already excellent reviews that have emphasized FPL and OKN measures of developing visual function.[10,32–35] In deciding which studies to include, emphasis has been placed on those results that have been replicated by more than one research group, wherever possible. Data from the other methods are selectively discussed when these data can help to fill in gaps or when they illustrate particularly sharp contrasts.

Spatiotemporal vision

The retinal images contain a precise spatiotemporal mapping of the visual scene onto two-dimensional surfaces. At the most basic level of processing, the visual system must extract the contrast of the retinal images as a function of time and spatial scale. Visual sensitivity is limited by both spatial and temporal factors. Infant developmental studies have tended to focus on sensitivity along one dimension at a time—by measuring contrast sensitivity as a function of spatial frequency for a fixed temporal frequency or vice versa. Sensitivity depends strongly on both parameters. Whereas the FPL technique can be used at any combination of spatiotemporal frequency, the eye movement and VEP measures each require temporally modulated stimuli. Given the fundamental importance of contrast sensitivity for subsequent visual processing, contrast sensitivity and the related function, grating acuity, are among the few visual functions to have been studied extensively with each of the major methods discussed previously.

Fig. 38.2 plots peak contrast sensitivity as a function of age as determined by the steady-state VEP,[36] DEM,[37–39] and FPL[38,40] methods. Each of these studies obtained peak sensitivity measures at a midrange of temporal frequencies (around 5–10 Hz). There is considerable development of contrast sensitivity in each of the techniques, but the absolute contrast sensitivity is higher with the VEP. By 10–14 weeks of age, infant peak contrast sensitivity over the 0.25 to 1 cpd range is approximately 200, which is within about a factor of 2 to 4 of adult levels when measured on the same apparatus.[36,41] Skoczenski and Norcia[42] found a factor of difference between 10-week-old infants and adults at 1 cpd. Shannon and coworkers[43] found sensitivities at 1.2 cpd that were a factor of about 6 lower than adults at 2 months, with the difference decreasing to a factor of 2.5 at 3 months. Contrast sensitivity measured with the steady-state reversal VEP develops over progressively longer intervals as spatial frequency increases,[36] as shown in Fig. 38.3.

In contrast to the VEP, several behavioral measurements of contrast sensitivity in this age range show values that are much lower (worse) than adult levels. Rasengane and colleagues[40] reported that low-spatial-frequency flicker sensitivity of 2-month-olds was a factor of 45 lower than adults, with 3- and 4-month-olds being a little less than 20 times less sensitive with FPL. Brown and colleagues[39] used a directional eye movement measure (0.31 cpd grating drifting at 15.5 deg/sec) and found that 3-month-olds were a factor of 100 less

sensitive than adults on the same measure. Dobkins and Teller[38] measured both FPL and DEM thresholds in 3-month-olds. They found that infants were almost 30 times less sensitive on the directional eye movement measure and about 60 times less sensitive when FPL and adults' forced-choice psychophysical thresholds were compared. FPL and DEM thresholds were within 20% of each other in the infants. In adults, DEM thresholds were higher than psychophysical thresholds by a factor of 2 to 3, depending on whether the subject's task was detection of the direction of motion or simple contrast detection. Peterzell and coworkers[44] measured contrast sensitivity for static gratings in 4-, 6-, and 8-month-olds using FPL and found that sensitivity increased from approximately 8 at 4 months of age to approximately 40 in 8-month-olds, again much lower than VEP sensitivity.

Hainline and Abramov[37] used DEM recorded by an infrared eye tracker to measure contrast sensitivity. The observer made a forced-choice judgment on the output of the tracker (noise level 0.5 degrees) rather than on naked-eye observation. Contrast sensitivity with this method develops to adult levels by 5 months of age (see Fig. 38.2). Absolute thresholds are lower than those measured with the VEP by a factor of about 4. Hainline and Abramov's contrast sensitivities are higher than those observed by Dobkins and Teller[38] or Brown and colleagues[39] who used naked-eye observation at substantially higher luminance. The difference in sensitivities obtained with naked eye and instrumented observation of eye movements suggests that at least some of the lower sensitivity seen in previous behavioral studies may have been due to information loss in the observer who is judging the infant's behavioral output.

Grating acuity

At the limit of the high spatial frequency limb of the contrast sensitivity function lies the observer's grating acuity. Grating acuity is limited by the optical quality of the eye, the spacing of the photoreceptors and the spatial pooling properties of the ganglion cells and subsequent receptive field mechanisms.[45–48] Grating acuity is also limited by temporal factors, being maximal at low temporal frequencies.

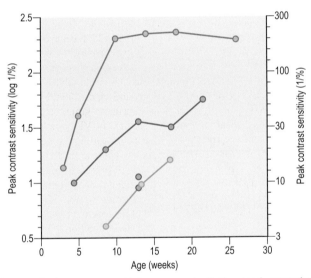

Fig. 38.2 Peak contrast sensitivity measured with the steady-state visual evoked potential (VEP), directional eye movement (DEM), and forced-choice preferential looking (FPL) methods. The VEP study (red circles) used grating patterns that were reversed in contrast at 6 Hz (mean luminance of 220 cd/m²). Peak sensitivity was derived from recordings over the 0.25 to 1 cpd range. The DEM studies (blue circles; half-filled circle) used 0.07- to 2.4-cpd gratings drifting at a constant velocity of 7 deg/sec or 0.25-cpd gratings drifting at 6 Hz. Dobkins and Teller measured FPL thresholds for 0.25 cpd/6 Hz reversing gratings, in addition (purple). Rasengane et al. measured contrast sensitivity for 10-degree luminance fields over the 1 to 25 Hz range (green circles). Peak sensitivity at any temporal frequency is plotted. Contrast sensitivity improves rapidly within each method. (From Norcia AM, Tyler CW, Hamer RD. Development of contrast sensitivity in the human infant. Vision Res 1990;30(10):1475–1486 (red circles); Hainline L. Conjugate eye movements of infants. In: K Simons, ed. Early visual development, normal and abnormal. New York: Oxford University Press, 1993. (blue circles); Dobkins KR, Teller DY. Infant contrast detectors are selective for direction of motion. Vision Res. 1996;36(2):281-294 (half-filled and purple circles); Rasengane TA, Allen D, Manny RE. Development of temporal contrast sensitivity in human infants. Vision Res. 1997;37(13):1747–1754 green circles.)

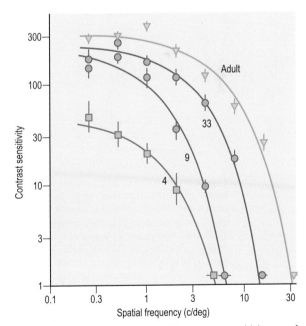

Fig. 38.3 Visual evoked potentials (VEP) contrast sensitivity as a function of spatial frequency and age for 6-Hz pattern reversal. Sensitivity development is progressively delayed at higher spatial frequencies. (Modified from Norcia AM, Tyler CW, Hamer RD. Development of contrast sensitivity in the human infant. Vision Res 1990;30(10):1475–1486.)

VEP grating acuity has been commonly measured using steady-state, pattern reversal targets in the frequency range of 5 to 10 Hz (10–20 contrast reversals per second). The acuity measurement is extrapolated from the high spatial frequency portion of the amplitude versus spatial frequency function. In this method, originally developed by Regan,[49] the spatial frequency of a temporally modulated pattern is systematically changed (swept) over a large range of spatial frequencies that span the expected acuity limit of the observer. Fig. 38.4 plots grating acuity as a function of age for such pattern reversal stimuli. Each study employed the swept spatial frequency technique. Acuity growth functions are similar across studies,[22,36,95,170,171,172,173,174] with acuity increasing from 4 to 6 cpd in 1-month-olds to about 15 to 20 cpd around 8 months of age, (e.g., within a factor of ~2 of the adult).

VEP acuity has also been measured with pattern onset-offset stimuli, in both transient and steady-state paradigms. Two studies of the transient on-off acuity growth function found that acuity improved from approximately 2 cpd at 1 month to 30 cpd by 5 months.[50,51] A third study that used checks rather than gratings[52] found an acuity of 2.3 cpd (corrected for Fourier fundamental spatial frequency of the checks) at 8 weeks, with an increase to 8 cpd at 24 weeks. When both transient onset-offset and 6 Hz contrast reversal stimuli were used to measure acuity in the same infants, two different rates of growth were found—transient onset-offset acuity increased 0.63 octaves per month versus 0.28 octaves per month with 6 Hz pattern reversal.[50] The observations that the rate at which acuity increases depends on the response component being measured suggests that different postreceptoral visual mechanisms have different rates of development.

Vernier acuity

Vernier acuity refers to a collection of spatial localization tasks requiring the detection of a misalignment relative to a reference. Adult Vernier thresholds are significantly better than would be predicted based on either the optical or anatomical properties of the eye. Therefore, Vernier acuity is considered one of the hyperacuities.[53-55] Because cortical processing is believed to be a critical factor limiting the hyperacuities,[56-58] the time course for the development of Vernier acuity has been investigated with great interest.

Most investigations of Vernier acuity during the first year of life have been cross-sectional, employing behavioral responses to moving stimuli.[59-62] However, two studies used stationary stimuli.[63,64] The

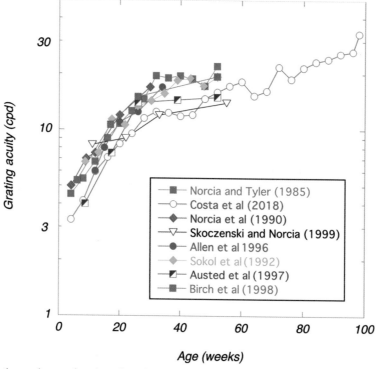

Fig. 38.4 Grating acuity as a function of age for 5- to 10-Hz pattern reversal stimuli. Each study employed the swept spatial frequency technique. Acuity growth functions are similar across studies, with acuity increasing from 4–6 cpd in 1-month-olds to around 15–20 cpd around 8 months of age. (Data are replotted as follows: Norcia AM, Tyler CW. Spatial frequency sweep VEP: Visual acuity during the first year of life. *Vision Res.* 1985;25(10): 1399–1408 (red squares); Norcia AM, Tyler CW, Hamer RD. Development of contrast sensitivity in the human infant. *Vision Res.* 1990;30(10):1475–1486 (green diamonds); Skoczenski AM, Norcia AM. Neural noise limitations on infant visual sensitivity. *Nature.* 1998;391(6668):697–700 (open triangles); Allen D, Norcia AM, Tyler CW. Comparative study of electrophysiological and psychophysical measurement of the contrast sensitivity function in humans. *Am J Optom Physiol Opt.* 1986;63(6):442–449 (purple circles); Sokol S, Moskowitz A, McCormack G. Infant VEP and preferential looking acuity measured with phase alternating gratings. *Invest Ophthalmol Vis Sci.* 1992;33(11):3156–3161 (cyan diamonds); Auestad N, Montalto MB, Hall RT, et al. Visual acuity, erythrocyte fatty acid composition, and growth in term infants fed formulas with long chain polyunsaturated fatty acids for one year: Ross Pediatric Lipid Study. *Pediatr Res.* 1997;41(1):1–10 (half-filled squares); Birch EE, Hoffman DR, Uauy R, et al. Visual acuity and the essentiality of docosahexaenoic acid and arachidonic acid in the diet of term infants. *Pediatr Res.* 1998;44(2):201–209 (magenta squares); and Costa MF, de Cassia Rodrigues Matos Franca V, Barboni MTS, Ventura DF. Maturation of binocular, monocular grating acuity and of the visual interocular difference in the first 2 years of life. *Clin EEG Neurosci.* 2018;49(3):159–170 (open circles).

results of several of these behavioral studies, plotted over the first 6 months of life, are summarized in Fig. 38.5. On average, Vernier acuity improves by about a factor of 6 to 8 over the first 6 months of life, with the best thresholds recorded to be around 200 seconds, 1.3 to 1.8 log units poorer than adults.

Zanker and colleagues[62] reported that after infancy, performance on their Vernier acuity task became comparable to that of adults by 5 years of age (see Fig. 38.6). However, others report that Vernier development is incomplete at age 5 years.[65–68] Based on the their data from preschool children, Carkeet and coworkers,[66] using a fitting procedure, calculated that Vernier acuity is two times lower than adult levels at 5.6 years of age (confidence interval 3.5 to 6.5 years, see data in Fig. 38.6). In a large study of secondary school students, psychophysical grating acuity was found not to change between 11 and 17 years of age, but Vernier acuity improved by a factor of 2.[68] Thus, there is some agreement in the literature that the development of Vernier acuity is incomplete during the early school years and may not fully mature until 18 to 20 years of age.[69–74]

As noted previously, the majority of infant behavioral paradigms used to investigate the development of Vernier acuity contained motion. Shoczenski and Aslin[75] have demonstrated that temporally modulated stimuli improve the Vernier thresholds of 3-month-old infants and suggest that Vernier thresholds obtained with moving stimuli may be governed by a local motion mechanism rather than a position-sensitive mechanism. Therefore, our understanding of the developmental time course of Vernier acuity and its relationship to the development of other visual functions is potentially confounded by some of the stimuli that have been used in behavioral paradigms to gain the infant's attention and interest in the task.

The VEP offers a unique solution to this problem. Norcia and colleagues[76] have suggested that by analyzing the separate Fourier components in the steady-state VEP, Vernier response components may be isolated from those arising from stimulus motion. The VEP response to the introduction of a Vernier offset (alignment/misalignment) differs from the response to the return to alignment (misalignment/

alignment). This asymmetric response to the introduction and then removal of a Vernier offset is reflected in the odd harmonics of the response to the stimulus modulation. The even harmonics in the evoked potential are produced in response to the symmetrical spatial aspects of the stimulus modulation (e.g., local motion of the offset grating) and may be used to examine *motion* acuity. The results obtained with a sweep VEP technique[77] are shown in Fig. 38.6. There is a rapid improvement in Vernier acuity over the first 4 months of life. By 6 months of age, Vernier acuity has improved by about a factor of 7, reaching a threshold of nearly 70 seconds, approximately 1 log unit poorer than the normal adult values obtained psychophysically. Between 6 months of age and 7.5 years, improvement occurs at a slower rate, reaching about 40 seconds, a 1.75 times improvement over the course of about 7 years. After the age of 7.5 years there is another, more rapid improvement in Vernier acuity. Although quantitatively better thresholds were obtained psychophysically by Carkeet and colleagues with stationary stimuli, there is a similar period during the early school years where no significant change in sensitivity was found, followed by a later increase at around age 10 years.

The developmental time course for Vernier acuity has been reported in several studies to be more prolonged than for grating acuity when measured within the same participants.[62,66,77] In each of these studies, Vernier acuity is worse in absolute terms in infancy and crosses over to become better than grating acuity, a trend also observed in a study restricted to the infant age range.[78] Vernier acuity also has a longer developmental sequence than grating acuity in macaque.[79] The more protracted development sequence for Vernier acuity is likely due to its critical limiting factors lying in cortex rather than in retinal sampling.

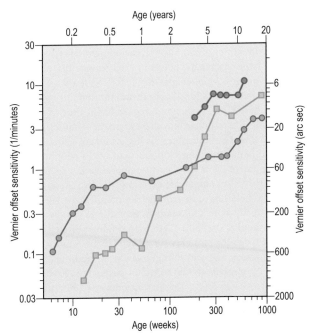

Fig. 38.6 Vernier acuity determined by the visually evoked potential *red circles*. Shown for comparison are behavioral data from Carkeet and coworkers *(blue circles)* and Zanker and colleagues *(squares)*. (From Skoczenski AM, Norcia AM. Late maturation of visual hyperacuity. *Psychol Sci.* 2002;13(6):537–541 (red circles); Carkeet A, Levi DM, Manny RE. Development of Vernier acuity in childhood. *Optom Vis Sci.* 1997; 74(9):741–750 (blue circles); and Zanker J, Mohn G, Weber U, et al. The development of vernier acuity in human infants. *Vision Res.* 1992; 32(8):1557–1564. (squares).)

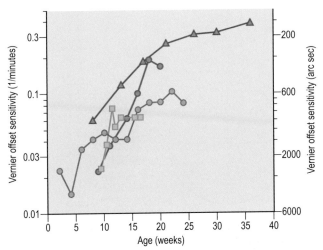

Fig. 38.5 Behaviorally determined Vernier sensitivity. (From Shimojo S, Birch EE, Gwiazda J, Held R. Development of vernier acuity in infants. *Vision Res.* 1984;24(7):721–728 (triangles); Shimojo S, Held R. Vernier acuity is less than grating acuity in 2- and 3-month-olds. *Vision Res.* 1987;27(1):77–86 (blue circles); Manny RE, Klein SA. The development of vernier acuity in infants. *Curr Eye Res.* 1984;3(3):453–462 (red circles); and Brown AM. Vernier acuity in human infants: rapid emergence shown in a longitudinal study. *Optom Vis Sci.* 1997;74(9):732–740 (squares).)

MOTION

The detection of motion involves the determination of speed and direction. The presence of direction selective mechanisms early in development has been demonstrated using each of the three major methods, FPL, VEP, and OKN. Directionally appropriate eye movements can be seen at term or even before.[10,101] Uncertainty remains as to whether these early ocular following responses are controlled by cortical or subcortical pathways. Direction selectivity has been demonstrated behaviorally using FPL and looking time–habituation methods by 6 to 8 weeks.[102,103] VEP responses associated with changes of direction have been recorded by 10 weeks of age.[19,21]

Motion direction asymmetries

On any measure, the adult visual system shows roughly equal sensitivity for all directions of motion.[104] Developing infants, on the other hand, show large, systematic biases in their monocular oculomotor and VEP responses. Monocular OKN (MOKN) is robust for nasalward motion but is weak for temporalward motion during the first 3 to 6 months of life[105–107] as shown in Fig. 38.7. The time to attaining a symmetric MOKN response may depend on the stimulus velocity,[107] with time to maturity being later for higher image velocities.

Young infants also show monocular VEPs response asymmetries suggestive of a nasalward/temporalward bias in cortical responses.[20,21,108–111] A comparable asymmetry is also present in infant macaques.[112] These response asymmetries manifest themselves in the monocular steady-state VEP made in response to rapidly oscillating gratings. In adults, oscillating gratings produce evoked responses primarily at twice the stimulus frequency (at the rate that stimulus direction changes, F2). In young infants, an additional response component is present at the stimulus frequency (first harmonic response, F1; see Fig. 38.8). The first harmonic is 180 degrees out of phase in the two eyes. This pattern of response—a significant first harmonic that is of opposite phase in the two eyes—is consistent with a response bias that is in opposite directions in the two eyes. The absolute direction of the bias, nasalward or temporalward, cannot be directly determined from the steady-state response. It is not known at present whether the cortical motion asymmetry tapped by the VEP causes the oculomotor asymmetry or whether the two phenomena represent immaturities in independent mechanisms with similar developmental sequences.

Symmetric cortical motion responses develop during the first 6 months of life (Fig. 38.9) for 6-Hz oscillatory motion of a

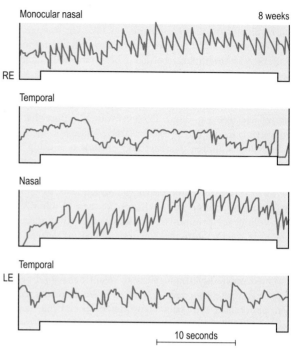

Fig. 38.7 Directional asymmetry of monocular optokinetic nystagmus (MOKN) adapted from reference.[105] MOKN is robust for nasalward stimulus motion (leftward motion in the right eye [*RE*] and rightward motion in the left eye [*LE*]) but is weak for temporalward motion. This directional asymmetry declines during the first few months of life.

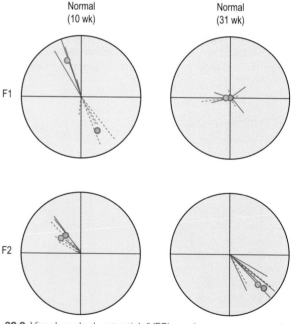

Fig. 38.8 Visual evoked potential (VEP) motion asymmetry, adapted from Norcia et al.[20] Steady-state VEPs to monocular oscillatory motion contain significant odd harmonics in young infants (F1). The phase of these components is shifted by 180 degrees between the two eyes in an 8-week-old infant (*top left* plot, individual trials are indicated by separate lines radiating from zero). The presence of odd harmonics suggests that the response to left and right motion is asymmetric and that the dominant direction is opposite in the two eyes. The odd-harmonic components decline in amplitude over the first 5–6 months of age as indicated by the data from a normal 31-week-old (*right panels*). Second harmonic response (F2) are present at both ages.

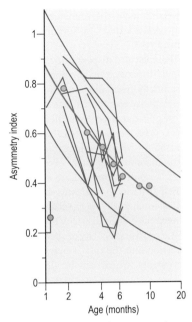

Fig. 38.9 Developmental sequence for symmetric motion VEPs. The degree of motion response asymmetry can be quantified by calculating the fraction of the total response (first plus second harmonic) that is contributed by the first harmonic (asymmetry index). The monocular oscillatory motion VEP is dominated by the first harmonic in early infancy (asymmetry index greater than 0.5), but the degree of asymmetry declines rapidly over the first 6 months for 6-Hz, 1-cpd targets. *Red circles* indicate mean responses for infants between 1.5 and 10 months. Longitudinal recordings are indicated by the *thin lines*. The smooth curves indicate a fit to the mean growth function ±1 standard deviation. The *blue circle* indicates the average asymmetry index for five infants between 0.5 and 1 month of age. (From Birch EE, Fawcett S, Stager D. Co-development of VEP motion response and binocular vision in normal infants and infantile esotropes. *Invest Ophthalmol Vis Sci.* 2000;41(7):1719–1723.)

low-spatial-frequency grating. Fig. 38.9 plots the ratio of amplitudes at the first harmonic to the sum of amplitudes at the first and second harmonics. This index runs from 1.0 for a completely asymmetric response to 0 for a completely symmetric response. Infants reach adult levels by about 5 months of age for low-spatial-frequency targets oscillating at 6 Hz.

The VEP motion asymmetry has been recorded in infants as young as 2 months of age,[21] suggesting that cortical direction selectivity is present at this time. Interestingly, the motion asymmetry was undetectable in infants younger than 8 weeks at 6 Hz, 1 cpd. Development of motion-specific VEPs over the neonatal period has been observed in a different stimulation paradigm[19] in which the age of first direction-specific responses was also earlier for lower stimulus velocities.

BINOCULAR VISION

This section explores the development of sensory fusion (the neurological combination of the images from each eye into a single percept) and stereopsis (the perception of depth based on a horizontal disparity between the retinal images in each eye). As with all visual processes, the parameters of the stimulus and the method of measurement may limit the infant's performance, as well as our understanding of the

developing visual system. Dichoptic stimulus presentations and the need to eliminate confounding monocular cues present unique challenges to studies of the development of fusion and stereopsis and have guided the selection of the studies reviewed.

Fusion

The most direct approach in determining the onset of sensory fusion in human infants has been to record a "cyclopean" VEP using one of two different paradigms. The first approach, popularized by Baitch and Levi[120] and applied to infants by France and Ver Hoeve,[121] presents a uniform field to each eye that is modulated at two different temporal frequencies (e.g., 8 Hz—right eye, 6 Hz—left eye). A cortical response recorded at either the sum (14 Hz) or the difference frequency (2 Hz, also termed the beat frequency) indicates the presence of binocular neurons that integrate and respond to the input from both eyes. Using this approach, France and Ver Hoeve[121] reported that a binocular response was present in the majority of typically developing infants by 2 months of age. The two-frequency approach has also been used to study the development of fusion and rivalry.[122] In that study, beat frequency responses were recordable only for stimuli that had the same orientation in the two eyes and were present in infants older than 5 months, the earliest age tested.

The second approach to identify the integration of information from the two eyes employs dynamic random-dot correlograms or stereograms. These stimuli consist of separate, dynamically updated fields of random dots presented dichoptically to the two eyes. Correlograms alternate between binocularly correlated and anticorrelated phases. In the correlated phase, the dot patterns are identical in the two eyes. In the anticorrelated phase, a dark dot in the pattern presented to one eye corresponds to a bright dot in the pattern presented to the fellow eye, and vice versa. A cortical response to the alternation between the two phases indicates successful binocular integration, as there are no monocular cues to the rate of stimulus alternation. The cyclopean VEP response to these correlated/anticorrelated stimuli has been interpreted as being indicative of fusion but not necessarily stereopsis because horizontal disparities are not present in the stimuli.[123–125] Using this approach, the onset of sensory fusion was initially reported to first occur between about 6 and 11 weeks of age.[23] Another study using the same display system[24] found a somewhat later age of onset (three of six 10- to 19-week-olds and eight of eight infants >19 weeks). A much larger study, again using the same display system, found a median onset age of 13 weeks.[126] Studies with other apparatus found a median onset age ~12 weeks[127] or 16 weeks.[128] This latter study found the same 16-week postnatal onset age for both term and preterm infants, indicating that the onset of binocularity is more tied to the extent of visual experience (time from birth) than it is from time from term.

Development of disparity sensitivity

Correlogram responses indicate the presence of binocular cells but do not directly index sensitivity to retinal disparity, the primary cue for depth. VEPs synchronized to the modulation of disparity in dynamic random-dot stereograms are first measurable between 3 and 5 months of age,[24,127,129] an age range similar to that for the onset of a correlogram response.

To further probe the developmental status of disparity mechanisms in infants, two hallmark features of adult stereopsis have been used to judge whether infant disparity-evoked VEPs are both qualitatively and quantitatively mature.[130] The first feature is that disparity sensitivity is much better for horizontal than vertical disparity. The second is that stereoacuity is much better in the presence of a disparity reference (relative disparity available) than in its absence (absolute disparity). Importantly, only horizontal disparity supports a percept of depth from disparity.

The existence of these markers of mature stereopsis was used as criteria for the developmental status of stereopsis in a study that measured VEP amplitude versus disparity functions for horizontal and vertical disparities and as a function of the quality of disparity reference cues.[130] Infants were recorded at 4–7 months of age, based on prior results reviewed previously indicating that disparity sensitivity should be well established at this age.

VEP disparity tuning functions for infants, children, and adults are shown in Fig. 38.10. Evoked responses for horizontal and vertical disparity are similar in 5-month-old infants but not in 6-year-olds or adults, in whom responses are much larger for horizonal disparity—a qualitative immaturity. Infant thresholds for horizontal disparity were approximately 10 times higher than those of adults, a quantitative immaturity, but those of 6-year-olds were similar to those of adults (0.55 arcmin vs. 0.45 arcmin, respectively). By contrast, infant thresholds for vertical disparity were only four times higher than those of adults. Quantitative and qualitative immaturities were also present in 5-month-old infants when tested with stimuli that moved in opposite directions in the two eyes.[131]

In addition to their elevated disparity thresholds and lack of a preference for horizontal disparity, the dynamics of the evoked response also differed substantially from adults and older children. In adults, the first harmonic response was approximately 5 times larger than the second harmonic response at large disparities, but in infants the ratio was 1.3.[130] Studies of correlogram responses have also reported that the response is dominated by the second harmonic in early infancy,[23,24,126] with the first harmonic emerging later.[24,128,132] Responses at the rate of disparity change (second harmonic) are consistent with transient rather than sustained disparity mechanisms that would manifest at the first harmonic. Transient disparity mechanisms contribute to vergence initiation,[133,134] whereas sustained disparity mechanisms are central to fine stereoacuity.[135] A relative precocity of absolute disparity sensitivity in infants may contribute to the early emergence of disparity-driven vergence eye movements, which can be demonstrated as early as 5 weeks.[136]

Age to maturity of disparity sensitivity

The full developmental sequence for sensitivity to disparity in random-dot stereograms has been studied in more detail using behavioral methods. First, there is remarkable consistency among laboratories concerning the onset of disparity sensitivity in random-dot patterns.[127,137–142] Second, a number of studies have measured horizontal disparity over wide age ranges.

Fig. 38.11 illustrates the development of global disparity sensitivity during infancy and later childhood years, as measured behaviorally. Beyond infancy, all studies show that continued improvement in stereo occurs during the preschool years. Two studies also report thresholds from normal adults under similar test conditions. Ciner

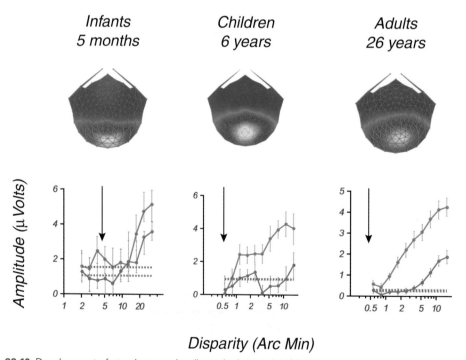

Fig. 38.10 Development of steady-state visually evoked potential (SSVEP) responses to changing horizontal *(blue)* and vertical disparity *(red)*. Disparity response functions are similar for horizontal and vertical disparity in 5-month-olds and threshold for horizontal disparity is ~4.5 arcmin *(arrow)*. Disparity response functions are dissimilar by 6 years of age, as are those of adults. Child threshold is ~0.55 arcmin and that of adults is ~0.45 arcmin.

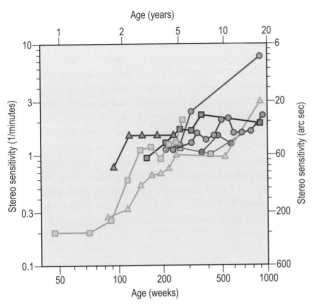

Fig. 38.11 The development of global stereopsis (seconds of arc) as a function of age (years). All studies are based on a behavioral response to a random-dot stereogram during the preschool years. (From Ciner EB, Schanel-Klitsch E, Scheiman M. Stereoacuity development in young children. *Optom Vis Sci.* 1991;68(7):533–536 (cyan triangles); Ciner EB, Schanel-Klitsch E, Herzberg C. Stereoacuity development: 6 months to 5 years. A new tool for testing and screening. *Optom Vis Sci.* 1996;73(1):43–48 green squares; Simons K. Stereoacuity norms in young children. *Arch Ophthalmol.* 1981;99(3):439–445 (tan circles); Birch EE, Hale LA. Operant assessment of stereoacuity. *Clin Vis Sci.* 1989;4:295–300. (blue triangles); Heron G, Dholakia S, Collins DE, McLaughlan H. Stereoscopic threshold in children and adults. *Am J Optom Physiol Opt.* 1985;62(8):505–515 (purple squares); Sloper JJ, Collins AD. Reduction in binocular enhancement of the visual-evoked potential during development accompanies increasing stereoacuity. *J Pediatr Ophthalmol Strabismus.* 1998;35(3):154–158 (gray squares); Williams S, Simpson A, Silva PA. Stereoacuity levels and vision problems in children from 7 to 11 years. *Ophthalmic Physiol Opt.* 1988;8(4):386–389 (olive circles); and Walraven J, Janzen P. TNO stereopsis test as an aid to the prevention of amblyopia. *Ophthalmic Physiol Opt.* 1993;13(4):350–356 (red circles).)

BOX 38.3   Sensitive and critical periods in visual development

Periods of rapid maturation in many sensory systems are associated with high levels of sensitivity to the quality and structure of the inputs from the environment.[151,152] Periods during development in which the effects of visual experience on development are particularly strong are referred to as "sensitive periods." If visual experience during a sensitive period is essential for development and permanently alters performance, this type of sensitive period is referred to as a "critical period."[153] Sensitive and critical periods differ in the extent to which experience has a permanent effect. If normal experience is not present during a critical period, restoration of normal input cannot rehabilitate normal function. Abnormal visual experience either before or after this period is not effective in disrupting development.

The presence and timing of a sensitive/critical period for the development of binocular vision in humans has been inferred from studies of explicitly binocular functions such as the interocular transfer of the tilt aftereffect[154] or stereoacuity[155] in patients who had strabismus with onset at different times after birth and in whom the strabismus persisted for different durations. Banks and coworkers[154] developed a simple descriptive mathematical model that they used to infer the time during development that the binocular visual system is most sensitive to disruption by strabismus. Using interocular transfer of the tilt aftereffect as the end point measure of binocular development, they found that abnormal visual experience around 1.7 years of age was maximally deleterious to final development for patients with infantile esotropia, but that the peak occurred at 1.0 years in patients with late-onset esotropia. The same model was used to locate the sensitive period for the development of stereopsis.[155] Patients with infantile esotropia showed peak sensitivity to abnormal experience around 0.36 years, but patients with accommodative esotropia had maximal sensitivity around 1.7 years. The fact that different outcome measures yield different estimates of the sensitive period, as do different kinds of strabismus, suggests that there are multiple binocular subsystems within the visual system, as a whole, and that these each have different developmental sequences. The existence of different sensitive periods for different visual functions is well established in both animal[156] and human models.[157]

and coworkers[143] (Fig. 38.11, filled circles) indicate that at age 5 years disparity sensitivity is still about a factor of 3 poorer than the adult. Simons[144] (Fig. 38.11, open circles) also found sensitivity was a factor of 3 poorer for 6-year-olds compared with adults.

Four studies that measured disparity sensitivity with the commercially available Nederlandse Organisatie voor Toegepast Natuurwetenschappelijk Onderzoek (TNO) test in school-aged children are also illustrated in Fig. 38.11. Wallraven and Jenzen[145] (Fig. 38.11, filled triangles) report that the ability to detect disparity in random-dot stereograms improves by a factor of 2 between the ages of 4 and 12 years. The data also suggest additional improvement up to 18 years of age, the oldest reported in the study. When the small number ($n = 4$) of 6- to 10-year-olds were tested[146] (Fig. 38.11, squares) and compared with 12 adults with normal vision, disparity sensitivity was a factor of 2 poorer than that measured in the adults. Heron and coworkers[147] (Fig 38.11, filled circles) report that disparity sensitivity as measured by the TNO was adult-like at 5 years of age. These investigators also noted that among the four stereotests evaluated in that report, the TNO gave the poorest thresholds and the largest variability in their sample. Using a real depth test, the Frisby Stereo Test, they found that disparity sensitivity was not yet adult-like at 7 years of age. Fox and coworkers[148] reported that with the Howard-Dolman real depth test, children 3 to 5 years of age were about 2.5 times less sensitive to disparity than adults (12.6 vs. 4.9 seconds of arc). The Howard-Dolman task involves a depth alignment judgment where the presence of stereopsis is indicated when the binocular threshold is better than the monocular threshold.

In summary, sensory fusion has been demonstrated as early as 2 months of age, while disparity sensitivity emerges no later than between 3 and 5 months of age, when tested with the VEP. When large-field, coarse-element stereograms are used, disparity-driven vergence can be measured even earlier, suggesting that it will be useful to measure VEP responses under similar conditions. Although there is considerable improvement in behavioral disparity sensitivity for globally defined targets over the first year of life, disparity sensitivity does not reach adult levels until after age 5 years. At age 5 or 6 years, disparity sensitivity is still about three times poorer than that of the adult.

Disparity-related responses in young infants may reflect the activity of early visual areas such as V1 that are sensitive to absolute but not relative disparity.[130] Responses to absolute disparity can be found very shortly after birth in macaque.[149,150] Robust sensitivity to relative disparity emerges in extrastriate visual areas, and development in these areas may limit the development of fine stereoacuity.

OBJECT-LEVEL PROCESSING

Recognition of objects lies at the top of the processing hierarchy of Fig. 38.1. Object recognition and the subprocess of object categorization is supported by a network of second-tier extrastriate visual areas located predominantly in ventral-temporal cortex,[158,159] with some mirroring of specializations in dorsal-occipito-temporal cortex.[160] Categorization implies, on the one hand, an ability to discriminate objects from different categories and, on the other hand, an ability to identify common attributes that members of the category share (see ref 161 for a broad review of the infant categorization literature).

Of all object categories, the developmental literature has emphasized the ecologically important object category of faces. A common approach in both transient event-related potential (ERP) and fMRI studies for detecting face processing–related activity is to contrast the evoked response to images of faces with those of other objects. ERP responses to images of faces typically elicit larger negative polarity responses in infants at around 290 ms when compared with response to other common objects, such as toys. The "N290" component is believed to be the precursor of the face-selective N170 component of

adults.[162] Many studies have used this approach, and the results are mixed with respect to the age of onset of a differential response.[163] Positive evidence for face selectivity has been found as early as 3 months of age in some studies but only later in others. Longitudinal data suggest that N290 selectivity for faces (vs. houses) is present and constant between 5 and 10 months.[163] Steady-state visually evoked potential (SSVEP) methods indicate face selectivity is present no later than 4 to 6 months.[164,165]

By using source-localization methods, it has been possible to show that the N290 component and its neuromagnetic counterpart have an underlying source distribution that is maximal in ventral surface areas previously associated with face-selective responses in fMRI studies.[166–168] ERP data from one of these studies[167] for infants between 4.5 and 12 months are shown on the scalp in Fig. 38.12A. The corresponding current density reconstructions (CDR) are shown

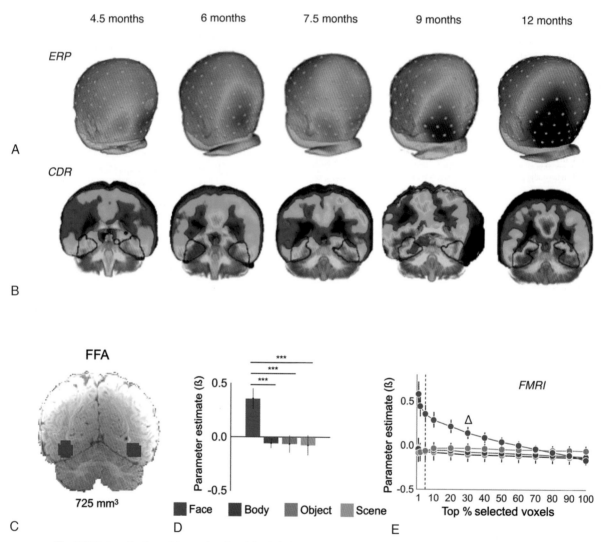

Fig. 38.12 Localization of face-related activity in infants. (A) Event-related potential (*ERP*) scalp topography for the N290 response component. (B) Recovered source distribution (current density reconstruction [*CDR*]) of the N290 response component. *Black outline* shows face-selective region of interest (*ROI*) derived from an adult atlas. Activity within this ROI increases with age. (C) Adult face-selective ROI in *purple* (fusiform face area, *FFA*) transferred to infant brain. (D) Beta weights for face, body, object, and scene conditions are selective for face-containing videos. (D) Beta weights in subsets of FFA voxels indicating that ~30% of voxels (*triangle*) are selective. (ERP data modified from Conte S, Richards JE, Guy MW, et al. Face-sensitive brain responses in the first year of life. *Neuroimage.* 2020;211:116602; fMRI data modified from Kosakowski HL, Cohen MA, Takahashi A, et al. Selective responses to faces, scenes, and bodies in the ventral visual pathway of infants. *Curr Biol.* 2022;32(2):265–274.)

within an atlas-based region of interest (ROI) in the fusiform gyrus (black outline) in Fig. 38.12B. Activity within this ROI becomes increasingly large for images of faces versus toys and houses between 4.5 and 6 months. The lower panel of Fig. 38.12 shows differential fMRI activations for videos containing faces, contrasted with videos containing bodies, objects, or scenes.[175] The activations were also measured within an ROI of face-selective voxels in adult visual cortex (fusiform face area [FFA], Fig. 38.12C) transferred to the infant brain.

Fig. 38.12D shows that average activation in this ROI in 6-month-olds is more strongly driven by videos containing faces compared with videos containing bodies, objects, or scenes. Fig. 38.12E indicates that about 30% of the voxels in this ROI are selective for faces. Other ROIs were found to be preferentially activated for the other categories in a fashion qualitatively similar to adults. Category specificity has also been demonstrated for snakes versus caterpillars or frogs in 7-month-olds using the SSVEP.[169]

SUMMARY

Maturation of visual function in humans occurs over very different time scales, depending on the particular aspect of function that is being measured. Within a particular visual function, development may proceed at quite different rates during different postnatal periods. In several of the functions reviewed in this chapter, there is an early, rapid period of development that is followed by a long, slow second phase that lasts into childhood or even adolescence. Low-spatial-frequency contrast sensitivity appears to be the most precocious function yet measured. Grating acuity measured with midfrequency contrast reversal has its initial rapid period of development during the first 8 months, while Vernier acuity appears to develop at a different rate over this period and is far from adult levels, as is stereoacuity.

Variations in the developmental sequences across visual functions presumably reflect limitations imposed at different levels of the visual hierarchy shown in Fig. 38.1. The critical immaturity limiting contrast sensitivity, grating acuity, and temporal resolution may lie in the early part of the pathway comprised of the retina and early cortical visual areas. Functions such as Vernier and stereoacuity are known to be quite sensitive to contrast in adults, and thus some of the immaturity in these functions is likely to be secondary to the reduced contrast sensitivity of the infant. However, other factors must also limit infant Vernier and stereoacuity, as their developmental sequences are longer than those underlying contrast sensitivity and grating acuity.

REFERENCES

1. Fantz R. A method for studying early visual development. Percept Motor Skills. 1956;6:13–15.
2. Fantz R. Pattern vision in young infants. Psychol Rec. 1958;8:43–47.
3. Teller DY. The forced-choice preferential looking procedure:a psychophysical technique for use with human infants. Infant Behav Develo. 1979;2:135–153.
4. Regan D. Human brain electrophysiology: Evoked potentials and evoked magnetic fields in science and medicine. New York: Elsevier; 1989.
5. Norcia AM, Appelbaum LG, Ales JM, et al. The steady-state visual evoked potential in vision research: A review. J Vis. 2015;15(6):4.
6. Ducati A, Fava E, Motti ED. Neuronal generators of the visual evoked potentials: intracerebral recording in awake humans. Electroencephalogr Clin Neurophysiol. 1988;71(2):89–99.
7. Noachtar S, Hashimoto T, Luders H. Pattern visual evoked potentials recorded from human occipital cortex with chronic subdural electrodes. Electroencephalogr Clin Neurophysiol. 1993;88(6):435–446.
8. Arroyo S, Lesser RP, Poon WT, et al. Neuronal generators of visual evoked potentials in humans: visual processing in the human cortex. Epilepsia. 1997;38(5):600–610.
9. Miles FA. Short-latency visual stabilization mechanisms that help to compensate for translational disturbances of gaze. Ann N Y Acad Sci. 1999;871:260–271.
10. Hainline L. Conjugate eye movements of infants. In: Simons K, ed. Early visual development, normal and abnormal. New York: Oxford University Press; 1993.
11. Leigh R, Zee D. The neurology of eye movements. 3 ed. Oxford University Press; New York, 1999.
12. Shupert C, Fuchs AF. Development of conjugate human eye movements. Vision Res. 1988; 28(5):585–596.
13. Jones PR, Kalwarowsky S, Atkinson J, et al. Automated measurement of resolution acuity in infants using remote eye-tracking. Invest Ophthalmol Vis Sci. 2014;55(12):8102–8110.
14. Hubel DH, Wiesel TN. Receptive fields, binocular interaction and functional architecture in the cat's visual cortex. J Physiol. 1962;160:106–154.
15. Barlow HB, Blakemore C, Pettigrew JD. The neural mechanism of binocular depth discrimination. J Physiol. 1967;193(2):327–342.
16. Schiller PH, Finlay BL, Volman SF. Quantitative studies of single-cell properties in monkey striate cortex. II. Orientation specificity and ocular dominance. J Neurophysiol. 1976;39(6):1320–1333.
17. Braddick OJ, Wattam-Bell J, Atkinson J. Orientation-specific cortical responses develop in early infancy. Nature. 1986;320(6063):617–619.
18. Manny RE. Orientation selectivity of 3-month-old infants. Vision Res. 1992;32(10):1817–1828.
19. Wattam-Bell J. Development of motion-specific cortical responses in infancy. Vision Res. 1991;31(2):287–297.
20. Norcia AM, Garcia H, Humphry R, et al. Anomalous motion VEPs in infants and in infantile esotropia. Invest Ophthalmol Vis Sci. 1991;32(2):436–439.
21. Birch EE, Fawcett S, Stager D. Co-development of VEP motion response and binocular vision in normal infants and infantile esotropes. Invest Ophthalmol Vis Sci. 2000;41(7):1719–1723.
22. Skoczenski AM, Norcia AM. Development of VEP Vernier acuity and grating acuity in human infants. Invest Ophthalmol Vis Sci. 1999;40(10):2411–2417.
23. Braddick O, Atkinson J, Julesz B, et al. Cortical binocularity in infants. Nature. 1980;288 (5789):363–365.
24. Petrig B, Julesz B, Kropfl W, et al. Development of stereopsis and cortical binocularity in human infants: electrophysiological evidence. Science. 1981;213(4514):1402–1405.
25. Cobb W, Morton H, Ettlinge G. Cerebral potentials evoked by pattern reversal and their suppression in visual rivalry. Nature. 1967;216(5120):1123–1125.
26. Lansing RW. Electroencephalographic correlates of binocualr rivalry in man. Science. 1964;146:1325–1327.
27. Brown RJ, Norcia AM. A method for investigating binocular rivalry in real-time with the steady-state VEP. Vision Res. 1997;37(17):2401–2408.
28. Wright KW, Fox BE, Eriksen KJ. PVEP evidence of true suppression in adult onset strabismus. J Pediatr Ophthalmol Strabismus. 1990;27(4):196–201.
29. Norcia AM, Harrad RA, Brown RJ. Changes in cortical activity during suppression in stereoblindness. Neuroreport. 2000;11(5):1007–1012.
30. Bach M, Meigen T. Similar electrophysiological correlates of texture segregation induced by luminance, orientation, motion and stereo. Vision Res. 1997;37(11):1409–1414.
31. Xie W, Nelson CA. A state-of-the-art review of pediatric EEG. Advances in Magnetic Resonance Technology and Applications. 2021;2:373–391.
32. Dobson V. The behavioral assessment of visual acuity in human infants. In: Berkeley MA, Stebbins WC, eds. Comparative Perception. Pittsburgh: Wiley; 1990.
33. Hamer R, Mayer L. The development of spatial vision. In: Albert DM, Jakobiec FA, eds. Principles and Practice of Ophthalmology:Basic Sciences. Philadelphia: WB. Saunders Co; 1994.
34. Daw N. Visual Development. 2 ed. Springer: New York, 1995.
35. Maurer D. Visual development. In: Lockman JJ, Tamis-LeMonda CS, eds. The Cambridge Handbook of Infant Development: Brain, Behavior, and Cultural Context. Cambridge University Press; Cambridge, 2020.
36. Norcia AM, Tyler CW, Hamer RD. Development of contrast sensitivity in the human infant. Vision Res. 1990;30(10):1475–1486.
37. Hainline L, Abramov I. Eye movement-based measures of development of spatial contrast sensitivity in infants. Optom Vis Sci. 1997;74(10):790–799.
38. Dobkins KR, Teller DY. Infant contrast detectors are selective for direction of motion. Vision Res. 1996;36(2):281–294.
39. Brown AM, Lindsey DT, McSweeney EM, Walters MM. Infant luminance and chromatic contrast sensitivity: Optokinetic nystagmus data on 3-month-olds. Vision Res. 1995;35(22):3145–3160.
40. Rasengane TA, Allen D, Manny RE. Development of temporal contrast sensitivity in human infants. Vision Res. 1997;37(13):1747–1754.
41. Kelly JP, Borchert K, Teller DY. The development of chromatic and achromatic contrast sensitivity in infancy as tested with the sweep VEP. Vision Res. 1997;37(15):2057–2072.
42. Skoczenski AM, Norcia AM. Neural noise limitations on infant visual sensitivity. Nature. 1998;391(6668):697–700.
43. Shannon E, Skoczenski AM, Banks MS. Retinal illuminance and contrast sensitivity in human infants. Vision Res. 1996;36(1):67–76.
44. Peterzell DH, Werner JS, Kaplan PS. Individual differences in contrast sensitivity functions: Longitudinal study of 4-, 6- and 8-month-old human infants. Vision Res. 1995;35(7):961–979.
45. Banks MS, Bennett PJ. Optical and photoreceptor immaturities limit the spatial and chromatic vision of human neonates. J Opt Soc Am A. 1988;5(12):2059–2079.

46. Wilson HR. Development of spatiotemporal mechanisms in infant vision. *Vision Res.* 1988;28(5):611–628.

47. Banks MS, Crowell JA. Front-end limitations to infant spatial vision:examination of two analyses. In: Simons K, ed. *Early Visual Develoment: Normal and Abnormal.* New York: Oxford; 1993.

48. Wilson HR. Theories of infant visual development. In: Simons K, ed. *Early Visual Develoment: Normal and Abnormal.* New York: Oxford; 1993.

49. Regan D. Speedy assessment of visual acuity in amblyopia by the evoked potential method. *Ophthalmologica.* 1977;175(3):159–164.

50. Orel-Bixler D, Norcia AM. Differential growth of acuity for steady-state pattern reversal and transient pattern VEPs. *Clin Visual Science.* 1987;2:1–9.

51. Marg E, Freeman DN, Peltzman P, Goldstein PJ. Visual acuity development in infants:Evoked potential measurements. *Invest Ophthalmol.* 1976;15:150–153.

52. DeVries-Khoe LH, Spekreijse H. Maturation of luminance and pattern EPs in man. *Doc Ophthalmol Proc Ser.* 1982;31:461–475.

53. Westheimer G. Editorial: Visual acuity and hyperacuity. *Invest Ophthalmol.* 1975;14(8):570–572.

54. Westheimer G. The spatial sense of the eye. Proctor lecture. *Invest Ophthalmol Vis Sci.* 1979;18(9):893–912.

55. Morgan M. Hyperacuity. In: Regan D, ed. *Spatial Vision, vol. 10: Vision and Visual Dysfunction.* Boca Raton, FL: CRC Press; 1991.

56. Barlow HB. Reconstructing the visual image in space and time. *Nature.* 1979;279(5710):189–190.

57. Westheimer G. The spatial grain of the perifoveal visual field. *Vision Res.* 1982;22(1):157–162.

58. Stanley OH. Cortical development and visual function. *Eye.* 1991;5(Pt 1):27–30.

59. Shimojo S, Birch EE, Gwiazda J, Held R. Development of vernier acuity in infants. *Vision Res.* 1984;24(7):721–728.

60. Manny RE, Klein SA. A three alternative tracking paradigm to measure vernier acuity of older infants. *Vision Res.* 1985;25(9):1245–1252.

61. Shimojo S, Held R. Vernier acuity is less than grating acuity in 2- and 3-month-olds. *Vision Res.* 1987;27(1):77–86.

62. Zanker J, Mohn G, Weber U, et al. The development of vernier acuity in human infants. *Vision Res.* 1992;32(8):1557–1564.

63. Manny RE, Klein SA. The development of vernier acuity in infants. *Curr Eye Res.* 1984;3(3):453–462.

64. Brown AM. Vernier acuity in human infants: rapid emergence shown in a longitudinal study. *Optom Vis Sci.* 1997;74(9):732–740.

65. Gonzalez EG, Steinbach MJ, Ono H, Rush-Smith N. Vernier acuity in monocular and binocular children. *Clin Vis Sci.* 1992;7:257–261.

66. Carkeet A, Levi DM, Manny RE. Development of Vernier acuity in childhood. *Optom Vis Sci.* 1997;74(9):741–750.

67. Kim E, Enoch JM, Fang MS, et al. Performance on the three-point Vernier alignment or acuity test as a function of age: Measurement extended to ages 5 to 9 years. *Optom Vis Sci.* 2000;77(9):492–495.

68. Bondarko VM, Semenov LA. Visual acuity and hyperacuity in 11- to 17-year-old secondary school students. *Human Physiology.* 2012;38:271–278.

69. Whitaker D, Elliot D, MacVeigh D. Variations in hyperacuity performance with age. *Ophthalmic Physiol Opt.* 1992;12:29–32.

70. Reich L, Lahshminarayanan V, Enoch JM. Analysis of the method of adjustment of testing potential acuity with the hyperacuity gap test:a preliminary report. *Clin Visual Science.* 1991;6:451–456.

71. Odom JV, Vasquez RJ, Schwartz TL, Linberg JV. Adult vernier thresholds do not increase with age; vernier bias does. *Invest Ophthalmol Vis Sci.* 1989;30(5):1004–1008.

72. Lakshminarayanan V, Aziz S, Enoch JM. Variation of the hyperacuity gap function with age. *Optom Vis Sci.* 1992;69(6):423–426.

73. Vilar E, Giraldez-Fernandez MJ, Enoch JM, et al. Performance on three-point vernier acuity targets as a function of age. *J Opt Soc Am A Opt Image Sci Vis.* 1995;12(10):2293–2304.

74. Li RW, Edwards MH, Brown B. Variation in vernier acuity with age. *Vision Res.* 2000;40(27):3775–3781.

75. Skoczenski AM, Aslin RN. Spatiotemporal factors in infant position sensitivity: single bar stimuli. *Vision Res.* 1992;32(9):1761–1769.

76. Norcia AM, Wesemann W, Manny RE. Electrophysiological correlates of vernier and relative motion mechanisms in human visual cortex. *Vis Neurosci.* 1999;16(6):1123–1131.

77. Skoczenski AM, Norcia AM. Late maturation of visual hyperacuity. *Psychol Sci.* 2002;13(6):537–541.

78. Skoczenski AM, Norcia AM. VEP measurements of form discrimination in human infants. *Investigative Ophthalmology & Visual Science.* 1994;35(4):2028–.

79. Kiorpes L. The puzzle of visual development: Behavior and neural limits. *J Neurosci.* 2016;36(45):11384–11393.

80. Ridder 3rd WH,, Rouse MW. Predicting potential acuities in amblyopes: predicting post-therapy acuity in amblyopes. *Doc Ophthalmol.* 2007;114(3):135–145.

81. Simon JW, Siegfried JB, Mills MD, et al. A new visual evoked potential system for vision screening in infants and young children. *J Aapos.* 2004;8(6):549–554.

82. Hou C, Good WV, Norcia AM. Validation study of VEP vernier acuity in normal-vision and amblyopic adults. *Investigative Ophthalmology & Visual Science.* 2007;48(9):4070–4078.

83. Hou C, Good WV, Norcia AM. Detection of amblyopia using sweep VEP vernier and grating acuity. *Invest Ophthalmol Vis Sci.* 2018;59(3):1435–1442.

84. Lim M, Soul JS, Hansen RM, et al. Development of visual acuity in children with cerebral visual impairment. *Arch Ophthalmol.* 2005;123(9):1215–1220.

85. Skoczenski AM, Good WV. Vernier acuity is selectively affected in infants and children with cortical visual impairment. *Dev Med Child Neurol.* 2004;46(8):526–532.

86. Watson T, Orel-Bixler D, Haegerstrom-Portnoy G. VEP vernier, VEP grating, and behavioral grating acuity in patients with cortical visual impairment. *Optom Vis Sci.* 2009;86(6):774–780.

87. Cavascan NN, Salomao SR, Sacai PY, et al. Contributing factors to VEP grating acuity deficit and inter-ocular acuity difference in children with cerebral visual impairment. *Doc Ophthalmol.* 2014;128(2):91–99.

88. Good WV, Hou C, Norcia AM. Spatial contrast sensitivity vision loss in children with cortical visual impairment. *Invest Ophthalmol Vis Sci.* 2012;53(12):7730–7734.

89. John FM, Bromham NR, Woodhouse JM, Candy TR. Spatial vision deficits in infants and children with Down syndrome. *Invest Ophthalmol Vis Sci.* 2004;45(5):1566–1572.

90. da Costa MF, Salomao SR, Berezovsky A, et al. Relationship between vision and motor impairment in children with spastic cerebral palsy: new evidence from electrophysiology. *Behav Brain Res.* 2004;149(2):145–150.

91. Hou C, Norcia AM, Madan A, et al. Visual cortical function in very low birth weight infants without retinal or cerebral pathology. *Invest Ophthalmol Vis Sci.* 2011;52(12):9091–9098.

92. Bradfield YS, France TD, Verhoeve J, Gangnon RE. Sweep visual evoked potential testing as a predictor of recognition acuity in albinism. *Arch Ophthalmol.* 2007;125(5):628–633.

93. Till C, Westall CA, Koren G, et al. Vision abnormalities in young children exposed prenatally to organic solvents. *Neurotoxicology.* 2005;26(4):599–613.

94. Hou C, Norcia AM, Madan A, Good WV. Visuocortical function in infants with a history of neonatal jaundice. *Investigative Ophthalmology & Visual Science.* 2014;55(10):6443–6449.

95. Birch EE, Hoffman DR, Uauy R, et al. Visual acuity and the essentiality of docosahexaenoic acid and arachidonic acid in the diet of term infants. *Pediatr Res.* 1998;44(2):201–209.

96. McKee SP, Levi DM, Movshon JA. The pattern of visual deficits in amblyopia. *J Vis.* 2003;3(5):380–405.

97. Birch EE, Swanson WH. Hyperacuity deficits in anisometropic and strabismic amblyopes with known ages of onset. *Vision Res.* 2000;40(9):1035–1040.

98. Bradley A, Freeman RD. Is reduced vernier acuity in amblyopia due to position, contrast or fixation deficits? *Vision Res.* 1985;25(1):55–66.

99. Levi DM, Klein S. Hyperacuity and amblyopia. *Nature.* 1982;298(5871):268–270.

100. Chandna A, Nichiporuk N, Nicholas S, et al. Motion processing deficits in children with cerebral visual impairment and good visual acuity. *Invest Ophthalmol Vis Sci.* 2021;62(14):12.

101. Dubowitz LM, Dubowitz V, Morante A, Verghote M. Visual function in the preterm and fullterm newborn infant. *Dev Med Child Neurol.* 1980;22(4):465–475.

102. Wattam-Bell J. Visual motion processing in one-month-old infants: Habituation experiments. *Vision Res.* 1996;36(11):1679–1685.

103. Wattam-Bell J. Visual motion processing in one-month-old infants: Preferential looking experiments. *Vision Res.* 1996;36(11):1671–1677.

104. Gros BL, Blake R, Hiris E. Anisotropies in visual motion perception: A fresh look. *J Opt Soc Am A Opt Image Sci Vis.* 1998;15(8):2003–2011.

105. Naegele JR, Held R. The postnatal development of monocular optokinetic nystagmus in infants. *Vision Res.* 1982;22(3):341–346.

106. Lewis TL, Maurer D, Chung JY, et al. The development of symmetrical OKN in infants: quantification based on OKN acuity for nasalward versus temporalward motion. *Vision Res.* 2000;40(4):445–453.

107. Roy N, Lachapelle P, Lepore F. Maturation of the optokinetic nystagmus as a function of the speed of stimulation in fullterm and preterm infants. *Clin Visual Science.* 1989;4:357–366.

108. Norcia AM, Hamer RD, Jampolsky A, Orel-Bixler D. Plasticity of human motion processing mechanisms following surgery for infantile esotropia. *Vision Res.* 1995;35(23–24):3279–3296.

109. Jampolsky A, Norcia AM, Hamer RD. Preoperative alternate occlusion decreases motion processing abnormalities in infantile esotropia. *J Pediatr Ophthalmol Strabismus.* 1994;31(1):6–17.

110. Bosworth RG, Birch EE. Direction-of-motion detection and motion VEP asymmetries in normal children and children with infantile esotropia. *Invest Ophthalmol Vis Sci.* 2007;48(12):5523–5531.

111. Mason AJ, Braddick OJ, Wattam-Bell J, Atkinson J. Directional motion asymmetry in infant VEPs—which direction? *Vision Res.* 2001;41(2):201–211.

112. Brown RJ, Norcia AM, Hamer RD, et al. Development of motion processing mechanisms in monkey and human infants. *Investigative Ophthalmology & Visual Science.* 1993;34(4):1356–.

113. Shea SJ, Chandna A, Norcia AM. Oscillatory motion but not pattern reversal elicits monocular motion VEP biases in infantile esotropia. *Vision Res.* 1999;39(10):1803–1811.

114. Kommerell G, Ullrich D, Gilles U, Bach M. Asymmetry of motion VEP in infantile strabismus and in central vestibular nystagmus. *Doc Ophthalmol.* 1995;89(4):373–381.

115. Anteby I, Zhai HF, Tychsen L. Asymmetric motion visually evoked potentials in infantile strabismus are not an artifact of latent nystagmus. *J Aapos.* 1998;2(3):153–158.

116. Hamer RD, Norcia AM, Orel-Bixler D, Hoyt CS. Motion VEPs in late-onset esotropia. *Clin Visual Science.* 1993;8(1):55–62.

117. Brosnahan D, Norcia AM, Schor CM, Taylor DG. OKN, perceptual and VEP direction biases in strabismus. *Vision Res.* 1998;38(18):2833–2840.

118. Gerth C, Mirabella G, Li X, et al. Timing of surgery for infantile esotropia in humans: effects on cortical motion visual evoked responses. *Invest Ophthalmol Vis Sci.* 2008;49(8):3432–3437.

119. Tychsen L, Wong AM, Foeller P, Bradley D. Early versus delayed repair of infantile strabismus in macaque monkeys: II. Effects on motion visually evoked responses. *Invest Ophthalmol Vis Sci.* 2004;45(3):821–827.

120. Baitch LW, Levi DM. Evidence for nonlinear binocular interactions in human visual cortex. *Vision Res.* 1988;28(10):1139–1143.

121. France TD, Ver Hoeve JN. VECP evidence for binocular function in infantile esotropia. *J Pediatr Ophthalmol Strabismus.* 1994;31(4):225–231.

122. Brown RJ, Candy TR, Norcia AM. Development of rivalry and dichoptic masking in human infants. *Invest Ophthalmol Vis Sci.* 1999;40(13):3324–3333.

123. Eizenman M, Westall CA, Geer I, et al. Electrophysiological evidence of cortical fusion in children with early- onset esotropia. *Invest Ophthalmol Vis Sci.* 1999;40(2):354–362.

124. Livingstone MS. Differences between stereopsis, interocular correlation and binocularity. *Vision Res.* 1996;36(8):1127–1140.

125. Poggio GF, Gonzalez F, Krause F. Stereoscopic mechanisms in monkey visual cortex: binocular correlation and disparity selectivity. *J Neurosci*. 1988;8(12):4531–4550.

126. Braddick O, Wattam-Bell J, Day J, Atkinson J. The onset of binocular function in human infants. *Hum Neurobiol*. 1983;2(2):65–69.

127. Birch E, Petrig B. FPL and VEP measures of fusion, stereopsis and stereoacuity in normal infants. *Vision Res*. 1996;36(9):1321–1327.

128. Jando G, Miko-Barath E, Marko K, et al. Early-onset binocularity in preterm infants reveals experience-dependent visual development in humans. *Proc Natl Acad Sci U S A*. 2012;109(27):11049–11152.

129. Skarf B, Eizenman M, Katz LM, et al. A new VEP system for studying binocular single vision in human infants. *J Pediatr Ophthalmol Strabismus*. 1993;30(4):237–242.

130. Norcia AM, Gerhard HE, Meredith WJ. Development of relative disparity sensitivity in human visual cortex. *J Neurosci*. 2017;37(23):5608–5619.

131. Kohler PJ, Meredith WJ, Norcia AM. Revisiting the functional significance of binocular cues for perceiving motion-in-depth. *Nat Commun*. 2018;9(1):3511.

132. Miko-Barath E, Marko K, Budai A, et al. Maturation of cyclopean visual evoked potential phase in preterm and full-term infants. *Invest Ophthalmol Vis Sci*. 2014;55(4):2574–2583.

133. Westheimer G, Mitchell DE. The sensory stimulus for disjunctive eye movements. *Vision Res*. 1969;9(7):749–755.

134. Jones R. Fusional vergence: sustained and transient components. *Am J Optom Physiol Opt*. 1980;57(9):640–644.

135. Harwerth RS, Rawlings SC. Viewing time and stereoscopic threshold with random-dot stereograms. *Am J Optom Physiol Opt*. 1977;54(7):452–457.

136. Seemiller ES, Cumming BG, Candy TR. Human infants can generate vergence responses to retinal disparity by 5 to 10 weeks of age. *J Vis*. 2018;18(6):17.

137. Birch EE, Salomao S. Infant random dot stereoacuity cards. *J Pediatr Ophthalmol Strabismus*. 1998;35(2):86–90.

138. Archer SM, Helveston EM, Miller KK, Ellis FD. Stereopsis in normal infants and infants with congenital esotropia. *Am J Ophthalmol*. 1986;101(5):591–596.

139. Shea SL, Fox R, Aslin RN, Dumais ST. Assessment of stereopsis in human infants. *Invest Ophthalmol Vis Sci*. 1980;19(11):1400–1404.

140. Fox R. Stereopsis in animals and human infants: A review of behavioral investigations. In: Aslin RN, Alberts J, Petersen M, eds. *Development of Perception: The Visual System*. New York: Academic Press; 1981.

141. Kavsek M. Infants' discrimination of crossed and uncrossed horizontal disparity. *Atten Percept Psychophys*. 2014;76(5):1429–1436.

142. Kavsek M. The onset of sensitivity to horizontal disparity in infancy: A short-term longitudinal study. *Infant Behav Dev*. 2013;36(3):329–343.

143. Ciner EB, Schanel-Klitsch E, Scheiman M. Stereoacuity development in young children. *Optom Vis Sci*. 1991;68(7):533–536.

144. Simons K. Stereoacuity norms in young children. *Arch Ophthalmol*. 1981;99(3):439–445.

145. Walraven J, Janzen P. TNO stereopsis test as an aid to the prevention of amblyopia. *Ophthalmic Physiol Opt*. 1993;13(4):350–356.

146. Sloper JJ, Collins AD. Reduction in binocular enhancement of the visual-evoked potential during preferential development accompanies increasing stereoacuity. *J Pediatr Ophthalmol Strabismus*. 1998;35(3):154–158.

147. Heron G, Dholakia S, Collins DE, McLaughlan H. Stereoscopic threshold in children and adults. *Am J Optom Physiol Opt*. 1985;62(8):505–515.

148. Fox R, Patterson R, Francis EL. Stereoacuity in young children. *Invest Ophthalmol Vis Sci*. 1986;27(4):598–600.

149. Chino YM, Smith 3rd EL,, Hatta S, Cheng H. Postnatal development of binocular disparity sensitivity in neurons of the primate visual cortex. *J Neurosci*. 1997;17(1):296–307.

150. Zhang B, Tao X, Shen G, et al. Receptive-field subfields of V2 neurons in macaque monkeys are adult-like near birth. *J Neurosci*. 2013;33(6):2639–2649.

151. Berardi N, Pizzorusso T, Maffei L. Critical periods during sensory development. *Curr Opin Neurobiol*. 2000;10(1):138–145.

152. Kiorpes L. Visual development in primates: Neural mechanisms and critical periods. *Dev Neurobiol*. 2015;75(10):1080–1090.

153. Knudsen EI. Sensitive periods in the development of the brain and behavior. *J Cogn Neurosci*. 2004;16(8):1412–1425.

154. Banks MS, Aslin RN, Letson RD. Sensitive period for the development of human binocular vision. *Science*. 1975;190(4215):675–677.

155. Fawcett SL, Wang YZ, Birch EE. The critical period for susceptibility of human stereopsis. *Invest Ophthalmol Vis Sci*. 2005;46(2):521–525.

156. Harwerth RS, Smith 3rd EL,, Duncan GC, et al. Multiple sensitive periods in the development of the primate visual system. *Science*. 1986;232(4747):235–238.

157. Lewis TL, Maurer D. Multiple sensitive periods in human visual development: evidence from visually deprived children. *Dev Psychobiol*. 2005;46(3):163–183.

158. Grill-Spector K, Weiner KS, Kay K, Gomez J. The functional neuroanatomy of human face perception. *Annu Rev Vis Sci*. 2017;3:167–196.

159. Margalit E, Jamison KW, Weiner KS, et al. Ultra-high-resolution fMRI of human ventral temporal cortex reveals differential representation of categories and domains. *J Neurosci*. 2020;40(15):3008–3024.

160. Hasson U, Harel M, Levy I, Malach R. Large-scale mirror-symmetry organization of human occipito-temporal object areas. *Neuron*. 2003;37(6):1027–1041.

161. Oakes L. Infant Categorization. In: Tamis-LeMonda JJLaCS, ed. . *The Cambridge Handbook of Infant Development: Brain, Behavior, and Cultural Context*. Cambridge University Press; Cambridge, 2020.

162. Halit H, Csibra G, Volein A, Johnson MH. Face-sensitive cortical processing in early infancy. *J Child Psychol Psychiatry*. 2004;45(7):1228–1234.

163. Di Lorenzo R, van den Boomen C, Kemner C, Junge C. Charting development of ERP components on face-categorization: Results from a large longitudinal sample of infants. *Dev Cogn Neurosci*. 2020;45:100840.

164. De Heering A, Rossion B. Rapid categorization of natural face images in the infant right hemisphere. *Elife*. 2015;4:e06564.

165. Farzin F, Hou C, Norcia AM. Piecing it together: infants' neural responses to face and object structure. *J Vis*. 2012;12(13):6.

166. Chen Y, Slinger M, Edgar JC, et al. Maturation of hemispheric specialization for face encoding during infancy and toddlerhood. *Dev Cogn Neurosci*. 2021;48:100918.

167. Conte S, Richards JE, Guy MW, et al. Face-sensitive brain responses in the first year of life. *Neuroimage*. 2020;211:116602.

168. Guy MW, Zieber N, Richards JE. The cortical development of specialized face processing in infancy. *Child Dev*. 2016;87(5):1581–1600.

169. Bertels J, Bourguignon M, de Heering A, et al. Snakes elicit specific neural responses in the human infant brain. *Sci Rep*. 2020;10(1):7443.

170. Norcia AM, Tyler CW. Spatial frequency sweep VEP: Visual acuity during the first year of life. *Vision Res*. 1985;25(10):1399–1408.

171. Allen D, Norcia AM, Tyler CW. Comparative study of electrophysiological and psychophysical measurement of the contrast sensitivity function in humans. *Am J Optom Physiol Opt*. 1986;63(6):442–449.

172. Sokol S, Moskowitz A, McCormack G. Infant VEP and preferential looking acuity measured with phase alternating gratings. *Invest Ophthalmol Vis Sci*. 1992;33(11):3156–3161.

173. Auestad N, Montalto MB, Hall RT, et al. Visual acuity, erythrocyte fatty acid composition, and growth in term infants fed formulas with long chain polyunsaturated fatty acids for one year. Ross Pediatric Lipid Study. *Pediatr Res*. 1997;41(1):1–10.

174. Costa MF, de Cassia Rodrigues Matos Franca V, Barboni MTS, Ventura DF. Maturation of binocular, monocular grating acuity and of the visual interocular difference in the first 2 years of life. *Clin EEG Neurosci*. 2018;49(3):159–170.

175. Kosakowski HL, Cohen MA, Takahashi A, et al. Selective responses to faces, scenes, and bodies in the ventral visual pathway of infants. *Curr Biol*. 2022;32(2):265–274.

Development of Retinogeniculate Projections

Melissa A. Lee and Carol Ann Mason

Introduction

The dorsal lateral geniculate nucleus of the thalamus (LGN) is the gateway through which visual information is transmitted from the retina to the cortex; therefore, conscious visual perception relies on the ability of LGN neurons to faithfully relay the specific features of the visual world that are encoded by the retina. Accordingly, the connections between retinal ganglion cells (RGCs) from each eye and LGN neurons are highly precise and organized.[1,2] A key feature of retinogeniculate organization that allows for binocular vision is that axons arising from each eye are segregated within the LGN.[1] Additionally, RGC projections are arranged such that neighboring cells in the retina innervate neighboring cells in the LGN, creating a retinotopic map in the thalamus that is capable of maintaining the spatial features of the visual scene.[3] The resolution of the retinal map is also maintained in the LGN; consequently, LGN receptive fields are similar to those of RGCs in their size and structure.[4] Finally, some cell type–specific organization also exists in the LGN, since different types of LGN neurons reside in distinct laminae and receive inputs from different subtypes of functionally distinct RGCs.[2,5–8]

How is such precise retinogeniculate circuitry established during development? First, RGC organization must be determined and maintained during the path from eye to brain. Numerous studies have demonstrated that upon RGC growth into the LGN, many aspects of retinogeniculate connectivity are initially imprecise, and that the immature circuit must subsequently undergo refinement to achieve its finely tuned mature form.[9–16] Much of this refinement occurs before the onset of vision.[10,11] It is now well established that this early refinement requires spontaneous retinal activity and molecular cues that are present throughout development, and that the non-neuronal cells of the brain, glia, are important players in sculpting the mature circuitry.[11,17–21]

FORMATION OF EYE-SPECIFIC TERRITORIES

Before reaching their eventual brain targets, RGCs exit the retina as a fasciculated bundle via the optic stalk, which then becomes the optic nerve. At the optic chiasm, the crucial choice point in RGC axon path determination, RGCs partially decussate: some RGC axons cross to the opposite-side hemisphere of the brain (contralateral RGCs) and other RGC axons remain on the same-side hemisphere of the brain (ipsilateral RGCs). Following partial decussation at the optic chiasm, when these axon populations are interleaved, RGCs regain topographic and eye-specific organization and refasciculate to form the optic tract, via which RGCs travel until they reach their final brain targets, including the LGN.

Decussation of ipsilateral and contralateral RGCs at the optic chiasm enables binocular vision by ensuring that each visual hemifield is adequately represented in both brain hemispheres. The extent of RGC decussation reflects evolution of eye placement—as organisms have evolved to have eyes more frontally positioned, the ratio of ipsilateral-to-contralateral axon projections has increased, with humans having a 45:55 ipsilateral-to-contralateral ratio, whereas animals with more laterally positioned eyes, such as fish, birds, and amphibians, have a much lower ipsilateral-to-contralateral ratio. In mice, the most utilized model system for studying visual pathway development, the ipsilateral-to-contralateral ratio is about 5:95.[22,23]

THE OPTIC CHIASM IS A CRUCIAL CHOICE POINT IN ESTABLISHING RGC AXON PROJECTIONS

The decision to cross onto the opposite side of the brain or to stay on the same side of the brain is molecularly guided. Developing RGC axons in the optic nerve grow among interfascicular glia.[24–26] At the optic chiasm midline, radial glia at the floor of the third ventricle form a palisade through which RGC axons extend.[27,28] This glial palisade is instructive for RGC navigation, as it expresses ligands to receptors on RGC growth cones that direct growing RGC axons to either cross or avoid the midline.

The receptor-ligand pairings that determine RGC midline choice at the optic chiasm are specific to each of these RGC axon subtypes, and RGC axon subtype is, in turn, dependent on the expression of distinct subtype-specific transcription factors that direct receptor expression. Ipsilateral RGC fate is principally determined by the transcription factor Zic2.[22] Zic2 drives the expression of the EphB1 receptor in ipsilateral RGCs, which interacts with radial glia–expressed EphrinB2 to drive RGC axon repulsion away from the midline and back into the ipsilateral optic tract.[29,30]

Determination of contralateral RGC identity and midline crossing is comparatively more complex, with contralateral RGC fate specified by a consortium of transcription factors including Islet2, Brn3a, and SoxC.[31–33] Midline glial and contralateral RGC axon signaling is similarly combinatorial, dependent on NrCAM, Sema6D, and Plexin-A1,[34] VEGF-A/Neuropilin1 signaling,[35,36] and noncanonical Wnt signaling, which functions dually in RGC sorting at the midline, playing a role in both ipsilateral midline repulsion and contralateral midline attraction.[37]

Intriguingly, axon-axon interactions have also been shown to mediate axon choice at the optic chiasm: Sonic hedgehog (Shh) is produced by contralateral RGCs at the retina and transported anterogradely along the axon to the optic chiasm, where it accumulates and repels ipsilateral RGCs via Boc receptor signaling.[38–40] Axon-axon interactions independent of midline crossing signals also mediate eye-specific axon organization in the optic tract, but the mechanisms guiding this interactions are still being elucidated.[41–45]

MOLECULAR MECHANISMS GUIDING THE FORMATION OF EYE-SPECIFIC AXONAL TERRITORIES

About 40% of all RGCs project to the LGN, where they are organized by eye specificity, topography, and subtype identity.[46–48] Although recent advances in single-cell genomics have allowed for increasingly greater resolution into RGC molecular identity and the subsequent delineation of additional RGC subtypes, little is known about the mechanisms underlying molecular RGC subtype-specific patterning in the LGN.[49–54] Indeed, eye-specific and topographic patterning in the LGN has been studied for far longer, although the mechanisms guiding RGC axon selection of appropriate eye-specific and topographic targets remain poorly understood. However, timing-based mechanisms and signaling via the Eph/Ephrins and homophilic Teneurin adhesion family members mediate retinotopic and eye-specific projections, respectively.[55–62]

RETINOGENICULATE PROJECTIONS ARE REFINED DURING DEVELOPMENT

Anatomical studies have shown that when the axons from the two eyes initially invade the LGN, their arbors extensively overlap, and functional studies have demonstrated that these overlapping projections give rise to binocularly innervated LGN neurons.[13,14,63,64] After this initial connectivity is established, there is a specific developmental window during which the axons from each eye segregate into nonoverlapping territories.[15,16] This eye-specific segregation results in a pattern of ipsilateral and contralateral projections that is highly stereotyped both in size and placement within the LGN.

Following the formation of eye-specific territories, RGCs undergo further refinement.[65] Whereas initially multiple retinogeniculate projections converge onto LGN target neurons, these projections have been understood canonically to refine to a near one-to-one ratio, with early studies showing that LGN neuron firing was nearly always preceded by the firing of a single, connected RGC.[66–72] Such a one-to-one view of the mature retinogeniculate synapse has been challenged in recent years, with studies using modern anatomical and electrophysiological recording techniques revealing a higher degree of anatomical convergence onto LGN relay neurons than previously understood.[73–76] These studies estimate an average of 10 to 14.5 RGCs per relay neuron in the mature LGN.[74–76] Importantly, these inputs are heterogeneous in strength, with only a minority of RGC inputs strong enough to drive postsynaptic firing alone, and functional convergence is limited, with most adult LGN neurons responding to dominant input from one and not both eyes.[76–78]

ACTIVITY-DEPENDENT REFINEMENT OF RETINOGENICULATE PROJECTIONS

Once it was appreciated that much of the initial development and refinement of retinogeniculate projections occurs before eye opening, these findings raised the question of whether synaptic transmission and/or neuronal activity are required for refinement (Fig. 39.1). The first demonstrations that action potentials are required for eye-specific segregation came from studies in which tetrodotoxin (TTX) was used to block sodium channels in fetal cat brain. This activity blockade

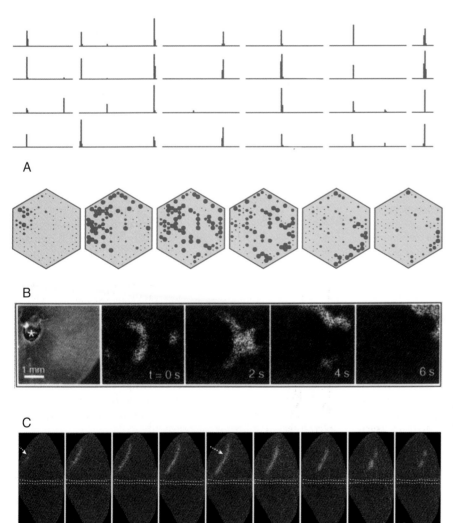

A

B

C

D

Fig. 39.1 The immature retina generates a pattern of synchronized bursting activity before vision. (**A**) Multielectrode recording of the spike activity from many cells in the isolated but intact ferret retina reveals the presence of rhythmic bursting in individual cells (*each line*). The bursts of four neighboring cells (shown by the *vertical histograms*) are correlated in time. (**B**) During a burst of activity, retinal ganglion cells (RGCs) are activated sequentially as a wave propagates across the recording electrodes. Shown here is an example of such a wave propagating across the hexagonal multielectrode array. *Left to right:* Sequential "snapshots" of the activity recorded every 0.5 second. Each dot is a cell, and the size of the dot is proportional to the spike rate. (**C**) Retinal waves are easily observed using calcium imaging. Changes in fluorescence intensity over time detected using a low-light camera show two waves that collide in a neonatal mouse retina. *First panel* shows the fluorescence labeling by fura-2, and *white regions* in the subsequent images show elevations in intracellular calcium. *, Optic nerve head. (**D**) Retinal waves in RGC axon arbor can be visualized and recorded in vivo via calcium imaging in the upper layers of the superior colliculus. Shown here is an example single-wave montage from a P3 WT mouse, with each frame shown at 2s intervals. *White arrows* show the onset and propagation of retinal wave front. (Panel D is from Burbridge TJ, Xu HP, Ackman JB, et al. Visual circuit development requires patterned activity mediated by retinal acetylcholine receptors. *Neuron.* 2014;84(5):1049–1064.)[108]

prevented the formation of eye-specific domains.[79,80] Further experiments found that spontaneous activity is generated in the retina during eye-specific segregation, and when spontaneous retinal activity is disrupted, eye-specific layers do not form and receptive fields are larger than normal.[81–84] Whereas the existence of spontaneous retinal waves was once controversial, the development of tools that enable these waves to be visualized and recorded in vivo have not only confirmed the existence of spontaneous waves in the retina but have also allowed for their characterization: waves propagate in a directionally biased manner, are weakly correlated between the two eyes, and produce corresponding waves of activity in postsynaptic neurons in the LGN, superior colliculus (SC), and visual cortex.[85]

WHAT PARAMETERS OF ACTIVITY DRIVE REFINEMENT?

Three stages of patterned wave activity have been described in the developing retina. The activity at each stage is mediated by distinct mechanisms and displays unique properties, such as the frequency of the activity, the area of the retina involved in the correlated activity, and the speed of the propagating wave.[51–53] These studies suggest that the unique features of these stages might contribute to the specific aspects of refinement that occur during each stage. The first stage of retinal activity, stage I, consists of infrequent bursts of patterned activity that appear embryonically and are largely mediated by communication through gap junctions.[86,87] The bulk of retinogeniculate refinement occurs during stage II waves. Stage II waves are mediated by acetylcholine release from starburst amacrine cells[88–90] and occur embryonically in mammals born with their eyes open and postnatally in mammals born with their eyes closed.[54,56] The final stage of patterned spontaneous activity, stage III, is mediated by glutamatergic transmission from bipolar cells, spans the period of eye opening, and is propagated, at least in part, due to glutamate spillover.[18,86,91–95]

Although most patterned spontaneous activity occur before eye opening, the developing retina responds to light passing through the closed eyelid. Intrinsically photosensitive RGCs (ipRGCs) emerge and respond to light during stage II cholinergic waves[96–99] and rod- and cone-mediated light responses are observed in RGCs with the onset of stage III glutamatergic waves.[100] Intriguingly, both stage II and stage III waves can be modulated by light, with effects on eye-specific segregation.[97,101]

A common mechanism that appears to underlie the development of connection specificity throughout the nervous system is activity-dependent competition among presynaptic inputs for postsynaptic space.[102,103] Evidence that eye-specific segregation involves competition among RGC inputs comes from studies in which activity was either blocked or enhanced in one eye, resulting in alterations to the pattern of ipsilateral and contralateral projections. In these studies when epibatidine was used to block cholinergic transmission in just one eye, the projections from the blocked eye lost territory in the LGN while the projections from the active eye expanded their coverage.[81] The converse was also true; that is, when activity was increased in one eye by intraocular administration of either forskolin or the cyclic AMP analog, CPT-cAMP (which increase the size, frequency, and speed of waves), the projections from the more active eye gained territory in the LGN at the expense of the nonenhanced eye's projections (Fig. 39.2).[104,105]

Both experimental and theoretical studies suggest that in addition to overall activity levels, specific aspects of patterned spontaneous activity may drive segregation through Hebbian mechanisms that strengthen and eliminate synaptic inputs over time.[106] The Hebbian model of synaptic competition predicts that ganglion cells that "fire together, wire

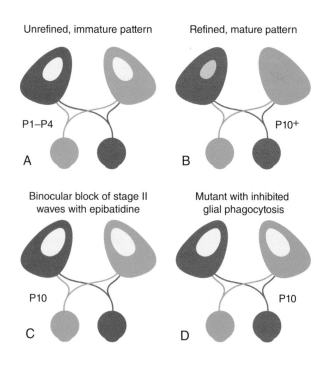

Unrefined, immature pattern   Refined, mature pattern

P1–P4   P10+

A   B

Binocular block of stage II waves with epibatidine   Mutant with inhibited glial phagocytosis

P10   P10

C   D

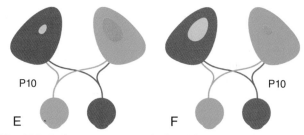

Epibatidine in one eye (green)   cAMP or forskolin in one eye (green)

P10   P10

E   F

Fig. 39.2 Both spontaneous retinal activity and ephrin signaling are required for the normal segregation of eye-specific inputs in the lateral geniculate nucleus (LGN). Diagram illustrates projection patterns in the rodent LGN. **(A)** Initially the projections from both eyes overlap in the LGN. In rodents this pattern can be seen between P1–P4. **(B)** During stage II retinal waves, the inputs from each eye segregate into nonoverlapping regions, with their mature pattern emerging around P10. **(C)** Pharmacologic ablation of stage II waves prevents segregation during this period. **(D)** In mutants with inhibited glial phagocytosis, such as the C3 KO and the Megf10 KO/Mertk KO, waves with altered correlation structure and frequency also prevent segregation during stage II. **(E, F)** Eye-specific segregation involves activity-dependent competition. **(E)** When stage II waves are blocked in one eye with epibatidine the projections from the blocked eye lose territory in the LGN while the projections from the normally active eye expand. **(F)** When stage II waves are increased in size and frequency in one eye, the projections from the enhanced eye gain territory in the LGN at the expense of the other eye's projections.

together." For Hebbian mechanisms to drive segregation, neighboring RGCs must fire in a correlated manner, while more distant RGCs or RGCs from different eyes must exhibit less correlated spiking, thereby allowing for the strengthening of the temporally correlated neighboring inputs and the weakening of the uncorrelated inputs. Indeed, these requirements are met as a consequence of wave propagation. For example, during a wave, neighboring RGCs are coactivated, causing their firing to become more synchronized than that of non-neighboring RGCs.

Selectively altering the spatiotemporal properties (i.e., bilateral synchrony,[107] frequency,[108] and directionality[109]) of waves can result in both improper topographic map formation and eye-specific segregation.[107,108,110] These studies indicate that certain characteristics of retinal waves are instructive for the proper development of RGC projections, with wave synchrony and frequency being particularly important for eye-specific segregation in the LGN.[107,108]

CELLULAR AND MOLECULAR MECHANISMS OF RGC AXON REFINEMENT

A major area of research is aimed at elucidating the molecular mechanisms that translate changes in synaptic drive into changes in synapse and axon morphology. Screening of transgenic mouse lines that display normal retinal waves yet have disrupted eye-specific segregation has demonstrated that several types of immune-related molecules are likely to be involved in this process. The first such example was the class I major histocompatibility complex (MHC). This protein is upregulated by activity in the LGN during the time of eye-specific segregation, and MHC I knockout mice display overlapping eye inputs.[111-115] RGCs in transgenic mice lacking expression of neuronal pentraxins (NPs) and the classical complement cascade initiating protein C1q also fail to fully segregate into eye-specific territories.[116,117]

Glia have emerged as major regulators of activity-dependent developmental refinement of RGC synapses. Transgenic mice independently lacking components of both microglial and astrocytic phagocytosis pathways show defects in eye-specific segregation.[20,21] Manipulation of stage II spontaneous activity via the induction of competition between ipsilateral and contralateral eyes resulted in the preferential engulfment of weaker inputs by both microglia and astrocytes.[20,21] Thus, both microglia and astrocytes contribute to eye-specific RGC segregation by actively engulfing weaker LGN synapses during early postnatal development.

Paralleling immune system phagocytes, microglia in the LGN appear to respond to "eat-me" or "don't-eat-me" signals from RGC synapses via activation or inhibition of the classical complement cascade.[118] Neuronal expression of C1q drives deposition of C3 ("eat-me") onto RGC synapses, which tags these synapses for microglial engulfment via binding of microglial CR3 receptors. This process can be blocked by neuronal expression of sushi repeat protein X-linked 2 (SRPX2), which binds C1q directly and inhibits its activity.[119] Conversely, microglial phagocytosis can be inhibited via neuronal expression of CD47 ("don't-eat-me"), which binds microglial SIRPα.[120] CD47 is preferentially expressed on more active RGC synapses, protecting these more active synapses from microglial phagocytosis.[120]

The molecular mechanisms regulating activity-dependent astrocyte phagocytosis of RGC synapses during eye-specific segregation are not yet fully defined but involve cooperation of the MERTK and MEGF10 signaling pathways.[21] Astrocyte phagocytosis of RGC synapses is also modulated by ApoE isoform in the LGN.[121] The apparent redundancy of microglial and astrocytic phagocytic pathways during activity-dependent eye-specific segregation underscores the importance of glial pruning, and whether or how these different pathways and cell types interact is an open area of investigation.

RGC synapse refinement is not exclusively the result of structural pruning within the proper eye-specific territory[122,123]—rather, labeling and detailed reconstruction of individual RGC arbors from P8 to P31 showed that spatial redistribution of axon boutons underlies late synapse refinement and experience-dependent plasticity at the retinogeniculate synapse, with average arbor size and complexity actually increasing during this period of time.[123] At P8, boutons are relatively evenly distributed across the RGC axon arbor. By P20, however, boutons have grouped into larger, dense clusters without restricted axon arbor regions, even while average number of boutons remains unchanged.[123] In mice that are deprived of light exposure from P20 to P31, axon size and complexity are unchanged, but bouton clusters are smaller and more spaced out along the axon arbor when compared with those in age-matched mice raised in standard light conditions, indicating that sensory experience may drive small-scale changes in axon bouton rearrangement.[123] This period of sensory experience–dependent synapse remodeling via bouton rearrangement is followed by a period of fine-scale structural pruning, with total axon length, complexity, and bouton density decreasing as remaining boutons grow in size from P31 to P60.[123]

Microglia and immune molecules have also been shown to be involved in RGC refinement during sensory experience in a non-phagocytic manner.[124] Concurrent with the latter phases of axon bouton rearrangement described previously, sensory experience–dependent retinogeniculate refinement is associated with the simultaneous strengthening of select synapses and elimination of weaker synapses. Mice lacking the cytokine receptor fibroblast growth factor–inducing protein (Fn14) have more, smaller synapses during this phase of refinement, indicating failure in both synapse strengthening and elimination.[125] Visual experience also induces the transcription of Fn14's ligand, TNF-associated weak induced of apoptosis (TWEAK), in a subset of microglia.[124] Fn14 expression alone function to increase the number of bulbous spines on LGN relay neurons, strengthening synapses in response to visual experience. However, when Fn14-expressing retinogeniculate connections are near TWEAK-expressing microglia, TWEAK suppresses this Fn14-dependent increase in spine number. This represents a phagocytosis-independent mechanism by which microglia shape synapse refinement.[124]

BEYOND EYE SPECIFICITY

Recent advances in single-cell sequencing have led to the identification of at least 40 different functional RGC subtypes,[49,50] with an estimated 75% of these subtypes projecting to the LGN.[78] In addition to eye-specific segregation, RGC axons undergo further restriction of their arbors into functionally distinct sublaminae. For example, major RGC classes can be subdivided into two subtypes: cells that are depolarized (ON ganglion cells) or hyperpolarized (OFF ganglion cells) by light onset.[126] At maturity these parallel ON and OFF pathways are segregated in the LGN at the level of single neurons; individual LGN neurons generally respond to increments or decrements in light but not both. In some species, such as the ferret, LGN neurons receiving ON input and OFF input reside in two distinct sublaminae within each eye-specific layer,[127] and these sublaminae develop just after eye-specific segregation and before opening.[128]

Other examples of functional classes of RGCs that project to the LGN are Y-cells, which process movement, X-cells, which are responsible for image acuity, and a heterogeneous population of W-cells.[2,10,129] Whether individual LGN neurons initially receive synaptic input from these multiple classes of ganglion cells is unclear. In the primate, however, magnocellular and parvocellular pathways project to distinct regions of the LGN from early stages as their axons innervate targets.[130-132] This suggests that during primate development single LGN neurons may receive inputs from just one class of RGC. This specificity could be due, at least in part, to the generation of different RGC classes at different times during development,[133] and to the fact that the axons of parvo cells reach the LGN before those of magno cells.[130] In addition, in primates the axons from the two eyes may initially innervate the LGN in a somewhat eye-specific manner; thus, the primate retinogeniculate connection may require less refinement than that of other mammals.[134]

Interestingly, studies also suggest that once the mature pattern of anatomical and functional connections has been established, they must be actively maintained.[91,135–137] Taken together, these data indicate that the mature retinogeniculate connection must be

sculpted out of an initially overconnected circuit, and that the extent of this refinement may vary from species to species. These data also suggest that retinogeniculate development occurs over several stages beginning with the segregation of eye-specific inputs, followed by a more fine-scale refinement phase that sharpens the retinotopic map, and a final maintenance phase during which this connection remains malleable.[138]

SUMMARY

The mature retinogeniculate pathway is highly organized in structure and function, and a clearer understanding of how this precise organization develops continues to emerge. Organized RGC growth and targeting, as well as axon refinement, shape this final organization. Specific features of spontaneous retinal activity appear to be critical, suggesting that activity may work in an instructive fashion. An important task for future studies will be to further elucidate the cellular and

molecular mechanisms, including participation by glial cells, that turn activity into structural changes in this pathway. The use of transgenic animals, additional genetic and molecular screens, and next-generation sequencing tools will allow for greater molecular insight into the mechanisms that underlie both the activity-dependent and -independent aspects of this process.

ACKNOWLEDGMENTS

The authors would like to thank the previous authors of this chapter, S.M. Koch and E.M. Ullian, for foundational contributions to this work.

REFERENCES

1. Kaas JH, Guillery RW, Allman JM. Some principles of organization in the dorsal lateral geniculate nucleus. *Brain Behav Evol.* 1972;6(1):253–299.
2. Rodieck RW. Visual pathways. *Annu Rev Neurosci.* 1979;2:193–225.
3. Roskies A, Friedman GC, O'Leary DD. Mechanisms and molecules controlling the development of retinal maps. *Perspect Dev Neurobiol.* 1995;3(1):63–75.
4. Bullier J, Norton TT. Comparison of receptive-field properties of X and Y ganglion cells with X and Y lateral geniculate cells in the cat. *J Neurophysiol.* 1979;42(1 Pt 1):274–291.
5. Leventhal AG, Rodieck RW, Dreher B. Central projections of cat retinal ganglion cells. *J Comp Neurol.* 1985;237(2):216–226.
6. Leventhal AG, Rodieck RW, Dreher B. Retinal ganglion cell classes in the Old World monkey: morphology and central projections. *Science.* 1981;213(4512):1139–1142.
7. Huberman AD, Manu M, Koch SM, et al. Architecture and activity-mediated refinement of axonal projections from a mosaic of genetically identified retinal ganglion cells. *Neuron.* 2008;59(3):425–438.
8. Huberman AD, Wei W, Elstrott J, Stafford BK, Feller MB, Barres BA. Genetic identification of an On-Off direction-selective retinal ganglion cell subtype reveals a layer-specific subcortical map of posterior motion. *Neuron.* 2009;62(3):327–334.
9. Constantine-Paton M, Cline HT, Debski E. Patterned activity, synaptic convergence, and the NMDA receptor in developing visual pathways. *Annu Rev Neurosci.* 1990;13:129–154.
10. Garraghty PE, Sur M. Competitive interactions influencing the development of retinal axonal arbors in cat lateral geniculate nucleus. *Physiol Rev.* 1993;73(3):529–545.
11. Goodman CS, Shatz CJ. Developmental mechanisms that generate precise patterns of neuronal connectivity. *Cell.* 1993;72(Suppl.):77–98.
12. Shatz CJ, Sretavan DW. Interactions between retinal ganglion cells during the development of the mammalian visual system. *Annu Rev Neurosci.* 1986;9:171–207.
13. Sretavan DW, Shatz CJ. Prenatal development of retinal ganglion cell axons: segregation into eye-specific layers within the cat's lateral geniculate nucleus. *J Neurosci.* 1986;6(1):234–251.
14. Shatz CJ, Kirkwood PA. Prenatal development of functional connections in the cat's retinogeniculate pathway. *J Neurosci.* 1984;4(5):1378–1397.
15. Sretavan DW, Shatz CJ. Prenatal development of cat retinogeniculate axon arbors in the absence of binocular interactions. *J Neurosci.* 1986;6(4):990–1003.
16. Sretavan DW, Shatz CJ. Axon trajectories and pattern of terminal arborization during the prenatal development of the cat's retinogeniculate pathway. *J Comp Neurol.* 1987;255(3):386–400.
17. Penn AA, Shatz CJ. Brain waves and brain wiring: the role of endogenous and sensory-driven neural activity in development. *Pediatr Res.* 1999;45(4 Pt 1):447–458.
18. Wong RO, Meister M, Shatz CJ. Transient period of correlated bursting activity during development of the mammalian retina. *Neuron.* 1993;11(5):923–938.
19. Pfeiffenberger C, Cutforth T, Woods G, et al. Ephrin-As and neural activity are required for eye-specific patterning during retinogeniculate mapping. *Nat Neurosci.* 2005;8(8):1022–1027.
20. Schafer DP, Lehrman EK, Kautzman AG, et al. Microglia sculpt postnatal neural circuits in an activity and complement-dependent manner. *Neuron.* 2012;74(4):691–705.
21. Chung WS, Clarke LE, Wang GX, et al. Astrocytes mediate synapse elimination through MEGF10 and MERTK pathways. *Nature.* 2013;504(7480):394–400.
22. Herrera E, Brown L, Aruga J, et al. Zic2 patterns binocular vision by specifying the uncrossed retinal projection. *Cell.* 2003;114(5):545–557.
23. Petros TJ, Rebsam A, Mason CA. Retinal axon growth at the optic chiasm: to cross or not to cross. *Annu Rev Neurosci.* 2008;31:295–315.
24. Bovolenta P, Mason C. Growth cone morphology varies with position in the developing mouse visual pathway from retina to first targets. *J Neurosci.* 1987;7(5):1447–1460.
25. Guillery RW, Walsh C. Changing glial organization relates to changing fiber order in the developing optic nerve of ferrets. *J Comp Neurol.* 1987;265(2):203–217.
26. Williams RW, Rakic P. Dispersion of growing axons within the optic nerve of the embryonic monkey. *Proc Natl Acad Sci U S A.* 1985;82(11):3906–3910.
27. Maggs A, Scholes J. Glial domains and nerve fiber patterns in the fish retinotectal pathway. *J Neurosci.* 1986;6(2):424–438.
28. Mason CA, Sretavan DW. Glia, neurons, and axon pathfinding during optic chiasm development. *Curr Opin Neurobiol.* 1997;7(5):647–653.
29. Williams SE, Mann F, Erskine L, et al. Ephrin-B2 and EphB1 mediate retinal axon divergence at the optic chiasm. *Neuron.* 2003;39(6):919–935.
30. Petros TJ, Bryson JB, Mason C. Ephrin-B2 elicits differential growth cone collapse and axon retraction in retinal ganglion cells from distinct retinal regions. *Dev Neurobiol.* 2010;70(11):781–794.
31. Pak W, Hindges R, Lim YS, Pfaff SL, O'Leary DD. Magnitude of binocular vision controlled by islet-2 repression of a genetic program that specifies laterality of retinal axon pathfinding. *Cell.* 2004;119(4):567–578.
32. Triplett JW, Wei W, Gonzalez C, et al. Dendritic and axonal targeting patterns of a genetically-specified class of retinal ganglion cells that participate in image-forming circuits. *Neural Dev.* 2014;9:2.
33. Kuwajima T, Soares CA, Sitko AA, Lefebvre V, Mason C. SoxC transcription factors promote contralateral retinal ganglion cell differentiation and axon guidance in the mouse visual system. *Neuron.* 2017;93(5):1110–1125. e5.
34. Kuwajima T, Yoshida Y, Takegahara N, et al. Optic chiasm presentation of Semaphorin6D in the context of Plexin-A1 and Nr-CAM promotes retinal axon midline crossing. *Neuron.* 2012;74(4):676–690.
35. Erskine L, Reijntjes S, Pratt T, et al. VEGF signaling through neuropilin 1 guides commissural axon crossing at the optic chiasm. *Neuron.* 2011;70(5):951–965.
36. Tillo M, Erskine L, Cariboni A, et al. VEGF189 binds NRP1 and is sufficient for VEGF/NRP1-dependent neuronal patterning in the developing brain. *Development.* 2015;142(2):314–319.
37. Morenilla-Palao C, Lopez-Cascales MT, Lopez-Atalaya JP, et al. A Zic2-regulated switch in a noncanonical Wnt/betacatenin pathway is essential for the formation of bilateral circuits. *Sci Adv.* 2020;6(46).
38. Fabre PJ, Shimogori T, Charron F. Segregation of ipsilateral retinal ganglion cell axons at the optic chiasm requires the Shh receptor Boc. *J Neurosci.* 2010;30(1):266–275.
39. Sanchez-Arrones L, Nieto-Lopez F, Sanchez-Camacho C, et al. Shh/Boc signaling is required for sustained generation of ipsilateral projecting ganglion cells in the mouse retina. *J Neurosci.* 2013;33(20):8596–8607.
40. Peng J, Fabre PJ, Dolique T, et al. Sonic Hedgehog is a remotely produced cue that controls axon guidance trans-axonally at a midline choice point. *Neuron.* 2018;97(2):326–340. e4.
41. Sitko AA, Kuwajima T, Mason CA. Eye-specific segregation and differential fasciculation of developing retinal ganglion cell axons in the mouse visual pathway. *J Comp Neurol.* 2018;526(7):1077–1096.
42. Bruce FM, Brown S, Smith JN, Fuerst PG, Erskine L. DSCAM promotes axon fasciculation and growth in the developing optic pathway. *Proc Natl Acad Sci U S A.* 2017;114(7):1702–1707.

43. Clements R, Wright KM. Retinal ganglion cell axon sorting at the optic chiasm requires dystroglycan. *Dev Biol*. 2018;442(2):210–219.
44. Cioni JM, Wong HH, Bressan D, Kodama L, Harris WA, Holt CE. Axon-axon interactions regulate topographic optic tract sorting via CYFIP2-dependent WAVE complex function. *Neuron*. 2018;97(5):1078–1093. e6.
45. Lee MA, Sitko AA, Khalid S, Shirasu-Hiza M, Mason CA. Spatiotemporal distribution of glia in and around the developing mouse optic tract. *J Comp Neurol*. 2019;527(3):508–521.
46. Martin PR. The projection of different retinal ganglion cell classes to the dorsal lateral geniculate nucleus in the hooded rat. *Exp Brain Res*. 1986;62(1):77–88.
47. Reese BE. 'Hidden lamination' in the dorsal lateral geniculate nucleus: the functional organization of this thalamic region in the rat. *Brain Res*. 1988;472(2):119–137.
48. Guido W. Development, form, and function of the mouse visual thalamus. *J Neurophysiol*. 2018;120(1):211–225.
49. Baden T, Berens P, Franke K, Roman Roson M, Bethge M, Euler T. The functional diversity of retinal ganglion cells in the mouse. *Nature*. 2016;529(7586):345–350.
50. Sanes JR, Masland RH. The types of retinal ganglion cells: current status and implications for neuronal classification. *Annu Rev Neurosci*. 2015;38:221–246.
51. Rheaume BA, Jereen A, Bolisetty M, et al. Single cell transcriptome profiling of retinal ganglion cells identifies cellular subtypes. *Nat Commun*. 2018;9(1):2759.
52. Laboissonniere LA, Goetz JJ, Martin GM, et al. Molecular signatures of retinal ganglion cells revealed through single cell profiling. *Sci Rep*. 2019;9(1):15778.
53. Peng YR, Shekhar K, Yan W, et al. Molecular classification and comparative taxonomics of foveal and peripheral cells in primate retina. *Cell*. 2019;176(5):1222–1237. e22.
54. Yan W, Laboulaye MA, Tran NM, Whitney IE, Benhar I, Sanes JR. Mouse retinal cell atlas: molecular identification of over sixty amacrine cell types. *J Neurosci*. 2020;40(27):5177–5195.
55. Osterhout JA, El-Danaf RN, Nguyen PL, Huberman AD. Birthdate and outgrowth timing predict cellular mechanisms of axon target matching in the developing visual pathway. *Cell Rep*. 2014;8(4):1006–1017.
56. Williams RW, Hogan D, Garraghty PE. Target recognition and visual maps in the thalamus of achiasmatic dogs. *Nature*. 1994;367(6464):637–639.
57. McLaughlin T, O'Leary DD. Molecular gradients and development of retinotopic maps. *Annu Rev Neurosci*. 2005;28:327–355.
58. Pfeiffenberger C, Yamada J, Feldheim DA. Ephrin-As and patterned retinal activity act together in the development of topographic maps in the primary visual system. *J Neurosci*. 2006;26(50):12873–12884.
59. Huberman AD, Murray KD, Warland DK, Feldheim DA, Chapman B. Ephrin-As mediate targeting of eye-specific projections to the lateral geniculate nucleus. *Nat Neurosci*. 2005;8(8):1013–1021.
60. Leamey CA, Merlin S, Lattouf P, et al. Ten_m3 regulates eye-specific patterning in the mammalian visual pathway and is required for binocular vision. *PLoS Biol*. 2007;5(9):e241.
61. Young TR, Bourke M, Zhou X, et al. Ten-m2 is required for the generation of binocular visual circuits. *J Neurosci*. 2013;33(30):12490–12509.
62. Leamey CA, Sawatari A. Teneurins: Mediators of complex neural circuit assembly in mammals. *Front Neurosci*. 2019;13:580.
63. Sretavan D, Shatz CJ. Prenatal development of individual retinogeniculate axons during the period of segregation. *Nature*. 1984;308(5962):845–848.
64. Ziburkus J, Guido W. Loss of binocular responses and reduced retinal convergence during the period of retinogeniculate axon segregation. *J Neurophysiol*. 2006;96(5):2775–2784.
65. Liang L, Chen C. Organization, function, and development of the mouse retinogeniculate synapse. *Annu Rev Vis Sci*. 2020;6:261–285.
66. Cleland BG, Dubin MW, Levick WR. Simultaneous recording of input and output of lateral geniculate neurones. *Nat New Biol*. 1971;231(23):191–192.
67. Kaplan E, Shapley R. The origin of the S (slow) potential in the mammalian lateral geniculate nucleus. *Exp Brain Res*. 1984;55(1):111–116.
68. Levick WR, Cleland BG, Dubin MW. Lateral geniculate neurons of cat: retinal inputs and physiology. *Invest Ophthalmol*. 1972;11(5):302–311.
69. Mastronarde DN. Two classes of single-input X-cells in cat lateral geniculate nucleus. II. Retinal inputs and the generation of receptive-field properties. *J Neurophysiol*. 1987;57(2): 381–413.
70. Mastronarde DN. Nonlagged relay cells and interneurons in the cat lateral geniculate nucleus: receptive-field properties and retinal inputs. *Vis Neurosci*. 1992;8(5):407–441.
71. Chen C, Regehr WG. Developmental remodeling of the retinogeniculate synapse. *Neuron*. 2000;28(3):955–966.
72. Jaubert-Miazza L, Green E, Lo FS, Bui K, Mills J, Guido W. Structural and functional composition of the developing retinogeniculate pathway in the mouse. *Vis Neurosci*. 2005;22(5):661–676.
73. Hammer S, Monavarfeshani A, Lemon T, Su J, Fox MA. Multiple retinal axons converge onto relay cells in the adult mouse thalamus. *Cell Rep*. 2015;12(10):1575–1583.
74. Morgan JL, Berger DR, Wetzel AW, Lichtman JW. The fuzzy logic of network connectivity in mouse visual thalamus. *Cell*. 2016;165(1):192–206.
75. Rompani SB, Mullner FE, Wanner A, et al. Different modes of visual integration in the lateral geniculate nucleus revealed by single-cell-initiated transsynaptic tracing. *Neuron*. 2017;93(4):767–776. e6.
76. Litvina EY, Chen C. Functional convergence at the retinogeniculate synapse. *Neuron*. 2017;96(2):330–338. e5.
77. Bauer J, Weiler S, Fernholz MHP, et al. Limited functional convergence of eye-specific inputs in the retinogeniculate pathway of the mouse. *Neuron*. 2021;109(15):2457–2468. e12.
78. Roman Roson M, Bauer Y, Kotkat AH, Berens P, Euler T, Busse L. Mouse dLGN receives functional input from a diverse population of retinal ganglion cells with limited convergence. *Neuron*. 2019;102(2):462–476. e8.
79. Sretavan DW, Shatz CJ, Stryker MP. Modification of retinal ganglion cell axon morphology by prenatal infusion of tetrodotoxin. *Nature*. 1988;336(6198):468–471.
80. Shatz CJ, Stryker MP. Prenatal tetrodotoxin infusion blocks segregation of retinogeniculate afferents. *Science*. 1988;242(4875):87–89.
81. Penn AA, Riquelme PA, Feller MB, Shatz CJ. Competition in retinogeniculate patterning driven by spontaneous activity. *Science*. 1998;279(5359):2108–2112.
82. Grubb MS, Rossi FM, Changeux JP, Thompson ID. Abnormal functional organization in the dorsal lateral geniculate nucleus of mice lacking the beta 2 subunit of the nicotinic acetylcholine receptor. *Neuron*. 2003;40(6):1161–1172.
83. Chandrasekaran AR, Plas DT, Gonzalez E, Crair MC. Evidence for an instructive role of retinal activity in retinotopic map refinement in the superior colliculus of the mouse. *J Neurosci*. 2005;25(29):6929–6938.
84. Mrsic-Flogel TD, Hofer SB, Creutzfeldt C, et al. Altered map of visual space in the superior colliculus of mice lacking early retinal waves. *J Neurosci*. 2005;25(29):6921–6928.
85. Ackman JB, Burbridge TJ, Crair MC. Retinal waves coordinate patterned activity throughout the developing visual system. *Nature*. 2012;490(7419):219–225.
86. Bansal A, Singer JH, Hwang BJ, Xu W, Beaudet A, Feller MB. Mice lacking specific nicotinic acetylcholine receptor subunits exhibit dramatically altered spontaneous activity patterns and reveal a limited role for retinal waves in forming ON and OFF circuits in the inner retina. *J Neurosci*. 2000;20(20):7672–7681.
87. Kahne M, Rudiger S, Kihara AH, Lindner B. Gap junctions set the speed and nucleation rate of stage I retinal waves. *PLoS Comput Biol*. 2019;15(4):e1006355.
88. Feller MB, Wellis DP, Stellwagen D, Werblin FS, Shatz CJ. Requirement for cholinergic synaptic transmission in the propagation of spontaneous retinal waves. *Science*. 1996;272 (5265):1182–1187.
89. Zheng JJ, Lee S, Zhou ZJ. A developmental switch in the excitability and function of the starburst network in the mammalian retina. *Neuron*. 2004;44(5):851–864.
90. Ford KJ, Feller MB. Assembly and disassembly of a retinal cholinergic network. *Vis Neurosci*. 2012;29(1):61–71.
91. Demas J, Sagdullaev BT, Green E, et al. Failure to maintain eye-specific segregation in nob, a mutant with abnormally patterned retinal activity. *Neuron*. 2006;50(2):247–259.
92. Syed MM, Lee S, Zheng J, Zhou ZJ. Stage-dependent dynamics and modulation of spontaneous waves in the developing rabbit retina. *J Physiol*. 2004;560(Pt 2):533–549.
93. Wong WT, Myhr KL, Miller ED, Wong RO. Developmental changes in the neurotransmitter regulation of correlated spontaneous retinal activity. *J Neurosci*. 2000;20(1):351–360.
94. Blankenship AG, Ford KJ, Johnson J, et al. Synaptic and extrasynaptic factors governing glutamatergic retinal waves. *Neuron*. 2009;62(2):230–241.
95. Maccione A, Hennig MH, Gandolfo M, et al. Following the ontogeny of retinal waves: pan-retinal recordings of population dynamics in the neonatal mouse. *J Physiol*. 2014;592(7): 1545–1563.
96. Tu DC, Zhang D, Demas J, et al. Physiologic diversity and development of intrinsically photosensitive retinal ganglion cells. *Neuron*. 2005;48(6):987–999.
97. Renna JM, Weng S, Berson DM. Light acts through melanopsin to alter retinal waves and segregation of retinogeniculate afferents. *Nat Neurosci*. 2011;14(7):827–829.
98. Kirkby LA, Feller MB. Intrinsically photosensitive ganglion cells contribute to plasticity in retinal wave circuits. *Proc Natl Acad Sci U S A*. 2013;110(29):12090–12095.
99. Arroyo DA, Kirkby LA, Feller MB. Retinal waves modulate an intraretinal circuit of intrinsically photosensitive retinal ganglion cells. *J Neurosci*. 2016;36(26):6892–6905.
100. Shen J, Colonnese MT. Development of activity in the mouse visual cortex. *J Neurosci*. 2016;36(48):12259–12275.
101. Tiriac A, Smith BE, Feller MB. Light prior to eye opening promotes retinal waves and eye-specific segregation. *Neuron*. 2018;100(5):1059–1065. e4.
102. Lichtman JW, Colman H. Synapse elimination and indelible memory. *Neuron*. 2000;25(2):269–278.
103. Sanes JR, Lichtman JW. Development of the vertebrate neuromuscular junction. *Annu Rev Neurosci*. 1999;22:389–442.
104. Stellwagen D, Shatz CJ. An instructive role for retinal waves in the development of retinogeniculate connectivity. *Neuron*. 2002;33(3):357–367.
105. Stellwagen D, Shatz CJ, Feller MB. Dynamics of retinal waves are controlled by cyclic AMP. *Neuron*. 1999;24(3):673–685.
106. Shatz CJ. Emergence of order in visual system development. *Proc Natl Acad Sci U S A*. 1996;
93(2):602–608.
107. Zhang J, Ackman JB, Xu HP, Crair MC. Visual map development depends on the temporal pattern of binocular activity in mice. *Nat Neurosci*. 2011;15(2):298–307.
108. Burbridge TJ, Xu HP, Ackman JB, et al. Visual circuit development requires patterned activity mediated by retinal acetylcholine receptors. *Neuron*. 2014;84(5):1049–1064.
109. Ge X, Zhang K, Gribizis A, Hamodi AS, Sabino AM, Crair MC. Retinal waves prime visual motion detection by simulating future optic flow. *Science*. 2021;373(6553).
110. Xu HP, Furman M, Mineur YS, et al. An instructive role for patterned spontaneous retinal activity in mouse visual map development. *Neuron*. 2011;70(6):1115–1127.
111. Goddard CA, Butts DA, Shatz CJ. Regulation of CNS synapses by neuronal MHC class I. *Proc Natl Acad Sci U S A*. 2007;104(16):6828–6833.
112. Huh GS, Boulanger LM, Du H, Riquelme PA, Brotz TM, Shatz CJ. Functional requirement for class I MHC in CNS development and plasticity. *Science*. 2000;290(5499):2155–2159.
113. Corriveau RA, Huh GS, Shatz CJ. Regulation of class I MHC gene expression in the developing and mature CNS by neural activity. *Neuron*. 1998;21(3):505–520.
114. Datwani A, McConnell MJ, Kanold PO, et al. Classical MHCI molecules regulate retino-geniculate refinement and limit ocular dominance plasticity. *Neuron*. 2009;64(4):463–470.
115. Lee H, Brott BK, Kirkby LA, et al. Synapse elimination and learning rules co-regulated by MHC class I H2-Db. *Nature*. 2014;509(7499):195–200.
116. Stevens B, Allen NJ, Vazquez LE, et al. The classical complement cascade mediates CNS synapse elimination. *Cell*. 2007;131(6):1164–1178.
117. Bjartmar L, Huberman AD, Ullian EM, et al. Neuronal pentraxins mediate synaptic refinement in the developing visual system. *J Neurosci*. 2006;26(23):6269–6281.
118. Kono R, Ikegaya Y, Koyama R. Phagocytic glial cells in brain homeostasis. *Cells*. 2021;10(6).

119. Cong Q, Soteros BM, Wollet M, Kim JH, Sia GM. The endogenous neuronal complement inhibitor SRPX2 protects against complement-mediated synapse elimination during development. *Nat Neurosci.* 2020;23(9):1067–1078.

120. Lehrman EK, Wilton DK, Litvina EY, et al. CD47 Protects synapses from excess microglia-mediated pruning during development. *Neuron.* 2018;100(1):120–134. e6.

121. Chung WS, Verghese PB, Chakraborty C, et al. Novel allele-dependent role for APOE in controlling the rate of synapse pruning by astrocytes. *Proc Natl Acad Sci U S A.* 2016;113(36): 10186–10191.

122. Dhande OS, Hua EW, Guh E, et al. Development of single retinofugal axon arbors in normal and beta2 knock-out mice. *J Neurosci.* 2011;31(9):3384–3399.

123. Hong YK, Park S, Litvina EY, Morales J, Sanes JR, Chen C. Refinement of the retinogeniculate synapse by bouton clustering. *Neuron.* 2014;84(2):332–339.

124. Cheadle L, Rivera SA, Phelps JS, et al. Sensory experience engages microglia to shape neural connectivity through a non-phagocytic mechanism. *Neuron.* 2020;108(3):451–468. e9.

125. Cheadle L, Tzeng CP, Kalish BT, et al. Visual experience-dependent expression of fn14 is required for retinogeniculate refinement. *Neuron.* 2018;99(3):525–539. e10.

126. Nelson R, Famiglietti Jr. EV, Kolb H. Intracellular staining reveals different levels of stratification for on- and off-center ganglion cells in cat retina. *J Neurophysiol.* 1978;41(2): 472–483.

127. Stryker MP, Zahs KR. On and off sublaminae in the lateral geniculate nucleus of the ferret. *J Neurosci.* 1983;3(10):1943–1951.

128. Cucchiaro J, Guillery RW. The development of the retinogeniculate pathways in normal and albino ferrets. *Proc R Soc Lond B Biol Sci.* 1984;223(1231):141–164.

129. Wingate RJ, Fitzgibbon T, Thompson ID. Lucifer yellow, retrograde tracers, and fractal analysis characterise adult ferret retinal ganglion cells. *J Comp Neurol.* 1992;323(4):449–474.

130. Meissirel C, Wikler KC, Chalupa LM, Rakic P. Early divergence of magnocellular and parvocellular functional subsystems in the embryonic primate visual system. *Proc Natl Acad Sci U S A.* 1997;94(11):5900–5905.

131. Snider CJ, Dehay C, Berland M, Kennedy H, Chalupa LM. Prenatal development of retinogeniculate axons in the macaque monkey during segregation of binocular inputs. *J Neurosci.* 1999;19(1):220–228.

132. Krahe TE, El-Danaf RN, Dilger EK, Henderson SC, Guido W. Morphologically distinct classes of relay cells exhibit regional preferences in the dorsal lateral geniculate nucleus of the mouse. *J Neurosci.* 2011;31(48):17437–17448.

133. Rapaport DH, Fletcher JT, LaVail MM, Rakic P. Genesis of neurons in the retinal ganglion cell layer of the monkey. *J Comp Neurol.* 1992;322(4):577–588.

134. Huberman AD, Dehay C, Berland M, Chalupa LM, Kennedy H. Early and rapid targeting of eye-specific axonal projections to the dorsal lateral geniculate nucleus in the fetal macaque. *J Neurosci.* 2005;25(16):4014–4023.

135. Chapman B. Necessity for afferent activity to maintain eye-specific segregation in ferret lateral geniculate nucleus. *Science.* 2000;287(5462):2479–2482.

136. Hooks BM, Chen C. Vision triggers an experience-dependent sensitive period at the retinogeniculate synapse. *J Neurosci.* 2008;28(18):4807–4817.

137. Hooks BM, Chen C. Distinct roles for spontaneous and visual activity in remodeling of the retinogeniculate synapse. *Neuron.* 2006;52(2):281–291.

138. Huberman AD. Mechanisms of eye-specific visual circuit development. *Curr Opin Neurobiol.* 2007;17(1):73–80.

40

Developmental Visual Deprivation

Yuzo M. Chino

INTRODUCTION

The vision of newborn infants is crude. As infants experience the normal visual environment, their vision rapidly improves, with different visual capabilities emerging at different ages. Determining the exact timing for the behavioral onset of specific visual functions and identifying the critical factors that limit their development have been the primary focus of perceptual and physiologic studies on vision development. Although immaturities of the physiologic optics and ocular motility are known to affect infant's vision soon after birth the maturation of the retina and, to a greater extent, the visual brain (i.e., the striate and extrastriate visual cortex) largely set a limit on their normal perceptual development.[1–3] The binocular and monocular receptive-field (RF) properties of neurons in the primary visual cortex (V1)[4–8] and secondary visual area V2[7–10] of infant monkeys are qualitatively "adult-like" near birth. However, the responsiveness of these neurons is quite low, reflecting, in part, retinal immaturity.[2,5,6,8,10] The weak and sluggish signaling of V1 and V2 neurons and the delayed maturation of higher-order visual areas are thought to be largely responsible for the slower perceptual development.[2,7–10]

The neuronal connections of the visual cortex are malleable for a considerable period of time after birth, the "critical" ("sensitive" or "plastic") period of development. The postnatal development of the visual cortex, therefore, requires normal visual experience and precise matching of the images in the two eyes. Experiencing binocularly discordant images early in life, *binocular imbalance*, has devastating effects on the development of the visual system because after eye opening, the neurons in the highly plastic visual cortex receive signals from the two eyes that do not match. Binocular imbalance commonly results from monocular form deprivation owing to congenital cataract or ptosis, chronic monocular defocus caused by large interocular differences in refractive power (anisometropia), and/or large misalignment of visual axes (strabismus). Experiencing binocular imbalance during early infancy causes binocular vision disorders, and, if untreated, amblyopia and/or abnormal binocular integration is likely to develop.

Topics in this chapter cover what we currently know about the perceptual consequences of early abnormal visual experience, the neural basis of altered vision, and the synaptic and molecular mechanisms of cortical plasticity. Macaque monkeys are ideal animal models for exploring the neural mechanisms underlying developmental vision disorders in humans. The anatomical and physiologic organizations of their visual system are nearly identical to humans. Perceptual studies in normal mature monkeys have documented extensively the striking similarities in monocular and binocular visual capabilities between macaque monkeys and humans.[3,11,12] The relative (scaled) time course of normal visual development in macaque monkeys parallels that of humans.[2,13–15] The primate visual cortex is structurally[16] and functionally[5–8] more developed at or near birth than the visual cortex in lower species. Many important discoveries on vision development have

been made on subprimate species.[17–23] However, in lower animals it is not always possible to establish a link between neural and perceptual deficits resulting from early abnormal visual experience. This chapter, therefore, primarily reviews studies on *nonhuman primates*. Studies with human infants are mentioned when appropriate, and research in subprimate species is described in detail mostly where the neural and molecular basis of cortical plasticity is discussed.

EFFECTS OF EARLY MONOCULAR FORM DEPRIVATION

Constant monocular form deprivation

Monocular form deprivation can result from an occlusion of the image in one eye or from a severely degraded image in the affected eye. Congenital dense cataracts and ptosis are the common causes of monocular form deprivation in human infants. To create primate models of monocular form deprivation, the eyelids of infant monkeys are surgically closed[24,25] or, more recently, by wearing diffuser lenses in front of one eye.[26]

Perceptual deficits

All binocular functions, including local/global stereopsis and binocular summation of contrast sensitivity, are severely compromised or lost following early monocular form deprivation.[25–27] The visual sensitivity of the deprived eye is dramatically reduced or virtually lost—form deprivation amblyopia (Fig. 40.1A).[25,27,28] Importantly, the severity of the contrast sensitivity loss resulting from monocular form deprivation is directly related to the degree of retinal image degradation during early infancy (Fig. 40.1B).[26]

Monocular deprivation also leads to an abnormal elongation of the eyes, hence the development of myopic refractive errors.[26,29,30] The deleterious effects of early monocular deprivation on spatial vision development are generally far more severe than the anomalies resulting from form deprivation in both eyes, bilateral form deprivation (Fig. 40.2).[31,32] As in monkeys with monocular form deprivation, bilateral form deprivation leads to a significant loss of binocular functions, including the detection of stereoscopic cues and binocular summation of contrast sensitivity (Fig. 40.2). In these binocularly deprived monkeys, the binocular contrast sensitivity function (Fig. 40.2, green square symbols) overlaps with the better eye's monocular sensitivity function (Fig. 40.2, blue circle symbols).[32]

Neural deficits

The most consistent effect of early monocular form deprivation on development is the anomalous changes in the ocular dominance distribution of V1 neurons (*ocular dominance plasticity*). During the *critical period* of development, the afferent fibers from the lateral geniculate nucleus (LGN) representing the two eyes compete for consolidation

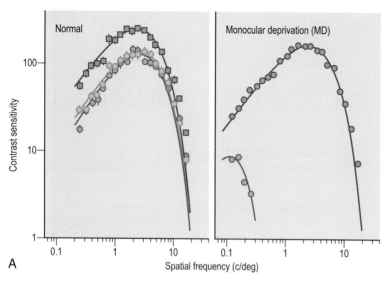

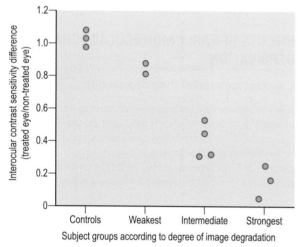

Fig. 40.1 Effects of early monocular form deprivation on contrast sensitivity in macaque monkeys. (**A**) Spatial contrast sensitivity functions (CSF) from normal (*left*) and monocularly form-deprived (*right*) monkeys. For the normal monkey, CSF under binocular viewing (*blue square*) and CSF for the right eye (*green circle*) and the left eye (*red circle*) are illustrated. Note large binocular summation of contrast sensitivity. For the MD monkey, CSF for the deprived eye (*red circle*) and CSF for the nondeprived eye (*purple circle*) are illustrated. (Redrawn from Harwerth RS, Crawford ML, Smith EL 3rd, Boltz RL. Behavioral studies of stimulus deprivation amblyopia in monkeys. *Vision Res.* 1981;21:779–789.) (**B**) Effects of the degree of image degradation on contrast sensitivity loss. (Redrawn from Smith EL 3rd, Hung LF. Form-deprivation myopia in monkeys is a graded phenomenon. *Vision Res.* 2000;40:371–381.)

of functional connections in V1 (*binocular competition*).[33,34] This early binocular competition is activity dependent, hence depriving normal signals from one eye puts the affected eye into competitive disadvantage and leads to a severe loss of functional connections in V1 from the deprived eye. The ocular dominance columns of the input layer in V1 (layer 4C) representing the deprived eye exhibit a substantial shrinkage.[24,34,35] The axon arbors of the afferent fibers from the LGN in the deprived columns show abnormal structural changes,[36] and the intrinsic long-range horizontal connections extending over multiple ocular dominance columns reorganize their wiring pattern in the cat primary visual cortex.[37,38]

Electrophysiological studies consistently report the severe loss of binocularly driven cells (i.e., neurons that can be activated by stimulation of either eye). Moreover, there is a clear shift in the ocular dominance distribution of cortical neurons away from the deprived eye. Specifically, the percentage of V1 neurons that can be activated or dominated by stimulation of the deprived eye is significantly decreased (Fig. 40.3).[24,34,39] The reduced functional innervation from the deprived eye is, at least in part, the neural basis for "undersampling" of visual scenes by the affected eye in form-deprivation amblyopia.[40]

For subcortical structures, there is a mild shrinkage of cell bodies of LGN neurons that receive input signals from the deprived eye.[33,34,41] However, the response properties of these primate LGN neurons are largely unaffected by early monocular form deprivation.[34,42,43] Interestingly, there is considerable evidence for functional alterations

in the cat LGN due to early abnormal visual experience.[17,44–46] In the primate retina there is no significant structural or functional abnormality due to early monocular form deprivation. Together, *major* neural changes resulting from early monocular form deprivations *in primates* occur beyond the LGN, that is, they begin in the primary visual cortex.

Intermittent monocular deprivation

Experiencing "normal vision" during early monocular form deprivation (*intermittent monocular form deprivation*) reduces some of the deleterious effects of early *constant* monocular form deprivation.[39,47–49] The effects of early intermittent deprivations have been studied using different rearing regimens including daily alternating monocular deprivation, reverse occlusion, and monocular form deprivation with daily brief periods of unrestricted vision.

Alternating monocular deprivation

Daily alternation of form deprivation between the two eyes has very little impact on the perceptual development of either eye in cats.[47,48] Consistent with this observation, the spatial RF properties such as orientation selectivity are normal. However, the same daily alternating deprivation devastates the development of binocular vision. Local stereopsis is lost and the proportion of binocularly driven neurons in area 17 is severely reduced. In monkeys, daily alternating monocular occlusion beginning *at birth* leads to a variety of abnormal eye positions and eye movements including strabismus and/or saccadic

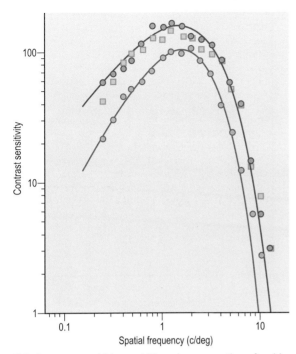

Fig. 40.2 Contrast sensitivity and binocular summation after binocular form deprivation. Spatial contrast sensitivity function of the right (*red circle*) and left (*blue circle*) eye after 16 weeks of deprivation beginning at 3 weeks of age. *Green square* symbols indicate contrast sensitivity under binocular viewing conditions. (Modified from Harwerth RS, Smith EL 3rd, Paul AD, Crawford ML, von Noorden GK. Functional effects of bilateral form deprivation in monkeys. *Invest Ophthalmol Vis Sci.* 1991;32:2311–2327.)

disconjugacy, that is, the amplitudes of saccades in the occluded eye are less than that in the viewing eye.[50–52]

Reverse occlusion

The effects of constant form deprivation in one eye, including spatial contrast sensitivity loss and ocular dominance shift in V1 away from the deprived eye, can be reversed if vision of the originally deprived eye is restored early in development and the fellow nondeprived eye is occluded—a *reverse occlusion*[53,54] (Fig. 40.4). The timing of the reverse occlusion is critical in determining the effectiveness of this procedure because the "recovery" of functions in the originally deprived eye may occur at the expense of the originally nondeprived eye. For example, contrast sensitivity can be restored if reverse occlusion occurs relatively early in the critical period, that is, if the original deprivation is short (e.g., 15 or 30 days). However, this early reversal leads to a loss of contrast sensitivity in the newly deprived (or originally nondeprived) eye (*red circles* in Fig. 40.4A)[53] and causes a corresponding shift in the ocular dominance distribution of V1 neurons favoring the initially deprived eye.[54] There is an optimal time for the reversal of monocular occlusion in order to achieve near-normal contrast sensitivity for both eyes (e.g., after 90 days of original monocular deprivation [Fig. 40.4B]).[53] In all cases, the binocular functions are diminished.[53] Similar effects of reverse occlusion have been studied extensively in cats, and the results have contributed to advancing our understanding of the neural mechanisms underlying the breakdown and recovery of visual functions from early monocular form deprivation.[19,55] The *clinical significance of these findings* is that this kind of animal study could provide key information for developing an effective clinical strategy for treating amblyopia with various *patching regimens*.

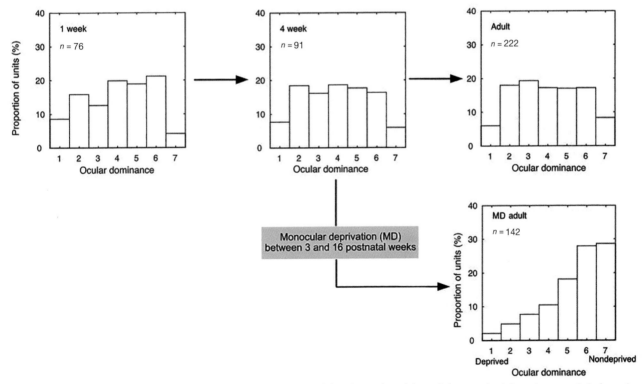

Fig. 40.3 Ocular dominance (OD) distributions of V1 neurons in normal infant (1 week and 4 weeks), normal adult, and monocularly form-deprived monkeys. Cells in OD 1 and 7 are exclusively driven by the contralateral or ipsilateral eye, respectively. Cells in OD 4 are binocularly balanced and neurons in OD 2 and 3 or OD 5 and 7 are dominated by the contralateral or ipsilateral eye, respectively. (Redrawn based on data from Chino YM, Smith EL 3rd, Hatta S, Cheng H. Postnatal development of binocular disparity sensitivity in neurons of the primate visual cortex. *J Neurosci.* 1997;17:296–307 and Sakai E, Bi H, Maruko I, Zhang B, Zheng J, Wensveen J, Harwerth RS, Smith EL 3rd, Chino YM. Cortical effects of brief daily periods of unrestricted vision during early monocular form deprivation. *J Neurophysiol.* 2006;95:2856–2865.)

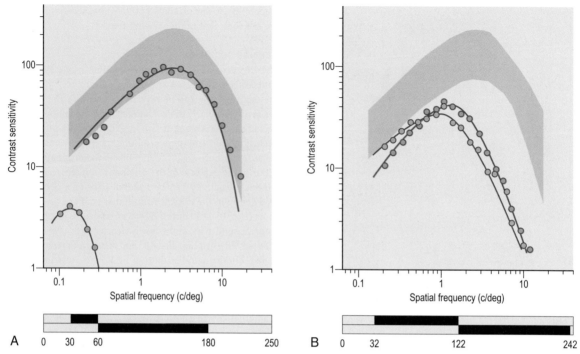

Fig. 40.4 Spatial contrast sensitivity functions (CSF) after reverse monocular occlusion. The functions for the originally deprived eye are illustrated with *blue circles.* The initial deprivation began at 21 days of age in all groups. (**A**) Reversal after 4 weeks of monocular deprivation. (**B**) After 3 months. *Shaded area* shows the normal range of contrast sensitivity in normal monkeys. (Modified from Harwerth RS, Smith EL 3rd, Crawford ML, von Noorden GK. The effects of reverse monocular deprivation in monkeys. I. Psychophysical experiments. *Exp Brain Res.* 1989;74:327–347.)

Brief unrestricted vision during monocular deprivation

Providing brief daily periods of normal vision (unrestricted vision) to the deprived eye during early monocular deprivation prevents or reduces the severity of form-deprivation amblyopia in monkeys.[49] Constant form deprivation (0 hour of unrestricted vision), as previously described, causes severe amblyopia of the deprived eye and a large shift in the ocular dominance of V1 neurons away from the deprived eye. However, only *1 hour* of unrestricted (normal) vision every day during the deprivation period (12 hours/day) dramatically improves the contrast sensitivity of the deprived eye, reducing the severity of form deprivation amblyopia. In these monkeys, the extent of abnormal ocular dominance shift in V1 is significantly reduced.[39] In stark contrast, the same "preventive" measure, even with 4 hours of daily unrestricted vision during the 12-hour deprivation period, does not prevent a severe loss of disparity-sensitive neurons, highlighting the extremely fragile nature of developing binocular connections in V1. Finally, constant monocular form deprivation leads to an elongation of the eye and thus the development of myopic refractive errors in the deprived eye.[56–58] However, a brief period of unrestricted vision during the deprivation period reduces the degree of myopic refractive error.[58] The *clinical relevance* of these studies is that the timely removal of the conditions that produce degradation of images or image occlusion (e.g., severe hyperopic anisometropia, cataract, or ptosis) is critically important for the prevention of amblyopia. If that is not immediately possible, "stopgap manipulations" such as lifting a drooping eyelid or keeping corrective lenses even for a short period of time every day are likely to have preventive effects against form-deprivation amblyopia and development of myopic refractive errors.[49]

Critical period

The critical (sensitive or plastic) period of vision development is traditionally defined as the postnatal period during which visual deprivation leads to long-term or permanent structural and/or functional changes of the visual system. The critical period differs substantially between species, the visual functions affected by deprivation, sites of neural alterations, and the nature of the visual deprivation (e.g., dark rearing, monocular form deprivation), monocular defocus, or ocular misalignment.[3,19,22,59] For example, the critical period for primates, unlike subprimate species, begins at or near birth.[27,35,60] Binocular functions are generally more readily disrupted by early visual deprivations than monocular spatial vision. The critical period for experience-dependent changes differs between cortical sites (e.g., V1, V2, V4, or MT [middle-temporal area or V5]), and between cortical layers within a given cortical site. The higher stages of processing (e.g., supra- and infragranular layers), compared with input layer within V1 or cortical sites later in the hierarchy of extrastriate visual areas, appear to have longer periods of plasticity.[2,19]

Critical period for monocular form deprivation

There are multiple "plastic" periods for different visual functions in macaque monkeys (Fig. 40.5).[27,60] Spectral sensitivity functions have relatively short critical periods that begin soon after birth and last for 3 months for scotopic spectral sensitivity and 6 months for photopic spectral sensitivity. The critical period for visual acuity loss is much longer, lasting over 24 months. Binocular vision development can be disrupted by monocular deprivation starting as late as 25 months of age (roughly equivalent to 8 years in humans).[27]

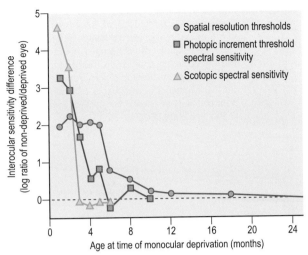

Fig. 40.5 The critical periods of development in macaque monkeys. Scotopic spectral sensitivity (*triangles*). Photopic spectral sensitivity (*square symbols*). Acuity (*circle symbols*). (Redrawn from Harwerth RS, Smith EL 3rd, Duncan GC, Crawford ML, von Noorden GK. Multiple sensitive periods in the development of the primate visual system. *Science.* 1986;232:235–238.)

Because the sensitivity of the visual cortex to deprivations varies substantially during the critical periods, the timing of deprivation (i.e., *onset and duration*) has significant effects on the severity of perceptual and neural deficits. At what age is monocular form deprivation likely to have the most damaging effects in monkeys? The perceptual development of contrast sensitivity and visual acuity in macaque monkeys is most vulnerable to monocular form deprivation during the first 5 postnatal months. A sharp drop of sensitivity to deprivation occurs after this initial period of heightened sensitivity, followed by a gradual decline over an extended period of time (i.e., >24 months) (Fig. 40.5).[27,60]

For ocular dominance plasticity in V1 of monkeys, the most severe shrinkage of ocular dominance columns for the deprived eye occurs with the *earliest*-onset age (e.g., 1 week of age).[35] The degree of shrinkage becomes progressively smaller as the onset of deprivation is delayed, and there is no obvious shrinkage if the onset is set at the 12th postnatal week. Thus, contrary to a classical observation,[24] the ocular dominance columns in layer 4C of monkey V1 are most sensitive to monocular deprivation right after birth.

These behavioral and anatomical studies reinforce the *clinical view* that the removal of dense congenital cataracts combined with high optical quality lenses or the correction of ptosis at the earliest possible postnatal time is essential to minimize the negative impact of monocular form deprivation in humans.[61–65]

The critical period for ocular dominance in cats begins at about 3 to 4 weeks of age when the optics of their eyes becomes relatively clear, peaks at around 6 to 8 weeks, and gradually decreases during the next 12 to 14 weeks.[33,66,67] Similar but earlier and shorter critical periods of plasticity for monocular deprivation have been reported for mice, rats, and ferrets, with minor variations.[68–70] The critical period is longer for monkeys than in lower species and appears to be generally correlated with animal life expectancy.[20,71] It is difficult to determine the precise critical period of vision development for humans, in part because of the difficulties associated with conducting experiments on human infants and dependence on clinical observations for data collection. Although the critical period for humans varies considerably for specific visual tasks and type of visual deprivation as evidenced in animal studies, the critical period for experience-dependent changes in human is thought to begin soon after birth (within 6 months or earlier), peak at around 1 to 3 years of age, and decline slowly until 7 to 8 years of age or later[19,72] (also see Chapter 38). Finally, recent evidence suggests that the "sensitive"/"plastic" period in human does not completely close during early development. Instead, "residual" cortical plasticity extends into adulthood, as it does in nonhuman primates and lower species.[22,72,73]

Molecular mechanisms of experience-dependent ocular dominance plasticity

The molecular mechanisms of experience-dependent ocular dominance plasticity have been extensively studied in rodents because the visual cortex of rodents is, in general, organized similarly to that of higher mammals[74–77] and a wide range of genetic manipulations are readily accessible in rodents.[19–21,55,76,78] As described previously for higher species, synaptic events following monocular deprivation (*binocular competition*) consist of an initial reversible reduction in functional connections to the deprived eye[69] and rewiring of the upper-layer long-range connections.[38] These are followed by extended periods of strengthening of the responses to the nondeprived eye and an eventual structural reorganization[20,21,33,79,80] (Fig. 40.6A).

Multiple cellular and circuit mechanisms are involved in ocular dominance plasticity in V1: Hebbian synaptic plasticity, homeostatic synaptic plasticity, and neuromodulator mechanisms (Fig. 40.6B).

Hebbian synaptic plasticity

The initial rapid changes occur as a result of *imbalance in the strength of the input signals* between the deprived and the nondeprived eyes. This imbalance disrupts the timing of the firing of action potentials between the presynaptic (LGN) and postsynaptic (V1) neurons for the deprived eye. Uncorrelated firing of action potentials between the presynaptic and postsynaptic neurons in V1 leads to a weakening of synaptic connections for the deprived eye while well-timed firing between the pre- and postsynaptic cells strengthens the synapses for the nondeprived eye.[21,81–84] The timing of presynaptic and postsynaptic neuronal spiking is also modulated by inhibitory neurons in the circuitry.[20–22,79,85,86] These activity-dependent changes in synaptic strength involve long-term potentiation (LTP) of input signals from the nondeprived eye and long-term depression (LTD) of signals from the deprived eye.[21,81,84,87–90]

Closely associated with LTP and LTD synaptic plasticity is the role of glutamate receptors in cortical neurons, in particular *n-methyl-D-aspartate* (NMDA), α-amino-3-hydroxy-5-methyl-4-isoxazolepropionic acid (AMPA), and γ-aminobutyric-acid (GABA) receptors (Fig. 40.6B). Excitatory synaptic transmission is mediated by NMDA and AMPA receptors, whereas inhibitory synaptic transmission is regulated by $GABA_{A\alpha}$ receptors. Each of these glutamate receptors has a broad range of critical roles in regulating the balance between excitation and inhibition and ocular dominance plasticity.[20–22,79,84,91]

NMDA receptors are made up of three types of subunits (NR1, NR2A, and NR2B). The normal postnatal changes in the expression of NR1 and NR2A or NR2B subunits (e.g., the NR2A/NR2B ratio being low at birth and gradually increasing during postnatal development) are also experience dependent. As a result, the developmental changes of the NMDA subunit expression owing to monocular deprivation (i.e., the activity-dependent regulation of the NR2A/NR2B ratios) are intimately involved in regulating the plasticity of the visual cortex. For example, an increase in the NR2A or NR2A/2B ratios leads to the induction of LTP and to a heightened sensitivity of synapses to modification.[92–94]

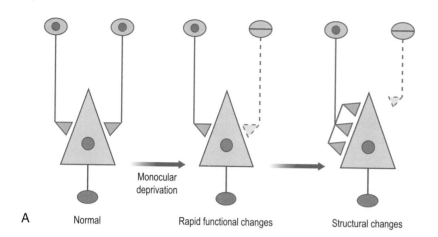

Fig. 40.6 Cortical mechanisms of ocular dominance plasticity. (**A**) Classic view of "binocular competition" in the primary visual cortex following early monocular form deprivation. (**B**) Schematic diagram illustrating the molecular mechanisms of experience-dependent cortical plasticity. (Redrawn from Tropea D, Van Wart A, Sur M. Molecular mechanisms of experience-dependent plasticity in visual cortex. *Philos Trans R Soc Lond B Biol Sci.* 2009;364:341–355)

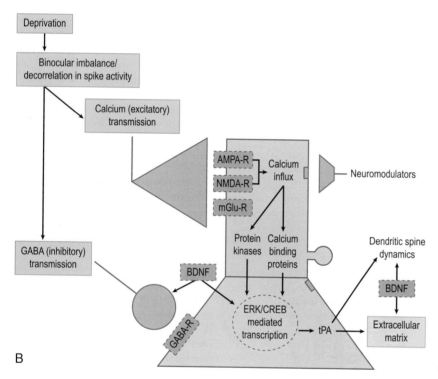

AMPA receptors, composed of GluR2 and either GluR1 or GluR3 subunits, are also involved in synaptic plasticity.[21,95–98] Synaptic strength is determined by the AMPA receptor density and calcium permeability. Repetitive activation of synapses leads to increased insertion of AMPA subunits into postsynaptic neuronal membrane, resulting in LTP, whereas reductions in synaptic activation (e.g., by monocular deprivation) remove AMPA receptors, leading to LTD.[19,21,99] Such redistribution of AMPA receptors is mediated by expression of the immediate gene Arc.[84] Prolonged LTD leads to structural changes (e.g., loss of synaptic contacts from the deprived eye).[84,85,89] Synaptic depolarization via activation of NMDA and AMPA receptors induces calcium influx and activates an intracellular signaling cascade. The second-messenger molecules that are directly involved in synaptic strength and ocular dominance plasticity include protein kinase (PKA), calcium/calmodulin-dependent protein kinase II (CaMKII), extracellular signal–regulated kinase 1,2 (ERK), cyclic AMP–responsive element-binding protein (CREB), and protein synthesis machinery. PKA, CaMKII, and ERK rapidly promote ocular dominance plasticity by modulating synaptic strength by phosphorylating plasticity-regulating molecules in glutamate or GABA receptors. This kinase signaling leads to the activation of CREB.[100–102] The changes initiated by activation of intracellular second-messenger molecules, along with the action of brain-derived neurotrophic factor (BDNF), leads to the enhanced expression of molecules that act on tissue plasminogen activation (tPA). BDNF and tPA can initiate the changes of dendritic spine motility,[84,103] spine density[84,104] and extracellular matrix[21] that ultimately result in rewiring of cortical circuits favoring the nondeprived eye.[85]

Homeostatic synaptic mechanisms

Because a single V1 neuron receives diverse multiple inputs, including the feedforward thalamic projection (e.g., intrinsic and feedback connections), Hebbian synaptic plasticity for a given neuron is strongly influenced by the level of past and current activity of all synapses in its neural circuit to maintain its stability (homeostatic synaptic plasticity).[21,23,85,98,105–107] There are two major theories on homeostatic plasticity. According to the "sliding threshold" or Bienenstock, Cooper, Munro (BCM) theory, a sustained period of high activity in neuronal network raises the threshold for LTP induction, resulting in LTD, whereas a prolonged period of low activity lowers the threshold and leads to LTP induction.[108-110] Another way that Hebbian synaptic plasticity can be influenced is to alter the "gain" of synapses (Scaling model).[106,107,111] Such gain control stabilizes the overall firing rate (i.e., prolonged high activity downscales excitatory synaptic events whereas prolonged low activity upscales them), thus adjusting average synaptic strength and maintaining the overall firing rate at a "normal" level.

Neuromodulator mechanisms

Another class of molecules involved in synaptic plasticity are the *neuromodulators*, including acetylcholine (Ach), noradrenaline (NA), and serotonin. These molecules are abundantly present throughout the cortex and have strong influence over ocular dominance plasticity.[21] For example, enhanced cholinergic or adrenergic systems facilitate LTP induction.[85,112-117] Changes in the expression of neuromodulators influence the level of LTP and/or LTD induction by modifying the intracellular calcium concentration by second-messenger pathways, resulting in the associated structural reorganizations of local connections to the visual cortex. Acetylcholine in V1 modulates the gain of geniculate inputs in layer 4C and exerts inhibitory influence over intracortical synaptic events, controlling the excitatory/inhibitory (E/I) balance in V1 during early development.[22,79,118] Cholinergic inputs facilitate the activity of somatostatin (SOM)-containing inhibitory neurons. SOM inhibitory neurons are known to inhibit parvalbumin-expressing inhibitory (PV) neurons and pyramidal neurons, leading to "disinhibition" by PV neurons over pyramidal neurons.[119,120] Such disinhibition influences ocular dominance plasticity[79] and the temporal dynamics of neuronal activity, leading to "improved" information processing in V1.[119] Finally, increasing evidence suggests that microglia (innate immune cells) modulate synaptic remodeling and plasticity by interacting with NE modulator and homeostatic synaptic mechanisms.[117,121-123]

GABA-mediated inhibition is important not only in maintaining the balance between cortical excitation and inhibition but also in regulating the *timing* of ocular dominance plasticity.[20,79,86,124,125] Manipulation of normal levels of GABAergic transmission by PV-expressing inhibitory neurons in the developing brain can delay or advance the onset of the critical period by altering E/I balance in V1.[22,79,125,126] Preventing the maturation of GABA-mediated transmission or dark rearing delays the critical period. Enhancing GABA transmission by infusing a GABA agonist (e.g., benzodiazepines)[125] or facilitating the growth of GABAergic interneurons by BDNF can advance the onset of critical period.[127-129] The *clinical significance* of these manipulations to "reset" the excitatory and inhibitory balance in V1 by various pharmacologic methods is that the results may provide new insights into the mechanisms underlying critical periods, and *potential* means to promote functional recovery in adults with developmental vision disorders[22,78,79] (but see further on "recovery from amblyopia").

EFFECTS OF EARLY MONOCULAR DEFOCUS

Constant monocular defocus

A less severe form of monocular image degradation results from large differences in refractive errors between the two eyes (*anisometropia*). Normal primates (including humans) begin their life with modest but binocularly balanced hyperopic refractive errors that decline to normal refractive state during early infancy (*emmetropization*).[130,131] If infants have large differences in refractive state between the two eyes, they are unable to focus with both eyes at the same time. To avoid experiencing binocularly discordant images, infants focus with one eye (typically with the eye with a less severe refractive error), and as a result the other eye experiences a defocused image (chronic defocus). Monkey

models of anisometropia are simulated by rearing infant monkeys with monocular defocusing lenses[130-132] or by monocular atropinization.[133]

Perceptual deficits

The perceptual consequences of untreated early anisometropia are generally similar to the anomalies found after early monocular form deprivation: impoverished binocular vision, reduced contrast sensitivity for high-spatial-frequency stimuli, and lower optotype acuity in the affected eye (*anisometropic amblyopia*).[133-140] However, the perceptual deficits in anisometropes are generally less severe than in monocular form deprivation and are spatial-frequency dependent (Fig. 40.7A). Anomalies vary substantially between individuals depending on the etiological factors and rearing histories (e.g., the degree of defocus).[140]

Neural deficits

Abnormal alterations in cortical physiology that result from early unilateral defocus are also similar to, but generally milder than, cortical deficits in monocularly form-deprived monkeys. The ocular dominance distribution of V1 neurons is marked by a substantial loss of binocularly balanced cells (ocular dominance between 3 and 5) and by a milder shift away from the affected eye[134,136-139,141,142] (Fig. 40.7B). The sensitivity of V1 neurons to binocular disparity is substantially reduced, and complex cells are more severely affected than simple cells in V1[136] (Fig. 40.7C). The spatial resolution and contrast sensitivity of V1 neurons for the affected eye of *severely* anisometropic monkeys are moderately lower than those for the fellow eye.[134,138,141]

In visual area 2 (V2), the ocular dominance shift away from the affected eye is more pronounced than that in V1 (Fig. 40.7B).[137,138] Under binocular viewing, the disparity sensitivity of V2 neurons is significantly reduced, and this disparity sensitivity loss in V2 is more severe than that in V1 (Fig. 40.7C). Also, binocular suppression is highly prevalent in V2[137] as in V1.[136] The monocular spatial RF properties of neurons driven by the affected eye (e.g., orientation bias, optimal spatial frequency, and RF center-surround sizes) are subnormal,[137] and the overall sensitivity of those V2 neurons is lower than that of normal cells.[138,139] Moreover, the RF spatial structure of V2 neurons, the "orderliness" in the spatial organization of RF "subfields," is severely disrupted, and the degree of such RF disorganization is directly correlated with the magnitude of binocular suppression[137] (see Fig. 40.16B). Neurons in V2 exhibit elevated and "noisy" spontaneous activity and contrast-dependent noisy spiking during visual stimulation, for example, increased variations in interspike intervals (spiking irregularity) and trial-to-trial fluctuations in spiking (Fano factor). This noisy spiking is well correlated with the strength of binocular suppression (Fig. 40.15C).[139] In MT of monkeys reared with monocular defocus, the ocular dominance distribution is shifted away from the affected eye, and the size of such shift is greater than that in V1.[143] The affected MT neurons show abnormal motion sensitivity (e.g., elevated coherent motion threshold, increased preferred stimulus speed) and shorter integration time.

Alternating defocus

Early monocular defocus can be alternated daily between the two eyes to prevent the development of monocular perceptual deficits (e.g., amblyopia).[132,144] If infant monkeys experience alternating defocus, the monocular response properties of V1 neurons, such as orientation selectivity, spatial-frequency tuning, and/or spatial resolution, do not show response alterations that favor one eye over the other, because each eye receives uninterrupted vision on alternate days during early infancy.[144] However, daily alternating defocus leads to a spatial frequency–dependent loss of local stereopsis (elevated disparity threshold) (Fig. 40.8B). This reduction of local stereopsis is exaggerated for high-spatial-frequency stimuli because larger

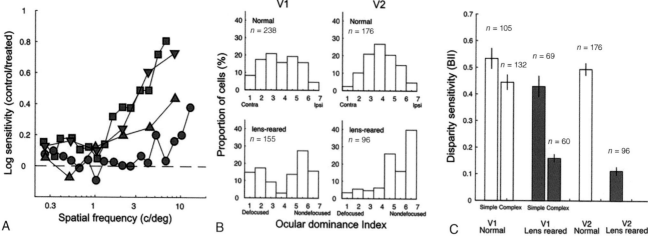

Fig. 40.7 Perceptual and neural deficits in anisometropic amblyopia. **(A)** Interocular differences in contrast sensitivity as a function of stimulus spatial frequency in four different monkeys reared with unilateral lens-defocus. **(B)** Ocular dominance distribution of V1 (*left*) and V2 (*right*) neurons in normal (*top*) and lens-reared (*bottom*) monkeys. **(C)** Disparity sensitivity loss in V1 and V2 of anisometropic monkeys. Note that complex cells had more severe deficits in V1. All V2 neurons are complex cells. (Redrawn from Smith EL 3rd, Harwerth RS, Crawford ML. Spatial contrast sensitivity deficits in monkeys produced by optically induced anisometropia. *Invest Ophthalmol Vis Sci.* 1985;26:330–342; Smith EL 3rd, Chino YM, N J, Cheng H, Crawford ML, Harwerth RS. Residual binocular interactions in the striate cortex of monkeys reared with abnormal binocular vision. *J Neurophysiol.* 1997;78:1353–1362; and Tao X, Zhang B, Shen G, et al. Early monocular defocus disrupts the normal development of receptive-field structure in V2 neurons of macaque monkeys. *J. Neurosci.* 2014;34:13840–13854.)

defocus generates greater conflicts between signals coming from the two eyes.[132] Moreover, the disparity sensitivities of V1 neurons are significantly reduced in these monkeys, and this reduction is also spatial-frequency dependent.[144]

These observations support the traditional view that local stereopsis is spatial-frequency dependent, and that binocular disparity information is processed by independent channels tuned to different spatial frequencies.[145,146] It is also evident that the local disparity processing mechanisms in V1 can be independently compromised by early abnormal visual experience depending on their spatial frequency–tuning properties. Finally, the effects of early alternating defocus on binocular vision development underscore the importance of having the normal presence of disparity-sensitive neurons in V1 for local stereopsis, although disparity-sensitive V1 neurons alone are not sufficient to support fine stereopsis (i.e., it requires further processing by extrastriate neurons). [147,148]

EFFECTS OF EARLY STRABISMUS

Strabismus is a chronic deviation of the visual axes that emerges shortly after birth.[149–152] The direction of the axis deviation can be convergent (esotropia), divergent (exotropia), or vertical (hypertropia). The etiology of infantile or congenital strabismus is not known. There is a clear familial tendency of developing strabismus, but the genetic factors responsible for infantile strabismus are not well understood.[151] In monkeys and humans, a high degree of uncorrected hypermetropia soon after birth is known to result in esotropia (accommodative esotropia).[153–156]

Perceptual deficits

Strabismic infants experience double vision (diplopia) immediately after the onset of misalignment. If "normal" alignment is not achieved in a timely manner, binocular vision anomalies, such as deficient stereoscopic vision (Fig. 40.9),[136,156–158] reduced binocular summation of

contrast sensitivity,[136] and clinical suppression,[159] are likely to develop. Amblyopia may develop if strabismus is not treated for an extended period of time during the critical period.[72,134,138,143,160]

Animal models of strabismus

The effects of experiencing early strabismus have been extensively studied in animals by artificially creating ocular misalignment shortly after birth. In monkey or cat models, human strabismus is commonly *simulated* by surgical[134,138,143,158,160–162] or optical[136,163–169] methods shortly after birth. The basic idea of either method is to disrupt binocular vision development. Also, alternating monocular occlusion (AOM) from birth leads to strabismus as mentioned previously, and these monkey models have served primarily for studies on ocular motility.[152,170] For the surgical method, the extraocular muscle of one eye (the medial rectus muscle for exotropia and the lateral rectus muscle for esotropia) is sectioned and the opposing muscle (the lateral or medial rectus muscle, respectively) is tied to induce the misalignment.[134,138,143,160] The surgical method creates a period of noncomitant or paralytic strabismus, that is, the angle of deviation changes with the field of gaze. This type of strabismus is less common in humans than comitant strabismus, that is, the angle of deviation does not change with the field of gaze. In monkeys with surgical strabismus, the manipulated eye is immediately placed at a competitive disadvantage and the nondeviating fellow eye becomes the "fixating" eye. As a result, the deviating eye is likely to develop amblyopia.[134,138,160,171]

For the optical method, infant monkeys are fitted with a helmet with a pair of base-in or base-out prisms around 3 to 4 weeks of age.[136,150,163–169] This method *simulates* comitant strabismus in humans. If the prism rearing begins at birth, ocular misalignment, exotropia or esotropia, develops.[152] Neither eye is disadvantaged because their fixation frequently alternates between the two eyes, and thus the prism-reared monkeys are less likely to develop amblyopia.[136,150,152,171] However, the effects of early surgical or optical strabismus are quite devastating on the perceptual and neural development of binocular vision.

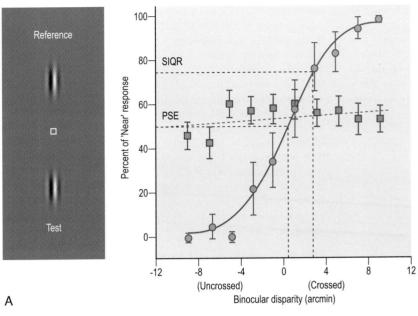

Fig. 40.8 Effects of early alternating defocus on disparity sensitivity. (**A**) Stimulus used to test local stereopsis in monkeys (*left*), and a psychometric function for binocular disparity discrimination (*right*). Stereoacuity is defined by disparity differences between the point of subject equality (*PSE*) and the semi-interquartile range (*SIQR*). Monocular control data are illustrated with *small squares*. (**B**) Disparity sensitivity loss as a function of spatial frequency in monkeys reared with 1.5-diopter alternating defocus (*left top*) and interocular differences (*left bottom*), and comparable values for monkeys reared with 3.0-diopter alternating defocus (*right column*). *Thick lines* signify the range of threshold values for normal monkeys. (Redrawn from Wensveen JM, Harwerth RS, Smith EL 3rd. Binocular deficits associated with early alternating monocular defocus. I. Behavioral observations. *J Neurophysiol.* 2003;90:3001–3011.)

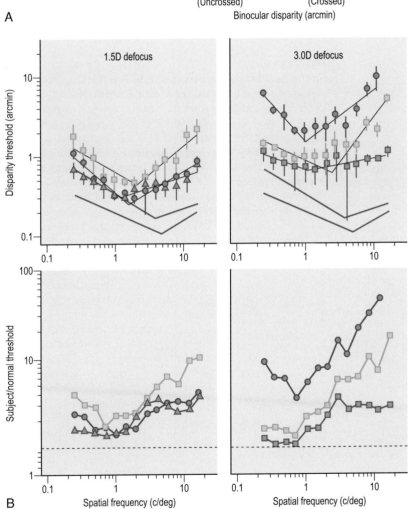

Neural deficits

The proportion of V1 and V2 neurons that can be activated by stimulation of either eye (classically defined as "binocular cells") is dramatically reduced in monkeys reared with surgical[134,138,152,160,172] or optical strabismus[136,150,169,173] (Fig. 40.10A). In monkeys reared with paralytic strabismus, the ocular dominance distribution of V1 neurons may slightly shift away from the deviating eye if strabismus is severe or does not shift at all (Fig. 40.10A).[134,138,160] Larger shifts in ocular dominance distribution are evident in V2 (Fig. 40.10A)[160] and the MT of monkeys with simulated paralytic strabismus.[143,174] The proportion of disparity-sensitive neurons is drastically reduced in V1[136,163,164,167,169] of stereo-deficient monkeys reared with optical strabismus (Figs. 40.10C,

40.11A, and 40.12B), and in both V1 and V2 of monkeys reared with surgical strabismus[160] (Fig. 40.10C).

Clinical suppression is a pervasive adaptive mechanism that humans with untreated strabismus develop to eliminate the disturbing impact of diplopia and visual confusion.[151] Monkeys reared with optical or surgical strabismus exhibit binocular suppression that is similar to clinical suppression in strabismic humans.[159] In strabismic

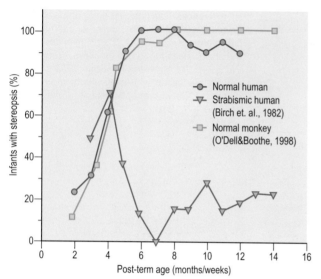

Fig. 40.9 Development of binocular vision. Development of stereopsis in normal human (*blue circles*) and monkey (*green square*) infants, and human infants with infantile esotropia (*red triangles*). (Redrawn based on data from Birch EE, Gwiazda J, Held R. Stereoacuity development for crossed and uncrossed disparities in human infants. *Vision Res.* 1982;22:507–513 and O'Dell C, Boothe RG. The development of stereoacuity in infant rhesus monkeys. *Vision Res.* 1997;37:2675–2684.)

monkeys and cats, V1 and V2 neurons exhibit robust binocular suppression (Figs. 40.10B, 40.12C, and 40.14B)[136,160,163–165,167,175–177] (but see Economides[178]), thus suggesting a potential link between abnormal binocular signal processing in V1 and V2 and binocular vision deficits for strabismic animals and humans.[160] Unless accompanied by consistent and extended periods of defocus in one eye, strabismus does not dramatically alter the monocular spatial response properties of V1 neurons.[134,160] Even if V1 neurons exhibit mild reductions in contrast sensitivity and/or spatial resolution for the deviating eye of severely amblyopic monkeys, such deficits in V1 are too small to account for their perceptual losses (Fig. 40.13).[3,59,160] However, the spatial resolution and orientation bias of V2 neurons in severely amblyopic monkeys are mildly but significantly lower than those in normal neurons.[160] In MT of strabismic monkeys exhibiting severe amblyopia, the neuronal responses to moving stimuli, especially preferred speed and integration time, are "subnormal."[143]

Effects of onset age and duration of strabismus

A critical issue for the management of infantile esotropia is the age at which corrective measures should be taken to preserve stereoscopic vision and establish alignment. The onset age and the duration of strabismus appear to play critical roles in determining the outcome.

Onset age

Several animal studies support the *clinical view* that surgical or optical correction should be considered as early as misalignment is detected, preferably around the time for the onset of stereopsis (4–6 months of age) (Fig. 40.9) for the preservation of fine binocular functions and later alignment[156,179–182] (but see ref 183) and reducing eye movement anomalies.[165,166,168,184] In monkeys, experiencing a brief period (2 weeks, equivalent to 2 months in humans) of optical strabismus beginning at 4 weeks of age (equivalent to 4 months in humans) drastically reduces the proportion of disparity-sensitive neurons and increases the prevalence of binocular suppression in monkey V1.[163] These binocular

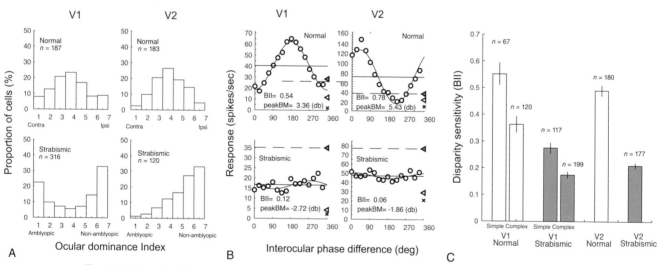

Fig. 40.10 Neural deficits in monkeys reared with optically induced strabismus. **(A)** Ocular dominance distribution of V1 (*left*) and V2 (*right*) neurons in normal (*top*) and strabismic (*bottom*) monkeys. **(B)** Representative disparity tuning functions of V1 (*left*) and V2 (*right*) neurons for normal (*top*) and strabismic (*bottom*) monkeys. Note that the neuron from a strabismic monkey exhibited a severe loss of disparity tuning and robust binocular suppression (binocular responses < dominant monocular response). **(C)** The average disparity sensitivity (BII) of V1 and V2 neurons in normal and strabismic monkeys. (Redrawn from Smith EL 3rd, Chino YM, N J, Cheng H, Crawford ML, Harwerth RS. Residual binocular interactions in the striate cortex of monkeys reared with abnormal binocular vision. *J Neurophysiol.* 1997;78:1353–1362 and Bi H, Zhang B, Tao X, Harwerth RS, Smith EL 3rd, Chino YM. Nuronal responses in visual area V2 (V2) of macaque monkeys with strabismic amblyopia. *Cereb Cortex.* 2011;21:2033–2045.)

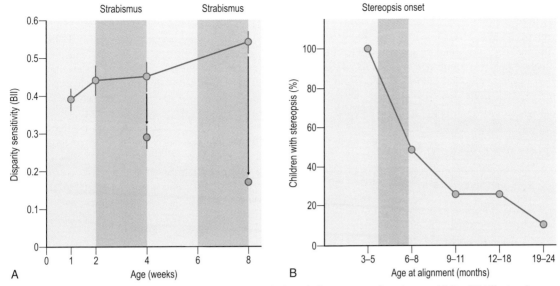

Fig. 40.11 Effects of onset age of strabismus and timing of alignment on disparity sensitivity. (**A**) Effects of onset age of strabismus on disparity sensitivity of V1 neurons in infant monkeys. Duration of optical strabismus was kept for 2 weeks while the onset age of strabismus was set either at 2 weeks or 6 weeks of age. Normal development of disparity sensitivity in V1 is also illustrated (*red circles*). Note that the reduction in disparity sensitivity is far greater for the late onset group than for the early onset group. (Redrawn based on data from Chino YM, Smith EL 3rd, Hatta S, Cheng H. Postnatal development of binocular disparity sensitivity in neurons of the primate visual cortex. *J Neurosci.* 1997;17:296–307 and Kumagami T, Zhang B, Smith EL 3rd, Chino YM. Effect of onset age of strabismus on the binocular responses of neurons in the monkey visual cortex. *Invest Ophthalmol Vis Sci.* 2000;41:948–954.) (**B**) Effects of alignment age on stereopsis in human strabismic infants. *Blue* area indicates the known onset age of stereopsis for normal human infants (i.e., between 4 and 6 months of age). (Redrawn from Birch EE, Fawcett S, Stager DR. Why does early surgical alignment improve stereoacuity outcomes in infantile esotropia? *J AAPOS.* 2000;4:10–14.)

response deficits are *more severe* when infant monkeys experience optical strabismus *after* 4 weeks of age (6–8 weeks) rather than *before* 4 weeks of age (2–4 weeks)[163,164] (Fig. 40.11A). Optical strabismus creates well-focused images that do not match between the two eyes. Consequently, unlike monocular deprivation, the most sensitive segment of the critical period for binocular disparity sensitivity is not immediately after birth when spatial vision is still very crude. Instead, it is soon after the known onset age of stereopsis around 4 to 8 weeks of age (equivalent to 4 to 8 months of age in humans) (Fig. 40.9). By this time of normal development, V1 and V2 neurons attain the qualitatively adult-like monocular spatial tuning properties.[5–8,185–188] Consequently, V1 and V2 neurons become more sensitive to smaller discrepancies in the images between the two eyes, and as a result their binocular response properties are more readily disrupted. The latest onset age of strabismus that can cause substantial binocular vision deficits and/or amblyopia is yet to be determined in primates. However, there are substantial perceptual deficits and anomalous alterations in the RF properties of V1 and V2 neurons even when surgical strabismus is induced as late as 6 months of age (roughly equivalent to 2 years of age in humans).[160]

Duration

In human infants, longer durations of strabismus result in greater deficits of binocular vision (stereopsis).[181,183] For infant monkeys reared with prisms, a similar relationship holds for disparity sensitivity deficits in V1. However the duration of optical strabismus has little impact on the disparity sensitivity loss of V1 neurons if it is longer than 2 weeks (Fig. 40.12B).[164] It is important to note that the effects of duration on disparity sensitivity reflect the combined effects of strabismus

duration and the timing of interocular alignment, that is, longer duration delays alignment and hence the restoration of unrestricted "normal" visual experience during the critical period for binocular vision development.

What is the *minimum* duration of misalignment required to alter the binocular response properties of V1 neurons in infant monkeys? Only 7 days of prism rearing (equivalent to 4 weeks in humans) beginning at 4 weeks of age are sufficient to disrupt the binocular disparity sensitivity of V1 neurons (Fig. 40.12B).[163,164,167] Three days of optical strabismus (equivalent to 12 days in human infants) does not significantly alter the disparity sensitivity. However, after only 3 days of experiencing optical strabismus, V1 neurons exhibit an abnormally high prevalence of binocular suppression (Fig. 40.12C). Importantly, binocular suppression in V1 after 3 days of prism rearing is as strong as suppression in monkeys that experience much longer durations (months or years) of strabismus. Thus, the very first neural alteration in V1 following the onset of strabismus is the emergence of robust binocular suppression.[167]

Eye movement anomalies in strabismus

Strabismic monkeys and humans exhibit substantial oculomotor anomalies.[152] Beside primary horizontal ocular misalignment, strabismic primates may exhibit dissociate vertical deviation (DVD),[189,190] alternate fixation,[190–192] fixation instability,[193–196] abnormal vergence, and temporal-to-nasal asymmetries in smooth-pursuit eye movement and visual tracking under monocular viewing,[51,151,174,193,197] similar to those found in normal infants.[197,198] Also strabismic humans and nonhuman primates often exhibit latent nystagmus or fusion maldevelopment nystagmus[152,168,199] and disconjugate eye movements.[51,152,200–203] Fixation

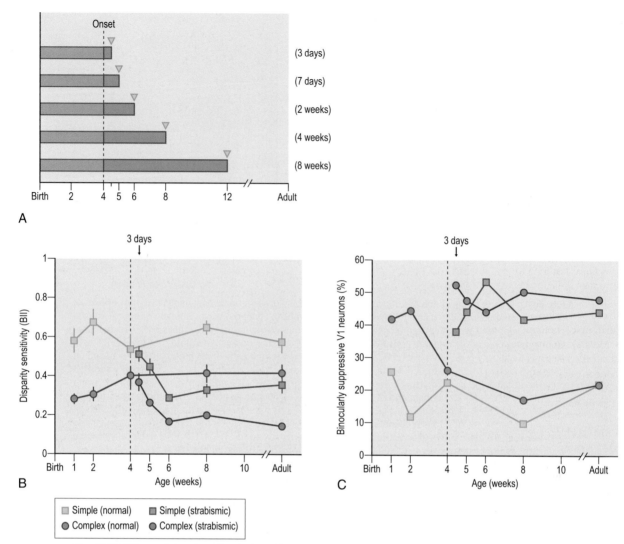

Fig. 40.12 Effects of duration of optical strabismus on binocular responses of V1 neurons. (**A**) Rearing regimen. The onset was kept at 4 weeks of age. The duration of prism rearing was varied between 3 days and 8 weeks. *Triangles* indicate the time of V1 recording experiments. (**B**) Effects of duration on disparity sensitivity of V1 neurons. Normal data are also illustrated. Data for strabismic adults come from monkeys reared with surgically induced strabismus. (**C**) Effects of strabismus duration on the prevalence of V1 neurons exhibiting binocular suppression. (Redrawn from Chino YM, Smith EL 3rd, Hatta S, Cheng H. Postnatal development of binocular disparity sensitivity in neurons of the primate visual cortex. *J Neurosci.* 1997;17:296–307; Mori T, Matsuura K, Zhang B, Smith EL 3rd, Chino YM. Effects of the duration of early strabismus on the binocular responses of neurons in the monkey visual cortex (V1). *Invest Ophthalmol Vis Sci.* 2002;43:1262–1269; and Zhang B, Bi H, Sakai E, et al. Rapid plasticity of binocular connections in developing monkey visual cortex (V1). *Proc Natl Acad Sci U S A.* 2005;102:9026–9031.)

instability in amblyopic monkeys and humans is characterized by frequent slow drifts, as well as the increased amplitude and frequency of microsaccades.[195,196] Also, fixation instability in amblyopes affects their visual acuity.[194,195] Finally, these eye movement deficits result from abnormal control of cortical neurons over the subcortical nuclei and the intrinsic nuclei of the cerebellum that support eye movements and visual tracking.[51,152,197,198,204–210]

The timing of corrective measures for infantile esotropia has significant impact on preventing eye movement anomalies.[152,165,168,184] In a series of studies by Tychsen and his colleagues, newborn monkeys were reared from birth with a goggle containing a 20-diopter prism in front of each eye until either 3 weeks of age ("early repair") or 3 to 6 months of age ("late repair"). Monkeys in late repair group exhibited temporal-to-nasal asymmetries of smooth-pursuit and optokinetic

nystagmus under monocular viewing, latent nystagmus, and persistent ocular misalignment. However, monkeys in the early repair group did not exhibit any of these motor deficits.[165,168,184] The motor deficits in the late repair group appeared to be linked to their abnormal visual cortical physiology and anatomy.[152,163,164,166,168,197] The *clinical implications* of these studies are that the earlier the corrective measures for infantile esotropia, the better the normal maturation of oculomotor functions[152,165] (but see ref 211).

AMBLYOPIA

Amblyopia is a developmental disorder of spatial vision. Amblyopia affects about 2% to 4% of children. Amblyopic primates exhibit reduced contrast sensitivity that is restricted to or exaggerated for mid- to high-spatial-frequency ranges of stimuli and also lower optotype acuity for the affected eye.[3,59,72,135,212] The nature and extent of visual anomalies in amblyopic children differ widely depending on the onset age, the status of binocular functions,[65,72,212–215] and the type of amblyopia, that is, strabismic, anisometropic, or form deprivation amblyopia.[65,72,212,215] Form deprivation amblyopia, the most frequently investigated type of amblyopia in animal studies, is far less prevalent among human infants in "developed" countries.[59,72]

Perceptual deficits

In addition to acuity and contrast sensitivity losses in all types of amblyopia, the visual system of strabismic and anisometropic amblyopes is known to be intrinsically "noisy," and their visual performance can be mimicked by introduction of noise in the stimuli.[216–218] The sensitivity of amblyopic humans to second-order stimuli is also reduced.[219,220] Strabismic and anisometropic amblyopes have difficulties in solving global perceptual tasks that require precise pooling of neighboring local feature information over extended ranges of space. These perceptual difficulties emerge in the form of abnormal contour integration, motion integration, and/or object segmentation.[59,72,221–224] Under binocular viewing, amblyopes frequently show impaired stereoscopic depth perception and robust suppression.[225–233] For strabismic and anisometropic amblyopes, many of the monocular deficits appear to be linked with their compromised binocular vision.[72,214,232–234]

As previously described for strabismic amblyopes, fixation instability, characterized by slow drift and frequent microsaccades,[152,194] is also observed in the affected eye of anisometropic amblyopes under monocular viewing.[195,199] Poor fixation may explain, at least in part, reduced acuity of the amblyopic eye[195] and could make the interpretation of testing and diagnostic results more difficult.[199] Also, saccadic reaction time is delayed in strabismic amblyopes.[235] Finally, amblyopic children may show impaired fine motor skills,[236,237] slow reading,[238] and reduced "quality of life."[234,239]

Neural deficits

Studies on the neural basis of *form deprivation amblyopia* have given us a relatively clear view of how the form-deprived eye loses its functional connections with the primary visual cortex (V1) and how the visual sensitivity of the affected eye is altogether lost even to the most basic, robust visual stimuli (Fig. 40.6).[3,19–21,59,67,72] For all types of amblyopic monkeys, lower sampling in V1 for the affected eye (e.g., ocular dominance shift away from the affected eye) and/or reduced spatial resolution and contrast sensitivity of V1 neurons are commonly invoked to explain the neural mechanisms underlying "low-level" perceptual deficits (i.e., reduction in contrast sensitivity and acuity).[3,4,33,34,59,67,72,134,138,160,172]

Unlike monocular form–deprived monkeys, however, a relatively small percentage of V1 neurons in strabismic or anisometropic monkeys exhibit reduced contrast sensitivity at high spatial frequencies and/or lower spatial resolutions.[134,138,160,240] As illustrated previously, a shift in ocular dominance distribution of V1 neurons away from the affected eye is relatively mild in anisometropic amblyopes and often absent in strabismic amblyopes.[59,134,138,160] Importantly, the magnitude of the V1 anomalies is too small to account for the severity of perceptual losses for anisometropic or strabismic amblyopes (Fig.40.13).[3,59,138,160,241] The most recent view on the neural basis of amblyopia, therefore, is that unlike in monocular form deprivation, the major cortical alterations that may limit a wide range of visual performance of anisometropic and strabismic amblyopes are likely to be present in areas downstream from V1, while milder but significant changes in monocular and binocular response properties begin in V1.[59,72,138,139,160] The neural deficits observed in extrastriate visual areas of amblyopic monkeys described

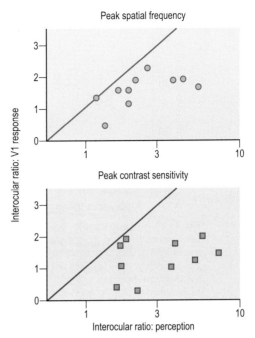

Fig. 40.13 Amblyopia and V1 cortical physiology in monkeys. The average optimal spatial frequency (*top*) and average peak contrast sensitivity (*bottom*) of V1 neurons as a function of perceptual differences in contrast sensitivity between the amblyopic and fellow eye of strabismic and anisometropic monkeys. Note that behavioral deficits are much greater than cortical deficits. (Redrawn from Kiorpes L, Movshon JA. Neural limitations on visual development in primates. In: *The Visual Neuroscience*. Chalupa LM, Werner SJ, eds. Cambridge, MA: MIT Press; 2004:159–173.)

further here and in previous sections may reflect the "amplification" of similar deficits in V1 (e.g., ocular dominance shift away from the amblyopic eye) (Fig. 40.7B),[143,160] contrast sensitivity loss,[139] enhanced spiking noise,[139,140] and binocular suppression (Fig. 40.14)[160] or deficits unique to extrastriate visual areas (e.g., disorganized RF structures in V2) (Fig. 40.16).[137]

Another important discovery on neural correlates of amblyopia is that binocular suppression, highly prevalent in V1 and V2 of strabismic or anisometropic monkeys, appears to play a significant role in the development of "basic" and complex perceptual deficits in amblyopia (Figs. 40.14–16)[72,136,139,160,232,234,242] The prevalence of binocularly suppressive V1 and V2 neurons is tightly correlated with the depth of amblyopia for individual strabismic or anisometropic monkeys (Fig. 40.14). The level of neural noise of V2 neurons (both spiking irregularity and trial-to-trial variability in spiking described in previous sections) is also positively correlated with the strength of binocular suppression (Fig. 40.15A).[139] Moreover, the level of neural noise in individual amblyopic monkeys is closely associated with the depth of amblyopia (Fig. 40.15B).[139]

The neural basis of more complex anomalies in amblyopic monkeys, such as excessive crowding and position uncertainty,[72,243] deficits in contour integration,[223,244] abnormal topographic mapping of visual space or topographic "jitter,"[245,246] and higher-order cognitive disorders,[247] had not been systematically investigated for monkeys until recent years. Such higher-order perceptual deficits in amblyopes are far more likely to involve abnormal signal processing in extrastriate visual areas.[3,59,72] As described previously, the RF structure of V2 neurons is severely disrupted in V2 of amblyopic monkeys.[137] The extent of such "disarray" of the RF structure for individual amblyopic monkeys is highly correlated with the prevalence of binocularly suppressive

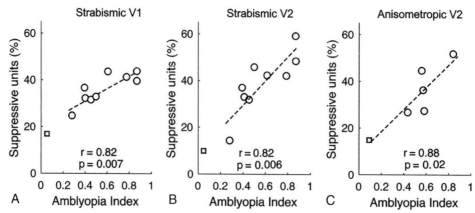

Fig. 40.14 Amblyopia and binocular suppression in monkeys. Relationship between the degree of amblyopia (amblyopia index) and the prevalence of V1 (**A**) and V2 (**B**) neurons exhibiting binocular suppression in strabismic monkeys. Similar relationships in V2 of anisometropic monkeys (**C**). *Square symbols* indicate normal control data. Note that monkeys with more severe amblyopia had a higher prevalence of suppression in V1 and V2. (Redrawn from Tao X, Zhang B, Shen G, et al. Early monocular defocus disrupts the normal development of receptive-field structure in V2 neurons of macaque monkeys. *J. Neurosci.* 2014;34:13840–13854 and Bi H, Zhang B, Tao X, Harwerth RS, Smith EL 3rd, Chino YM. Neuronal responses in visual area V2 (V2) of macaque monkeys with strabismic amblyopia. *Cereb Cortex.* 2011;21:2033–2045.)

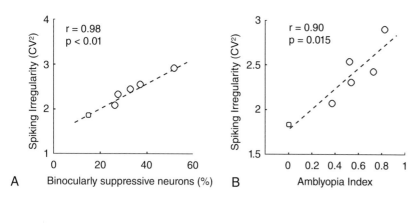

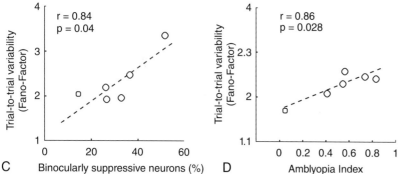

Fig. 40.15 High correlations between degree of amblyopia, suppression, and "neural noise" in monkeys with anisometropic amblyopia. Relationship between spiking irregularity and prevalence of binocularly suppressive V2 neurons (**A**) and the degree of amblyopia (**B**). Similar relationships between trial-to-trial variability (Fano factor) and binocular suppression (**C**) and severity of amblyopia (**D**). *Square symbols* indicate normal controls. (Redrawn from Wang Y, Zhang B, Tao X, Wensveen JM, Smith EL 3rd, Chino YM. Noisy spiking in visual area V2 of amblyopic monkeys. *J Neurosci.* 2017;37:922–935.)

neurons and also with the depth of amblyopia (Fig. 40.16). Finally, the inability of V2 neurons to integrate signals over extended space is also strongly correlated with the depth of amblyopia in anisometropic or strabismic monkeys.[135,137,139]

Improved visual performance in children and adults with developmental disorders

Although the impact of early binocular imbalance on the visual system development becomes increasingly small with age, the mature visual brain is not completely hard-wired and exhibits a wide range

of plasticity.[22,72,78,248–253] However, the nature and the extent of plasticity in the "mature" primary visual cortex (V1) of higher species have been a matter of considerable debate.[72,253–257] As mentioned previously, the level of plasticity in the mature visual cortex of rodents remains relatively high if the "molecular brake" that reduces or eliminates cortical plasticity is removed by drug application or manipulations of "homeostatic synaptic plasticity" (e.g., by dark exposure, TTX application in the eye, or retinal lesions).[72,78,218,249] However, amblyopia therapies or drug treatments based on such discoveries in rodent V1 are either not possible to apply to human infants (e.g., dark exposure, TTX

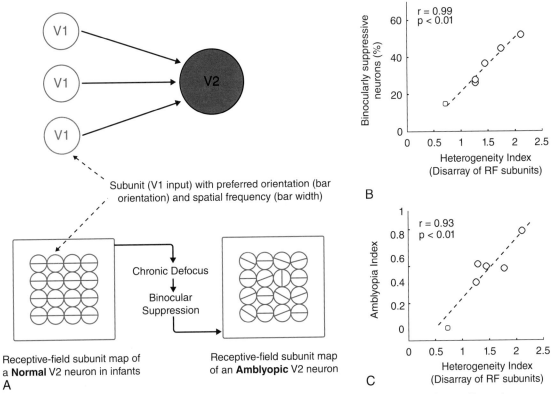

Fig. 40.16 Amblyopia and receptive-field (*RF*) structure of V2 neurons. **(A)** Schematic diagram illustrating a model of how the RF structure of an infant monkey made up of V1 inputs may be disorganized by chronic defocus owing to early anisometropia. **(B)** High correlation between binocularly suppressive V2 neurons and the degree of disarray in receptive-field subunit map. **(C)** High correlation between the severity of amblyopia and the degree of disarray in RF subunit maps. *Square symbols* indicate normal controls. (Panels B and C redrawn from Tao X, Zhang B, Shen G, et al. Early monocular defocus disrupts the normal development of receptive-field structure in V2 neurons of macaque monkeys. *J. Neurosci.* 2014;34:13840–13854.)

application, or retinal lesions) or have not been effective in promoting recovery in higher species including humans.[72,258–261]

Another form of "adult plasticity" that has gained much attention is "perceptual learning" where visual performance improves with repeated practice.[65,72,218,234,253,262] Perceptual learning appears to occur as a result of alterations of functional connections in the primate visual brain (i.e., V1 and higher-order visual areas).[253,263–265] These discoveries have raised the possibility that visual performance of amblyopic children and adults could be improved by training and practice. Indeed, repeated practice significantly improves the performance of amblyopic children and adults for a variety of visual tasks in laboratory settings.[72,262,266,267] The effectiveness of perceptual learning, however, is often limited by the "nature" of the tasks (e.g., highly repetitive and "boring"), low compliance, and/or performance improvement specific to trained stimuli, although improvement transfer has been observed for certain visual tasks.[266–268] To reduce the potentially "negative" impact of the "traditional" perceptual learning approach, amblyopia therapies using *videogames* (action or nonaction) have been widely employed with notable success in improving visual acuity,[234,269,270] stereoacuity,[271,272] and higher cognitive functions.[72,273] The effectiveness of perceptual learning or the videogame application, however, has not been extensively tested in large-scale randomized clinical trials.[72]

Finally, based on studies in V1 and V2 of amblyopic monkeys described previously[137,139,160] and perceptual studies in human amblyopes that demonstrated strong relationships between binocular suppression and monocular perceptual impairments,[229,232,233,274] the "novel" binocular approach has been adopted to treat amblyopia in children, *binocular therapy*.[65,72,234,275–279] The basic idea is to reduce effectively the impact of binocular suppression by training amblyopic children with balanced dichoptic stimuli (e.g., by stimulating the amblyopic eye with "stronger" or more effective stimuli while *simultaneously* stimulating the fellow eye with proportionately less effective stimuli). The outcome of the binocular therapy is somewhat "mixed" depending on testing conditions (e.g., laboratory testing vs. randomized clinical trials), the degree of compliance, and the age of amblyopic children.[72,234,280] Improvement of acuity is generally observed in all settings if the treatment begins at younger ages[234] (but see ref 280). Also, improvement in acuity comparable to that from traditional patching can be achieved by binocular therapies for much shorter periods of treatment time.[234] Importantly, binocular therapy is quite effective in improving binocular functions (e.g., stereoacuity).[234,276,279,281] It is still a matter of considerable debate, however, whether the binocular therapy is *more effective* in improving visual acuity of amblyopic children than traditional patching.[72,234,282,283] Considered together, although the early intervention of abnormal visual conditions during infancy is critical in preventing or minimizing the impact of binocular vision disorders, children of all ages and adults with amblyopia may benefit from well thought out treatment regimens.

SUMMARY

Newborn primates open their eyes and begin to see the world. Because their developing visual brain is highly malleable during early infancy, the maturation of visual functions requires clear unrestricted images in each eye and precise matching of the images of the two eyes. If one eye is deprived of clear vision during the critical period of development causing binocular imbalance, the infant's visual brain is abnormally reorganized. Binocular imbalance commonly results from monocular form deprivation, chronic monocular defocus, and/or large misalignment of visual axes. Anomalous reorganization of the visual brain begins largely in the primary visual cortex (V1), but not in the retina. Neural deficits resulting from early abnormal visual experience are thought to be extensive in visual areas beyond V1. Binocular visual capacities, such as stereopsis and binocular summation of contrast sensitivity, are compromised, and suppression often dominates the developing visual brain under binocular viewing. If the visual conditions responsible for binocular imbalance are untreated during early development, amblyopia is likely to emerge in the affected eye. Animal studies are designed to give insight into the neural basis of developmental vision anomalies and provide key information that is beneficial for establishing effective strategies for the prevention and treatment of binocular vision disorders.

REFERENCES

1. Chino YM, Bi H, Zhang B. The postnatal development of the neuronal response properties in primate visual cortex. In: Kaas J, Collins C, eds. *Primate vision*. Boca Raton: CRC Press, 2004:81–108.
2. Kiorpes L. Visual development in primates: neural mechanisms and critical periods. *Dev. Neurobiol.* 2015;75:1080–1090.
3. Kiorpes L. The puzzle of visual development: behavior and neural limits. *J Neurosci.* 2016;36:11384–11393.
4. Wiesel TN. Postnatal development of the visual cortex and the influence of environment. *Nature.* 1982;299:583–591.
5. Chino YM, Smith 3rd EL, Hatta S, Cheng H. Postnatal development of binocular disparity sensitivity in neurons of the primate visual cortex. *J Neurosci.* 1997;17:296–307.
6. Zhang B, Smith 3rd EL, Chino YM. Postnatal development of onset transient responses in macaque V1 and V2 neurons. *J. Neurophysiol.* 2008;100:1476–1487.
7. Zheng J, Zhang B, Bi H, Watanabe I, Nakatsuka C, Smith 3rd EL, Chino YM. Development of temporal response properties and contrast sensitivity of V1 and V2 neurons in macaque monkeys. *J. Neurophysiol.* 2007;97:3905–3916.
8. Maruko I, Zhang B, Tao X, Tong J, Smith 3rd EL, Chino YM. Postnatal development of disparity sensitivity in visual area 2 (V2) of macaque monkeys. *J Neurophysiol.* 2008;100:2486–2495.
9. Zhang B, Zheng J, Watanabe I, Maruko I, Bi H, Smith 3rd EL, Chino Y. Delayed maturation of receptive field center/surround mechanisms in V2. *Proc Natl Acad Sci U S A.* 2005;102:5862–5867.
10. Zhang B, Tao X, Shen G, Smith 3rd EL, Ohzawa I, Chino YM. Receptive-field subfields of V2 neurons in macaque monkeys are adult-like near birth. *J. Neurosci.* 2013;33:2639–2649.
11. Harwerth RS, Smith 3rd EL. Binocular summation in man and monkey. *Am. J. Optom. Physiol.* 1985;62:439–446.
12. Boothe RG, Dobson V, Teller DY. Postnatal development of vision in human and nonhuman primates. *Annu Rev. Neurosci.* 1985;8:495–545.
13. Birch EE, Gwiazda J, Held R. Stereoacuity development for crossed and uncrossed disparities in human infants. *Vision Res.* 1982;22:507–513.
14. O'Dell C, Boothe RG. The development of stereoacuity in infant rhesus monkeys. *Vision Res.* 1997;37:2675–2684.
15. Kiorpes L. Development of vernier acuity and grating acuity in normally reared monkeys. *Vis Neurosci.* 1992;9:243–251.
16. Horton JC, Hocking DR. An adult-like pattern of ocular dominance columns in striate cortex of newborn monkeys prior to visual experience. *J Neurosci.* 1996;16:1791–1807.
17. Sherman SM, Spear PD. Organization of visual pathways in normal and visually deprived cats. *Physiol Rev.* 1982;62:738–855.
18. Mitchell DE. In: Chalupa LM, Werner JS, eds. *The effects of selected forms of early visual deprivation on perception: The Visual Neuroscience.* Cambridge, MA: MIT Press; 2004:189.
19. Daw NW. *Visual Development.* 3rd ed. New York: Springer; 2013.
20. Hensch TK. Critical period plasticity in local cortical circuits. *Nat Rev Neurosci.* 2005;6:877–888.
21. Tropea D, Van Wart A, Sur M. Molecular mechanisms of experience-dependent plasticity in visual cortex. *Philos Trans R Soc Lond B Biol Sci.* 2009;364:341–355.
22. Hensch TK, Quinlan EM. Critical period in amblyopia. *Vis. Neurosci.* 2018;35:E014.
23. Lee H-K, Kirkwood A. Mechanisms of homeostatic synaptic plasticity *in vivo*. *Front. Cell. Neurosci.* 2019;13:520.
24. LeVay S, Wiesel TN, Hubel DH. The development of ocular dominance columns in normal and visually deprived monkeys. *J Comp Neurol.* 1980;191:1–51.
25. Harwerth RS, Crawford ML, Smith 3rd EL, Boltz RL. Behavioral studies of stimulus deprivation amblyopia in monkeys. *Vision Res.* 1981;21:779–789.
26. Smith 3rd EL, Hung LF. Form-deprivation myopia in monkeys is a graded phenomenon. *Vision Res.* 2000;40:371–381.
27. Harwerth RS, Smith 3rd EL, Crawford ML, von Noorden GK. Behavioral studies of the sensitive periods of development of visual functions in monkeys. *Behav Brain Res.* 1990;41:179–198.
28. Boothe RG, Dobson V, Teller DY. Postnatal development of vision in human and nonhuman primates. *Annu Rev. Neurosci.* 1985;8:495–545.
29. Wiesel TN, Raviola E. Myopia and eye enlargement after neonatal lid fusion in monkeys. *Nature.* 1977;266:66–68.
30. Smith 3rd EL, Harwerth RS, Crawford ML, von Noorden GK. Observations on the effects of form deprivation on the refractive status of the monkey. *Invest Ophthalmol Vis Sci.* 1987;28:1236–1245.
31. Crawford ML, Blake R, Cool SJ, von Noorden GK. Physiological consequences of unilateral and bilateral eye closure in macaque monkeys: some further observations. *Brain Res.* 1975;84:150–154.
32. Harwerth RS, Smith 3rd EL, Paul AD, Crawford ML, Von Noorden GK. Functional effects of bilateral form deprivation in monkeys. *Invest Ophthalmol Vis Sci.* 1991;32:2311–2327.
33. Hubel DH, Wiesel TN. The period of susceptibility to the physiological effects of unilateral eye closure in kittens. *J Physiol.* 1970;206:419–436.
34. Hubel DH, Wiesel TN, LeVay S. Plasticity of ocular dominance columns in monkey striate cortex. *Philos Trans R Soc Lond B Biol Sci.* 1977;278:377–409.
35. Horton JC, Hocking DR. Timing of the critical period for plasticity of ocular dominance columns in macaque striate cortex. *J Neurosci.* 1997;17:3684–3709.
36. Antonini A, Stryker MP. Plasticity of geniculocortical afferents following brief or prolonged monocular occlusion in the cat. *J Comp Neurol.* 1996;369:64–82.
37. Trachtenberg JT, Trepel C, Stryker MP. Rapid extragranular plasticity in the absence of thalamocortical plasticity in the developing primary visual cortex. *Science.* 2000;287:2029–2032.
38. Trachtenberg JT, Stryker MP. Rapid anatomical plasticity of horizontal connections in the developing visual cortex. *J Neurosci.* 2001;21:3476–3482.
39. Sakai E, Bi H, Maruko I, Zhang B, Zheng J, Wensveen J, Harwerth RS, Smith 3rd EL, Chino YM. Cortical effects of brief daily periods of unrestricted vision during early monocular form deprivation. *J Neurophysiol.* 2006;95:2856–2865.
40. Levi DM. Visual processing in amblyopia: human studies. *Strabismus.* 2006;14:11–19.
41. Vital-Durand F, Garey LJ, Blakemore C. Monocular and binocular deprivation in the monkey: morphological effects and reversibility. *Brain Res.* 1978;158:45–64.
42. Blakemore C, Vital-Durand F. Effects of visual deprivation on the development of the monkey's lateral geniculate nucleus. *J Physiol.* 1986;380:493–511.
43. Levitt JB, Schumer RA, Sherman SM, Spear PD, Movshon JA. Visual response properties of neurons in the LGN of normally reared and visually deprived macaque monkeys. *J Neurophysiol.* 2001;85:2111–2129.
44. Chino YM, Kaplan E. Abnormal orientation bias of LGN neurons in strabismic cats. *Invest Ophthalmol Vis Sci.* 1988;29:644–648.
45. Chino YM, Cheng H, Smith 3rd EL, Garraghty PE, Roe AW, Sur M. Early discordant binocular vision disrupts signal transfer in the lateral geniculate nucleus. *Proc Natl Acad Sci U S A.* 1994;91:6938–6942.
46. Cheng H, Chino YM, Smith 3rd EL, Hamamoto J, Yoshida K. Transfer characteristics of X LGN neurons in cats reared with early discordant binocular vision. *J Neurophysiol.* 1995;74:2558–2572.
47. Blake R, Hirsch HV. Deficits in binocular depth perception in cats after alternating monocular deprivation. *Science.* 1975;190:1114–1116.
48. Tieman DG, McCall MA, Hirsch HV. Physiological effects of unequal alternating monocular exposure. *J Neurophysiol.* 1983;49:804–818.
49. Wensveen JM, Harwerth RS, Hung LF, Ramamirtham R, Kee CS, Smith 3rd EL. Brief daily periods of unrestricted vision can prevent form-deprivation amblyopia. *Invest Ophthalmol Vis Sci.* 2006;47:2468–2477.
50. Das VE, Mustari MJ. Correlation of cross-axis eye movements and motoneuron activity in non-human primates with "A" pattern strabismus. *Invest Ophthalmol Vis Sci.* 2007;48:665–674.
51. Fu L, Tusa RJ, Mustari MJ, Das VE. Horizontal saccade disconjugacy in strabismic monkeys. *Invest Ophthalmol Vis Sci.* 2007;48:3107–3114.
52. Das VE. Strabismus and the oculomotor system: insight from macaque models. *Annu Rev Vis Sci.* 2016;2:37–59.
53. Harwerth RS, Smith 3rd EL, Crawford ML, von Noorden GK. The effects of reverse monocular deprivation in monkeys. I. Psychophysical experiments. *Exp Brain Res.* 1989;74:327–347.
54. Crawford ML, de Faber JT, Harwerth RS, Smith 3rd EL, von Noorden GK. The effects of reverse monocular deprivation in monkeys. II. Electrophysiological and anatomical studies. *Exp Brain Res.* 1989;74:338–347.
55. Mitchell DE, Sengpiel F. Neural mechanisms of recovery following early visual deprivation. *Phil Trans R Soc Lond B Biol Sci.* 2009;364:383–398.
56. Smith 3rd EL, Hung LF. The role of optical defocus in regulating refractive development in infant monkeys. *Vision Res.* 1999;39:1415–1435.
57. Smith 3rd EL, Hung LF, Harwerth RS. The degree of image degradation and the depth of amblyopia. *Invest Ophthalmol Vis Sci.* 2000;41:3775–3781.
58. Smith EL, Hung LF, Kee CS, Qiao Y. Effects of brief periods of unrestricted vision on the development of form-deprivation myopia in monkeys. *Invest Ophthalmol Vis Sci.* 2002;43:291–299.

59. Kiorpes L. Understanding the development of amblyopia using macaque monkey models. *Proc Natl Acad Sci USA.* 2019;116:26217–26223.

60. Harwerth RS, Smith 3rd EL, Duncan GC, Crawford ML, von Noorden GK. Multiple sensitive periods in the development of the primate visual system. *Science.* 1986;232:235–238.

61. Birch EE, Stager DR. Prevalence of good visual acuity following surgery for congenital unilateral cataract. *Arch Ophthalmol.* 1988;106:40–43.

62. Drummond GT, Scott WE, Keech RV. Management of monocular congenital cataracts. *Arch Ophthalmol.* 1989;107:45–51.

63. Wright KW, Matsumoto E, Edelman PM. Binocular fusion and stereopsis associated with early surgery for monocular congenital cataracts. *Arch Ophthalmol.* 1992;110:1607–1609.

64. Holmes JM, Lazar EI, Melia BM, et al. Effect of age on response to amblyopia treatment in children. *Arch. Ophthalmol.* 2011;129:1451–1457.

65. Birch EE. Amblyopia and binocular vision. *Prog. Retin. Eye Res.* 2013;33:67–84.

66. Olson CR, Freeman RD. Profile of the sensitive period for monocular deprivation in kittens. *Exp Brain Res.* 1980;39:17–21.

67. Wiesel TN, Hubel DH. Single-cell responses in striate cortex of kittens deprived of vision in one eye. *J Neurophysiol.* 1963;26:1003–1017.

68. Fagiolini M, Pizzorusso T, Berardi N, Domenici L, Maffei L. Functional postnatal development of the rat primary visual cortex and the role of visual experience: dark rearing and monocular deprivation. *Vision Res.* 1994;34:709–720.

69. Gordon JA, Stryker MP. Experience-dependent plasticity of binocular responses in the primary visual cortex of the mouse. *J Neurosci.* 1996;16:3274–3286.

70. Issa NP, Trachtenberg JT, Chapman B, Zahs KR, Stryker MP. The critical period for ocular dominance plasticity in the ferret's visual cortex. *J Neurosci.* 1999;19:6965–6978.

71. Berardi N, Pizzorusso T, Maffei L. Critical periods during sensory development. *Curr Opin Neurobiol.* 2000;10:138–145.

72. Levi DM. Rethinking amblyopia 2020. *Vision Res.* 2020;176:118–129.

73. Gilbert CD, Li W. Adult visual cortical plasticity. *Neuron.* 2012;75:250–264.

74. Wang Q, Burkhalter A. Area map of mouse visual cortex. *J Comp Neurol.* 2007;502:339–357.

75. Niell CM, Stryker MP. Highly selective receptive fields in mouse visual cortex. *J Neurosci.* 2008;28:7520–7536.

76. Hooks BM, Chen C. Critical periods in the visual system: changing views for a model of experience-dependent plasticity. *Neuron.* 2007;56:312–326.

77. Van den Bergh G, Zhang B, Arckens L, Chino YM. Receptive-field properties of V1 and V2 neurons in mice and macaque monkeys. *J Comp Neurol.* 2010;518:2051–2070.

78. Morishita H, Hensch TK. Critical period revisited: impact on vision. *Curr Opin Neurobiol.* 2008;18:101–107.

79. Hooks BM, Chen C. Circuitry underlying experience-dependent plasticity in the mouse visual system. *Neuron.* 2020;106:21–36.

80. Antonini A, Stryker MP. Rapid remodeling of axonal arbors in the visual cortex. *Science.* 1993;260:1819–1821.

81. Frenkel MY, Bear MF. How monocular deprivation shifts ocular dominance in visual cortex of young mice. *Neuron.* 2004;44:917–923.

82. Song S, Miller KD, Abbott LF. Competitive Hebbian learning through spike-timing-dependent synaptic plasticity. *Nat Neurosci.* 2000;3:919–926.

83. Bi G, Poo M. Synaptic modification by correlated activity: Hebb's postulate revisited. *Annu Rev Neurosci.* 2001;24:139–166.

84. El-Boustanin S,I,J,P,K, Brenton-Provencher V, Knott GW, Okuno H, Bito H, Sur M. Locally coordinated synaptic plasticity of visual cortex neurons in vivo. *Science.* 2018;360:1349–1354.

85. Liesman J. Glutamatergic synapses are structurally and biochemically complex because of multiple plasticity: long-term potentiation, long-term depression, short-term potentiation and scaling. *Phil. Trans. R. Soc. B.* 2017;372:20160260.

86. Heinen K, Baker RE, Spijker S, Rosahl T, van Pelt J, Brussaard AB. Impaired dendritic spine maturation in GABAA receptor alpha1 subunit knock out mice. *Neuroscience.* 2003;122:699–705.

87. Artola A, Brocher S, Singer W. Different voltage-dependent thresholds for inducing long-term depression and long-term potentiation in slices of rat visual cortex. *Nature.* 1990;347:69–72.

88. Heynen AJ, Yoon BJ, Liu CH, Chung HJ, Huganir RL, Bear MF. Molecular mechanism for loss of visual cortical responsiveness following brief monocular deprivation. *Nat Neurosci.* 2003;6:854–862.

89. Espinosa JS, Stryker MP. Development and plasticity of the primary visual cortex. *Neuron.* 2012;75:230–249.

90. Lambo ME, Tarringlano GG. Synaptic and intrinsic homeostatic mechanisms cooperate to increase L2/3 pyramidal neuron excitability during the late phase of critical period plasticity. *J. Neurosci.* 2013;33:8810–8819.

91. Sur M. Mechanisms of plasticity in the developing and adult visual cortex. *Prog. Brain Res.* 2013;207:243–254.

92. Liu L, Wong TP, Pozza MF, Lingenhoehl K, Wang Y, Sheng M, Auberson YP, Wang YT. Role of NMDA receptor subtypes in governing the direction of hippocampal synaptic plasticity. *Science.* 2004;304:1021–1024.

93. Massey PV, Johnson BE, Moult PR, Auberson YP, Brown MW, Molnar E, Collingridge GL, Bashir ZI. Differential roles of NR2A and NR2B-containing NMDA receptors in cortical long-term potentiation and long-term depression. *J Neurosci.* 2004;24:7821–7828.

94. Cho KK, Khibnik L, Philpot BD, Bear MF. The ratio of NR2A/B NMDA receptor subunits determines the qualities of ocular dominance plasticity in visual cortex. *Proc Natl Acad Sci U S A.* 2009;106:5377–5382.

95. Daw NW, Reid SN, Beaver CJ. Development and function of metabotropic glutamate receptors in cat visual cortex. *J Neurobiol.* 1999;41:102–107.

96. Wang XF, Daw NW. Long term potentiation varies with layer in rat visual cortex. *Brain Res.* 2003;989:26–34.

97. Dolen G, Bear MF. Role for metabotropic glutamate receptor 5 (mGluR5) in the pathogenesis of fragile X syndrome. *J Physiol.* 2008;586:1503–1508.

98. Rodoriguez G, Mesik L, Gao M, Parkins S, Saha R, Lee HK. Disruption of NDMA receptors function prevents normal experience-dependent homeostatic synaptic plasticity in mouse primary visual cortex. *J. Neurosci.* 2019;39:2117–2118.

99. Jiang B, Trevino M, Kirkwood A. Sequential development of long-term potentiation and depression in different layers of the mouse visual cortex. *J Neurosci.* 2007;27:9648–9652.

100. Pham TA, Impey S, Storm DR, Stryker MP. CRE-mediated gene transcription in neocortical neuronal plasticity during the developmental critical period. *Neuron.* 1999;22:63–72.

101. Mower AF, Liao DS, Nestler EJ, Neve RL, Ramoa AS. cAMP/Ca2+ response element-binding protein function is essential for ocular dominance plasticity. *J Neurosci.* 2002;22:2237–2245.

102. Cancedda L, Putignano E, Impey S, Maffei L, Ratto GM, Pizzorusso T. Patterned vision causes CRE-mediated gene expression in the visual cortex through PKA and ERK. *J Neurosci.* 2003;23:7012–7020.

103. Majewska A, Sur M. Motility of dendritic spines in visual cortex in vivo: changes during the critical period and effects of visual deprivation. *Proc Natl Acad Sci U S A.* 2003;100:16024–16029.

104. Oray S, Majewska A, Sur M. Dendritic spine dynamics are regulated by monocular deprivation and extracellular matrix degradation. *Neuron.* 2004;44:1021–1040.

105. Fox K, Stryker MD. Integrating Hebbian and homeostatic plasticity: introduction. *Phil. Trans. R. Soc. B.* 2017;372:20160413.

106. Bridi MCD, De Pasquale Lantz GI, Gu Y, Borrell A, Choi SY, He K, Tran T, Hong SZ, Dykman A, Lee K, Quinlan EM, Kirkwood A. Two distinct mechanisms for experience-dependent homeostasis. *Nat. Neurosci.* 2018;21:843–850.

107. Lee H-K, Kirkwood A. Mechanisms of homeostatic synaptic plasticity in vivo. *Front. Cell. Neurosci.* 2019;13:520.

108. Kirkwood A, Riout MC, Bear MF. Experience-dependent modification of synaptic plasticity in visual cortex. *Nature.* 1996;381:526–528.

109. Cooper LN, bear MF. The BCM theory of synaptic modification at 30: interaction of theory with experiment. *Nat. Rev. Neurosci.* 2012;13:798–810.

110. Guo Y, Huang S, Pasquale R, McGehrin K, Zao K, Kirkwood A. Dark exposure extends the integration window for spike-timing-dependent plasticity. *J. Neurosci.* 2012;32:15027–15035.

111. Turringlano GG, Nelson SB. Homeostatic plasticity in the developing nervous system. *Nat. Rev. Neurosci.* 2004;5:97–107.

112. Kasamatsu T, Pettigrew JD. Depletion of brain catecholamines: failure of ocular dominance shift after monocular occlusion in kittens. *Science.* 1976;194:206–209.

113. Bear MF, Singer W. Modulation of visual cortical plasticity by acetylcholine and noradrenaline. *Nature.* 1986;320:172–176.

114. Gu Q, Singer W. Involvement of serotonin in developmental plasticity of kitten visual cortex. *Eur J Neurosci.* 1995;7:1146–1153.

115. Stackman RW, Hammond RS, Linardatos E, Gerlach A, Maylie J, Adelman JP, Tzounopoulos T. Small conductance Ca2+ activate K+ channels modulate synaptic plasticity and memory encoding. *J. Neurosci.* 2002;22:10163–10171.

116. Giessel AJ, Sabatini BI. M1 Muscarinic receptors boost synaptic potential and calcium influx in dendritic spines by inhibiting postsynaptic SK channels. *Neurons.* 2010;68:936–947.

117. Stowell RD, Sipe GO, Dawes RP, Batchelor HN, Lordy KA, Whitelaw BS, Stoessel M, Bladiak JM, Brown E, Sur M, Majewska AK. Noradrenergic signaling in the wakeful state inhibits microglial surveillance and synaptic plasticity in the mouse visual cortex. *Nat. Neurosci.* 2019;22:1782–1792.

118. Obermayer J, Verhoog MB, Luchicchi A, Mansvelder HD. Cholinergic modulation of cortical microcircuits is layer-specific: evidence from rodent, monkey, and human brain. *Front. Neural Circuits.* 2017;11:100.

119. Chen N, Sugihara H, Sur M. An acetylcholine activated microcircuit drives temporal dynamics of cortical activity. *Nat Neurosci.* 2015;18:892–902.

120. Sugihara H, Chen N, Sur M. Cell specific modulation of plasticity and cortical state by cholinergic inputs to the visual cortex. *J. Physiol. Paris.* 2016;110:37–43.

121. Schafer DP, Lehrman EK, Stevens B. The "quad-partite" synapses: microglia-synapse interactions in the developing and mature CNS. *Glia.* 2013;61:24–36.

122. Parkhurst CN, Yang G, Ninan I, et al. Microglia promote learning-dependent synapse formation through brain-derived neurotrophic factor. *Cell.* 2013;155:1596–1609.

123. Sipe GO, Lowery RL, Tremblay M-E, Kelly EA, Lamantia CE, Majewaska AK. Microglia P2Y12 is necessary for synaptic plasticity in mouse visual cortex. *Nature Commun.* 2016;7:10905.

124. Mataga N, Mizuguchi Y, Hensch TK. Experience-dependent pruning of dendritic spines in visual cortex by tissue plasminogen activator. *Neuron.* 2004;44:1031–1041.

125. Fagiolini M, Fritschy JM, Low K, Mohler H, Rudolph U, Hensch TK. Specific GABAA circuits for visual cortical plasticity. *Science.* 2004;303:1681–1683.

126. Yaeger CE, Ringach D, Trachtenberg JT. Neuromodulatory control of localized dendritic spiking in critical period cortex. *Nature.* 2019;567:100–104.

127. Huang ZJ, Kirkwood A, Pizzorusso T, Porciatti V, Morales B, Bear MF, Maffei L, Tonegawa S. BDNF regulates the maturation of inhibition and the critical period of plasticity in mouse visual cortex. *Cell.* 1999;98:739–755.

128. Hanover JL, Huang ZJ, Tonegawa S, Stryker MP.) Brain-derived neurotrophic factor overexpression induces precocious critical period in mouse visual cortex. *J Neurosci.* 199919: p. RC40 (1–5).

129. Kirkwood A, Rozas C, Kirkwood J, Perez F, Bear MF. Modulation of long-term synaptic depression in visual cortex by acetylcholine and norepinephrine. *J Neurosci.* 1999;19:1599–1609.

130. Smith 3rd EL, Hung LF, Harwerth RS. Effects of optically induced blur on the refractive status of young monkeys. *Vision Res.* 1994;34:293–301.

131. Smith 3rd EL. Spectacle lenses and emmetropization: the role of optical defocus in regulating ocular development. *Optom Vis Sci.* 1998;75:388–398.

132. Wensveen JM, Harwerth RS, Smith 3rd EL. Binocular deficits associated with early alternating monocular defocus. I. Behavioral observations. *J Neurophysiol.* 2003;90:3001–3011.

133. Kiorpes L, Boothe RG, Hendrickson AE, Movshon JA, Eggers HM, Gizzi MS. Effects of early unilateral blur on the macaque's visual system. I. Behavioral observations. *J Neurosci.* 1987;7:1318–1326.

134. Kiorpes L, Kiper DC, O'Keefe LP, Cavanaugh JR, Movshon JA. Neuronal correlates of amblyopia in the visual cortex of macaque monkeys with experimental strabismus and anisometropia. *J Neurosci.* 1998;18:6411–6424.

135. Smith 3rd EL, Harwerth RS, Crawford ML. Spatial contrast sensitivity deficits in monkeys produced by optically induced anisometropia. *Invest Ophthalmol Vis Sci.* 1985;26:330–342.

136. Smith 3rd EL, Chino YM, NJ, Cheng H, Crawford ML, Harwerth RS. Residual binocular interactions in the striate cortex of monkeys reared with abnormal binocular vision. *J Neurophysiol.* 1997;78:1353–1362.

137. Tao X, Zhang B, Shen G, et al. Early monocular defocus disrupts the normal development of receptive-field structure in V2 neurons of macaque monkeys. *J. Neurosci.* 2014;34:13840–13854.

138. Shooner C, Hallum LE, Kumbhani RD, Garcia-Marin V, Kelly JG, Majaj NJ, Movshon JA, Kiorpes L. Population representation of visual information in area V1 and V2 of amblyopic monkeys. *Vision. Res.* 2015;114:56–67.

139. Wang Y, Zhang B, Tao X, Wensveen JM, Smith 3rd EL, Chino YM. Noisy spiking in visual area V2 of amblyopic monkeys. *J. Neurosci.* 2017;37:922–935.

140. Smith 3rd EL, Hung L-F, Arumugan B, Wensveen JM, Chino Y,M, Harwerth RS. Observations on the relationship between anisometropia, amblyopia and strabismus. *Vison Res.* 2017;134:26–42.

141. Movshon JA, Eggers HM, Gizzi MS, Hendrickson AE, Kiorpes L, Boothe RG. Effects of early unilateral blur on the macaque's visual system. III. Physiological observations. *J Neurosci.* 1987;7:1340–1351.

142. Kiorpes L, Daw N. Cortical correlates of amblyopia. *Vis. Neurosci.* 2018;35:E016.

143. El-Shamayleh Y, Kiorpes L, Kohn A, Movshon JA. Visual motion processing by neurons in area MT of macaque monkeys with experimental amblyopia. *J. Neurosci.* 2010;30:12198–12209.

144. Zhang B, Matsuura K, Mori T, Wensveen JM, Harwerth RS, Smith 3rd EL, Chino Y. Binocular deficits associated with early alternating monocular defocus. II. Neurophysiological observations. *J Neurophysiol.* 2003;90:3012–3023.

145. Schor CM, Wood IC, Ogawa J. Spatial tuning of static and dynamic local stereopsis. *Vision Res.* 1984;24:573–578.

146. Yang Y, Blake R. Spatial frequency tuning of human stereopsis. *Vision Res.* 1991;31:1177–1189.

147. Cumming BG, Parker AJ. Responses of primary visual cortical neurons to binocular disparity without depth perception. *Nature.* 1997;389:280–283.

148. Cumming BG, Parker AJ. Local disparity not perceived depth is signaled by binocular neurons in cortical area V1 of the Macaque. *J. Neurosci.* 2000;20:4758–4767.

149. Birch EE. Stereopsis in infants and its developmental relation to visual acuity, in *Early.* In: Simons K, ed. *Development: Normal and Abnormal.* Oxford, U.K: Oxford University Press; 1993.

150. Crawford MI, von Noorden GK. Optically induced concomitant strabismus in monkeys. *Invest. Ophthalmol. Vis Sci.* 1980;19:1105–1109.

151. von Noorden GK. *Binocular Vision and Ocular Motility: Theory and Management.* 5th ed. St. Louis: Mosby; 1996.

152. Das VE. Strabismus and the oculomotor system: Insight from macaque models. *Annu Rev Vis. Sci.* 2016;2:37–59.

153. Quick MW, Eggers HM, Boothe RG. Natural strabismus in monkeys: convergence errors assessed by cover test and photographic methods. *Invest Ophthalmol Vis Sci.* 1992;33:2986–3004.

154. Fawcett SL, Birch EE. Risk factors for abnormal binocular vision after successful alignment of accommodative esotropia. *J AAPOS.* 2003;7:256–262.

155. Birch EE, Fawcett SL, Morale SE, Weakley Jr. DR, Wheaton DH. Risk factors for accommodative esotropia among hypermetropic children. *Invest Ophthalmol Vis Sci.* 2005;46:526–529.

156. Birch EE, Wang J. Stereoacuity outcomes after treatment of infantile and accommodative Esotropia. *Optom Vis Sci.* 2009;86:647–652.

157. Crawford ML, Harwerth RS, Smith 3rd EL, von Noorden GK. Loss of stereopsis in monkeys following prismatic binocular dissociation during infancy. *Behav Brain Res.* 1996;79:207–218.

158. Harwerth RS, Smith 3rd EL, Crawford ML, von Noorden GK. Stereopsis and disparity vergence in monkeys with subnormal binocular vision. *Vision Res.* 1997;37:483–493.

159. Wensveen JM, Harwerth RS, Smith 3rd EL. Clinical suppression in monkeys reared with abnormal binocular visual experience. *Vision Res.* 2001;41:1593–1608.

160. Bi H, Zhang B, Tao X, Harwerth RS, Smith 3rd EL, Chino YM. Neuronal responses in visual area V2 (V2) of macaque monkeys with strabismic amblyopia. *Cereb Cortex.* 2011;21:2033–2045.

161. Chino YM, Shansky MS, Jankowski WI, Banser FA. Effects of rearing kittens with convergent strabismus on development of receptive-field properties of striate cortex neurons. *J. Neurosci.* 1983;50:265–286.

162. Scholl B, Tan AY, Priebe NJ. Strabismus disrupts binocular synaptic integration in primary visual cortex. *J. Neurosci.* 2013;33:17108–17120.

163. Kumagami T, Zhang B, Smith 3rd EL, Chino YM. Effect of onset age of strabismus on the binocular responses of neurons in the monkey visual cortex. *Invest Ophthalmol Vis Sci.* 2000;41:948–954.

164. Mori T, Matsuura K, Zhang B, Smith 3rd EL, Chino YM. Effects of the duration of early strabismus on the binocular responses of neurons in the monkey visual cortex (V1). *Invest Ophthalmol Vis Sci.* 2002;43:1262–1269.

165. Wong AM, Foeller P, Bradley D, Burkhalter A, Tychsen L. Early versus delayed repair of infantile strabismus in macaque monkeys: I. Ocular motor effects. *J AAPOS.* 2003;7:200–209.

166. Tychsen L, Wong AM, Foeller P, Bradley D. Early versus delayed repair of infantile strabismus in macaque monkeys: II. Effects on motion visually evoked responses. *Invest Ophthalmol Vis Sci.* 2004;45:821–827.

167. Zhang B, Bi H, Sakai E, et al. Rapid plasticity of binocular connections in developing monkey visual cortex (V1). *Proc Natl Acad Sci U S A.* 2005;102:9026–9031.

168. Richards M, Wong A, Foeller P, Bradley D, Tychsen L. Duration of binocular decorrelation predicts the severity of latent (fusion maldevelopment) nystagmus in strabismic macaque monkeys. *Invest Ophthalmol Vis Sci.* 2008;49:1872–1878.

169. Nakatsuka C, Zhang B, Watanabe I, Zheng J, Bi H, Ganz L, Smith 3rd EL, Harwerth RS, Chino YM. Effects of perceptual learning on local stereopsis and neuronal responses of V1 and V2 in prism-reared monkeys. *J. Neurophysiol.* 2007;97:2612–2626.

170. Das VE, Mustari MJ. Correlation of cross-axis eye movements and motor neuron activity in non-human primates with "A" pattern strabismus. *Invest. Ophthalmol. Vis. Sci.* 2007;48:665–674.

171. Harwerth RS, Smith 3rd EL, Boltz RL, Crawford ML, von Noorden GK. Behavioral studies on the effect of abnormal early visual experience in monkeys: spatial modulation sensitivity. *Vision Res.* 1983;23:1501–1510.

172. Crawford ML, von Noorden GK. The effects of short-term experimental strabismus on the visual system in Macaca mulatta. *Invest Ophthalmol Vis Sci.* 1979;18:496–505.

173. Crawford ML, von Noorden GK, Meharg LS, Rhodes JW, Harwerth RS, Smith 3rd EL, Miller DD. Binocular neurons and binocular function in monkeys and children. *Invest Ophthalmol Vis Sci.* 1983;24:491–495.

174. Kiorpes L, Walton PJ, O'Keefe LP, Movshon JA, Lisberger SG. Effects of early-onset artificial strabismus on pursuit eye movements and on neuronal responses in area MT of macaque monkeys. *J Neurosci.* 1996;16:6537–6553.

175. Chino YM, Smith 3rd EL, Yoshida K, Cheng H, Hamamoto J. Binocular interactions in striate cortical neurons of cats reared with discordant visual inputs. *J. Neurosci.* 1994;14:5050–5067.

176. Sengpiel F, Blakemore C, Kind PC, Harrad R. Interocular suppression in the visual cortex of strabismic cats. *J. Neurosci.* 1994;14:6855–6871.

177. Adams DL, Economides JR, Sincich LC, Horton JC. Cortical metabolic activity matches the pattern of visual suppression in strabismus. *J. Neurosci.* 2014;33:3752–3759.

178. Economides JR, Adams DL, Horton JC. Interocular suppression in primary visual cortex in strabismus. *J. Neurosci.* 2021;41:5522–5533.

179. Wright KW. Strabismus management. *Curr Opin Ophthalmol.* 1994;5(5):25–29.

180. Birch EE, Stager DR, Everett ME. Random dot stereoacuity following surgical correction of infantile esotropia. *J Pediatr Ophthalmol Strabismus.* 1995;32:231–235.

181. Birch EE, Fawcett S, Stager DR. Why does early surgical alignment improve stereoacuity outcomes in infantile esotropia? *J AAPOS.* 2000;4:10–14.

182. Fawcett S, Birch EE. Factors influencing stereoacuity in accommodative esotropia. *JAAPOS.* 2000;4:15–20.

183. Ing MR, Okino LM. Outcome study of stereopsis in relation to duration on misalignment in congenital esotropia. *JAAPOS.* 2002;6:3–8.

184. Hasany A, Wong A, Foeller P, Bradley D, Tychsen L. Duration of binocular decorrelation in infancy predicts the severity of nasotemporal pursuit asymmetries in strabismic macaque monkeys. *Neuroscience.* 2008;156:403–411.

185. Hatta S, Kumagami T, Qian J, Thornton M, Smith 3rd EL, Chino YM. Nasotemporal directional bias of V1 neurons in young infant monkeys. *Invest Ophthalmol Vis Sci.* 1998;39:2259–2267.

186. Endo M, Kaas JH, Jain N, Smith 3rd EL, Chino Y. Binocular cross-orientation suppression in the primary visual cortex (V1) of infant rhesus monkeys. *Invest Ophthalmol Vis Sci.* 2000;41:4022–4031.

187. Zhang B, Bi H, Sakai E, Maruko I, Zheng J, Smith 3rd EL, Chino YM. Rapid plasticity of binocular connections in developing monkey visual cortex (V1). *Proc. Nat. Acad Sci.* 2005;102:9026–9031.

188. Das VE, Fu LN, Mustari MJ, Tusa RJ. Incomittance in monkeys with strabismus. *Strabismus.* 2005;13:33–41.

189. Guyton DL. Dissociated vertical deviation: etiology, mechanisms, and associated phenomena. Costenbarder lecture. *J AAAPOS.* 2000;4:131–134.

190. Das VE. Alternating fixation and saccade behavior in non-human primates with alternating occlusion induced exotropia. *Invest. Ophthalmol. Vis. Sci.* 2009;50:3703–3710.

191. Economides JR, Adams DI, Joeson CM, Horton JC. Oculomotor behavior in macaque with surgical exotropia. *J. Neurophysiol.* 2007;98:3411–3422.

192. Agaoglu MN, LeSage SK, Joshi AC, Das VE. Spatial pattern of fixation switch behavior in strabismic monkeys. *Invest. Ophthalmol. Vis. Sci.* 2014;55:1259–1268.

193. Tusa RJ, Mustari MJ, Burrows AF, Fuchs AF. Gaze-stabilizing deficits and latent nystagmus in monkeys with brief, early onset visual deprivation: eye movement recordings. *J. Neurophysiol.* 2001;86:651–661.

194. Subramanian V, Jost RM, Birch EE. A quantitative study of fixation stability in amblyopia. *Invest. Ophthalmol. Vis. Sci.* 2013;54:1998–2003.

195. Chung ST, Kumar G, Li RW, Levi DM. Characteristics of fixation eye movements in amblyopia: limitation on fixation stability and acuity? *Vision Res.* 2015;114:87–99.

196. Pirdanka OH, Das VE. Influence of Target parameters on fixation stability in normal and strabismic monkeys. *Invest. Ophthalmol. Vis. Sci.* 2016;57:1087–1095.

197. Bosworth RG, Birch EE. Direction-of-motion detection and motion VEP asymmetries in normal children and children with infantile esotropia. *Invest Ophthalmol Vis Sci.* 2007;48:5523–5531.

198. Brown RJ, Wilson JR, Norcia AM, Boothe RG. Development of directional motion symmetry in the monocular visually evoked potential of infant monkeys. *Vision Res.* 1998;38:1253–1263.

199. Zhang B, Stevenson SS, Cheng H, Laron M, Kumar G, Tong J, Chino YM. Effects of fixation instability on multifocal VEP (mfVEP) responses in amblyopes. *J Vis.* 2008;8(16):1–14.
200. Kapoula Z, Bucci MP, Egger T, Garraud I. Impairment of the binocular coordination of saccades in strabismus. *Vis. Res.* 1997;37:2757–2766.
201. Walton MM, Ono S, Mustari MJ. Vertical and oblique saccadic disconjugacy in strabismus. *Invest. Ophthalmol. Vis. Sci.* 2014;55:275–290.
202. Ghasia FF, Shaikh AG, Jacobs J, Walker MF. Cross-coupled eye movement supports neural origin of pattern strabismus. *Invest. Ophthalmol. Vis Sci.* 2015;56:2855–2866.
203. Tycshen L, Wong AM, Burkhalter A. Paucity of horizontal connections for binocular vision in V1 of naturally strabismic macaques: Cytochrome oxidase compartment specificity. *J. Comp. Neurol.* 2004;474:261–275.
204. Watanabe I, Bi H, Zhang B, Sakai E, Mori T, Harwerth RS, Smith 3rd EL, Chino YM. Directional bias of neurons in V1 and V2 of strabismic monkeys: temporal-to-nasal asymmetry? *Invest Ophthalmol Vis Sci.* 2005;46:3899–3905.
205. Tychsen L. Causing and curing infantile esotropia in primates: the role of decorrelated binocular input (an American Ophthalmological Society thesis). *Trans Am Ophthalmol Soc.* 2007;105:564–593.
206. Mustari MJ, Tusa RJ, Burrows AF, Fuchs AF, Livingston CA. Gaze-stabilizing deficits and latent nystagmus in monkeys with early onset visual deprivation: role of the pretectum NOT. *J. Neurophysiol.* 2001;86:662–675.
207. Mustari MJ, Ono S, Vitolleo KC. How disturbed visual processing early in life leads to disorders of gaze-holding and smooth pursuit. *Prog. Brain Res.* 2008;171:487–495.
208. Tychsen L, Richards M, Wong A, Foeller P, Bradely D, Burkhalter A. The neural mechanisms for latent (fusion maldevelopment) nystagmus. *J. Neuroophthalmol.* 2010;30: 276–283.
209. Mustari MJ, Ono S. Neural mechanisms for smooth pursuit in strabismus. *Ann. N. Y. Acad. Sci.* 2011;1233:187–193.
210. Joshi AC, Das VE. Muscimol inactivation of caudal fastigial nucleus and posterior interposed nucleus in monkeys with strabismus. *J. Neurophysiol.* 2013;110:1882–1891.
211. Simmonsz HJ, Kolling GH. Best age for surgery for infantile esotropia. *Eur. J. Paediatr Neurol.* 2011;15:205–208.
212. McKee SP, Levi DM, Movshon JA. The pattern of visual deficits in amblyopia. *J Vis.* 2003;3: 380–405.
213. Levi DM, McKee SP, Movshon JA. Visual deficits in anisometropia. *Vision Res.* 2011;51: 48–57.
214. Levi DM, Knill DC, Bevelier D. Stereopsis and amblyopia: a mini-review. *Vision Res.* 2015; 114:17–30.
215. Maurer D, McKee SP. Classification and diversity of amblyopia. *Visual Neurosci.* 2018;35:E012.
216. Levi DM, Klein SA. Noise provides some new signals about the spatial vision of amblyopes. *J. Neurosci.* 2003;23:2522–2526.
217. Pelli DG, Levi DM, Chung ST. Using visual noise to characterize amblyopic letter identification. *J Vis.* 2004;4:904–920.
218. Levi DM, Klein SA, Chen I. What limits performance in the amblyopic visual system: seeing signals in noise with an amblyopic brain. *J. Vision.* 2008;8:1–23.
219. Wong EH, Levi DM, McGraw PV. Is second-order spatial loss in amblyopia explained by the loss of first-order spatial input? *Vision Res.* 2001;41:2951–2960.
220. Chung STL, Li RW, Levi DM. Identification of letters from perceptual learning in adults with amblyopia. *Vision Res.* 2006;46:3853–3861.
221. Chandna A, Pennefather PM, Kovacs I, Norcia AM. Contour integration deficits in anisometropic amblyopia. *Invest Ophthalmol Vis Sci.* 2001;42:875–878.
222. Mussap AJ, Levi DM. Orientation-based texture segmentation in strabismic amblyopia. *Vision Res.* 1999;39:411–418.
223. Kozma P, Kiorpes L. Contour integration in amblyopic monkeys. *Vis Neurosci.* 2003;20: 577–588.
224. Kiorpes L, Tang C, Movshon JA. Sensitivity to visual motion in amblyopic macaque monkeys. *Vision Res.* 2006;39:4125–4160.
225. Westheimer G, McKee SP. Stereoscopic acuity with defocused and spatially filtered retinal images. *J. Opt. Soc. Am.* 1980;70:772–778.
226. Legge GE, Gu Y. Stereopsis and contrast. *Vision Res.* 1989;29:989–1004.
227. Hess RF. The site and nature of suppression in squint amblyopia. *Vision Res.* 1991;31:111–117.
228. Harrad RA, Hess RF. Binocular integration of contrast information in amblyopia. *Vision Res.* 1992;32:2135–2150.
229. Massouri B, Thompson B, Hess RF. Measurements of suprathreshold binocular interactions in amblyopia. *Vision Res.* 2008;48:2775–2784.
230. Ding J, Klein SA, Levi DM. Binocular combination in abnormal binocular vision. *J. Vision.* 2011;13:14.
231. Ding J, Levi DM. Rebalancing binocular vision in amblyopia. *Ophthal. Physiol. Opt.* 2014; 34:199–213.
232. Hess RF, Thompson B, Baker DH. Binocular vision in amblyopia: structure, suppression, and plasticity. *Ophthal. Physiol. Opt.* 2014;34:146–162.
233. Hess RF, Thompson B. Amblyopia and binocular approach to its therapy. *Vision Res.* 2015; 114:4–16.
234. Birch EE. Recent advances in screening and treatment for amblyopia. *Ophthalmol. Ther.* 2021;10:815–830.
235. Gambacorta C, Ding J, McKee SP, Levi DM. Both saccadic and manual responses in the amblyopic eye of strabismics are irreducibly delayed. *J. Vision.* 2018;18:20.
236. Grant S, Suttle C, Melmoth DR, Conway ML, Sloper JJ. Age- and stereovision-dependent eye-hand coordination deficits in children with amblyopia and abnormal binocularity. *Invest. Ophthalmol. Vis. Sci.* 2014;55:5687–5701.
237. NiechwieJ-Szwedo E, Goltz HC, Colpa L, Chandrakumar M, Wong AMF. Effects of reduced acuity and stereoacuity on saccades and reaching movements in adults with amblyopia and strabismus. *Invest. Ophthalmol. Vis. Sci.* 2017;58:60–65.
238. Kelly KR, Jost RM, De La Cruz A, Birch EE. Amblyopic children read more slowly than controls under natural binocular reading conditions. *J. AAPOS.* 2015;19:515–520.
239. Hatt SR, Leske DA, Castaneda YS, Wernimont SM, Lieberman L, Cheng-Patel CS, Birch EE, Holmes JM. Understanding the impact of residual amblyopia on functional vision and eye-related quality of life using the Ped EyeQ. *Am. J. Ophthalmol.* 2020;218:173–181.
240. Acar K, Kiorpes L, Movshon JA, Smith MA. Altered functional interactions between neurons in primary visual cortex of macaque monkeys with experimental amblyopia. *J. Neurophysiol.* 2019;122:2243–2258.
241. Kiorpes L, Movshon JA. Neural limitations on visual development in primates. In: Chalupa LM, Werner SJ, eds. *The Visual Neurosciences*. Cambridge, MA: MIT Press; 2004:159–173.
242. Hallum LE, Shooner C, Kumbhani RD, Kelly JG, Garcia-Martin V, Majaj NJ, Movshon JA, Kiorpes L. Altered balance of receptive field excitation and suppression in visual cortex of amblyopic macaque monkeys. *J. Neurosci.* 2017;37:8216–8226.
243. Levi DM. Crowding—an essential bottleneck for object recognition: a mini review. *Vision Res.* 2008;48:635–654.
244. Chandna A, Pnnefather PM, Kovacs I, Norcia AM. Contour integration deficits in anisometropic amblyopia. *Invest. Ophthalmol. Vis. Sci.* 2001;42:875–878.
245. Hess RF, Field DJ. Is the spatial deficit in strabismic amblyopia due to loss of cells or an uncalibrated disarray of cells? *Vision Res.* 1994;34:3397–3406.
246. Levi DM, Klein SA, Sharma V. Position jitter and undersampling in pattern perception. *Vision Res.* 1999;39:445–465.
247. Sharma V, Levi DM, Klein SA. Undercounting features and missing features: evidence for a high-level deficit in strabismic amblyopia. *Nat Neurosci.* 2000;3:496–501.
248. Kaas JH, Krubitzer LA, Chino YM, Langston AL, Polley EH, Blair N. Reorganization of retinotopic cortical maps in adult mammals after lesions of the retina. *Science.* 1990;248:229–231.
249. Chino YM, Kaas JH, Smith 3rd EL, Langston AL, Cheng H. Rapid reorganization of cortical maps in adult cats following restricted deafferentation in retina. *Vision Res.* 1992;32:789–796.
250. Chino YM, Smith 3rd EL, Kaas JH, Sasaki Y, Cheng H. Receptive-field properties of deafferentated visual cortical neurons after topographic map reorganization in adult cats. *J Neurosci.* 1995;15:2417–2433.
251. Giannikopoulos DV, Eysel UT. Dynamics and specificity of cortical map reorganization after retinal lesions. *Proc Natl Acad Sci U S A.* 2006;103:10805–10810.
252. Darian-Smith C, Gilbert CD. Topographic reorganization in the striate cortex of the adult cat and monkey is cortically mediated. *J Neurosci.* 1995;15:1631–1647.
253. Gilbert CD, Li W. Adult visual cortical plasticity (2012). *Neuron.* 2012;75:250–264.
254. Smirnakis SM, Brewer AA, Schmid MC, Tolias AS, Schuz A, Augath M, Inhoffen W, Wandell BA, Logothetis NK. Lack of long-term cortical reorganization after macaque retinal lesions. *Nature.* 2005;435:300–307.
255. Calford MB, Chino YM, Das A, Eysel UT, Gilbert CD, Heinen SJ, Kaas JH, Ullman S. Neuroscience: rewiring the adult brain. *Nature. 438: E3; discussion.* 2005:E3–4.
256. Horton JC, Fahle M, Mulder T, Trauzettel-Klosinski S. Adaptation, perceptual learning, and plasticity of brain function. *Graefes Arch Clin Exp Ophthalmol.* 2017;255:435–447.
257. Maya Ventencourt JF, Sale A, Viegi A, Baroncelli L, De Pasquale R, O'Leary OF, Castren E, Maffei L. The antidepressant fluoxetin restores plasticity in adult visual cortex. *Science.* 2008;320:385–388.
258. Chung ST, Li RW, Silver MA, Levi DM. Donopenzil does not enhance perceptual learning in adults with amblyopia. *Front Neurosci.* 2017;11:448.
259. Holman KD, Duffy KR, Mitchell DE. Short periods of darkness fail to restore visual or neural plasticity in adult cats. *Vis Neurosci.* 2018;35:E002.
260. Lagas AK, Black JM, Russell BR, Kydd RR, Thompson B. The effect of combined patching and citraloparam on visual acuity in adults with amblyopia: a randomized, crossover, placebo-controlled trial. *Neural Plast.* 2019;2019:5857243.
261. Campana G, Fongoni L, Astle A, McGraw PV. Does physical exercise and congruent visual stimulation enhance perceptual learning? *Ophthal Physiol Opt.* 2020;40:680–691.
262. Dosher B, Lu ZI. Visual perceptual learning and models. *Ann Rev Vis Sci.* 2017;3:343–363.
263. Yang T, Maunsell JH. The effect of perceptual learning on neuronal responses in monkey visual area V4. *J Neurosci.* 2004;24:1617–1626.
264. Chowdhury SA, DeAngelis GC. Fine discrimination training alters the causal contribution of macaque area MT to depth perception. *Neuron.* 2008;60:367–377.
265. Nakatsuka C, Zhang B, Watanabe I, Zheng J, Bi H, Ganz L, Smith 3rd EL, Harwerth RS, Chino YM. Effects of perceptual learning on local stereopsis and neuronal responses of V1 and V2 in prism-reared monkeys. *J Neurophysiol.* 2007;97:2612–2626.
266. Levi DM, Li RW. Improving the performance of the amblyopic visual system. *Philos Trans R Soc Lond B Biol Sci.* 2009;364:399–407.
267. Levi DM. Prentice award lecture 2011: removing the brakes on plasticity in the amblyopic brain. *Opt. Vision Sci.* 2012;89:827–838.
268. Tsirlin I, Copla L, Giltz HC, Wong AM. Behavioral training as a new treatment for adult amblyopia: a meta-analysis and systematic review. *Invest Ophthalmol Vis Sci.* 2015;56: 4061–4075.
269. Li WR, Ngo CV, Nguyen J, Levi DM. Video-game play induces plasticity in the visual system of adults with amblyopia. *Plos Biology.* 2011;9e1001135.
270. Li WR, Ngo CV, Levi DM. Relieving the attentional blink in the amblyopic brain with video games. *Sci Rep.* 2015;5:8483.
271. Vedamurthy I, Knill DC, Huang SJ, Yung A, Ding J, Kwon O-S, Bavelier D, Levi DM. Recovering stereovision by squashing virtual bugs in virtual reality environment. *Philos Trans R Soc Lond B Bio Sci.* 2016;37120150264.
272. Li RW, Tran KD, Bui JK, Atonucci MM, Ngo CV, Levi DM. Improving adult vision with stereoscopic 3-dimensional video games. *Ophthalomol.* 2018;125:1660–1662.
273. Bavelier D, Green CS, Ponget A, Schrater P. Brain plasticity through the life span: learning to learn and video games. *Ann. Rev. Neurosci.* 2012;30:14964–14971.
274. Birch EE, Morale SE, Jost RM, De La Cruz A, Kelly KR, Wang YZ, Bex PJ. Assessing suppression in amblyopic children with a dichoptic chart. *Invest Ophthalmol Vis Sci.* 2015;57:5649–5654.

275. Li SL, Jost RM, Morale SE, Stager DR, Dao L, Stager D, Birch EE. Binocular iPad treatment for amblyopic children. *Eye (Lond).* 2014;28:1246–1253.

276. Vedamurthy I, Nahum M, Huang SJ, Zheng F, Bayliss J, Vavelier D, Levi DM. A dichoptic custom-made action video game for treatment of adult amblyopia. *Vision Res.* 2015;114:173–187.

277. Gambacorta C, Nahum M, Vedamurthy I, Bayliss J, Jordan J, Bavelier D, Levi DM. An action video game for the treatment of amblyopia in children: a feasibility study. *Vision Res.* 2018;148:1–14.

278. Kelly KR, Jost RM, Dao L, Beauchamp CL, Leffler JN, Birch EE. Binocular iPad game vs patching for treatment of amblyopia in children: a randomized clinical trial. *JAMA Ophthalmol.* 2016;134:1402–1408.

279. Jost RM, Kelly KR, Hunter JS, Stager DR, Luu B, Lefler JN, Dao L, Beauchamp CL, Birch EE. A randomized clinical trial of contrast increment protocols for binocular amblyopia treatment. *J AAPOS.* 2020;24282e.1–282e7.

280. Holmes JM, Levi DM. Treatment of amblyopia as a function of age. *Visual Neurosci.* 2018;35:E015.

281. Kelly KR, Jost RM, Wang Y-Z, Dao L, Beauchamp CL, Leffler JN, Birch EE. Improved binocular outcomes following binocular treatment for childhood amblyopia. *Invest. Ophthalmol Vis Sci.* 2018;59:1221–1228.

282. Pineles SL, Aakalu VK, Hutchinson AK, Galvin JA, Heidary G, Binenbaum G, VanderVeen DK, Lambert SR. Binocular treatment of amblyopia: a report by the American Academy of Ophthalmology. *Ophthalmology.* 2020;127:261–272.

283. Birch EE, Jost RM, Kelly KR, Lefler JN, Dao L, Beauchamp CL. Baseline and clinical factors associated with response to amblyopia treatment in a randomized clinical trial. *Optom. Vis. Sci.* 2020;97:316–323.

41

The Effects of Visual Deprivation After Infancy

Ione Fine, Valenteen Savage, and Woon Ju Park

INTRODUCTION

Over the last three decades it has been well documented that visual deprivation, especially when it occurs early in life, results in fundamental alterations of neural function across more than 25% of cortex—changes that range from metabolism to behavior and collectively represent one of the most dramatic examples of plasticity in the human brain. As schematized in Fig. 41.1, blindness has massive impact across multiple neuroanatomical levels, from molecules to function.

"Blindness" is an extremely broad term, with a variety of definitions that vary across common usage and the legal, medical, rehabilitation, and scientific literatures (Box 41.1). In this review we primarily focus on early congenital or late severe (light perception [LP] or worse) blindness because these forms of blindness are the most heavily studied. Scientists studying the effects of early blindness have generally focused on relatively homogenous groups of individuals with LP or no LP (NLP) vision occurring either at or within a year of birth. Scientists studying late blindness have, similarly, often focused on groups of individuals with a normal visual history until adulthood, followed by NLP and LP. However, these groups represent a relatively small proportion of blind individuals. Most blind individuals have significant residual vision, and many have a complex medical history that involves worsening vision over many years (Fig. 41.2).

NEUROANATOMICAL DEVELOPMENT

Fig. 41.3 shows a schematic of the major milestones for white matter, neuronal, and biochemical development within visual pathways before and after eye opening.

White matter pathways

In the normally developing brain, the early wave of migrating neurons that provides a first rough blueprint of cerebral organization is primarily governed by intrinsic signaling, controlled in part by graded expression of transcription factors.[1] These pathways begin to form well before the onset of visual experience, beginning around postconception (PC) day 80. By PC day 200 the major visual white matter tracts linking occipital cortex to other regions of the brain and the connectivity patterns underlying the retinotopic topography of early visual areas (V1-V2-V3) have begun to develop, well before the axons from the optic radiations innervate cortex.

However, although major white matter pathways are established relatively early in development, these prenatal tracts are initially unmyelinated, with the elaboration of the myelin sheath around neuronal axons only beginning at birth. Myelination of posterior tracts is rapid in the first year or two of life, and continues throughout childhood.[2,3]

Both human and animal models (for a review of the early literature, see ref[4]) find that early blindness leads to atrophy of the pathways from the retina to early visual cortex. Several animal models have shown atrophy of the connections between the eye and V1 after early-onset blindness.[5,6] Similarly, a variety of studies in humans have consistently found decreased white matter volume, decreased axial diffusivity, and increased radial diffusivity in the optic nerve and radiations within both early-blind[7-9] and anophthalmic[10] individuals.

In contrast to these subcortical pathways, the effects of blindness on corticocortical pathways are relatively subtle. Consistent with the evidence that the macrostructure of these pathways develops before the onset of retinal input, neither the strength nor the macroscale topographic organization of callosal connections are dramatically affected by early blindness, and retinotopic organization seems to persist in the absence of visual experience.[11,12] The main changes in corticocortical white matter that have been observed as a result of early blindness using diffusion-weighted imaging suggest attenuation of occipital to temporal connections, and enhanced connectivity between occipital and frontal cortex (for review, see ref[13]).

Neurochemistry and microstructure

Extensive literature on animal models suggests that the development of local excitatory and inhibitory networks is strongly mediated by visual experience. Visual deprivation, especially early in development, substantially changes the balance of this intricate system, altering the timeline of occipital cortex development.

The local microstructure and neurochemical balance of cortex is in an immature state at birth. At eye opening, all excitatory neurons appear pyramidal, with a prominent apical dendrite and few small basal dendrites. Excitatory synaptic activity is heavily mediated by N-methyl-D-aspartate (NMDA); over 50% of synapses lack α-amino-3-hydroxy-5-methyl-4-isoxazolepropionic acid (AMPA) receptors and are consequently "silent"—functionally inactive.[14,15] Inhibitory neurons are similarly immature.

Excitatory pyramidal cell properties mature rapidly after eye opening, including pyramidal spine density[16] and the conversion of pyramidal cells to their mature stellate form.[17] Expression of NMDA receptor subunit GluN1[15] and the shape of the excitatory postsynaptic potential[18] become close to adult-like within the first postnatal year.

This early synaptic activity within the excitatory system triggers the development of inhibitory pathways. Excitatory activity triggers the downregulation of polysialic acid on neural cell adhesion molecule (PSA-NCAM) expression, thereby releasing a brake on precocious plasticity.[19] Excitatory activity also triggers the production of brain-derived neurotrophic factor,[20] which, in conjunction with neural activity, facilitates the maturation of both inhibitory parvalbumin (PV)-containing interneurons and silent synapses.[21] The onset of visual experience triggers the transport of orthodenticle homeobox 2 (Otx2) from retinal to PV cells, where it promotes PV cell maturation.[22] As a result, inhibitory PV cells increase in complexity, and the number of inhibitory connections increases,[15,23] reaching adult levels by 1.5 years of age.

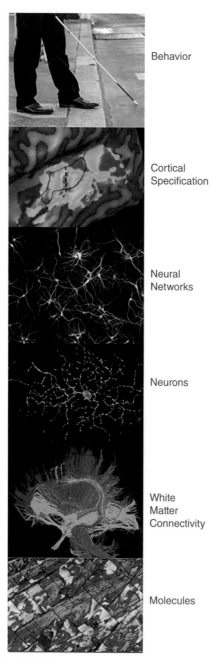

Behavior

Cortical
Specification

Neural
Networks

Neurons

White
Matter
Connectivity

Molecules

Fig. 41.1 Early blindness changes brain organization across multiple scales. These alterations include neurotransmitter regulation, local synaptic connectivity, neural network organization, white matter pathways, cortical specification, and behavioral abilities, as discussed in the main text.

This changing balance between excitatory/inhibitory (E/I) responses in neural circuitry[24,25] seems to be partially responsible for controlling the onset and end of the sensitive period. Early in development, excitation dominates cortical circuits, and the resulting neural activity acts as a maturational trigger. As inhibitory processes approach maturation, synaptic drive transitions from dominant excitation to dominant inhibition, helping to trigger the end of the sensitive period.[26]

Overall, in normal development, the number of excitatory synapses continues to increase for several months postnatally, but within the occipital cortex the number of synapses asymptotes at the surprisingly early age of 8 months.[27] However, some of these excitatory synapses lack AMPA and remain functionally silent.[14,15] It is not until the second

BOX 41.1   Blindness

- Legally blind (US definition): Vision worse than 20/200, or a field of view smaller than 20 degrees in the better eye.
- Finger counting: An individual can tell how many fingers the ophthalmologist is holding up.
- Hand motion: An individual can tell that the ophthalmologist is waving a hand in front of their eyes.
- Light perception (LP): An individual can tell if the lights in a room are on or off (roughly similar to a normally sighted individual's vision with their eyes closed).
- No light perception (NLP): An individual cannot tell whether the lights in a room are on or off.

postnatal year that most remaining excitatory synapses contain both AMPA and NMDA receptors, rendering them functionally active. Studies suggest a tight relationship between visual experience, the maturation of these silent synapses, and the refinement of local network connections.[28] Between 8 months and 11 years, pruning occurs, with the loss of about 40% of synapses; synapse numbers then remain stable through most of adulthood.[29]

This developmental timeline is fundamentally altered by deprivation. One key mechanism thought to influence the sensitive period is the changing balance between excitatory and inhibitory responses in neural circuitry.[24,25] In darkness, the excitatory drive is reduced, slowing maturation. As a consequence, visual deprivation delays, prolongs, or "reawakens" developmental levels of plasticity for many processes, including BDNF expression,[30] maturation of inhibitory PV cells,[31] silent synapse maturation,[14] the remodeling of layer 4 pyramidal cells into spiny neurons,[17] neuronal tuning,[32,33] and visual acuity.[32]

Consistent with the hypothesis that visual deprivation slows or halts development, there is evidence of elevated neurochemical concentrations of excitatory choline and *myo*-inositol, with indications of reduced inhibitory gamma-aminobutyric acid (GABA) in early-blind[34] and anophthalmic[35] individuals. Elevated levels of both choline and *myo*-inositol are characteristic of immature cortex; concentrations of both neurochemicals, as measured by magnetic resonance spectroscopy (MRS), are high at birth and gradually decrease in the first few years of life.[36]

Alternatively, higher levels of choline and *myo*-inositol might possibly reflect long-term upregulation of cholinergic phospholipid pathways consequent on early blindness, as has been found in one animal model.[37] While acetylcholine is a very small component of the MRS choline peak, MRS ¹H choline measurements are a surprisingly reliable surrogate marker of acetylcholine: in animal models the correlation across individuals between measured choline and acetylcholine levels is above 0.8 across multiple brain regions.[38] In the case of *myo*-inositol, cholinergic activity might stimulate phosphoinositide hydrolysis and thereby raise the level of intracellular inositol.[39] Elevated levels of *myo*-inositol might also reflect increased astrocyte density; dark-reared animals given access to both an enriched multisensory environment and voluntary exercise show enhanced astrocyte densities compared with control rats or rats dark reared in a nonenriched environment.[40,41]

Deprived cortex is not simply immature cortex. Total creatine levels in V1 are significantly higher in anophthalmic[35] and early-blind individuals,[34] whereas total creatine levels are lower in infants than in adulthood.[36] As a potential marker of energetic metabolism, increased levels of total creatine in anophthalmia and early blindness are consistent with evidence of upregulated metabolic processing in the occipital cortex of early-blind subjects at rest and during auditory and tactile tasks[42–45] and animal studies showing increased neuronal excitability.[46]

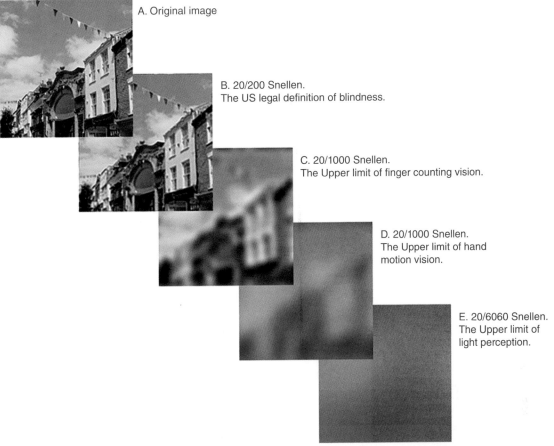

A. Original image

B. 20/200 Snellen.
The US legal definition of blindness.

C. 20/1000 Snellen.
The Upper limit of finger counting vision.

D. 20/1000 Snellen.
The Upper limit of hand
motion vision.

E. 20/6060 Snellen.
The Upper limit of
light perception.

Fig. 41.2 Blindness is a broad term, characterizing a wide range of visual impairments. (**A**) Original picture, representing a 20-degree field of view. (**B**) The upper limit of the legal definition of blindness. 20/200 Snellen acuity, simulated by removing frequencies above 3 cycles/degree (cpd). (**C**) The upper limit of finger-counting vision. 20/1000 Snellen acuity, simulated by removing frequencies above 0.6 cpd. (**D**) The upper limit of hand motion vision. 20/2500 Snellen acuity simulated by removing frequencies above 0.24 cpd. (**E**) The upper limit of light perception vision. 20/6060 Snellen acuity, simulated by removing frequencies above 0.1 cpd. (The conversion from "finger counting" and "hand motion" to Snellen acuity based on Schulze-Bonsel K, Feltgen N, Burau H, Hansen L, Bach M. Visual acuities "hand motion" and "counting fingers" can be quantified with the freiburg visual acuity test. *Invest Ophthalmol Vis Sci.* 2006;47(3):1236–124; Photo from Sarah. (August 7, 2021). York, UK. https://unsplash.com/photos/CGfOBE1E2oA.)

Gray matter and neuronal tuning

Early enucleation leads to atrophy of the lateral geniculate nucleus (LGN) in both animal models[47,48,49,50,51] and individuals with anophthalmia,[10] as well as to atrophy of cortical input layer 4 in animal models.[48,49,50,51]

Early blindness and anophthalmia has also been shown to result in a permanent increase in cortical thickness[10,52,53] and a decrease in occipital cortical folding in anophthalmic and early-blind individuals.[54,55] Although this increase in cortical thickness has generally been attributed to a lack of experience-dependent cortical pruning after birth, it is likely that other mechanisms may contribute. Cortical expansion relies heavily on a special type of progenitor cell that generates a fiber scaffold (at around human prenatal day 120), which promotes tangential dispersion of radially migrating neurons and thereby facilitates surface area growth within the cortical sheet.[56] This cortical expansion has a prolonged developmental timeline; for example, in humans, the area of V1 does not reach its adult size until more than 2 years of age. Enucleation in ferrets reduces the density of these progenitor cells, and the resulting lack of tangential dispersion leads to an increase in cell density and

cortical thickness, along with a reduction in cortical surface area.[56] It is also possible that the *apparent* increases in cortical thickness as a result of blindness, as measured using T1-weighted MRI, represent increased T1 contrast owing to reduced myelination within the stria of Gennari (the input layer of V1) rather than a genuine increase in cortical thickness.[57] Increases in cortical thickness and reductions in surface area are more pronounced in anophthalmic than early-blind individuals, suggesting that both prenatal and postnatal developmental mechanisms contribute to these anatomical differences.[55]

However, many aspects of cortical synaptic microstructure seem to be driven by molecular signaling, and develop relatively normally in the absence of visual experience. For example, the retinotopic organization of local connections across V1-V2-V3, whereby a region in V1 precisely connects with regions in V2 that represent the same retinal patch, occurs around prenatal day 200, only shortly after LGN axons innervate the cortex (prenatal day 180). Retinotopic maps in the dorsal LGN and cortex have been shown to persist when retinal waves are disrupted, albeit with reduced precision.[12,58–61] More generally, feature-specific microcircuits in layers 2 and 3 develop even in the absence of

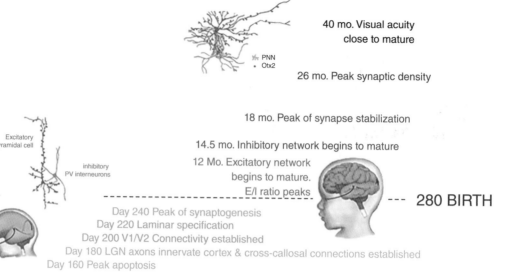

Fig. 41.3 The time course of milestones of developmental plasticity, measured across a variety of species. We normalized postconception (PC) and postnatal (PN) days for each species to a timeline based on human development using the Workman translating time model. Prenatal events are reported as days PC; PN dates are shown as months PN. *E/I*, excitatory/inhibitory; *LGN*, lateral geniculate nucleus. (Reproduced with permission from the Annual Review of Vision Science, Volume 4 © 2018 by Annual Reviews, http://www.annualreviews.org. Park WJ, Fine I. New insights into cortical development and plasticity: From molecules to behavior. *Curr Opin Physiol.* 2020;16:50–60. https://doi.org/10.1016/j.cophys.2020.06.004.)

visual experience.[62–64] Cells sharing the same stimulus preferences are preferentially connected to each other even in dark-reared animals.[63] Visual experience sculpts and refines these existing feature-based circuits to form microstructures that represent ocular dominance columns, receptive-field orientation and size, direction, and disparity tuning.[4,47,65–67] Sight-recovery subjects blinded at an early age with sight restored in adulthood have low acuity[68] but retain retinotopic organization,[11] and motion-selective responses can be measured within the visual motion area human middle temporal complex (hMT+).[69] Thus, visual experience does not establish neural response selectivities but rather sculpts and refines neural microcircuits that are established well before the onset of visual experience.

THE PERCEPTUAL AND NEURAL EFFECTS OF EARLY VISION LOSS

Early blindness has traditionally been used as a model system for examining sensory plasticity, with the assumption that the behavioral and neural differences found in early-blind individuals are primarily the consequence of sensory deprivation. However, in recent years it has become increasingly apparent that many of the effects of blindness may be due to the strikingly different perceptual and cognitive demands posed by blindness.

There are good reasons to believe that much of the plasticity that occurs as a result of early blindness reflects the development or hyperdevelopment of cognitive rather than sensory processes. For instance, the critical learning period for early blindness extends into the teenage years when sensory processes are adult-like, but cognitive processes are still developing.[70] As described further, blind individuals also show enhanced capacities within many tasks that are clearly cognitive. However it remains unclear whether these enhanced capacities reflect simple excellence through expertise or uniquely heightened capacities available only after sensory loss.

There is now an increased appreciation for the capacity of the developing brain to generate novel cortically specialized areas (e.g., areas specialized for reading and numerosity) in childhood, by "repurposing" on evolutionarily older circuits evolved for other functions.[71] It seems plausible that the same mechanisms that permit this "neuronal recycling" may underlie cross-modal plasticity and compensatory hypertrophy as a result of blindness. If so, gaining traction on how the brain responds to early blindness is likely to provide important insights into the mechanisms that underlie the complex developmental plasticity that permits novel neurocognitive specializations through training.

Touch and Braille
Behavior

It is often suggested that blind subjects may have enhanced tactile abilities. However, it is still unclear to what extent there are differences in tactile performance between sighted and blind subjects and, if so, whether this improved performance should be attributed to blindness per se rather than the effects of extensive practice with Braille.

In many (but not all[74]) studies, blind individuals do not show improved tactile acuity compared with sighted individuals for

Braille-like stimuli, especially after sighted individuals undergo some training,[72,73] With grating orientation and detection judgments, results are similarly inconsistent, with some[75-77] but not all[72,74] studies finding enhanced tactile acuity in the blind.

The reasons for these inconsistencies remain unclear. As discussed by Voss et al.[78] the age and gender of the individuals play a role. Results may also depend on how blind individuals read Braille. Not only do individuals differ widely in fluency, but they also vary in whether they read with one or multiple fingers. In individuals who read Braille with more than one finger, the cortical representation linked to the fingers used in Braille appears to merge. Although this may result in greater tactile acuity,[77] it can also result in a topographical uncertainty, which leads to worse performance when asked to discriminate which finger was being lightly stimulated.[79] Whether sensory adaptations designed to enhance Braille reading lead to better or worse performance on a given tactile task may depend on both the particular tactile task and which fingers are tested.

Neural responses

Numerous neuroimaging studies have demonstrated that early-blind subjects consistently show large neural responses for both tactile stimuli[80] and Braille words in V1, extrastriate, and lateral occipital cortices.[81-86]

One region consistently activated by Braille is the ventral occipitotemporal cortex (vOTC)—a region selectively associated with visual reading in sighted individuals.[87] These responses are likely to reflect feedback from higher-level language areas. The magnitude of blood oxygen level dependent (BOLD) responses to Braille is highly correlated on an individual basis with verbal memory ability,[81] and these vOTC responses in blind, but not sighted, individuals are sensitive to grammatical structure.[87] transcranial magnetic stimulation (TMS) applied to occipital cortex interferes with Braille processing,[88] but only after a delay of 50 to 80 ms, compared with shorter periods of 20–40 ms when applied to somatosensory cortex.[73]

Despite reflecting feedback from language areas, occipital cortex may play a functional role in Braille reading in early-blind subjects: there is the interesting case study of an early-blind woman who, following an occipital stroke, lost the ability to read Braille without loss of her ability to detect Braille letters or loss of her other somatosensory abilities.[89]

BOLD responses in vOTC can be also elicited after extensive training in Braille in sighted individuals,[90] suggesting that these feedback responses may be mediated by practice with Braille, rather than the loss of visual input per se.

Auditory processing
Pitch

Behavior. One of the fundamental unanswered questions in blindness is whether blind individuals "hear" better. Blind individuals are more likely to have careers that utilize their auditory abilities (e.g., piano tuner or musician, Fig. 41.4), which leads to a common perception that blindness results in an improved sensitivity to auditory information.

Several studies have noted enhanced pitch and timbre perception in early-blind but not late-blind individuals,[91-93] although others have not.[94,95] It is reported that more blind than sighted musicians (~57% vs. <20%) have absolute pitch.[96] Similarly, early-blind individuals are also better at discriminating pitch in both speech-related sounds (vowels) and musical instruments.[97] These enhanced auditory abilities cannot be attributed to blind individuals having more extensive musical experience; blind individuals showed improved pitch discrimination performances even when prior music training was accounted for.[92,93]

Neural responses. The neural substrates underlying enhanced pitch perception following blindness remain largely unknown. Traditionally, it has been thought that the recruitment of visual occipital areas may contribute to pitch processing in blind individuals. One blind musician has been demonstrated to show occipital responses in a pitch memory task that were not observed in sighted musicians,[98] and an exploratory study found that cortical thickness in certain occipital areas was correlated with scores on a melody task in early-blind individuals.[92]

A number of studies have reported an attenuated response to pure tone stimuli in the temporal lobe of blind individuals compared with sighted controls.[95,99] This has been interpreted as reduced participation in auditory processing, perhaps owing to increased "efficiency" of processing within the intact modality or owing to function being "usurped" by a reorganized occipital cortex. An alternative explanation is that these previous results might have reflected narrower tuning rather than reduced responsiveness—narrower tuning would be

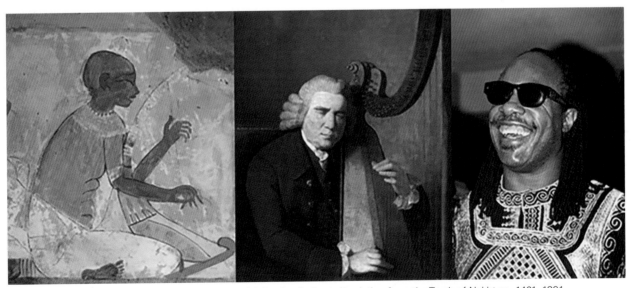

Fig. 41.4 (A) A blind musician playing a harp detail of a wall painting from the Tomb of Nakht ca. 1401–1391 BC. **(B)** The Blind Harpist, John Parry (d. 1782). **(C)** Stevie Wonder Smith. (**C**, from Washington D.C. National Assoc. of black owned broadcasters March 1994 © copyright John Mathew Smith 2001", and listed as being licensed under a creative commons license.

expected to result in a smaller population of neurons responding to any given narrow-band stimulus, which would reduce the measured activation in a sound versus silence comparison. Consistent with this, early-blind individuals are shown to have narrower auditory frequency tuning, as estimated by population receptive-field mapping, within primary auditory cortex.[100]

Space

Behavior. Early-blind individuals seem to have a similar or enhanced ability to localize single sound sources,[101,102] and perform similarly or better than sighted individuals when determining which of two sounds is further to the right or slightly higher,[103,104] especially in the periphery. A variety of other studies similarly suggest an improved ability to process auditory spatial cues, including greater sensitivity to monaural, and spectral cues for spatial location and distance.[105–108]

However, early-blind participants who are not echolocators[109] have deficits in auditory bisection tasks (deciding which of two speakers an intermediate speaker is closer to), suggesting a weaker representation of allocentric[110,111] auditory space. This is thought to be due to a lack of visual calibration: auditory localization and bisection performance for sighted individuals is analogously worse for the back than the front plane—presumably owing to lacking eyes in the back of our heads.[103,112]

This absence of visual calibration may also explain why blind individuals show superior *monaural* localization abilities in the horizontal plane,[107] but inferior localization abilities in the vertical plane[113,114]; monaural cues can be calibrated against binaural auditory cues in the horizontal but not the vertical plane.

Interestingly, a small study ($n = 3$) in individuals with central vision loss showed evidence of a selective impairment of central auditory localization abilities,[101,115] once again suggesting an important role for visual calibration.

Neural responses. Occipital responses during auditory spatial tasks have been reported using PET,[116,117] event-related potentials,[118] and functional magnetic resonance imaging (fMRI)[119] in early-blind individuals. These cross-modal responses as a result of blindness appear to be right lateralized, within dorsal regions associated with subserving visuospatial and motion processing in sighted individuals.[116,119] Responses also tend to be larger in those early-blind individuals with superior auditory localization performance,[117,118]

The recruitment of the occipital visual areas during auditory spatial localization tasks seem to play a functional role: when transcranial magnetic stimulation is applied to the right occipital cortex, it selectively disrupts the ability of blind individuals to localize sounds in space, while not affecting performance for pitch or intensity.[120]

One possibility is that these cortical responses reflect direct auditory cortex input. If so, we would expect these responses to be limited to peripheral stimuli, given that in primates, anatomical connections from the auditory cortex to occipital areas primarily project to the areas that respond to visual periphery.[121] Alternatively (although not exclusively), these responses may reflect feedback driven by connections from higher-level areas normally associated with visuospatial processing.[122] This is consistent with the right hemisphere lateralization that has been observed for these auditory spatial responses—in sighted individuals only lesions of the right hemisphere result in impairments in visuospatial processing.[123]

Motion

Behavior. A variety of studies have suggested recruitment of hMT+, a region strongly associated with visual motion processing in sighted individuals, for auditory motion as a result of early blindness.[124–128] However relatively few studies have examined the auditory

motion perceptual abilities in blind individuals. Early-blind individuals have been shown to outperform sighted individuals both in a simple auditory motion discrimination—the minimum audible movement angle,[129] and in a more complex task requiring judging the overall direction of multiple moving sources.[130]

Neural responses. As noted previously, cross-modal plasticity within the deprived "visual" motion area hMT+ has been extensively studied. In sight-recovery subjects and early-blind[125] individuals hMT+ responds selectively to auditory motion but not to other complex auditory stimuli.[127,130,131] In blind individuals, cross-modal responses in hMT+ appear to be direction selective, and are correlated with direction of perceived motion in ambiguous stimuli.[130]

These auditory responses in hMT+ are accompanied by a *loss* of selectivity to auditory motion in the right planum temporale, an area associated with auditory motion processing in sighted individuals,[124,125] suggesting that the recruitment of hMT+ may result from competition between cortical areas, as discussed further in the chapter.

Auditory language and cognition

Behavior. Early studies on language acquisition in blind children demonstrate both delays and differences in language development compared with their sighted peers. One noticeable area of delay is in extending meaning to new referents; when a toddler first learns the word "doggie" she may think it only refers to *her* dog, but she will learn quickly that this word belongs to a class of objects.[132] There is also evidence that, perhaps unsurprisingly, blind children learn concepts of time before space, whereas space before time is more usual in sighted children.[133] Blind children may also be slower to develop the ability to maintain a shared coherent topic in conversation[132]; one possibility is that this is due to the lack of visual cues to shared attention, another is that caregiver-initiated exchanges with blind children tend to be somewhat impoverished, focusing on labels rather than description ("two buttons" vs. "that button is bigger and it has more holes").

These difficulties seem to represent delays rather than permanent deficits—recent studies in adults suggest similar or even enhanced abilities to process auditory language in early individuals: blind individuals demonstrate superior performances in verbal fluency, sentence comprehension, and verbal working memory tasks[134,135] and even show similar levels of conceptual understanding for verbs that have "visual" meanings when compared with sighted controls.[136]

Neural responses. An increasing number of studies suggest responses within occipital areas in auditory language processing following blindness.[85,118,137–141] The recruitment of the occipital cortex for language seems to be associated with higher-level cognitive (rather than phonological or sensory) processing, and appears to be independent of the ability to read Braille.[140] Activity within the occipital areas to spoken language is greater when blind individuals perform a task that involves attending to the meaning (vs. rhyme) of words[141] and is modulated by the semantic content and grammatical structure of the stimuli.[137,139] There is some evidence that these responses play a functional role: transcranial magnetic stimulation applied to the anatomical location of V1 disrupts performances in a verb-generation task in blind, but not in sighted, individuals, leading to more semantic errors when producing verbs related to cueing-nouns.[142]

Cross-modal responses in the visual areas have also been observed for other tasks that are primarily cognitive, including verbal working memory,[81] retrieval of episodic memory,[143] cognitive load,[144] and numerical processing.[145,146] Some functional segregation has been observed: the areas that respond to numbers seem to be anatomically distinct from those that respond to auditory language.[145,146]

It is not yet entirely clear how or why early areas in the visual processing hierarchy respond during high-level tasks involving auditory language or cognition. As described previously, anatomical evidence suggests that these responses must be primarily mediated by preexisting white matter connections, rather than via major novel cortical connections.

Similarly to the recruitment of hMT+ for auditory motion, the recruitment of occipital cortex for auditory language/cognition seems to require blindness onset to occur during early childhood. Responses to spoken language in the occipital cortex appear to develop by age 4 years following blindness[140] and are not observed in late-blind individuals,[147] suggesting the existence of a sensitive period that extends beyond infancy.

WHAT ARE THE MECHANISMS THAT UNDERLIE CROSS-MODAL PLASTICITY?

As described previously, blindness leads to a striking reorganization in which regions of the brain that are normally driven primarily by visual input begin to respond to auditory and tactile input and/or cognitive and language tasks. The source, role, and mechanisms underlying cross-modal plasticity following blindness are still largely mysterious.

Given the early prenatal development of white matter tracts, and the failure to find major tract differences as a result of blindness, it seems increasingly likely that white matter structure constrains functional role, rather than the other way around.[148]

One important question is the degree to which occipital cortex responses are driven by low-level sensory signals from subcortical or primary auditory or somatosensory cortex, versus receiving more elaborated top-down signals from higher-level cognitive areas. There is some evidence that the superior colliculus, a "visual" subcortical structure, is recruited by the auditory system in congenital and early-onset blindness,[149] and there is some evidence of direct connections between auditory and occipital cortex.[121,150] It has been suggested that cross-modal connectivity and correspondences between auditory and visual perception may be stronger in young children,[151] and that in the absence of vision these cross-modal connections are not subject to competitive pruning over development. However, as described previously, there is also strong evidence that cross-modal responses in occipital cortex, especially in earlier visual areas such as V1, may reflect top-down language and/or cognitive processes.

According to the strong form of the "supramodal" or "metamodal" hypothesis, even traditionally unimodal brain areas are carrying out modality-independent tasks whose computations are not inextricably visual.[152,153] Thus, the role of hMT+ is to determine the motion of objects in space, the role of the visual word form area (VWFA) is to decode structured spatial information for language information, and the role of the fusiform face area is to identify the presence and identity of individuals. Importantly, it is assumed that these supramodal capacities exist in both sighted and early-blind individuals, and merely require either temporary deprivation[154] or training,[90] to be "unmasked."

A variety of studies have demonstrated auditory and tactile sensory responses within visual areas in sighted individuals, as predicted by the metamodal hypothesis. However, across all these studies, the observed cross-modal responses might also be attributed to known cross-modal modulatory influences or difficulties in accurately identifying particular brain areas. For example, spatial attention to one location is known to "spread" cross-modally—attention to the right visual field increases left hemisphere neural responses within both early visual and auditory areas, and vice versa.[155] Visualization is also known to operate

cross-modally,[156] which likely explains why occipital BOLD responses to embossed Roman letters[157] are seen in both blind and sighted individuals. Finally, in some studies the use of group averaging techniques and/or probabilistic atlases may accidentally include neighboring/adjacent regions that are genuinely multimodal. For example, whereas several studies have found auditory and tactile responses within hMT+ in sighted individuals, those studies that rigorously control for cross-modal attentional influences and define hMT+ with extreme caution do not.[125,127,130,158]

An alternative hypothesis is that the cross-modal plasticity in hMT+ observed in early-blind individuals shares many of the same underlying mechanisms as "neuronal recycling" whereby heavily trained skills (such as reading in sighted individuals), rely on the "recycling" of evolutionarily older circuits that originally evolved for different, but similar, functions.[71] Novel functions can "colonize" circuits that are sufficiently close to the required function and sufficiently plastic to reorient a significant fraction of their neural resources to this novel use. This thereby explains the relatively tight homologies of cross-modal function that have been found for many specialized areas within early-blind individuals, as described previously.

This novel specialization is not simply driven by competition between inputs for cortical representation, but also by corticocortical competition *across* cortical areas for functional role. The first suggestion of corticocortical competition for functional role came from a study of Sadato et al.[159] who found that secondary somatosensory areas were less activated by Braille reading in blind individuals than in sighted controls. More recently, recruitment of hMT+ for auditory motion processing in early-blind individuals has been shown to be accompanied by a *loss* of selectivity for auditory motion in the right planum temporale[130,160] (Fig. 41.5).

Perhaps the most mysterious aspects of cross-modal plasticity are the auditory and tactile responses that are found in early visual areas such as V1 and V2. As described previously, an increasing number of studies suggest that regions near the occipital pole may be involved in abstract cognitive tasks, such as Braille reading, verbal working memory, language, and even mathematics.[81,82,139,146]

One possibility is that the exuberant reciprocal feedback connectivity between high-level (e.g., lateral occipital cortex [LOC]) and low-level (e.g., V1) visual areas may be repurposed to perform an analogous role as the feedforward connections from LOC to higher-level cortex—further elaborating and abstracting information.[148] Thus, early visual areas become involved in cognitive processes such as verbal working memory, language, and mathematics. One concern with this theory is that it requires assuming that these connections, despite being formed prenatally, are "content neutral" and can be repurposed from their original modulatory purpose (e.g., focusing selective attention and providing an "error signal" within selected subgroups of lower-level neurons[161]) to subserve the complex computations that would be required in a "reverse hierarchy."

An alternative explanation is that these cross-modal activations within early visual areas represent an indiscriminate amplification of both intrinsic noise within early visual areas and feedback signals from higher-level visual areas. As described previously, both animal models[51,162–164] and measurements in humans[39,165] show that visually deprived cortex undergoes a shift in the E/I balance toward greater excitation. These feedback signals, in the absence of meaningful feedforward input, do not play a functional role. According to this theory, repetitive transcranial magnetic stimulation (rTMS) interference with cognitive processes such as verbal memory[166] might be due to the shift toward greater excitation increasing the effective amplitude of the rTMS signal, resulting in downstream interference within higher-level areas that are functionally involved in the task.

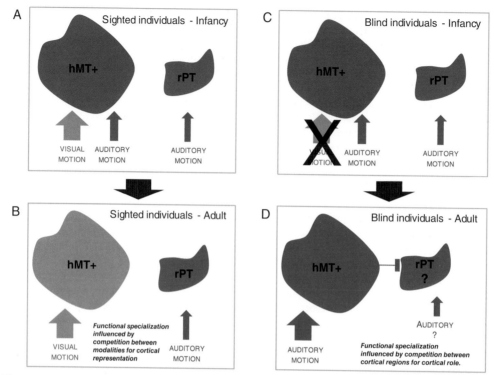

Fig. 41.5 (**A**) It is hypothesized that early in development hMT+ receives both auditory and visual input. (**B**) In sighted individuals, it is believed that auditory inputs are pruned as a result of competition between auditory and visual input. (**C**) In the absence of vision, auditory inputs into hMT+ are strengthened. (**D**) However, it has also been observed that the right planum temporale (rPT) loses selectivity for auditory motion, presumably owing to competition between cortical areas for functional role.

RECOVERY OF SIGHT AFTER EARLY BLINDNESS

Cases of sight recovery after extended periods of congenital blindness provide windows into the functional consequences of early visual deprivation on visual development and brain plasticity. These cases are extremely rare in high-income countries, so until the last decade, insights into the effects of early visual deprivation were primarily based on a handful of case studies.[167,168] However, in the last decade a series of recent projects have focused on removing congenital cataracts in children in lower-income countries (Project Prakash[169] and Project Eye Opener[170]). These programs, because their motivations are medical as well as scientific, have resulted in a shift in scientific emphasis away from characterizing visual deficits or abnormalities, toward an emphasis on the ability of these children to make use of visual information in daily life, despite striking differences in the processing of visual information.

Unsurprisingly, given the role of visual experience in fine-tuning synaptic connectivity, early visual deprivation leads to severe losses in the ability to process fine detail (binocular amblyopia).[69,70,171] When congenital cataracts (which often permit a small amount of form vision) are removed in children (aged 8–17 years) significant recovery of function occurs in the months after surgery, but acuity remains poor, with Snellen acuity levels generally being worse than 20/120.[69]

Once these acuity losses are accounted for, sight-recovery individuals seem to have little difficulty on most two-dimensional (2D) form or color tasks.[70,124,170,171]

Similarly, provided acuity losses are accounted for, sight-recovery participants do not show significant impairments in motion processing,[70] including being able to understand biological motion.[70,172] Robust

responses to visual motion are seen in hMT+.[127] The retention of visual motion processing in these subjects might be considered somewhat surprising, given the evidence that after early blindness hMT+ selectively processes auditory motion, as described previously. However, data suggest that in cases of sight recovery, visual and cross-modal responses coexist within hMT+.[125,127] It remains to be seen whether neurons in these areas are jointly tuned for both properties, but stronger transfer of adaptation from auditory to visual motion stimuli has been noted in sight-recovery individuals.[173]

The most striking losses observed in sight-recovery patients seem to be related to three-dimensional (3D) visual inference, including difficulties integrating parts of an object passing behind an occluder over time,[174] Kaniza shapes, an inability to interpret pictorial cues or shape from shading, difficulties recognizing 3D objects from novel viewpoints, and difficulty with more complex face identification tasks.[70,170,175] Although performance can improve dramatically in these tasks, the bulk of the evidence suggests that even after decades of restored sight, many aspects of high-level processing remain impaired.[176] Some (although not all) of these improvements in performance likely reflect improvement in the ability to interpret a world that is primarily 2D, rather than the development of a true 3D visual representation of the world.

Consistent with these behavioral studies, fMRI and visual evoked potential (VEP) studies suggest a dramatic and persistent disruption of neural responses within category-selective extrastriate areas.[70,176,177]

Finally, several studies have addressed the question of whether an "amodal" conception of objects common to both senses exists a priori, or whether this concept requires experience to develop. Immediately after cataract removal, participants have difficulty matching seen and felt objects, but performance improves rapidly.[178] In a case report of a child who recovered her sight after removal of her dense bilateral cataracts, accurate reaching and grasping behavior was observed within half an hour of her first sight, while visual recognition of previously felt objects required a few days to develop.[179] A more quantitative study found that within months of surgery, visual and haptic integration behavior in sight-recovery individuals became comparable to those who are normally sighted, once visual acuity was accounted for.[180] One interpretation of these initial difficulties in matching seen and felt objects is that there is no "immediate" transfer of amodal knowledge after sight restoration. However, another possibility is that these difficulties do not reflect lack of amodal transfer, but rather simply reflect the known difficulties these individuals have in interpreting 3D objects visually.[181]

LATE BLINDNESS

The most dramatic behavioral adaptations to blindness are restricted to individuals who become blind early in life. Late-blind subjects tend to be much less fluent at skills such as Braille and use of a cane than early-blind subjects, though there are many individual exceptions. Understanding the reason for this is clinically important because for 87% of blind individuals globally, the onset of blindness occurs after the age of 14, and individuals above the age of 50 contribute over 80% of the global prevalence of blindness.[182]

One reason for this may be that adaptive skills are easier to learn at an early age, when cortex is more plastic. However, the enhanced skills of early-deprived individuals may also be partially due to behavioral and cultural factors—early-blind subjects tend to learn Braille and cane use at school, and as a result learn to rely on Braille and independent navigation skills more heavily than those deprived at a later age. What is most likely is that these two factors may reinforce each other: Early-blind subjects may learn sensory substitution skills more easily than those deprived later in life. This makes them rely on these skills more heavily, giving them practice and thereby further improving those skills; this, in turn, increases the amount of cross-modal plasticity that occurs. In those deprived later in life, this "circle of competency" may be much more difficult to establish.

Behavior

Despite showing far less cross-modal plasticity (as described further) late-blind individuals—even those who undergo loss later in life, or who undergo only partial visual loss—do show enhanced auditory behavior abilities across many tasks.[129,183–186]

Interestingly, in bisection auditory tasks thought to rely heavily on visual feedback for calibration,[187–189] late-blind individuals appear to retain the sighted advantage suggesting that this calibration is robust to prolonged deprivation.

It is perhaps somewhat surprising that late-blind individuals show similar behavioral enhancements as early-blind individuals across many tasks, given the strong evidence for different underlying neural activation patterns. Although both early- and late-blind individuals must learn to rely on auditory and tactile information, and therefore show comparable improvements in performance (perhaps reaching the limit of the available sensory information), they may reach these performance asymptotes via different neural mechanisms. It is easy to overlook the ability of the brain to produce analogous functional behavior through divergent methods of neuroplastic adaptation. However, the presence of similar auditory behavioral skills in late- and early-blind people does raise the concern that the cross-modal responses that are observed in early-blind individuals may be less critical for the auditory enhancements in performance observed in these individuals than has previously been assumed.

Neural responses

Although both early- and late-blind individuals show novel activations in typically visual brain areas, activation patterns within these areas in late-blind individuals are not only generally weaker, but often involve activation of slightly different neural areas.[82,83,94,157,184,185,190] Thus, although neural functional plasticity is maintained late into life, plasticity later in life is likely driven by different underlying mechanisms.

As described previously, even in early-blind individuals, plasticity is likely heavily constrained by white matter pathways that are established early in development. In late-blind individuals, plasticity presumably must occur within a visual architecture that is fully established.

One possibility is that late-blind cross-modal responses reflect top-down processes such as cross-modal feature-based attention,[155] attentional filling-in,[191,192] and visualization.[156,193,194] One fundamental difference between these two groups is that late-blind individuals may rely heavily on "visualization"—translating tactile and auditory information into a remembered visual sketchpad, whereas it is difficult to even conceive of "visualization" in the context of congenital blindness.

SENSORY SUBSTITUTION

Blind individuals must adapt and thrive in a world designed primarily by and for sighted individuals. To meet this challenge, blind and visually impaired individuals have access to a range of technological and behavioral tools, known collectively as sensory substitution technologies.

The range of skills and technologies that can be described as sensory substitution is immensely broad, ranging from learning to estimate when a drinking glass is full by the sound of the liquid and the weight of the glass, to smartphone apps used to navigate, to fully technological wearable prostheses that transmute visual information into verbal descriptions of the world.

Until recently, there were three sensory substitution technologies that were standardly used by blind individuals: Braille (invented in the early 1800s) for reading/writing, and the white cane and guide dog (both established in the early 1900s) for navigation. However, the last few decades have seen a rapid transformation in the field of sensory substitution that has impacted both literacy and navigation.

After decades of being the standard in blind education, Braille is being swiftly replaced by text-to-speech technologies. Over the last few decades, as most written materials have become available in a digital format and dictation software has improved, there has been a precipitous drop in the use of Braille. Digital technologies are less expensive, more accessible (it is much easier to download a book then send it to be transcribed), and support faster "reading" rates. Indeed in the blind community there is a heated debate currently about "the end of literacy" that bibliophile sighted individuals might consider an ominous foreshadowing.[195]

As far as navigation is concerned, the revolution is just beginning. Until recently, most attempts to improve on the guide dog and white cane focused on converting relatively low-level visual information into auditory or tactile cues. Examples include transducing a camera's image onto a 10 × 10 grid of electrodes placed on the tongue,[196] an echolocation device that transduces ultrasonic echoes containing information about object distance into auditory signals,[197] or the use of auditory frequencies and timbres over time to represent 2D spatial patterns.[198,199] Although participants could be successfully trained to high performance levels using these devices in the laboratory, to date none has been widely adopted by the blind community. It is not clear whether this is due to the amount of training that is needed to successfully use these devices,[200] the fact that using these devices necessarily interferes

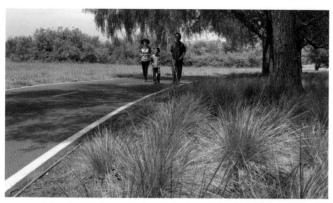

Fig. 41.6 Daniel Kish teaches visually-impaired student Nathan the skills of perception cane navigation and human echolocation. ©World Access For The Blind.

with natural auditory input, or it being impossible to transmit enough low-level visual information via audition or touch to be useful outside the laboratory context, in the cluttered visual world.

More recently, huge advances in artificial intelligence (AI) have permitted a radical new approach. First, the improved ability of AI to recognize faces, objects, and text mean that new apps for the blind no longer focus on presenting low-level sensory information—it is now possible to provide detailed auditory cues: "Pyrenees shepherd," "Fred," "Waitrose cocktail gherkins."[201] Second, vast improvements in GPS mapping and navigation technologies and databases provide an infrastructure for providing wayfinding information for blind individuals that was not previously available.[202]

Finally, there is a reawakened interest in a very low-tech solution - human echolocation. Using either the sound of a clicking tongue, or a simple handheld clicker, practitioners are able to navigate complex, novel environments, discern the layout of multiple objects and even identify simple objects. Echolocation can be used to judge the distance of objects, estimate their shape and size, and is sensitive to the unique acoustic absorption characteristics of different objects and materials in the environment .[203] Although scientists were aware of the potential of what was termed "facial vision" since the mid-1700s, blind children were often discouraged from 'clicking', which was misinterpreted as a repetitive behavior or a 'blindism'. Recent activism from within the blind community has led to renewed scientific interest[204,205] and an increased availability of training in echolocation (Fig. 41.6).

CONCLUSIONS

Over the last two decades a wide variety of studies have established that blindness results in remarkable changes in the response properties of

the human occipital cortex and have further shown that these changes in response properties underlie a variety of skill differences between blind and sighted subjects.

However, the neurophysiological substrates of human cross-modal plasticity remain frustratingly mysterious. It is still not clear whether the sources of cross-modal responses in occipital cortex include thalamic input, direct input from primary auditory or somatosensory areas, and/or feedback connections from polysensory extrastriate cortex. It does seem fairly clear that these connections are either mediated by preexisting anatomical pathways, or deviations in developmental "pruning," with little evidence for the existence of entirely novel anatomical pathways in early-blind individuals. Nor are the mechanisms underlying development of novel functional cortical specializations clear—although evidence does suggest that competition between inputs for cortical representation and intracortical competition both play a role.

A deeper understanding of how neural deterioration as a result of blindness and cross-modal plasticity might interact will also prove increasingly important as new sight restoration procedures (such as retinal implants, epithelial stem cell replacements, gene therapies, and retinal transplants) become available. The cross-modal plasticity that occurs as a result of sensory deprivation may well be of benefit to the blind individual, playing an important role in allowing them to make better use of his or her remaining senses. It is important therefore to be aware that restoring vision may have the unintended consequence of interfering with cross-modal abilities. This is of particular concern because, as described earlier, the neural deterioration that occurs as a result of early blindness does seem to severely limit an individual's ability to make use of restored vision.

Take, for example, the classic description of sight-recovery subject SB's inability to deal with crossing the road after sight restoration[169]:

He found the traffic frightening, and would not attempt to cross even a comparatively small street by himself. This was in marked contrast to his former behavior, as described to us by his wife, when he would cross any street in his own town by himself. In London, and later in his home town, he would show evident fear, even when led by a companion whom he trusted, and it was many months before he would venture alone.

Clearly, new visual information interfered with SB's ability to use cross-modal skills that he had relied on preoperatively. Thus, the decision to implant a prosthetic device or carry out a restorative surgery needs to consider not only the potential loss to any residual vision or hearing but also the potential of the device to interfere with the use of auditory and tactile skills. Given that the ability to make use of the restored sense will often be limited, any potential deterioration in a patients' ability to navigate with a cane or read Braille must be treated as a serious concern.

ACKNOWLEDGMENTS

Many thanks to Geoffrey Boynton for comments on this manuscript. W.P. was supported by Weill Neurohub Postdoctoral Fellowship. T.S. and I.F. were supported by an NIH National Eye Institute and Office of Director, Office of Behavioral and Social Sciences Research award R01EY014645 (to I.F.)

REFERENCES

1. Dubois J, Dehaene-Lambertz G, Kulikova S, Poupon C, Hüppi PS, Hertz-Pannier L. The early development of brain white matter: a review of imaging studies in fetuses, newborns and infants. *Neuroscience.* 2014;276:48–71.
2. Lebel C, Deoni S. The development of brain white matter microstructure. *Neuroimage.* 2018;182:207–218.
3. Brody BA, Kinney HC, Kloman AS, Gilles FH. Sequence of central nervous system myelination in human infancy. I. An autopsy study of myelination. *Journal of Neuropathology & Experimental Neurology.* 1987;46(3):283–301.
4. Movshon JA, Van Sluyters RC. Visual neural development. *Annu Rev Psychol.* 1981;32:477–522.
5. Kahn DM, Krubitzer L. Massive cross-modal cortical plasticity and the emergence of a new cortical area in developmentally blind mammals. *Proc Natl Acad Sci U S A.* 2002;99(17):11429–11434.

6. Karlen SJ, Kahn DM, Krubitzer L. Early blindness results in abnormal corticocortical and thalamocortical connections. *Neuroscience.* 2006;142(3):843–858.
7. Noppeney U, Friston KJ, Ashburner J, Frackowiak R, Price CJ. Early visual deprivation induces structural plasticity in gray and white matter. *Curr Biol.* 2005;15(13):R488–490.
8. Ptito M, Schneider FCG, Paulson OB, Kupers R. Alterations of the visual pathways in congenital blindness. *Exp. Brain Res.* 2008;187:41–49.
9. Shimony JS, Burton H, Epstein AA, McLaren DG, Sun SW, Snyder AZ. Diffusion tensor imaging reveals white matter reorganization in early blind humans. *Cereb Cortex.* 2006;16(11):1653–1661.
10. Bridge H, Cowey A, Ragge N, Watkins K. Imaging studies in congenital anophthalmia reveal preservation of *brain architecture in 'visual' cortex. Brain.* 2009;132(Pt 12):3467–3480.
11. Levin N, Dumoulin SO, Winawer J, Dougherty RF, Wandell BA. Cortical maps and white matter tracts following long period of visual deprivation and retinal image restoration. *Neuron.* 2010;65(1):21–31.
12. Bock AS, Binda P, Benson NC, Bridge H, Watkins KE, Fine I. Resting-state retinotopic organization in the absence of retinal input and visual Experience. *J Neurosci.* 2015;35(36):12366–12382.
13. Bock AS, Fine I. Anatomical and functional plasticity in early blind individuals and the mixture of experts architecture. *Front Hum Neurosci.* 2014;8971–971.
14. Favaro PD, Huang X, Hosang L, Stodieck S, Cui L, Liu Y-z, Schlüter OM. An opposing function of paralogs in balancing developmental synapse maturation. *PLoS biology.* 2018;16(12):e2006838.
15. Huang X, Stodieck SK, Goetze B, Cui L, Wong MH, Wenzel C, Schlüter OM. Progressive maturation of silent synapses governs the duration of a critical period. *Proc Natl Acad Sci U S A.* 2015;112(24):E3131–3140.
16. Boothe RG, Greenough WT, Lund JS, Wrege K. A quantitative investigation of spine and dendrite development of neurons in visual cortex (area 17) of Macaca nemestrina monkeys. *J Comp Neurol.* 1979;186(3):473–489.
17. Callaway EM, Borrell V. Developmental sculpting of dendritic morphology of layer 4 neurons in visual cortex: influence of retinal input. *J Neurosci.* 2011;31(20):7456–7470.
18. Iwakiri M, Komatsu Y. Postnatal development of NMDA receptor-mediated synaptic transmission in cat visual cortex. *Brain Res Dev Brain Res.* 1993;74(1):89–97.
19. Di Cristo G, Chattopadhyaya B, Kuhlman SJ, Fu Y, Bélanger MC, Wu CZ, Huang ZJ. Activity-dependent PSA expression regulates inhibitory maturation and onset of critical period plasticity. *Nat Neurosci.* 2007;10(12):1569–1577.
20. Huang ZJ, Kirkwood A, Pizzorusso T, Porciatti V, Morales B, Bear MF, Tonegawa S. BDNF regulates the maturation of inhibition and the critical period of plasticity in mouse visual cortex. *Cell.* 1999;98(6):739–755.
21. Nakata H, Nakamura S. Brain-derived neurotrophic factor regulates AMPA receptor trafficking to post-synaptic densities via IP3R and TRPC calcium signaling. *FEBS Lett.* 2007;581(10):2047–2054.
22. Sugiyama S, Di Nardo AA, Aizawa S, Matsuo I, Volovitch M, Prochiantz A, Hensch TK. Experience-dependent transfer of Otx2 homeoprotein into the visual cortex activates postnatal plasticity. *Cell.* 2008;134(3):508–520. doi:.
23. Berardi N, Pizzorusso T, Ratto GM, Maffei L. Molecular basis of plasticity in the visual cortex. *Trends Neurosci.* 2003;26(7):369–378.
24. Tatti R, Swanson OK, Lee MSE, Maffei A. Layer-specific developmental changes in excitation and inhibition in rat primary visual cortex. *eNeuro.* 2017;4(6).
25. Hensch TK, Quinlan EM. Critical periods in amblyopia. *Vis Neurosci.* 2018;35:E014.
26. Hensch TK. Critical period plasticity in local cortical circuits. *Nat Rev Neurosci.* 2005;6(11):877–888.
27. Huttenlocher PR, Dabholkar AS. Regional differences in synaptogenesis in human cerebral cortex. *J Comp Neurol.* 1997;387(2):167–178.
28. Huang X. Silent synapse: A new player in visual cortex critical period plasticity. *Pharmacol Res.* 2019;141:586–590.
29. Huttenlocher PR, de Courten C. The development of synapses in striate cortex of man. *Hum Neurobiol.* 1987;6(1):1–9.
30. Castrén E, Zafra F, Thoenen H, Lindholm D. Light regulates expression of brain-derived neurotrophic factor mRNA in rat visual cortex. *Proc Natl Acad Sci U S A.* 1992;89(20):9444–9448.
31. Feese BD, Pafundo DE, Schmehl MN, Kuhlman SJ. Binocular deprivation induces both age-dependent and age-independent forms of plasticity in parvalbumin inhibitory neuron visual response properties. *J Neurophysiol.* 2018;119(2):738–751.
32. Kang E, Durand S, LeBlanc JJ, Hensch TK, Chen C, Fagiolini M. Visual acuity development and plasticity in the absence of sensory experience. *J Neurosci.* 2013;33(45):17789–17796.
33. Fagiolini M, Pizzorusso T, Berardi N, Domenici L, Maffei L. Functional postnatal development of the rat primary visual cortex and the role of visual experience: dark rearing and monocular deprivation. *Vision Res.* 1994;34(6):709–720.
34. Weaver KE, Richards TL, Saenz M, Petropoulos H, Fine I. Neurochemical changes within human early blind occipital cortex. *Neuroscience.* 2013;252:222–233.
35. Coullon GS, Emir UE, Fine I, Watkins KE, Bridge H. Neurochemical changes in the pericalcarine cortex in congenital blindness attributable to bilateral anophthalmia. *J Neurophysiol.* 2015;114(3):1725–1733.
36. Bluml S, Wisnowski JL, Nelson Jr. MD,, Paquette L, Gilles FH, Kinney HC, Panigrahy A. Metabolic maturation of the human brain from birth through adolescence: insights from in vivo magnetic resonance spectroscopy. *Cereb Cortex.* 2013;23(12):2944–2955. https://doi.org/10.1093/cercor/bhs283.
37. Fosse VM, Heggelund P, Fonnum F. Postnatal development of glutamatergic, GABAergic, and cholinergic neurotransmitter phenotypes in the visual cortex, lateral geniculate nucleus, pulvinar, and superior colliculus in cats. *J Neurosci.* 1989;9(2):426–435.
38. Wang XC, Du XX, Tian Q, Wang JZ. Correlation between choline signal intensity and acetylcholine level in different brain regions of rat. *Neurochem Res.* 2008;33(5):814–819.
39. Wess J. Molecular biology of muscarinic acetylcholine receptors. *Crit Rev Neurobiol.* 1996;10(1):69–99.
40. Argandona EG, Bengoetxea H, Lafuente JV. Physical exercise is required for environmental enrichment to offset the quantitative effects of dark-rearing on the s-100beta astrocytic density in the rat visual cortex. *J Anat.* 2009;215(2):132–140.
41. Bengoetxea H, Ortuzar N, Rico-Barrio I, Lafuente JV, Argandoña EG. Increased physical activity is not enough to recover astrocytic population from dark-rearing. *Synergy with multisensory enrichment is required. Front Cell Neurosci.* 2013;7:170.
42. De Volder AG, Bol A, Blin J, Robert A, Arno P, Grandin C, Veraart C. Brain energy metabolism in early blind subjects: Neural activity in the visual cortex. *Brain Res.* 1997;750:235–244.
43. Uhl F, Franzen P, Podreka I, Steiner M, Deecke L. Increased regional cerebral blood flow in inferior occipital cortex and cerebellum of early blind humans. *Neurosci Lett.* 1993;150(2):162–164.
44. Veraart C, De Volder AG, Wanet-Defalque MC, Bol A, Michel C, Goffinet AM. Glucose Utilization in human visual cortex is abnormally elevated in blindness of early onset but decreased in blindness of late onset. *Brain Res.* 1990;510:115–121.
45. Wanet-Defalque MC, Veraart C, De Volder A, Metz R, Michel C, Dooms G, Goffinet A. High metabolic activity in the visual cortex of early blind human subjects. *Brain Res.* 1988;446(2):369–373.
46. Benevento LA, Bakkum BW, Port JD, Cohen RS. The effects of dark-rearing on the electrophysiology of the rat visual cortex. *Brain Res.* 1992;572(1–2):198–207.
47. Wiesel TN, Hubel DH. Effects of visual deprivation on morphology and physiology of cells in the cats lateral geniculate body. *J Neurophysiol.* 1963;26:978–993.
48. Dehay C, Giroud P, Berland M, Killackey H, Kennedy H. Contribution of thalamic input to the specification of cytoarchitectonic cortical fields in the primate: effects of bilateral enucleation in the fetal monkey on the boundaries, dimensions, and gyrification of striate and extrastriate cortex. *J Comp Neurol.* 1996;367(1):70–89.
49. Dehay C, Giroud P, Berland M, Killackey HP, Kennedy H. Phenotypic characterisation of respecified visual cortex subsequent to prenatal enucleation in the monkey: development of acetylcholinesterase and cytochrome oxidase patterns. *J Comp Neurol.* 1996;376(3):386–402.
50. Karlen SJ, Krubitzer L. Effects of bilateral enucleation on the size of visual and nonvisual areas of the brain. *Cereb Cortex,* 1996;19(6):1360–1371.
51. Rakic P, Suner I, Williams RW. A novel cytoarchitectonic area induced experimentally within the primate visual cortex. *Proceedings of the National Academy of Sciences.* 1991:88(6);2083–2087.
52. Anurova I, Renier LA, De Volder AG, Carlson S, Rauschecker JP. Relationship between cortical thickness and functional activation in the early blind. *Cereb Cortex.* 2015;25(8):2035–2048.
53. Jiang J, Zhu W, Shi F, Liu Y, Li J, Qin W, Jiang T. Thick visual cortex in the early blind. *J Neurosci.* 2009;29(7):2205–2211.
54. Guerreiro MJ, Erfort MV, Henssler J, Putzar L, Röder B. Increased visual cortical thickness in sight-recovery individuals. *Hum Brain Mapp.* 2015;36(12):5265–5274.
55. Andelin AK, Olavarria JF, Fine I, Taber EN, Schwartz D, Kroenke CD, Stevens AA. The effect of onset age of visual deprivation on visual cortex surface area across-species. *Cereb Cortex.* 2019;29(10):4321–4333.
56. Reillo I, de Juan Romero C, Garcia-Cabezas MA, Borrell V. A role for intermediate radial glia in the tangential expansion of the mammalian cerebral cortex. *Cereb Cortex.* 2011;21(7):1674–1694.
57. Natu VS, Gomez J, Barnett M, Jeska B, Kirilina E, Jaeger C, Grill-Spector K. Apparent thinning of human visual cortex during childhood is associated with myelination. *Proc Natl Acad Sci U S A.* 2019;116(41):20750–20759.
58. McLaughlin T, Torborg CL, Feller MB, O'Leary DD. Retinotopic map refinement requires spontaneous retinal waves during a brief critical period of development. *Neuron.* 2003;40(6):1147–1160.
59. Striem-Amit E, Ovadia-Caro S, Caramazza A, Margulies DS, Villringer A, Amedi A. Functional connectivity of visual cortex in the blind follows retinotopic organization principles. *Brain.* 2015;138(Pt 6):1679–1695.
60. Cang J, Renteria RC, Kaneko M, Liu X, Copenhagen DR, Stryker MP. Development of precise maps in visual cortex requires patterned spontaneous activity in the retina. *Neuron.* 2005;48(5):797–809.
61. Grubb MS, Rossi FM, Changeux JP, Thompson ID. Abnormal functional organization in the dorsal lateral geniculate nucleus of mice lacking the beta 2 subunit of the nicotinic acetylcholine receptor. *Neuron.* 2003;40(6):1161–1172.
62. Ishikawa AW, Komatsu Y, Yoshimura Y. Experience-dependent emergence of fine-scale networks in visual cortex. *The Journal of Neuroscience.* 2014;34(37):12576–12586.
63. Ko H, Mrsic-Flogel TD, Hofer SB. Emergence of feature-specific connectivity in cortical microcircuits in the absence of visual experience. *The Journal of Neuroscience.* 2014;34(29):9812–9816.
64. Rizzi M, Russell L, Powell K. Do visual circuits mature without visual stimuli? *The Journal of Neuroscience.* 2014;34(48):15833–15835.
65. Ackman JB, Crair MC. Role of emergent neural activity in visual map development. *Curr Opin Neurobiol.* 2014;24(1):166–175.
66. Sherman SM, Spear PD. Organization of visual pathways in normal and visually deprived cats. *Physiol Rev.* 1982;62(2):738–855.
67. Wiesel TN, Hubel DH. Comparison of the effects of unilateral and bilateral eye closure on cortical unit responses in kittens. *J Neurophysiol.* 1965;28(6):1029–1040.
68. Kalia A, Lesmes LA, Dorr M, Gandhi T, Chatterjee G, Ganesh S, Sinha P. Development of pattern vision following early and extended blindness. *Proc Natl Acad Sci U S A.* 2014;111(5):2035–2039.
69. Fine I, Wade AR, Brewer AA, May MG, Goodman DF, Boynton GM, MacLeod DI. Long-term deprivation affects visual perception and cortex. *Nat Neurosci.* 2003;6(9):915–916.
70. Sadato N, Okada T, Honda M, Yonekura Y. Critical period for cross-modal plasticity in blind humans: a functional MRI study. *Neuroimage.* 2002;16(2):389–400.
71. Dehaene S, Cohen L. Cultural recycling of cortical maps. *Neuron.* 2007;56(2):384–398.

72. Grant AC, Thiagarajah MC, Sathian K. Tactile perception in blind Braille readers: A psychophysical study of acuity and hyperacuity using gratings and dot patterns. *Percept Psychophys.* 2000;62(2):301–312.

73. Pascual-Leone A, Torres F. Plasticity of the sensorimotor cortex representation of the reading finger in Braille readers. *Brain.* 1993;116(1):39–52.

74. Alary F, Duquette M, Goldstein R, Chapman CE, Voss P, La Buissonnière-Ariza V, Lepore F. Tactile acuity in the blind: a closer look reveals superiority over the sighted in some but not all cutaneous tasks. *Neuropsychologia.* 2009;47(10):2037–2043.

75. Goldreich D, Kanics IM. Tactile acuity is enhanced in blindness. *J Neurosci.* 2003;23(8):3439–3445.

76. Goldreich D, Kanics IM. Performance of blind and sighted humans on a tactile grating detection task. *Percept Psychophys.* 2006;68(8):1363–1371.

77. Van Boven RW, Hamilton RH, Kauffman T, Keenan JP, Pascual-Leone A. Tactile spatial resolution in blind braille readers. *Neurology.* 2000;54(12):2230–2236.

78. Voss P, Collignon O, Lassonde M, Lepore F. Adaptation to sensory loss. *WIREs Cognitive Science.* 2010;1(3):308–328.

79. Sterr A, Müller MM, Elbert T, Rockstroh B, Pantev C, Taub E. Perceptual correlates of changes in cortical representation of fingers in blind multifinger Braille readers. *J Neurosci.* 1998;18(11):4417–4423.

80. Uhl F, Franzen P, Lindinger G, Lang W, Deecke L. On the functionality of the visually deprived occipital cortex in early blind persons. *Neurosci Lett.* 1991;124(2):256–259.

81. Amedi A, Raz N, Pianka P, Malach R, Zohary E. Early 'visual' cortex activation correlates with superior verbal memory performance in the blind. *Nat Neurosci.* 2003;6(7):758–766.

82. Burton H. Visual cortex activity in early and late blind people. *J Neurosci.* 2003;23(10):4005–4011.

83. Burton H, Snyder AZ, Conturo TE, Akbudak E, Ollinger JM, Raichle ME. Adaptive changes in early and late blind: a fMRI study of Braille reading. *J Neurophysiol.* 2002;87(1):589–607.

84. Noppeney U, Friston KJ, Price CJ. Effects of visual deprivation on the organization of the semantic system. *Brain.* 2003;126(Pt 7):1620–1627.

85. Roder B, Stock O, Bien S, Neville H, Rosler F. Speech processing activates visual cortex in congenitally blind humans. *Eur J Neurosci.* 2002;16(5):930–936.

86. Sadato N, Pascual-Leone A, Grafman J, Ibanez V, Deiber MP, Dold G, Hallett M. Activation of the primary visual cortex by Braille reading in blind subjects. *Nature.* 1996;380(6574):526–528.

87. Kim JS, Kanjlia S, Merabet LB, Bedny M. Development of the visual word form area requires visual experience: Evidence from blind Braille readers. *The Journal of neuroscience: the official journal of the Society for Neuroscience.* 2017;37(47):11495–11504.

88. Cohen LG, Celnik P, Pascual-Leone A, Corwell B, Falz L, Dambrosia J, Hallett M. Functional relevance of cross-modal plasticity in blind humans. *Nature.* 1997;389(6647):180–183.

89. Hamilton R, Keenan JP, Catala M, Pascual-Leone A. Alexia for Braille following bilateral occipital stroke in an early blind woman. *Neuroreport.* 2000;11:237–240.

90. Siuda-Krzywicka K, Bola Ł, Paplińska M, Sumera E, Jednoróg K, Marchewka A,, Szwed M. Massive cortical reorganization in sighted Braille readers. *Elife.* 2016;5e10762-e10762.

91. Gougoux F, Lepore F, Lassonde M, Voss P, Zatorre RJ, Belin P. Neuropsychology: pitch discrimination in the early blind. *Nature.* 2004;430(6997):309.

92. Voss P, Zatorre RJ. Occipital cortical thickness predicts performance on pitch and musical tasks in blind individuals. *Cereb Cortex.* 2012;22(11):2455–2465.

93. Wan CY, Wood AG, Reutens DC, Wilson SJ. Early but not late-blindness leads to enhanced auditory perception. *Neuropsychologia.* 2010;48(1):344–348.

94. Collignon O, Dormal G, Albouy G, Vandewalle G, Voss P, Phillips C, Lepore F. Impact of blindness onset on the functional organization and the connectivity of the occipital cortex. *Brain.* 2013;136(9):2769–2783.

95. Watkins KE, Shakespeare TJ, O'Donoghue MC, Alexander I, Ragge N, Cowey A, Bridge H. Early auditory processing in area V5/MT+ of the congenitally blind brain. *J Neurosci.* 2013;33(46):18242–18246.

96. Hamilton RH, Pascual-Leone A, Schlaug G. Absolute pitch in blind musicians. *Neuroreport.* 2004;15(5):803–806.

97. Arnaud L, Gracco V, Ménard L. Enhanced perception of pitch changes in speech and music in early blind adults. *Neuropsychologia.* 2018;117:261–270.

98. Gaab N, Schulze K, Ozdemir E, Schlaug G. Neural correlates of absolute pitch differ between blind and sighted musicians. *Neuroreport.* 2006;17(18):1853–1857.

99. Stevens AA, Weaver KE. Functional characteristics of auditory cortex in the blind. *Behav Brain Res.* 2009;196:134–138.

100. Huber E, Chang K, Alvarez I, Hundle A, Bridge H, Fine I. Early blindness shapes cortical representations of auditory frequency within auditory cortex. *J Neurosci.* 2019;39(26):5143–5152.

101. Lessard N, Pare M, Lepore F, Lassonde M. Early-blind human subjects localize sound sources better than sighted subjects. *Nature.* 1998;395(6699):278–280.

102. Roder B, Teder-Salejarvi W, Sterr A, Rosler F, Hillyard SA, Neville HJ. Improved auditory spatial tuning in blind humans. *Nature.* 1999;400(6740):162–166.

103. Battal C, Occelli V, Bertonati G, Falagiarda F, Collignon O. General enhancement of spatial hearing in congenitally blind people. *Psychological Science.* 2020;31(9):1129–1139.

104. Gori M, Sandini G, Martinoli C, Burr DC. Impairment of auditory spatial localization in congenitally blind human subjects. *Brain.* 2014;137(Pt 1):288–293.

105. Kolarik AJ, Cirstea S, Pardhan S. Evidence for enhanced discrimination of virtual auditory distance among blind listeners using level and direct-to-reverberant cues. *Exp Brain Res.* 2013;224(4):623–633.

106. Nilsson ME, Schenkman BN. Blind people are more sensitive than sighted people to binaural sound-location cues, particularly inter-aural level differences. *Hear Res.* 2016;332:223–232.

107. Doucet ME, Guillemot JP, Lassonde M, Gagné JP, Leclerc C, Lepore F. Blind subjects process auditory spectral cues more efficiently than sighted individuals. *Exp Brain Res.* 2005;160(2):194–202.

108. Dufour A, Després O, Candas V. Enhanced sensitivity to echo cues in blind subjects. *Exp Brain Res.* 2005;165(4):515–519.

109. Vercillo T, Milne JL, Gori M, Goodale MA. Enhanced auditory spatial localization in blind echolocators. *Neuropsychologia.* 2015;67:35–40.

110. Vercillo T, Tonelli A, Gori M. Early visual deprivation prompts the use of body-centered frames of reference for auditory localization. *Cognition.* 2018;170:263–269.

111. Voss P. Auditory spatial perception without vision. *Front Psychol.* 2016;7:1960.

112. Aggius-Vella E, Campus C, Gori M. Different audio spatial metric representation around the body. *Sci Rep.* 2018;8(1):9383.

113. Voss P, Tabry V, Zatorre RJ. Trade-off in the sound localization abilities of early blind individuals between the horizontal and vertical planes. *J Neurosci.* 2015;35(15):6051–6056.

114. Zwiers MP, Van Opstal AJ, Cruysberg JR. A spatial hearing deficit in early-blind humans. *J Neurosci.* 2001;21(9):RC142: 141–145.

115. Ahmad H, Setti W, Campus C, Capris E, Facchini V, Sandini G, Gori M. The sound of scotoma: Audio space representation reorganization in individuals with macular degeneration. *Frontiers in integrative neuroscience.* 2019;13:44.

116. Weeks R, Horwitz B, Aziz-Sultan A, Tian B, Wessinger CM, Cohen LG, Rauschecker JP. A positron emission tomographic study of auditory localization in the congenitally blind. *J Neurosci.* 2000;20(7):2664–2672.

117. Gougoux F, Zatorre RJ, Lassonde M, Voss P, Lepore F. A functional neuroimaging study of sound localization: visual cortex activity predicts performance in early-blind individuals. *PLoS Biol.* 2005;3(2):e27.

118. Leclerc C, Saint-Amour D, Lavoie ME, Lassonde M, Lepore F. Brain functional reorganization in early blind humans revealed by auditory event-related potentials. *Neuroreport.* 2000;11(3):545–550.

119. Collignon O, Vandewalle G, Voss P, Albouy G, Charbonneau G, Lassonde M, Lepore F. Functional specialization for auditory-spatial processing in the occipital cortex of congenitally blind humans. *Proc Natl Acad Sci U S A.* 2011;108(11):4435–4440.

120. Collignon O, Lassonde M, Lepore F, Bastien D, Veraart C. Functional cerebral reorganization for auditory spatial processing and auditory substitution of vision in early blind subjects. *Cereb Cortex.* 2007;17(2):457–465.

121. Falchier A, Clavagnier S, Barone P, Kennedy H. Anatomical evidence of multimodal integration in primate striate cortex. *J Neurosci.* 2002;22(13):5749–5759.

122. Clavagnier S, Falchier A, Kennedy H. Long-distance feedback projections to area V1: implications for multisensory integration, spatial awareness, and visual consciousness. *Cogn Affect Behav Neurosci.* 2004;4(2):117–126.

123. Heilman KM, Bowers D, Valenstein E, Watson RT. The right hemisphere: Neuropsychological functions. *J Neurosurg.* 1986;64(5):693–704.

124. Dormal G, Rezk M, Yakobov E, Lepore F, Collignon O. Auditory motion in the sighted and blind: Early visual deprivation triggers a large-scale imbalance between auditory and "visual" brain regions. *Neuroimage.* 2016;134:630–644.

125. Jiang F, Stecker GC, Boynton GM, Fine I. Early blindness results in developmental plasticity for auditory motion processing within auditory and occipital cortex. *Front Hum Neurosci.* 2016;10:324.

126. Poirier C, Collignon O, Scheiber C, Renier L, Vanlierde A, Tranduy D, De Volder AG. Auditory motion perception activates visual motion areas in early blind subjects. *Neuroimage.* 2006;31(1):279–285.

127. Saenz M, Lewis LB, Huth AG, Fine I, Koch C. Visual motion area MT+/V5 responds to auditory motion in human sight-recovery Subjects. *J Neurosci.* 2008;28(20):5141–5148.

128. Strnad L, Peelen MV, Bedny M, Caramazza A. Multivoxel pattern analysis reveals auditory motion information in MT+ of both congenitally blind and sighted individuals. *PLoS ONE.* 2013;8(4):e63198. =.

129. Lewald J. Exceptional ability of blind humans to hear sound motion: implications for the emergence of auditory space. *Neuropsychologia.* 2013;51(1):181–186.

130. Jiang F, Stecker GC, Fine I. Auditory motion processing after early blindness. *J Vis.* 2014;14(13):4.

131. Bedny M, Konkle T, Pelphrey K, Saxe R, Pascual-Leone A. Sensitive period for a multimodal response in human visual motion area MT/MST. *Curr Biol.* 2010;20(21):1900–1906.

132. Andersen ES, Dunlea A, Kekelis L. The impact of input: Language acquisition in the visually impaired. *First Language.* 1993;13(37):23–49.

133. Dunlea A, Andersen ES. The emergence process: Conceptual and linguistic influences on morphological development. *First Language.* 1992;12(34):95–115.

134. Loiotile R, Lane C, Omaki A, Bedny M. Enhanced performance on a sentence comprehension task in congenitally blind adults. *Language, cognition and neuroscience.* 2020;35(8):1010–1023.

135. Occelli V, Lacey S, Stephens C, Merabet LB, Sathian K. Enhanced verbal abilities in the congenitally blind. *Experimental brain research.* 2017;235(6):1709–1718.

136. Bedny M, Koster-Hale J, Elli G, Yazzolino L, Saxe R. There's more to "sparkle" than meets the eye: Knowledge of vision and light verbs among congenitally blind and sighted individuals. *Cognition.* 2019;189:105–115.

137. Lane C, Kanjlia S, Omaki A, Bedny M. "Visual" cortex of congenitally blind adults responds to syntactic movement. *J Neurosci.* 2015;35(37):12859–12868.

138. Watkins KE, Cowey A, Alexander I, Filippini N, Kennedy JM, Smith SM, Bridge H. Language networks in anophthalmia: maintained hierarchy of processing in 'visual' cortex. *Brain.* 2012;135(Pt 5):1566–1577.

139. Bedny M, Pascual-Leone A, Dodell-Feder D, Fedorenko E, Saxe R. Language processing in the occipital cortex of congenitally blind adults. *Proc Natl Acad Sci U S A.* 2011;108(11):4429–4434.

140. Bedny M, Richardson H, Saxe R. "Visual" cortex responds to spoken language in blind children. *j neurosci.* 2015;35(33):11674–11681.

141. Burton H, Diamond JB, McDermott KB. Dissociating cortical regions activated by semantic and phonological tasks: a FMRI study in blind and sighted people. *J Neurophysiol.* 2003;90(3):1965–1982.

142. Amedi A, Floel A, Raz N, Cohen L, Zohary E. Combining fMRI and TMS to assess the functional role of the blinds occipital cortex in verbal tasks: TU 335. *Neuroimage.* 2004:22.

143. Raz N, Amedi A, Zohary E. V1 activation in congenitally blind humans is associated with episodic retrieval. *Cereb Cortex.* 2005;15(9):1459–1468.

144. Kanjlia S, Loiotile RE, Harhen N, Bedny M. 'Visual' cortices of congenitally blind adults are sensitive to response selection demands in a go/no-go task. *Neuroimage.* 2021;236:118023.

145. Kanjlia S, Feigenson L, Bedny M. Neural basis of approximate number in congenital blindness. *Cortex.* 2021;142:342–356.

146. Kanjlia S, Lane C, Feigenson L, Bedny M. Absence of visual experience modifies the neural basis of numerical thinking. *Proc Natl Acad Sci U S A.* 2016;113(40):11172–11177.

147. Pant R, Kanjlia S, Bedny M. A sensitive period in the neural phenotype of language in blind individuals. *Dev Cogn Neurosci.* 2020;41:100744.

148. Bedny M. Evidence from blindness for a cognitively pluripotent cortex. *Trends Cogn Sci.* 2017;21(9):637–648.

149. Coullon GS, Jiang F, Fine I, Watkins KE, Bridge H. Subcortical functional reorganization due to early blindness. *J Neurophysiol.* 2015;113(7):2889–2899.

150. Gurtubay-Antolin A, Battal C, Maffei C, Rezk M, Mattioni S, Jovicich J, Collignon O. Direct structural connections between auditory and visual motion-selective regions in humans. *J Neurosci.* 2021;41(11):2393–2405.

151. Spector F, Maurer D. Synesthesia: a new approach to understanding the development of perception. *Dev Psychol.* 2009;45(1):175–189.

152. Pascual-Leone A, Hamilton R. The metamodal organization of the brain. *Prog Brain Res.* 2001;Vol. 134:427–445.

153. Cecchetti L, Kupers R, Ptito M, Pietrini P, Ricciardi E. Are supramodality and cross-modal plasticity the yin and yang of brain development? From blindness to rehabilitation. *Front Syst Neurosci.* 2016;1089–89.

154. Merabet LB, Hamilton R, Schlaug G, Swisher JD, Kiriakopoulos ET, Pitskel NB, Pascual-Leone A. Rapid and reversible recruitment of early visual cortex for touch. *PLoS ONE.* 2008;3(8):e3046.

155. Ciaramitaro VM, Buracas GT, Boynton GM. Spatial and cross-modal attention alter responses to unattended sensory information in early visual and auditory human cortex. *J Neurophysiol.* 2007;98(4):2399–2413.

156. Kourtzi Z, Kanwisher N. Activation in human MT/MST by static images with implied motion. *J Cogn Neurosci.* 2000;12(1):48–55.

157. Burton H, McLaren DG, Sinclair RJ. Reading embossed capital letters: an fMRI study in blind and sighted individuals. *Hum Brain Mapp.* 2006;27(4):325–339.

158. Jiang F, Beauchamp MS, Fine I. Re-examining overlap between tactile and visual motion responses within hMT+ and STS. *Neuroimage.* 2015;119:187–196.

159. Sadato N, Pascual-Leone A, Grafman J, Deiber MP, Ibanez V, Hallett M. Neural networks for Braille reading by the blind. *Brain.* 1998;121(Pt 7):1213–1229.

160. Dormal G, Lepore F, Harissi-Dagher M, Albouy G, Bertone A, Rossion B, Collignon O. Tracking the evolution of crossmodal plasticity and visual functions before and after sight restoration. *J Neurophysiol.* 2015;113(6):1727–1742.

161. Siu C, Balsor J, Merlin S, Federer F, Angelucci A. A direct interareal feedback-to-feedforward circuit in primate visual cortex. *Nat Commun.* 2021;12(1):4911–4911.

162. Kätzel D, Miesenböck G. Experience-dependent rewiring of specific inhibitory connections in adult neocortex. *PLoS Biol.* 2014;12(2):e1001798.

163. Morales B, Choi SY, Kirkwood A. Dark rearing alters the development of GABAergic transmission in visual cortex. *J Neurosci.* 2002;22(18):8084–8090.

164. Desgent S, Ptito M. Cortical GABAergic interneurons in cross-modal plasticity following early blindness. *Neural Plast.* 2012;2012:590725.

165. Boroojerdi B, Battaglia F, Muellbacher W, Cohen LG. Mechanisms underlying rapid experience-dependent plasticity in the human visual cortex. *Proc Natl Acad Sci U S A.* 2001;98(25):14698–14701.

166. Amedi A, Floel A, Knecht S, Zohary E, Cohen LG. Transcranial magnetic stimulation of the occipital pole interferes with verbal processing in blind subjects. *Nat Neurosci.* 2004;7(11):1266–1270.

167. Cheselden W. An account of some observations made by a young gentleman, who was born blind, or who lost his sight so early, that he had no remembrance of ever having seen, and was couch'd between 13 and 14 years of age. *Phil. Trans.* 1728;402:447–450.

168. Gregory RL, Wallace JG. *Recovery from early blindness: A case study. Experimental Psychological Society Monograph 2.* Cambridge: Heffer and Sons; 1963.

169. Sinha P. Once blind and now they see. *Sci Am.* 2013;309(1):48–55.

170. McKyton A, Ben-Zion I, Doron R, Zohary E. The limits of shape recognition following late emergence from blindness. *Curr Biol.* 2015;25(18):2373–2378.

171. Ostrovsky Y, Andalman A, Sinha P. Vision following extended congenital blindness. *Psychol Sci.* 2006;17(12):1009–1014.

172. Bottari D, Troje NF, Ley P, Hense M, Kekunnaya R, Röder B. The neural development of the biological motion processing system does not rely on early visual input. *Cortex.* 2015;71:359–367.

173. Guerreiro MJS, Putzar L, Röder B. Persisting Cross-Modal Changes in Sight-Recovery Individuals Modulate Visual Perception. *Current Biology.* 2016;26(22):3096–3100.

174. Orlov T, Raveh M, McKyton A, Ben-Zion I, Zohary E. Learning to perceive shape from temporal integration following late emergence from blindness. *Curr Biol.* 2021;31(14):3162–3167. e3165.

175. Gandhi TK, Singh AK, Swami P, Ganesh S, Sinha P. Emergence of categorical face perception after extended early-onset blindness. *Proc Natl Acad Sci U S A.* 2017;114(23):6139–6143.

176. Huber E, Webster JM, Brewer AA, MacLeod DI, Wandell BA, Boynton GM, Fine I. A lack of experience-dependent plasticity after more than a decade of recovered sight. *Psychol Sci.* 2015;26(4):393–401.

177. Sourav S, Bottari D, Kekunnaya R, Röder B. Evidence of a retinotopic organization of early visual cortex but impaired extrastriate processing in sight recovery individuals. *Journal of Vision.* 2018;18(3):22–22.

178. Held R, Ostrovsky Y, de Gelder B, Gandhi T, Ganesh S, Mathur U, Sinha P. The newly sighted fail to match seen with felt. *Nature Neuroscience.* 2011;14(5):551–553.

179. Chen J, Wu ED, Chen X, Zhu LH, Li X, Thorn F, Qu J. Rapid integration of tactile and visual information by a newly sighted child. *Curr Biol.* 2016;26(8):1069–1074.

180. Senna I, Andres E, McKyton A, Ben-Zion I, Zohary E, Ernst MO. Development of multisensory integration following prolonged early-onset visual deprivation. *Current Biology.* 2021;31(21):4879–4885. e4876.

181. Schwenkler J. On the matching of seen and felt shape by newly sighted subjects. *Iperception.* 2012;3(3):186–188.

182. WHO. *Global Data on Visual Impairments 2010.* Geneva: World Health Organization; 2012.

183. Paré S, Bleau M, Djerourou I, Malotaux V, Kupers R, Ptito M. Spatial navigation with horizontally spatialized sounds in early and late blind individuals. *PLoS ONE.* 2021;16(2):e0247448.

184. Tao Q, Chan CCH, Luo Y-J, Li J-J, Ting K-H, Wang J, Lee TMC. How does experience modulate auditory spatial processing in individuals with blindness? *Brain Topography.* 2015;28(3):506–519.

185. Voss P, Gougoux F, Zatorre RJ, Lassonde M, Lepore F. Differential occipital responses in early- and late-blind individuals during a sound-source discrimination task. *Neuroimage.* 2008;40(2):746–758.

186. Voss P, Lassonde M, Gougoux F, Fortin M, Guillemot JP, Lepore F. Early- and late-onset blind individuals show supra-normal auditory abilities in far-space. *Curr Biol.* 2004;14(19):1734–1738.

187. Amadeo MB, Campus C, Gori M. Impact of years of blindness on neural circuits underlying auditory spatial representation. *Neuroimage.* 2019;191:140–149.

188. Esposito D, Bollini A, Gori M. (1–5 Nov. 2021). The link between blindness onset and audiospatial processing: testing audiomotor cues in acoustic virtual reality. Paper presented at the 2021 43rd Annual International Conference of the IEEE Engineering in Medicine & Biology Society (EMBC).

189. Finocchietti S, Cappagli G, Gori M. Encoding audio motion: spatial impairment in early blind individuals. *Front Psychol.* 2015;6:1357.

190. Burton H, McLaren DG. Visual cortex activation in late-onset, Braille naive blind individuals: an fMRI study during semantic and phonological tasks with heard words. *Neurosci Lett.* 2006;392(1–2):38–42.

191. Masuda Y, Dumoulin SO, Nakadomari S, Wandell BA. V1 projection zone signals in human macular degeneration depend on task, not stimulus. *Cereb Cortex.* 2008;18(11):2483–2493.

192. Masuda Y, Horiguchi H, Dumoulin SO, Furuta A, Miyauchi S, Nakadomari S, Wandell BA. Task-dependent V1 responses in human retinitis pigmentosa. *Invest Ophthalmol Vis Sci.* 2010;51(10):5356–5364.

193. Williams MA, Baker CI, Op de Beeck HP, Shim WM, Dang S, Triantafyllou C, Kanwisher N. Feedback of visual object information to foveal retinotopic cortex. *Nat Neurosci.* 2008;11(12):1439–1445.

194. Hsieh PJ, Vul E, Kanwisher N. Recognition alters the spatial pattern of FMRI activation in early retinotopic cortex. *J Neurophysiol.* 2010;103(3):1501–1507.

195. Aviv R. *Listening to Braille. The New York Times;* Jan 3, 2010.

196. Chebat D-R, Schneider FC, Kupers R, Ptito M. Navigation with a sensory substitution device in congenitally blind individuals. *Neuroreport.* 2011;22(7):342–347.

197. De Volder AG, Catalan-Ahumada M, Robert A, Bol A, Labar D, Coppens A, Veraart C. Changes in occipital cortex activity in early blind humans using a sensory substitution device. *Brain Res.* 1999;826(1):128–134.

198. Meijer PB. An experimental system for auditory image representations. *IEEE Trans Biomed Eng.* 1992;39(2):112–121.

199. Arno P, De Volder AG, Vanlierde A, Wanet-Defalque MC, Streel E, Robert A, Veraart C. Occipital activation by pattern recognition in the early blind using auditory substitution for vision. *Neuroimage.* 2001;13(4):632–645.

200. Buchs G, Haimler B, Kerem M, Maidenbaum S, Braun L, Amedi A. A self-training program for sensory substitution devices. *PLoS ONE.* 2021;16(4):e0250281.

201. Nishajith A, Nivedha J, Nair SS, Shaffi JM. (2018). Smart cap-wearable visual guidance system for blind. Paper presented at the 2018 International Conference on Inventive Research in Computing Applications (ICIRCA).

202. May M. (2000). Accessible GPS navigation and digital map information for blind consumers. Paper presented at the Proceedings of the 13th International Technical Meeting of the Satellite Division of The Institute of Navigation (ION GPS 2000).

203. Norman LJ, Dodsworth C, Foresteire D, Thaler L. Human click-based echolocation: Effects of blindness and age, and real-life implications in a 10-week training program. *PLoS ONE.* 2021;16(6):e0252330.

204. Thaler L, Arnott SR, Goodale MA. Neural correlates of natural human echolocation in early and late blind echolocation experts. *PLoS ONE.* 2011;6(5):e20162.

205. Thaler L, Reich GM, Zhang X, Wang D, Smith GE, Tao Z, Antoniou M. Mouth-clicks used by blind expert human echolocators – signal description and model based signal synthesis. *PLoS Comput Biol.* 2017;13(8):e1005670.

INDEX

Notes:

vs. indicates a comparison or differential diagnosis
Page numbers followed by *t* indicate tables, by *f*
  indicate figures, by *b* indicate boxes.
To save space in the index, the following
  abbreviations have been used:
IPL – inner plexiform layer
ipRGCs - intrinsically photosensitive retinal
  ganglion cells
LGN – lateral geniculate nucleus
RGC – retinal ganglion cells
RPE – retinal pigment epithelium

A

ABCA4 mutations, 411*b*
ABCA4 gene, Stargardt's disease, 425*b*, 426
ABCD1 transporter, 411*b*
Abducens nerve (cranial nerve VI), 350*f*
  anatomy, 192*f*
  extraocular muscle innervation, 54
  eye movements, 213, 239*f*
  orbit, 351–352, 352*f*
  orbital apex, 349
  route of, 192–193
Aberration-free system, 28
Aberrations
  representation of, 30–31
  visual acuity, 652–653
Aberrometer
  evolution of, 33–34, 33*f*
  Shack-Hartmann, 33–34, 34*f*
Abnormal retinal correspondence, binocular
  vision. *See* Binocular vision
Absolute disparity, 707, 707*f*
Absorption spectra
  rhodopsin, 421–422, 428*f*
  rods *vs.* cones, 428, 428*f*
ACAs. *See* Anterior ciliary arteries (ACAs)
Accommodation, 8
  age-related changes, 8
  anatomy, 39–52.
    see also specific anatomical features
  basic mechanism of, 62–64
  birds, 37
    diving birds, 37
  carnivores, 37
  comparative anatomy, 37
  definition, 37–38
  herbivores, 37
  historical aspects, 37
  mammals, 37
  measurement, 55–56, 55*b*
    dynamic measurement, 55
    illumination levels, 55
    optical refractive power, 55
    static measurement, 55
    subjective, 55
  mechanism of, 38*b*, 38*f*, 45*f*, 52–53, 53*f*
    ciliary muscle, 52–53
    crystalline lens, 50–52
    lens capsule, 49–50, 52*f*

Accommodation *(Continued)*
  optical changes, 40*f*, 53–54
    lens, 53–54
    lens anterior surface, 53–54
  optical requirements, 39
  pharmacology, 54–55
    acetylcholine neurotransmitters, 54–55
    muscarinic antagonists, 54–55
    pilocarpine, 54–55
  pupil near reflex, 532–533
  stimulus, 54
    blur cues, 54
    convergence, 54
    Edinger–Westphal nucleus, 54
    focusing efforts, 54
    intraocular muscles, 54
    longitudinal chromatic aberration, 54
    pharmacology, 54
    postganglionic ciliary nerves, 54
  tension spikes, 64–65
  See also Presbyopia
Accommodative amplitude
  definition, 39
  measurement, 55
Accommodative movements, age-related changes
  in, 58, 60*f*
AC conventional fast synapses. *See* Retinal
  synaptic organization
AC efferent slow transmitter synapses. *See* Retinal
  synaptic organization
Acetylcholine, 750
  accommodation, 54–55
  aqueous tear film layer secretion, 370
  conjunctival goblet cells, 366
  receptors, extraocular muscles, 193
Achromatism. *See* Chromatic aberrations
Achromatopsia, 627
Acinar cells, 373
Acinar electrolyte/water secretion, tear film,
  aqueous layer. *See* Tear film, aqueous layer
Actin cytoskeleton, 135
Actin filaments, aqueous humor drainage, 264, 265*f*
Action potentials
  ipRGC depolarizing photoresponse, 552–553
  optic nerve axonal conduction, 585–586
Action spectra
  photoreceptors, 437
  rods, 437, 440*f*
Active immune barrier, 343–344, 344*b*
Active phase, corneal stroma wound healing, 86
Activity-dependent refinement, of retinogeniculate
  projection development, 749–750, 749*f*
Activity drive refinement, retinogeniculate
  projection development, 750–751, 750*f*
Adaptation
  light. *See* Light adaptation
  paradigm, 638
  spatial form, 640, 640*f*
Adaptive optics scanning laser ophthalmoscopy
  (AO-SLO), 284, 285*f*
Adenosine, retinal vasodilator, 306
Adie's tonic pupil, 544*f*, 545–546, 545*f*
  anisocoria, 540*t*

Adie's tonic pupil *(Continued)*
  causes, 545–546
Adie syndrome, 546
  diagnosis, 543–544
Adipose tissue. *See* Fat tissue
α-Adrenergic receptors
  α1-adrenergic agonists, 253
  α2-adrenergic agonists, aqueous humor
    drainage, 265
β-Adrenergic receptors
  antagonists, aqueous humor formation
    regulation, 253
  aqueous humor drainage, 264–265
  $β_1$-adrenergic agonists, aqueous humor
    regulation, 253
  $β_2$-adrenergic receptors, 43
Adrenergic supersensitivity, 542
Adrenoleukodystrophy, 411*b*
Adult eye, 6–10.
  see also specific systems
Adult plasticity, 769
Advanced Glaucoma Intervention Study (AGIS), 687
Adversarial attacks, 633
AE (Cl^-/HCO_3^-) exchanger, tear film, aqueous
  production, 373
Aerobic metabolism, 141
Afferent sensory nerves, lacrimal glands, 370
Age of onset
  disparity sensitivity, 742–743, 743*f*
  strabismus, 764–765
Age-related cataracts, GSH delivery to lens
  nucleus, 143–146, 144*f*
Age-related changes, 22–24
  accommodation, 8
  cataracts, 22
  in ciliary muscle
    accommodative movements, 58, 60*f*
    human, 57–58, 59*f*
    rhesus, 56–57
  cornea, 69–106
  lens, 49–50, 129*f*, 151–156
  motion processing, 731
  presbyopia, 56
  sclera, 106–118
  visual acuity. *See* Visual acuity
  vitreous body. *See* Vitreous body
  in zonule, 58–60
Age-related macular degeneration (AMD),
  180–181, 343*b*
  ocular blood flow, 310–311, 310*f*, 311*f*
Age-related maculopathy (ARM), slowed dark
  adaptation, 462*b*
Age-related nuclear cataracts
  GSH levels, 155
  pathophysiology, 154–156, 155*f*
Agnosia, 627
AK (astigmatic keratotomy), 105
Akinetopsia, 633
Alertness, lateral geniculate nucleus, 607, 609–610
Aliasing, visual acuity, 654–656
All-*trans*-retinol (vitamin A)
  corneal stromal wound healing, 84–86
  deficiency, slowed dark adaptation, 462

788

All-*trans*-retinol (vitamin A) (*Continued*)
  re-isomerization, visual cycle, 341
  retinal pigment epithelium, 339
ALS (amyotrophic lateral sclerosis), extraocular
    muscle sparing, 207
Alternate bar patterns, 12, 13*f*
Alternating intermittent monocular form
    deprivation, 756–757
Alzheimer disease, motion processing, 731
Amacrine cells
  bilingual, 495–496
  dendritic compartments, 498
  ipRGC synaptic input, 558–560
  polyaxonal, 495
  visual processing, inner retina, 495–496
Amblyopia, 665–666, 665*b*, 766–770
  anisometropic. *See* Anisometropic amblyopia
  and binocular suppression, 767, 768*f*
  crowding, 665–666
  deprivation, 756
  form deprivation, 755, 767
  functional losses, 665, 666*f*
  incidence, 665
  neural deficits, 767–768, 769*f*
  patching regimens, 757
  perceptual deficits, 767
  and receptive-field (RF) structure of V2
      neurons, 769*f*
  severity, 665
  strabismic. *See* Strabismic amblyopia
AMD. *See* Age-related macular degeneration (AMD)
α-Amino-3-hydroxy-5-methyl-4-
    isoxazolepropionic acid (AMPA), 775
Ammonium ions, honeybee retina in vitro studies,
    331*f*
Amodal conception, 782–783
AMPA receptors, 481–482
  developmental visual deprivation, 759–760
  horizontal cells, 465
  outer retinal signal processing, 481–482
  retinal synaptic organization, 470–471
Amphetamines, 542
Amyotrophic lateral sclerosis (ALS), extraocular
    muscle sparing, 207
Anatomical barriers, corneal drug delivery,
    104–105, 109*f*
Anatomy
  development, 1–4.
  see also specific anatomical structures
Anesthesia, pupil reflex dilation, 533
Angle-closure glaucoma, mydriasis, 545
Angular artery, eyelids, 359*f*
Angular vestibulo-ocular reflex, 224–225
Animal models
  developmental visual deprivation, 755
  glaucoma, 588
  ipRGCs, 555
  ischemic optic neuropathy, 587
  optic neuritis, 587
  strabismus. *See* Strabismus
  white matter pathways, 775
Aniseikonia, 711–713, 711*f*, 712*b*
Anisocoria, 539, 539*f*
  Adie's tonic pupil, 540*t*
  bright light, 532*f*, 538*t*, 543
  causes, 531, 540*t*
  contraction, 531
  in dark, 539

Anisocoria (*Continued*)
  definition, 527
  Horner's syndrome *vs.*, 539
  physiologic, 540*t*
  simple, 539
Anisometropia, 711–713, 711*f*, 761
Anisometropic amblyopia, 645, 761
  constant monocular defocus, 761
  neural deficits, 767–768
Anisotropies, visual acuity, 658*f*, 659, 659*f*, 660*f*
Annulus of Zinn, 349, 350*f*
Anomalous binocular correspondence (ABC), 714
  anomalous motor fusion mechanisms in, 717
  anomalous sensory fusion mechanisms, 717
  binocular fusion in, 717
  computation of binocular disparity in, 715–716,
      715*f*, 716*f*
  visual directions and horopter in, 714–715
Anomalous motor fusion mechanisms, in ABC, 717
Anomalous posterior detachment, vitreous body,
      180, 181*f*
Anomalous sensory fusion mechanisms, ABC, 717
Anterior ciliary arteries (ACAs), 246*f*, 247*f*
  episcleral vasculature, 116
Anterior cortex, vitreous body, 167–168
Anterior ethmoidal arteries, 353*f*
  orbit, 353
Anterior ethmoidal nerve, 192*f*
Anterior hyaloid, 49, 51*f*
Anterior ischemic optic neuropathy (AION), 530,
      538*t*
Anterior lamella, eyelid margin, 356
Anterior scleral foramen, 110–112
Antioxidant defense systems, metabolic
      determinants of lens, 141
Antioxidants delivery, lens core, 143–146
APE, rhodopsin phosphorylation, 426
Aperture size, visual acuity, 654–656
Apoptosis
  corneal ultraviolet light filtration, 106
  RGC death, 588–589
Apparent, 777
Apparent frontoparallel plane (AFPP), 703–704, 712
Apparent motion, 730
Applanation tonometry techniques, 116
Apraclonidine, Horner's syndrome diagnosis, 542
Aquaporin(s)
  aqueous humor drainage, 249–250
  electrolyte/water secretion regulation, tear film,
      mucous production, 369
Aquaporin-1, 270–271
Aqueous humor, 245–283
  composition, 246–251, 248*t*
  definition, 6
  drainage. *See* Aqueous humor drainage
  flow pathways, 245, 247*f*
  formation, 245, 246*f*, 252*b*
    active secretion, 248–250, 249*f*
    blood–aqueous barrier, 250–251, 251*t*
    chloride ions, 249–250
    diffusion, 248
    organic molecules transport, 251
    physiology, 248
    pigmented and nonpigmented epithelium
        coordination, 250
    sodium ions, 249–250
    sodium-potassium-activated ATPase,
        249–250

Aqueous humor (*Continued*)
    ultrafiltration, 248
  formation regulation, 251–255, 252*f*
    adrenergic control, 253
    carbonic anhydrase inhibitor effects, 254–255
    cholinergic control, 253
    pharmacological strategies, 254–255
  intraocular pressure, 245
  pharmacology, corneal drug delivery, 104
  production, 245
  secretion, 248–250, 254*t*
  structure, 125*f*, 245–246
    ciliary body, 245–246
    ciliary epithelium, 245–246
    trabecular meshwork, 245
Aqueous humor drainage, 255–262
  adrenergic effects
    conventional outflow, 264
    unconventional outflow, 264–265
  cell volume effects, 270–271
    aquaporins, 270–271
    chloride channels, 271
    Na-K-Cl cotransporter, 270
  cholinergic effects
    conventional outflow, 263
    unconventional outflow, 263–264, 264*f*
  conventional outflow dysfunction, 268
  conventional outflow pathway
    anatomy, 256–258
    IOP homeostasis, 258–262, 259*f*, 260*f*, 261*f*
    juxtacanalicular tissue, 257*f*, 258*f*, 262
    mechanosensation, 261*f*, 264
    TM movement, 258–259, 260*f*
    TM role, 258, 259*f*
  corticosteroid effects, 265–267
    11β-hydroxysteroid dehydrogenase, 267
    crosslinked actin networks, 268, 268*f*
    dexamethasone, 267–268
    ethacrynic acid effects, 267
    microtubules, 267
    myocilin, 268
    TM cytoskeleton, 268
  cytoskeletal/cell junctional mechanisms,
      265–267, 265*b*
    actin filaments, 265–266, 265*f*
    caldesmon, 266–267
    cytochasin effects, 266
    H-7 effects, aqueous humor drainage,
        266–267
    latrunculin effects, 266
    myosin light chain kinase inhibition, 266–267
    Y-27632 effects, 266–267
  fluid mechanics, 255–256
    choroidal detachment, 255–256
    Goldmann equation, 255
    Schlemm's canal, 255, 256*f*
    TM, 255
    uveovortex flow, 255–256
  glaucoma, 262
  hyaluronidase effects, 271
  outflow obstruction, 262–263
    cells, 262–263
    extracellular matrix accumulation, 262
    particulates, 262–263
  pharmacology, 263–271
  prostaglandin effects, 269–270, 269*b*, 269*t*
    deficient mice models, 269–270
    plasmin generation, 269

Aqueous humor drainage *(Continued)*
uveoscleral outflow system, 269t, 270t
protease effects, 271
renin-angiotensin effects, 271
nitric oxide, 271
Aqueous layer, tear film. *See* Tear film, aqueous layer
Aqueous vein, 246f
Arachidonic acid, endothelium-derived retinal vasodilator, 303–305
Arcuate scotomas, 684
Area, pupil size, 536t
Area summation curve, 645–646, 646f
Argyll–Robertson pupils, 546
Aristotle, 701
ARM. *See* Age-related maculopathy (ARM)
Arousal, LGN. *See* Lateral geniculate nucleus (LGN)
Arrangement tests, 669–670
Arrestin
dark-adapted rod recovery phase, 419f, 425f, 426
mutations, Oguchi disease, 437b
Arterial supply
orbit, 352–353, 353f.
see also specific arteries
Arteriovenous ratio, 289–290
Artifactual visual field, 692–697, 694f, 695f, 697f, 698f
Artificial intelligence (AI), 784
Ascorbate, in aqueous humor, 248
Ascorbic acid (vitamin C), 141
corneal ultraviolet light filtration, 106
Associated phoria, 705
Asthenopia, 706b, 708
Astigmatic keratotomy (AK), 105
Astigmatism, 24, 711–713, 711f
irregular, 28–30
mechanism, 27, 29f
transient, 4
Astrocytes, 581
axonal conduction, 586
development, 584
phagocytosis, 751
retinal vasodilator, 302–303
Astrocytoma, 581
Astrogliosis, optic nerve injury, 590
Asymmetries
motion detection development, 739
vergence, foveal gaze shift. *See* Foveal gaze shift
ATP-binding cassette (ABC) transporters, 405–406, 406t, 407f.
see also under ABC
Atropine
aqueous humor drainage, 263
myopia, 1
Attentional modulation, of LGN, 609
Attention, primary visual cortex, 622
A-type horizontal cell, 483
Auditory language and cognition, 780–781
behavior, 780
neural responses, 780–781
Auditory processing, 779–781
auditory language and cognition, 780–781
motion, 780
pitch, 779–780
space, 780
Autoimmune diseases, sclera, 118b
Automated static perimetry
advantages of, 677

Automated static perimetry *(Continued)*
disadvantages of, 677
Automatic gain control (AGC), 706
Autophagy, lens transparency, 131
Autoregulation, ocular circulation regulation, 296–300
Autosomal recessive retinitis punctata albescens, 342
a-wave, electroretinograms, 506
Axial anisometropia, 711
Axial elongation in myopia, 110
Axial length, development, 1–3
Axon(s)
counts, 580
depolarization, 585
development, 583–584
dimensions, 580
guidance, 584–585
injury signaling, RGC death, 589
number, 584
optic nerve. *See* Optic nerve (cranial nerve II)
regeneration, failure. *See* Optic nerve injury
repolarization, 585–586
transport, 586
Axonal cells (AxCs)
conventional fast synapses. *See* Retinal synaptic organization
efferent slow transmitter synapses. *See* Retinal synaptic organization
sensory neuroepithelium, 464
Axon-axon interactions, 748
Axonless cells, sensory neuroepithelium, 465

B

Background intensity, scotopic vision, 453
Bagolini striated lenses, 714
Bailey–Lovie chart, 10, 13f
Ball-and-socket joints, lens fiber cells, 131, 134f
Baron-Cohen, Simon, 6
Barrier properties, cornea, 86–98
Basal epithelial cells, corneal epithelium, 87, 92f
Basement membrane, corneal endothelium. *See* Corneal endothelium
Bathorhodopsin, 423
Bayesian approach, 711
Bayesian test strategy, 687
BC ribbon synapses. *See* Retinal synaptic organization
BCRP. *See* Breast cancer resistance protein (BCRP)
BCs. *See* Bipolar cell(s) (BCs)
BEB (benign essential blepharospasm), 358, 358b
Behavioral measurements, spatio-temporal vision development, 737
Benign essential blepharospasm (BEB), 358, 358b
Bicarbonate, modulation of flash response by, 433–434
Bilateral corrugator supercilii muscles, 354
Bilateral form deprivation, 755, 757f
Binocular combination, 706–707, 706f
Binocular competition
constant monocular form deprivation, 755–756
developmental visual deprivation, 759
Binocular consequences, 242–243
eye movements, 242–243
search zones, 242
Binocular constraints, eye movements. *See* Eye movements, neural control

Binocular disparity, in ABC, 715–716
Binocular (retinal) disparity and depth perception, 707–711
absolute and relative disparity, 707, 707f
combining depth cues, 711
depth and distance, nonstereoscopic cues to, 710
retinal disparity, perceptual constancy and perceived depth, 709–710, 710f
stereoacuity, 707f, 708–709, 708f, 709b
stereopsis and the "matching problem", 709
See also Binocular vision
Binocular eye movements, 703
Binocular fusion, in ABC, 717
Binocular horopter, 705f
Binocular imbalance, 755
Binocularity, 616
Binocular neuron, 701–702
Binocular over monocular, superiority of, 706
Binocular primary visual cortex neurons, 701–702
Binocular rivalry, 707
Binocular suppression, 706–707, 706f
amblyopia and, 767, 768f
Binocular therapy, 769
Binocular vision, 701–720
ABC
anomalous motor fusion mechanisms in, 717
anomalous sensory fusion mechanisms, 717
binocular fusion in, 717
computation of binocular disparity in, 715–716, 715f, 716f
visual directions and horopter in, 714–715
anomalies of, 711–714
anisometropia, astigmatism and aniseikonia, 711–713, 711f
anomalous binocular correspondence, 714
strabismic suppression, 713–714
strabismus, 713, 713f
binocular combination and binocular suppression, 706–707, 706f
binocular (retinal) disparity and depth perception, 707–711
absolute and relative disparity, 707, 707f
combining depth cues, 711
depth and distance, nonstereoscopic cues to, 710
retinal disparity, perceptual constancy and perceived depth, 709–710, 710f
stereoacuity, 707f, 708–709, 708f, 709b
stereopsis and the "matching problem", 709
binocular eye movements, 703
infant vision development. *See* Infant vision development
normal retinal correspondence and horopter, 703–705, 703f
natural environment, disparities in, 704, 705f
Panum's fusional area, 705, 706b
perceived distance, subclasses of anomalous correspondence and errors, 717
single percept, mapping two eye's images into, 701–702
stereoacuity. *See* Stereoacuity
stereopsis. *See* Stereopsis
two eyes, 701
visual direction, 702–703, 702f
Biomechanical properties, lens, 140
Biomechanical testing, cornea, 112b
Biomechanics, lens fiber cells morphology, 137–140, 137f

Bipolar cell(s) (BCs), 480
  axon terminals, 496–497, 497b
  ipRGC synaptic input, 558, 559f
  mammalian diversity, 465
  off-center (hyperpolarizing), 480
  on-center (depolarizing), 480
  output synapses, outer retinal signal processing.
    See Signal processing, outer retina
  sensory neuroepithelium, 464
  signaling, inner plexiform layer signal
    processing. see Signal processing, inner
    plexiform layer
  signal processing, outer retina, 486–490, 489f
  visual pathways, 486–490, 489f
  visual processing, inner retina, 495
Birds, accommodation, 37
Bitemporal visual field deficits, 684
Black curved line, 703–704, 704f
Black-white circuitry. See Color vision
Bleaching adaptation. See Dark adaptation
Blindness, 775, 776b, 777f
See also Visual deprivation
Blindsight, 576b, 598, 604b, 635
Blind spot, historical aspects, 549
Blinking, 358
  involuntary, 83
Bloch's law, 721, 722f
Blood–aqueous barrier, 410
  aqueous humor. See Aqueous humor
Blood flow, retinal, 285–289, 288f
Blood-oxygen-level-dependent functional
    magnetic resonance imaging (BOLD
    fMRI), 332
Blood–retina barrier (BRB), 287f, 324, 331
  outer, 409–410, 409f
    BCRP, 410
    MRP, 410
    P-glycoprotein, 409–410
  passive permeability, vitreous body. See Vitreous
    body
Blood supply, optic nerve. See Optic nerve (cranial
    nerve II)
Blood vessels, retina, 8
Blue-yellow color vision
  circuitry. See Color vision
  defects, 671
Blur cues, accommodation stimulus, 54
Blurring, 709
Boerhaave, Herman, 612
Bone morphogenetic protein 4 (BMP4), 201–202
Bothnia dystrophy, slowed dark adaptation, 462
Botulinum toxin studies, extraocular muscle
    remodeling, 200
Bowman's layer. See Cornea
Bradyopsia, 427b
  R9AP mutation, 461b
  RGS9-1 mutation, 461b
  transducin shutoff, 437b
Braille, 778–779
  behavior, 778–779
  neural responses, 779
Brainstem
  eye sensory innervation, 391–392
  lateral geniculate nucleus inputs from, 601
  modulation, LGN, 609–610
  oculomotor coordinates, 239–241
Branch retinal artery occlusion (BRAO), relative
    afferent pupillary defect, 538t

Branch retinal vein occlusion (BRVO), relative
    afferent pupillary defect, 538t
BRAO (branch retinal artery occlusion), relative
    afferent pupillary defect, 538t
BRB. See Blood–retina barrier (BRB)
Breast cancer resistance protein (BCRP), 405, 410
Brief unrestricted vision, intermittent monocular
    form deprivation, 758
Bright light, anisocoria, 532f, 538t, 543
Bright light responses, photoreceptor junctional
    conductances, 441–449, 444f
Brillouin microscopy, 112b
Brillouin optical scattering system (BOSS), 112b
Bruch's membrane, 118
  primary vitreous, 173–174
Brücke brightness enhancement effect, 728
BRVO (branch retinal vein occlusion), relative
    afferent pupillary defect, 538t
B-type horizontal cell, 483
Bullae, corneal edema, 96
Bunazosin, aqueous humor drainage, 265
Burian Allen electrode, electroretinograms, 507f,
    509
b-wave, electroretinograms, 506

C

CACNA1F gene, 446b, 447f
N-cadherin, lens fiber cells, 131, 135
Calcitonin gene-related peptide (CGRP)
  aqueous humor regulation, 251–252
  meibomian gland regulation, 375
Calcium-activated anion current ($I_{Cl(Ca)}$), 448, 448f
Calcium-activated calmodulin, 471
Calcium-activated potassium channel, tear film,
    373
Calcium-activated potassium current ($I_{K(Ca)}$),
    446–448
Calcium-dependent mechanisms, light adaptation.
    See Light adaptation
Calcium ions
  cytoplasmic, phototransduction, 458
  dark-adapted rod recovery phase, 426
  dark-adapted rod resting state, 417
  extraocular muscles, 197
  intracellular
    aqueous tear film layer secretion, 371
    neuron–glial cell interactions, 324
  permeability, dark-adapted rod resting state,
    416–417
Caldesmon, 267
Callosal connections, white matter
    pathways, 775
Calmodulin, calcium-activated, 471
Campana cell, 465–466
Canaliculus, common, 349f
Capillary plexus, ocular circulation, 285f
Carbonic anhydrase inhibitor effects, aqueous
    humor regulation, 254–255
Carboplatin, scleral permeability, 117t
Cardinal points, 2–3, 3f
Carnivores, accommodation, 37
Carotid plexus, 379f
Cartesian coordinate arrangement, 677
Cataracts
  age-related changes, 22–24
    nuclear. See Age-related nuclear cataracts
  development, 152–156

Cataracts (Continued)
  epidemiology, 152–153
  glare and contrast sensitivity, 16
  pathophysiology
    diabetic cortical, 153–154, 154f
    nuclear cataract, 154–156, 155f
  progress measurement, 15
  surgery, 152b, 152f, 153b, 153f
    corneal stromal wound healing, 105
    See also Intraocular lenses (IOLs)
  visual acuity, 16
  vitreous oxygen and, 182–183, 183f
Cation chloride cotransporter (CCC) transporters,
    147
Cation flow, CNG channel, 438
Caveolin-1 knockout, retinal vasodilator, 303,
    304f
CCC (Cation chloride cotransporter) transporters,
    147
CCDD (congenital cranial dysinnervation
    disorders), 205
CCM, structure, 246f, 247f
CD47, 751
Cell(s)
  aqueous humor outflow obstruction, 262–263
  LGN. See Lateral geniculate nucleus (LGN)
  orientation, radial current flow, 506, 507f
  primary visual cortex (V1). See Primary visual
    cortex (V1)
  volume, aqueous humor drainage. See Aqueous
    humor drainage.
  see also specific cells
Cell culture models, retinal glycolysis, 328–329
Cellular architecture, lens fiber cells, 131, 132f
Cellular organelles, lens transparency, 130–131
Cellular organization, of human lens, 124–126,
    126f
Cellular retinaldehyde binding protein (CRALBP),
    visual cycle, 341
Cellular retinol binding protein (CRBP), visual
    cycle, 341
Center-surround antagonistic receptive field
    (CSARF) organization. See Signal
    processing, outer retina
Center-surround organization, retinal synapses,
    472–474, 473f
Central cornea, corneal reference points, 71, 72f–73f
Central projections, ipRGCs. See Retinal ganglion
    cells, intrinsically photosensitive (ipRGCs)
Central retinal arterial equivalent (CRAE),
    289–290
Central retinal artery (CRA), 284, 353f
  optic nerve head blood supply, 581
Central retinal artery occlusion (CRAO), 538t
Central retinal vein (CRV), 284
Central retinal vein occlusion (CRVO), 538t
Central retinal venular equivalent (CRVE),
    289–290
Central scotomas, 684
Central serous retinopathy (CSR), 538t
Central visual field damage, 531
Central visual pathways, 571–577
  retinal projection targets, 571–573, 572f, 574f,
    576b
  dorsal terminal nucleus, 573
  Edinger–Westphal nucleus, 573
  lateral terminal nucleus, 573
  LGN, 571–573

Central visual pathways (Continued)
   medial terminal nucleus, 573
   paraventricular nucleus, 573
   pretectum, 571
   pulvinar nucleus of thalamus, 573
   superior colliculus, 571
   suprachiasmatic nucleus, 573
   supraoptic nucleus, 573
   visual field lesions, 573–576, 575f
      diffusion tensor imaging, 575f, 576b
      homonymous hemianopia, 574, 575f, 576b
      LGN, 574, 575f
      one optic nerve, 573
      optic chiasm, 573, 575f
      temporal hemifield of contralateral eye, 573–574, 575f
Centrocecal scotomas, 684
Cerebral cortex
   contrast sensitivity. See Contrast sensitivity
   magnification factor, 656f, 657
CFF. See Critical flicker fusion (CFF) frequency
cGMP
   CNG channel binding, 438
   dark-adapted rod recovery phase, 426
   dark-adapted rod resting state, 417
   light adaptation, 459
cGMP-dependent cation channels, RPE, 340–341
cGMP-gated channel, dark-adapted rod resting state, 416–417
CGRP. See Calcitonin gene-related peptide (CGRP)
Chart contrast, visual acuity testing, 10–11
Chart luminance, visual acuity testing, 10
Chemical substances, vitreous body, 167
   plasma gradients, 167
   regional differences, 167
Chiasmal compression, relative afferent pupillary defect, 538t
Childhood Horner's syndrome. See Horner's syndrome
Chloride/bicarbonate (AE) exchanger, tear film, aqueous production, 373
Chloride channels
   aqueous humor drainage, 271
   retinal pigment epithelium, 340
Chloride ions
   aqueous humor formation, 249–250
   electrolyte/water secretion regulation, 368
   electroretinogram glial currents, 508
   lacrimal gland fluid composition, 373–374
   retinal pigment epithelium transport, 340, 341f
Chloride reversal potential, 472
Cholecystokinin, iris, 534
Cholinergic agonists, 366–367, 373
   aqueous production of tear film, 370–371, 371f
Cholinergic mechanisms, aqueous humor drainage. See Aqueous humor drainage
Cholinergics, aqueous humor drainage, 263
Chondroitin sulfate, 164
Choroid, 39–40, 41f
   pressure-flow relationship, 296, 298f
   sensory nerves, 379
   structure, 125f
Chromatic aberrations, 20–21, 27, 28f
   visual acuity, 652–653
Chromaticity, critical duration, 723, 724f
Chromatic pupillary light responses, 530

Chromatic sensitivity
   spatial form processing. See Spatial form, early processing
   temporal sensitivity, 725
Chromatic visual processing, 485–486, 488f
Chromophore recycling pathways, 461
Chronic progressive external ophthalmoplegia (CPEO), 207–208, 208b
Ciliary body, 40–41
   contraction, emmetropization, 3
   pars plana, 40–41, 245
   pars plicata, 40–41
   sensory nerves, 388f, 391
   structure, 125f
   vasculature, 247f
Ciliary epithelium, aqueous humor structure, 245–246
Ciliary ganglion, anatomy, 192f, 379f
Ciliary muscle, 41–52, 41f, 42f, 43f
   accommodation, 52–53
   age-related changes
      accommodative movements, 58, 60f
      in human, 57–58, 59f
      in rhesus, 56–57
   anatomy, 41f, 42f
   anterior longitudinal region of, 64–65
   β2-adrenergic receptors, 43
   boundaries, 41–42
   longitudinal fibers, 42–43
   M3 muscarinic receptors, 43
   muscle groups, 42–43
   presbyopia. See Presbyopia
   radial fibers, 42–43
   by ultrasound biomicroscopy, 42f
Ciliary nerve, 378–379
   distribution, 379
Ciliary process, structure, 246f, 247f
Circadian photoentrainment, ipRGC central projections, 563–564, 564f
Circuits for surround modulation, 619–620, 619f
Circulation. See Ocular circulation
Cisplatin, scleral permeability, 117t
cis-trans isomerization, rhodopsin phosphorylation, 424–426
Classical receptive field, V1, 615–616, 615f, 617f
Classification systems, assessing visual field progression, 687
Clearance mechanisms, scleral drug delivery, 107f, 118
Cl⁻/HCO3⁻ (AE) exchanger, tear film, aqueous production, 373
Clinical judgment, 686
Clinical slit-lamp examination, 76–78
Clinical suppression, 764
Clonidine, aqueous humor formation, 253
Cloquet's canal, 176, 176f
Cloverleaf visual field, 698f
CME (cystoid macular edema), 538t
CNG channels. See Cyclic nucleotide gated (CNG) channels
Coarse stereopsis, 710
Cocaine eye drops
   childhood Horner's syndrome diagnosis, 543
   Horner's syndrome diagnosis, 541–542
Cochet–Bonnet esthesiometer, 83–84
Cochlin, transforming growth factor-β, 262
Coding of disparity, binocular eye movements, 222–224

Cold-sensitive sensory nerves, 391
Cold thermoreceptors, corneal sensory nerves, 386f, 387b, 391
Collaborative Initial Glaucoma Treatment Study (CIGTS), 687
Collagen(s)
   Bowman's layer, 78
   corneal light transmission, 78–79, 80f, 81f, 82f, 83f
   degradation, sclera development, 108
   scleral mechanical properties, 112–113
   vitreous, 165–166
      aging, 177
      type II, 165, 166f
      type IX, 165–166
      type VI, 166
      type VII, 166
      type V/XI, 166
Collagen fibrils, corneal ectasia, 102, 107f
Collagen type I, cornea, 78, 79f
Collagen type IV, cornea, 78, 82f
Collector channel, 246f
Color, iris, 534–535
Color blindness. See Color vision defects
Color Doppler imaging, ocular blood flow measurement, 290–291, 290f
Color polarity switching, visual processing, inner retina, 498
Color vision, 641, 668–674
   black-white circuitry, 671–673, 672f
      LGN, 671–673
      L/M cones, 671–673
      primary visual cortex, 671–673
   blue-yellow circuitry, 477, 671
      fovea, 671
      H2 horizontal cells, 671
      midget ganglion cells, 671
      OFF-center midget ganglion cells, 671
      ON-center midget ganglion cells, 671
      output pathways, 671
      S-cone-specific ON bipolar cells, 671
      small bistratified ganglion cells, 671
   future work, 673
   historical aspects, 668
   ipRGC synaptic input, 560, 560f
   long-(L) wavelength sensitive cones, 668
   middle-(M) wavelength sensitive cones, 668
   molecular genetics, 668–669
   neural circuitry, 670–671.
   see also specific circuits
   red-green circuitry, 476f, 477, 671, 672f
   short-(S) wavelength sensitive cones, 668, 669f
   tests of, 669–670
Color vision defects, 668, 669b
   blue-yellow defects, 671
   CNG channel mutations, 443b
   deutan defects, 668
   deuteranomaly, 669b
   deuteranopia, 669b
   L opsin gene deletions, 668
   M opsin gene deletions, 668
   nomenclature, 669b
   protan defects, 668
   protanomaly, 669b
   protanopia, 669b
   red-green defects, 669
   tritan defects, 668–669, 669b

Color visual field tests, 688b
Common canaliculus, 349f
Comparative anatomy, accommodation, 37
Complete congenital stationary night blindness, 511
Complex cells, 616
Compliance loss, presbyopia, 62
Compressive optic neuropathy, 578
 relative afferent pupillary defect, 538t
Computerized pupillography, 538
Computerized pupillometry, 537f, 538, 539f
Cornea
 nerve injury, 396–400, 398f, 399f
 sensitivity, 396, 397f
Cone photoreceptor, 668
Cone pigment regeneration, 461
Cone-rod dystrophy, 445b
Cones
 action spectra, 437, 440f
  population differences, 440b, 441f
 compartmentalization, 414, 415f–416f, 417f
 density, visual acuity eccentricity, 655f, 656
 flash photovoltage responses, 432
 light adaptation. See Light adaptation
 location, 414
 minimum resolvable acuity, 649
 NCKX2 exchanger, 440–441
 opsins, 669b
 photopic vision, 452
 steady light photocurrent responses, 437
  bleaching effects, 437
  pigment regeneration, 437
 SWS1, 465
Confocal microscopy, 76–78
Congenital cranial dysinnervation disorders (CCDD), 205
Congenital fibrosis, extraocular muscles, 206b
Congenital Horner's syndrome, 543
Congenital stationary night blindness (CSNB), 425b, 513–514
 electroretinograms, 421f
Congenital stationary night blindness type 2 (CSNB2), 481
Congruous visual field loss, 684
Conjunctiva
 efflux transport, 408f
 epithelium barrier, 410–411
 goblet cells, tear film. See Tear film, mucous layer
 sensory nerves, 399f
  functional characteristics, 387–392, 388f
  See also Corneal sensory nerves
Connexin(s), lens fiber cells. See Lens fiber cells
Connexin 36 gap junction proteins, outer retinal signal processing, 480, 481f
Conscious vision, ipRGC central projections, 565
Constant monocular defocus. See Visual deprivation, developmental
Constant monocular form deprivation. See Visual deprivation, developmental
Contact lenses, 86b
 corneal endothelial cell injury, 111b–112b
Contact lens, glare and contrast sensitivity, 16
Context of vision. See Primary visual cortex (V1)
Continuous flash suppression (CFS), 707
Contour integration, 619
Contraction, anisocoria, 531
Contralateral eye (nasal retina), LGN layers and maps, 598

Contralateral RGCs, 748
 axon signaling, 748
Contrast
 definition and units, 11
 enhancements. See Contrast enhancement
 visual acuity, 658, 659f
Contrast borders, temporal sensitivity, 727–728
Contrast constancy, 638
 spatial form, 643–644, 643f, 644f
Contrast enhancement, 22–24, 23f
 edge sharpening, 22, 23f
 Vernier acuity, 22–23, 24f
Contrast gain, 644
 control, 646
Contrast luminance, 16
Contrast sensitivity, 641, 642f, 645, 661f, 688b
 clinical conditions, 16–20
  corneal conditions, 16–18
  optical conditions, 16.
  see also specific diseases/disorders
 definition and units, 11–12
 development, 664
 foveal viewings, 660f, 661f
 glare, 15–16
 illumination vs., 15
 lowest contrast, 660f, 661
 measurement, 661
 peripheral vision, 661–662, 662f
  low spatial frequencies, 662, 662f
  magnification theory, 661–662, 662f
  receptive fields, 662
 spherical aberration impact on, 32
 testing, 10–11
  recording of, 14–15, 14f
  sine waves, 15–16
  targets, 12–13
 tissue light scattering, 15–16
 window of visibility, 660–661, 660f
Contrast sensitivity function (CSF), 638, 639f, 640
Contrast sensitivity loss, 645
Convective flow, vitreous body, 173
Conventional outflow, aqueous humor drainage
 adrenergic effects, 264
 cholinergic effects, 263
Conventional outflow pathway, aqueous humor drainage, 256–258
Convergence accommodation, stimulus, 54
Convolutional neural networks (CNNs), 632b, 633
Cookie cutter punched-out deficits, 685
Copper mydriasis, anisocoria, 540t
Cornea, 69–106
 aging, 69–71
 anatomy, 69–71, 70f
 asphericity, 74
 barrier properties, 86–98
 Bowman's layer, 69
  collagens, 78
  development, 69–71
 composition, 76t
 dehydration, metabolic pump function, 92
 Descemet's membrane, 69
 development, 69–71, 72f
 diseases of, 69
 drug delivery, 102–105, 109f
  anatomical barriers, 104–105, 109f
  aqueous humor, 102–104
  hydrophilic drugs, 104–105
  intracameral injections, 105, 109f
  intrastromal injections, 105, 109f

Cornea (Continued)
 lipophilic drugs, 104–105
 physicochemical properties, 102
 physiological barriers, 104–105
 subconjunctival injections, 105, 109f
 topical, 104–105, 104f
 transconjunctival, 105, 109f
 vitreous cavity, 104, 109f
 ectasia, 101–102
  collagen fibrils, 102, 107f
  ultimate tensile stress, 101–102
 edema, 16, 93–97
  bullae, 96
  epithelium, 97
  functional effects, 95
  imbibition pressure, 95, 99f
  progress measurement, 15–16, 15f
  proteoglycans, 96–97
  stroma, 97, 99f
  swelling pressure, 93–97
  transparency loss, 96
 efflux transport, 408f, 409
 embryology, 69–71
 emmetropization, 3
 endothelium. See Corneal endothelium
 epithelial barrier properties, 86–98, 90f
  basal epithelial cells, 87, 92f
  cytoskeletal intermediate filaments, 86
  gel-forming mucins, 86–87
  hemidesmosomes, 86, 90f, 91f
  immune cells, 84f, 89
  Langerhans cells, 89
  membrane-associated mucins, 86–87, 91f
  transient amplifying cells, 87–89, 92f
  X,Y,Z hypothesis, 87
  zonula occludens tight junctions, 86–87, 90f
 epithelium, 69
  basement membrane, 71
 fiber arrangement, 7
 glycosaminoglycans, 6
 growth, 69–71
 injury sensitivity, 383t, 397f
 mechanical properties, 80f, 98–102, 103f
  biomechanical testing, 112b
  deformability, 100
  stiffness. see below
  strength extensibility, 100–101
  stress. see below
  toughness, 100–101
 nerves
  light transmission. See Corneal light transmission
  sensory. See Corneal sensory nerves
  stromal nerves, 379–381, 380f
 optical properties. See Corneal optical properties
 P-glycoprotein, 408
 reference points/measurements, 71–74, 72f–73f
  central cornea, 71
  corneal apex, 71–74, 72f–73f
  corneal sighting center, 74
  device's axis point, 71–74
  limbus, 71
  peripheral optical zone, 71
  posterior chamber intraocular lens, 74
  sulcus, 71
  thinnest corneal point, 74
 role of, 6–7
 sclera vs., 106

Cornea (Continued)
  stiffness, 100–101
    ex vivo experiments, 101
    inflation studies, 101
    primary creep, 101
    secondary creep, 101
    structure effects, 101, 103f
    uniaxial strip extensiometry, 101
    viscoelastic properties, 100–101
  stress, 100–102, 103f, 104f
    crushing, 100
    piercing, 100
    transmural pressure, 100
  stroma proper, 69
    development, 70–71
  structure, 125f
  thickness, 69
  tomography, 78b
  topography, 78b
  transplantation, endothelial cell injury, 111
  ultraviolet light filtration, 105–106
    apoptosis, 106
    ascorbic acid, 106
    epithelial damage, 106
    exposure variability, 105–106, 110f
    reactive oxygen species, 106
    "snow blindness", 105
Corneal ablations, 33
Corneal apex, 71–74, 72f–73f
Corneal endothelium, 69
  barrier properties, 89–98, 93f, 94f
    development, 91, 98f
    pump-leak hypothesis, 89–91
  basement membrane, 97
    characteristics, 97
    deposition, 93f, 97
    structure, 97
  cell injury, 111b–112b
    pharmacologic injury, 99t, 111–112
    surgery, 111
  development, 70–71
  endothelial cell density, 91
    ethnic differences, 91–92, 98f
  glycocalyx, 97
  leaky barrier function, 92, 94f
    nutrients, 92
  metabolic pump function, 92–93, 95f–96f
    alteration, 92–93, 98f
    corneal dehydration, 92
    Na$^+$/K$^+$-ATPase, 92
Cornea limbus, 106
Corneal light transmission, 76–86
  clinical slit-lamp examination, 76–78
  collagen, 78–79, 80f, 81f, 82f, 83f
  confocal microscopy, 76–78
  corneal nerves, 82–84
    disease, 84
    electrophysiology, 82
    health measure, 83–84
    involuntary blinking, 83
    microneuromas, 84
    trigeminal nerve, 82, 88f
  dendritic cells, 81, 84f
  keratocytes, 79–81, 84f
  light scattering, 76–78, 79f
  proteoglycans, 81–82, 85f
    decorin, 81–82, 85f
    dermatan sulfate, 81–82, 87f
    glycosaminoglycans, 81

Corneal light transmission (Continued)
    keratan sulfate, 81–82
    lumican, 81–82
    mimecan, 81–82
    structure, 81
  stroma, 76–78, 76t
  stromal wound healing, 84–86
    active phase, 86
    cytokines, 84–86
    growth factors, 84–86
    keratocyte apoptosis, 84–86
    remodeling phase, 86
    variation, 105b
  transparency, 76
  ultraviolet light, 76–78, 79f
Corneal optical properties, 74–86
  contrast sensitivity, 16
  light refraction, 74–76, 75f
    corneal asphericity, 74
    total corneal dioptric power, 74
  light transmission. See Corneal light
      transmission
  optical power, 38–39
  power, refractive power, 654
  transparency, 7, 7f
  visual acuity, 10
Corneal reflex, 683
Corneal sensory nerves, 379–382
  corneal stromal nerves, 379–381, 380f, 381f
  density, 382
  development, 385–387, 386f
  dynamic remodeling, 385, 386f, 387b
  functional characteristics, 387–392, 388f
  intraepithelial nerve terminals, 381f, 382
  reduced/enhanced sensitivity, 383t
  regeneration, 386f, 387
  sub-basal nerve plexus, 381–382, 381f
  subepithelial nerve plexus, 380f, 381, 381f
Corneal sighting center (CSC), 74
Corneal Visualisation Scheimpflug Technology
    (Corvis ST), 112b
Correction, myopia, 654
Cortex adhaerens, lens fiber cells, 131
Cortex, vitreous body, 167
Cortical and reticular modulation, LGN, 609, 609f
Cortical blindness, 635
Cortical circuit, in V1, 615
Cortical expansion, 777
Cortical plasticity cortical plasticity, 778
Corticocortical feedback connections, in V1, 620
Corticocortical outputs, V1, 620
Corticosteroid mechanisms, aqueous humor
    drainage. See Aqueous humor drainage
Cortisol, aqueous humor drainage, 267
Corvis Biomechanical Index (CBI), 112b
Covert attention (without eye movement),
    531–532
CP49/Bfsp2 mutation, hereditary cataract, 135
CPEO (chronic progressive external
    ophthalmoplegia), 207–208, 208b
CPT-cAMP, 750
C1q, 751
CRA. See Central retinal artery (CRA)
Craik–Cornsweet–O'Brien illusion, 22, 23f
CRALBP (cellular retinaldehyde binding protein),
    visual cycle, 341
Cranial motor nerve innervation, extraocular
    muscles. See Extraocular muscles (EOMs)
Cranial nerve II. See Optic nerve (cranial nerve II)

Cranial nerve III. See Oculomotor nerve (cranial
    nerve III)
Cranial nerve IV. See Trochlear nerve (cranial
    nerve IV)
Cranial nerve V. See Trigeminal nerve (cranial
    nerve V)
Cranial nerve VI. See Abducens nerve (cranial
    nerve VI)
Cranial nerve VII. See Facial nerve (cranial nerve
    VII)
CRAO (central retinal artery occlusion), 538t
CRBP (cellular retinol binding protein), visual
    cycle, 341
Critical duration, 721–723
  affecting factors, 721–723
  definition, 721
Critical flicker fusion (CFF) frequency, 723, 723f
  definition, 723
  eccentricity, 723
  measurement of, 729
  stimulus chromaticity, 723, 724f
  stimulus luminance, 723, 723f
  stimulus size effects, 723–724, 723f
Critical period, 622
  developmental visual deprivation. See Visual
      deprivation, developmental
Critical spacing, reading, 659
"Crossed" diplopia, 702–703
Crossed disparities, 707
Cross-modal plasticity, mechanisms, 781
Crowding
  amblyopia, 665–666
  peripheral vision, visual acuity, 657–658, 657b,
      658f
Crushing, corneal stress, 100
CRVO (central retinal vein occlusion), 538t
Crystalline lens, 50–52
See also Lens
  role of, 7–8
Crystallins, 7
See also Lens crystallins
β Crystallins, 139
γ Crystallins, 139
CSARF (center-surround antagonistic receptive
    field) organization. See Signal processing,
    outer retina
CSF. See Contrast sensitivity function (CSF)
CSNB. See Congenital stationary night blindness
    (CSNB)
CSNB2. See Congenital stationary night blindness
    type 2 (CSNB2)
CSR (central serous retinopathy), 538t
C-type cone horizontal cells, 485–486
Cuboid cells, lens, 125
Current density reconstructions (CDR), 744–745
Current source density, dark-adapted a-wave, 510
Current-to-voltage relationship, rod CNG channel,
    438–439, 443f
Customized ablation, 33
Cutoff spatial frequency, visual acuity, 652
c wave, electroretinograms, 508, 508f
Cx46, lens fiber cells, 131
Cx50, lens fiber cells, 131
Cyclic AMP analog, 750
Cyclic nucleotide gated (CNG) channels, 437–441
  cation flow, 438
  cGMP binding, 438
  closure, 438–439
    rod hyperpolarization, 438–439

Cyclic nucleotide gated (CNG) channels (Continued)
  flash photocurrent responses, 432
  light response activation, 423
  mutations, color blindness, 443b
  rods, 438
    current-to-voltage relationship, 438–439, 443f
    structure, 437–438, 442f
Cyclopean, 709
Cyclopean eye
  gaze direction of, 702
  retina of, 702
Cycloplegia, 54–55
Cysteine, 145
Cystoid macular edema (CME), 538t
Cytochalasin, 266
Cytochrome oxidase (CO) blobs, 617–619, 618f
Cytokines
  corneal stromal wound healing, 84–86
  RPE secretion, 343
Cytoplasmic calcium, phototransduction, 458
Cytoskeletal/cell junctional mechanisms. See Aqueous humor drainage
Cytoskeletal protein changes, lens differentiation, 135–137
Cytoskeleton
  intermediate filaments, corneal epithelium, 86
  lens fiber cells. See Lens fiber cells

D

DAP (device's axis point), 71–74
Dark adaptation
  definition, 427, 451, 462
  light adaptation vs., 451
  pupil light reflex, 529
  rods. See Dark-adapted rods
  slowed, 462b
Dark-adapted a-wave. See Electroretinograms, full-field dark-adapted (Ganzfeld) flash
Dark-adapted b-wave. See Electroretinograms, full-field dark-adapted (Ganzfeld) flash
Dark-adapted rods, 414–428, 462–463, 462f
  amplification, 426–427
  changing light adaptation, 427
  guanine nucleotide turnover, 427
    PDE6, 427
  light adaptation vs., 461–462
  light response activation, 421–424
    CNG channel, 424
    G-protein activation, 423
    neurotransmitter release, 424
    PDE6 activation, 424
    rhodopsin photoisomerization. See Rhodopsin
  recovery phase, 424–426
    arrestin binding, 419f, 426
    calcium ions, 426
    cGMP restoration, 426
    G-protein inactivation, 426
    guanylate cyclase, 426
    guanylate cyclase activation, 426
    PDE6 inactivation, 426
    retinoid recycling, 424–426
    retinoid regeneration, 424–426
    RGS9-1 actions, 423f, 426, 427b
    rhodopsin phosphorylation. See Rhodopsin
  resting state, 414–421

Dark-adapted rods (Continued)
    calcium ions, 417
    calcium permeability, 416–417
    cGMP-gated channel, 416–417
    cGMP levels, 417
    dark current, 416–417
    G_t protein (transducin), 421, 422f
    guanylate cyclase, 417–418
    lipids, 421, 422f, 423f
    membrane potential, 414–416
    Na^+/Ca^+-K^+ exchanger protein, 417
    PDE6, 417–418
    potassium channels, 414–416
    rhodopsin, 418–420
    sodium-potassium-ATPase, 414–416
    saturating light level response, 427
Dark, anisocoria, 539
Dark circulating current, flash photocurrent responses, 434f
Dark current, dark-adapted rod resting state, 416–417
Dark-field microscopy, vitreous body, 177–178
Darkness, single photon detection, 434
Dark oxygen consumption, retina, 326
Decibel scale, 681–682
Decorin, corneal light transmission, 81–82, 85f
Deep convolutional neural networks, 638
Deep lamellar endothelial keratoplasty (DLEK), corneal endothelial cell injury, 111
Deep sleep, pupil reflex dilation, 533
Deformability
  cornea, 100
  decline, presbyopia, 61
Degenerative remodeling, vitreous body, 179
Dehydration, sclera, 116
Delayed rectifier potassium current (I_{KV}), 441–443, 445f
DEM (direction of eye motion), ocular following movements, 735
Demyelinating diseases, 530
Dendritic cells, corneal light transmission, 81, 84f
Depolarizing photoresponse, ipRGCs. See Retinal ganglion cells, intrinsically photosensitive (ipRGCs)
Depressor supercilii muscle, 354
Deprivation amblyopia, intermittent monocular form deprivation, 758
Deprivation of vision in development. See Visual deprivation, developmental
Deprivation timing, critical period, 758
Deprived cortex, 776
Depth of field, 39
  definition, 39
Depth of focus, 17–18, 18f, 19f, 20f
  development, 2
  pupil, 527
  pupillary aperture, 17, 20f
  spherical aberration impact on, 32
Dermatan sulfate, corneal light transmission, 81–82, 87f
Descemet's membrane, 69
Descemet's membrane endothelial keratoplasty (DMEK), 111
Descemet's stripping automated endothelial keratoplasty (DSAEK), 111
Descemet's stripping endothelial keratoplasty (DLEK), 111
Descending parasympathetic pathway, 363

Desensitization
  light adaptation electrical responses, 454
  scotopic vision, 453, 453f
  Weber's law, 452
Destructive interference, 19
Deutan color vision defects, 669b
Deuteranomaly, color vision defects, 668
Deuteranopia, color vision defects, 669b
Development of vision
  infant vision. See Infant vision development
  visual deprivation. See Visual deprivation, developmental
Device's axis point (DAP), 71–74
Dexamethasone
  aqueous humor drainage, 267–268
  scleral permeability, 117t
D-glucuronic acid, 164
Diabetes mellitus, ocular blood flow disease, 308–310, 309f
Diabetic cortical cataracts
  osmotic and oxidative stress, 154
  pathophysiology, 153–154
  STZ treatment, 153–154
Diabetic retinopathy, 308–310, 309f, 310f
Differential light threshold. See Increment (differential) light threshold
Diffraction, visual acuity, 652, 654f
Diffractive lens, 27
Diffusing media opacity, relative afferent pupillary defect, 538t
Diffusion, aqueous humor formation, 248
Diffusion barrier function, vitreous body. See Vitreous body
Diffusion tensor imaging (DTI), 575f, 576b
Diffusion, vitreous body, 172–173, 173f
Dilation failure, pupil, 546–547, 547t
Diltiazem, CNG channel inhibition, 440
Diopters, 39
Diplopia, 703f, 716
  of nonfixated objects lying, 703
Direct-current electroretinograms, 509
Directional eye movements, spatio-temporal vision development, 737
Directionally sensitive retinal ganglion cells. See Retinal ganglion cell(s) (RGCs)
Direction of eye motion (DEM), ocular following movements, 735
Direction preference map, 616
Direction-selective neurons, motion neural encoding, 730
Direction selectivity, 616
  circuit, 499–500, 501f
Disconjugate shifts, foveal gaze shift. See Foveal gaze shift
Disjunctive saccadic eye movements, 222, 223f
Disparity sensitivity, 742–743
  age of onset, 742–743, 743f
  development, 742–743, 742f
    global disparity, 742–743, 743f
    studies, 742
Disrupted phototransduction shut-off, light adaptation, 461b
Dissociated vertical deviation (DVD), 229
Divalent block, 438
Divergence eye movements, 707
Diving birds, accommodation, 37
DLEK (Descemet's stripping endothelial keratoplasty), 111

DLEK (deep lamellar endothelial keratoplasty), corneal endothelial cell injury, 111

DMEK (Descemet's membrane endothelial keratoplasty), 111

Dominant time constant changes, rod light adaptation, 461

Donder's law, three-dimensional rotations, 237, 238f

Dopamine, 560
  AC efferent slow transmitter synapses, 468
  interplexiform cells, 483
  retinal synaptic organization, 470–471

Dopamine D1 receptors, retina, 469–471

Dopamine D2 receptors, retina, 469–471

Doppler OCT, ocular blood flow measurement, 292, 292f, 293f

Dorsal lateral geniculate nucleus of the thalamus (dLGN)
  See also Retinogeniculate projection development

Dorsal midbrain lesion studies, pupil light reflex, 531b

Dorsal midbrain syndrome, 546

Dorsal nasal arteries, 353f, 359f

Dorsal streams, extrastriate visual cortex. *See* Extrastriate visual cortex (V2)

Dorsal terminal nucleus (DTN), retinal projection targets, 573

Dorsal visual network, 633–635
  link to perception and action, 634
  receptive fields and visual selectivity, 633
  subconscious vision, 634–635
  subcortical inputs, 634–635

Doxil, scleral permeability, 117t

Doxohexanaenoic acid, retinal pigmented epithelium transport, 339

Doxorubicin, scleral permeability, 117t

Droplet sequencing methods, 598, 600b

Drosophila, phototransduction cascade, 551

Drug delivery
  cornea. *See* Cornea
  sclera. *See* Sclera

Dry eye disease
  associated conditions, 374b
  definition, 366b
  MUC1 mucin, 366

Dry eyes, 395, 395b

Dryness sensation, 395, 395b

DSAEK (Descemet's stripping automated endothelial keratoplasty), 111

DTI. *See* Diffusion tensor imaging (DTI)

DTN (dorsal terminal nucleus), retinal projection targets, 573

Dual feedback control system, 147f

Duchenne muscular dystrophy, 205

Ductal electrolyte/water secretion. *See* Tear film, aqueous layer

Duration
  pupil size, 536t
  strabismus, 765

d-wave, electroretinograms, 506

Dye-based angiography, 289

Dynamic corneal response (DCR) parameters, 112b

Dynamic measurement, accommodation, 55

Dynamic random dot correlograms, 741

Dynamic remodeling, corneal sensory nerves, 385, 386f, 387b

E

EAC (episcleral arterial circle), 114f–115f, 116

Early blindness, recovery of sight after, 782–783

Early manifest glaucoma treatment (EMGT), 687

Early processing of spatial form. *See* Spatial form, early processing

Early Treatment of Diabetic Retinopathy Study (ETDRS) chart, 663

Early vision loss, perceptual and neural effects of, 778–781
  auditory processing, 779–781
  touch and braille, 778–779

Early vision, visual processing hierarchy, 735–736

ECCE (extracapsular cataract extraction), 111

Eccentricity
  critical flicker fusion frequency, 723, 724f
  function of, 641–642
  visual acuity. *See* Visual acuity
  visual fields, 675

Eccentricity and polar angle, in visual space, 630, 630f

ECD (endothelial cell density). *See* Corneal endothelium

Echolocation, 784

Echothiophate, aqueous humor drainage, 263

ECM. *See* Extracellular matrix (ECM)

Ectasia, cornea. *See* Cornea

Edema
  cornea. *See* Cornea
  corneal, 16–18
  progress measurement, 15–16, 15f
  sclera, 116

Edge-to-edge spacing, for foveal targets, 657–658

Edinger–Westphal nucleus
  accommodation stimulus, 54
  pupil light reflex, 528
  pupil near reflex, 533
  pupil reflex dilation, 533
  retinal projection targets, 573

Efferent arm, pupil light reflex, 532, 533b

Efferent defects, pupil, 539–547

Efflux transporters, 405–406, 406t
  cornea outward transport, 408–409, 408f
  genetic variation and ocular diseases, 411, 411t
    ABCA4, 411b
    ABCD1, 411b
    adrenoleukodystrophy, 411b
    MRP6, 411b
    multidrug resistance, 411b
    pseudoxanthoma elasticum (PXE), 411b
    sterol homeostasis, 411b
  methods, 406–408
    ocular cell and tissue models, 407–408
    overexpressing cells, 407
    proteomic analysis, 406–407
    in vivo animal experiments, 408
  species-dependent expression, 408–409, 408f. *see also specific types*

EGF. *See* Epidermal growth factor (EGF)

Egocentric direction, 702–703

Egocentric localization, 702

Elastic modulus, lens, 61

Elastin, scleral mechanical properties, 112–113

Electrical coupling, photoreceptor junctional conductances
  calcium-activated anion current ($I_{Cl(Ca)}$), 448, 448f

Electrical coupling, photoreceptor junctional conductances (*Continued*)
  calcium-activated potassium current ($I_{K(Ca)}$), 446–448
  electrotonic coupling, 448

Electrical microstimulation, 532

Electrical responses
  cone light adaptation, 454, 455f
  light adaptation. *See* Light adaptation

Electrolyte secretion regulation
  tear film, aqueous layer. *See* Tear film, aqueous layer
  tear film, mucous layer. *See* Tear film, mucous layer

Electrophysiological recording techniques, 749

Electrophysiology
  constant monocular form deprivation, 756, 757f
  corneal nerves, 82
  neuron–glial cell interaction, 325–326
  optic nerve, 585
  photoreceptor–Müller cell interaction, 332

Electrophysiology perimetry, 688b

Electroretinogram(s) (ERGs), 506–526
  amplitude, dark-adapted b-wave, 514, 516f
  component definition, 509
  congenital stationary night blindness, 421f
  c-wave, 509
  definition, 506
  direct-current, 509
  extracellular, retinal glycolysis, 328, 328f
  flash type, 506, 507f
  generation, 506–509
    stimulus conditions, 507f, 508–509
  glial currents, 506–508
    Cl⁻ ions, 508
    c-wave, 508, 508f
    extracellular K⁺ ions, 508
    inward rectifying K⁺ channels, 508
    Müller cells, 508
    Na⁺ ions, 508
    negative scotopic threshold response, 508
    photopic negative response, 508
    slow PIII, 508, 508f
    time course, 513–514, 514f, 516f
  ipRGC intraretinal output, 561
  light-adapted, cone-driven. *See* Electroretinograms, light-adapted, cone-driven
  local, 506
  multifocal, 523
    definition, 523
    glutamate analog studies, 523, 523f
    retinal cells, 523b
    technique, 523
  negative, dark-adapted a-wave, 510–511
  noninvasive recording, 509
    Burian Allen electrode, 506–509, 507f
    H-K loop electrodes, 509
  radial current flow, 506–508
    a-wave, 506
    b-wave, 506
    cell orientation, 506, 507f
    d-wave, 506
  slow PIII, 508–509, 508f
  stimulus conditions, 507f, 508–509

Electroretinograms, full-field dark-adapted (Ganzfeld) flash, 510–516
  dark-adapted a-wave, 510–514

Electroretinograms, full-field dark-adapted (Ganzfeld) flash (Continued)
current source density, 510
mixed rod-cone a-wave, 510f, 512, 513f
modeling, 511, 512f
negative ERGs, 510–511
rod response time course, 513–514, 514f
dark-adapted b-wave, 511f, 514, 515f
ERG amplitude, 514, 516f
GABA, 514
PII, 514, 516f
human vs. macaque, 510, 510f
mouse, 510
scotopic threshold response, 510, 511f, 514–516, 515f, 516f
NMDA receptor agonist studies, 514
retinal cells, 523b
Electroretinograms, light-adapted, cone-driven, 516–523
flicker ERG, 507f, 519
mice vs. primates, 519
Nob1 mice, 519
ON- and OFF-pathway interactions, 519
isolating cone-driven responses, 513f, 516–517, 517f
genetically-manipulated mouse models, 517
stimulus wavelength, 516–517
light-adapted a-wave, 517–518, 518f
PDA-sensitive postreceptoral neurons, 517, 518f
retinal cells, 523b
light-adapted b-wave, 518–519, 518f, 521f
retinal cells, 513b
TTX studies, 519
light-adapted d-wave, 507f, 518f, 519
intraretinal analysis, 518–519, 518f
retinal cells, 513b
oscillatory potentials, 507f, 519–521
feedback mechanisms, 521
generation, 521
inner retinal neurons, 519–520
retinal cells, 513b
TTX studies, 519–520
pattern ERG, 522–523
glaucoma, 522
retinal cells, 506
photopic negative response, 521f, 522, 522f
electroretinogram glial currents, 508
primary open angle glaucoma, 522
retinal cells, 524b
stimulus conditions, 507f, 508–509
spatial extent, 509
Electrotonic coupling, photoreceptor junctional conductances, 448
bright light responses, 441, 444f
delayed rectifier potassium current (I_{KV}), 441–443, 445f
hyperpolarization-activated current (I_H), 443, 446f
voltage-activated calcium current (I_{Ca}), 443–445, 446b, 446f, 447f
Elongated eyes, myopia, 1
Embryology
cornea, 69–106
vitreous body. See Vitreous body
Embryonic lens development, 126–127, 128f
Emmetropia
ciliary body contraction, 3

Emmetropia (Continued)
definition, 29f, 653
development, 24
lens power changes, 3
refractive power loss, 3
sclera development, 108
Emmetropization, 761
Endothelial cell density (ECD). See Corneal endothelium
Endothelial cell injury, cornea. See Cornea
Endothelial nitric oxide synthase (eNOS/NOS-3), 371
Endothelins, retinal vasodilator, 303–305, 305f
Endothelium
cornea. See Cornea
retinal vasodilator, 303–305, 304f, 305f
retinal vasculature. See Retinal vasculature
Energy substrate compartmentalization, neuron–glial cell interaction. See Neuron–glial cell interaction
"En grappe" endings, extraocular muscle neuromuscular junctions, 193, 194f
Enhanced S cone syndrome, 437b
eNOS. See Endothelial nitric oxide synthase (eNOS/NOS-3)
"En plaque" endings, extraocular muscle neuromuscular junctions, 193, 194f
Enucleation, side effects, 550b
EOMs. See Extraocular muscles (EOMs)
Ephrin signaling, 750f
Epidermal growth factor (EGF)
conjunctival goblet cells
proliferation, 367
signaling pathway, 367
protein secretion regulation, tear film, aqueous production, 372
transforming growth factor (TGFα), 367
Epinephrine
aqueous humor drainage, 264
electrolyte/water secretion regulation, 369
Episclera, 106, 110–112
scleral mechanical properties, 113, 114f–115f
vasculature. See Sclera
Episcleral arterial circle (EAC), 114f–115f, 116
Episcleral vein, 246f
Episcleral venous pressure (EVP), scleral mechanical properties, 113
Epithelial cells, lens, 50–52
Epithelial plugs, corneal stromal wound healing, 86
Epithelium
cornea. See Cornea
corneal edema, 96–97
damage, corneal ultraviolet light filtration, 106
lens, 125
ERGs. See Electroretinogram(s) (ERGs)
ERK1/2 inhibitory pathway, aqueous tear film layer secretion, 371, 372f
Esthesiometry, 378
Estropia, 229
ETDRS (Early Treatment of Diabetic Retinopathy Study) chart, 663
Ethacrynic acid (ECA), aqueous humor drainage, 267
Ethacrynic acid effects, aqueous humor drainage, 267
Ethmoid bone, 347, 348f
Ethnic differences, endothelial cell density, 91–92, 98f

Event analysis, visual field, assessing visual field progression, 687
Event-related potential (ERP), 744, 744f
Evisceration, side effects, 550b
Evolution of aberrometers, 33–34, 33f
Evolution of eye, 22
EVP (episcleral venous pressure), scleral mechanical properties, 113
Excimer laser-based keratorefractive surgery, 111
Excitatory amino acid transporter (EAAT), 324, 325f
Excitatory/inhibitory (E/I) responses, 776
Excitatory signals, inner plexiform layer. see Signal processing, inner plexiform layer
Exfoliation glaucoma, 262
Exotropia, 229
Explainable artificial intelligence (XAI), 633
Extracapsular cataract extraction (ECCE), 111
Extracellular ATP, photoreceptors, 324
Extracellular diffusion barrier, lens fiber cells, 133
Extracellular electroretinograms, retinal glycolysis, 328, 328f
Extracellular lactate
retinal blood flow, 334
retinal nitric oxide, 335
Extracellular matrix (ECM)
aqueous humor outflow obstruction, 262
lens development, 127, 128f
Extracellular potassium ions, electroretinogram glial currents, 508
Extraclassical receptive field, in V1, 619
Extraocular muscles (EOMs), 189–211
anatomy, 189–203
associated diseases, 207–208, 207t
congenital fibrosis, 206b
development, 201–203, 203f–204f
diseases/disorders, 203, 207t
See also Eye movements. specific diseases/ disorders
eye movements, neural control, 212–215, 213f
histological anatomy, 193–197
fast fibers, 193, 197f
fiber polymorphism, 195–197, 199f
fiber variation, 193–194, 198f
global layers, 193–194
heavy chain expression, 193
layers, 193, 197f
limb muscle vs., 193–194
mismatched myofibers, 197, 199f
orbital layers, 193–194
slow fibers, 193
horizontal eye movements, 190
innervation, 54, 192–193, 192f, 194f
acetylcholine receptors, 193
individual nerves, 193.
see also specific nerves
neuromuscular junctions, 193, 194f
intorsion, 190, 192f
metabolism, 197–200
calcium, 197
glutathione reductases, 197–199
mitochondria, 197
superoxide dismutases, 197–199
muscle diseases, spared in, 205–207, 207t
orbital connective tissue, 193, 195f, 196f, 207t
orientation, 190, 191t
physiology, 193–197
proprioception, 200–201, 201f, 202f

Extraocular muscles (EOMs) *(Continued)*
  remodelling, 200, 200*f*
    botulinum toxin studies, 200
    denervation/reinnervation animal models, 200
    Pitx2, 200
  saccades, 189
  smooth pursuit, 189
  vertical eye movements, 190.
  see also specific muscles
Extraretinal signals
  gaze stabilization. *See* Gaze stabilization
  LGN. *See* Lateral geniculate nucleus (LGN)
Extrastriate cortex regions, 627
Extrastriate visual cortex (V2), 627–637
  dorsal visual network, 633–635
    link to perception and action, 634
    receptive fields and visual selectivity, 633
    subconscious vision, 634–635
    subcortical inputs, 634–635
  plasticity and rehabilitation, 635
    cortical blindness, 635
    prospects for vision rehabilitation, 635
  ventral visual network, 627–633
    applications, 633
    distributed coding, 631
    hierarchical processing, 630, 630*f*
    invariance, 632–633
    receptive fields and visual selectivity, 630–631
    topographical features, 629–630
    ventral stream, 632.
  see also specific methods
Extravascular intraretinal acidosis, retinal blood
    flow, 334
Ex vivo experiments, corneal stiffness, 101
Eye(s)
  elongation, myopia, 1
  movements. *See* Eye movements
  young. *See* Young eye
Eyebrows, 354
  muscles, 354, 354*f*
Eye-head gaze shifts, 228–229
Eye-in-head motion, 236–237
Eyelids, 355–357
  anatomy, 354–357, 357*f*
  fat tissue, 358
  innervation, 359–360, 360*f*
  lymphatics, 359
  margin, 355–357
    anterior lamella, 356
    Lockwood's ligament, 356–357
    meibomian glands, 357
    Moll glands, 356
    orbicularis muscle, 349*f*, 356
    palpebral conjunctiva, 357
    posterior lamella, 356–357
    tarsal plates, 357
    Whitnall's ligament, 356–357
    Zeis glands, 356
  musculature, 357–360
  vasculature, 359, 359*f*
Eye movements
  anomalies, strabismus, 765–766
  diseases, 203–205.
    see also specific diseases/disorders
  foveal gaze shift. *See* Foveal gaze shift
  functional classification. *see specific movements*
  gaze stabilization. *See* Gaze stabilization
  horizontal

Eye movements *(Continued)*
    extraocular muscles, 190
    medial rectus muscles, 190
  kinematics, 236
  monitoring of, development, 6
  neural control. *see below*
  three-dimensional, 236–244
Eye movements, neural control, 212–235
  abducens nerve (cranial nerve VI), 213
  biomechanics, 215–216
    force, 215
    oculomotor plant, 215, 215*f*
  classification, 212, 213*t*
  disjunctive saccades, 222, 223*f*
  disorders. *see specific diseases/disorders*
  final common pathways, 212–217
    extraocular eye muscles, 212–215, 213*f*
    hierarchy of, 212, 213*b*
    oculomotor nerve (cranial nerve III), 213
    trochlear nerve (cranial nerve IV), 213
  interactions, 227–229
    eye-head, 228–229
    gaze pursuit, 229
    gaze shifts, 227, 228*f*
  motor neurons, 213, 214*f*
    relationships, 215–216, 216*f*
  premotor neurons, 213, 214*f*
    gaze redirection, 217–224
  saccades, 212, 217–220, 217*f*
    main sequence, 217*b*
    microsaccades control, 220
    motor map, 217, 218*f*
    omnipause neurons role, 220
    premotor circuit, 217, 218*f*
    pulse-step command, 216–217, 216*f*
  smooth pursuit, 220–221, 221*f*
  smooth vergence, 221–222, 222*f*
  voluntary binocular, 221–224
    coding of disparity, 222–224.
  see also specific movements
Eye movements, three-dimensional
  Donders' law, 237, 238*f*
  eye-in-head motion, 236–237
  head-unrestrained gaze shift, 237–238, 238*f*
  Listing's law, 236–237
Eye-specific axonal territories, molecular
    mechanisms guiding formation of, 748–749
Eye-specific segregation, 750, 750*f*
Eye-specific territories, formation of, 748–749

F

Face perception, 631
Facial anatomy, 354–357
Facial artery, eyelids, 359, 359*f*
Facial nerve (cranial nerve VII)
  differential diagnosis, 355
  eyebrow, 354
  eyelids, 359
  paralysis, 355, 356*b*
  route of, 192–193
Facial recognition, 4–5, 5*f*
Facial vein, eyelids, 359
FACT (Functional Acuity Contrast Test), 664
FAK (focal adhesion kinase), 342–343
False torsion, Listing's law, 236–237
Fast fibers, extraocular muscles, 193, 197*f*

Fast focal neurochemistry, retinal synaptic
    organization, 470
Fat tissue
  eyelids, 358
  orbit, 351
FAZ. *See* Foveal avascular zone (FAZ)
FDT. *See* Frequency-doubling technology
    (FDT)
Feedback connections, in V1, 619–620
Feedback pathways
  negative, light adaptation, 459, 459*f*
  retinal synaptic organization, 472
Feedback synapses, horizontal cell output
    synapses, 484, 485*f*, 486*f*, 487*f*
Feedforward pathways
  retinal synaptic organization, 472
  in V1, 614, 614*f*
Feedforward synapses, horizontal cell output
    synapses, 484–485, 488*f*
FEF (frontal eye fields), saccades, 223–224
Femto-laser-assisted in situ keratomileusis
    (LASIK), 31
Ferrier, David, 612
Ferry-Porter law, 723, 723*f*
FGF (fibroblast growth factor), lens fiber cell
    differentiation, 128–129, 130*f*
Fiber cell compaction, nuclear fiber cells, 133
Fiber cells, lens, 125
Fibril-associated collagens with interrupted
    terminals (FACIT), 78
Fibrillins, 166
Fibroblast growth factor (FGF), lens fiber cell
    differentiation, 128–129, 130*f*
Fibronectin, transforming growth factor-β, 262
Fibrosis, congenital, extraocular muscles, 206*b*
Fibrous liquefaction, vitreous body, 177–178, 177*f*
Fibulins, 166
Field progression determination, visual field. *See*
    Visual field
Filensin proteins, 136
Filter-rectify- filter (FRF) arrangement, 641
Finite element modeling, scleral mechanical
    properties, 113, 114*f*–115*f*
First-order information, 640
Fixation disparity, 705
Fixed immobile pupil, 527
Flank-to-target interactions, 706
Flash photocurrent responses
  photoreceptors. *See* Photoreceptor(s)
  rods, 433, 435*f*
Flash photovoltage responses
  cones, 432
  photoreceptors. *See* Photoreceptor(s)
  rods, 432
Flash strength effects, flash photocurrent
    responses, 433, 435*f*, 436*f*
Flash type electroretinograms, 506, 507*f*
Flicker
  retinal vasodilator, 300, 301*f*, 304*f*
  temporal sensitivity, 728
Flicker electroretinograms. *See*
    Electroretinograms, light-adapted,
    cone-driven
Flicker-sensitivity experiments, temporal contrast
    sensitivity, 724
Floccular lobe, 221
Fluid mechanics, aqueous humor drainage. *See*
    Aqueous humor drainage

Fluorescein tracer studies
    scleral permeability, 117t
    vitreous body. See Vitreous body
fMRI. See Functional magnetic resonance imaging (fMRI)
Focal adhesion kinase (FAK), 342–343
Focus, depth of. See Depth of focus
Focusing efforts, accommodation stimulus, 54
Following movements
    direction of eye motion, 735
    infant vision development, 735
    visual processing hierarchy, 735–740, 736f
Forced-choice preferential looking (FPL), 735
    motion detection development, 740
    visual processing hierarchy, 735
Force, eye movements, 215
Forehead, 354
    muscles, 354f.
        see also specific muscles
Form deprivation amblyopia, 755–761, 766–767
FORUM, 677
FOS (frequency of seeing curve), 675–676
Foster, Russell, 549–550
Foucault gratings, 13
Fourier transformation, 13
Fourth root summation, 645–646
Fovea, 4, 612
    blue-yellow circuitry, 671
    photoreceptors, 9
    structure, 125f
    yellow pigment, 19
Foveal avascular zone (FAZ), 293–294
Foveal gaze shift, rapid conjugate shifts (saccadic eye movements). See Saccades
Foveal reflex, 6
Foveal viewings, contrast sensitivity, 660f, 661f
Foveal window of visibility. See Spatial form, early processing
Foville's syndrome, 230–231
FPL. See Forced-choice preferential looking (FPL)
Fractures, 616
Fractures, orbit lateral wall, 348, 349f
Frequency-doubling technology (FDT), 678–679, 688–691, 691f
Frequency of seeing curve (FOS), 675–676
Fresh tonic pupil, 543
Frisby Stereo Test, 743
Frontal bone, 189, 347, 348f
Frontal eye fields (FEFs), saccades, 223–224
Frontal nerve, 350f, 378–379
Frontal sinus, 347
Fuchs' endothelial corneal dystrophy, 16
Functional Acuity Contrast Test (FACT), 664
Functional architecture, primary visual cortex (V1). See Primary visual cortex (V1)
Functional architecture, V1, 616–619
    columns and maps, 616–617, 618f
    cytochrome oxidase blobs, 617–619, 618f
Functional imaging, retinal glycolysis, 327
Functional magnetic resonance imaging (fMRI), 629, 638
    early blindness, recovery of sight after, 782
    space, 780
Functional neuronal activity, neuron–glial cell interaction, 330–331
Fundus albipunctatus, slowed dark adaptation, 462
Fusion, binocular vision development, 741

G

GABA
    dark-adapted b -wave, 514
    horizontal cell
        feedback, 484, 485f, 486f, 487f
        feedforward, 484–485, 488f
        synaptic output, 484
    inner plexiform layer signal processing. see Signal processing, inner plexiform layer
    ipRGC synaptic input, 558–560
    Müller glial cells, 330
    receptors, developmental visual deprivation, 759, 760f
    ribbon synapses, 468
    transmitter receptors, 481
Gain control suppression, 646
Gamma-aminobutyric acid (GABA), 776
γ-tropomyosin (γTM), 135
Ganglion cell fibers, 676
Ganglion-cell photoreceptors. See Retinal ganglion cells, intrinsically photosensitive (ipRGCs)
Ganglion cell responses, horizontal cell output synapses, 486
Ganglion cells. See Retinal ganglion cell(s) (RGCs)
Gangliosides, 363
Ganzfeld electroretinograms, 536
Gaze disorder, 230–231, 230b, 230f
Gaze pursuit, 229
Gaze shifts, 227, 228f
    eye-head, 228–229
    head-unrestrained, 237–238
    upstream control, 228–229
Gaze stabilization, 224–227
    nerve control, vestibulo-ocular reflex. See Vestibulo-ocular reflex (VOR)
Gaze tracking, 683
GCAP1 protein, 460
GCAPs (guanylyl cyclase activating proteins), 458
Genetic testing, color vision tests, 670
Gennari, Francesco, 612
Geometric effect, 712
Geometric vertical horopter, 705f
Germinative zone, lens, 125
Giant cell arteritis, 546
Glare
    contrast sensitivity, 15–16
    testing, 15–16, 16f
    visual acuity, 664
Glaucoma, 696f
    angle-closure, mydriasis, 545
    animal models, 588
    aqueous humor drainage, 262
    exfoliation, 262
    glucocorticoid, 267
    hemolytic, 262
    ocular blood flow disease, 306–308, 307f, 308f
    optic nerve injury, 587–588, 588f
    pattern ERG, 522
    phacolytic, 262
    primary open-angle. See Primary open-angle glaucoma (POAG)
    relative afferent pupillary defect, 538t
    temporal sensitivity, 729
    uveitic, 262
Glaucoma hemifield test (GHT), 682
Glia, 751
Gliaform neurons, 464–465

Glial cells
    biochemistry, 329–330
    electroretinograms. See Electroretinogram(s) (ERGs)
    neuronal sensing, 324
Glial (astrocyte)- neuron–lactate shuttle hypothesis, 332
Glial palisade, 748
Gliotoxic L-2-aminoadipic acid (LAA), 300
Glucocorticoid glaucoma, 267
Glucose
    metabolism enzymes, 327
    retinal glycolysis, 327
    retinal vasodilator, 306
    transport
        Müller glial cells, 329–330
        retinal pigmented epithelium, 339
Glucose metabolism, metabolic determinants of lens, 140–141
Glucose transporters (GLUTs), 334
GluR6 knockout mice, negative ERG, 511
Glutamate, 324, 481
    analog studies, multifocal electroretinograms, 523, 523f
    BC ribbon synapses, 468
    excitotoxicity, 470b
    honeybee retina in vitro studies, 331f
    Müller glial cells, 330
    outer retinal signal processing. See Signal processing, outer retina
    photoreceptor ribbon synapses, 467, 469f
Glutamatergic monopolar interneurons (GluMIs), 465–466
Glutamate transporters, 145, 146f
Glutamine synthetase (GS), 324
Glutathione (GSH)
    age-related nuclear cataracts, 155
    levels maintenance, 141, 142f
    synthesis, 145
Glutathione reductases, extraocular muscles, 197–199
GLUT1, retinal pigmented epithelium, 339
GLUT3, retinal pigmented epithelium, 339
Glycine, 145
    inner plexiform layer signal processing. see Signal processing, inner plexiform layer
    Müller glial cells, 330
Glycocalyx
    corneal endothelium, 97
    tear film. See Tear film
Glycogen
    neuron–glial cell interaction, 330
    photoreceptor–Müller cell interaction, 332
Glycolysis
    hexokinase, 326
    retina. See Retina
Glycosaminoglycans (GAGs), 164–165
    aqueous humor drainage, 271
    chondroitin sulfate, 164
    cornea, 6
    corneal light transmission, 81
    heparan sulfate, 164
    hyaluronan, 164
    scleral mechanical properties, 113
Gnostic cell, 631
Goblet cell mucin production, regulation of, 366–368
    proliferation, 367–368, 368f

Goblet cell mucin production, regulation of (Continued)
    secretion in disease, 367
    secretion in health, 366–367, 367f, 368f
Goblet cell mucous secretion, 366
Goldmann applanation tonometer, 116
Goldmann equation, aqueous humor drainage, 255
Goldmann-like perimeter, 677
G$_t$ protein. See Transducin
G-proteins
    activation, light response activation, 423
    inactivation, dark-adapted rod recovery phase, 426
    subunits, rods vs. cones, 428
Graded hyperpolarizations, flash photovoltage responses, 432, 433f, 434f
Gradient of refractive index, lens, 124, 138–140, 138f
Gradient refractive index, lens, 38–39
Grandmother cell, 631
Granit–Harper law, 723–724, 723f
    foveal revision, 723, 723f
Grating acuity, infant vision development. See Infant vision development
Grating stimuli, 616
Grave's ophthalmopathy, 587
Gray matter, 777–778
Greater sphenoid wing, 348f
Growth factors
    corneal stromal wound healing, 84–86
    oligodendrocyte development, 583
    RPE secretion, 343.
    see also specific growth factors
Guanine nucleotide turnover, dark-adapted rods. See Dark-adapted rods
Guanylate cyclase
    activation, 426
    dark-adapted rod recovery phase, 426
    dark-adapted rod resting state, 417–418
Guanylyl cyclase activating proteins (GCAPs), 458
Guanylyl cyclase activation, 459–460, 459f
GUCY2D gene, 426
Guided progression analysis (GPA), 687

H

H-7 effects, aqueous humor, 266–267
H2 horizontal cells, blue-yellow circuitry, 671
Half angle rule, Listing's law, 237, 239f
Halobacterium halobium, 8
Haplopia, 703f
Hardy, Rand and Rittler (HRR) pseudoisochromatic plates, 670–671
HCAR1, lactate and, 331–332, 334
Head-unrestrained gaze shift, 237–238, 238f
Heavy chain expression, extraocular muscles, 193
Hebbian model, 750–751
Hebbian synaptic plasticity, developmental visual deprivation, 759
Hemianopia
    homonymous, 574, 575f, 576b
    nasal, 573–574, 575f
Hemidesmosomes, corneal epithelium, 86, 90f, 91f
Hemolytic glaucoma, 262
Hemorrhage, intraocular, 538t
Heparan sulfate, 164

Herbivores, accommodation, 37
Hering-Bielschowsky afterimage test, 714
Hering-Hillebrand deviation, 703–704
Herpes zoster iritis, 545
Heterocellular coupling
    RGCs, 474
    retinal synaptic organization, 469–470
Heterotropia, 713, 713f
Hexokinase, glycolysis, 326
Higher-order aberrations (HOAs)
    corrections with, 33
        contact lenses, 33
        intraocular lenses (IOLs), 33
        spectacles, 33
    impact on vision, 31–32
        treatments to alleviate, 32–33
    phase function reduction from, 33
    spherical aberration and, 31.
    see also specific aberrations
High-resolution light microscopic autoradiography, 329f, 331–332
H-K loop electrodes, electroretinograms, 509
HOA. See Higher-order aberrations (HOA)
"Hockey stick" approach, 687
Homeostatic synaptic mechanisms, 760–761
Homeostatic synaptic plasticity, 768–769
Homocellular coupling, retinal synaptic organization, 469–470
Homonymous hemianopia, 574, 575f, 576b
Homonymous semicongruous visual field deficit, 684
Homonymous visual field loss, 684
Horizontal binocular disparity, 707
Horizontal cell(s) (HCs), 465, 480
    AMPA receptors, 465
    bipolar cell output synapses and, 481, 482f
    non-canonical signaling, 468–469
    outer retinal signal processing. See Signal processing, outer retina
    photoreceptor signaling, 482–483
    phylogenetics, 465
Horizontal connections, in V1, 619–620
Horizontal eye movements. See Eye movements
Horizontal meridian, 684
Hormonal regulation, meibomian glands, 375
Horner's syndrome, 541b
    anisocoria vs., 539
    childhood, 543
        cocaine eye drops, 543
    congenital, 543
    pharmacologic diagnosis
        apraclonidine, 542
        cocaine, 542
        denervation localization, 542
    pupil asymmetry, 539
    pupil dilation lag, 539, 542f
Horopter, 703–705, 703f
    in ABC, 714–715
Howard-Dolman real depth test, 743
HSD-1 (11β–Hydroxysteroid dehydrogenase), 267
Hubbard, Ruth, 428
Hubel, David, 612
Human models
    cone light adaptation, 458f, 461
    white matter pathways, 775
Human retina, 326
Human visual system, 527
Humoral mechanisms, pupil reflex dilation, 534

Humphrey Field Analyzer. See Static perimetry
Humphrey field analyzer, 677, 680, 681f
Humphrey matrix (second-generation) frequency-doubling technology (FDT), 691, 692f
Hyalocytes, vitreous body, 167–168, 170f
Hyaloid vascular system, regression of, 174–176, 174f, 175f
Hyaluronan, 164
    collagen binding, 164
    lipid binding, 164, 170f
Hyaluronic acid, vitreous body, 164
    aging, 177
Hyaluronidase, aqueous humor drainage, 271
Hydrogen clearance, ocular circulation measurement, 289
Hydrogen peroxide, 141
Hydrophilic drugs, corneal drug delivery, 104–105
3-Hydroxykynurenine (3-OHK), 142
3-Hydroxykynurenine O-β-D-glucoside (3-OHKG), 142
11β–Hydroxysteroid dehydrogenase (HSD-1), 267
Hyperactive signaling diseases/disorders, photoreceptors, 437b
Hyperacuities, 708
    definition, 651–652
    development, 664–665
Hypercolumn, 616
Hypercomplex or end-stopped cells, 616
Hyperopia
    development, 24
    mechanism, 27, 29f
Hyperpolarization, 484
Hyperpolarization current (I$_H$), photoreceptors, 443, 446f
Hypertropia, 229
Hypothalamus, SCN, ipRGC circadian photoentrainment, 563–564
Hypotropia, 229

I

I$_{Ca}$ (voltage-activated calcium current), 443–445, 446b, 447f
I$_{Cl(Ca)}$ (calcium-activated anion current), 448, 448f
Identical visual directions (IVDs), 714–715
Idiopathic infantile nystagmus (INS), 205
Idiopathic intracranial hypertension (IIH), 530
Idiopathic optic neuritis, 587
IGF. See Insulin-like growth factor (IGF)
IGF-1 (insulin-like growth factor 1), RPE secretion, 343
iGluRs. See Ionotropic glutamate receptors (iGluRs)
I$_H$ (hyperpolarization current), photoreceptors, 443, 446f
I$_{K(Ca)}$ (calcium-activated potassium current), 446–448
I$_{KV}$ (delayed rectifier potassium current), 441–443, 445f
Illumination
    accommodation measurement, 55
    contrast sensitivity vs., 15
    photoreceptor–Müller cell metabolic interactions, 332
Image-degrading defenses, retina, 19
Image plane, 27–28

Image quality
   polychromatic, 27
   pupil, 527
Image segmentation, 728–729
Image, visual acuity, 652, 653*f*
Imbert-Fick principle, 116
Immature retina, 749*f*
Immortalized human meibomian gland epithelial
   cells, 375
Immune molecules, 751
Immune response
   corneal epithelium, 84*f*, 89
   optic nerve injury, 589–590
Immunoglobulin A (IgA), secretory, tear film, 370
Immunohistochemistry, vitreous body, 174, 176*f*
INC (Interstitial nucleus of Cajal), 230–231, 241
Incomplete Schubert–Bornstein congenital
   stationary night blindness, 446*b*
   CACNA1F gene, 446*b*, 447*f*
Incongruous visual field loss, 684
Incremental light detection, 688*b*
Increment (differential) light threshold, visual
   fields, 675–676
Infantile strabismus syndrome, 229*b*
Infant vision development, 735–747
   assessment, 735
   binocular vision, 741–743
     disparity sensitivity. *See* Disparity sensitivity
     fusion, 741
     stereopsis, 742
   grating acuity, 737–738
     pattern onset-offset stimuli, 738
     visual evoked potentials, 738
   motion detection, 740–741
     asymmetries, 740, 740*f*
     FPL, 740
     optokinetic nystagmus, 740, 740*f*
     symmetric cortical motion, 740–741
     visual evoked potentials, 740
   object-level processing, 743–745, 744*f*
   ocular following movements, 735
   preferential looking, 735
   spatiotemporal vision, 736–737
     behavioral measurements, 737
     directional eye movements, 737
     peak-contrast sensitivity, 737, 737*f*
     steady-state visual evoked potentials, 737,
     737*f*
   Vernier acuity, 738–740
   visual evoked potentials, 735
   visual processing hierarchy, 735–740
     early vision, 735–736
     FPL, 736
     middle vision, 736
     object recognition, 735–736
     ocular following movements, 736
     visual evoked potentials, 736
Inferior division III nerve, anatomy, 192*f*
Inferior oblique muscles, 190, 357*f*
   anatomy, 191*f*, 192*f*
   paths of, 190, 191*f*, 192*f*
Inferior oculomotor nerve, 350*f*
Inferior ophthalmic vein, 350*f*
Inferior orbicularis muscle, 357*f*
Inferior orbital fissure, 189
   orbital apex, 349
Inferior orbital vein, 353–354
Inferior rectus muscles, 189, 350*f*

Inferior oblique muscles *(Continued)*
   anatomy, 191*f*, 192*f*
   eyelids, 358
Inferior tarsal muscle, 357*f*
Inferior trochlear nerve, 192*f*
Inferior visual field, 676
Inferomedial strut, orbit, 349
Inflation studies, corneal stiffness, 101
Inflation testing, scleral mechanical properties,
   113, 114*f*–115*f*
Infraorbital artery, 359, 359*f*
Infraorbital nerve, 379, 379*f*
Inhibited glial phagocytosis, 750*f*
Inner blood–retina barrier. *See* Blood–retina
   barrier (BRB)
Inner plexiform layer (IPL)
   signal processing. *see* Signal processing, inner
     plexiform layer
   visual processing, inner retina, 496–498
     amacrine cell dendritic compartments, 498
     bipolar cell axon terminals, 496–497, 497*b*
     dendritic retinal ganglion cells, 498
Inner retina, 326
   bipolar cells, 324
   See also Retina
Innervation
   eyelids, 359–360, 360*f*
   iris, 534
   sensory. *See* Sensory innervation (of eye).
   see also specific anatomical structure. specific
     nerves
INO (Internuclear ophthalmoplegia), 230–231
Inputs, primary visual cortex. *See* Primary visual
   cortex (V1)
Insulin-like growth factor (IGF), lens fiber cell
   differentiation, 128–129
Insulin-like growth factor-1 receptor (IGF-1R),
   351
Insulin-like growth factor 1 (IGF-1), RPE
   secretion, 343
Insulin, photoreceptor–Müller cell interaction, 332
Integrin αvβ5, photoreceptor outer segment
   phagocytosis, 342–343
Intensity discrimination, 16
Intergeniculate leaflet (IGL), ipRGC circadian
   photoentrainment, 563–564
Interlaminar circuitry and cell types, V1, 614–615
   cortical circuit, 615
     feedforward pathways, 614, 614*f*
     intralaminar and feedback pathways, 614, 614*f*
     parallel streams, 614–615, 614*f*
Intermediate filaments, lens fiber cell architecture,
   135, 136*f*
Intermittent monocular form deprivation. *See*
   Visual deprivation, developmental
Internal carotid artery, 353*f*
   intracranial optic nerve, 583
International Society for Clinical
   Electrophysiology of Vision (ISCEV), 509,
   513*b*
Interneurons, pupil light reflex. *See* Pupil light
   reflex
Internuclear ophthalmoplegia (INO), 230–231
Interphotoreceptor matrix retinal binding protein
   (IRPB), 341
Interplexiform cells, 483
   retinal neuron modulation, 483
Interpretation guide. *See* Visual field

Interpupillary distance (IPD), 709
Interstitial nucleus of Cajal (INC), 230–231, 241
Intorsion
   extraocular muscles, 190, 192*f*
   superior oblique muscles, 190, 192*f*
Intracameral injections, corneal drug delivery,
   105, 109*f*
Intracranial optic nerve, 579
   blood supply, 583
Intraepithelial nerve terminals, corneal sensory
   nerves, 381*f*, 382
Intralaminar and feedback pathways, in V1, 614,
   614*f*
Intraocular hemorrhage, relative afferent pupillary
   defect, 538*t*
Intraocular lenses (IOLs)
   spectral design, 552*b*
   spherical aberrations, 21
Intraocular muscles, accommodation stimulus, 54
Intraocular pressure (IOP)
   aqueous humor, 245
   ciliary body sensory nerves, 391
   dependent mechanosensation model, 261*f*
   homeostasis, 258–262, 259*f*, 260*f*, 261*f*
   iris sensory nerves, 391
   ocular circulation regulation, 299, 300*f*
   scleral mechanical properties, 113–116
   scleral sensory nerves, 391
   transforming growth factor-β, 262
Intraorbital optic nerve, 578, 579*f*
   blood supply, 582–583
Intraretinal output, ipRGCs, 561–562, 561*f*
Intrascleral optic nerve, 578
Intrastromal injections, corneal drug delivery,
   105, 109*f*
Intravitreal accommodative movements, 50*t*
Intravitreal injections
   retinal blood flow, 334
   scleral drug delivery, 109*f*, 116
Intrinsically photosensitive retinal ganglion cell
   (ipRGC), 530
Intrinsically photosensitive RGCs (ipRGCs), 750
Inverse syneresis, 149*b*, 149*f*
Invertebrate-like phototransduction cascade,
   ipRGCs, 551–552
Involuntary blinking, corneal nerves, 83
Inward rectifying K+ channels (Kir),
   electroretinogram glial currents, 508
Iodoacetate studies, retinal glycolysis, 328
IOLs. *See* Intraocular lenses (IOLs)
Ionotropic glutamate receptors (iGluRs)
   differential expression, 470
   retinal synaptic organization, 470
Ion transport
   RPE. *See* Retinal pigment epithelium (RPE).
   specific ions
IOP. *See* Intraocular pressure (IOP)
IPD. *See* Interpupillary distance (IPD)
IPL. *See* Inner plexiform layer (IPL)
ipRGCs. *See* Retinal ganglion cells, intrinsically
   photosensitive (ipRGCs)
Ipsilateral eye (temporal retina), LGN layers and
   maps, 598
Ipsilateral RGCs, 748
Ipsilateral-to-contralateral ratio, 748
Iridoplegia, traumatic, mydriasis, 544
Iris
   anatomy, 42*f*

Iris *(Continued)*
  color, 534–535
  dilator, 534–535
  ischemia, 543
  neuronal input, 534
  sensory nerves, 388f, 391
    cold-sensitive, 391
    intraocular pressure, 391
  slit-lamp biomicroscope examination, 543
  structure, 125f, 534–535, 535f
Iris sphincter, 534–535
  cholinergic drug response, 543–545, 544f
    supersensitivity, 543–544
    undersensitivity, 544–545
  damage, anisocoria, 540t
Iron mydriasis, anisocoria, 540t
IRPB (interphotoreceptor matrix retinal binding protein), 341
Irregular astigmatism, 28–30
ISCEV (International Society for Clinical Electrophysiology of Vision), 509, 513b
Ischemic optic neuropathy, 587
  animal models, 587
Ishihara's test of color vision, 669
Isolated cat retina studies, photoreceptor–Müller cell interaction, 332
Isolated cell models, neuron–glial cell interaction, 330f, 331–332
Isotope studies, retinal glycolysis, 328

J

Jerk nystagmus, 232, 232b
Juxtacanalicular tissue (JCT), aqueous humor drainage, 256, 257f, 258f

K

Kainate receptors, 481–482
KCCl (potassium–chloride symporter), 373
KCC2, retinal synaptic organization, 472
K cells, LGN. *See* Lateral geniculate nucleus (LGN)
Kearns–Sayre syndrome, 207–208
Keeler, Clyde, 549
Kelman phacoemulsification (KPE), 111
Keratan sulfate, corneal light transmission, 81–82
Keratectomy, photoreactive. *See* Photorefractive keratectomy (PRK)
Keratitis, neurotrophic, 392–393
Keratoconus, 16
Keratocytes
  apoptosis, 84
  corneal light transmission, 79–81, 84f
Keratometry, 78b
Keratoplasty
  penetrating, 16
  posterior lamellar, 111
Keratotomy
  astigmatic, 105
  radial, 105
Kinematics, 3D, 236
Kinetic perimetry, 677–678
Kinetics, ipRGCs. *See* Retinal ganglion cells, intrinsically photosensitive (ipRGCs)
Kir (inward rectifying K+ channels), electroretinogram glial currents, 508
K layers (koniocellular), LGN layers and maps, 605

K LGN axons, 612
Knockout animals, α-crystallins, 139
KPE (Kelman phacoemulsification), 111
Krebs cycle, 334
Kynurenine (Kyn), 142

L

Lacrimal artery, 353f, 359f
Lacrimal bone, 189, 347, 348f, 349f
Lacrimal gland, 370
  afferent and efferent neural regulation of, 365f
  anatomy, 364f
  fluid composition, 373–374
    chloride ions, 373–374
    potassium ions, 373–374
    sodium ions, 373–374
  innervation, 370
  structure, 369
Lacrimal nerve, 350f, 378–379
  anatomy, 192f
Lacrimal sac, 349f
Lacrimal sac fossa, 349, 349f
Lacritin, 374
Lactate
  extracellular. *See* Extracellular lactate
  Müller glial cells, 330, 330f
  neuron–glial cell interaction, 331
  photoreceptor–Müller cell metabolic interactions, 332–333
  retinal pigment epithelium transport, 341f
L-Lactate injection studies, retinal blood flow, 334
Lamina cribosa, 110–112
Lamina fusca, 69
Langerhans cells, corneal epithelium, 89
Large gap junction, lens fiber cells differentiation, 133
Large pupil, 527
LASEK (laser-assisted subepithelial keratectomy), 97
Laser-assisted subepithelial keratectomy (LASEK), 97
Laser Doppler flowmetry (LDF), ocular blood flow measurement, 290
Laser Doppler velocimetry, ocular blood flow measurement, 290
Laser in situ keratomileusis (LASIK), 97
  corneal stromal wound healing, 89f, 105
Laser speckle flowgraphy, ocular blood flow measurement, 291–292, 291f
LASIK. *See* Laser in situ keratomileusis (LASIK)
Late blindness
  behavior, 783
  neural responses, 783
Lateral canthal region, eyelid, 358
Lateral geniculate nucleus (LGN), 598–611, 701–702, 777
  anatomy, 598, 599f
  axons, 603, 612
  black-white circuitry, 671–673
  bottom-up visual inputs to V1 from, 612, 614f
  circuitry, 602
    drivers and modulators, 602
    proximal dendrites of LGN neurons, 602, 602f
    retinal and local interneuron synapses, 602
    retinal ganglion cells, 602, 602f

Lateral geniculate nucleus (LGN) *(Continued)*
  constant monocular form deprivation, 755–756
  development and cellular taxonomy, 598–599
  firing mode of, 610
  gateway to conscious visual perception, 598
  inputs, 599–602, 601f
    from brain stem, 601
    cortical, 600
    from local interneurons, 601–602
    retinal, 599–600, 601f
    superior colliculus, 601
    from thalamic reticular nucleus, 600–601
  ipRGC central projections, 565
  layers and maps
    contralateral eye, 605
    ipsilateral eye (temporal retina), 605
    K layers (koniocellular), 605
    M layers (magnocellular), 605
    P layers (parvocellular), 605, 606f
    visual space, 605, 608f
  modulation of, 609–610, 609f
    brainstem, 609–610
    cortical and reticular, 609, 609f
  outputs, 602–604, 603f
    primary visual cortex. *See* Primary visual cortex (V1)
  primary visual cortex, 603–605, 603f
  receptive fields, 604–605, 606f
    K layers (koniocellular), 605
    M layers (magnocellular), 605
    P layers (parvocellular), 605, 606f
  retinal projection targets, 571–573
  retinogeniculate transmission, 605–607, 608f
  of thalamus, 598
  visual field lesions, 574, 575f
Lateral geniculate nucleus of the thalamus (LGN), 748
Lateral habenula, ipRGC central projections, 565
Lateral intraparietal area (LIP), saccades, 223–224
Lateral occipital cortex (LOC), 781
Lateral posterior ciliary arteries, orbit, 352
Lateral rectus muscle, 350f, 357f
  anatomy, 191f, 192f
  horizontal eye movements, 190
  myofiber type, 189–190
Lateral short posterior ciliary arteries, optic nerve, head blood supply, 581–582
Lateral terminal nucleus (LTN), retinal projection targets, 573
Lateral wall, orbit, 347–348
Latrunculin, aqueous humor drainage, 266–267
LCA. *See* Leber's congenital amaurosis (LCA)
LCA (longitudinal chromatic aberration), 54
LDF (laser Doppler flowmetry), ocular blood flow measurement, 290
Leaky barrier function, corneal endothelium. *See* Corneal endothelium
Leber's congenital amaurosis (LCA), 342
  GUCY2D gene, 426
  ipRGCs, 551b
  RPE65 mutations, 440f, 443b
Leber's hereditary optic neuropathy (LHON), 530
Lens, 39–40, 124–163
  accommodative movements of, 64
  age-dependent changes, 151–156
    cataract development, 152–156
    presbyopia development, 151–152
    refractive power, 151

Lens (Continued)
  age-related changes, 49–50, 129f
  anatomy, 42f
  anterior surface, accommodation, 53–54
  antioxidants, 143–146
  ball-and-socket joints, 131, 134f
  biomechanical properties, 140
  CCC transporters, 148
  cellular organization of human, 124–126, 126f
  crystalline, 50–52
  development and growth, 124–129, 125f, 126f
  differentiation, 128–129
    composition and ultrastructure, 131–132
    cortex adhaerens, 131
    EphA2, 129
    fibroblast growth factor, 128–129, 130f
    insulin-like growth factor, 128–129
    membrane junction changes, 131, 134f
    N-cadherin, 131
    phrin-A5, 129
    planar cell polarity, 129
  diffractive, 27
  dual feedback control system, 147f
  elongation and, 125–126, 127f
  embryonic, 126–127, 128f
    extracellular matrix, 127, 128f
    lens pit, 127, 128f
    lens placode, 127, 128f
    Pax6 transcription factor, 126
    primary fiber cells, 127
  epithelium, 50–52, 125
  equatorial diameter, presbyopia, 60
  fiber cells. See Lens fiber cells
  germinative zone, 125
  glutathione (GSH)
    delivery to nucleus, 144f
    maintenance, 141, 142f
    synthesis, 145
  gradient of refractive index, 124, 138–140, 138f
    α-crystallins, 139
    β/γ crystallins, 139
    membrane fusion, 140
  growth of, 124–129, 125f
  loss of ability. See Presbyopia
  mass, 149
  metabolic determinants, 140–142
    antioxidant defense systems, 141
    glucose metabolism, 140–141
    glutathione (GSH) levels maintenance, 141, 142f
    pentose phosphate pathway, 141
    UV protection, 142
  microcirculation system, 143, 143f
  nutrients, 143–146
    and anitioxidants delivery, 143–146
  optical changes, 53–54
  optical power, 38–39
    changes in emmetropization, 3
    gradient refractive index, 38–39
  ordered cellular architecture, 131, 132f
  physiological determinants, 142–151
  posterior surface curvature, 38–39
  presbyopia, 56, 56b, 151–152
  refraction, 124, 129–132
    lens nucleus, 149
    metabolic determinants, 140–142
    physiological determinants, 142–151
  regional differences, 131, 133t

Lens (Continued)
    extracellular diffusion barrier, 133
    fiber cell compaction, 133
    large gap junction, 133
    membrane fusions, 133
  role of, 7–8
  spherical aberrations, 21, 124, 125b, 125f
  stiffness. See Presbyopia
  structure, 19, 125f
    regional differences, 132–137
  tongue-and-groove interdigitations, 131–132, 134f
  transparency, 124, 129–132
    autophagy, 131
    metabolic determinants, 140–142
    nuclei and cellular organelles loss, 130–131
    organelle-free zone, 130–131
    physiological determinants, 142–151
    vasculature loss, 130
  UV protection, 142
  water content regulation, 146–149
    lens nucleus, 149, 150f
    lens power regulation, 149–150
    outer cortex, 147–149
    volume/pressure regulation, 148–149
Lens capsule, 39–40, 49–50
  accommodation, 49–50, 52f
  accommodative movements of, 64
  changes, 60
Lens crystallins
  α-crystallins, 138
    knockout mice, 139
  β/γ crystallins, 139
Lens fiber cells
  cytoskeletal protein changes, 135–137
    actin, 135
    cytoskeletal interactions, 136–137
    intermediate filaments, 135, 136f
    microtubules, 135–137
  differentiation
    glutamate transporters, 145, 146f
  regional differences
    biomechanics, 137–140, 137f
    lens transparency, 137–140, 137f
    optics, 137–140, 137f
Lens paradox, presbyopia, 61
Lens pit, 127, 128f
Lens placode, 126
Lens rim artifact, 695f
Lens transparency, lens fiber cells morphology, 137–140, 137f
Lenticular sclerosis, presbyopia, 62
Leptomeninges, optic nerve, 581
Lesser sphenoid wing, 348f
Levator aponeurosis, eyelids, 357f
Levator muscle, 350f, 357f
Levator palpebrae superioris muscle, 192f, 357–358
LGN. See Lateral geniculate nucleus (LGN)
Light absorption, 21
  RPE, 339
Light adaptation, 451–463
  calcium-dependent mechanisms, 458–460
    cGMP turnover, 458
    channel reactivation, 460
    guanylyl cyclase activation, 459–460, 459f
    negative feedback loop, 459, 459f
    shortened activated rhodopsin lifetime, 460

Light adaptation (Continued)
  cones, 437, 453
    electrical responses, 454, 455f, 457, 457f
    human models, 458f, 461
    molecular basis, 457t, 458f, 460
    saturation avoidance, 460–461
  dark adaptation vs., 451
  definition, 427, 451
  disrupted phototransduction shut-off, 461b
  electrical responses, 453–458, 453f
    acceleration of, 454, 455f, 456f
    cone recovery, 456–457, 457f
    desensitization, 454
    recovery, 455, 456f
    saturation in rods, 453–454, 454f
    sensitivity on background intensity, 455–456, 455f
    See also Weber's law
  molecular basis, 458–461.
    see also specific mechanisms
  pupil size, 536t
  purposes of, 451
  rods, 453, 453f
    dark adaptation vs., 462
    dominant time constant changes, 461
    electrical response saturation, 453–454, 454f
    protein translocation, 461–462
Light-adapted a-wave. See Electroretinograms, light-adapted, cone-driven
Light-adapted b-wave. See Electroretinograms, light-adapted, cone-driven
Light-adapted d-wave. See Electroretinograms, light-adapted, cone-driven
Light increments, visual fields, 676
Light intensity, pupil size, 536t
Light-near dissociation, 533b
Light oxygen consumption, retina, 326
Light refraction, cornea. See Corneal optical properties
Light response activation, dark-adapted rods. See Dark-adapted rods
Light scattering, 19
  corneal light transmission, 76–78, 79f
  natural defences, 19–20
Light transmission, cornea. See Corneal light transmission
Limbal plexus nerves, 379
Limbus, corneal reference points, 71
Linear correlation analysis, ocular circulation, 287–289, 288f
Line orientation receptor development, 5–6
Lipid(s)
  dark-adapted rod resting state, 421, 422f, 423f
  meibomian glands, 374–375, 375f
Lipid layer, tear film. See Tear film
Lipophilic drugs, corneal drug delivery, 104–105
LIP (Lateral intraparietal area), saccades, 223–224
Listing's law, 236–237
L/M cones, black-white circuitry, 671–673
Local electroretinograms, 506
Local interneurons, lateral geniculate nucleus inputs from, 601–602
Local stereopsis, spatial frequency, 761–762
Lockwood's ligament, 356–357, 357f
LogMAR
  minimum recognizable acuity, 650–651, 651t
  visual acuity, 10–22
Log Visual Acuity, 650–651

Long ciliary nerve, 192*f*, 379*f*
Long posterior ciliary arteries (LPCA), 116, 246*f*, 247*f*
Long-range horizontal connections, in V1, 619–620
Long-term depression (LTD), developmental visual deprivation, 759
Long-term potentiation (LTP), developmental visual deprivation, 759
Longitudinal chromatic aberration (LCA), 27, 54
Longitudinal fibers, ciliary muscle, 42–43
L opsin gene deletions, color vision defects, 668
Lower bar deflections, 683
Low spatial frequencies, peripheral vision contrast sensitivity, 662, 662*f*
LPCA (long posterior ciliary arteries), 116, 246*f*, 247*f*
LRAT (lecithin:retinol transferase), visual cycle, 341
LTN. *See* Lateral terminal nucleus (LTN)
L-type cone horizontal cells, 485–486
Lumican, corneal light transmission, 81–82
Luminance
    spatial form, early processing. *See* Spatial form, early processing
    temporal sensitivity, 727
    visual acuity. *See* Visual acuity
Luminance-pedestal, 728
Lumirhodopsin, 423
Lutein, photo-oxidative damage defense, 339
Lymphatics
    eyelids, 359
    orbit, 354
    sclera, 98*f*, 106
    scleral mechanical properties, 112–113, 114*f*–115*f*

M

M3 muscarinic receptors, ciliary muscle, 43
Magnetic resonance imaging (MRI)
    functional. *See* Functional magnetic resonance imaging (fMRI)
    presbyopia, 61, 62*f*
Magnification theory, peripheral vision contrast sensitivity, 661–662, 662*f*
Magnocellular system, temporal sensitivity measurement, 729
Major arterial circle, 246*f*, 247*f*
Major histocompatibility complex (MHC), 751
Mammals, accommodation, 37
MAR. *See* Minimum Angle of Resolution (MAR)
MAR (minutes of arc), 10, 12*t*
Matrix metalloproteinases (MMPs), 271
    tear film glycocalyx, 363
    transforming growth factor-β effects, 262
Maxilla, 348*f*
Maxillary bone, 189, 347, 349*f*
Maxillary temporal arteries, 353
M cells, LGN. *See* Lateral geniculate nucleus (LGN)
MCT1 (monocarbohydrate transporter 1), 340
MCT3 (monocarbohydrate transporter 3), 340
Mean deviation (MD), 682
Mechanical stretching studies, lens in presbyopia, 61, 62*f*
Mechanonociceptors, corneal sensory nerves, 387, 388*f*, 389*f*–390*f*

Medial canthal region, eyelid, 358
Medial palpebral arteries, 353*f*
Medial posterior ciliary arteries, 352
Medial rectus capsulopalpebral fascia, 358
Medial rectus muscles, 189–190, 350*f*
    anatomy, 191*f*, 192*f*
    horizontal eye movements, 190
    myofiber type, 190
Medial retinaculum, 358
Medial superior temporal area (MST), 634, 634*f*
Medial terminal nucleus (MTN), retinal projection targets, 573
Medial wall, orbit, 348
Meibomian glands
    anatomy, 364*f*
    diseases, 375*b*
    eyelid margin, 357
    hormonal regulation, 375
    lipid production, 374–375, 375*f*
    meibum, 374–375
    neural regulation, 375
    structure, 374–375
Meibum, 374–375
Melanin, photo-oxidative damage defense, 339
Melanopsin, 550–551
    discovery, 550
    gene therapy, 557*b*, 558*f*
    knockout mice, ipRGCs pupillary light reflex, 563
    signal transduction, 551–552
    visual cycle, 550–551
Melanopsin ganglion cells, pupil light reflex, 530, 530*b*
Membrane-associated mucins, 86–87, 91*f*
Membrane fusions
    gradient of refractive index, 140
    lens fiber cells, 133
Membrane junction changes, lens fiber cells, 131, 134*f*
Membrane potential
    dark-adapted rod resting state, 414–416
    flash photovoltage responses, 432
Membranes, rods, 414, 417*f*
Meninges, optic nerve development, 584
Meningothelial cells, optic nerve, 581
Merocrine, tear film, aqueous production, 370
MERRF (myoclonic epilepsy associated with ragged red fibers), 207–208
Mesopic vision, 452
Metabolic buffer function. *See* Vitreous body
Metabolic energy, 324
Metabolic pump function, corneal endothelium. *See* Corneal endothelium
Metabolism
    compartmentation, honeybee retina in vitro studies, 330*f*
    photoreceptor–Müller cell interaction. *see* Photoreceptor–Müller cell interaction
    scleral drug delivery, 118
Metabotropic glutamate receptors (mGluRs), 481
    differential expression, 470
    mGluR1, 470
    mGluR4, 470
    mGluR5, 470
    mGluR6, 465*b*, 481
    mGluR7, 470
    mGluR8, 470
    retinal synaptic organization, 470

"Metamodal" hypothesis, 781
Metarhodopsin I, 423
    catalytic activity, 424
    rhodopsin photoisomerization, 421–422
Methotrexate, scleral permeability, 117*t*
mGluRs. *See* Metabotropic glutamate receptors (mGluRs)
Microcirculation system, lens, 143, 143*f*
Microglia, 751
    optic nerve, 581
Microneuromas, corneal nerves, 84
Microplicae, lens fiber cells, 131–132, 134*f*
Microscopy, confocal, 76–78
Microsphere technology, ocular circulation measurement, 289
Microstrabismus, 709*b*
Microstructure, neuroanatomical development, 775–776
Microtubules
    aqueous humor drainage, 267
    lens fiber cells differentiation, 135–137
Midbrain
    pupil light reflex, 531
    tectal damage, relative afferent pupillary defect, 538*t*
Middle temporal area (MT), 634
    lesion studies, motion processing, 730
    motion neural encoding, 730
        lesion studies, 730
    strabismus, 763–764
Middle vision, visual processing hierarchy, 736
Middle-(M) wavelength sensitive cones, color vision, 668, 669*f*
Midface, 354–355
    definition, 354
    facial mimetic muscles, 355
    See also Superficial musculoaponeurotic system (SMAS)
Midget ganglion cells, 671
Midline glial RGC axon signaling, 748
Mimecan, corneal light transmission, 81–82
Minimal resolvable acuity, 649
Minimum Angle of Resolution (MAR), minimum recognizable acuity, 650–651, 651*t*
Minimum discriminable acuity. *See* Visual acuity
Minimum recognizable acuity. *See* Visual acuity
Minimum resolvable acuity. *See* Visual acuity
Minimum visual acuity. *See* Visual acuity
Minutes of arc (MAR), 10, 12*t*
Mitochondria, 427
    extraocular muscles, 197
Mitomycin C, topical, 111
Mitoxantrone-resistance protein (MRP). *See* Breast cancer resistance protein (BCRP)
Mixed rod-cone a-wave, 510*f*, 512, 513*f*
M layers (magnocellular), LGN layers and maps, 605
MMPs. *See* Matrix metalloproteinases (MMPs)
Modeling, dark-adapted a-wave, 511, 512*f*
Modified binary search (MOBS) procedure, 688–690
Modulation transfer function (MTF), 17, 31
    visual acuity, 652, 653*f*, 654*f*
Molecular genetics, color vision, 668–669
Molecular mechanisms, of eye-specific axonal territories, 748–749
Moll glands, eyelid margin, 356
Monocarbohydrate transporter 1 (MCT1), 340

Monocarbohydrate transporter 3 (MCT3), 340
Monochromatic aberrations, 28–30, 29*f*
Monocular consequences, 242, 243*f*
Monocular defocus, developmental visual deprivation, 761
Monovision, 708
  unwanted effect of, 708
Mood modulation, ipRGC central projections, 565
M opsin gene deletions, color vision defects, 668, 669*f*
Motion, 780
  apparent, 730
  behavior, 780
  directionally selective RGC, 475–477, 475*f*
  infant vision development. *See* Infant vision development
  neural responses, 780
  pupil size, 536*t*
  retinal synaptic organization, 475–477
Motion adaptation, 730
Motion aftereffects, 730
Motion-in-depth, binocular vision. *See* Binocular vision
Motion perception, 634–635
Motion perimetry, 688*b*
Motion processing, 730
  clinical applications, 731
  MT lesion studies, 730–731
  neural encoding, 730–731
  perceptual evidence, 730
  psychophysical evidence, 730
  superior temporal cortical region lesions, 731
Motion recognition, development, 6
Motoneuron innervations, eye movements neural control, 212–215, 213*f*
Motoneurons, eye movements, 238–239, 239*f*
Motor innervation, orbit, 351–352, 352*f*
Motor neurons, eye movements, 213, 214*f*
Motor nuclei, eye movements. *See* Eye movements, neural control
Motor planning, LGN. *See* Lateral geniculate nucleus (LGN)
Moxifloxacin, 544
M pathways, contrast sensitivity. *See* Contrast sensitivity
MRI. *See* Magnetic resonance imaging (MRI)
MRP. *See* Breast cancer resistance protein (BCRP); Multidrug resistance associated protein (MRP)
MRP1, 408
MRP2. *See* Multidrug resistance associated protein (MRP)
MRP5, 408
MRP6, 411*b*
MRPs. *See* Multidrug resistance-associated proteins (MRPs)
MT. *See* Middle temporal area (MT)
MTF. *See* Modulation transfer function (MTF)
MTN. *See* Medial terminal nucleus (MTN)
Mucin(s)
  gel-forming, corneal epithelium, 86–87
  membrane-associated, 86–87, 91*f*
  membrane-spanning, 363, 365*f*
  secreted, 365*f*
  tear film glycocalyx, 363, 364*f*
Mucin MUC1
  dry eye disease, 366
  tear film, 363

Mucin MUC5AC, tear film, mucous production, 366
Mucin MUC4, tear film, 363
Mucin MUC16, tear film, 363
Mucous layer, tear film. *See* Tear film, mucous layer
Müller glial cells, 328–330, 461
  distribution, 326
  electroretinogram glial currents, 508
  functions in inner retina, 325*f*
  GABA, 330
  glucose transport, 329–330
  glutamate, 330
  glycine, 330
  lactate release, 330, 330*f*
  morphology, 329–330, 329*f*
  photoreceptor interactions. *see* Photoreceptor–Müller cell interaction
Multidrug resistance associated protein (MRP)
  BRB, 410
  MRP3, 408
  MRP5, 408
Multidrug resistance-associated proteins (MRPs), 405
Multifocal electroretinograms. *See* Electroretinogram(s) (ERGs)
Multifocal electroretinography (MERG), 688*b*
Multifocal pupillographic objective perimetry, 539
Multifocal visual evoked potentials (MVEP), 688*b*
Multipolar neurons, 464–465
Munk, Hermann, 612
Muscarinic receptor(s)
  antagonists, accommodation, 54–55
  aqueous humor drainage, 263
  conjunctival goblet cells, 366
Muscle groups, ciliary muscle, 42–43
Muscle spindles, extraocular muscles, 200, 201*f*
Muscular arteries, 353*f*
Muscular dystrophies, extraocular muscle sparing, 205
Myasthenia gravis
  extraocular muscles, 208
  treatment, 208*b*
Mydriasis
  angle-closure glaucoma, 545
  anticholinergic, 544–545
  causes, 544–545
  copper, 540*t*
  pharmacologic, anisocoria, 540*t*
Myelination
  oligodendrocytes, 583–584
  optic nerve, 580–581, 582*f*
  of posterior tracts, 775
  vision development, 4, 4*f*
myf5
  extraocular muscle development, 202–203
Myocilin, aqueous humor drainage, 268
Myoclonic epilepsy associated with ragged red fibers (MERRF), 207–208
MyoD, extraocular muscle development, 202–203
Myofiber type, medial rectus muscles, 190
Myogenic mechanisms
  defined, 296
  ocular circulation regulation, 296
Myo-inositol, 776
Myonuclear addition, 199–200
Myopia, 24
  atropine use, 1
  characteristics, 37–38

Myopia (*Continued*)
  correction, 654
  development, 24
  elongated eyes, 1
  mechanism, 27, 29*f*
  pathologic, 24
  prevalence, 24
  sclera development, 108

N

Na$^+$/Ca^{2+}-K$^+$ (sodium-potassium-calcium) exchanger protein 1 (NCKX1), 440–441
N-acetyl-D-glucosamine, 164
Na$^+$/H$^+$ exchanger. *See* Sodium-proton (Na$^+$/H$^+$) exchanger
Na$^+$/K$^+$-ATPase. *See* Sodium-potassium-ATPase (Na$^+$/K$^+$-ATPase)
Na, K-ATPase transport, in aqueous humor, 249
Na$^+$-K$^+$-2Cl$^-$ symporter. *See* Sodium-potassium-chloride (Na$^+$-K$^+$-2Cl$^-$) symporter (NKCCl)
Na$^+$/K$^+$ pumps, 143
Narcotic tolerance, pupil, 527–528
Nasal bone, 348*f*
Nasal field, pupil light reflex, 531
Nasal hemianopia, 573–574, 575*f*
Nasal retina, LGN layers and maps, 598
Nasal steps, 684
Nasal visual field, 676
Nasociliary nerve, 349, 350*f*, 378–379, 379*f*
NCKX1 (Na$^+$/Ca^{2+}-K$^+$/sodium-potassium-calcium exchanger protein 1), 440–441
NCKX2. *See* Sodium-potassium-calcium (Na$^+$/Ca^{2+}-K$^+$) exchanger protein 2 (NCKX2)
N290 component, 744
Near pupil response. *See* Pupil light reflex
Negative electroretinogram, dark-adapted a-wave, 510–511
Negative feedback loop, light adaptation, 459, 459*f*
Negative scotopic threshold response (nSTR), 508
Neovascularization, VEGF, 335, 343
Nerve fiber layer, optic nerve, 578, 579*b*, 579*f*
Nerve fiber separation
  perimetry, 676
  visual fields, 676
Nerve growth factor (NGF), 84–86
N-ethylmaleimide (NEM), 154
Neural activity
  development, 4, 4*f*
  meibomian glands, 375
  motion processing, 730–731
Neural control
  retinal vasodilator, 305–306, 306*f*
  three-dimensional eye movements, 240*f*
Neural density filters, relative afferent pupillary defect, 537–538
Neural responses, 779
Neurite extension inhibition, axon regeneration failure, 590
Neuroanatomical development, 775–778, 778*f*
  gray matter and neuronal tuning, 777–778
  neurochemistry and microstructure, 775–776
  white matter pathways, 775
Neurochemistry
  LGN. *See* Lateral geniculate nucleus (LGN)
  neuroanatomical development, 775–776

Neuroenhancement, optic nerve repair, 591
Neurogenic inflammation, 378
Neuro-glial activity, retinal vasculature. See Retinal vasculature
Neuromodulators
  developmental visual deprivation, 761
  inner plexiform layer signal processing. see Signal processing, inner plexiform layer
Neuromuscular junctions (NMJs), extraocular muscles, 193, 194f
Neuronal pentraxins (NPs), 751
Neuronal recycling, 781
Neuronal tuning, 777–778
Neuron–glial cell interaction, 324–338
  electrophysiology, 325–326
  energy substrate compartmentalization, 331–332
    endogenous lactate, 331
    glial (astrocyte)- neuron–lactate shuttle hypothesis, 332
    high-resolution light microscopic autoradiography, 329f, 331–332
    isolated cell models, 330f, 331–332
  functional neuronal activity, 330–331
  glycogen, 330
  intracellular calcium, 324
  metabolism division, 330–331, 331f
  retinal whole-mount studies, 324
  See also Glial cells; Retina
Neuron-intrinsic limitations, axon regeneration failure, 590–591
Neurons in primary visual cortex, 638
Neurons/nerves
  color vision, 670–671
  injury, sensory innervation. See Sensory innervation (of eye)
  orbit. See Orbit
  sclera, 88f, 106
Neuropeptides
  eye sensory innervation, 393, 393b
  retinal synaptic organization, 471
  trigeminal ganglion neurons, 378
Neuroprotection, optic nerve repair, 591
Neurotransmitters
  light response activation, 424
  optic nerve vasculature, 583
  see also specific neurotransmitters
Neurotrophic keratitis, 392–393
Neurovascular coupling, 300–303, 301f
  flicker stimulation, 300, 301f, 304f
NGF (nerve growth factor), 84–86
Night blindness, 428
  defective rod synapses, 446b
  rhodopsin mutations, 420
Night vision
  circuit, 498–499, 499f
  spherical aberration impact on, 32
Nitric oxide
  aqueous humor drainage, 271
  endothelium-derived retinal vasodilator, 303, 304f
  retina, 334
    blood flow, 335
    extracellular lactate, 335
    local factors, 335
    vascular endothelial growth factor, 335
  retinal synaptic organization, 471
  retinal vasodilator, 302–303

Nitric oxide synthase (NOS), 334–335
  aqueous humor drainage, 259–260, 261f, 271
  endothelium-derived retinal vasodilator, 303
  ocular circulation regulation, 299–300, 300f
  retinal vasodilator, 303.
  see also specific types
NKCC1 (Sodium-potassium-chloride cotransporter) activity, 146–147
NKCCl. See Sodium-potassium-chloride (Na+-K+-2Cl−) symporter (NKCCl)
NMDA receptors agonist studies, scotopic threshold response, 514
N-methyl-D-aspartate (NMDA), 775
NMJs (neuromuscular junctions), extraocular muscles, 193, 194f
nob1 mice
  flicker ERG, 519
  negative ERG, 511
Nodal point, 2, 3f
Non-collagenous structural proteins, 166–167
  fibrillins, 166
  fibulins, 166
  opticin, 167
  versican, 166
Nonfixated objects lying, diplopia of, 703
Non-invasive techniques
  electroretinograms. See Electroretinogram(s) (ERGs)
Nonmammalian photoreceptor ribbon synapses, 468, 468f
Nonstrabismic binocular anomalies, 717
Norepinephrine, aqueous humor drainage, 264
Normal binocular vision, 701
Normal retinal correspondence, binocular vision. See Binocular vision
NOS-3. See Endothelial nitric oxide synthase (eNOS/NOS-3)
Notations, minimum recognizable acuity, 651t
Novel cells, 465–466
nSTR (negative scotopic threshold response), 508
Nuclear cataract, 154–156, 155f
Nuclei loss, lens transparency, 130–131
Nutrients, corneal endothelium, 92
Nutrients delivery, lens core, 143–146
Nyctalopin (NYX), 481
Nyquist limit, 650f, 654–656, 655f
Nystagmus, 205, 232, 232b
  definition, 205
  optokinetic. See Optokinetic nystagmus (OKN)
  surgery, 205b

O

OA. See Ophthalmic artery (OA)
Object boundaries, spatial form, 638
Object-level processing, infant vision development, 743–745, 744f
Object motion sensitivity circuit, 499, 500f
Object recognition, visual processing hierarchy, 735–736
OCTA. See Optical coherence tomography angiography (OCTA)
OCT angiography, ocular blood flow measurement, 292–294, 293f, 294f
Ocular blood flow measurement
  invasive technology, 289
    hydrogen clearance, 289

Ocular blood flow measurement (Continued)
  microsphere technology, 289
  oxygen-sensitive electrodes, 289
  noninvasive technology, 289–295
    color Doppler imaging, 290–291, 290f
    Doppler OCT, 292, 292f, 293f
    dye-based angiography, 289
    laser Doppler flowmetry, 290
    laser Doppler velocimetry, 290
    laser speckle flowgraphy, 291–292, 291f
    OCTA, 292–294, 293f, 294f
    retinal vessel diameter, 289–290, 289f
    spectroscopic oximetry, 294–295, 294f
Ocular circulation, 284–323
  age-related macular degeneration, 310–311, 310f, 311f
  anatomy, 286f
  blood-retinal barrier, 287f
  in disease, 306–308
    diabetes mellitus, 308–310, 309f
    diabetic retinopathy, 308–310, 309f, 310f
    glaucoma, 306–308, 307f, 308f.
    see also specific diseases
  linear correlation analysis, 287–289, 288f
  regulation, 295–313, 295f
    autoregulation, 296–300, 297f
    choroidal pressure-flow relationship, 296, 298f
    IOP, 299, 300f
    metabolic control, 295–296, 295f
    neurovascular coupling, 300–303, 301f
    NO synthase inhibition, 299–300, 300f
    ONH pressure-flow relationship, 299–300, 301f
    retinal blood flow, 296, 298f
  retinal blood flow, 285–289, 288f
  retinal oxygenation, 285–289, 288f
  systemic disease, 311–313, 312f, 313f
  vascular system, 284–285
    capillary plexus, 285f
    optical coherence tomography angiography (OCTA), 284, 285f
  Zinn-Haller ring, 287f.
  see also specific vessels
Ocular counterroll, Listing's law, 237
Ocular dominance, 616
  bands, 616
  constant monocular form deprivation, 755–756
  intermittent monocular form deprivation, 757
  plasticity, 755–756
    primary visual cortex, 622, 622f
Ocular following movements, 735
Ocular kinematics, 3D, 236
Ocular noniceptive nerve fibers, 394b
Ocular pain. See Pain
Ocular perfusion defect, 311, 313f
Ocular Response Analyzer (ORA), 112b
Ocular surface sensitivity testing, 395–396
  Belmonte esthesiometer, 396
  Cochet–Bonnet esthesiometer, 395
  von Frey filaments, 395
Oculocentric directions, 702–703
Oculomotor imbalance, 706b
Oculomotor nerve (cranial nerve III)
  aberrant regeneration, 546, 546f
  anatomy, 379f
  congenital cranial dysinnervation disorders, 205
  extraocular muscle innervation, 54
  eyelids, 359
  eye movements, 213

Oculomotor nerve (cranial nerve III) *(Continued)*
  orbit, 351, 352*f*
  orbital apex, 349
  palsy
    anisocoria, 540*t*, 543–544
    pupil involvement, 532*b*, 546
  route of, 193
Oculomotor plant, eye movements, 215, 215*f*
Oculomotor system, neurologic disorders,
    229–232, 229*b*
  gaze disorder, 230–231, 230*b*, 230*f*
  nystagmus, 232, 232*b*
  saccade disorder, 231–232, 231*b*, 231*f*
  strabismus, 229–230
OFF bipolar cells, 480
OFF-center midget retinal ganglion cells, blue-
    yellow circuitry, 671
OFZ (Organelle-free zone), lens transparency,
    130–131
Oguchi disease
  arrestin mutations, 437*b*
  rhodopsin mutations, 437*b*
OKN. *See* Optokinetic nystagmus (OKN)
Oligodendrocyte precursor cells (OPCs), 583
Oligodendrocytes
  development, 583–584
    myelination, 583–584
  optic nerve, 580–581, 582*f*
    axonal conduction, 586
    development, 583–584
OMAG. *See* Optical microangiography (OMAG)
Omnipause neurons, saccadic eye movement, 220
ON bipolar cells, 480
  ipRGC synaptic input, 558, 559*f*
ON-center midget retinal ganglion cells, blue-
    yellow circuitry, 671
Opacified posterior capsules, glare and contrast
    sensitivity, 16*f*, 17
Opaqueness, definition, 15
Ophthalmic artery (OA), 284, 350*f*, 353*f*
  orbit, 352
  route of, 192–193
Ophthalmic nerve, 352
Ophthalmoplegic migraine, 546
OPN1LW, 669*b*
OPN1MW, 669*b*
OPN1SW, 669*b*
Opsins
  cones, 669*b*
  rhodopsin phosphorylation, 426
Optical aberrations, 18–20, 27–31
  chromatic aberrations, 27, 28*f*
  monochromatic aberrations, 28–30, 29*f*
  representations of, 30–31.
  see also specific aberrations
Optical coherence tomography angiography
    (OCTA), 284, 285*f*, 313*f*
Optical defocus, on stereoacuity, 708
Optical microangiography (OMAG), 292–293
Optical nerve head (ONH), 284
  ocular circulation regulation, 296–299, 299*f*
Optical quality, standard metrics of, 30–31
Optical quality of the eye. *See* Visual acuity
Optic artery, 192*f*
Optic canal, blood supply, 583
Optic chiasm, 748
  blood supply, 583
  optic nerve, 579

Optic chiasm *(Continued)*
  temporal retina RGC axons, 579
  visual field lesions, 573, 575*f*
Optic disc
  effects, vitreous body, 180
  intrascleral optic nerve, 578, 579*f*
  structure, 125*f*
Optic foramen, 192–193
  orbit, 190
  orbital apex, 349
Opticin, 167
Optic nerve (cranial nerve II), 350*f*, 578–597, 676
  anatomy, 192*f*, 578–580
    intraorbital, 578, 579*f*
    intrascleral, 578, 580*f*
    optic chiasm, 579
    optic tract, 579
    RGC axons, 578, 579*b*, 579*f*
  axonal conduction, 585–586
    action potentials, 585–586
    astrocytes, 586
    oligodendrocytes, 586
  axonal transport, 586
  axon counts, 580
  axon dimensions, 580
  axons, 580
  blood supply, 581–583
    intracranial optic nerve, 583
    intraorbital optic nerve, 582–583
    optic canal, 582–583
    optic chiasm, 583
    optic nerve head, 581–582, 583*f*
    optic tract, 583
    vascular biology, 583
  development, 583–585
    astrocytes, 584
    axon growth, 584
    axon guidance, 584–585
    axon number, 584
    meninges, 584
    oligodendrocytes, 583–584
  diameter, 580
  electrophysiology, 585
    axonal conduction. *see above*
  glioma, 581
  injury. *See* Optic nerve injury
  intracranial. *See* Intracranial optic nerve
  intraorbital. *See* Intraorbital optic nerve
  microscopic anatomy/cytology, 580–581
    astrocytes, 581
    axons, 580
    meninges, 581
    meningothelial cells, 581
    microglia, 581
    myelin, 580–581, 582*f*
    oligodendrocytes, 580–581, 582*f*
  oligodendrocytes. *See* Oligodendrocytes
  orbit, 351
  physiology, 585–586
  repair. *See* Optic nerve repair
  structure, 125*f*
  synaptic transmission, 585
Optic nerve head, blood supply, 581–582, 583*f*
Optic nerve injury, 586–591
  astrogliosis, 590
  axon regeneration failure, 590–591
    neurite extension inhibition, 590
    neuron-intrinsic limitations, 590–591

Optic nerve injury *(Continued)*
  clinical implications, 586
  compressive optic neuropathy, 587
  glaucoma, 587–588, 588*f*
  immune activation, 589–590
  ischemic optic neuropathy, 587
  papilledema, 588
  phagocytosis, 589–590
  RGC death
    apoptosis, 588–589
    axonal injury signaling, 589
    time course, 589
  traumatic optic neuropathy, 586–587
  types, 586–588.
  see also specific types
Optic nerve repair, 591
  neuroenhancement, 591
  neuroprotection, 591
  remyelination, 591
  RGC axon regeneration, 591
  RGC survival, 591
Optic neuritis, 645
  animal models, 587
  relative afferent pupillary defect, 538*t*
Optic neuropathy
  compressive. *See* Compressive optic neuropathy
  ischemic. *See* Ischemic optic neuropathy
  traumatic, 586–587
Optics, lens fiber cells morphology, 137–140, 137*f*
Optics of the eye, 1–26, 38–39
  development, 1–6
  focusing, 39
  pupil, 529*b*
Optic tract
  blood supply, 583
  lesions, relative afferent pupillary defect, 538*t*
  optic nerve, 579
Optimized ablation, 33
Optokinetic nystagmus (OKN), 735
  AOS, 573
  motion detection development, 740
  ocular following movements, 735
  visual acuity testing, 664
Optokinetic reflex (VOR), 224–227
  neural control, 225–227, 227*f*
Optokinetic reflex (OKR) eye movements, 212
Ora sclerata, 41*f*
Orbicularis muscle, 356–357
Orbit, 190, 190*f*
  anatomy, 347–354
  connective tissue, extraocular muscles, 193,
      195*f*, 196*f*, 207*t*
  fat tissue, 351
  geometry of, 189, 190*f*
  lymphatic drainage, 354
  nerves, 351–352
    abducens nerve, 351–352, 352*f*
    motor innervation, 351–352, 352*f*
    oculomotor nerve, 351–352, 352*f*
    ophthalmic nerve, 352
    optic nerve, 351
    parasympathetic fibers, 352
    sympathetic fibers, 352
    trigeminal nerve, 351
    trochlear nerve, 352, 352*f*
  orbital apex, 349, 350*b*, 350*f*
    abducens nerve, 349
    inferior orbital fissure, 349

Orbit *(Continued)*
  nasociliary nerve, 349
  oculomotor nerve, 349
  optic foramen, 349
  superior orbital fissure, 349
  osteology, 347–349, 348f
    bones, 347
    frontal sinus, 347
    inferomedial strut, 349
    lacrimal sac fossa, 349, 349f
    lateral wall, 348
    medial wall, 348
    orbital floor, 348
    orbital rim, 347, 348f
    orbital roof, 347
  periorbital fascia, 349–351
    Tenon's capsule, 350–351, 351f
  soft tissues, 349–352.
    see also specific tissues
  vasculature, 352–354
    arterial supply, 352–353, 353f
    venous drainage, 353–354
Orbital apex. *See* Orbit
Orbital floor, 348
Orbital rim, 347, 348f
Orbital roof, 347
Ordinary least squares (OLS) linear regression, 687
Organelle-free zone (OFZ), lens transparency, 130–131
Organic molecules, active transport, 251
Orientation selectivity, 615–616
  circuit, 500, 502f
Orthodenticle homeobox 2 (Otx2), 775
Oscillatory potentials. *See* Electroretinograms, light-adapted, cone-driven
Outer blood–retina barrier. *See* Blood–retina barrier (BRB)
Outer cortex, water content regulation, 147–149
Outer retina, 326
Outflow obstruction, aqueous humor drainage. *See* Aqueous humor drainage; Glaucoma
Output pathways
  blue-yellow circuitry, 671
  primary visual cortex. *See* Primary visual cortex (V1)
Outward-directed transport, 405–413
  corneal, 408–409, 408f
  future aspects, 412
  genetic variation and ocular diseases, 411, 411t
  pharmacology, 411–412, 411b
  tissue eye barriers, 405, 406f
  See also Efflux transporters. *specific transporters*
Oxidative Stress Response Kinase 1 (OXSR1), 147–148
OXSR1 (Oxidative Stress Response Kinase 1), 147–148
Oxygenation, retina, 285–289, 288f
Oxygen consumption (QO$_2$)
  retina. *See* Retina
  RPE, 326
Oxygen-sensitive electrodes, 289
Oxygen transport, vitreous body, 182

P

PACAP. *See* Pituitary adenylate cyclase-activating peptide (PACAP)
PAI-1(plasminogen activator inhibitor), 262

Pain, 396
  definition, 378
Paired frontalis muscles, 354
Palatine bone, 347, 348f
Palisade endings, extraocular muscles, 201, 202f
Palpebral conjunctiva, 357
Panum's fusional area (PFA), 705, 706b
Parallel feedback streams, from V2 to V1, 621–622
Paralleling immune system phagocytes, 751
Parallel inputs/outputs, primary visual cortex. *See* Primary visual cortex (V1)
Parallel input streams, V1, 620–621
Parallel output streams, V1, 620–621
Parallel pathways from V1, 620, 621f
Parallel retinal ganglion cell output pathways. *see* Signal processing, inner plexiform layer
Parallel streams
  within V1, 614–615, 614f
  from V1 to V2, 620, 621f
Paramedian pontine reticular formation (PPRF), 241
  saccadic eye movements, 217–218
Parasympathetic and sympathetic innervation, 252f
Parasympathetic nervous system
  conjunctival goblet cells, 366
  lacrimal glands, 370, 370f
  orbit, 351–352
Paraventricular nucleus, retinal projection targets, 573
Paraxial mesoderm, extraocular muscle development, 201–202
Paraxial vergence calculations, 53–54
Pars plana, 40–41
Pars plicata, 40–41
Parvalbumin (PV)-containing interneurons, 775
Parvalbumin-expressing (PV) interneurons, 615
Parvocellular retinal ganglion cells, 727
Passive diffusion, scleral drug delivery, 117–118
Patch-clamp analysis, dry eye, 367
Patching regimens, amblyopia, 757
Pathologic myopia, 24
Pattern Deviation plot, 683
Pattern electroretinograms (PERG). *See* Electroretinograms, light-adapted, cone-driven
Pattern onset-offset stimuli, grating acuity development, 738
PAX7 cells, 199–200
Pax3 transcription factor, extraocular muscle development, 201–202
Pax6 transcription factor, lens development, 127, 128f
PCAs (posterior ciliary arteries), 284, 352
P cells. *See* Lateral geniculate nucleus (LGN)
PCIOL (posterior chamber intraocular lens), 74
PDA-sensitive postreceptoral neurons, light-adapted a-wave, 517, 518f
PDE6
  activation, light response activation, 424
  dark-adapted rod resting state, 417–418
  guanine nucleotide turnover, 427
  inactivation, dark-adapted rod recovery phase, 426
  subunits, rods *vs.* cones, 428
Peak-contrast sensitivity, spatio-temporal vision development, 737, 737f
PEDF (pigment epithelium derived factor), 182

Pelli–Robson CS chart, 664, 664f
Penetrating keratoplasty, 16
Penicillin G, scleral permeability, 117t
Pentose phosphate pathway, retinal glycolysis, 328
Perceived depth, 709–710, 710f
Perceived distance, subclasses of anomalous correspondence and errors, 717
Perceived visual direction, 702f
Perception of static stimuli, 633
Perception of visual motion, 634
Perceptual constancy, 709–710, 710f
Perceptual deficits
  amblyopia, 767
  strabismus, 762
Perceptual evidence, motion processing, 730
Perceptual learning, 769
Perfusion pressure calculation, ocular circulation regulation, 296
PERG (pattern electroretinograms). *See* Electroretinograms, light-adapted, cone-driven
Peribulbar injections, scleral drug delivery, 109f, 116–117
Perimeter bowl
  blurred image of, 692
  surface of, 692
Perimetric location, pupil size, 536t
Perimetry
  advantages of, 676
  forms of, 677–680
    kinetic perimetry, 677–678
    static perimetry, 677
    suprathreshold static perimetry, 678–680, 680f
    frequency-doubling technology, 678–679, 688–691, 691f
  kinetic. *See* Kinetic perimetry
  physiologic basis for, 676
  psychophysical basis for, 675–676
  short wavelength automated. *See* Short wavelength automated perimetry (SWAP)
  static. *See* Static perimetry
  suprathreshold static. *See* Suprathreshold static perimetry
Periodic stimuli, temporal sensitivity to, 723–730
Periorbital fascia. *See* Orbit
Peripheral fundus, 178–179
  and vitreous base, 171
Peripheral ganglion cells
  eyelids, 359
  optic nerve axons, 578, 579f
Peripheral optical zone, corneal reference points, 71
Peripheral vision, contrast sensitivity. *See* Contrast sensitivity
Peripheral window of visibility, spatial form, early processing. *See* Spatial form, early processing
Permanent suppression, 707
Persistent fetal vasculature (PFV) syndrome, 176–177
PFA. *See* Panum's fusional area (PFA)
PFV (Persistent fetal vasculature) syndrome, 176–177
P-glycoprotein (P-gp), 405
  BRB, 409–410
  cornea, 408
  rabbit cornea, 408

P-gp. *See* P-glycoprotein (P-gp)
Phacoemulsification, 152
Phacolytic glaucoma, 262
Phagocytosis, optic nerve injury, 589–590
Phalloidin, aqueous humor drainage, 264
Pharmacologic ablation of stage II waves, 750*f*
Pharmacologically selective actuator module-
    glycine receptors (PSAM-GlyR), 486
Pharmacologic mydriasis, anisocoria, 540*t*
Pharmacology
    accommodation stimulus, 54–55
    corneal endothelial cell injury, 99*t*, 111–112
    eye sensory innervation. *See* Sensory
        innervation (of eye)
Phospholipase Cβ, aqueous tear film layer
    secretion, 370
Phosphorylation, rhodopsin. *See* Rhodopsin
Photic modulation of the pineal, ipRGC central
    projections, 563–564
Photoisomerization, rhodopsin. *See* Rhodopsin
Photo-oxidative damage, RPE, 339
Photopic negative response (PhNR). *See*
    Electroretinograms, light-adapted, cone-
    driven
Photopic vision, 452
    cones, 452
    scotopic vision *vs.*, 452, 453*f*
Photopigments, 669
    gene designations, 669*b*
    regeneration, cones, 437
Photoreceptor(s), 676
    action spectra, 437
    CNG channel. *See* Cyclic nucleotide gated
        (CNG) channels
    development, 3–4
    extracellular ATP, 324
    flash photocurrent responses, 432–433
        cyclic nucleotide gated channels, 432
        dark (circulating) current, 434*f*
        duration of, 433, 435*f*
        flash strength effects, 433, 435*f*
    flash photovoltage responses, 432
        graded hyperpolarizations, 432, 433*f*, 434*f*
        membrane potentials, 432
    fovea, 9
    hyperactive signaling diseases/disorders, 437*b*.
        see also specific diseases/disorders
    mammalian, 465
    Na⁺/K⁺, Ca²⁺ exchanger protein. *see specific*
        receptors
    outer retinal signal processing. *See* Signal
        processing, outer retina
    oxygen consumption
        in dark, 326
        in light, 326
    photoresponses, 432–450
    pupil light reflex, 528–529
    ribbon synapses. *See* Retinal synaptic
        organization
    sensory neuroepithelium, 464
    single photon detection, 434–435
        darkness, 434
        response constancy, 434, 434*f*
        rhodopsin limitations, 437
    size and spacing, 9–10
        visual acuity, 654–656, 655*f*
    steady light photocurrent responses, 437, 438*f*
    See also Cones; Rod(s)

Photoreceptor outer segment (POS), phagocytosis,
    342–343
    reactive oxygen species, 342
    receptors, 342, 343*f*
Photorefractive keratectomy (PRK), 97
    corneal stromal wound healing, 89*f*, 105
Phototransduction, 414–431, 458, 458*f*, 551–552
    cytoplasmic calcium, 458
    dark-adapted rods. *See* Dark-adapted rods
    definition, 414
    diseases/disorders, 428.
        see also specific diseases/disorders
    Drosophila, 551
    guanylyl cyclase activating proteins, 458
    ipRGCs, 551–552, 553*f*
    rods *vs.* cones, 428
        absorption spectra, 428, 428*f*
        G-protein subunits, 428
        molecules, 428
        PDE6 subunits, 428
        phototransduction molecules, 428
        physiology, 428
Physiological barriers, corneal drug delivery, 104–105
Physiologic anisocoria, 540*t*
Piercing, corneal stress, 100
Pigmented and nonpigmented epithelium
    coordination, 250
Pigment epithelium derived factor(PEDF), 182
Pigment function, retina, 19
PII, dark-adapted b -wave, 514, 516*f*
PIII, slow. *See* Slow PIII
Pilocarpine
    accommodation, 54–55
    aqueous humor drainage, 263
    iris response, 543–544, 544*f*
Pinwheel-like organization, 616
Pitch, 779–780
    behavior, 779, 779*f*
    neural responses, 779–780
Pituitary adenylate cyclase-activating peptide
    (PACAP)
    aqueous humor regulation, 251–252
Pitx2 transcription factor, 202
    extraocular muscle development, 202
Pitx3 transcription factor, extraocular muscle
    development, 203*f*–204*f*
Placenta-specific ABC protein. *See* Breast cancer
    resistance protein (BCRP)
Plasmin, aqueous humor drainage, 269
Plasminogen activator inhibitor (PAI-1), 262
Plasticity and rehabilitation, extrastriate visual
    cortex, 635
    cortical blindness, 635
    prospects for vision rehabilitation, 635
P layers (parvocellular), LGN layers and maps,
    605, 606*f*
PLK (posterior lamellar keratoplasty), 111
POAG. *See* Primary open-angle glaucoma (POAG)
Point spread function (PSF), 31, 31*f*
Polarity, retinal synaptic organization, 472
Polychromatic image quality, 27
Polymodal nociceptors, corneal sensory nerves,
    387–391, 388*f*, 389*f*–390*f*
Polymyxin B, scleral permeability, 117*t*
Polynomials, Zernike, 30, 30*f*
Polysialic acid on neural cell adhesion molecule
    (PSA-NCAM), 775
Population receptive field (pRF), 642, 643*f*

Position judgements, minimum discriminable
    acuity, 652
Position-vestibular pause (PVP) neurons, 224
Posterior capsule opacification (PCO), 153*b*, 153*f*
Posterior chamber intraocular lens (PCIOL), 74
Posterior ciliary arteries (PCAs), 284, 352
Posterior cortex, vitreous body, 167–168
Posterior draining-dural cavernous fistulae, 546
Posterior ethmoidal arteries, 353, 353*f*
Posterior lamella, 356–357
Posterior lamellar keratoplasty (PLK), 111
Posterior scleral foramen, 110–112
Posterior segment pharmacotherapy, 181–182
Posterior surface curvature, lens, 37–38
Posterior vitreous detachment (PVD), 179–180
Postganglionic ciliary nerves, accommodation
    stimulus, 54
Post-ganglionic parasympathetic nerves, 363
Postgeniculate damage, relative afferent pupillary
    defect, 538*t*
Postillumination pupil response (PIPR), 530
Post-natal growth, sclera development, 108
Post-translational modifications, rhodopsin, 420,
    420*f*
Potassium channels
    calcium-activated, tear film, 373
    dark-adapted rod resting state, 414–416
    tear film, aqueous production, 373
Potassium–chloride symporter (KCCl), 373
Potassium ions
    extracellular, electroretinogram glial currents, 508
    lacrimal gland fluid composition, 373–374
    RPE, 340–341
P pathways, contrast sensitivity. *See* Contrast
    sensitivity
PPRF. *See* Paramedian pontine reticular formation
    (PPRF)
PPRF (Paramedian pontine reticular formation), 241
P2 receptors, 373
Prechordal mesoderm, extraocular muscle
    development, 201–202
Preferential looking (PL)
    infant vision development, 735
    visual acuity testing, 664
Premotor neurons, eye movements, 213, 214*f*
Premotor saccadic neurons, 220
Prenyl-binding protein, 421
Presbyopes, 708
Presbyopia, 24, 56, 56*b*, 706
    age-related changes, 55.
        see also specific changes
    ciliary muscle changes
        accommodative movements, 58, 60*f*
        capsule, 60
        human, 57–58, 59*f*
        rhesus model, 56–57, 57*f*, 58*f*, 59*f*
    contributing factors, 56–65.
        see also specific factors
    definition, 37, 56
    development, 151–152
    lens capsule changes, 60
    lens elastic modulus, 61
    lens growth, 60–61
        equatorial diameter, 60
        lens paradox, 61
        refractive power, 61
    lens loss of ability, 61
        deformability decline, 61

Presbyopia *(Continued)*
elastic modulus, 61
magnetic resonance imaging, 61, 62*f*
mechanical stretching studies, 61, 62*f*
lens stiffness, 61–62, 63*f*
compliance loss, 62
lenticular sclerosis, 62
progression of, 38*f*
tension spikes, 64–65
zonule changes, 58–60
centripetal pulling, 58–60
Pressure regulation, lens, 148–149, 148*f*
Pretectum neurons, pupil light reflex, 531
Pretectum, retinal projection targets, 571
pRF. *See* Population receptive field (pRF)
Primary creep, corneal stiffness, 101
Primary fiber cells, lens development, 127
Primary open-angle glaucoma (POAG)
aqueous outflow obstruction, 262
extracellular matrix, 262
photopic negative response, 522
Primary visual cortex (V1), 612–626
attention, 622
black-white circuitry, 671–673
constant monocular form deprivation, 755–756
critical period, 622
interlaminar circuitry and cell types, 614–615
cortical circuit, 615
feedforward pathways, 614, 614*f*
intralaminar and feedback pathways, 614, 614*f*
parallel streams, 614–615, 614*f*
ocular dominance plasticity, 622, 622*f*
orientation and spatial frequency tuning in, 616, 617*f*
other inputs to, 613–614
outputs to other cortical areas, 620
output streams from, 620–622
corticocortical outputs, 620
parallel feedback streams from V2 to V1, 621–622
parallel input streams, 620–621
parallel output streams, 620–621
subcortical outputs, 620
possible rehabilitation strategies, 624, 624*f*
processing in, 615–620
circuits for surround modulation, 619–620, 619*f*
classical receptive field, 615–616, 615*f*, 617*f*
extraclassical receptive field, 619
functional architecture, 616–619
responses
attention affects, 622
behavioral context affects, 622–623
expectation affects, 623
learning affects, 622, 623*f*
visual field in, 612, 613*f*
visual inputs, 612–615
bottom-up, 612–615, 614*f*
Primary visual cortex, lateral geniculate nucleus, 603–605, 603*f*
Primate anterior ocular segment, anatomy, 246*f*
Primate color coding, 477
PRK. *See* Photorefractive keratectomy (PRK)
Projected visual directions, 702
Prolonged light flashes, ipRGC kinetics, 554
Proprioception, extraocular muscles, 200–201, 201*f*, 202*f*

Prosopagnosia, 627
Prostaglandin(s)
aqueous humor drainage. *See* Aqueous humor drainage
retinal vasodilator, 302–303
Protan color vision defects, 668
Protanomaly, 669*b*
Protein(s)
secretion regulation, tear film. *See* Tear film, aqueous layer
translocation, rod light adaptation, 461.
see also specific proteins
Protein kinase C (PKC), 366
aqueous tear film layer secretion, 371
Protein-protein disulfides (PSSP), 154–155
Proteoglycans, 363
cornea. *See* Corneal light transmission
corneal edema, 96–97
scleral mechanical properties, 112–113
Proteomic analysis, efflux transporters, 406–407
Proximal sublamina b, 464
PSAM-GlyR. *See* Pharmacologically selective actuator module-glycine receptors (PSAM-GlyR)
Pseudoisochromatic plate tests, 670
Pseudoxanthoma elasticum (PXE), 411*b*
PSF. *See* Point spread function (PSF)
PSSP (protein-protein disulfides), 154–155
Psychophysical basis, visual fields. *See* Visual field
Psychophysical evidence, motion processing, 730
Pterygopalatine ganglion, 379*f*
Ptolemy, 701
Pulfrich effect, 708
Pulse-step command, saccadic eye movement, 216–217, 216*f*
horizontal saccades, 219–220, 219*f*
vertical/torsional, 220
Pulvinar nucleus of thalamus, retinal projection targets, 573
Pump-leak hypothesis, corneal endothelium, 89–91
Pupil
aperture, depth of focus, 17, 20*f*
asymmetry, Horner's syndrome, 539
clinical assessment, 527, 529*f*
defects, 536–539
efferent defects, 539–547.
see also specific diseases/disorders
depth of focus, 527
dilation failure, 546–547, 547*t*
dilation lag, Horner's syndrome, 539, 542*f*
functions, 527, 528*f*
image quality, 527
inequality. *See* Anisocoria
involvement in third nerve palsies, 546
large, 527
light regulation, 527–548
light properties, 535–536, 535*f*, 536*t*
See also Pupil light reflex
movement, 527
narcotic tolerance, 527–528
optics, 528*b*
perimetry, 539
pharmacology, 527–528
reflex dilation, 533–534
anesthesia, 533
deep sleep, 533
Edinger–Westphal nucleus, 533

Pupil *(Continued)*
humoral mechanisms, 534
supranuclear inhibition, 533
sympathetic innervation, 533, 534*f*
retinal illumination, 527
size
duration, 536*t*
reduction, 32
Pupillary responses, 527–528
Pupil light reflex, 528–534, 530*f*
afferent arm, 528–531
dark adaptation, 529
melanopsin ganglion cells, 530, 530*b*
midbrain pathway, 531
photoreceptors, 528–529
Purkinje shift, 528–529
RGCs, 530
clinical observation, 536–538, 537*f*
in diagnosis, 563*b*
dorsal midbrain lesion studies, 531*b*
Edinger–Westphal nucleus, 528
efferent arm, 532, 532*f*
interneuron arm, 531–532
central visual field damage, 531
ganglion cell axons, 531
nasal field, 531
pretectal neurons, 531
temporal field, 531
uncrossed pathway, 531
ipRGC central projections, 563, 563*f*
See also Pupil near reflex
Pupil near reflex, 528–534, 530*f*
accommodation, 532–533
definition, 532–533
Edinger–Westphal nucleus, 533
evaluation, 546
supranuclear control, 533
Purinergic agonists, 372–373
Purkinje shift, pupil light reflex, 528–529
Pursuit, smooth. *See* Smooth pursuit
PVD. *See* Posterior vitreous detachment (PVD)
PVZ-INS LE strand, 45
P2X receptors, 373
P2X$_7$ receptors, 367, 373
Pyruvate, retina, 326

Q

QO$_2$. *See* Oxygen consumption (QO$_2$)
Qualitative stereopsis, 710
Quantitative stereopsis, 710

R

Radial current flow, electroretinograms. *See* Electroretinogram(s) (ERGs)
Radial fibers, ciliary muscle, 42–43
Radial keratotomy (RK), 105
Random-dot stereogram (RDS), 709, 709*f*
RAPD. *See* Relative afferent pupillary defect (RAPD)
Raphe interpositus nucleus (RIP), 217–218
R9AP mutation
Bradyopsia, 461*b*
transducin shutoff, 443*b*
Rayleigh color match, 670
Rayleigh limit, 652, 653*f*

Reactive oxygen species (ROS)
    corneal ultraviolet light filtration, 106
    photoreceptor outer segment phagocytosis, 342–343
    RPE, 339
Reading, visual acuity. *See* Visual acuity
Receptive field(s), 629–630
    ipRGCs, 556
    lateral geniculate nucleus, 604–605, 606*f*
        K layers (koniocellular), 605
        M layers (magnocellular), 605
        P layers (parvocellular), 605, 606*f*
    LGN. *See* Lateral geniculate nucleus (LGN)
    peripheral vision contrast sensitivity, 662
    primary visual cortex. *See* Primary visual cortex (V1)
    spatial form, visual processing of, 642
    and visual selectivity, 630–631
Receptive-field (RF) structure, of V2 neurons, 769*f*
Receptor-ligand pairings, 748
Red-green circuitry
    color vision, 671, 672*f*
    defects, 671
Reference frame transformation, 241
Reference points/measurements, cornea. *See* Cornea
Refraction, lens. *See* Lens
Refractive errors, 24
    prevalence, 24
    spherical aberration impact on, 32
    visual acuity, 653.
    see also specific diseases/disorders
Refractive index, sclera, 106, 114*f*
Refractive power
    accommodation measurement, 55
    cornea, 654
    emmetropization, 3
    presbyopia, 61
Refractive surgery, 75*f*, 97*b*
    glare and contrast sensitivity, 16–17.
    see also specific methods
Regional differences
    lens fiber cells morphology
        biomechanics, 137–140, 137*f*
        lens transparency, 137–140, 137*f*
        optics, 137–140, 137*f*
    vitreous body, 167
Regional differences, lens fiber cells, 131, 133*t*
Region of interest (ROI), 744–745
Relative afferent pupillary defect (RAPD), 527, 529*b*
    clinical disorders, 538*t*
    management, 538*b*
    quantification, 537
    visual field damage, 537–538, 537*f*
Relative disparity, 707, 707*f*
Relative egocentric direction, 702–703
Relay cells, LGN, 599
Remodeling phase, corneal stroma wound healing, 86
Remyelination, optic nerve repair, 591
Renin-angiotensin effects, aqueous humor drainage, 271
Representation of aberrations, 30–31
Resolution, definition and units, 11, 11*f*
Response constancy, single photon detection, 434, 434*f*
Resting state, dark-adapted rods. *See* Dark-adapted rods

Retina, 527
    blood vessels. *See* Retinal vasculature
    cells
        multifocal electroretinograms, 524*b*
        photopic negative response, 524*b*
        scotopic threshold response, 524*b*
    cone positioning, 19
    of cyclopean eye, 702
    detachment, relative afferent pupillary defect, 538*t*
    diseases/disorders, 429*b*
        degeneration, 428
        detachment. *see above.*
        see also specific diseases/disorders
    eccentricity, critical duration, 721–723
    energy metabolism, 325–326, 333*f*
    gaze stabilization. *See* Gaze stabilization
    glycolysis, 326–329
        cell culture models, 328–329
        extracellular electroretinogram, 328, 328*f*
        functional imaging, 327
        glucose metabolism enzymes, 327
        glucose supply, 327
        intact retinal studies, 328
        iodoacetate studies, 328
        isotope studies, 328
        pentose phosphate pathway, 328
    illuminance, temporal contrast sensitivity, 725
    illumination, pupil, 527
    image-degrading defenses, 19
    inner
        oxygen distribution/consumption, 326–327, 327*f*
        signal processing. *see* Signal processing, inner plexiform layer
        visual processing. *See* Visual processing, inner retina
    inputs, LGN. *See* Lateral geniculate nucleus (LGN)
    ipRGCs, 556, 556*f*, 557*f*
    ischemia, negative ERG, 511
    light waves, 324
    neurons, 464–467
        gliaform cell phenotype, 465
        gliaform neurons, 464
        multipolar neuron phenotype, 465
        multipolar neurons, 464
        novel cells, 465–466
        sensory neuroepithelium, 464–465
        true glia, 466–467.
        see also specific types
    outer, signal processing. *See* Signal processing, outer retina
    oxygen distribution/consumption, 326–327
        dark oxygen consumption, 326
        inner retina, 326, 327*f*
        light oxygen consumption, 326
        photoreceptor QO_2 in dark, 326
        photoreceptor QO_2 in light, 326
    pigment function, 20
    predominant function of, 324
    projection targets. *See* Central visual pathways
    pyruvate, 326
    role of, 8–10
    structure, 125*f*
    synaptic organization. *See* Retinal synaptic organization
    topography, visual acuity eccentricity, 655*f*, 657
    vasculature. *See* Retinal vasculature

Retina (*Continued*)
    vitreous body support function. *See* Vitreous body
    vitreous interface. *See* Vitreo-retinal interface
    whole-mount studies, neuron–glial cell interaction, 324
Retinal correspondence, 703–705, 703*f*
Retinal disparity, 616, 709–710, 710*f*
Retinal ganglion cell(s) (RGCs), 324–325, 325*f*, 598, 602, 602*f*, 701–702, 748, 749*f*
    apoptosis, 588–589
    axon injury signaling, 589
    axon regeneration, 591
    axons, optic nerve (cranial nerve II), 578, 579*b*, 579*f*
    death. *See* Optic nerve injury
    directionally selective motion, 475–477, 475*f*
    midget ganglion cells, 671
    parallel RGC output pathways. *see* Signal processing, inner plexiform layer
    parvocellular retinal ganglion cells, 727
    peripheral. *See* Peripheral ganglion cells
    pupil light reflex, 530
    regeneration, neurotrophic factors, 591
    small bistratified, blue-yellow circuitry, 671
    small bistratified RGC, blue-yellow circuitry, 671
    survival
        neurotrophic factors, 591
        optic nerve repair, 591
        time course, 589
    visual processing, inner retina, 498
Retinal ganglion cells, intrinsically photosensitive (ipRGCs), 549–570
    activity regulation, 565
    central projections, 562–566, 562*f*
        circadian photoentrainment, 563–564, 564*f*
        conscious light perception, 565
        lateral habenula, 565
        LGN, 565
        mood modulation, 565
        photic modulation of the pineal, 563–564
        pupillary light reflex, 563, 563*b*, 563*f*
        sleep regulation, 565, 565*b*
    depolarizing photoresponse, 552–553
        action potentials, 552–553, 554*f*
        voltage-gated sodium channels, 552–553
    development, 566
    discovery, 550
    functional properties, 550–558
    gene therapy, 557*b*, 558*f*
    historical roots, 549–550
    invertebrate-like phototransduction cascade, 551–552
    kinetics, 554
        prolonged light flashes, 554
        termination, 554
    morphology, 554–556, 555*f*
    pathological state resistance, 556–557
    phototransduction cascade, 551–552, 553*f*
    receptive field, 556, 556*f*
    resistance, 556–557
    retinal distribution, 556, 556*f*, 557*f*
    sensitivity, 553–554
    spectral tuning, 551, 552*b*, 552*f*
        output behavior, 551
    synaptic input, 558–560, 559*f*
        amacrine cells, 558–560

Retinal ganglion cells, intrinsically photosensitive (ipRGCs) (Continued)
  bipolar cells, 558, 559f
  ON bipolar cells, 558, 559f
  extrinsic versus intrinsic photoresponses, 560, 560f
  synaptic output, 560–566
    central projections. see above
    intraretinal output, 561–562, 561f.
    see also Non-image-forming vision
Retinal illumination, 527
Retinal metabolism and function, 332
  experimental models of, 329f
    ammonium ions, 331f
    glutamate, 331f
    metabolic compartmentation, 330f
  metabolic interactions, 329f, 330f, 332–333, 333f
    blood-oxygen-level-dependent functional magnetic resonance imaging, 331f, 333, 333f
    electrophysiology, 332
    glycogen, 332
    illumination, 332
    insulin, 332
    isolated cat retina studies, 332
    lactate, 332
    "missing lactate", 332–333, 333b
    relative compartmentalization, 331f, 333, 333f
Retinal oculocentric directions, 702
Retinal pigment epithelium (RPE), 339–346, 340f, 405
  active immune barrier, 343–344, 344b
  as barrier, 331
  definition, 339
  diseases by genetic defects, 342b
  ion transport, 340–341
    cGMP-dependent cation channels, 340–341
    potassium, 340–341
    sodium-bicarbonate cotransporter, 341
    sodium-potassium ATPase, 341
    sodium-potassium-chloride cotransporter, 341
    sodium-proton exchanger, 341
  light absorption, 339
  oxygen consumption, 326
  photo-oxidative damage, 339
  phototransducers, 414, 415f–416f
  retinal detachment, 341b
  scleral embryology, 106–108
  secretion, 343
    cytokines, 343
    growth factors, 343
    insulin-like growth factor 1, 343
    tissue inhibitors of matrix metalloproteases, 343
    tumor necrosis factor-α, 343
    vascular endothelial growth factor, 343
  structure, 339
  transepithelial transport, 339–340
    blood to photoreceptors, 339
    retina to blood, 339–340
  visual cycle, 341–342, 342f
    all-trans-retinol re-isomerization, 341
    CRALP (cellular retinaldehyde binding protein), 341
    CRBP (cellular retinol binding protein), 341
    IRPB (interphotoreceptor matrix retinal binding protein), 341

Retinal pigment epithelium (RPE) (Continued)
    light vs. dark, 341–342
    LRAT (lecithin:retinol transferase), 341
Retinal points, 704f
Retinal synaptic organization, 464–479, 466f, 468f
  AC conventional fast synapses, 468
    acetylcholine, 468
  AC efferent slow transmitter synapses, 468
    dopamine, 468
  AxC conventional fast synapses, 468
    acetylcholine, 468
  AxC efferent slow transmitter synapses, 468
    dopamine, 468
  BC ribbon synapses, 468
    GABA signaling, 468
    glutamatergic signaling, 468
  coupling patterns, 469–470
  coupling types, 469–470
  fast focal neurochemistry, 470
  global neurochemistry, 470–471
    calcium-activated calmodulin, 471
    dopamine, 470–471
    feedback, 472
    feedforward, 472
    nested feedback/feedforward, 472
    neuropeptides, 471
    nitric oxide, 471
    polarity, 472
    signal processing, 471–472
    sign-conserving transfers, 466f, 471–472
    sign-inverting transfers, 466f, 471–472
    synaptic chains, 472
    transporter modulation, 471
  HC non-canonical signaling, 468–469
  networks, 472–477
    center-surround organization, 472–474, 473f
    disease reversal, 477
    mammalian rod pathways, 474–475
    motion, 475–477
    primate color coding, 477
    rod-cone crossover networks, 475, 475f
    signaling mechanisms, 464
    transmission electron microscopy, 464
  photoreceptor ribbon synapses, 467–468
    glutamate release, 467, 469f
    nonmammalians, 468, 468f
Retinal vasculature, 466–467
  blood flow, 334
    extracellular lactate, 334
    extravascular intraretinal acidosis, 334
    intravitreal injection studies, 334
    L-lactate injection studies, 334
    sodium lactate injection studies, 334
Retinal vasodilator
  endothelial factors, 303–305, 304f, 305f
  humoral control, 306
  neural control, 305–306, 306f
  neurovascular coupling, 300–303, 301f
    caveoilin-1 knockout, 303, 304f
    cellular mechanisms, 302–303, 303f
    endothelial factors, 303–305, 304f, 305f
    flicker stimulation, 300, 301f, 304f
    molecular mechanisms, 302–303, 303f
    nanotube, 303, 303f
    nitric oxide, 302–303, 303f
    prostaglandins, 302–303
  ocular circulation regulation, 296, 298f
  oxygenation, 285–289

Retinal vasodilator (Continued)
Retinal vessel diameter, 289–290, 289f
Retinal waves, 749f
Retinitis pigmentosa, 429b, 477
Retinogeniculate circuitry, 748
Retinogeniculate connections, 607
Retinogeniculate projection development, 748–754
  activity-dependent refinement of, 749–750, 749f
  activity drive refinement, parameters of, 750–751, 750f
  beyond eye specificity, 751–752
  eye-specific territories, formation of, 748
  molecular mechanisms, 748–749
  optic chiasm, 748
  refined during development, 749
  RGC axon projections, crucial choice point in, 748
  RGC axon refinement, cellular and molecular mechanisms of, 751
Retinogeniculate synapses, 605–607
Retinogeniculate transmission, 605–607, 608f
Retinoid
  recycling, 424–426
  regeneration, 424–426
Retino-RPE-scleral visual signaling pathway, 108–110
Retinotopic map, 627
Retrobulbar injections, 109f, 116–117
Retrograde transport, optic nerve, 586
Reverse occlusion, intermittent monocular form deprivation, 757, 758f
RGC axon projections, crucial choice point in, 748
RGC axon refinement, cellular and molecular mechanisms of, 751
RGCs. See Retinal ganglion cell(s) (RGCs)
RGS9-1 mutation
  bradyopsia, 461b
  dark-adapted rod recovery phase, 423f, 426, 427b
  transducin shutoff, 443b
Rhesus ciliary muscles, 56–57, 57f, 58f, 59f
Rhodamine, scleral permeability, 117t
Rhodopsin, 8–9
  absorption spectrum, 421–422, 428f
  dark-adapted rod resting state, 418–420
  inactivation, rhodopsin kinase, 460
  mutations, 420
    Oguchi disease, 443b
  phosphorylation, 424–426
    APE, 426
    cis-trans isomerization, 424–426
    opsin, 426
    rhodopsin kinase, 424
  photoisomerization, 418f, 419f, 420f, 421–423
    metarhodopsin II formation, 423
    structural changes, 423
  post-translational modifications, 420, 420f
  single photon detection, 437
  structure, 418–420, 418f, 419f, 420f
Rhodopsin kinase
  rhodopsin inactivation, 460
  rhodopsin phosphorylation, 424
Right hand rule, 238f
riMLF (rostral interstitial medial longitudinal fasciculus), 217–218, 241
Ring scotomas, 683
RK (radial keratotomy), 105

RNA sequencing, 615
Rod(s)
  action spectra, 437, 440f
  CNG channel. See Cyclic nucleotide gated
    (CNG) channels
  compartmentalization, 414, 415f–416f, 417f
  cone coupling, 480
  dark-adapted. See Dark-adapted rods
  defective synapses, night blindness, 446b
  flash photocurrent responses, 433, 435f
  flash photovoltage responses, 432
  hyperpolarization, CNG channel closure,
    438–439
  light adaptation. See Light adaptation
  location, 414
  membrane systems, 414, 417f
  minimum resolvable acuity, 649
  modulation of flash response by bicarbonate,
    433–434
  NCKX1 exchanger, 440–441
  positioning, retina, 19
  response time course, dark-adapted a-wave,
    513–514, 514f
  single photon detection, 434–435
    aberrant responses, 435, 436f, 443b
    rhodopsin limitations, 437
  steady light photocurrent responses, 437, 438f
    bleaching effects, 437, 438f
  visual acuity eccentricity, 656
Rod-cone crossover networks, 475, 475f
Rod outer segments (ROS), 414
  photoreceptor–retinal pigment epithelia
    interactions, 333–334
Rod photoreceptors, 498
Rod signal pathways, 498, 499f
Root-mean-squared (RMS) WFE, 30
ROS. See Reactive oxygen species (ROS); Rod
    outer segments (ROS)
Rostral interstitial nucleus of medial longitudinal
    fasciculus (riMLF), 217–218, 241
Rotational kinematics, 236
RPE. See Retinal pigment epithelium (RPE)
RPE metabolic interactions, 333–334
  glucose transporters, 334
  Krebs cycle, 334
  rod outer segments, 333–334
RPE65 mutations, Leber's congenital amaurosis,
    440f, 443b
Rupture, scleral mechanical properties, 113

S

Saccades, 212
  disorders, 231–232, 231b, 231f
  extraocular muscles, 189
  zero torsion, 241
SAD (seasonal affective disorder), 565
Saturating light level response, dark-adapted rods,
    427
Saturation constant, 644
SBK (sub-Bowman's keratomileusis), 97
SC. See Superior colliculus (SC)
Scaling model, 760–761
Scheiner, Christopher, 33–34
Scheiner's disc, 33f
Schlemm's canal (SC), 64–65, 246f
  aqueous humor drainage, 256f

Schwalbe's line, 64–65
Sclera, 49, 51f, 106–118
  aging, 106–110
  anatomy, 41f, 72f–73f, 106, 110f
  aqueous humor drainage, 269
  autoimmune diseases, 118b
  composition, 76t
  cornea vs., 106
  dehydration and edema, 116
  development, 106–110
    collagen degradation, 108
    elderly, 110
    emmetropization, 108
    intra-ocular pressure, 108
    myopia, 108
    post-natal growth, 108
    retino-RPE-scleral visual signaling pathway,
      108–110
    visual feedback mechanisms, 108
  drug delivery, 116–118
    clearance mechanisms, 107f, 118
    intravitreal injections, 109f, 116
    metabolism, 118
    passive diffusion, 117–118
    peribulbar injections, 109f, 116–117
    periocular, 109f, 116–117
    permeability of drugs, 117t
    retrobulbar injections, 109f, 116–117
    subconjunctival injections, 109f, 116–117
    sub-Tenon's injections, 109f, 116–117
    topical drugs, 116
    trans-scleral pathway, 109f, 116–117
    vascular endothelial growth factor, 117
  embryology, 106–110
    RPE, 106–108
  episcleral vasculature, 69, 116
    anterior ciliary arteries, 116
    episcleral arterial circle, 114f–115f, 116
    long posterior ciliary arteries, 116
  growth, 106–110
  lamina fusca, 69
  lymphatic layers, 98f, 106
  mechanical properties, 112–116
    collagen, 113
    elastin, 113
    episclera, 113, 114f–115f
    episcleral venous pressure, 113
    finite element modeling, 113, 114f–115f
    glycosaminoglycans, 112–113
    inflation testing, 113, 114f–115f
    intraocular pressure, 116
    lymph vasculature, 113, 114f–115f
    proteoglycans, 113
    rupture, 113
    stress–strain curves, 113–116
  nerve supply, 88f, 106
  reference points and measurements, 109f,
    110–112
    anterior scleral foramen, 110–112
    posterior scleral foramen, 110–112
  refractive index, 106, 114f
  scleral stroma, 69
  sensory nerves, 388f, 391
  structure, 125f
  thickness, 69
  wound healing, 116
Scleral spur, 64–65
Scleral thickness, 110–112

Scleral vein, 246f
SCN of hypothalamus, ipRGC circadian
    photoentrainment, 563–564
S-cone-specific ON bipolar cells, blue-yellow
    circuitry, 671
Scotopic threshold response (STR). See
    Electroretinograms, full-field dark-adapted
    (Ganzfeld) flash
Scotopic vision, 452–453, 453f
  background intensity, 452
  desensitization, 452, 453f
  photopic vision vs., 452, 453f
Seasonal affective disorder (SAD), 565
Secondary cataracts. See Cataracts
Secondary creep, corneal stiffness, 101
Second-generation Humphrey matrix perimeter,
    690–691
Second-order information, 641
Second-order vision, 638, 641, 642f
Secretory immunoglobulin A (sIgA), tear film,
    aqueous production, 370
Selective adaptation, temporal sensitivity, 726–727
Sensitivity
  to chromatic information, 641–642
  spatial form, 641–642, 642f, 643f
Sensitivity loss, detection of, 680–683, 681f, 682f,
    683f
Sensory innervation (of eye), 378–404
  anatomy, 378–385, 379f
    trigeminal ganglion neurons, 378
  central pathways, 382–385, 384f, 391–392
    brainstem, 391–392
    thalamus, 392
  distribution, 379
  dryness, 395, 395b
  functional characteristics, 387–392, 388f
    cold thermoreceptors, 388f, 391
    mechanonociceptors, 387, 388f, 389f–390f
    polymodal nociceptors, 387–391, 388f, 389f–390f
  inflammation, 393–394
    CGRP, 394
    mediators, 389f–390f, 393–394
    morphology, 393–395
    sensitization, 389f–390f, 393–394
    SP, 394
    spontaneous pain, 393–394
  nerve injury, 394–395
  sensations, 395–400, 397f, 398f, 399f
    corneal, 396, 397f
    ocular surface sensitivity testing, 395–396
    systemic conditions, 396–400
  trophic effects, 392–393, 393b.
  see also specific nerves
Sensory neuroepithelium, retinal neurons, 464
Sensory substitution, 783–784, 784f
Shack-Hartmann aberrometer, 33–34, 34f
Shack-Hartmann sensor, 34f
Shear stress, retinal vasodilator, 305
Shh (Sonic Hedgehog), extraocular muscle
    development, 201–202
Short ciliary arteries (SCAs), 284
Short ciliary nerve, 379f
Short-(S) wavelength sensitive cones, color vision,
    465, 668, 669f
Short wavelength automated perimetry (SWAP),
    688, 690f
Shortened activated rhodopsin lifetime, light
    adaptation, 460

Sight recovery, 777–778, 782
Signaling pathways
    conjunctival goblet cells, 366, 368f
    protein secretion regulation, 370
    retinal synaptic organization, 464
Signal processing
    inner retina. *see* Signal processing, inner plexiform layer
    LGN. *See* Lateral geniculate nucleus (LGN)
    outer retina. *See* Signal processing, outer retina
    retinal synaptic organization, 471–472
Signal processing, outer retina, 480–494
    bipolar cells, 486–490, 489f
        amacrine cell, 486–487
        cone, 490
        IPL, 488
        rod, 489f, 490
        visual pathways, 486–490, 489f
    horizontal cell, 483–486
        A-type, 483
        B-type, 483
        center-surround antagonistic receptive field, 484
        chromatic visual processing, 485–486, 488f
        coupled networks, 483–484
        feedback, 484, 485f, 486f, 487f
        GABAergic synapses, 484, 485f, 486f, 487f
        ganglion cell responses, 486
        interneurons inhibition, 483
        morphology, 483f
        synaptic GABA output, 484
    interplexiform cells, 483
        retinal neuron modulation, 483
    photoreceptor electrical synapses, 454f, 480–481
        bipolar cell output synapses, 481, 482f
        connexin 36 gap junction proteins, 480, 481f
        horizontal cell output synapses, 481, 482f
        horizontal cells signaling, 482–483
        OFF-cone bipolar cells, 481–482
        ON-cone bipolar cells, 481, 482f
        resolution, 480
        rod–cone coupling, 480
        signal-to-noise ratio, 480–481
Signal-to-noise ratio, outer retinal signal processing, 480–481
Signal transduction, melanopsin, 551–552
Sign-conserving pathways, retinal synaptic organization, 466f, 471–472
Sign-inverting pathways, retinal synaptic organization, 466f, 471–472
Silent synapses, 775
Simple anisocoria, 539
Simple cells, 615–616, 615f
Simulation program and integrated circuit emphasis (SPICE), 513–514
Sine waves, contrast sensitivity testing, 13–14, 15f
Single binocular vision, 701
Single cortical cells. *See* Contrast sensitivity
Single photon detection
    photoreceptors. *See* Photoreceptor(s)
    rods. *See* Rod(s)
Sinusoidal gratings, 653f, 659–660
SITA Faster visual field tests, 687–688, 689f
SITA SWAP, 688
SKI study, visual acuity age-relation, 665, 665f
Sleep-arousal, LGN modulation by, 598
Sleep regulation, ipRGC central projections, 565, 565b

Slit-lamp biomicroscope examination, 543
Slowed dark adaptation, 462b
Slow fibers, extraocular muscles, 193
Slow PIII
    electroretinogram glial currents, 508, 508f
    electroretinograms, 508–509, 508f
Small bistratified retinal ganglion cells, blue-yellow circuitry, 671
Small-incision lenticule extraction (SMILE), 77f, 97
SMAS. *See* Superficial musculoaponeurotic system (SMAS)
Smooth pursuit
    extraocular muscles, 189
    eye movements, 212
Smooth vergence eye movements, 212
    neural control, 221–222, 222f
Snellen acuity charts, 10, 13f, 650, 651f
Snellen, Hermann, 10
"Snow blindness", corneal ultraviolet light filtration, 105
SN60WF, 33
Social seeing, 6
Sodium-bicarbonate cotransporter, RPE, 341
Sodium ions
    aqueous humor formation, 248–249
    electrolyte/water secretion regulation, tear film, mucous production, 368
    electroretinogram glial currents, 508
    lacrimal gland fluid composition, 373–374
Sodium lactate injection studies, retinal blood flow, 334
Sodium-potassium-ATPase (Na$^+$/K$^+$-ATPase)
    corneal endothelium, 92
    dark-adapted rod resting state, 414–416
    electrolyte/water secretion regulation, tear film, mucous production, 369
    retinal pigmented epithelium transport, 340–341
    tear film, aqueous production, 373
Sodium-potassium-calcium (Na$^+$/Ca^{2+}-K$^+$) exchanger protein 1 (NCKX1), 440–441
Sodium-potassium-calcium (Na$^+$/Ca^{2+}-K$^+$) exchanger protein 2 (NCKX2)
    cones, 440–441
    dark-adapted rod resting state, 417
Sodium-potassium-calcium (Na$^+$/K$^+$, Ca^{2+}) exchanger protein(s), 437–441
Sodium-potassium-chloride cotransporter (NKCC1) activity, 146–147
Sodium-potassium-chloride (Na$^+$-K$^+$-2Cl$^-$) symporter (NKCCl), 341
    electrolyte/water secretion regulation, tear film, mucous production, 369
    tear film, aqueous production, 373
Sodium-proton (Na$^+$/H$^+$) exchanger, 484
    RPE, 341
    tear film, aqueous production, 373
Soft tissues, orbit, 349–352
Somatostatin-expressing (SST) interneurons, 615
Sonic hedgehog (Shh), 748
Sorsby fundus dystrophy, 462
Space, 780
    behavior, 780
    neural responses, 780
SPAK (Ste-20-like Proline Alanine Rich Kinase), 147–148
Spatial attention, 622

Spatial contrast sensitivity, intermittent monocular form deprivation, 757
Spatial effects, temporal sensitivity, 725, 726f
Spatial form, early processing
    contrast sensitivity. *See* Contrast sensitivity
Spatial form, visual processing of, 638–648
    adaptation, 640, 640f
    contrast constancy, 643–644, 643f, 644f
    distributed representation, 646–647
    early visual mechanisms, 638–640, 639f
    effect of disease on, 644–645, 645f
    sensitivity and receptive field size *vs.* eccentricity, 641–643, 642f
    spatial changes in luminance, color, contrast, and texture, 640–641, 641f
    summation and suppression of signals, 645–646, 646f
    suprathreshold vision, 643–644, 643f, 644f
Spatial frequency, 616, 708
    local stereopsis, 761–762
    pupil size, 536t
    visual acuity, 652, 654f
Spatial pooling, 646
Spatial vision, effect of disease on, 644–645, 645f
Spatial vision with low contrast. *See* Visual acuity
Spatial visual field tests, 688b
Spatiotemporal contrast sensitivity function, 725
Spatiotemporal transformation, eye movements, 241
Spatiotemporal vision, infant vision development. *See* Infant vision development
Spatiotemporal visual field tests, 688b
Specialized proresolving mediators (SPMs), 367
Spectral composition, temporal summation, 721–723
Spectral sensitivity, pupil size, 536t
Spectral tuning, ipRGCs. *See* Retinal ganglion cells, intrinsically photosensitive (ipRGCs)
Spectroscopic oxymetry, ocular blood flow measurement, 294–295, 294f
Sphenoid bone, 347
Spherical aberration, 21, 21f
    HOAs and, 31
    impact on contrast sensitivity, 32
    impact on depth of focus, 32
    impact on night vision, 32
    impact on refractive error, 32
    impact on vision, 31–32
    impact on visual acuity, 32
    intraocular lenses, 21
    lens, 21, 124, 125b, 125f
    visual acuity, 652–653
Split spectrum amplitude decorrelation (SSADA), 292–293
Spontaneous pain, inflammation, 393–394
Spontaneous retinal activity, 749–750, 750f
Square waves, 13
Squint, 713
SSADA. *See* Split spectrum amplitude decorrelation (SSADA)
Stargardt's disease, 342, 425b
    ABCA4 gene, 425b, 426
Static measurement, accommodation, 55
Static perimetry, 677
    suprathreshold. *See* Suprathreshold static perimetry
Steady light photocurrent responses, 437, 438f
    cones. *See* Cones
    rods. *See* Rod(s)

Steady-state visual evoked potentials, spatiotemporal vision development, 737, 737f
Steady state visually evoked potential (SSVEP), 744
Ste-20-like Proline Alanine Rich Kinase (SPAK), 147–148
Stereoacuity, 707f, 708–709, 708f, 709b
    optical defocus on, 708
Stereo-contrast paradox, 708
Stereo-fusion, 706
Stereogram, 708, 709f
Stereopsis, 708
    binocular vision development, 742
    coarse and, 710
    local, spatial frequency, 761–762
    and "matching problem", 709
    quantitative and qualitative, 710
Sterol homeostasis, 411b
Stiffness, cornea. See Cornea
Stimulation, accommodation measurement, 55–56
Stimulus chromaticity, 723, 724f
Stimulus conditions, electroretinograms, 507f, 508–509
Stimulus luminance, critical flicker fusion frequency, 723, 723f
Stimulus size effects, critical flicker fusion frequency, 723–724
Stimulus to accommodation, 54
STR. See Electroretinograms, full-field dark-adapted (Ganzfeld) flash
Strabismic amblyopia, 644–645
    neural deficits, 767–768, 769f
Strabismic suppression, 713–714
Strabismus, 204–205, 229–230, 713, 713f, 762–766
    animal models, 204–205, 762
        optical methods, 762
        surgical methods, 762
    definition, 762
    duration effects, 764–765
    eye movement anomalies, 765–766
    motion asymmetries, 741
    muscle structure, 204–205
    neural changes, 763–764
    onset age effects, 764–765, 764f
    perceptual deficits, 762
    retinal correspondence and suppression in, 713f
    treatment, 204–205, 205b
Strength extensibility, cornea, 100–101
Streptozotocin (STZ) treatment, cataract, 153–154
Stress, cornea. See Cornea
Stress–strain curves, scleral mechanical properties, 113–116
Striate cortex. See Primary visual cortex (V1)
Stroma
    corneal edema, 95, 99f
    corneal light transmission, 76–78, 76t
Sub-basal nerve plexus, corneal sensory nerves, 381–382, 381f
Sub-Bowman's keratomileusis (SBK), 97
Subconjunctival injections
    corneal drug delivery, 105, 109f
    scleral drug delivery, 109f, 116–117
Subcortical disorder, 230f
Subcortical outputs, V1, 620
Subcortical pathways, white matter pathways, 775
Subcortical structures, constant monocular form deprivation, 756
Subepithelial nerve plexus, 381

Subjective measurement, accommodation, 55
Substance P
    inflammation, 394
    meibomian gland regulation, 375
Sub-Tenon's injections, scleral drug delivery, 109f, 116–117
Sulcus, corneal reference points, 71
Superficial musculoaponeurotic system (SMAS), 354–355, 355b, 355f
    bony attachments, 355, 355f, 356f
Superficial temporal arteries
    eyelids, 359, 359f
    orbit, 353
Superior colliculus (SC), 598
    lateral geniculate nucleus inputs from, 601
    retinal projection targets, 573
    saccadic eye movements, 218, 218f
Superior division III nerve, 192f
Superior muscle of Riolan, 349f
Superior oblique muscles, 190, 350f
    anatomy, 191f, 192f
    intorsion, 190, 191t, 192f
    paths of, 190, 191f, 192f
Superior oculomotor nerve, 350f
Superior ophthalmic veins, 350f
    route of, 192–193
Superior orbital fissure, 192–193, 349
Superior rectus muscles, 190, 191f, 192f, 350f
Superior tarsal muscle, 357–358, 357f
Superior temporal cortical region, lesions, 731
Superoxide dismutases, extraocular muscles, 197–199
Suppression, 706
Suppression, binocular vision. See Binocular vision
Suppression scotoma, 713–714
Suprachiasmatic nucleus, retinal projection targets, 573
"Supramodal" hypothesis, 781
Supramolecular organization, vitreous body, 167
Supranuclear regions
    pupil near reflex, 533
    pupil reflex dilation, 533
Supraoptic nucleus, retinal projection targets, 573
Supraorbital artery, 353f
    eyelids, 359f
    orbit, 353
Supraorbital nerve, 192f, 359, 360f
Suprathreshold static perimetry, 678–680, 680f
Suprathreshold vision, spatial form, 643–644, 643f, 644f
Supratrochlear artery, 359f
Supratrochlear nerve, 378–379
Surgery
    corneal endothelial cell injury, 111
    nystagmus, 205b.
    see also specific techniques
Surround effects, temporal sensitivity, 727–728, 728f, 729f
Surround modulation, in V1, 616, 619
    circuits for, 619–620, 619f
Surround suppression, 616
Sushi repeat protein X-linked 2 (SRPX2), 751
SWAP. See Short wavelength automated perimetry (SWAP)
Swelling pressure, corneal edema, 93–95
SWS1, cones, 465
Symmetric cortical motion, motion detection development, 740–741

Sympathetic nervous system
    conjunctival goblet cells, 366
    lacrimal glands, 370
    orbit, 352
    pupil reflex dilation, 533, 534f
Symptomatic posterior detachment, vitreous body, 179–180, 179f
Synaptic chains, retinal synaptic organization, 472
Synaptic pathways
    ipRGCs. See Retinal ganglion cells, intrinsically photosensitive (ipRGCs)
    optic nerve, 585
Synechiae, mydriasis, 545
Syneresis, 149b
Systemic disease, ocular blood flow, 311–313, 312f, 313f

T

Talbot–Plateau law, 728
Target-to-flank interactions, 706
Tarsal plates, eyelid margin, 357
TASS (toxic anterior segment syndrome), 112
TBNC (trigeminal brainstem nuclear complex), 382–383
TCP (thinnest corneal point), 74
TDRD7 mutation, pediatric cataract, 135
Tear film, 363–377
    glycocalyx, 363–366
        mucins, 363, 365f
        ocular surface, function on, 363–366
        regulation, 363
        structure, 363
    lipid layer, 363, 374–376
        function, 375–376
        See also Meibomian glands
    mucous layer. see below
    secretion, 363
    structure, 363, 364f
    thickness, 363
Tear film, aqueous production, 363, 369–374
    acinar electrolyte/water secretion, 373, 373f
        Cl^-/HCO_3^- (AE) exchanger, 373
        Na^+/H^+ (NHE) exchanger, 373
        Na^+-K^+-2Cl^- symporter (NKCCl), 373
        NKA, 373
    ductal electrolyte/water secretion, 373
        calcium-activated K^+ channel, 373
        K^+-Cl^- symporter (KCCl), 373
        potassium channels, 373
    electrolyte/water secretion regulation, 373
        neural activation, 373, 374f
    function, 374, 374b
    protein secretion regulation, 370–373
        cholinergic agonists, 370–371, 371f
        EGF, 372
        merocrine secretion, 370
        purinergic agonists, 372–373
        secretory IgA, 370
        signaling pathways, 370
        VIP, 371, 371f
Tear film, mucous production, 363, 366–369
    conjunctival goblet cells, 366
        proliferation, 367, 368f
        regulation, 366–368, 367f
        signaling pathways, 366, 368f
    electrolyte/water secretion regulation, 368–369, 369f

Tear film, mucous production (Continued)
  aquaporins, 369
  chloride ions, 368
  epinephrine, 369
  sodium ions, 368
  sodium-potassium-ATPase, 369
  sodium-potassium-chloride cotransporter
    (NKCCl), 369
  stimulation, 369
  function, 369
  structure, 365f, 366
    MUC5AC mucin, 366
Tear secretion, 363
Tecnis-Z9000, 33
Temporal contrast sensitivity, 724–725, 726f
  measurement of, 727, 728f
Temporal field, pupil light reflex, 531
Temporal frequency, pupil size, 536t
Temporal hemifield of contralateral eye, visual
  field lesions, 573–574, 575f
Temporal phase separation, temporal sensitivity,
  728–729
Temporal properties of vision, 721–734
Temporal retina, LGN layers and maps, 598
Temporal sensitivity
  chromatic temporal sensitivity, 725
  flicker effects, 728
  measurement applications, 729
  mechanisms, 725–727, 727f
  periodic stimuli, 721–723
    critical flicker fusion frequency. See Critical
      flicker fusion (CFF) frequency
    temporal contrast sensitivity, 724–725, 726f
  to periodic stimuli, 723–730
  spatial effects, 725
  surround effects, 727–728
  temporal phase separation, 728–729
Temporal summation, 721–723
  definition, 721
Temporal visual field, 676
  tests, 688b
Tendinous annulus, 189–190
Tenon's capsule, 349–350, 351f, 357f
Tension spikes, 64–65
Teprotumumab, 351
Tetrodotoxin (TTX), 749–750, 768–769
  light-adapted b-wave, 519
Text-to-speech technologies, 783
TGF-β. See Transforming growth factor-β (TGF-β)
Thalamic reticular nucleus (TRN), 600–601
Thalamus
  eye sensory innervation, 392
  of lateral geniculate nucleus, 598
TH1 dopaminergic, 465
TH1 dopaminergic axonal cells, 465
Thinnest corneal point (TCP), 74
Three-dimensional eye movements, 236–244
  brainstem oculomotor coordinates, 239–241
    damage symptoms, 241
    transformation, 241
  consequences
    binocular, 242–243
    monocular, 242, 243f
    perceptual, 241
  control mechanisms, 238–239
    motoneurons and muscles, 238–239, 239f
  eye-in-head motion, 236–237
  head-unrestrained gaze shift, 237–238, 238f

Three-dimensional eye movements (Continued)
  kinematics, 236
  Listing's law, 236–237
    false torsion, 236–237
    half angle rule, 237
    ocular counterroll, 237
    vestibulo-ocular reflex, 237
  neural control, 240f
  transformation
    higher, 240f, 241, 242f
    reference frame, 241
    spatiotemporal, 241
    two-dimensional to three-dimensional, 241
Three-dimensional (3D) visual inference, 782
Thyroid eye disease (TED), 351
  extraocular muscles, 207, 208f
  optic neuropathy, 208b
Time course
  electroretinogram glial currents, 513–514, 514f,
    516f
  RGC death, 589
Timolol, aqueous humor drainage, 265
TIMP (tissue inhibitors of matrix
    metalloproteinase), 343
Tissue inhibitors of matrix metalloproteinase
    (TIMP), 343
Tissue light scattering, contrast sensitivity, 15–16
Tmod1 (Tropomodulin 1), lens fiber cells, 135
TMS. See Transcranial magnetic stimulation (TMS)
TNF-associated weak induced of apoptosis
    (TWEAK), 751
Tolosa-Hunt syndrome, 546
Tomographic Biomechanical Index (TBI), 112b
Tomography, cornea, 78b
Tongue-and-groove interdigitations, lens fiber
    cells, 131–132, 134f
Topical drugs
  cornea, 102–104, 109f
  sclera, 116.
  see also specific drugs
Topical mitomycin C, corneal endothelial cell
    injury, 111
Topographic mapping, 701–702
Topography, cornea, 78b
Torsional pulse-step command, saccades, 220
Total corneal dioptric power, 74
Total Deviation plots, 682
Touch, 778–779
  behavior, 778–779
  neural responses, 779
Toughness, cornea, 100–101
Toxic anterior segment syndrome (TASS), 112
Trabecular meshwork (TM), 64–65
  aqueous humor, 245
  aqueous humor drainage, 258–259, 260f
Trafficking, 145
Transcellular aqueous transport theory,
    259f
Transconjunctival injections, corneal drug
    delivery, 105, 109f
Transcranial magnetic stimulation (TMS),
    646–647
Transducin
  bradyopsia, 443b
  dark-adapted rod resting state, 421, 422f
  R9AP mutations, 443b
Transepithelial transport, RPE. See Retinal
    pigment epithelium (RPE)

Transforming growth factor-β (TGF-β)
  cochlin production, 262
  corneal stromal wound healing, 84–86
  fibronectin, 262
  intraocular pressure, 262
  matrix metalloproteinase, 262
  plasminogen activator inhibitor, 262
Transient amplifying (TA) cells, corneal
    epithelium, 87–89, 92f
Transient astigmatism, 4, 5f
Transient visual evoked potentials, 735
Transition zone, lens fiber cell differentiation, 128–129
Translational vestibulo-ocular reflex, 224–225
Transmission electron microscopy, retinal synaptic
    organization, 464
Transmural pressure, corneal stress, 100
Transparency
  cornea, 7, 7f
  corneal light transmission, 76
  lens. See Lens
Transporter modulation, retinal synaptic
    organization, 471
Trans-scleral drug delivery, 109f, 116
Transverse chromatic aberration (TCA), 27
Traumatic iridoplegia, mydriasis, 544
Traumatic optic neuropathy, 586–587
Trend analysis visual field, assessing visual field
    progression, 687
Treviranus, 549
Trigeminal brainstem nuclear complex (TBNC),
    382–383
Trigeminal ganglion neurons, 387–391
  anatomy, 379f
  eye sensory innervation, 378
Trigeminal nerve (cranial nerve V)
  corneal nerves, 82–84, 88f
  eyelids, 359, 360f
  ophthalmic division
    iris innervation, 534
    route of, 193
  orbit, 351
Trigger-happy, 693, 697f
Tritan defects, 668
TRN. See Thalamic reticular nucleus (TRN)
Trochlea, anatomy, 191f, 192f
Trochlear nerve (cranial nerve IV), 350f
  anatomy, 192f
  congenital cranial dysinnervation disorders, 205
  extraocular muscle innervation, 54
  eye movements, 213
  orbit, 352, 352f
  route of, 192–193
Tropomodulin 1 (Tmod1), lens fiber cells, 135
True glia, retinal neurons, 466–467
Tumor necrosis factor-α (TNF-α), RPE secretion, 343
Two eye's images, mapping, 701–702
Tyndall effect, 246–247
Type II collagen, vitreous body, 165, 166f
Type VI collagen, vitreous body, 166
Type VII collagen, vitreous body, 166
Type IX collagen, vitreous body, 165–166
Type V/XI collagen, vitreous body, 166

U

Uhthoff's phenomenon, 587
Ultimate tensile stress (UTS), corneal ectasia,
    101–102

Ultrafiltration, aqueous humor formation, 248
Ultrasound biomicroscopy
  of ciliary muscle, 42*f*
  of vitreous, 45–49, 46*f*
Ultraviolet light
  corneal filtration. *See* Cornea
  corneal light transmission, 76–78, 79*f*
Unconventional outflow, aqueous humor drainage
  adrenergic effects, 264–265
  cholinergic effects, 263–264, 264*f*
Uncorrected astigmatism, 706*b*
Uncrossed disparities, 707
Uncrossed pathway, pupil light reflex, 531
Uniaxial strip extensiometry, corneal stiffness, 101
Unilateral functional visual field loss, relative
  afferent pupillary defect, 538*t*
Unilateral optical defocus, 708
Upper bar deflections, 683
Upper eyelid, 692
Urrets–Zavalia syndrome, 545
Utilize lactate, 326
UTS (ultimate tensile stress), corneal ectasia, 101–102
Uveitic glaucoma, 262
Uveoscleral outflow, aqueous humor, 269*t*, 270*t*
Uveovortex flow, aqueous humor drainage, 255–256

V

V1. *See* Primary visual cortex (V1)
V2. *See* Extrastriate visual cortex (V2)
V5. *See* Middle temporal area (MT)
Vancomycin, scleral permeability, 117*t*
Vascular endothelial growth factor (VEGF)
  neovascularization, 335
  retinal nitric oxide, 335
  RPE secretion, 343
  scleral drug delivery, 117
Vascular system, 284–285
  central retinal artery, 284
Vasculature, 583
  optic nerve, 583
  retina, 466–467
  See also Ocular circulation. *specific vessels*
Vasculature loss, lens transparency, 130
Vasoactive intestinal peptide (VIP), 366
  aqueous humor regulation, 251–252
  conjunctival goblet cells, 366
  protein secretion regulation, 371, 371*f*
Vasoactive intestinal peptide–expressing (VIP)
  cells, 615
VEGF. *See* Vascular endothelial growth factor
  (VEGF)
Venous drainage, orbit, 353–354
Ventral and dorsal processing streams, 627, 629*f*
Ventral occipitotemporal cortex (vOTC), 779
Ventral pathway, 631
Ventral stream, 631
  extrastriate visual cortex. *See* Extrastriate visual
    cortex (V2)
Ventral visual network, 627–633
  applications, 633
  distributed coding, 631
  hierarchical processing, 630, 630*f*
  invariance, 632–633
  receptive fields and visual selectivity, 630–631
  topographical features, 629–630
  ventral stream, 632
VEPs. *See* Visual evoked potentials (VEPs)

Vernier acuity
  contrast enhancement, 22–24, 23*f*
  definition, 738
  infant vision development, 738–740
  luminance, 658
  minimum discriminable acuity, 651
Versican, 166
Vertebrate experimental models, photoreceptor–
    Müller cell interaction. *see* Photoreceptor–
    Müller cell interaction
Vertical eye movements, extraocular muscles, 190
Vertical horopter, 704
Vertical meridian, 684
Vertical pulse-step command, saccades, 220
Vestibulo-ocular reflex (VOR), 212, 224–227, 225*f*,
    226*f*
  angular, 224–225
  Listing's law, 237
  neural control, 224–225
  suppression, 227
  translational, 224–225
Vieth-Muller circle (VMO), 703–704, 704*f*
Vimentin filaments, lens fiber cell architecture,
    135, 136*f*
Vinblastine, scleral permeability, 117*t*
VIP. *See* Vasoactive intestinal peptide (VIP)
Viscoelastic properties, corneal stiffness, 100–101
Visible light waves, 7
Vision degrading myodesopsia, 183
Vision, spherical aberration impact on, 31–32
Vision rehabilitation, prospects for, 635
Vision restoration, visual deprivation. *See* Visual
    deprivation
Visual acuity, 39, 649–667
  age-relation, 665
    SKI study, 665, 665*f*
  aliasing, 654–656
  anisotropies, 658*f*, 659, 659*f*, 660*f*
  aperture size, 654–656
  children, 654
  clinical testing, 662–664
    Bailey–Lovie chart, 663, 663*f*
    chart design, 651*f*, 662–664, 663*b*
    Early Treatment of Diabetic Retinopathy
      Study chart, 663
    Functional Acuity Contrast Test, 664
    optokinetic nystagmus, 664
    Pelli–Robson CS chart, 664, 664*f*
    preferential looking, 664
    visual-evoked potentials, 664
  cone to RGC convergence, 656
  contrast, 658, 659*f*
  crowding in peripheral vision, 657–658, 657*b*,
    658*f*
  definition, 649–652, 650*b*
  development, 1, 2*f*, 664
  eccentricity, 655*f*, 656–657, 656*f*, 657*f*
    cone density, 655*f*, 656
    cortical magnification factor, 656, 656*f*
    inverse cortical magnification, 656*f*, 657
    retinal topography, 655*f*, 657
    rods, 656
  forms of, 650*t*.
    see also specific forms
  glare, 664
  limiting factors, 652–659.
    see also specific factors
  log MAR, 10–22

Visual acuity (*Continued*)
  luminance, 658, 658*f*
    Vernier acuity, 658
  minimum discriminable acuity, 649, 651–652,
    651*f*
    definition, 651
    position judgements, 652
    Vernier acuity, 651
  minimum recognizable acuity, 649–651
    logMAR, 650–651, 651*t*
    Log Visual Acuity, 650–651
    Minimum Angle of Resolution, 650–651, 651*t*
    notations, 651*t*
    Snellen acuity charts, 650, 651*f*
  minimum resolvable acuity, 649
    assessment, 649, 650*f*
    cones, 649
    definition, 649
    rods, 649
  minimum visual acuity, 649
    historical aspects, 649
    target size, 649
  motion, 658–659
  Nyquist limit, 650*f*, 654–656, 655*f*
  optical quality of the eye, 652–654
    aberrations, 652–653
    chromatic aberrations, 652–653
    cutoff spatial frequency, 652
    diffraction, 652, 654*f*
    modulation transfer function, 652, 653*f*, 654*f*
    Rayleigh limit, 652, 653*f*
    refractive errors, 653
    retinal image, 652, 653*f*
    spatial frequency, 652, 654*f*
    spherical aberrations, 652–653
  photoreceptor size/spacing, 654–656, 655*f*
  reading, 659, 660*f*
    critical spacing, 659
  spatial vision with low contrast, 659–666
    measurement, 659–660
    sinusoidal gratings, 653*f*, 659–660
    See also Contrast sensitivity
  specificity, 649–652
  spherical aberration impact on, 32
  testing, 10
    chart contrast, 10–11
    chart luminance, 10
  time, 658
Visual cortex. *See* Primary visual cortex (V1)
Visual cortical areas, 627, 628*f*–629*f*
Visual cycle
  melanopsin, 550–551
  RPE. *See* Retinal pigment epithelium (RPE)
Visual deprivation, 775–787
  cross-modal plasticity, mechanisms, 781
  early blindness, recovery of sight after, 782–783
  early vision loss, perceptual and neural effects
    of, 778–781
    auditory processing, 779–781
    touch and braille, 778–779
  late blindness, 783
    behavior, 783
    neural responses, 783
  neuroanatomical development, 775–778, 778*f*
    gray matter and neuronal tuning, 777–778
    neurochemistry and microstructure, 775–776
    white matter pathways, 775
  sensory substitution, 783–784, 784*f*

Visual deprivation, developmental, 755–774
  alternating defocus, 761–762
  animal models, 755
  constant monocular defocus, 761
    neural changes, 761, 762f
    perceptual deficits, 761
  constant monocular form deprivation, 755–756
    neural changes, 755–756
    perceptual deficits, 755
  critical period, 755–756, 758
    deprivation timing, 758–759
  early monocular, 755–761
  intermittent monocular form deprivation, 756–758
    alternating, 756–757
    brief unrestricted vision, 758
    reverse occlusion, 757, 758f
  molecular mechanisms, 759–761
    AMPA receptors, 759–760
    binocular competition, 759
    GABA receptors, 759, 760f
    Hebbian synaptic plasticity, 759–760
    homeostatic synaptic mechanisms, 760–761
    long-term depression, 759
    long-term potentiation, 759
    neuromodulators, 761
    NMDA receptors, 759
  monocular defocus, 761–762.
    see also specific types
  visual performance improvement, 768–769
Visual development. See Development of vision
Visual direction
  in ABC, 714–715
  binocular vision, 702–703, 702f
  See also Binocular vision
Visual evoked potentials (VEPs)
  early blindness, recovery of sight after, 782
  infant vision development, 735
  motion detection development, 740
  transient, 735
  Vernier acuity, 738–740
  visual acuity testing, 664
  visual processing hierarchy, 736
Visual feedback mechanisms, sclera development, 108
Visual field, 675–700, 676f
  alternative and new visual field test procedures, 687–691
    frequency-doubling technology perimetry, 688–691
    short wavelength automated perimetry, 688, 690f
    SITA Faster and 24-2 C visual field tests, 687–688, 689f
  artifactual, 692–697, 694f, 695f, 697f, 698f
  constriction, 683
  damage, relative afferent pupillary defect, 536–539, 537f
  detection of sensitivity loss and interpretation, 680–683, 681f, 682f, 683f
  interpretation guidelines, 685–686, 686b
  nasal, 676
  patterns created by various pathologies, 683, 685f
  physiological basis, 675–676
  progression, assessment, 686–687
    classification systems, 687
    clinical judgment, 686

Visual field (Continued)
    event analysis, 687
    hybrid combined event and trend analysis, 687
    trend analysis, 687
  psychophysical basis, 675–676
    eccentricity, 675
    frequency of seeing curve, 675–676
    increment (differential) light threshold, 675–676
    light increments, 675–676
    Weber's law, 675
  tablets and virtual reality headsets, 691, 692f
  temporal, 675
  visual field loss, patterns of, 683–685
  See also Perimetry
Visual field, aberrations vary across, 27–28
Visual field index (VFI), 683
Visual field loss
  central scotomas, 684
  congruous, 684
  generalized/widespread, 683
  homonymous, 684
  horizontal wedge, 684
  incongruous, 684
  patterns of, 683–685
  pie in the sky, 684
  pie on the floor, 685
  shape and location of, 686
Visual field printout, 683
Visual field tests
  advantages of, 676
  24-2 C test, 687–688, 689f
Visualization, 783
Visual pathways, central. See Central visual pathways
Visual performance improvement, developmental visual deprivation, 768–769
Visual pigments. See Photopigments
Visual processing, infant vision development. See Infant vision development
Visual processing, inner retina, 495–505
  computational principles, 495, 496f
  example circuits, 498–501
    color polarity switching, 498
    direction selectivity circuit, 499–500, 501f
    night vision circuit, 498–499, 499f
    object motion sensitivity, 499, 500f
    orientation selectivity circuit, 500, 502f
  IPL, 496–498
    amacrine cell dendritic compartments, 498
    bipolar cell axon terminals, 496–497, 497b
    dendritic retinal ganglion cells, 498
  players, 495–496
    amacrine cells, 495–496
    bipolar cells, 495
    retinal ganglion cells, 496
Visual word form area (VWFA), 781
Visuomotor transformation, smooth pursuit, 220–221, 221f
Vitamin A. See All-trans-retinol (vitamin A)
Vitamin C. See Ascorbic acid (vitamin C)
Vitreo-macular interface, 172
Vitreo-papillary interface, 172
Vitreo-retinal adhesion, 171
  full-thickness, 180
  partial-thickness, 180
  weakening, 178

Vitreo-retinal interface, 168–171, 171f
  extracellular matrix, 169–171
  ILM, 168–169, 171f, 172f
  Müller cells, 168–169, 172f
  Weiss ring, 169
Vitreo-retinovascular bands, 172
Vitreoschisisy, 180
Vitreous body, 164–188
  aging, 177–180, 177f
    anomalous posterior detachment, 180, 181f
    epidemiology, 179
    fibrous liquefaction, 177
    molecular mechanism, 177
    posterior detachment, 179–180
    structural changes, 177–179, 177f, 178f
    symptomatic posterior detachment, 179–180, 179f
  anatomy, 42f, 167–172, 168f
    anterior cortex, 167–168
    base, 168, 171f
    posterior cortex, 167–168, 169f
  biochemistry, 164–167, 165f
    chemical substances, 167, 167t
    collagens, 165–166, 166f
    glycosaminoglycans, 164–165
    non-collagenous structural proteins, 166–167
    supramolecular organization, 167
  biophysics, 172–173
    convective flow, 173
    diffusion, 172–173, 173f
    transvitreous transport, 172–173
  developmental anomalies, 174
  embryology, 173–177, 176f
  growth, 176
  human, 165f
  immunohistochemistry, 174, 176f
  oxygen cataracts, 182–183, 183f
  physiology, 180–183
    diffusion barriers, 180–182
    metabolic buffer, 182–183
    optical transparency, 183
    oxidative stress, 182–183, 183f
    oxygen transport, 182
    structural support, 180
  primary, 173–174
  proteomics, 174, 176f
  retinal support function, posterior vitreous detachment. See Posterior vitreous detachment (PVD)
  rheology, 177f
  secondary, 174–176
  structure, 125f, 172f
  topographic variations, 171–172
    peripheral fundus and vitreous base, 171
    vitreo-retinal adhesion, 171
  ultrastructure, 164, 165f
Vitreous cavity, corneal drug delivery, 104, 109f
Vitreous membrane, 45–49
  accommodative posterior movement of, 45–49, 49f, 50f
  by ultrasound biomicroscopy, 46f
Vitreous zonule, 45
Voltage-activated calcium current (I_{Ca}), photoreceptor junctional conductances, 443–445, 446b, 447f
Voltage-gated sodium channels, ipRGC depolarizing photoresponse, 552–553
Volume regulation, lens, 148–149, 148f

Voluntary binocular eye movements, neural control, 221–224
Voluntary gaze shifts, 227
von Graefe, Albrecht, 612
Von Helmholtz, H H, accommodation, 37
VOR. *See* Vestibulo-ocular reflex (VOR)

W

Wald, George, 428
Water balance, retinal pigmented epithelium transport, 339
Water content regulation, lens, 146–149
Water secretion regulation
  tear film, aqueous layer. *See* Tear film, aqueous layer
  tear film, mucous layer. *See* Tear film, mucous layer
Wavefront-customized ablations, 33
Wavefront error (WFE), 30, 30*f*
Wavefront-guided ablations, 33
Wavefront-optimized ablations, 33
Wavefront sensing, 33–35
  evolution of aberrometers, 33–34, 33*f*
Wavefront-sensing devices, 35
Weber region, 453
Weber's law, 455–456, 456*f*
  desensitization, 452
  visual fields, 675
Weiss ring, vitreo-retinal interface, 169, 178*f*
Westheimer, 708
White matter pathways, 775

Whitnall's ligament, 357–358
  eyelid margin, 355–357
  eyelids, 355–357, 357*f*
Wiesel, Torsten, 612
Willis, Thomas, 612
Window of visibility, contrast sensitivity, 660–661, 660*f*
With No Lysine Kinases (WNK), 147–148
Wnt3a, 201–202
Wnt/Frz signaling, 129
Worth four-dot test, 714
Wound healing, sclera, 116

X

X,Y,Z hypothesis, corneal epithelium, 87

Y

Y-27632, aqueous humor drainage, 266–267
Y-cells, 751–752
Yellow pigment, fovea, 19
Young eye, 1–6
  physiology, 4–6.
  see also specific systems
Young, Thomas, accommodation, 37

Z

Zeaxanthin, 339
Zebrafish cones, 460

Zeis glands, 356
Zernike polynomials, 30, 30*f*
Zero-disparity reference, 716
Zero torsion saccades, 241
Zinn, annulus of, 350*f*
Zinn-Haller ring, 287*f*
Zone of clear single binocular vision (ZCSBV), 717
Zonula occludens tight junctions, corneal epithelium, 86–87, 90*f*
Zonular fibers, 43–45, 45*f*
  anatomy, 41*f*
  anterior, 43–45, 45*f*
    as tool, 45
  posterior, 45
  PVZ-INS LE strand, 45
  vitreous, 45
  zonular plexus, 45
Zonular plexus and posterior zonule, 45
Zonules
  age-related changes in, 58–60
  lens and, 124, 125*f*
  presbyopia. *See* Presbyopia
  structure, 125*f*
Zygoma, orbit, 189
Zygomatic bone, 348*f*
  orbit, 189, 347